The Wondrous Story of Anesthesia

Edmond I Eger II
Lawrence J. Saidman
Rod N. Westhorpe

Editors

The Wondrous Story
of Anesthesia

To Steve
With best regards
Ted Eger
15 Sept 14

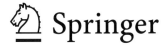 Springer

Editors

Edmond I Eger II, MD
Emeritus Professor, Department of Anesthesia
    and Perioperative Care
University of California, San Francisco
    San Francisco, CA, USA

Lawrence J. Saidman, MD
Emeritus Professor
Department of Anesthesia
Stanford University, Stanford, CA, USA

Rod N. Westhorpe, OAM, MB, BS FRCA, FANZCA
Former Honorary Curator, Geoffrey Kaye
    Museum of Anaesthetic History
Australian and New Zealand College
    of Anaesthetists, Melbourne, VIC, Australia

ISBN 978-1-4614-8440-0   ISBN 978-1-4614-8441-7 (eBook)
DOI 10.1007/978-1-4614-8441-7
Springer New York Heidelberg Dordrecht London

Library of Congress Control Number: 2013948224

Printed on acid-free paper

Springer is part of Springer Science+Business Media (www.springer.com)

To those responsible for the discovery and evolution of anesthesia.

Preface

This story describes events in three succeeding eras: first, events during the time preceding and immediately after the demonstration of anesthesia; then those in the subsequent 90 years of slow evolution of the specialty, ending in the 1950s; and finally those from the 1950s to the present, a period of explosive growth. Our lives span the last of these, the era in which modern anesthesia evolved from empiricism—"doing what worked"—to a practice relying on science and evidenced-based medicine. We sought to tell this story before too many grand participants died or were unable to tell their story. Many died in the past decade: Safar (2003); Marx (2004); Greene (2005)—including since we began this project in 2007—Haglund, Ibsen and Keats (2007); Gray (2008); Parsloe (2009); Smith and Terrell (2010); Gordh, Morris and Pierce (2011). We would have lost too many opportunities had we failed to act.

We enlisted 100 authors to construct 53 chapters (The Individual Stories) describing specific aspects of the evolution of anesthesia: people, countries, drugs, science, organizations, education, and more, each a thread in the tapestry of a larger story, each chapter written by anesthetists and others who lived this history. These 53 chapters make up the second part of our book. The first part wove stories from these chapters into chronologies described in 14 additional chapters (The Woven Stories) which provide a coherent picture of the development of anesthesia, a framework that facilitates an understanding of how events and people described in the second part of the book jointly shaped the development of the specialty.

Our contributors represent the Americas, Europe, the Middle and Far East, and Australia and New Zealand. They were chosen because of demonstrated expertise and/or actual participation in the development of a specific subject or of the specialty in a specific geographic area. Several chapter titles may seem idiosyncratic for a history book and were chosen because the subjects seemed to represent existing trends that were likely to influence the future.

A book of this breadth could not have been produced without the help supplied by our 100 contributors. Each endured multiple suggestions, changes, requests for no fewer than four revisions and a gentle nagging for more and more and more that in retrospect probably bordered on abuse. A few did not tolerate our intrusiveness and withdrew before completing their assignments. Fortunately, replacements were found and despite a shortened timeline for completion they met our deadlines. To all of these dear friends we offer our gratitude—we are in your debt!

The book is a story, not a recitation of pharmacology or physiology. It is not intended to educate the student in techniques or mechanisms. It describes the issues that shaped anesthesia, the incidents and humor, the anecdotes that put a human face to this wonderful specialty. We hope it shows the interactions between diverse forces that made this great specialty grow, and provides a sense of where those forces may take us in the future.

We three editors (Fig. 1) and many of our contributors hail from English speaking countries. While our respective forms of English are nearly identical they do differ slightly in spellings, e.g., an(a)esthesia, vapo(u)r, (o)esophagus, antagoni(s)ze, and many more. Rather than dictating the use of American English throughout, we elected to use the spelling common to the country of the chapter's author(s).

Redundancy in the descriptions of subjects, persons, and events is a frequent complaint lodged against multi-authored books, especially those like ours wherein the stories span centuries. Rather than purging the text of such repetitions, we allowed them to remain where and

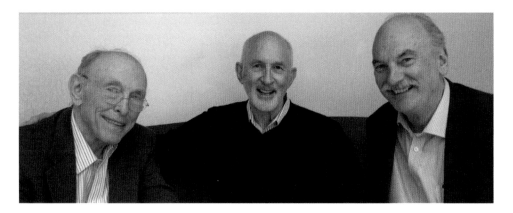

Fig. 1 The three editors, from left to right: Edmond (Ted) Eger, Lawrence J. Saidman, and Rod N. Westhorpe

whenever they obviously belonged. The largest example, the discussion of Danish anesthesiologist Bjørn Ibsen's impact upon intensive care medicine, intensive care units, and associated issues appears in five chapters, each with its own focus.

Finally, a tribute to **The Power of Three** (Fig. 1). As might have been expected, in the 6 years over which we wrote and re-wrote this book, we disagreed regarding the how, who, when, where, why, and whether of many things. We settled each of these disputes (mostly) without rancor by taking a vote. For anyone anticipating a similar future exercise, we advise avoiding an even number of participants.

It has been a wonderful journey that has allowed us to re-live lives we loved.

San Francisco, CA, USA   Edmond I Eger II
Stanford, CA, USA   Lawrence J. Saidman
Melbourne, VIC, Australia   Rod N. Westhorpe

Contents

Contributors

David Baker, DM FRCA Hôpital Necker-Enfants Malades, Paris, Club de l'histoire de l'anesthésie et de la réanimation français, Souillac, France

Diane Biehl, MD, FRCPC Department of Anesthesia, University of Manitoba, Winnipeg, Canada

John G Brock-Utne, MA, MD, PhD, FFA (SA) Department of Anesthesia, Stanford University Medical Center, Stanford, CA, USA

Robert Byrick, FRCPC Department of Anesthesia, University of Toronto, St. Michael's Hospital, Toronto, Ontario, Canada

Michael Cahalan, MD Department of Anesthesiology, University of Utah, Salt Lake City, UT, USA

James E. Caldwell, MBChB Department of Anesthesia and Perioperative Medicine, University of California, San Francisco, San Francisco, CA, USA

Selma Harrison Calmes, MD The David Geffen School of Medicine at UCLA, Los Angeles, CA, USA

William Camann, MD Department of Anesthesiology, Brigham and Women's Hospital, Boston, MA, USA

Daniel B. Carr, MD, DABPM, FFPM ANZCA (Hon.) Program on Pain Research, Education and Policy, Tufts University School of Medicine, Boston, MA USA

Susan S. Caulk, CRNA, MA (Retired) Director of Continuing Education, Certification, Recertification, American Association of Nurse Anesthetists, Park Ridge, IL, USA

Jean-Bernard Cazalaà, MD Hôpitaux de Paris, Club d'histoire de l'anesthésie et de la réanimation (CHAR) français, Paris, France

Davy C. H. Cheng, MD, MSc, FRCPC, FCAHS Department of Anesthesia & Perioperative Medicine, University of Western Ontario, London Health Science Centre & St Joseph's Health Care, London, ON, Canada

Marie-Thérèse Cousin, MD Anesthésiologiste des Hôpitaux de Paris, Club de l'histoire de l'anesthésie et de la réanimation France, Buc, France

Michael J Cousins, AM, MB, BS, MD, DSc, FANZCA, FRCA, FFPMANZCA, FAChPM (RACP), DSc (Hon.) Department of Anaesthesia and Pain Management, Royal North Shore Hospital, University of Sydney Sydney, Australia

Douglas Craig, MDCM, FRCPC Department of Anesthesia, University of Manitoba, MB, Winnipeg, Canada

Karen B. Domino, MD, MPH Department of Anesthesiology and Pain Medicine, University of Washington, Seattle, WA, USA

Jerry A. Dorsch Mayo Clinic Jacksonville, Jacksonville, FL, USA

Susan E. Dorsch Orange Park, FL, USA

Kenneth Drasner, MD Department of Anesthesia and Perioperative Care, San Francisco General Hospital, University of California, San Francisco, San Francisco, CA, USA

Edmond I Eger II, MD Department of Anesthesia and Perioperative Care, University of California, San Francisco, San Francisco, CA, USA

Jan Eklund, MD, PhD Department of Anesthesiology and Intensive Care, Karolinska Institute and Hospital, Karolinska vägen, Solna, Sweden

Xiaomei Feng, M.D., Ph.D. Department of Anesthesiology, Shanghai Ruijin Hospital, School of Medicine, Shanghai Jiaotong University, Shanghai, China

Dennis M. Fisher, MD P Less Than, San Francisco, CA, USA

Prof. Nicholas P. Franks, FRCA, FMedSci Biophysics Section, Blackett Laboratory, Imperial College, South Kensington, London, UK

Elizabeth A. M. Frost, MB ChB, DRCOG Department of Anesthesiology, Icahn Medical Center at Mount Sinai, New York, NY, USA

Amna A. Ghouse, MD Department of Anesthesiology, The University of Texas Medical School at Houston, Houston, TX, USA

John (Iain) Glen, BVMS, DVA, PhD, FRCA Oaklands, Knutsford, Cheshire WA, UK

Michael Goerig, MD Department Anesthesia and Intensive Care, University Hospital Hamburg-Eppendorf, Hamburg, Germany

George Gregory, MD Department of Anesthesia, University of California, San Francisco, San Francisco, CA, USA

Carin A. Hagberg, MD Department of Anesthesiology, The University of Texas Medical School at Houston, Houston, TX, USA

Martin H:son Holmdahl, MD, PhD Uppsala University, Uppsala, Sweden

Prof. Harriet W. Hopf, MD Department of Anesthesiology, University of Utah School of Medicine, East, Salt Lake City, UT, USA

Yuguang Huang, MD, PhD Department of Anesthesiology, Peking Union Medical College Hospital, Dongcheng District, Beijing, China

Francis P. Hughes, PhD The Villages, FL, USA

Dawn G. Iannucci, BA, CCRC School of Public Health, The University of Texas Health Science Center at Houston and Department of Anesthesiology, University of Texas Medical School, Houston, TX, USA

Stephen H. Jackson, MD Department of Anesthesiology, Good Samaritan Hospital of San Jose, San Jose, CA, USA

Ron Jones, MD Imperial College of Science, Technology and Medicine, University of London, London, UK

Christopher D. Kent, MD Department of Anesthesiology and Pain Medicine, University of Washington, Seattle, WA, USA

Jerry Kim, MD Department of Anesthesiology & Pain Medicine, Seattle Children's Hospital, University of Washington, Seattle, WA, USA

Bruce Evan Koch, CRNA, MSN Clinical Nurse Anesthetist, Kootenai Medical Center, Spirit Lake, Coeur d'Alene, Idaho, USA

Colleen G. Koch, MD, MS, MBA Department of Cardiothoracic Anesthesia (J-4), Cleveland Clinic Lerner College of Medicine of Case Western Reserve University, Cleveland, OH, USA

John C. Kraft, BSc Department of Anesthesiology & Pain Medicine, University of Washington, Seattle, WA, USA

Ruth Landau, MD Obstetric Anesthesia & Clinical Genetics Research, Department of Anesthesiology & Pain Medicine,University of Washington, Seattle, WA, USA

Richard Leazer, BBA, MBA Verona, WI, USA

Jin Liu, MD Department of Anesthesia and Critical Care, West China Hospital, Sichuan University, Chengdu, Sichuan, China

Prof. Edward Lowenstein, MD Dept. of Anesthesia, Critical Care and Pain Medicine, Massachusetts General Hospital, Boston, MA, USA

Peter L. McDermott, MD, PhD Camarillo, CA, USA

Kathryn E. McGoldrick, MD Society for Ambulatory Anesthesia, New York Medical College, Valhalla, NY, USA

Estela Melman, MD Department of Anesthesia, American British Cowdry Medical Center, Mexico City, Mexico

Alan F. Merry, MBChB, FANZCA, FFPMANZCA, FRCA Department of Anaesthesiology, University of Auckland, Auckland, New Zealand

M. R. Meyer, MD, JD, LLM Department of Anesthesia, Massachusetts General Hospital, Boston, MA, USA

Donald C. Morris, MSc The Washington Group, Inc., Seattle WA, USA

Lucien E. Morris, MD, FRCA, FFARACS (Hon) DSc Anesthesiology, Medical College of Ohio, Toledo OH, USA

Michael Mulroy, MD Faculty Anesthesiologist, Department of Anesthesiology, Virginia Mason Medical Center, Seattle, WA, USA

David Needham, BSc (Eng), ACGI, PhD Villa Sainte Marie, Vence, France

Gail Van Norman, MD Department of Anesthesiology and Pain Medicine, Department of Biomedical Ethics, University of Washington Medical Center, Seattle, WA, USA

Manuel Pardo, Jr. MD Department of Anesthesia and Perioperative Care, University of California, San Francisco, San Francisco, CA, USA

Prof. Thomas Pasch, MD, FRCA Anaesthesiology, University Hospital Zurich, Zurich, Switzerland

Karen Plaus, PhD, CRNA, FAAN National Board on Certification and Recertification of Nurse Anesthetists (NBCRNA), Chicago, IL, USA

Cedric Prys-Roberts, MA, DM, PhD, FRCA, FANZCA, FCMSA (Hon), FCAI (Hon) Past President, Royal College of Anaesthetists, Emeritus Professor, University of Bristol, Foxes Mead, Cleeve, Bristol, UK

Prof. J. G. Reves, MD Medical University of South Carolina, Charleston, SC, USA

William B. Runciman, BSc (Med), MBBCh, FANZCA, FJFICM, FHKCA, FRCA, PhD School of Psychology, Social Work and Social Policy, Sleep Research Centre, University of South Australia City East Campus, North Terrace, Adelaide, SA, Australia

Lawrence J. Saidman, MD Department of Anesthesia, Stanford University, Stanford, California, USA

Debra A. Schwinn, MD The University of Iowa 212 CMAB, Iowa, USA

Steven L. Shafer, MD School of Medicine, Stanford University, Stanford, CA, USA

William Silen, MD Department of Surgery, Harvard Medical School, Boston, MA, USA

Peter Simpson, MD, FRCA, FRCP Royal College of Anaesthetists, London, UK

Robert N. Sladen, MBChB MRCP, FRCPC, FCCM Division of Critical Care, Department of Anesthesiology, College of Physicians & Surgeons of Columbia University, New York, NY, USA

Stephen Slogoff, MD Department of Anesthesiology, Stritch School of Medicine, Loyola University, Chicago, IL, USA

Prof. Theodore H. Stanley, MD Department of Anesthesiology, School of Medicine, University of Utah, Salt Lake City, UT, USA

Eugene P. Steffey Department of Surgical and Radiological Sciences, School of Veterinary Medicine, University of California, Davis, Davis, CA, USA

Robert K. Stoelting, MD Department of Anesthesia, Indiana University School of Medicine, Anesthesia Patient Safety Foundation, Indianapolis, IN, USA

Kjell Erik Stromskag, MD, PhD Department of Anesthesiology and Intensive Care, Molde Hospital, Molde, Norway

Kunio Suwa, MD Department of Lifecare, Section of Medical Engineering, Teikyo Junior College, Shibuya, Tokyo, Japan

Keith Sykes, MA, MB BChir (Cantab), FRCA, Hon, FANZCA, Hon, FCA(SA) Emeritus Professor, University of Oxford, Oxford, UK

Jukka Takala, MD, PhD Department of Intensive Care Medicine, University Hospital Bern (Inselspital) and University of Bern, Switzerland

Jeanette Thirlwell, MB, BS, FFARACS, FANZCA Executive Editor, *Anaesthesia and Intensive Care*, Australian Society of Anaesthetists, Sydney, Australia

Paul Thomas, BS, MBA Bridgewater, NJ, USA

Dr. Adolfo Héctor Venturini Faculty of Medicine, University of Buenos Aires, Nueva York, Argentina

John G. Wade, MD, FRCPC Faculty of Medicine, Department of Anesthesia, University of Manitoba, Winnipeg, Canada

Guolin Wang, MD Department of Anesthesiology, Tianjin Medical University General Hospital, Tianjin, China

Rod N. Westhorpe, OAM, MB, BS, FRCA, FANZCA Melbourne, Australia

Paul F. White, PhD, MD, FANZCA Department of Anesthesia, Cedars-Sinai Medical Center in Los Angeles, Los Angeles, USA

Jeanine P. Wiener-Kronish, MD Department of Anesthesia, Critical Care and Pain Medicine, Massachusetts General Hospital, Harvard Medical School, Boston, MA, USA

Buwei Yu, MD, PhD Department of Anesthesiology, Shanghai Ruijin Hospital, School of Medicine, Shanghai Jiaotong University, Shanghai, China

Xuerong Yu, MD, PhD Department of Anesthesiology, Peking Union Medical College Hospital, Beijing, China

Part I

The Woven Story of Anesthesia: Eras, Exemplars, and Looking Forward

History to 1798

Edmond I Eger II, Lawrence J. Saidman and Rod N. Westhorpe

Summary

Surgeons in ancient times undertook diverse operations, usually at great speed to diminish the duration of suffering. Skulls from 5,000 BCE show trephination, the removal of a piece of bone from the head. Egyptians in 3,600 BCE performed circumcisions and tracheotomies. In 1700 BCE, Babylonians excised tumors. Egyptians cauterized breast tumors and excised peripheral aneurysms. The Roman surgeon, Galen, in the second Century CE, treated cataracts to restore sight, and he cut out the uvula to cure chronic coughing. Surgeons in Europe might be physicians, monks or barbers who in the thirteenth and fourteenth centuries wrote books on surgery. They gained recognition by their study of the anatomy of cadavers. Thus, in 1543 Vesalius published *"On the Fabric of the Human Body"*, demolishing centuries of errors, and opening the door to the performance of accurate surgery.

The horrors of pain, shock, and infection hindered surgeons. Operations brought infection, an added threat to life. Surgeons had surprising remedies, some desperately wrong (e.g., venesection), and some perhaps surprisingly wise (e.g., irrigating wounds with alcohol).

Before the advent of anesthesia, humans used diverse means to diminish pain, including pressure or ice to numb extremities. They administered herbal potions including mandragora, hemp-marijuana, opium, and alcohol. The Incas may have known of the topical effect of coca/cocaine, but they had no way to inject it other than spit coca-laced saliva into the wound. That might have some effect, but the amount of active cocaine was small and the effect probably too little to produce anesthesia.

Some potions contained hallucinogens, particularly scopolamine. Some prescriptions with wonderful names had unknown components: In 500 BCE, Hua Tuo gave "mafeisan" or "cannabis boil powder". In the Middle Ages, patients might suck liquid or breathe vapors from soporific sponges. And since the 1700s, we knew that we could produce immobility with a curare tipped dart, but we now know that would not eliminate pain.

Practitioners applied positive thinking and forms of suggestion, including modern magical rings, necklaces, and charms for the parturient. Greeks applied oils and warm compresses during labor, anticipating the warm compresses, massage and herbal teas used today. Were they placebos (which can have positive effects)? Mesmer's late eighteenth century creation of animal magnetism may have also relied on suggestion, perhaps a form of hypnosis that inconsistently assuaged surgical pain.

World Events Before 1798

The Jews credited 3761 BCE as the date of creation, but scientists suggest it was billions of years earlier. By 4000–3000 BCE, civilizations had arisen in China, Korea, Japan, Mesopotamia, and Egypt, aided by the development of agriculture, domestication of animals, invention of the wheel (including the potter's wheel), and writing. The Bronze Age appeared in 3000–2000 BCE, and the Egyptians constructed the pyramids. Parallel great kingdoms ruled Egypt and China, and an egalitarian civilization arose in the Indus Valley. In 2000–1000 BCE, Central Asian Indo-European invaders on horse-powered chariots overran Egypt and Babylonia. The Iron Age appeared in 1000–0 BCE, and Judaism, Zoroastrianism, Hinduism, Jainism and Buddhism developed. Greece conquered Persia, and the Romans conquered Greece and established the Roman Republic. In the first century CE, Rome dominated Europe, North Africa and the Near East, and the Han Dynasty ruled China. In the second century, Cai Lun invented paper, and Roman civilization peaked. The Prophet Muhammad began the Muslim conquests in 622 CE. In this century, India gave smallpox to Europe, and the world's population shrank to 200 million. In the eighth century, Arabian expansion continued,

E. I Eger II (✉)
Department of Anesthesia and Perioperative Care,
University of California, San Francisco, CA, USA
e-mail: egere@anesthesia.ucsf.edu

L. J. Saidman
Department of Anesthesia, Stanford University,
Stanford, CA, USA
e-mail: lsaidman@stanford.edu

R. N. Westhorpe
Melbourne, Australia
e-mail: westhorpe@netspace.net.au

E. I Eger II et al. (eds.), *The Wondrous Story of Anesthesia,* DOI 10.1007/978-1-4614-8441-7_1, © Edmond I Eger, MD 2014

and Charlemagne came to power. Vikings repeatedly invaded Britain in the ninth century. The eleventh century saw the worst of Europe's Dark Ages (500–1500 CE), but great advances in science took place in China. Gutenberg invented mechanical movable type printing about 1439. The Spanish Inquisition began in 1492 the same year that Columbus landed in America. Copernicus proposed the sun as center of the universe in the 1540s. In the seventeenth century, Newton invented the calculus and his Laws of Motion. The eighteenth century saw French, American, and industrial revolutions, including invention of the steam engine.

Ancient Approaches to Pain Relief

We cringe, thinking of Galen, a prominent physician and surgeon in ancient Rome, [1] performing uvulectomy, cataract extractions, caesarean sections, and amputations in unanesthetized patients. We cringe, thinking of children forcibly restrained to allow surgery to proceed. Despite the absence of any clear path to pain-free surgery, surgeons in ancient times undertook diverse operations, usually at great speed to diminish the duration of suffering. How did these ancient surgeons deal with the issue of pain?

Ancient civilizations may have used pressure or ice to numb extremities. Magical herbs, including marijuana, might have been given. Perhaps the first known use of anesthesia came from China, where in 500 BCE, Hua Tuo combined herbs and wine into a concoction known as "mafeisan" or "cannabis boil powder".

In 40–90 CE, the Greek, Pedanius Dioscorides, used opium or mandragora to minimize pain during surgery. However, such therapies might be lethal or ineffective, or both. Opium could cause patients to stop breathing. Belladonna drugs in mandragora might lead to a fatal increase in temperature. Other surgeons experimented with opioids, alcohol, or a blow to the head—imperfect techniques that did not offer the control and reversibility required for anesthesia. Alcohol, for example, needed to be consumed in precisely the right quantity to cause unconsciousness, but not death. Persuading the underdosed inebriate to drink more might be impossible, and in the meantime, their irrational behavior and propensity to vomit made such a remedy ineffective.

Some remedies may have anticipated modern approaches. South American Indians may have chewed coca leaves and spat into the surgical field, thereby applying the first local anesthetic. However, the lack of cocaine alkaloids available in raw coca leaves may have limited its effectiveness [1].

---

[1] In the second century CE, Galen treated cataracts to restore sight and cut out the uvula to cure the chronic cough.

Surgery Without Anesthesia: A Painful Proposition

The Earliest Surgeries

A history of anesthesia is not complete without a discussion of the history of surgery. Anesthesia is a recent invention relative to surgery. Brutality attended the earliest surgeries. One early procedure appeared in all parts of the world except the Far East. Called "trephination," it involved making a hole through the patient's skull to expose the brain. Archeologists have unearthed skulls dating to 10,000 BCE, that show evidence of the practice. Some such skulls had healed, indicating that the holes resulted from a deliberate surgical act. The purpose of trephination remains a matter of speculation. Did it have religious implications? Did it release evil spirits?

Even in ancient times, humans performed complex surgical procedures. By 3,600 BCE, Egyptians performed tracheotomies, cutting a hole in a patient's windpipe to ease airflow. In 1,700–1,600 BCE, Egyptian surgeons operated on tumors and aneurysms. They used cautery to remove breast cancers and treat other ailments, literally burning away the offending body part.

So common were surgical procedures, that the 1,700 BCE Code of Hammurabi (Babylon) dictated the cost of surgeries, including incisions of tumors, giving discounts for operations on slaves. The Code dealt harshly with surgical failure: "if a physician make a large incision with the operating knife, and kill him, or open a tumor with the operating knife, and cut out the eye, his hands shall be cut off." We may assume that malpractice was rare.

Egyptian and Greek surgical practices may have anticipated modern therapies. *The Edwin Smith Papyrus*, an Ancient Egyptian medical text and the oldest known surgical treatise on trauma, described the healing of injuries in 3,000 BCE, and suggested the application of meat to wounds to decrease bleeding, possibly using tissue clotting factors to achieve hemostasis. The ancient Greeks treated wounds with wine, perhaps acting to sterilize the incisions.

Records indicate the types of care given to wounds during this period, and the diversity of surgical procedures, but few records indicated attempts to dull the pain of surgery. How did ancient humans endure having a quarter-sized hole bored into their skull, the extraction of tumors, and the destruction of maladies by burning? The agony is difficult to imagine.

As the new millennium approached, surgeries became more complex, and the center of progress shifted from Greece to Rome. The Romans contributed to the knowledge essential for conducting surgery. The ancient Roman physician, Celsus (25 BCE-CE 50), accurately described the body's response to trauma or infection, using terms characteristic of inflammation—redness, swelling, heat and pain. The great Roman surgeon, Galen (CE 129–199), performed cataract extractions, perhaps by displacing the opaque lens into the vitreous humor with a needle. A surgeon to gladiators, he made major contributions to the knowledge of anatomy through his observations of normal and abnormal structure. He dissected pigs and apes because human dissection was forbidden. However, by relying on dissection of animals, some of his extrapolations to human anatomy initiated errors that continued for centuries, errors sustained because of Galen's fame.

Ancient Jews in the Middle East also conducted surgeries. The Talmud described the suturing of wounds, the reduction of dislocations, the amputation of limbs, and the performance of Caesarian sections. The Jews had quaint remedies including the application of onions to wounds, a therapy for preventing infection that has modern support [2].

Dealing with the Pain of Surgery in the Ninth Through Twelfth Centuries

Church edicts during the Middle Ages, particularly the Dark Ages, diminished the use of surgery, and in 1163, the church forbade monks from shedding blood—and thus from performing surgery. Enter the barbers, men taught surgery by the monks before the Church's prohibition. These barber-craftsmen continued performing surgeries. They repaired hernias, removed bladder stones and cataracts, among other procedures, thereby preserving a modicum of surgical craft.

Pain always accompanied surgery; what to do about the pain? In the Middle Ages, patients might suck liquid or breathe vapors from sponges which offered mandrake, henbane or other hallucinogens such as hyoscine and scopolamine [3]. It sounds wonderful, a sponge to cause sleep, to shield its beneficiaries from the cruelty of the knife.

> "The most popular method of inducing narcosis was the so-called soporific sponge, *spongia somnifera*. Historians have found descriptions of it in manuscripts dating to the ninth century. Nicholas of Salerno described its ingredients in the twelfth century as opium, hyoscyamine, mulberry juice, lettuce seed, hemlock, mandrake and ivy. A fresh sea-sponge was to be soaked in the mixture and allowed to dry 'in the sun during the dog-days until all the liquid is consumed.' When required for use, the concoction was re-constituted by dipping the sponge in water. Because the medieval manuscripts recommended applying the sponge to the subject's nostrils, it has been thought that this was meant to be a form of inhalation anesthesia, but there is good evidence that the potion was usually administered as a drink [4]."

Medieval physicians even thought of an antidote: "Reversal of the narcotizing effect was to be attained with the juice of fennel-root or with vinegar [4]." But the soporific sponge probably could not produce anesthesia. Patients given scopolamine may not remember the agony of surgery, but they would move in response to the inflicted pain, and they might move vigorously [5].

Thirteenth–Fourteenth Centuries: Ether is Synthesized and Surgery Grows

In 1275, Spaniard Raymond Lully (Fig. 1.1) created a compound that, centuries later, would become the world's most important anesthetic. He combined sulfuric acid with wine to produce ethyl ether, which he called sweet oil of vitriol. But Lully did nothing further with his discovery, and patients everywhere would have to wait nearly 600 years for ether to be used to produce anesthesia.

Italian and French surgery resumed, growing as the Middle Ages ended. Published in Salerno, the earliest book on operations, the Bamberg Surgery, elevated the prestige of Italian surgery. Italian and French barber-surgeon guilds competed with each other and with so-called "masters of surgery", for royal recognition and support. Italian master surgeon, Lanfranc of Milan, irrigated wounds with wine (as had Greek physicians 1,500 years earlier) before closure of the wounds. In 1,290, Lanfranc left for France, thereby transferring considerable surgical authority from Italy to France. His 1296 book, *Practice and Art of All of Surgery*, further inspired French surgery.

French master surgeon Guy de Chauliac's 1368 book, *Inventory of the Complete Works of Surgery,* supplemented Lanfranc's work. Both Lanfranc's and de Chauliac's books appeared in Latin, and thus were inaccessible to most barber-surgeons until translated into French and other European languages. This contributed to the stiff competition between the master surgeons (who were likely to speak Latin) and the barber-surgeon guilds. The books guided surgery in France, and to some extent in England, for two centuries. They advised treatment of tumors, sores, and fractures, and prescribed antidotes and drugs. England however, remained a backwater controlled primarily by barber-surgeons, who competed with the less numerous military surgeons.

Fifteenth and Sixteenth Centuries

The 1425 translation of Guy de Chauliac's book from Latin into French and English, aided the barber-surgeons (known as the "surgeons of the short gowns") in their mounting competition with Latin-educated university surgeons (the "long gown" academic surgeons). Barber-surgeons grew more numerous than their long-gown counterparts, in part because the barber surgeon was more accessible. Although the barber-surgeons lacked social status or academic rank, the public found them to be more approachable, and eventually recognized that they also possessed superior skills that decreased complications and mortality.

Two self-educated Frenchmen, Pierre Franco and Ambroise Paré, advanced surgery in France and the reputation of such surgery in the world. They learned to perform surgery

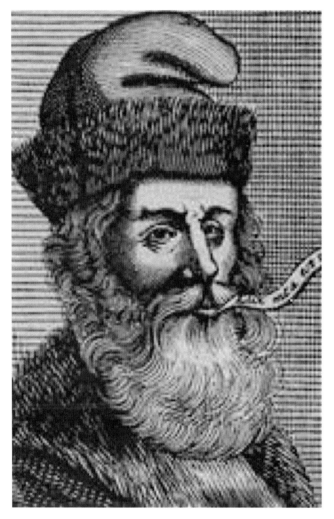

Fig. 1.1 In 1275, Raymond Lully (pictured with words coming from his mouth) synthesized diethyl ether ("ether") by mixing wine and sulphuric acid, calling it sweet oil of vitriol, but he made nothing of it

from itinerant lithotomists and herniotomists (Franco), and barber-surgeons (Paré). Franco is thought to have fought charlatans, and Paré helped bridge the divide between the barber-surgeons and academic surgeons.

The Renaissance generated a new era of discovery in surgery. The Renaissance diminished the power of the Church and thereby limited its power to prevent human dissection. As a consequence, surgeons gained important new insights into anatomy that materially advanced surgery. In 1543, 29 year-old Andreas Vesalius published his classic book *On the Fabric of the Human Body*, demolishing centuries of errors based on Galen's dissections of animals, or ignorant imaginings [6, 7].

A half-century later, in 1597, Gaspare Tagliacozzi published *The Surgery of Defects by Implantations*, a treatise on the management of mutilating injuries–plastic surgery in 1597. Tagliacozzi precisely instructed surgeons on the reconstruction of noses and ears. The uncomplaining immobilized

patient waited for two or three weeks for the skin graft from the arm to gain circulation from the nose [6, 7]. Plastic surgery without a drop of anesthesia.

It was not for lack of an anesthetic. It was not for lack of an observation that the anesthetic might block pain. As Lully had done three centuries earlier, in 1540, 25 year-old Valerius Cordus (Fig. 1.2a) once again produced ether (sweet oil of vitriol) by adding sulfuric acid to wine [8, 9]. About the same time, Theophrastus Bombastus von Hohenheim (Fig. 1.2b), better known as Paracelsus [10] noted that ether "has associated with it such a sweetness that it is taken even by chickens, and they fall asleep from it for a while but awaken later without harm." Paracelsus continued, "On this sulphur no other judgment should be passed than that in diseases which need to be treated with anodynes (pain killers) it quiets all suffering without any harm, and relieves all pain, and quenches all fevers, and prevents complications in all illnesses [8]."

Why did no one notice? A potent painkiller, ether would eventually be widely used as an anesthetic, but Paracelsus died in 1541 without demonstrating this possibility. Had anyone tumbled to the possibilities inherent in Paracelsus' observation that ether put chickens to a reversible sleep, one which relieves all pain, anesthesia might have been discovered three centuries sooner.

Perhaps Italian scholar, polymath and playwright, John Baptista Porta, had discovered the anesthetic potential of ether. In his 1597 work on "*Natural Magic*," Porta noted:

> At last shall be related a wonderful method by which any sleeping person may inhale a soporific medicine. From what we have said, any one will easily know that he is liable to suffer severely after sleep caused by medicine, and to have his suspicions aroused [11]."

> "But the quintessence is extracted from a number of the above named medicines by somniferous (sleep-inducing) menstrual. This is put into leaden vessels perfectly closed, lest the least aura should escape, for the medicine would vanish away. When it is used, the cover being removed, it is applied to the nostrils of the sleeping person, he draws in the most subtile (sic) power of the vapour by smellings, and so blocks up the fortress of the senses that he is plunged into the most profound, sleep, and cannot be roused without the greatest effort. After the sleep, no heaviness of the head remains nor any suspicion of trick or fraud. These things are plain to the skilful physician, but unintelligible to the wicked [11]."

Although he does not describe what chemicals he uses, Porta (who sometimes was called a "professor of secrets") could have been describing ether. Much later, John Snow (author of *On Chloroform and other Anaesthetics: Their Action and Administration*) reflects on Porta's 1597 book and makes his own astute observations concerning Porta's description. Snow states,

> "The author [Porta] does not make known what the 'somniferous menstrual' were, with which the 'quinta essentia' were

Fig. 1.2a Using the approach used by Lully nearly three centuries earlier, Valerius Cordus (I.2) synthesized ether in 1540.
1.2b However, this time someone—Paracelsus (I.3)—made observations on pharmacological qualities of the new compound: "…it quiets all suffering without any harm, and relieves all pain…"

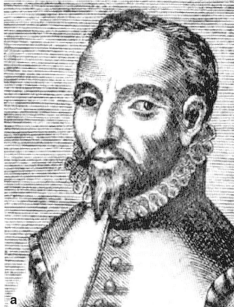 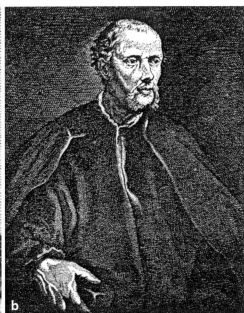

extracted. As sulphuric ether had been described more than fifty years before he published his work, it is not improbable that this was the evanescent substance which required the vessel be carefully closed up, and that the profound sleep was simply caused by this, as the narcotic principles dissolved in it would remain in the bottle in the form of extracts…Porta does not say that operations were performed under the influence of the inhalation, or in fact, that it was applied to any useful purpose whatever [11]".

Why didn't Porta apply his observations to relieve the pain of surgery? Why didn't Paracelsus do the same? As Winston Churchill observed: "Men stumble over the truth from time to time, but most pick themselves up and hurry off as if nothing happened."

And what of possibilities other than ether might there been to diminish pain? Shakespeare reminds us of remedies such as the Mandrake root:

"Not poppy, nor mandragora,
Nor all the drowsy syrups of the world,
Shall ever medicine thee to that sweet sleep
Which thou ow'dst yesterday."
Shakespeare: Othello III.iii

Just like the soporific sponge, the Mandrake root contains deliriant hallucinogenic tropane alkaloids, such as hyoscyamine and scopolamine [12]. Those who take sufficient hyoscyamine (an alkaloid precursor of scopolamine) may lapse into a coma, one that adds a risk of lethal increases in temperature because scopolamine can prevent sweating [13]. Enormous doses of scopolamine or its sister, atropine, have been used in the treatment of depression, so they are relatively safe as long as the ambient temperature does not require

sweating to keep cool [14, 15]. As already noted, although such doses may eliminate the remembrance of surgery, they do not produce anesthesia. They do not produce a patient who is immobile in the face of noxious stimulation [5].

The Seventeenth Century

By the turn of the seventeenth century, surgical procedures became more complex (and thus more painful), and the practice of medicine more professional. The scientific revolution was in full swing, and experimentation began to replace speculation. William Harvey's 1628 book, *An Anatomical Exercise on the Motion of the Heart and Blood in Living Beings*, described his momentous discoveries concerning the anatomy and physiology of the circulation of blood, how blood moved from heart to artery to vein and back again [7]. And Hieronymous Fabricius ab Aquopendente, a teacher to Harvey, not only demonstrated venous valves but also used a technique for tracheotomies—puncturing the windpipe to allow passage of air—that is similar to the approach used today. Adding to Harvey's contribution, in 1661, Marcello Malpighi described the capillaries and their function.

In the 1500s–1600s, Colleges of Physicians arose in England, Scotland and Ireland, acquiring the Royal prefix by the 1600s. This brought prestige to physicians (internists), but little to the surgeons. Surgeons continued to struggle for recognition in their field. French barber-surgeons eventually received the legal right to treat all wounds. As is the case today, the "private practice" barber-surgeons received higher fees than their academic competition, the master surgeons. Even so, to make ends meet, in addition to doing surgery, barber-surgeons performed bloodletting and mundane wound care. They became more technically proficient than the academicians but did not contribute to advances in knowledge.

The seventeenth century saw the first demonstration of the possibility of intravenous anesthesia. In 1656, Christopher Wren (the architect for St. Paul's cathedral and a founder of the Royal Society) infused wine and ale from a syringe made of dog's bladder, through a goose quill needle into the vein of a dog [16, 17]. Wren wrote "I have injected wine and ale in a living dog into the mass of blood by a veine (sic), in good quantities, till I have made him extremely drunk, but soon after he pisseth it out." The dog survived the experiment. The dog, incidentally, was provided by Robert Boyle, author of Boyle's law.. Wren later gave opium intravenously via a quill to dogs, causing unconsciousness in some animals but killing others [17]. Wren's experiment was the first known injection to produce anesthesia.

The Eighteenth Century: The Verge of Discovery

The eighteenth century brought the professionalization of medicine to Europe and eventually, to the US. By the 1700s, academic surgeons gradually became recognized as professionals equal to physicians, largely because they demonstrated the importance and interdependence of pathological (diseased) anatomy and pathophysiology (diseased function). French surgical training increasingly included teaching an accepted body of knowledge in courses and schools. Two events moved French surgery closer to a profession. One was the 1731 establishment of the Royal Academy or College of Surgery. Second was a 1743 Royal Declaration, forbidding master surgeons to work as barbers. Laws promulgated after the initiation of the French Revolution in 1789, added to the rise of surgery in France. The Faculty of Medicine and the College of Surgery were abolished in 1792, replaced in 1794 by the School of Health that imposed identical educational requirements for those practicing medicine and surgery [6, 7].

In the last half of the eighteenth century, surgery in Great Britain also progressed rapidly. In 1745, the British Parliament separated surgeons from the barber guilds by enacting a bill that formed a Corporation of Surgeons. Led by Percival Pott and John Hunter, [6, 7] Britain displaced France as the most important European center for surgical education and training. Pott and Hunter's knowledge of anatomy advanced surgery as a scientific discipline. Hunter made important observations, describing, for example, the pathophysiology of surgical diseases, and supplying observations on malignant tumors and the growth of collateral circulation after arterial occlusion. This information was particularly important to

treatment of aneurysms.[2] Pott connected the occupation of chimneysweeps with their development of scrotal cancer.

Medicine and surgery were stagnant in North America from 1600 to 1750, and self-educated "physicians" served most medical needs. As 1800 approached, Americans increasingly admired physicians, prompting progressive numbers of Americans to obtain training from the more advanced European system of medical education.

Eighteenth century internal medicine sped forward in diagnosis and treatment. The parallel development of eighteenth century pathological anatomy and experimental physiology strengthened the connection of internal medicine and surgery. Surgeons increasingly correlated disease with anatomical (pathological) changes. This reflected the view long held by physicians, that disease processes had physiologic consequences. Regardless of these developments, without anesthesia and antisepsis, surgery advanced slowly.

Several important discoveries were made during this period. One was by Englishman Joseph Priestly, who had committed himself to the ministry, but believed that understanding nature would further the aims of religion. Priestly's experiments resulted in the discovery of new gases or "airs", among them oxygen and nitrous oxide. He produced nitrous oxide by heating iron filings with nitric acid in 1772, publishing his studies three years later. However, like Paracelsus' oversight about the possibilities of ether two and a half centuries earlier, Priestly missed the significance of his discovery and little was then made of the new air.

Perhaps the most important discovery of the time originated from a 1735 expedition, led by French explorer Charles de la Condamine into South America's Amazon River region, where he observed the natives using blowpipes to propel poisonous arrows with lethal effects while hunting [18]. In 1769, while in South America, English physician Edwin Bancroft wrote of his observations of the natives concentrating the poisonous mix of bark and roots, noting that they avoided exposing wounds in their skin to the confection [19]. Bancroft brought samples of the poison, known as curare, back to England.

In 1811, English surgeon Benjamin Brodie, reported that although the poison caused breathing to cease in a donkey, the heart continued to beat, [20] and beating could be sustained if ventilation was supported [21]. In an 1814 demonstration, Brodie and Sewell, a veterinary surgeon, dramatically demonstrated the innocuousness of curare if ventilation

---

[2] Ironically, Hunter had angina pectoris, presciently noting that "my life is in the hands of any rascal who chooses to annoy and tease me." A fatal heart attack at age 65 followed an argument at St. Georges Hospital on 14 October 1793. Pott described the anatomy of congenital inguinal hernias in his "Treatise on Ruptures." He advocated emergent operations for incarcerated hernias. Most famous was his 1775 Chirurgical Observations, a 5-page essay correctly connecting scrotal cancer in chimney sweeps to their exposure to tars.

was supported. Sykes, a well-known surgeon described the experiment as follows [22]:

> A she-ass received the wourali poison in the shoulder, and died apparently in 10 min. An incision was made in its windpipe, and through it the lungs were regularly inflated for two hours with a pair of bellows. Suspended animation returned. The ass held up her head and looked around; but the inflating being discontinued, she sunk once more in apparent death. The artificial breathing was immediately recommenced, and continued without intermission for two hours more. This saved the ass from final dissolution; she rose up, and walked about; she seemed neither in agitation nor in pain. The wound, through which the poison entered, was healed without difficulty…and by Midsummer (the ass) became fat and frisky…The kind hearted reader will rejoice on learning that Earl Percy, pitying her misfortunes, sent her down from London to Walton Hall, near Wakefield. There she goes by the name Wouralia. Wouralia shall be sheltered from the wintry storm; and when the summer comes she shall feed in the finest pasture. No burden shall be place on her and she shall end her days in peace."

To survive the paralytic effects of curare, Wouralia the donkey had a tracheotomy and ventilation with a bellows. Wouralia did just as Sykes described, and lived another 25 years in peace. The local paper supplied an obituary.

Prior to Brodie and Sewell's experiments, interest had already developed in approaches to secure the airway. As a result, their efforts built on the practice of earlier surgeons like Hooke, Kite, Herholdt and Rafn. In 1667, Robert Hooke performed an extraordinary and cruel sequel to Vesalius' 1550s experiment. Hooke showed that blowing air down the windpipe and out through multiple punctures in the lungs of an awake dog sustained life, even though the lungs were still. In 1788, Kite ventilated a drowning victim's lungs through a tube he placed blindly through the oropharynx and into the windpipe. Nearly a decade later, Herholdt and Rafn described blind digitally assisted tracheal intubation, to resuscitate drowning victims.

Some aspects of modern surgery and management of the airway arose early. Concentrating cohorts of war casualties or victims of epidemics in one place enhances their monitoring and care—in ancient or modern times—anticipating the development of hospitals. The Bible implies the use of mouth-to-mouth respiration (2 Kings, iv, 34), and midwives used it to revive the new-born. Slowly, science and medicine would bring together the airway and ventilatory necessities, the concentrating of patients to supply the intensive care that became part of modern anesthesia.

And What About Positive Thinking?

Other than Priestly's discovery of nitrous oxide, little else anticipated the approaching demonstration of anesthesia in 1846 besides the mind control that physicians and others long had practiced. Practitioners have seemingly forever applied positive thinking and various forms of suggestion, including modern magical rings, necklaces and charms for the parturient. Greeks applied oils and warm compresses during labor, anticipating the warm compresses, massage and herbal teas used today. Were these placebos (which can have positive effects)? In the latter part of the eighteenth century, Franz Mesmer created "theories of animal magnetism," perhaps a form of hypnosis. Mesmerism provided an inconsistently effective management of the pain of surgery. The scientific establishment noted the absence of any rationale for Mesmerism's effectiveness.

Reprise

By the nineteenth century, the surgeon had become a full member of the medical community, contributing to the knowledge of human anatomy and pathology, and to an elaboration of surgical procedures. The operations performed included amputations, cataract removal, cesarean sections, cosmetic surgery, removal of bladder stones, ligation of major arteries, excision of superficial tumors, excision of anal fistulas, and repair of hernias. The range staggers the imagination, more so, given the absence of anesthesia. Surgeons focused on acute processes, conditions requiring immediate care: simple fractures, dislocations, and abscesses. Infection compromised treatment and was a constant threat to life. But most of all, pain limited the number of surgeries that might be performed, and thus limited progress in surgery.

Acknowledgment The authors appreciate the editorial suggestions made by Ms. Shawnee Shahroody Spitler.

References

1. Plowman T, Rivier L. Cocaine and cinnamoylcocaine content of thirty-one species of Erythroxylum (Erythroxylaceae). Ann Botony (Lond) 1983;51:641–59.
2. Draelos ZD The ability of onion extract gel to improve the cosmetic appearance of postsurgical scars. J Cosmet Dermatol. 2008;7:101–4.
3. Juvin P, Desmonts JM. The ancestors of inhalational anesthesia: the Soporific Sponges (XIth–XVIIth centuries): how a universally recommended medical technique was abruptly discarded. Anesthesiology. 2000;93:265–9.
4. Nuland SB. The origins of anesthesia. Birmington: Adams, Jr.; 1983. p. 11.
5. Eger EI II, Zhang Y, Laster MJ, Flood P, Kendig JJ, Sonner JM. Acetylcholine receptors do not mediate the immobilization produced by inhaled anesthetics. Anesth Analg. 2002;94:1500–4.
6. Rutkow IM. The origins of modern surgery, surgery-basic science and clinical evidence. New York: Springer; 2001. pp. 2–19.
7. Haeger K The Illustrated 2 of surgery. Houston: Bell Publishing Co.; 1988.
8. Keys TE. The history of surgical anesthesia. Park Ridge: Wood Library-Museum of Anesthesiology; 1996. p. 9.

9. Ball C, Westhorpe R. Ether before anaesthesia. Anaesth Intensive Care. 1996;24:3.

10. Gallucci JM. Who deserves the credit for discovering ether's use as a surgical anesthetic? J Hist Dent. 2008;56:38–43.

11. Snow J. On chloroform and other anaesthetics: their action and administration. London: John Churchill; 1858. pp. 1–443.

12. Roberts MF, Wink M. Alkaloids. Biochemistry, ecology, and medicinal applications. New York: Plenum Press; 1998. p 34.

13. Beach GO, Fitzgerald RP, Holmes R, Phibbs B, Stuckenhoff H. Scopolamine poisoning. N Engl J Med. 1964;270:1354–55.

14. Brichcin S, Filipova A. Atropine coma therapy and a proposal for using scopolamine in psychiatric treatment. Act Nerv Super (Praha). 1965;7:248.

15. Brichcin S, Filipova A. [2 years of experience with cholinergolytic comas]. Cesk Psychiatr. 1967;63:248–51.

16. Major DJ. Chirurgia infusoria placidis CL: vivorium dubiis impugnata, cun modesta ad Eadem, Responsione. Kiloni, 1667.

17. Dagnino J. Wren, Boyle, and the origins of intravenous injections and the Royal Society of London. Anesthesiology. 2009;111:923–4. (author reply 924).

18. de la Condamine M. Relation abrégée d'un Voyage fait dans l'intérieur de l'Amérique de, dpuis 1 Côte de la Mer du Sud, jusques aux Côtes du Brésil et de la Guiane, en descendant la rivière des Amazones. Histoire de l'académie Royale des Sciences 1745:391–492.

19. Bancroft E. An essay on the natural history of Guiana and South America. London: T Becket & PA De Hont. 1769.

20. Brodie BC. Experiments and observations on the different modes in which death is produced by certain vegetable poisons. Philos Trans Roy Soc Lond. 1811;102:178–208.

21. Brodie BC. Further experiments and observations on the action of poisons on the animal system. Philos Trans Roy Soc Lond. 1812;102:205–27.

22. Sykes K. Harold Griffith memorial lecture. The Griffith legacy. Can J Anaesth. 1993;40:365–74.

The Half Century Before Ether Day

Edmond I Eger II, Rod N. Westhorpe and Lawrence J. Saidman

Summary

The gases and vapors later known as anesthetics had been synthesized or isolated before (ether, nitrous oxide and carbon dioxide) or would be synthesized in (chloroform) the period from 1798 through 1846. They served various purposes. In 1798–1800, Humphry Davy used nitrous oxide for recreation and research, noting its capacity to diminish or even abolish pain. He suggested its use for surgery, but no one noticed. In 1823, Hickman used carbon dioxide to cause what he called "suspended animation", a state that permitted apparently painless surgery in animals. But no one noticed. In the 1840s, Clarke, Long, and Smilie each administered ether in amounts sufficient to permit surgery to be undertaken without pain. But they thought too little of what they had done, or didn't know what they had done, to request public credit for their accomplishment. And no one noticed.

As indicated in the preceding chapter, despite the absence of anesthesia, despite the agony of surgery, despite the great risk of infection and death from infection, surgery intruded into any immediately accessible structure thought to need attention. The exemptions might be abdominal, thoracic, and intracranial operations, but surgeons might go even there. The agony of remembrance of surgery was expressed vividly, revealing what we know today as post-traumatic stress disorder (PTSD).

World Events in the Half Century Before Ether Day

In 1799 Napoleon staged a coup d'état, becoming First Consul of France, five years later crowning himself Emperor. With the 1803 Louisiana Purchase, the US more than doubled its size, buying The West. The steam engine appeared in 1804. Nelson defeated Napoleon's fleet at Trafalgar in 1805, and winter defeated Napoleon's army in Russia in 1812. After his defeat he was exiled to Elba (1814), but he escaped the next year, and began the Hundred Days leading to his final defeat at Waterloo. In 1820, a Russian expedition discovered Antarctica. Three years later, James Monroe declared his eponymous Doctrine (any effort by European nations to interfere with governance in North or South America or colonize land would be viewed by the US as an act of aggression). The first electric motor appeared in 1829 and in 1836, Samuel Colt

manufactured his six shooter. Several inventors made "telegraphs", the one by Samuel Morse in the late 1830s being the most successful. Rowland Hill introduced the postage stamp in 1840. The first publicly funded telegraph line in 1844 sent Morris' message: 'What hath God Wrought?" Two Opium Wars waged from 1839 to 1860 forced China to make many concessions to France, the UK, the US, and Russia, greatly weakening China's power.

A Chronology of Major Themes up to Ether Day

1798–1800: Humphry Davy Misses the Gold Ring

In Bristol, England, Thomas Beddoes established the Pneumatic Institution to treat pulmonary tuberculosis with "new airs", various gases including nitrous oxide. Traveling in 1798, he met the precocious 20-year-old Humphry Davy (1778–1829) and recruited him to superintend his laboratory. Davy (Fig. 2.1) vigorously pursued his charge, particularly in studies of nitrous oxide, studies involving self-experimentation to the point of addiction. Well, we might say, of course, but Keys points out that this took a bit of courage: "...an American chemist and physician, Samuel Latham Mitchill, administered nitrous oxide to animals with such dire results that he came to the conclusion that this gas was very poisonous [1]." We know now, that lack of oxygen rather than the nitrous oxide itself caused death, but who knew that then? "He (Mitchill) also believed that nitrous oxide

E. I Eger II (✉)
Department of Anesthesia and Perioperative Care, University of California, San Francisco, CA, USA
e-mail: egere@anesthesia.ucsf.edu

R. N. Westhorpe
Melbourne, Australia
e-mail: westhorpe@netspace.net.au

L. J. Saidman
Department of Anesthesia, Stanford University, Stanford, CA, USA
e-mail: lsaidman@stanford.edu

E. I Eger II et al. (eds.), *The Wondrous Story of Anesthesia,* DOI 10.1007/978-1-4614-8441-7_2, © Edmond I Eger, MD 2014

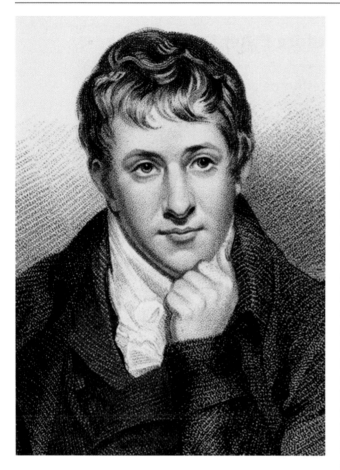

Fig. 2.1 Humphry Davy, the precocious superintendent of the Pneumatic Institution in Bristol, described the capacity of nitrous oxide to prevent pain, suggesting its use in surgical procedures, but no one took up his suggestion

repose and consistent action. On the day when the inflammation was most troublesome, I breathed three large doses of nitrous oxide. The pain always diminished after the first four or five respirations; the thrilling came on as usual, and uneasiness was for a few minutes swallowed up in pleasure. As the former state of mind returned, the state of organ returned with it; and I once imagined that the pain was more severe after the experiment than before."

Part of this fits with what we now believe about the effects of nitrous oxide. It may decrease the perception of pain (i.e., cause analgesia), in part, by activating the receptors turned on by opioids such as morphine [4]. Tolerance (a decreased effectiveness) develops with nitrous oxide, especially with repeated administration, possibly explaining enhanced pain on recovery [5].

On page 556 of his book, we find Davy's famous quotation suggesting the possibility of surgical anesthesia: "As nitrous oxide in its extensive operation appears capable of destroying physical pain, it may probably be used with advantage during surgical operations in which no great effusion of blood takes place [3]." His suggestion went unnoticed. This meteor of a man went on to discover several elements including sodium, and construct the miners' safety lamp, but his inaction regarding nitrous oxide cost him anesthesia's gold ring, the greatest discovery in all of medicine. He was immortalized by Edmund Clerihew Bentley's poem (a *clerihew* is a poetic 4-line verse that takes the form AA, AA, BB, BB). The first-ever clerihew was perhaps written during a particularly boring chemistry lecture:

> Sir Humphry Davy
> Was not fond of gravy
> He lived in the odium
> Of having discovered sodium.

1800–1810

As the nineteenth century began, the US had but 4 medical schools. Benjamin Rush (1745–1813), professor at the foremost school, the University of Pennsylvania, had attempted to minimize labor pain by applying leeches to remove blood. Since the pain of childbirth caused stimulation, he reasoned that bloodletting would offer relief by producing an opposing depression. In defense of higher learning in the US, note that Rush obtained his medical education at the University of Edinburgh and St Thomas' Hospital in London. Others shared his belief in the curative power of the removal of blood by venesection (Stanley, p 54) [6]: "In 1809, The Times reported on an American, Captain James Niblett, who over two months had been bled of 600 ounces of blood, more than fifty instances in addition to leeches."

In 1803, Serturner isolated morphine from opium.

might possibly be the contagium for the spread of epidemics [1]." In addition, 5 years before Davy's discoveries, Mitchill described the "anesthesia" produced by inhalation of nitrous oxide [2]. Thus, a mixture of courage, bravado, foolishness and addictive behavior probably underlay Davy's inhalation of nitrous oxide. Keys wrote that "instead of dying, he (Davy) experienced many pleasurable sensations; he felt an agreeable sense of giddiness, a relaxation of the muscles, noticed his hearing to be more acute, and in general felt so cheerful that he was compelled to laugh." By 1800, Davy had written a 580 page book describing his adventures [3], displaying more than a passing fondness for its properties: "… a desire to breathe (nitrous oxide) is always awakened in me by the sight of a person breathing, or even by that of an air-bag or an air-holder." His is an early example of the potential of anesthetics to produce addiction.

On page 465 of Davy's book, he described his self-treatment for the pain associated with eruption of a wisdom tooth:

> "In cutting one of the unlucky teeth called dentes sapientiae, I experienced an extensive inflammation of the gum, accompanied with great pain, which equally destroyed the power of

Fig. 2.2 The agony of surgery without anesthesia and the violence of the response to surgery are readily imagined

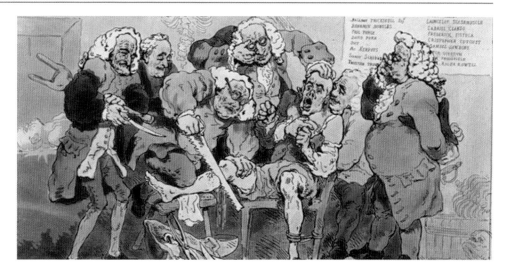

1810–1820

Numerous reports describe the agony of surgery and the lingering after effects, what we might now call post traumatic stress disorder (PTSD). Columnist David Brooks wrote [7]: "In 1811, the popular novelist Fanny Burney learned that she had breast cancer and underwent a mastectomy without anesthesia:

"'I felt the instrument—describing a curve—cutting against the grain, if I may so say, while the flesh resisted in a manner so forcible as to oppose & tire the hand of the operator who was forced to change from the right to the left,..I began a scream that lasted intermittingly during the whole time of the incision—& I almost marvel that it rings not in my ears still.' The surgeon removed most of the breast but then had to go in a few more times to complete the work: 'I then felt the Knife rackling against the breast bone—scraping it! This performed while I yet remained in utterly speechless torture.'"

Brooks noted that Burney wrote about more than the immediate experience. She described the recurring impact on her emotions. "Not for days, not for weeks, but for months I could not speak of this terrible business without nearly again going through it!… I dare not revise, nor read, the recollection is still so painful." PTSD, indeed!

A patient of Scottish surgeon James Simpson provided another vivid description of the agony of remembrances of surgery [8]:

"Suffering so great as I underwent cannot be expressed in words…but the blank whirlwind of emotion, the horror of great darkness, and the sense of desertion by God and man, which swept through my mind, and overwhelmed my heart, I can never forget…Those are not pleasant remembrances. For a long time they haunted me, and even now they are easily resuscitated; and though they cannot bring back the suffering attending the events which gave them a place in my memory, they can occasion a suffering of their own, and be the cause of a disquiet which favors neither mental nor bodily health."

It might have been nearly impossible for four strong men to restrain a terrified woman or man subjected to the knife (Fig. 2.2). And the struggles of the consenting patient could be sufficient to cause the operating table to disintegrate [9].

Yet surgery continued despite the woe it induced, despite the agony, despite the haunting memories. For some, pain was something to be borne, a misery that nonetheless did not preclude surgery or surgical advancement.

In 1818, Michael Faraday noted parallels between the effects of ether and nitrous oxide [10, 11]:

"When the vapour of ether mixed with common air is inhaled, it produces effects very similar to those occasioned by nitrous oxide…In trying the effects of the ethereal vapour on persons who are peculiarly affected by nitrous oxide, the similarity of sensation produced was very unexpectedly found to have taken place. One person who always feels a depression of spirits on inhaling the gas, had sensation of a similar kind produced by inhaling the vapour."

Faraday raised a caution regarding ether [10]: "By the imprudent inspiration of ether, a gentleman was thrown into a very lethargic state, which continued with occasional periods of intermission for more than 30 hours, and a great depression of spirits; for many days the pulse was so much lowered that considerable fears were entertained for his life."

Surgeons used counter-irritants "to inflict pain in the hope of healing [6]." They would apply blistering agents. They would remove blood with lances and leeches. In 1819, Sir Walter Scott, plagued with stomach cramps was subjected to

"profuse bleeding and liberal blistering" causing him to scream "without interval through the night, terrifying his family and servants…Looking back on the ordeal Scott reflected wryly that his doctors had told him that 'mere pain cannot kill'…The suffering inseparable from treatment before or besides surgery, however, explains how the acute pain of surgery was perhaps merely an intensification of a regime in which prolonged pain was seen as an inevitable part of healing [6]." (p 56)

1820–1830

In the first half of the nineteenth century, surgeons devised operations of increasingly greater complexity, invasiveness and duration. Stanley [6] reported (pp 64–5) that in 1822,

> "Working in a cottage in poor light Liston excised a tumour beneath McNair's shoulder blade…'I began by making an incision of a foot long…I felt my finger and knife dip into the body of the tumour…I immediately thrust my sponge into the cavity, so as to command the haemorrhagy. The patient, who had borne the operation well…now dropped his head off the pillow, pale, cold, and almost lifeless. I then…saw that nothing but a bold stroke of the knife could save the boy from immediate death. Pulling out the sponge, therefore, with one rapid incision I completely separated the upper edge of the tumour…After removing the tumour, I found it necessary to saw off the ragged and spongy part of the scapula, so as to leave only a fourth part of that bone….' Liston's patient survived the operation but died four months later…."

The Lancet was first published in 1823. Five years later, the *Boston Medical and Surgical Journal* (later the *New England Journal of Medicine*) began publication. Such journals plus newspapers described medical discoveries, including ether's anesthetic properties just two decades later.

In 1823 and 1824, a young English surgeon, Henry Hickman (1800–1830), gave animals carbon dioxide to breathe, causing a "suspended animation" that allowed apparently painless amputation. Hickman reported his observations to the Royal Society and to Charles X in France, but neither responded. Well, he tried and then died of tuberculosis. Credit him with advancing the idea that surgery might be undertaken painlessly by the inhalation of an agent whose elimination could rapidly reverse the pain-relieving effect. This idea may have been crucial to the discovery of anesthesia. Otherwise the widespread belief of the inevitability of pain would prevent a search for a remedy.

In 1829, Babbington viewed the glottis, the opening to the larynx, using indirect laryngoscopy, i.e., viewing the larynx using mirrors. Increasingly we shall see attempts to control the freedom of the passage of air to the lungs. Viewing the larynx was important to such attempts.

1830–1840

The great surgeon, James Syme, operated on 95 patients in Minto House in 1830 [6]: 10 major amputations of the legs; 9 minor amputations of fingers or toes; 7 novel excisions of elbows or knees (i.e., removal of a diseased portion of the knee or elbow, thus avoiding amputation); 4 breast resections for cancer; excision of an upper jaw; removal of 11 tumors; 4 lithotomies (for bladder stone); ligation of 2 aneurysms; and repair of a strangulated hernia. He performed several minor operations: 6 for hemorrhoids; 4 for anal fistulas; 3 nasal polyps; and 1 for cataract. All this in 1 year when Syme was aged 30.

In 1831, von Liebig, Soubeiran and Guthrie independently discovered chloroform.

1840: The State of Medicine and Surgery

By 1840, the US had 30 medical schools. The curriculum typically occupied two four-month blocks, and covered seven courses. Ability to pay entrance fees determined admission to most schools. Physicians supplemented their training with apprenticeships, the "house pupil" experience, or they traveled to Europe for advanced training. No medical students were women.

Latin American surgeons undertook operations in homes, hospitals, or local inns. In Europe, surgery and delivery might be accomplished in hospitals. Despite the absence of anesthesia, there seemed little that surgeons would not do. Nordic surgeons performed major operations; they removed the mandible, performed gastrectomies, and repaired inguinal hernias and cleft lips. In Chap. 3, Stanley [6] noted the many major procedures done in Great Britain that were improved upon in the first half of the nineteenth century, including trephination, amputation, herniotomy and lithotomy, each with multiple surgical approaches. The rectum offered 23 operable conditions.

> "By the 1840s over twenty arteries could be ligated (for aneurism consequent to the considerable incidence of syphilis), most frequently the aorta, the popliteal (in the thigh), the inguinal (in the groin), the subclavian (near the collarbone), and the carotid (in the neck)…In 1832 in the distant colony of New South Wales, Australia, William Bland, one of Sydney's most prominent surgeons attempted to ligate a subclavian aneurism of William Mullen, a convict. Mullen, whose wife had paid Bland twenty pounds, died after eighteen days. Bland attempted a second operation in 1837, keeping the patient on the table for five-and-a-half hours." (Stanley pp 76–7)

Fergusson performed more than 200 cleft palate repairs in unanesthetized children – with a mortality rate of only 1% [12]. Most procedures were accomplished with dispatch. In London, Liston famously said before he began surgery: "Time me, gentlemen, time me!" Infection and mortality were ever present.

What could be done to diminish the agony of surgery? Latin American clergy and shamans used opium, herbal extracts, and alcohol to decrease surgical pain. Patients required restraint. In Australia and New Zealand, neither the aborigines nor the Maori used "anesthesia", although aborigines chewed "pituri" or "pedgery", herbs producing intoxication or hallucination. Pituri could cause respiratory arrest and death in animals.

Stanley (p 203) [6] argued that courage supported the surgeon as well as the patient. The surgeon dreaded the pain he (no female surgeons) inflicted. He knew the immediate, sometimes bloody, disasters that awaited his actions. Loss of blood might kill the patient sooner, and infection later. "The desire to finish an operation quickly (whether from concern for the patient or for reputation) imposed a peculiar strain on operators. Some expressed this tension by shouting at the patient, colleagues or dressers. The tension showed in the haste with which, as Samuel Cooper said, surgeons sawed through bone with 'short, very rapid, and almost convulsive strokes'." Operations were done speedily to diminish the anguish of the patient. Amputations of the upper or lower extremities might be accomplished in 15 to 30 seconds with closure to follow (Stanley, pp 226–7) [6]. Although the operation might be accomplished with dispatch, cleaning up and closure could impose an hour of great misery: "As dressers wiped a sponge over the raw surface 'perhaps studded by the truncated ends of large nerves,' patients would twitch and gasp. At each 'catch of the forceps and noosing of the ligature' the patient might shriek" (Stanley, p 229) [6].

"The surgeon might lament what he had to do, ending surgery with tears in his eyes or retiring to vomit in solitude. Surgeons were known to faint mid-operation and their assistants had to supervene. Appetite lessened and sleep came hard." (Stanley, p 205) [6] A tension existed between the necessity of surgical pain and the desire to heal. The focus of the surgeon might be intense: "After performing an amputation by transfixion in the Adelaide Hospital, (George Mayo) remarked 'How quiet the patient has been!' A colleague, startled at his absorption, retorted 'Why, man, he was screaming all the time'" [6].

But there was a certain resignation. As the French surgeon Alfred Velpeau said in 1839, "The abolishment of pain in surgery is a chimera. It is absurd to go on seeking it…knife and pain are two words in surgery that must forever be associated in the consciousness of the patient." Again, note this impediment to the discovery of anesthesia, the remedy that Velpeau said could not exist.

One also sees the foolishness of physicians in this time. In the early 1840s, surgeons treated stuttering by operation: "Yearsley…excised the patients' uvula and tonsils…(giving) the patients 'instantaneous' relief.' Patients previously 'scarcely able to articulate half a dozen words' became able to speak 'with a wonderful degree of fluency'." (Stanley, p 248) [6]—shades of Galen.

1840–1846: The Non-discovery of Ether Anesthesia

In the 1840s, several physicians/dentists discovered the anesthetic effects of ether before Ether Day, but either didn't publicize their findings at the time, or didn't appreciate what they had found. They knew of the inebriating effects of ether and employed it in one or a few patients. These early timid

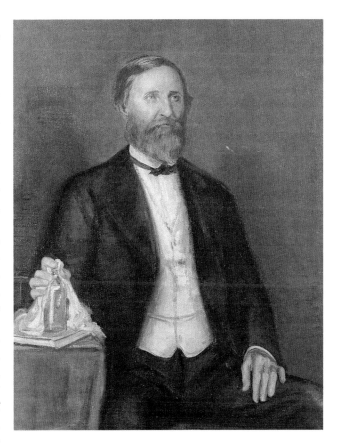

Fig. 2.3 In 1842, Crawford Long used ether to deliberately provide anesthesia. He did not report this, despite his repeated successful application of ether for anesthesia. Like many others, he missed the gold ring. (Courtesy of the University of Pennsylvania Art Collection, Philadelphia, PA)

successes illustrate the caution and apprehension of those who didn't realize that they had succeeded. Perhaps success required audacity, a daredevil ego, and greed. In 1842, William Clarke, who "was in the habit of entertaining his companions with inhalations of ether," anesthetized a Miss Hobbie with ether poured on a towel [13]. Dr. Elijah Pope then extracted a tooth from Miss Hobbie "without pain" [13]. "This would appear to be the first use of ether anesthesia on record; it antedated the work of Crawford Long (1815–1878) by at least two months. Apparently Clarke considered his contribution of no importance, for it is not mentioned in an account of his life in Stone, RF: Biography of Eminent American Physicians and Surgeons, Indianapolis, Carlon and Hollenbeck, 1894, p. 89" [13]. Clarke's failure to publicize his discovery cost him his place in history.

Like Clarke, Long (Fig. 2.3) had engaged in ether frolics; he knew the inebriation it produced and that ether might be safe to breathe, at least to levels that produced inebriation.

"The first patient to whom I administered ether in a surgical operation, was Mr. James M. Venable, who…consulted me on several occasions in regard to the propriety of removing two small tumours situated on the back part of his neck, but would postpone from time to time having the operations performed, from dread of pain. At length I mentioned to him the fact of my receiving bruises while under the influence of the vapour of ether, without suffering, and as I knew him to be fond of, and accustomed to inhale ether, I suggested to him the probability that the operations might be performed without pain and proposed operating on him while under its influence. …The ether was given to Mr. Venable on a towel; and when fully under its influence I extirpated the tumour….The patient continued to inhale ether during the time of the operation; and when informed it was over, seemed incredulous, until the tumour was shown him. He gave no evidence of suffering during the operation, and assured me, after it was over, that he did not experience the slightest degree of pain from its performance. This operation was performed on the 30th March, 1842" [14].

Long anesthetized and operated on several additional patients, including a child for an amputation. So he was both an adult and pediatric anesthetist. But he did not report his findings until 1849 [14]. As with Clarke, Long's delay cost him his provenance as the discoverer of anesthesia.

In 1846, Elton Romeo Smilie (1819–1889) also gave ether and produced anesthesia, not realizing that ether had caused the anesthesia [15, 16]. He sought to diminish the coughing of a tubercular clergyman by administering opium. Thinking to vaporize the opium with ether, he did not realize that the ether and not the opium would vaporize – leaving the opium behind. This worked well for the good clergyman. Smilie published his findings, including the use of the mixture for the lancing of an abscess [16]. But because he reported that the opium caused the effect, he gained no credit for the discovery.

Smilie's efforts also indicated the concern that he had regarding the potential for untoward effects of his treatment with ether or opium. Wolfe wrote (pp 187–8) [17]:

"After the patient had inhaled the mixture (of opium and ether), Smilie sent him home, but when calling upon him a few hours later, he found that the patient had fainted and had bumped his head on a table while falling; thus he gave him no more…Smilie's enthusiasm for continuing his use of this panacea was soon deflated by his medical friends, who dissuaded him, telling him that opium had been used extensively in surgery and had been found to be dangerous in large doses that were effective."

Reprise

So close were all these–Clarke, Long, and Smilie, or, Humphry Davy, or Hickman. But not close enough. We might think that they should have been driven by the need to relieve the agony of surgery. But they were not. Surgery and pain were inseparable partners, and always had been. Anesthesia was a chimera. The stories of those who made the discovery are told in Chap. 3.

References

1. Keys TE. The history of surgical anesthesia. Park Ridge: Wood Library-Museum of Anesthesiology; 1996. pp. 15–6.
2. Bergman NA. Samuel Latham Mitchill (1764–1831). A neglected American pioneer of anesthesia. JAMA 1985;253:675–8.
3. Davy H. Researches, chemical and philosophical; chiefly concerning nitrous oxide or dephlogisticated nitrous air and its respiration. Bristol: Biggs and Cottle, 1800. pp. 1–580.
4. Gillman MA. Analgesic (sub anesthetic) nitrous oxide interacts with the endogenous opioid system: a review of the evidence. Life Sci. 1986;39:1209–21.
5. Ramsay DS, Leroux BG, Rothen M, Prall CW, Fiset LO, Woods SC. Nitrous oxide analgesia in humans: acute and chronic tolerance. Pain. 2005;114:19–28.
6. Stanley P. For fear of pain. British surgery, 1790–1850. New York: Rodopi; 2003.
7. Brooks D. New York Times, 23 August, 2010, p. A23.
8 Ashurst J. Surgery before the days of anesthesia, Massachusetts General Hospital: The semicentennial of anesthesia. Oct. 16, 1846-Oct. 16, 1896. Edited by Warren JC WJ, Richardson WL, Beach HH, Shattuck FC, Bigelow WS. Cambridge: H.O. Houghton & Co.; 1897. pp. 27.
9. Skey F. Operative surgery. London: John Churchill; 1850. p. 9.
10. Keys TE. The history of surgical anesthesia. Park Ridge: Wood Library-Museum of Anesthesiology; 1996. pp. 18–19.
11. Bergman NA. Michael Faraday and his contribution to anesthesia. Anesthesiology. 1992;77:812–6.
12. Bruce J. The footprints of Scottish paediatric surgery. J R Coll Surg Edinb. 1976;21:133–47.
13. Keys TE. The history of surgical anesthesia. Park Ridge: Wood Library-Museum of Anesthesiology; 1996. pp. 21–2.
14. Long CW. An account of the first use of sulphuric ether by inhalation as an anaesthetic in surgical operations. Southern Med Surg J. 1849;5:705–13.
15. McMechan FH. An early investigator in anesthesia. Boston Med Surg J. 1915;172:239.
16. Smilie ER. Insensibility produced by the inhalation of the vapor of the ethereal solution of opium. Boston Med Surg J. 1846;35:263–4.
17. Wolfe RJ. Tarnished Idol: William Thomas Green Morton and the introduction of surgical anesthesia: a chronicle of the ether controversy. San Francisco: Norman Publishing; 2001.

1844–1846: The Discovery and Demonstration of Anesthesia

3

Edmond I Eger II, Lawrence J. Saidman and Rod N. Westhorpe

Summary

Gardner Colton, a Columbia University medical student, began the discovery of anesthesia by offering (for pay) a public entertainment, a demonstration of the intoxicating effect of nitrous oxide. The dentist Horace Wells attended a demonstration in Hartford, observing that while inebriated, Samuel Cooley injured himself, apparently not feeling the injury as it occurred. Seeking a means to practice painless dentistry, Wells asked Colton to attend his office the next day, and to administer nitrous oxide to Wells while an associate, John Riggs, pulled one of Wells' teeth. Wells felt no pain, and then gave nitrous oxide to several of his patients, practicing painless dentistry on most of them. His success prompted him to approach the great surgeon Warren at the Massachusetts General Hospital (MGH), requesting that he allow Wells to attempt a public demonstration at the Harvard Medical School. The demonstration failed, the audience denouncing Wells for his "humbug".

Two men claimed to have thought of ether anesthesia. Charles Jackson alleged that he supplied the dentist William Morton, an associate and pupil of Wells, with the idea. Morton had observed Wells' early success with nitrous oxide and recalled that ether given in ether frolics had effects similar to those of nitrous oxide and thus might substitute for nitrous oxide. Morton anesthetized his father's dog and other small farm animals with ether. Subsequently he breathed ether, himself, noting the numbness and sedation it produced. On the evening of 20 Sept 1846, Morton put ether on a handkerchief and applied the handkerchief to a patient, Eban Frost, from whom he then painlessly extracted a bicuspid. On subsequent days, he gave ether to several more patients. Success with these patients, and the notion that money might be made from the discovery emboldened Morton who attempted a public demonstration in what became known as the Ether Dome. The demonstration succeeded. Warren announced: "Gentlemen, this is no humbug"; and the news quickly went around the world.

World Events, 1844–1846

In 1844, Morse patented the telegraph in the US, and George Williams founded the YMCA in London. Parliament passed the Factory Act, imposing a maximum 12 h working day for women, and a 6 h day for children aged 6 to 13. In 1845, British inventor Stephen Perry patented the rubber band. But the big year was 1846. In that year, the US acquired the Oregon Territory and began the Mexican-American War.

Mexico lost, ceding Texas, California, Arizona, New Mexico, Utah, and Nevada to the US. Richard March Hoe invented the rotary printing press, and Elias Howe invented the sewing machine. The potato famine caused 1.6 million Irish to immigrate to the US. The illegitimate son of the Duke of Northumberland, James Smithson, established the Smithsonian Institution with a grant of $ 500,000. Orson Squire Fowler published his bestseller, *Matrimony: Or, Phrenology and Physiology Applied to the Selection of Congenial Companions for Life*. British Prime Minister, Robert Peel, repealed the Corn Laws, replacing the Colonial mercantile trade system with Free Trade. Finally, the first recorded baseball game was played in Hoboken, New Jersey on 9 June under the Cartwright Rules. The New York Nine beat the Knickerbockers 29 to 1, even though the Knickerbockers' owner, Alexander Cartwright, served as umpire.

And 16 October 1846, William Morton demonstrated ether anesthesia in what came to be called the Ether Dome.

E. I Eger II (✉)
Department of Anesthesia and Perioperative Care,
University of California, San Francisco, CA, USA
e-mail: egere@anesthesia.ucsf.edu

L. J. Saidman
Department of Anesthesia, Stanford University,
Stanford, CA, USA
e-mail: lsaidman@stanford.edu

R. N. Westhorpe
Melbourne, Australia
e-mail: westhorpe@netspace.net.au

E. I Eger II et al. (eds.), *The Wondrous Story of Anesthesia,* DOI 10.1007/978-1-4614-8441-7_3, © Edmond I Eger, MD 2014

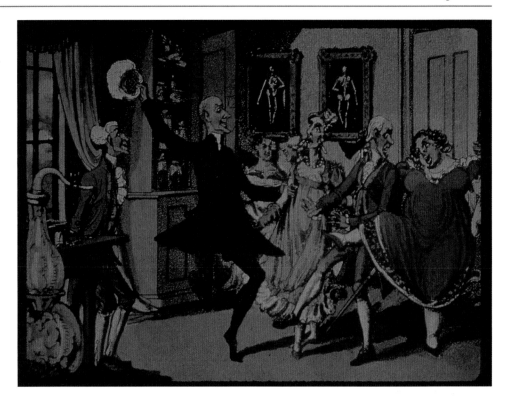

Major Themes Leading to and Following Ether Day

Where previous chapters covered decades, centuries or millennia, the present chronology spans two years. Where previous chapters described incremental steps, the present story is of men in 10-league boots who discovered anesthesia. These disparate men argued, each with some justification, that they deserved credit for the discovery of anesthesia: the honorable dreamer-dentist Horace Wells; the snobbish, brilliant, knowledgeable, self-aggrandizing chemist Charles Jackson; and the unscrupulous, rapacious scoundrel, dentist William Morton—whom most credit for the discovery. All three died unhappily; Wells a suicide, Jackson a cripple, and Morton impoverished.

A larger group facilitated but never claimed the discovery. For the most part, these men came to happy ends. They included the showman-medical student Gardner Quincy Colton, whose public exhibition prompted Wells' test of nitrous oxide, and the elderly distinguished surgeon John Collins Warren who facilitated two attempts at a demonstration of anesthesia although he likely had little faith that either would work. The surgeons Henry Bigelow and George Hayward arranged Morton's appearance at the Massachusetts General Hospital operating theatre on 16 Oct 1846, Ether Day. Glassmakers Joseph Wightman and Nathan Chamberlain made the globe that Morton used to deliver ether to the patient. Augustus Gould advised Morton on how to avoid asphyxiating the patient during ether administration (Morton

boarded with Gould who was a physician). And Gilbert Abbott "volunteered" to be the first patient publically anesthetized with ether (etherized).

Several books detail the circumstances of the discovery: Fenster's lyrical "Ether Day" [1], Wolfe's scholarly "Tarnished Idol" [2], and Wolfe and Patterson's defense in "The Head Behind the Hands" [3] of Jackson's role come immediately to mind. There are more: Keys' classic "The History of Surgical Anesthesia" [4], and Thorwald's riveting (but sometimes inaccurate) fictionalized description in "The Century of the Surgeon" [5]. We cheerfully acknowledge that much of the present chapter draws on these books.

The Dentist Deserves Credit

The story of the discovery, and the first public demonstration that inhaled gases could make painless surgery possible, began with Horace Wells, the Vermont son of affluent parents. Having completed a dental apprenticeship in 1836, the 21 year-old Wells moved to Hartford Connecticut. His practice flourished, and he worried that wealth might compromise his morality. Fenster (p. 54) quotes him [1]: "It is my sincere desire to do as much good as possible, and I hope and pray that no selfish motive may ever influence me to go contrary to this principle." This good and trusting, but naïve man, became a chicken amongst the foxes.

Many had used the long-known inebriating effects of nitrous oxide and ether for recreational purposes (Fig. 3.1) and

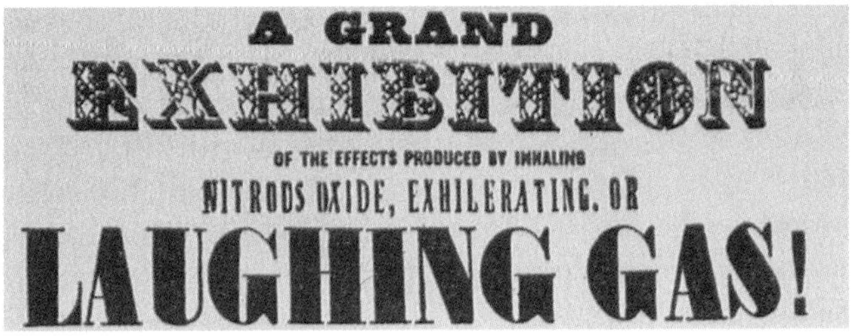

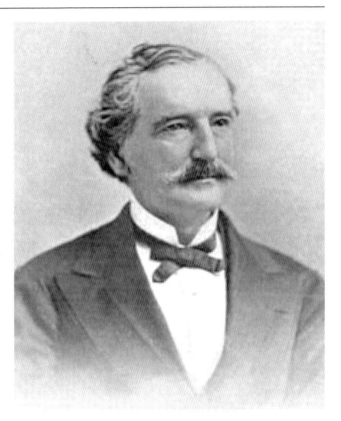

Fig. 3.2 Replication of a poster advertising an exhibition of the inebriation produced by nitrous oxide. (From a larger picture broadcast on the internet by general-anaesthesia.com.)

public entertainments (Fig. 3.2). Gardner Colton (Fig. 3.3) was an enterprising medical student seeking funds to put himself through what today would be Columbia University. He advertized in the Hartford Courant [6]:

> "A grand exhibition of the effects produced by inhaling nitrous oxide, exhilarating or laughing gas! will be given at Union Hall this (Tuesday) evening, Dec 10th, 1844. Forty Gallons of Gas will be prepared and administered to all in the audience who desire to inhale it.
>
> "Twelve Young Men have volunteered to inhale the Gas, to commence the entertainment.
>
> "Eight Strong Men are engaged to occupy the front seats to protect those under the influence of the Gas from injuring themselves or others. This course is adopted that no apprehension of danger may be entertained. Probably no one will attempt to fight.
>
> "The Effect of the Gas is to make those who inhale it either Laugh, Sing, Dance, Speak or Fight, etc., etc., according to the leading trait of their character. They seem to retain consciousness enough to not say or do that which they would have occasion to regret…Those who inhale the Gas once, are always anxious to inhale it the second time. There is not an exception to this rule.
>
> "Entertainment to commence at 7 o'clock. Tickets 25 cents."

Samuel Cooley gave his remembrances of the evening's events to a Congressional Committee charged with determining who had priority in the discovery of anesthesia. The resulting Walker Report found that Cooley,

> "while under the influence of the gas did run against and throw down several of the settees (benches) in the…hall and thereby throwing himself down, and causing several severe bruises upon his knees and other parts of his person; and that after the peculiar influence of said gas had subsided, his friends then present asked if he had not injured himself, and then directed his attention to the acts which he had committed unconsciously while under the operation of said gas. He then found by examination that his knees were severely injured, and he then exposed his knees to those present, and found that the skin was severely abraised (sic) and broken…(Cooley) 'believed that if a person could be restrained, that he could undergo a severe surgical operation without feeling any pain at the time.' Dr. Wells then remarked, 'that he believed that a person could have a tooth extracted while under its influence and not feel any pain.'"

That attracted Horace Wells' attention. He was looking for a way to practice painless dentistry.

Fig. 3.3 Gardner Colton. (Courtesy of Wikipedia.)

The Walker Report continued, noting that Wells (Fig. 3.4) seized on this idea and convinced Colton to come to his office the succeeding day, to administer nitrous oxide. With Wells under its influence, an associate, John Riggs, pulled one of Wells' teeth. Wells claimed he felt no pain. In the ensuing weeks, Wells learned to produce nitrous oxide and applied it successfully in more than a dozen patients for the extraction of teeth. He then sought to demonstrate this discovery. George Hayward acted as an intermediary between Wells and the Hershey Professor of Anatomy and Surgery at Harvard, John Collins Warren.

In a later defense of his claim to be the discoverer of anesthesia, Wells wrote a letter to the editor (published 9 Dec 1846) of the Hartford Courant:

> "I was so much elated with this discovery, that I started immediately for Boston, resolving to give it into the hands of proper persons, without expecting to derive any pecuniary benefit therefrom. I called on Drs. Warren and Haywood (in fact Dr. George Hayward) and made known to them the result of the experiments I had made. They appeared to be interested in the matter, and treated me with much kindness and attention. I was invited by Dr. Warren to address the Medical Class upon the subject, at the close of his lecture. I accordingly embraced the opportunity, and took occasion to remark that the same result would be produced, let the nervous system be excited sufficiently by any means whatever; that I had made use of nitrous oxide gas or protoxide of nitrogen as being the most harmless. I was then invited to administer it to one of their patients who was expecting to have a limb amputated. I remained some two or three days in Boston for this purpose, but the patient decided not to have the operation performed at that time. It was then

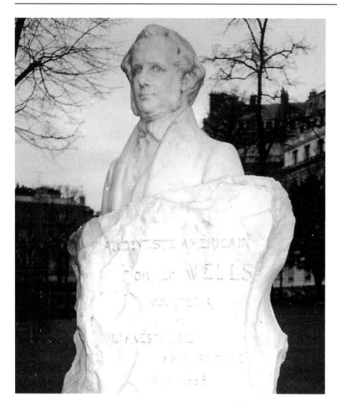

Fig. 3.4 Horace Wells statue in the Place des États-Unis in Paris. (Courtesy of Rod N. Westhorpe.)

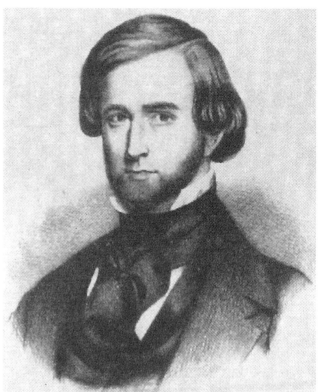

Fig. 3.5 A young, perhaps foppish, William Morton. Image from a portrait by William Hudson, Jr., in 1844. (From the Wellesley Historical Society)

proposed that I should administer it to an individual for the purpose of extracting a tooth. Accordingly a large number of students, with several physicians, met to see the operation performed—one of their number to be the patient. Unfortunately for the experiment, the gas bag was by mistake withdrawn much too soon, and he was but partially under its influence when the tooth was extracted. He testified that he experienced some pain, but not as much as usually attends the operation. As there was no other patient present, that the experiment might be repeated, and as several expressed their opinion that it was a humbug affair, (which in fact was all the thanks I got for this gratuitous service), I accordingly left the next morning for home. While in Boston, I conversed with Drs. Charles T. Jackson and W.T.G. Morton, upon the subject, both of whom admitted it to be entirely new to them. Dr. Jackson expressed much surprise that severe operations could be performed without pain...."

Wells had the reasoning wrong. Anesthesia doesn't result from excitation (although excitation may appear in the transition from the awake to anesthetized states). It results from a depression of the nervous system. But his reasoning would have been irrelevant had he succeeded in his demonstration. He nearly did.

Fenster (p. 64) [1] summarized observations made later by CA Taft who was present at the attempted demonstration:

"The students in the audience...jeered at their laughing-gas man. He heard the word 'humbug,' called out over and over again. No one took much notice when the patient awoke fully and protested that he had experienced almost no pain."

The medical profession's skepticism had been confirmed.

With Considerable Help, a Scoundrel Succeeds

Now to William Morton (Fig. 3.5). Wolfe noted (Chap. 2) [2], that Morton was born in August 1819 in Charlton Massachusetts, son to a Quaker, James Morton a well-off farmer, then merchant, who fell on hard times in the mid-1830s. Early in life, Morton demonstrated what might be thought of as psychopathic behavior, including the story that he had "nearly killed his young sister Elizabeth by forcing 'some unearthly compound down her throat, as she lay asleep in her cradle'." He attended several educational academies within a few years and his "separation from these schools may not have been entirely voluntary."

With the collapse of his father's finances, Morton headed west to seek his fortune, but not entirely from honest work. In large part, Morton's activities were uncovered by his competitor for the discovery of anesthesia, Jackson, who sought to discredit Morton. From 1836 to 1839, Morton lived in Rochester, New York, where initially he worked as a clerk in the dry-goods trade. Morton used his knowledge to swindle several thousand dollars from Loren Ames, with whom he had formed a partnership. He next swindled Phineas Cook, again in Rochester. He was expelled for profanity and dis-honesty from the Brick Church. Finally, he swindled Sarah Seward who ran a private seminary, indicating he would support his sister's schooling but failing to do so.

Morton's unsavory reputation made Rochester inhos-pitable, so early in 1839 Morton decamped for Cincinnati, where he spent 9 months. He now swindled Charles Pom-roy (yet another dry goods merchant) and several customers of Pomroy and Company, becoming increasingly proficient at various forms of lying, forgery and false accounting. He stole from his own company. George Bates (swindled by Morton) noted (Wolfe, p. 27): "The cunning unscrupulous-ness & boldness with which he carried on his operation, in my belief, mark his career as being without parallel among the swindlers who from time to time have infested our city."

On to St. Louis where through lies and forgeries, Mor-ton attempted to swindle James Sickles, but was discovered and foiled. Deposed years after the demonstration of ether anesthesia, Mordicai DeLange gave an additional view of Morton, one repeated in various guises (Wolfe, p. 30): "…in Morton I had discerned a degree of general ignorance which would make a scientific discovery by him, appear to me to be no less than miraculous." A newspaper in 1839 (Wolfe, p. 32) described Morton as

"…about five feet, ten or eleven inches high, well made, a slouching gait. His features are well formed, his complexion is fair and ruddy, his hair light and rather coarse, and pushed up from his head. His eyes are blue, his teeth white and perfect… He dresses in good clothes, but rather foppishly…His voice is coarse and loud; he is remarkably ignorant of matters of general knowledge, and is very apt to betray his ignorance, by the silli-ness of his remarks."

This public rebuke pushed Morton back to Cincinnati. While in Cincinnati, Morton became engaged to the daughter of a wealthy Jewish merchant and apparently in furtherance of this relationship underwent circumcision—without anesthe-sia (Fenster, p. 87) [1]. Morton traveled from Cincinnati to Baltimore in 1840 where he narrowly failed to swindle a Mr. NS Jacobs. An attempt at arrest was made too late; Morton escaped, leaving behind materials he used to commit forgery.

By the early 1840s, Morton realized that his actions might soon lead to imprisonment. He transiently disappeared, per-haps to Charlton, while the heat cooled. His next activities suggested a more cautious approach to amassing a fortune. He turned to dentistry, in 1843 attaching himself to Wells as an apprentice and then as a business partner. Consistent with his previous behavior, he did not live up to his bargain with Wells. He enrolled at Harvard Medical School (admissions were slightly more lax than at present) with Charles Jackson (Fig. 3.6) as his preceptor in medicine.

According to Keys (p. 25) [7], Morton developed a pro-cess for making artificial teeth that required removal of the patients teeth, including the roots. The pain associated with

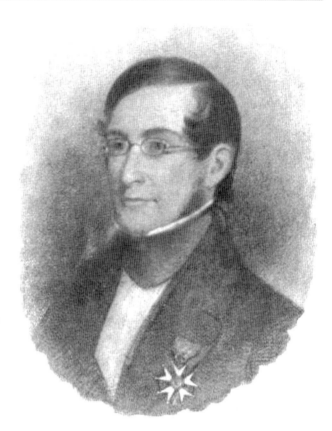

Fig. 3.6 Charles Jackson. (Courtesy of Wikipedia.)

removal of the teeth limited the number of interested pa-tients. Jackson recommended that Morton sprinkle ether in the area surrounding the operative site, apparently envision-ing a local effect. In July 1844, a Miss Parrott asked to have a tooth filled. Morton applied the ether as recommended by Jackson and found it effective in minimizing the pain from his procedure.

Considerably after the demonstration of ether anesthesia, Jackson argued that he had known about ether's effects since 1842 when he experienced irritation of his airway from the accidental breathing of chlorine gas (Fenster, pp. 124–7) [1] and self-medicated with inhalation of ether. He obtained relief and repeated the experiment on himself finding that his body became numb. He thought (in 1842, he said) that this might serve as an anesthetic. Why didn't he then advertise his thought to the world or try its demonstration? We recall from Chapter 2 that Crawford Long privately demonstrated anesthesia, albeit failing to publicize his results. Jackson nei-ther experimented nor publicized "his" idea. He had oppor-tunities: he was an apprentice physician, and he had connec-tions to the greatest surgeons in Boston (he was a personal friend of Warren). But nothing. He left such trivial matters to Morton.

Jump forward to Sept 1846. Morton knew of Well's successes and failures with nitrous oxide. He approached

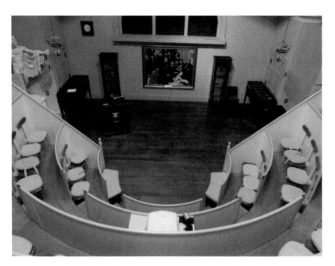

Fig. 3.7 Inside the Ether Dome. The statue of Apollo (left) and the mummy in the case were there in the room on Ether Day. Warren and Lucia Prosperi created the painting seen in the background depicting the surgery on Ether Day [8]. (Courtesy of Dr. Rajesh Haridas, Australia.)

Jackson for advice. Morton indicated that he approached Jackson for help with details, and Jackson obliged, in particular suggesting the use of pure ether (ether adulterated with alcohol, for example, might be ineffective because the presence of the alcohol would diminish the vapor pressure—the concentration—of ether). Jackson also suggested a delivery system consisting of a rubber bag containing ether connected to a glass tube from which a patient might breathe. Jackson contended that he told Morton that ether might be used to impart insensibility sufficient to allow the performance of surgery without pain. Each man may have lied. Morton reported that he experimented with ether using himself and his dog as subjects, finding that numbness and unconsciousness ensued. On 30 Sept 1846, he gave ether to Eben Frost. With Frost under the influence of the ether, Morton painlessly removed an abscessed tooth from Frost, a success reported the next day in the Boston Transcript (Fenster, p. 74) [1]. Jackson attended neither this demonstration nor any other that he claimed to have prompted.

Morton continued to experiment with ether in his patients. The surgeon, Henry Bigelow (who ultimately facilitated the demonstration of anesthesia with ether), encouraged Morton. Morton's motives were clear. He wanted to patent (and he did patent) the discovery of anesthesia in order to gain a fortune. Through Bigelow, he applied to Warren to demonstrate the insensibility produced by his new discovery, and on 16 Oct 1846, he was scheduled to do just that in what would become known as the Ether Dome (Fig. 3.7). Morton arrived late, being delayed by the glassmaker who had modified his inhaler for ether. Warren greeted him testily: "Well, sir, your patient is ready!" Morton prepared his inhaler and had the patient, Gilbert Abbott, breathe the ether until unconscious-

ness supervened. Morton then turned to Warren, repeating the earlier taunt: "Your patient is ready, sir!"

Warren's matter of fact report described the next few moments that changed the world.

> "The patient being prepared for the operation, the apparatus was applied to his mouth by Dr. Morton for about three minutes, at the end of which time he (Abbott) sank into a state of insensibility. I immediately made an incision about 3 inches long through the skin of the neck, and began a dissection among important nerves and blood vessels without any expression of pain on the part of the patient. Soon after he began to speak incoherently, and appeared to be in an agitated state during the remainder of the operation. Being asked immediately afterwards whether he has suffered much, he said that he had felt as if his neck had been scratched; but subsequently, when inquired of by me, his statement was, that he did not experience pain at the time, although aware that the operation was proceeding."

The demonstration was later posed and photographed (Fig. 3.8). In 2001, Warren and Lucia Prosperi created a painting of the event (seen in the background of Fig. 3.7) [8].

Warren's report understates this arguably greatest of all medical discoveries. It also doesn't repeat what is anesthesia's most famous quotation. Recalling the audience's jeering of Wells nearly two years earlier, immediately after the conclusion of the procedure, Warren is alleged to have said: "Gentlemen—This is no humbug."

One other postscript: It seems that the first successful demonstration of anesthesia was, in fact, a demonstration of ether analgesia (freedom from pain in a conscious patient), something Artusio applied to patients a century later [9, 10].

The Name

What should this new state, this release from the agony of surgery be called? Morton favored *Letheon*, a name he devised for his patented ether. *Anesthesia* came from Oliver Wendell Holmes in a 21 November letter to Morton (Keys, p. 30) [4]:

> "My Dear Sir: Everybody wants to have a hand in a great discovery. All I will do is give you a hint or two as to names–or the name–to be applied to the state produced and the agent.

> "The state should, I think, be called 'Anaesthesia.' This signifies insensibility–more particularly (as used by Linnaeus and Cullen) to objects of touch…."

The word was not new, but its meaning in the context used by Holmes was new. Hippocrates used anesthesia to indicate a "loss of the power of feeling" as a consequence of a severe disease process, one usually anticipating death [11]. Holmes' use of "anesthesia" was for a drug-induced reversible state.

Fig. 3.8 A posed photograph after the fact with Morton appearing to give ether while Warren and his colleagues stand by. (From Harvard University and pub.acsorg.)

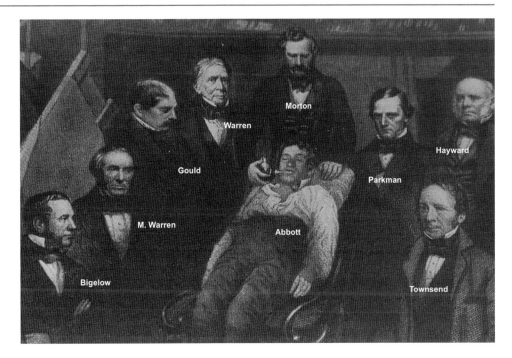

Squabbles and Sadness

None of the claimants to the discovery fared well after 16 October. The ever-ambitious Morton patented (with Jackson) ether, naming it Letheon, but found the patent to be unenforceable. Even the US government violated the patent. The use of ether quickly spread, with little money flowing to Morton whose expenses exceeded his income. Morton returned to dentistry and land speculation, borrowing money to support his activities, money rarely repaid. For a decade-and-a-half after 1849, Morton turned to another cash source, Congress. Morton claimed that he was the sole discoverer of anesthesia, and because of the failure of the government to protect his patent rights, he deserved a compensation of $ 100,000–$ 200,000. A select committee took up the issue, agreeing with Morton and recommending to the full Congress, an award of $ 100,000. Through publicity and lobbying, Morton tried but failed to convince Congress to approve the recommendation. True to form, Morton's lobbying was underwritten by funds embezzled by William Tuckerman from the Eastern Railroad (Wolfe, Chapter 21) [2]. Tuckerman was later caught for stealing from the US mails and imprisoned.

Despite the illegal base which supported Morton, he might have succeeded in his appeal to Congress had Charles Jackson and the Connecticut legislature (below) not intervened. Learning of the possibility of an award to Morton, Jackson wrote to senator Charles Sumner, asserting that he, Jackson, deserved the award. Jackson noted that the patent for ether named him as a co-discoverer of ether's anesthetic effects. He also detailed Morton's crooked dealings as proof of Morton's undeserving character, but this went nowhere as relevant to who might have discovered anesthesia.

As noted above, Jackson claimed to have thought of the application of ether as an anesthetic in 1842—but then did nothing to demonstrate its properties. What strength had such a claim? It was clearly less than that of Crawford Long who had the idea and put it into practice but also failed to broadcast his discovery to the world.

Wells might have tried again to persuade the surgeon Warren to allow a second demonstration. Had he succeeded, the prize would have been his. Even so, the Connecticut legislature designated him posthumously as the discoverer, an act that compromised Morton's efforts for recognition and reward. As Fenster notes (p. 174) [1], "…the emergence of Horace Wells and his eloquent defenders was a godsend for all those in the U.S. Congress who just didn't want to give one hundred thousand dollars to anybody for anything, least of all to Morton for Letheon." Wells drifted from dentistry (which would have nicely supported him), to dealing with minimal success in the sale of reproductions of art. He dabbled with chloroform, inhaling the vapors, himself. He descended into madness and addiction to chloroform, ending with his arrest in New York City in January 1848 for throwing sulfuric acid at several ladies of ill repute. In his cell he inhaled chloroform, slashed his femoral artery, and died. He did not deserve such an end.

Morton and Jackson continued squabbling, to the financial detriment of both in their efforts before Congress. In 1861, the Civil War began and Morton provided anesthesia to Union soldiers to bolster his case, but to no avail. He tried lecturing, but his lectures were disasters.

On 15 June 1868, New York City was exceptionally warm. Morton had come to the city, seeking help to rebut an article in the prestigious Atlantic Monthly that had accorded

Jackson the honor of anesthesia's discovery. Morton fell ill, became increasingly irrational, and died soon thereafter.

In contrast to Morton, for most of his life Jackson enjoyed financial stability, a consequence of an inheritance and his work as a geologist/surveyor. In 1868, he discovered that a cousin had seized his inheritance (Fenster, p. 233) [1]. In May 1873, he suffered a stroke which left him incapacitated for the remaining seven years of his life.

Who Deserves Credit?

Who deserves credit for the discovery/demonstration of anesthesia? Wells and Jackson contributed—and so did many other people. In the late 1840s, France's Académie des Sciences (one of the leading arbiters of science) adjudicated the claims of Jackson, Morton and Wells for the discovery of anesthesia, first giving the honor to Jackson. Then in 1850, the Academy changed its mind, awarding the prize equally to Jackson and Morton, while the Medical Society of Paris gave it to Wells (the news arriving in Hartford a few days after his suicide). The details of the protagonists' lobbying of French academia may be found in Chapter 28.

But it was Morton, Morton the rogue, the greedy scoundrel, the crook looking for the fast buck, the man who lived on the edge of being jailed for his crimes and misdemeanors who showed the world. Of the discovery, Julie Fenster said wonderfully (pp. 126–7) [1]:

> "(Morton) had to travel fast and he knew it; he was standing in the operating theater of the Massachusetts General Hospital demonstrating etherization within seventeen days of the emergence of the discovery of September 30 (Morton's first use of ether in Eben Frost)…Morton threw it like a paper airplane into the future. It happened to land on October 16."

Most, including the editors of this book, credit him with the discovery.

Why Wasn't Anesthesia Discovered Earlier? …and Why Boston?

The means to produce anesthesia had been at hand long before the discovery. That ether and/or nitrous oxide could diminish or abolish pain, could produce unconsciousness, was known. Lully synthesized ether in 1275. Cordus repeated the synthesis in 1540, and Paracelsus noted its soporific and analgesic properties in 1541. Priestly synthesized nitrous oxide in the early 1770s, and Davy wrote of its anesthetic properties in 1800. In his Chapter 16, Norman Bergman (1926–1999) detailed the considerable numbers of observations on narcotic and other effects of ether before 16 Oct 1846 [12]. These included soporific, analgesic and inebriating effects that paralleled the effects of nitrous oxide. In the US, Guthrie

had discovered chloroform in 1831. He described it as "a grateful diffusive stimulant, and that…it may be probably introduced into medicine", although there is doubt that he had any inkling as to its soporific effect [13]. He was actually seeking a pesticide.

So why the delay in the discovery of anesthesia? Several possibilities jointly provide an explanation:

- Pain is God's will, His punishment for sin
- Pain is natural and beneficial, essential to healing
- Individual suffering is unimportant; only the group is important
- The production of insensibility is too dangerous
- Anesthesia isn't needed to perform surgery
- Anesthesia can't possibly exist.

Pain is God's Will, His Punishment for Sin

Campagna echoed this explanation, the view that pain should not be avoided lest the guilty party incur God's wrath [14]. Campagna further argued that the religious injunction against the abolition of pain, a conservative view supporting the status quo, explained why anesthesia was first demonstrated in Boston. At the time of the demonstration of the anesthetic effects of ether, Boston was a medical backwater, ceding first place to cities such as Philadelphia. Supporting this view, Campagna [14] quoted a wonderfully snooty letter written at that time on behalf of the University of South Carolina in petitioning their state legislature for a medical school: "…I say nothing respecting those [hospitals and medical schools] of New England, because they have furnished no manifest occasion for peculiar notice, nor have they risen beyond the level of mediocrity." Many in the New World considered that pain and sickness were manifestations of sin to be enjoyed as a means of expurgation. They were visitations of God's will and thus to be welcomed. But Boston's clerics/physicians, particularly Cotton Mather, were not so sure that ills were God's punishment. When smallpox struck the Boston area in 1721, Mather urged a Dr. Boylston to practice variolation—the inoculation of uninfected persons with effluent from sores on infected patients. The practice was clearly effective, making God's will suspect, yet not convincing the townsmen who often violently opposed variolation for religious reasons (God's will, again).

The Revolutionary War diminished Boston's population by 75%, particularly physicians because they actively supported the revolution. A new medical community arose, one intimately acquainted with the injuries and diseases of war. In the 1780s, Harvard College opened a medical school with John Collins Warren as the first Hersey Professor of Anatomy and Surgery. Warren helped in the formation of the Boston Medical Society and the Journal which became the New England Journal of Medicine.

Smallpox struck again in 1799–1801, but this time an acceptance of variolation began in Boston and spread to other parts of the country. Campanga argued that by 1820–1846,

"To variable degrees, the millennium-old belief that sickness was a punishment that had origin in God's anger had dissipated. The seemingly innate 'urge' to relieve pain, an urge that was sanctioned neither by social nor theological premises, became a tenable thought amenable to critical analysis and scientific experimentation. Slowly but assuredly, medical traditions of dubious value came under the scrutiny of the medical practitioners of Boston and elsewhere. With each success, physicians and their patients solidified their belief that the thoughtful application of scientific reasoning could improve man's lot in the world and that men were not powerless against diseases long considered evidence of God's will."

Pain is Natural and Beneficial, Essential to Healing

Stanley noted (p. 288) [15] that even after the demonstration of the anesthetic effects of ether and chloroform some surgeons abjured their use. This may have derived from the

"belief that pain, far from being undesirable, was natural and beneficial…Its very absence, a surgeon asserted, was itself 'a symptom of disease…Patients could read devotional works offering, for example, *Motives and Encouragements to Bear Afflictions Patiently* which suggested 'the more Pains…the greater glory'".

An Individual's Suffering is Unimportant; Only the Group is Important

Papper proposed that a focus on the importance of the group as opposed to the individual delayed the discovery of anesthesia. If the individual was unimportant, then the individual's suffering also was unimportant [16], but the romantic movement, the belief that mankind has the right to pursue happiness, succeeded in convincing society that the individual was important.

The Production of Insensibility is too Dangerous

We previously noted the finding that nitrous oxide could kill and ether could produce prolonged somnolence that gave fear for the health of the sleeper. Such observations perhaps tempered enthusiasm for their use to abolish the pain of surgery. Adding to the sometimes untoward findings with nitrous oxide and ether was the unwarranted connection to the known dangers of alcohol and opium (the competing anesthetics). Alcohol and opium might blunt the perception of pain, and patients had used both in anticipation of surgery. However, the production of anesthesia with alcohol or opium presented extraordinary dangers and did not permit control of the anesthetic state. Alcohol and opium had to be swallowed. Ingest too little and anesthesia didn't result—but the inebriated—yet insufficiently anesthetized—patient might be too sedated to ingest more alcohol or opium. What about the other extreme? Ingesting an excess of alcohol or opium presented enormous risks and, in the case of opium, an inadequate return on investment. An overdose of opium alone, even an enormous dose, does not produce anesthesia (the recipient still may move in response to surgery), and doses of opium too small to adequately blunt pain could cause patients to stop breathing—and die. Stanley (p. 285) [15] quotes Moore: "The strongest dose we dare venture has little or no effect in mitigating the sufferings of the patient during the operation." And opioids caused vomiting, which some surgeons felt was a harbinger of death.

Alcohol wasn't much better, although a sufficient dose of alcohol produced anesthesia. One problem was that "zero order kinetics" underlay the metabolism (elimination) of alcohol—the rate of metabolism is constant per minute regardless of whether there is a large or small amount of alcohol in the body. Ingest too much alcohol and it takes a long time to recover, and it may kill by excessively depressing breathing before recovery can occur (note the examples of alcohol poisoning among college students at fraternity initiations). And all that fluid that goes with the alcohol may come rushing back up the gullet and flood the lungs, quickly strangling the patient. Bergman (p. 350) called it "anesthesia by deadly intoxication" [12].

So the physician, the surgeon, and the patient might view these alternatives to the agony of surgery as unpredictable in effect and likely lethal. The common view probably held that nitrous oxide and ether were no better than opium and alcohol. Fenster (p. 39) [1] added that nitrous oxide (and ether) may have fared poorly because they were fads ridiculed by satirists. As noted above, when Mitchill gave 100 % nitrous oxide he quickly killed animals, and the "imprudent inspiration" of ether produced prolonged narcosis that caused Faraday to fear for the patient's life. Better to suffer and live.

What wasn't appreciated was how greatly ether and nitrous oxide differed from alcohol and opium. Both ether and nitrous oxide could be added to effect without assistance from the patient. The patient didn't have to swallow to take in more anesthetic, just keep breathing. And unlike alcohol and opium, neither ether nor nitrous oxide depressed breathing at anesthetic concentrations [17, 18]. And first order, not zero order kinetics governed the elimination of both ether and nitrous oxide; that is, the more anesthetic present, the greater the rate of elimination (i.e., an overdose could be eliminated quickly). Elimination always occurred as long as breathing continued. Thus ether and nitrous oxide were inherently safer anesthetics, far safer than alcohol or opium. But who knew that in 1600 or 1700, or 1800?

Anesthesia is not Needed to Perform Surgery

The observation that surgery advanced despite the absence of anesthesia tells us something contrary to conventional wisdom. Dreadful and dangerous as surgical pain might be, it did not preclude progress. Stanley [15] (p. 73): "The popular modern view, that surgeons were able to perform only 'a small number' of procedures before the introduction of anaesthesia, is simply wrong." This speaks to the fifth reason why anesthesia was not discovered earlier; it wasn't necessary!

Anesthesia Cannot Possibly Exist

We suggest that the most likely explanation for the delay in the discovery of anesthesia was the belief that it did not, could not, exist. If it did not exist, then a search for this dragon would be fruitless. French surgeon Velpeau said in 1839, "The abolishment of pain in surgery is a chimera. It is absurd to go on seeking it…knife and pain are two words in surgery that must forever be associated in the consciousness of the patient" [19]. One bit of circumstantial evidence further supports the credibility of this explanation—that no one believed that anesthesia could exist—as the most plausible reason for the delay in the discovery of anesthesia. The immediate, worldwide acceptance of anesthesia suggests that the first five explanations carried little weight. As Snow noted (p. 19) [20], "No great improvement in the practice of medicine was probably ever established so readily as the inhalation of ether for the prevention of pain." Why would anesthesia be immediately accepted, if pain is God's will or pain is beneficial, or individual suffering is unimportant (undermining explanations 1 through 3)? One or two successes should convince surgeon or patient that anesthesia is safe (eliminating explanation 4). And if anesthesia isn't needed to perform surgery then why did so many take it up (demolishing explanation 5)? The simplest plausible explanation for the failure to search for anesthesia is that no one thought it could exist (Occam's razor).

Reprise

Three people vied for the honor of having discovered anesthesia: Wells, Jackson, and Morton. Wells produced anesthesia privately but failed in his attempt at a public demonstration. Jackson never attempted a public demonstration, and his claim is as valid as his bogus claim to have invented the telegraph. The fearless, greedy, ignorant, embezzling, fraud and thief Morton demonstrated the idea (no matter that he may or may not independently have thought of it), and rightly claimed the prize. None of these men died well. Several who facilitated the discovery, particularly Warren and Colton, led admirable lives fully and well. And why wasn't anesthesia discovered sooner? We supply several possibilities, but favor the notion that too few interested parties thought it could exist.

References

1. Fenster J. Ether day: the strange tale of America's greatest medical discovery and the haunted men who made it. New York: Harper Collins; 2001.
2. Wolfe RJ. Tarnished idol: William Thomas Green Morton and the introduction of surgical anesthesia: a chronicle of the ether controversy. San Francisco: Norman Publishing; 2001.
3. Wolfe RJ, Patterson RW. Charles Thomas Jackson, "the head behind the hands": applying science to implement discovery and invention in early nineteenth century America. Novato, CA: J. Norman History of Science.com; 2008.
4. Keys TE. The history of surgical anesthesia. Park Ridge: Wood Library-Museum of Anesthesiology; 1996.
5. Thorwald J. The century of the surgeon. New York:Pantheon Books, Inc.; 1956.
6. Nuland SB. Chapter VII. Nitrous oxide: a discovery in vain. The origins of anesthesia. Birmington: Leslie B. Adams, Jr.; 1983.
7. Garraway SM, Xu Q, Inturrisi CE. siRNA-mediated knockdown of the NR1 subunit gene of the NMDA receptor attenuates formalin-induced pain behaviors in adult rats. J Pain. 2009;10:380–90.
8. Desai SP, Desai MS, Maddi R, Battit GE. A tale of two paintings: depictions of the first public demonstration of ether anesthesia. Anesthesiology. 2007;106:1046–50.
9. Artusio JF Jr. Di-ethyl ether analgesia: a detailed description of the first stage of ether anesthesia in man. J Pharmacol Exp Ther. 1954;111:343–8.
10. Artusio JF Jr. Ether analgesia during major surgery. J Am Med Assoc. 1955;157:33–6.
11. Astyrakaki E, Papaioannou A, Askitopoulou H. References to anesthesia, pain, and analgesia in the Hippocratic Collection. Anesth Analg. 2010;110:188–94.
12. Bergman NA. The genesis of surgical anesthesia. Park Ridge, IL: Wood Library-Museum of Anesthesiology; 1998. pp. 1–448.
13. Hatfield MP. Lest we forget: a tribute to Dr. Samuel Guthrie, the American discoverer of chloroform. Chic Clin Pure Water J. 1905;18:179–83.
14. Campagna JA. The end of religious fatalism: Boston as the venue for the demonstration of ether for the intentional relief of pain. Surgery. 2005;138:46–55.
15. Stanley P. For fear of pain. British surgery, 1790–1850. New York: Rodopi; 2003.
16. Papper EM. The influence of romantic literature on the medical understanding of pain and suffering—the stimulus to the discovery of anesthesia. Perspectives Biol Med. 1992;35:401–15.
17. Larson CP Jr, Eger EI II, Muallem M, Buechel DR, Munson ES, Eisele JH. The effects of diethyl ether and methoxyflurane on ventilation: II. A comparative study in man. Anesthesiology. 1969;30:174–84.
18. Hornbein TF, Eger EI II, Winter PM, Smith G, Wetstone D, Smith KH. The minimum alveolar concentration of nitrous oxide in man. Anesth Analg. 1982;61:553–6.
19. Wikiquote: en.wikiquote.org/wiki/Incorrect_predictions
20. Snow J. On Chloroform and other Anaesthetics: their action and administration. London: John Churchill; 1858. pp. 1–443.

1846–1860: Following the Discovery of Anesthesia

4

Edmond I Eger II, Rod N. Westhorpe and Lawrence J. Saidman

Summary

Four things soon followed the discovery of ether anesthesia. First, within weeks to months, ether was used in distant and disparate parts of the world—Europe, Australia, Mexico and Latin America. Second, for the moment, nitrous oxide was abandoned. Third, in 1847 Simpson discovered the anesthetic properties of chloroform that, for a time, replaced the pungent, flammable ether, especially in the UK. Fourth, the discovery of anesthesia was one thing, but how to deliver it safely was another. We needed a guidebook, a description of the clinical characteristics of anesthesia that might allow control of the anesthetic state. In 1847, Snow supplied just that for ether. In 1858, he similarly described the degrees of chloroform anesthesia, in the process analyzing the dangers of this more dangerous anesthetic and teaching how to avoid disaster. He, more than anyone, laid the groundwork for the specialty we call anesthesiology.

World Events, 1846–1860

The 1848 Revolution in France established the Second French Republic and led to political instability in Europe. In that year, Brigham Young led the Mormons to Utah, Marx and Engels published the Communist Manifesto, and gold was discovered at Sutter's Mill in California. In 1851, a miner luckless in California returned to Australia and found gold, initiating a gold rush that swelled the population six-fold by 1856. The 1850 Taiping Rebellion in China led to civil war and 20 million deaths over the ensuing 15 years. In 1855, the world's first transcontinental railroad was completed—across the Isthmus of Panama. The Crimean War began, ending a year later but not before Florence Nightingale built the foundation for professional nursing. In 1859, Darwin published *On the Origin of Species*, and construction of the Suez Canal began.

E. I Eger II (✉)
Department of Anesthesia and Perioperative Care,
University of California, San Francisco, CA, USA
e-mail: egere@anesthesia.ucsf.edu

R. N. Westhorpe
Melbourne, Australia
e-mail: westhorpe@netspace.net.au

L. J. Saidman
Department of Anesthesia, Stanford University,
Stanford, CA, USA
e-mail: lsaidman@stanford.edu

A Chronology of Events Soon After the Discovery of Anesthesia

1846

The news of Morton's 16 October 1846 demonstration (Ether Day) traveled fast. A successful trial of ether took place in Paris on 16 December 1846, followed by anesthesia in both Scotland and London on 19 December, the one in London "…by a dentist named James Robinson (1813–1862). Within a few days, John Snow had heard of the subject and was sufficiently interested to make arrangements to see the process first hand."[1] More on Snow in a moment. Liston used ether on 21 December 1846 in London, for an amputation, supposedly remarking "*This Yankee dodge beats mesmerism hollow.*"

How famous, how important was this discovery? Pretty famous, pretty important. As we shall note, it revolutionized surgery. The citations that the report of its discovery received in the *New England Journal of Medicine* suggest its fame and worth. The most cited of all *New England Journal of Medicine* reports is Bigelow's 1846 description of the discovery [2]. And the second most cited is Warren's report, also in 1846 [3]. Two more reports on ether anesthesia make the top ten: Cox's essay, also in 1846 [4], and Hayward's 1847 essay [5].

1847: Ether Is Given Around the World

On 23 January 1847, Heyfelder gave ether anesthesia in Germany. It was also given in Argentina, Brazil, Cuba,

Guatemala, Mexico, Peru, Uruguay, and Venezuela in 1847. In that year, Peter Parker introduced ether anesthesia into China, using an apparatus supplied by Charles Jackson. Relying on news arriving in Hobart and Sydney via London, Australians William Pugh and John Belisario both gave ether on 7 June. A New Zealand instrument maker (no medical man, he), James Marriott, gave the first surgical anesthetic to a Wellington Gaol inmate on 27 September. Prompted by Edward Barton, US and Mexican forces used ether anesthesia in 1847 in the Mexican-American war. The world did not hesitate to employ this amazing discovery.

Simpson Looks for Something Better

Scottish obstetrician, James Simpson, used ether to produce anesthesia, but soon searched for something better than the pungent ether for his delicate ladies. As described by his colleague, a Professor Miller, Simpson found chloroform on 4 November 1847 [6]:

> "…(O)n returning home after a weary day's labour, Dr. Simpson with his two friends and assistants, Drs. Keith and Duncan, sat down to their somewhat hazardous work in Dr. Simpson's dining-room. Having inhaled several substances, but without much effect, it occurred to Dr. Simpson to try a ponderous material … that happened to be a small bottle of chloroform. It was searched for and recovered from beneath a heap of waste paper. And with each tumbler newly charged, the inhalers resumed their vocation. Immediately an unwonted hilarity seized the party—they became brighteyed, very happy, and very loquacious—expatiating on the delicious aroma of the new fluid. The conversation was of unusual intelligence, and quite charmed the listeners— some ladies of the family and a naval officer, brother-in-law of Dr. Simpson. But suddenly there was a talk of sounds being heard like those of a cotton mill louder and louder; a moment more and then all was quiet—and then crash! On awakening Dr. Simpson's first perception was mental—'This is far stronger and better than ether,' said he to himself. His second was to note that he was prostrate on the floor, and that among the friends about him there was both confusion and alarm. Hearing a noise he turned round and saw Dr. Duncan beneath a chair—his jaw dropped, his eyes staring, his head bent half under him; quite unconscious, and snoring in a most determined and alarming manner. More noise still and much motion. And then his eyes overtook Dr. Keith's feet and legs making valorous attempts to overturn the supper table, or more probably to annihilate everything that was on it. By and by Dr. Simpson having regained his seat, Dr. Duncan having finished his uncomfortable and unrefreshing slumber, and Dr. Keith having come to an arrangement with the table and its contents, the *sederunt* was resumed. Each expressed himself delighted with this new agent, and its inhalation was repeated many times that night…until the supply of chloroform was fairly exhausted."

Miller probably embellished the circumstances of discovery. And several contributors to the discovery of the anesthetic effects of chloroform in addition to Simpson have been suggested [7]. With minor resistance from clergy and others, Simpson introduced chloroform into practice. It became the "British" anesthetic while ether remained the "Yankee dodge".

As with ether, chloroform, a more easily given but more dangerous anesthetic, was quickly accepted in countries most influenced by the UK. By the end of 1847, chloroform replaced ether in France as the anesthetic of choice despite sudden and inexplicable fatalities with its use. More countries joined up in succeeding years. Chloroform displaced ether in Argentina, Brazil, Chile, Peru, Uruguay, and Venezuela. Soon ether and chloroform were used everywhere— slowly or quickly overcoming religious objections and medical skepticism. In 1847, Fanny Longfellow, wife of the poet, received ether to aid in delivery. Simpson gave ether to relieve the pain of childbirth for a woman with a deformed pelvis. And in 1853, Queen Victoria received chloroform to relieve the pain of childbirth. The anesthetist was John Snow.

The First Theory of Narcosis

In 1847, Harless and von Bibra noted that ether and chloroform could dissolve lipids. They proposed that anesthetics acted by removing lipids from the brain. Anesthetics drycleaned the neurons. That perhaps explained how anesthesia was produced. But it didn't explain how recovery from anesthesia occurred, and occurred so rapidly. What returned the lipids to the brain and put them in the proper place?

Anesthetic Choice Affects Anesthetic Practice

Nicholas Greene argues that the US discovery of ether anesthesia led to pride of ownership. This proprietary position hindered the advancement of the specialty of anesthesia in North America [8]. The relative safety of ether did not demand that someone make a career from its delivery. In contrast, chloroform was the UK discovery. They owned that anesthetic. The dangerous chloroform made anesthesia more interesting. Quoting Valpeau: "*On the subject of ether, that it is a wonderful and terrible agent, I will say of chloroform, that it is still more wonderful and more terrible*"[9]

Near the time when Eger thought to become an anesthetist in the US, Lundy advised that only incompetent physicians became anesthetists [10]. Henry Beecher made a similar, if more politic, observation: "…anesthesia technique can be mastered by ordinary men who are ordinarily deft, with only a modest requirement of intelligence and of knowledge and judgment."[11] Ether delivery required little skill. What a difference from the British world besot with chloroform! And lucky Britain immediately found the greatest anesthetist that ever lived. The US had William Morton who didn't understand what he was doing, and England had John Snow (Fig. 4.1) who knew exactly what he was doing—and told the world. Snow's work anticipated many elements of modern anesthesia.

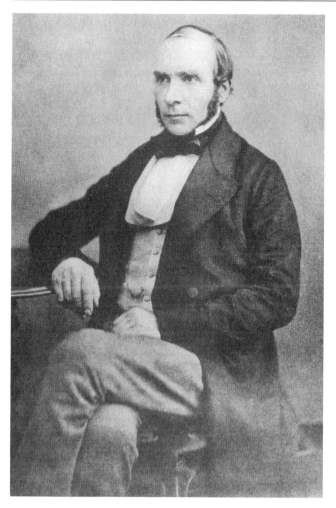

Fig. 4.1 John Snow

Snow Tells How to Give Anesthesia

In 1847, the medical community needed to know how to deliver anesthesia smoothly and safely and how to control the depth of anesthesia with as much precision as the available anesthetics and extant equipment permitted. Expressions such as a greater depth or level of anesthesia indicated achievement of a greater anesthetic effect. Enter Snow's classic book on the delivery of ether [12]. A decade later, he supplied his second classic book—on the delivery of chloroform [13]. To digress a moment: Snow's genius extended beyond anesthesia. He was the father of epidemiology, famously diagnosing the cause of an 1854 cholera epidemic in London that killed 500 people in 10 days (in the preface of the referenced book) [13]. To deal with the epidemic, Snow told the vestrymen of St. James district to remove the handle from the Broad Street pump (p xxi). His studies revealed that the dead had drawn from the Broad Street well. The vestrymen of St. James's (the district containing the well) were "incredulous, but had the good sense to carry out the advice. The pump-handle was removed, and the plague was stayed."

Snow, born in York, on 15 June 1813, was the eldest son of a farmer. In 1827 he was apprenticed to a surgeon. Other apprenticeships followed. For a few years Snow became a vegetarian (he determined later that it was not healthful) and temperance advocate. He came to London to study at the Hunterian School of Medicine, becoming a physician in 1838. His friend Richardson described Snow as "Not particularly quick of apprehension, or ready in invention, he yet always kept in the foreground by his indomitable perseverance and determination in following up whatever line of investigation was open to him (p v)."[13]

John Snow's observations on anesthesia were as brilliant (although not as flamboyant) as his prescription for stopping the cholera epidemic. Regarding ether [12], Snow described 5 degrees (i.e., stages) of anesthesia, anticipating by more than half a century, Guedel's classic four Stages (and many Signs) of anesthesia [14]. Snow observed (p 1): "In the first degree of etherization I shall include the various changes of feeling that a person may experience, whilst he still retains a correct consciousness…and a capacity to direct his voluntary movements." Aha! So in the first degree, the patient is awake, aware, and remembers.

Snow continued (p 2): "In…the second degree, mental functions may be exercised, and voluntary actions performed, but in a disordered manner." The patient is still awake and aware—but there may be no memory of that awareness.

Snow (p 10) noted that anesthesia produces amnesia and described much of MACawake (the anesthetic concentration preventing awareness in half of subjects who, however, respond appropriately to commands such as "open your eyes") [15] a century before the concept was developed: "…and if…the patient is allowed to recover still further during the operation, it will probably happen that in the second degree he will either lie perfectly calm, or talk in his dreams about subjects totally unconnected with pain, or the operation which is still going on."

Snow repeatedly returned to the notion of dreams occurring in the second degree of anesthesia but "there can be no dreams or ideas of any kind in the third and fourth degrees…." (p 11). This accords with the modern determination that dreams occur during recovery from anesthesia and not during anesthesia [16]. "In the third degree, there is no evidence of any mental function being exercised, and consequently no voluntary motions occur; but muscular contractions, in addition to those concerned in respiration, may sometimes take place" (pp 1–2) [12]. Thus, in the third degree, the patient may respond to surgery with movement.

Snow, like Morton, noted another component of the third or even the second degree, one that anticipated Joseph Artusio's 1950s publications [17, 18] on ether analgesia (p 10). Unlike Morton, the far more perceptive Snow knew what he had. "I believe that pain is seldom felt in the stage of which we are treating–the third degree succeeding the fourth (i.e., during recovery from the fourth degree)—and of course never remembered afterwards, as there is no knowledge or mental perception of it."

The analgesia noted above for the second or third degree, seemed to be most obvious during recovery from anesthesia and not during induction of anesthesia. Snow speculated that this might be the result of ether acting on peripheral nerves rather than on the central nervous system, an intriguing idea that might fit with the known lesser blood flow to nerves and the greater affinity of anesthetics for nerves as compared to brain. The smaller flow and the greater affinity would delay the establishment of a sufficient ether concentration in the nerves, and hence delay the appearance of analgesia. Snow's idea remains to be tested.

"In the fourth degree, no movements are seen except those of respiration, and they are incapable of being influenced by external impressions."

Snow's description of movement with incision in the third degree, and its absence in the fourth degree, anticipated by a century, the discovery of MAC (the minimum alveolar concentration preventing movement in response to incision in 50% of patients) [19]. Indeed, Snow wrote: "Ether contributes other benefits besides preventing pain. It keeps patients still, who otherwise would not be" (p 53) [12]. And (p 6): "If this degree of etherization is not well established when the operation begins, the first cut may cause a sudden contraction of the whole muscular system." And thus Snow appreciated the need for equilibration of the site of action with the ether delivered to that site. And (p 7): "In (the fourth) degree of etherization the patient always remains perfectly passive under every kind of operation; and…the muscles are completely relaxed…." He even described the use of a supramaximal stimulus as important to a test of the efficacy of anesthesia (p 36) [12]: "…there may be insensitivity to a slight lesion—as a suture in the skin, for instance—at a time when a greater wound would cause signs of pain." Thus Snow observed that one level of anesthesia may permit a muscular response to a supramaximal stimulus, but one degree deeper prevented that response once equilibrium had been obtained. Snow only needed the ability to measure the concentration of ether in the lungs (the alveoli) to have described MAC, the modern standard by which the unit depth of anesthesia is defined [20].

"In the fifth degree…respiratory movements are more or less paralysed and become difficult, feeble, or irregular." Snow advised against entering the fifth degree, concerned that undue depression of breathing and the heart might follow.

Snow described eye signs, changes that allow the assessment of anesthetic depth (p 5) [12]: "The patient may have moved his eyes about in the second degree, and even directed them to objects, but in this degree (deeper anesthesia) they are stationary, or if they do move, their motions have nothing of a voluntary character…The eyelids may be either open, or partly or tightly closed, but in either case, if lifted or moved by the finger, the orbicularis palpebrarum (the eyelid) contracts." These degrees (or Guedel's variation on them) were used to define depth of anesthesia for the next century.

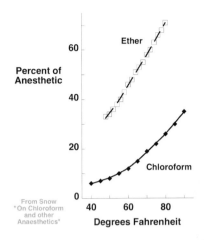

Fig. 4.2 Snow found that as temperature of an anesthetic increased, so did the concentration in the air overlying the anesthetic. (From Snow J: On the Inhalation of the Vapour of Ether in Surgical Operations: Containing a Description of the Various Stages of Etherization, and a Statement of the Result of Nearly Eighty Operations in Which Ether Has Been Employed In St. George's and University College Hospitals. London: John Churchill; 1847. pp 1–88.)

Snow was amazingly perceptive. He anticipated that ether might be metabolized (p 84) [12]: "It is not improbable that some of the ether inhaled is decomposed in the body; but this does not alter the question of de-etherization…for assuredly by far the greater portion of the ether escape by the breath exhaled." Actually, he may have erred there because by far the lesser portion of some inhaled anesthetics escape by exhalation [21, 22]. We don't know about ether.

He recognized that age and breathing affected ether kinetics (the movement of ether into and out of the body; p 43) [12]: "Elderly people are slower in recovering than young ones as their respiration is less active, and the ether takes a longer time to evaporate in the breath. For the same reason, if sickness has been caused by the ether, the patient is longer in recovering, as it depresses the respiratory movements."

Snow recognized the importance of control over the concentration of ether and the connection between concentration and the degree of anesthetization (p 15) [12]: "I have spoken of a knowledge of the strength of the vapour as being essential to a correct determination of the state of the patient at all times: and this brings us to the apparatus for the administration of the vapour, as, without a suitable one, the proportions of air and of vapour cannot be determined." He recognized the importance of controlling the temperature of the vaporizer (with a water jacket) to avoid changes in the concentration of anesthetic (Figs. 4.2 and 4.3). He recognized the need to supply sufficient surface area to assure the saturation of the gas passing through the vaporizer with anesthetic. His vaporizer allowed for the introduction of air to dilute the ether stream (anticipating the modern "variable bypass vaporizer" by more than a century.)

Snow made the inspiratory tube leading from his vaporizer large enough to minimize resistance to breathing. And

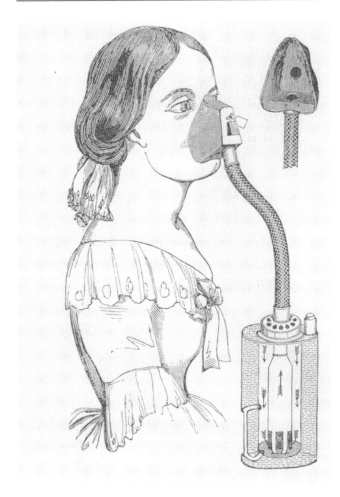

Fig. 4.3 A genteel lady breathes ether or chloroform from a vaporizer constructed to ensure the fullest concentration of anesthetic. A jacket filled with water buffers the vaporizer against temperature changes and thus against changes in the anesthetic concentration issuing from the vaporizer. A valve on the mask may be slipped more or less to one side to allow room air to dilute the anesthetic drawn from the vaporizer. When in place over the hole exiting from the mask, the valve allows no room air in but allows easy exit of the gases inspired by the patient (p 82) [12]. (From Snow J: On the Inhalation of the Vapour of Ether in Surgical Operations: Containing a Description of the Various Stages of Etherization, and a Statement of the Result of Nearly Eighty Operations in Which Ether Has Been Employed In St. George's and University College Hospitals. London: John Churchill; 1847. pp 1–88.)

he provided a mask covering mouth and nose and a valve that produced a non-rebreathing system (Fig. 4.3).

> He noted (p 21) that "…many of the apparatuses at first invented did not allow of easy respiration, but offered obstructions to it, by sponges, by the ether itself, by valves of insufficient size, but more particularly by tubes of too narrow caliber; and there is reason to believe that, in many instances, this was the cause of failure, and that in others the insensibility, when produced, was partly due to asphyxia…." His valves were "…made of vulcanised India rubber; they (were) light, (were) attached so as to rise with the least appreciable force and they closed again, of themselves, in any posture in which the patient can be required to be placed."

Snow was a plodding sedulous genius.

Simpson Disagrees with Snow

Simpson disagreed with Snow's complex approach to anesthetic delivery. Simpson preferred delivery by a few drops of chloroform on a handkerchief. And, in various forms, much of the world agreed with him well into the twentieth century. The handkerchief approach precluded a calibrated delivery, a precision of control over anesthesia depth. Thus it demanded the evaluation of anesthetic effect found in Snow's degrees to guide anesthetic delivery, but those degrees had a subjective element that made them imperfect guides.

More Observations by Snow

Snow recognized that impurities might compromise the delivery of the ether and described how to secure a purer ether (pp 23–4) [12], particularly by using water to remove the alcohol that was frequently a contaminant. He observed that the water that therefore also entered the ether was salutary (pp 22–3) [12]. "I…allow this small quantity of water to remain in the ether, in order that the air which is inhaled with the vapour of ether may be always saturated also with vapour of water, when it will be more bland, and less irritating, than if it contained but little moisture…", a finding duplicated a century later with another kind of ether [23]. What a clever fellow.

Snow developed an understanding and delivery of anesthesia with powers of observation and carefully thought out rudimentary apparatus. He had the endearing arrogance of the great anesthetist (p 33) [12]: "…there is no person who cannot be rendered insensible by ether…." No one can resist; no one.

Snow Turns to Chloroform

Like Ross Terrell a century later [24], Simpson and Snow sought the better anesthetic. In 1847, Snow turned his attention to Simpson's "British" anesthetic. His resulting classic book compared ether and chloroform [13]. The five degrees of anesthesia were essentially unchanged. Snow experimented with animals, making discoveries confirmed a century later. Like later investigators [25], Snow (pp 72–3) [13] found that a greater body temperature increased anesthetic requirement.

Snow Explains Why Chloroform Kills

More than 50 reports of deaths associated with chloroform use appeared in the 10 years following its discovery. Hannah Greener, aged 15, was first, dying at Winlaton, near Newcastle on 28 Jan 1848. Reports came from North America (first, Cincinnati), France (Boulogne), India (Hyderabad), Ger-

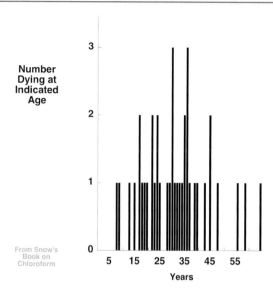

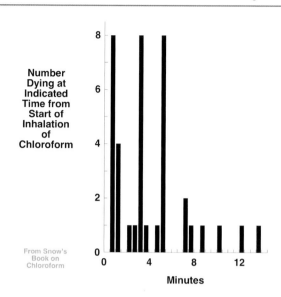

Fig. 4.4 In those cases of death in association with the use of chloroform where the age of the patient was known, death appeared most frequently in young adults. (From Snow J: On the Inhalation of the Vapour of Ether in Surgical Operations: Containing a Description of the Various Stages of Etherization, and a Statement of the Result of Nearly Eighty Operations in Which Ether Has Been Employed In St. George's and University College Hospitals. London: John Churchill; 1847. pp 1–88.)

Fig. 4.5 Snow found that deaths associated with chloroform usually occurred soon after initiation of anesthesia, a timing we now know [25] to be consistent with ventricular fibrillation secondary to sensitization of the heart to the increased sympathetic activity associated with excitation.

many (Berlin), Jamaica (Kingston), Sweden (Stockholm), Austria (Vienna), and on the high seas near Mauritius. But mostly from Great Britain. Snow recognized that chloroform was more dangerous than ether, believing "…that ether is altogether incapable of causing the sudden death by paralysis of the heart, which has caused the accidents which have happened during the administration of chloroform" (p 362) [13]. He thought that the chloroform deaths were preventable, often a consequence of the excessive use of chloroform, producing what he called cardiac syncope. "…accidents from this agent would arise by its suddenly paralyzing the heart, if it were not sufficiently diluted with air; and a careful review of all the recorded cases of fatal accident shows that nearly every one of them has happened in this way…." (p 251) [13].

Snow recognized that death associated with chloroform correlated with age in an unexpected manner. He believed that the incidence of surgery increased with increasing age, but he found that deaths occurred in younger patients (Fig. 4.4). We now know that younger patients should be more resistant to cardiac arrest from depression of the heart but may be more susceptible to lethal rhythms such as ventricular fibrillation, a condition in which the heart contracts in an uncoordinated manner because of a flaw in the electrical impulses prompting the heart to beat. Snow also found that sudden death occurred early in the administration of anesthesia (Fig. 4.5), presumably during a time of heightened sympathetic activity, something that would predispose to ventricular fibrillation.

Chloroform is an alkane, and alkanes predispose to ventricular fibrillation, while ethers do not [26].

Snow may also have failed to adequately recognize one other crucial limitation of chloroform. Chloroform depresses breathing whereas ether does not [27], at least in the range of concentrations needed for surgical anesthesia. Snow knew quite a bit about breathing but didn't appreciate the consequence of the small reserve of oxygen available to his patients. Todays' patients may breathe 100 % oxygen, making depression of respiration a minor matter, but Snow's patients breathed room air—21 % oxygen—and were at risk of inadequate oxygenation. Snow recognized that breathing could become partially obstructed ("stertorous") but didn't advise what to do until complete obstruction of the airway occurred—in which case he would pull the tongue forward. He resuscitated two patients in that manner (pp 254–5) [13].

Snow beat back the attacks on chloroform, taking heart from his statistics showing that the introduction of chloroform did not increase mortality. If he had not defended it as cogently as he had, one wonders whether chloroform would have survived the adverse publicity. Part of his defense lay in his observation that "…chloroform possesses advantages over ether, in being more convenient and less disagreeable…." (p 23) [13], but his greatest defense was his summary recitation of his anesthetization of nearly 5,000 patients without a death from "cardiac syncopy." You just had to do it right! As Greene observed [9], giving chloroform anesthesia safely required skill, while less skill was required to give ether safely.

Snow's contributions are today commemorated in many ways, one being the John Snow Society. Membership is open to anyone who has visited the John Snow pub in Broadwick Street, Soho, adjacent to the site of the original water pump. It is the only ale house in the world, named after an anesthetist.

In 1847, one more inhaled anesthetic was discovered [28]. Flourens described the anesthetic properties of ethyl chloride, and a year later, Heyfelder gave it to three patients. Although administered occasionally, it languished for the next half century because of the inconvenience associated with its containment and use: it boiled at room temperature (boiling point 12.5 °C). It also didn't help that it cost more than chloroform and ether to make.

1849

In 1849, Elizabeth Blackwell received her medical degree from Geneva Medical College in NY. Blackwell was the first woman physician in modern times to receive a medical degree, and she led the entry of women into medicine throughout the world. And also in that year, facilitated by the discovery of anesthesia, the great US surgeon James Sims repaired a vesicovaginal fistula, a passage for leakage from the bladder to the vagina, and the first major surgical advance after the discovery of anesthesia.

1850

In 1850, John Warren addressed the American Medical Association, describing what constituted adequate anesthesia care: Have a dedicated person continuously deliver anesthesia to a fasting supine patient. Administer anesthesia sufficient to produce relaxation. Beware of obstructing breathing, and don't set fire to the operating room. Yes, that should do it.

1853

In 1853, Perry's battleships opened Japan to western influences, including anesthesia. And Queen Victoria chose chloroform to relieve labor pain during the birth of Prince Leopold. She thereby ended any lingering moral opposition to the relief of pain during childbirth, and her request for chloroform at the births of two of her children, accelerated the acceptance of anesthesia.

The hollow needle devised by Francis Rynd in 1844, and the hypodermic syringe introduced by Charles Pravaz in 1853 enabled additions to anesthesia such as premedication. They were essential to the later development of regional (local) anesthesia and the intravenous approach to anesthesia.

1854

Veterinarians hesitantly adopted anesthesia, some considering that excitation during induction indicated suffering or pain. Others were concerned by reports of accidents and deaths. Veterinarians initially used anesthesia as much to prevent struggling during surgery as to prevent pain. US physician and veterinarian George Dadd described his use of ether and chloroform in animals to prevent pain from surgery in animals, incidentally recognizing the greater safety of ether. Dadd's book, Modern Horse Doctor [29], recommended that (p 252): "…in all operations of this kind, the subject be etherized, not only in view of preventing pain, but that we may, in the absence of all struggling on the part of our patient, perform the operation satisfactorily, and in much less time after etherization has taken place than otherwise."

1855

In Japan, Sugita gave the first ether anesthetic, for a patient having a mastectomy, and ether anesthesia reached Iceland.

1858

Acting on the need for purer ether, physician Squibb formed Squibb Pharmaceutical.

Snow died 16 June 1858 at age 45 while composing the last portion of his book on chloroform. Autopsy revealed that he died from the untoward effects of failure of his kidneys (p xliv) [13]. The immediate cause of death appears to have been a stroke. Snow's friend, BW Richardson, completed Snow's book On Chloroform and other Anaesthetics. Snow's summaries of his cases (pp 271–318) [13], most from the 1850s, tell us about the surgical needs for anesthesia (Table 4.1). The surgeries that Snow listed, were the surgeries that had been done before anesthesia's discovery, including repairs of cleft lips, ligation of arteries, and lots of teeth pulled without pain. It took decades for surgeons to fully use Morton's gift.

The brevity of most procedures in the 1850s informed the delivery of anesthesia. So did Snow's description of the degrees of anesthesia. Anesthesia was like a ball bounced on the pavement, a descent into oblivion and then a partial recovery following by second and third descents and recoveries. This may have been the safest method for delivery of anesthesia, especially with chloroform because of the profound

Table 4.1 Some operations for which Snow gave chloroform, 1848–58

Operation	Number
Bladder stone removal	246
Urethral operations	137
Amputation of the thigh, leg, arm, ankle, or miscellaneous	109
Operations for necrosis	197
Excisions: head of the femur, elbow, knee, or wrist	43
Removal of tumors of the jaw	24
Tumors of the female breast	222
Tumors behind the angle of the jaw	41
Cysts	71
Fatty tumors	66
Miscellaneous tumors	87
Nevi	116
Ligature of arteries	14
Hare-lip	147
Division of nerves	28
Operations on the eye	158
Removal of foreign bodies and polyps from the ear or nose	22
Operations in the mouth	24
Plastic operations	50
Raising depressed sections of skull	4
Operations for ununited fractures	7
Reduction of dislocations	27
Forcible movement of stiff joints	22
Tenotomy	78
Operation for strangulated hernia	19
Operations for hemorrhoids or fissure of the anus	215
Fistula involving the anus	218
Ovarian tumors	9
Operations for cancer of the vagina	18
Operations for rupture of the perineum (prolapse)	14
Removal of testicle or penis	27
Operations for phymosis	76
Removal of enlarged bursa	6
Evulsion of the nails	28
Laryngectomy for croup (!)	2
Extraction of teeth	867
Total	3439

Snow gave more anesthetics, including those for childbirth, but with a few exceptions (e.g., for two of Queen Victoria's deliveries) those for childbirth were not recorded

depression of breathing, and because without supplemental oxygen there was a great risk of asphyxia. But it was also employed with ether—down and up and down again—far different from the later approach that produced a sustained level of anesthesia, one appropriate to longer surgical procedures.

Reprise

Morton's discovery, perhaps the greatest discovery in all of medicine, began an enormous change in patient care, one that continues to this day. Snow transformed Morton's clumsy beginnings into an art, and a science. Snow's science dominated anesthetic delivery for the better part of a century. His work anticipated modern vaporizers and concepts such as MAC, pharmacokinetics (what the body does to drugs), and pharmacodynamics (what drugs do to the body).

References

1. Ellis RH. The case books of Dr. John Snow. Med Hist Suppl. 1994;14:xviii.
2. Bigelow HJ. Insensibility during surgical operations produced by inhalation. Boston Med Surg J. 1846;35:309–17.
3. Warren JC. Inhalation of ethereal vapor for the prevention of pain in surgical operations. Boston Med Surg J. 1846;35:375–9.
4. Cox AL. Experiments with the Letheon in New York. Boston Med Surg J. 1846;35:456–9.
5. Hayward G. Some account of the first use of sulphuric ether by inhalation in surgical practice. Boston Med Surg J. 1847;36:229–34.
6. Gordon HL. Sir James Young Simpson and chloroform (1811–1870). In: Masters of Medicine, edited by Ernest Hart. Available in The Project Gutenberg EBook. The original book was of the above title, published by T. Fisher Unwin, Paternoster Square, London; 1897.
7. Defalque RJ, Wright AJ. The discovery of chloroform: has David Waldie's role been exaggerated? Anesthesiology. 2011;114:1004–5.
8. Greene NM. A consideration of factors in the discovery of anesthesia and their effects on its development. Anesthesiology. 1971;35:515–22.
9. en.wikipedia.org/wiki/Alfred-Armand-Louis-Marie_Velpeau.
10. Lundy JS. Factors that influenced the development of anesthesiology. Anesth Analg. 1946;25:38–43.
11. Beecher HK. The specialty of anesthesia and its application in the Harvard University-Massachusetts General Hospital Department. Ann Surg. 1947;126:486–99.
12. Snow J. On the inhalation of the vapour of ether in surgical operations: containing a description of the various stages of etherization, and a statement of the result of nearly eighty operations in which ether has been employed in St. George's and University College Hospitals. London: John Churchill; 1847. pp. 1–88.
13. Snow J. On chloroform and other anaesthetics: their action and administration. London: John Churchill; 1858. pp. 1–443.
14. Guedel AE. Inhalation anesthesia: a fundamental guide. New York: Macmillan; 1937. pp. 1–172.
15. Stoelting RK, Longnecker DE, Eger EI, II. Minimal alveolar concentrations on awakening from methoxyflurane, halothane, ether and fluroxene in man: MAC awake. Anesthesiology. 1970;33:5–9.
16. Leslie K, Skrzypek H, Paech MJ, Kurowski I, Whybrow T. Dreaming during anesthesia and anesthetic depth in elective surgery patients: a prospective cohort study. Anesthesiology. 2007;106:33–42.
17. Artusio JF, Jr. Di-ethyl ether analgesia: a detailed description of the first stage of ether anesthesia in man. J Pharmacol Exp Ther. 1954;111:343–8.
18. Artusio JF, Jr. Ether analgesia during major surgery. J Am Med Assoc. 1955;157:33–6.
19. Saidman LJ, Eger EI, II. Effect of nitrous oxide and of narcotic premedication on the alveolar concentration of halothane required for anesthesia. Anesthesiology. 1964;25:302–6.
20. Merkel G, Eger EI, II. A comparative study of halothane 2 halopropane anesthesia. Including a method for determining equipotency. Anesthesiology. 1963;24:346–57.
21. Carpenter RL, Eger EI, II, Johnson BH, Unadkat JD, Sheiner LB. Pharmacokinetics of inhaled anesthetics in humans: measurements during and after the simultaneous administration of enflurane, halothane, isoflurane, methoxyflurane, and nitrous oxide. Anesth Analg. 1986;65:575–82.

22. Carpenter RL, Eger EI, II, Johnson BH, Unadkat JD, Sheiner LB. The extent of metabolism of inhaled anesthetics in humans. Anesthesiology. 1986;65:201–5.

23. Wilkes AR, Hall JE, Wright E, Grundler S. The effect of humidification and smoking habit on the incidence of adverse airway events during deepening of anaesthesia with desflurane. Anaesthesia. 2000;55:685–9.

24. Burns WB, Eger EI, 2nd. Ross C. Terrell, PhD, an anesthetic pioneer. Anesth Analg. 2011;113:387–9.

25. Eger EI, II, Saidman LJ, Brandstater B. Temperature dependence of halothane and cyclopropane anesthesia in dogs: correlation with some theories of anesthetic action. Anesthesiology. 1965;26:764–70.

26. Johnston RR, Eger EI, II, Wilson C. A comparative interaction of epinephrine with enflurane, isoflurane, and halothane in man. Anesth Analg. 1976,55:709–12.

27. Larson CP, Jr, Eger EI, II, Muallem M, Buechel DR, Munson ES, Eisele JH. The effects of diethyl ether and methoxyflurane on ventilation: II. A comparative study in man. Anesthesiology. 1969;30:174–84.

28. Kim J, Yao A, Atherley R, Carstens E, Jinks SL, Antognini JF. Neurons in the ventral spinal cord are more depressed by isoflurane, halothane, and propofol than are neurons in the dorsal spinal cord. Anesth Analg. 2007;105:1020–6.

29. Dadd GH. The modern horse doctor. Boston: JP Jewett; 1854.

1860–1910: The Specialty of Anesthesia Develops Slowly

5

Edmond I Eger II, Lawrence J. Saidman and Rod N. Westhorpe

Summary

The discovery of anesthesia ultimately enabled remarkable advances in surgical care, but did not immediately change operations. At first, surgeons still pulled teeth, managed injuries, amputated limbs, and performed brief operations requiring momentary but deep levels of anesthesia. So the anesthetist drove the level of anesthesia down and then allowed it to "bounce" up, the surgeon operating at deeper levels of anesthesia. Further advances required improvements.

First, appreciating anesthesia's potential, surgeons devised longer operations that required steadier levels of anesthesia. Less bouncing up and down. This mandated the development of delivery systems allowing increasingly precise control of the anesthetic; it prompted the invention of the anesthetic machine, bringing together compressed gases in iron cylinders, a means to blend the gases, control their flow, and add vapors in some ordered, better known manner.

Second, immediately after anesthesia's discovery no anesthetists existed. A surgeon became surgeon *and* anesthetist, something undesirable for lengthy, procedures. So the surgeon engaged an assistant to supply anesthesia, in the UK another physician, but in much of the world nurses or technicians (a euphemism for secretaries, orderlies, medical students)—part-time anesthetists with little skill. The resulting morbidity and mortality were initially ignored, perhaps because operations were few in number (few patients died), or perhaps because infections killed more than did anesthesia. Surgeons developed antisepsis and asepsis, and then anesthetic deaths did matter.

Third, with Koller's 1884 demonstration of cocaine's local anesthetic effects, some surgeons again became both anesthetist and surgeon. German speaking surgeons seized the opportunity to develop regional anesthesia and remain in charge. But still, things could go awry. Someone best keep an eye on the patient.

Fourth, increasing surgical complexity and increasing demands for better anesthetic delivery mandated the rise of professional anesthetists, sooner in the US and the UK than in other countries. Nurses led the way in the US (with physicians not far behind), and physicians/surgeons supplied anesthesia in the UK, some of the Commonwealth, and Europe. Much of the world relied on technicians and nurses directed by surgeons.

Anesthesia increased surgical possibilities, resulting in formal residencies to educate surgeons, but formal programs lagged for nurse and physician anesthetists. Between the 1850s and early 1900s, women in the US founded 17 medical schools. All but Drexel closed shortly after the turn of the century.

World Events, 1860–1910

More than 500,000 combatants died in the 1861–1865 American Civil War. In 1865, Lewis Carroll published Alice's Adventures in Wonderland. A year later, Gregor Mendel reported his laws of inheritance, beginning the modern study of genetics. In 1876, Alexander Graham Bell patented the telephone, and Mark Twain published *The Adventures of Tom Sawyer*. Thomas Edison patented the light bulb in 1879. In 1884–1885, Chicagoan William Le Baron Jenney oversaw the construction of the first skyscraper. Karl Benz patented and produced the first gasoline-powered automobile, a 1-cylinder beauty, in 1885. Two years later, Heinrich Hertz discovered the photoelectric effect. In 1888, Louis Le Prince produced the first movie (*Roundhay Garden Scene*), and the first edition of the *Oxford English Dictionary* was published. New Zealand gave women the right to vote in 1893– a first. In 1894, Emile Zola wrote *J'accuse*, attacking anti-Semitism in the Dreyfus Affair. Wilhelm Roentgen discovered X-rays in 1895, and for this received the first Nobel Prize in physics. Svante Arrhenius and Thomas Chamberlin connected CO_2 emissions to global warming in 1896, but no one noticed

E. I Eger II (✉)
Department of Anesthesia and Perioperative Care, University of California, 94143-0464, San Francisco, CA, USA
e-mail: egere@anesthesia.ucsf.edu

L. J. Saidman
Department of Anesthesia, Stanford University, Stanford, CA, USA
e-mail: lsaidman@stanford.edu

R. N. Westhorpe
Melbourne, Australia
e-mail: westhorpe@netspace.net.au

E. I Eger II et al. (eds.), *The Wondrous Story of Anesthesia*, DOI 10.1007/978-1-4614-8441-7_5, © Edmond I Eger, MD 2014

for a half-century. In 1897, Karl Braun invented the modern cathode ray tube. HG Wells created science fiction with his 1898 *War of the Worlds*. In 1903, the Wright Brothers flew a heavier than air craft at Kitty Hawk, North Carolina, and Marie Curie shared the Nobel Prize in Physics with her husband Pierre Curie and Henri Becquerel. France failed in their attempted 1890–1903 construction of the Panama Canal. The US took up the challenge in 1904, completing the Canal in 1914. In 1905, Albert Einstein proposed his theory of special relativity. In 1907, Pablo Picasso painted Les Demoiselles d'Avignon, beginning cubism. In 1908, Ford initiated mass production with his Model T Ford.

Introduction

Several parallel, yet connected, stories unfolded in the half-century that followed 1860. The present chapter provides these stories, noting how each might have influenced the other. They are stories of growth, of wars, of visionaries and visions, sometimes advancing by reason, often by trial and error, but always advancing.

The Development of Surgery

The Surgeon Before the Discovery of Anesthesia

The discovery of anesthesia facilitated enormous changes in surgery and the surgeon. The surgeon Frederick Treves described the surgeon in the days before anesthesia [1]:

> We find him an ignorant, illiterate, sordid creature, not above the allurements of money-grubbing, and not without suspicion of dishonest practices and of a leaning towards the bottle. He was to a large extent a mere retailer of physic, and in the public eye he ranked with the quacks and nostrum-sellers with whom he competed…The training of the surgeon was paltry, casual, and inefficient.

Lest we smile, let us remember that the early anesthetist, particularly in the US, had much the same defects. Then Treves described the impact of the discovery of anesthesia on surgery and surgeons [1].

> The changes that the discovery has wrought in the personality of the surgeon, in his bearing, in his methods, and in his capabilities are as wondrous as the discovery itself. The operator is undisturbed by the harass of alarms and the misery of giving pain. He can afford to be leisurely without fear of being regarded as timorous. To the older surgeon every tick of the clock upon the wall was a mandate for haste, every groan of the patient a call for hurried action, and he alone did best who had the quickest fingers and the hardest heart. Time now counts for little, and success is no longer to be measured by the beatings of a watch. The mask of the anaesthetist has blotted out the anguished face of the patient, and the horror of a vivisection on a fellow-man has passed away. Thus it happens that the surgeon has gained dignity, calmness, confidence, and, not least of all, the gentle hand.

> Anaesthetics have, moreover, greatly extended the domain of surgery by rendering possible operations which before could only have been dreamt about, and by allowing elaborate measures to be carried out step by step.

> The introduction of anaesthetics has not only developed surgery, but it has engendered surgeons. It has opened up the craft to many, for in the pre-anaesthetic days the qualities required for success in operating were qualities to be expected only in the few.

So surgery grew because ether and chloroform anesthesia had been discovered. The discovery sufficed for all surgical requirements—and so, apart from Snow telling us how to do it safely (along the way devising an anesthetic delivery system including a stable-delivery vaporizer, making astute observations on the cardiorespiratory effects of anesthetics, and telling us how chloroform killed patients), nothing more seemed necessary. The greater need was to improve the surgeon and what he might do (there were no she surgeons) [1]:

> The surgeon at the commencement of the (nineteenth) century appears to have lacked most of what we now consider to be the essentials of the art, and we can only view with amazement the scantiness of his learning and the poverty of his equipment. He knew little more of inflammation than that it was represented by swelling, heat, redness, and pain. His knowledge of the causes of inflammation and of those dangers which follow upon open wounds was scarcely in advance of that professed in the days of Hippocrates. He had no glimmer of the possibilities of asepsis. He had no anaesthetic, no hypodermic syringe, no clinical thermometer and no practical means of investigation in clinical chemistry. The very name bacteriology did not exist, and the treatment of disease by prepared serums would have appeared to him as wild as the wildest therapeutic dream of ancient days. Although vaccination had been introduced in the last year of the eighteenth century, the magnitude and nature of the principle it involved had not been appreciated.

> The microscope as an aid to diagnosis played no part in the equipment of the surgeon. He had neither laryngoscope nor ophthalmoscope, and his acquaintance with otology, skin affections, and the diseases of women was at the best rudimentary and indistinct. He had only rude mediaeval orthopedic appliances, and he knew nothing of the lithotrite (an instrument for crushing a kidney stone) nor of the array of instruments which are now in daily use in connection with ophthalmic, laryngeal, cranial, and abdominal surgery. It would seem indeed that there was little for him to do but to open abscesses and sow the seeds of chronic septicemia, to excise tumours of the structure of which he talked much and knew little, to amputate limbs for diseases he could not mend, and to draw blood whenever doubt existed as to what was best to be done.

In sum, Treves tells us that in the nineteenth century, the surgeon had mountains to climb, the biggest of which had been the absence of anesthesia. Once anesthesia was discovered, once every patient could be anesthetized, once that colossal step was taken, nothing more was immediately required of the anesthetist or of anesthesia.

Brutal procedures could be accomplished at a leisurely pace without agony. Patients who had rejected surgery because of the anticipation of unbearable pain now allowed surgery, increasing the numbers of surgical procedures undertaken. Surgeons could improve everyday operations (e.g., pulling/restoring teeth, amputations, removing bladder stones.) A thousand and one minor modifications might be tried to advance the quality of surgical outcomes. And the surgeon could quickly learn which approaches gave the best results because many more patients would accept surgery—all because of anesthesia. No Committees on Human Research slowed what the good and bad surgeon might try. Surgery grew, limited only by the numbers, ingenuity, energy and skill of surgeons. The economic attractiveness of surgery expanded the numbers of increasingly more qualified physicians into the practice, compounding the rate at which surgical knowledge grew. All because ether and chloroform anesthesia had been discovered.

Antisepsis and Asepsis are Invented

The picture wasn't quite as rosy as the last paragraph implies. Anesthesia enabled an expansion of surgery, but the most elegant operation was useless if the patient died from infection. Elegance was the mark of a successful surgeon, striding to the operating table, pausing to remove his top hat and leather gloves. His frock coat might bear dried blood from previous operations, and the lapel served as a convenient place to hold surgical needles ready-threaded with silk. His hands might carry infection from one patient to the next. Anesthesia only solved one problem; infection carried enormous risk, even for the simplest operation.

In 1867, Joseph Lister published a series of articles in The Lancet (March-September 1867) under the title *Antiseptic Principle of the Practice of Surgery*, urging surgeons to wash their hands before operations with 5 % carbolic acid (phenol) solutions, to wash instruments in the same solution, and to spray the solution in the operating theatre. The resulting reduction in infection decreased morbidity and mortality and thereby encouraged the use of hospitals for surgery. Hospitals had rightly been thought of as a source of a dangerous contagion.

In 1886, Ernst von Bergmann (1836–1907) added to Lister's remedy. von Bergmann developed steam sterilization, thereby ensuring the sterility of instruments, an essential ingredient of asepsis. Other rituals such as the use of masks, operating gowns, hats, and sterile gloves evolved rapidly thereafter. The addition of asepsis to antisepsis further decreased infections, and accordingly increased surgical care in hospitals. But a few surgeons aided by anesthetists (e.g., Nicoll [2] in Scotland and Waters [3] in the US) bucked this trend in the first 70 years of the twentieth century, harbingers of outpatient surgery that would become 80 % of US practice by the end of the twentieth century.

The Great, Heroic Surgeons Appear

Surgeons arose to seize the opportunity offered by anesthesia, with or without infection. First (Table 5.1), in 1849 the US gynecologist, J. Marion Sims, successfully repaired a vesico-vaginal fistula, that disastrous connection between bladder and vagina plaguing and ostracizing many young African post partum women that Abraham Verghese described in his beautiful story, *Cutting for Stone*. Two decades later, German surgeon Theodor Billroth began a series of innovative operative procedures, beginning with perineal prostatectomy in 1867. In 1873 he added laryngectomy, and in 1881 gastrectomy, ultimately in two flavors (Billroth I and Billroth II).

In 1881, US surgeon William Halsted performed the first emergency blood transfusion—on his sister. In 1889, he introduced rubber surgical gloves, less to avoid sepsis than to protect the hands of his fiancée who just happened to be his scrub nurse. In the mid 1890s, he established the US model for training surgeons (including the pyramid system that kept budding surgeons in servitude for what must have seemed like a lifetime) and developed the radical mastectomy. This unnecessarily mutilating operation would eventually be abolished, but not for nearly a century. Indeed, in 1899 the American Surgical Association established Halsted's mastectomy and inguinal hernia repair as gold standards. He was not a quick surgeon. Will Mayo is said to have remarked after two hours of observing Halsted work: "My God, this is the first time I have seen the wound healing at the upper end while it is still being operated upon at the lower end [4]."

From the 1880s to the 1900s, Swiss surgeon Theodor Kocher removed thyroid glands for goiter and hyperthyroidism, receiving the Nobel Prize for Medicine in 1909, for showing the importance of thyroid secretion. He also won fame for abdominal, orthopedic, and intracranial operations, and for contributions to antisepsis.

Surgeons started to go places where they had never gone, in the process increasing demands on anesthesia, forcing anesthesia to grow. In 1896, Rehn in Frankfurt sutured a wound of the heart, one of the first operations on the heart, up to then an off-limits organ for the surgeon. In 1902, Hill in Montgomery, Alabama repeated the feat. In 1901, Norwegian surgeon Christian Igelsrud performed the first successful open cardiopulmonary resuscitation. The world took little note. In 1910, Harvey Cushing drove to the base of the brain to remove pituitary tumors.

The last half of the nineteenth century saw the surgeon become the equal of other physicians, become an admired

Table 5.1 Great Surgical and Surgical Adjunct Developments in the Nineteenth and Twentieth Centuries

Date	Contribution	Surgeon/Scientist
1849	Repair, vesico-vaginal fistula	J. Marion Sims
1867	Perineal prostatectomy for cancer	Theodor Billroth
1867	Antisepsis	Joseph Lister
1871	Esophagectomy	Theodor Billroth
1873	Total removal of the larynx for cancer	Theodor Billroth
1875	Suprapubic bladder tumor removal	Theodor Billroth
1881–1885	Gastrectomy for stomach cancer (Billroth I and II)	Theodor Billroth
1882	Radical mastectomy for breast cancer	William Halsted
1882	Successful open cholecystectomy	Carl Langenbush
1882	Drainage of a pancreatic cyst	Carl Gussenbauer
1886	Steam sterilization (asepsis)	Ernst von Bergmann
1888	Repair of aneurysm	Rudolph Matas
1889	Improved inguinal hernia repair—the gold standard	William Halsted
1891	Hemipelvectomy	Theodor Billroth
1895	X-rays discovered	William Roentgen
1901	Discovery of human blood groups	Karl Landsteiner
1901	Visualization of the abdominal contents through a tube	George Kelling
1906	Direct blood transfusion	George Crile
1909	Development of surgery for thyroid disease	Theodor Kocher
1909	Tracheal insufflation for aeration	Rudolf Matas
1910	Pituitary tumor removal through the nose	Harvey Cushing
1912	Suturing of blood vessels	Alexis Carrel
1913	Resection of cancer of the esophagus	Franz Torek
1923	Treatment of aortic obstruction	Rene Leriche
1924	X-ray visualization of the gall bladder	Evarts Graham
1928	Observation of effect of penicillin	Alexander Fleming
1932	First sulfonamide	Gerhard Domagk
1933	Pneumonectomy for cancer	Evarts Graham
1935	Resection for pancreatic cancer	Allan Whipple
1938	Closure of a patent ductus arteriosis	Robert Gross
1941	Hormonal influence on prostate cancer	Charles Huggins
1945	Resection of an aortic coarctation	Robert Gross
1946	Endarterectomy for arterial occlusions	J. Cid Dos Santos
1948	Repair of a mitral valve	Harken & Bailey
1951	Resection and graft replacement of aortic aneruysm	Charles Dubost
1953	Successful cardiopulmonary bypass	John Gibbon
1954	Successful transplant of a kidney between two humans	Harrison & Murray
1983	Cause and treatment of peptic ulcer discovered	Marshall & Warren
1991	Laparoscopic cholecystectomy	Erich Muhe

Table 5.2 Surgeon Nobel Larueates in Medicine and Physiology, 1901–2005

Year	Laureate	Reason for Prize Award
1909	Theodor Kocher	Contributions to thyroid physiology and surgery
1911	Allvar Gullstrand	Dioptrics of the eye
1912	Alexis Carrel	Blood vessel suturing
1914	Robert Barany	Pathophysiology of the vestibular apparatus
1922	Frederick Banting	The discovery of insulin
1949	Walter Hess	The importance of the diencephalon to the circulation
1956	Werner Forssmann	Heart catheterization and circulatory pathology
1966	Charles Huggins	Hormonal treatment of prostatic cancer
1990	Joseph Murray	Organ transplantation

physician-scientist. Fredrick Treves was Sir Frederick Treves. And in the twentieth century, surgeons repeatedly won the Nobel Prize for their work (Table 5.2) [5]. Surgeons and surgery had arrived, primarily because anesthesia had been discovered.

Anesthesia Practice Evolved in Disparate Ways Across the World

The Evolving Practice of Anesthesia in the US

The staggering numbers of wounded produced by the Civil War (1861–1865) engendered the development of surgeons, but did nothing to develop anesthetists or further anesthetic delivery:

> …ether or chloroform poured or dropped on a towel, a rag, or other vaporizer was the accepted method for anesthetizing the many wounded soldiers of the Union and Confederate armies during the Civil War, and for most patients during the rest of the nineteenth and the early twentieth centuries in America. Surgeons directed all aspects of treatment of their patients. They recruited anesthetists from the operating room personnel, such as nurses, hospital porters (orderlies), janitors, and even the surgeons' secretaries…the anesthetist was regarded as the 'low man on the totem pole' during the late 1800s and the early 1900s [6].

The surgeon supervised anesthetic delivery, a demanding responsibility that distracted from his primary task. Anesthesia continued to be dangerous as suggested by an 1885 survey by the Scandinavian Society of Surgeons giving an anesthetic mortality of 1 in 2,000–3,000, perhaps more with chloroform than ether [7]. Concerns regarding the safety and the availability of anesthetic service may have prompted US surgeons in the Midwest to employ Catholic Sisters (nurses) to provide anesthesia on a full-time basis. Thus Mary Bernard at St. Vincent's Hospital in Erie Pennsylvania, was recruited in 1877. At first directed by the surgeon, these anesthetists increasingly gained experience by trial and error. Unlike the part-time anesthetist, they had the advantage of frequently repeated opportunities to learn their craft.

By the 1880s, more than 90 Midwest Catholic hospitals used sisters for anesthesia, thereby providing a more consistent and likely safer service than did the part-time anesthetist, physician or not. Most famously, in the late 1880s, sisters Edith and Dinah Graham became the first nurse anesthetists at the Mayo Clinic. In 1893, the Mayo brothers recruited Alice Magaw, the most celebrated nurse anesthetist of the nineteenth century. Magaw replaced the Graham sisters. The Mayo brothers soon added Florence Henderson.

> The Mayos had given the job to Miss (Edith) Graham and then to Miss (Alice) Magaw in the first place through necessity; they had no interns. And when the interns came, the brothers decided that a nurse was better suited to the task because she was more likely to keep her mind on it, whereas the intern was naturally more interested in what the surgeon was doing [8].

Although the brothers provided initial training, Magaw and Henderson then independently perfected the smooth and safe delivery of anesthesia with ether.

The situation differed in other parts of the US. Anesthesia in the US had no distinction in the medical community. Training of physicians in anesthesia and the reputation of the physician anesthetist (in contrast to the nurse anesthetist) was abysmal. The 1894 experience of Harvey Cushing, later the father of neurosurgery, as a student at Harvard illustrates anesthesia's low standing and the disasters that ignorance brought [9]:

> My first giving of an anaesthetic was when, a third-year student, I was called down from the seats and sent in a little side room with a patient and an orderly and told to put the patient to sleep. I knew nothing about the patient whatsoever, merely that a nurse came in and gave the patient a hypodermic injection. I proceeded as best I could under the orderly's directions, and in view of the repeated urgent calls for the patient from the amphitheatre it seemed to be an interminable time for the old man, who kept gagging, to go to sleep. We finally wheeled him in. I can vividly recall just how he looked and the feel of his bedraggled whiskers. The operation was started and at this juncture there was a sudden great gush of fluid from the patient's mouth, most of which was inhaled, and he died. I stood aside, burning with chagrin and remorse. No one paid the slightest attention to me, although I supposed I had killed the patient. To my perfect amazement, I was told it was nothing at all, that I had nothing to do with the man's death, that he had a strangulated hernia and had been vomiting all night anyway, and that sort of thing happened frequently and I had better forget about it and go on with the medical school. I went on with the medical school, but I have never forgotten about it.

This terrible event embodied the state of anesthesia in some parts of the US: an orderly directed a third year medical student in the administration of an anesthetic to a seriously ill and ill-prepared patient. As he promised, Cushing never forgot about it. Moreover, to the benefit of anesthesia, he

did something about it. With Codman, in 1895 he developed the anesthetic record with intraoperative recording of heart rate and blood pressure (itself, a new measurement in medicine) in that record at five-minute intervals. That record persists to the present, albeit now in an electronic form [10, 11]. The record was adopted in the US, but its use in other countries might vary. In the UK, use of anesthetic records, indeed, measurement of heart rate and blood pressure in the operating room, only began in the last half of the twentieth century.

Thus, by the beginning of the twentieth century in the US, the quality of anesthesia had a tri-modal distribution. First, nurse anesthetists, particularly in the Midwest, pursued anesthesia as a full-time occupation and honed their skills by regular practice. They took pride in what they did and did it well. They might know little about the science of anesthesia, but they were likely to give anesthesia safely and smoothly, and they taught other nurses how to do the same. Second, the part-time anesthetist, physician, medical student, nurse, orderly, or secretary, was also likely to know little about the science of anesthesia, but in contrast to the full-time nurse anesthetist was unpracticed in the art, and relied on the equally limited surgeon to provide direction. Anesthesia given by such persons was neither smooth nor safe (note Cushing's experience, above). Third, a small, but growing, number of physicians elected to pursue a full time practice of anesthesia, and like the Midwest nurses, might acquire skill in anesthetic delivery. Unlike nurses, these physicians might be driven to a career in anesthesia by their ineptness as physicians. In the 1900s, we find that "… the dean of Harvard Medical School wrote to the president of Harvard that the practice of anesthesia '…is so narrow a subject that a good man would not want to tie himself down to that and would hardly be willing to do so.' [12, 13]" But some of them, particularly women, would be leaders. For example, in the latter part of the 1890s, Isabella Herb practiced anesthesia at Augustana Hospital in Chicago, in 1922 becoming president of the first nationwide US anesthesia society, the American Association of Anesthetists (AAA). In 1898, Mary Botsford practiced anesthesia at the Children's Hospital of San Francisco. In 1922, she led the effort to found the Anesthesia Section of the California Medical Association, and was its first president.

The Evolving Practice of Anesthesia in the UK

Soon after the 1846 demonstration of ether anesthesia and the 1847 demonstration of chloroform anesthesia, Great Britain embraced anesthesia as part of the practice of medicine. Physicians, not nurses or orderlies, gave anesthesia. Perhaps this resulted from a preference for the use of the more dangerous anesthetic, chloroform, possibly a provincial response to chloroform's discovery as an anesthetic in Scotland. Perhaps this resulted from the power of John Snow's studies and writings and those of other giants (Simpson, Clover and more) who accompanied him.

Regardless of the reason, a cadre of physicians gave anesthesia in the UK from the beginning of the history of anesthesia. Buxton advocated the compulsory study of anesthetics in medical curricula. Hospital residents or family doctors gave most anesthetics in Australia where deaths associated with chloroform repeatedly brought calls for full-time chloroformists, calls that were ignored. Commonly the surgeon invited the referring general practitioner to be the "chloroformist". The low professional and economic status of anesthetists impeded the attraction of young doctors into the specialty as full-time practitioners, a condition that continued worldwide to the mid-twentieth century

The World's First Anesthetic Society Forms in the UK

In the UK, the number of physicians principally practicing anesthesia became sufficient to merit the formation of a society. Frederick Silk noted that "for some years…the subject of anaesthetics had occupied a very prominent position in the professional controversies of the period and its importance as a branch of medical education and special practice was becoming more generally recognised. It seemed to me therefore that…an attempt should be made to form a special Society of Anaesthetists [14]." And so in 1893, 40 founding members established the Society of Anaesthetists in London, electing Woodhouse Braine as President, Silk as secretary and Dudley Buxton as treasurer. George Oliver made the first presentation to the Society: "The size of the radial pulse under anaesthesia". This first true anesthetic society soon gathered members from Europe, North America, South Africa and Australia, and by 1900, grew to more than 100 members, many of them women. Indeed, it was the first medical society admitting women as full members. That it arose in the UK, and that so many members were to be found, indicated the pre-eminence of British anesthesia.

Surgeons Outside the US and UK Might Give and Direct Anesthesia

Surgeons were not fools. They realized the risks imposed by the inept or ignorant anesthetist. In the early 1900s, they popularized regional anesthesia with enthusiastic reports and textbooks describing virtually all modern block techniques in some form. By using regional anesthesia, they could continue to control anesthetic delivery and give safer anesthesia into the bargain. In 1901, Cleveland Clinic founder, surgeon George Crile, showed that regional techniques blocked "surgical shock", presaging "pre-emptive analgesia".

Unlike the situation in GB, where physician-anesthetists controlled anesthetic delivery, in Germany, surgeons directed anesthesia and devised methods for anesthetic delivery. In 1894, Schleich unsuccessfully advocated specialization in anaesthesia. In 1895, Witzel continuously dripped liquid ether or chloroform from bottles onto masks invented by Esmarch and Schimmelbusch, progressively increasing the anesthetic concentration, a technique used for the next half century or more. The direction by the German surgeon of part-time anesthetists, was the model for much of the anesthetic world outside of the US and the UK. In summary, by the 1900s, the anesthetic world consisted of three kinds: the nurse anesthetist/physician anesthetist/surgeon-directed model used in the US; the part-time/full-time physician-anesthetist model adopted in the UK and Commonwealth; and the surgeon-directed model used in most other places.

The First Anesthetic Society in the US

A few but growing number of physicians in the US took a small step, an advance that would grow in importance. The step indicated how far anesthesia had come. On 6 October 1905, nine physician-anesthetists met at Long Island College Hospital in Brooklyn at the invitation of Adolf Erdmann "because, as he put it, 'there are a few physicians practising (sic) anesthesia in the area, and these men ought to get together and form a society' [15]." Thus was formed The Long Island Society of Anesthetists (LISA). This new society would "promote the art and science of anesthetics" [15]. An excellent goal since the practice often possessed little art and less science. Bringing practitioners together allowed the sharing of experiences and enabled the cultivation of outside wisdom (e.g., bring in a speaker; appropriate for a society but hard to justify for just one person.)

These worthy goals alone, could explain the formation of what became the American Society of Anesthesiologists. However, one wonders whether other incentives prompted this convening. Given that anyone could administer anesthesia, the title of anesthetist provided little status. Surgeons (who now had a considerable cachet) often regarded anesthetists with disdain, even contempt. An anesthetic (or any) society, bestowed an authority onto its members, an armor against disdain and contempt. It allowed its members to argue that they possess something of value.

LISA morphed into the New York Society of Anesthetists in 1911, then into the American Society of Anesthetists in 1936, and finally to the American Society of Anesthesiologists in 1945. As with the formation of the Society of Anaesthetists in the UK in 1893, the establishment of LISA twelve years later indicated that a critical mass had been reached in the US. Both organizations would supply the specialty with educational, political, and economic powers that would grow progressively. These would provide a positive feedback that would increase the attractiveness and influence of the specialty. But it would take several decades to produce major changes. This was the first trickle in what was destined to become a world-wide torrent.

The First Anesthesia Journal

In 1891, dentist Samuel Hayes began a vanity press quarterly publication, 'Dental and Surgical Microcosm'. This might be considered the first anesthesia journal, for it discussed anesthetic matters and preached against 'asphyxial (nitrous oxide) anesthesia' without the provision of oxygen. Hayes died in 1897 and so did Microcosm. And why a dentist? Perhaps because dentists used anesthesia, especially nitrous oxide, more than did surgeons. They were interested in the safe and convenient delivery of anesthesia, and as we shall see, they disproportionately contributed to the early evolution of the anesthetic machine.

Anesthesiologists and other Scientists Consider How Drugs Act

How Does Curare Produce Paralysis?

In the 1860s, Claude Bernard showed that curare neither depressed conduction along nerves, nor prevented muscles from contracting when they were directly stimulated. Curare, he determined, caused paralysis by preventing the nerve impulse from traveling to the muscle through the junction between nerve and muscle, the myoneural junction [16].

How Do General Anesthetics Work?

Bernard proposed that a reversible coagulation of nerves underlay the production of anesthesia by some means that applied to all forms of life—a unitary mechanism of anesthesia. In contrast, two years later, LR Hermann suggested that the solution of anesthetics in brain lipids might be the basis for how they acted.

At the turn of the century, Meyer and Overton recognized that the theory proposed by von Bibra and Harless in 1847 (ether and chloroform acted by dissolving neural lipids) could not explain the rapid reversibility of narcosis, adding the further problem that dilute aqueous solutions of ether would not dissolve lipids although they could cause anesthesia. Like Hermann, Meyer and Overton proposed instead that anesthetics produced their effect by dissolving in the lipids. In support of this idea, they showed that anesthetic potency correlated with partitioning of the anesthetic between water and lipid. Partitioning that favored the lodgment of the anesthetic in lipid also favored greater potency.

Another Revolution; the Application of Local Anesthetics

Koller Discovers Local Anesthesia

The discovery of the anesthetic effects of ether and chloroform revolutionized the practice of surgery. A second, quieter revolution was to come with the discovery of local anesthesia.

In 1862, von Schroff reported that cocaine numbed the tongue but did not apply his observation to surgery. What a chance missed! It was not the last. In 1873, Alexander Bennett demonstrated the anesthetic properties of cocaine (Keys, p. 108) [17], but little was made of this. In 1880, von Anrep recommended testing cocaine as a local anesthetic but like von Schroff, von Anrep did not apply his suggestion. He, too, missed his chance.

Subsequently, Sigmund Freud and Carl Koller experimented with cocaine while both were in residence at the Vienna General Hospital, where Koller was intent on becoming an ophthalmologist. On one occasion, when Freud was away, Koller's colleague, Engel, licked some cocaine off the blade of his penknife and remarked that his tongue was numb. Koller wrote:

> I realized that I had in my possession the local anaesthetic which I had previously been searching for. I went at once to Striker's laboratory, made a solution of cocaine and instilled a drop in the eye of a frog, and afterward of a guinea pig, I found the cornea and conjunctiva anesthetic—that is, insensitive to mechanical, chemical, thermic and faradic stimulation. Afterwards I repeated these experiments on myself, some colleagues and many patients [18].

Koller prepared a report for the Heidelberg Ophthalmological Society meeting to be held in September, 1884, but could not afford to attend. Instead, his friend Joseph Brettauer presented his paper. Koller's report that cocaine produced corneal insensibility for ophthalmological procedures was a sensation, a second anesthetic revolution that marked the birth of local anesthesia. The news spread as quickly as had the news of ether some 38 years previously. Recognition of cocaine's ability to induce insensibility led to application for topical and then other forms of anesthesia. In 1887 Corning produced regional anesthesia by injecting cocaine into a specific nerve (Keys, p. 109) [17]. Ordinary and great (e.g., William Halsted) surgeons used cocaine to produce peripheral nerve blocks.

Surgeons seized on Koller's discovery, partly because it enabled them to control both anesthesia and surgery. It encouraged operations in the surgeon's office. However, in the late 1880s and the 1890s, reports of central nervous system and cardiac toxicity attended cocaine's expanded use. Concerns regarding these factors and an increased knowledge of chemistry prompted a search for new local anesthetics. As cocaine was a benzoic acid ester, synthetic efforts focused on this class of compounds, and in 1890, Ritsert identified benzocaine. But benzocaine's poor water solubility made it suitable only for topical anesthesia, a sunburn remedy. In 1904 a better benzoic acid ester was made: procaine.

Bier Produces Spinal Anesthesia with Cocaine

Although Corning developed spinal anesthesia using cocaine in 1885, it remained for Bier in the late 1890s to make spinal anesthesia popular. In 1897, Bier gave the first spinal "block" in Germany. Obstetricians and gynecologists implemented this form of anesthesia. German surgeons first rejected the method because of reported side effects. Bier's work led most of the world to adopt spinal anesthesia. From 1898 into the 1900s, spinal blocks were produced with cocaine, while after 1903, Amylocaine (stovaine) briefly became the agent of choice. However, stovaine was identified as a nerve irritant and was displaced in 1904 by procaine, synthesized by the German Alfred Einhorn. Procaine suffered from two limitations. Its duration of action was brief (perhaps 45 minutes), and allergic sensitivity to its metabolite, para-aminobenzoic acid, appeared. These limitations notwithstanding, spinal anesthesia was performed in Argentina, Brazil, Chile, Colombia, Ecuador, Peru, Uruguay, and Venezuela. Spinal anesthetics were given in Mexico, Cuba, Guatamala, El Salvador and Nicaragua, and probably Panama. They were given in Europe and North America. Spinal anesthesia was increasingly adopted because it cost little, made minimal equipment demands, and allowed surgeons to give the anesthetic and then attend to the surgery.

In 1907, AE Barker solved a problem that Bier had noted, the tendency for spinal anesthesia to be uncontrolled in the extent to which the level of anesthesia spread [19]. Barker showed that the spread could be controlled by controlling the baricity—the weight—of the anesthetic-containing liquid injected into spinal fluid. Inject liquid heavier than spinal fluid and the liquid would sink to the part of the spinal canal that was most dependent.

Intravenous Regional Anesthesia

In 1908, Bier described "intravenous regional anesthesia", a technique in which a tourniquet was used to isolate a limb from its circulation while local anesthetic was injected into the venous portion of the isolated limb. The technique continues to be used today.

Addiction

Many who gave cocaine found it addicting. Indeed, addiction had been a problem for anesthetists from the beginning of its history (e.g., remember Wells' addiction to chloroform). From 1883 to 1900, 35% of male morphine addicts in an Ontario treatment center were physicians (not just anesthetists).

Commercialism in the 1890s increased the potential for addiction to cocaine. Both Coca Cola and "vin Mariani", a "tonic wine" to "fortify and refresh body and brain, restoring health and vitality" contained cocaine. In 1892, William Osler noted that physicians injecting morphine to control pain had a greater incidence of morphine addiction. In 1894, Jansen Mattison reported that physicians comprised 70% of the morphine-addicted patients in his Home for Habitues. Some medical literature characterized opioid addiction as a loss of "moral will" or a problem affecting susceptible, weak individuals. Mattison disagreed: "… talk about weak will as a reason why strong men succumb to morphia …is twaddle." Whether addiction to drugs was a disease or a sign of weak will remained a question for many societies and individuals.

More on Inhaled Anesthetics

Ethyl chloride anesthetized skin, the nearby anesthetist, and the patient

Carlson used ethyl chloride in 1894 for local anesthesia [20]. Spray it on the skin and its evaporation made the skin cold to the point of anesthesia. The evaporation might also anesthetize the nearby anesthetist. It produced a rapid pleasant induction of general anesthesia and allowed a rapid recovery, but it was hard to control since it boiled at 12.5 °C and it was costly. It was used mainly for brief procedures or for induction prior to ether anesthesia [21]. In 1922, Oldenbourg listed its contraindications: "It is not suitable for prolonged administration on account of its dangers, expense, and great strain on the anesthetist." He added: "It should not be used in alcoholists and neurotics, and is decidedly contra-indicated in mechanical and inflammatory respiratory obstruction; in cardio-vascular degenerations and all conditions giving rise to marked dyspnoea [22]."

Whatever Happened to Chloroform?

From the year of its discovery forwards, deaths attended the use of chloroform. They continued to plague the practice of anesthesia, and increasingly provoked mention in the medical, and even the daily press. There were two schools of thought as to causation: the Edinburgh school, based on Professor of Surgery, James Syme's (1799–1870) belief that death was due to paralysis of respiration, and the English school, convinced that the heart stopped first.

Syme was a great friend and supporter of James Simpson, and advocated the use of chloroform, with the dictum (not based on any evidence) that one should "attend to the respiration, never mind the pulse." Flourens in France, and Snow in England, studied animals to determine why the heart stopped. Flourens proposed that chloroform was so dangerous that it should not be used at all. Snow, with limited means, found that death resulted from excessive percentages of chloroform, and that although respiration usually ceased first, sometimes it was the heart that stopped.

In 1855, a Chloroform Commission was held in Paris, concluding that in animals, the respiration ceased first. Snow went further. He divided the vagus nerves and found that at low percentages of chloroform given for long periods, the respiration failed first, while at high percentages, the circulation often failed first. Still the dispute raged.

In 1864, the Royal Medical and Chirurgical Society appointed a committee that confirmed Snow's findings. In addition they found that the blood pressure always fell before the respiratory arrest. They advised the use of an alcohol, chloroform, ether mixture, the A.C.E. mixture as a safer alternative. Other experiments tended to support Snow's findings, and most suggested that chloroform was primarily a heart poison. Views remained divided. The English school advised close observation of the circulation and the respiration, while the Scottish school, following Syme's dictum, believed that watching the respiration was all that was necessary, and that watching the circulation may distract from the more important observation.

Enter Surgeon Lieutenant Colonel Lawrie, Syme's former pupil, with apparently a great admiration for his former teacher. Lawrie convinced the Nizam of Hyderabad to fund research that might answer the question once and for all. The commission of 1888 was dismissed as being inadequately conducted. A second commission was sought by Lawrie, again funded by the Nizam. A large number of experiments, all carefully documented with chart recordings etc. showed that:

- Chloroform has no direct injurious effect on the heart
- Chloroform anaesthesia is absolutely free from risk if attention be paid to the respiration.
- The danger in chloroform anaesthesia rests entirely with respiratory interference.
- Respiration always fails before the heart.
- Slowing or arrest of the heart by nervous interference under chloroform is beneficial.
- Fall of blood pressure from the administration of chloroform is beneficial.

This convinced many, but some skeptics questioned the science. Starting with cross circulation studies in animals by Gaskell and Shore, demonstrating that chloroform caused cardiac arrest in an animal which had not inhaled the agent. Many researchers around the world entered the fray. Lawrie attacked them all with vitriol, asserting faulty technique.

Leonard Hill in London repeated the Hyderabad commission's experiments in 1897 and could not support their conclusions. Many others, in different countries, found that death was primarily due to cardiac arrest. In 1901, a British Medical Association report also suggested that the cause was cardiac. Lawrie commenced a concerted and sometimes bitter campaign in the journals of the day to sway others to his view.

In the meantime, Edward Embley, anesthetist, and part time researcher in the pathology department at Melbourne University, conducted experiments in dogs [23]. He showed that cardiac syncope, due to vagal stimulation, caused death on induction, and that general depression, and a fall in blood pressure, followed by respiratory failure caused later death. His research was published in the British Medical Journal in 1902, over 33 pages and three sequential issues. Embley cleverly chose dogs, whose vagal and cardiac responses to chloroform are similar to those in humans, while several of the previous studies used cats. In cats, chloroform causes excitability. Embley also monitored the dogs throughout the experiment. Lawrie's dogs were anesthetized outside the laboratory, and deaths during induction were ignored. In 1912–1914, A Goodman Levy showed that the cardiac syncope was due to ventricular fibrillation…but he had the advantage of the use of an electrocardiogram [24, 25].

Controlling Anesthetic and Oxygen Delivery to the Patient

Evolution of the Use of Nitrous Oxide

Colton, the showman whose exhibition prompted Wells' 1844 failed demonstration of nitrous oxide anesthesia, traveled to California in search of gold. Not finding any, he returned to New England where, in 1863, he took up dental anesthesia with nitrous oxide (Keys, p. 108) [17]. He kept a casebook indicating the administration of 100,000 anesthetics without a fatality—a world record for the next century. His successful use revived the fortunes of nitrous oxide, at least for dental practice or for brief procedures. It could only be given continuously for one or two minutes because the use of pure nitrous oxide excluded oxygen—not a safe thing to do.

In 1868, the surgeon Edmund Andrews suggested the solution to the problem of hypoxia when giving nitrous oxide: add oxygen [26]. This is obvious now, but was less so then. John Snow cavalierly said in 1847: "If the skin becomes inclined to purple, the face-piece may be removed for half a minute…but there need be no alarm [27]." Andrews was ahead of his time, but his solution presented logistic difficulties resulting from the inability to store compressed gases. Imagine going to the patient with an enormous balloon filled with nitrous oxide and oxygen. Adding oxygen demanded the production and storage of compressed gases, a means of mixing those gases, and a method of presenting them to the patient. Thus Andrews' suggestion did not produce an immediate change, for no anesthetic machine existed to deliver nitrous oxide combined with oxygen. The delivery of 100% nitrous oxide with occasional breaths of fresh air continued for several years.

In early 1870, Coxeter and Son supplied refillable cylinders with liquefied nitrous oxide, at a cost of 3 pence per gallon. Soon after, Johnston Brothers of New York supplied the American market with liquefied nitrous oxide [17]. This was an essential step in the practical deployment of nitrous oxide.

In 1879, Paul Bert showed that Andrews was correct. Nitrous oxide safely produced anesthesia if given in a hyperbaric pressure chamber with sufficient oxygen [28]. A century later, Hornbein showed that such anesthesia was less than ideal [29]. Using a hyperbaric chamber, Hornbein found in volunteers, that anesthetic partial pressures of nitrous oxide caused muscle rigidity and considerable post anesthetic nausea and vomiting.

In 1885, nearly two decades after Andrews' suggestion, industry added high-pressure oxygen cylinders to the cylinders already built to hold liquid nitrous oxide. The SS White Company then patented what might be recognized as an anesthetic machine. In 1886, Viennese dentist Hillischer produced a machine dispensing the combination of nitrous oxide (he called it Schlafgas or sleeping gas) and oxygen. The SS White Co. machine and Hillischer's machine provided a rough control of oxygen concentrations.

In 1887, Frederick Hewitt invented a machine to concurrently administer nitrous oxide and oxygen—but not ether [30]. Other machines for the delivery of nitrous oxide and oxygen followed, and ultimately ether delivery was added in various ways, some safer than others. Hewitt explained why the combination of nitrous oxide with ether was so useful: "It is obvious that if the etherisation be preceded by the administration of nitrous oxide, the taste and odour of ether, and the other objections here referred to, will be completely relieved. It may indeed be said that nitrous oxide supplies the deficiencies of ether just as ether supplies the deficiencies of nitrous oxide" [31]. This form of anesthetic delivery continued for more than a half-century.

> As a resident (1956–1958), the primary anesthetic I (EIE) gave was nitrous oxide plus ether in a background of oxygen, the so-called 'gas-oxygen-ether' (GOE) mixture. I also gave 'open-drop' ether, ether dripped onto a gauze-covered mask without nitrous oxide. The difference from GOE anesthesia was considerable.

Premedication Becomes Part of Anesthetic Delivery

In the late 1800s, clinicians increasingly injected morphine and scopolamine or atropine before ether anesthesia. The combination shortened induction and decreased anesthetic requirement. Scopolamine blocked the production of secretions resulting from the irritant effects of ether, and had

the added benefits of decreasing preoperative apprehension and providing amnesia for the unpleasantness attending induction of anesthesia. Morphine accelerated induction (by providing some of the anesthesia before the first drop of ether was poured) and minimized perception of ether's irritant effects. The capacity of morphine to depress breathing was of limited concern because ether itself did not depress breathing.

Beyond their use for premedication, morphine plus scopolamine were given in increased amounts to produce "twilight sleep" providing analgesia and amnesia for surgical procedures and obstetric deliveries. This technique was largely, but not completely, abandoned in the US in 1914 because of associated morbidity and mortality. LJS remembers in 1961 being bitten by a patient in which the combination had been used. The patient did not remember the event, but LJS did.

Control Over the Delivered Concentration of Volatile Anesthetic

Snow had invented a vaporizer that delivered a known and constant partial pressure of ether or chloroform, the saturated vapor pressure. Such a high partial pressure/concentration greatly exceeded that needed clinically. Joseph Clover solved the problem of delivering a precisely known, *clinical* concentration of chloroform to a patient. He devised a large, air-tight bag into which he added a known quantity of liquid chloroform and a known amount of air. Beyond the cumbersomeness of such a solution was the problem of adjustment of the delivered concentration. Only the originally concocted concentration was known with precision.

Another approach provided little to no control over the delivered concentration but might induce anesthesia rapidly. In 1880, Danish Surgeon Oskar Wancher introduced his airtight bag. He added 50 mL of liquid ether plus the exhaled air of the patient to the bag. The patient then breathed and rebreathed this mixture, producing increasing hypercapnia and hypoxia. The danger from breathing too little oxygen and too much carbon dioxide was partially countered by the hyperventilation that they produced. The approach accelerated the induction of anesthesia because of the hyperventilation, complimented by the anesthetic effect of hypoxia.

Improved Anesthetic Machines and the Addition of Ventilators

In 1902, dentist Teter developed a gas machine that delivered a variable mixture of oxygen and nitrous oxide, each controlled by separate but inaccurate valves, and without an indication of percentage or flow. Still we were making progress, and dentists like Teter often led the way. A year later, Dragerwerk developed a device to absorb carbon dioxide from rebreathed gases using soda lime (mostly calcium hydroxide spiked with a bit of sodium and potassium hydroxide). Another step forward.

The increasing demands of surgery for a safe sustained delivery of anesthesia, led to the invention of new devices. In 1906, US dentist (yes, another dentist!) Jay Heidbrink, modified Teter's machine to produce an oxygen-nitrous oxide anesthesia machine. In that year, Green and Janeway began building machines to deliver intermittent positive pressure ventilation (IPPV) and demonstrated the advantages of controlled (as opposed to assisted) ventilation. However, they prematurely discontinued their groundbreaking work. A year later, Dräger produced the Pulmotor, a compressed-gas powered IPPV ventilator designed to breathe for rescued miners, later applied to the anesthetized patient.

In 1908, Kuppers introduced the rotameter to deliver a precisely measured gas flow. Gas (oxygen or nitrous oxide, perhaps) lifted a rotating cylinder within a tube that broadened with increasing height (i.e., was tapered); a greater height of the cylinder indicated a greater flow, and this could be determined and the rotameter thereby calibrated. Neu subsequently used it in an anesthesia apparatus. The rotameter became the primary gauge of flow in the last half of the twentieth century. Also in 1908, Ombré-danne devised his inhaler for ether. It became the favored method for anesthetic delivery in France and Latin America for a half century, the French reluctantly parting from it in the 1950s.

Development of Standards

As might be imagined, because of the flammable nature of ether, the major anesthetic of the time, the National Fire Protection Association, formed in 1896, became the first of several organizations to set standards for anesthesia and anesthesia equipment. Other organizations included the US Food and Drug Administration (1906); the US Compressed Gas Association (1913); and the American Standards Institute (1918). These dry developments would materially increase the safety of anesthetic delivery.

Studies of Oxyhemoglobin

Uptake of Oxygen by Blood Changes the Absorption of Light

In 1862, Hoppe-Seyler crystallized the pigment that supplies blood's color, naming it hemoglobin. Oxygen and hemoglo-bin, he found, form a dissociable compound he called oxy-hemoglobin. He proved that hemoglobin caused the absorption of green and blue light, the "Soret band," and that this absorption changed when he shook the solution with air (the air delivering oxygen to the blood). He thereby gave us the beginnings of oxyhemoglobin percent saturation measurement in the blood, the beginnings of oximetry.

In 1876, von Vierordt found that stopping circulation in the finger, caused the two bands of reflected light representing oxyhemoglobin to disappear and that of deoxygenated hemoglobin to appear. He measured the finger's oxygen consumption by timing this change. His observations brought us another step closer to oximetry.

In the 1890s, Danneel, in Nernst's laboratory, found that dissolved oxygen reacts with a negatively charged metal (cathode) in proportion to the oxygen pressure. Although he identified the principle of the polarographic electrode, organic substances "poisoned" the cathode surface, making it useless for the determination of oxygen partial pressures in protein-containing solutions like blood.

Assuring an Unobstructed airway

Pulling or Pushing the Tongue Forward

The obstructed airway was increasingly recognized as a source of danger during anesthesia. One might pull the tongue forward with a forceps to relieve obstruction, but that often caused tongue injury. In 1873, Norwegian Heiberg invented the "jaw thrust" (pulling the jaw, and thus the tongue, forward) to remove airway obstruction. Esmarch advocated the technique 5 years later and was credited with the invention, but Heiberg should get the credit. Jaw thrust continues to the present as an effective way to maintain an open airway.

However, maintenance of a patent airway by jaw thrust required two hands to lift the jaw. In 1880, Howard suggested an alternative, head tilt and extension, something that might be done with one hand, a technique still used to relieve obstruction by the tongue. But head tilt and extension concurrently moved the tongue, jaw and head en bloc; so why should such a maneuver relieve obstruction? The contemporary answer is that the extension lifts the hyoid cartilage, the bony structure just above the Adam's Apple portion of the larynx. Extending the head tightens the muscles attached from jaw tip to hyoid cartilage and from cartilage to sternum, thereby pulling the hyoid cartilage forward. Since the tongue attaches to the hyoid, this maneuver lifts the tongue from the back of the pharynx and relieves obstruction. As already noted, part of the magic is that head tilt and extension can also be accomplished with just one hand, a great advantage to the anesthetist who already has too few hands.

Put a Tube in the Trachea

Pulling or pushing the tongue didn't always solve the problem. Enter the Scot, William Macewen, who intubated the trachea with a metal tube in awake patients, blindly guiding the tube with his fingers. He then might deliver anesthesia through the tracheal tube. Although Macewen pioneered blind orotracheal intubation for anesthetic delivery, he abandoned this approach in 1880 when a patient died during the use of intubation associated with induction of anesthesia. However and under different circumstances, in 1882, New York surgeon O'Dwyer blindly put a metal tube into the glottic opening to bypass the suffocating pseudo membranes of diphtheria in children. In 1887, Fell used intermittent positive pressure ventilation (IPPV) from a bellows delivered via a face mask to inflate the lungs. Combining the O'Dwyer tube with the Fell bellows produced the Fell-O'Dwyer apparatus. In 1894, Alfred Kirstein reported looking at the larynx with his "autoscope", and a year later, Killian used Kirstein's autoscope to visualize and extract a foreign body from a patient's bronchus. In 1899. van Stockum constructed a metal tracheal tube fitted with an inflatable cuff.

Or Use an Oral Airway

In 1908 Hewitt devised a simple but vital advance –an oropharyngeal artificial airway to relieve airway obstruction in patients in whom the trachea is not intubated. Such an artificial airway relieved obstruction by providing a clear passage to the rear of the pharynx. The artificial airway continued to evolve and save patients' lives for the rest of the century, passing through the Waters and Guedel versions of the oropharyngeal airway in the 1930s to the remarkable laryngeal mask airway in the 1980s.

Respiratory physiology

Control of Ventilation

In 1876, Woillez described a manual ventilator that applied intermittent negative pressure to the chest, a forerunner to the iron lung. However, this approach was cumbersome and would present a barrier to operations on the chest or lung. In 1899, Matas reported the successful use of intermittent positive pressure ventilation applied to the airway during an operation to remove a chest wall tumor.

In 1902, Tuffier and Hallion reported on "Intrathoracic operations with artificial respiration by insufflation"—blowing oxygen containing anesthetic into the airway (e.g., the oropharynx)—in animals using a rhythmic inflation method. This solved the "Pneumothorax problem" the problem of lung collapse when the chest is opened, a problem that leads to insufficient oxygen in the blood [32], and like Matas' method, allowed access to the chest.

In 1909, Meltzer and Auer repeated Tuffier and Hallion's insufflation. This technique continued in use for a half century. Eger remembers its frequent application in the late 1950s during tonsillectomies, blowing oxygen laden with ether into children's mouths. The happy surgeons and slightly less happy anesthetists would go home partially anesthetized from the fumes they inhaled. Incorrectly, surgeons also thought that insufflation supplied "ventilation."

German surgeon, Sauerbruch, had another solution to the pneumothorax problem. He wanted to perform thoracic surgery, but opening the chest caused lung collapse, hypoxia and death. To prevent lung collapse, in 1903 he built a giant chamber having a negative pressure of about 5 cm of water. It enclosed the patient's body with the head protruding from the chamber. The surgeons joined the patient in the chamber, but they kept their heads inside. This maintained inflation of the patient's lungs, but it did not supply ventilation. Sauerbruch demonstrated its use in 1904, and could not be convinced that ventilation also needed to be supplied. That would have been unphysiologic, he said.

Reprise

Morton's demonstration of ether anesthesia on 16 October 1846 (ether day) accelerated progress in surgery, enabling both increased numbers of surgeries and new operations. Such increases affected the demand for superior education and training of surgeons. Germany, Austria, the UK and the US soon led as centers of surgical knowledge. Formal organizations were established to further surgical learning and to improve standards of care in Britain (The Royal College of Surgeons 1815), Germany (Deutsche Gesellschaft fur Chirurgie 1872), France (College of Surgery 1880) and the US (American Surgical Association 1880) [33]. The last half of the nineteenth century produced an age of giants: James Sims (1813–1883) and William Halsted (1852–1922) in the US; Theodor Billroth (1829–1894) in Austria; and Theodor Kocher (1841–1917) in Switzerland. A need arose for the communication of the dramatic increase in the number and type of procedures, giving rise to new journals such as Archiv fur Klinische Chirurgie (1860) and Annals of Surgery (1885). These supplemented or displaced the textbooks and treatises that had been the foundation of medical writing.

Snow extended Morton's and Simpson's discoveries as much into science as could be done in that age, and his work was little improved upon for decades. Ether and chloroform, supplemented by nitrous oxide and oxygen, remained the mainstays of anesthetic practice for the next century. Anesthesia failed to advance or it advanced slowly, primarily in improved methods of delivery and ways to keep the airway open. Ether and chloroform are gone now, and nitrous oxide may disappear, too [34]. But anesthesia with ether and then chloroform constituted a colossal advance that enabled the development of surgery without further advances in anesthesia. It took surgeons a half, perhaps a whole century, to catch up to and then demand more of anesthesia [35].

References

1. Treves F. Address in surgery. Br Med J. 1900;2:284–9.
2. Nicoll JH. The surgery of infancy. Br Med J. 1909;18:753–4.
3. Waters RM. The down-town anesthesia clinic. Am J Surg. 1919;39(suppl):71–3.
4. Rankin JS. William Stewart Halsted: a lecture by Dr. Peter D. Olch. Ann Surg. 2006;243:418–25.
5. Cosimi AB. Surgeons and the Nobel Prize. Arch Surg. 2006;141:340–8.
6. Bacon DR, McGoldrick KE, Lema MJ. The american society of anesthesiologists: a century of challenges and progress. Park Ridge: Wood Library-Museum of Anesthesiology; 2005, pp. 1–225.
7. Lindh A. Sammanställning af narkosstatistiken från de nordiska länderna för året 1 mars 1894 till 1 mars 1895. Nordiskt Medicinskt Arkiv. 1895;23:1–27.
8. Clapesattle HB. The Doctors Mayo. Rochester, MN, Mayo foundation for medical education and research. 1969. pp. 13, 256–7.
9. Shephard DAE. Harvey Cushing and anaesthesia. Can Anaes Soc J. 1965;12:431–42.
10. Cushing H. On routine determinations of arterial tension in operating room and clinic. Boston Med Surg J. 1903;148:250–6.
11. Cushing HW. Anaesthesia Charts of. Letter to F. A. Washburn. Boston: Treadwell Library, Massachusetts General Hospital; 1895.
12. Waisel DB. The role of World War II and the European theater of operations in the development of anesthesiology as a physician specialty in the USA. Anesthesiology. 2001;94:907–14.
13. Bunker JP. The Anesthesiologist and Surgeon: Partners in the Operating Room. Boston: Little, Brown and Company; 1972.
14. Dinnick OP. The first anaesthetic society. Progress in Anaesthesiology. Excerpta Medica International Congress Series 200. 1968. pp. 181–6.
15. Betcher AM, Ciliberti BJ, Wood PM, Wright LH. The jubilee year of organized anesthesia. Anesthesiology. 1956;17:226–64.
16. Sykes K. Harold Griffith memorial lecture. The Griffith legacy. Can. J Anaesth [Journal canadien d'anesthesie]. 1993;40:365–74.
17. Keys TE. The history of surgical anesthesia. Park Ridge: Wood Library-Museum of Anesthesiology; 1996.
18. Koller C. Historical notes on the beginning of local anesthesia. JAMA. 1928;90:1742–3.
19. Barker AE. Clinical experiences with spinal analgesia in 100 cases. Br med J. 1907;1:665.
20. Kim J, Yao A, Atherley R, Carstens E, Jinks SL, Antognini JF. Neurons in the ventral spinal cord are more depressed by isoflurane, halothane, and propofol than are neurons in the dorsal spinal cord. Anesth Analg. 2007;105:1020–6.
21. Dederer C. The induction of anesthesia and ethyl chloride. Cal State J Med. 1914;12:421–2.
22. Oldenbourg LA. Preliminary report on ethyl chloride anethesia in minor operations. Cal State J Med. 1922;20:394–5.
23. Embley EH. The causation of death during the administration of chloroform. Br Med J. 1902;2:817–21.
24. Levy A. A cardiac effect of adrenalin in chloroformed subjects. Br Med J. 1912;2:627–30.
25. Levy AG. Sudden death under light chloroform anaesthesia. Proc Roy Soc Med. 1914;7:57–84.
26. Lichtenstein ME, Method H. Edmund Andrews, M.D., a biographical sketch with historical notes concerning nitrous oxide anesthesia. Q Bull Northwest Univ Med Sch. 1953;27:337–52.
27. Snow J. On the inhalation of the vapour of ether in surgical operations: containing a description of the various stages of etherization, and a statement of the result of nearly eighty operations in which ether has been employed in St. George's and University College Hospitals. London: John Churchill; 1847. pp. 1–88.
28. Bert P. Anesthesie par de protoxyde d'azote melange—d'oxygene et employ sour prission. Compt Rendu Acad Sci (Paris). 1879;89:132–5.
29. Hornbein TF, Eger EI II, Winter PM, Smith G, Wetstone D, Smith KH. The minimum alveolar concentration of nitrous oxide in man. Anesth Analg. 1982;61:553–6.
30. Smith WD. A history of nitrous oxide and oxygen anaesthesia. IX. The introduction of nitrous oxide and oxygen anaesthesia. Br J Anaesth. 1966;38:950–63.
31. Hewitt F. The administration of nitrous oxide and ether in combination or succession. Br Med J. 1887;2(1391):452–4.
32. Tuffier T, Hallion L. Opérations intrathoraciques avec respiration artficielle par insufflation. CR Soc Biol. 1896;22:951, 1047, 1085.
33. Rutkow IM. American surgery: an illustrated history. Philadelphia: Lippincott; 1998.
34. Myles PS, Leslie K, Chan MT, Forbes A, Paech MJ, Peyton P, Silbert BS, Pascoe E. Avoidance of nitrous oxide for patients undergoing major surgery: a randomized controlled trial. Anesthesiology. 2007;107:221–31.
35. Greene NM. Anesthesia and the development of surgery (1846–1896). Anesth Analg. 1979;58:5–12.

1910–1950: Anesthesia Before, During, and After Two World Wars

Edmond I Eger II, Rod N. Westhorpe and Lawrence J. Saidman

Summary

Who gave anesthesia from 1910 to 1950? Physicians in GB and the British Commonwealth, a mix of nurse anesthetists and physicians in the US, and surgeons directing part-time anesthetists in Europe and the rest of the world. Anesthetic societies arose, in GB (1893), the US (1905), France and Australia (1934), Canada and South Africa (1943), and Argentina (1945). And societies published Anesthesia & Analgesia (1922), the British Journal of Anaesthesia (1923), Anesthésie et Analgésie (1935), Revista Argentina de Anestesia y Analgesia (1939), Anesthesiology (1940), and Anaesthesia (1946). In the US and France, nurse anesthetists vied with physician anesthetists, conflicts not yet ended. Societies also governed formal training and certification, a tangible recognition of the quality care that a diplomate could provide.

The first nurse anesthesia school opened in Portland in 1909, with four others added before World War I. Supported by surgeon Crile, Hodgins opened her nurse school at the Cleveland Clinic in 1915, spawning 54 similar schools in the next two decades. In 1927 at the University of Wisconsin, Waters initiated the world's first academic department of anesthesia. In 1936, Beecher, not trained in anesthesia, became Anaesthestist-In-Chief at the Massachusetts General Hospital. In 1937, Macintosh became the Nuffield Professor of Anaesthetics in Oxford. In World War II, the US armed services ordered many drafted physicians to give anesthesia, greatly increasing the pool of US physician anesthetists.

With the rise in formal training, came the first subspecialties: Robson developed pediatrics in 1919; Lundy set up the first US blood bank in1935; Labat and Rovenstine established elements of pain medicine and regional anesthesia in the 1930s, further pursued in the 1940s by Moore and Bonica; and in the 1940s and 1950s, Hershenson, Apgar and Marx promoted obstetrical anesthesia.

Rudimentary anesthetic machines from the 1860s to 1910s evolved in the 1910s to 1950s to provide greater control and safety. Morris' 1948 Copper Kettle allowed precisely delivered volatile anesthetics. New drugs accompanied advances in equipment: cyclopropane (1929), divinyl ether and meperidine (1932), thiopental (1934), curare (1942), lidocaine (1948), and succinylcholine (1949).

In 1918–1920, Magill and Rowbotham insufflated ether through rubber tracheal tubes to anesthetize patients with facial injuries. In 1926, Starling invented a piston pump ventilator. In the 1930s, Waters and Guedel introduced oral airways that are still used to maintain an airway. With Nosworthy in Great Britain, Waters and Guedel applied intubation and controlled ventilation during anesthesia. In 1931, Waters and Gale used one lung ventilation to supply a quieter operative field for pulmonary surgery. Luft invented the infrared analyzer in 1937. In the 1940s, Cournand and Forssmann advanced special catheters into the pulmonary artery and got the Nobel prize. In the 1940s, Miller and Macintosh described their blades for laryngoscopy. In 1949, Carlens invented the double-lumen tube.

World Events Before, During, and After Two World Wars

In 1912, the Royal Mail Steamer (RMS) Titanic struck an iceberg in the North Atlantic and sank. World War I (1914–18) devastated Europe and nearby countries, including Russia. In 1915, TS Eliot published The Love Song of J. Alfred Prufrock. Between 1918 and 1920, the Spanish flu killed 20 to 100 million people. In the 1920s, women gained the right to vote in multiple countries (US, 1920). In 1922, James Joyce published Ulysses, and the Soviet Union

E. I Eger II (✉)
Department of Anesthesia and Perioperative Care,
University of California, San Francisco, CA, USA
e-mail: egere@anesthesia.ucsf.edu

R. N. Westhorpe
Melbourne, Australia
e-mail: westhorpe@netspace.net.au

L. J. Saidman
Department of Anesthesia, Stanford University, Stanford, CA, USA
e-mail: lsaidman@stanford.edu

E. I Eger II et al. (eds.), *The Wondrous Story of Anesthesia*, DOI 10.1007/978-1-4614-8441-7_6, © Edmond I Eger, MD 2014

was created. The Great Depression followed the 1929 stock market crash. Mohandas Gandhi led the 1930 non-violent Satyagraha movement in India. Movies and radio became dominant means of communication and entertainment in the 1930s. Franklin Roosevelt was elected in 1932, beginning the New Deal. In 1933, Hitler and the National Socialist German Worker's Party (the Nazi Party) seized power. Between 1935 and 1938, Germany annexed Austria, Czechoslovakia, and the Saar, leading to the Munich appeasement ("Peace in our time"). Between 1936 and 1939, Franco's army fought and won the Spanish Civil War, Pablo Picasso painted "Guernica", and Japan invaded China, starting the Second Sino-Japanese War. In 1938, Robert Watt invented radar. In 1939, Germany invaded Poland, initiating World War II (1940–1945), the most destructive armed conflict in human history. The US destroyed Hiroshima and Nagasaki in 1945 with atomic bombs, leading to the Japanese surrender. In 1947, the Cold War and the Marshal plan (which enabled the economic recovery of Europe) began. Arthur Miller's play, Death of a Salesman, premiered in 1949. In 1950, Joseph McCarthy began his witch-hunt for communist sympathizers.

Introduction

The US, GB, and Europe provided major anesthetic developments from 1910 to 1950. Several small events laid a base for the gigantic leaps forward that anesthesia took after 1950. These included growth in the numbers of full-time physician and nurse anesthetists, and the development of societies and associated journals (science), subspecialties, formal training, and certification. The presence of greater numbers of anesthesiologists gave rise to the earlier development of societies. Part of the base for the leap into modern anesthesia included advances in drugs and airway management, and an increasing sophistication in control over anesthetic delivery. Chapter 6 provides its stories as a group of parallel evolving, chronological streams that often touched each other.

Surgical and Surgical Adjuvant Advances and Demands on Anesthesia

Surgeons Develop New Surgical Procedures

The great surgeons of the previous half century had already devised procedures familiar to us today (see Table 5.1). In 1910, US surgeon Harvey Cushing developed hypophysectomy (removal of pituitary tumors), safely accessing the pi-

tuitary which lies at the base of the brain through an ingenious route, the nose.

Increasingly, surgeons ventured into hitherto forbidden sites, particularly the lung and heart, aided and abetted by increasingly skilled anesthetists, both physicians and nurses. In 1933, US surgeon, Evarts Graham excised a cancerous lung from a fellow physician [1]. The patient was cured, the first such patient. Graham, a smoker, however, died from lung cancer, but not before reporting that cigarette smoking had carcinogenic effects [2].

Children also benefited. In 1936, surgeon William Ladd began development of pediatric surgery at Boston Children's Hospital, happily dependent on Betty Lank, the chief nurse anesthetist. Lank gave ether or cyclopropane via mask, even to prone patients breathing spontaneously. She was an exceptional anesthetist, talented and fearless. Lank gave anesthesia for several surgical firsts. In 1938, unsupervised, resident surgeon Robert Gross closed a congenital defect, a blood vessel between the aorta and the pulmonary artery (a patent ductus arteriosus), a connection of major blood vessels. In that year, Ladd repaired an abnormal congenital connection between the esophagus and trachea (a tracheoesophageal fistula). Mortality usually exceeded 70 % for such procedures. In Sweden, Clarence Crafoord repaired a coarctation (narrowing) of the aorta in 1944. A year later, Robert Gross, now a "real" surgeon, resected an aortic aneurysm (a dilation of the aorta), again with the aid of Lank. At this time, Merel Harmel (a mere resident) and Austin Lamont gave open drop ether to Alfred Blalock's patient for the first Blalock-Taussig shunt treatment of the combination of congenital abnormalities constituting the tetralogy of Fallot. They described what they did in the first cardiac anesthesiology paper [3]. Truly a giant step into an unknown world described in Chapter 61. Lank later taught Harmel and Lamont to use cyclopropane and tracheal intubation.

In 1948, Smithy devised and accomplished the first commissurotomy for mitral stenosis, blindly opening the deformed valve with a finger inserted through a small hole in the left atrium. Ironically, he suffered from mitral stenosis and pleaded that his operation be applied to him. To no avail; Smithy died at age 34 from his disease.

The Price of Advances in Surgery?

In an "Anaesthetic Number" of the 1938 Medical Journal of Australia, Geoffrey Kaye published results from a survey of nearly 400,000 anesthetics at 14 hospitals, finding a mortality from anesthesia of around 1:1,000. Over subsequent years, the College of Anesthetists continued the tradition of reviewing and publishing mortality data for Australian anesthesia, becoming a major worldwide advocate of measures to decrease mortality and morbidity from anesthesia.

The Surgeon as Anesthetist

Local anesthesia was thought to be safer than general, particularly chloroform anesthesia. The use of local anesthesia minimized respiratory problems associated with general anesthesia, and allowed a control over anesthesia by the surgeon. Accordingly, surgeons, particularly European surgeons, physicians with a love of anatomy, quickly seized on the possibilities offered by Koller's 1884 discovery of the local anesthetic properties of cocaine, devising many regional anesthetic techniques still used (see Chapter 5). This approach to anesthesia continued in the 1910s. In 1911, Hirschel invented the axillary approach to the brachial plexus while Kulenkampff described the supraclavicular approach.

Tools that Furthered the Cause of Surgery

In the 1920s, physicist William Bovie developed the electrocautery [4], a device that stopped bleeding by burning blood vessels. Harvey Cushing first used the "Bovie" in 1927 [4]. Surgeons used it because it hastened the conduct of surgery. But surgeons and anesthetists alike used it with apprehension (justified, it turns out, by the occasional report of explosion killing all in the vicinity) or not at all in the presence of flammable and explosive anesthetics such as ether, ethylene and cyclopropane.

Further Attacks on the Problem of Infection

For millennia, two colossal problems had limited the advance of surgery: pain and infection. General anesthesia with ether or chloroform from the 1840s, and regional anesthesia from the 1880s, had overcome the first, and antisepsis and asepsis from the 1860s had done much to counter the second. However antisepsis and asepsis sometimes failed both surgeon and patient. Something was needed to manage infection that eluded antisepsis and asepsis.

In 1928, Alexander Fleming discovered the antibiotic penicillin. He couldn't make sufficient pure quantities, and so for a time penicillin remained a laboratory curiosity. In 1938, Howard Florey and Ernst Chain began the work that eventually supplied the world with penicillin, and with Fleming, in 1945 they won the Nobel prize in Medicine. Add the 1932 discovery by Gerhard Domagk, a German biochemist, that the sulfanilamide Prontosil had antibiotic properties. The age of antibiotics had arrived, making surgery—and thus anesthesia—yet safer.

Socioeconomic Factors from 1910 to 1950 Affect Progress in Anesthesia

The Flexner Report

Abraham Flexner's report, *Medical Education in the United States and Canada*, described the shortcomings of North American medical education compared to European education. Over the next 10 years, the Flexner report contributed to closure of approximately one-third of US medical schools. Sixteen of the 17 schools devoted to the education of women closed for lack of support for the scientific underpinnings that the Flexner report revealed and demanded.

World War I

The Great War (World War I) that ravaged Europe began in 1914. In that year, surgeon George Crile and his personal and chief nurse anesthetist, Agatha Hodgins, provided service in Europe in an American "ambulance" (hospital), delivering and perfecting anesthesia with nitrous-oxide/oxygen after belladonna plus morphine premedication (Crile termed the result anoci-association, a state in which patients did not perceive pain. It foreshadowed balanced anesthesia.) In Europe, nurses provided anesthesia in American Hospitals before and during World War I, using the Crile-Hodgins approach. This was thought to be particularly useful in soldiers who had lost considerable blood. Three years earlier, Crile had reported before the American Surgical Association on 10,787 operations anesthetized under Hodgins' supervision with no anesthetic death [5].

World War I involved many nations, and killed 5 to 10 million participants. Few physicians in the American Expeditionary Force (active from 1917 through 1919) had trained in anesthesia (no formal training programs for physicians existed), and anesthetic equipment was primitive, often delivered with open drop ether or chloroform. How did the anesthetist safely provide anesthesia for vast numbers of American surgical casualties when orderlies and secretaries and stretcher-bearers provided part-time anesthetic care?

Enter Arthur Guedel, the motorcycle anesthetist. Guedel rode his motorcycle from hospital to hospital to train diverse "anesthetists" and direct the administration of ether anesthetics. His system was so effective that it became a standard, one that EIE used 40 years later. It was so profoundly ingrained that it was applied to new anesthetics that appeared five decades later, although it really only applied to ether [6].

Guedel understood the need to train and supervise a cadre of orderlies, secretaries and stretcher-bearers. His genius recognized the need for simplification, for the construction of a scheme whereby anyone, even those with little training, might assess the degree of anesthetization and use the degree to guide anesthetic delivery (see Fig. 39.2, [7]). Guedel's scheme had the elements described by John Snow 70 years earlier [8], but Guedel made it more accessible to someone with limited training by supplying a chart to guide the anesthetist. Breathing and the eyes told the anesthetist everything needed to gauge how much anesthetic to give or withhold. There were 4 "stages" of anesthesia, akin to Snow's 5 degrees:

In the first stage, the patient might respond to command and although not anesthetized might have considerable analgesia. Breathing would be regular. The patient controlled movement of the eyes. The pupils were normal in size and constricted in response to light.

Hallmarks of stage 2, or "excitation" included irregular breathing and roving of the eyes. The pupils might vary in size but would constrict if exposed to light. Movement, sometimes violent movement requiring restraint of the patient might occur in this stage during induction of anesthesia. Such movement was less likely during recovery from anesthesia.

Stage 3, the stage of surgical anesthesia, had 4 "planes". In plane 1, breathing was deep and regular. Movement of the eyes might occur, particularly at the upper end of this plane. Pupils were normal in size and constricted to light. Plane 2 scarcely altered breathing, but eye movement ceased and the pupils dilated slightly—but still constricted in response to light. In plane 3, breathing decreased and became "jerky". The pupils now dilated and incompletely responded to light. In plane 4, breathing progressively decreased, and the pupils dilated widely and did not respond to light.

In stage 4, breathing ceased. The heart might stop beating in stage 4 or even in plane 4 of stage 3. As with Snow's fifth degree, the anesthetist was encouraged to avoid stage 4 or even plane 4 of stage 3.

Perhaps the quality of anesthetic care provided by the British exceeded that provided by the American Expeditionary Force because a physician (rather than the better trained nurse) was designated as the anesthetist—although he (there were no females-see below) might not have engaged in anesthesia since medical school [9]. But the tasks overwhelmed even the full-time physician anesthetists. The wounded poured into casualty clearing stations (CCS) at a sometimes ferocious rate: "At the Battle of the Somme, for example, some 14,000 casualties moved through the CCSs on the first day, and CCS number 29 at Gezaincourt alone received 11,186 wounded soldiers in the first 3 days of conflict." [9]

The British also tried various approaches to anesthesia, discovering that spinal anesthesia resulted in excessive hypotension in patients already suffering from shock. They discovered that nitrous oxide combined with ether improved survival and applied the combination increasingly as the war progressed. This, of course, necessitated the production of anesthetic machines. Geoffrey Marshall and Henry Boyle, both working in France, independently devised a portable anesthesia apparatus, using bubble flowmeters as developed by James Gwathmey of New York. Coxeter and Son produced commercial versions of both. Thus, the use of anesthetic machines began in earnest (e.g., in GB, Boyle introduced his anesthetic machine with the Boyle's bottle for vaporization of anesthetic in 1917). Delivery of anesthetic from machines increasingly displaced the gauze mask-open drop ether approach to anesthetic delivery. The Americans joined in this move.

Both British and American anesthetists/surgeons in World War I studied the management of shock [9]. Giving salt-water solutions (normal saline) provided short-lived benefit. German surgeon Hercher used hypertonic solutions for fluid resuscitation in wounded soldiers. Gum-acacia solutions had a longer effect than saline. The best result came from applying the new knowledge of blood types and preservation of blood, with the consequence that the war accelerated the development of transfusion medicine.

The beleaguered Germans in World War I probably had the worst time of all. "In the German Army, it was proposed by Professor Schleich that (ether) be carried mixed with some ethyl chloride, so as to be self-administered after injury in order to allow the regimental medical officer to concentrate solely on treatment." [9]

World War II Advances Anesthesia in the US but Detracts Elsewhere

World War II severed European contact with advances in anesthesia in the US and GB. This and the demands of the war hindered progress in Europe and much of the world. The approach of the War increased the pressure in GB to educate anesthetists. The Association of Anaesthetists of Great Britain and Ireland (AAGBI) trained full-time anesthetists.

World War II dramatically accelerated the growth of physician anesthesia, nurse anesthesia, and women in medicine in the US. The number of schools of nurse anesthesia approved by the American Association of Nurse Anesthetists (AANA) increased. On the debit side, the war delayed implementation of the first nurse anesthesia qualifying examination until 1945. The urgent need to enlarge the pool of anesthetists, particularly anesthesiologists (physician anesthetists) to manage great numbers of casualties resulted in "crash" training programs for drafted physicians, who were ordered to become anesthesiologists. By the war's end, many such drafted anesthesiologists discovered that they liked the associated technical demands and opportunities.

Women in Medicine

In 1914, 8 women were members of the American Association of Anesthetists (AAA), 9 % of membership. By 1916, 15 women (9 %) were members. In 1915, 3.6 % of physicians were women. Among women, only gynecology exceeded anesthesia in popularity. World War I opened a 19-month window of increased opportunities for American women to enter medical schools and internships. It also offered opportunities that comedian-commentator Jon Stewart would have seized. In 1917, the US Army's Judge Advocate General ruled that since women cannot vote, they were not "citizens," and could not be commissioned medical officers.

By 1920, 5.0 % of US physicians were women, an increase consequent on the vacancies in medical schools left by men who were fighting in World War I. By 1930, this had decreased to 4.4 %. When World War II began, the US had 7,708 women physicians, less than in 1910. In 1920, three women headed anesthesia "departments" in the US: Herb at Rush, Botsford at UCSF, and her trainee Palmer at Stanford. Passage of the nineteenth amendment in 1920 gave US women the right to vote. In 1922, at the University of Iowa, Mary Ross became the first woman anesthesia resident. In that year, Isabella Herb became president of the first nationwide US anesthesia society, the American Association of Anesthetists (AAA). Also in 1922, Mary Botsford, who practiced anesthesia at the Children's Hospital of San Francisco, led the effort to found the Anesthesia Section of the California Medical Association, and was its first president. In 1930, Botsford became president of the Associated Anesthetists of the United States and Canada, an organization that evolved from the AAA.

In 1938, working in Peking Union Medical College in Beijing, Ma Yueqing became the first Chinese anesthesiologist. In that year, the fourth female trained by Ralph Waters, Virginia Apgar, became Director of the Division of Anesthesia and Attending Anesthetist at Columbia. There is a "delicious irony" in that Waters had earlier commented to Guedel: "…M.D. ladies…are useless in the profession. I am through with them. Ladies are nice socially but not (as) professionals" (from Selma Calmes in Chapter 16).

During World War II, 10 million men were inducted into the armed services. The resulting shortage of civilian male candidates opened medical school, internship and residency opportunities for women. And anesthesia was attractive to these new female physicians. In 1940, 87 (12 %) of ASA members were women. In 1949, 251 (9.9 %) were women, becoming 11 % in 1963, nearly twice the percent of females in the physician population (6 %). Ironically, the armed services excluded female anesthesiologists. In 1942, Surgeon General James Magee proclaimed that "Women should not belong" and only six served as anesthesiologists in World War II. Nine had served in World War I.

Evolution of US Anesthetic Organizations

American Society of Anesthesiologists (ASA)

The London Society of Anaesthetists, the first anesthetic society, was founded in 1893. A dozen years later, 9 professional brothers founded the second society, the Long Island Society of Anesthetists (LISA). Membership grew to 23 in 1911, and the enlarged society changed its name to the grander New York Society of Anesthetists (NYSA), reflecting the broader geographical distribution of its membership [10]. At the last meeting of the old society, Yandell Henderson of Yale spoke of the importance of physiological chemistry to the anesthetist, and Max Verworn from the University of Bonn lectured on Narcosis, suggesting that anesthesia resulted from an inadequate supply or use of oxygen. The establishment of LISA and the NYSA reflected the growing numbers of anesthetists and the interest in their craft. A new constitution reaffirmed the notion that the purpose of the society was "the advancement of the science and art of anesthesia." The yearly dues tripled, from $ 1 to $ 3. The NYSA sought but was denied recognition by the American Medical Association (AMA). The NYSA Fellowship Committee certified candidates in oral, written and practical examinations.

In the ensuing two decades, other anesthetic societies arose in the US: the American Association of Anesthetists (1912), the Interstate Association of Anesthetists (1915), the American Society of Regional Anesthesia (1923), and the International Anesthesia Research Society (IARS, 1925). These and local and regional societies focused on the education and competitive practices of this developing medical specialty. They sought to create a certifying system for practitioners. In the early 1930s, Ralph Waters, Paul Wood, and John Lundy unsuccessfully lobbied for creation of a Section of Anesthesiology within the American Medical Association. In support of the evolution of the NYSA to a national organization, in 1936 the NYSA changed its name to the American Society of Anesthetists. In 1945, the American Society of Anesthetists changed its name to the American Society of Anesthesiologists (ASA). This and the appearance of other new societies reflected the increasing numbers of physicians engaged in anesthesia.

These activities reflected the growing numbers of physician anesthetists in the US, but it should be noted that the number of nurse anesthetists was increasing concurrently. The increases in both accelerated in the 1940s.

We do not know the motivations that led physicians to enter anesthesia, but the need to strengthen their status seems clear, and this likely added to the desire to form societies. A lowly status may have been deserved: In 1947, John Lundy wrote that "there was a tendency for only those physicians who were incompetent in general practice or in other branches to limit themselves to the practice of anesthesia." [11] Why the incompetent? Did the study of anesthesia lack depth, lack challenge? Perhaps. Consider the letter that the Dean of Harvard Medical School wrote to the President of Harvard in 1906: "The practice of anesthesia is so narrow a subject that a good man would not want to tie himself down to that and would hardly be willing to do so." [12] Keith Sykes and John Bunker described many anesthetists of the time as perhaps "…simply attempting to escape from the responsibilities of an unsuccessful or bothersome practice." [13] What a dismal state! And finally Beecher (yes that one) stated that "anesthesia technique can be mastered by ordinary men who are ordinarily deft, with only a modest requirement of intelligence and of knowledge and judgment." [14]

Membership in societies supplied one route to status. Societies also provided forums for developing a body of knowledge that might certify the value of anesthesia and the anesthetist. Both the IARS and the ASA held yearly national meetings to advance the causes of education and research in anesthesia, meetings that gradually grew in size and quality. The IARS had offered such meetings for decades; the first Annual Session of the ASA was held in 1945.

As indicated above, Societies first formed in GB (1893) and the US (1905). No national societies were added for 3 decades thereafter. Societies developed in Australia and France in the 1930s. World War II transiently slowed additions, and then began a flood of societies that subsequently continued for 6 decades.

Waters had established the first anesthesia residency training program with his arrival at the University of Wisconsin in 1927. By 1943, 45 US anesthesia residency training programs were approved, increasing to 213 by 1950—with only 107 residents. This grew to 5,556 residents in 132 programs in 2010.

With the ending of World War II in 1945, the ASA created a "Committee on Postgraduate Education" to define how to educate returning physicians who had served as anesthetists during the war, and new physicians seeking training in anesthesia. Approximately a half decade later, the Committee issued "Recommendations for a Curriculum in Anesthesiology", prescribing a minimum of 2 years of training for candidates with no prior instruction, but crediting the experience of those who had received "on the job" training.

In 1949, Paul Wood's collection of historical materials became the Wood Library-Museum (WLM). The WLM found a permanent home at the Park Ridge ASA offices in 1963.

The International Anesthesia Research Society (IARS)

One charismatic anesthesiologist, Francis McMechan, shaped much of the history of anesthesia, particularly the story of the IARS, from 1910 to 1939. In 1911, rapidly progressing rheumatoid arthritis prevented McMechan from continuing his medical/anesthetic practice. McMechan joined the American Association of Anesthetists, formally organized in 1912, and quickly became its leader and the "union organizer" for anesthesia, encouraging the development of several regional societies. The Interstate Association of Anesthetists (Ohio and Kentucky) formed in 1915, in 1925 morphing into the Mid-Western Association of Anesthetists. McMechan encouraged development of the Canadian Society of Anesthetists in 1921, the Pacific Coast Society of Anesthetists in 1922; the Southern Association of Anesthetists in 1922; and the Eastern Society of Anesthetists in 1923. McMechan organized a parallel National Anesthesia Research Society (NARS) in 1919 that became the International Anesthesia Research Society (IARS) in 1925. The IARS became the umbrella society for McMechan's other organizations in 1941.

In 1925, The IARS limited membership to physicians, dentists and researchers with advanced degrees, and offered certification to anesthesiologists. Through written communications and travel promoting anesthesiology, McMechan attracted authors, society members and subscribers to Current Researches, a vehicle for scientific communication and IARS announcements. Commercial advertising was introduced. McMechan's wife, Laurette McMechan, acted as Assistant Editor, an indispensible assistance to the wheelchair-bound McMechan.

In the early 1930s, rheumatoid arthritis increasingly crippled McMechan, and Laurette McMechan assumed a growing role in the management of the IARS and Current Researches in Anesthesia and Analgesia. McMechan intentionally had placed himself in a seated position so that as his joints fused he retained visual contact with others during his travels [15]. McMechan died on 29 June 1939.

The American Association of Nurse Anesthetists (AANA) and Training of Nurse Anesthetists

Before 1910, informal training programs for nurse anesthesia had developed in the Midwest US, particularly at the Mayo Clinic and Cleveland's Lakeside Hospital, strongly supported by their respective surgical leaders, the Mayo brothers and George Crile. The threat of The Great War (World War I) prompted St. Vincent's Hospital, Portland, OR (1909); St. John's Hospital, Springfield, IL (1912); The New York Post-Graduate Hospital, New York City, NY (1912); and Long Island College Hospital, Brooklyn, NY (1914) to train nurses in anesthesia in 6 month on-the-job programs. A diploma was issued upon completion, but there was no mention of an assessment or a graduation examination.

In 1915, with Crile's support, Hodgins opened her influential school for nurse anesthetists at Lakeside

Hospital (later part of the Cleveland Clinic). By 1940, Hodgins' school had spawned 54 schools of nurse anesthesia. Training of nurse anesthetists thus began decades before the major development of physician anesthesia training in the US.

In 1916, McMechan unsuccessfully made legislative efforts to prohibit nurse anesthesia, arguing that it allowed nurses to practice medicine. Subsequent statutes in numerous states legalized nurse anesthesia practice, but specified physician supervision of nurse anesthetists. The recent Bush administration modified the supervisory limitation, allowing states to "opt out" of the requirement for physician supervision. By 2012, 17 of 31 eligible states had opted out.

Efforts to suppress nurse anesthesia turned to the courts. In 1917, surgeon Louis Frank with nurse anesthetist Margaret Hatfield sued the Kentucky State Board of Health to test the contention that Hatfield was practicing medicine. Frank and Hatfield won.

In 1923, Agatha Hodgins fostered the formation of the Lakeside Alumni of nurse anesthetists. The Lakeside Alumni would grow, and in 1931 became the National Association of Nurse Anesthetists (NANA) through the efforts of pioneers Hodgins, Helen Lamb, and Gertrude Fife. The NANA was the first specialty nursing organization in the US. Formal education at this time required 4 months training. State nurse anesthetist societies arose concurrently in the US (e.g., Ohio first in 1931). In 1933, the National Association of Nurse Anesthetists published a report (now the 'AANA Journal') of their first annual meeting. And NANA president Fife proposed establishing a national board examination for nurse anesthetists.

Before World War II, the American Board of Surgery pressured the NANA to meet with the ABS and the American Board of Anesthesiology, to consider having the ABA approve a training curriculum and certification for nurse anesthetists. Distrust however, caused the discussions to founder, losing an opportunity to strengthen the physician-nurse relationship.

In 1939, the NANA concluded that training required a minimum of 6 months, and that a NANA curriculum needed development, but insistence on specific curriculum content and durations were set aside for the duration of the war. In that year, the NANA changed its name to the American Association of Nurse Anesthetists (AANA).

In 1941, AANA President Shupp suggested that passage of a qualifying examination should define eligibility for AANA membership, and by the mid 1940s, new members were qualified by examination, except for those grandfathered in. In 1945, the first AANA qualifying examination was administered, leading in 1956 to the appellation Certified Registered Nurse Anesthetist (CRNA).

Certification of Physician-Anesthetist Competency: Evolution of the American Board of Anesthesiology (ABA)

In 1931, the NYSA established a Committee on Fellowships, initiating development of a certification process. The Committee incorporated in New York as the "American Board of Anesthesiology" (ABA). The ABA initially only certified local practitioners, precluding recognition by the nationally-based American Medical Association (AMA). In 1935, the ABA accepted anesthetists from 17 states for examination.

Anesthesiology in the US sought recognition by the medical establishment, including recognition of its capacity to certify competency. In 1936, the New York Society became the American Society of Anesthetists. Despite this change, the American Medical Association, the official grantor of certification, would not recognize it as a "regional" society. The next maneuver bypassed the AMA. In 1938, the AMA's Advisory Board for Medical Specialties (ABMS) approved the affiliation of an American Board of Anesthesiology (ABA) with the American Board of Surgery (ABS), a move proposed by Erwin Schmidt, Chief surgeon at the University of Wisconsin, and a friend to Ralph Waters. That is, the ABA became an affiliate board of the already approved ABS. The ABA proposed to examine and certify the fitness of those who met certain standards, and to establish standards for training in anesthesia. Ralph Tovell, Henry Ruth, Emery Rovenstine, John Lundy, Paul Wood, Ralph Waters and others guided this birth of the ABA. In 1939, the AMA Council on Scientific Assembly recommended establishment of a Section on Anesthesia, a recommendation approved by the AMA House of Delegates in 1940. Anesthesia had arrived in the US!

More broadly to the issue of medical education in the US, in 1937 the ABMS created the Commission on Graduate Medical Education, with a mandate to "formulate the educational problems and principles involved in the continuation of medical training for a period of years after graduation and the adequate training of specialists, and to make recommendations for methods whereby those in practice, general and limited, may keep abreast of new developments in diagnosis, treatment and prevention."

While McMechan was alive, he had promoted certification of specialists in anesthesia by the IARS. This and the condemnation of non-physician anesthetists had separated his and ASA organizations, and precluded collaboration in forming the ABA. Once the ABA was formed, IARS certification gradually became irrelevant. The IARS Board rejected a proposed amalgamation with the ASA, continuing two societies, two annual meetings and, ultimately, two journals.

In 1939, the American Board of Anesthesiology became an independent board and certified 9 diplomats by examination. This number would increase to 105 by 1940 and 706 by 1950.

The ABMS now required at least three years of postgraduate training, a few years in practice, and the successful completion of written, oral, and practical examinations to achieve diplomate status. Thus, while medical schools and teaching hospitals controlled US undergraduate educational experience, the professions themselves governed graduate medical education.

In 1944, the ABA made two years of approved anesthesia training mandatory for credentialing—except that credit was given for military anesthesia practice. Saklad questioned the reliability of ABA essay examinations. The horde of military anesthesiologists returning to civilian practice after World War II made the issue moot; grading essay examinations became impractical.

In 1945, Meyer Saklad also questioned the validity of ABA oral examinations because the examiners chose the questions asked. This issue recurred over the years, causing a transition to a Guided Question (all candidates are questioned about the same clinical scenario) format in the 1960s. One of the editors of this book (LJS) recalls fondly his oral exam taken before the development of the Guided Question. Fully one half of his exam dealt with inhaled anesthetic pharmacokinetics, this occurring after he had spent a year as research fellow with Ted Eger. In the 2000s, computers applied algorithms that compensated for the bias imposed by harsher versus more lenient examiner grading and by more difficult questions.

Veterinary Anesthesia

Initially, some veterinarians hesitated applying anesthesia, viewing the struggles during induction of anesthesia as reflecting pain. In addition, large struggling animals might endanger both animal and veterinarian. Once past the induction, however, animals became quiescent, and veterinarians increasingly used anesthesia, doing so initially as much to immobilize as to relieve pain. Although they initially questioned whether anesthesia prevented or caused pain, veterinarians came to accept that anesthesia prevented the perception of pain. The 1876 Cruelty to Animals Act restricted the use of animals in experiments to licensed persons who had obtained Home Office permission for particular procedures.

In 1915, Louis Merillat noted the increased use of anesthesia to relieve pain rather than produce restraint. In the same year, Frederick Hobday published the first English textbook devoted exclusively to veterinary anesthesia, *Anaesthesia and Narcosis of Animals and Birds*. In 1919, the British Parliament enacted an Anaesthetics Bill for Animals, specifying that anesthesia must "…prevent the animal feeling pain". A much later (1964) Anaesthetics Bill allowed flexibility in anesthetic choice as long as it produced "adequate anaesthesia".

In 1924, Bemis and colleagues published a summary of contemporary regional nerve blocks in horses [16]. Smithcors noted that, "It remained for veterinarians Retzgen of Berlin [and also Pape and Pitzch] in 1925, and Franz Benesch of Austria in 1926, to demonstrate in horses and cattle respectively, that epidural anesthesia with the needle introduced distal to the spinal cord proper, was a safe technique." [17] Other reports of regional anesthesia appeared later, surprisingly, for surgery in large animals.

In 1937, one of the giants of veterinary medicine, Wright, first used thiopental intravenously in animals. In 1941, Wright's first edition of Veterinary Anaesthesia laid the foundations of *modern* veterinary anesthesia. It was a well-received book. In 1961, Wright and LW Hall (of Cambridge University) co-authored the 5th edition.

Anesthesia Subspecialties

Obstetric Anesthesia

Twilight sleep, the state resulting from the intramuscular injection of scopolamine and morphine, had been introduced in Europe in the first decade of the twentieth century, for use in labor and delivery. In 1914, US women organized the National Twilight Sleep Association in the US, successfully bringing this popular European technique to North America. However, the amounts of morphine were often insufficient to minimize pain. Laboring women might thrash and scream yet reported a pain free birth experience because the scopolamine suppressed memory. In 1915, a prominent advocate of the approach died during childbirth, having received twilight sleep. This brought the National Twilight Sleep Association to an end. Nonetheless, twilight sleep remained in use in a few US hospitals until the 1960s.

In the 1920s, one in two hundred (0.5 %) British women died during childbirth. This unacceptable mortality led a group of British women in 1928 to form the National Birthday Trust Fund, that aimed to reduce the mortality and make modern pain relief during childbirth available for all women.

In 1940, Bert Hershenson was the only full-time obstetrical anesthesiologist in the US. He established the first US Division of Obstetric Anesthesia at the Boston Lying-In Hospital in 1942, and wrote the first textbook devoted solely to obstetric anesthesia. Weiss, a successor to Hershenson in Boston, advocated the use of epidural analgesia. Also in 1940, continuous spinal anesthesia developed in the US with William Lemmon's malleable needle that could be left in place after insertion. And Virginia Apgar became treasurer of the ASA, the last woman to serve as an ASA Officer for the next 27 years.

In 1942, Robert Hingson and Waldo Edwards adapted Lemmon's malleable needle for injections into the caudal canal and for extended analgesia for labor and delivery. Hingson later taught the technique to Gertie Marx, the grand dame of obstetrical anesthesia.

Pediatric Anesthesia

Returning from service in World War I, Charles Robson, became Anaesthetist-in-Chief at Toronto's Hospital for Sick Children in 1919, continuing in that role for 3 decades. Recognized as the father of pediatric anesthesia, he defined the major problems extant in pediatric anesthesia—and their solutions.

In 1945, Bob Smith became head of pediatric anesthesia at Boston Children's Hospital, noting that chief nurse anesthetist Elizabeth Lank "made me a pediatric anesthesiologist." Smith's program changed the world of pediatric anesthesia.

Regional Anesthesia and Pain Management

In 1921, Spanish surgeon Fidel Pagés-Miravé described the lumbar epidural injection of local anesthetic. A decade later, Italian Achille Dogliotti popularized the technique. It may have been more than that. A colleague of Cedric Prys-Roberts claimed that he saw Dogliotti operating on the thyroid gland under cervical epidural anesthesia (personal communication, 15 Nov 2012).

In 1924, William Mayo invited John Lundy to develop the anesthesia department at the Mayo Clinic. The changes that he introduced included the increased application of regional anesthesia. In 1935, Emery Rovenstine succeeded Gaston Labat at Bellevue and applied regional techniques to treat pain, initiating a movement that gained momentum in the second half of the century.

Thus, in the 1920s and 1930s, regional anesthesia had begun with Lundy, Labat and Rovenstine in the Eastern and Midwest portions of the US. Earlier it had been advanced by European surgeons. Perhaps the biggest boost came in the US Northwest after World War II. In 1947, John Bonica was appointed chief of the Department of Anesthesiology at Tacoma General Hospital where he established a multidisciplinary team to manage chronic pain. He subsequently pioneered regional anesthesia techniques for labor pain relief, later writing arguably the most comprehensive textbook on regional anesthesia [18]. He devoted the last part of his career to the relief of chronic pain, a deeply personal endeavor. More about that later. At approximately the same time, senior surgeons at the Virginia Mason Clinic in Seattle hired Daniel Moore to supply anesthesia for increasingly complex surgical procedures. Moore established a residency in anesthesia in 1948, and by 1953, 50 % of patients undergoing surgery at the Clinic received regional anesthesia.

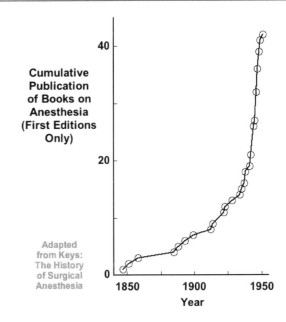

Fig. 6.1 The cumulative increase in the number of books (first editions) on anesthesia accelerated after World War II. (Data from Keys' History of Surgical Anesthesia.)

Books and Journals

Books

Books can be the repositories of accrued knowledge, and as such reflect the growth in knowledge. They may also indirectly reflect the numbers of parties interested in a field of knowledge. Keys' History of Surgical Anesthesia indicates first editions of published books focused on anesthesia. A cumulative graph of their numbers (Fig. 6.1) suggests a rough parallel to the growth in the number of anesthetists.

The following gives a chronology of some of the books published between 1910 and 1950: In 1915, Frederick Hobday published the first English textbook devoted exclusively to veterinary anesthesia, *Anaesthesia and Narcosis of Animals and Birds*. A year later, Norwegian Nils Groendahl published the first Nordic anesthesia textbook—for nurses—and by 1920, nurse anesthetists gave most anesthetics in Nordic countries. In 1920, Charles Mayo recruited Frenchman Gaston Labat, to the Mayo's clinic where Labat wrote his famous textbook on regional anesthesia. At the clinic and later at Bellevue Hospital, Labat introduced the regular use of regional anesthesia. In 1923, The first pediatric anesthesia textbook "Anesthesia in Children" was published in GB. Bert Hershenson at the Boston Lying-In Hospital published the first textbook devoted solely to obstetric anesthesia in 1942. "Anaesthetic Methods" was published in 1946. Written by Geoffrey Kaye, Robert Orton, and Douglas Renton, it was the second and most important anesthesia textbook in Australia and New Zealand.

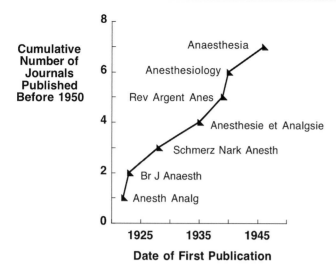

Fig. 6.2 The cumulative number of anesthetic journals launched between 1910 and 1950 rectilinearly increase. (Data from Chapter 34)

Journals

Individuals and anesthetic societies contributed to advancement of knowledge by the publication of such knowledge in journals as well as books. Seven or more journals were launched in the period between 1910 and 1950 (Fig. 6.2).

In the 1910s, Joseph McDonald, managing editor of the 'American Journal of Surgery', had mentored Francis McMechan who edited a 'Quarterly Supplement' 'Anesthesia and Analgesia'. When McDonald died in 1922, McMechan created the National Anaesthesia Research Society (later the International Anesthesia Research Society) which in August 1922 first published '*Current Researches in Anesthesia and Analgesia*', the predecessor of Anesthesia & Analgesia, the worlds' first major anesthetic journal. In 1925, the International Anesthesia Research Society (IARS) succeeded the National Anesthesia Research Society, becoming the owner and publisher of Current Researches in Anesthesia and Analgesia.

Hyman Cohen, a soldier in the US Army, married a Manchester girl in 1904, entered medical school at St Bartholomew's Hospital in London, graduated in 1916 and became a full-time anesthetist. In 1923 he initiated the *British Journal of Anaesthesia* "devoted entirely to the interests of anaesthesia and its practitioners", continuing as editor from 1923 to 1928.

The journals, *Der Schmerz*, and *Narkose und Anaesthesie*, formed in 1928, merging to *Schmerz, Narkose und Anaesthesie* in 1929, and lasting until 1943. These added to pressures in Germany to specialize in anesthesia, but influential surgeons rejected the idea, and World War II stopped discussion and publication. In 1935, The French Society of Anaesthesia and Analgesia launched '*Anesthésie et Analgésie*'. In 1939, '*Revista Argentina de Anestesia y Analgesia*', perhaps the first multinational anesthesia journal, began publication in Buenos Aires.

Out of respect for McMechan, the ASA had refrained from publishing a journal that would compete with Anesthesia & Analgesia, but with his death in 1939, publication of *Anesthesiology* soon followed. The first edition appeared in June 1940 with Henry Ruth as editor.

The Jan—Feb 1940 issue of *Current Researches in Anesthesia and Analgesia* announced Howard Dittrick's appointment as Directing Editor. He was a physician (a gynecologist) with a background in medical editing, but was not an anesthesiologist. With Dittrick's appointment, the IARS Board of Governors became the Editorial Board and confirmed Laurette's continuing roles as Assistant Executive-Secretary-Editor. Anesthesiology provided stiff competition to Current Researches in Anesthesia and Analgesia, dominating it as a repository for important clinical and basic research for the next 50 years. World War II added to Current Researches in Anesthesia and Analgesia's difficulties. The Journal continued bimonthly publication throughout the 1940s, but the numbers of society members and subscribers declined. Having a non-anesthesiologist serve as Editor-in-Chief may have contributed to the diminished position of the Journal.

Anaesthesia, the Journal of the Association of Anaesthetists of Great Britain and Ireland was founded in 1946.

The Rise of Academic Departments

At the Turn of the Century

In the latter part of the 1890s, a few US anesthesiologists assumed teaching and leadership roles. Two women established the beginnings of what might be thought of as departments in the early 1900s. Isabella Herb practiced anesthesia at Augustana Hospital in Chicago, in 1922 becoming president of the first nationwide anesthesia society, the American Association of Anesthetists (AAA). In 1898, Mary Botsford practiced anesthesia at the Children's Hospital of San Francisco. In 1922, she led the effort to found the Anesthesia Section of the California Medical Association, and was its first president. In 1930, Botsford became president of the Associated Anesthetists of the United States and Canada, an organization that evolved from the AAA.

Three World Leaders in Anesthesia

Although many giants contributed to the development of the specialty in the 1930s, three stand out, leaders who dramatically expanded the depth of training, clinical care, and research in anesthesia. These were Ralph Waters, Henry Beecher, and Robert Macintosh.

A chance visit by Ralph Waters to the University of Wisconsin, and the desire of the then chair of surgery, Erwin Schmidt, to improve the quality of anesthetic delivery at Wisconsin, led to Waters' appointment as an Assistant Professor of Anesthesia in January 1927. Surgery was beginning to repay its debt to anesthesia! Waters thus chaired the first department of anesthesia (as opposed to a division of a department of surgery) in the US [13]. ([1]However, an alternative "first" may exist.) [19]

Waters developed an academic department dedicated to optimum patient care, education of medical students and interns, post-graduate education, and research into the scientific foundations of anesthesia. Roughly following the example set by departments of surgery, he created a 3-year post-graduate residency program. He expected graduating residents to serve as leaders, thereby imposing his vision for academic anesthesia across the country. His graduates, and, in turn, graduates of their programs established most US academic programs. For example, Saidman, an editor of this book, held the chair at the University of California, San Diego. He traced his academic heritage back through Stuart Cullen (UCSF), through Emory Rovenstine (Bellevue), and then to Waters (U Wisconsin). The University of Wisconsin residency program also served as a model for early programs in GB and Canada.

In contrast to Waters' emphasis on clinical care, the second great department in the US emphasized research. In 1936, Harvard appointed a partially trained surgeon, Henry Beecher, as an instructor in anesthesia and, incidentally, the Anesthetist-in-Chief in the Division of Surgery. That is, Harvard designated someone with no training in anesthesia to oversee anesthetic delivery.

> "Beecher responded to the challenge by teaching himself how to give anesthetics, by writing a textbook on The Physiology of Anaesthesia, and by introducing the basic principles of laboratory research to the clinical practice of anesthesia. His efforts were rewarded when he was appointed Henry Isaiah Dorr Professor of Research and Teaching in Anaesthetics and Anaesthesia, a Chair that had been funded originally in 1917. In 1938, he thus became the first incumbent of the first Chair to be endowed in anesthesia." [13]

"Dr. Beecher's 'hands on' clinical performance was not the cause of many accolades."[2] Conversely, Beecher was a superb investigator whose work reflected well on anesthesia. He advanced our understanding of the power of the placebo [20]. He observed that the brain controlled the perception of pain [21]. He gave us one of the first outcome studies (more about that later), a study that stands today as one of the best of its kind, one showing that anesthesia could kill patients [22]. And finally, he established ethics as an important arm of anesthesia and medicine (more about that, too, later) [23]. He truly was a giant.

Academic anesthesia in GB owes much to bicycles built by William Morris (Lord Nuffield) [13]. His successful business morphed into the profitable production of automobiles, first the Morris Bullnose that went 50 mph, got 50 miles to the gallon, and defeated Ford in Great Britain. Fortunately for anesthesia, Morris enjoyed golf and purchased the Huntercombe Golf Club, a club frequented by physicians, including New Zealand born anesthetist, Robert Macintosh. Morris wished to found a school of medicine at Oxford and told his physician friends that he intended to underwrite the establishment of chairs in medicine, surgery, and obstetrics, the then dominant triumvirate. Macintosh smiled and asked why anesthesia had been omitted? Morris had been pleasantly anesthetized by his friend Macintosh, and after a bit of reflection, Morris added a fourth—an anaesthetic—chair to his potential bequest. Oxford first refused (anesthesia was unworthy) but relented when Morris threatened to withdraw his offer for all of the endowment. He also sweetened the bequest from 1.2 million pounds to 2.0 million pounds. So was born the Nuffield Chair of Anaesthetics in 1937, the first occupant being Macintosh, later Sir Robert. World War II dictated a clinical direction for the first years of the department, and only after that war did Oxford contribute information vital to the basis for anesthesia, continued under the guidance of Sir Keith Sykes, one of the contributors to the present history.

Why Waters, Beecher, and Macintosh? Is it the Willie Sutton Principle? Recall that Sutton, a bank robber, was asked why he robbed banks? Answer: "Because that's where the money is!" Waters, Beecher, and Macintosh because that's where the physician-anesthetists of the world were—half in the US and much of the rest in GB.

1910–1950: Diverse Anesthetic Developments in Various Parts of the World

Australia-New Zealand

In 1929, in Australia only Rupert Hornabrook and Fred Green in Melbourne, and Gilbert Brown in Adelaide were full time anesthetists. Geoffrey Kaye, a young and enthusiastic doctor had shown a keenness for anesthesia, despite it being considered "suitable only for the physically unfit or

---

[1] Dr. Jane Fitch and her associate, Dr. Vaidy Rao, noted to EIE that the University of Oklahoma should be given recognition as one of the earliest—if not the first—departments of anesthesia. "This department was not organized until 1930, at which time John Alfred Morrett, M.D., became its head, from 1930 to 1938…Floyd Jackson Bolend, M.D… (was)…head of the hospital Department of Anesthesia until 1930, at which time the School of Medicine's Department of Anesthesiology was formed."

[2] George E. Battit: Henry K Beecher and the Early Years of the Anesthesia Service. Chapter 5 in the privately published book "This is No Humbug!" edited by Richard J. Kitz.

the unambitious". He attended the Australasian[3] Medical Congress, which had newly established a section of anaesthetics, and met Francis McMechan. He was to become McMechan's protégé leading to lifelong communication with Waters, McKesson, Lundy and others. In 1932, *Practical Anaesthesia*, the collated work of several anaesthetists, edited by Kaye, appeared in Australia.

In 1934, the Australian Society of Anaesthetists was founded. A diploma course began at Sydney University in 1944, and at Melbourne University in 1946. In 1946, Kaye established the teaching centre at Melbourne University, together with a library and museum, and in 1948, Kaye assisted in forming The New Zealand Society.

In 1949, Harry Daly, President of the Australian Society of Anaesthetists, negotiated with the College of Surgeons (representing both Australia and New Zealand) to establish the Australian Faculty of Anaesthetists.

Great Britain and Ireland

In 1932, Henry Featherstone and Ivan Magill guided the founding of the Association of Anaesthetists of Great Britain and Ireland (AAGBI).

In 1935, Magill assisted in the inauguration of the Diploma in Anaesthesia (DA), awarded by the Anaesthetic Section of the Royal Society of Medicine. The Diploma was not quite awarded by anesthetists [13]. Magill and the Association of Anaesthetists of Great Britain and Ireland struggled to provide the diploma, but it could not be awarded by the Association because the Association was not "an Examining Body". To bypass this impediment, a Conjoint Board of the Royal Colleges of Physicians and Surgeons (surgeons again to the rescue) conducted the examination. Anesthetists gained control of the process after World War II, in 1948.

Soon after the conclusion of World War II, universities at Bristol (1946), Newcastle-upon-Tyne (1949), Cardiff (Welsh National School of Medicine; 1952) and Liverpool (1959) created Departments of Anaesthesia. Cecil Gray and his colleagues popularized the use of curare (d-tubocurarine), creating the 'Liverpool technique' a forerunner of balanced anesthesia. Research blossomed in support of new surgeries that required controlled ventilation and circulation.

In 1948, AAGBI Diplomates were in place when anesthesia was recognized as a medical specialty in GB. The Faculty of Anaesthetists formed within the Royal College of Surgeons, and the Fellowship Diploma was instituted (FFARCS). AAGBI representations to the Spens Committee led to equal status and pay of the all-too-few anesthetists with other hospital-based specialists.

---

[3] Australasia refers to Australia and New Zealand, as in the Royal Australasian College of Surgeons.

France

In 1934, the French Society of Anesthesia and Intensive Care (originally the Société Française d'Etude de l'Anesthésie et de l'Analgésie—name changed to the current one after 1957) was founded, but became inactive during World War II. It was reborn in 1946, the Société Française d'anesthésie et d'analgésie (SFAA) with 117 members, mostly French surgeons but including 17 anesthetists.

Until 1947, surgeons directed anesthesia and received all fees, with about 10 % given to "assistants". Anesthetists provided all drugs and equipment, prompting the use of the least expensive approaches to anesthesia. In 1947, the newly created Chair of Surgical Techniques in Paris assembled a 6-week course supplemented by a 6-month hospital assignment supervised by surgeons or physicians. Students (doctors and nurses) completing this course received a "Certificate of Anaesthesia". Article 45 of the code of practice gave the French "*surgeon… the right to choose his operating assistants as well as the anaesthestist.*" Anesthesia was only a "competence". From 1947, "Special anaesthesia" given by a qualified anesthetist was paid separately from the surgeon's fee. Progress!

In 1948, examinations were added to the 6-month course for doctors, leading to award of the Diplôme d'Anesthésie-Réanimation (Diploma in Anaesthesia and post-operative care). French nurse anesthetists continued to receive the Certificate of Anaesthesia, which now required successful completion of a written examination. From 1948 to 1973, nurse anesthetist training schools opened in France and trained 1500 students. From 1960, almost all cities with universities had a nurse-anesthetists school. Passage of an examination led to the *Certificat d'Aptitude aux Fonctions d'Aide Anesthésiste*. Like physicians, nurse anesthetists organised training programs and trade unions, and worked in accordance with statutes that they had devised. They competed with doctors, producing antagonisms yet to be resolved. However, in contrast to the case in the US, they could not work independently.

Nordic Countries

Having trained with Beecher in 1938, in 1940, Torsten Gordh introduced anesthesia training in Sweden, occupying the first position established for an anesthesiologist in Scandinavia and mainland Europe, at the Karolinska Hospital in Stockholm. Then and in subsequent years, nurses (learning from on-the-job experiences) gave anesthesia in Nordic countries and surgeons carried the responsibility. Many surgeons argued that anesthesia should be established as a medical specialty, and positions for physician anesthetists were increasingly funded in major hospitals. Pioneer Nordic anesthesiologists usually trained abroad. They included Trier Mørch and Ole Secher (Denmark); Eero Turpeinen (Finland); Elias Eyvindsson (Iceland); Otto Mollestad and Ivar Lund (Norway); and Gordh (Sweden).

Nordic societies were established soon after World War II: the Swedish Society of Anesthesiologists was founded in 1946; the Norwegian Association and the Danish Anesthesia Association in 1949; the Finnish Society of Anesthesiologists in 1952; and the Icelandic Society of Anesthesia and Intensive Care in 1960. In 1949, Nordic pioneers founded the Scandinavian Association of Anesthesiologists.

And in Other Parts of Europe

With the return to peace after World War II, 1-to-3 year anesthesia training programs arose in Europe. The average mandated period was 2 years, matching that in the US and focusing on anesthetic delivery. In 1947, the Dutch organized a national training curriculum, and the Unitarian Service Committee sent American anesthesiologists to Austria, to lecture on and demonstrate modern anesthetic techniques.

In 1948, the Netherlands Society of Anesthesiologists was founded and anesthesia was recognized as a specialty. The Belgians and Italians began training courses.

In 1949, the World Health Organization (WHO) and Denmark (Copenhagen) jointly established a one-year course for anesthesiologists in theoretical and practical techniques of delivering anesthesia. This successful course was repeated 23 times, continuing to 1972.

While working in Germany, in 1949, American anesthetist Jean Henley completed the first modern German anesthesia textbook, *Einführung in die Praxis der modernen Inhalationsnarkose* (*Introduction to the Practice of Modern Inhalation Anaesthesia*). German authors soon followed suit. In 1981, the German Society of Anesthesiology and Intensive Care Medicine awarded Henley an honorary membership.

Latin America

The Mexican Society of Anesthetists was founded in 1934. In Brazil, aspects of training in anesthesia were established and expanded to the first Brazilian specialty school in 1941. By 1946, Mexico was sufficiently large to organize its own congresses, while other Latin American countries joined regional organizations. In 1947, Marín founded the first "*School of Anesthesia*" for Columbian physicians, and teaching of clinical anesthesia began in Uruguay. In 1948, Vicente García Olivera created the first center for pain treatment in Mexico.

Far East

In 1934, the Nippon Dental Junior College initiated the first anesthesia department in Japan.

World War II and the following civil war had devastated China. Anesthesiology had to rebuild from the basic delivery of open-drop ether or chloroform or regional/spinal anesthesia. It spread outward from Shanghai and Beijing. Physicians, students, nurses, nuns, and technicians, and only a few professional anesthesiologists (e.g., Yueqing Ma from Peking Union Medical College) delivered anesthesia. The founders of Chinese anesthesiology (Jone Wu and Xingfang Li from Shanghai; Deyan Shang, Rong Xie and Huiying Tan from Beijing) returned from the US and Europe with modern ideas concerning anesthetic delivery. Shang established the first Department of Anesthesiology in China in the National Lanzhou Hospital.

New Delivery Systems and Drugs

Devices for Delivery of Nitrous Oxide (with or without Ether) Anesthesia

The first anesthetic by Horace Wells delivered 100 % nitrous oxide from a bag, thereby imposing hypoxia—interrupted by periods of inadequate anesthesia while the patient breathed room air. The former of these troublesome limitations could be dealt with as Edmund Andrews suggested in the 1860s, by adding oxygen to the nitrous oxide. Over the succeeding 30–40 years various advancements led to gas machines, such as that invented by Teter (a dentist) in 1902, that delivered a variable mixture of oxygen and nitrous oxide, each controlled by separate but inaccurate valves and without an indication of percentage or flow. Kuppers' 1908 invention of the rotameter allowed delivery of a precisely measured gas flow and known oxygen/nitrous oxide concentrations. The German, Neu, used rotameters to precisely deliver readable flows of anesthetic gases from the Rotameter Company's new anesthesia machine. Other machines in the 1900s allowed the addition of ether or chloroform to compensate for the limited potency of nitrous oxide.

In 1915–16, Dennis Jackson described a carbon dioxide absorption system for delivery of rebreathed anesthetic gases [24, 25]. This was not immediately widely applied but laid the groundwork for modern anesthetic delivery. Jackson had suggested the use of the circle absorption system but used a solution of base to accomplish carbon dioxide absorption—an impractical solution.

By 1920, Dräger machines could deliver nitrous-oxide-oxygen-ether (the so-called gas-oxygen ether or GOE anesthetic). Gauss gave acetylene as an anesthetic, but explosions limited its acceptance. The high import costs of nitrous-oxide

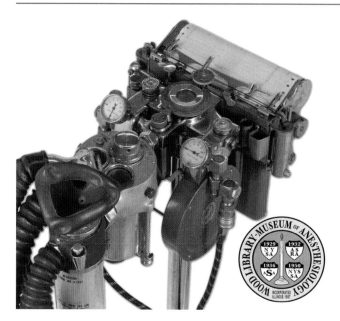

Fig. 6.3 A photograph of a later version of the McKesson Nargraf machine. (Courtesy of the Wood Library-Museum of Anesthesiology, Park Ridge, IL)

led to the use of rebreathing to minimize its consumption. In 1923, Waters introduced the to-and-fro carbon dioxide absorption system allowing low gas flows and rebreathing.

In 1925, Drägerwerk of Germany developed the first circle breathing system for use in their Model A anesthesia machine. There were separate hoses for inhalation and exhalation; large, low resistance, thin mica unidirectional valves that forced the gases to move in a circle; a cartridge for the soda lime; a reservoir bag, and a pressure-limiting valve—all the ingredients found in modern circle systems.

However, in 1930, McKesson departed from the direction of anesthetic equipment development described above by introducing the McKesson-Nargraf machine (Fig. 6.3). It could (deliberately) deliver lethal concentrations of oxygen, as suggested by an experience reported by Gerald Zeitlin [26]:

> "Let's return to the Whittington Hospital on the high and leafy hills of North London. The Senior Consultant in Anaesthesia was named Otto by his parents, the Belams. I called him 'Sir'. One quiet afternoon Dr. Belam asked me if I would kindly replace him at a dental surgeon's office in a shopfront in nearby Holloway Road.
>
> "'All she needs for her extractions is some gas from a McKesson machine. She keeps open on Wednesday evenings for the working men. She is very quick. Get there just before six.'
>
> "The dentist was a middle-aged lady with frosty hair. She met me in her empty waiting room.
>
> "'Otto phoned me you'd be coming. Go in there and fiddle with his machine. The first one'll be here in ten minutes. No fillings. Just exodontia on Wednesday evenings.'
>
> "I had never seen such an anesthesia machine before. I 'fiddled' with it. I peered at the dial at the top. This indicated that by turning the dial one could deliver a mixture of two gases, in precise percentages from zero to one hundred; or from one hundred to zero. Very ingenious. And it made sense, to be able to vary

precisely the percentage of oxygen the patient breathes. I read an engraved label indicating that the McKesson Company in Toledo, Ohio, had made it. I had never encountered an American machine before. I stood back to gain perspective.

> "Then I saw the ugliness of my situation. The only two gas cylinders attached were one each of nitrous oxide and oxygen. Nitrous oxide is a very weak anesthetic agent: so feeble at rendering people unconscious that it has become known as 'laughing gas', that is, it makes you drunk and giggly. Never before had I given it without adding something more potent, ether and more recently, halothane.
>
> "Dr. Frosty the dentist introduced me to the first patient, a muscular builder still in his paint-covered overalls. He was sweating, not from exertion but fear. Anesthesia for dental surgery requires the patient to breathe a gas mixture from a mask that fits over the nose but leaves the mouth accessible. I cursed myself for not even thinking of asking Dr. Belam about taking some Pentothal for intravenous use. I must have been mesmerized by that phrase so rarely used by anesthesiologists about surgeons, 'She's quick.'
>
> "I applied the nasal mask and dialed a 90% nitrous, 10% oxygen mixture.
>
> "'Please take some deep breaths through your nose,' I said. And he did. He closed his eyes but continued to sweat. My free hand counted his pulse rate: about 110 beats per minute. He was not frightened. He was terrified.
>
> "'Shall I begin?' she asked.
>
> "'Yes,' I said because I did not know enough to choose between 'yes' or 'no' and 'yes' seemed more optimistic. I am known as an optimist.
>
> "'I can't even open his mouth. Anyway he's too pink. Otto gets them very black and then they relax and I can get the bite-block in—to keep his mouth open,' she said kindly.
>
> "I cut the oxygen to 5%. To put it another way, I increased the nitrous oxide to 95%. I felt nervous. My hand holding the nose mask felt shaky.
>
> "'What are you going to do? He's still pink and his teeth are clenched,' she said less kindly.
>
> "'I dare not give him any less oxygen. I'm afraid to.'
>
> "'Well Otto is not, so why are you? You are no use to me. Go back to the hospital and tell Otto not to send me people without experience. I'll use local, but all these big men hate needles,' she said without any kindness at all."

Zeitlin continued, describing McKesson's technique of "secondary saturation", a euphemism for producing profound hypoxia by administration of 100% nitrous oxide for a few minutes and then supplying sufficient oxygen to sustain life. The combination of nitrous oxide and hypoxia was akin to a blow to the head and rendered the patient unconscious, relaxed, and, sometimes brain injured as Zeitlin found in his reading of Courville's book [27]. EIE remembers the urban legend suggesting that the IQ of the citizens of Toledo where McKesson built his machines, was less than that in other parts of the US.

A Simple Anesthetic System with Wide Application

In 1937, Ayre in GB described his use of a simple "T"-piece for endotracheal anesthesia in children. Patients breathed spontaneously from this device although a "sigh" could be provided by occluding the expiratory limb. (Care was needed, however, to avoid overexpansion of the lungs). Ayre had a cleft lip and palate, speaking with a "honking" sound that mesmerized children when he induced anesthesia. Later, this simple device was modified by Jackson Rees by adding tubing and a bag—a modification commonly used today to provide anesthesia for children or to provide supplemental oxygen to patients in transit from the OR to the PACU or ICU.

The Heyday of the In-circuit Vaporizer

In a circle system, the vaporizer can be located inside the breathing system ("in-circuit") or outside the system. Produced and sold from the late 1930s to the 1960s, the Ohio #8 bottle was the most popular in-circuit vaporizer in North America. Its sister, the Goldman, was used throughout the rest of the world. Both were potentially dangerous because increased ventilation increased the passage of circulating gases through the vaporizer. That was fine if ventilation were spontaneous and if the anesthetic depressed breathing because the depressed ventilation would prevent the delivery of more anesthetic. But if the anesthetist controlled ventilation manually, then all bets were off and the anesthetist could rapidly deliver sufficient anesthetic to produce cardiac arrest. This potential risk increased when using anesthetics having relatively low blood solubility, high potency, and high vapor pressure (halothane for example) were employed in the in-circle device in a patient whose ventilation was being controlled. With controlled ventilation a delivered concentration approaching the saturated vapor concentration (33 % in the case of halothane) could theoretically be delivered within seconds or minutes, potentially leading to cardiac arrest [28].

A New Vaporizer, the Copper Kettle

In 1943, Lucien Morris graduated from Western Reserve Medical School. Chance and personal interest lead him to chemistry and medicine, to Ralph Waters and an anesthesia residency that he pursued after World War II, and to the invention of the Copper Kettle.

In 1947, during his second year of residency, Lucien Morris participated in the ongoing departmental study of chloroform as though it were a new anesthetic agent. The poor control over chloroform vapor concentration frustrated him, and he foolishly lamented that "anyone ought to be able to make a better vaporizer than this". Waters took him up on his complaint and persuaded him to deal with the issue. Morris applied the principles that John Snow used a century earlier: adequate anesthetic vaporization and control over vapor pressure. He added the goals of delivery of a known con-

centration of anesthetic at a measured fresh gas inflow rate. As did Snow, Morris controlled the anesthetic temperature, and thus its vapor pressure, by housing it in a copper sump. He delivered two precisely known flows—one to the sump and the other bypassing the sump. Flow through the sump passed through a sintered bubbler, ensuring complete vapor equilibration with the flow. Knowing the liquid anesthetic temperature and the two flows allowed a precise calculation of the anesthetic concentration delivered to the circle system. In 1948, the Foregger Company of New York delivered the first prototype Copper Kettle to Morris.

New Inhaled Anesthetics Are Developed and Old Ones Studied

Ethylene

The development of the anesthetic machine enabled the use of anesthetics not heretofore applied. Having noted that ethylene in illuminating gas "put carnations to sleep", Arno Luckhardt demonstrated that it also put animals to sleep. In 1923, Luckhardt and Carter introduced ethylene as an inhaled anesthetic at Presbyterian Hospital in Chicago [29]. "I (EIE) gave this smelly (like garlic) gas in that hospital only three decades later, perhaps in the same room. I wonder." Ethylene was sufficiently more potent than nitrous oxide, such that at an effective concentration, e.g. MAC [30], normoxia (normal hemoglobin oxygen saturation) could be maintained. It may therefore have satisfied Dr Frosty without scaring Dr Zeitlin. However, it was explosive, and that combined with its disagreeable odor resulted in a relatively short life as a clinical anesthetic.

Divinyl Ether, the Designer Anesthetic

Most anesthetics were discovered by happenstance, but a few were discovered by design. In 1930, pharmacologist Chauncy Leake (with M-Y Chen) noted that ether (diethyl ether) consisted of two ethanes joined by an oxygen. Further, he noted that ethylene (an ethane from which two hydrogens had been removed) was more potent than ethane. How about, he thought, substituting ethylenes for the ethanes in diethyl ether? [31] The resulting compound, divinyl ether, was more pleasant and far more rapid-acting than diethyl ether [32]. It was typically used to induce anesthesia, followed by diethyl ether to maintain anesthesia. EIE used divinyl ether for more than a decade. No matter that it also caused mutations [33], and was probably a carcinogen (who knew?) And there are stories about convulsions with divinyl ether. Leake was a character, beloved by some and sneered at by a few.

Cyclopropane

In 1933, Waters gave cyclopropane in clinical practice [29, 34], using his to-and-fro rebreathing technique for carbon dioxide absorption [35] so that he could deliver just a small volume of this expensive and explosive gas. Cyclopropane became the "champagne" of anesthetics: It had no pungency, it was potent (could cause anesthesia all by itself), and it produced anesthesia rapidly, in part because it had a limited solubility in blood. The low solubility meant that the body didn't soak up a lot of molecules before becoming sufficiently full. Unlike most inhaled anesthetics, cyclopropane did not depress blood pressure—desirable in patients at risk of hypotension from hemorrhage or decreased cardiac function. However, hypotension (also called cyclopropane shock) might appear at the end of surgery as the cyclopropane was withdrawn, perhaps because the removal of cyclpropane decreased the stimulation of sympathetic tone.

The low solubility and absence of pungency made cyclopropane a marvelous induction anesthetic. When faced four decades later with a need to anesthetize volunteers with ether for studies of that anesthetic's effects on breathing and the circulation [36, 37], EIE used cyclopropane to induce anesthesia, telling the volunteers that if they just took 10 breaths, they would be asleep (and then he'd turn on the smelly, pungent ether with no problem). He lied. It only took 3 breaths. Wham! What a neat anesthetic—except that if a spark happened nearby it blew up, killing patient and anesthetist, too. Even so, cyclopropane continued as one of the significant anesthetics in the US through the 1950s.

The Atomic Bomb Advanced Fluorine Chemistry and Made Modern Inhaled Anesthetics Feasible

From 1943 to 1945, fluorine chemistry advanced consequent to the need for separation and purification of uranium isotopes to make an atomic bomb in the Manhattan project. The process attached 6 fluorines to each uranium atom and thereby converted the uranium into gases. The gaseous isotopes then were separated by centrifugation. The knowledge gained in fluorine chemistry ultimately enabled development of what we call the modern inhaled anesthetics, compounds halogenated with fluorine to eliminate flammability. Methoxyflurane was synthesized incidentally as part of the Manhattan project but was not thought of as an anesthetic. However, we did get halothane, enflurane, isoflurane, desflurane, and sevoflurane–and Teflon®.

New Local Anesthetics and Their Uses

Dibucaine

In 1925, the local anesthetic dibucaine, was synthesized to overcome difficulties with procaine, allergy and short duration. It was clinically useful but displayed a narrow therapeutic ratio. Dibucaine later found a use in the diagnosis of the cause of prolonged neuromuscular blockade from succinylcholine (the dibucaine number).

Lidocaine

Swedes Nils Löfgren and Bengt Lundqvist synthesized lidocaine in 1943, and Torsten Gordh studied it in volunteers and patients in 1945, leading to its clinical release. Lidocaine acted faster with longer anesthetic effects than procaine, and did not produce allergic reactions. As we shall see, Swedish scientists developed new local anesthetics into the last half of the twentieth century and were key to increasing the use of regional techniques.

Local Anesthetics as General Anesthetics

In Buenos Aires, Gregorio Aranés and Ivar Castellanos reported "*Brief observations on anesthesia with Pentothal Sodium and Procaine*" in 1949. The effectiveness, low cost and compactness of this Latin American technique led to its widespread application. In later years, lidocaine replaced procaine.

New Barbiturates

Pentobarbital

In 1928, pentobarbital was synthesized. Pentobarbital might be substituted as premedication for or added to morphine. It offered two advantages over morphine: greater sedation and much less postoperative nausea and vomiting [38]. It was also used before regional anesthesia to increase the threshold to local anesthetic-induced seizures. Of course this might also obscure the fact that an intravenous injection of local anesthetic had occurred.

Hexobarbital

In 1932, the great German chemist Helmut Weese and Walther Scharpff synthesized the first water-soluble, short-acting barbiturate, hexobarbital, briefly used worldwide—until displaced in many countries by the release of thiopental two years later. In 1943, Weese invented 4 % polyvinyl pyrrolidone, which was used successfully as a plasma substitute during the German North African campaign and later to manage hemodynamic instability during surgery.

Thiopental

In 1934, Waters gave thiopental (Pentothal®) to a patient [39]. So did Lundy a few months later [40]. The introduction of this induction anesthetic into clinical practice was widely accepted as a major advance, although its advantages vis-à-vis hexobarbital were not great. Hexobarbital was the "German" drug while thiopental had been discovered by chemists working at Abbott Laboratories in the US. Hexobabital administration was sometimes associated with muscle movement. Both barbiturates altered the induction process for the better. Induction of anesthesia with ether had been an unpleasant process for anesthetist and patient. EIE remembers (as a patient) such an induction with horror. A choking swirling down into a vortex of descending blackness, much as one might imagine dying to be. Induction with a barbiturate produced a quick and pleasant transformation from wakefulness to sleep. "Count backwards, please, from one hundred…." Sleep came before 90, arriving effortlessly and without claustrophobia and terror.

The First Synthetic Opioid

The approach of World War II and a possible interruption to the supply of anticholinergic (belladonna) drugs led the German government to underwrite the synthesis of meperidine (Demerol) in 1932. Meperidine had weak anticholinergic properties, but better yet, it was soon found to be a good synthetic opioid, and the supply of opium was also tenuous. One of the initial claims touting the advantages of meperidine was that it spared respiration (but then the same was said about other opioids). In 1947, after induction with thiopental, Neff used meperidine and nitrous oxide to produce "balanced anesthesia".

Neuromuscular Blockade Comes to Anesthesia

Although surgeon Arthur Lawen gave curare in 1912 to facilitate tracheal intubation and assisted ventilation for surgical procedures, the idea did not catch on—perhaps because the curare was impure and its effects difficult to predict. But what an opportunity missed. In the 1930s, Richard Gill brought curare from South America to the US in large amounts, offering a supply to pharmacologist AR McIntyre who with Squibb chemists partially purified the crude extract. Horace Holaday devised the rabbit head drop test to assay the potency and thereby standardize the concentration, allowing its consistent use for studies as Intocostrin (partially purified curare).

In 1939, US psychiatrist Abram Bennet reported that Intocostrin prevented compression fractures from convulsive therapy. Bennet neither supported ventilation nor reversed residual neuromuscular blockade. Like Goldilocks, he gave just enough.

In the early 1940s, Stuart Cullen gave Intocostrin to dogs, and because it appeared to cause bronchospasm said it has "no place in anesthesia". He should have read Lawen's work. In 1942, with no IRB approval, no oversight, and no previous experience, Harold Griffith and Enid Johnson at the Homeopathic Hospital of Montreal successfully administered Intocostrin to 25 patients anesthetized with cyclopropane [41]. They described "complete muscle relaxation" lasting 10–15 min without serious effects on respiration pulse or blood pressure and no artificial respiration was used! Goldilocks, again. This description notwithstanding, curare's introduction ultimately mandated the control of ventilation and stimulated the development of ventilators in the 1940s. These developments increased the reach of surgeons into the chest and heart.

In 1949, Daniel Bovet observed the paralytic effect of succinylcholine which quickly became a popular means to rapidly produce transient paralysis. This relaxant soon became the standard for inducing complete muscle relaxation, relaxation sufficient to allow tracheal intubation. Because of unwanted side effects however, the search for a rapid acting relaxant of short duration has proceeded for more than 40 years. Although several held promise, none acted with the rapidity of succinylcholine.

Pharmacokinetic/Pharmacodynamic (PK/PD), Mechanisms, and Genetics

In 1924, Howard Haggard began the study of anesthetic pharmacokinetics (what does the body do to drugs?) with his examination of ether pharmacokinetics in dogs. However, unlike the 1950s when the specialty was ready for PK/PD (pharmacodynamics: what do drugs do to the body?) information, Haggard's research did not result in clinically useful practice changes at that time.

In 1935, Meyer's son, Kurt, reformulated the Meyer-Overton theory: "Narcosis commences when any chemically indifferent substance has attained a certain molar concentration in the lipoids of the (brain)" [42]. The most parsimonious theory that followed from this observation was that changes to membrane lipids caused anesthesia. A few souls (but only a few) still believe there may be something to this.

In 1941, building on Archibald Garrod's identification of inborn errors of metabolism as a recessive trait, Beadle and Tatum proposed their 'one gene, one enzyme' theory [43].

Why These New Drugs and New Theories?

What prompted this burst of new anesthetics after a near century of limited inactivity? World War I and the development of anesthetic machines made some of it possible. And the recruitment of some giants into the practice of anesthesia didn't hurt. Another factor might have been simply an increase, albeit still small, in the numbers of anesthetists who thought of anesthesia as more than just a job. Such physicians and nurses might look for new agents, for better ways, to provide anesthesia to an increasing patient base and to meet broadening surgical demands.

In this endeavor they were sometimes helped, sometimes hindered, by their surgical colleagues. As Ralph Waters' surgical colleague, Erwin Schmidt wrote in the Annals of Surgery in 1937:

> "Anesthesia was gladly welcomed, but received little aid or stimulation either as an art or a science, by the surgical profession….attempts to improve the status of anesthesia by medical men were frowned on by the surgical profession, and often deliberately hindered. This attitude placed anesthesia in the hands of young assistants who looked upon it as a necessary evil, a step, or stage on their way to become a surgeon, or into the hands of a technician." [44]

Looking Down the Airway; Providing an Airway; Ventilating the Lungs

Looking

In 1910, Chevalier Jackson had invented a direct laryngoscope, and two years later, Charles Elsberg used it to enable tracheal intubation. In 1939, Noel Gillespie developed a pediatric laryngoscope. In 1941, Robert Miller described his straight blade for laryngoscopy by direct elevation of the epiglottis. Two years later Robert Macintosh added his blade for indirect elevation. These simple inventions remained the mainstays of anesthetic laryngoscopy from then to the present.

Tubes in the Trachea

In 1919, Ivan Magill and Stanley Rowbotham inserted a narrow-bore rubber tube into the trachea for insufflation, later complimenting that with an exit tube. Merging these produced the rubber tracheal tube. In 1940, Sydney Leader founded Portland Plastics (eventually Portex). As World War II progressed, he promoted the change from harder rubber tubes to softer polyvinyl chloride tubes, tubes used to the present.

Artificial Oral and Tracheal Airways

In 1908, Frederic Hewitt described his oropharyngeal airway, little more than a slightly curved tube that provided a conduit to the posterior oropharynx. Karl Connell introduced a curved metal airway in 1913, that in 1933, Guedel copied in hard black rubber. Waters added an insufflation port. Oral airways contoured to fit the oropharynx, remain the present gold standard. They were a marvelous advance in airway management, as much for their time as the laryngeal mask airway introduced a half century later. Contributing further to airway management, these two pioneers in the US, and Michael Nosworthy in GB popularized Macewen and Matas' principles of tracheal intubation and positive pressure ventilation during anesthesia. In 1935, in GB, Francis Shipway attacked the problem of aspiration with a cuffed oropharyngeal airway, thereby anticipating the development of the laryngeal mask airway by a half-century.

Although essential to the advancement of thoracic surgery, positive pressure ventilation required thoracic surgeons to operate on moving lungs. Waters and Joseph Gale solved this problem in 1931 by ventilating only the non-operated lung. Better yet, in 1949, Swede Eric Carlens invented the double-lumen tube for use in bronchospirometry and a year later for use in anesthetized patients. Now the surgeon had the luxury of operating on immobile lungs and other intrathoracic structures (esophagus, aorta, diaphragm).

Ventilate the Lungs

In 1916, K Giertz described the advantages of intermittent positive pressure ventilation (IPPV) over Ferdinand Sauerbruch's method of simply inflating the lungs, but Giertz' publication was in Swedish, and the world did not read it. In 1929, Philip Drinker and Charles McKann produced the iron lung, a mechanical external ventilator that applied intermittent negative pressure to the chest wall (and the rest of the body, excluding the head) and cost $ 3,000. In 1931, John (Jack) Emerson manufactured a machine similar to Drinker and McKann's from standard parts, and costing $ 1,000. Drinker sued pleading infringement but Emerson prevailed. Over the next 30 years these "iron lungs" saved many lives, but cumbersomeness and cost, even at $ 1,000, limited their availability and usefulness. In 1933, the Swedish company AGA with surgeon Paul Frenckner (A Swedish ENT physician) constructed the respirator (Spiropulsator), described by Giertz in 1916, and improved by Crafoord in 1938 who used it for ventilatory support during pneumonectomy. In 1947, a motor engineer, JH Blease, in England produced a prototype mechanical ventilator with a commercial model realized in 1950.

In 1938, polio broke out in GB. Seeing a need for machines to support breathing, Lord Nuffield turned to Macintosh for advice, Nuffield offering to provide a tank ventilator for every Commonwealth hospital requesting one. Australian Ted Both, had designed a simple wooden version of the Drinker "iron lung" and allowed Nuffield to use his design. By 1947, the Morris car factory had built 1,750 of Both's ventilators.

In 1948, Albert Bower and Ray Bennett provided ventilatory support as needed to nearly 300 cases of patients in California suffering from polio. For unclear reasons they supported ventilation with a combination of a tank (Drinker) ventilator and intermittent positive pressure ventilation (via mask or tracheostomy) [45, 46]. They analyzed blood to assess the adequacy of their management [47]. Their work antedated Bjørn Ibsen's similar 1952 management of the great polio epidemic in Copenhagen, which led to the worldwide development of intensive care units. Ibsen gave credit to them in his description of his work.

In Germany, in 1935, W Capelle gave continuous postoperative subcutaneous injection of local anaesthetics into abdominal areas to facilitate deep breathing and decrease the incidence of postoperative pneumonia [48]. This technique has gained favor intermittently over the years, the most recent version being the On-Q PainBuster® Post-op Pain Relief System providing continuous infusions of dilute local anesthetic through subcutaneously implanted perforated cannulae.

Monitoring Respiratory Gases

In 1932, Corning Glass marketed the first precise pH glass capillary electrode.

In 1935, Matthes constructed the first device to continuously measure the hemoglobin oxygen saturation of human blood in vivo by transillumination of an ear. In 1941, Millikan developed a lightweight ear oxygen meter he called an oximeter. Wood made calibration possible by adding a capsule to Millikan's oximeter to squeeze the blood out of the tissue to set zero, then letting the blood back in. Closer yet were we to the pulse oximeter.

In 1937, in Germany, Luft invented the principle underlying the infrared anesthetic and carbon dioxide analyzers so ubiquitous today. The Germans later used it for tracking V-bombs, the ram-jets and rockets that rained down on GB towards the end of World War II.

Using the EEG to Monitor Anesthesia

In 1937, in humans, Gibbs in the US documented the effects of various drugs on the electroencephalogram (EEG). From 1949 to 1952, anesthesiologist Albert Faulconer and neurologist Reginald Bickford at the Mayo Clinic used the electroencephalogram to define depth of anesthesia and brain well-being. Faulconer showed that inhaled anesthetics and thiopental produced an EEG pattern that changed in a roughly predictable manner with increasing anesthetic concentrations [49–52]. Twenty years later while at UCSD, Bickford continued his involvement with anesthesiologists, when he developed the Compressed Spectral Array—a processed form of the EEG, simplifying identification of decreased blood flow to the brain during cardiopulmonary bypass [53].

Physicians and the Problem of Drug Abuse

In the 1930s, Federal treatment of addiction began with the establishment of drug addiction treatment hospitals by the US Public Health Service, facilities with features of both hospitals and prisons, consistent with a view of addiction as a disease and a vice. In 1947, the UK Home Office found that 21 % of addicts were physicians; 23 % in 1956. It was not long before it was recognized that anesthesiologists were represented in drug abuse facilities at a far greater rate than expected, based on their percentage among all physicians.

Reprise

A renaissance in anesthesia, particularly in the US and GB, occurred between 1910 and 1950. World War I drew physicians into anesthesia and forced some technical improvements such as the Boyles anesthetic machine and use of blood transfusions. Guedel developed his technique for defining depth of anesthesia. As the numbers of anesthetists grew in the US, two societies arose: the American Society of Anesthesiologists and the International Anesthesia Research Society, and in Great Britain the Association of Anaesthetists of Great Britain and Ireland. Academic departments developed at the University of Wisconsin (Waters chair); Harvard (Beecher) and Oxford (Macintosh). In combination, the societies and academic departments increased recognition of the role of the anesthetist and improved quality through education and examination for certification/credentialing. Similar developments occurred in the rest of the world in subsequent years.

New anesthetics, especially thiopental, ethylene, divinyl ether, and cyclopropane, came into being. And the invention of the Bovie and the discovery of antibiotics helped the surgeon, the patient, and, thereby, anesthesia. The development of the atomic bomb required increased knowledge of fluorine chemistry, leading to Teflon® and modern inhaled anesthetics. Chance and interest led Lucien Morris to the invention of a device that allowed the precise delivery of those anesthetics, the Copper Kettle.

World War II dramatically increased the numbers of anesthesiologists in the US. Many of those drafted into anesthesia discovered an attraction to the specialty. Their service eased their requirements for credentialing, and the advent of health insurance ensured a reasonable compensation. Similar changes occurred in other countries but because of the devastation of World War II and civil wars, did not occur immediately, but at times delayed by decades.

References

1. Graham EA, Singer JJ. Successful removal of an entire lung for carcinoma of the bronchus. JAMA. 1933;101:371–4.
2. Wynder EL, Graham EA. Tobacco smoking as a possible etiologic factor in bronchiogenic carcinoma; a study of 684 proved cases. JAMA. 1950;143:329–36.
3. Harmel MH, Lamont A. Anesthesia in the surgical treatment of congenital pulmonic stenosis. Anesthesiology. 1946;7:477–98.
4. Pollack SV, Carruthers A, Grekin RC. The history of electrosurgery. Dermatol Surg. 2000;26:904–8.
5. Bankert M. Watchful care: a history of America's nurse anesthetists. New York: Cintinuum; 1989. pp. 1–58.
6. Cullen DJ, Eger EI II, Stevens WC, Smith NT, Cromwell TH, Cullen BF, Gregory GA, Bahlman SH, Dolan WM, Stoelting RK, Fourcade HE. Clinical signs of anesthesia. Anesthesiology. 1972;36:21–36.
7. Guedel AE. Inhalation anesthesia: a fundamental guide. New York: Macmillan; 1937. pp. 1–172.

8. Snow J. On the inhalation of the vapour of ether in surgical operations: containing a description of the various stages of etherization, and a statement of the result of nearly eighty operations in which ether has been employed in St. George's and University College Hospitals. London: John Churchill; 1847. pp. 1–88.

9. Metcalfe NH. The effect of the First World War (1914–1918) on the development of British anaesthesia. Eur J Anaesthesiol. 2007;24:649–57.

10. Betcher AM, Ciliberti BJ, Wood PM, Wright LH. The jubilee year of organized anesthesia. Anesthesiology. 1956;17:226–64.

11. Lundy JS. Factors that influenced the development of anesthesiology. Anesth Analg. 1946;25:38–43.

12. Bunker JP. The anesthesiologist and surgeon: partners in the operating room. Boston: Little, Brown and Company; 1972.

13. Sykes K, Bunker J. Anaesthesia and the practice of medicine: historical perspectives. London: Royal Society of Medicine Press Ltd.; 2007. pp. 1–303.

14. Beecher HK. The specialty of anesthesia and its application in the Harvard University-Massachusetts General Hospital Department. Ann Surg. 1947;126:486–99.

15. Bacon DR. Special article: Francis Hoeffer McMechan, MD: creator of modern anesthesiology? Anesth Analg. 2012;115:1393–400.

16. Bemis HE, AGuard WF, Covault CH. Anesthesia, general and local. J Am Vet Med Assoc. 1924;64:413–39.

17. Smithcors JF. History of veterinary anesthesia. In: Soma LR, editor. Textbook of veterinary anesthesia. 1 ed. 1971; pp. 1–23.

18. Bonica JJ. The management of pain, with special emphasis on the use of analgesic block in diagnosis, prognosis and therapy. Philadelphia: Lea & Febiger; 1953. pp 1–1533.

19. Everett MR. Medical education in Oklahoma. The University of Oklahoma School of Medicine and Medical Center 1900–1931. Norman: University of Oklahoma Press. 1972. pp. 279–80.

20. Beecher HK. The powerful placebo. JAMA. 1955;159:1602–6.

21. Beecher HK. Pain in men wounded in battle. Ann Surg. 1946;123:96–105.

22. Beecher HK, Todd DP. A study of the deaths associated with anesthesia and surgery. Based on a study of 599,548 anesthesias in 10 institutions, 1948–1953, inclusive. Publication Number 254, American Lecture Series, edited by John Adriani. Charles C. Thomas. Springfield, Illinois;1954. pp. 3–66.

23. Beecher HK. Experimentation in man. JAMA. 1959;169:461–78.

24. Jackson DE. A new method for the production of general analgesia and anesthesia with a description of the apparatus used. J Lab Clin Med. 1915;1:1–12.

25. Jackson DE. The employment of closed ether anesthesia for ordinary laboratory experiments. J Lab Clin Med. 1916;2:94.

26. Zeitlin G. Laughing and crying about anesthesia: a memoir of risk and safety. Noth Charleston: CreateSpace; 2011. pp. 1–260.

27. Courville CB. Untoward effects of nitrous oxide anesthesia; with particular reference to residual neurologic and psychiatric manifestations. Mountain View: Pacific Press Association; 1939. pp. 1–174.

28. Gibbons RT, Steffey EP, Eger EI, II. The effect of spontaneous versus controlled ventilation on the rate of rise of alveolar halothane concentration in dogs. Anesth Analg. 1977;56:32–4.

29. Adriani J. The pharmacology of anesthetic drugs. Springfield: Charles C Thomas; 1952.

30. Miller RD, Wahrenbrock EA, Schroeder CF, Knipstein TW, Eger EI, II, Buechel DR. Ethylene-halothane anesthesia: addition or synergism? Anesthesiology. 1969;31:301–4.

31. Leake CD, Chen M-Y. The anesthetic properties of certain unsaturated ethers. Proc Soc Exp Biol Med. 1930;28:151–4.

32. Gelfan S, Bell IR. The anesthetic action of divinyl oxide on humans. J Pharm Exp Ther. 1933;47:1–3.

33. White AE, Takehisa S, Eger EI II, Wolff S, Stevens WC. Sister chromatid exchanges induced by inhaled anesthetics. Anesthesiology. 1979;50:426–30.

34. Waters RM. Present status of cyclopropane. Br Med J. 1936;2:1013–7.

35. Waters RM. Clinical scope and utility of carbon dioxid filtration in inhalation anesthesia. Anesth Analg. 1924;3:20–2.

36. Larson CP Jr, Eger EI, II, Muallem M, Buechel DR, Munson ES, Eisele JH. The effects of diethyl ether and methoxyflurane on ventilation: II. A comparative study in man. Anesthesiology. 1969;30:174–84.

37. Gregory GA, Eger EI, II, Smith NT, Cullen BF, Cullen DJ. The cardiovascular effects of diethyl ether in man. Anesthesiology. 1971;34:19–24.

38. Eger EI, II, Kraft ID, Keasling HH. A comparison of atropine, or scopolamine, plus pentobarbital, meperidine. or morphine as pediatric preanesthetic medication. Anesthesiology. 1961;22:962–9.

39. Pratt TW, Tatum AL, Hathaway HR et al. Sodium ethyl (1-methyl butyl) thiobarbiturate: preliminary experimental and clinical study. Am J Surg. 1936;31:464–6.

40. Lundy J, Tovell R. Some of the newer local and general anesthetic agents. Methods of their administration. Northwest Med (Seattle). 1934;33:308–11.

41. Griffith HR, Johnson E. The use of curare in general anesthesia. Anesthesiology. 1942;3:418–20.

42. Meyer HK, Hemmi H. Beiträge zur theorie der narkose. III. Biochem Z. 1935;277:39–71.

43. Beadle GW, Tatum EL. Genetic control of biochemical reactions in neurospora. Proc Nat Acad Sci (USA). 1941;27:499–506.

44. Waters RM, Schmidt ER. Anesthesia and surgery. Ann Surg. 1937;106:788–94.

45. Bower AG, Bennett VR, Dillon JB, Axelrod B. Investigation on the care and treatment of poliomyelitis patients. Ann West Med Surg. 1950;4:561–82.

46. Bower AG, Bennett VR, Dillon JB, Axelrod B. Investigation on the care and treatment of poliomyelitis patients. II. Physiological studies of various treatment procedures and mechanical equipment. Ann West Med Surg. 1950;4:686–716.

47. Dail CW, Bennett VR, Bower AG. Measurement of respiratory deficiencies in poliomyelitis. Arch Phys Med Rehabil. 1950;31:276–80.

48. Capelle W. Die Bedentung des Wundschmerzes und seiner ausschaltung fur dan Ablauf der Atmungbei Laparotl-mierten. Dtch Z Chi. 1935;246:466.

49. Courtin RF, Bickford RG, Faulconer A, Jr. The classification and significance of electro-encephalographic patterns produced by nitrous oxide-ether anesthesia during surgical operations. Proc Staff Meet Mayo Clin. 1950;25:197–206.

50. Faulconer A, Jr. Correlation of concentrations of ether in arterial blood with electro-encephalographic patterns occurring during ether-oxygen and during nitrous oxide, oxygen and ether anesthesia of human surgical patients. Anesthesiology. 1952;13:361–9.

51. Faulconer A, Pender JW, Bickford RG. The influence of partial pressure of nitrous oxide on the depth of anesthesia and the electroencephalogram in man. Anesthesiology. 1949;10:601–9.

52. Kiersey DK, Bickford RG, Faulconer A, Jr. Electro-encephalographic patterns produced by thiopental sodium during surgical operations; description and classification. Br J Anaesth. 1951;23:141–52.

53. Stockard JJ, Bickford RG, Schauble JF. Pressure-dependent cerebral ischemia during cardiopulmonary bypass. Neurology. 1973;23:521–9.

History Reflected in the Evolving Approaches to Anesthesia for a Patient Undergoing Cholecystectomy

Lawrence J. Saidman, Rod N. Westhorpe and Edmond I Eger II

Cholecystectomy in the 1880s

The evolving management of today's second most common procedure [1], cholecystectomy, the simple removal of the gall bladder, illustrates the history of anesthesia and surgery, ancient and modern. Cholecystectomy is not part of the numerous operations conducted before the discovery of anesthesia in 1846 because the gall bladder could not be accessed in the living unanesthetized human. Nor did cholecystectomy occur immediately after Morton's demonstration, because the operation wasn't invented. Credit Berlin surgeon Carl Langenbuch at the Lazarus Hospital for his 1882 report of a cholecystectomy [2]. Given the date, we might surmise that he might or might not have premedicated his spontaneously breathing patient with morphine and scopolamine. He directed the anesthesia, given by a nurse or student who dropped ether (or chloroform) onto a Schimmelbusch gauze mask. The anesthetist sought deeper levels of ether to produce the muscle relaxation needed to access the gall bladder. This was heading into dangerous territory, and the awakening would have been slow, especially following a "deep" ether anesthetic. Lister's carbolic acid spray would have provided antisepsis during the procedure. The chances of survival would have been around 80%, a 20% mortality

L. J. Saidman (✉)
Department of Anesthesia, Stanford University,
Stanford, CA, USA
e-mail: lsaidman@stanford.edu

R. N. Westhorpe
Melbourne, Australia
e-mail: westhorpe@netspace.net.au

E. I Eger II
Department of Anesthesia and Perioperative Care,
University of California, San Francisco, CA 94143-0464, USA
e-mail: egere@anesthesia.ucsf.edu

from the combined risk of the anesthesia and postoperative infection.

Approaching the 1950s

The three editors of this book have been clinical anesthesiologists during most of the 60+ years described in this essay characterizing the changing nature of anesthesia care since 1950. Just imagine the experience (and challenge) of beginning a career as an "etherist" and ending it using a videolaryngoscope. Yet one aspect of our careers that made leaving clinical medicine so difficult has not changed—the wonder of the "miracle" of anesthesia—and the amazing sensation that occurs after telling your patient to "just take a few breaths" while you inject a drug allowing you to assume responsibility for that patient's very existence. Few physicians appreciate how addictive that can be.

As the 1950s approached, the care provided by anesthetists expanded, and ether (or cyclopropane) was increasingly supplemented by the use of IV agents, tracheal intubation, and sometimes, muscle relaxation. The next 60 years saw a revolution in anesthesia care, resulting from many incremental changes, including the development of new anesthetics (Fig. 7.1). These played out in different ways in different regions of the world, largely influenced by the aftermath of World War II and local economics. The greatest diversity in development was in the 30 years from 1950 to 1980, after which advances continued in parallel, particularly in the developed world.

In the early 1950s, Europe was recovering from the physical and economic devastation of World War II, and Great Britain was essentially broke. The British Commonwealth, including Australia, New Zealand, Canada, and South Africa, all endured delayed economic recovery. Asia and Japan were similarly affected, and other countries depended on Britain, Europe or the US for experience and training in anesthesia. In the immediate post war period, only the US had the financial resources to make major investments in health

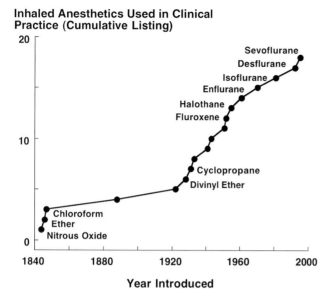

Inhaled Anesthetics Used in Clinical Practice (Cumulative Listing)

Year Introduced

Fig. 7.1. Ether, chloroform and nitrous oxide served most of the world's needs for general anesthesia for a century. The increasing importance of anesthesia was associated with the development of inhaled anesthetics (e.g., cyclopropane) that competed with these original anesthetics in the 1920s and 1930s. Advances in fluorine chemistry resulting from the need to purify uranium in the 1940s for the atomic bomb led to the development of modern anesthetics (anesthetics containing fluorine; agents noted to the left of the cumulative graph.)

care. There was another confounding factor. Clinical anesthesia in the US greatly depended on nurse anesthetists, and they followed protocols, unlike physicians, who were more inclined to do it "their way".

Thus, developments in anesthesia tended to occur first in the US, where they could be afforded, and subsequently were adopted elsewhere. The following descriptions of practice, discuss US practice, noting differences from practice in other parts of the world.

As we approached the 1950s, the anesthesia for a cholecystectomy might have been similar in many parts of the world. Events flowing from World War II were about to shape anesthesia in different ways, in different countries, but they hadn't done so yet. Ether, even after 100 years, was still the mainstay of anesthesia care (Fig. 7.1). The male patient, who at this time was almost certainly a smoker with a chronic cough, would have his preoperative care managed entirely by the surgeon, and might not see the anesthetist until he reached the operating room. Anesthesia would be induced, thankfully, by an intravenous (IV) injection of thiopental, after premedication with morphine and scopolamine. It is unlikely that IV fluids would have been administered, and in the unlikely event that the new muscle relaxant, Intocostrin, had been available, it probably would not have been used. Ether was still the usual anesthetic, perhaps assisted by some additional morphine. It likely would be given by mask, but

in a few patients the trachea would have been intubated with a red rubber tracheal tube. In some cases cyclopropane might be used, with a circle absorption circuit to limit its escape and minimize the risk of explosion.

Postoperatively, the patient returned to their hospital room, and would likely spend two weeks recuperating. Pain would be managed by intramuscular or subcutaneous injections of morphine, administered sparingly by nurses according to a routine prescribed by the surgeon. Vomiting would be managed by the provision of a bowl. The diet would consist of weak tea, graduating to thin soup, and eventually something more substantial. The risk of dying was about 1:1000, a risk that would decrease by two orders of magnitude by the 2000s.

The 1950s Anesthetic

The patient requiring a cholecystectomy was still a smoker, and, reflecting the diet of the time, was lean. The anesthesiologist visited the patient in hospital the evening before surgery, reviewed the laboratory and chest X-ray results, took a rudimentary history, examined the chest, and described the likely anesthetic course to the patient. Pentobarbital was given to encourage sleep the night before surgery. As before, morphine and scopolamine were injected intramuscularly, an hour before surgery. A nasogastric tube was inserted before the patient left for the operating room (OR).

In the OR, 5% dextrose in water was infused IV via a steel needle inserted into a vein on the back of the hand, which was carefully padded to avoid infiltration. In the UK, no IV infusion was initiated preoperatively, only as necessary once the surgery had begun. Induction began with an injection made directly through a standard hypodermic needle taped in place. In the US, blood pressures were obtained manually using Riva Rocci's method and palpation of the superficial temporal artery allowed monitoring of heart rate. The US anesthetist manually recorded these vital signs every 5 minutes on a chart devised a half century earlier by Codman and Cushing [3]. Elsewhere, the anesthetist might neither measure nor record such details. Oxford's Macintosh famously argued that "The pulse is of little value as a guide to nitrous oxide anaesthesia [4]." The anesthetist injected thiopental from a glass syringe to induce anesthesia which was then sustained with nitrous oxide plus diethyl ether vaporized from an in-circuit Ohio 8 bottle in the US or a Goldman bottle elsewhere. In Great Britain and the Commonwealth, a Boyle's machine might be used, with ether vaporized into a Mapleson "A" circuit from a Boyle bottle. As always, the anesthetist judged the amount of ether to give by the patient's responses to the ether given [5]. Small doses of d-tubocurarine (Intocostrin) facilitated relaxation yet permitted continuing spontaneous, manually-assisted, ventilation via a hard conductive-rubber mask. Others might have given open drop ether via a Schimmelbusch mask just as in 1882 or provided anesthesia with cyclopropane.

The surgeon made a right subcostal incision. No antibiotics were given, nor was temperature monitored. The surgeon's satisfaction and the anesthesiologist's observation of the abdomen defined relaxation. OR personnel wore cotton clothing and shoes having conductive soles, and anesthetic circuits were conductive to reduce the likelihood of static electricity igniting the ether, or more importantly, the cyclopropane. The flammability of ether and cyclopropane usually precluded the use of electrocautery. As the fascia was closed, the anesthetist augmented relaxation by controlling ventilation (still by mask) and increasing the ether concentration, and then with fascial closure complete ceased ether delivery and control of ventilation. The UK anesthetist antagonized residual effects of curare, but the US anesthetist might not give neostigmine for fear of stopping the heart.

No supplemental oxygen was given during transport to the hospital room unless cyanosis was evident. Blood pressure and pulse rate might be monitored. The surgeon prescribed intramuscular injections of morphine to manage postoperative pain. Postanesthetic visits were rarely performed and notes documenting complications were written into the chart. A junior surgical house officer visited the patient twice daily to provide postoperative care. Recovery in hospital might exceed a week with no prophylaxis for deep vein thrombosis.

The 1960s Anesthetic

In the 1960s, the work of surgeon Thomas Shires prompted the use of salt-containing IV fluids [6]. Succinylcholine followed induction of anesthesia with thiopental, and the trachea was intubated with a cuffed red rubber tracheal tube cleansed with soap and water after its use in a prior patient.

Anesthesia was established and maintained with halothane in 70 % nitrous oxide, and might but usually did not include intermittent IV doses of morphine or meperidine. Small doses of d-tubocurarine sustained relaxation. Later in the 1960s, (the 1970s in many countries) these changed to disposable polyvinylchloride tracheal tubes, enflurane, fentanyl, and pancuronium. Given the conversion to halothane or enflurane, the surgeon now used the electrocautery. OR personnel still wore shoes having conductive soles to reduce the likelihood of static electricity igniting cyclopropane or ether if they were used—an increasingly rare occasion. Ventilation was controlled either manually or with the aid of a mechanical ventilator. The effects of curare were empirically antagonized using neostigmine and atropine (toward the end of the decade, twitch height might be monitored).

Once spontaneous ventilation and patient movement began, the tracheal tube was removed. The patient was transported to the Post Anesthesia Care Unit (PACU) rather than immediately to their room. Recovery took several days with no prophylaxis for deep vein thrombosis. Pain was controlled by intramuscular injection of opioid at prescribed intervals with allowance for additional doses at the patient's request. Persistent vomiting, now much less common with the demise of ether, might invite an intramuscular injection of prochlorperazine.

The 1970s Anesthetic

The patient's IV fluids flowed through a disposable plastic catheter. Enflurane displaced halothane in the US because of concern regarding halothane hepatotoxicity, and flammable agents disappeared. Fear of bowel distension from nitrous oxide administration diminished or eliminated the use of that anesthetic [7]. Monitoring of blood pressure might use an oscillotonometer in GB and other countries, where a pulse meter might be attached to a patient finger, giving a needle deflection with each heartbeat, but no sound. An electrocardiogram CRT waveform might be displayed, with leads attached to all four limbs by small gel covered metal plates, each secured by a rubber strap.

Postoperative pain management might include an opioid infusion. Intermittent leg compression supplied deep vein thrombosis prophylaxis. Nausea and vomiting was still a problem.

The 1980s Anesthetic

Major changes have occurred. The patient arrived at the hospital in the morning for afternoon surgery, clutching a folder of X-rays, including his/her chest film. Apart from a slice of toast and a cup of tea early this morning, he/she had fasted since dinner the previous night. An electrocardiogram and blood tests for hemoglobin and electrolytes were performed as an outpatient. The anesthesiologist saw the patient at noon, obtained a short medical and anesthesia history, examined the heart and lungs, and briefly discussed the anesthetic process. Midazolam and fentanyl were given for anxiolysis and preparation for induction of anesthesia.

In the operating room, if one of the new pulse oximeters was available, the sensor was applied before induction of anesthesia. Electrocardiogram electrodes were placed on the patient using disposable adhesive discs with conductive gel. A blood pressure cuff was applied and connected to an automated device measuring blood pressure and heart rate every five minutes. A lower thoracic epidural catheter was placed under local anesthesia and might be used for intraoperative anesthesia. It would be used to supply postoperative analgesia. Some centers would have used this approach in previous decades. The patient breathed oxygen from a soft clear disposable facemask while awaiting induction of anesthesia. Thiopental, succinylcholine, atracurium (the newly available muscle relaxant), and fentanyl were drawn into unlabeled disposable plastic (no more reused glass) syringes. Following the relaxation produced by thiopental and succinylcholine, the anesthetist inserted a new disposable PVC tracheal tube. Isoflurane in oxygen-enriched air was administered from an absorption circuit. A mechanical ventilator supplied intermittent positive pressure ventilation (IPPV). The anesthesiologist didn't need to squeeze the sphygmomanometer bulb, but still had to write heart rate, blood pressure, and hemoglobin oxygen saturation (SpO2) values by hand.

The monitored ECG had a heart rate alarm. An expensive new analyzer might measure end-tidal CO_2. A disconnect and high-pressure alarm were attached to the ventilator circuit. Temperature was not controlled nor was a prophylactic antibiotic given.

Following emergence from anesthesia, the patient was placed on their side and covered with a warm blanket before transport to the PACU while breathing supplemental oxygen. Blood pressure and pulse rate were monitored, and oxygen supplied until return to the ward.

Postoperatively, an epidural infusion or Patient Controlled Analgesia device might be used. Metoclopramide would be prescribed in case of nausea or vomiting. It was unlikely that the anesthesiologist visited the patient again. Regular mechanical, intermittent lower extremity compression supplied deep vein thrombosis prophylaxis.

The 1990s Anesthetic

Little change occurred in the preoperative preparation for what now would be a laparoscopic cholecystectomy in a patient who verged on morbid obesity. In the operating room, the patient reclined on a wedge that raised the chest and head. The anesthetist gave cefazolin IV as per hospital guidelines [8]. Preoxygenation via a soft, clear, disposable plastic mask increased SpO_2 to 100 %. Induction of anesthesia with fentanyl, propofol (which has replaced thiopental), and rocuronium, decreased SpO_2 which returned to normal with tracheal intubation and positive pressure ventilation. Tracheal intubation was confirmed by the CO_2 waveform measured with a stand-alone infrared analyzer that also measured end-tidal anesthetic concentrations. Isoflurane or desflurane in O_2 was administered and IPPV provided to produce slight hypocapnia. A neuromuscular monitor indicated the extent of muscle paralysis. Delivered anesthetic in 60 % O_2 (balance N_2) was increased to produce an end-tidal concentration of 1 MAC. A remifentanil infusion was initiated. Blood

pressure decreased to 105/65 mmHg (heart rate 69), and the end-tidal anesthetic concentration was decreased to 0.5 to 0.7 MAC. Both arms were padded and strapped to boards set at 90° to the body. Esophageal temperature was 36 °C and was maintained above this level by forced air warming to minimize the risk of postoperative infection [9]. The wedge was removed.

The head of the table was angled upward, and blood pressure decreased to 85/55 mmHg but increased to 110/65 mmHg with infusion of phenylephrine. The surgeon used videoscope guided instruments to enter the abdomen and attend to gall bladder removal laparoscopically [10]. The abdominal cavity was inflated with carbon dioxide, to enable the surgeon to operate. Anesthesia continued with inhaled anesthetic at half MAC or slightly more, supplemented with an infusion of remifentanil. Ventilation was increased to compensate for the increased end-tidal CO_2 produced by absorption of CO_2 from the peritoneal cavity. As the end of surgery approached, the remifentanil infusion was decreased and ventilation was slowed to permit end-tidal CO_2 to rise. Neostigmine and atropine were given despite no measurable neuromuscular blockade. With placement of the last cutaneous sutures, the anesthetist halted anesthetic delivery, increased O_2 inflow, deflated the tracheal tube cuff, and stopped the remifentanil infusion. If desflurane was used, as expected from its low solubility and rapid elimination, in 3 minutes, the patient's eyes would open, breathing began, and the tracheal tube was removed.

On awakening, the patient was transported to the PACU breathing supplemental oxygen from a bag and mask. He or she was able to respond verbally to questions regarding comfort, pain and nausea. The patient spent the night in the PACU, monitored for episodes of apnea. A PCA device dispensing small doses of morphine easily controlled pain. Prophylaxis for deep vein thrombosis included subcutaneous heparin and compression stockings. The patient was discharged the following day.

The 2000s Anesthetic

As in the 1990s, our patient was seen for a preoperative assessment at the Anesthesia Perioperative Medicine Center the day before surgery. Examination revealed a normal patient except for a Mallampati 3 value with limited forward displacement of the mandible but normal flexion-extension of their neck. Additional laboratory testing was not performed. Surgery in an Outpatient Surgery facility adjacent to a full service hospital was planned. Preanesthetic preparation was identical to that provided in the 1990s except that our anesthesia machine now incorporated an electronic anesthesia record, and while the patient breathed oxygen, the circulating nurse conducted a "time out" to confirm the name of the patient, the proposed surgery and its intended site, and queried the anesthesiologist regarding known drug allergies. The time-out might also have covered concerns about airway management, availability of blood, and when the prophylactic antibiotic was administered. Following induction of anesthesia with fentanyl and propofol (both given, as were all drugs, from labeled syringes), the ability to ventilate the lungs was confirmed and rocuronium, and sevoflurane in O_2 were administered. Once an elicited twitch was eliminated, laryngoscopy using a video-laryngoscope allowed easy tracheal intubation and anesthesia was maintained using remifentanil, sevoflurane, oxygen, and air to produce an FiO_2 of 80 %, the greater FIO_2 nominally sought to minimize postoperative infection [11]. With closure of the fascia, the neuromuscular block was antagonized using neostigmine and atropine, and ketorolac was injected for postoperative analgesia. Triple antiemetic therapy was administered to diminish postoperative nausea and vomiting in this patient who was at high risk for PONV [12]. Postoperative notes were recorded electronically.

The anesthesia for our 2000s patient might differ in other developed countries, particularly in some parts of Europe where total intravenous anesthesia (TIVA) had become popular, especially TIVA using target controlled infusions based on Schwilden's algorithm [13]. In the US and some other parts of the world, because of concern regarding awareness, and despite some disagreement regarding the efficacy of computer-processed electroencephalograms, the sedative element of TIVA might be guided by on-line computer analysis of the electroencephalogram. And some anesthetists used a hybrid combination of techniques applying a modest concentration, perhaps 0.5 MAC, of a poorly soluble inhaled anesthetic with infusions of propofol and an opioid and one of the programs supplying the result of a computer-processed electroencephalogram [14].

Reprise

Our patient illustrates the evolving nature of modern anesthesia, showing the progression of drugs used (inhaled anesthetics, induction agents, anxiolytics, opioids, neuromuscular blocking drugs), the means of their delivery (for both injected and inhaled agents), approaches to anesthetic and surgical practice (in patient vs. out patient; long stay vs. short stay), control over the anesthetic state and postoperative pain, and means to manage the airway and postoperative nausea and vomiting. They hint at the evolution of patient, surgeon, and anesthetist and the interactions among the three. But beyond surface appearances, they do not show the profound changes wrought in the quality and education of the anesthetist and surgeon, the improvement in outcomes, the amazing decreases in mortality and morbidity. They do not consider the implications of those changes to the future of the specialty.

References

1. Karam J, Roslyn JR. Cholelithiasis and cholecystectomy. Maingot's abdominal operations. 12th edn. Prentice Hall International Inc.; 1997. vol 2 pp. 1717–38.
2. Servetus M. Christianismi restitutio and other writings. Birmingham [O'Malley CD, trans]. The Classics of Medicine Library; 1989. p. 115.
3. Beecher HK. The first anesthesia records (Codman, Cushing). Surg Gynecol Obstet. 1940;71:689–95.
4. Macintosh RR, Bannister FB. Essentials of general anaesthesia. Oxford: 5th Blackwell Scientific Publications; 1952.
5. Guedel AE. Inhalation anesthesia: a fundamental guide. New York: Macmillan Co.; 1937. pp. 1–172.
6. Shires T, Williams J, Brown F. Acute change in extracellular fluids associated with major surgical procedures. Ann Surg. 1961;154:803–10.
7. Eger EI II, Saidman LJ. Hazards of nitrous oxide anesthesia in bowel obstruction and pneumothorax. Anesthesiology. 1965;26:61–6.
8. Waddell TK, Rotstein OD. Antimicrobial prophylaxis in surgery. Committee on Antimicrobial Agents, Canadian Infectious Disease Society. CMAJ. 1994;151:925–31.
9. Kurz A, Sessler DI, Lenhardt R. Perioperative normothermia to reduce the incidence of surgical-wound infection and shorten hospitalization. Study of Wound Infection and Temperature Group. N Engl J Med. 1996;334:1209–15.
10. Consensus conference NIH. Gallstones and laparoscopic cholecystectomy. JAMA. 1993;269:1018–24.
11. Greif R, Akca O, Horn EP, Kurz A, Sessler DI. Supplemental perioperative oxygen to reduce the incidence of surgical-wound infection. Outcomes Research Group. N Engl J Med. 2000;342:161–7.
12. Apfel CC, Korttila K, Abdalla M, Kerger H, Turan A, Vedder I, Zernak C, Danner K, Jokela R, Pocock SJ, Trenkler S, Kredel M, Biedler A, Sessler DI, Roewer N IMPACT, Investigators. A factorial trial of six interventions for the prevention of postoperative nausea and vomiting. N Engl J Med. 2004;350:2441–51.
13. Schwilden H. A general method for calculating the dosage scheme in linear pharmacokinetics. Eur J Clin Pharmacol. 1981;20:379–86.
14. Whitlock EL, Villafranca AJ, Lin N, Palanca BJ, Jacobsohn E, Finkel KJ, Zhang L, Burnside BA, Kaiser HA, Evers AS, Avidan MS. Relationship between bispectral index values and volatile anesthetic concentrations during the maintenance phase of anesthesia in the B-Unaware trial. Anesthesiology. 2011;115:1209–18.

Major Anesthetic Themes in the 1950s

8

Edmond I Eger II, Lawrence J. Saidman and Rod N. Westhorpe

Summary

World War II and subsequent local conflicts (e.g., the Chinese Civil War) left Europe and much of the Far East in tatters while the US applied its great military, economic and scientific strengths to diverse purposes, including support for the development of anesthesia. Anesthesia in some regions (South-Central America and Mexico) and countries (Switzerland, Sweden) progressed because they had not participated in the War. Despite limited resources, discoveries changing the face of anesthesia arose in Europe. Suckling, at Imperial Chemical Industries in England, synthesized 12 compounds in his search for a better anesthetic, striking gold on the ninth try, halothane, the first successful modern (fluorinated) inhaled anesthetic. In Copenhagen, with meager equipment and a willingly dragooned rag-tag corps of students, physicians and dentists, Bjørn Ibsen successfully fought a virulent epidemic of polio, in the process inventing intensive care medicine and intensive care units, and hastening the development of ventilators and blood gas analysis. 1955 marked the founding of the World Federation of Societies of Anaesthesiologists in London.

The 1950s saw a doubling of US nurses and physicians dedicated to a career in anesthesia. Bonica continued his contribution to the management of pain. With American Medical Association (AMA) support, the American Society of Anesthesiologists (ASA) demanded that anesthesiologists practice on a fee-for-service basis, leading to unforeseen increases in the attractiveness and economic power of anesthesia as a specialty and in the support of anesthetic research. The quick-on-quick-off neuromuscular blocking drug succinylcholine was released for use in 1951. In 1953, Apgar published her simple score, remarkably advancing our immediate estimate of a newborn's well-being. In 1954, Beecher and Todd described their monumental outcomes study, reporting that the use of curare increased mortality 6-fold, but (amazingly) not realizing that the probable cause was lack of reversal of residual relaxant effect. The release of the Copper Kettle (1953) and Fluotec® variable bypass (1956) vaporizers allowed a precise control over the delivered concentrations of inhaled anesthetics. They enabled the safer delivery of the new anesthetic, halothane. Beecher promoted the use of the placebo and controlled trials. In the next decade, these led to the development of informed consent and Institutional Review Boards to protect subject rights, laying the basis for modern ethical human experimentation. Finally, in 1959, Webb and Graves described their results for patients cared for on an outpatient basis, presaging the development of modern ambulatory surgery.

World Events in the 1950s

Global wars disappeared when World War II ended in 1945, only to be replaced by undeclared wars like the Cold War, the 1950–1953 Korean War, and civil conflicts in Cuba and elsewhere. Joseph McCarthy began a witch-hunt revealing the presence of communists in the highest levels of the US government but also destroying the lives of many innocents despite their contributions to society. McCarthy forced the US to the right and towards isolationism. So did Russia's launch of Sputnik 1 which pushed the US to put humans on the moon in the next decade. It was a decade of stunning scientific-medical advances: Crick, Watson, and Franklin discovered the helical structure of DNA; the first organ transplants were done in Boston and Paris; and Jonas Salk's polio vaccine ended the terror of that dread disease. There were memorable (some might say trivial) cultural shifts in this decade. Elvis Presley began his superstar career, Hemingway wrote The Old Man and the Sea, Nabokov wrote Lolita, and Pasternak wrote Doctor Zhivago. Hugh Hefner launched Playboy magazine. Hula Hoops and the Frisbee appeared. Toward the end of the decade, six countries signed the Treaty of Rome, leading to the European Union and great hope for a better economic and social future.

E. I Eger II (✉)
Department of Anesthesia and Perioperative Care,
University of California, San Francisco, CA, USA
e-mail: egere@anesthesia.ucsf.edu

L. J. Saidman
Department of Anesthesia, Stanford University,
Stanford, CA, USA
e-mail: lsaidman@stanford.edu

R. N. Westhorpe
Melbourne, Australia
e-mail: westhorpe@netspace.net.au

E. I Eger II et al. (eds.), *The Wondrous Story of Anesthesia*, DOI 10.1007/978-1-4614-8441-7_8, © Edmond I Eger, MD 2014

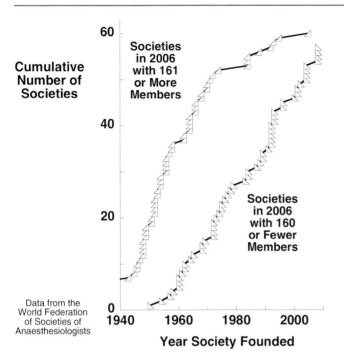

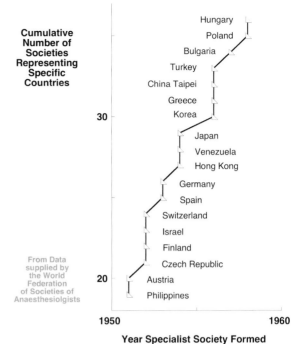

Fig. 8.1 Countries with more anesthetists than the median in 2006, of 160 members, formed societies roughly one-and-a-half to three decades sooner than those having less than the median. (Data from the World Federation of Societies of Anaesthesiologists.)

Fig. 8.2 The rapid growth in societies that began in the 1940s continued in the 1950s with the addition of 22 new societies, 12 in Europe, 5 in Central-South America-Caribbean, and 5 in the Far East-Asia. (Data from the World Federation of Societies of Anaesthesiologists.)

Generalizations

As with all history, each new era builds on the preceding ones. By the 1950s, a sufficiency in the numbers of interested anesthesiologists enabled the formation of societies and journals in various countries. For reasons partly related to an abiding interest in anesthesia, US and European countries had larger numbers of anesthesiologists, and such numbers likely facilitated the earlier development of anesthetic societies and associated instruments (Fig. 8.1). The rapid growth in anesthetic societies in specific countries began in the 1940s and continued in the 1950s with the addition of 23 new societies (Fig. 8.2), 12 in Europe, 5 in Central-South America-Caribbean, and 5 in the Far East/Asia.

As may be apparent from the preceding figures and discussion, anesthesia societies arose at different rates in different parts of the world (Fig. 8.3). Despite the devastation wreaked on Europe by World War II, anesthesia societies in Western Europe appeared in the late 1940s and early 1950s, a decade before they appeared in less affluent, more slowly reconstructed, Russian-controlled Eastern Europe. Western European countries benefited from the Marshall plan. Societies in South America appeared at times between these extremes. Having fewer resources and fewer anesthesiologists, Central American and Caribbean Island societies arose a decade after those in South America.

World War II Unevenly Affected the Geographic Growth of Anesthesia

At the beginning of the War, few trained anesthetists existed in any part of the world, and most of those few were from English-speaking countries. Countries who were slow to recover from the war could not support a major development of a trained cadre of anesthetists; their goal was survival and rebuilding of their infrastructure and industry. Furthermore, in much of the world, anesthesia had been, and continued to be, viewed as something anyone could undertake. Anyone could give anesthesia. No anesthesiologists? What's the problem?

Thus, despite the enormous increase in the numbers of operations imposed by war, anesthesia made few advances in numbers or status in Eastern Europe, the USSR, and Asia. In the UK, physicians had long been the providers of anesthesia and a subset of UK physicians practiced only anesthesia. The US had responded to the increase in surgeries in World War II by forcing physicians into the delivery of anesthesia. Why physicians? Well, they were men, and men could be drafted. More trained anesthetists were nurses, but most of these were women [1]. Compounding the problem, if a nurse anesthetist volunteered for service, she was not guaranteed to practice anesthesia! [That wasn't unique to nurses. Following residency in 1958 I (EIE) was drafted into

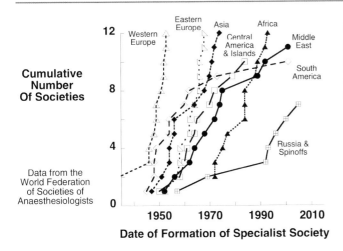

Fig. 8.3 The relationship seen in Fig. 8.1 partly explains the differences seen in Fig. 8.3. Larger numbers of anesthesiologists in Western Europe led to an earlier development of societies than in South America, Eastern Europe, Asia, Central America, the Caribbean islands and the Middle East. Economic advancement may add to the explanation of differences in the appearance and growth of anesthesia in different regions. (Data from the World Federation of Societies of Anaesthesiologists.)

the army more than a decade after the end of World War II. Although I was the Chief of the Anesthesia and Operative Section (in charge of 1 operating room and a closet), I was also a general duty medical officer who did a lot of physical examinations. I remember finding a thyroid nodule during a routine examination one day and giving anesthesia to the patient the next day for removal of his cancer.] The spectacular increases in the numbers of US physicians forced to practice anesthesia imply something else. These were young anesthetists with the energy and ambition that comes with youth. They made their way against established but older specialists.

Drafted US Physicians Become Anesthesiologists

In the early phases of World War II, waves of US physicians trained to become anesthetists in programs lasting up to 3 months, the products of these courses calling themselves 90-day wonders. In 1942, (Col.) Ralph Tovell surveyed American military hospitals in England and found that insufficiently trained physicians provided anesthesia services. In the following year, this led 99 officers to receive 1 month or more training in the better-prepared British hospitals. Parallel courses for the 90-day wonders were given in the US.

"Until the war, there had been only one military course in anesthesia. Stevens J. Martin, M.D., who trained in Wisconsin under Ralph M. Waters, M.D., organized the first Army course in anesthesia in July 1941 at Tilton General Hospital, Fort Dix, New Jersey. This course became the model used for the anesthesia courses developed by The Subcommittee on Anesthesia of the National Research Council….Courses began in the summer of 1942." [1]

Because of the great need for anesthetists, many physicians pressed into service as anesthetists did not even have the limited training described above. They were self-taught. In 1944, the Army recognized a need for upgrading their skills and knowledge and

"gave four intensive courses in anesthesia taught by 'the outstanding physician-anesthetist in the theater.' (the military theater of operations)…A fourth cohort was an amalgam of on-the-job training and informal and formal apprenticeships by medical officers in the theater. In American units with adequately experienced medical officers, training and apprenticeship programs for local and rotating officers were established. The newly trained physician-anesthetists then returned to their own hospitals to train more medical officers…in anesthesia,,.As the war continued, required apprenticeships were implemented to address the increasingly inadequate number of physician-anesthetists. In fact, because of the shortage, in November 1944, it was determined that a trained replacement was required before an anesthetist could move out." [1]

The unintended effect of the War was an enormous increase in the number of anesthesiologists dedicated to the specialty. In 1940, there were 568 ASA members, of which 105 were ABA diplomats. By 1950, these numbers had increased to 3,393 and 706. They were to double again in the 1950s. This forced growth in the number of US physician-anesthetists presented unexpected opportunities, while other factors imposed by the war augmented the effects of those opportunities.

First, physicians pressed into administering anesthesia often discovered that they liked what they did, finding that anesthesia presented surprising pleasures and challenges such as the use of regional anesthesia—more than half of the operations were performed under regional anesthesia [1]. General anesthesia was increasingly administered through a tracheal tube, demanding the acquisition of a technical skill [1]. And the anesthesiologist assumed the role of perioperative physician, responsible for the patient before and after as well as during anesthesia.

Second, surgeons supported by physician-anesthetists, found that they liked what they got.

"…surgeons have made or will make their first contacts with competent anesthesiologists in the armed forces and work under such improved conditions provided by them. After such an experience, it is to be seriously doubted whether many of them will be content on their return to civilian practice to retrogress to the inferior type of unsupervised technician anesthesia, where, as the law requires…the surgeons…must assume full responsibility for the anesthesia, even though fully occupied with the technical requirements of the surgery…." [2]

In Great Britain and its Commonwealth countries however, surgeons had been used to anesthesia being provided by physicians, but that didn't stop them from maintaining their place at the top of the tree.

A third factor encouraged physicians forced into anesthesia to continue as anesthesiologists. The American Board of Anesthesiology credited such physicians with a year of residency—i.e., half the time mandated to complete a residency. Take just one year of residency and become (if you passed your exams) a board-certified anesthesiologist.

Waisel noted a fourth factor supporting the growth of anesthesia as a specialty during and after World War II: wage and price controls [1]. These controls were imposed to limit inflation. To compensate for this limitation to recruitment of workers, corporations increased benefits, including health insurance, something that prompted the increased use of medical/surgical services and, ultimately, the demand for anesthesia and anesthetists. As an aside, one might note that this means of paying for health care partly underlies our present health care crisis. Outside the US, anesthetists continued to be remunerated at a fraction of the rate pertaining to surgeons. Many were actually paid a moiety out of the surgeons' fee. In GB, the National Health Service ensured that all doctors were paid the same—within the service.

To summarize, several factors contributed to what became the basis for a remarkable growth in physician-anesthetists and nurse-anesthetists. Physicians drafted into anesthesia discovered that it was more challenging and rewarding than they had anticipated. Many surgeons became supporters of such physician-anesthetists. The financial base for anesthesia increased in the US. And board certification was made easier to acquire for those with on-the-job training. One might add the reasons given by residents today: the attractions of acute care, of seeing an immediate effect of anesthetic ministrations, the everyday application of principles of physiology and pharmacology.

But I (EIE) believe there is a sixth reason, one more powerful than the above five incentives to a career in anesthesia. My conversion to anesthesia provides an illustration.

"My career in anesthesia began on a pleasant spring day in 1952 as a newly minted first year medical student who wished to make money as an anesthesia extern. After a two-month summer apprenticeship in anesthesia, I would take call for my mentor, who could rest secure at home knowing that the care of emergency patients was in my capable hands! On that first day, he showed me how to start an intravenous infusion of 0.2 % thiopental, dial a 70 % concentration of nitrous oxide, properly hold a rubber mask to the patient's face, and watch the rebreathing bag. Then he left the room. And I was in trouble. The rebreathing bag moved less and less and finally stopped. I knew little of anesthesia, just information supplied in a couple of lectures in pharmacology. But I knew that breathing was good and not breathing was bad. In a squeaky voice I told the surgeon that the patient had stopped breathing. With great presence of mind, and instead of berating me for obvious incompetence, he asked if I wanted him to give artificial respiration. "Yes, please." I responded, voice still high-pitched. The surgeon squeezed the chest, the rebreathing bag now moved, and the circulating nurse fetched my mentor—who noted that the rebreathing bag could be used to ventilate the patient's lungs. I finished the

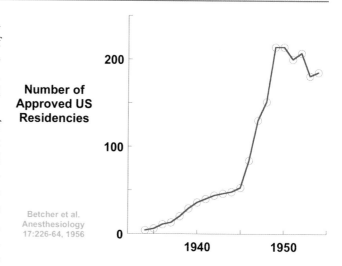

Fig. 8.4 The increasing numbers of residency programs in the US after World War II in part reflected the demand for training in anesthesia. This demand stabilized, as did the number of approved residencies, in the 1950s. The increase may also have reflected the desire by hospitals to access anesthetic services at low cost. (Data from Betcher et al. Anesthesiology 17:226–64, 1956.)

day exhausted and smelling of terror. The epiphany came as I sat thinking of the day's events. To that moment I'd dreamed of becoming a second Robert Koch, a country physician who would make great medical discoveries as a general practitioner. A wonderfully naïve dream that suddenly vanished as I thought 'You nearly killed a patient, today, and if you chose anesthesia as a career, you could do that every day. Every day you could take a patient's life in your hands. Every day.' To a control freak (me) that image was as seductive as seduction comes." [3]

I'm probably not alone. Anesthesia confers enormous power. With each anesthetic, the anesthetist takes a patient's life in their hands, exerts complete control over another human being, over the brain, breathing, the circulation, the muscles. Enormous power, and with it, enormous responsibility, an addictive and intoxicating mix.

Worldwide Training in Anesthesia

These diverse forces dramatically increased the numbers of physicians and nurses who chose anesthesia as a career in the US. Training programs increased, particularly after World War II, to accommodate this career choice (Fig. 8.4). Parallel growth occurred worldwide, but as noted above, the timing and rate of growth differed as a function of social and economic factors. South America had been spared the horrors of World War II, and in the 1950s–1960s, residencies arose in Bolivia, Brazil, Colombia, Peru, Uruguay and Venezuela, some of 2 years duration. Between 1948 and 1973 in France, nurse anesthesia training schools opened in most cities, training 1500 students who on passing an examination, received a *Certificat d'Aptitude aux Fonctions d'Aide*

Anesthésiste. As in the US, the graduating nurse anesthetists established their own institutions and competed with anesthesiologists, resulting in continuing antagonisms.

The length of formal training varied enormously worldwide, particularly soon after World War II. By the 1950s, with internship, it would be 3 years in the US. It was already 3 years in GB, including internship, and it started as 3 years in Australia and New Zealand in 1952. Given that World War II had placed the US as leader in many ways, much of the world initially might use 3 years as a standard. The 1950s were a time of great diversity and change in the perception of the appropriate duration of training. Limited economic resources and an immediate need for trained anesthetists might favor shorter periods of training. In the 1950s in Europe, the minimum prescribed periods differed by an order of magnitude. But by the 1980s this had narrowed to between 4 and 7 years, with most European countries agreeing that 5 years were needed.

It is a cruel irony that training in anesthesia, and anesthesia societies, developed slowly in the USSR and China, countries suffering most from World War II, countries that had contributed the most human lives, whose infrastructure had been devastated, and who had access to fewer resources that might assist rebuilding. Isolated by the cold war, devoting limited resources to strengthening military power, continuing to bleed from civil war (China) and government tyranny (in the USSR; and note China's Cultural Revolution), these countries educated few anesthesiologists and had but limited and diverse durations of training. Contrast this with growth in Japan which had also lost substantial human life and infrastructure, but was occupied by what turned out to be a benevolent force, imposing a stability that allowed rebuilding to occur. The Japanese Society of Anesthesiologists was established in 1954, whereas the Russian Federation of Anaesthesiologists and Reanimatologists was not established until 1972, and the Chinese Society of Anesthesiologists began in 1988.

Fee-for-Service and the Association of University Anesthesiologists (AUA)

The Association of University Anesthetists, later the Association of University Anesthesiologists, perhaps the leading organization for anesthetic academicians in the US, developed in the early 1950s. Emanuel Papper played a crucial role in its birth, a role he described in a witty, self-deprecating history [4]. A stated purpose of the AUA was "…to promote and discuss research and teaching in Anesthesia." [5] The larger truth was a bit seamier [4]. In 1950, organized anesthesia (namely the American Society of Anesthesiologists—the ASA) pressured practitioners to not accept a salary for their anesthetic services. The ASA argued that anesthesia was the practice of medicine and a hospital (the management paying the salary) could not practice medicine. The ASA appeared to adopt the Hess Report of the American Medical Association: "A physician should not dispose of his professional attainments or services to any hospital, lay body, organization, group or individual, by whatever name called, or however organized, under terms or conditions which permit exploitation of the services of the physician for the financial profit of the agency concerned." Papper believed that the ASA and the Directors of the American Board of Anesthesiology (ABA) interpreted this section of the Hess Report to mean that salaried forms of the practice of anesthesiology were unethical. He contended that "Attentive reading of the approved Hess Report does not support this interpretation so clearly." What a diplomat was our Papper. The concern regarding fee-for-service was peculiar to the US. In other countries in the world, salaried medical practice, in hospitals, was and continues to be an accepted practice.

The pressure applied by the ASA included the threat of loss of ASA/AMA membership and Board certification. It never was clear that the ASA would broadly impose sanctions on salaried academics, many of which were—and are—quite happy with a salaried arrangement, unconcerned with any ethical implications. But we know of one case where pressure was supposedly brought to bear on an anesthesiologist for accepting a salaried arrangement. In the Ellensburg Daily Record, June 10, 1954 the report reads:

> "**Physician Sues Medical Society In King County**. SEATTLE (UP)—Claiming he has been socially ostracized and denied membership in the King County Medical Society because he works for a salary rather than for fees, Dr. Lloyd H. Mousel has filed suit against the society and seven other medical groups. The doctor, formerly of Washington, D.C., and the Mayo Clinic, has worked at Seattle's Swedish Hospital since 1949 as director of anesthesiology on a salary basis. This, he said, has resulted in rejection of his application to transfer his membership from the District of Columbia to the King County Medical Society."

Papper argued that "Little recognition was given then, or for that matter now, on the dangerous irrelevancy of linking ethical behavior of a physician in practice to the manner in which he or she earned a living as a matter of principle. It is *how* these practices are used that determines whether the method leads to inequities and to abuse of patient care rather than the process itself."

The potential intrusions of the ASA distressed four academics. Perhaps most distressed was the ethicist Henry Beecher—joined by Papper, Austin Lamont, and Robert Dripps, anesthetic giants of the period. Over several months, these four constructed an organization that might voice the views of academia. The organization, of course, would have research and education as its stated primary purpose, but in fact, the underlying purpose would be to keep the ASA from dictating the economics of anesthetic academia.

The AUA has served academic anesthesia and the specialty well. It initially had elitist pretensions. The original

Table 8.1 A comparison of median annual salaries of some specialties in the USA in 2011

Speciality	Median Salary
Orthopedic Surgeon	$ 500,672
Gastroenterologist	$ 405,000
Invasive Cardiologist	$ 402,000
Anesthesiologist	**$ 370,500**
General Surgeon	$ 357,091
Obstetrician-Gynecologist	$ 275,152
Emergency Medicine	$ 267,293
Ophthalmologist	$ 238,200
Neurologist	$ 236,500
Urologist	$ 222,920
Pediatrician	$ 209,873
Family Medicine	$ 208.861

Data from SK&A, A Cegedim Company. 2601 Main St, Suite 650, Irvine, CA 92614; 800-752-5478. U.S. Physician Compensation Trends. Revised August 2011

by-laws mandated a membership that was not to exceed 100. Tom Hornbein and John Bonica challenged this with the argument that the membership needed to be broadly based if it were to truly represent academia. Their egalitarian view prevailed, and in 1971 the 100 member limit was removed.

Further to elitist pretensions, at the AUA meeting in 1973, the membership discussed the possibility of awarding some honor for the best research done during that year. I (EIE) was all for it. However, Papper demolished the proposal by suggesting that it was "OK, but it really was like little boys who gave each other medals and epaulets." Immediately after the day's meeting ended, Hornbein and I found an army-navy supply store and bought the biggest, gaudiest pair of epaulets available and attached double-sided tape to each. Before that evening's formal black-tie (more elitist stuff) AUA banquet, we convinced the AUA President, Nick Greene, that this was the time to put Papper's suggestion to work. At the banquet, after reading the usual announcements, Greene, intoned that this evening he would reveal the First Manny Papper Awardee for Excellence in Research. "Would Dr. Papper please stand for the Award?" Papper hesitantly rose. Hornbein and I strode up from behind and clapped the epaulets onto his shoulder. Ruefully, Papper commented that he "should have kept his mouth shut." This was the first and last Manny Papper Award.

The AUA has grown, with 613 active and 176 senior members as of 2012 (Email from Annie DeVries, AUA Administrative Assistant, 15 Nov 12). Beyond a research mission, it has a larger focus on educational and political matters. Despite its initial hostility to the ASA, it has a present cordial and cooperative relationship with the ASA.

In 1978, the Federal Trade Commission required that the ASA sign a Consent Decree agreeing, "…that an anesthesiologist is free to choose whatever arrangement he prefers for compensation of his professional services." A demand for a fee-for-service arrangement could no longer be imposed by the ASA or the ABA. Nonetheless, the nearly three decades over which fee-for-service had been the main method of compensation had, with other factors (see above), made anesthesiology an economically attractive specialty in the US, an attraction that continues to this day (Table 8.1). This attraction had several consequences. It added to the ease of recruitment into the specialty, including physicians from outside the US. It enabled academic departments to support research with time and seed money. This luxury helped make US anesthesiology a world leader in anesthesia research for much of the 1950s to the 1980s.

New Inhaled Anesthetics and New Vaporizers for Their Delivery

The Development of Modern Inhaled Anesthetics

The anesthesia provided by ether and chloroform in 1846 and 1847 was an enormous step forward. It enabled unheard-of, unthought-of surgeries. For a century, it sufficed for most purposes that surgeons could imagine. Advances were not required until surgeons began to push boundaries for which ether and chloroform, and the technology and skills needed for anesthetic delivery, were insufficient. Surgery demanded more. The benefits of the electrocautery (the Bovie, first used by Cushing in 1926) and other electrical equipment, encouraged development of new nonflammable anesthetics. Chloroform was nonflammable but too toxic. The coincidence of this need, plus the new fluorine chemistry required for development of the atomic bomb, gave rise to modern inhaled anesthetics, compounds halogenated with fluorine.

Why fluorine? Because this smallest of halogens clings with greater strength to other atoms, particularly carbon atoms. The chlorine in chloroform can be torn from its carbon mate and this underlies the toxicity of chloroform; prevent the separation of the two atoms and you prevent hepatic injury [6]. Fluorine-carbon combinations are usually less vulnerable than chlorine-carbon combinations to degradation by carbon dioxide absorbents or to metabolism, and thus are usually less subject to the sometimes-toxic consequences of degradation or metabolism. Fluorination had another virtue. It made compounds less soluble and thus more readily eliminated; patients awoke sooner after anesthesia.

The first of these modern inhaled anesthetics was fluroxene, synthesized by Julius Shukys in the late 1940s and released in 1953. I (EIE) had come into anesthesia at this time in Chicago, having suddenly decided on a career direction change from general practitioner to anesthesiologist (see above). This caused me to try to learn all that I could about anesthesia. It wasn't hard to do because there wasn't much to learn. I sought out the teaching venues in Chicago. The head of the University of Illinois program, Max Sadove, led one of these. Each week he presided over the morbidity and mortality sessions (now portentously called Grand Rounds), cigar in hand, calling for cases to present. It was not a formal enterprise. I remember a discussion of fluroxene, ending with Sadove's paraphrased comment that "We've tried it now in humans; perhaps we should test it in dogs." Lucky they went in that direction because it is toxic to many animals (including dogs), [6] but not to humans [7]. Fluroxene enjoyed a minor vogue and commercial success, but it caused cardiovascular stimulation, [8] was irritating to breathe, and produced substantial postoperative nausea and vomiting. Its trade name was Fluromar, but it sometimes disparagingly was called Vomomar or Flurobarf.

The first truly successful modern inhaled anesthetic was halothane, synthesized in 1951 by Charles Suckling of Imperial Chemical Industries in England. He was acting on an inspired guess by his boss, John Ferguson, who had studied fluorine-containing agrochemical agents for fumigation of grain silos, noting that some of the agents knocked out weevils and beetles who recovered quite nicely [9]. After testing by James Raventos in animals, Michael Johnstone used halothane clinically in 1956 [10]. Halothane was less soluble in blood and thus allowed a more rapid awakening from anesthesia than did chloroform. However, the bigger concern was injury to the liver (hepatotoxicity). Chloroform was a classic hepatotoxin. If you gave it to an animal, it injured the liver. The more you gave, the greater the injury [11]. At least in the beginning, halothane didn't do that in humans. Chance favored halothane. The first patient scheduled to be anesthetized with halothane had her surgery cancelled because of a slight illness that subsequently became manifest as jaundice due to hepatitis. Had she received halothane, the subsequent hepatic illness would surely have been considered to be due to the anesthetic. But the gods smiled on halothane, and the next patient survived uneventfully.

Michael Johnstone was not the only one to test the new anesthetic. Cedric Prys-Roberts (personal communication to EIE, 15 Nov 12) remembered that

"it was also sent to Roger Bryce-Smith in Oxford, and to George Ellis at St Bartholomews Hospital. As a medical student early in 1957 I did an anaesthetic attachment for one month, mostly with George Ellis. He used halothane in a Marrett head (vaporizer within a circle system with CO_2 absorption) with spontaneous breathing after a thiopentone induction. He taught me to anaesthetize patients for retropubic prostatectomy (open abdomen, slight head down tilt) with this technique—his admonitions: 1) never squeeze the bag! (for obvious reasons)[1]—if the patient

stops breathing—leave them alone so long as they are pink—they will start breathing again when they are ready; 2) don't take the blood pressure—you will only be worried because it will be low, and; 3) don't turn down the halothane vaporizer setting unless you can feel an irregular pulse"

The University of Iowa was one of the clinical test centers for this new anesthetic. I (EIE) remember its arrival in large brown-glass bottles in 1956. We would smell it, impressed with the absence of pungency that the familiar ether imposed. Unwittingly, we found that it also dulled the sense of smell. Having sniffed from one of the new bottles, I found that there was scarcely any odor on sniffing a second time. My fellow residents ran this test on the new bottle with the same result. We concluded that it came from a weakened batch and poured the contents down the drain! How easy it was to induce anesthesia with this potent, non-flammable, non-pungent anesthetic that appeared to spare the liver from harm. And so it succeeded, in the process making hundreds of millions of dollars for ICI. By 1960, halothane had mostly swept the decks clear, largely displacing chloroform, ether, and cyclopropane from clinical practice.

The introduction of halothane did more than decrease the use of other inhaled anesthetics; it changed the practice of anesthesia. Because it had no pungency, was potent, and had a low solubility, anesthesia with halothane could be induced rapidly and without untoward airway responses such as excessive secretions, coughing and laryngospasm. Gone was the advantage of premedication with morphine (to hasten induction, decrease the need for inhaled anesthetic, and depress the response to airway irritation) and scopolamine (to minimize the appearance of secretions and decrease the remembrance of the terror of induction of anesthesia). Add to this that morphine imposed disadvantageous effects: unlike ether, halothane decreased breathing, an effect that administration of morphine enhanced. In addition, morphine increased postoperative nausea and vomiting. Thus the elimination of morphine-scopolamine premedication occurred, but surprisingly it did not occur immediately. Inertia is a powerful force, even in the face of fact and reason.

New Vaporizers

Although the earliest great anesthetists understood the need to control the concentration of anesthetic delivered to the patient, such control was usually unknown or ignored in favor of looking for and being guided by the patient's responses to the anesthetic being delivered—the signs of anesthetic depth so beautifully described by Snow, [12] and later, Guedel [13]. These signs could however lead the anesthetist astray. The art of deciphering these signs was less than perfect, even in the best of hands. Compounding the problem was a lack of knowledge of the anesthetic

---

[1] The ventilation would potentially increase the inspired and alveolar halothane concentrations to lethal levels because of the use of the in-circuit vaporizer.

concentration that the patient breathed. The patient breathing from a gauze mask wetted with ether or chloroform breathed a concentration that might be anything! A few "non-rebreathing" vaporizers might deliver a known concentration, but these were part of wasteful systems, systems in which all the flow of gases went through the vaporizer and the patient did not breathe the gas again. Some vaporizers delivered a graded concentration (e.g., the Boyles vaporizer), but with these the anesthetist knew only that he/she delivered more or less anesthetic when the vaporizer dial was adjusted up or down. Where a vaporizer was used in a rebreathing system (a system in which the patient rebreathed the anesthetic after carbon dioxide had been extracted from the rebreathed gases), again the control was up or down but the specific concentration remained unknown. The importance of rebreathing with such a system was doubly risky. Not only was the amount added by the vaporizer unknown, the extent of rebreathing was also unknown.

The anesthetic gases (nitrous oxide, ethylene, and cyclopropane), gases as opposed to the vapor anesthetics like halothane, could be delivered in known concentrations. The concentration of cyclopropane delivered to a rebreathing system could be accurately calculated from the readings on the flowmeters delivering oxygen and cyclopropane: if the cyclopropane flowmeter indicated a flow of 200 ml/min and the oxygen flowmeter indicated 800 ml/min, then the delivered concentration of cyclopropane was 20%. But these gases were either on their way out (ethylene and cyclopropane), or had insufficient potency to be used by themselves (nitrous oxide).

The Copper Kettle

The ease of calculation of concentrations of gaseous anesthetics like cyclopropane did not apply to volatile liquids and their vapors, such as ether or chloroform. In the late 1940s, Lucien Morris saw that it could. If a known flow of oxygen could be delivered through a liquid anesthetic such as ether, that anesthetic would be added to the stream in a known concentration, a concentration determined by the vapor pressure of the anesthetic relative to barometric pressure.

In the late 1940s, Morris began work on his invention of the Copper Kettle, with delivery of the first commercial version in 1951 [14]. Why copper? For the same reason that Snow had made his vaporizer of copper—great heat conductivity and thus stability of temperature in the face of cooling by vaporization of anesthetic. The Copper Kettle enabled the precise prediction of the anesthetic concentration delivered to the anesthetic circuit (the rebreathing system). Many anesthetists disliked the Copper Kettle because it required a calculation to apply properly, but, my, it did work.

It arrived at a propitious time. Although it was invented to allow a precise delivery of chloroform, it could be used for

the precise delivery of any volatile anesthetic. The discovery and release of halothane followed soon after the introduction of the Copper Kettle—and the Copper Kettle could be (and was) used to deliver halothane. The safe use of halothane demanded more control over the delivery of anesthesia than did ether. Halothane was far more dangerous because it was more potent, [15] and less soluble in blood [16, 17]. Add to this the absence of pungency and a high vapor pressure, and it is easy to understand that halothane could produce anesthesia with dangerous rapidity. Dangerous because it depressed breathing [18] and the circulation [7, 19] whereas ether might not, or even do the opposite [7, 20, 21]. There were imitations (equally good) of the Copper Kettle (e.g., the Vernitrol®—perhaps from "vernier control"). They, too, were used for the safer delivery of halothane and other modern inhaled anesthetics.

The Variable Bypass Vaporizer

The Cyprane Company circumvented the anesthetist's fear of algebra—of having to calculate the concentration produced by the Copper Kettle. In the last half of the 1950s, Cyprane introduced (at great expense and profit) the variable bypass vaporizer, the Fluotec®, to accompany the introduction of halothane (with the commercial name Fluothane®). The algebra-challenged anesthesia community in the US welcomed the Fluotec®. The variable bypass vaporizer dial gave an immediate reading of the delivered anesthetic concentration (no calculations needed), largely unaffected by inflow rate or room temperature. That, alone, would probably have ensured the success of the Fluotec® (and its imitations). In the US, Ayerst Laboratories, the purveyor of halothane, added to the incentive by offering the Fluotec® free with a minimum purchase of halothane. The same approach was not used in the worldwide promotion of halothane where less safe vaporizers (e.g., Boyles) continued in use. The decision by Ayerst to donate Fluotecs to institutions purchasing halothane accelerated the acceptance of halothane. It also hastened the demise of the competing Copper Kettle and Vernitrol®.

Polio Prompts the Development of Intensive Care Medicine (ICM) and Intensive Care Units (ICUs)

A Plague Strikes Copenhagen Poliomyelitis (polio) has afflicted humans since the dawn of history. It comes and goes, is sometimes mild and is sometimes crushing, with a substantial fraction of the population severely affected. In the last 5 months of 1952, Copenhagen, a city of 1.2 million, was struck by such a severe attack [22]. The Blegdam Hospital of 500 beds received approximately 3000 patients suffering from polio, roughly a third of whom evidenced paralysis, including a "high incidence of respiratory insufficiency with or without impairment of swallowing". Over 300 patients had this "bulbar polio." [22] At the peak of the epidemic in early September, 50 cases were admitted daily with 10% of them breathing inadequately. Death was erroneously considered to result from viral infection of the base of the brain [23, 24].

Compare these circumstances with those from previous times. From 1934 through 1944, Blegdam had admitted 76 cases of polio with respiratory failure requiring use of cuirass ventilators. Of these patients, 80% died [22]. Blegdam was unprepared to deal with the 1952 onslaught, having one tank respirator (an Emerson) and 6 largely ineffective cuirass ventilators. HC Lassen, the Chief Physician, gave his estimate of the grave situation in which he found his patients:

> "I do not want to dramatize the state of affairs existing in the middle of August 1952, but it certainly was desperate! Nearly all our patients with bulbar poliomyelitis had died! On August 25 we decided to call into consultation our anaesthetist colleague, Dr. Bjørn Ibsen…." [22]

The Ibsen Plan and Its Consequences Ibsen had trained in anesthesia for a year at the Massachusetts General Hospital, learning and applying the principles of positive pressure ventilation. He saw this as the best approach to dealing with the critical situation. Lassen agreed, and together they implemented a program designed by Ibsen. A tracheotomy was performed on each patient evidencing bulbar polio, a cuffed tube was inserted through the tracheotomy, and manual positive pressure ventilation was maintained via a bag connected to a humidified source of 50% oxygen/50% nitrogen through a to-and-fro canister. But who would supply the ventilation? "At the height of the epidemic the staff of doctors permanently on the job was 35–40; we had about 600 trained nurses and 250 medical students coming in daily, working in relays." [22] At times, dental students were added to the work force. Working 6-hour shifts, each had to supply continuous positive pressure ventilation, monitor the patient, manage tracheal secretions that might accumulate, and alert attending physicians to problems. The mortality rate in this cohort with bulbar polio decreased from 90% to 25%-still high but a rate that was less than it probably would have been without Ibsen's intervention.

The principles learned in the 1952 Copenhagen polio epidemic revolutionized the management of sick patients requiring intensive care. An appreciation of the therapeutic power of intensive care, of gathering similarly sick patients in one area for treatment such as ongoing support of ventilation, in short order led to intensive care medicine (ICM) and intensive care units (ICUs). Ibsen opened the first ICU a year later.

Part of the management of Ibsen's patients included the evaluation of the effectiveness of ventilation through analysis of respiratory gases (e.g., CO_2) in arterial blood, with an approach specifically devised during the epidemic by Poul Astrup [25]. Blood-gas analysis could be done, with cumbersome, time-consuming methods that could never have met the needs of Ibsen's far too numerous patients. Astrup's work shortened and simplified the process. It was a major step in the evolution of blood gas analysis, culminating in Severinghaus' 1958 construction of the first 3-function (O_2, CO_2, pH) blood gas apparatus that is used in some form in every modern hospital [25].

And, of course, the epidemic and the need for controlled ventilation prompted the development of automatic ventilators devised specifically to provide continuous intermittent positive pressure ventilation without fail, 24 hours a day, 7 days a week. It seemed as though an infinite number of anesthetists and engineers came to see what happened in Copenhagen and went home and made a newer, better IPPV ventilator. Many were primitive yet enjoyed widespread and long use (e.g., the Radclifffe ventilator introduced in 1953). Engström in Sweden invented one of the world's most successful mechanical ventilators, tested in the 1952 Copenhagen epidemic and the 1953 Swedish polio epidemic. The British parallel to the Engstrom was the Smith-Clarke ventilator. Diverse and often less expensive ventilators followed (e.g., the Howells, the Manley, and the Barnet ventilators). US Engineers Bird and Bennett developed ventilators powered by compressed gas. And all the above led to a need for and the development of personnel to manage the ventilator. This took two general forms. In the US, the respiratory therapist with specific training and credentials managed respiratory care. Elsewhere, ICU nurses with special additional training managed the ventilator. All of the above developed because of the confluence of a polio epidemic and a few visionaries.

A postscript. In 1954, Lassen [26] and Honey [27] reported survival of patients with severe tetanus who received curare and mechanical ventilation. They applied the lessons learned in the 1952 polio epidemic.

The First Massive Anesthesia Outcome Study

Curare Has a Dark Side

Like today's consortiums studying cancer and other medical problems, consortiums have studied anesthetic-related outcomes, sometimes with surprising results. Beecher and Todd led the first major consortium in anesthesia to study a serious outcome, an investigation of the factors predicting death after anesthesia in 599,500 patients in 10 university institutions. They concluded that curare had a dark side, an unexpected association with a 6-fold increase in mortality [28, 29]. 1:2100 deaths occurred in the absence of curare and 1:370 in cases in which curare was given (see Beecher and Todd,

Table 8.2 Severity of surgery and increased death rates associated with curare

Curare	Surgery	Total Number of Patients	Number of Anesthetic Deaths	Anesthetic Death Rate	Increased Death Rate With Curare
No	Minor	349,939	69	1:5071	
Yes	Minor	205,519	162	1:1270	4.0-fold
No	Major	27,777	12	1:2314	
Yes	Major	16,313	85	1:192	12-fold

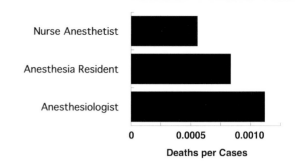

Fig. 8.5 Beecher and Todd [28, 29] found a lower mortality associated with the administration of anesthesia by nurse anesthetists. (Data from their Table XIX B)

Table 13) [28, 29]. Many of the cases not given curare were minor cases and critics might have suggested that this skewed the results. But dividing the cases into minor and major gave qualitatively similar findings (Table 8.2). Similarly, physical status did not affect the ratio: Those with PS 1, 2, and 5 had death rates of 1:660 if given curare and 1:3100 if not, whereas those with PS 3, 4, 6, and 7 had respective death rates of 1:96 versus 1:560. Beecher and Todd's Table 16 demonstrates that over the five years of the study, deaths associated with the use of thiopental progressively decreased when not accompanied by curare (from 1:720 to 1:3400) whereas they remained constant when curare was given (1:380 to 1:420).

An additional subanalysis examined the effect of ether vs cyclopropane, with and without curare, on mortality. In the absence of curare, mortality was similar with ether (1:2500) and cyclopropane (1:3300). But when curare was added, mortality was greater with ether (1;250) than with cyclopropane (1:1200). We know that awakening occurs far slower after anesthesia with the more soluble ether, and perhaps this exaggerated any residual effect of curare in the partially paralyzed patient lying unattended in the recovery room or ward, They thereby might have had a greater likelihood of airway obstruction, hypoxia or other untoward respiratory event.

Initial Rejection of the Beecher-Todd Results

The anesthesia community did not immediately embrace Beecher and Todd's conclusions, perhaps because the results were published in a surgical journal [28], and surgeons then sometimes suggested to anesthetists that they were doing something dangerous. Some surgeons insisted that anesthetists refrain from using the "deadly" curare.

Abajian and colleagues faulted Beecher and Todd's study [30]. A primary concern was Beecher and Todd's failure to gather data concerning "…site of operation, depth of relaxation required, duration of anesthesia and operation, and severity of surgical trauma." Indeed, such confounding variables might have explained the results without resort to a consideration of the effect of muscle relaxants. Abajian et al. also noted statistical lapses and anomalies. For example, over the course of this 5-year study "…the use of 'curare' was increas-

ing by 64 per cent (from 1:18 to 1:11) (Table XII), (while) the total anesthesia death rate was falling by 23 per cent (from 1:1440 to 1:1880) (Table XXVIII)." [30] They emphasized the likelihood of an associative rather than a causal relationship of curare and death. Nowhere did they raise a question concerning reversal of neuromuscular blockade.

In a further rebuttal, Dripps et al. performed a retrospective study for a 10-year period (1947–1957) from which they culled 33,224 patients who had either spinal anesthesia or general anesthesia with muscle relaxants [31]. No deaths

> "attributable to anesthesia (arose) in the 16,000 physically fit patients anesthetized by either technique. As the patients' physical condition worsened, deaths related to anesthesia increased in incidence…No evidence of an inherent toxicity of muscle relaxants could be found. When deaths were related to the use of muscle relaxants, errors of omission or commission were always apparent."

Relaxant was thought to contribute to death in 12 patients; in 8 of these, death occurred because of "failure to provide adequate pulmonary exchange." The death rate in those receiving relaxants was 1:536. Nowhere did they raise a question concerning reversal of neuromuscular blockade.

Some of Beecher and Todd's findings seemed to fly in the face of reason. Training as a physician anesthetist did not appear to decrease mortality (Fig. 8.5). Beecher and Todd explained:

> "Common observation indicates that the physician specialist on the average cares for the patient faced with the more trying and difficult operation than does the nurse, even though both groups work with a comparable number of patients in poor physical status. This is supported by the data of Table XIX, where it can be seen that although the physician specialist anesthetizes only half as many patients as the nurse, he is charged with an equal number of anesthesia deaths. In the light of this, to deny the greater difficulty of the physician specialist's cases is to reduce the matter to an absurdity where one would be obliged to argue that the physician's learning was a dangerous thing."

But Beecher and Todd's data did not show that the nurse anesthetists were assigned less major surgery (this wasn't stated) or less vulnerable patients. Regarding the latter point, of the patients anesthetized by nurse anesthetists, 14% were listed as Physical Status 3, 4, 6, or 7 (PS 6 corresponds to the current Physical Status 3E and 4E and 7 corresponds to 5) whereas only 12% of those anesthetized by anesthesiologists were given such a PS. Thus, if anything, the nurses anesthetized sicker patients. For a moment consider another possibility that might explain the lower mortality associated with anesthesia given by nurse anesthetists. By the late 1940s, over 50 schools for the formal training of nurse anesthetists had come into existence [32]. Anesthesiologists and nurse anesthetists may have been trained differently, but training was given to many nurse anesthetists. Perhaps because of their lesser medical background, nurse anesthetists were trained to follow "cookbook" guidelines, faithfully giving anesthesia by prescribed methods, an approach that we now appreciate may have certain safety advantages, particularly when less options are available [33, 34]. They may have been less flexible in their approach to anesthesia, but perhaps as Mies van der Rohe said, sometimes "Less is more."

Residual Blockade Probably Underlay the Greater Mortality

The increased mortality associated with curare in Beecher and Todd's study was probably due to the inadequate reversal of residual paralysis. We knew how to reverse the paralysis with drugs such as neostigmine, but often we didn't. Perhaps we thought, "Well, the patient can breathe and move; isn't that enough?" The patient could move, could breathe, but had less than normal strength. Perhaps full strength was needed to deal with vomit that might appear in the back of the throat or to cough sufficiently to expel mucous deep within the lungs. Have we learned from this? Maybe less than completely. A 2005 outcomes study of a cohort derived from 870,000 patients, again suggested the potential lethality of the residual effects of muscle relaxants whose effects have not been antagonized [35].

Research in Anesthesia

The preceeding discussions suggest the clinical focus of research in anesthesia in the 1950s. Attention was paid to the development of new anesthetics (e.g., halothane) and anesthetic adjuvants (succinylcholine) and to increasing the control over their delivery and safety (Copper Kettle and variable-bypass vaporizer). Attention was paid to the new clinical management of disasters such as the Copenhagen polio epidemic, the associated clinical research leading to intensive care medicine, new ventilators, and modern blood gas analysis. Attention was paid to outcomes as in Beecher and Todd's controversial massive study.

In largest part, research support came from industry or the personal contributions of individuals who gave their time and thought. Support also came from government agencies, not necessarily those we think of today. For example, the Medical Research and Development Board, Office of the Surgeon General, Department of the Army underwrote Beecher and Todd's study. Private sources also supplied support. The Wellcome Trust gave $140,000 to support anesthesia research at McGill University. "The Trust award is seen by McGill as a great breakthrough for the specialty, which is unsupported by British Research Councils and other grant-giving agencies at this time." (At http://www.wellcome.ac.uk/timeline/, type in Anaesthesia in the search box.) The Trust also gave $69,000 to fund a Chair of Anesthesiology in New York. The considerable increase in support for anesthesia research by the National Institutes of Health began in the next decade.

Other Important Events in the 1950s

1950

Pain Management At mid-century, interest in regional anesthesia waned, partly because new drugs producing general anesthesia made general anesthesia more attractive, and partly because of issues of duration and safety of regional anesthesia (e.g., the development of paralysis after spinal anesthesia) [36]. Notwithstanding this view, the 1950s saw the rise to prominence of giants in regional anesthesia, leaders such as John Bonica and Daniel Moore. They followed in the footsteps of previous giants in the US (e.g., John Lundy and Emery Rovenstine) and the largely German approaches to methods of peripheral and neuraxial (think August Bier) nerve block developed within 2-3 decades of the discovery of the local anesthetic properties of cocaine in 1884. Bonica enlarged the importance of regional anesthesia and particularly the management of pain control, including the development of pain clinics. At mid-century, both Moore and Bonica published now classic books on regional anesthesia and pain management.

Dogs and Cats Benefit, Too Humans were not the only beneficiaries of the growth in the specialty. UK veterinarians Barbara Weaver and Leslie Hall became the first veterinarians to exclusively practice anesthesia. Weaver wrote: "In the 1950s when Leslie and I became interested in anaesthesia, realizing we were some 50 years behind the 'medics' we adapted human techniques for our patients." (Personal communication to Eugene Steffey, 2010).

Management of Postoperative Nausea and Vomiting (PONV) The earliest anesthetics, nitrous oxide and ether, produced PONV, perhaps in part as a consequence of their capacity to stimulate the sympathetic nervous system. For the first century of anesthesia, PONV was accepted as an inevitable byproduct of anesthesia, but then some questioned whether patients really needed to suffer this side effect. By 1950, the antihistamine dramamine had been discovered and was used to treat motion sickness. A natural extension was to apply this remedy to the management of PONV [37]. Thus began the discovery and application of a series of antiemetics including the antihistamine cyclizine (1955); phenothizines (1960): the dopamine receptor antagonist droperidol (1961); and the serotonin antagonist ondansetron (1980s).

1951

A New Rapid and Short-acting Muscle Relaxant Daniel Bovet had noted the paralytic effect of succinylcholine in 1949, and this neuromuscular blocking drug was released for clinical use in 1951. It had qualities that anesthetists sought in a drug to produce relaxation, particularly a rapid onset (more rapid than any other neuromuscular blocking drug) and a faster offset than the long lasting curare. It seemed just right for the anesthetist wanting a brief period of relaxation such as that needed for the insertion of a tracheal tube. Indeed, at first it seemed perfect: "*Its use is not accompanied by unwanted side-effects and the incidence of post-operative complications after its use is low.*" [38] Its rapid offset was due to its degradation by plasma cholinesterase. But it wasn't perfect. It could cause prolonged neuromuscular blockade after being used for prolonged periods of time, or in patients who (it was subsequently discovered) lacked the ability to break the drug down. The lack of the enzyme, plasma cholinesterase, was genetically determined and unraveling this mystery led to a new appreciation of the potential pharmacological consequences of genetic abnormalities, and to the development of a new science called pharmacogenetics, a term Freidrich Vogel invented in 1959 [39].

1952

Chloroprocaine, a New Local Anesthetic Released for clinical use in 1951, the local anesthetic chloroprocaine did not receive immediate acclaim. It was an ester-linked local anesthetic and seemed therefore to be a reversion to anesthetics like tetracaine and procaine, each of which had drawbacks, including toxic reactions or allergic responses to p-amino benzoic acid. Many considered that these had been minimized with the release for clinical use of the amide-linked local anesthetic, lidocaine. But chloroprocaine had an underappreciated advantage, a vulnerability to rapid degradation

by plasma cholinesterases. It remained intact as long as it wasn't in blood, but once in blood it was degraded and its local anesthetic toxicity removed. This benefit led to its resurrection decades later.

Beecher and Human Experimentation In the 1950s, Henry Beecher made several influential suggestions regarding human experimentation. In 1952, noting the powerful effect that placebos have, he argued for their use in human trials as an essential control [40]. In 1959, his thoughts about controlled experiments led him to argue for informed consent for all participants in studies on humans. To oversee the imposition of informed consent required the development of Institutional Review Boards in the succeeding decade. All of these developments govern the conduct of human research today.

1953

Virginia Apgar Scores Virginia Apgar, then the leader of obstetrical anesthesia at Columbia University, was at breakfast with a medical student who asked her how she would evaluate the physical status of a newborn child. "Easy" she is reported to have said, immediately writing the five elements of her 10-point Score on a cafeteria napkin. After a bit more work, she published her eponymous score, "the Apgar", which defines the condition of all babies born in the world today, correlating closely with the immediate well-being of the newborn [41]. Later in her career, "Ginny" worked to prevent crippling birth defects, becoming president of the March of Dimes Foundation. She received the ASA Distinguished Service Award in 1961.

Also in 1953, Bonica published the first edition of his classic book, "The Management of Pain", and Gibbons successfully applied a heart-lung machine, allowing greater time for surgeons to work in a bloodless field without injury to the brain.

1954

An Invention of War Becomes One of Peace Luft invented the infrared analyzer in Germany in 1937 [42]. It had been put to various war-time purposes (e.g., tracking the V-bombs). Liston-Becker used the invention to manufacture and sell an infrared analyzer in the early 1950s [43]. Ultimately, this device became a ubiquitous bit of operating room furniture, and a savior to many patients. It allowed a breath-by-breath estimate of the adequacy of breathing (by the measurement of CO_2) [44] and the adequacy of anesthesia (by measurement of the vapors causing the anesthesia). Perhaps most importantly, it certified the presence of respired gases by the detection of CO_2, and thereby guaranteed the placement of a tracheal tube into the trachea rather than the esophagus.

Were Neuroaxial Blocks Safe? For various reasons, by mid-century, concern had been raised regarding the safety of local anesthetics, particularly when delivered to the spinal canal. Cases of paralysis had been reported [36]. In 1954, Dripps and Vandam reported the results of a prospective study of 10,098 patients given spinal anesthesia with tetracaine, finding no severe neurologic problem [45]. Coupled with the introduction of aminoamide local anesthetics such as lidocaine, their findings supported a resurgence of interest in regional techniques in the US.

And Incidentally in 1954 … Hall and Weaver introduced balanced anesthesia including curare to the clinical management of dogs and cats, not finding the bronchospasm in dogs that had troubled Stuart Cullen. US surgeons Harrison and Murray successfully transplanted a human kidney.
James Elam showed that medically untrained individuals taught to maintain a clear airway without a tracheal tube could provide normal levels of oxygen and carbon dioxide for prolonged periods with Expired Air Resuscitation (mouth to mouth breathing). Elam persuaded Peter Safar to join a crusade to promote Expired Air Resuscitation. By 1958, Safar had demonstrated that laypersons could relieve obstruction of the airway by the tongue, by thrusting the jaw forwards and tilting the head backwards. Also in 1958, Safar developed the first ICU in the US.

In one of anesthesia's most quoted articles, Mapleson described how systems not using carbon dioxide absorption (open systems) worked to assure normal carbon dioxide levels in the patient breathing from such systems [46]. Such systems rely on a sufficient inflow rate to eliminate carbon dioxide. Mapleson told us what those flows were.

1955

The Birth of the World Federation of Societies of Anaesthesiologists (WFSA) Although still in disarray consequent to the ravages of World War II, remnant members of the Société d'études sur l'anesthésie et l'analgésie (SEAA) organized an international congress in Paris in 1951. Societies from 32 countries considered founding an international society. Marcel Thalheimer, Secretary of the Société des Etudes, persisted in pursuing the organization of such a society, advancing the idea at the September 1951 Congress of Anaesthesia in London. Representatives of 32 societies elected an interim committee tasked with constructing the structure of a new international organization of anesthesiologists. From this came the WFSA, with its first meeting in Scheveningen, The Netherlands, in 1955. Societies from 28 countries contrib-

uted to the founding, including the International Anesthesia Research Society (IARS) from the US, one of Francis McMechan's creations. The IARS represented the US on the planning committee since the ASA preferred to remain an "Official Observer". Harold Griffith (then Chair of the Board of Trustees of the IARS) was elected as the first WFSA President. Establishment of the WFSA achieved McMechan's dream of an international organization of anesthesiologists.

1956

Nitrous Oxide Can Be Lethal In 1956, Lassen et al. attempted to minimize pain in patients suffering from tetanus by having them breathe nitrous oxide [47]. The therapy decreased pain, but over the course of days, the continued inhalation of nitrous oxide produced severe bone marrow depression and death. Was it something to do with prolonged administration of anesthetics or was there something peculiar to nitrous oxide (or both)? Decades later, the capacity of nitrous oxide to uniquely destroy a vital enzyme, methionine synthase, was shown [48]. The inactivation of methionine synthase led to a decreased availability of the essential amino acid methionine and decreased production of folate, essential for the production of DNA.

Also in 1956 The initials CRNA (Certified Registered Nurse Anesthetist) came into use in the US. At this time, a year was required to complete training in nurse anesthesia. This would more than double in subsequent years.

Methohexital (Brevital), a shorter-acting barbiturate was introduced. Because it stimulated the central nervous system, it competed poorly with thiopental—except for the anesthetic management of patients undergoing electroconvulsive therapy. It remains popular today for the management of such patients because it has less capacity to suppress the induction of convulsions.

1957: An Important Political Change that Ultimately Influenced Anesthesia

Six countries signed the Treaty of Rome, creating the European Economic Community (EEC) that grew to today's European Union (EU) of 27 member states with lots of opportunities and problems. Increasing mutual recognition of medical qualifications and harmonization of medical education accompanied this political process.

1959

Modern Outpatient Anesthesia Begins Canadian anesthetists Eric Webb and Horace Graves reported their 6-month experience with 494 surgical patients cared for as outpatients [49]. Others had earlier provided anesthesia to outpatients. In 1909, a Scot, James Nicoll, reported his experiences with this approach in approximately 9000 children [50]. Indeed, he may be the father of outpatient anesthesia. Ralph Waters had provided outpatient anesthesia in the 1910s [51], but it is Webb and Graves who started the modern move to this approach to anesthetic delivery, a move that expanded in the next decade.

Late 1950s

Resusci-Anne Norwegian toy-manufacturer, Åsmund Laerdal developed the mannequin "Resusci-Anne", used to teach cardiopulmonary resuscitation (CPR). Resusci-Anne was released in 1960. Laerdal's work complemented the thrust of the research by Peter Safar and James Elam on cardiopulmonary resuscitation. Resusci-Anne began the modern movement towards teaching with simulators.

Manufacturers Make Anesthesia Safer The late 1950s saw a mundane addition to the safety of anesthetic delivery, the invention of the Pin Index Safety System and Diameter Index Safety System by Wayne Hay and Harold May, employees of the Ohio Medical and Surgical Equipment Co. Prior to the invention and application of this system, a tank of nitrous oxide might be attached to the place normally occupied by an oxygen cylinder—with disastrous results from the delivery of gases lacking oxygen. Hay and May donated the resulting 1963 patents to the Compressed Gas Association facilitating the use of the system by all manufacturers, internationally. All patients having general anesthesia potentially benefited from their generous act.

Reprise

The effects of World War II accelerated—and retarded—the rise of modern anesthesia. It arrested development in Europe, the USSR, and Asia, but hastened development in the US. The recruitment (drafting) of physicians into the US Armed Services for a brief period of training in anesthesia, followed by a mandated practice of anesthesia, caused this acceleration. Physicians forced to learn and practice anesthesia often discovered that the calling pleased them. Succinylcholine became available in 1951. Perhaps the most important advance of the 1950s arose from Bjørn Ibsen's management of the 1952 polio epidemic in Copenhagen. His work led to the establishment of Intensive Care Medicine and Intensive Care Units, and to the development of ventilators and blood-gas analysis. The World Federation of Societies of Anaesthesiologists was founded in 1955. The advances in fluorine chemistry, needed to develop the atomic bomb paved the way for

Suckling's synthesis of the inhaled anesthetic halothane. Released for clinical use in 1956, halothane soon displaced essentially all its predecessors. Important to the safe delivery of halothane, our ability to control the delivery of inhaled anesthetics increased enormously with the invention of the Copper Kettle and variable bypass vaporizers. Muscle relaxants were first used in humans in 1942. In 1954 Beecher and Todd's outcomes research indicated that muscle relaxants could be a mixed blessing if not managed properly, if their residual effects were not reversed. In the 1950s we had two new drugs in addition to halothane—succinylcholine and chloroprocaine. Beecher successfully argued for the use of placebo-controlled experimentation, for the use of informed consent, and ultimately for the establishment of Institutional Review Boards (IRBs). Finally, in 1959, Webb and Graves reported their results with the first modern outpatient anesthesia.

References

1. Waisel DB. The role of World War II and the European theater of operations in the development of anesthesiology as a physician specialty in the USA. Anesthesiology. 2001;94:907–14.
2. Ruth HS. Postwar planning in anesthesiology. N Engl J Med. 1944;231:669–672.
3. Eger EI, 2nd. After you, please: the second Annual John W. Severinghaus Lecture on Translational Science. Anesthesiology. 2010;112:786–93.
4. Papper EM. The origins of the association of University Anesthesiologists. Anesth Analg. 1992;74:436–53.
5. Introduction to the 1964 Directory of the Association of University Anesthetists.
6. Scholler KL. Modification of the effects of chloroform on the rat liver. Brit J Anaesth. 1970;42:603–5.
7. Fiserova-Bergerova V. Metabolism and toxicity of 2,2,2-trifluoroethyl vinyl ether. Environ Health Perspect. 1977;21:225–30.
8. Eger EI, 2nd, Smith NT, Cullen DJ, Cullen BF, Gregory GA. A comparison of the cardiovascular effects of halothane, fluroxene, ether and cyclopropane in man: a resume. Anesthesiology. 1971;34:25–41.
9. Raventos J. The action of Fluothane—a new volatile anaesthetic. Br J Pharmacol. 1956;11:394–410.
10. Johnstone M. The human cardiovascular response to Fluothane anaesthesia. Br J Anaesth. 1956;28:392–410.
11. Anand SS, Soni MG, Vaidya VS, Murthy SN, Mumtaz MM, Mehendale HM. Extent and timeliness of tissue repair determines the dose-related hepatotoxicity of chloroform. Int J Toxicol. 2003;22:25–33.
12. Snow J. On the inhalation of the vapour of ether in surgical operations: containing a description of the various stages of etherization, and a statement of the result of nearly eighty operations in which ether has been employed in St. George's and University College Hospitals. London: John Churchill; 1847. pp. 1–88.
13. Guedel AE. Inhalation anesthesia: a fundamental guide. New York: Macmillan Co; 1937. pp. 1–172.
14. Morris LE. A new vaporizer for liquid anesthetic agents. Anesthesiology. 1952;13:587–93.
15. Quasha AL, Eger EI, II, Tinker JH. Determination and applications of MAC. Anesthesiology. 1980;53:315–34.
16. Larson CP, Jr, Eger EI, II, Severinghaus JW. The solubility of halothane in blood and tissue homogenates. Anesthesiology. 1962;23:349–55.

17. Eger EI, II, Shargel RO, Merkel G. Solubility of diethyl ether in water, blood and oil. Anesthesiology. 1963;24:676–8.

18. Munson ES, Larson CP, Jr, Babad AA, Regan MJ, Buechel DR, Eger EI, II. The effects of halothane, fluroxene and cyclopropane on ventilation: a comparative study in man. Anesthesiology. 1966;27:716–28.

19. Eger EI, II, Smith NT, Stoelting RK, Cullen DJ, Kadis LB, Whitcher CE. Cardiovascular effects of halothane in man. Anesthesiology. 1970;32:396–409.

20. Larson CP, Jr, Eger EI, II, Muallem M, Buechel DR, Munson ES, Eisele JH. The effects of diethyl ether and methoxyflurane on ventilation: II. A comparative study in man. Anesthesiology. 1969;30:174–84.

21. Gregory GA, Eger EI, II, Smith NT, Cullen BF, Cullen DJ. The cardiovascular effects of diethyl ether in man. Anesthesiology. 1971;34:19–24.

22. Lassen HC. The epidemic of poliomyelitis in Copenhagen, 1952. Proc R Soc Med. 1954;47:67–71.

23. Wackers GL. Modern anaesthesiological principles for bulbar polio: manual IPPR in the 1952 polio-epidemic in Copenhagen. Acta Anaesthesiol Scand. 1994;38:420–31.

24. Lassen HC. A preliminary report on the 1952 epidemic of poliomyelitis in Copenhagen with special reference to the treatment of acute respiratory insufficiency. Lancet 1953;1:37–41.

25. Severinghaus JW, Astrup PB. History of blood gas analysis. Int Anesthesiol Clin. 1987;25:1–224.

26. Lassen HC, Bjorneboe M, Ibsen B, Neukirch F. Treatment of tetanus with curarisation, general anaesthesia, and intratracheal positive-pressure ventilation. Lancet. 1954;267:1040–4.

27. Honey GE, Dwyer BE, Smith AC, Spalding JM. Tetanus treated with tubocurarine and intermittent positive-pressure respiration. Brit Med J. 1954;2:442–3.

28. Beecher HK, Todd DP. A study of the deaths associated with anesthesia and surgery: based on a study of 599, 548 anesthesias in ten institutions 1948–1952, inclusive. Ann Surg 1954;140:2–35.

29. Beecher HK, Todd DP. A study of the deaths associated with anesthesia and surgery. Based on a study of 599,548 anesthesias in 10 institutions, 1948–1953, inclusive. Publication Number 254, American Lecture Series, edited by John Adriani. Charles C. Thomas, Springfield, Illinois, 1954, pp. 3–66.

30. Abajian J, Arrowood JG, Barrett RH, Dwyer CS, Eversole UH, Fine JH, Hand LV, Howrie WC, Marcus PS, Martin SJ, Nicholson MJ, Saklad E, Saklad M, Sellman P, Smith RM, Woodbridge PD. Critique of "A study of the deaths associated with anesthesia and surgery". Ann Surg. 1955;142:138–41.

31. Dripps RD, Lamont A, Eckenhorr JE. The role of anaesthesia in surgical mortality. J Am Med Assoc. 1961;178:261–6.

32. Richards L. Second award of appreciation. J Am Assoc Nurs Anesth. 1948;16:331–3.

33. Pronovost P, Jenckes M, Dorman T, Garrett E, Breslow MJ, Rosenfeld BA, Lipsett PA, Bass E. Organizational characteristics of intensive care units related to outcomes of abdominal aortic surgery. J Amer Med Assoc. 1999;281:1310–7.

34. Pronovost PJ. We need leaders: The 48th Annual Rovenstine Lecture. Anesthesiology. 2010;112:779–85.

35. Arbous MS, Meursing AE, van Kleef JW, de Lange JJ, Spoormans HH, Touw P, Werner FM, Grobbee DE. Impact of anesthesia management characteristics on severe morbidity and mortality. Anesthesiology. 2005;102:257–68.

36. Kennedy F, Effron AS, Perry G. The grave spinal cord paralyses caused by spinal anesthesia. Surg Gynecol Obstet. 1950;91:385–98.

37. Rudolph CJ, Park DD, Hamilton C. Treatment of postanesthesia nausea and vomiting. J Am Med Assoc. 1950;144:1283.

38. Foldes FF, McNall PG, Borrego-Hinojosa JM. Succinylcholine: a new approach to muscular relaxation in anesthesiology. N Engl J Med. 1952;247:596–600.

39. Vogel F. Moderne problem der humangenetik. Ergeb Inn Med U Kinderheilk. 1959;12:52–125.

40. Beecher HK. Experimental pharmacology and measurement of the subjective response. Science. 1952;116:157–62.

41. Apgar V. A proposal for a new method of evaluation of the newborn infant. Curr Res Anesth Analg. 1953;32:260–7.

42. Luft K. Über eine neue Methode der registrierenden Gasanalyse mit Hilfe der Absorption ultraroter Strahlen ohne spektrale Zerlegung. Ztschrf Techn Phys. 1943;24:97–104.

43. Siebecker KL, Mendenhall JT, Emanuel DA. Carbon dioxide in anesthetic atmospheres as measured by the Liston-Becker (infrared aborption) gas analyzer; preliminary report. J Thorac Surg. 1954;27:468–76.

44. Dubois AB, Fowler RC, Soffer A, Fenn WO. Alveolar CO_2 measured by expiration into the rapid infrared analyzer. J Appl Physiol. 1952;4:526–34.

45. Dripps RD, Vandam LD. Long-term follow-up of patients who received 10,098 spinal anesthetics: failure to discover major neurological sequelae. J Am Med Assoc. 1954;156:1486–91.

46. Mapleson WW. The elimination of rebreathing in various semi-closed anaesthetic systems. Br J Anaesth. 1954;26:323–32.

47. Lassen HCA, Henriksen E, Neukirch F, Kristensen HS. Treatment of tetanus. Severe bone-marrow depression after prolonged nitrous-oxide anaesthesia. Lancet. 1956;1:527–30.

48. Deacon R, Lumb M, Perry J, Chanarin I, Minty B, Halsey MJ, Nunn JF. Selective inactivation of vitamine B12 by nitrous oxide. Lancet. 1978;2:1023–4.

49. Webb E, Graves HB. Anesthesia for the ambulant patient. Anesth Analg. 1959;38:359–63.

50. Nicoll JH. The surgery of infancy. Br Med J. 1909;18:753–4.

51. Waters RM. The down-town anesthesia clinic. Am J Surg. 1919;39(suppl):71–3.

Major Anesthetic Themes in the 1960s

Lawrence J. Saidman, Rod N. Westhorpe and Edmond I Eger II

Summary

Several developments dominated progress in anesthesia in the 1960s. Consistent with the maturing of a clinical specialty, anesthesia related research began to emerge in selected departments—mostly within the US and Europe. Emanuel Papper's actions as special consultant to the Institute of General Medical Sciences facilitated greater NIH funding earmarked for anesthesiology, particularly for studies examining inhaled anesthetic pharmacokinetics, pharmacodynamics, and toxicity. Investigations of toxicity culminated in the National Halothane Study largely exonerating halothane as a hepatotoxin. Pharmaceutical companies introduced several new anesthetic drugs (pancuronium ketamine, fentanyl, droperidol, bupivacaine, and enflurane), advancing patient care and facilitating faculty development via interactions between academia and industry, largely in the US and Europe. Surgical subspecialty development spurred parallel developments in anesthesiology, promoting targeted research efforts in obstetrical, neurosurgical, and cardiac anesthesia.

Expanding clinical research increased concerns regarding the ethical treatment of human subjects. Beecher's landmark article in 1966 exposed questionably ethical clinical research performed without informed consent, and led to the requirement for prior review and approval by Institutional Review Boards (IRBs), revolutionizing clinical research practices. Manpower concerns about the specialty in the US, as a result of a relatively small number of American medical graduates (AMGs) selecting training in anesthesiology, resulted in an ASA program underwriting medical student anesthesia preceptorships. This program was ultimately associated with a tripling in the number of graduates electing anesthesiology as a career choice. It also helped that several factors increased economic opportunities in anesthesia, including support from Medicare.

International development of the specialty was reflected by formation of the Latin American Confederation of Societies of Anesthesiologists in Lima Peru in 1962 and the first International Training Center of Anesthesiologists of the World Federation of Societies of Anaesthesiologists (WFSA) in Caracas in 1967. In 1963, the European Union of medical Specialists stipulated training requirements for anesthesiologists and in the 1960s formal training programs were established in many European countries for nurse anesthetists.

World Events in the 1960s

Theodore Maiman's demonstration of a working laser and release of the oral contraceptive opened the decade. Regarding the increasing use of LSD, Jefferson Airplane's Paul Kantner famously said "If you can remember anything about the sixties, you weren't really there." Soviet cosmonaut Yuri Gagarin orbited the Earth, and Kennedy established the Peace Corps. Then, a series of near-cataclysmic events descended. In 1961, the US invasion of Cuba (The Bay of Pigs) failed.

In 1962, the USSR deployed ballistic missiles in Cuba aimed toward the US, provoking a crisis that came within days of initiating a nuclear war. LJS remembers becoming temporarily deranged and stocking up on Dinty Moore Stew the night before the missiles were to fly. In the course of 15 years (mainly the 1960s), the US progressively increased its commitment to South Vietnam in its War with North Vietnam, at its peak sending more than 500,000 troops. In the US, assassinations of President John F Kennedy (1963), Senator Robert Kennedy (1968), and civil rights leader Dr. Martin Luther King (1968) caused extreme political and social unrest. Combined with protests against the Vietnam war, these events destroyed the presidency of Lyndon Johnson and caused the election of Richard Nixon. The 1967 Six Day War between Israel and Egypt, Syria, and Jordan changed the military balance of power in the Middle East and increased the West's dependency upon OPEC. But it didn't matter because this was The Summer of Love in San Francisco. In 1965, Richard Feynman was awarded the Nobel prize in physics. He paved the way to a greater understanding of the quantum

L. J. Saidman (✉)
Department of Anesthesia, Stanford University, Stanford, CA, USA
e-mail: lsaidman@stanford.edu

R. N. Westhorpe
Melbourne, Australia
e-mail: westhorpe@netspace.net.au

E. I Eger II
Department of Anesthesia and Perioperative Care,
University of California, San Francisco, CA, USA
e-mail: egere@anesthesia.ucsf.edu

E. I Eger II et al. (eds.), *The Wondrous Story of Anesthesia,* DOI 10.1007/978-1-4614-8441-7_9, © Edmond I Eger, MD 2014

nature of the atom, and pioneered far-reaching advances in chemistry. Finally, Neil Armstrong and Buzz Aldrin walked on the moon, ending the 1960s on a positive note by opening the age of Space exploration.

Anesthetic-Induced Organ Toxicity and Metabolism of Inhaled Anesthetics

The decade opened with concerns regarding halothane-induced morbidity following sporadic reports of post anesthetic hepatic toxicity [1]. These reports prompted the Committee on Anesthesia of the National Academy of Science-National Research Council (NAS-NRC) to conduct a retrospective, 34-institution 850,000-patient study (the National Halothane Study) [2] to assess the risk of hepatic injury and death from anesthesia with halothane [3]. The study showed that halothane did not increase the overall risk of hepatic injury or death, decreasing the immediate level of concern.

Nonetheless, reports of rare, otherwise unexplained cases of injury sustained concerns regarding halothane hepatotoxicity. These led some anesthetists to avoid using halothane in patients undergoing liver surgery or in patients with prior signs of hepatic injury following halothane…or using halothane at all. Supporting a causal relationship between halothane administration and hepatic injury, shortly after publication of the National Halothane Study, Rehder et al demonstrated significant hepatic metabolism of halothane [4]. Once the patent on halothane expired, its low cost and many advantageous properties dictated its continued use through the next several decades, especially in less developed countries. In developed countries, its use in adults decreased with the introduction of the less hepatotoxic enflurane in the late 1960s. The decrease in the use of halothane occurred more rapidly in the litigious US than in other developed countries. In Europe, enflurane, and later isoflurane, were slow to be adopted. Because of issues of pungency and because hepatotoxicity in children was thought to be less evident, halothane continued to be used in children until sevoflurane was introduced in the 1990s.

Similar concerns regarding methoxyflurane resulted in a rethinking of criteria used to assess the potential risks of newer volatile anesthetics. Methoxyflurane metabolism resulted in high blood and urine concentrations of free fluoride ion, potentially causing renal injury [5–7]. The discovery of the renal lesion associated with the administration and metabolism of methoxyflurane, significantly curtailed its continued use. Anesthesiologists had also become increasingly sophisticated, recognizing that the high blood and lipid solubility slowed the rate of induction, slowed emergence, and prolonged postoperative somnolence. The development of enflurane, a safer (less metabolized to noxious metabolites)

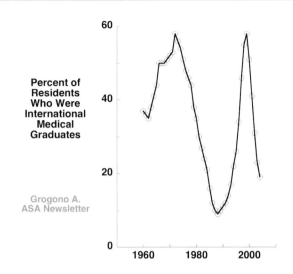

Fig. 9.1 The percent of anesthesiology residents who were IMGs increased to 58 % in 1972, falling to a nadir of 9 % two decades later. A second peak followed Clinton's focus on the development of primary care physicians in the 1990s

and kinetically advantageous (much less soluble) alternative, added to the incentive to abandon methoxyflurane.

Anesthesia Manpower in the US and the ASA Preceptor Program

In 1960, International Medical Graduates (IMGs) filled 38 % of anesthesiology residency positions in the US (Fig. 9.1), a percentage that exceeded that for other specialties and subsequently increased to nearly 60 % by 1972. While not necessarily reflecting resident quality, this characterization of the specialty diminished its prestige among American Medical Graduates (AMGs), such that, in 1964, ASA President Al Betcher, convinced the ASA to survey the status of the specialty in education, research, and teaching. Completed in 1967, the survey prompted the formation of a Council of Education that included a Committee on Medical Student Preceptorships. This committee developed a Preceptorship Program that provided an 8 week paid experience to medical students who had completed two years of medical school. During the 8 weeks, they were assigned to an anesthesiologist in private practice or academia, observing, and where feasible participating, in day-to-day care of patients. Between the initiation of this program in 1966, and 1969, more than 1100 students participated. The number of American Medical Graduates (AMGs) electing anesthesiology as a career tripled following the implementation of the program. While the percentage of IMGs in anesthesia training programs continued to increase, it peaked in 1972, and was followed by a progressive decline, reaching a nadir of 9 % by 1988 (Fig. 9.1) [8].

My (LJS) experience as a medical student predicted success of the Preceptorship Program. If you exposed students to the specialty, "they will come". As a 1960 junior medical student at the University of Michigan, I chose anesthesia to satisfy the requirement for a 6 week surgical subspecialty rotation. My choice was determined when I drew an ace of diamonds from a worn deck of cards used to decide medical student surgical rotation assignments. Anesthesia was a "plum assignment" because the assigned student actively participated in patient care…and because there were no student night call obligations. Although the anesthesia department at the University of Michigan conducted little if any laboratory research, the staff anesthetists were attentive to students, perhaps giving a bit more responsibility than was warranted. I remember accompanying a young staff anesthesiologist to Jackson prison—at the time the largest penal institution in the US—and while caring for three patients requiring tracheal intubation, deftly inserted the tracheal tube…into the esophagus. My mentor calmly suggested the tube be removed and assured me that all would be well and that this was not an uncommon event for the budding anesthesiologist. I found the experience of caring for patients whose lives depended upon me exhilarating, and my life was serendipitously changed forever. In retrospect, I wonder if providing care for some really rough desperados might also have inspired my career choice….

Returning to the issue of IMGs versus AMGs, in the 1990s, the number of AMGs selecting anesthesia again decreased when following Bill Clinton's election to the US Presidency in 1992, he appointed his wife, Hilary Clinton in 1993, to Chair a task force charged with developing a program that would provide universal health care. Passage of this program was doomed however when Conservatives, Libertarians, organized medicine, and the health insurance industry suggested that such a new bureaucratic structure that incorporated universal coverage, mandating purchase of insurance, would limit patient choice and adversely affect medical care. In addition, medical school deans/administrators may have advised medical students that practice opportunities might not be available in anesthesia while there would be a large increase in positions for primary care physicians. The number of AMGs electing anesthesia upon graduation decreased to zero in many programs with a reciprocal increase in the percentage of IMG anesthesia residents to 58% by 1999 before declining once again to less than 20% (Fig. 9.1)

Anesthesiology Grew Worldwide

In the 1960s, societies continued to grow worldwide. Eastern Europe, Asia, Central America and the Middle East experienced an increase in the numbers of trained anesthetists who hungered for collegial interactions and education. This

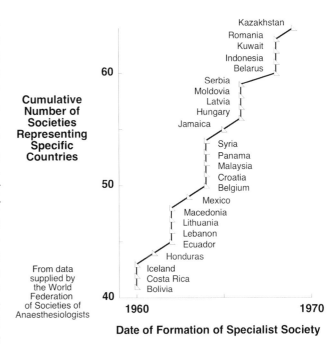

Fig. 9.2 Worldwide, large numbers of anesthetic societies continued to be added in the 1960s, two dozen in all

growth was superimposed on that achieved in the previous decades in Western Europe, Latin America, and the English-speaking countries. Altogether in the 1960s, two dozen anesthesia societies were founded worldwide (Fig. 9.2).

Emergence of Research in Academic Anesthesia Departments

As the 1960s began, anesthesiology worldwide was a specialty short of trained physicians. In the US, fewer than 2500 board-certified anesthesiologists served a country of 180 million or approximately 1.4/100,000 population. Many US medical schools had anesthesia divisions rather than departments, divisions housed within departments of surgery. Most were consumed by large clinical responsibilities. Only a handful of academic departments (e.g., Harvard, Columbia, Pennsylvania, Iowa, Wisconsin, UCSF, University of Washington) supported research activities with mature trained investigators. Fewer yet had NIH-supported research grants. There were hardly any trained subspecialists. This began to change in the 1960s, starting a transformation of the specialty in the US from one dominated by empiricism to one employing the tools of modern science, spreading its clinical involvement from the operating room to the delivery suite, intensive care unit, post anesthetic care unit, ambulatory surgery suite and acute and chronic pain management departments.

Between 1960 and 1971, 15 new university departments headed by chairs, were established in GB. While clinical anesthesia was their primary responsibility, several of these became the spearheads of research, encouraging higher academic qualifications. In 1968, the Anaesthetic Research Society was formally established out of a less formal group that had begun in 1958.

In the 1960s, research in anesthesiology was largely "phenomenological" (a term now considered pejorative), observational studies lacking a mechanism explaining the cause of the observation. The titles of typical research papers began with "The effect of" rather than "Here is the reason for the effect of". But "we needed to walk before we could run". We first needed to provide observations. These would lead to questions such as why and how.

A confluence of factors was needed to enable the first steps. These included devices capable of accurately and rapidly measuring small amounts of anesthetic drugs, research funds sufficient to support talented but unproved academics who were freed from clinical responsibilities, and prescient department leaders in and out of the specialty who recognized the need to develop a scientific base leading to important questions. IS Ravdin, a surgeon at the University of Pennsylvania, had addressed this issue nearly 20 years earlier. stating that "While the importance of the technical advances in a young field is not to be minimized, it is the fundamental contributions which lead to a better understanding of anesthesia that will mark the real maturity of anesthesiologists [9]." Robert Dripps, Chairman of Anesthesia also at the University of Pennsylvania, stated in 1949 that "Talented young men in the specialty of anesthesiology must be encouraged and supported if their inclinations are toward investigation" and "once trained, these young scientists will require budgets, laboratories, and time free from clinical responsibilities [10]". Finally, in an editorial in 1950, Salter (a non-anesthesiologist) stated:

> "There must be trained a group of so-called academic anesthesiologists. They must have the special training and sufficient leisure to advance the basic concepts of applied science. They must not be run ragged with routine assignments but must be protected from the irate surgeon who demands "service now" in the name of all humanity and the trustees". [11]

Although several factors accounted for the delayed development of anesthesiology as a specialty in Asia and much of Europe, the factor that was undeniably of greatest importance was World War II, with its horrific devastation, millions killed, destruction of physical and governmental infrastructure, and the resulting revisions of social order and scientific institutions—a complete reordering of society. With democracy replacing authoritarianism in Japan and German speaking countries, virtually every institution required restructuring. Combined with the fact that the specialty had been slow to develop before the war, these factors delayed its development until nearly the 1960s. For example and as nicely described by Goerig in Chapter 29, up to the 1950s, tracheal intubation was still performed digitally and under topical anesthesia and it was not until the clinical use of muscle relaxants well into the 1950s that laryngoscopes were used. Goerig observed that in 1959, German nursing authorities officially refused to perform "intravenous anaesthesia methods, intubation procedures, controlled ventilation or use of curare".

In Japan, the specialty was slow to develop, partly because of the impact of World War II and partly because anesthesia even by the middle 1950s was not considered a recognized specialty. Of importance was the number of leaders trained in the US in the 1950s, returning to Japan as professors in key universities. Suwa notes (Chapter 31) that this system initially allowed permanent qualification as a specialist following two years of training and/or experience administering general anesthesia to 300 patients. This has changed to a far more demanding system today.

1960s Research Themes: Pharmacokinetics, Pharmacodynamics and MAC

In the 1920s, Haggard investigated the absorption, distribution, and elimination of diethyl ether in dogs [12, 13], and 30 years later Severinghaus measured nitrous oxide uptake in humans [14]. Those were the sum of the pharmacokinetic work up to the 1960s, work that dominated much of research in anesthesia in that decade. Some might add that the great Seymour Kety supplied the first paper explaining the pharmacokinetics of inhaled anesthetics [15], but he missed the importance of the differential distribution of tissue blood flow. In 1960, Henry Price published the first pharmacokinetic paper providing insight into why drugs distribute as they do, using a physiological-anatomical model. Price described the distribution of thiopental in humans (Fig. 9.3) [16], in the process correcting Kety's error.

Now go back two decades. The attack upon Pearl Harbor in 1941 killed thousands of Americans. It was asserted (apocryphally) that more deaths resulted from intravenous thiopental than from bombs or other projectiles. The simulation provided by Price explained this statement. Traumatic injury and blood loss decreased the volume of the central blood compartment. Thiopental injected into this smaller volume would produce a greater concentration which, when delivered to highly perfused tissues (viscera such as the heart and brain) would result in greater anesthetic depth, cardiac depression, hypotension…and death. This simple explanation would apply to any intravenous medication and was a cornerstone of non-inhaled PK principals over the remainder of the decade. Obviously, this effect could be mitigated by decreasing the dose, and or restoring blood volume with blood transfusion and or intravenous fluid.

However, while the theory may have been convincing and the explanation logical, it appears that the facts conflicted

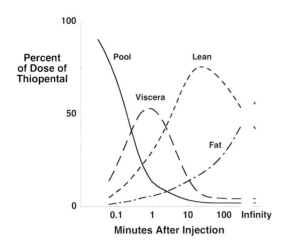

Fig. 9.3 Using an analogue model, Price convincingly argued that thiopental nearly immediately redistributed from the central pool of blood into which it was injected into the viscera where it acted, and that its evanescent effect depended on further redistribution, first and most importantly to muscle and later to fat. Until publication of his work, fat had been considered the cause of the evanescence. (From Price HL: A dynamic concept of the distribution of thiopental in the human body. Anesthesiology 1960; 21: 40–5, with permission.)

with both. In Chapter 47, Paul White comments that: "… an analysis by FE Bennetts suggested that…despite shortages of oxygen and transfusion supplies, thiopental caused few deaths [17]."

Early in the 1960s, interest in pharmacokinetics flourished. The 1962 symposium on this topic sponsored by the New York Academy of Medicine and the National Research Council-National Academy of Sciences, illustrates the intense focus. Thirty five scientists from around the world (four from the UK, one from Canada, and the remainder from the US) presented the results of largely unpublished research, using measurements and simulations to define what was then known about the pharmacokinetics of inhaled and intravenous agents [18]. The simulations might apply electrical analogs or complicated mathematical models. The contributors speculated on and provided indirect evidence for the inter-tissue diffusion of inhaled anesthetics. They set the stage for further measurements and simulations that continued for the next four decades. For the inhaled anesthetics, research was initially dominated by researchers at UCSF led by Edmond Eger and his many colleagues and trainees in the US, Europe, and Asia. The results from these studies informed our understanding of clinical pharmacokinetics for the subsequent 40 years. Many of the ideas were gathered in Eger's 1974 book, Anesthetic Uptake and Action [19].

Before the 60s, empiricism ruled both practice and research in the specialty. Little could be measured accurately, and clinical experience rather than evidence based medicine drove clinical care. A typical anesthetic, reflecting the changing nature of the specialty between 1950 and 2013, for an adult in the US, undergoing major abdominal or thoracic

surgery is described in Chapter 7. The amount of inhaled agent delivered was driven by the vital signs and surgical requirements such as control of blood loss or the relaxation required to perform surgery. But what was the needed dose/concentration, and how did one define "needed"? How did altered physical status, associated co-morbidities, and physiological changes (e.g., body temperature or blood gases) influence this dose? Up to the late 1950s, the volatile anesthetic dose could not easily be measured, and an agreed upon response was not available. Should it be a change in blood pressure or pulse rate or respiratory rate? Of course, patient condition and surgical circumstances would affect these responses. On the other hand, how about an end point that everyone could agree upon, one that made clinical sense? And thus was born MAC—the minimum alveolar concentration preventing movement in response to a noxious (surgical incision) stimulus—perhaps the most utilized metric of anesthetic dose ever! A bit of irony—the study first describing MAC used both halothane and halopropane—the latter an anesthetic *never released* for clinical use [20].

Edmond (Ted) Eger trained in anesthesia at the University of Iowa, and following two years in the US Army stationed at Ft Leavenworth Kansas, joined Stuart Cullen and John Severinghaus in the anesthesia department at the University of California San Francisco (UCSF). Eger's interest in pharmacokinetics, and ultimately MAC, began in 1957 while he was a first year resident. Severinghaus (then a second-year resident at Iowa) lectured on the uptake of inhaled anesthetics, using Kety's ideas and Severinghaus' results from his study of nitrous oxide uptake. He said that uptake of greater amounts of anesthetic (as with the highly soluble anesthetic ether) would slow the induction of anesthesia. To Eger (and most anesthesia residents yet today hearing this for the first time) it seemed obviously incorrect. A greater uptake would deliver more anesthetic to the blood and brain, so how could Severinghaus be right? Eger argued with Severinghaus for an hour after the lecture, but Severinghaus wouldn't budge. Higher solubility, greater uptake, slower onset of action. It just didn't seem correct…but it was. Severinghaus was always correct.

And now Eger was hooked. The more he thought about the reason that ether acted slowly, the more he was drawn to the beauty of the relationships that led to that idea. He spent days, weeks, and years dreaming about the relationships. Finally, it was time to put pen to paper. During his two years in the US Army (1958-1960), Eger used algebra and iterations to develop his descriptions of inhaled anesthetic pharmacokinetics. Along with parallel ideas from others in the field, Eger's thoughts opened a new era of understanding as to why we do what we do, and how to logically conduct inhaled anesthesia taking into account hemodynamic and respiratory perturbations. The ideas and thoughts opened new ways to assess the worth of new inhaled anesthetics prior to FDA approval. The principles elucidated over this decade revised

Fig. 9.4 The three investigators who developed the notion of MAC, John Severinghaus, Giles Merkel, and Edmond Eger. (From UCSF departmental photographs from the early 1960's)

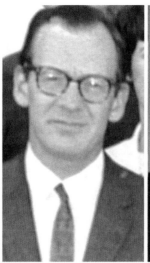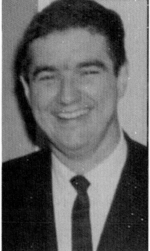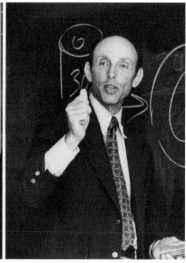

the way in which anesthetics were administered, and more importantly, enhanced understanding of pharmacokinetics by those responsible for delivery of anesthesia.

Equally important and influential was the development of the above-noted MAC by Eger and his colleagues (Fig. 9.4). The two crucial components in the definition of MAC were "alveolar" concentration and "muscular response" to a noxious stimulus such as a skin incision. Alveolar concentration (or its surrogate, partial pressure) was crucial because it approximated the anesthetic partial pressure in arterial blood, that in turn is presumed to approximate the partial pressure at the anesthetic site of action preventing movement in response to surgery. While this site of action was initially opined to be the brain, subsequent findings by Antognini and Schwartz at UC Davis [21] and Rampil et al at UCSF [22] established the spinal cord as the major site of action.

Movement was the second crucial component of MAC because preventing movement is the principal responsibility of the anesthetist to both the patient and to the surgeon. And it was an easily recognized and unambiguous response occurring in every experimental subject and species (avoidance to noxious stimulation), and was thus as applicable in the laboratory as it was in the operating room.

MAC-related research quantified clinically important physiological and physical effects of inhaled anesthetics. In particular, it allowed a comparison of these effects by different agents at multiples of equipotent concentrations, with the reasonable assurance that the results of a study performed at one site anywhere in the world could reasonably be compared with results performed elsewhere, as long as the MAC multiples were the same. Similarly, employing MAC as a measure of anesthetic depth simplified the study of new anesthetics. This meant that when enflurane (late 1960s), isoflurane (1980s), sevoflurane and desflurane (1990s) were released for clinical use, similar studies at similar anesthetic

depths had been performed at different institutions with reasonable assurance that nearly identical conditions had been present for each agent.

Serendipity: MAC and Malignant Hyperthermia

The first study measuring MAC in humans was conducted at UCSF in 1962-63 using surgical patients anesthetized with halothane with or without nitrous oxide or opiate premedication [23]. In each patient a predetermined alveolar concentration was achieved and held steady for at least 15 minutes prior to the skin incision to allow equilibration of the end-tidal anesthetic concentration to its site of action in the central nervous system. Following incision, the patient was observed for purposeful movement. MAC was based on the combined responses from a group of patients. The investigators decided to validate the accuracy of this measurement by studying the response of four patients, each serving as their own control. In these patients, following induction of anesthesia with halothane and oxygen, needles were inserted subcutaneously in the forearm and attached to a stimulator that could provide a supra-maximal stimulus. Similar to the method described above, once a predetermined alveolar halothane concentration had been achieved, the stimulus was applied and the response—movement or not—was noted. If movement occurred, the alveolar concentration was increased in steps until movement was abolished, and the process repeated in the opposite direction. Thus several "cross-overs" were achieved and the midpoint of the concentrations allowing and preventing movement was designated as MAC.

The first patient studied was an obese (BMI 33) 47 year-old man scheduled for repair of a ventral hernia by a surgeon noted for his insistence on profound muscle relaxation. After completing the MAC study, Saidman and Eger relinquished care of the patient to the resident and staff anesthetist and departed for the lab. However, shortly after, they were recalled to the OR because the patient's temperature had increased. Temperature was not routinely monitored in 1963, but fortuitously and fortunately it was monitored in this case because of the MAC determination. Although a succinylcholine infusion had been and was being used, the surgeon complained that abdominal rigidity interfered with his work. The patient was sweating and breathing deeply, the color of the carbon dioxide absorbent indicated exhaustion, and the succinylcholine infusion was running rapidly. The temperature of the patient now exceeded 107 F, ultimately increasing to 108.5 F. One of the original blood-gas machines assembled by John Severinghaus and Freeman Bradley [24] was available and an arterial sample revealed a pH of 6.82, a pCO_2 of 179 mmHg, a pO_2 of 143 mmHg and a severe metabolic acidosis (base deficit—14.3 meq/L). Blood pressure decreased from 110/70 mmHg to 40/0 mmHg and was treated with metaraminol. The surgeon was asked to quickly complete the procedure, the patient was packed in ice, 3000 ml of lactated Ringer's solution were rapidly infused, and bicarbonate was given to correct the metabolic acidosis. Within 30 minutes, the temperature decreased to103 F and in another 30 minutes to 97.2 F. The blood pressure increased to 110/70 without further therapy, and the patient survived without any apparent neurological deficit. Dantrolene, a muscle relaxant presently used in the management of malignant hyperthermia, was not available in 1963.

This case was presented before the anesthesia section of the 1964 AMA meeting held in San Francisco and when the moderator queried the audience if any had experienced a similar case, several replied that they had in patients who, similarly, had also been anesthetized with halothane and paralyzed with succinylcholine. This patient had likely suffered from malignant hyperthermia and provided the first ever determination of the metabolic aberration associated with this syndrome [25]. An earlier paper by Denborough highlighted the fact that a similar syndrome had been noted in many relatives (some of whom had died) within a family. Because the title of the paper did not mention temperature, it escaped notice when the UCSF patient was being reviewed [26].

Variations of these MAC studies also allowed other clinically relevant metrics to be defined including the concentration at which awareness is likely (MAC Awake) [27], the concentration at which coughing in response to endotracheal intubation is likely (MAC EI) [28], the concentration which blocks an adrenergic response to surgical stimulation (MAC-BAR) [29], and MAC as a function of age [30]. In addition, because MACs were later shown to be additive, the substitution of a fractional MAC concentration of an anesthetic with less cardiovascular depression, for a portion of a second anesthetic, permitted the anesthetist to provide an equal

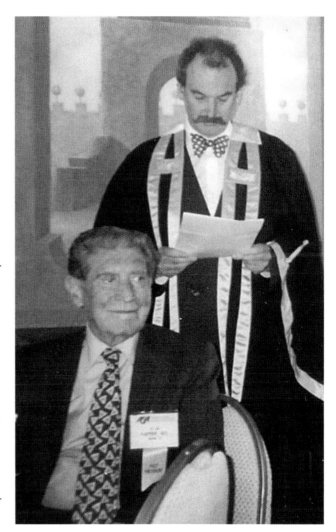

Fig. 9.5 Photograph of a young Rod N. Westhorpe conferring an Honorary FANZCA on Emmanuel Papper in 1996. (Courtesy of Rod N. Westhorpe.)

anesthetic depth while causing less total cardiovascular depression.

Emanuel Papper Goes to Washington

As mentioned earlier, anesthesia research in the first half of the 1960s in the US was largely phenomenological, and research funding for the specialty was limited, few departments receiving support. Emanuel (Manny) Papper (Fig. 9.5) the Chairman of the anesthesia department at Columbia University took a leave of absence to serve as Principal Consultant to Fred Stone, the Director of the Institute of General Medical Sciences of the NIH. Papper acted to assist Stone in developing programs especially targeting young academic anesthesiologists. Commenting on Papper's performance, Stone opined that "In his six months as Principal Consultant for the Institute, Doctor Papper accomplished what it would have taken staff three years to accomplish [31]".

Subspecialties and the Evolution of Specialty Research and Training

Except for pediatric anesthetists and perhaps a few obstetrical anesthetists, as the 1960s approached, most anesthesia practitioners were "generalists", caring for all patients regardless of age, surgical procedure, or gender. However, during this decade several factors increasingly led to subspecialization in anesthesia and surgery. Increasing numbers of certified anesthesiologists allowed time for a few to train in subspecialty academic programs pursuing a body of knowledge unique to that subspecialty (e.g. obstetric related physiology and pharmacology), and those who performed research on problems related to a specific cohort of patients (parturients or perhaps pregnant ewes) similarly increased. Although there is little evidence describing a cause-effect for this change, one might speculate that a key factor included surgical advances demanding more of anesthesia and anesthesiologists. Moreover, increased interest, knowledge and training evolved into discrete clinical specialty rotations, and subsequently to specialty (fellowship) training programs for trainees. Small cohorts of practitioners then provided care to patients having a limited spectrum of diseases (Neurosurgical, Obstetrical, Cardiac, Thoracic).

Initially, generalists resisted subspecialty development. It would narrow options for generalists, perhaps affecting income. It might lessen their worth, and it would alter call-schedules, relegating the generalists to what may be thought of as less interesting work than those working in more "exotic" specialties. However, the tide toward sub-specialization moved inexorably forward, leading to discrete work groups within departments concentrating on cardiac, obstetric, pediatric, neurosurgical, regional anesthesia, critical care, anesthesia for ambulatory surgery, and, more recently, management.

These groups increasingly grew in the 1960s, forming formal societies in the 1970s that in turn sponsored scientific and educational meetings, published scientific journals, defined educational goals and requirements for certification, and finally became exclusionary, constricting practice opportunities of generalists especially in teaching hospitals. Remarkably, specialty societies in both the US and the UK grew at a nearly simultaneous rate during the 1970s and beyond (see Fig. 10.2).

Initial research among the specialties largely remained phenomenological, describing effects, rather than explaining why they occurred. Thus, neurosurgical anesthesiologists measured the effect of volatile anesthetics on cerebral blood flow and metabolism to define the "best" combination of drugs to use in patients with increased intracranial pressure.

Obstetric anesthesiologists noted the effect of different vasoactive drugs on fetal lamb well being, or in humans comparing Apgar scores, or in-utero heart rate patterns. Great excitement accompanied the NEJM article from the MGH group of cardiac anesthesiologists in 1969, showing "high dose morphine" to be associated with greater cardiovascular stability, especially in patients with valvular disorders, but it, too, was phenomenological [32]. Of course as with many, *innovative* (including phenomenological) discoveries, this had been suggested earlier [33]. Unfortunately, the use of high-dose morphine anesthesia was sometimes associated with patient awareness.

Differential Solubility and Gas Transfer into and from Gas Filled Spaces in the Body

In 1936, Aird suggested that if a space in the body were filled with a gas of blood solubility greater than nitrogen, the space would decrease in size because the gas would be removed from the space faster than nitrogen could be brought into the space (and even faster if oxygen rather than air was breathed). This also assumed that the same gas was not being simultaneously breathed [34]. An appreciation of the more rapid elimination of more soluble gases from body spaces was applied to accelerate the removal of the gas used for pneumoencephalography and thereby shorten the duration of the headache associated with this procedure [35]. In 1953, it was recognized that the converse would occur if a closed space within the body was filled with a gas of blood solubility less than that of nitrogen. Such a space would increase in size if the walls were compliant [36, 37].

These effects of differential solubility were applied during the 1960s to prevent increases in the size of, or pressure within, gas filled spaces in the bodies of patients. Thus anesthetists might avoid using nitrous oxide during surgery for which the risk of air embolism was increased, such as intracranial surgery in a patient in the sitting position [38], a patient with a large emphysematous bullous, or a patient with intestinal obstruction (Fig. 9.6) [39]. Conversely nitrous oxide might be used to **deliberately** provoke an increase in the size of the space to provide an "early warning" that air has been entrained in this same patient in the sitting position. Also in 1965, Saidman and Eger demonstrated that the administration of the more soluble gas, nitrous oxide, would increase the pressure in a non-compliant space (e.g., the intracranial space) containing the less soluble gas, nitrogen [40]. Such a potentially dangerous change arose in patients undergoing pneumoencephalography or any procedure in which air was allowed within the skull. More recently, ophthalmologists used the principle to maintain pressure within gas filled spaces (injecting a bubble of very low solubility sulfur-hexafluoride into the posterior chamber of the eye to "stent the retina"

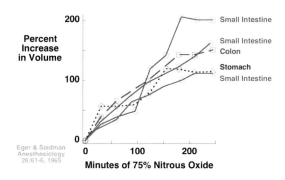

Fig. 9.6 The administration of 75 % nitrous oxide to dogs increases the volume of gas contained in various portions of the intestinal tract by approximately equal amounts. Data from Eger and Saidman who in their report did not indicate why they studied 3 loops of small bowel but only one stomach and one colon. (From Eger EI, II, Saidman LJ: Hazards of nitrous oxide anesthesia in bowel obstruction and pneumothorax. Anesthesiology 1965; 26: 61–6, with permission.)

following surgery for retinal detachment). This incurred a risk of a great increase in intraocular pressure if such a patient then breathed nitrous oxide. The resulting increase in pressure could lead to retinal ischemia and blindness [41].

Other Important Changes in the1960s

Physiology An understanding of cardiorespiratory physiology and pharmacology underlay advances in pharmacokinetics and patient care. One of the great pioneers in this field from the late 1950s to the 1980s was the British anesthesiologist, John Nunn. He began work at the Royal College of Surgeons, then became Professor in Leeds, and subsequently assumed the directorship of the Medical Research Council unit at Northwick Park Hospital. Initially his studies centered on lung ventilation/perfusion relationships during anesthesia and surgery [42], and their effects on oxygenation during, and especially after, anesthesia [43, 44]. Such studies led to his world-renowned book on Applied Respiratory Physiology [45]. He had a special affection for diverse aspects of inhaled anesthetic pharmacology, ranging from the effects of volatile anesthetics on depolymerisation in cellular microtubules [46], to the toxic effects of nitrous oxide [47]. His prodigious output led to receipt of the ASA Excellence in Research Award in 1991. He retired in the 1990s to pursue his lifelong love and study of Egyptian hieroglyphics.

Pharmacogenetics It was the rare anesthesiologist who had not at some time been confronted by a patient experiencing prolonged paralysis following an intravenous injection of succinylcholine. The 1950s discovery of genetic polymorphism of the esterase responsible for the metabolism of succinylcholine, led to Kalow's work on dibucaine numbers [48], and his classic 1962 monograph [49].

New Drugs Pancuronium. In 1960, d-tubocurarine (curare) was the most frequently used muscle relaxant. Unless the initial dose far exceeded that required for relaxation during surgery, its onset was relatively slow and thus unsuitable for rapid sequence induction. In addition, use of a large dose risked substantial hypotension due to histamine release, and delayed the ability to pharmacologically reverse its effect. Thus, when concerned about a patient considered at risk of vomiting and aspiration during induction of anesthesia, and if for some reason succinylcholine was contraindicated, awake tracheal intubation, unpleasant for both patient and anesthetist, was often employed.

Curare was essentially replaced in 1967 when pancuronium, an amino steroid, was released for clinical use [50]. Its principal advantages compared with curare were that 1) side effects related to histamine were rare; and 2) the onset of action was faster making it more suitable for use during a rapid-sequence induction. However, pancuronium increased heart rate. Indeed, the use of pancuronium might be preferred to prevent the bradycardia associated with a large dose of fentanyl.

Fentanyl also came to the market in the 1960s. Initially it was combined with droperidol as "Innovar", in a fixed 50:1 dose ratio (2.5 mg droperidol:0.050 mg fentanyl), producing what had been popularized as neurolept-analgesia, a term according to Paul White, that Oliver Wendell Holmes considered prior to coining "anaesthesia". Initially used as premedication, Innovar could produce a panic like effect that might cause an occasional cancellation of surgery [51]. Because of this side effect and a dislike for fixed dose combinations of drugs, Innovar was soon abandoned. Fentanyl on the other hand was increasingly adopted for use, first in small doses and then in larger ones. It continues (when not in short supply) as a nearly universally used rapid-onset, relatively short acting opioid during most types of surgery, sedation, and as an adjunct for spinal and epidural anesthesia.

Ketamine, introduced during the1960s, was developed for clinical use by Gunter Corssen and Ed Domino [52]. It had two distinguishing differences. First, its sympathomimetic actions recommended it as a suitable substitute for thiopental for the induction of anesthesia in patients displaying hemodynamic instablility, particularly those scheduled for a rapid induction of anesthesia. This benefit was shared by etomidate which has more recently largely replaced ketamine for this purpose. Second, given at doses that cause anesthesia, ketamine caused undesirable psychomimetic after-effects, at times lasting for days and distressing patients and their caregivers. Lesser doses, however, appeared to not produce such effects, yet had the capacity to produce analgesia. Because of these analgesic effects, ketamine has more recently been used as an anesthesia adjunct especially in patients with long standing chronic pain problems for which they take "industrial" sized maintenance doses of opioids [53].

Bupivacaine, a longer-acting, lipid-soluble anesthetic was released into clinical practice in Scandinavia in 1963. As Drasner points out in chapter 51, in laboratory studies, bupivacaine's systemic toxicity appeared to be equivalent to that of tetracaine and four times greater than that of mepivacaine, paralleling their relative potency [54]. However, in the 1970s, several clinical reports suggested the potential for cardiac toxicity. Prentiss suggested that toxicity resulted from a direct effect of this lipid- soluble, highly-bound anesthetic [55]. By 1982, concerns regarding toxicity led to elimination of the 0.75 % formulation, the widespread use of a test dose, and incremental injections as standard anesthetic practice. These modifications provided effective, but not foolproof, protection of the patient.

Beecher: Science and Ethics—A Giant Astride Medicine

As described in Chapter 8, during the 1950s, Henry Beecher published two landmark contributions. In conjunction with Donald Todd, in 1954 Beecher reported the first large prospective anesthesia outcome study, providing the incidence of anesthesia related mortality including the finding that administration of curare increased mortality [56]. In the same year, Beecher described the importance of the placebo response [57]. It is difficult to imagine two more important papers shaping anesthesia research and clinical care for generations.

Beecher was not yet done however. During the 1960s, he continued to make momentous contributions to medicine in general and the specialty in particular. Subsequent to the original Nuremberg trials in 1947, the Doctors Trial resulted in convictions of German physicians accused of medical experimentation on human beings. Ultimately ten principles evolving from the trial became known as the Nuremberg Code, and defined the principles governing future human experimentation. These principles included:

1. The voluntary consent of the human subject is absolutely essential. This means that the person involved should have legal capacity to give consent;
2. The experiment should potentially yield fruitful results for the good of society, be unprocurable by other methods or means of study, and not be random and unnecessary in nature.
3. The experiment should be based on the results of animal experimentation and knowledge of the natural history of the disease.
4. The experiment should be so conducted as to avoid all unnecessary physical and mental suffering and injury.
5. No experiment should be conducted where there is a prior reason to believe that death or disabling injury will occur.

6. The degree of risk to be taken should never exceed that determined by the humanitarian importance of the problem to be solved by the experiment.
7. Proper preparations should be made and adequate facilities provided to protect the experimental subject against even remote possibilities of injury, disability, or death.
8. Only scientifically qualified persons should conduct the experiment.
9. During the course of the experiment the human subject should be at liberty to bring the experiment to an end.
10. During the course of the experiment the scientist in charge must be prepared to terminate the experiment at any stage, if he has probable cause to believe…that a continuation of the experiment is likely to result in injury, disability, or death to the experimental subject.

Although these principles were a foundation for the Helsinki Principles initially published in 1964, it seems that they had not been sufficiently codified to prevent abuses described in the now historic paper by Beecher. The paper was probably instrumental in the NIH requirement that local institutional review boards (IRBs) approve all human experimentation supported by NIH funds [58]. Beecher stated in his paper (rejected for publication in JAMA) that "Evidence is at hand that many of the patients in the examples to follow never had the risk satisfactorily explained to them. And it seems obvious that further hundreds have not known that they were the subjects of an experiment although grave consequences have been suffered as a direct result of experiments described here". Beecher examined "100 consecutive human studies published in 1964, in an excellent journal; 12 of these seemed to be unethical". Examples of these 100 studies were classified as either: Withholding Effective Treatment, Study of Therapy, Physiologic Studies, Studies to Improve the Understanding of Disease, Technical Study of Disease, or Bizarre Study. Selected examples from among these studies included: injection of melanoma from a daughter into an informed and volunteering mother, who died from metastatic melanoma nearly 15 months later; performing a placebo vs penicillin controlled study in patients with streptococcal respiratory infections in spite of the known efficacy of penicillin—2 of the controls developed acute rheumatic fever and in one, acute nephritis occurred; and in order to define the toxicology of chloramphenicol, 2 G vs 6 G were given to randomly selected patients with aplastic anemia subsequently developing in 10 % and 86 % respectively.

In his second 1960s initiative, Beecher attempted to define brain death [59]. The burden posed by brain-injured patients on the family (both social as well as economic), the need for hospital beds, and "the obsolete criteria for the definition of death that can lead to controversy in obtaining organs for transplantation" prompted the initiative. In the absence of anesthesia, hypothermia, or drug intoxication, four criteria defined brain death: Unawareness and unresponsiveness; lack of movement or breathing; absent reflexes; and absent EEG activity. This assessment must be made by a physician. When completed and discussed by the attending physicians and all other care givers (all of whom must concur with the conclusions), the respirator may be turned off. Commenting on the issues surrounding creation and promulgation of these criteria, Ed Lowenstein observed that "it seems likely that the whole brain criteria for brain death promulgated by Henry K Beecher and the Harvard Ad Hoc Committee 40 years ago will remain the standard for the foreseeable future [60]."

Thus this body of work in the two decades following World War II shaped the conduct of human research in ways not previously imagined. Although only the Beecher-Todd report is solely applicable to the specialty, we take enormous pride in acknowledging Beecher as "one of ours".

Reprise

The decade of the 1960s might be described as the "Golden Age of Anesthesia" because of the changes throughout the world profoundly influencing all aspects of the specialty and some that reached beyond the specialty. Research into the pharmacokinetics and pharmacodynamics of anesthesia grew to maturity in this and the next decade. In a search for "why and what", phenomenological research increasingly turned into basic "how and where" research. New drugs appeared (bupivacaine, enflurane, fentanyl, ketamine, etomidate, pancuronium) or disappeared (Innovar, methoxyflurane), and their effects were investigated. Sub-specialization was soon accompanied by worldwide specialty societies, and specialty oriented journals facilitated training of experts and spurred targeted research contributing to improved anesthetic care. In the US, recruitment into the specialty grew out of an ASA initiative aimed at exposing medical students to the specialty while still early in their careers. Also in the US, passage of the Medicare Act in 1965 included anesthesiologists in Part B, stipulating reimbursement on a fee for service basis (similar to that for most physicians), improving salaries for anesthesiologists, and coinciding with a nearly exponential growth in anesthesiologist numbers in every subsequent decade.

References

1. Brody GL, Sweet RB. Halothane anesthesia as a possible cause of massive hepatic necrosis. Anesthesiology. 1963;24:29–37.
2. Bunker JP, Forrest WH, Moesteller F, Vandam L. The National Halothane Study. Bethesda: National Institutes of Health; 1969.
3. Summary of the National Halothane Study. Possible association between halothane anesthesia and postoperative hepatic necrosis. Report by Subcommittee on the National Halothane Study of the Committee on Anesthesia, National Academy of Science. JAMA. 1966;197:775–88.
4. Rehder K, Forbes J, Alter H, Hessler O, Stier A. Halothane biotransformation in man: A quantitative study. Anesthesiology. 1967;28:711–5.
5. Crandell WB, Macdonald A. Nephropathy associated with methoxyflurane anesthesia. A follow-up report. JAMA. 1968;205:798–9.
6. Pezzi PJ, Frobese AS, Greenberg SR. Methoyflurane and renal toxicity. Lancet. 1966;287:823.
7. Austin WH, Villandry PJ. Methoxyflurane and renal function. Anesthesiology. 1967;28:637.
8. Betcher AM. Historical development of the American Society of Anesthesiologists. In: Volpitto PP, Vandam LD, Thomas CC, Editors. The genesis of contemporary American anesthesiology. Springfield: IL; 1982.
9. Ravdin IS. A surgeon comments on the speciality of anesthesiology. Anesthesiology. 1941;2:207–8.
10. Dripps RD. Research and its relationship to clinical anesthesiology. Anesthesiology. 1949;10:690–5.
11. Salter WT. The leaven of the profession. Anesthesiology. 1950;11:374–6.
12. Haggard AW. The absorption, distribution and elimination of ethyl ether. II. Analysis of the mechanism of absorption and elimination of such a gas or vapor as ethyl ether. J Biol Chem. 1924;59:753–96.
13. Haggard AW. The absorption, distribution and elimination of ethyl ether. III. The relation of the concentration of ether, or any similar volatile substance in the central nervous system to the concentration in the arterial blood and the buffer action of the body. J Biol Chem. 1924;59:797–832.
14. Severinghaus JW. The rate of uptake of nitrous oxide in man. J Clin Invest. 1954;33:1183–9.
15. Kety SS. Theory and application of exchange of inert gas at the lungs and tissues. Pharmacol Rev. 1951;3:1–41.
16. Price HL. A dynamic concept of the distribution of thiopental in the human body. Anesthesiology. 1960;21:40–5.
17. Bennetts FE. Thiopentone anaesthesia at Pearl Harbor. Br J Anaesth. 1995;75:366–8.
18. Papper EM, Kitz RJe. Uptake and Distribution of Anesthetic Agents. New York: McGraw-Hill; 1963.
19. Eger EI II. Anesthetic uptake and action. Baltimore: Williams and Wilkins; 1974. pp. 1–371.
20. Merkel G, Eger EI II. A comparative study of halothane and halopropane anesthesia. Including a method for determining equipotency. Anesthesiology. 1963;24:346–57.
21. Antognini JF, Schwartz K. Exaggerated anesthetic requirements in the preferentially anesthetized brain. Anesthesiology. 1993;79:1244–9.
22. Rampil IJ, Mason P, Singh H. Anesthetic potency (MAC) is independent of forebrain structures in the rat. Anesthesiology. 1993;78:707–12.
23. Saidman LJ, Eger EI II. Effect of nitrous oxide and of narcotic premedication on the alveolar concentration of halothane required for anesthesia. Anesthesiology. 1964;25:302–6.
24. Severinghaus JW, Bradley AF. Electrodes for blood pO2 and pCO2 determination. J Appl Physiol. 1958;13:515–20.
25. Saidman LJ, Havard ES, Eger EI II. Hyperthermia during anesthesia. JAMA. 1964;190:1029–32.
26. Denborough MA, Forster JF, Lovell RR, Maplestone PA, Villiers JD. Anaesthetic deaths in a family. Br J Anaesth. 1962;34:395–6.
27. Stoelting RK, Longnecker DE, Eger EI II. Minimal alveolar concentrations on awakening from methoxyflurane, halothane, ether and fluroxene in man: MAC awake. Anesthesiology. 1970;33:5–9.
28. Yakaitis RW, Blitt CD, Anjiulo JP. End-tidal halothane concentration for tracheal intubation. Anesthesiology. 1977;47:386–8.
29. Roizen MF, Horrigan RW, Frazer BF. Anesthetic doses blocking adrenergic (stress) and cardiovascular responses to incision—MAC BAR. Anesthesiology. 1981;54:390–8.

30. Gregory GA, Eger EI II, Munson ES. The relationship between age and halothane requirement in man. Anesthesiology. 1969;30:488–91.
31. Stone FL. Some observations on anesthesiology in transicion. In: Bunker JP, Editor. Education in anesthesiology. New York: Columbia University Press; 1967.
32. Lowenstein E, Hallowell P, Levine FH, Daggett WM, Austen WG, Laver MB. Cardiovascular response to large doses of intravenous morphine in man. N Engl J Med. 1969;281:1389–93.
33. Wynands JE, Sheridan CA, Kelkar K. Coronary artery disease and anaesthesia (experience in 120 patients for revascularization of the heart). Can J Anaesth. 1967;14:382–98.
34. Aird RB. Experimental encephalography with anesthetic gasses. Arch Surg. 1936;32:193.
35. Newman HW. Encephalography with ethylene. JAMA. 1937;108:461.
36. Tenney SM, Carpenter FG, Rahn H. Gas transfers in a sulfur hexafluoride pneumoperitoneum. J Appl Physiol. 1953;6:201–8.
37. Hunter AR. Problems of anaesthesia in artificial pneumothorax. Proc Roy Soc Med. 1955;48:765.
38. Munson ES, Merrick HC. Effect of nitrous oxide on venous air embolism. Anesthesiology. 1966;27:783–7.
39. Eger EI II, Saidman LJ. Hazards of nitrous oxide anesthesia in bowel obstruction and pneumothorax. Anesthesiology. 1965;26:61–6.
40. Saidman LJ, Eger EI II. Change in cerebrospinal fluid pressure during pneumoencephalography under nitrous oxide anesthesia. Anesthesiology. 1965;26:67–72.
41. Wolf GL, Capuano C, Hartung J. Nitrous oxide increases intraocular pressure after intravitreal sulfur hexafluoride injection. Anesthesiology. 1983;59:547–8.
42. Campbell EJ, Nunn JF, Peckett BW. A comparison of artificial ventilation and spontaneous respiration with particular reference to ventilation-bloodflow relationships. Br J Anaesth. 1958;30:166–75.
43. Nunn JF. Factors influencing the arterial oxygen tension during halothane anaesthesia with spontaneous respiration. Br J Anaesth. 1964;36:327–41.
44. Nunn JF, Bergman NA, Coleman AJ. Factors influencing the arterial oxygen tension during anaesthesia with artificial ventilation. Br J Anaesth. 1965;37:898–914.
45. Nunn JF. Applied respiratory physiology with special reference to anaesthesia. London: Butterworth; 1969.
46. Allison AC, Nunn JF. Effects of general anaesthetics on microtubules: a possible mechanism of anaesthesia. Lancet. 1968;2:1326–9.
47. Deacon R, Lumb M, Perry J, Chanarin I, Minty B, Halsey MJ, Nunn JF. Selective inactivation of vitamine B12 by nitrous oxide. Lancet. 1978;2:1023–4.
48. Kalow W. Staron N: On distribution and inheritance of atypical forms of human serum cholinesterase, as indicated by dibucaine numbers. Can J Biochem Physiol. 1957;35:1305–20.
49. Kalow W. Pharmacogenetics; heredity and the response to drugs. Philadelphia: W.B. Saunders Co.; 1962.
50. Baird WL, Reid AM. The neuromuscular blocking properties of a new steroid compound, pancuronium bromide. A pilot study in man. Br J Anaesth. 1967;39:775–80.
51. Briggs RM, Ogg MJ. Patients' refusal of surgery after innovar premedication. Plast Reconstr Surg. 1973;51:158–61.
52. Corssen G, Domino EF. Dissociative anesthesia: further pharmacologic studies and first clinical experience with the phencyclidine derivative CI-581. Anesth Analg. 1966;45:29–40.
53. Loftus RW, Yeager MP, Clark JA, Brown JR, Abdu WA, Sengupta DK, Beach ML. Intraoperative ketamine reduces perioperative opiate consumption in opiate-dependent patients with chronic back pain undergoing back surgery. Anesthesiology. 2010;113:639–46.
54. Henn F, Brattsand R. Some pharmacological and toxicological properties of a new long-acting local analgesic, LAC-43 (marcaine), in comparison with mepivacaine and tetracaine. Acta Anaesthesiol Scand Suppl. 1966;21:9–30.
55. Prentiss JE. Cardiac arrest following caudal anesthesia. Anesthesiology. 1979;50:51–3.
56. Beecher HK, Todd DP. A study of the deaths associated with anesthesia and surgery: based on a study of 599,548 anesthesias in ten institutions 1948–1952, inclusive. Ann Surg. 1954;140:2–35.
57. Beecher HK. Experimental pharmacology and measurement of the subjective response. Science. 1952;116:157–62.
58. Beecher HK. Ethics and clinical research. N Engl J Med. 1966;274:1354–60.
59. A definition of irreversible coma. Report of the Ad Hoc Committee of the Harvard Medical School to examine the definition of brain death. JAMA. 1968;205:337–40.
60. Lowenstein E. Defining brain death: motivations and future directions. In: Lowenstein E, McPeek B, Editors. Enduring contributions of Henry K. Beecher to medicine, science and society. Alphen aan den Rijn, Netherlands: Wolters Kluwer/Lippincott Williams & Wilkins; 2007.

Major Anesthetic Themes in the 1970s

10

Rod N. Westhorpe, Lawrence J. Saidman and Edmond I Eger II

Summary

Specialist anesthesiologists increased in numbers and influence, in the process creating subspecialty societies and jour-nals. In some countries (e.g., Cuba and Panama), numbers of nurse anesthetists decreased dramatically, but in others (e.g., the US) they increased. Continuing a trend initiated in the 1960s, investment in anesthesia research expanded.

In the 1960s, halothane displaced ether as the volatile anesthetic agent of choice. However, postoperative liver dysfunction attributed to halothane led many anesthesiologists of the time to prematurely abandon its use in favor of probably inferior alternatives. Methoxyflurane and trichloroethylene had their champions, but neither matched the advantageous features of halothane. The search was on for a replacement. By the mid 1970s, enflurane supplanted halothane in many developed countries (especially the US) except in children because of halothane's absence of pungency.

Understanding of neuromuscular blocking drug pharmacokinetics and pharmacodynamics led to more rational use and monitoring of muscle relaxants. Dantrolene was used to treat malignant hyperthermia.

Anesthesia expanded from the operating room to support the use of new imaging technology. Outpatient surgery greatly increased in the US—fifty years after Ralph Waters' "Downtown Anesthesia Clinic" began this trend. New understanding of pain pathways, and the introduction of new methods of pain relief moved anesthesiologists into post-operative pain management. Opioid receptors were discovered, and opioids were given intrathecally to provide analgesia. Regional anesthesia became established as an integral part of everyday anesthesia practice. Led by their respective champions, Alon Winnie and John Bonica, the subspecialties of regional anesthesia and pain medicine established an international presence.

In 1978, Cooper and colleagues published the results of their study of critical incidents during anesthesia. Having obtained taped interviews from anesthesiologists, and making use of new developments in computer technology, they looked objectively at the roles of human factors and equipment failure in the causation of incidents during anesthesia. This study began the worldwide "safety movement" in anesthesia.

"You, you may say I'm a dreamer" said John Lennon, and for anesthesia, some of those dreams came true.

World Events in the 1970s

"Imagine," John Lennon's immortal song, released in 1971, epitomised the aspirations of younger people for a safer and better world. It was not all to be. The 1970s heralded myriad changes in the world. Science, technology and the social fabric of society were to be altered forever. In 1970, people wrote letters by hand, using a ballpoint pen, a Bic©. The first microprocessor appeared in 1971, and IBM released a mini-computer, the 5100, in 1975. It was a complete pro-grammable system designed for professional and scientific problem-solvers. It was also expensive—up to $ 20,000. Apple computer Inc. was founded in 1976. Writing letters changed after 1979, when a word processing system was in-troduced (Wordstar), turning illegible hand-written letters to clearly written documents. And we placed these in stamped envelopes and waited, and waited, for a reply. The next step, transmission via the internet, arose in the 1980s. The coun-terculture movement that began in the late 1960s, epitomized social change in the 1970s. The long running Vietnam War ended in 1973 with the US and its allies withdrawing their troops after loud and sometimes bloody public protests. In the aftermath of the 1972 burglary of the Watergate offic-es of the Democratic National Committee, Richard Nixon resigned his presidency in 1974. Urban terrorism raised its profile with the murder of Israeli athletes at the 1972 Munich

R. N. Westhorpe (✉)
Melbourne, Australia
e-mail: westhorpe@netspace.net.au

L. J. Saidman
Department of Anesthesia, Stanford University, Stanford, CA, USA
e-mail: lsaidman@stanford.edu

E. I Eger II
Department of Anesthesia and Perioperative Care, University of California, San Francisco, CA, USA
e-mail: egere@anesthesia.ucsf.edu

E. I Eger II et al. (eds.), *The Wondrous Story of Anesthesia,* DOI 10.1007/978-1-4614-8441-7_10, © Edmond I Eger, MD 2014

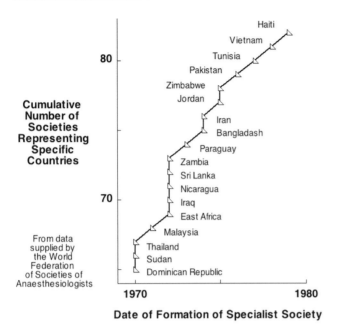

Cumulative Number of Societies Representing Specific Countries

Haiti
Vietnam
Tunisia
Pakistan
Zimbabwe
Jordan
Iran
Bangladash
Paraguay
Zambia
Sri Lanka
Nicaragua
Iraq
East Africa
Malaysia
Thailand
Sudan
Dominican Republic

From data supplied by the World Federation of Societies of Anaesthesiologists

1970   1980

Date of Formation of Specialist Society

Fig. 10.1 The cumulative number of anesthetic societies in the world continued to grow—by 18—in the 1970s. Most arose in developing countries

Olympics, and in 1973, the Arab-Israeli conflict (the Yom Kippur War) once again led to a crisis in the price and availability of oil. China remained in the paralyzing grip of Mao's cultural revolution until 1976. In 1979 under Ayatollah Khomeini, the Iranian revolution transformed Iran from the Shah-led autocracy into a theocracy. And Russia occupied Afghanistan, much to its later regret.

Anesthesia, a Child of the 1970s

The previous two decades set the scene for the massive changes in the specialty that would occur in the remainder of the twentieth century. Most developed countries and many others had established training programs in anesthesia. Countries with lesser numbers of anesthesiologists per head of population lagged behind in the development of anesthesia societies (see Fig. 8.1), particularly those in Africa, Central America, the Middle East, China and the USSR. Many of these countries added anesthetic societies in the 1970s (Fig. 10.1). Most developed countries established societies to enable this new breed of medical specialists to share knowledge and advance their status (see Fig. 8.3). It was still a "junior" specialty, but was starting to flex its muscles. A specialty that was perceived to immediately connect physiology and pharmacology to patient care attracted increasing numbers of doctors.

Anesthesia also attracted women into the specialty. The proportion of women as medical students in the US greatly increased in the 1960s and 1970s. Title IX of the 1972

Higher Education Act banned discrimination in admissions and salaries in any institution receiving federal government funding. Although the number of women accepted into medical school almost tripled from 1971 to 1975, it would be some time before women fully achieved senior roles in specialist medical organisations. There were exceptions. In Australia, women assumed leading roles in the specialty as early as the 1950s. Mary Burnell became the first woman President of the Australian Society of Anaesthetists in 1955, and in 1966, she became Dean of the Faculty of Anaesthetists, just as Patricia Mackay (nee Wilson) was elected President of the Society. In the US, before the 1980s, few women had assumed major roles in anesthesia since Virginia Apgar and Gertie Marx, had done so some 20 or more years earlier.[1]

Professionalism and Consolidation

At the beginning of the 1970s, many surgeons recognised the value of an anesthesiologist to their own practice but were reluctant to acknowledge the place of another senior physician in the operating room. The operating room is referred to as the operating "theatre" and surgeons had long relished their place in (or at least under) the spotlights as "the captain of the ship."

In his February 1976 editorial in Anesthesiology, Nick Greene noted that the traditional approach to anesthesia—"the best anesthetic is the one the anesthetist is most familiar with"—was no longer acceptable. He argued that the goal should be to administer an anesthetic optimizing the patient's care. The growth of professionalism accompanied the maturation of anesthesia departments and societies, with a gradual rejection of subservience of the anesthesiologist to the surgeon. There was a significant economic imperative in this process, since in countries where private practice predominated, there were substantial fee differentials between anesthesiologists and surgeons. Although some societies divested the responsibility for training to sister organisations in the form of Faculties (notably of Colleges of Surgeons or Physicians), most societies maintained a primary educational role while developing an increased profile in political negotiation for better conditions and remuneration.

By 1980, the place of the specialty was firmly established. Younger surgeons recognised the value of a productive working relationship with the emergent specialty, and placed increasing trust in the anesthesiologist, including their involvement in preoperative assessment and postopera-

---

[1] Judy Donegan became the first woman ABA Director in 1983, and Betty Stephenson, the first woman ASA President in 1991. Jane Fitch became President-elect of the ASA in 2012.

tive care. Still, some of the "old guard's" influence remained, and sometimes their prejudices rubbed off on their trainees.

Non-specialist Anesthesia

In many countries, the 1970s saw the gradual disappearance of non-specialists in anesthesia practice. As training programs generated more specialists, full-time anesthesia practice replaced the part-time anesthetist in general practice. In some European (especially Nordic) countries and many developing countries, as well as in the US, nurses continued to play an important role in the provision of anesthesia services. In the US, the traditional place of the nurse anesthetist came under threat when in 1974, the US Office of Education required that a body independent of the American Association of Nurse Anesthetists (AANA) would be needed to accredit training centers. The AANA had been the training and certifying organisation since 1931, and proposed an independent body comprised of Certified Registered Nurse Anesthetists (CRNAs), anesthesiologists and members of the public. The American Society of Anesthesiologists (ASA) sought to establish a competing Faculty of Nurse Anesthesia to accredit CRNAs. The ASA did not succeed in gaining control over CRNA accreditation which was ultimately entrusted to the Council on Accreditation of Nurse Anesthesia Programs (CANAP), as proposed by the AANA.

Sub-specialization

Although most anesthesiologists in 1970 were "generalists", as the specialty matured and the scope and complexity of anesthesia grew, some developed skills and enthusiasm for particular branches of the specialty. These involved obstetric, pediatric, neurosurgical, cardiac, and regional anesthesia, and intensive care. The desire to share information, and advance the quality of care through focussed research and education, led to the formation of sub-specialty organisations, or special interest groups. The establishment of these groups required sufficient numbers of practitioners to sustain them, and this was initially only possible in places like the US and Great Britain, where formal specialty training and certification had been in place for sufficient time. (Fig. 10.2). The Society of Obstetric Anesthesia and Perinatology (SOAP) was established in 1968, and in the following year, the Obstetric Anaesthetist Association was established in Great Britain. By 1970, Great Britain had also established a society for anesthetic research. Then, in the 1970s, several new subspecialist societies or associations formed in both the US and Great Britain, paving the way for the establishment of similar groups in the 1980s and 1990s in other regions of the world. Although there might have been sufficient numbers

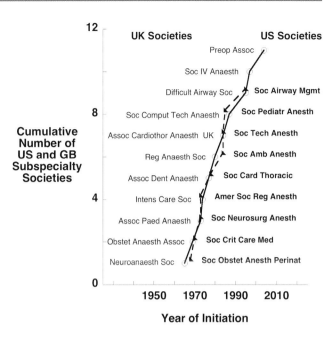

Fig. 10.2 The cumulative increase in the number of subspecialty anesthesia societies occurred linearly and in parallel in the US and UK

of European anesthesiologists to sustain the creation of subspecialty anesthesia organisations, they did not arise until the 1980s. This probably reflected the later establishment of formal training programs. The subspecialty societies or associations formed in Great Britain during the 1970s encompassed critical care, pediatric, cardiovascular, dental and regional anesthesia with several parallel organizations arising in the US (Fig. 10.2).

Training and Examinations

Between 1970 and 1980, most countries in Europe established formal training programs in anesthesia with durations commonly of 3 to 5 years. Not all imposed a formal examination process.

Since the 1950s, training in the US had been overseen by the Anesthesiology Residency Review Committee (RRC) comprising representatives of the AMA Council on Medical Education and Hospitals, and the American Board of Anesthesiology. Attempts to rationalise all postgraduate medical training in the late 1960s had failed and in 1972, five bodies, the AMA, the Association of American Medical Colleges, the American Board of Medical Specialties, American Hospital Association, and the Council on Medical Specialty Societies convened to resolve matters. This resulted in two accrediting bodies, only one of which was to survive, the Liaison Committee on Graduate Medical Education.

A further complication arose because there were two examining bodies, the American Society of Anesthesiologists' American College of Anesthesiology (ACA), and the

American Board of Anesthesiology (ABA). The ACA certified some practitioners whom the ABA considered unsuitable, or who had failed the ABA examination. This created uncertainty for hospitals and credentialing committees. Arthur Keats led the resolution of the impasse. In 1971, he became chairman of the ABA examinations committee while he was also editor in chief of *Anesthesiology*. Through his efforts, the ACA ultimately ceased awarding certificates. At the same time, Keats led a revision of the examination system, creating the Guided Question (intended to provide a more standardized exam), and a comprehensive analysis of the then scope of anesthesiology practice. Both written and in-service training examinations were revised, and a computerized analysis of the results of the exam was introduced. Further, the ABA (using the Rasch model), oversaw the introduction of analysis of the written examination, to ensure that it was a valid test of required knowledge, and would enable feedback to both examiners and residents.

In Great Britain, the Association of Anaesthetists of Great Britain and Ireland established a formal training program in 1932, some time after Waters established his program in 1923. The first formal examination took place in 1935, the Diploma in Anaesthetics, awarded by the Anaesthetic Section of the Royal Society of Medicine. By the 1970s, the Faculty of Anaesthetists within the Royal College of Surgeons, was well established. Training was of four years duration with one year of "higher professional training" to be undertaken after successful completion of the primary and final examinations. Both examinations had written and oral components.

In Europe, the six signatories to the Treaty of Rome in 1957, established the Union Européenne des Médecins Spécialistes (UEMS) in 1958. Intended as a source of discussion and consultation for European Economic Community (EEC) legislation, it eventually became the umbrella organization for national medical specialist organizations in all EEC countries, as well Norway and Switzerland. Specialist sections were created and the Section of Anesthesiology first met in 1962. In 1963, the Section stipulated a minimum training of 3 years, at a time when training in the six member countries varied from 2 to 7 years. The Section reviewed the directive in 1969, agreeing on a minimum training period of 4 years. In 1973, the periods of training still varied between 3 and 7 years in EEC countries, and between 2 and 6 years in non-EEC countries.

In Canada, the Royal College of Physicians and Surgeons of Canada (RCPSC) was established in 1929, and began by recognizing the need to give recognition to doctors engaged in "special work". The qualification was initially gained by invitation, with an examination introduced in 1931, leading to the title "Fellow". It was primarily aimed at physicians and surgeons in an academic role, while anesthesiologists were not considered in the "same league". In 1937, a less

rigorous program of "certification" was introduced, however anesthesia was still not considered as a specialty, although it was eventually included in 1942. Until 1971, the dual system of certification and fellowship persisted, with both fellows and certificants being recognized as specialist anesthesiologists. In 1971, a single training, examination and accreditation system was instituted. This and the four-year training program meant that Canadian specialists were at last treated as equal to other specialists within the RCPSC.

In Australia and New Zealand, the training and examination process for certification as a Fellow of the Faculty of Anaesthetists of the Royal Australasian College of Surgeons, was similar to that in Great Britain, without the requirement for a year of higher professional training.

In Japan in the 1960s, two years training and/or experience in administering anesthesia to 300 patients resulted in a permanent qualification that once obtained, remained in force indefinitely. The duration of training has increased to at least 4 years at the first step of certification (see Chapter 31).

Medical practice in China recovered slowly from the 1966–1976 Cultural Revolution, which had forced many doctors to perform non-medical manual work. Despite these hindrances, in 1979, the Chinese Society of Anaesthesiology was formed with 44 members.

In Mexico, and Central and South America, development of anesthesia lagged behind that in the US, Canada, and Europe. Nevertheless, by 1970, most countries in this region had established specialist societies (see Figs. 6.2, 8.2, and 9.2), and some had instituted training programs. Through the 1970s, with growth in the number of academic departments of anesthesia, more training programs were established. The 1970s also saw the disappearance of nurse anesthetists from many countries in the region.

Academic Development

In Great Britain, during the 1960s, 15 new academic departments of anesthesia were created, consolidating the advancement of academic anesthesia. Several university research departments were created, and several anesthesiologists acquired MDs or PhDs. This enhanced the status of anesthesia in the region and had the effect of attracting many anesthesiologists from current and former British Commonwealth countries (Australia, Canada, India, New Zealand, Pakistan, and South Africa) to Great Britain. Many of these anesthesiologists returned to their countries of origin to assist in establishing academic departments, although in most cases it took some years before university research departments were created.

In the US, funded academic departments were well established, and the 1970s saw an expansion of anesthesia research, championed by enthusiastic and dedicated people.

Theirs was the model that many other countries wished to emulate, but few could afford.

This was also a period when collaboration between academic anesthesiologists and industry reached a new peak. Several companies enthusiastically pursued the development of anesthesia equipment and drugs—Ohio (enflurane), Cyprane (variable bypass, tec-type vaporizers), ICI (propofol), Glaxo (althesin), Burroughs Wellcome (atracurium), Organon (pancuronium), to name a few, and all had close ties with research anesthesiogists.

Journals

By 1970, many of the major anesthesia journals of the world were well established (e.g., see Fig. 6.1), and the only further one to appear during the decade was *Anaesthesia and Intensive Care*, first published by the Australian Society of Anaesthetists in 1972. The 1970s did however see the appearance of subspecialty journals. As might be expected, the earliest subspecialty journals to appear were consistent with the first subspecialties to create organisations, except for obstetric anesthesia. *Critical Care Medicine* was first published in 1973, and following the formation of the International Association for the Study of Pain (IASP) in 1974, *Pain* was published in 1975, with Patrick Wall as its first editor-in-chief. *Pain* eventually achieved the highest impact factor of all anesthesia-related journals in 2011. In 1976, *Regional Anesthesia* was first published, later to be renamed *Regional Anesthesia and Pain Medicine*. In 1978, another journal dedicated to regional anesthesia appeared as a supplement to *Der Anaesthesist,* named *Regionale Anaesthesie.*

The Beginning of the End for Halothane

At the beginning of the 1970s, anesthesia commonly relied on the use of thiopental, nitrous oxide, and halothane, with the probable addition of a muscle relaxant and opioid. The notation on many anesthetic records of the time "GOH", signified the mainstay of practice; "Gas (nitrous oxide), Oxygen and Halothane".

The documentation of cases of liver dysfunction following halothane had led to widespread investigation in the 1960s. The detailed results, published in 1969, pointed to a rare but real mortality rate from hepatotoxicity of some 1:120,000 [1]. This was enough to reassure some, especially pediatric anesthetists, but the coming demise of halothane was established. In many cases it was not anesthesiologists who condemned it, but physicians (internists), who quickly blamed any episode of postoperative jaundice on halothane, often without justification. Outside the US, some anesthesiologists chose to use alternatives, either methoxyflurane or

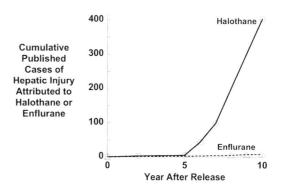

Fig. 10.3 Few cases of hepatic injury were reported in the first 5 years following the release of halothane, but after 5 years, a dramatic increase in published reports of injury followed. This biphasic response would be expected if an allergic response underlay injury. The steep increase would require an initial "sensitization" to halothane. In contrast to halothane, no dramatic increase in published reports of injury occurred in the first 10 years after the release of enflurane for clinical use

trichloroethylene, and some even clung to ether. All had their problems, and were to disappear from general use by the mid 1970s. The possibility of renal failure as result of free fluoride ion from degradation of methoxyflurane had been described previously, but was characterised by Mazze and Cousins in 1973 [2]. The search was on for a replacement.

Ross Terrell had identified enflurane in the mid-1960s, a fluorinated methyl ethyl ether with characteristics likely to make it safer than halothane, an alkane. He noted that the ethers had less propensity to cause arrhythmias and that only 2–3 % of enflurane was metabolised, resulting in fewer potentially toxic metabolites. Introduced in the early 1970s, enflurane was the answer to many prayers, only to be tarnished by the appearance of tonic and clonic muscle movement, associated with EEG epileptiform activity. This was not a major impediment, and in the US and some other developed countries around the world, enflurane displaced halothane from the operating room. With increasing use of enflurane, it was clear that hepatotoxicity was much less than with halothane [3]. In particular, the number of cases reported in the years after release appeared at a far slower rate than after the release of halothane (Fig. 10.3).

The Trouble with Isoflurane

Ross Terrell synthesized the isomer of enflurane, isoflurane, in 1965. It was more difficult to produce and purify, delaying its development. Once a suitable method was found, and animal tests had been done, clinical trials began in 1971. Initial results were encouraging. Isoflurane met many of the criteria of the ideal inhalational agent; it was stable, had low blood solubility, low level of biodegradation (0.2 %), and was nonflammable. It was also devoid of epileptogenic activity and allowed a rapid recovery. Just as it was about to be released in 1975, a study by Tom Corbett at the University of Michigan suggested that isoflurane was a carcinogen in mice [4].

Corbett phoned Eger with the news. Eger, Terrell and Jim Vitcha from Ohio Medical (the manufacturer of isoflurane) went to the University of Michigan to discuss the experiment with Corbett, finding several key flaws in the study. In particular, there were too few negative control animals, no dose-response relationship had been determined, and Corbett had not blinded his examination of animals for tumor [4]. Even more frighteningly, there were no control animals given alternative anesthetics. Corbett had assumed the problem was limited to isoflurane, but other anesthetics were far more vulnerable to metabolism and the production of potentially toxic metabolites that might have produced genetic changes. Still, that magic word "cancer" made such objections moot. Clearly the test would have to be repeated with the flaws eliminated. Everyone involved knew this.

But Eger also knew that Ohio would dither while it decided whether to fight the findings or support (at great cost) the required study. Not willing to wait for what they knew would be a long-delayed decision, the impatient Eger and his colleague, Wendel Stevens, elected to initiate the study using discretionary funds Eger had gathered from previous work, believing that Ohio would be forced to pursue and support the study. They would sponge off the university for a few months.

For a time, it went as planned. Ohio capitulated nearly a year later and asked Eger and Stevens to proceed with the study, now clandestinely underway, a study of thousands of animals. But for a phone call requesting a small change in the protocol, the conspirators would have pulled it off, covering up their early start. Vitcha called Eger asking if the study animals might be kept alive three months longer than originally planned after their in utero exposure to the anesthetics, 18 rather than 15 months. Too late; the animals were already in formaldehyde! Eger and Stevens flew to Chicago to meet with their friends from Ohio Medical and confess their sins.

The conspirators then completed the study, convincing Corbett to join them, this time as a blinded examiner of the tissues of the study animals for cancer. The result was that none of the study anesthetics, none of the modern anesthetics, caused cancer except that the most metabolized anesthetic, methoxyflurane tended to show a trend towards an increased incidence [5].

Published in 1978, this negative result allowed the clinical release of isoflurane to proceed. Isoflurane was marketed in another year or two, becoming the dominant inhaled anesthetic of the 1980s.

In the 1970s, pediatric anesthesiologists continued using halothane because it was less pungent than enflurane, and did not have the stigma of epileptogenicity. Anesthesia was commonly induced in children by inhalation, and their in-

duction and recovery was as fast with halothane despite the modestly lower solubility of enflurane. In addition, halothane had not been incriminated in the causation of liver injury in children.

Calibrated Vaporizers

Both the Copper Kettle and the Fluotec Mark 2 (the Mark 1 was recalled shortly after release because of a problem with the control knob) had been available since the 1950s. The Copper Kettle could be accurately used with any volatile inhalation agent, and would be used for halothane, methoxyflurane, and enflurane until it was superseded by variable bypass vaporisers. The Fluotec Mark 2 was a modification of the Tritec, the first temperature compensated vaporiser produced by Cyprane in England, for use with trichloroethylene. The "tec" vaporiser was later modified to accommodate methoxyflurane (Pentec), and enflurane (Enfluratec). There was also an Ethertec designed for use in developing countries.

Despite the availability of calibrated, temperature compensated vaporisers, at the beginning of the 1970s, many anesthetics were still given using the old Boyle bottles, particularly outside North America. Because the Copper Kettle and the Vernitrol had an established place in the US as universal vaporisers that could be used with either ether or halothane (albeit requiring some mathematical calculations on the part of the anesthesiologist), the initial marketing of halothane in the US was accompanied by an aggressive joint campaign by Ayerst Laboratories marketing halothane, and Fraser Sweatman, the agents for the Cyprane "Fluotec" vaporiser. This ensured that hospitals procuring a supply of halothane would receive free vaporisers. Boyle bottles and the Ohio #8 vaporizer quickly became obsolete, and the Copper Kettles and Vernitrols gradually disappeared.

In Germany, Drager had introduced the "Vapor" temperature compensated vaporiser, but elsewhere outside North America, where there was no competition for the Fluotec, Boyle bottles were still in use, as there was no incentive for hospitals to equip their operating rooms with new and expensive devices. These had originally been used for ether, were uncalibrated, and could deliver high concentrations of halothane. Producing new glass bottles labelled "Fluothane" or "Trilene" served to identify them as "new" vaporisers, but they were little better than dripping the agent onto a towel—the anesthesiologist had no idea how much was being administered. The recent establishment of the principle of MAC by Eger and colleagues had little meaning to those forced to use such equipment by the lack of investment by hospitals in the emerging specialty. Boyle bottles were of course convenient for many anesthesiologists in private practice who had to supply their own halothane, allowing them to empty the remaining contents back into their personal container at the end of a case. This advantage was also somewhat dangerous if the anesthesiologist did not label and/or empty the "bottle" and a second person filled it with a different agent.

Cyprane introduced the "Tec" 3 vaporiser in 1969. It had several advantages over the "Tec 2" models. The output was linear at all flow rates, and it eliminated the "pumping" effect of positive pressure ventilation that could silently increase output. By the end of the 1970s, all inhalation agents were delivered through calibrated, temperature compensated vaporisers, usually the Tec 3 or similar devices manufactured by Ohio or Drager. The concept of MAC had informed the 1970s anesthesiologist as to the concentration of anesthetic agent required for elimination of a response to the surgeon's knife, but until the end-tidal concentration was routinely monitored, could only be interpreted in terms of the inhaled concentration. At least by the end of the decade, the anesthesiologist had a calibrated vaporiser to help.

Induction with Steroids

Thiopental retained its place as the primary induction agent at the beginning of the 1970s, but was to be challenged by alternatives. Thiopental found an additional role after Michenfelder and Theye showed in 1973 that it reduced cerebral metabolism and might protect the brain against hypoxic injury [6]. The use of the drug for cerebral protection by "induced coma" continued for many years. Such virtues notwithstanding, the search was on for a replacement for thiopental, for a drug that avoided the cardio-respiratory depression so characteristic of induction, especially in the patient with vascular disease.

Etomidate, a carboxylated imidazole derivative rather than a barbiturate, was released in the mid 1970s. Because it was hydrophobic, it was formulated in propylene glycol, however the pain and irritation on injection, and myoclonic movements after injection, limited its popularity. It did nevertheless provide greater cardiovascular stability than its rival, thiopental.

Glaxo released a new anesthetic induction agent in Europe in 1973, comprising a mixture of two steroid molecules. Althesin included alphaxalone as the anesthetic, accompanied by alphadolone to increase the solubility in a Cremophor EL solution. Althesin provided a smooth painless induction accompanied by little cardiovascular effect and rapid recovery. It gained a firm place in outpatient anesthesia until reports of allergic reactions began to appear, reactions largely related to the presence of Cremophor EL. Althesin was never released in the US.

Ketamine, a phencyclidine derivative was developed in 1962. It was first used clinically on American soldiers in the Vietnam War in 1970, and although it was devoid of cardiovascular depressant effects, its hallucinogenic tendency,

a consequence of its chemical heritage, resulted in what was to be called "dissociative anesthesia". Such a label was of little comfort to those who experienced the less desirable manifestations including perceived loss of their arms or legs. Ketamine found a place in field use in civil disasters and in low dose infusions for pain management, but that was after the 1970s.

Thus, by the end of the 1970s, thiopental had defended its place as the induction agent of choice. It was now only available as a 2.5 % formulation (requiring mixing of powder and sterile water before use) because the previously available 5 % solution had been shown to cause skin necrosis after extravasation, and ischemia after arterial injection. Use of the 2.5 % solution largely eliminated these complications. The drug was available in multi-dose bottles, commonly 100 or 250 ml. The fear of disease transmission was unheard of, and anesthesiologists of the time recall prepared solutions being used for several days on subsequent patients. Perhaps that wasn't quite as foolish as it might sound. Alkalinity of thiopental solutions (pH 10–11) made them sterile. By 1970, in most countries, metal intravenous cannulae (needles) had been replaced by plastic disposable cannulae (catheters), often still with a metal hub.

Relaxed about Relaxants

In 1970, the available muscle relaxants included succinylcholine for rapid action and short procedures, and d-tubocurare (curare) or pancuronium for prolonged effect. The 1970s will not be remembered for new relaxants, but for the increased understanding of their pharmacology and pharmacokinetics, and the introduction of routine methods of monitoring the depth of neuromuscular blockade.

As the decade began, the ways in which injected drugs acted on the body (pharmacodynamics) and how they were affected by the body (pharmacokinetics), were little understood. In 1973, Leslie Benet and colleagues created the concept of "clearance" in landmark research that led to greater understanding of individual dosage and toxicity of drugs [7]. At the same time, Lewis Sheiner introduced the concept of "concentration—effect" relationships, leading Sheiner and Stuart Beal to develop NONMEM, a computer program for modelling of pharmacokinetics [8]. Using these tools, Ronald Miller and colleagues, also at UCSF, studied the action of curare. Measuring the concentration of a drug at its effect site (the neuromuscular junction in the case of curare) is not feasible. But Miller and Sheiner recognised that the effect (and the concentration) at the effect site always lagged behind what the anesthesiologist had given (i.e., the blood concentration) to induce paralysis, and that the opposite was true during recovery [9]. This enabled an estimation of drug concentration at the effect site, and from this they could infer the effects of such things such as hepatic or renal failure on drug concentration and clearance. Their work enabled a new understanding of the pharmacodynamics and pharmacokinetics of curare, and indeed, of many other drugs used in anesthesia.

In 1970, Hassan Ali and colleagues applied a series of four identical stimuli to the ulnar nerve via surface electrodes at half second intervals. The response of the pollcis longus muscle to the fourth stimulus was compared to the first. Ali determined that a ratio of less than 0.7 indicated residual paralysis from a muscle relaxant. The "Train of Four" did not require a baseline measurement, and therefore could be applied after injection of the neuromuscular blocking drug, and could even be used in awake patients with minimal discomfort. Crude estimation of the ratio could be performed by the anesthesiologist manually sensing the twitch response. The use of surface electrodes also eliminated the need for needles. The ability to monitor the depth of neuromuscular block, and the adequacy of reversal was a great advance in the prevention of postoperative hypoventilation due to residual paralysis [10].

Alon Winnie Promoted Regional Anesthesia

Although no new local anesthetic agents appeared in the 1970s, the polio-stricken Alon Winnie championed the use of regional plexus blocks, in particular of the brachial, cervical and lumbar plexuses. Anesthesiologists embraced these new techniques for intraoperative use as part of the expanding armamentarium of anesthesia practice. Fine, high quality disposable spinal needles were developed, and epidural anesthesia benefited from the development of precise loss of resistance syringes, encouraging a greater use of these techniques as part of anesthesia care.

Beyond his clinical contributions, Winnie's great legacy from the 1970s was his re-establishment, with colleagues, of the American Society of Regional Anesthesia (ASRA). The Society was dedicated to the promotion, investigation and teaching of regional anesthesia. The first congress of the Society was held in 1976, soon followed by the publication of the first issue of the journal *Regional Anesthesia*. The formation of ASRA, and Winnie's international profile, encouraged the establishment of similar organisations elsewhere in the world, with the European Society beginning in 1979.

In 1976, Danish gastrointestinal surgeon Henrik Kehlet's observations of stress responses to surgery convinced him that epidural regional anesthesia imposed before surgery and continued postoperatively could attenuate the catabolic (i.e., protein-wasting) effects of surgery. The notion was to prevent "central sensitization", to block afferent nociceptive traffic completely. To avoid central sensitization required a sufficient density of neural afferent blockade for a sufficient time, over a sufficient number of spinal segments [11].

A cautionary note on regional anesthesia appeared in 1979, with the first report of the cardiotoxic effects of bupivacaine, ultimately leading to revised guidelines on dosage [12].

The Painful Truth

The 1970s brought a change in the way anesthesiologists approached pain management, intraoperatively at first, and later postoperatively. Just before the start of the decade, high dose morphine anesthesia became popular in patients having valvular heart surgery because it blocked the hemodynamic and metabolic responses to surgical stress. Outcome studies suggested however, that such patients had incomplete amnesia and suffered from greater histamine release, consequent venodilation, and prolonged postoperative respiratory depression. Venodilation also resulted in greater transfusion requirements. High dose fentanyl, introduced in the late 1960s, offered a suitable alternative, with less histamine release and less hypotension. Fentanyl began to displace morphine (and meperidine) from routine anesthesia practice, although its propensity to lead to respiratory depression was recognised as a limitation. Anesthesiologists had to "learn" how to use a new analgesic with quite different pharmacokenetics. Most importantly, fentanyl (and its later sisters alfentanil, sufentanil, and remifentanil) easily passed through the blood-brain barrier whereas morphine did not. The result was that fentanyl acted quickly—within minutes from the time of its injection—and its effect disappeared as it left the blood consequent to hepatic metabolism. In contrast, morphine's effect came on slowly, reaching a peak in perhaps 45 minutes. And although the blood level might decrease, morphine remained in the brain and its blood levels might not reflect its continuing effect.

Anesthesiologists took an increasing interest in acute pain management, and in particular, in postoperative pain. John Bonica led this movement, no doubt stimulated by his personal problems with pain imposed by the result of injuries suffered in his earlier career as a professional wrestler. In 1972, he initiated a global organization to establish pain as a differentiated field of study. He oversaw the organisation of an international meeting in 1973 that attracted 102 international speakers. As noted earlier, attendants at that meeting established the International Association for the Study of Pain (IASP), and planned a new journal, *Pain*.

The 1970s saw the introduction of acute pain services, usually led by anesthesiologists. Surgeons and other clinicians saw the benefits of such services and compounded the enthusiasm. Sechzer reported the first patient controlled analgesia (PCA) system for postoperative pain in 1968 [13]. In this manually controlled system, a nurse administered small increments of morphine or meperidine according to patient demand. Forrest and colleagues described the first automated device in 1970 [14]. Increasingly sophisticated devices appeared through the 1970s, culminating in Hull's On Demand Analgesia Computer (ODAC) in 1979 [15].

The idea that opioids might act on specific receptors emanated from Wall's and Melzack's 1965 gate control theory. In 1973, Pert and Snyder discovered specific opioid receptors in neural tissue [16]. In 1976, neuroscientists Arthur Duggan and Tony Yaksh provided unequivocal evidence of a spinal site of action of morphine [17, 18]. Wall, while visiting Israel, convinced Florella Magora and her colleagues to administer morphine epidurally for various types of pain. Their results were published in a letter to *The Lancet* on 10 March 1979 [19]. The ensuing publication by Behar et al. encouraged Michael Cousins and colleagues to issue a preliminary report of their study of intrathecal morphine and meperidine, and epidural meperidine. They had been prompted to embark on the study after Wang published the results of a small 1978 study of intrathecal morphine [20]. Matas had described his use of intrathecal morphine in 1900 [21], but at that time the dangers of cephalic spead of the drug were not recognized. The blood and CSF pharmacodynamic and pharmacokinetic data, and neurological assessment, strongly suggested a spinal site, with sparing of normal non-noxious sensation, motor power and sympathetic function. Cousin's Letter, titled "Selective Spinal Analgesia", was accepted 24 hours after receipt and published in May 1979 [22].

Anesthesia Machines: Still the Same, But Not for Long

In any 1970s operating room, the anesthesiologist's main tool-in-trade, the anesthesia machine, had remained largely unchanged for two decades. In many instances, the machine was likely to be 20 years old. The only major improvement was the attachment of a calibrated vaporiser, when administrative and funding support were available. It was still possible however, to administer two different inhalation agents in series, and guidelines were in place suggesting the order in which the vaporisers should be positioned to minimize the danger of this arrangement.

The conduct of anesthesia was however changing. By the 1970s, anesthetists usually routinely measured blood pressure, and pulse meters had appeared in GB (Fig. 10.4). ECG devices with their "beep" provided the alternative in the US. Pulse meters were small devices attached to the patient's fingertip, using a pressure sensor to create a deflection of an ammeter needle and later a flashing light or audible beep. They alleviated the need for the anesthesiologist to constantly palpate the patient's radial or superficial temporal artery. The

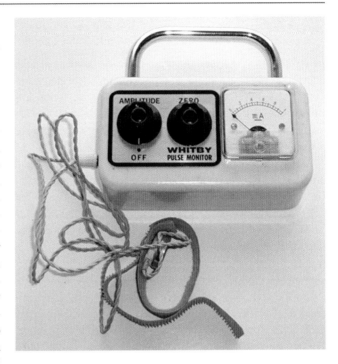

Fig. 10.4 The pulse meter, a simple device supplying a continuous visual (but not auditory) measure of pulse rate. (Courtesy of Rod N. Westhorpe.)

anesthesiologist's task was increasingly demanding! Often holding a face mask on a patient, watching an electrocardiograph, taking the occasional blood pressure (one handed if one could afford an oscillotonometer), and manually recording events. The pulse meter was a great innovation.

Another great innovation was the 1976 introduction of an automated non-invasive blood pressure device, the "Dinamap" by Maynard Ramsey III. Ramsey, who graduated first in chemistry, then in medicine, and then obtained a doctorate in biomedical engineering, described his career as "satisfying, challenging, rewarding and much of the time, lots of fun" [23]. He developed his first disposable intra-arterial pressure device while still a medical student. Using newly available miniature electronic components, he developed the model 825 Dinamap (Device for Indirect Non-invasive Mean Arterial Pressure). It measured only mean arterial pressure, Ramsey considering that the measurement was more informative as an indication of tissue perfusion than systolic and diastolic pressures. He may have been correct, but anesthesiologists were not ready to accept his reasoning, and he responded with the model 845 in 1978, which measured systolic, diastolic and mean pressures as well as heart rate [24].

Another change that occurred in the 1970s was the disappearance of the flammable anesthetics ether, ethylene, and cyclopropane, thus eliminating the need for conductive rubber, and other antistatic measures in the operating room. Nevertheless, there was a long lag time before all protective measures were eliminated…just in case.

How Safe?

In 1971, Scurr described the trend of deaths associated with anesthesia in Great Britain, in relation to the increased number of anesthesia services being performed. He found improvement, and that this had started in the mid 1930s. He suggested the improvement related to "proper education and training in anesthesia" [25].

The 1970s revealed a watershed in the recognition and study of the factors involved in the generation of anesthesia-induced morbidity and mortality. In his paper "There, but for the grace of God…" Wylie commented on the analysis of 66 cases of cardiac arrest during anesthesia reported to the Medical Defence Union in Britain from 1964 to 1973, noting that the number of deaths associated with anesthesia had been falling dramatically since the 1950s, coinciding "with the early days of modern anaesthesia and of specialization…" Wylie determined that about 50% of the cardiac arrests were preventable and 18% resulted from negligence. He suggested that the latter might have been prevented had a proper preoperative assessment been made by an anesthetist or had the anesthetist maintained direct responsibility in the immediate postoperative period [26].

But, it was reasoned that counting the dead was not necessarily a good way to assess the safety of anesthesia, especially when the number of deaths was falling.

Jeffrey Cooper promoted a new approach to this problem. Cooper graduated with a Masters in biomedical engineering and a PhD in chemical engineering in 1972, and joined the bioengineering unit of the Department of Anesthesia at the Massachusetts General Hospital. His close contact with anesthesiologists at work led to his talk at a NATO conference on Human Factors in Healthcare in 1974, entitled "The Anesthesia Machine; An Accident Waiting to Happen". An audience member suggested that he use the Critical Incident Technique described in the 1950s by Flanagan, to study operating room accidents [27, 28]. So began Cooper's landmark studies leading to minimum monitoring standards and the analysis of human factors in the safety of anesthetic delivery. The patient safety movement was born and would ultimately be embraced by all of healthcare.

In their first paper, in 1978 Cooper and his colleagues analysed 359 critical incidents identified at interview with staff anesthesiogists and residents. Human error was involved in 82% of incidents, and equipment failure could only be blamed in 14%. The most frequent incidents were breathing circuit disconnections, inadvertent changes in gas flow, and "syringe swap" [29].

These results led the team to look at preventive strategies in both anesthesia practice, and in the design of equipment. They developed a prototype anesthetic machine, "The Boston Anesthesia Machine", that was displayed at the 1976 annual meeting of the ASA. It was the first application of microprocessor technology, replacing rotameters with solenoid valves and representing gas flows by bar graph displays. An injector system (from a Volkswagen) introduced volatile agents into the breathing system, each agent having a separate non-interchangeable canister. A microprocessor controlled oxygen concentrations in breathing gas, and the actual percentage and circuit pressure were measured automatically. Alarms were applied to various machine parameters, and could be set by the user. The display included messages regarding system faults and corrective strategies. Although never used in patients, the machine gave a foretaste of what was to come [30].

In 1978, Canada became the first country to have a comprehensive standard for anesthetic gas machines. Because both Left (British) and Right handed (American) machines were in common use, sometimes in the same hospital, instances had occurred where the oxygen knob was inadvertently turned off instead of nitrous oxide.

The most important outcome of Cooper's studies was the adoption in 1979 of the anesthesia machine standard, the American National Standards Institute standard Z79.8–1979. The standard aimed to eliminate or warn of serious problems. The requirements included flowmeters in series instead of in parallel, fluted oxygen flow control knobs for tactile feedback, and a means to prevent administration of a hypoxic mixture. Machines manufactured after publication of this standard needed to meet all its requirements.

Soon, some colleagues also began to examine the anesthesiologist's workplace. Ergonomics entered anesthesia in the late 1970s with studies of the anesthesiologist at work. The spatial activity of the anesthesiologist had extended to 360 degrees, and the traditional arrangement of the anesthetic machine behind the anesthesiologist was no longer an efficient one. These studies would direct changes in the operating room over the following two decades.

Safely Anesthetizing the Patient with Cardiovascular Disease

In the 1980s and 1990s, several study results argued that controlling heart rate with beta sympathetic blocking drugs decreased morbidity and mortality, and these will be discussed in succeeding chapters. In 1972, one view held that therapy with beta-receptor blocking drugs for treatment of severe angina should be halted because patients receiving such drugs tolerated anesthesia poorly and had impaired cardiovascular responses to stresses such as hemorrhage [31]. In 1973, Prys-Roberts' group presented an alternative view, suggesting that "hypertensive patients are protected (by pretreatment with a beta-receptor antagonist) from the undesirable sequelae of laryngoscopy and intubation, and from myocardial ischemia associated with arterial hypotension…" [32] Validation and an expansion of such work by Mangano, Wallace and others was yet to come.

Poison in the Air

Perhaps more than patients were at risk from anesthesia. A 1967 study by Vaisman, published in Russian, alerted anesthesiologists and operating room personnel to the potential hazard of breathing trace concentrations of volatile agents for long periods [33]. Vaisman surveyed Russian anesthesiologists and found an increased incidence of poor health, miscarriages and neurological problems, problems associated with exposure to volatile agents, long working hours, emotional stress, and excessive attention to their work.

Many supporting reports followed. In 1971, Ellis Cohen et al surveyed operating room nurses and found an increased incidence of miscarriage, followed by Knill-Jones et al in 1972, who showed that female anesthesiologists had an increased incidence of miscarriage and of congenital anomalies in their offspring. In 1973, Corbett et al showed an increased incidence of cancer in anesthetic nurses, and later, an increase in congenital anomalies in offspring. Although a study by Ericson and Kallen in 1979 failed to confirm the results of the earlier studies, the die was cast [34]. The National Institute for Occupational Safety and Health (NIOSH) had initiated the ASA National Health Survey of Operating Room Personnel, but before completing the study, it released its recommendations in 1977, believing that sufficient circumstantial proof had been gathered. Standards on safe practice and scavenging were produced, along with recommendations on maximum safe levels of all inhaled agents—all arbitrarily determined.

These studies and reports led to the worldwide introduction of stringent measures to minimize or even eliminate trace levels of anesthetic gases from the operating room. Many persist to this day. This despite Spence and colleagues' publication in 1987 [35]. Spence surveyed all female UK medical school graduates under the age of 40 working in hospitals from 1977 to 1984. They surveyed 11,500 women and found that there was no difference in the incidence of infertility, miscarriage, cancer, neuropathy or congenital anomalies in offspring, in anesthesiologists compared with unexposed female hospital doctors.

Ventilators

In the early 1970s, there was still some support for the use of Negative End Expiratory Pressure (NEEP) during the expiratory phase, in the belief that a reduced intrathoracic pressure would improve venous return. Many ventilators of the era included the option of NEEP, but PEEP soon superseded NEEP when it was realised that NEEP could impair alveolar gas exchange while PEEP might do the opposite. The notion that PEEP might help followed the paper by Ashbaugh et al in the Lancet in 1967 [36]. Ventilation improved in patients with what would be called Acute Respiratory Distress Syndrome, when they were treated with 5 to 10 cm H_2O of PEEP. PEEP was applied in anesthesia by the end of the 1970s, initially to critically ill patients. Anesthesia ventilators came to be fitted with a PEEP option as standard.

Most anesthesia ventilators of the time were simple devices. In Great Britain, the Manley ventilator, designed by Roger Manley in 1959 while he was a House Officer, was virtually ubiquitous. It was powered by the fresh gas flow of the anesthetic machine, and was used to provide ventilation from a non-rebreathing circuit. The Manley ventilator had no alarms, and had a maximum inspiratory pressure of 30 cm H_2O.

In the US, the Bird and Air Shields Ventilators were commonly used, usually with a "bag-in-bottle" arrangement driving a rebreathing circuit with CO_2 absorption. When not enough ventilators were available, the anesthesiologist squeezed the rebreathing bag. Anesthesiologists in Australia and New Zealand largely relied on the latter method, although some used the "auto hand", a simple electrically driven device comprising two boards hinged at one side, with the rebreathing bag placed between them.

Europeans were more sophisticated. They used the Engström ventilator and a variety of others developed as a consequence of the 1952 Copenhagen polio epidemic. Although originally designed for use in intensive care, or in thoracic surgery, they found their way into the operating room. In 1971, the Elema-Schönander company introduced the first Servo ventilator, a microprocessor controlled device designed for intensive care, but ultimately used by anesthesiologists. The new ventilator was so quiet that during one early trial, the company representative found the ventilator pushed into a corner each morning. The staff were convinced that the lack of noise indicated the ventilator wasn't working. Another hospital asked the company to insert a window in the ventilator so that they could see the bellows move [37].

Early ventilators had to be equipped with autoclavable patient circuits. However in the mid 1970s, sterilisable low volume bacterial filters became available. Although these could be placed in the patient circuit and decreased the threat of infection, they did not eliminate the need for sterilization.

Rubbered Out

Although polyvinyl chloride tubes had been on the market since World War II, in 1970, many countries still used red rubber tracheal tubes. The reason was simple. The sterile and individually pre-packed PVC tubes were expensive when compared with the reusable rubber tubes. The cuffs on reusable tubes did not last as long as they used to, because now they were subject to disinfection by autoclaving or high temperature washing [38–40].

Disposable PVC tubes with an inflatable cuff were introduced in 1964, with thick cuff material mirroring the design of rubber cuffs. In 1969, Geffin and Pontopiddan stretched the standard PVC cuff in boiling water to make it thinner, and the result was considered less likely to cause compression injury to the tracheal wall [41]. Through the 1970s, the manufactured cuff became even thinner, with a larger diameter, enabling lower cuff inflation pressures. The use of disposable PVC tubes also decreased or eliminated the standard test of cuff competency before each use when it was realised that the practice was largely a waste of time.

In 1975, a revolutionary new tracheal tube was designed to replace the "Oxford" pattern red rubber tube, often used for oral or nasal surgery. The Oxford tube had a 90-degree bend, and could then be attached to a right angle connector to produce a 180 degree turn, allowing the patient circuit to be placed parallel to the patient's chest and chin. This ensured that the anesthetic circuit was away from the surgical field. Ring, Adair and Elwin performed 10,000 intubations with their prototype before publishing their results, and introduced the RAE pre-formed tube in 1975 [42].

Disposable anesthetic circuits were sold in the US in the 1970s. Much of the remainder of the world did not adopt their use, at least immediately, because of the additional cost. EIE remembers Henrik Bendixen (then Chair at the University of California, San Deigo) rejecting their use, saying that it would increase the landfill problem.

Plastic disposable facemasks also appeared in the 1970s in the US. Again, the cost was prohibitive for most countries to introduce them to routine practice, and the traditional black antistatic rubber masks continued in use.

Ikeda reported on a new flexible fiberoptic bronchoscope in 1971. Stiles et al published the first 100 cases using the device for tracheal intubation, demonstrating that intubation could be performed in less than 60 seconds [43].

Outpatient Anesthesia

Nicoll initiated outpatient anesthesia with 7000 Scottish children undergoing surgery for various conditions between 1899 and 1909 [44]. The first free-standing surgical outpatient clinic was Ralph Waters' "Downtown Anesthesia Clinic", described in 1919 [45]. Charles Hill followed Waters in establishing a free-standing outpatient facility in Providence, Rhode Island in 1968. The facility included a fully-equipped operating suite and a recovery room. However it failed due to lack of financial support from government

and insurers. In 1970, free-standing units within hospital settings were established at the Hammersmith Hospital in London, and the Gulson Hospital in Coventry, England [46]. In Phoenix, Arizona, Ford and Reed, learning from Hill's experience, obtained clearance from local authorities, and sought funding approval from insurers before opening their Surgicenter® in 1970. In 1976, Ford and Reed described how they had treated more than 33,000 patients without a death or malpractice suit [47]. Others, both in the United States and internationally followed their lead. By the 1980s, outpatient anesthesia caught the eye of the accountants and blossomed.

Anesthesiology Outside the Operating Room

Anesthesiologists also began moving away from the operating room. The first computerized tomography (CT) scanner (called the EMI Scanner) was installed at a hospital in London. It is said that EMI funded the development and early commercial production of the scanner through their association with The Beatles. So began an increasing demand for anesthesia in CT facilities, usually in circumstances that were not anesthesiologist-friendly. Although many applauded the passing of pneumoencephalograms, early CT devices took up to 30 minutes to complete a set of images. With improved technology, the scan time diminished to the point where anesthesia would rarely be needed, except in children. The first magnetic resonance imaging scan of a human being was performed in 1977. That's another story.

And also in the 1970s

A Test and a Treatment for Malignant Hyperthermia

Werner Kalow, who had been instrumental in defining the dibucaine test for pseudocholinesterase variants, and had effectively established the science of pharmacogenetics, tested some muscle samples for contractile force in vitro. In 1970, he and Britt noted that muscle from malignant hyperthermia (MH) patients contracted with abnormal strength in the presence of caffeine [48]. They thereby created the first test for susceptibility to MH. In 1971, Ellis and colleagues further demonstrated that halothane augmented muscle contraction in such patients [49].

Dantrolene was first proposed as a new type of muscle relaxant in 1967, and it was used to treat spasticity in the 1970s. In 1975, Gainsford Harrison reported that dantrolene treatment minimized the MH response induced by halothane in susceptible pigs. This provided the only effective pharmacological treatment so far identified [50].

Anesthetics and How They Act

Before the 1960s, the Meyer Overton theory of anesthetic action provided a major basis for our notion of how anesthetics acted. The theory suggested that the solution of anesthetic agents in the lipids of neural cell membranes caused anesthesia. The 1970s saw the rejuvenation of lipid theories. The best known one was the "Critical Volume Hypothesis" originally proposed by Mullins and refined by Miller and Smith. It had the advantage of providing an explanation for the experimental "pressure reversal" of anesthesia (i.e., pop an anesthetized mouse into a hyperbaric chamber and raise the pressure to 100 atmospheres and the mouse would wake up). A popular theory held that anesthetics induced a thickening in the lipid bi-layer of neural cell membranes, thus altering permeability. Nick Franks and William Lieb had opposing views about the thickening or thinning of the layer. In 1975 they used X-ray and neutron diffraction to show that neither was correct—there was no change (see Chapter 45). There were other problems with the lipid theories, for example, how to explain the absence of anesthesia with some lipid soluble drugs, and the variation in anesthetic effect with enantiomer drugs. Despite all the theories, we were little the wiser.

Aoyagi and the Oximeter

Japanese Takuo Aoyagi was working as a research engineer with Nihon Khoden in Japan in 1971, seeking to non-invasively measure cardiac output by a dye dilution technique using an ear densitometer. The pulsatile variations in the transmitted light signal produced an artefact that prevented accurate measurement. In attempting to eliminate the artefact, Aoyagi realised that the variation in transmitted light with red and infrared light was analogous to the principle underlying hemoglobin oxygen saturation measurement by previously described oximeters. He selected two wavelengths, 630 nm and 900 nm, the latter being insensitive to the dye he was using, and the former known to be sensitive to oxygen saturation. He found that the 900 nm wavelength was also sensitive to oxygen but in the opposite direction. This serendipitous result led him to further investigate the phenomenon, and by late 1973, he had developed a prototype ear oximeter. In 1974, he presented the "improved earpiece oximeter" to the Japanese Society of Medical Electronics and Biological Engineering. A first commercial version was produced, but the company decided not to pursue further development and did not patent the device. Aoyagi was transferred to another division within the company and the pulse oximeter was to become the story of the next decade.

Reprise

Increasing anesthesiologist numbers and diversity in the 1970s led to subspecialty societies and journals. Women constituted a rising fraction of anesthesiolgists. The practice of anesthesia became more diverse with an expanding application of outpatient surgery, establishment of regional anesthesia in everyday practice, and a rising use of anesthesia outside the operating room.

Our understanding of anesthetic drugs and how to best use them changed. In the US, and to a lesser extent elsewhere, the minimally hepatotoxic enflurane replaced halothane. We explored neuromuscular pharmacokinetics and clinically defined recovery from neuromuscular blockade. Dantrolene treatment of malignant hyperthermia was initiated. We incorrectly thought we might understand how inhaled anesthetics acted. We found opioid receptors in the spinal cord, leading to intrathecal opioid administration to provide analgesia. Patients received opioid analgesia on demand.

The worldwide "safety movement" in anesthesia started in the 1970s, growing rapidly in succeeding decades. Part of this resulted from an examination of the underlying causes of injury. Part probably resulted from the increasing application of automated monitoring of simple things such as pulse rate, ECG, blood pressure, and blood oxygen saturation, and increasing precision in inhaled anesthetic delivery and ventilation. Safety also likely followed from greater numbers of highly trained anesthetists. These trends continued in succeeding decades.

References

1. Bunker JP, Forrest WH, Moesteller F, Vandam L. The national halothane study. Bethesda: National Institutes of Health; 1969.
2. Mazze RI, Cousins MJ. Renal toxicity of anaesthetics: with specific reference to the nephrotoxicity of methoxyflurane. Canad Anaesth Soc J. 1973;20:64–80.
3. Eger EI II, Smuckler EA, Ferrell LD, Goldsmith CH, Johnson BH. Is enflurane hepatotoxic? Anesth Analg. 1986;65:21–30.
4. Corbett TH. Cancer and congenital anomalies associated with anesthetics. Ann NY Acad Sci. 1976;271:58–66.
5. Eger EI II, White AE, Brown CL, Biava CG, Corbett TH, Stevens WC. A test of the carcinogenicity of enflurane, isoflurane, halothane, methoxyflurane, and nitrous oxide in mice. Anesth Analg. 1978;57:678–94.
6. Michenfelder JD, Theye RA. Cerebral protection by thiopental during hypoxia. Anesthesiology. 1973;39:510–7.
7. Rowland M, Benet L, Graham G. Clearance concepts in pharmacokinetics. J Pharmacokinet Biopharm. 1973;1:123–36.
8. Sheiner LB, Beal SL. Evaluation of methods for estimating population pharmacokinetics parameters. I. Michaelis-Menten model: routine clinical pharmacokinetic data. J Pharmacokinet Biopharm. 1980;8:553–71.
9. Sheiner LB, Stanski DR, Vozeh S, Miller RD, Ham J. Simultaneous modeling of pharmacokinetics and pharmacodynamics: application to d-tubocurarine. Clin Pharmacol Ther. 1979;25:358–71.

10. Ali HH, Utting JE, Nightingale DA, Gray C. Quantitative assessment of residual curarization in humans. Br J Anaesth. 1970;42:802–3.
11. Kehlet H. Clinical course and hypothalamic-pituitary-adrenocortical function in glucocorticoid-treated patients. Copenhagen: FADL's Forlag; 1976.
12. Prentiss JE. Cardiac arrest following caudal anesthesia. Anesthesiology. 1979;50:51–3.
13. Sechzer PH. Objective measurement of pain. Anesthesiology. 1968;29:109–10. (abstract).
14. Forrest WH Jr, Smethurst PW, Kienitz ME. Self-administration of intravenous analgesics. Anesthesiology. 1970;33:363–5.
15. White WD, Pearce DJ, Norman J. Postoperative analgesia: a comparison of intravenous on-demand fentanyl with epidural bupivacaine. Br Med J. 1979;2:166–7.
16. Pert CB, Snyder SH. Opiate receptor: demonstration in nervous tissue. Science. 1973;179:1011–4.
17. Duggan AW, Hall JG, Headley PM. Morphine, enkephalin and the substantia gelatinosa. Nature. 1976;264:456–8.
18. Yaksh TL, Rudy TA. Analgesia mediated by a direct spinal action of narcotics. Science. 1976;192:1357–8.
19. Behar M, Magora F, Olshwang D, Davidson JT. Epidural morphine in treatment of pain. Lancet. 1979;1:527–9.
20. Wang JK, Nauss LA, Thomas JE. Pain relief by intrathecally applied morphine in man. Anesthesiology. 1979;50:149–51.
21. Matas R. Local and regional anesthesia with cocain and other analgesic drugs, including the subarachanoid method, as applied in general surgical practice. Philadelphia Med J. 1900;6:820–43.
22. Cousins MJ, Mather LE, Glynn CJ, Wilson PR, Graham JR. Selective spinal analgesia. Lancet. 1979;1:1141–2.
23. Szeto A. Mike Ramsey—A medical device entrepreneur. Engineering Med Biol. 2002;21:12–3.
24. Ball CM, Westhorpe RN. Historical notes on anaesthesia and intensive care. 2–12. Sydney: Australian Society of Anaesthetists; 2012. pp 228–9.
25. Scurr CF. Evolution and revolution in anaesthetic training. Ann R Coll Surg Engl. 1971;48:274–92.
26. Wylie WD. There, but for the grace of God...'. Ann R Coll Surg Engl. 1975;56:171–80.
27. Vassalo SA. Lewis H Wright memorial lecture. ASA Newsletter. 2001;75:22–4.
28. Cooper JB, Newbower RS. The anesthesia machine—an accident waiting to happen. In: Pickett M, Triggs TJ, editors. Human factors in health care. Lexington: DC Heath & Co; 1975. pp. 345–58.
29. Cooper JB, Newbower RS, Long CD, McPeek B. Preventable anesthesia mishaps: a study of human factors. Anesthesiology. 1978;49:399–406.
30. Cooper JB, Newbower RS, Moore JW, Trautman ED. A new anesthesia delivery system. Anesthesiology. 1978;49:310–8.
31. Viljoen JF, Estafanous FG, Kellner GA. Propranolol and cardiac surgery. J Thorac Cardiovasc Surg. 1972;64:826–30.
32. Prys-Roberts C, Foex P, Biro GP, Roberts JG. Studies of anaesthesia in relation to hypertension. V. Adrenergic beta-receptor blockade. Br J Anaesth. 1973;45:671–81.
33. Vaisman AI. [Working conditions in the operating room and their effect on the health of anesthetists]. Eksp Khir Anesteziol. 1967;12:44–9.
34. Ericson A, Kallen B. Survey of infants born in 1973 or 1975 to Swedish women working in operating rooms during their pregnancies. Anesth Analg. 1979;58:302–5.
35. Spence AA. Environmental pollution by inhalation anaesthetics. Br J Anaesth. 1987;59:96–103.
36. Ashbaugh DG, Bigelow DB, Petty TL, Levine BE. Acute respiratory distress in adults. Lancet. 1967;2:319–23.
37. http://www.maquet.com/content/Documents/Site_Specific/MAQUETcom/GENERAL_The_Servo_Story.pdf
38. Watson WF. Development of the PVC endotracheal tube. BioMaterials. 1980;1:41–6.
39. Calverley RK. Intubation in anaesthesia. In: Atkinson RS, Boulton TB, editors. The History of Anaesthesia. London: Royal Society of Medicine; 1989. pp. 333–41.
40. Russell CA. Developments in thermoplastic tracheal tubes. In: Barr AM, Boulton TB, Wilkinson DJ, editors. Essays on the History of Anaesthesia. London: Royal Society of Medicine; 1996. pp. 94–7.
41. Geffin B, Pontoppidan H. Reduction of tracheal damage by the pre-stretching of inflatable cuffs. Anesthesiology. 1969;31:462–3.
42. Ring WH. RAE (Ring, Adair, Elwyn) endotracheal tubes: wallace Harold Ring (1932-). In: Maltby JR, editor. Notable Names in Anaesthesia. London: Royal Society of Medicine; 2002. pp. 167–9.
43. Stiles CM, Stiles QR, Denson JS. A flexible fiber optic laryngoscope. JAMA. 1972;221:1246–7.
44. Nicoll JH. The surgery of infancy. Br Med J. 1909;18:753–4.
45. Waters RM. The down-town anesthesia clinic. Am J Surg. 1919;39 (suppl):71–3.
46. Berrill TH. A year in the life of a surgical day unit. Br Med J. 1972;4:348–9.
47. Reed WA, Ford JL. Development of an independent outpatient surgical center. Int Anesthesiol Clin. 1976;14:113–30.
48. Kalow W, Britt BA, Terreau ME, Haist C. Metabolic error of muscle metabolism after recovery from malignant hyperthermia. Lancet . 1970;2:895–8.
49. Ellis FR, Harriman DG, Keaney NP, Kyei-Mensah K, Tyrrell JH. Halothane-induced muscle contracture as a cause of hyperpyrexia. Br J Anaesth. 1971;43:721–2.
50. Harrison GG. Control of the malignant hyperpyrexic syndrome in MHS swine by dantrolene sodium. Br J Anaesth. 1975;47:62–5.

Rod N. Westhorpe, Lawrence J. Saidman and Edmond I Eger II

Summary

The 1980s were anesthesia's "adolescence". The specialty became increasingly independent and self-assured, ceasing subservience to surgeons or any specialist. Part-time anesthetic practitioners diminished in numbers or vanished.

The anesthetist's acknowledged love of "gadgets" enlarged, the specialty embracing technology, applying it to the delivery and control of anesthesia. More importantly it underlay a revolution in patient monitoring.

Anesthesia benefited from two new drugs, isoflurane and propofol, as well as from new analgesics, local anesthetics, muscle relaxants and antiemetics. The benzodiazepine, midazolam, nearly foundered after causing deaths from respiratory depression, particularly in the elderly, because of inadequate supervision. Archie Brain invented the Laryngeal Mask Airway, the most important new airway device since Hewitt's invention of the oral airway in 1908.

Arguably, the greatest change came in the examination of safety and outcomes in routine practice. Partly stimulated by medico-legal attention given to adverse outcomes, the specialty instituted processes to examine and prevent potential failures in patient care. The "patient safety" movement was established, and pervaded all of health care by the century's end.

Michael Jackson said it in his 1988 song, "The Man in the Mirror": We needed to change ourselves to make the world a better place.

World Events in the 1980s

The 1980s expanded the benefits and drawbacks of technological advances. Ted Turner founded CNN in 1980, and by mid-decade, the PC, the MAC, and Windows were released, altering how we work, play, and communicate. The 1988 opening of the internet added to the revolution. Events and international politics proceeded in unexpected directions, all under the watchful gaze of television and international media. We learned of John Lennon's 1980 assassination. We learned that a toxic gas leak killed 16,000 people in Bhopal, that an earthquake devastated Mexico City, that an oil spill from the Exxon Valdez contaminated hundreds of miles of pristine Alaskan coastline, and that a meltdown occurred in the Chernobyl nuclear energy plant. Thousands of spectators and millions on television saw the space shuttle Challenger explode shortly after launch. The world watched the brutal suppression of protest in Tiananmen Square in 1989.

In 1979, the Iron Lady, Margaret Thatcher, became Britain's first woman Prime Minister. With Helmut Kohl and Ronald Reagan, in the 1980s she revived right-wing politics in the West. The Soviet Union disintegrated, several eastern European countries found new democratic freedoms, and the Berlin Wall fell in 1989. The 1980–1988 Iran—Iraq war ended in an uneasy peace, but not before chemical weapons made their ugly entrance. Russia departed Afghanistan, opening the way for a resurgent fundamentalist Taliban. The AIDS epidemic began in earnest, and Michael Jackson rose to international fame.

Anesthesia Flexes Its Muscles

By 1980, the number of non-specialists providing anesthesia in developed countries had diminished and would largely disappear by 1990, as specialist training and certification solidified around similar worldwide standards. Departments of anesthesia became independent of surgical departments, following the lead established in the US and GB. Regional societies flourished with increasing membership bases, allowing some to exert political influence.

R. N. Westhorpe (✉)
Melbourne, Australia
e-mail: westhorpe@netspace.net.au

L. J. Saidman
Department of Anesthesia, Stanford University, Stanford, CA, USA
e-mail: lsaidman@stanford.edu

E. I Eger II
Department of Anesthesia and Perioperative Care, University of California, San Francisco, CA, USA
e-mail: egere@anesthesia.ucsf.edu

E. I Eger II et al. (eds.), *The Wondrous Story of Anesthesia*, DOI 10.1007/978-1-4614-8441-7_11, © Edmond I Eger, MD 2014

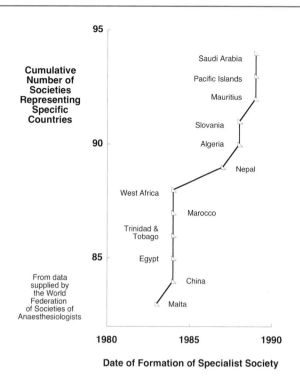

Cumulative Number of Societies Representing Specific Countries

95

Saudi Arabia

Pacific Islands

Mauritius

Slovania

90

Algeria

Nepal

West Africa

Marocco

Trinidad & Tobago

85

Egypt

From data supplied by the World Federation of Societies of Anaesthesiologists

China

Malta

1980   1985   1990

Date of Formation of Specialist Society

Fig. 11.1 Anesthetic societies continued to accumulate, a dozen in the 1980s

More and Larger Societies

Many smaller and developing nations established societies in the 1980s, as did some Middle Eastern countries such as Saudi Arabia and Egypt (Fig. 11.1). The two French societies that had supported opposing views about anesthesia practice reconciled in 1982. In 1960, a disagreement regarding the election of a non-anesthetist to the presidency of the Société Française d'Anesthésie, d'Analgésie et Réanimation (SFAAR) followed an ongoing controversy over the method of anesthesia. There were two camps. Pierre Huguenard led the "Laboritiens" who followed the teachings of Henri Laborit (1914–1995) favouring neurolept anesthesia. They were at odds with those embracing inhalation anesthesia, led by Jean Lassner. Lassner had also established an alternative journal to the official Society journal (edited by Huguenard). Huguenard left the Society and with Jean Bimar, founded l'Association des Anesthésistes Français, with a new journal. Following the reconciliation, the new society, la Société Française d'Anesthésie et Réanimation (SFAR) established the still published journal *Annales Francaises d'Anesthésie Réanimation*.

In South America, in 1987, the societies in Argentina, Brazil, Paraguay and Uruguay formed the Federation of South American Societies of Anesthesiology (FASA), later to be joined by Bolivia, Chile, and Colombia. In the same year, the larger Latin American Confederation of Societies of

Anesthesiologists (CLASA) that had been established in 1962, became the South American Regional Section of the World Federation of Societies of Anaesthesiologists (WFSA). The Pan Arab Section and the African Section remained to be created in 1990 and 1997 respectively.

The American Society of Anesthesiologists (ASA) continued to grow in numbers and influence. Membership increased from just under 17,000 in 1980, to 27,000 in 1990. It came into conflict with government and non-government agencies in the 1980s. In the late 1970s, the Federal Trade Commission questioned the billing practices of anesthetists, citing curtailment of competition through the use of a common guide to fee setting, the Relative Value Guide. The ASA was large enough to take on the FTC, and in 1979 successfully defended use of the RVG. Predictably, the FTC did not go away, and targeted groups and individuals for uncompetitive practices and in particular, relationships with nurse anesthetists. These matters and others kept the ASA busy for the whole decade, prompting the Society to establish a permanent Office of Government Affairs (OGA) in Washington DC, in 1984. The decision was vindicated in 1985. Congress passed a bill giving nurse anesthetists the right to practice independently in the care of government employees, but through the efforts of the OGA, the ASA secured a Presidential veto of the legislation.

The ASA perceived that the public did not appreciate the contributions and importance of anesthesia delivered by anesthesiologists. Accordingly, the ASA began a public education program in 1981, utilizing the media, videos and brochures, with media tours targeting major cities. A 1985 review of the program for its effectiveness found that "the man in the street in this country is not the least bit concerned about anesthesiology, let alone anesthesiologists". As a result, by 1987, the program had been substantially curtailed, targeting only hospital administrators and legislators [1]. Several other countries failed to learn from this experience, and spent large sums of money on media-based public education programs (National Anaesthesia Days) in the early 2000s, only to abandon them within a few years of their commencement.

Through the 1980s, women increasingly influenced the specialty. They accepted leadership roles in the US including 3 academic chairs in 1986 (but this out of more than 100 programs). In 1988, Gertie Marx received the ASA Distinguished Service Award. Nevertheless, their rate of board certification was less, and academic advancement appeared to be slower. This prompted a request by a group of women activists to the ASA for the formation of an ad hoc committee on women's issues and a panel to discuss such issues at the Annual Meeting. The request was denied. In 1986, ASA delegate Betty Stephenson proposed a resolution that the ASA bylaws be degendered. The resolution also failed approval by the ASA House of Delegates, but ASA President, Peter McDermott later administratively degendered the ASA's bylaws and documents. As noted in Chapter 2: "In October 1992, I (McDermott) became ASA president and issued an order degendering the language of ASA bylaws and other documents. It would have been embarrassing to have the issue debated (in the House of Delegates) by old white men."

Subspecialty Societies

The burgeoning specialty spawned subspecialty organizations in Europe for regional anesthesia (1980), intensive care (1982), cardiothoracic anesthesia (1985), and pediatric anesthesia (1986). International societies established in the previous decade accommodated subspecialty interest in obstetrics, neuroanesthesia, and pain. The European Society of Intensive Care Medicine created the European Diploma in Intensive Care (EDIC) in 1988, and this became widely accepted.

In Canada, Australia, and New Zealand, subspecialty societies or "special interest groups" began to appear under the auspices of the major organisations, the Faculty of Anaesthetists (Australia and New Zealand), and the Canadian Anaesthesiologists Society. International subspecialty organisations for pain, obstetric anesthesia, neuroanesthesia, and regional anesthesia supported membership from all countries.

In the US, the Society for Ambulatory Anesthesia (SAMBA) was established in 1984, reflecting the increasing focus on outpatient surgery and anesthesia, and the Society for Pediatric Anesthesia (SPA) was established in 1986.

The Growth of Education

The 1980s saw further expansion and consolidation of basic and advanced education in anesthesia.

In the US, in 1980, after years of disagreement between the organizations involved in undergraduate and postgraduate medical education, the Coordinating Council on Medical Education (CCME) was disbanded. The Liaison Committee on Graduate Medical Education had been accrediting postgraduate programs since 1975, and in 1981 was renamed the Accreditation Council for Graduate Medical Education (ACGME) under the auspices of the American Medical Association (AMA), the American Hospital Association (AHA) and the Advisory Board for Medical Specialties (ABMS). The ACGME continues to be the accrediting body for all medical internship and residency training programs.

The American Board of Anesthesiology refined the examination process, in particular determining means to diminish variability in both questions and assessment of oral examinations. During the 1980s, the Board initiated internal discussions regarding the introduction of recertification and the number of Board certified diplomats increased from 9800 to 19000.

The Society for Education in Anesthesia (SEA) was formed in the early 1980s with an aim of engaging consultant anesthetists in the education of medical students and residents. A founder, Philip Liu, wrote in the first newsletter in 1984 of his hope that that "members of this Society will develop a genuine sense of fellowship, so that individuals with an interest and vocation in the teaching of anesthesiology will find a network of support and a resource for communication." The Society has continued its educational role, and has never sought a political one.

In 1977, Jean Lassner established the European Academy of Anesthesiology (EAA) in Paris, to promote meetings and exchange of ideas between European anesthetists, with a particular emphasis on teaching methods. The Academy established the *European Journal of Anaesthesiology* in 1984, edited by British anesthetist, John Zorab. In the same year, the European Diploma in Anaesthesia and Intensive Care (EDA) was introduced.

The Diploma comprised a two part multi-lingual examination, with the second part to be taken after completing 6 years of post graduate medical practice,[1] including 4 years in anesthesia. This was at a time when the Anaesthesiology Section of the Union Européenne des Médecins Spécialistes (UEMS), established in 1962, was the official body under the European Union for recommending minimum training times, but without any formal power. The Diploma, although not officially recognized, provided evidence that the diplomate had met uniform educational standards. Nevertheless, it did not replace individual national accreditation, and did not provide for cross-border portability. In 1989, the EAA also created a voluntary Hospital Recognition Program, primarily for those countries that did not have their own hospital accreditation system. Although not accepted by the UEMS, the program was supported by the Anaesthesiology Section.

During the 1980s, several European countries adopted all or part of the EDA as a mandatory part of their accreditation process for specialist recognition. In 1980, the Section recommended a minimum training time of 5 years. However during the decade, the minimum duration in most western and eastern European countries was 4 years (see Fig. 38.1). In contrast, training in Russia varied from less than one, to two years. In Paris, in 1989, a new Diploma, the Diplôme d'études supérieures en anesthésié-réanimation (DESA) was created, requiring 5 years of postgraduate anesthesia training.

In 1986, anesthetists in The Netherlands, France and Belgium established the Fondation Européenne d'Enseignement

---

[1] Practice, as in medical practice after graduation as a doctor.

en Anesthésiologie (FEEA) to provide continuing medical education (CME) in anesthesia, through the conduct of refresher courses. FEEA extended its activity to more countries as the size of the European Union grew.

Matters were further confused by the establishment of the European Society of Anaesthesiologists (ESA) in 1992, the European Board of Anaesthesiology (EBA) in 1993, and the Confederation of European National Societies of Anaesthesiology (CENSA) that had evolved from the WFSA regional section. These anesthesia-related educational bodies functioned independently, but co-operatively, and in the 2000s were brought under the joint umbrella of the ESA and EBA.

In Great Britain, while functioning within the Royal College of Surgeons, the Faculty of Anaesthetists had long provided training, accreditation and examination for Fellowship. Reflecting the earned status of the specialty, in 1988, the Faculty became an independent College of Anaesthetists. By this time the period of training was 7 years including basic, intermediate and specialised training. Because these requirements exceeded those for European qualification, few European anesthetists could practice as specialist consultants in Great Britain. Reciprocal arrangements were to be resolved during the next decade.

In other areas of the globe, anesthesia training was either being established or extended. By the end of the 1980s, all major Latin American countries had formal training programs in place with a minimum period of 3 years.

Despite the short time since the 1976 end of the Cultural Revolution, Chinese anesthetists had established the Chinese Society of Anesthesiology in 1979 and several Colleges in the succeeding decade. The first College was in Xuzhou Medical School in 1987, with three more founded in 1988, at Harbin, Hunan, and Tongji medical universities. These were undergraduate medical courses, offering major studies in anesthesia, critical care and pain management. In the 1980s, three new journals were launched, the *Chinese Journal of Anesthesiology*, the *Foreign Medical Sciences (Anesthesiology and Resuscitation)*, and *The Journal of Clinical Anesthesiology*. Despite this, in many hospitals, anesthesia was often considered a technical rather than a clinical (i.e., professional) practice. This changed in 1989, when the Ministry of Public Health formally defined the criteria for a department of anesthesiology: "The department of anesthesiology should be a clinical department rather than a technical department. More emphasis should be showed on personnel training, instrument and equipment. The working level should be improved to meet the demands of medical development."

Intensive (Critical) Care Training

Beginning with Bjørn Ibsen's management of the 1952 polio epidemic in Copenhagen, anesthesiologists have been at the forefront of the development of intensive care medicine, utilizing their skills in respiratory and emergency care. Accordingly, anesthesia training programs increasingly stipulated training in intensive care. In 1982, the European Society of Intensive Care Medicine (ESICM) was founded, and 6 years later the Society created the European Diploma in Intensive Care (EDIC). At the time, the specialty was not recognized as a separate section under the UEMS, partly due to its multidisciplinary nature. This was to occur in 1999. It remains separate from the ESA.

In the US, critical care medicine had been one of several subspecialties, in which experience was required as part of the formal accreditation process by the American Board of Anesthesiology (ABA). Critical care experience was distinguished by being the only subspecialty for which a minimum time was stipulated (2 months). In 1985, the ABA introduced the first subspecialty certificate—in critical care medicine.

Nurse Anesthetists

In few countries is the presence of nurse anesthesia of greater importance to anesthetic delivery than in the US. In the US, during the late 1970s, the intertwined relationship between the certification process for nurse anesthetists, and the political role of the American Association of Nurse Anesthetists (AANA) was finally separated. After 1982, the independent Council on Certification issued a certificate (Certified Registered Nurse Anesthetist—CRNA) that no longer required membership in the association. Through the remainder of the 1980s, the Council embarked on a process to standardize and validate the large number of training programs, and introduce an objective standardized examination process.

In 1989, a meeting of nurse anesthetists in Switzerland, representing 11 countries, founded the International Federation of Nurse Anesthetists.

Academic Anesthesia

In Great Britain, Margaret Thatcher's conservative government curtailed funding for academic support, and anesthesia research suffered. Universities relied largely on public funding for their operation, applying it to both teaching and research within their own jurisdiction. After reviewing the method of funding, in 1986, funding for research was redistributed to research councils. Universities, or their research staff, now had to compete for grants. Universities became business enterprises, competing in a marketplace for research funds. Suddenly, anesthesia researchers contended against everyone else for a portion of a diminished pool. Fields of investigation that had greater perceived or real benefit to the population were at a distinct advantage. Anesthesia became a victim of its own success; too few patients died or were injured by anesthesia. For anesthetists who were partly academic and partly clinical and teaching practitioners, the situation was worse as they did not have the same time or level of support in writing grant applications as did their full time academic colleagues.

The Japanese Society of Anaesthesiology began publication of the *Journal of Anaesthesia* in 1987, an English language journal that would compete with Masui.

Isoflurane Finally Makes It

After being cleared of the reported carcinogenic risk that had thwarted its planned release in the mid 1970s, isoflurane was introduced to clinical anesthesia in 1981, It soon replaced its structural isomer, enflurane, having the benefits of faster induction and recovery, absent epileptogenicity, and only 0.2 % biodegradation. Seemingly, the only drawback was a mild pungency, making it less suitable as an inhaled induction agent. The pungency ensured the persistence of halothane in pediatric practice.

Was it too good to be true? Soon a potential issue appeared. Isoflurane caused a dose-related decrease in blood pressure, due to vascular dilation, rather than myocardial depression, as with halothane. The dilation also affected coronary vessels, and a debate began about "coronary artery steal", diverting blood flow away from collateral vessels that were unable to dilate. Subsequent studies showed the fears to be unfounded.

Japan Tries a Reject

Ross Terrell had synthesized sevoflurane and desflurane in the 1960s. Both had been set aside as unsuitable for further study, sevoflurane because it was unstable in soda lime, and desflurane because it was difficult to make, had a low potency and high saturated vapour pressure. Increasingly, the extent of metabolism and the absence of degradation by CO_2 absorbants were considered crucial properties of desirable modern inhaled anesthetics. Less was better, dictating subsequent development of enflurane, isoflurane, and desflurane, all agents with progressively less metabolic degradation than halothane or methoxyflurane.

Despite these concerns, sevoflurane was transiently resurrected in the 1970s. Animal studies suggested that it might show promise as an "ideal" inhalation agent. Minimal cardiorespiratory stimulation accompanied a low pungency and rapid induction. However, in addition to the instability in soda lime, the potential for fluoride-induced renal failure (as with methoxyflurane) was raised on the basis of experiments in rats. Baxter and ICI shelved sevoflurane in the late

1970s, although human trials in the early 1980s, confirmed sevoflurane's suitability from a clinical, if not a laboratory perspective.

Anaquest resurrected desflurane in the 1980s, as part of a search for a better anesthetic for outpatient surgery. The first human subject, Jeremy Cashman, received desflurane at Guy's hospital in 1988. He survived and went on to an academic career in anesthesia. Meanwhile, Baxter offered the rights to Anaquest, for development of sevoflurane for the North American market. Anaquest took an option for one year while they considered the matter.

Anaquest thus had the rights to desflurane, the option from Baxter on sevoflurane, and a difficult choice: which one to develop for the anesthesia market? Despite the difficult and expensive manufacturing process, the need for a radically new vaporiser, and its airway irritability, desflurane had a long patent life, was more stable and less soluble than sevoflurane and underwent negligible metabolism. It was a close decision, but sevoflurane lost.

Enter Maruishi, a Japanese pharmaceutical company operating in a less regulated environment. They bought the rights to sevoflurane from Baxter and succeeded with its commercialization in Japan in the late 1980s. Maruishi licensed the international rights to sevoflurane to Abbott Laboratories, in 1992.

Two Out of Five

The 1980s saw the release of five new muscle relaxants, only two of which survived. Vecuronium was released in 1980 as the first "designer" relaxant. Once the exact structure of curare was known, and the cause of the vagolytic and neuromuscular blocking effects of pancuronium could be defined at a molecular level, the new monoquaternary drug, vecuronium was conceived. It had the same potency as pancuronium, one twentieth of the vagolytic action, and an effect that lasted half as long. The latter property resulted from its dual elimination via both the liver and kidney, unlike pancuronium's dependence on renal elimination.

Not long afterwards, another new relaxant, atracurium appeared. Its advantage over other relaxants was that its elimination was partly by Hofmann spontaneous degradation in plasma and tissue, as well as by ester hydrolysis and organ metabolism. Atracurium became popular worldwide. There was however, widespread caution because the drug was known to cause histamine release with resulting hypotension and tachycardia. Except in rare circumstances, these effects were mild and transient, and were often overstated [2].

An additional atracurium related concern was raised due to laudanosine, a by-product of the metabolism of atracurium, that if present in sufficient concentrations may cause seizures due to a decreased seizure threshold. However, because

Hofmann degradation reduces the atracurium concentration, it was unlikely that laudanosine would reach concentrations capable of causing seizures—also the case for the isomer of atracurium, cisatracurium.

John Savarese introduced mivacurium in 1984, as a relaxant with a short duration of action, resulting from its hydrolysis by plasma cholinesterase, just like succinylcholine. But it lasted twice as long as succinylcholine, and more importantly, it also took twice as long to act. It never achieved great popularity but continues to be available in some countries. Doxecurium and pipecuronium were also released in the 1980s, but offered no advantages over vecuronium and atracurium, and failed to find a market.

The advent of neuromuscular blocking drugs having fewer side effects and kinetics allowing easier reversal, encouraged their use in critical care units for the control of patients requiring mechanical ventilation. This reflected the increased use of long-term ventilation, and a mistaken view among some critical care physicians that muscle relaxants possessed analgesic and/or anxiolytic properties. (As far as the authors know, this view was not expressed in print and may just be an urban legend. But it has a curious support in the 2003 finding that muscle relaxant administration can decrease the BIS value, albeit with no decrease in consciousness [3].) An unforseen result of long term paralysis was prolonged muscle weakness after tracheal extubation, identified in 1985 [4]. Use of smaller and intermittent doses solved the problem.

A Problem with Bupivacaine

A 1979 editorial in *Anesthesiology*, by Albright, brought attention to six cases of cardiac arrest associated with the use of the local anesthetics, bupivacaine and etidocaine [5]. Several additional cases were soon reported. Many were fatal, and were associated with the use of 0.75% bupivacaine in obstetrics. In 1983, the US FDA banned the use of 0.75% solution in obstetrics. These cases also resulted in the recommendation of a test dose in epidural anesthesia as well as incremental dosing. Studies suggested that bupivacaine affects voltage-gated sodium channels in cardiomyocytes, but the exact mechanism is yet to be defined.

Intravenous MAC

During the 1980s, three groups chased the automatic control of total intravenous anaesthesia, Prys-Roberts' group in Bristol, the Schwilden/Schuttler group in Germany, and the Stanford group in the US. In 1980, Cedric Prys-Roberts conceived of a "MAC" for intravenous anesthetics. His group determined EC_{50} and EC_{95} values for quasi-steady state in-

fusions of methohexital and althesin [6], and for the new emulsion formulation of propofol [7]. While others used the Dixon up-and-down method (which is parsimonious in terms of numbers of patients required) to provide the EC_{50}, Prys-Roberts and colleagues used a probit analysis, arguing that such analysis allowed determination of both the EC_{50} and EC_{95}. Prys-Roberts' group opted to develop closed-loop control systems knowing that they probably would not be able to control anesthesia precisely (because no single variable or parameter can accurately differentiate between consciousness and unconsciousness, let alone the more complex so-called "depth of anaesthesia" paradigm.) The Germans followed a similar approach, and the Stanford group went the pharmacokinetic route. All reached similar conclusions. Prys-Roberts' group determined the pharmacokinetic and pharmacodynamic model in small children using probit analysis [8], and joined forces with an engineering group in Oxford to develop a neural network approach using parametric modelling and on-line statistical pattern recognition of the EEG during anesthesia. Prys-Roberts wrote to LJS (personal note 16 Nov 2012): "I am as convinced now as I was then that it is no more difficult to control total intravenous anaesthesia (e.g., propofol/alfentanil/relaxant) using a manually controlled set of pumps [9] than it is to control inhalational anaesthesia by adjusting the setting of a vaporiser."

Regarding the parallel development in Germany, pharmacologist, Ekkehard Krüger-Thiemer devised mathematical models for drug uptake in the 1960s. Using these, Bonn anesthetist and mathematician, Helmut Schwilden, in 1981, developed a theoretical pharmacokinetic model to achieve a target plasma concentration. With colleagues, he then developed a programmable infusion pump called CATIA, or Computer Assisted Titration of Intravenous Anesthesia. This was the first "Target Controlled Infusion" or "TCI" device [10, 11].

During the early to mid 1980s, Stanski and colleagues at Stanford used power spectral analysis of the EEG to study the pharamacokinetics of hypnotics and opioids. Their studies with thiopental supported the feasibility of TCI. The release of propofol in 1986, with its faster biodegradation, lent itself to TCI. Audrey Shafer and Paul White performed much of the early work in determining the pharmacokinetic and pharmacodynamic profile for propofol at Stanford University. Using this and additional information, Gavin Kenny and Colleagues in Glasgow developed a TCI device in 1990, which was released commercially in 1993 [12, 13].

Brain's Brilliant Idea

After many years of development, British anesthetist, Archie Brain introduced the first completely new airway device since Hewitt introduced his airway in 1908. Using and modifying rubber nasal masks to fit snugly around the laryngeal inlet, and connecting the mask to a tube, he developed the Laryngeal Mask Airway. He tried around 100 prototypes in over 6000 patients, before approaching a major commercial endotracheal tube manufacturer. Brain's confidence in the device led him to establish the Laryngeal Mask Company, and the commercial version was made of autoclavable silicone and introduced to the market in 1988 (1992 in the US, due to delays in FDA approval). It has since been made in disposable PVC, and has proven to revolutionize airway management, largely eliminating "mask anesthesia" while adding to the armamentarium for dealing with difficult airway issues.

The acceptance of the "LMA" was not immediate, and might have taken much longer had it not been for the concurrent introduction of propofol which replaced the use of thiopental. Propofol was introduced in 1986, first in New Zealand, after considerable effort to find a suitable vehicle for intravenous use. Propofol displaced thiopental because of its rapid degradation, its lower incidence of postoperative nausea and vomiting, and its depression of upper airway reflexes. The depression of these reflexes facilitated the insertion of the LMA that would often have induced gagging after thiopental. Thus two new products synergised each other's adoption into clinical practice. Propofol did not gain approval from the FDA in the US until 1989.

Airway Management Advanced in Other Ways

In the early 1980s, Roger Bullard introduced a rigid fibreoptic intubation laryngoscope. In 1982, Hiroshi Inoue invented the "Univent" tube, a disposable reinvention of the bronchus blocker and endotracheal tube described by Macintosh in 1935. In 1987, Frass and colleagues in Austria invented the "Combitube" and Mizus invented a tube exchanger, the Mizus Endotracheal Tube Replacement Obturator (METTRO), superseded by the Cook exchanger in 1990. Ikeda and the Asahi Corporation developed a flexible video endoscope.

Outpatient Anesthesia

Outpatient anesthesia had become popular by 1980, receiving several boosts during the decade. In 1984, the Society for Ambulatory Anesthesia (SAMBA) was established, just when surgeons embraced endoscopic or minimally invasive surgery. The introduction in the late 1980s of propofol and the LMA added to the rise in outpatient anesthesia. Rapid recovery to full wakefulness, less nausea and vomiting, and new methods of airway management without the need for tracheal intubation facilitated the management of patients on a day only basis.

In the US, the number of "Office-based" procedures also increased, from 2 to 5 % of all procedures, over the period from 1984 to 1990.

Anesthesia Embraces Technology

Several technological advances introduced in the 1990s improved the practice of anesthesia, although the improvement was not validated statistically. Intuitive application correlating with dramatically reduced mortality inspired the confidence of the specialty in those advocating the changes. Monitoring of respired gases (carbon dioxide, oxygen, and inhalation agent concentrations), and of oxyhemoglobin saturation (oximetry) added to the existing armoury of modalities that informed the anesthetist as to the status of the patient and the anesthesia delivery system. The delivery system also began to change from the traditional "gas machine" to an integrated workstation.

Capnometry

John Severinghaus and colleagues installed a mass spectrometer in a 10 room operating suite in the mid 1970s. Using multiplexed sampling through 30 metre nylon catheters, they monitored respiratory gases at 1-minute intervals. It was expensive to install and maintain, but gave the anesthetist and researcher a taste of what could be done. Indeed, those who used the device became addicted to the minute-by-minute arrival of the latest end-tidal anesthetic and carbon dioxide values, and when the mass spectrometer "went down" (which it sometimes did) they felt uneasy. This led to the increasing adoption of stand-alone infrared analysis. The development of the infrared CO_2 analyzer began with the "Luft" cell, described in Chapter 55. The first clinically usable infrared capnometer was the 1950s Beckman LB1. The sampling head of this large and cumbersome device needed to be pressurized by a bicycle pump to prevent ingress of potentially flammable anesthetic gases. EIE commented that "It may have 'needed' to be pressurized but rarely was, and no explosion ever resulted that I knew of. It would be difficult to imagine how an explosive concentration could have been achieved within the device."

Both Hewlett-Packard and Siemens-Elema developed mainstream infrared capnometers in the late 1970s. The HP47210A, a spin-off from a contract to develop an exhaust gas analyser for General Motors, was designed for use in the operating room, while the Siemens–Elema 930 was designed specifically for use with the series 900 ventilators. The 930 was released around 1976, and the HP47210A in 1980. The HP47210A was the first practical infrared analyser for use in anesthesia, displaying end-tidal and instantaneous CO_2 measurements and respiratory rate, with alarms. It also could measure transcutaneous CO_2 using a heated electrode.

Although there was no waveform display, over 50,000 units were sold.

Datex Instrumentarium, a Finish company, developed a sidestream capnometer, the CD-101, at about the same time. It had an analogue needle display showing the instantaneous CO_2 on a percentage scale. As with the HP device, interference from nitrous oxide was countered by a switch, introducing an electrical adjustment. Similarly, all early devices required regular calibration, both at zero and with a known sample gas. The Netherlands was probably the first country to recommend capnometry as a monitor for all patients undergoing controlled ventilation, in 1978. By the end of the 1980s, capnometers with waveform displays, of both sidestream and mainstream variety were readily available, but were not yet routinely used.

Oxygen Gas Monitoring

Oxygen Analysers. By 1980, polarographic oxygen monitors were readily available. They were easily calibrated and accompanied by alarm functions, and ideal for verifying that the gas emanating from the anesthetic machine when oxygen was turned on, was indeed oxygen. Surprisingly, they did not find their way into routine use until later in the decade, when they became part of the first minimum monitoring standards. (See below)

Pulse Oximetry. Takuo Aoyagi's discovery of pulse oximetry in 1971, led his employer, the Nihon Kohden company, to develop a commercial model in 1974, primarily for use in respiratory physiology laboratories. They patented the technology in Japan but not elsewhere, and did not pursue further development. Minolta produced another commercial version in 1977, but it was not a commercial success and was sensitive to movement. Biox Technology refined and marketed the device in the US in 1980, again for respiratory laboratories. Another Minolta was tested at Stanford University by Bill New and colleagues. Soon, two pulse oximeters were marketed primarily for use in anesthesia, the Biox 3700 (now owned by the Ohmeda Corporation) and the Nellcor N100 (developed by a new company named after its founders, Bill New, Jack Lloyd, and Jim Corenham). A feature of the Nellcor N100 was the modulated sound signifying a changing oxygen saturation, and was patented by Nellcor. However, recognizing the potential value to patient safety, Nellcor elected to not enforce its patent rights [14].

Pulse oximeters assumed an increasing place in routine anesthesia monitoring, and some anesthetists considered it to be the major advance in the specialty during the 1980s. Nevertheless, it took some time for oximeters to be adopted universally. Many anesthetists doubted their value relative to their initial high cost. The industry was not entirely confident either. The Nellcor company looked to become a public company listed on the stock exchange, but were told that they needed more than oximetry. Accordingly, they developed the Nellcor N1000 that combined capnometry with pulse oximetry, and success was assured [15].

Transesophageal Echocardiography. In the mid 1980s, two-dimensional transesophageal echocardiography was introduced to the cardiac operating room. Cardiologists were first to employ the technology, but anesthetists were quick to embrace it.

Cooper, Harvard and Standards

In 1978, Jeff Cooper and his colleagues from the Massachusetts General Hospital, published the preliminary studies of critical incidents in anesthesia, suggesting that human error played a significant role in their causation. In the years following, they collected further data, resulting in the landmark publication in 1984 of "*An analysis of major errors and equipment failures in anesthesia management: Considerations for prevention and detection*". Collection of the new data was crucial; as the last sentence in the paper states, "Awareness of the problems is a necessary first step". Equipment failure explained only 4% of incidents leading to substantive negative outcomes; human error was the dominant factor in causation of incidents. To address human factors in prevention, the authors suggested strategies that tackled training, supervision, organization, ergonomics, and monitoring [16].

At the same time, the medical malpractice insurer for the Harvard group of 9 hospitals had noticed an increase in the number and cost of anesthesia-related claims, out of proportion to any increase in the number of anesthesia providers. The Harvard Risk Management Committee was established, with Cooper as a member, to review all cases reported over the years 1976 to 1984. The committee determined that the majority of incidents involved failures of ventilation or oxygenation that might be preventable by the institution of appropriate monitoring and practices. The anesthesia chairs of the 9 hospitals endorsed the recommendations and these were published in the Journal of the American Medical Association in August 1986, to become universally known as the "Harvard Monitoring Standards" [17]. The standards advised the continued presence of an anesthetist, measuring and recording the heart rate and blood pressure at least at five-minute intervals. They recommended continuous monitoring of ventilation and circulation (by any means), the continuous use of an electrocardiogram, continuous monitoring (with alarm capability) of oxygen concentration in gas delivery, and use of a breathing circuit disconnect alarm during mechanical ventilation. Temperature monitoring was to be available.

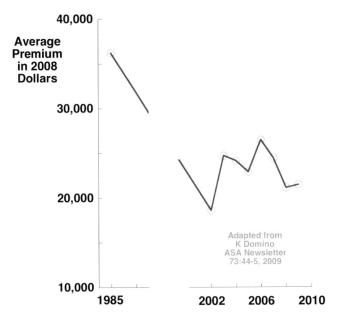

Fig. 11.2 Karen Domino's report in the 2009 ASA Newsletter provided data suggesting that 1980s and later efforts to increase the safety of anesthesia bore fruit. Implementation of various reforms was associated with a decrease in malpractice costs by approximately 40%

No previous attempt, anywhere, had set mandatory guidelines for medical practice, and opposition from anesthetists in practice was therefore anticipated. To this end, staff in the 9 hospitals were consulted in the development of realistic standards that were technically achievable and affordable, recognising that some practices would need to change and some equipment would need to be upgraded. Widespread acceptance followed, and within a short time, excellent compliance with the standards occurred within the Harvard group. Eichhorn and colleagues noted at the end of their paper that "Insurance carriers may provide the impetus, but physician leadership is required" [17].

In October 1986, the American Society of Anesthesiologists adopted a set of standards, based on the Harvard standards, but augmented by the non-mandatory addition of pulse oximetry, capnography, and a monitor of airway gas flow or volume. Many anesthetists reacted negatively, claiming that they had practiced safely for years without new and expensive technology. But they were gradually outnumbered. The rest is history, as they say, as the standards were repeatedly updated, and both anesthesia-related mortality, and malpractice premiums declined (Fig. 11.2).

Anesthesia Patient Safety Foundation (APSF)

In parallel with the adoption of standard guidelines, the President of the American Society of Anesthesiologists, Ellison ("Jeep") Pierce, together with Cooper and Richard Kitz, organised a 1984 International Symposium on Preventable Anesthesia Mortality and Morbidity. From that initiative came the APSF, founded in 1986. The APSF became the model for the National Patient Safety Foundation (NPSF) founded in 1997 with its headquarters in Boston.

Safety Sought in Australia, New Zealand, and Other Countries

In Australia and New Zealand, the potential consequences of the "Harvard Standards" were soon appreciated. Malpractice insurance was becoming a growth industry, and limitations on hospital funding restricted expenditure on new technology, especially in anesthesia. The standards prompted a legal misinterpretation that if a patient had been injured or had died as a result of anesthesia, and an electrocardiogram had not been used, then the anesthetist would be considered culpable. It was widely believed that although electrocardiographic monitoring was vitally important in many patients, it was not a good monitor of circulatory integrity, was not the most appropriate monitor in young and healthy patients [18]. Indeed, in many instances it was not used correctly as an indicator of myocardial ischemia. It was also clear that pulse oximetry was a useful monitor of circulatory integrity, but was expensive. These thoughts prompted Bill Runciman to convene a meeting of some 60 anesthetists in Adelaide in 1987, to discuss monitoring and safety. From that meeting came the Anaesthesia Incident Monitoring Study (AIMS) in 1988, the promulgation of Australian and New Zealand anesthesia monitoring standards in 1988, and the Australian Patient Safety Foundation (APSF) in 1989.

The 1988 anesthesia monitoring standard in Australia and New Zealand, endorsed by the Faculty of Anaesthetists of the Royal Australasian College of Surgeons, was similar to the Harvard standards, differing in the mandatory continuous presence of a physician anesthetist, the availability (not mandatory use) of an electrocardiogram, and the recommendation that a pulse oximeter should be available for every patient. They were revised in 1990, to institute mandatory use of pulse oximetry in every anesthetised patient by the beginning of 1992.

Other countries introduced similar standards, some making the electrocardiogram mandatory, others not. In all cases, the standards have been repeatedly updated in the context of the country in which they are used, and in 2008, the World Federation of Societies of Anaesthesiology published "International Standards for the Safe Practice of Anaesthesia".

Did these efforts influence the malpractice crisis that prompted their initiation? We cannot tell for certain, but in succeeding years, the cost of malpractice insurance in the US decreased by roughly 40% (Fig. 11.2). In Australia, the cost never reached the dizzying heights seen in the US, but has nevertheless also decreased substantially. This surrogate measure of morbidity and mortality suggests the value of the efforts.

Counting the Dead

The 1980s also saw an increasingly concerted effort to collect data on mortality related to anesthesia. The first report of the Confidential Enquiry into Perioperative Deaths (CEPOD), in 1987, was a joint initiative of anaesthetists and surgeons in Great Britain. The recommendation that practitioners audit their practices in a quest to improve patient care was an important stimulus to the introduction of quality assurance into anesthesia. Collection of morbidity and mortality data has continued to be an important contribution to education and safe practice.

Critical Incidents and Simulation

The AIMS study in Australia and New Zealand applied the critical incident analysis, pioneered in anesthesia by Cooper, to the collection of data. The resulting enormous body of data could be used to validate the usefulness of various monitors and processes, and to confirm the appropriateness of published minimum monitoring standards. The data were also used to develop crisis management algorithms that could be applied in every day anesthesia practice. This was an application of the system used in the aviation industry to eliminate subjective and intuitive solutions to a rapidly emerging crisis. Some physicians found it difficult to adopt this concept, having spent all their formative education based on deductive reasoning. The failure of such a process in the midst of a crisis prompted Runciman and colleagues to develop the algorithms [19, 20].

Building on the information provided by critical incident analysis, and also following the lead of the aviation industry, David Gaba established a mannequin-based anesthesia simulator at Stanford in 1988. Nik Gravenstein established a similar simulator in Gainsville, Florida, shortly afterwards.

First applied in health care to the specialty of anesthesia, critical incident analysis is now the mainstay for the review of patient safety in all fields.

Machine Design

Critical review of the anesthetist's workplace began in the 1970s. Studies of the operational environment and Cooper's investigations from the early 1970s led to the publication of the American National Standards Institute's ANSI Z79.8-1979 standard for anesthetic machines. It focused on the design and placement of controls and displays, taking into account human factors engineering. One of the principals, Leslie Rendall-Baker, had co-designed the Fraser-Harlake "line of sight" machine in 1976 by adapting a standard machine and aligning the breathing bag, flowmeters, monitors, ventilator and vaporisers, adjacent to the patient's head. In 1980, Boquet et al published their study of the anesthetist's activity during normal practice, using these data to develop

a mock-up design. Rendall-Baker published "Problems with Anesthetic Machines and Their Solutions" in 1982. This was the era of change from the standard design of the previous 40 or more years to today's anesthesia workstation [21, 22].

In the early 1980s, two commercial designs heralded what was to come. The Engstrom series 2000 was a modular vertical component machine, mirroring Boquet's proposal, and the Ohio Modulus Wing reflected the Fraser Harlake design. Neither was commercially successful, partly because of entrenched user resistance. Part of the issue was also the serial adoption of new monitors (pulse oximetry, capnography and others) as separate units with distinctive displays, alarms and connections, additions stacked onto a traditional machine in a haphazard, often unstable manner, reminiscent of a "Christmas tree". Not until the end of the 1980s were controls, monitors, displays and alarms ergonomically integrated [23].

Two novel anesthesia machines appeared in the 1980s. In 1986, the Swedish Engström company introduced the "Elsa" machine with digital flowmeter displays, and an integrated capnometer, oxygen analyser, anesthetic agent monitor, and ventilator. The machine had three ports for the connection of standard factory bottles of halothane, isoflurane, or enflurane. Liquid agent was withdrawn and injected into the gas stream under electronic control. It had a quirky bistable valve to change from spontaneous to controlled ventilation, that many anesthetists found difficult to use at first.

The "Physioflex" machine, developed by the Dutch company, Physio BV, was a radical design based on a closed circuit where gases were circulated by a blower. Based on a constant combined circuit and lung volume, ventilation was achieved by changing the machine circuit volume. Like the "Elsa", standard bottles of volatile anaesthetic agent were attached to indexed ports. Anaesthetic agent was added to the gas stream by liquid injection, and the selected end-tidal concentration of the agent was then servo controlled, during both spontaneous and controlled ventilation, using a charcoal filter to extract the agent from the circuit if necessary. The "Physioflex" was eventually bought by Drager, and an agent port for sevoflurane added [23]. Both machines were confined to the European market, and did not find widespread acceptance. They were at least a decade ahead of their time.

Recognizing an Old Problem

Substance abuse and drug addiction are ancient problems. The experiences of people participating in "nitrous oxide parties and ether frolics" engendered the discoveries of the anesthetic properties of nitrous oxide and ether. The bad news was that those who might know better, knowledgable physicians and nurses, abused drugs. Horace Wells' suicide directly resulted from his addiction to chloroform, and self-experimentation with morphine and cocaine. Self-administration, usually by intravenous injection, of opioids, CNS stimulants and depressants led many early and late anesthetists unwittingly into a life of addiction. Misuse of almost every opioid, sedative-hypnotic, and anesthetic drug has continued, and some of the brightest anesthesiologists and other physicians have died from overdoses or from taking other drugs to ease their withdrawal symptoms. The problem increased, in parallel with the rise in illicit drug use in the community.

In 1975, the Georgia Medical Association instituted the Impaired Physician Program. In 1983, it was reported that of the first 507 patients admitted to the program, 9.6 % were anesthesiologists, yet anesthesiologists comprised only 4 % of physicians. In parallel surveys, 13 % of physicians in impaired physician programs were anesthesiologists. Success of treatment varied, and a high relapse and death rate accompanied the use of parenteral opioids. In the 1980s, Gravenstein anonymously surveyed 31 academic departments of anesthesia, reporting in 1983 that for the years 1974 to 1979, between 1 and 2 % of anesthetists had misused drugs, with 47 associated deaths [24].

Lecky and colleagues, at the University of Pennsylvania provided advice on the recognition and management of potentially impaired colleagues, through a staff educational program [25]. This anticipated the many prospective programs to assist in the early recognition of colleagues at risk from substance abuse or other issues including stress, depression, and physical health. Today, the most common cause of physician impairment is the abuse of alcohol and other mood altering drugs. Recovery programs are offered throughout the US, and the addicted physician is mandated to enter them as a condition for retaining his or her medical license.

Pain Management Made Disparate Advances

In 1980, "Project Pain" was established at MGH and Shriners Burn Institute, to study pain in burned children. The results led to greater recognition of pain in burned children, and the use of subcutaneous lidocaine and adrenaline during grafting procedures. In 1983, Clifford Woolf confirmed that spinal anesthesia given before injury can prevent central sensitization. In 1984, Cousins and Mather published a review of intrathecal and epidural opioids that became the most cited anesthesia paper in the literature [26]. In 1988, Brian Ready reported on the first formally established Acute Pain Service.

And in the 1980s

Slogoff and Keats published their study "Does perioperative myocardial ischemia lead to postoperative myocardial infarction?" [27], linking intraoperative tachycardia to post-

operative myocardial infarction and leading to widespread use of ß-blockers. Around the same time, Franks and Lieb developed an experimental model using luciferase (a protein) from firefly tails to demonstrate competitive binding by anesthetics to protein binding sites, thereby undercutting support for lipid theories of anesthetic action [28]. Bernie Wetchler published "*Anesthesia for Ambulatory Surgery*", and in 1990, Paul White published "*Outpatient Anesthesia*", such books reflecting the importance that "same day" anesthesia and surgery had achieved.

Reprise

The 1980s could arguably be described as the modern decade of greatest change in anesthesia practice. Change was largely driven by anesthesiologists, anesthesiologists aided and abetted by other specialists and by industry invention and investment. Anesthetists were offered new anesthetics (isoflurane, sevoflurane, desflurane and propofol) and a new sedative drug (midazolam) that remain today's standards. Anesthetists could use newer, safer muscle relaxants, vecuronium and atracurium. Safety continued its wondrous advance through the development of organizations focused on decreasing mortality and morbidity from anesthesia, and through the rise of subspecialties. Safety was furthered by the increasing use of infrared analysis of respiratory and anesthetic gases and by the development and application of the pulse oximeter. Airway management improved marvelously, adding to safety, most notably through the release of the Laryngeal Mask Airway. Gadgets were introduced to clinical practice that promised great control over the anesthetic delivery, including Target Controlled Infusions. Anesthetists and surgeons could be guided by transesophageal echocardiography. Outpatient anesthesia reached maturity. Altogether, the 1980s could be called the decade in which modern anesthesia came of age.

References

1. Smith BE. The 1980s: a decade of change. In: Bacon DR, McGoldrick KE, Lema MJ, editors. The American society of anesthesiologists—a century of challenges and progress. Wood Library-Museum of Anesthesiology. 2005. pp. 173–91.
2. Fisher DM, Canfell PC, Fahey MR, Rosen JI, Rupp SM, Sheiner LB, Miller RD. Elimination of atracurium in humans: contribution of Hofmann elimination and ester hydrolysis versus organ-based elimination. Anesthesiology. 1986;65:6–12.
3. Messner M, Beese U, Romstock J, Dinkel M, Tschaikowsky K. The bispectral index declines during neuromuscular block in fully awake persons. Anesth Analg. 2003;97:488–91.
4. Op de Coul AA, Lambregts PC, Koeman J, van Puyenbroek MJ, Ter Laak HJ, Gabreels-Festen AA. Neuromuscular complications in patients given Pavulon (pancuronium bromide) during artificial ventilation. Clin Neurol Neurosurg. 1985;87:17–22.

5. Albright GA. Cardiac arrest following regional anesthesia with etidocaine or bupivacaine. Anesthesiology. 1979;51:285–7.

6. Sear JW, Prys-Roberts C, Phillips KC. Age influences the minimum infusion rate (ED50) for continuous infusions of Althesin and methohexitone. Eur J Anaesthesiol. 1984;1:319–25.

7. Spelina KR, Coates DP, Monk CR, Prys-Roberts C, Norley I, Turtle MJ. Dose requirements of propofol by infusion during nitrous oxide anaesthesia in man. I: Patients premedicated with morphine sulphate. Br J Anaesth. 1986;58:1080–4.

8. Browne BL, Prys-Roberts C, Wolf AR. Propofol and alfentanil in children: infusion technique and dose requirement for total i.v. anaesthesia. Br J Anaesth. 1992;69:570–6.

9. Roberts FL, Dixon J, Lewis GT, Tackley RM, Prys-Roberts C. Induction and maintenance of propofol anaesthesia. A manual infusion scheme. Anaesthesia. 1988;43 Suppl:14–7.

10. Schwilden H. A general method for calculating the dosage scheme in linear pharmacokinetics. Eur J Clin Pharmacol. 1981;20:379–86.

11. Schuttler J, Schwilden H, Stoekel H. Pharmacokinetics as applied to total intravenous anaesthesia. Practical implications. Anaesthesia. 1983;38 Suppl:53–6.

12. Shafer A, Doze VA, Shafer SL, White PF. Pharmacokinetics and pharmacodynamics of propofol infusions during general anesthesia. Anesthesiology. 1988;69:348–56.

13. Hudson RJ, Stanski DR, Saidman LJ, Meathe E. A model for studying depth of anesthesia and acute tolerance to thiopental. Anesthesiology. 1983;59:301–8.

14. Westhorpe RN, Ball C. The pulse oximeter. Anaesth Intensive Care. 2008;36:767.

15. Jaffe MB. Infrared measurement of carbon dioxide in the human breath: "breathe-through" devices from Tyndall to the present day. Anesth Analg. 2008;107:890–904.

16. Cooper JB, Newbower RS, Kitz RJ. An analysis of major errors and equipment failures in anesthesia management: Considerations for prevention and detection. Anesthesiology. 1984;60:34–42.

17. Eichhorn JH, Cooper JB, Cullen DJ, Maier WR, Philip JH, Seeman RG. Standards for patient monitoring during anesthesia at Harvard Medical School. JAMA. 1986;256:1017–20.

18. Runciman WB. Monitoring and patient safety: an overview. Anaesth Intensive Care. 1988;16:11–3.

19. Runciman WB. Crisis management. Anaesth Intensive Care. 1988;16:86–8.

20. Runciman WB, Webb RK, Klepper ID, Lee R, Williamson JA, Barker L. The Australian incident monitoring study. Crisis management–validation of an algorithm by analysis of 2000 incident reports. Anaesth Intensive Care. 1993;21:579–92.

21. Rendell-Baker L. Problems with anesthetic gas machines and their solutions. Int Anesthesiol Clin. 1982;20:1–82.

22. Boquet G, Bushman JA, Davenport HT. The anaesthetic machine–a study of function and design. Br J Anaesth. 1980;52:61–7.

23. Westhorpe RN. The anesthetic machine in the 1990s. Anesthesiol Rev. 1992;19:46–55.

24. Ward CF, Ward GC, Saidman LJ. Drug abuse in anesthesia training programs. A survey: 1970 through 1980. JAMA: the j Am Med Assoc. 1983;250:922–5.

25. Lecky JH, Aukburg SJ, Conahan TJ 3rd, Geer RT, Ominsky AJ, Gross J, Muravchick S, Wollman H. A departmental policy addressing chemical substance abuse. Anesthesiology. 1986;65:414–7.

26. Cousins MJ, Mather LE. Intrathecal and epidural administration of opioids. Anesthesiology. 1984;61:276–310.

27. Slogoff S, Keats AS. Does perioperative myocardial ischemia lead to postoperative myocardial infarction? Anesthesiology. 1985;62:107–14.

28. Franks NP, Lieb WR. Do general anaesthetics act by competitive binding to specific receptors? Nature. 1984;310:599–601.

Significant Developments in the 1990s

12

Edmond I Eger II, Rod N. Westhorpe and Lawrence J. Saidman

Summary

Advances and retreats in the 1990s often appeared in pairs. Two rapid acting neuromuscular blocking drugs, rocuronium, and the isomer of atracurium, cisatricurium, came onto the market. Unlike rocuronium, elimination of cisatricurium did not require hepatic degradation. The inhaled anesthetics, desflurane and sevoflurane, were released for clinical use. Although possessing greater stability and lower solubility, desflurane stimulated cardiorespiratory systems while sevoflurane did not, ultimately causing the popularity of sevoflurane to eclipse that of desflurane.

Several studies focused on the safety of regional anesthesia. Injection of 5% lidocaine through intrathecal microbore catheters could produce spinal cord injury, probably by confining the injected lidocaine to a small area. Lidocaine injected intrathecally could also produce transient neurological injury. Ropivacaine, an enantiomer of bupivicaine, was developed to decrease systemic local anesthetic toxicity. If toxicity arose anyway, intravenous infusion of lipid could decrease the availability and thus toxicity of a local anesthetic. The 1990s saw the use of ultrasound to guide local anesthetic placement, adding to safety by decreasing the amount of anesthetic needed, and adding to patient comfort by avoiding the earlier use of paresthesias to guide needle placement.

Various initiatives such as application of evidence-based algorithms and checklists decreased anesthesia-related morbidity and mortality in the decades leading to the 1990s. The WFSA adopted the multi-language online journal '*Update in Anaesthesia*', spreading knowledge of the science and safe practice of anesthesia in developing countries. Adding to anesthetic safety, 1990s studies found that the slow heart rate produced by beta blocking drugs could protect the heart from ischemia. Later research demonstrated that potent inhaled anesthetics protected the ischemic heart by a mechanism akin to that with ischemic preconditioning. Other studies showed that a normal temperature, and maybe more oxygen, prevented wound infection.

In the 1990s, new anesthesia machines combined all needed components into a lovely, albeit costly, "anesthesia workstation". The Engstrom-General Electric version included the computer-controlled Anesthesia Delivery Unit (ADU) that precisely delivered any anesthetic, including desflurane. Except for the US, the world approved machines to provide a Target Controlled Infusion of propofol.

Experiments in the 1990s advanced our appreciation of how inhaled anesthetics acted. To the surprise of many, investigators reported that the spinal cord (not the brain) mediates the immobility produced by inhaled anesthetics. Further decreasing the notion that inhaled anesthetics acted by altering the lipid bilayer, many highly halogenated compounds were found to disobey the Meyer-Overton correlation. The argument that proteins were the site of anesthetic action thereby gained traction. The finding of stereospecific effects of isoflurane isomers on MAC and ion channels added support to that notion.

World Events in the 1990s

The decade began hopefully with Germany's reunification, but the first Gulf War cast a pall. CNN covered the war with an immediate presence, establishing that network as the major television source for world news. Instability and advances marked 1991 with the Soviet Union disintegrating and the Cold War and the Warsaw Pact ending. A series of positive world events followed: The internet arrived. In 1992, Bill Clinton signed the North American Free Trade Agreement (NAFTA), beloved by capitalists and despised by US unions. The 1993 Treaty of Maastricht established

E. I Eger II (✉)
Department of Anesthesia and Perioperative Care,
University of California, San Francisco, CA, USA
e-mail: egere@anesthesia.ucsf.edu

R. N. Westhorpe
Melbourne, Australia
e-mail: westhorpe@netspace.net.au

L. J. Saidman
Department of Anesthesia, Stanford University, Stanford, CA, USA
e-mail: lsaidman@stanford.edu

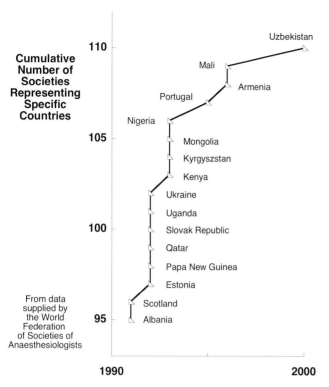

Cumulative Number of Societies Representing Specific Countries

Uzbekistan
Mali
Armenia
Portugal
Nigeria
Mongolia
Kyrgyszstan
Kenya
Ukraine
Uganda
Slovak Republic
Qatar
Papa New Guinea
Estonia
Scotland
Albania

From data supplied by the World Federation of Societies of Anaesthesiologists

1990   2000

Date of Formation of Specialist Society

Fig. 12.1 Sixteen new anesthesia societies appeared in the 1900s, several from the new countries that arose from the ashes of the Soviet Union

the European Union, a mixed blessing. The Global Positioning System (GPS) became fully operational. To the world's astonishment and applause, in 1994, South Africa peacefully elected Nelson Mandela as its first black President. In the next year, protease inhibitors were released, markedly decreasing AIDS mortality. The search engine Google appeared in 1997. About then, things took a turn for the worse. The Taliban seized control of Afghanistan in 1996, the year that the First Chechen War began, lasting until 1998, the year that India and Pakistan acquired nuclear weapons. In 1999, the Euro became the official currency for 12 countries. It seemed like such a good idea at the time.

Still More Anesthesia Societies

The 1991 disintegration of the Soviet Union into individual countries resulted in the appearance of several new anesthesia societies. These joined with societies that arose in other countries in the 1990s, in which the numbers of anesthesiologists had reached a critical mass (Fig. 12.1). Altogether, 16 new societies appeared.

Better Neuromuscular Blocking Drugs? Yes and No

The search for better neuromuscular blocking drugs continued, particularly the search for a drug with a faster onset and an assured termination of effect. Succinylcholine fitted that description but it caused muscle pain, untoward increased potassium release, and prolonged effects in patients with pseudocholinesterase deficiency. So the search went on. Organon synthesized rocuronium, and in 1989, the first report of its use in animals appeared [1]. Within a year, results in humans were published, [2] leading to its release for clinical use in 1994. It appeared to have a faster onset than the then competitor, vecuronium and many anesthetists used it. A competing company, Burroughs Wellcome (now GlaxoSmithKline) had manufactured the rapid-acting drug atracurium. However, atracurium caused histamine release/allergic reactions, making it less than perfect. A stereoisomer of atracurium, cisatricurium avoided these side effects. In 1995, cisatricurium dosing and recovery characteristics were reported for humans, [3] and it became clinically available soon thereafter. Like atracurium, cisatracurium elimination did not require renal or hepatic function, instead depending on Hofmann elimination (hydrolysis). Recovery was therefore assured and many anesthetists felt more secure with its use.

But neither rocuronium nor cisatracurium were perfect; neither produced paralysis as rapidly as did succinylcholine. In 1999, Organon reported synthesis of a drug with these properties, rapacuronium [4]. Initial uses in hundreds of patients gave promising results. Unfortunately, when hundreds of thousands of patients were given rapacuronium, a few (especially children) developed severe bronchospasm, [5] and in 2001 rapacuronium was removed from the market.

The Continuing Advance of Inhaled Anesthesia

In much of the world, halothane was the inhaled anesthetic of the 1960s; enflurane, the 1970s; and isoflurane, the 1980s. By the 1980s, the practice of surgery increasingly turned from a hospital-based to an ambulatory-based practice, taking with it or being led by anesthesia. The "come-and-go" nature of ambulatory surgery increased the need for anesthetics with more transient effects, anesthetics that allowed a more rapid recovery, and safe release of patients to go home. Thus the shift to propofol in the 1980s. In the 1990s, desflurane and sevoflurane, poorly soluble inhaled anesthetics that complimented the rapid recovery from propofol, were released for clinical use.

In 1990, Ron Jones described some of desflurane's effects in volunteers [6]. Other studies in humans concurrently detailed desflurane's cardiorespiratory, neuromuscular, metabolic and cerebral effects. Anaquest pursued the commercialization of desflurane, with presentations to the FDA in 1991 that gained desflurane's approval and allowed marketing in 1992—at the same time that isoflurane's patent expired and its profitability to Anaquest declined (as told in Chapter 10, isoflurane had been synthesized by Anaquest employee, Ross Terrell, in the 1960s and commercialized by Anaquest in the 1980s).

Sevoflurane was resurrected at about the same time as was desflurane. Terrell had also synthesized sevoflurane in the 1960s but had not pursued its development because it was unstable in the presence of a base, as found in CO_2 absorbents. Bernard Regan at Travenol Laboratories had independently synthesized sevoflurane. Studies by Richard Wallin detailed some of sevoflurane's pharmacology [7, 8]. Wallin appreciated but was less deterred by the vulnerability of sevoflurane to degradation. In 1981, Duncan Holiday reported that sevoflurane induced anesthesia rapidly and smoothly in volunteers [9]. For a time, that was as far as it got; Some laboratory studies had found toxic effects of sevoflurane in rats [10, 11], and so it was put aside.

Baxter (successor to Travenol) approached Anaquest in 1987 to discuss licensing of sevoflurane by Anaquest. After a year of considering that possibility, Anaquest rejected Baxter's offer, reasoning that their then-being-developed desflurane's lesser solubility and greater stability made it superior. Furthermore, by a fortunate oversight, desflurane had patent protection. In the 1960s, Terrell had made desflurane using a process that required elemental fluorine. It was dangerous and expensive to make, and its lesser potency (a third that of isoflurane) meant that much more would have to be produced—adding to the expense. Terrell thought so little of desflurane's prospects that no patent had been obtained and no publication had detailed its properties. The absence of public declarations meant that desflurane could be patented as though it had been discovered yesterday. In contrast, sevoflurane had been in the public domain for decades and had, at most, a 5-year exclusivity protection. Rebuffed by Anaquest, Baxter sold sevoflurane to Maruishi, a small Japanese pharma, who after further study brought sevoflurane to market in Japan in 1990 where it was a success…without reports of injury. Maruishi then turned to Abbott Laboratories which in 1992 accepted an offer to license sevoflurane for worldwide sales excluding Japan and China [12]. In 1993, Abbott made sevoflurane available.

The proponents of sevoflurane and desflurane had grand struggles in the 1990s. Statistically significant differences were found that didn't always translate to meaningful clinical differences. In 1991, Nobu Yasuda showed that the kinetics of desflurane were superior to those of sevoflurane [13, 14]. Studied by Richard Weiskopf in volunteers in 1992, desflurane did not produce evidence of renal injury [15], but

five years later, Eger showed that prolonged anesthesia with sevoflurane at 2 L/min inflow rate could produce nephrotic levels of albumin in the urine of volunteers [16], a finding confirmed in studies of patients by Higuchi et al. in 1998 [17]. Such transient injury correlated with the amount of a degradation product of sevoflurane, compound A, that the subject breathed [16–19]. These findings appeared to confirm Anaquest's decision to pursue desflurane rather than sevoflurane. However, although injury might be produced (and even that was not accepted by many sevoflurane proponents), the injury required prolonged (8-hour) exposure at relatively high sevoflurane concentrations (1.25 MAC) with fresh Baralyme® absorbent (which produced greater amounts of compound A from sevoflurane degradation than did other absorbents or partially used absorbents). And the injury was transient. Thus the proponents of sevoflurane might reasonably dismiss any injury as clinically unimportant.

There is a delicious irony to this story. In response to Eger's (yes the same Eger as the editor of this book) compelling testimony to the FDA regarding the potential for renal injury, sevoflurane administration in humans in the US was limited by the FDA to 2 MAC hours at 1 L/min for two hours after which the fresh gas flow had to be increased to 2 L/min. Because of this proscription, however, most anesthetists used the higher flow (2 L/min—or even 3 L/min) thus generating greater profits for Abbott (the licensee from Maruishi), the rival company to that producing desflurane, the anesthetic favored by Eger. Who would have guessed?

More relevant was the finding that desflurane, but not sevoflurane, might stimulate the cardiovascular system [20, 21], and irritate the airway (Fig. 12.2) [22]. Such clinically important unwanted effects of desflurane ultimately caused the popularity of sevoflurane to eclipse that of desflurane. Too late, it was appreciated that such unwanted effects of desflurane only became apparent at concentrations exceeding 1 MAC [6, 23], and that the concurrent use of opioids like fentanyl diminished or abolished such effects [24].

Dexmedetomidine and Mivazerol

The alpha2-adrenoceptor agonist dexmedetomidine had been developed in the late 1980s, and this continued to its approval for human use in the 1990s. In 1988, Vickery et al showed that it decreases anesthetic requirement (MAC) in dogs, and if given in sufficient dosage could suffice, alone, for anesthesia [25]. It does more than just affect anesthetic requirement. It decreases heart rate, and as shown in the late 1990s, it and a sister drug, mivazerol could protect the heart with coronary artery disease from ischemic injury [26, 27].

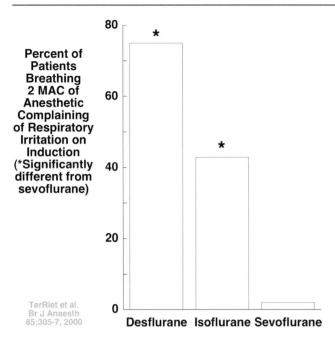

Fig. 12.2 Ter Riet et al. induced anesthesia in patients with 2 MAC of desflurane, isoflurane, or sevoflurane, finding postoperatively that few if any complained of irritation of the airway when anesthetized with sevoflurane [22]

Advances in Local Anesthetics and Their Delivery

Placement of catheters in the cerebrospinal fluid of the spinal canal requires making a hole in the arachnoid membrane of a size that predisposed to leakage of cerebrospinal fluid and thereby increased the potential for "spinal headache". It seemed obvious that the smaller the catheter, the better. Animated by this notion, in 1991, Rigler and Drasner used such catheters to produce spinal anesthesia with lidocaine. To their surprise, they found an associated spinal cord injury [28]. Studies suggested that this resulted because the slow injection, forced by the narrowness of the microbore catheter, concentrated the injected lidocaine, and because lidocaine had a greater inherent toxicity than previously appreciated. Further study led to the 1993 observation that even when a microbore catheter was not used, the subtle neurotoxicity of lidocaine produced a "transient neurological syndrome" (TNS) [29]. This effect was not seen with bupivacaine [30]. The TNS peculiarly associated with lidocaine, plus the rare serious injury, markedly decreased the use of lidocaine as a spinal anesthetic.

Local anesthetics also have a dose-dependent capacity to cause untoward effects from their systemic presence. In particular, bupivacaine can cause profound cardiac depression [31]. Investigators attacked such toxicity in several ways. One effective strategy proposed in the 1980s decreased bupivacaine dosage, using a smaller concentration as well as smaller incremental volumes [31]. A less effective one took advantage of potential differences in bupivacaine's two enantiomers, leading to the 1996 marketing of ropivacaine [levobupivacaine, the S (−) enantiomer] which has less affinity for cardiac sodium channels than the R (+) mirror image [32]. But the differences in toxicity between bupivacaine's enantiomers were small and probably of little clinical significance. Weinberg described another strategy for dealing with toxicity, in 1998 finding that lipid infused intravenously could absorb and thereby decrease the availability and toxicity of bupivacaine [33].

Finally, accurate placement of local anesthetic to achieve anesthesia enhances the safety of local anesthetics/regional anesthesia by minimizing the amount of local anesthetic required and by avoiding injection of anesthetic in blood vessels. In 1994, University of Vienna investigators described ultrasound identification of peripheral nerves (specifically the brachial plexus) [34]. This advance revolutionized regional anesthesia, not only decreasing the amount of anesthetic required and potentially reducing complications, but also decreasing patient discomfort since it avoided the use of paresthesias to guide needle placement. To that time, paresthesias or anatomical landmarks had been the standard approaches to identifying the correct position of the tip of the needle used to inject the local anesthetic.

Outcomes Studies and Mundane Checklists Add to Safety

Various 1990s outcomes studies increased the safety of anesthesia. Several studies built on the 1985 observation by Slogoff and Keats that a slower heart rate protected against postoperative myocardial infarction in patients having coronary artery bypass operations [35]. In the late 1990s–2000s, Mangano [36] and Wallace [37] found that administration of atenolol or clonidine to decrease beta adrenergic activity, decreased mortality in patients having operations for cardiac disease.

Inhaled anesthetics could also play a protective role. In 1997, Cason's group showed that isoflurane administration produced cardioprotection akin to protection produced by "ischemic preconditioning" [38]. Other potent inhaled anesthetics had this effect, a cardioprotection that long (days) outlasted the presence of the anesthetic [39]. Thus in 2003, De Hert showed that the use of anesthetics such as desflurane or sevoflurane could greatly decrease myocardial injury from the myocardial ischemia inherent to coronary artery surgery [40]. On the other hand, injected anesthetics could sometimes play an untoward role. In 1992, Parke et al. found that prolonged (days) infusion of propofol produced a profound acidosis, lipidemia, and myocardial failure that could be lethal to children [41]. Whether this resulted from the vehicle used to deliver propofol, to propofol itself, or to some other factor was unclear.

The ability of the anesthetist to control physiological variables could increase patient welfare. In 1996, Kurz, Sessler and Lenhardt showed that maintaining normal body temperature protected against wound infection after colon resection [42]. This study profoundly influenced practice in the US and worldwide. Use of forced air warmers to maintain normothermia in all but brief procedures became standard. In 1997, Hopf and Hunt demonstrated that breathing greater concentrations of oxygen decreased wound infection and hastened healing [43]. It is not clear that this prompted the use of greater inspired concentrations of oxygen.

The US Institute of Medicine report "To Err Is Human" published in 1999, suggested that anesthesia-related mortality decreased from 2 deaths per 10,000 anesthetics in the 1980s to about 1 death per 200,000 a decade later [44]. This admirable increase in safety resulted from numerous worldwide initiatives. For example, in 1991, Gaba convened a conference focused on human error in anesthesia, leading to the introduction of algorithms and checklists similar to those used to ensure safety in commercial aviation. In 1999, Pronovost et al. reported on the use of such an approach to decrease morbidity and mortality from venous catheter induced infection [45]. Not everyone agreed that the decreased overall rate of mortality was as dramatic as suggested [46].

Safety advanced worldwide. To do this, less developed countries relied on proven simple approaches to safety, approaches disseminated by means that such a world could access and afford. In 1992, the World Anaesthesia Society, a Specialist Society of the Association of Anaesthetists of Great Britain and Ireland, funded 'Update in Anaesthesia' the international journal of the World Federation of the Societies of Anaesthesiologists (WFSA), with supplemental funding by the UK Overseas Development Administration.[1] The WFSA adopted 'Update in Anaesthesia' to spread knowledge of the science and safe practice of anesthesia in developing countries. Free copies were sent to 3,000 English-speaking anesthetists. Free download from the internet was available in English, French, Mandarin, and Spanish.

Electroconvulsive therapy (ECT) remains as the primary therapy for major depression. It comes at a price. Patients correctly apprehend that such therapy can decrease mental function and can be associated with prolonged memory loss. With his anesthesia colleagues in Vienna, psychiatrist Langer hypothesized that the electrical silence that followed convulsions, rather than the convulsions, themselves, produced the desired effect, resetting the brain. For those with limited to no computer expertise, this notion is similar to the underlying cure of computer woes sometimes magically achieved by turning the computer off and then on again. Langer continues

with his proposal: Perhaps using inhaled anesthetics to achieve electrical silence might produce the same effect as convulsions without causing memory loss. Consistent with that hypothesis, in 1985, they demonstrated that deep anesthesia with isoflurane, inducing a period of 'electrocerebral silence,' reduced depression in 9 of 11 subjects [47]. They confirmed these results in 1995 [48].

In 1993, a separate group from Wurzburg confirmed that burst-suppression-level isoflurane was as effective as ECT [49], with the caveat that anesthesia required more time and monitoring than ECT. Perhaps this explains why the use of isoflurane for management of major depression has not become routine. Or perhaps anesthetic management of depression is not used because psychiatrists make treatment decisions and because the evidence supporting treatment with isoflurane came from small studies, only some of which were randomized and controlled. But it seems a pity this isn't resolved. We'd rather have a brief anesthesia than ECT for our depression.

Advances in Equipment

Before the 1990s, hospitals and anesthetists purchased anesthesia machines and monitors separately, this offering the advantage of modular selection of the "best" device. However, displays, controls and alarms varied, predisposing to confusion. In the 1990s, purveyors of anesthetic equipment integrated the anesthesia machine, ventilator and monitors into an "anesthesia workstation" in which all modalities were displayed in one place, with alarms coordinated and prioritized. But the cost of the new machines could approach $ 100,000.

Engstrom (later Datex-Engstrom and then General Electric) released the Anesthesia Delivery Unit (ADU), incorporating a new form of the variable bypass vaporizer, in 1995. This was the first anesthesia machine where gas flows through the bypass versus the vaporizer sump were controlled by a computer. The computer control-module was separate from the anesthetic sump. The former was programmed to deal with any of the anesthetics (including desflurane) while the latter (the sump) was specific to the anesthetic. Based on feedback from agent monitors, the computer-controlled flows were adjusted to deliver the agent concentration dialed on the anesthesia machine. Any anesthetic, including desflurane, could be used with this variable bypass vaporizer. As suggested in the previous paragraph, the vaporizer was integrated into a complete anesthesia machine, the ADU.

In 1981, Schwilden supplied an analysis that suggested the feasibility of a computer-controlled infusion of an anesthetic or anesthetic adjuvant drug in a manner that achieved a targeted concentration at the effect site of the drug, wherever that might be [50]. By the 1990s, several investigators had applied Schwilden's approach (e.g., see Raemer et al. [51]

[1] Information may be accessed at update.anaesthesiologists.org/.

and Shafer et al. [52]) By 1995, machines to provide a Target Controlled Infusion of propofol (e.g., the 'Diprifusor') [53] were approved in much of the world…but not in the US.

SIM 1 the first computer-controlled anesthesia-dedicated mannequin simulator was made for use at the University of Southern California in the 1960s [54]. Although it appeared promising, it was never released commercially. In the 1980s, David Gaba at Stanford University [55], and Michael Good and JS Gravenstein at the University of Florida created simulators for investigating human performance, training and safety in anesthesia [56]. And from the late 1990s through to 2010, training and recertification with computerized simulators grew rapidly despite limited evidence of sustained efficacy. In 2000, there were less than 200 computerized mannequin simulators, but by 2011 this had increased to more than 7000 (see Chapter 37).

How do Anesthetics Work?

Our appreciation of the mechanisms underlying the action of inhaled anesthetics advanced in the 1990s. In 1993, to the surprise of many anesthetists, Antognini and Schwartz [57], and Rampil [58] reported that the spinal cord and not the brain mediated the immobility produced by inhaled anesthetics. And in a further blow to the notion that inhaled anesthetics acted by altering the lipid bilayer, Koblin et al. reported in 1994, that many polyhalogenated and perfluorinated compounds disobeyed the Meyer-Overton correlation [59]. If not lipids, then perhaps proteins were the site of anesthetic action—as Franks and Lieb argued [60]. In support of that notion, Lysko et al. found stereospecific effects of isoflurane isomers on MAC [61], and, similarly, Franks and Lieb showed stereospecificity for actions of isoflurane on nerve ion channels [62].

Also in the 1990s

Increasingly, the anesthesiologist, sometimes deliberately and sometimes by chance, has become a perioperative physician with responsibilities that extend beyond the operating room [63]. Consistent with this concept was Fischer's 1996 argument that anesthesiologists should establish and supervise clinics for the preoperative evaluation and preparation of patients for surgery [64].

In 1998, a mandated increase to 2.5 years duration of training was imposed on US Nurse anesthesia training programs and all graduates had to earn a master's degree. Further increases were programmed for the future, including a requirement that graduates earn a doctorate. For now, that development has been postponed to 2025.

In 1983, Gualtieri et al. suggested that drug addicted anesthesia residents should seek work in another specialty because of the poor success rate for re-entry into anesthesia [65]. A 1991 study by Pelton and Ikeda suggested however that up to 70% of health care professionals, including anesthesiologists, successfully return to medical practice [66]. Paris and Canavan reported a similar finding in 1999 [67]. No evidence indicated that anesthesia providers in recovery returning to anesthetic delivery posed an increased risk to patient safety.

Reprise

The 1990s advanced safety, control and understanding of clinical anesthesia. Two new, poorly soluble inhaled anesthetics, sevoflurane and desflurane allowed a more precise control over the anesthetic state. Sevoflurane did so without cardiorespiratory stimulation. Both protected the heart from hypoxia. An older anesthetic, isoflurane, could reverse mental depression. We learned that all these anesthetics acted on central pattern generators in the ventral spinal cord to make patients immobile despite ongoing surgery. We also learned that the Meyer-Overton theory correlating lipophilicity and anesthetic potency didn't always work, indirectly suggesting that inhaled anesthetics operated on proteins. Two new muscle relaxants, recuronium and cis-atracurium added to safety by acting more rapidly and for shorter times. On the other hand, the historically "safe" local anesthetic lidocaine, was found to be mildly or severely neurotoxic, particularly when given through an intrathecal microbore catheter. In another blow to local anesthetics, higher doses of bupivicaine produced cardiovascular collapse. We dealt with this problem by giving less bupivicaine (helped by the development of ultrasound guidance which allowed more accurate placement of the bupivicaine) and giving it more slowly. We might switch to the less toxic enantiomer of bupivicaine, ropivicaine, and if all else failed we treated toxicity with intravenous lipid which swept up the local anesthetic. More to safety, we applied checklists to decrease infection. We prevented hypothermia, and that, too, decreased infection. In Europe and other places outside the US, we used machines to give target controlled infusions to maximize the kinetic advantages of propofol. It was a good decade for anesthesia.

References

1. Muir AW, Houston J, Green KL, Marshall RJ, Bowman WC, Marshall IG. Effects of a new neuromuscular blocking agent (Org 9426) in anaesthetized cats and pigs and in isolated nerve-muscle preparations. Br J Anaesth. 1989;63:400–10.

2. Wierda JM, de Wit AP, Kuizenga K, Agoston S. Clinical observations on the neuromuscular blocking action of Org 9426, a new steroidal non-depolarizing agent. Br J Anaesth. 1990;64:521–3.

3. Prielipp RC, Coursin DB, Scuderi PE, Bowton DL, Ford SR, Cardenas VJ Jr., Vender J, Howard D, Casale EJ, Murray MJ. Comparison of the infusion requirements and recovery profiles of vecuronium and cisatracurium 51W89 in intensive care unit patients. Anesth Analg. 1995;81:3–12.

4. Fleming NW, Chung F, Glass PS, Kitts JB, Kirkegaard-Nielsen H, Gronert GA, Chan V, Gan TJ, Cicutti N, Caldwell JE. Comparison of the intubation conditions provided by rapacuronium (ORG 9487) or succinylcholine in humans during anesthesia with fentanyl and propofol. Anesthesiology. 1999;91:1311–7.

5. Rajchert DM, Pasquariello CA, Watcha MF, Schreiner MS. Rapacuronium and the risk of bronchospasm in pediatric patients. Anesth Analg. 2002;94:488–93.

6. Jones RM, Cashman JN, Mant TGK. Clinical impressions and cardiorespiratory effects of a new fluorinated inhalation anaesthetic, desflurane (I-653), in volunteers. Br J Anaesth. 1990;64:11–5.

7. Wallin RF, Napoli MD, Regan BM. Laboratory investigation of a new series of inhalational anesthetic agents: the halomethyl polyfluoroisopropyl ethers. In: Fink BR, editor. Cellular Biology and Toxicity of Anesthetics. Baltimore: Williams & Wilkins Co; 1972. pp. 286–95.

8. Wallin RF, Regan BM, Napoli MD, Stern IJ. Sevoflurane: a new inhalational anesthetic agent. Anesth Analg. 1975;54:758–65.

9. Holaday DA, Smith FR. Clinical characteristics and biotransformation of sevoflurane in healthy human volunteers. Anesthesiology. 1981;54:100–6.

10. Cook TL, Beppu WJ, Hitt BA, Kosek JC, Mazze RI. A comparison of renal effects and metabolism of sevoflurane and methoxyflurane in enzyme-induced rats. Anesth Analg. 1975;54:829–35.

11. Hitt BA, Mazze RI, Cook TL, Beppu WJ, Kosek JC. Thermoregulatory defect in rats during anesthesia. Anesth Analg. 1977;56:9–14.

12. Brown BR Jr. Sevoflurane: introduction and overview. Anesth Analg. 1995;81:S. 1–3.

13. Yasuda N, Lockhart SH, Eger EI II, Weiskopf RB, Johnson BH, Freire BA, Fassoulaki A. Kinetics of desflurane, isoflurane, and halothane in humans. Anesthesiology. 1991;74:489–98.

14. Yasuda N, Lockhart SH, Eger EI II, Weiskopf RB, Liu J, Laster M, Taheri S, Peterson NA. Comparison of kinetics of sevoflurane and isoflurane in humans. Anesth Analg. 1991;72:316–24.

15. Weiskopf RB, Eger EI II, Ionescu P, Yasuda N, Cahalan MK, Freire B, Peterson N, Lockhart SH, Rampil IJ, Laster M. Desflurane does not produce hepatic or renal injury in human volunteers. Anesth Analg. 1992;74:570–4.

16. Eger EI II, Koblin DD, Bowland T, Ionescu P, Laster MJ, Fang Z, Gong D, Sonner J, Weiskopf RB. Nephrotoxicity of sevoflurane vs. desflurane anesthesia in volunteers. Anesth Analg. 1997;84:160–8.

17. Higuchi H, Sumita S, Wada H, Ura T, Ikemoto T, Nakai T, Kanno M, Satoh T. Effects of sevoflurane and isoflurane on renal function and on possible markers of nephrotoxicity. Anesthesiology. 1998;89:307–22.

18. Gonsowski CT, Laster MJ, Eger EI II, Ferrell LD, Kerschmann RL. Toxicity of compound A in rats. Effect of a 3-hour administration. Anesthesiology. 1994;80:556–65.

19. Gonsowski CT, Laster MJ, Eger EI II, Ferrell LD, Kerschmann RL. Toxicity of compound A in rats. Effect of increasing duration of administration. Anesthesiology. 1994;80:566–73.

20. Ebert TJ, Muzi M, Lopatka CW. Neurocirculatory responses to sevoflurane in humans. A comparison to desflurane. Anesthesiology. 1995;83:88–95.

21. Weiskopf RB, Eger EI II, Noorani M, Daniel M. Repetitive rapid increases in desflurane concentration blunt transient cardiovascular stimulation in humans. Anesthesiology. 1994;81:843–9.

22. Ter Riet MF, De Souza GJA, Jacobs JS, Young D, Lewis MC, Herrington C, Gold MI. Which is most pungent: isoflurane, sevoflurane or desflurane? Br J Anaesth. 2000;85:305–7.

23. Rampil IJ, Lockhart SH, Zwass MS, Peterson N, Yasuda N, Eger EI 2nd, Weiskopf RB, Damask MC. Clinical characteristics of desflurane in surgical patients: minimum alveolar concentration. Anesthesiology. 1991;74:429–33.

24. Weiskopf RB, Eger EI 2nd, Noorani M, Daniel M. Fentanyl, esmolol, and clonidine blunt the transient cardiovascular stimulation induced by desflurane in humans. Anesthesiology. 1994;81:1350–5.

25. Vickery RG, Sheridan BC, Segal IS, Maze M. Anesthetic and hemodynamic effects of the stereoisomers of medetomidine, an alpha 2-adrenergic agonist, in halothane-anesthetized dogs. Anesth Analg. 1988;67:611–5.

26. Oliver MF, Goldman L, Julian DG, Holme I. Effect of mivazerol on perioperative cardiac complications during non-cardiac surgery in patients with coronary heart disease: the European Mivazerol Trial (EMIT). Anesthesiology. 1999;91:951–61.

27. Talke P, Li J, Jain U, Leung J, Drasner K, Hollenberg M, Mangano DT. Effects of perioperative dexmedetomidine infusion in patients undergoing vascular surgery. The Study of Perioperative Ischemia Research Group. Anesthesiology. 1995;82:620–33.

28. Rigler ML, Drasner K, Krejcie TC, Yelich SJ, Scholnick FT, DeFontes J, Bohner D. Cauda equina syndrome after continuous spinal anesthesia. Anesth Analg. 1991;72:275–81.

29. Schneider M, Ettlin T, Kaufmann M, Schumacher P, Urwyler A, Hampl K, von Hochstetter A. Transient neurologic toxicity after hyperbaric subarachnoid anesthesia with 5 % lidocaine. Anesth Analg. 1993;76:1154–7.

30. Pollock JE, Neal JM, Stephenson CA, Wiley CE. Prospective study of the incidence of transient radicular irritation in patients undergoing spinal anesthesia. Anesthesiology. 1996;84:1361–7.

31. Adverse Reactions with Bupivacaine. FDA Drug Bull. 1983;13:23.

32. Valenzuela C, Snyders DJ, Bennett PB, Tamargo J, Hondeghem LM. Stereoselective block of cardiac sodium channels by bupivacaine in guinea pig ventricular myocytes. Circulation. 1995;92:3014–24.

33. Weinberg GL, VadeBoncouer T, Ramaraju GA, Garcia-Amaro MF, Cwik MJ. Pretreatment or resuscitation with a lipid infusion shifts the dose-response to bupivacaine-induced asystole in rats. Anesthesiology. 1998;88:1071–5.

34. Kapral S, Krafft P, Eibenberger K, Fitzgerald R, Gosch M, Weinstabl C. Ultrasound-guided supraclavicular approach for regional anesthesia of the brachial plexus. Anesth Analg. 1994;78:507–13.

35. Slogoff S, Keats AS. Does perioperative myocardial ischemia lead to postoperative myocardial infarction? Anesthesiology. 1985;62:107–14.

36. Mangano DT, Layug EL, Wallace A, Tateo I. Effect of atenolol on mortality and cardiovascular morbidity after noncardiac surgery. Multicenter Study of Perioperative Ischemia Research Group. N Engl J Med. 1996;335:1713–20.

37. Wallace AW, Galindez D, Salahieh A, Layug EL, Lazo EA, Haratonik KA, Boisvert DM, Kardatzke D. Effect of clonidine on cardiovascular morbidity and mortality after noncardiac surgery. Anesthesiology. 2004;101:284–93.

38. Cason BA, Gamperl AK, Slocum RE, Hickey RF. Anesthetic-induced preconditioning: previous administration of isoflurane decreases myocardial infarct size in rabbits. Anesthesiology. 1997;87:1182–90.

39. Zaugg M, Lucchinetti E, Spahn DR, Pasch T, Schaub MC. Volatile anesthetics mimic cardiac preconditioning by priming the activation of mitochondrial KATP channels via multiple signaling pathway. Anesthesiology. 2002;97:4–14.

40. De Hert SG, Cromheecke S, ten Broecke PW, Mertens E, De Blier IG, Stockman BA, Rodrigus IE, Van der Linden PJ. Effects of propofol, desflurane, and sevoflurane on recovery of myocardial function after coronary surgery in elderly high risk patients. Anesthesiology. 2003;99:314–23.

41. Parke TJ, Stevens JE, Rice AS, Greenaway CL, Bray RJ, Smith PJ, Waldmann CS, Verghese C. Metabolic acidosis and fatal myocardial failure after propofol infusion in children: five case reports. BMJ. 1992;305:613–6.

42. Kurz A, Sessler DI, Lenhardt R. Perioperative normothermia to reduce the incidence of surgical-wound infection and shorten hospitalization. Study of Wound Infection and Temperature Group. N Engl J Med. 1996;334:1209–15.

43. Hopf HW, Hunt TK, West JM, Blomquist P, Goodson WH 3rd, Jensen JA, Jonsson K, Paty PB, Rabkin JM, Upton RA, von Smitten K, Whitney JD. Wound tissue oxygen tension predicts the risk of wound infection in surgical patients. Arch Surg. 1997;132:997–1004. (discussion 1005)

44. Kohn LT, Corrigan JM, Donaldson MS. To err is human: building a safer health system. Washingon, DC: National Academy Press (Institute of Medicine); 2000.

45. Pronovost P, Jenckes M, Dorman T, Garrett E, Breslow MJ, Rosenfeld BA, Lipsett PA, Bass E. Organizational characteristics of intensive care units related to outcomes of abdominal aortic surgery. J Amer Med Assoc. 1999;281:1310–7.

46. Lagasse RS. Anesthesia safety: model or myth? A review of the published literature and analysis of current original data. Anesthesiology. 2002;97:1609–17.

47. Langer G, Neumark J, Koinig G, Graf M, Schoenbeck G. Rapid psychotherapeutic effects of anesthesia with isoflurane (ED narcotherapy) in treatment-refractory depressed patients. NeuropsychoBiology. 1985;14:118–20.

48. Langer G, Karazman R, Neumark J, Saletu B, Schoenbeck G, Gruenberger J, Dittrich R, Petricek W, hoffmann P, Linzmayer L, Anderer P, Steinberger K. Isoflurane narcotherapy in depressive patients refractory to conventional antidepressant drug treatment. A double-blind comparison with electroconvulsive treatment. NeuropsychoBiology. 1995;31:182–94.

49. Engelhardt W, Carl G, Hartung E. Intra-individual open comparison of burst-suppression-isoflurane-anaesthesia versus electroconvulsive therapy in the treatment of severe depression. Eur J Anaesthesiol. 1993;10:113–8.

50. Schwilden H. A general method for calculating the dosage scheme in linear pharmacokinetics. Eur J Clin Pharmacol. 1981;20:379–86.

51. Raemer DB, Buschman A, Varvel JR, Philip BK, Johnson MD, Stein DA, Shafer SL. The prospective use of population pharmacokinetics in a computer-driven infusion system for alfentanil. Anesthesiology. 1990;73:66–72.

52. Shafer SL, Varvel JR, Aziz N, Scott JC. Pharmacokinetics of fentanyl administered by computer-controlled infusion pump. Anesthesiology. 1990;73:1091–102.

53. Glen JB. The development of 'Diprifusor': a TCI system for propofol. Anaesthesia. 1998;53 Suppl 1:13–21.

54. Denson JS, Abrahamson S. A computer-controlled patient simulator. JAMA. 1969;208:504–8.

55. Gaba DM, DeAnda A. A comprehensive anesthesia simulation environment: re-creating the operating room for research and training. Anesthesiology. 1988;69:387–94.

56. Cooper JB, Taqueti VR. A brief history of the development of mannequin simulators for clinical education and training. Qual Saf Health Care. 2004;13 Suppl 1:i11–8.

57. Antognini JF, Schwartz K. Exaggerated anesthetic requirements in the preferentially anesthetized brain. Anesthesiology. 1993;79:1244–9.

58. Rampil IJ, Mason P, Singh H. Anesthetic potency (MAC) is independent of forebrain structures in the rat. Anesthesiology. 1993;78:707–12.

59. Koblin DD, Chortkoff BS, Laster MJ, Eger EI II, Halsey MJ, Ionescu P. Polyhalogenated and perfluorinated compounds that disobey the Meyer-Overton hypothesis. Anesth Analg. 1994;79:1043–8.

60. Franks NP, Lieb WR. Molecular and cellular mechanisms of general anaesthesia. Nature. 1994;367:607–14.

61. Lysko GS, Robinson JL, Casto R, Ferrone RA. The stereospecific effects of isoflurane isomers in vivo. Eur J Pharmacol. 1994;263:25–9.

62. Franks NP, Lieb WR. Stereospecific effects of inhalational general anesthetic optical isomers on nerve ion channels. Science. 1991;254:427–30.

63. Saidman LJ. The 33rd Rovenstine Lecture. What I have learned from 9 years and 9,000 papers. Anesthesiology. 1995;83:191–7.

64. Fischer SP. Development and effectiveness of an anesthesia preoperative evaluation clinic in a teaching hospital. Anesthesiology. 1996;85:196–206.

65. Gualtieri AC, Cosentino JP, Becker JS: The California experience with the diversion program for impaired physicians. JAMA. 1983;249:226–9.

66. Pelton C, Ikeda RM. The California Physicians Diversion Program's experience with recovering anesthesiologists. J Psychoactive Drugs. 1991;23:427–31.

67. Paris RT, Canavan DI. Physician substance abuse impairment: anesthesiologists vs. other specialties. J Addict Dis. 1999;18:1–7.

Major Anesthesia-Related Events in the 2000s and Beyond

13

Lawrence J. Saidman, Rod N. Westhorpe and Edmond I Eger II

Summary

The dramatic scientific and technologic advances of anesthesia in preceding decades slowed in the 2000s, with maturation of the specialty and associated subspecialties. Certificates attesting expertise in anesthesiology and subspecialities now require or will require recertification.

Except for sugammadex, no new anesthesia-related drugs were released for use, and few new drugs are on the horizon. New uses for old drugs were found such as administering ketamine to lessen postoperative dependence on opioids, and substituting intrathecal 2-chloroprocaine for lidocaine to avoid lidocaine-associated transient neurologic syndrome. The 2000s saw technical advances such as the GlideScope, the first of many video-laryngoscopes, and increased adoption of ultrasound-assisted regional anesthesia. Several societies recommended ultrasound guidance for insertion of central venous catheters.

Fears that increased risk precluded outpatient surgery for ASA PS III patients were shown to be unfounded, and approximately 80 % of elective surgical and diagnostic procedures in the US were performed on an outpatient basis. However, office-based sedation appeared to increase risk relative to that in free-standing ambulatory surgery centers (ASCs), probably because of less oversight and training of those delivering sedation. The Lifebox Foundation promoted the 2004 Global Oximetry initiative of the WFSA, to make oximetry and capnography available and thereby diminish mortality in low-income regions of the world.

Three major worldwide instances of plagiarism, fraud, and lack of informed consent by anesthesiologists were revealed, resulting in retraction of a record number of publications, and prosecution and incarceration of at least one investigator.

The percentage of women anesthesia residents in the US increased from 27 % in 2000 to 38 % in 2010, women increasingly chaired Departments of Anesthesia, and 9 of 22 SAMBA Presidents were women. In the 2000s, governing agencies in the US and Europe progressively limited duty hours of residents in all specialties. In 2005, Pandit noted that only 6 of 23 UK universities sustained departmental or divisional structures for anesthesia.

Several analyses suggested that anesthesia safety reached new heights with death rates attributable to anesthesia of less than 1:100,000. If immediate mortality has reached an irreducible minimum, future efforts may aim to decrease long-term morbidity and mortality and associated health care costs. Consistent with this thought, Mark Warner as President of the American Society of Anesthesiologists in 2011 described the "Perioperative Surgical Home" proposing that anesthesiologists coordinate all matters relating to the in-hospital care of surgical patients. Now that would be a game changer!

L. J. Saidman (✉)
Department of Anesthesia, Stanford University, Stanford, CA, USA
e-mail: lsaidman@stanford.edu

R. N. Westhorpe
Melbourne, Australia
e-mail: westhorpe@netspace.net.au

E. I Eger II
Department of Anesthesia and Perioperative Care, University of California, San Francisco, CA, USA
e-mail: egere@anesthesia.ucsf.edu

World Events Shaping the 2000s

The decade began with the controversial 5:4 ruling by the US Supreme Court, delivering the US presidency to George W Bush. On 11 September 2001, commercial airliners became weapons of mass destruction (WMDs) deliberately destroying the World Trade Center in NYC, killing more than 3000 people. The subsequent "War on Terror" produced the US invasion of Afghanistan in search of Osama bin Laden and presaged the 2003 Iraq War justified by a search for never-to-be-found WMDs. SARS and Bird flu epidemics interfered with world travel in 2002 and 2006. Hurricane Katrina and the Indian Ocean Tsunami convincingly demonstrated the power of Mother Nature, nearly destroying a city of 500,000 and killing more than 240,000. In 2008, at the Beijing Olympics and again in 2012 in London, Usain Bolt and Michael Phelps became household names. So did Lance Armstrong after winning the Tour de France for seven consecutive years. In 2012 he was banned for life from racing for using banned substances. Barack Obama became the first African-American US President. In the early months of his presidency, the deregulated finance industry's ability to create mortgages for people who could not afford them, and then sell the debt for a profit, led the housing market "bubble" to burst, bringing near collapse of the world's economy. Bernard Madoff created the largest ever "Ponzi" scheme cheating investors out of 60 billion dollars. China and India developed into new economic powerhouses epitomizing the best and the worst of globalization. Google became the search engine of choice, and Facebook and Twitter emerged, creating a vast industry called "social media". The smart phone revolutionized communications and Apple became the world's most valuable company. Finally, in the US in 2010, proponents of the Affordable Care Act overcame enormous political opposition, providing access to medical care to 30 million previously uninsured American citizens, the US joining the rest of the developed world in offering (nearly) universal health care.

Pharmacology: Where are the Drugs?

One new medication pertinent to anesthesia, sugammadex, gained approval for clinical use in the 2000s in much of the world, but was not approved for use in the US. In contrast, at least 6-to-13 new medications had appeared in each of the six previous decades (Fig. 13.1).

Released for clinical use in the late 1990s, the ultra-short acting non-depolarizing neuromuscular blocking agent rapacuronium received an enthusiastic reception because the time to onset of action was similar to that of succinylcholine, succinylcholine-like side effects were absent, and neostigmine easily antagonized residual neuromuscular block. It was considered advantageous for use in patients at risk of aspiration and requiring a rapid sequence induction. However, Organon voluntarily withdrew rapacuronium from the market in 2001, due to concern regarding unexplained fatalities and severe bronchospasm occurring during post-marketing surveillance.

In the 2000s, Organon developed a radically new approach to reverse neuromuscular blockade. By "surrounding" a molecule of a neuromuscular blocking drug (particularly rocuronium), the cyclodextrin sugammadex could inactivate the action of the relaxant. A major advantage of sugammadex was the ability to immediately antagonize "deep" neuromuscular block, including that following rapid sequence induction. Like rapacuronium however, sugam-

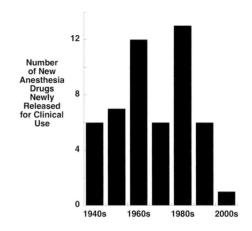

Fig. 13.1 Six to thirteen new anesthesia related drugs were introduced in each decade between 1940 and 2000. But from 2000 to 2013 only a single medication, sugammadex was introduced (while not available in the US, it was approved in more than 50 countries worldwide.)

madex was also associated with occasional cases of hypersensitivity reactions [1, 2], and while available throughout much of the world, as of 2013 it had not been approved by the FDA for clinical use. Interestingly, case reports describing the use of sugammadex to successfully treat severe rocuronium-induced bronchospasm (presumably by inactivating the molecule provoking the anaphylaxis) provided support for an otherwise unintended use of the drug in patients with anaphylaxis from rocuronium not responsive to other treatment [3].

A neuromuscular blocking drug, gantacurium, is in phase three trials. Like atracurium, gantacurium produced a nondepolarizing blockade, but rather than undergoing Hofmann degradation, inactivation occurred by adduct formation with L-cysteine. Exogenously administered L-cysteine could accelerate inactivation, independent of blood pH, temperature, or depth of block [4].

Reasons for the dearth of new anesthesia related medications in the 2000s included the enormous cost of drug development and the relatively small market for anesthesia related medications. Increasing cost controls placed by third party payers and/or governmental decision makers may have also exerted an effect. But the primary limitation may have been the proven efficacy and safety of already available drugs. Improving on the excellence of presently available anesthetics and anesthetic adjuvants proved difficult. Contrast these circumstances with those in the 1950s to 1970s, a period of considerable drug development. The increasing use of electrocautery reduced the suitability of ether and cyclopropane, and an appreciation of the importance of decreased blood solubility and lesser metabolism, stimulated synthesis of new inhaled agents, first halothane, then methoxyflurane (a mistake) then enflurane, isoflurane, sevoflurane, and desflurane. While none were perfect, it is difficult to imagine development of additional volatile agents. The same might be said of propofol, the intravenous induction/maintenance drug that replaced thiopental, or the anxiolytic drug midazolam that replaced diazepam, or the present array of opioids. Neuromuscular blocking drugs in the 1950s included d-tubocurarine, metacurine, decamethonium, gallamine, and succinylcholine, all relaxants with notable limitations that led to the "oniums" and "uriums" of the 1960s–1990s. While also not perfect, these drugs advanced the field so far that safety and efficacy were less problematic, and other than searching for a faster-shorter-acting non-depolarizer, further "tinkering" would seem to have a low benefit/cost ratio.

Thus safety and pleasantness of anesthetic delivery, rather than newness remained the principal concerns of the anesthesiologist. Improving safety might not depend upon newer and better medications. Instead of developing new drugs, newer applications of older drugs occurred in the 2000s. These included administration of small doses of ketamine at induction of anesthesia and at intervals during surgery to supply analgesia, especially in patients with chronic pain who otherwise required large doses of opioids [5].

Postoperative nausea and vomiting (PONV) has long concerned patient and anesthetist. In the 2000s and before, anesthetists increasingly appreciated the factors predisposing to PONV. Various remedies had been shown to be effective up to a certain dose, beyond which further doses added little to a reduction in PONV. Apfel et al. added another dimension, in 2004 showing that combining 2 or 3 such remedies increased their antiemetic effect [6]. The implication of this finding was not that more drug was effective, but that PONV resulted from effects on multiple receptors. Thus the use of remedies influencing multiple receptors was more effective than increasing the dose affecting a single receptor.

In the 1980s, 2-chloroprocaine (CP) was nearly abandoned because of concern regarding spinal cord injury associated with inadvertent intrathecal injection of a large dose for epidural anesthesia [7]. CP use at much lower doses returned for spinal anesthesia in patients undergoing relatively brief surgery [8]. However, such delivery represents an off label application, and the difficulty of "obtaining FDA approval or exemption to study the use of spinal CP in a randomized-controlled manner, (means that) the safety of CP will likely be determined by large scale clinical practice"[9].

Awareness during anesthesia has long been acknowledged as a risk in severely injured patients not tolerating the circulatory effects of amnestic concentrations of inhaled anesthetics [10]. A parallel concern has arisen from the increased use of total intravenous anesthesia (TIVA), especially for patients receiving neuromuscular blocking agents in doses that prevent movement reflecting pain or awareness. Providing an end tidal anesthetic concentration slightly exceeding MAC-Awake is considered sufficient to prevent awareness in most patients [11]. With TIVA, a surrogate matching MAC-Awake has been sought, developing an advocacy for

so-called awareness monitors [the bispectral index (BIS) or entropy monitors] to assure the presence of amnesia [12]. The value of these devices continues to be debated.

Ultrasound-Guided Procedures in Anesthesia—I Can See it Now!

Ultrasound technology has had a place in anesthesia since the 1980s with the introduction of transesophageal echocardiography [13]. Its origins as an adjunct to anesthesia-based procedures began in the 1990s [14, 15], but in the 2000s the promise of ultrasound assisted techniques blossomed. Anesthesiologists with their roots in the 1960s remember the anxiety associated with "walking the needle along the first rib" while performing supraclavicular brachial plexus blocks (pray, don't let me pierce the dome of the pleura!), or drawing lines on the buttocks before sciatic-femoral blocks (where were those nerves anyway?) Remember too, instructing an inexperienced resident in the use of surface landmarks to cannulate the internal jugular vein (especially nerve racking in a small child and still more problematic when the surgeon was nearby). Such terrors receded in the 2000s. More than 95 % of the 1200 papers published describing ultrasound assistance for regional blocks, jugular vein and other vessel cannulation (and all papers describing training in these techniques) appeared after 2000.

The 2000s' use of ultrasound guidance in regional anesthesia increased the ability to observe intravascular or intraneural injection of local anesthetic, lessened local anesthetic systemic toxicity (because a smaller volume of local anesthetic was needed, particularly advantageous in smaller children), and decreased patient discomfort relative to the previous method of nerve identification (paresthesias from nerve stimulation). Studies comparing landmark vs. ultrasound assistance for internal vein cannulation showed that ultrasound assistance led to a more rapid completion of the procedure, a greater frequency of successful performance, fewer attempts, and less morbidity (carotid puncture or hematoma formation) [16]. Recommendations from several societies including the Society Of Cardiovascular Anesthesiologists [17], and the American Society of Anesthesiologists [18] regarding its use, have recently emerged.

While these advantages appeared to indicate the usefulness of ultrasound assistance, many studies used as part of a recent American Society for Regional Anesthesia—Evidence Based Assessment were too small and the complications too infrequent to provide statistically significant evidence of superiority [19]. They relied on surrogate measures such as onset time and number of nerves anesthetized rather than more clinically relevant criteria including the ability to complete surgery without block supplementation or general anesthesia. Furthermore, experts performed many of the randomized control trials included in this assessment and their results may not reflect the success rate of anesthetists occasionally using regional anesthesia. As this clinical area matures, a specific period of training and experience may be expected, perhaps similar to that currently required for certification in trans-esophageal echocardiography. 3-D simulation trainers, with tactile feedback, are being developed.

Scientific Misconduct

The known frequency and magnitude of scientific misconduct increased enormously in the 2000s. Plagiarism and fraud accounted for most of these reports, the latter composed of "made-up" data and patient-related research lacking patient consent and/or Investigational Review Board (IRB) approval. Plagiarism detection probably increased because of newly available software that laid bare the use of another's words without proper attribution. Shafer, described a taxonomy of plagiarism varying in seriousness from Intellectual Theft (use of ideas, analysis, and large blocks of words without proper attribution—unacceptable) to Self Plagiarism (use of one's own words to describe perhaps a technical analysis or method not easily lending itself to restatement—OK) [20]. As Shafer stated, "it is unrealistic to expect an author working in a field to generate a novel description every time he or she chooses to write about it (but) extremes of self plagiarism including that approaching duplicate publication are clearly unethical and may be subject to manuscript retraction." (see cited references as an example) [21, 22].

Shafer also described "Plagiarism for Scientific English" used by authors uncomfortable expressing their thoughts in English. While understandable, this is not justifiable and if excessive may also be grounds for retraction [23]. Given that scientific journals increasingly screen every submission for plagiarism, the frequency of retraction for plagiarism will probably approach but not reach zero because plagiarism can escape detection by the detection software [24] It is tempting to speculate on the incidence of plagiarism before the "plagiarism detection software" era. This remains for others to explore.

Alas, no scientific fraud-detecting software comparable to plagiarism-detecting software exists. In the 2000s three major scandals revealed fraudulent anesthesia-related research published over the past several decades. First, Scott Reuben an investigator at Baystate Medical Center in Springfield Massachusetts published numerous papers describing the benefits of postoperative multimodal pain management. In 2009, more than 20 published papers and abstracts were retracted when individuals in his institution discovered that Reuben fabricated the data in these reports. Importantly, the falsity of the results cast doubt on recommendations regarding several clinically important treatments [25]. Reuben was sentenced for health care fraud to 6 months in prison, fined $ 50,000 and ordered to repay more than $ 300,000 to several pharmaceutical companies.

German investigator Joachim Boldt published more than 200 papers over the past 25 years, many comparing efficacy and safety of colloids, including hydroxyethyl starch and albumin, in humans. In early 2010, several readers noted suspicious data appearing in a paper published in 2009 [26]. The data, particularly the variability in the measurements of several cytokines and of blood gas data was too small. This led to an investigation revealing that no study had been performed! Further investigation of all of Boldt's research resulted in retraction of 88 papers, most for lack of evidence that patient consent had been obtained. At the time, this comprised the greatest number of retracted papers by a single author.

But wait! Not to be outdone, Yoshitaka Fujii a Japanese anesthesiologist has been accused of falsifying data in 172 (126 supposedly randomized control studies) of 212 papers published between 1993 and 2011. Fujii's credibility had been questioned in a 2000 Letter to the Editor [27] commenting on one of his published papers [28], that the data were "incredibly nice". In March 2012, John Carlisle a British anesthesiologist reported that the likelihood "of the data from all of Fujii's published papers being generated experimentally—as opposed to by fraud—(was) implausibly small, in the order of $1:1 \times 10^{30}$ [29]." Using a meta-analysis, Carlisle subsequently assessed the impact of deleting Fujii's research papers on our understanding of the impact of several antiemetics, showing far less antiemetic effect and a lack of synergy between these medications [30].

Assuming that the concerns regarding Fujii's reports hold up, of the 2,200 papers retracted from the literature since 1970, anesthesiologists authored nearly 13 %. In addition to diminishing the credibility of our specialty, such fraud could adversely affect patient care, if clinicians were misled by the recommendations emanating from the fraudulent papers.

Anesthesia Safety Through the 2000s: Is it a Snake or a Tree?

Defining anesthetic safety is akin to the parable in which blind men touch an elephant and describe what they have touched. "It is like a snake" says the man grabbing the tail. Oh no, says the man hugging the leg, "it is just like a tree". Context is important in describing the shape of an elephant and in describing the past and present history of anesthesia safety.

Anesthesia-related death rates of 1:500 to 1:2,000 were reported in the 1920s 1930s and 1940s (Fig. 13.2) [31–33]. We and others argue that by the 2000s, the safety of anesthesia

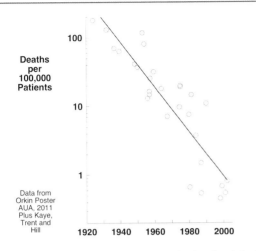

Fig. 13.2 Observational data describing anesthesia related death rate suggest a progressive decrease in mortality of two orders of magnitude during the history of modern anesthesia

had dramatically increased. Today's low mortality probably represents the cumulative result of multiple factors.

In 1954, Beecher and Todd published their landmark report of anesthesia-related mortality in a surgical journal [34]. Some fellow anesthesiologists dismissed the study [35]. Nonetheless, it illustrated some of the forces leading to today's amazing record of safety. Beecher and Todd prospectively studied 600,000 patients receiving various anesthetics. The mortality attributed to anesthesia as the primary cause was 1:2680 and contributory in 1:1560. The authors indicted curare as an important cause of death, finding many more deaths in patients receiving curare, with the greatest incidence of anesthesia-related death occurring in patients given both curare and ether (1:250). A plausible explanation of the greater mortality in this latter group is that patients reached the recovery room still partially anesthetized (because of the high blood solubility of ether), partially paralyzed (by curare and the synergistic effect produced by residual ether and hypercapnia secondary to hypoventilation), and breathing room air rather than air supplemented with oxygen. That is the explanation Cecil Gray supplied in an interview at Oxford in 1996:[1]

"… when he (Beecher) published the paper it was quite obvious these patients were returned to bed still curarised, and lying there. Now, the secret was when they were still curarised, breathing ineffectively, not only was that not good for them, from the point of view of the collapse of the lung and so forth, but also they accumulated carbon dioxide. Their carbon dioxide tension went up, which potentiated any residual curare, so it became a thing called residual curarisation, which was a thing unknown to us".

[1] The Royal College of Physicians and Oxford Brookes University, Medical Sciences Video Archive MSV A 145, Professor Cecil Gray CBE KCSG FRCP FRCS FRCA in interview with Dr Max Blythe, Oxford, 25th November 1996, Interview Two.

Gray also explains the difference between of the results with curare in the US and England:

"Now, the Americans were frightened of prostigmine because of its effect on the heart: give enough of it and it will just stop the heart, you see. But if you give atropine, atropine blocked that action but didn't block the action on the muscles, the reversal of the tubocurarine. And we worked out the technique in which we were giving atropine and prostigmine, feeling our way until we got the right sort of dose. Then over the months, I suppose it was—yes it was certainly months—we came to give it absolutely routinely, because there was no trouble."

Further to the elimination of the problem, monitoring of neuromuscular block began in the 1960s and became increasingly routine by the 1970s.

Subsequent observational studies (counting bodies) in the 1970s and 1980s reported anesthesia related death rates approaching 1:10,000 [36], decreasing further in the 1990s and 2000s to between 1:100,000 and 1:200,000 [37, 38]. In 1994, Lucien Leape commented "Whereas mortality from anesthesia was one in 10,000–20,000 just a decade or so ago, it is now estimated at less than one in 200,000. Anesthesiologists have led the medical profession in recognizing system factors as causes of errors in designing fail-safe systems in training to avoid errors [39]." The Institute of Medicine singled out the specialty for its success in reducing anesthesia related mortality [40].

Not all parties (including the authors of one of the essays in this book) accepted a two orders of magnitude decrease in anesthetic related mortality [41, 42], and many factors (including variations in surgical care, severity and number of co-morbidities and use or non-use of antibiotics) make comparisons of death rates between different eras difficult. But other measures—perhaps only surrogates of quality—lend support to the conclusion that a remarkable improvement has occurred, attributable to what we do and how we do it. For example, liability insurance rates—corrected for inflation—have decreased by forty percent over the last 40 years (Fig. 11.1).

Several factors may have decreased mortality over the more than 6 decades of outcome data portrayed in Fig. 13.2. Most of these factors would produce a gradual, progressive improvement. They include better training programs incorporating the use of simulators, recruitment of higher quality trainees, successive introduction of inhaled anesthetics, hypnotics and opioids with more favorable pharmacokinetic and dynamic profiles, the application of specific antagonists of neuromuscular blocking drugs, more effective preoperative and postoperative management, and the increased use of electronic medical records. They might also include the invention of monitors with proper alerts, anesthetic machines preventing delivery of hypoxic gas mixtures, and the influence of national and international patient safety organizations. Some factors such as perioperative "check lists"

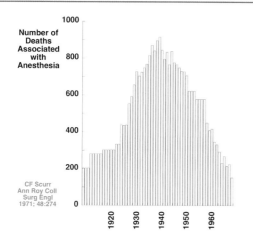

Fig. 13.3 Anesthesia-related deaths in England from 1908 to 1968 increased to a peak in the late 1930s and then dramatically decreased by nearly an order of magnitude. (Data from Scurr et al [43])

lated issues have the greater need? In 2009, Daniel Sessler commented:

> "An unfortunate consequence of our improvement is that some consider anesthetic safety a more-or-less solved problem. At the very least, the number of intraoperative deaths is now so small that policymakers might reasonably conclude that resources would be better invested elsewhere. This thought process may contribute to the dismally small amount of funding that the National Institutes of Health provides for anesthesiology research" [44].

Sessler also noted that compared with anesthesia-related deaths as defined by death within days following surgery, "mortality in the year after surgery is about 10,000 times more common than preventable anesthetic mortality." Increasingly anesthesiologist-directed initiatives and research efforts should focus on factors influencing long-term surgical outcomes. An early example was the 1996 study of Mangano et al. demonstrating a beneficial effect on long-term outcome of beta blockers in patients undergoing non-cardiac surgery [45].

Similar to the remarkable safety record in hospital-based surgery, outpatient surgery experienced a safety record greater than that originally anticipated. Dillon in 1967, opined that ASA PS III patients with diabetes, vascular insufficiency and anemia were unsuitable for surgery in an outpatient center [46]. But in 1976, as described by McGoldrick (Chapter 59), "Reed and Ford reported on 33,000 cases without a single death or malpractice suit [47], and in 2004 Ansell and Montgomery reported that ASA PS III patients had no obvious increase in morbidity or mortality relative to ASA PS I or II patients [48]."

Why should this be a surprise? Assuming a quality of care in an ambulatory surgery center similar to that in a tertiary care hospital, no reason suggests that the death rate for the two should differ. Of course this depends upon proper patient selection, upon suitable patient care at home, and upon availability of transport to a tertiary care facility if needed. And the patient treated at an outpatient surgery center may be at less risk of encountering infections.

On the other hand, office based surgery, another surgical site favored by patients and surgeons because of convenience and lower cost, may have a greater rate of both mortality and morbidity than that associated with ambulatory surgery centers [49]. Reasons for this seem obvious: a lack of oversight resulting in excessive sedation by the surgeon performing surgery while simultaneously providing sedation; lack of training (as well as practice) of the surgeon in airway management and other emergency procedures; limited familiarity with the consequences of the administration of potent opioids and sedative hypnotics; and poor selection of patients undergoing what may be lengthy and painful procedures. Consistent with this reasoning, mortality decreased by 58 % in the year following implementation of a standard

(time outs), response to malpractice liability crises (including adoption of monitoring standards), analysis of outcomes from malpractice cases (closed claims studies), and publication of evidence based practice parameters, guidelines, and advisories, might impose more immediate, step-like decreases in mortality because they are rapidly adopted.

Consider the anesthesia-related deaths data from England from 1908 to 1968 (Fig. 13.3). Consistent with an increasing number of operations (data not provided), deaths increased during the first thirty years, reaching a peak in the late 1930s. The number of anesthesia-related deaths declined over the next 30 years, doing so by nearly an order of magnitude. It seems unlikely that this would be explained by a decrease in the number of surgeries per year; if anything, the contrary would be likely. During this latter time, departments of anesthesia arose, anesthesia attracted better students, and halothane with a precision vaporizer for delivery was introduced [43]. None of these explanations provide a provable cause and effect relationship, but we submit that together they provide a compelling story supporting an actual improvement in patient safety meriting the comments of Leape and the Institute of Medicine.

In the 1930s, mortality from anesthesia might have killed 1:1000 patients anesthetized. If that applied to an annual delivery of 50 million anesthetics, anesthesia would have killed 500,000 patients, a mortality demanding attention. But assuming a present mortality of 1:100,000 to 1:200,000 and again an annual delivery in the 2000s of 50 million anesthetics, only 250-to-500 people would die in the US from anesthesia-related causes. In contrast, 400,000 people die yearly from smoking, alcohol-related automobile accidents and gunshot related deaths, 800–1,600 times the number of anesthesia-related deaths. Should additional resources be expended to achieve further decreases in anesthesia-related mortality when other more pressing health care re-that required an anesthesiologist in attendance for any case during which either general anesthesia, deep sedation, or regional anesthesia was used [50].

Perioperative Medicine and More

Originally proposed as a term defining the "job description" of anesthesia departments [51], Mark Warner reintroduced perioperative medicine as the Perioperative Surgical Home.®[2] In this role, anesthesiologists would manage and coordinate all in-hospital care related to the surgical patient. This differs from the current practice in many hospitals wherein surgeon, anesthesiologist, primary care physician, hospitalist, physician assistant, nurse practitioner, and intensivist (as needed) independently (and not necessarily in a coordinated manner) provide perioperative care.

More specifically, Warner states "The Perioperative Surgical Home is proposed as a demonstration project to evaluate whether anesthesiologists supported by Medicare, Medicaid and private health plans will be able to achieve the following goals:"

- "Reduce unjustified variation in utilization and expenditures.
- Improve the safety, effectiveness, timeliness and efficiency of health care.
- Increase the ability of beneficiaries to participate in decisions concerning their care.
- Provide delivery of care that is consistent with evidence-based guidelines in historically underserved areas.
- Decrease unjustified variation in utilization and expenditures under the Medicare program."

"If anesthesiologists' efforts reduce length of stays, numbers of transfusions and the complications that accompany them, and improve patient satisfaction and safety, it is logical that the medical center and facility administrators will find value in this extension of anesthesia practice". For example, anesthesiologists understand and are in a position to manage the factors underlying surgical site infections (SSIs), a complication estimated by Edmiston et al to be responsible for more than 1.6 billion dollars in cost, and 3.7 million extra hospital days [52]. As Mauermann and Nemergut point out, factors influencing SSIs and under the control of the anesthesiologist include the maintenance of body temperature [53], the amount and timing of antibiotics, the FiO_2 (greater than 80%) [54], intravenous fluid administration, decisions regarding blood transfusions, and prevention of hyperglycemia [55]. Additional long term outcomes in the anesthesiologist's purview include cognitive effects of

inhaled anesthetics in infants and small children [56], and the effects or lack of effects of inhaled vs regional anesthesia on cancer recurrence [57, 58].

An extended role for the anesthesiologist as envisioned by The Perioperative Surgical Home has counterparts in other countries. In France for example, anesthesiologists have via SAMU (Service d'Aide Médicale Urgente), assumed control of all emergency out of hospital care. In the 1970s, anesthesiologists Cara, Huguenard, Lareng and Serre, developed SAMU, reasoning that "in emergencies the hospital should go to the patient and not the contrary." Doctors (anesthesiologists) "dispatch and control the emergency response teams and unlike many emergency medical services, SAMU is an extension of the hospital service itself." And in 2006 " The development of SAMU demonstrates the widening borders of anesthesiology, a specialty only relatively recently recognised in France. In 2006, the SAMU received 15 million calls" (Chapter 27).

But is the Perioperative Surgical Home preempted by today's Hospitalist? The arguments for The Perioperative Surgical Home seem cogent and compelling, but may compete with the present implementation and control of patient's hospital care by Hospitalists. Hospitalists, a growing arm of medicine, already govern the care of patients entering hospitals, facilitating patient care from entry to departure. Can and will anesthesiologists compete with this group?

Kapur in her 2011 Rovenstine lecture addresses this question this by listing qualifications needed by anesthesiologists to assert the dominant role envisioned by Warner [59].

1. "Determine quality benchmarks and equal or exceed them".
2. "Oversee and solve perioperative, periprocedural, intensive care, and pain issues throughout the health system, utilizing a cost-effective mix of providers appropriate for the severity of the cases".
3. "Facilitate procedural through-put at all levels, including critical care".
4. "Become integral to the management of all areas where acute care and pain services are being delivered".
5. "Become the acute care go-to people, the acute care solution, for each of our clinical sites".

Further, Kapur comments that as "Miller and Hannenberg stated in 2005 [60], None of the existing medical specialties is fully equipped to provide comprehensive care in all of these areas, but anesthesiology is a strong contender for the best qualified". We regret that we will not be part of this evolving role for this specialty but look forward as observers to the fulfillment of the exciting possibilities described above.

Regarding the anesthesiologist's role as a perioperative physician, Merlin Larson commented that "the perioperative period is the ideal time to counsel patients about bad habits such as smoking and over-eating. The perioperative

---

[2] As Taken from a report [310-3.2] submitted to the ASA House of Delegates on Aug. 21, 2011, by then ASA President Mark Warner, M.D., entitled "Surgical Home Draft Proposal,".

period initiates a major disruption in patient's lives and it provides the ideal time for them to change how they live. We should take full advantage of this time—and use our special skills to help them recover with elation instead of depression. If we don't as a specialty look closely at how to help patients during this stressful period in their lives, then we will always be turning around to see if someone (such as a CRNA) is catching us". (Personal communication October 10, 2012).

Accordingly and in furtherance of the objectives of the Surgical Home is the recently announced program instituted at Monash University in Melbourne Australia and providing a Masters Degree in Perioperative Medicine (http://masters.periopmedicine.org.au/). As stated in the program description

> "Surgical patients are getting older and sicker. Many clinicians caring for surgical patients are challenged by the growing complexity of these patients, particularly their perioperative management. Pre-admission clinics are responding, and perioperative medicine is becoming an emerging field. This course will be conducted by Monash University (Academic Board of Anaesthesia and Perioperative Medicine and Department of Epidemiology and Preventative Medicine), in conjunction with the Alfred Hospital's Department of Anaesthesia and Perioperative Medicine (Director Prof Paul Myles).
> Key objectives of the perioperative medicine component are:
> 1. Provide clinicians with information to care for the growing complexity of surgical patients.
> 2. Provide a greater understanding of the importance and functioning of the pre-admission clinic.
> 3. Equip the perioperative physician to risk stratify and optimize care of the patient in the perioperative period.
> 4. Collaboratively manage the patient in the perioperative period, in particular the perioperative management of patients with acute medical, cardiac, and other organ dysfunction.
> 5. Equip the perioperative physician with the managerial skills to lead a multidisciplinary perioperative management team.
> 6. Equip the perioperative physician with basic research skills to further perioperative medicine research."

These objectives mirror the qualifications outlined by Kapur in her 2011 Rovenstine lecture [59], suggesting that worldwide support for this concept may be building.

Some Reflections

Over the previous 60 years (and more), the quality of personnel needed to deliver anesthesia, and their skills, tools, and medications have vastly improved. So has anesthesiology's position in the medical hierarchy. We increasingly occupy senior positions in our medical schools, hospitals, and medical societies and participate at all levels in national and international initiatives reforming medical care and extending this miracle of anesthesia to less developed areas of the world. Worldwide, anesthesia continues to grow. The numbers of anesthesiologists increase, and surprisingly, there seems to be no decrease in the rate of addition of anes-

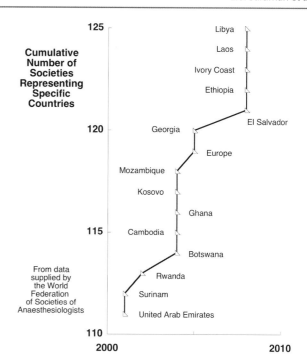

Fig. 13.4 Fifteen more anesthesia societies arose between 2000 and 2010, there seeming to be no decrease from the rates of addition in previous decades

thesia societies (Fig. 13.4). Is further advancement needed; shall we declare victory and go home; or should we seek new challenges?

And what might those challenges be? Here's one. Although we might think we know how anesthetic agents produce unconsciousness, we have but a vague idea of the mechanisms underlying injected drugs and a still vaguer notion of how inhaled anesthetics act to produce unconsciousness, unawareness, and immobility. Why pursue that challenge? Because it might tell us how the brain works.

References

1. Godai K, Hasegawa-Moriyama M, Kuniyoshi T, Kakoi T, Ikoma K, Isowaki S, Matsunaga A, Kanmura Y. Three cases of suspected sugammadex-induced hypersensitivity reactions. Br J Anaesth. 2012;109:216–8.
2. Motoyama Y, Izuta S, Maekawa N, Chuma R. [A case of anaphylactic reaction caused by sugammadex]. Masui. 2012;61:746–8.
3. McDonnell NJ, Pavy TJ, Green LK, Platt PR. Sugammadex in the management of rocuronium-induced anaphylaxis. Br J Anaesth. 2011;106:199–201.
4. Lien CA, Savard P, Belmont M, Sunaga H, Savarese JJ. Fumarates: unique nondepolarizing neuromuscular blocking agents that are antagonized by cysteine. J Crit Care. 2009;24:50–7.
5. Laskowski K, Stirling A, McKay WP, Lim HJ. A systematic review of intravenous ketamine for postoperative analgesia. Can J Anaesth. 2011;58:911–23.
6. Apfel CC, Korttila K, Abdalla M, Kerger H, Turan A, Vedder I, Zernak C, Danner K, Jokela R, Pocock SJ, Trenkler S, Kredel M,

Biedler A, Sessler DI, Roewer N. IMPACT Investigators: a factorial trial of six interventions for the prevention of postoperative nausea and vomiting. N Engl J Med. 2004;350:2441–51.

7. Reisner LS, Hochman BN, Plumer MH. Persistent neurologic deficit and adhesive arachnoiditis following intrathecal 2-chloroprocaine injection. Anesth Analg. 1980;59:452–4.

8. Casati A, Danelli G, Berti M, Fioro A, Fanelli A, Benassi C, Petronella G, Fanelli G. Intrathecal 2-chloroprocaine for lower limb outpatient surgery: a prospective, randomized, double-blind, clinical evaluation. Anesth Analg. 2006;103:234–8.

9. Pollock JE. Intrathecal chloroprocaine–not yet "safe" by US FDA parameters. Int Anesthesiol Clin. 2012;50:93–100.

10. Bogetz MS, Katz JA. Recall of surgery for major trauma. Anesthesiology. 1984;61:6–9.

11. Dwyer R, Bennett HL, Eger EI, II, Heilbron D. Effects of isoflurane and nitrous oxide in subanesthetic concentrations on memory and responsiveness in volunteers. Anesthesiology. 1992;77:888–98.

12. Avidan MS, Jacobsohn E, Glick D, Burnside BA, Zhang L, Villafranca A, Karl L, Kamal S, Torres B, O'Connor M, Evers AS, Gradwohl S, Lin N, Palanca BJ, Mashour GA. Prevention of intraoperative awareness in a high-risk surgical population. N Engl J Med. 2011;365:591–600.

13. Cahalan MK, Kremer P, Schiller NB et al. Intraoperative monitoring with two dimendional transesophageal echocardiography. Anesthesiology. 1982;57:A–152.

14. Kirvela O, Svedstrom E, Lundbom N. Ultrasonic guidance of lumbar sympathetic and celiac plexus block: a new technique. Reg Anesth. 1992;17:43–6.

15. Kapral S, Krafft P, Eibenberger K, Fitzgerald R, Gosch M, Weinstabl C. Ultrasound-guided supraclavicular approach for regional anesthesia of the brachial plexus. Anesth Analg. 1994;78:507–13.

16. Serafimidis K, Sakorafas GH, Konstantoudakis G, Petropoulou K, Giannopoulos GP, Danias N, Peros G, Safioleas M. Ultrasoundguided catheterization of the internal jugular vein in oncologic patients; comparison with the classical anatomic landmark technique: a prospective study. Int J Surg. 2009;7:526–8.

17. Troianos CA, Hartman GS, Glas KE, Skubas NJ, Eberhardt RT, Walker JD, Reeves ST. Special articles: guidelines for performing ultrasound guided vascular cannulation: recommendations of the American Society of Echocardiography and the Society Of Cardiovascular Anesthesiologists. Anesth Analg. 2012;114:46–72.

18. Rupp SM, Apfelbaum JL, Blitt C, Caplan RA, Connis RT, Domino KB, Fleisher LA, Grant S, Mark JB, Morray JP, Nickinovich DG, Tung A. Practice guidelines for central venous access: a report by the American Society of Anesthesiologists Task Force on Central Venous Access. Anesthesiology. 2012;116:539–73.

19. Neal JM, Brull R, Chan VW, Grant SA, Horn JL, Liu SS, McCartney CJ, Narouze SN, Perlas A, Salinas FV, Sites BD, Tsui BC. The ASRA evidence-based medicine assessment of ultrasound-guided regional anesthesia and pain medicine: executive summary. Reg Anesth Pain Med. 2010;35:S1–9.

20. Shafer SL. You will be caught. Anesth Analg. 2011;112:491–3.

21. Neligan PJ, Malhotra G, Fraser M, Williams N, Greenblatt EP, Cereda M, Ochroch EA. Continuous positive airway pressure via the Boussignac system immediately after extubation improves lung function in morbidly obese patients with obstructive sleep apnea undergoing laparoscopic bariatric surgery. Anesthesiology. 2009;110:878–84.

22. Neligan PJ, Malhotra G, Fraser M, Williams N, Greenblatt EP, Cereda M, Ochroch EA. Noninvasive ventilation immediately after extubation improves lung function in morbidly obese patients with obstructive sleep apnea undergoing laparoscopic bariatric surgery. Anesth Analg. 2010;110:1360–5.

23. Bhatnagar S. Request for retraction. Anesth Analg. 2010;111:1560.

24. Eldawlatly A, Shafer SL. Caveat lector. Anesth Analg. 2012;114:1160–2.

25. Shafer SL. Tattered threads. Anesth Analg. 2009;108:1361–3.

26. Boldt J, Suttner S, Brosch C, Lehmann A, Rohm K, Mengistu A. Cardiopulmonary bypass priming using a high dose of a balanced hydroxyethyl starch versus an albumin-based priming strategy. Anesth Analg. 2009;109:1752–62.

27. Kranke P, Apfel CC, Roewer N, Fujii Y. Reported data on granisetron and postoperative nausea and vomiting by Fujii et al. Are incredibly nice! Anesth Analg. 2000;90:1004–7.

28. Fujii Y, Saitoh Y, Tanaka H, Toyooka H. Comparison of ramosetron and granisetron for preventing postoperative nausea and vomiting after gynecologic surgery. Anesth Analg. 1999;89:476–9.

29. Carlisle JB. The analysis of 168 randomised controlled trials to test data integrity. Anaesthesia. 2012;67:521–37.

30. Carlisle JB. A meta-analysis of prevention of postoperative nausea and vomiting: randomised controlled trials by Fujii et al. compared with other authors. Anaesthesia. 2012;67:1076–90.

31. Kaye G. Anaesthetic deaths in Melbourne 1929–1934. Br J Anaesth. 1936;13:110–27.

32. Trent JC, Gaster E. Anesthetic Deaths in 54,128 Consecutive Cases. Ann Surg. 1944;119:954–8.

33. Hill EF, Hunter AR. Death on the operating table. Br J Anaesth. 1948;21:24–31.

34. Beecher HK, Todd DP. A study of the deaths associated with anesthesia and surgery: based on a study of 599,548 anesthesias in ten institutions 1948–1952, inclusive. Ann Surg. 1954;140:2–35.

35. Abajian J, Arrowood JG, Barrett RH, Dwyer CS, Eversole UH, Fine JH, Hand LV, Howrie WC, Marcus PS, Martin SJ, Nicholson MJ, Saklad E, Saklad M, Sellman P, Smith RM, Woodbridge PD. Critique of "A Study of the Deaths Associated with Anesthesia and Surgery". Ann Surg. 1955;142:138–41.

36. Tiret L, Desmonts JM, Hatton F, Vourc'h G. Complications associated with anaesthesia–a prospective survey in France. Can Anaesth Soc J. 1986;33:336–44.

37. Li G, Warner M, Lang BH, Huang L, Sun LS. Epidemiology of anesthesia-related mortality in the United States, 1999–2005. Anesthesiology. 2009;110:759–65.

38. Lienhart A, Auroy Y, Pequignot F, Benhamou D, Warszawski J, Bovet M, Jougla E. Survey of anesthesia-related mortality in France. Anesthesiology. 2006;105:1087–97.

39. Leape LL. Error in medicine. JAMA. 1994;272:1851–7.

40. Kohn LT, Corrigan JM, Donaldson MS. To err is human: building a safer health system. Washingon, DC, National Academy Press (Institute of Medicine), 2000.

41. Lagasse RS. Anesthesia safety: model or myth? A review of the published literature and analysis of current original data. Anesthesiology. 2002;97:1609–17.

42. Lagasse RS. Innocent prattle. Anesthesiology. 2009;110:698–9.

43. Scurr CF. Evolution and revolution in anaesthetic training. Ann R Coll Surg Engl. 1971;48:274–92.

44. Sessler DI. Long-term consequences of anesthetic management. Anesthesiology. 2009;111:1–4.

45. Mangano DT, Layug EL, Wallace A, Tateo I. Effect of atenolol on mortality and cardiovascular morbidity after noncardiac surgery. Multicenter Study of Perioperative Ischemia Research Group. N Engl J Med. 1996;335:1713–20.

46. Dillon JB. Anesthetic management of the outpatient. Anesth Rounds. 1967;2:1–15.

47. Reed WA, Ford JL. Development of an independent outpatient surgical center. Int Anesthesiol Clin. 1976;14:113–30.

48. Ansell GL, Montgomery JE. Outcome of ASA III patients undergoing day case surgery. Br J Anaesth. 2004;92:71–4.

49. Vila H Jr, Soto R, Cantor AB, Mackey D. Comparative outcomes analysis of procedures performed in physician offices and ambulatory surgery centers. Arch Surg. 2003;138:991–5.

50. Vila H, Soto RG, Miguel RV et al. 2003 update: outcomes analysis of procedures performed in Florida physician offices and ambulatory surgery centers. Anesthesiology. 2003;99:A1364.

51. Saidman LJ. The 33rd Rovenstine Lecture. What I have learned from 9 years and 9,000 papers. Anesthesiology. 1995;83:191–7.

52. Edmiston CE, Spencer M, Lewis BD, Brown KR, Rossi PJ, Henen CR, Smith HW, Seabrook GR. Reducing the risk of surgical site infections: did we really think SCIP was going to lead us to the promised land? Surg Infect (Larchmt). 2011;12:169–77.

53. Kurz A, Sessler DI, Lenhardt R. Perioperative normothermia to reduce the incidence of surgical-wound infection and shorten hospitalization. Study of Wound Infection and Temperature Group. N Engl J Med. 1996;334:1209–15.

54. Hopf HW, Hunt TK, West JM, Blomquist P, Goodson WH III, Jensen JA, Jonsson K, Paty PB, Rabkin JM, Upton RA, von Smitten K, Whitney JD. Wound tissue oxygen tension predicts the risk of wound infection in surgical patients. Arch Surg 1997;132:997–1004; discussion 1005.

55. Mauermann WJ, Nemergut EC. The anesthesiologist's role in the prevention of surgical site infections. Anesthesiology 2006;105:413–21;quiz 439–40.

56. DiMaggio C, Sun LS, Li G. Early childhood exposure to anesthesia and risk of developmental and behavioral disorders in a sibling birth cohort. Anesth Analg. 2011;113:1143–51.

57. Lai R, Peng Z, Chen D, Wang X, Xing W, Zeng W, Chen M. The effects of anesthetic technique on cancer recurrence in percutaneous radiofrequency ablation of small hepatocellular carcinoma. Anesth Analg. 2012;114:290–6.

58. Gottschalk A, Ford JG, Regelin CC, You J, Mascha EJ, Sessler DI, Durieux ME, Nemergut EC. Association between epidural analgesia and cancer recurrence after colorectal cancer surgery. Anesthesiology. 2010;113:27–34.

59. Kapur PA. Leading into the future: the 50th annual Rovenstine lecture. Anesthesiology. 2012;116:758–67.

60. Miller R, Hannenberg A. Anesthesiology's choices for the next century. ASA Newsletter 2005; (Centennial Issue):36–7.

Predicting the Future

14

Lawrence J. Saidman, Rod N. Westhorpe and Edmond I Eger II

"The future ain't what it used to be."—Yogi Berra, famous American baseball player and manager

We asked each editor-in-chief of 16 anesthesia journals to supply a 500-word (or less) essay predicting their respective vision of local or worldwide anesthesia in 2023. Each was asked to ignore the great risk of being wrong. They were enjoined not to use "may be" or "might be" but to make definitive statements ("will be"). Some took this to heart and made grand, adventuresome predictions while others were more cautious. The reader will have to judge the likelihood of each being correct. In 10 years we all will know for sure… maybe.

Allan Basbaum, PhD, Editor-in-Chief, *Pain*

Plus ça change, plus ça reste. In 2023, NSAIDs will remain the treatment of choice for pain associated with tissue injury and inflammation. Despite the generally unavoidable side effects of morphine and other opioids, I also predict that they will still be the drugs of choice to treat the most severe pain, particularly the most intractable pain (e.g. in cancer). For the near future, gabapentenoids will remain the first line approach for neuropathic pain, despite the accepted mantra that the efficacy is roughly 30% relief of pain in 30% of patients. However, given the focus of basic and clinical research on neuropathic pain, I expect that new entities will appear and replace gabapentenoids by 2023.

L. J. Saidman (✉)
Department of Anesthesia, Stanford University, Stanford, CA, USA
e-mail: lsaidman@stanford.edu

R. N. Westhorpe
Melbourne, Australia
e-mail: westhorpe@netspace.net.au

E. I Eger II
Department of Anesthesia and Perioperative Care,
University of California, San Francisco, CA, USA
e-mail: egere@anesthesia.ucsf.edu

Paralleling the continued use of NSAIDS, is the likely introduction of antibodies directed against nerve growth factor (NGF), which in clinical trials proved remarkably effective against osteoarthritis. I expect that before 2023, these antibodies, or some variation, will overcome the serious limitations that arose during their development, namely deleterious effects on non-target joints. I do not expect that these antibodies will be routinely used for pain induced by tissue injury, including post-operative pain, but they will be introduced and be effective for severe arthritic conditions—possibly even for back pain. Most importantly, studies of anti-NGF provided what I consider the most convincing evidence that animal models used to study clinical pain conditions are predictive of the clinical condition. Unfortunately, many large pharmaceutical companies doubted the utility of animal models and accordingly decreased their discovery efforts. That decision will slow the development of new entities, which of course will contribute to the continued use of existing analgesic therapies.

Crystal balls are hard to come by, so predictions must also be based on the many new targets that molecular and genetic analyses revealed in recent years. Unfortunately, despite the discovery of numerous molecules that predominate and, in some cases, reside exclusively in nociceptors, I am not optimistic about the development of effective antagonists against these highly localized channels/receptors. The problem is that blockade of a single entity will not effectively silence the nociceptor, which is required to produce generalized pain control. My skepticism is not because of lack of efficacy or selectivity of the antagonists, but rather because of the heterogeneity of the nociceptor channels that underlie the generation of pain. Thus, I believe that a more generalized blockade of "pain" transmission is required, which is precisely what occurs with existing agents, notably those acting at sodium or calcium channels. For the same reason, I expect that a drug targeting the NaV1.7 subtype of voltage gated sodium channels will be in use by 2023. Whether it will be targeted with a small molecule or a virus carrying an siRNA that knocks down NaV1.7 messages is not known, but development of a successful drug is likely.

Mario J. Da Conceicao, MD, MSc, PhD, Editor-in-Chief, *Brazilian Journal of Anesthesiology*

Anesthesiologists have increasingly moved beyond the operating room to a more diversified role in the perioperative care of surgical patients. They play central roles in delivering analgesia, and lead acute pain control teams; they deliver and provide guidelines for sedation services for diagnostic and therapeutic procedures outside the operating room, and at times outside the hospital as part of home care services. They have assumed roles in hospital administration and critical care services. These activities will expand in the next decade.

Molecular biology has increased our understanding of the mechanism of action of anesthetic drugs, particularly facilitating investigations of the role of receptor subunits in anesthetic end points. $GABA_A$, glycine, NMDA, and acetylcholine receptors are likely targets for various anesthetic prototypes. The creation of animals lacking particular receptor subunits ("knockouts") or possessing subunits that act normally except for their response to anesthetics ("knockins") will find increasing use in studies of anesthetic actions.

There may be advances in treatment of local anesthetic overdose with lipid or hypertonic saline solutions, but other than this we are unlikely to see many advances in anesthetic drugs or devices. Drug and device development requires enormous investments, with few new products reaching the market in a process that can take as long as 20 years—other markets are more attractive than the anesthesiology market.

Important in vitro pharmacological effects require confirmation in vivo. And important in vivo findings in animals must be confirmed in humans. One important question that requires an answer is: "Are anesthetics dangerous to developing brains?" They seem to be in rodents. Is in vitro apoptosis a danger in animals and more importantly in humans? This issue will be resolved in the next decade by epidemiological outcome studies. I predict that the findings will indicate minimal danger to humans.

Thousands of papers are now submitted to dozens of journals dedicated to anesthesia. I do not foresee a decrease.

Finally, unlike many South American countries, Brazil prohibits delivery of anesthesia by non-physicians. However, economic and supply issues preclude continuation of this practice. Reimbursement of anesthesiologists by insurance companies and salaries of public health care providers are under increasing pressure, decreasing the attractiveness of a career in anesthesia and thus the number of anesthesiologists. Consequently, non-physician-delivered anesthesia will arise in the next decade in Brazil. This will be a still greater problem in other South American countries, especially those lacking training programs.

James Eisenach, MD, PhD; Editor-in-Chief, *Anesthesiology*

My guess is that anesthesia research in 2023 will continue the existing model of a relatively small number of investigators, either singly or in small, local groups, examining highly focused physiologic/ pharmacologic questions. This model will incrementally increase our knowledge and care of patients, particularly with technology-focused research, such as implantable devices, portable imaging approaches to procedures, and targeted drug delivery. A dearth of commercial interest in developing better drugs for anesthesia might be countered by academic development, exemplified by recent work on etomidate derivatives. I predict that in 10 years we will only rarely apply genetic testing clinically, confining it to a few highly specific circumstances.

We will see the universal application of electronic medical records and the development of large clinical registries and databases. Whether these will revolutionize our practice is unclear but complications (unexpected difficult airway management, malignant hyperthermia, position related injury) from prior anesthetics and surgeries will be more easily and uniformly made known. We will have greater confidence in the prevalence and antecedents of both common and rare clinical problems, and the findings from these approaches will generate more hypotheses than they will test. Disparities across hospitals and practice systems will trigger interventions, oftentimes with arguably weak scientific evidence.

On a positive note, I am encouraged by the number of anesthesiologists around the globe who partner with others in and outside the specialty to organize large, multi-center observational and interventional clinical trials. We arrived to this approach late compared with our medical colleagues. Major problems in perioperative morbidity and mortality, problems arising nearly exclusively outside the operating room, can best be approached using methods that collect information on large populations, and we will increasingly apply such methods.

In summary, we have a modest chance of advancing technology and, perhaps, pharmacology in anesthesiology over the next 10 years. By 2023 we will have recognized that perioperative and acute critical care periods remain dangerous. We will replace an emphasis on the cult of safety regarding rare morbid events from anesthesia delivery in the operating room, with a focus on more frequent major perioperative problems. We will be guided by results from multi-center, large clinical trials that use electronic, registry, and database findings in a responsible and scientific manner to address problems like perioperative myocardial infarction, stroke, and renal impairment, as well as postoperative cognitive dysfunction and chronic pain.

Neville M. Gibbs, MBBS, MD, FANZCA, Chief Editor, *Anaesthesia and Intensive Care*

In 10 years, anaesthesiologists will scan their patient's identification number and procedure code into their hand held computer or phone, and obtain a list of anaesthesia risks specific to the patient. Risks considered will include the likelihood of anaphylaxis, awareness, post-operative cognitive dysfunction, tumour recurrence, thrombosis (and other cardiovascular events), pain, and postoperative nausea and vomiting. Links to evidence-based data will support each item. Advice on risks and their management will consider the patient's physiological, biochemical, pharmacological and pathological data, including genomic information, all accessed wirelessly from linked databases. These data will inform the options, also delivered wirelessly, for optimal anaesthetic management, including the best options for prevention of untoward effects. Other links will offer instruction on specific aspects of anaesthesia care, including vascular access, airway maintenance, and regional blocks. A phone-based video camera may be used to obtain advice from a colleague or supervisor at a different site, and to record procedures into the medical record. Algorithms that consider intraoperative data will automatically collect such data, apply trend analysis, take into account pre-operative patient data, and will supply early warning of potential complications.

Anaesthesiologists will routinely use their ultrasound imaging equipment and skills to guide vascular access, perform nerve blocks, assess the patient's airway, and confirm airway device position. Transthoracic echocardiography using portable or hand held devices will be used routinely for real-time simple and complex hemodynamic assessments.

The role of the anaesthesiologist will not change significantly, but the procedures requiring anaesthesia services will continue the current trend to less invasive procedures performed more often outside the traditional operating room. Subspecialisation will become essential to ensure adequate training and maintenance of skills, and to meet expectations in relation to accreditation, expertise, and safety. This will prompt the development of novel methods for competency assurance and assessment, with greater emphasis on both simulation and multi-rater feedback.

Anaesthetic research will emphasize risk stratification, pre-operative optimisation and postoperative care. Research into risk stratification will include the identification of biomarkers or genotypic predictors of adverse outcomes (e.g. postoperative cognitive dysfunction, major cardiovascular

events) to better inform patients, and to prompt consideration of lower risk alternatives where necessary. There will be a focus on decreasing human error to improve safety rather than on a search for safer agents. Pharmacological research will develop shorter acting drugs, drugs offering novel reversal mechanisms (e.g. cyclodextrins), and drugs that minimise adverse responses to tissue injury (e.g. inactivation of mediators by monoclonal antibodies).

Accessibility to safe anaesthesia will increase in less developed countries and remote areas through: collaborative education programmes that increase the skills and numbers of physicians and non-physicians providing anaesthesia in these areas, sponsorship of essential monitors and equipment (e.g. pulse oximetry, and purpose built simple/inexpensive/portable anaesthesia machines) and greater use of telemedicine for teaching and advice regarding individual patients.

Overall, changes will be related more to rapid advances in technology and better application of knowledge than to paradigm shifts in basic science concepts…but paradigm shifts are inherently unpredictable.

Ghassan E. Kanazi, MD, Editor-in-Chief, *Middle East Journal of Anesthesiology*

In the next decade, anesthesiologists will assume greater roles in the preoperative evaluation and perioperative management of surgical patients. Preoperatively, they will work to improve the ability of patients to withstand the impact of surgery and improve surgical outcome, often doing so without the aid of consultants—the anesthesiologist becoming the "medical" consultant. Technological advances will allow anesthesiologists to monitor intraoperative care from a distance. Nurse anesthetists who will provide bedside monitoring and immediate intervention will replace anesthesiologists in the operating room. Postoperatively, anesthesiologists will be charged with the responsibility for pain management. Improvements in anesthetic-surgical outcomes will be accomplished by application of outcomes-based research led by anesthesiologists.

There will be quantum leaps in monitoring. Blue tooth technology will supplant hard wiring and tangled monitoring wires. Non-invasive monitoring will largely replace the need for percutaneous catheters for arterial and central venous blood pressure measurements. Non-invasive monitors will also routinely provide measurement of tissue perfusion, and oxygen delivery and extraction during anesthesia.

Closed loop systems that monitor and titrate anesthetic and adjuvant drug delivery (as anesthetic depth and hemodynamic requirements prescribe) will displace human control. Such increased automation will ultimately (perhaps in 2 decades rather than 1) eliminate the need for the presence of either an anesthesiologist or nurse in the operating room.

The anesthesiologist will provide supervision and intervene to manage critical incidents.

Debate will continue concerning the use of inhalational versus intravenous agents as the mainstay for maintenance of anesthesia. Need will prompt the development of safer and better inhalational agents (e.g., one that does not produce postoperative agitation or laryngospasm on induction of anesthesia) and/or intravenous agents. I think that both will continue to be used. Evaluating depth of anesthesia will be seen to potentially influence morbidity and mortality. Accordingly we will develop monitors that will enable titration of anesthetics to minimize overdose, improve emergence and decrease cost, as noted above, using such monitors in closed loop systems.

The role of anesthesiologists will continue to expand outside the Operating Room especially for moderate and deep sedation for office-based procedures, endoscopies, magnetic resonance imaging procedures and more. There may be an expansion in the role of hypnosis as a technique that anesthesiologists will use as a less expensive and safer alternative to pharmacological sedation.

Anesthesiologists will increasingly resume the postoperative care of critically ill patients and will have a large role in Critical Care Medicine. The anesthesiologist is the most suitable person for the application of pharmacological advancements for the treatment of chronic pain and palliative care and will continue to be involved in Pain Medicine and palliative care.

Ailun Luo, MD, Editor-in-Chief, *Chinese Journal of Anesthesiology* (with Professors Qinchen Jin, Jing Zhao, and Zhonghuang Xu)

In 2011, the Chinese Society of Anesthesiology promulgated 5 goals: 1) assure patient safety; 2) develop "healthcare with comfort"; 3) improve hospital efficiency; 4) coordinate relationships among different departments; and 5) achieve community awareness of the importance of anesthesiology. Directly and indirectly, these goals will dictate developments in the next decade.

In the twentieth century, large differences between rural and urban economies produced an uneven distribution of medical development, and in much of China, anesthesia did not catch up with the rest of the world until the twenty-first century. Although acupuncture and traditional Chinese medicine are still applied in China, most anesthetic theories, techniques and drugs are now the same as those found in western countries. Remaining differences are predicted to decrease.

In ten years, Chinese anesthesiologists will increasingly act as perioperative physicians with active roles in ICU and pain management. In addition to caring for patients undergoing surgery, they will support more patients outside of the operating room undergoing cardiac catheterization, endoscopy, interventional radiology, and arrhythmia surgery. Improvement in the Chinese economy, and an accompanying increase in the number of anesthesiologists will promote healthcare with comfort (e.g., painless upper endoscopy under general anesthesia.)

Over the past 30 years, an imposed family planning has decreased the birth rate and increased the percentage of patients older than 60 from 10.3 % in 2000 to 13.3 % in 2010 with further increases predicted. In ten years surgical (e.g., transplantation) and anesthetic (e.g., ultrasound guidance for nerve blocks and TEE) techniques widely available in the West will be commonly adopted in China. Similarly, newer anesthetic techniques (e.g., general anesthesia combined with regional anesthesia, the latter also used for postoperative pain control), short-acting drugs producing rapid onset and relative hemodynamic stability (e.g., sufentanil and rocuronium), and other drugs recently introduced in the West (e.g., levobupivacaine, parecoxib sodium, and new analgesics) will become widely available.

In ten years, we will widely use fiberoptic and similar techniques in airway management. Reliable noninvasive or minor invasive techniques will increasingly replace invasive techniques. Anesthesia will increasingly adopt TIVA, prompting improved monitoring of anesthesia depth, leading to closed-loop (auto-control) delivery of anesthesia.

Presently, anesthesiologists in major cities such as Beijing and Shanghai provide modern anesthetic delivery, but differences in delivery in other regions can be huge. Establishment of standard requirements for anesthesia monitoring will minimize regional differences and will lead to the use of automatic anesthesia data input systems and related databases.

China's huge population and increasing amounts of surgery have caused shortages of allogenic blood despite increasing donation of blood. Within ten years indications for transfusion will be stricter, component transfusion will be broadly applied, and new plasma substitutes will be developed and used. Prevention of blood-borne transmitted diseases will receive extensive attention because of an increasing incidence of hepatitis C and AIDS.

In summary, China's current level of medicine, including anesthesiology, has unevenly approached that in advanced countries. The remaining differences are expected to narrow or disappear in ten years.

Donald R Miller, MD, FRCPC, Editor-in-Chief, Canadian Journal of Anesthesia

Globalization notwithstanding, in 2023, large inter-country and inter-continental variations will persist within anesthesiology. One example of variations that will continue is differences in the scope of practice of anesthesiologists as perioperative physicians. Increasing funding constraints and accountability within publicly funded systems will profoundly impact clinical practice. A 6–7% annual increase in health care expenditures in Canada, or elsewhere, cannot be sustained. An increasing burden of illness in aging, obese, or more medically compromised patients undergoing increasingly complex (and expensive) operations must be served. One result will be less taxpayer funding and increased privatization with proportionately more anesthesia services provided outside publicly funded hospitals. Although some will bemoan a loss in autonomy in elements of clinical decision-making, perioperative decisions will be governed by funding constraints, increasingly stringent guidelines and/or evidence-based clinical care maps supported by pharmacoeconomic data, optimization of human resources, and shortest possible hospital length of stay. Routine pharmacogenetic testing will support evidence-based guidelines for drug dosage, improving therapeutic efficacy and enhancing patient safety.

To enhance operating room efficiency, anesthesiologsts will increase their roles as operating room managers. Parallel processing will be increased to maximize OR efficiency. Examples include induction of anesthesia while surgical trays are being prepared, and use of centralized induction and block rooms to minimize case turnover time. Anesthesiologists will continue to deliver anesthesia services as a medical act, with increasing support by anesthesia assistants. Technological advances and cost constraints will prompt hospitals to become "critical care and emergency towers" offering short (ambulatory) stays for 85% of patients undergoing major elective and emergency cases requiring delivery of complex anesthesia care. Electronic anesthetic/medical records will become ubiquitous, having established their value for critical incident review and quality assurance. Technology and data processing advances will produce wireless, smart and compact monitoring systems and iPad-like devices and will provide online algorithms for patient management.

Team-based, interdisciplinary research will replace the individual researcher in most academic health science centres. Such research will produce new intravenous, and/or local anesthetics with higher therapeutic ratios (LD50/ED50) and fewer side effects than existing drugs provide. Results of studies of anesthetic mechanisms will facilitate development of drugs imposing minimal postoperative respiratory depression and postoperative neurocognitive dysfunction. New insights into neuronal network behaviour will result in an improved monitor of anesthetic depth.

Despite the many challenges, the future of the specialty is bright, albeit qualitatively and quantitatively changed. By 2023, anesthesiology will emerge from relative undersupply. High ranking medical students who routinely extend their training through fellowships, and postgraduate degrees in education and clinical epidemiology will continue to apply to this competitive specialty. The scope of clinical practice will continue to expand beyond the operating room and intensive care unit, for example, by provision of home care services for chronic pain, regional blocks and infusion therapy. Medical simulation will be integrated into anesthesia education, certification and re-certification. By 2023, hard copy publications of anesthesia journals and textbooks will have disappeared, and participants at scientific congresses will view presentations in the comfort of their home or office.

Joseph M. Neal, MD, Editor-in-Chief, *Regional Anesthesia and Pain Medicine* (with James P. Rathmell, Associate Editor-in-Chief for Pain Medicine)

Although anesthesiologists and pain medicine specialists both treat pain and use regional anesthetic techniques, within a decade anesthesiologists will assume sole responsibility for managing acute postoperative pain, while pain medicine specialists will focus on the care of patients with chronic and cancer pain. Rather than continuing as a subspecialty of parent disciplines (including anesthesiology, physical medicine, neurology, psychiatry), pain medicine will become an independent specialty in the US, as it has in many parts of the world.

Indications for thoracic epidural analgesia will decrease as advances in minimally-invasive surgery, multimodal analgesia, and receptor-specific opioid antagonists negate its traditional benefits, and potent irreversible anticoagulants limit its applicability. Peripheral regional techniques will replace neuraxial approaches, and development of sustained release, sensory neuron-specific local analgesics, will allow single-injection to replace continuous techniques. The "ultrasound revolution" will evolve to 3-dimensional ultrasonography with exquisite image resolution. Both anesthesiologists and pain medicine specialists will use new imaging modalities such as light impedance to accurately identify vascular and neural structures, and both will use new radiologic guidance-systems.

Minimally invasive methods will be developed to treat many painful disorders now requiring open operative intervention. The first to appear will be those to treat chronic spinal pain. Targeted biologic therapies will attain common usage, including monoclonal antibodies directed against specific inflammatory mediators that sustain pain, and specific growth factors and ion-channel inhibitors that directly influence the establishment and maintenance of neuronal plasticity that leads to persistent pain. These treatments will require precisely placed drug or devices accurately deployed percutaneously to get therapeutic agents to their site of action in high concentrations. Several future biologics (e.g., monocloncal antibodies against tumor necrosis factor alpha) will work poorly when given systemically, but will be effective when placed next to their target (e.g., a nerve root inflamed from disc herniation). Similarly, accurate device deployment will increase the likelihood of effective therapy. The roots of pain medicine specialists in anesthesiology and their expertise in image-guided intervention place them ideally to lead the application of these minimally invasive techniques.

Intense pressure to control increasing healthcare costs will profoundly impact both regional anesthesia and pain medicine. We will use approaches that decrease hospitalization and accelerate recovery. A present case in point: we combine numerous modalities (we decrease the amount of local anesthetic; add a long-acting opioid; arrange for early involvement of physical therapy, and ensure assistance at home on day two) to decrease recovery time after total joint arthroplasty from 4 days to 2 days. In 2023, the disciplines of regional anesthesia and pain medicine will supply more effective care at a lower cost.

Benoît Plaud, MD, PhD, Editor-in-Chief, *Annales Françaises d'Anesthésie et de Réanimation*

Imagination… is the preview of life's coming attractions— Albert Einstein

When I began my anesthesia residency in the 1980s, my mentors suggested that the greatest challenge confronting the specialty was to decrease anesthesia-related mortality and severe morbidity, particularly permanent brain damage. They succeeded in this enterprise in France, and so did anesthesiologists worldwide. With an associated mortality of approximately 1:200,000, anesthesia is one of medicine's safer endeavors. To further improve upon this by 2023 will require control of human factors by methods similar to those applied in commercial aviation. Because of its direct influence on outcome, the anesthesia team rather than a new drug or new device will be of primary importance. By 2023, we will have improved perioperative health status and life expectancy simply by applying protocols defined by evidence-based safety rules. Further, we will have decreased surgical mortality by increasing cooperation between treating physicians, using multifaceted medical team training, simulation, ongoing coaching, and checklists to trigger operating room briefings and debriefings.

As with the rest of the population, aging of the medical population will decrease the numbers of physician and nurse anesthetists who in turn will care for a greater number of older patients requiring more complex care. Cost controls will be accomplished by anesthesiologists who will delegate care of less difficult cases to yet better trained non-physicians under the supervision of anesthesiologists. With a proper evolution of the roles of anesthesiologists and nurse anesthetists, this will not decrease the attractiveness of our specialty.

Anesthesiologists have contributed to the safety of the perioperative process through better pre-operative evaluation, and better delivery of anesthesia and postoperative care. We will not have new anesthetic drugs or adjuvants in 2023. The key to improving outcome will be to apply evidence-based guidelines to current drugs and monitoring.

Although research is the cornerstone of the specialty, research in anesthesia will decrease because of governmental fiscal constraints However, by 2023 we will have an understanding of the genetic basis for inter-patient variability that will provide improved outcomes… via tailoring individual medical strategies… to specific patient genotypes. These strategies will apply to the entire anesthesia process, including preoperative evaluation, anesthetic management, and postoperative care.

Lars Rasmussen, MD, PhD, Editor-in-Chief, *Acta Anaesthesiologica Scandinavica*

Anesthesia will adapt to surgical advances and changing patient characteristics. By 2023, a greater proportion of procedures will be performed endoscopically, percutaneously, or via small surgical incisions. These less invasive techniques may be implemented in combination with robotic surgery, leading to less tissue trauma, less fluid shifts, and minimal blood loss. The result will decrease the need for fluid administration, postoperative opioids, and extensive monitoring. Infiltration anesthesia and light sedation will suffice for many procedures, reducing the need for general anesthesia.

In 10 years, patients having elective surgery will rarely stay in hospital overnight afterwards. Non-opioid analgesia will suffice for many patients, reducing opioid related postoperative complications. Preoperative identification of high pain responders will be identified by genetic profiling. They will be offered regional anesthesia for pain relief.

Titration of anesthetic drugs will be facilitated by improved monitoring of brain function, by rapid spontaneous degradation of injected drugs, by specific reversal agents, or by the rapid pulmonary elimination of poorly soluble inhaled anesthetics.

The proportion of elderly surgical patients will increase, and they will actively contribute to decisions about their anesthesia management. Because of their greater knowledge of medical care and of their own health status and medications, they will expect to choose the type of anesthesia such as general versus regional technique, and elements of their postoperative care. Fewer older patients will retire from work, and most will expect to resume usual activities—including a return to work—soon after surgery. The decreased impact of surgery and anesthesia on their general physical status, and a shortened recovery period, will facilitate the fulfilling of this expectation. This will demand that anesthetists adopt regimens that allow early mobilization and discharge. Invasive anesthetic techniques, such as neuraxial blocks and peripheral nerve blocks that produce motor block and urinary retention, will be disadvantageous in this respect.

The mismatch between demand for anesthesia services and provider capacity will necessitate more widespread implementation of nurse anesthetists or anesthetic assistants. This will enable anesthesiologists to focus on the challenging cases but it will also require good communication skills and team management capability.

Charles Reilly, MB ChB (Glasgow), MD (Glasgow), FRCA, Editor-in-Chief, *British Journal of Anaesthesia*

Projecting what may change in anaesthesia by 2023 might begin with a reflection on the changes I have seen in my years as an anaesthetist, appreciating that this carries the temptation to think that the big developments have already happened. Maybe they have. By the 1980s we had in practice nearly all the agents we use currently, and in the 1980s and 1990s we added major developments in monitoring. Current trainees find it hard to believe that in 1990, automated non-invasive blood pressure measurement was not customary, pulse oximetry was a new experimental monitor, and transesophageal echocardiography was far from routine.

I do not foresee further developments in general anaesthesia drugs. However, an increased understanding of the cellular and molecular mechanisms of pain and of the inflammatory process will lead to the invention and introduction of specifically targeted analgesic agents and agents for the treatment of sepsis.

By 2023, we will devise a reliable, universally accepted monitor of depth of anaesthesia. While the manufacturers of the BIS and entropy instruments should be applauded for their efforts, their devices have considerable limitations, are unevenly accepted and used, and compare poorly with the example of pulse oximetry which in a few years went from development to acceptance as a minimum standard. Results with new depth monitors will provide real-time values that closely correlate with gold-standard measures of anaesthetic depth. They will find particular application when end-tidal analysis cannot be used to certify adequacy of anaesthesia.

At present, we might predict that the perioperative complication rate and mortality for a *group* of patients undergoing surgical procedure X is Y% and Z%. In 2023, preoperative assessment of the cardiovascular and respiratory systems will enable the anaesthetist to say with accuracy that this *individual* patient has a 1 in A risk of specific complication B. This process follows closely from our current interests in preoperative optimisation, fast-tracking and multimodal analgesia. In 10 years' time we will increasingly play

the role of a perioperative physician who co-ordinates the preoperative preparation, intra-operative care and postoperative management for each patient.

Making predictions is a risky business, with a greater chance of getting it wrong than appearing prescient. Perhaps the most certainly correct prediction is that the now large gap between anaesthesia provision in developed and underdeveloped countries will widen. This will include differences in availability of trained personnel, choice of drugs, and type of equipment. I hope that the anaesthetic community will respond to these disparities with the ingenuity and intelligence that it has shown in meeting challenges in preceding decades.

Professor Dr. Rolf Rossaint and Professor Dr. Bernhard Zwißler, Co-Editors-in-Chief, *Der Anaesthesist*

By 2023, the present focus of German anesthesiologists on anesthesia, intensive care, out-of-hospital physician based emergency systems, and pain management will be expanded. For example, anesthesiologists will increasingly assume responsibility for all surgical intensive care patients. Moreover, the anesthesiologist will direct the immediate perioperative phase of patient treatment. Increasingly, anesthesiologists will manage Emergency Departments and/or Departments of Palliative Medicine.

Although nearly 900 physicians complete anesthesiology training every year, the additional clinical activities indicated above will lead to a shortage, in part because German law dictates that physicians must provide anesthesia (nurse anesthetists may support but not replace anesthesiologists). The shortage may even be great enough to threaten the existence of some hospitals. Compounding the problem, 70 % of medical students are females who will demand and receive new working time options. To overcome this shortage, as is the case today, university anesthesiology departments will continue to aim to be ranked by medical students as the best teaching departments, in part by a continuing investment in and the use of simulators in teaching.

Due to stricter legal requirements and related insurance costs governing clinical studies, anesthesia research in 2023 will emphasize basic investigations, using modern molecular biology techniques in animals or in vitro, often involving topics at boundaries with other disciplines. National or international research foundations will fund this basic research. The resulting papers will be of higher quality than today's papers, and will follow the requirements of specific writing guidelines such as those found in CONSORT (Consolidated Standards of Reporting Trials) and PRISMA (Preferred Reporting Items for Systematic Reviews). In 2023 there will be fewer innovations in devices or drugs, and those that are developed will be evaluated in hospitals with good infrastructures for performing clinical studies, and will be financed by industry. In 2023, clinical researchers will supplement the fewer, well performed Research Clinical Trials with observational studies and studies using comparative effectiveness research methods. Comparative effectiveness research will allow for a holistic view (i.e., more than just anesthesia) of our patients to reduce morbidity and mortality. Examples are management of anemia with preoperative intravenously administered iron, and improvement of long-term cancer outcome using particular anesthesia techniques.

By 2023, improvement in patient outcomes will result by adopting clinical pathways developed from guidelines that avoid/reduce medical errors. Avoidance of medical errors will require use of computerized checklists reflecting the most important items of the guidelines. Finally, by 2023, there will be centers for telemedicine where specialized physicians (including anesthesiologists) will care for patients with out-of-hospital emergencies or emergencies in smaller ICUs, or will support anesthesiologists in the operating room.

Steve Shafer, MD, Editor-in-Chief, *Anesthesia & Analgesia*

Anesthesia in 2023 in the US will look like anesthesia today. Four factors weigh against the introduction of new drugs and drug delivery systems: small market size, high cost of development, lack of regulatory enthusiasm, and complacency within the anesthesia community because of the high quality of drugs and devices currently available. We will provide general anesthesia with propofol, sevoflurane, fentanyl, succinylcholine, rocuronium, vecuronium, and nitrous oxide, with minor amounts of ketamine, desflurane, remifentanil, dexmedetomidine, and cisatracurium. However, some "standard" generic injectable drugs will vanish due to the small market and high regulatory burden for such drugs. These factors will also make drug shortages more common. Our European colleagues will continue their transition towards intravenous anesthesia because of the availability of target controlled drug delivery, a technology unavailable in the United States.

We will see minor improvements in monitors of ventilation and oxygenation. Oximetry-based monitoring of total hemoglobin, carboxyhemoglobin, and methemoglobin will become routine, as will plethysmographic monitoring of intravascular volume. Brain function monitoring will not improve, a consequence of our inexplicable opposition to EEG monitoring. Nearly every operating room will be equipped with ultrasound monitors. These will be routinely used for placing peripheral and central venous, arterial, and spinal and epidural catheters. Small, inexpensive TEE devices may become common.

Our practice will be less fun. In years past I challenged residents to induce anesthesia with the smallest possible volume containing intravenous agents. The winner was a 1 ml "dart" holding 0.5 mls (50 mg) of ketamine plus 0.5 mls (25 µg) of sufentanil which was used to draw up 10 mg of vecuronium. I taught residents how to induce anesthesia with isoflurane via mask, and how to titrate ketamine and methadone. Future administrators will be less tolerant of "let's try this today". Our employers, our payers, and our patients will expect practice uniformity.

Our research will focus on outcomes driven by public demand for the best healthcare for the least money. Preoperative screening and triage will improve. Less expensive anesthesia providers will care for low risk patients, allowing anesthesiologists to focus on high-risk patients.

Our practice will become increasingly transparent. Anesthesia information management systems and video recorders will capture every drug, dose, and clinical decision. Algorithms will assess our care in real time. Although our vigilance may lapse, the supervisory software in our information management systems will not—and will alert us to deviations in vital signs or clinical practice that presage a problem. Algorithms will identify areas where our skills need to improve.

Information management systems will document our compliance with "best practices", which will be reviewed by our employers and payers. Practice incentives will be structured to compel us to provide anesthesia in a manner that enforces best practices. We will chafe at the lack of autonomy, but ensuring conformity with standards of care will likely enhance care.

Koh Shingu, MD, Editor-in-Chief, *Journal of Anesthesia*

In the next decade, Japan must confront physician shortages in anesthesia, emergency medicine, pediatrics, and obstetrics, and must face problems of mal-distribution, especially in provincial areas. The revised resident training system initiated in 2004 may compound the problem. Previously, most residents trained in hospitals associated with the universities from which they graduated. In 2003, these represented 72.5 % of new residents. In the new matching system, residents may choose any hospital certified by the government for training for 2 years. In 2010, the percent of new residents trained in the university hospitals from which they graduated decreased to 47.2 %. They now tend to select residencies in larger cities and in departments imposing less burdensome schedules.

The Japanese government has increased the capacity of medical university faculties to train the greater number of physicians needed to care for an increasingly aged population. The intake of medical students increased from 7,625 in 2006 to 8,923 in 2011. In 2021, this will raise the number of physicians per 100,000 patients to 260—from 215 today. But will this 21 % increase keep pace with demand? I think not. In 2011, 7,000 anesthesiologists will administer about 2,000,000 general anesthetics in Japan. Over the next decade, an aging population will require an increased number of procedures. An increased need for critical care facilities and pain clinics will further raise the need for anesthesiologists. Combined with a low birth rate (i.e., a decreasing support base) an increased financial burden will be imposed upon Japanese society (peaking in 2035), further limiting the ability to pay for more anesthesiologists. Ironically, the resulting increasing burden on anesthesiologists will hinder recruitment of new trainees.

I predict that a financially feasible solution to meeting this impending shortage of anesthesiologists will require introducing nurse anesthetists having competencies similar to those in other countries. The Japanese Society of Anesthesiologists proposes "perioperative nurses" directed by anesthesiologists. These perioperative nurses will enable anesthesiologists to make greater use of their abilities in anesthesia, including research, training, and education, over the coming decade.

Martin R. Tramèr, MD, DPhil, Editor-in-Chief, *European Journal of Anaesthesiology*

Three major changes will affect the anesthetic world in the forthcoming decade: a change in patient demographics, a change in surgical techniques, and an increase in out-of-theatre care. These changes will significantly increase workload.

Anesthesiologists will adapt to increasing numbers of older and sicker patients. Such polymorbid high-risk patients taking a multitude of drugs will need care during the entire perioperative period, starting with preoperative risk assessment allowing for rational preparation and triage. Intraoperative care and postoperative rehabilitation will focus on prevention and therapy of the main complications of surgery and anesthesia such as infection, postoperative cognitive dysfunction, and pain including acute and chronic postsurgical neuropathic pain. To reduce perioperative mortality, anesthesiologists will focus on postoperative care. Intermediate care units will be mandatory to achieve that goal.

Surgery will move towards minimal invasive approaches combining multidisciplinary interventions, and the use of high-tech aids, like robots. Thus, surgical interventions will become still more complex and lengthy. Surgeons will increasingly perform surgery from outside the operating theatre, connected wirelessly to a patient. As a consequence, anesthesiologists will work in huge, dark, hybrid theatres, caring for increasingly older and sicker patients requiring increasingly prolonged anesthesia. Communication with surgeons will become more difficult as they increasingly perform surgery without entering the operating theatre. Anesthesiologists will become theatre managers, key players in controlling this most expensive environment in healthcare. They will facilitate communication between surgeons, will organize smooth transitions between operations, and will ensure perioperative safety.

Anesthesia workload for non-surgical tasks outside the theatre will continue to increase, with obstetricians, radiologists, cardiologists, gastroenterologists and chest physicians as regular customers of anesthesiologists. Patients will expect comfort, safety, and professional care during labor, cerebral aneurysm coiling, colonoscopic polyp resection, catheter-based renal sympathetic denervation for resistant hypertension, and implantation of lung volume reduction coils for the treatment of severe emphysema. The anesthesiologist's main dilemma will be to match an ever-increasing workload with limited human resources. Workload will increase about 30 % during the next 10 years. Not all anesthesiology departments will be able to respond to all exigencies. Intraoperative care of low-risk surgical patients will often be delegated to nurse anesthetists who work under the supervision of anesthesiologists. Non-anesthesiologists will perform out of theatre sedation. Countries that have practiced anesthesia with doctor-nurse anesthesia teams will be better prepared to face this challenge. To ensure safety, anesthesiologists will define standards of care and will teach and supervise non-anesthesiologists and nurse anesthetists.

I believe that pharmacogenetic research and high-tech monitoring will not significantly affect our working environment in the next 10 years—perhaps in 20 years or more, but not in 10. The main challenges by the end of the next decade will be logistic in nature; the anesthesiologist team will have to cope with a changing, challenging working environment and an increasing workload.

Steve M. Yentis, BSc, MBBS, FRCA, MD, MA, Editor-in-Chief, *Anaesthesia*

Bah humbug

Many changes I foresee in the UK over the next decade relate to organisational factors, particularly how services are delivered. As I write, a severe financial 'squeeze' grips much of the world, and the British Government is currently on a mission of cost-curtailment, from which healthcare and science are anything but immune. Concurrently, the National Health Service (NHS) is embarking on a major and controversial reconfiguration, accompanied by decreased public sector pensions and pay, and increased retirement age. Such gloomy realities influence my predictions.

Service delivery

Over the last decade or two, hospital care in the NHS has moved from a largely consultant-led but trainee-delivered service, to a consultant-delivered service (conflicting with the need to control costs). Anaesthetists have been among those leading this trend. However, continued expansion in consultant numbers is not considered sustainable. Accordingly, a major shortfall in hospital consultant positions will occur within the next decade—one possible outcome being a sub-consultant grade or its semantic equivalent, with (lower) salary to match. Anaesthetists may be especially vulnerable because everyone who isn't an anaesthetist sometimes still views them as technicians not requiring consultant (let alone medical) status. Unlike some countries, the UK has no tradition of anaesthesia provision by non-medical personnel, and the Physicians' Assistants programme, developed over the last decade to solve the predicted shortage of specialists, is unlikely to be sustained. Instead, the merging of NHS services is becoming the preferred option (despite the accompanying and politically unpalatable closure of departments or even hospitals that this brings).

Training

The traditional UK model of apprenticeship, by which consultants closely supervise junior trainees who assume increasing responsibility as they acquire and develop appropriate skills and attitudes, is likely to continue, as is the recent trend towards earlier subspecialisation. Whilst the latter may be cheaper and therefore more 'efficient', it also produces practitioners with a narrower range of experiences (and perhaps capabilities). Restrictions on working hours imposed by the European Working Time Directive exacerbate this trend: trainees do less (which may not be a bad thing) but can do less (which probably is).

Research

The most obvious current trend is a reduction in time, resources, and enthusiasm to pursue the clinically-orientated research that has fuelled our specialty's development. An increasing emphasis on fewer, larger, 'proper' (and very expensive) randomised trials compounds this limitation. Many feel this is short-sighted. Support for the development of new anaesthetic drugs, machines, and devices will continue but will be limited and will be more targeted than in the past (probably an improvement). Fewer UK studies are likely to fill our journals.

The Only Way is Up

I was attracted to anaesthesia because anaesthetists seemed more capable and nicer people than those in other specialties. I see no evidence that this is changing, and am encouraged by the continuous inflow of enthusiastic, clever, conscientious people into our specialty. *Dum spiro spero*.

A Synthesis of Opinions from Editors of Sixteen Anesthesia Jounals

Table 14.1 summarizes the points made by 4 or more of the editors-in-chief. The number of editors who made a comment is given in the second column and the percent of those agreeing with the stated item appears in the third column. Thus, four editors thought that research funding for anesthesia would decrease over the next decade. Twelve editors weighed in on whether new drugs will be made for use by anesthetists, but only half of these thought they would be made, the other half suggesting that they would not or that at best but a few would be made. The following discussion supplies further detail.

New Drugs, Devices, and Safety

Fifty percent of editors discussing drug development predicted (item 3) a continuation of the 2000s when only one new drug (sugammadex) was introduced, pointing to the huge costs associated with new drug development, the relatively small market for anesthetic drugs, and of greatest importance, the proven efficacy and safety of currently available volatile agents, opioids, hypnotics, and neuromuscular blocking agents.

These medications are safe in trained hands. Future increases in safety will not be achieved by developing new drugs but by improving training, especially training of non-physicians, and by supplementing that training with devices that guide the less-trained individual. A case in point concerns a device (Sedasys System) available in Europe but not the US facilitating the safe administration of propofol for patients undergoing endoscopic and other out-of-operating room procedures. The Sedasys System links a propofol infusion to the pulse oximeter, capnograph, and blood pressure signals, and patient responsiveness.

Some editors would apply the information revolution to enhance safety. The ubiquitous ID band worn by hospital patients will more than just identify the 2023 patient. When scanned, the band will reveal drug allergies and the patient's prior incidence of postoperative cognitive dysfunction, nausea and emesis, deep venous thrombosis, and difficult airway. It will provide risk stratification and suggestions including optimal anesthetic management for each problem.

Table 14.1 Editors' Predictions of Changes over the Next Decade[1]

Item	Number with a Comment	Percent Agreeing
1. Research funding will decrease	4	100%
2. Clinical research will focus on outcome trials	4	100%
3. New drugs will be made	12	50%
4. New devices will be made (esp brain function)	9	56%
5. Molecular biology will be used in research	5	100%
6. The perioperative role of the anesthesiologist will increase	7	100%
7. Particularly in pain management	6	100%
8. A shortage of anesthesiologists will exist	8	88%
9. More non-anesthesiologists will deliver anesthesia	7	86%
10. Genetic testing will be used preoperatively	6	67%
11. Non-invasive monitoring will increase	5	100%
12. Checklists will guide clinical care	4	100%
13. Anesthetists will use electronic records	4	100%
14. Differences among countries in the quality of anesthesia will decrease	4	50%

[1] Putting the editors' comments in particular categories sometimes required interpreting what they meant. Thus, the results in Table 14.1 probably should be considered but semi-quantitative. And, of course, the table ignores imaginative comments made by several editors because we only summarized those comments where four (25%) or more editors had addressed a particular issue.

Anesthesia Personnel, Scope of Practice, and the Cost of Care

The editors predict an increased use of less trained individuals (i.e. more non-physicians; item 9) in locations and patients requiring a lower intensity of care. Three factors underlay this prediction: First, the increasing cost of medical care associated with new technology. Second, a demand for greater care by a vulnerable subset of patients such as those found in an aging population having greater co-morbidities. And third, an increasing number of patients in developed as well as less developed countries requiring care. The use of non-physicians to care for less vulnerable patients will allow physicians trained in perioperative medicine to care for those requiring a higher intensity of care such as patients in critical care units, emergency rooms, and pain management centers. Thus, even in countries presently providing anesthesia services using only physicians, acceptance of non-physicians as supervised assistants is predicted to accommodate the increasing need for diverse services such as care in endoscopy and radiology suites, infusion services, home care of patients with implanted regional block catheters, and preoperative assessment clinics.

The anesthesiologist will increasingly take on the role of perioperative care manager (item 6), especially where patients have many or complex co-morbidities.

Research

Some editors predicted fewer investigators pursuing highly focused laboratory based projects, and more globally-united investigators pursuing both observational and interventional large-scale clinical trials (item 2). And rather than concentrating on decreasing the vanishingly small number of perioperative deaths, these studies will use comparative effectiveness methods to examine the impact of anesthesia and surgery on long-term outcomes including stroke, myocardial infarction, cognitive dysfunction in the elderly patient and small children, metabolic dysfunction, and cancer recurrence. A few editors predicted that we will look to biomarkers or genotypes to control outcome, cautioning, however, that genetic testing in 10 years will be applied in only a few highly specific circumstances (item 10).

Pain Management

Because of their limited efficacy in the treatment of neuropathic pain (efficacy of 30% in 30% of patients), gaba-pentenoids will be replaced by 2023 by a drug yet to be created. NSAIDS will remain the treatment of choice in the treatment of pain associated with tissue injury and inflammation, especially important because increased minimally invasive surgery (robotic and laparoscopic) should lessen the need for opioids. There will be fewer thoracic epidurals (because of concern regarding concomitant use of anti-coagulants) and greater use of multi-modal analgesic techniques. By 2023, targeted biologic therapies against specific inflammatory mediators that sustain pain including monoclonal antibodies directed against nerve growth factor (proven effective against osteoarthritis in clinical trials) will be available. "High pain" responders will be identified and offered regional anesthesia techniques permitting earlier mobilization and discharge. Finally, Pain Medicine as a primary specialty will assume management of patients with chronic painful conditions. Anesthesiologists will represent one of several specialties that compete in this arena. However, anesthesiologists will likely dominate in the arena of acute pain management as follows surgery (item 7).

International Outreach

The editors suggested that the international community would address the uneven availability of medical resources throughout the world. This is presently an intra- and inter-national issue depriving huge populations of even basic anesthesia and surgical care. For example, non-availability of obstetric anesthesia support for high risk pregnancies increases fetal and maternal mortality and morbidity (e.g., urogenital fistulae). And lack of cosmetic surgery for children born with disfiguring congenital abnormalities condemns this cohort to a life of abuse and exclusion. Programs and international organizations providing expert patient care and training of indigenous personnel will greatly increase by 2023. This may be accomplished by the use of non-physician anesthesia providers and telemedicine educational programs. While half of the editors raising this issue thought that such measures would decrease differences among countries in the quality of anesthesia (item 14) half had the opposite view.

Reprise: two views of the future

Given the diversity of their interests and locations, not surprisingly, our editors provide sometimes common, sometimes dissimilar views of the future (Table 14.1). Some opt for a pessimistic ("Bah, humbug") view of things to come. They foresee less support for research and clinical enterprises with a resulting decrease in the development of new information and new investigators essential to academia. They believe that fewer (if any) new drugs or devices will appear. Shortages of highly-trained professionals and increasing clinical demands (more surgeries in diverse places for sometimes prolonged procedures) will force reliance on less expensive anesthetists with more limited training to give clinical anesthesia to an older, sicker, fatter patient population. To sustain the safety that modern anesthesia has so carefully cultivated will mandate anesthesia dictated by mind-numbing checklists. Adding insult to injury, departments of anesthesia may be subsumed by larger enterprises, the name "anesthesia" sometimes disappearing and programs directed by someone with no immediate expertise in anesthesia. We will lose, or have now lost, control of areas of medicine we developed (e.g., intensive care medicine; management of chronic pain.) This has already occurred in some parts of the world.

Not so fast says the optimists. The anesthesiologist has and will evolve into the leader of Perioperative Medicine, the physician best equipped by history and training to manage the perioperative care of the surgical patient from admission through procedure (sometimes surgical, sometimes not) and postoperative care in the PACU or ICU and home again. We will continue to control the management of acute pain and with that advantage, compete with other specialties for the management of chronic pain. We already vie for control of intensive care medicine, particularly as it deals with surgical care. Our immediate relationship with our surgical colleagues stands us in good stead there. With superb drugs and devices already at hand, we need but a few new devices (e.g., a 3-D ultrasound device; a more precise depth monitor) and fewer drugs (perhaps ones that guarantee reversal of paralysis or ones that supply anesthesia with neither circulatory depression nor stimulation). Cutting edge bench research employing molecular biology will be applied in a limited number of institutions as has been the case in the past. We will increase safety, but not by adding to what already is a marvelous record for the immediate intra and postoperative period, one that admittedly must make use of those checklists. The gold for increasing safety lies in avoiding problems weeks, months or years after surgery. Thus, clinical research will increasingly shift to multicenter long-term outcomes research. No need to think doom and gloom. Although demanding, the future is bright.

Surgery Before and After the Discovery of Anesthesia

15

William Silen and Elizabeth A. M. Frost

Summary

Long before the advent of anesthesia, operations relied on a detailed knowledge of anatomy gained by dissection of the dead. Morton's demonstration of ether anesthesia on 16 Oct 1846 made planned surgery possible, that is surgery in a silent motionless patient. Thus began the era of the great surgeons of Europe (Billroth, Kocher, Torek) and the US (Sims, Halsted, Cushing). Supporting discoveries added to the advances: Lister used antisepsis with carbolic acid spray (1867); Macewen intubated the trachea (1870s); Roentgen discovered X-rays (1895); Landsteiner identified blood groups (1900) and Domagk synthesized sulfonamides (1932).

For a century, the anesthetic properties and simple methods of delivery of ether, chloroform and nitrous oxide sufficed for most surgical needs. By the 1950s however, surgical advances demanded manipulation of vital functions such as controlled ventilation and deliberate hypotension. Advances such as electrocautery and cardiopulmonary bypass machines required the safe nonflammable anesthetics developed in the 1950s and later. The 1950s and 1960s saw the initiation of immunosuppression making organ transplantation feasible. None of this reflected the myriad expansions of other kinds of operations—orthopedic, gynecologic, urologic, bariatric, orthodontic and more. The perturbations produced by surgery became enormous—and anesthesia had to contribute more. That's another story.

More recently, the demands of surgery changed in ways few had foreseen. Surgeons fearlessly tackled problems in unfit patients—obese, elderly, debilitated, and diseased. Surgeons in the 1980s practiced in new venues, ambulatory care centers or even in their offices, again demanding more of anesthesia—quicker awakening and fewer side effects. Some operations are not done by surgeons—radiologists now intervene in many vital organs, and cardiologists stent coronary arteries. Less invasive operations such as laparoscopic procedures (Muhe performed a laparoscopic cholecystectomy in 1991), and robotic surgery place sometimes less and sometimes just different, demands on anesthesia. Surgery is a brave new world.

Introduction

The reader may wonder at the inclusion of a history of surgery in a book detailing the history of anesthesia, thinking that the story of surgery runs parallel to but is separate from the story of anesthesia. Not so: Surgery existed long before the demonstration of anesthesia with most surgeons doing little to assuage the pain resulting from their work. But surgeons (including dentists) discovered general (Horace Wells and William Morton) and local (Carl Koller) anesthesia. They became the first anesthetists, quickly morphing into directors of anesthesia, usually both performing surgery and controlling the delivery of anesthesia. They developed various aspects of the safe delivery of anesthesia, including airway management, and they devised diverse approaches to regional anesthesia. They were the captains of the ship, the leaders of the operative enterprise. Anesthesia initially was a surgical subspecialty or "competence". Surgeons reluctantly relinquished their direction of anesthesia, only surrendering control more than a century after Morton's demonstration. As surgeons advanced their reach they demanded more of anesthesia, and the resulting advances in anesthesia facilitated the growth of surgery. So did the genius of anesthetists who independently made advances that supported surgery. The resulting complexity of anesthesia made it impossible for surgeon to be both surgeon and anesthetist. And yet, the two specialties always were joined at the hip, part of the same enterprise.

Mythology

Chiron the Centaur, born in Thessaly, celebrated for applying herbs to wounds, is presumed to have been the father of surgery. Aesculapius, the son of Apollo, thought by some

E. A. M. Frost (✉)
Department of Anesthesiology, Icahn Medical Center at Mount Sinai, New York, NY, USA
e-mail: elzfrost@aol.com

W. Silen
Department of Surgery, Harvard Medical School, Boston, MA, USA

E. I Eger II et al. (eds.), *The Wondrous Story of Anesthesia,* DOI 10.1007/978-1-4614-8441-7_15, © Edmond I Eger, MD 2014

to be Chiron's pupil, and by others his predecessor, may have outdone Chiron. Of course, perhaps neither existed. Apollo, himself the son of almighty Zeus, was the original Greek God of Physic and Healing, but he resigned in favor of his son, Apollo God of the Sun, whose temples became the repository for all medical and surgical knowledge. Even Celsus testified that Aesculapius was the most ancient authority in surgery. Homer's Iliad immortalized Podalirius and Machaon, the 2 sons of Aesculapius, as they followed Agamemnon to the Trojan wars and cared for the sick and wounded. Podalirius was reputed to be the first phlebotomist.

Ancient Civilizations

The first surgical operations probably took place in the Mesolithic period (10,000 BCE–5,000 BCE). Skulls with rounded, often multiple defects suggesting trephination have been excavated from graves in all countries of the world except China, Japan, the Malay Peninsula and Australia. Many intact skulls showed evidence of healing, without infection, indicating deliberate surgery [1].What prompted these interventions? Perhaps it was for epilepsy, headache, a passage into manhood or spiritual or religious reasons. Trephination persisted in primitive civilizations in some form until the early 20th century [2]. How was pain minimized for these operations? Coca leaves were widely used in Peru. Perhaps an early anesthetist was the assistant who chewed the leaves and spat in the wound, a technique used and described for centuries in South America—but the concentration of cocaine in such saliva may have been too small to be effective [3].

Despite its advanced culture and influence, little physical evidence indicates that Babylonians practiced surgery. However, the Code of Hammurabi, perhaps the first law book, defined physician practice, (not unlike what may happen today). Laws 215–223, set out rewards and punishments for surgeons. "If a physician make a large incision with an operating knife and cure it, or if he open a tumor (over the eye) with an operating knife, and saves the eye, he shall receive 10 shekels in money." This sum decreased to 5 shekels if the patient was the son of a plebian, to 2 shekels if the patient was a slave (fee to be paid by the owner). However, "if a physician make a large incision with the operating knife, and kill him, or open a tumor with the operating knife, and cut out the eye, his hands shall be cut off." If he killed a slave, then he had to replace him. Broken bones and soft tissue injury repair were to be compensated with 5 shekels [4].

The Edwin Smith papyrus is the earliest written record of surgical practice, and is an incomplete copy of an earlier treatise composed about 3,000 BCE. It describes 48 cases that may have been records from the Egyptian architect-

physician, Imhotep. Fifteen cases concerned head injury, 12 related to facial wounds and fractures, and 7 to vertebral injuries. The remaining 14 cases involved pathology of the thorax. The author described healing of wounds, and advised placing traumatized skin edges together, and using fresh meat for its hemostatic value as the usual dressing for the first day. It might be a stretch to say that this recommendation anticipated the tissue clotting factors discovered in modern times. The author recognized that the injury caused pain and that movement and examination exacerbated the pain. But the physician was advised to "palpate his wound although he shudders exceedingly…. cause him to lift his face; if it is painful for him to open his mouth, his heart beats feebly" (from case 7, a depressed skull fracture.) [5] The author was probably differentiating injuries that could and could not be treated. The feeble pulse and shuddering suggested a fatal wound, and the physician could not make it worse. As the patient with a fatal wound was most likely not responsive, then the response to palpation would help the clinician to decide whether or not the wound was treatable.

Several medical records survive from ancient Egypt (circa 2000–1600 BCE). The Ebers manuscript (University of Leipzig) describes medical recipes and incantations. It also identifies peripheral arterial aneurysms, recommending the following: "treat it with a knife and burn it with a fire so that it bleeds not too much."

Greeks, Romans and Jews

The Homeric poems, the Iliad and the Odyssey (800 to 700 BCE) [1] provide the first Greek allusions to surgical subjects. They presented realistic descriptions of battle wounds and attempts to treat them. Between 800 BCE and 700 BCE, "schools" of medicine and associations of philosophers, priest-physicians and practitioners arose throughout Greece. Hippocrates (circa 460–370 BCE) "the father of modern medicine," born on the Greek island of Cos, worked to disentangle medicine from religious mysticism. He rejected the prevailing thought that credited supernatural and divine forces as the cause of disease, claiming instead that environmental factors, diet and living habits caused illness. Stimulated by Hippocrates, several authors compiled some 72 works, the Corpus Hippocraticum. The Hippocratic School (actually two schools, the Knidian and Koan Schools) focused on patient care and prognosis rather than diagnosis. The Koan School believed that an imbalance of the 4 humors (blood, black bile, yellow bile and phlegm) caused illness. These teachings contrasted with those of the Knidian School, which sought diagnoses and specific treatments. Surgical sections from Hippocrates' writings [6] describe the treatment of hemorrhoids, fistulas, wounds, injuries of the head, and fractures, as well as prognosis of various wounds. For example,

"Only wine should be used to moisten the wound unless it is on a joint. Sparse food, and no drink but water, are important for all injuries—and more so with fresh wounds than old, with wounds that have somehow become or risk becoming inflamed, with joint injuries, or when cramps may occur but also with abdominal wounds and most of all, with injuries of the head or thigh bone or any other bone." [6]

Trephination was recommended for skull fractures, epilepsy, blindness and headache. The practitioner was advised to avoid suture lines and the temporal area for fear of arterial (? middle meningeal artery) damage, which might cause contralateral convulsions. Advice also directed that the inner table of the skull should be preserved to protect the dura.

Cornelius Celsus (25 BCE–CE 50) in his De Medicina described the characteristics of inflammation, including redness, swelling, heat and pain (rubor, tumor, calor and dolor) and the use of the ligature to control bleeding [1, 7]. He also wrote of the signs and symptoms of head injuries, noting that fractures of the base of the skull were usually fatal. He recommended incinerated egg yolk as a styptic powder for treatment of meningeal hemorrhage [7].

The famous Roman (but of Greek ethnicity) Galen (CE 129–199) is generally regarded as second only to Hippocrates as a physician [1], and he repeated much of the latter's teachings. He was an accomplished technical surgeon who served for many years as chief surgeon to the Roman gladiators. Galen carried out detailed anatomical dissections in pigs and apes rather than humans (human dissection was forbidden). His detailed discussion of pathologic swellings and inflammation is probably his greatest contribution. It came close to modern views of such lesions. Galen had a pugnacious personality and presented his views and ideas with a force that convinced many, including the Church and its leaders, of their veracity. Galen treated blindness due to opaqueness of the lens by performing cataract surgery. Perhaps he loosened the opaque lens from its bindings and displaced it into the vitreous rather than extracted the lens. Indeed, it is difficult to see how the lens might be extracted without destroying the eye. However, Galen was far from the perfect physician. He practiced venesection (blood letting or bleeding), perhaps to rebalance the humors, to the detriment of untold numbers of patients. Because of the respect for his authority, blood letting continued for nearly two thousand years. He became wealthy by performing uvulectomies (removal of the uvula in the back of the throat) for chronic cough, an irrational, ineffective—and painful—procedure.

By this time, many surgical instruments were developed. Scalpels were made with blades of steel and handles of bronze. Probes, directors, guards and elevators were known. Tissue and bone forceps, drills (whirled by a thong) chisels and gouges were part of a surgeon's armamentarium [8].

It is difficult today, to conceive of Galen and other surgeons performing uvulectomies, cataract extractions, cae-sarean sections, or amputations in unanesthetized patients. What enabled patient tolerance of these procedures—and others? The ancients knew of the hypnotic and analgesic effects of alcohol, herbs, including mandrake, henbane, cannabis and opium, and the saliva from the chewing of coca leaves as mentioned previously. The speed and dexterity of the surgeons must also have played a part. Anecdotal reports suggest that they performed these procedures in 2–3 minutes or less, although it is difficult to imagine that extensive trephinations could have been performed in less than 30 minutes.

Pedanius Dioscorides (40–90 CE), a Greek surgeon in Nero's army in the 1st century CE, described the use of many herbs. His work, De Materia Medica, was the standard pharamocopeia for some 1500 years. He wrote "sleeping potions such as opium or mandragora are applied to such people as shall be cut or cauterized…for they do not apprehend pain because they are overcome with dead sleep…but used too much they make men speechless (i.e., dead)." He described how wine made from mandragora could induce "anesthesia", an absence of sensation in people about to undergo surgery. The Greeks may also have recognized that pressure on the carotid artery causes loss of consciousness (Karoun, from which carotid is derived, means "to fall into sleep"). Dioscorides' use of the word "anesthesia", anticipated Holmes recommendation to Morton by almost 1800 years [9].

The Talmud (200–500 CE) describes many surgical procedures undertaken by the ancient Jews including the suture of wounds, reduction of dislocations, amputations, and Caesarian sections [1]. The care of wounds also received attention: "To treat a wound, one applies cotton or lint, and sponge as well as garlic and onion peels which are secured by a thread (Tosefta Shabbat 5:3–4)". That such advice was avant garde, is supported by a recent clinical study demonstrating the benefits of a gel of onion extract on the appearance of post-surgical scars [10]. The Talmud discussed the relief of pain for many conditions. For example: "If one's loins pain him, he must NOT rub them with wine or vinegar, but he may anoint them with oil, yet not rose oil".

The Middle Ages

The Middle Ages began with the fall of Rome to the Goths in 476 CE, and continued until the Turks conquered Constantinople in 1453 CE. Widespread ignorance and lack of social progress in the early Middle Ages (476–814 CE), caused it to be named the Dark Ages. The high esteem accorded surgery during Greco-Roman times disappeared during this period.. In the 12th century, the Roman Catholic Church declared that shedding of blood was incompatible with holy office (the Ecclesia abhoret a sanguine edict of 1163), thereby prohibiting monks (the "educated class") from performing surgery. The clergy treated surgeons with contempt because they believed that incising or cutting another human body, and touching such wounds with one's hands was unclean and unholy. Enter the barbers as surgeons. The barbers had shaved the monks and cut their hair according to styles of specific religious orders. They had also assisted the monks in the performance of surgical procedures. The withdrawal of monks from surgery left a vacuum that the barbers filled. They used the training they had received by assisting the monks, and applied it in the performance of operations for hernias, bladder stones (seemingly violating the Hippocratic oath stating, "I will not use the knife, not even on sufferers from stone"), and even cataracts.

Although these barber-craftsmen ensured the survival of surgery, the shift in responsibility from monks to barbers, diminished the craft of surgery in the 12th and 13th centuries. There was a relatively transient resurgence in Western Europe at the School of Salerno near Naples (founded in the 9th century CE), sparked by an important surgical manuscript, the Bamberg Surgery, which covered in detail the management of all types of wounds (Corner GW. Salernian surgery and especially the "Bamberg Surgery" with an account of a previously undescribed manuscript of the Bamberg Surgery, in the possession of Harvey Cushing) [11].

By the end of the 13th century, Italian leadership in surgical education had declined substantially because of civil war. During this war, Matteo I Viscenti exiled a leader in Italian surgery, Guido Lanfranc of Milan (1250–1306), in 1290. Lanfranc went first to Lyons and later to Paris. There he completed his Practica Quae Dicitur Ars Completa Totius Chirurgiae (Practice and Art of All of Surgery) in 1296, a compilation of teachings from the Arab world and his master, William de Saliceto. The work became the foundation of French surgical teaching for many years, and reached 70 editions. Lanfranc made an interesting observation regarding the diagnosis of skull fractures (some 500 years before the invention of X rays): He would place a violin string between a patient's rear molars. Plucking the string caused the skull to vibrate with a musical note. If the sound was bright and clear, the skull was intact and healthy. If the sound was dim and muffled, it indicated the presence of a fracture. He also argued against the separation of surgery and medicine (advocated since the time of Avicenna), noting that a good surgeon should also be a good physician. In France he associated with the Confraternity of Saints Cosmos and Damian, named after twin brothers who were martyred in 287 CE and who were recognized as the patron saints of surgery for services to the needy—they did not accept payment for their services [1].

In addition to the Confraternity, a guild of Parisian barber surgeons came into existence. Lanfranc bitterly criticized the barber surgeons [12]. A great jealousy arose between them and the Confraternity, leading Phillip IV of France to order,

in 1311, that only "masters of surgery" who passed a royally authorized examination could practice surgery in Paris. The edict disenfranchised the barber surgeons. Unwelcome in the Confraternity, the barber surgeons obtained a royal charter in 1372, legalizing their position. They received the designation "barber-surgeon", but were not allowed to treat any wounds thought to be non-mortal! Such would seem a pyrrhic victory. A desire to protect ill-defined professional territorial boundaries (turf) underlay the evolution of the Confraternity and guilds of barber-surgeons. How much does this differ from modern times?

A contemporary of Lanfranc, Henri de Mandeville (1260–1320), became prominent as a strong opponent of surgical quackery. In his book, Chirurgie, he describes as quackery, the barber-surgeons' practice of placing noxious and corrosive substances in wounds, rather than cleaning them. As Mandeville's career came to an end, the University at Montpellier in France began to rival Paris as the center of European medical and surgical education. The most prominent of its graduates, Guy de Chauliac (1300–1380), authored a 7-part work, Inventarium Sive Collectorium Cyrurgie (Inventory of the Complete Works of Surgery), published in 1368, describing methods dominating surgery in France, and to some extent in England, for the next three centuries. The texts dealt with tumors and sores as well as fractures, antidotes and drugs [1, 12]. Of special importance were descriptions of splinting and traction for fractures of the limbs. Because the work was written in Latin, it was not immediately accessible to the less educated barber-surgeons. Over the next century, it was translated into English (about 1425 CE), French and other languages, allowing the non-Latin-educated barber-surgeons access to surgical teachings, aiding their struggle against the more educated university surgeons.

English surgery during the Middle Ages lagged behind that in France and Italy. In 13th and 14th century London, guilds or companies were established to control various trades. Initially, barber-surgeons were allowed almost exclusive control of the practice of surgery in the City, and this antagonized the smaller number of military surgeons, causing them financial harm. The barber-surgeons and military surgeons fought economic and political battles for the right to supervise anyone practicing surgery. The London city corporation sided sometimes with one group and sometimes with the other, creating recurring indecision.

The Renaissance

An understanding of anatomy underlies modern surgery. Fundamental changes in the study of anatomy, changes enabled by the weakening of the Church's ban on human dissection in the 14th century, prompted a resurgence of surgery during the Renaissance. Removal of impediments to dissection and

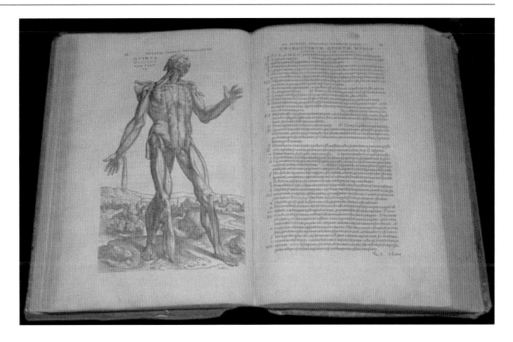

Fig. 15.1 From Vesalius' De Humani Corporis Fabrica. (lane. stanford.edu/portals/history/ves-alius.htm; lane.stanford.edu/.../vesaliusSketchfull.jpg)

autopsy enabled Andreas Vesalius (1514–1564) to become proficient in human dissection. His work at the University of Padua, as Professor in Anatomy, culminated in his publication in 1543 (at the age of 29) of De Humani Corporis Fabrica (On the Fabric of the Human Body; Fig. 15.1). Many errors arising from Galen's reports from dissections of animals, or simply from baseless misconceptions, were revealed and corrected [1, 12]. Vesalius was in good company. Italian surgeons, unlike their less literate German and Swiss counterparts, were often university educated, and some achieved academic distinction. Vesalius' friend, Bartolomeo Eusta-chius, described the inner ear and the process of dentition. He also discovered the adrenal glands in 1563. Guido Guidi (1508–69) described many anatomical structures, such as the Vidian artery, nerve and vein [3]. Gaspare Tagliacozzi (1547–99), perhaps the father of plastic surgery, provided detailed methods for treating mutilating injuries in his De Curtorum Chirurgia per Insitionem Libri Duo (1597; Fig. 15.2).

The last great Italian Renaissance surgeon, Hierony-mus Fabricius ab Aquapendente (1533–1620) became so popular as a teacher, anatomist, and surgeon, that he felt compelled to build (at his own expense) in Padua, the first known permanent amphitheater for anatomy demonstrations [1, 12]. Contributions to the development of surgery by Fabricius include techniques in tracheostomy, thoracentesis, and urethral stricture repair, and the development of many surgical instruments. Perhaps his most important discovery was that of venous valves, later used by his pupil William Harvey to explain the circulation of blood. Also from the University of Padua, Johannes Vesling, professor of anatomy, published Syntagma Anatomicum, which became the most widely used illustrated anatomical book of the 17th century. He also corresponded with Harvey, and

his manual was one of the first to accept the circulation of blood impelled by the heart.

Other countries contributed to the renaissance. European surgery owed much to two Frenchmen, Pierre Franco (1500–1561) and Ambroise Paré (1510–1590) [1, 12]. Their achievements were noteworthy because both had risen from poverty, and neither was university educated. Itinerant lithotomists and herniotomists trained Franco, whereas Paré emerged from a barber-surgeon apprenticeship. Franco acted to remove surgery from the grip of charlatans, and to place it under the auspices of trained practitioners. He successfully repaired hernias and removed bladder stones. In 1541, Paré passed an examination to become a "master barbersurgeon" and a member of the guild. Despite protests over his background as a barber's apprentice and his vernacular rather than Latin speech, and with the support of an academic French surgeon Jacques Dalechamps (1513–88), Paré was granted membership of the College of St. Como (1554). This membership was important because it facilitated a later union of the barber-surgeons and the academic surgeons. Paré rose to become the official royal surgeon to Henry II, Francis II, Charles IX and Henry III. He was instrumental in moving surgical practice towards the modern model and helped abolish some erroneous techniques of the ancients, such as the use of the cauterizing iron to stop hemorrhage, encouraging the use of ligatures, especially of arteries. He designed a "bec de corbin" or crow's beak which was a predecessor to the hemostat. He treated wounds with egg yolk, oil of roses and turpentine rather than with boiling oil [13]. In his famous statement, "I treated him. God cured him", Paré demonstrated great humility.

The struggle between university surgeons and the barber-surgeons mounted. The barber-surgeons moved beyond the

The Seventeenth Century

In the 17th century, experimentation began to replace speculation, and the scientific revolution changed the history of medicine. William Harvey (1518–1657) discovered the fundamental anatomy and physiology of the circulation of the blood [11]. His book Exercitatio Anatomica De Motu Cordis Et Sanguinis In Animalbus (An Anatomical Exercise on the Motion of the Heart and Blood in Living Beings; 1628) may be the most important book in the history of medicine. We now take for granted his great insights, but at the time, they were revolutionary. In addition to Harvey's contribution, Marcello Malpighi (1628–94) described the capillaries and their function in 1661.

However, surgery did not progress in the 17th century as rapidly as did anatomy, physiology and internal medicine. Despite their limitations, barber-surgeons in France were given the legal right to treat all wounds. In the second half of the 17th century, the barber-surgeons continued to favor their own union for financial reasons; and began to command higher fees than their academic counterparts (shades of modern surgery). Because it was difficult to make a living practicing only "surgery", barber-surgeons provided "barber work" such as bloodletting and mundane wound care. By the end of the 17th century, the activities of barber-surgeons and academic surgeons diverged, and this disjunction produced alterations in the character of surgery that became more evident in the 18th century. Although the surgeons of the late 17th century, particularly the barber-surgeons, developed increasing technical proficiency and surgical dexterity, they contributed little to fundamental advances in knowledge. Rather, medical and herbal therapies were developed. One of the first medical texts in English, The Physician's Practice, was published in 1639: "wherein are contained all inward diseases from the head to the foot by that famous and worthy Physician, Walter Bruel". Surgery was not recommended and gave place to bleeding from the nose to let the evil out, leeches to the temporal artery, bathing in water from flayed foxes, and diuretics. What wonderful fun.

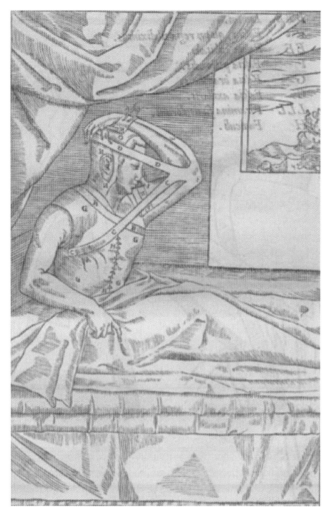

Fig. 15.2 " Gaspar Tagliacozzi, (1546–99) professor of surgery and anatomy at the University of Bologna, published De Curtorum Chirurgia to instruct surgeons on all they needed to know about reconstructing noses and ears. It is the first published work on plastic surgery. The work's twenty-two plates depict every step of the process of rhinoplasty and are among the best-known illustrations in the history of medicine. Shown here is the patient, immobilized in a vest of Tagliacozzi's devising, waiting for the skin graft taken from the arm to adhere to the nose. The process was supposed to take two to three weeks." [1, 12] (From De Curtorum Chirurgia per Insitionem Venice, Bindoni, 1597.)

The Eighteenth Century

Anatomic research by academic surgeons continued during most of the 18th century. By the end of the century, surgeons rose above their past station as technicians, and received ever more acceptance as professionals equal to physicians. At the beginning of the century, surgical training in France increasingly included the teaching of an accepted body of knowledge in courses and schools. The establishment of the Royal Academy or College of Surgery in 1731, together with a Royal Declaration in 1743 forbidding master surgeons to work as barbers, transformed French surgery from a craft to a profession.

legal limitations that had earlier been placed on their practices. They became known euphemistically as the "surgeons of the short gowns", in contradistinction to the "long gowns" or academic surgeons (cf residents and senior physicians). Barber-surgeons grew more numerous than their "long-gown" counterparts probably because of the elitist and exclusionist attitude of the latter. For the average Parisian, the "short-gown" barber surgeon was more accessible, cheaper, and more pleasant than his academic counterpart. Although the barber-surgeons had a lesser social status and academic rank, the public eventually recognized them as having superior skills, fewer complications, and lower morbidity and mortality.

The French Revolution (~1780–1793) profoundly changed medicine and surgery. In 1792, by law, the Faculty of Medicine and College of Surgery were abolished, and in 1794 the creation of the Ecole de Sante (School of Health) inextricably united medicine and surgery [1, 12]. Educational requirements to practice either medicine or surgery were now identical, and only one degree, that of Doctor of Medicine, was awarded. The first surgical periodical, Journal de Chirurgie, appeared in 1791, edited by Pierre-Joseph Desault, an anatomist and surgeon trained in part by barber surgeons. Desault established a school of anatomy in 1776, and became surgeon major to the Hopital de la Charite in 1782. A renowned lecturer, he developed the journal as a means for his students to publish their most interesting cases. These 18th century events came about in part because surgeons and others had shown the importance and interdependence of pathological anatomy and pathophysiology.

In 1745, the British Parliament passed a bill forming an independent Company or Corporation of Surgeons, thereby divorcing surgeons from the barber guilds. Unfortunately, the Company failed to uphold standards for admission and to adequately organize surgical education. Despite these limitations, by the last decade of the century, Britain displaced France as the most important European center for surgical education and training.

This transition occurred largely because of Percivall Pott (1714–1788) and John Hunter (1728–1793) [1, 12]. Pott's reputation as a fine clinician exceeded that of his pupil, Hunter. Sustaining a compound fracture of his femur in 1756 (not the injury subsequently called Pott's fracture), Pott prevailed on his attending surgeons to splint his leg rather than amputate it. He recovered completely and published his own experiences and observations in 1769, in an influential work translated into French and Italian [14]. He described the anatomy of congenital inguinal hernias in a "Treatise on Ruptures", arthritic tuberculosis of the spine (Pott's disease) and was an enthusiastic advocate of early operations for incarcerated hernias [15]. Perhaps most importantly, he observed an association between exposure to soot and a high incidence of scrotal cancer (later identified as squamous cell carcinoma). His 1775 Chirurgical Observations, an essay five pages long, discussed cancer among chimney sweeps—the first identification of an environmental carcinogen. His investigations contributed to epidemiology and the Chimney Sweeper's Act of 1788. (Bernardino Ramazzini had published "Diseases of Workers", [16] a work anonymously translated into English in 1705 as Diseases of Tradesmen. Chimney sweeps and occupationally induced cancer were not described.)

John Hunter, the youngest of 10 children, was born at Long Calderwood, 10 miles from Glasgow. He followed his brother William, who was also a surgeon and anatomist, to London and served an apprenticeship with the latter for many years before being appointed as surgeon to St. George's Hospital. He had a large practice and was considered a dexterous surgeon, but his main contributions to medicine and surgery were his lectures and writings, especially those concerning the pathophysiology of surgical diseases and comparative anatomy. He studied animals from leeches to elephants. He had difficulty overcoming a natural dislike of speaking and although he gave extensive courses, he "never gave the first lecture without taking 30 drops of laudanum to take off the effects of his uneasiness". [17] [The source for this is found in Mr. Home's introduction in John Hunter's book [17]. Home had lived and worked with Hunter for most of Hunter's life.] In addition to observations on malignant tumors, he studied the development of collateral circulation after occlusion of major arteries leading to improved treatment of aneurysms. He also wrote extensively on the development of the teeth [18].

Hunter had angina pectoris and frequent transient ischemic attacks. He said "my life is in the hands of any rascal who chooses to annoy and tease me". His prediction was accurate. He went to St. Georges Hospital on 16 October 1793 in his usual state of health (Mr. Home p lxi) and "meeting with some things which irritated his mind, he withheld his sentiments, in which state of restraint he went into the next room and turning round to Dr. Robertson, he dropt dead". He was 65. An autopsy indicated severe valvular disease and evidence of several old myocardial infarctions. A contributing factor may have been his self-inoculation with syphilis because he was sure he could cure himself, believing that no two diseases could coexist in one organism. Both Pott and Hunter dignified surgery by stressing the importance of making it a scientific discipline, one largely based on precise anatomical dissection and understanding. The Hunterian Museum at the Royal College of Surgeons in London has retained a large collection of Hunter's anatomical dissections.

The London Company of Surgeons encouraged the study of anatomy, and from 1752, was granted the corpses of all executed felons. The Surgeons' Hall dissections were formal affairs and students were relegated to the role of spectators [19]. This encouraged the development of private anatomy instructors, securing bodies from alternative sources. In his book "The London Tradesman" Robert Campbell wrote in 1747 of the young surgeon that "it is not sufficient for him to attend anatomy lectures, and to see two or three subjects cursorily dissected; but he must put his hand to it himself, and be able to dissect every part, with the same accuracy that the Professor performs."

The medical school in Edinburgh began to outshine those in England. In 1726, Alexander Monro (1697–1767), a surgeon trained in Leiden, was appointed as professor of anatomy. His son, Monro II (1733–1817), and grandson Monro III (1773–1859), followed him, thus holding the chair in the family for 120 continuous years. Training in Edinburgh focused on educating a doctor to be well-rounded in surgery and medicine. In 1778, the school of surgery became the Edinburgh Royal College of Surgeons. In England, most medical education took place outside the universities, and the Hunterian anatomy school was one of many similar schools training surgeons. The London Company of Surgeons eventually secured legitimacy by being granted a Royal charter in 1800.

Military and socioeconomic strife prompted inconsistent surgical practices in Germany. Formal surgical education and training were limited, and local barbers and quacks dispensed most surgical treatment. In North America, medicine and surgery made minimal advances from 1600 to 1750. Few actual physicians or surgeons existed, and self-educated "physicians" served most medical needs. By the late 18th century, society began to hold physicians in higher regard, and increasing numbers of Americans obtained their medical degrees in Europe, returning to the colonies with valuable clinical acumen and technical skills. By the end of the 18th century, the role of surgery within the overall context of medicine became clearer. An increasing interdependence of internal medicine and surgery followed the parallel development of 18th century pathological anatomy and experimental physiology. For thousands of years, surgeons attempted to connect disease to an objective anatomical diagnosis. With the advent of the understanding of pathology, surgeons could regard disease from a viewpoint long prevalent among physicians, one that considered disease processes and their physiologic consequences, rather than the effect of these on anatomy.

However, meaningful gains in surgery required the advent of anesthesia and antisepsis. By contrast, 18th century internal medicine yielded more impressive results in diagnosis and treatment. A better understanding of both anatomy and pathology, allowed surgeons to conduct procedures more expeditiously and accurately, but with the suffering that only anesthesia would abolish.

The Nineteenth Century Before the Discovery of Anesthesia

During the first half of the 19th century, the scope of surgery slowly increased. Surgeons treated simple fractures and dislocations, drained abscesses, sutured wounds, and performed amputations. Stimulated by the improved education and training described above, surgeons could ligate major arteries, treat aneurysms and excise some superficial tumors. Some treated anal fistulae, hernias and cataracts. Compound fractures (the broken bone extending through skin) remained mostly unmanageable because resulting severe infections produced a staggering morbidity and mortality, and were thus still treated mainly by amputation, which itself had a high mortality rate. Trephination continued in vogue. In the textbook "The Principles of Surgery", published by Lea and Blanchard, Philadelphia in 1848, [20] no mention is made of pain relief during operations. Only 1 page of Malgaigne's

Operative Surgery addresses pain control, [21] and the operator is encouraged to use narcotics. Malgaigne notes that animal magnetism does not work, and that it is better to distract the patient, work quickly or crush or cut the nerve to the area (pp 42–3).

The anticipation of pain caused some patients to refuse surgery, but some (many?) were amazingly stoic. John Hunter was summoned to Downing Street by the Prime Minister, William Pitt the Younger, in 1786, to excise an "encysted tumour" (perhaps a sebaceous cyst) Pitt would not allow Hunter to tie his hands as was the custom, asserting that he would not move during the operation. He asked how long the operation would take, and Hunter gave an estimate of six minutes. Pitt fixed his eyes on the Horse Guards' clock, and remained motionless until the operation was over, whereupon he remarked: "You have exceeded your time by half a minute." [22]

Changes in the education and training of surgeons were among the most important advances during the early and mid-portions of the 19th century. By the mid-19th century, Germany, Austria and soon after, the US, supplanted France as centers of surgical knowledge. William Halsted (1852–1922) adopted the German "pyramid" system of clinical training for interns and residents at the Johns Hopkins Hospital. Surgical journals such as Archiv fur Klinische Chirurgie (1860), Annals of Surgery (1885), and other periodicals supplemented the textbooks and treatises that had been the foundation of medical writing.

The Royal College of Surgeons of Ireland was founded in 1784 by charter from George III, with a supplemental charter from Queen Victoria in 1844. The College was formed along the lines of the College de St Cosme in Paris, created by Royal charter from Louis IX in 1255. Surgical organizations followed in Britain (The Royal College of Surgeons 1815), Germany (Deutsche Gesellschaft fur Chirurgie 1872), and the US (American Surgical Association 1880) [23]. The US Civil War (1861–1865) introduced many physicians to the basic principles of surgery and the limited use of anesthetic agents. American surgical practice evolved expeditiously with on-site education and training.

Mid-Late Nineteenth Century and Early 20th Century

In the last half of the 19th century, surgical practice changed more abruptly than in all of its previous history. Pivotal events, namely the discovery of anesthesia and the establishment of antisepsis, enabled an amazing transformation.

In 1844, Horace Wells (1815–1848), a dentist from Hartford Connecticut, discovered the anesthetic effects of nitrous oxide, but failed in an attempted public demonstration of those effects. He shared his findings with another dentist, William Morton (1819–1868). On 16 October 1846, Morton gave the first public demonstration of the effects of sulfuric ether anesthesia on Gilbert Abbott from whom, John Warren (1778–1856), professor of surgery at Harvard Medical School, removed a vascular tumor of the neck. Greatly impressed with the new discovery, Warren uttered his famous words: "Gentlemen, this is no humbug". A new epoch in surgery had begun. Operations could be performed more efficaciously, and haste was no longer of primary concern [23].

Word of the discovery of the use of ether to allow for painless surgery spread around the world in weeks. James Simpson in Edinburgh heard of this and applied it in his practice. He found the pungency less than desirable. In a search for something better than ether, he enticed his colleagues to sniff several vapors after dinner, including chloroform. They all fell asleep. Simpson used chloroform the next day in his obstetrical practice. (4 November 1847). Six days later, he reported to the Edinburgh Medico Chirurgical Society on more than 30 painless deliveries [24].

The Scottish Church opposed the use of chloroform, for God said, "Unto the woman, I will greatly multiply thy sorrow and thy conception; in sorrow thou shalt bring forth children; and thy desire shall be to thy husband and he shall rule over thee." (Genesis 111:16) In Edinburgh in 1591 A young lady, Euphemia Maclean, had asked a midwife, Agnes Samson, known as the Wise Woman of Keith, for relief from labor pains. She was publicly burned by order of King James as a warning to any woman who wished to be relieved of God's judgment.

Simpson was denounced from some Scottish pulpits and in pamphlets. One clergyman proclaimed that "Chloroform is a decoy of Satan, apparently offering itself to bless women; but in the end it will harden society and rob God of the deep, earnest cries which arise in time of trouble for help." [25] Simpson countered in "Answers to the religious objections against the employment of anesthetic agents in midwifery and surgery" in 1847. He argued that the Hebrew word "sorrow" could be translated as "toil" or "labor". Because of their erect position, childbirth in humans is much more laborious than in animals and the Bible was only recognizing a physiologic fact [25].

Queen Victoria scuttled this thinking when she insisted, on the advice of her physician, James Clark, that the surgeon/anesthetist, John Snow, administer chloroform for the birth of Prince Leopold in 1853. The lady was obviously satisfied and invited Snow back in 1857, to attend during the birth of Princess Beatrice. Snow, who had studied at the Hunterian school, was admitted to the Royal College of Surgeons in 1838. Snow figured in the initial safe development of anesthesia and was arguably the greatest anesthetist that ever lived. His broad use of both ether and chloroform led to his publication of two books which, incidentally might be said to describe office based anesthesia [26, 27]. He was also known for his insights as an epidemiologist, one leading to

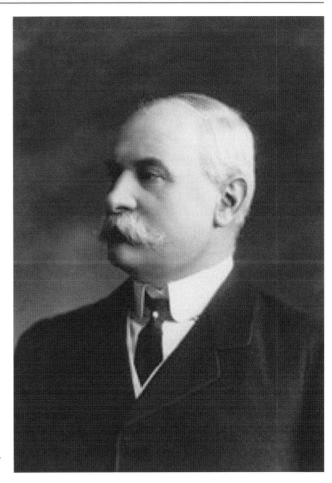

Fig. 15.3 Frederick Treves. (From Wikipedia.)

control of the cholera epidemic in Soho in London. His study led him to believe that the Broad Street well was contaminated. He assisted in halting the epidemic by persuading the City Council to remove the handle from the Broad Street water pump.

In 1900, Frederick Treves (Fig. 15.3) described the impact of the discovery of anesthesia on surgery and surgeons [28]:

"The changes that the discovery has wrought in the personality of the surgeon, in his bearing, in his methods, and in his capabilities are as wondrous as the discovery itself. The operator is undisturbed by the harass of alarms and the misery of giving pain. He can afford to be leisurely without fear of being regarded as timorous. To the older surgeon every tick of the clock upon the wall was a mandate for haste, every groan of the patient a call for hurried action, and he alone did best who had the quickest fingers and the hardest heart. Time now counts for little, and success is no longer to be measured by the beatings of a watch. The mask of the anaesthetist has blotted out the anguished face of the patient, and the horror of a vivisection on a fellow-man has passed away. Thus it happens that the surgeon has gained dignity, calmness, confidence, and, not least of all, the gentle hand."

"Anaesthetics have, moreover, greatly extended the domain of surgery by rendering possible operations which before could only have been dreamt about, and by allowing elaborate measures to be carried out step by step."

In 1886, for the first time, a surgical textbook dedicated an entire chapter to anesthesia [29].

A Century of Surgical and Other Giants

James Sims (1813–1883), was one of the first "giants" in surgery [23]. He is thought of as the father of modern gynecology. After many unsuccessful attempts to repair vesicovaginal fistulae (a tunnel between bladder and vagina), he achieved a cure on November 12 1849, in a patient who had undergone thirteen prior unsuccessful procedures. He attributed his success partly to positioning the patient on her left side with the thigh bent upward toward the abdomen, which allowed excellent visualization of the fistula. This position is now known as the Sims position. Sims' surgical expertise became famous, his practice grew, and he initiated research on menstrual problems, sterility, and artificial insemination. He founded the Women's Hospital in New York in 1855, with the aid of several prominent citizens, in particular their wives. Sims' interests extended beyond gynecology. He performed the first successful cholecystostomy for gallstone removal, in 1878. In 1882, Carl Langenbush performed the first successful cholecystectomy (gall bladder removal).

Theodor Billroth (1829–1894; Fig. 15.4), was born in Rugen on the Baltic coast. Billroth liked music more than books as a youngster. However, after his father died, his mother persuaded him to study medicine. He settled in Vienna at the completion of his training, because of Vienna's reputation in music. But nary a patient came in the first two months. Then he stumbled upon a job assisting the greatest surgeon of the day, Bernhard von Langenbeck (1810–1887), the founder of Archiv fur Klinische Chirurgie. Billroth used a microscope to examine the large collection of tumors at the Charite Hospital, classifying them and writing a dissertation on his findings. He was made an associate professor of surgery and histology in 1856, and four years later, his scientific and clinical skills became renowned throughout German-speaking lands. He was appointed professor in Zurich. Interested mainly in infection and healing of wounds, he was the first to use regular temperature measurement post-operatively, and to recognize that a rising temperature is often the initial sign of complications, an observation of vital importance to this day.

Billroth returned to Vienna as the professor of surgery when the chairman retired. He created one of the finest schools in the history of surgery and his legacy continues. Billroth performed the first total removal of the larynx for cancer (1873), the first hemipelvectomy (1891), the first

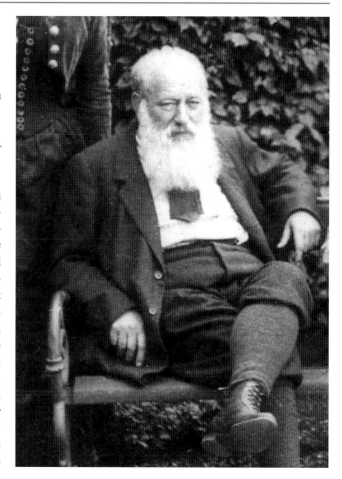

Fig. 15.4 Theodor Billroth (1829–1894) (From Wikipedia.)

perineal prostatectomy for cancer (1867), and the first suprapubic removal of a bladder tumor (1875). His boldness and technique made him a pioneer in abdominal surgery. On 29 January 1881, Billroth performed the first removal of a cancerous stomach in an operation taking one hour and thirty minutes [30]. The operation attached the remaining proximal stomach to the duodenum and became known as the Billroth I procedure. Unfortunately, the cancer returned, causing obstruction at the junction of the stomach and duodenum. Billroth recognized that he needed to connect the stomach with the intestine in a position less likely to become obstructed, even with recurrence of the tumor. On 15 January 1885, he removed another stomach cancer, closing the duodenum and connecting the stomach with the jejunum. This "Billroth II" procedure is used today.

Theodor Kocher (1841–1917; Fig. 15.5) greatly influenced American surgery in the second half of the 19th century, not only because of his impact on the understanding and treatment of thyroid disease but also because Halsted studied with him. Halsted returned to the US, bringing Kocher's precise, gentle and meticulous technique. Kocher was born and educated in Bern, Switzerland, where he became professor at the

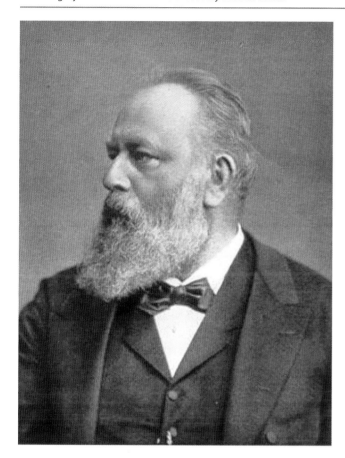

Fig. 15.5 Theodor Kocher (1814–1917). (From upload.wikimedia. org/wikipedia/commons/thumb/...)

age of 31. Bern was the center of the goiter district, and the prevalence of goiter spurred Kocher to investigate the regulation of thyroid function. In 1850, the mortality rate for thyroid surgery was about 50 %, usually from uncontrolled bleeding. With his meticulous technique, Kocher decreased the mortality rate to 0.2 % in some 4000 thyroidectomies. For this and his other contributions he received the Nobel Prize in Medicine in 1909. Good surgeons obey Kocher's rule: "a surgeon is a doctor who can operate and who knows when not to." [11]

The recognition of antisepsis, without which major surgical procedures often ended in infection and death, equals the discovery of anesthesia in importance to the advancement of surgery. *Joseph Lister* (1827–1912), Professor of Surgery at the Royal Infirmary in Glasgow, recognized that air-borne microorganisms caused surgical infections. In wards next to the cemetery where bodies awaiting burial were tossed from the windows (tale heard by EAMF as a student), the infection rate was higher than in the wards at the opposite end of the hospital. The Glasgow necropolis is immediately adjacent to the Royal Infirmary. In 1867, after two years of testing his theory, Lister described the use of a carbolic acid spray to minimize infection (Fig. 15.6). Gradually, Lister's principles of antisepsis gave way to those of asepsis, the complete

elimination of bacteria. Ernst von Bergmann (1836–1907), developed steam sterilization (1886) that ensured the sterility of instruments, an essential ingredient of asepsis. Other antiseptic rituals such as the use of masks, operating gowns, hats, and sterile gloves evolved rapidly thereafter [23].

Another Scot and successor to Lister at the Royal Infirmary in Glasgow, advanced both surgery and anesthesia by developing tracheal intubation. *William Macewen* was Medical Superintendent of the Glasgow Fever Hospital where he dealt with many deaths from respiratory obstruction due to diphtheria. He developed metal tubes that could be inserted into the tracheas of cadavers, following the observations of Desault some 100 years previously. He reported the case of a Glasgwegian who rushed up to his flat after work. Boiling water had just been poured from the potatoes prepared for his dinner, and he picked one up and popped it into his mouth. The potato lodged in his throat and was expelled with great difficulty. A few hours later and after some libation, he had trouble breathing. A note from a Dr. McMillan read "Urgent case, probably requiring operation." Rather than proceeding to tracheostomy, Macewen passed a gum elastic No 12, and successively larger catheters into the man's trachea, thereby relieving the obstruction. The catheters were maintained for 36 hours and the patient went home on the 6th day [31].

On July 5th 1878, Macewen passed a tube into the larynx of a patient, before induction of chloroform anesthesia, for removal of an epithelioma from the base of the tongue [32–33]. He was also dedicated to the teaching of anesthesia, unlike Lister, who vehemently opposed the emergence of specialists devoted to anesthesia, believing that his own clerks were superior to other chloroformists [34]. Macewen mandated practical instruction and certification in anesthetics for students and residents who worked in his wards. After an anesthetic death and much national publicity, the Board of Managers at the Glasgow Royal Infirmary adopted a resolution (Board of Managers Reports Glasgow Royal Infirmary 1882–3 Archives, University of Glasgow) on 7 March 1883, that required training in anesthetics for all medical students and clerks [35].

Macewen was offered the Chair of Surgery at Johns Hopkins in 1889. He refused the offer because the trustees would not grant him supervision and training of nurses, instead electing to wait for appointment as the Regius Professor at the University of Glasgow in 1892. He might have added considerably to American surgery—and anesthesia [36].

Victor Horsley (1857–1916), Macewen's concurrent neurosurgical counterpart in London, investigated the effects of several anesthetic agents on himself. While a house surgeon to John Marshall at University Hospital, London, he had his friends anesthetize him or he self-administered anesthetics some 50 times. He devised several means to monitor and record his sensations, developing pain charts linked to the percentage of anesthetic administered. The hospital authorities

Fig. 15.6 An operation in which Joseph Lister uses his carbolic acid spray

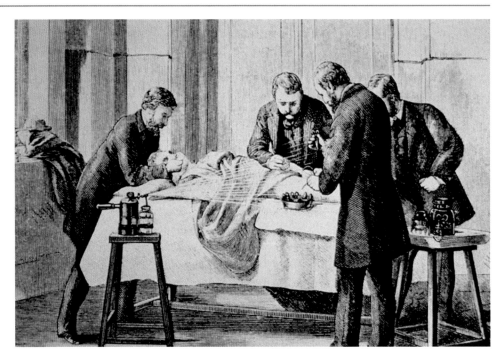

reported that the amount of anesthetic used increased during his apprenticeship. He recognized the value of hypotension obtained with increasing concentrations of chloroform. Ether was not to be used as it caused hypertension, increased blood viscosity, produced excessive bleeding, and resulted in severe postoperative vomiting. While he initially advocated a combination of chloroform and morphine, he later abandoned morphine because of its respiratory depressant effects. Chloroform was administered at that time by applying a cloth on which the liquid had been sprinkled. Insisting that control of the concentration was essential, Horsley used a vaporizer developed by a physical chemist, Vernon Harcourt. He added oxygen, believing that oxygen would reduce capillary bleeding [37, 38].

William Halsted (1852–1922; Fig. 15.7) influenced surgical development in the US. He began his work in 1889, in the newly opened Johns Hopkins Hospital in Baltimore, advancing surgery by emphasizing physiology as well as anatomy (and what might have happened had Macewen accepted the post—see above?) He was a meticulous surgeon who moved surgery from the heroic operating "theater" to the relative sterility of the operating room and the privacy of the research laboratory. His development of radical mastectomy for breast cancer, in 1898, became the gold standard for the treatment of that malignancy [39]. In the late 1970s, when local excision and radiotherapy were found to yield equivalent outcomes, those who advocated the less radical option had to overcome considerable doubt, sometimes including doubts concerning their surgical skill. While less mutilating

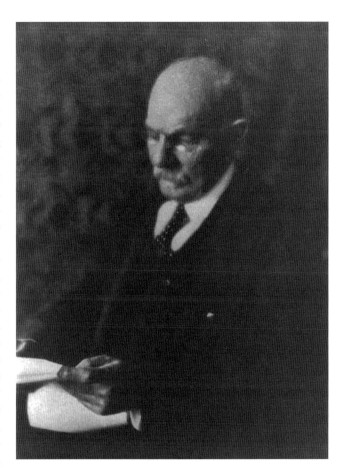

Fig. 15.7 William Halsted (1852–1922). (From en.wikipedia.org/wiki/File:WilliamHalsted.jpg)

procedures have supplanted radical mastectomy, Halsted's teachings on the spread of malignancies to regional lymph nodes (in this case, axillary nodes) guides today's practice.

Halsted's training program was patterned on the German model that required a dedication to meticulous care of the patient with graded and increasing responsibility over a period of at least five years—or until the professor deemed the trainee to be an independent and safe surgeon. Today this is called a pyramid system, a system in which five or six candidates begin at a first year level, but with only one or two completing the full five years. The aspiring resident surgeon lived in the hospital for 24 hours a day, hence the terms "resident" and "residency". Graduates of Halsted's training program were highly regarded, and increasingly populated teaching hospitals, promulgating Halsted's principles. The "Halstedian" residency became the standard for training. Modifications are imposed now by limited-hour work-week rules, rules passed by the Residency Review Committee, and its equivalent elsewhere, as a result of concern regarding resident fatigue and consequent errors. The successful trainee in a 5 or 6 year program who ultimately achieves the esteemed status of chief resident, is well prepared for a career as an independent physician and surgeon. He or she may now also be married during training.

A German obstetrician, Walbaum, described a hand cover for operations in 1758, [40] However Halsted deserves credit for popularizing the use of gloves throughout the world. His interest in gloves was accidental. The mercury-bichloride solution used to sterilize instruments had produced an incapacitating eczema on the hands of his favorite nurse—who happened to be his fiancée. He urged her to try rubber gloves. They worked and were soon adopted by him and his staff. "Venus had come to the aid of Aesculapius."

Halsted began self-experimentation with cocaine when he learned of its topical anesthetic properties, and became addicted. He was treated with morphine and then struggled with addiction to morphine for much of his life.

Surgeons immediately applied the 1895 discovery of X-rays [11] to the diagnosis and location of fractures, dislocations and the removal of foreign bodies. *Wilhelm von Roentgen* (1845–1923), whose name was given to these rays, actually belonged to the world of physics. Educated in Holland and Switzerland, he held professorships at Strasbourg, Giessen, and Wurzburg, studying heat and electricity. In November 1895, while experimenting with current through a vacuum in a tube, he made a chance observation of a greenish glow from a screen on a nearby shelf. This glow continued even when he stopped the current. He found that the screen was painted with a phosphorescent substance, and it was this that glowed when struck by invisible "rays" from the vacuum tube. He proved that the invisible rays generated by his tube could pass through wood, and other materials, unlike light and heat waves. Sometimes he noticed an image of his

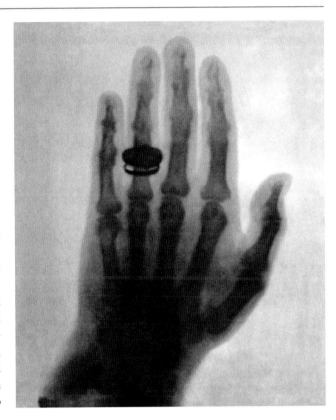

Fig. 15.8 Roentgen's image of his wife's hand. (From www.cs.brown. edu/.../cs024/images/canon/37.jpg)

own hand on the phosphorescent screen. Being an avid photographer, he set up a film before the screen, laid his wife's hand on the plate, and produced the world's first X-Ray picture, showing bones and a wedding ring (Fig. 15.8). Weeks later, he reported to the scientific academy in Wurzburg, "On a New Kind of Radiation". Few discoveries, apart from anesthesia, spread as fast as this one. He refused a Bavarian title but accepted the first Nobel Prize in physics in 1901, and lived on as a professor in Munich [11].

Roentgen's discovery profoundly altered surgery, but in more subtle ways than anesthesia and antisepsis. Before X-rays, doctors had to rely on their five senses. The advent of X-rays facilitated more precise diagnoses and therefore more definitive therapy. Soon it was realized that soft organs could be visualized by X-rays using a "contrast material", such as that developed by Graham and Cole for imaging the gall bladder. Injection of such material into the nipples of amputated breasts demonstrated how cancer changed them. X-ray mammography, without injection of contrast material, became an important tool in the diagnosis of breast cancer in 1962. It is difficult to envision modern medicine and surgery without X-rays.

Harvey Cushing (1869–1939; Fig. 15.9) was another American pioneer of surgery—and anesthesia. He studied at Yale and Harvard, and trained at Johns Hopkins Hospital

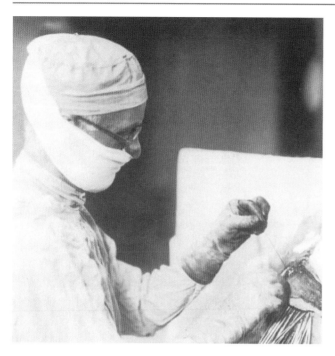

Fig. 15.9 Harvey Cushing operating. (From l.murugan.tripod.com/Murugan/id22.html.)

with Halsted. During his residency with Halsted, he became interested in neurosurgery and determined to give it better diagnostic methods, becoming one of the first in American surgery to employ X-rays.

As a medical student in the 1890s, Cushing was asked to stand in for the anesthetist Frank Lyman, in the process killing the patient he had been instructed to anesthetize [41]. This terrible event illustrates the then low state of anesthesia in the US: an orderly directed a third year medical student (Cushing) in the administration of an anesthetic to a seriously ill patient (a different arrangement from that in Great Britain where physicians gave the anesthetic). Cushing never forgot about it. Moreover, to the benefit of anesthesia, he did something about it [42]. The disaster led to the development of closer attention paid to the anesthetized patient. It led to Codman and Cushing's development of the anesthetic record under the urging of his chief, FB Harrington, and the setting down of the patient's heart rate and blood pressure in that record at five minute intervals, still a standard in anesthetic records (Fig. 15.10). Cushing had seen blood pressure measured in Europe when he visited the Ospidale di St Matteo in Padua where he was impressed with an adaptation of Scipione Riva Rocci's device. Later, in 1930, Cushing was to write:

"...I am not so sure that the general use of a blood pressure device in clinical work has done more good than harm. Just as Floyer's pulse watch led to two previously unknown diseases, tachycardia and bradycardia, so the sphygmomanometer has led to the uncovering of the diseases (God save the mark) of hypertension and hypotension, which have vastly added to the number of neurasthenics in the world." [43]

Cushing barely tolerated the weaknesses of lesser individuals. Consorting with females, and certainly marriage, were not allowed among his (male) residents. (Dr. Davidoff, wife of the neurosurgeon, Professor Davidoff, told EAMF, how she had to creep into her husband's quarters to see him. Both lived in fear that their marriage would be discovered). A Johns Hopkins nurse told a second anecdote. An inexperienced student nurse was substituting for the anesthetist. At a tense moment, Cushing ordered her to take a blood pressure. A few moments later he felt a tug on his pants as the nurse place the pneumatic cuff around his leg [43].

Cushing became professor of surgery at Harvard Medical School (and chief of surgery at the Peter Bent Brigham Hospital in Boston) in 1912. A perfectionist, he brought to neurosurgery the ultimate refinements in pre-operative preparation and operative technique. He introduced silver clips to occlude blood vessels in tissues (the brain) that could not be ligatured or pressed to staunch bleeding. He played an important role in the development of the Bovie electrocautery, a standard method today, of halting bleeding. Cushing's skill reduced the mortality rate in patients undergoing brain operations, from 50–60% to about 10%, by 1930 [44].

Inspired by Halsted's work with local anesthesia and by observations of deaths under ether anesthesia, Cushing applied local infiltration of cocaine for hernia and thyroid operations in 1898, [45] and for amputation somewhat later [46]. He kept meticulously detailed records of all of his work, insisting that records similar to current anesthetic records (see above) be maintained on his patients. He wrote extensively on his studies of brain tumors and developed a classification for these lesions, especially meningiomas. His finest work was "The Pituitary Body and Its Disorders" (1912), describing the syndrome which now bears his name. He developed the present operation for removal of pituitary tumors by an approach through the nose (trans-sphenoidal hypophysectomy), [47] entering the brain at its base rather than the more dangerous approach, traversing the brain from above.

Cushing was also a bibliophile. Antique book dealers everywhere knew of—and doubtless profited by—his friendly race with the Swedish surgeon Erik Waller, to collect the world's best library of medical history. Whether Waller or Cushing won may be debated. Later in life, he wrote a biography of William Osler (1849–1919), a Canadian and teacher whom he worshipped. His biography of Osler won Cushing the Pulitzer Prize in 1926.

Alexis Carrel (1873–1944), a Frenchman who came to the US in 1905, was another major innovator. He worked first in Chicago, and from 1906–1939 at the Rockefeller Institute for Medical Research in New York City. He revolutionized surgery of the vascular system with his technique for suturing blood vessels end-to-end with fine needles and suture material. He investigated grafting of organs, including the transplantation of organs from animal to animal; he replaced

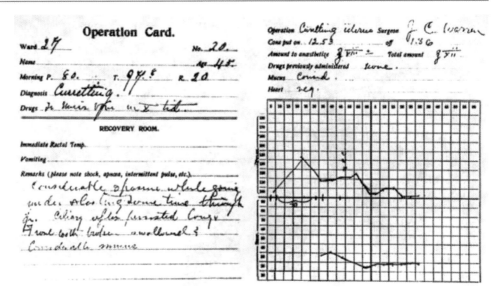

Fig. 15.10 An anesthetic record kept by EA Codman in November 1894. (From Beecher HK. The first anesthesia records (Codman, Cushing). 1940. Surg Gynecol Obstet 71:689, with permission.)

arteries with veins. In 1938, he crowned his long research on transplantation by keeping organs alive outside the body with a pump built by Charles Lindbergh (1902–1974). His work provided the foundation for today's organ transplantation, and for the treatment of arterial occlusive disease, of aneurysms, and of coronary artery disease. He well deserved his 1912 Nobel Prize in Medicine but failed to mention Charles Guthrie (1880–1963), an important collaborator during a two-year period at the Rockefeller Center.

Carrel developed the "Carrel-Dakin" solution used in World War I, an antiseptic still used. He also wrote, "Man the Unknown" (1935), arguing that a "utopia" run by geniuses should replace democracy. He played a role in French politics, particularly with the fascist Parti Populaire Francais during the 1930s, and may have helped implement eugenics policies in Vichy France. He was accused of helping the Nazis—whose physicians tarnished the reputation of medicine by performing inhumane experiments on individuals in concentration camps. He died in 1951, before his trial for collaboration. His suture technique came into practice three years later when his countryman, Charles Dubost, removed an aneurysm and sutured the two cut ends together [48].

The introduction of anesthesia profoundly altered the practice of surgery. Painless surgery was regarded as bold therapy, and the theatricality of the event was not lost on increasing numbers of surgeons who were emboldened to devise new and more technically complex operations. Some of these procedures provided little more than a poor excuse for the act of surgery. Thoughtful members of the surgical community became alarmed with what was considered to be the exploitation of surgery for financial gain. John Watson (1807–1863), a well known New York City surgeon, expressed concern more emphatically. "Surgery…..is a good thing, a useful, an excellent thing in its way, but too much of it is a great evil. And the sooner you find this out for yourself, the better for your patients".

Rudolph Matas (1860–1957) of New Orleans, was an imaginative surgeon who performed the world's first known aneurysmorrhaphy (correction of a ballooning of an artery) in 1888 [49]. Matas' activities and his innovations impacted on more than vascular surgery. During the 1890s, he performed some of the earliest successful pre-planned attempts at intraspinal cocainization (spinal anesthesia) [50]. With 3 colleagues, Larue, Gessner, and Allen, he successfully used intrathecal cocaine for a hemorrhoidectomy in a 32 year old Argentinian, on 18 December 1899. Earlier attempts on November 10, using intrathecal eucaine B to relieve pain in a man with a tuberculous knee joint, did not succeed.

At the turn of the century, Matas developed a test to determine the adequacy of the collateral circulation before performing surgery on the great vessels. He is also credited with introducing tracheal insufflation (blowing gases, particularly oxygen, into the trachea), a technique perfected by Samuel Melzer and John Auer in 1909 who, working on a suggestion made by Vesalius 350 years previously, applied positive pressure to the lungs, allowing the chest to be opened.

Notwithstanding these wonderful contributions, American physicians were slow to separate surgery from general medical practice. Some surgeons such as Samuel Gross (1805–1884) of Jefferson Medical College in Philadelphia, himself highly regarded by colleagues and patients, wrote and campaigned against specialization [23]. Influenced by Gross, the 1866 Committee on Medical Ethics of the American Medical Association carefully considered the advantages and disadvantages of specialization, and concluded that the disadvantages could only be overcome if the specialist were to begin his career as a generalist physician-surgeon, and slowly adopt his new specialty. Consequently, in the US, the rise of surgery as both a scientific and well-regulated profession did not begin in earnest until the late 1880s. At that time, it became evident that theoretical concepts and valid applications would be necessary to demonstrate the scientific basis of surgery, not only to non-surgical medical colleagues, but especially to the lay public. Surgeons needed to allay society's fear of the surgical unknown, and present surgery as an accepted part of the established medical armamentarium. The results obtained by surgeons treating the wounded in World War I, played an important role in convincing the public of the value of surgery in the treatment of non-war related conditions.

Evarts Graham (1883–1957) performed the first successful pneumonectomy for lung cancer in 1933, on a patient who himself was a physician [51]. Years later, Graham, a heavy smoker, recognized the role of cigarette smoking in the pathogenesis of carcinoma of the lung, and to the surprise and dismay of conservative physicians and surgeons, he openly decried smoking during conventions and meetings. Today, such a stance is standard, but in the 1950s, it was unusual. Graham succumbed to cancer of the lung some years later. His first patient, the physician with the same disease, outlived him.

Graham was not only a pioneer in pulmonary surgery, but also in X-Ray studies of the gall bladder. In 1924, he and a young resident in his surgical training program, Warren Cole, collaborated with Mallinckrodt Chemical Works in St. Louis, to develop a compound excreted and concentrated in the bile, enabling the gall bladder to be visualized by X-Ray. This test is still used today.

Graham loved music and wrote that

> "… surgery is like music, which has its great artists and its great composers. The great musical artists are like the great surgeons. They often perform before large audiences with great technical skill, and they have large incomes. But what they accomplish is the work of the composers, the creative men who have made it possible for them to perform and who often have received only modest economic rewards. What our present surgeons need is more men of the composer type".

Antibiotics Greatly Impact Surgery in the Twentieth Century

Paul Ehrlich (1854–1915), a German bacteriologist, was the first to employ "antimicrobial chemotherapy". He synthesized several "magic bullets" that would target specific disease-causing organisms, and was responsible for the development of arsenicals to treat syphilis. For those discoveries, he shared a Nobel Prize in Medicine in 1908.

In the early 1930s, *Gerhard Domagk* (1888–1964) invented a red dye which protected mice against streptococcus bacteria, and which was patented as Prontosil in 1932. Although Prontosil was effective in mice, it was not clear that the same effect would be obtained in humans. Domagk's daughter fell seriously ill of a streptococcal infection, and in desperation, Domagk gave her Prontosil. She recovered completely. Prontosil and its many relatives, known as sulfonamides,

proved to be effective against infections in wounds, lungs, urinary tract and other organs—earning for Domagk a Nobel Prize in Medicine in 1939. The Nazis forbade him to accept it and even arrested him. This bizarre outcome resulted because Carl von Ossietzky, who had won the Nobel Peace Prize in 1935, angered the Nazis by his criticism of the German government. German nationals were prohibited by law from accepting the prize [52]. Domagk finally received the prize in 1947.

In 1928, the Scot, *Alexander Fleming* (1881–1955), while studying staphylococcus bacteria, noticed that no bacteria grew around mold that developed in old culture plates. He inferred that the mold, Penicillium notatum, contained an antibacterial substance that he called penicillin. Nothing further was done until World War II when Howard Florey (1898–1968) from Australia, and Ernst Chain (1906–1979) from Germany, discovered how to obtain useful amounts of penicillin from the mold. All three were knighted and shared a Nobel Prize in Medicine in 1945. The discovery of penicillin is one of the most important breakthroughs in medicine.

Fleming's discovery inspired *Selma Waksman* (1888–1973), a world authority on microbes in soil, to look there for substances similar to penicillin, and he found streptomycin. In 1952, he too received a Nobel Prize in Medicine. Streptomycin provided the first medical cure for tuberculosis, which previously often required removal of portions of the lung containing an infected cavity, or which necessitated removal of multiple ribs to collapse cavities in the thorax infected with tuberculosis.

Antibiotics revolutionized surgery. They prevented surgical (wound) site infections after operations for appendicitis, diverticulitis, colonic and intestinal resections, and peritonitis, and are now given routinely before surgery. They had an unexpected effect on the common operation for peptic ulcer disease. In 1982, Australians *Barry Marshall* and *J. Robin Warren*, demonstrated that the bacterium Helicobacter pylori caused peptic ulceration [53]. Their finding was met with skepticism, a skepticism Marshall countered by drinking a culture of Helicobacter with resulting stomach inflammation. Antibacterial agents eradicated H. pylori, and with that, the need for operations to treat perforated ulcers and persistent ulcerative disease of the stomach and duodenum. Prior to this, stomach operations for intractable peptic ulcerations kept surgeons busy. Marshall and Warren were awarded the 2005 Nobel Prize in Medicine.

Later in the Twentieth Century

World War II greatly expanded surgery as a specialty, and increased the number of surgeons throughout the country. Many of these individuals, newly indoctrinated in the rigors of technically complex operations for trauma, became leaders in the construction and improvement of hospitals, multispecialty clinics, and surgical facilities in their home-towns. Large urban and community hospitals established surgical training programs, and increasing numbers of students graduating from medical school sought surgical residencies. The trend toward specialization became so great that extinction of the general practitioner became a threat. The change in the demographics of the American doctor was most dramatic for the surgical specialties. In 1930, 10 % of the medical profession considered themselves surgeons, but by 1975 over one third of all physicians were full time practitioners of either general surgery or one of the surgical specialties.

The greater number of surgeons loosened the indications for surgery. In 1970, John Bunker, an anesthesiologist at Stanford University, reported that not only were there twice as many surgeons in the average American city as in an English city, but twice as many surgical procedures were performed per capita—without any demonstrable short or long term health-related benefits [54]. Parallel studies undertaken recently showed similar results, and such findings are likely to profoundly change surgical practice and the delivery of health care in the US.

American Cardiothoracic and Transplant Surgery after World War II

World War II undermined the economies of most countries of the world. The diversion of resources to war undercut the growth of medicine, including surgery—but not the US. This ended European surgical superiority and North Americans became the leaders of world surgery. Two developments emphasized the importance of post-World War II American surgery: the maturation of cardiac surgery as a new surgical specialty, and the emergence of organ transplantation. As the first president of the US to undergo a major abdominal operation (ileotransverse anastomosis for intestinal obstruction due to Crohn's disease) Dwight Eisenhower (1890–1969) enhanced the fascination with surgery, especially since he experienced an uneventful postoperative course. This example of a leader setting an example for a country is similar to the popularizing of epidural analgesia in Japan after the Emperor underwent abdominal surgery, anesthetized in part with epidural analgesia (see Chapter 31 on the History of Anesthesia in Japan).

Robert Gross (1905–1988), at the Boston Children's Hospital, initiated modern cardiac surgery. While still a surgical resident, he successfully repaired a congenital defect, a patent ductus arteriosus (an abnormal opening between the left pulmonary artery and the aorta) in a seven year old girl [55]. In 1945, he resected a coarctation (narrowing) of the aorta and reconstructed anatomic continuity with an end to end anastomosis [56]. In 1948, Dwight Harken (1910–1993), a Boston based surgeon, and Charles Bailey (1910–1993) of Jefferson Medical College, independently carried out suc-

cessful operations for mitral stenosis (narrowing of the intra cardiac mitral valve). These procedures challenged the long-held medical myth of the heart as an organ so vital and complex that it could not withstand surgical intervention.

Yet, technically complex cardiac repair procedures could not be developed further until the operative field could be rendered free of blood, and the unrelenting beating of the heart could be stopped while circulation to the body was maintained. *John Gibbon, Jr.* (1903–1973), whose tenacity in the research laboratory became legendary, worked with engineers for six years to develop a heart-lung machine which he employed to successfully repair an atrial septal defect in the heart of an 18 year old woman, in May 1953 [57].

Substituting a healthy organ for a sick one is a surgeon's dream. Carrel's suture method caused a wave of enthusiasm for transplantation after initial experience with long-lived "auto-transplants" (i.e., take out a kidney and put it back into the same animal and the kidney and animal survive). Enthusiasm dimmed when it became apparent that a host animal would reject a guest organ from another animal! The body's immunity "defense mechanism" killed such foreign cells.

Peter Medawar (1915–1987) in London, showed during the 1940s, that a guest organ's life was shorter in a host animal that had previously received a graft from the same donor [58]. The same was true in a host previously receiving white blood cells from the donor. These prior "transplants" activated the immune system, preparing it for hostile action when confronted by invasion of similar subsequent transplants. The immune response protects us all from infections (e.g., once we have measles, the immune system defends us from a subsequent infection by the measles virus), but the immune system does not stop when faced with an organ transplant. Medawar discovered that cortisone could increase the life of the transplant, thus providing an "immunosuppressive" weapon against rejection. Medawar received the Nobel Prize in Medicine in 1960. Other investigators subsequently developed better immunosuppressive agents.

In 1954, Bostonians *J. Hartwell Harrison* (1909–1984) and *Joseph Murray* (1919–2012), performed the first successful human kidney transplantation between identical twins [59]. Identity of the twin's tissue types made chemical immunosuppression unnecessary. Harrison and Murray followed that feat in 1959, with a kidney from a non-identical twin. Whole body radiation was given to provide immunosuppression [60]. In 1962, a transplant was completed between unrelated individuals using drug immunosuppression, thus opening the door to such operations on a large scale [61]. The world has now seen hundreds of thousands of kidney transplants, allowing people with severe renal damage an alternative to chronic dialysis treatment. Over 85 % of patients who receive cadaver kidneys live and function normally, albeit with suppressed immune systems.

In 1963, *Thomas Starzl* (1926–) in Denver began transplantation of human livers [62]. His progress report in 1981 heightened interest in the method, and today it is well established for adults with primary cancer or chronic inflammation of the liver, and for children born with narrowed bile ducts. Whole organ pancreatic transplantation for the treatment of diabetes soon followed, as did cardiac, intestinal and bone marrow transplants.

In New York, Adrian Kantrowitz practiced transplanting hearts in puppies for years. He had planned a human operation but was prevented at the last minute because the donor infant, an anencephalic, had not been declared brain dead. His next opportunity came on December 6th 1967, just 3 days after the first heart transplant performed at Groote Schuur Hospital in Cape Town, South Africa, by *Christiaan Barnard* (1922–2001). Kantrowitz' patient lived for 6.5 hours, Barnard's for 18 days. Kantrowitz found ways to supplement the work of the natural heart, developing the left ventricular assist device (1972), the intra aortic balloon pump (1967), and the implantable pacemaker (1962; designed with General Electric).

Gender and Race in American Surgery

Gender and racial bias have affected the evolution of American surgery. African-Americans and women were innocent victims of prejudice well into the mid-twentieth century, forcing unending struggles to attain competency in surgery. Fortunately, these barriers have been largely erased, and today, women and African-Americans hold important positions, including chairmanships of departments of surgery, throughout the US. Overall, of those who consider themselves to be general surgeons, roughly 10% are women of whom 90% are under 44 years of age. African-American general and thoracic surgeons constitute 1.7–3% of general surgeons in the US but these percentages continue to increase [23].

Blood Transfusion: A Pillar of Support for Today's Surgery

The idea that blood transferred from a healthy person to an old or sick person can convey youth and vitality is ancient, noted in Egyptian medicine as early as 2000 BCE. We do not know when the first blood transfusion from one human to another was successfully accomplished. In the early-mid 19th century, the London physiologist and obstetrician, James Blundell, began the process that led to modern transfusion. Animal experiments convinced him that transfusions could save the lives of bled-out patients, and that this could help women in childbirth. His success was limited because he did not understand that blood from one person might or might not be transferable to another. Successful transfusions—

those without reaction—probably resulted from good luck, but by 1868, transfusions had caused many deaths, and the practice disappeared.

The turning point came with *Karl Landsteiner*'s (1868–1943) discovery of blood groups. In a modest article in 1901, in his native Vienna's Klinische Wochenschrift, [63] Landsteiner and his group at the Rockefeller Institute argued that humans had one of three blood groups, called A, B, and O. A year later, a fourth group (AB) was discovered. They proved that blood normally contains antibodies (antibodies are proteins that combine with and incapacitate other specific proteins called antigens) that are directed at antigen proteins in particular types of blood cells. If blood with the wrong antigen is given to a person possessing antibodies directed against it, the red blood cells clump together (agglutinate) and are destroyed. By giving blood of the person's own blood group, this great danger can be avoided. Landsteiner also found that type O blood cannot be agglutinated (no one has type O antibodies) and thus can be given to anybody—the universal donor. He was awarded the Nobel Prize in Medicine in 1930.

Early transfusions transferred blood directly from one individual to another. There were no bottles or bags of blood. A pioneer in direct transfusion, George Crile (1864–1943) of Cleveland, described his method in 1906 [64]. His stature and advocacy continued person-to-person transfusion until the blood banks that evolved in the mid 20th century made this obsolete. The availability of banked blood enormously impacted on surgery. Complex operations for vascular conditions, malignancies and many surgical procedures, including organ transplantation, could scarcely have been accomplished without this remarkable development.

Entering the Twenty-First Century

Over 100 years ago, Georg Kelling described the establishment of a pneumoperitoneum, and placement of a trochar through which a cystoscope could be introduced into the abdomen for viewing (laparoscopy) of the abdominal contents. Heinz Kalk, in the early 1930s, popularized laparoscopy using room air to create a pneumoperitoneum [65]. Initially employed by gynecologists, it was not until 1991, that general surgeons began to use laparoscopy. *Erich Muhe* (1938–2005) carried out the first laparoscopic cholecystectomy (gallbladder removal) in Germany [66]. CO_2 replaced room air to create the pneumoperitoneum, CO_2 providing greater safety than air by avoiding catastrophic gas embolism.

As surgeons became more adept with laparoscopic cholecystectomy, the use of laparoscopy for nearly every intra-abdominal operation grew explosively, and it is now the preferred approach for almost all surgeries, including bariatric procedures. Even resections of the liver, which in the absence of cirrhosis can be carried out by open techniques with a mortality rate as low as 3 %, are now done laparoscopically. Clearly, well-controlled prospective trials to compare open with laparoscopic treatment are required, and many are ongoing today. The primary advantage of laparoscopy is that multiple tiny incisions replace the larger incisions of open procedures, which cause greater post-operative pain and incisional complications such as dehiscense (wound edge separation) and herniation. Lessened post-operative pain is the clearest advantage of laparoscopy and thoracoscopy, often allowing earlier discharge from the hospital and return to work. On the other hand, laparoscopic procedures may be longer and are more costly than open procedures. Robotic surgery has now entered operating rooms and, perhaps driven by marketing, is the method of choice for prostatic surgery. Evidence based medical reports have not uniformly supported better outcomes [67]. It is too early to determine its ultimate role in surgery.

The goal to use ever-smaller incisions has impacted surgeries such as thyroid and parathyroid procedures. Scientific studies are needed to determine whether these are superior to more conventional approaches, or whether their increased use is simply a reflection of the "macho" surgeon.

Anesthesia has increasingly affected surgical practice—and vice versa. Advances in anesthesia made possible the move from in-patient to out-patient and office-based surgery. Advances in anesthesia have enabled performance of even the most difficult surgery in the sickest patients. Drugs with evanescent effect have been developed, drugs that allow precise control of the anesthetic state, including a fast recovery that would have seemed miraculous to the 19th century surgeon—and anesthetist. Computerized records ensure accurate and contemporaneous collection of patient data. Intraoperative monitoring, especially with continuous pulse oximetry and capnography, has ensured an amazing level of safety [68].

Other changes may not be viewed by members of the surgical and anesthetic communities as advances. Increasingly, it seems that surgical practice is dictated by insurance carriers and the legal profession. How these trends will affect the public and medical profession remains to be seen.

Although we cannot describe all who significantly contributed to the development of surgery in the late 19th and 20th centuries, certain important events require mention. These are summarized in Table 15.1.

Integration of Surgery and Anesthesia

Anesthesiologists, in concert with surgeons, have revolutionized post-operative care, especially for patients requiring the special services of an intensive care unit. Anesthesiologists contribute to the origination, development and management

Table 15.1 Surgical Developments in the late 19th and 20th centuries

Date	Contribution	Surgeon/Scientist
1849	Repair, vesico-vaginal fistula	James Sims
1867	Antisepsis	Joseph Lister
1867	Perineal prostatectomy for cancer	Theodor Billroth
1871	Esophagectomy	Theodor Billroth
1873	Total removal of the larynx for cancer	Theodor Billroth
1875	Suprapubic bladder tumor removal	Theodor Billroth
1878	Tracheal intubation	William Macewin
1881	Gastrectomy for stomach cancer (Billroth I)	Theodor Billroth
1882	Radical mastectomy for breast cancer	William Halsted
1882	Successful open cholecystectomy	Carl Langenbush
1882	Drainage of a pancreatic cyst	Carl Gussenbauer
1885	Gastrectomy for stomach cancer (Billroth II)	Theodor Billroth
1886	Asepsis/steam sterilization	Ernst von Bergmann
1888	Repair of aneurysm	Rudolph Matas
1889	Improved inguinal hernia repair becomes the gold standard	William Halsted
1889	Use of surgical rubber gloves	William Halsted
1891	Hemipelvectomy	Theodor Billroth
1894	First use of the anesthetic chart	Codman & Cushing
1895	X-rays discovered	William Roentgon
1901	Discovery of human blood groups	Karl Landsteiner
1901	Visualization of the abdominal contents through a tube	George Kelling
1906	Direct blood transfusion	George Crile
1908	The magic bullet for syphilis	Paul Erlich
1909	Development of surgery for thyroid disease	Theodor Kocher
1909	Tracheal insufflation for aeration	Matas & Melzer & Auer
1910	Pituitary tumor removal through the nose	Harvey Cushing
1912	Nobel prize for suturing of blood vessels	Alexis Carrel
1913	Resection of cancer of the esophagus	Franz Torek
1923	Treatment of aortic obstruction	Rene Leriche
1924	X-ray visualization of the gall bladder	Evarts Graham
1928	Observation of effect of penicillin	Alexander Fleming
1932	First sulfonamide	Gerhard Domagk
1933	Pneumonectomy for cancer	Evarts Graham
1935	Resection for pancreatic cancer	Allan Whipple
1939	Closure of a patent ductus arteriosis	Robert Gross
1941	Hormonal influence on prostate cancer	Charles Huggins
1943	Streptomycin discovered	Selman Waksman
1945	Resection of an aortic coarctation	Robert Gross
1946	Endarterectomy for arterial occlusions	J. Cid Dos Santos
1948	Repair of a mitral valve	Harken & Bailey
1951	Resection and graft replacement of aortic aneurysm	Charles Dubost
1953	Successful cardiopulmonary bypass	John Gibbon
1954	Successful transplant of a kidney between two humans	Harrison & Murray
1963	Human liver transplantation	Thomas Starzl
1967	Human heart transplantation	Christiaan Barnard
1983	Cause and treatment of peptic ulcer discovered	Marshall & Warren
1991	Laparoscopic cholecystectomy	Erich Muhe

of intensive care units. Similarly, successful pain management is integral to the early return to normal daily living, and anesthesiologists, again in concert with surgeons, have made major contributions in this area.

Roughly 50–60 years ago, most anesthesiologists were members of a department of surgery, or were hired by surgeons or surgical departments to carry out their work. This lack of independence seriously hampered their ability to rise academically. It became apparent that for anesthesiology to realize its potential, independent departments led by excellent scientists and clinicians were necessary. Many chairmen of surgical departments fought this trend, and when one of the authors of this essay (WS) at the Harvard Medical School elected to recruit a first-class professor of anesthesia, to establish an independent department of anesthesia at the Beth Israel Hospital in 1966, an eminent colleague at another Harvard hospital chastised him for his effort. The attitude exemplified by that surgeon and others, slowed the progress and development of anesthesiology. Fortunately, more thoughtful surgeons properly concluded that the life of the patient was as much in the hands of the anesthesiologist as in those of the surgeon. Today, surgeons and anesthesiologists in separate administrative departments, work effectively in a collegial and supportive manner to the benefit of all, most importantly for the patients they serve.

References

1. Rutkow IM. The origins of modern surgery, surgery-basic science and clinical evidence. New York: Springer Verlag, Inc.; 2001. pp. 2–19.
2. Bandelier AF. Aboriginal trephining in Bolivia. Am Anthrpol. 1904;6:440–6.
3. Fairley HB. Anesthesia in the Inca empire. Rev Esp Anestesiol Reanim. 2007;54:556–62.
4. The Code of Hammurabi Trans LW King Yale Law School. http.//Avalon.lawyale.edu/ancient/hamframe.asp Accessed: 31 January, 2010.
5. Breasted JHT. Edwin Smith Papyrus. University of Chicago Oriental Institute, Chicago: University of Chicago Press; 1930. p. 177.
6. Adams F. Hippocrates on injuries of the head. In: The genuine works of Hippocrates in 2 vols. London: The Sydenham Society; 1849.
7. Celsus AC. De Medicina. Book 8, Chapter 4. WG Spencer, translator. Cambridge: Harvard University Press; 1935.
8. Milne JS. Surgical instruments in Greek and Roman times. Oxford: Clarendon Press; 1907.
9. Nuland SB. The classics of anesthesia. The classics of medicine library. Birmingham, Alabama: Div. of Gryphon Editions, Ltd; 1983: 9.
10. Draelos ZD. The ability of onion extract gel to improve the cosmetic appearance of postsurgical scars. J Cosmet Dermatol. 2008;7:101–4.
11. Haeger K. The illustrated history of surgery. Houston, Texas: Bell Publishing Co.; 1988.
12. Corner GW. The rise of medicine at Salerno in the 12th century. Yale Univ Library call # Hist R 141 933C; 1933.
13. Pare A. Method of curing wounds with egg yolk and oil of roses and turpentine reather than with boiling oil. In: Keynes G. The apologie and treatise of ambroise pare. London: Falcon Educational Books; 1951. p 138.
14. Pott P. Some few general remarks upon fractures and dislocation. L. Hawes, W. Clarke, and R. Collins. 1769.
15. Pott P. Chirurgical Works (in 3 volumes), Vol 3, pp. 267-330. London: T Lowndes et al., 1783.
16. Ramazzini B. De morbis artificum (diseases of workers). Translated by Wright WC. Chicago: University of Chicago Press; 1713/1940.
17. Hunter J. The natural history of the human teeth. London, J Johnson, No. 72, St. Paul's Church-Yard; 1778.
18. Porter R. The greatest benefit to mankind. London: HarperCollins; 1997. pp. 1–831.
19. Mr. Home's introduction (the life of the author, p xxiv) in John Hunter's book, A treatise on the blood, inflammation and gunshot wounds. London: John Richardson; 1794.
20. Miller J. The principles of surgery. Philadelphia: Lea and Blanchard; 1848.
21. Malgaigne JF. Manual of operative surgery (Translated from the French by F. Brittan). 356 Strand, London: Henry Renshaw; 1846.
22. Ehrman J. The Younger Pitt. Volume 1—years of acclaim. London: Constable & C.; 1969. p. 594.
23. Rutkow IM. American surgery: an illustrated history. Philadelphia: Lippincott; 1998.
24. Simpson JY. On a new anaesthetic agent, more efficient than sulphuric ether. Lancet. 1847;2:549–50.
25. Haggard HA. Devils, drugs and doctors. New York: Blue Ribbon Books; 1929. pp 107–9.
26. Snow J. On chloroform and other anaesthetics: their action and administration. New Burlington Street, London: John Churchill; 1858. pp. 1–443.
27. Snow J. On the inhalation of the vapour of ether in surgical operations: containing a description of the various stages of etherization, and a statement of the result of nearly eighty operations in which ether has been employed in St. George's and University College Hospitals. London: John Churchill; 1847; pp. 1–88.
28. Treves F. Address in surgery. Br Med J. 1900;2:284–9.
29. Mills J. Anaesthesia. In: Treves F Editor. Manual of surgery (in 3 volumes). Philadelphia: Lea Brothers; 1886. pp. 103–26.
30. Billroth T. Gastrectomie. Wien Med Wochenschr. 1881;31:162–5.
31. Bowman AK. The life and teaching of Sir William Macewen. London: William Hodge and Co; 1942. pp. 98–9.
32. Macewen W. The introduction of tubes into the larynx through the mouth instead of tracheotomy and laryngotomy. Glasgow Med J. 1879;9:72.
33. Macewen W. The introduction of tubes into the larynx through the mouth instead of tracheotomy and laryngotomy. Glasgow Med J. 1879;12:218.
34. Watt OM. Glasgow anaesthetists 1846–1946. Clydebank: James Pender; 1962.
35. Frost E. The contributions of Sir William Macewen, a pioneer neurosurgeon, to an early quality assurance survey in anesthesia. J Neuro Anesth. 1991;3:28–33.
36. Walker AE. A history of neurological surgery. New York: Hafner Pub Co; 1967. p. 178.
37. Paget S. Sir Victor Horsley. A study of his life and work. London: Constable; 1919. p. 184.
38. Horsley V. On the technique of surgical operations on the central nervous system. Totonto Lancet. 1906;2:484–8.
39. Halsted WS. I. The results of radical operations for the cure of carcinoma of the breast. Ann Surg. 1907;46:1–19.
40. Miller JM. William Stewart Halsted and the use of the surgical rubber glove. Surgery. 1982;92:541–3.
41. Shephard DAE. Harvey cushing and anaesthesia. Can Anaes Soc J. 1965;12:431–42.
42. Cushing HW. Anaesthesia Charts of 1895. Letter to F.A. Washburn. Treadwell Library, Massachusetts General Hospital, Boston, MA.
43. Fulton J. Harvey cushing, a Biography. Oxford: Blackwell; 1946. p. 216.

44. Bliss M. Harvey cushing: a life in surgery. Oxford: Oxford University Press; 2005.
45. Cushing HW. Cocaine anesthesia in the tretment of certain cases of hernia and in operations for thyroid tumors. Johns Hopkins Bulletin. 1898;9:192–3.
46. Cushing H. I. On the avoidance of shock in major amputations by cocainization of large nerve-trunks preliminary to their division. With observations on blood-pressure changes in surgical cases. Ann Surg. 1902;36:321–45.
47. Koltai PJ, Goldstein JC, Parnes SM, Price JC. External rhinoplasty approach to transsphenoidal hypophysectomy. Arch Otolaryngol. 1985;111:456–8.
48. Dubost C, Allary M, Oeconomos N. Resection of an aneurysm of the abdominal aorta: reestablishment of the continuity by a preserved human arterial graft, with result after five months. AMA Arch Surg. 1952;64:405–8.
49. Matas R. Traumatic aneurysm of the left brachial artery. Incision and partial excision of the sac-recovery. Med News NY. 1888;53:462–6.
50. Simmons GH, (Editor). Medical News. JAMA. 1899;33:1659.
51. Graham EA, Singer JJ. Successful removal of an entire lung for carcinoma of the bronchus. JAMA. 1933;101:371–4.
52. Schück H, Sohlman R, Österling A, Liljestrand G, Westgren A, Siegbahn M, Schous A, Ståhle NK. The prize in physiology and medicine: the nobel prizes in wartime. In: Nobel foundation. Nobel: the man and his prizes. Stockholm: Klara Civiltryckeri; 1950. pp. 167–79.
53. Marshall BJ, Warren JR. Unidentified curved bacilli in the stomach of patients with gastritis and peptic ulceration. Lancet. 1984;1:1311–5.
54. Bunker JP. Surgical manpower. A comparison of operations and surgeons in the United States and in England and Wales. N Engl J Med. 1970;282:135–44.
55. Gross RE, Hubbard JP. Landmark article Feb 25, 1939: surgical ligation of a patent ductus arteriosus. Report of first successful case. By Robert E. Gross and John P. Hubbard. JAMA. 1984;251:1201–2.
56. Gross RE. Surgical correction for coarctation of the aorta. Surgery. 1945;18:673–8.
57. Gibbon JH, Jr. Application of a mechanical heart and lung apparatus to cardiac surgery. Minn Med. 1954;37:171–85.
58. Medawar PB. The behaviour and fate of skin autografts and skin homografts in rabbits: a report to the War Wounds Committee of the Medical Research Council. J Anat. 1944;78:176–99.
59. Harrison JH, Merrill JP, Murray JE. Renal homotransplantation in identical twins. Surg Forum. 1956;6:432–6.
60. Merrill JP, Murray JE, Harrison JH, Friedman EA, Dealy JB, Jr, Dammin GJ. Successful homotranplantation of the kidney between non-identical twins. N Eng J Med. 1960;262:1251–60.
61. Murray JE, Wilson RE, Tilney NL, Merrill JP, Cooper WC, Birtch AG, Carpenter CB, Hager EB, Dammin GJ, Harrison JH. Five years' experience in renal transplantation with immunosuppressive drugs: survival, function, complications, and the role of lymphocyte depletion by thoracic duct fistula. Ann Surg. 1968;168:416–35.
62. Starzl TE, Groth CG, Brettschneider L, Penn I, Fulginiti VA, Moon JB, Blanchard H, Martin AJ, Jr., Porter KA. Orthotopic homotransplantation of the human liver. Ann Surg. 1968;168:392–415.
63. Landsteiner K. Ueber Agglutinationserscheinungen normalen menschlichen Blutes. Wiener Klinische Wochenschrift. 1901;14:1132–4.
64. Crile G. I. The technique of direct transfusion of blood. Ann Surg. 1907;46:329–32.
65. Kalk H. Erfahrungen mit der Laparoskopie. Z Klin Med. 1929;111:303–48.
66. Muhe E. [Laparoscopic cholecystectomy—late results]. Langenbecks Arch Chir Suppl Kongressbd. 1991:416–23.
67. Lepor H. Status of radical prostatectomy in 2009; Is there medical evidence to justify the robotic approach? Rev Urol. 2009;11:61–70.
68. Kohn LT, Corrigan JM, Donaldson MS. To err is human: Building a safer health system. Washingon, DC: National Academy Press (Institute of Medicine); 2000.

A History of Women in American Anesthesiology

16

Selma Harrison Calmes

Summary

Women came slowly to medicine and anesthesia. The first modern woman physician, Elizabeth Blackwell, received her degree in 1849. The University of Zurich Medical School enrolled women in 1867. To increase their opportunities, American women founded 17 medical schools and 7 hospitals in the 19th century, but the move to scientific medicine prompted by the Flexner Report caused closure of all but one after 1910. Men avoided anesthesia because it offered minimal pay and status in the 19th century, but that presented an opening for women such as Herb in Chicago and Botsford in San Francisco at the turn of the century. In 1916, women constituted 19% of the American Association of Anesthetists (AAA) membership, but only 3.6% of physicians were women.

American women physicians were rejected for service as regular officers in both World Wars. In 1920, 3 women chaired anesthesia departments, and the first anesthesia resident, Mary Ross, completed training at the University of Iowa in 1923. Between World Wars, men were favored over women for internships and residencies. Only 4% to 5% of physicians were women. Waters established his residency program in anesthesia at the University of Wisconsin in 1927. Of his first 6 trainees, 3 were women, and one, Apgar, published her eponymous Score, in 1953. Marx entered anesthesia in the late 1930s, becoming the "Mother of Obstetric Anesthesia."

The Armed Forces in World War II drafted male physicians into anesthesia, many finding that they liked it, leading to competition with females after the war. Industry provided free health insurance during World War II, making anesthesia financially attractive, and further increasing competition from males. And then the tide slowly changed, equalizing the competition. Title IX of the 1972 Higher Education Act banned discrimination in admissions. Female medical students increased from 824 in 1964–65, to 1,295 in 1970–71 and 3,392 in 1974–75. In 2000, 27% of residents in anesthesia were females, but in 2010, 38%.

In 2004, 5 of the 7 major medical specialty organizations (not anesthesia) had female presidents. The ASA's only woman president, Stephenson, served in 1991, but the President elect for 2013 is Jane Fitch. In the 1980s, 6.5% of female anesthesiology faculty, but 17.7% of male faculty, were full professors, a difference not materially changed in the 2000s. Comparing the 2000s to the 1980s, the number of female American Board of Anesthesiology examiners increased. By 2010 the number of female Directors of the Board had increased to 3/12. Women became editors of modern anesthesia journals in 1980 (*Anesthesia and Analgesia*) and 1987 (*Anesthesiology*). By 2011, 4 were editors at Anesthesia and Analgesia and 2 at Anesthesiology. In 2010, women chaired anesthesia departments at more than a dozen prestigious medical schools. One became dean at the University of Iowa in 2012. This US-focused history had its counterpart in other developed countries, particularly the UK and Australia where women sometimes played greater and earlier roles in governance of anesthesia than did women in the US.

Introduction

No women were physicians when surgical anesthesia was demonstrated in 1846, and few existed as anesthesiology initially developed. By the 20th century however, lack of manpower combined with acceptance of female anesthetists provided an opening that women physicians filled. They be-

came leaders; three women served as presidents of national anesthesia organizations from 1922–1930, when women could not belong to many specialty societies. In 2013, more women than men graduated as physicians, and although an increased number now selected anesthesia, proportionately fewer women became leaders. This story illustrates how history and society affected the place of women in the practice of medicine and anesthesiology. The chapter focuses on the US, because in the modern era, women first became physicians in the US, and because more information documents women's activities in anesthesiology.

S. H. Calmes (✉)
The David Geffen School of Medicine at UCLA,
Los Angeles, CA, USA
e-mail: shcmd@ucla.edu

E. I Eger II et al. (eds.), *The Wondrous Story of Anesthesia*, DOI 10.1007/978-1-4614-8441-7_16, © Edmond I Eger, MD 2014

A Brief History of Women in Medicine

In 2700 BCE, Egyptian Merit Ptah is said to be the earliest recorded woman physician. For the most part, universities excluded women, although some mediaeval Italian universities trained female physicians. The first modern woman to be awarded a medical degree, US citizen Elizabeth Blackwell (1821–1910), received her degree, in 1849 after a long and difficult struggle [1]. This set the pattern for future women in medicine [2]. Women battled against perceptions of lesser physical and mental competence (smaller brain size), difficulties during menstruation, and conflicts with their traditional roles as wives and mothers. In the 19th century, women felt that they might improve a profession that applied foolish remedies such as bleeding and purging. "Why not *prevent* disease?"

Women also entered medicine for economic reasons; medicine offered an alternative to a career as a poorly paid teacher, their other major option. Early women physicians were usually unmarried, and they paid for their medical education by teaching. Women could pursue medicine as a career because the youthful US lacked the rigid traditions of European medicine [3]. Medical schools, particularly the many marginal ones, in mid-19th century America had lax admissions policies. It was also easy to establish a medical school. American women founded 17 medical schools and 7 hospitals in the 19th century, providing opportunities for women in medical education that included internships, which became important after the turn of the century [2]. Because these schools and hospitals facilitated the entry of women into medicine, they also facilitated women physicians' entry into anesthesia. There was geographic skewing of the distribution of women physician anesthetists, California having the most through the 1930s, in no small part because of Mary Botsford (1865–1939), who pioneered the development of anesthesia in the San Francisco Bay Area from 1910 to 1930 [4].

The opportunities for women in America's medical institutions became known worldwide, and hundreds came to the US for medical training. Such competition may have motivated changes in Europe. In 1867, the University of Zurich became the first modern European school to enroll female medical students. L'École de Médicine in Paris followed in 1868. Such openings prompted some American women to train in the scientifically superior European schools [3].

Regardless of the school's location, women studying medicine were isolated. Separate lectures for women and men were common in "coeducational" schools, as was social segregation [3]. Women were usually unable to join medical societies. Their professional lives *had* to center on the women's medical institutions where they had studied.

The Flexner Report of 1910 affected all medical schools and was a crucial factor leading to subsequent closure of all but one of the women's medical schools (the Woman's

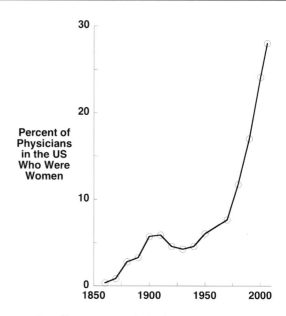

Fig. 16.1 Overall we see two periods of rapid growth in women physicians as a percentage of the total number of physicians. The first began in the latter part of the nineteenth century and peaked at approximately 1910. The plateau lasted for a half century. Growth increased dramatically with the evolution of the feminist and civil rights movements in the 1960s

Medical College of Philadelphia, now Drexel University College of Medicine, survived) [2]. This report documented the deficiencies of existing medical schools, prompting the transformation of American medical training into the present science-based institutions. Most women's medical schools could not provide the laboratories, equipment (such as microscopes), or faculty necessary to teach scientific medicine. Few of the remaining medical schools accepted women, and the proportion of women physicians decreased from 6.0 % of the physician population in 1910, to 4.4 % in 1930 and only returned to 6.1 % in 1950 (Fig. 16.1) [2]. During this time, anesthesiology became a specialty. One of the editors of this book (LJS) remembers 9 women in a University of Michigan class of 209 in 1961.

1846 to the End of World War I

The Suitability of Women for Anesthesia

Medical specialization languished until the end of the 19th century, and anesthesia offered minimal attraction. Few operations were done, and anesthetic agents hadn't changed in a half century. In the US almost anyone (untrained physicians, nurses, medical students, and orderlies) could—and did—give anesthesia. Because anesthesia seemed like a nurse's job, it had low status and reimbursement was poor. It was difficult therefore, to interest physicians in anesthesia. These issues were summed up in the discussion after a 1918 talk on professional anesthesia by Ralph Waters (1883–1979), who would lead the move to modern anesthesia. An audience member stated:

"If you get a nurse to give an anesthetic, there is really no inducement for a doctor to make a specialty of it…The reason we have not better men or a larger number of good men giving general anesthetics is that we do not see that they are properly paid." He added: "I think the main reason that we are having nurses give anesthetics…is the question of money…I am going to pay out anywhere from one hundred to one hundred and fifty dollars a month for anesthesia (by physicians), and if I can hire a girl who will keep my instruments clean, and who will do my office book-keeping, work, etc (as well as give anesthesia), I can get her for about sixty-odd dollars a month." [5]

Some surgeons thought that women physicians combined the desirable characteristics of nurses—submissiveness and acceptance of lower pay—with the medical knowledge needed to improve surgical outcomes. Albert Ochsner (1861–1943) wrote in his 1920 surgical text that: "The best anesthesias are conducted by women at the present time, because it is possible to select women with the highest degree of intelligence and judgment for this work, while medical men possessing these qualities can almost never be induced to elect anesthesia as a specialty [6]."

It gets worse. Hugh Cabot, Professor of Surgery at the University of Michigan, and Surgeon-in-Chief at University Hospital, Ann Arbor, Michigan, closed the 1927 American Surgical Association meeting with

"I would lay particular stress upon the importance of the selection of (anesthetists). They should always be good-looking… Half of the anesthetic effect, when no anesthesia is used, depends upon the appearance of the anesthetist…." [7]

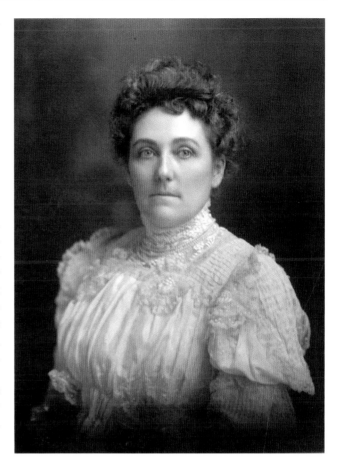

Fig. 16.2 Isabella Herb was the first woman physician known to specialize in anesthesia. She began her career in 1897 and was the first physician anesthetist at the Mayo Clinic, 1899–1904. (Courtesy of the Olmstead County Historical Society, Rochester, MN.)

The First Women Physician Anesthetists

Two women physicians, Isabella Herb (1863–1943) (Fig. 16.2) and Mary Botsford (1865–1939) (Fig. 16.3), committed themselves to anesthesia in the 1890s. Botsford graduated in 1897 from the coeducational Medical Department of the University of California (now the University of California at San Francisco, UCSF), one of 8 women in a class of 59 [8]. She then studied at the Children's Hospital of San Francisco (CHSF) founded by women physicians in 1875 [5], first as one of 6 interns, and later as a resident [9]. By 1898, she held the title of Anesthetist [10].

Herb graduated in 1892 from the Woman's Medical College of Chicago. She interned at the Mary Thompson Hospital (founded in 1865 by women physicians), remaining there in various roles, including Superintendent, until 1897 when she moved to the Augustana Hospital in Chicago to practice anesthesia and pathology [11]. The hospital's surgeon was Oschner, as noted above, an advocate for female anesthetists. By 1900, 13.0 % of Chicago's physicians and 13.8 % of San Francisco's physicians were female, training or practicing at

the women's hospitals. Nationally, only 5.6 % of physicians were female [2].

As a student rotating to San Francisco's City and County Hospital (the medical school did not have its own hospital then), Botsford was appalled by the illness that patients suffered with chloroform. Interning at CHSF, she saw equally bad results with ether. A close friend wrote:

"…Botsford…followed me in the surgical service (at CHSF)… She saw patients return from the operating room so saturated from ether that they were ill for a week from the effect of the anesthetic. She told one of the surgeons that she was going to specialize in anesthesia. He replied that she was crazy and could never make a success of it." [12]

Few operations were done then. For example, CHSF did only 3 operations in December 1903 and 4 the following month [13]. Both women pursued other medical work to survive. Herb practiced pathology, and Botsford maintained a general medical practice [14]. Herb was a widow [11], and Botsford separated from her physician-husband before entering medical school. Until her death, Botsford supported her niece and grand-niece [15].

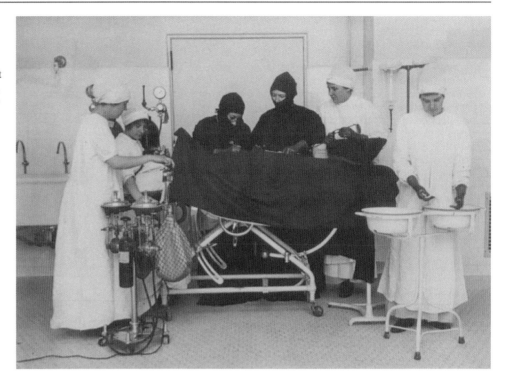

Fig. 16.3 Mary Botsford, the second known woman physician specializing in anesthesia, at left, instructing an intern at CHSF. (Courtesy of The Bancroft Library, University of California, Berkeley. Call number 1989.058-pic ctn 1)

Herb began her anesthesia career at the Augustana Hospital in 1897, working with Lawrence Prince (1859–1946), a pioneer of open drop ether and chloroform. She was also the hospital's pathologist [11]. She probably earned no income from giving anesthesia because Augustana Hospital was a charitable institution [16]. Similarly, Botsford earned no anesthesia fees from her first five years in practice [12].

Herb published the first paper on anesthesia by a woman physician in 1898 [17]. In 1899, she became the first physician anesthetist (and the pathologist) at the Mayo Clinic. She left anesthesia to pursue pathology in 1904, studying in Europe and conducting research in Chicago, but in 1909 she was appointed chief anesthetist at Presbyterian Hospital and Rush Medical College in Chicago. Arthur Bevan, another surgeon-advocate for women physicians in anesthesia, was chief of surgery. Herb was the first woman on the medical school faculty [11].

No one taught Botsford anesthesia. Making careful observations, she learned by herself what was safe and effective. In 1910, Botsford became "Assistant in Surgery" (responsible for anesthesia) at the new UCSF hospital in San Francisco [18], the city's only officially appointed anesthetist. This, the most prominent hospital in the state, had a single operating room. She received no salary from her academic position, but did develop a lucrative practice among San Francisco's elite at a nearby private hospital. She also continued as anesthetist at CHSF. Unlike many at that time, she recognized the need to add supplemental oxygen to nitrous oxide, and specialized in nitrous oxide-oxygen anesthesia

[19]. She published her first article, on nitrous oxide-oxygen anesthesia, in 1916 [20].

Internships became more important, but after 1900 few hospitals accepted women interns, channeling female medical graduates into the few hospitals that did, primarily the women's hospitals. Working in such institutions, in a specialty "suitable" for women, Herb and Botsford attracted these interns. After anesthesia training with Herb in Chicago, women interns later assumed faculty positions at Rush and the University of Chicago. Anesthesia training with Botsford led interns to positions at UCSF, Stanford, or private hospitals in the San Francisco Bay Area. Stanford, then Cooper Medical School, had a Botsford-trained physician anesthetist, Caroline Palmer (1867–1947), from 1909 [21]. By the 1920s, Botsford or Palmer had trained women physician anesthetists for all but one of the major San Francisco Bay Area hospitals [4]. Herb's and Botsford's efforts attracted a disproportionately large number of women physician anesthetists to Chicago and San Francisco, a skewing of geographic distribution that continued until the 1940s (Fig. 16.4) [4].

Herb and Botsford were also active in the development of local, state, and national anesthesia societies. In 1922, Botsford led the effort to found the Anesthesia Section of the California Medical Association, and was the first president. She successfully lobbied for a state law requiring all interns to learn anesthesia [4]. In 1922, Herb became president of the first nationwide anesthesia society, the American Association of Anesthetists (AAA, founded in 1912 by Francis McMechan) [11]. and in 1930, Botsford was president of the Associated Anesthetists of the United States and Canada, an

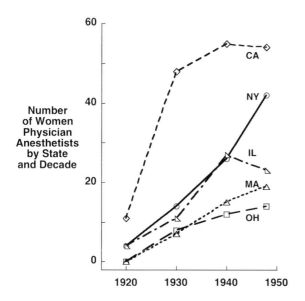

Fig. 16.4 The number of women physician anesthetists increased in the figured states after World War I. Note that Herb taught in Chicago and Botsford in San Francisco

organization that evolved from the AAA [4]. Eleanor Seymour (1877–1961) of Los Angeles, was another woman AAA president, in 1922–23 [22]. A 1903 University of Southern California medical graduate, Seymour interned at CHSF in 1903–1904, where she would have been influenced by Botsford. Like Herb, she had also practiced pathology [23]. She led a bitter legal fight in California against nurse anesthetists, and organized the first anesthesia society in Los Angeles, the Southern California Society of Anesthetists [24, 25].

Herb and Botsford were widely known, respected, and a little feared. When considering a move from Indiana to California in 1928, Arthur Guedel (1883–1956) asked Ralph Waters if he should go to Los Angeles or San Francisco. Waters replied,

> "Now about San Francisco. I can give you a bit of dope. San Francisco and all the territory around is the private property of Botsford. It's female and doubtless will remain so, but as I understand it, extremely well handled. She is a bit of a czar on her throne at least that is the impression I have…make friends (but) don't try to invade her territory." [26]

Guedel wisely went to Los Angeles.

The Women of the First Anesthesia Organization [27]

A woman physician, Emilie (also Amelia) Schirmer (1872–1951) of Brooklyn, was present in 1905, at the first general meeting in Brooklyn of the Long Island Society of Anesthetists (LISA), the predecessor of the present American Society of Anesthesiologists (ASA). Schirmer practiced pathology as well as anesthesia until the late 1940s. Four more women joined LISA early enough to be Charter Members. All five graduated from a women's medical college or trained at a

women's hospital and then practiced at a women's medical institution. Reflecting the America of that time, all were immigrants (two from Germany, and one each from Austria, Sweden and England). Three were married.

As evidenced by their accomplishments, these were inquisitive and talented, self-taught women. In 1923, 6 months after the discovery of ethylene's anesthetic properties, Schirmer gave a clinical demonstration of ethylene anesthesia at a joint meeting of East Coast anesthesia societies. Charter member Alma Vedin (1863–1925), was the first female officer of LISA, elected to the Executive Committee in 1918 and later serving as vice president—the first woman officer of a professional anesthesia society. She graduated in 1899 from the Women's Medical College of the New York Infirmary (NYI), founded by Elizabeth Blackwell, the first modern woman physician. She served as anesthetist at the NYI and, after 1915, at the New York Hospital. That year, she reported 115 cases of endotracheal anesthesia, including thoracic cases [28], at a time when endotracheal anesthesia was seldom used and chest surgery was rare. How she learned these advanced anesthetic techniques is unknown.

The Women Physician Anesthetists of World War I

As measured by membership in professional anesthesia organizations, increasing numbers of woman physicians practiced anesthesia in the decades before World War I. The need to pay membership dues endorsed their commitment to professional anesthesia. Other women physicians also practiced anesthesia, therefore numbers from membership directories probably underestimate the actual number of female physician anesthetists. The American Medical Association's (AMA) annual directories of physicians began recording who was an AAA member in 1914, when 8 women were AAA members, 9% of AAA membership. Two years later, 15 women were members, 19% of AAA membership [29]. In 1915, only 3.6% of all physicians were women [30]. These data illustrate the relative popularity of anesthesia for women physicians, a popularity confirmed by a survey undertaken by the Council of National Defense's Committee on Women Physicians, in preparation for World War I. Among women, only gynecology was more popular than anesthesia [31].

World War I revealed an ambivalence concerning recruitment of women physician anesthetists. By 1916, the Army and the Red Cross had organized base hospitals centered at major university hospitals where the staff worked together daily. Surgical units, with nurse or physician anesthetists, were the core of these base hospitals. When the US entered the war in April, 1917, 33 base hospitals were nearly ready; 6 sailed for Europe that month [32]. However, there were no physician anesthetists in the Army [33]. Although women physicians wanted to serve, the Army's Judge Advocate

General ruled in August 1917 that the term "citizens," used in 1916 legislation to expand the Army Medical Corps, did not include women. Because they could not vote, they were not considered to be citizens, and because they were not citizens, women could not be commissioned medical officers [31].

Increasing casualties made the Army desperate for anesthetists. Male physician anesthetists were still rare. Nurses were trained in anesthesia as rapidly as possible, but these efforts were insufficient. In March 1918, the Army reconsidered its position, and women physician anesthetists were offered employment as "contract surgeons," medical specialists hired temporarily. This lowly position had no rank or benefits, no command authority and the pay of a first lieutenant [31].

The Army advertised that: "women between the ages of 23 and 45, born in the United States, who are graduates of reputable medical schools and who are skilled in the administration of anaesthesia, are eligible for employment...." Recruitment was actually broader. If not trained already, women physicians could be sent to "an intensive course of instruction in the administration of anesthetics [34]." Only five of the 16 women physician anesthetists recruited had practiced anesthesia before the war. Only 2 were sent for training, one to the Mayo Clinic and the other to an Army general hospital. Eleven went overseas, at least 2 to forward combat units. Anesthetists were the only female contract surgeons sent overseas [31].

Anne Tjomsland (1880–1968) and Frances Haines (1882–1966) were the first female physician anesthetists to go overseas, both with units formed in 1916: Tjomsland for Bellevue's Base Hospital No. 1 and Haines for Rush-Presbyterian's Base Hospital No. 13. Both of these essential members of their units were refused commissions because they were female. Their Base Hospitals' chief surgeons battled Army bureaucracy to no avail, and both women had to sign on as contract surgeons [31].

There is little information on Tjomsland, but Haines wrote of her war-time experiences. A 1913 graduate of the University of Nebraska College of Medicine, she interned at Chicago's Mary Thompson Hospital and became an anesthetist in Herb's department in 1916 [35]. Arriving in France on June 10, 1918, she oversaw anesthesia at a 1,500 bed hospital in Limoges [36]. Ether was in short supply and to conserve the agent, she developed a technique that used its analgesic effects only, something not normally done at the time. This was done with open drop ether, demonstrating Haines' considerable skill:

> "One night in Limoges at 10 PM, I began the anesthetic for the removal of the entire left lung of a soldier whose large arteries, wounded in battle, bled whenever the sterile gauze packing was even partially removed. His heart kept actively beating, right in the field of operation. Had he taken one sudden deep breath, the surgeons' instruments could have slipped and punctured more blood vessels. I kept the patient breathing quietly and smoothly throughout the operation. The surgeons commended me. The patient recovered."

Haines also trained enlisted men and corpsmen to give anesthesia. She served for 16 months as a contract surgeon, the second-longest serving female contract surgeon [31]. Haines published her anesthesia experiences in collections of World War I anesthesia articles [37]. Reports in the medical women's literature [38]. and testimony at Congressional hearings [39] document the expertise of these female physician anesthetists.

After her return, Haines practiced anesthesia in Chicago. She served as president of the Mid-Western Association of Anesthetists in 1926 [40]. Poor health ended her anesthesia practice, and a 1964 radio show on her effort to get an Army pension described a surreal tragedy:

> "...Dr. Haines still maintains a tiny, cramped office in downtown Chicago, where, if she's lucky, she may treat two patients a day. Often she earns as little as a dollar a day. These small fees are hardly worth her making the long bus trip from her small north side apartment each day. But she has no choice. If she doesn't, she will starve."

Her Army pension was denied, and she died destitute in 1966 [41].

Finally convinced of women physician anesthetists' usefulness, the Army established Anesthetic Unit I in September 1918, the only time such a unit title was used. Once overseas, its 7 women physician anesthetists and 2 male medical officers relieved anesthesia staff in various units, especially Base Hospital No. 15 stationed in the Argonne [31].

On home territory, the women contract surgeons were assigned to various Army hospitals, where they gave anesthesia and taught others (primarily nurses) to give anesthesia. Botsford served as a contract surgeon at San Francisco's Letterman Army Hospital, in addition to teaching anesthesia at the Medical Department of the University of California [42]. This assignment allowed her to continue her private practice and provide for her two dependents. Another woman physician, Rose Bowers of Indiana, was ordered "to report to the Surgical Unit as Anesthetist" at Camp Grant in Rockford, Illinois, just as the 1918 influenza epidemic hit. Within 6 days, the number of hospital beds increased from 610 to 4,102. All military functions ceased, and Bowers spent the rest of the war caring for patients with influenza [43].

World War I provided opportunities for the women physician anesthetists to prove their skills, and they did. Many of these women continued in anesthesia after the war.

1920 to World War II

World War I opened a 19 month window of opportunities for American women to enter medical school and pursue internships, opportunities that lessened with the end of the war. Several other factors also decreased the number of women physicians after the war. American medical schools decreased from 166 in 1904, to 76 by 1930, as marginal schools closed in the accelerating move to scientific medicine. Most schools imposed a quota, usually 5% or less, for women and minorities such as Jews and African Americans. Admission increasingly required baccalaureate degrees, and the cost of medical education increased, making it unaffordable for many women. In 1920, 5.0% of physicians were women; by 1930, this had decreased to 4.4% (Fig. 16.1). When World War II began, the US had 7,708 women physicians, fewer than in 1910 [44] And women had trouble obtaining the increasingly required internships. In 1921, 40 of 482 AMA approved hospitals accepted women interns. In the 1930s, 250 female medical graduates competed annually for the 185 internships open to women, while 4,844 male graduates competed for 6,154 positions [30].

Discouraging though this inter-war period was for most women physicians, it seemed attractive for women physician anesthetists. Women were there at the founding of anesthetic institutions and served as leaders in those institutions. Three chaired anesthesia departments in 1920: Herb at Rush, Botsford at UCSF, and her trainee Palmer at Stanford, and these important leaders influenced the geographic distribution of women physician anesthetists, as previously noted (Fig. 16.4). But women physician anesthetists spread throughout the country, appearing in smaller towns, from Oregon to Texas to New York [45].

One change having little immediate effect was passage of the 19th amendment to the Constitution of the US on August 26, 1920, giving women the right to vote. In 1918, the Senate refused to pass the amendment, but women began feeling their power. The National Woman's Party responded by attacking anti-suffrage Senators, suggesting that they should not be re-elected. In 1919, the Senate passed the amendment by 56 votes to 25.

First Resident: Mary Ross of Iowa

Anesthesia residencies as we know them today did not officially exist until 1927, but some physicians sought training in anesthesia. The year after her 1922 medical school graduation from the University of Iowa, Mary Ross (later Gillespie, 1895–1980) trained in anesthesia with Louis Harding (1866–1959), the self-taught physician in charge of anesthesia at Iowa. She received a Certificate of Residency Training in Anesthesia in 1923. This training is considered to be the first formal residency in anesthesia [46].

Dorothy Diamond (also spelled Dimond) (1896–1975), a 1922 medical graduate of the University of Minnesota, interned in 1922–1923 at CHSF, where she would have been taught by Botsford [47]. In 1924–1926, she followed Ross' example of training with Harding. Diamond replaced Harding in 1930 as chief of anesthesia at Iowa, until September 1937. Stuart Cullen, assumed the chair (a Division of Surgery) at Iowa in 1938 [46].

Residents: The Women of Wisconsin

Ralph Waters, considered the father of academic anesthesia in the US, began the residency in anesthesia at the University of Wisconsin (UW) in 1927. This pivotal residency, directly or through its heirs, trained most future leaders of academic anesthesia in the US and several other countries. In the years Waters reigned, women made up 16.4 percent of the anesthesiology residents, a percent exceeded only by women in pediatrics (Fig. 16.5). Waters' first 2 trainees were women, and 3 of the first 6 were women. At the time, this differed from other UW departments which had nearly all male trainees, except for pediatrics [48]. The first 2 anesthesia trainees were single but married while in practice, and could not be traced further in anesthesia [49]. As then expected, they probably stopped practice after marrying.

The third woman trainee, Martha Kohl (1901–1985), illustrates the difficulties then faced by married professional women. She was accepted because of an outstanding recommendation from Waters' close friend, pharmacologist Chauncey Leake (1896–1978), who had recently moved from Madison to San Francisco to chair the pharmacology department at UCSF. After 2 years at the University of Wisconsin medical school, Kohl got a masters' degree in pharmacology working under Leake [50]. She then transferred to Rush in Chicago for her remaining years of medical school and her internship. (Internship was required at Rush before the MD was granted [51].) She wrote to Waters to say that, she was "on the anesthesia service as an intern at Presbyterian Hospital under the direction of Dr. Isabella Herb for four and a half months. I have arranged for at least a month of work in my present internship (at CHSF) in anesthesia under the direction of Dr. Mary Botsford… [52]." She obtained her MD in 1931 [51].

Leake's recommendation also indicated that Kohl had a husband and a child, something not mentioned in Kohl's own letter. She reached Madison on April 4, 1931, but left on July 1, 1932. Writing to Leake in June 1932, Waters observed "she is somewhat uncertain about her family affairs…" and asked if there were opportunities for Kohl in San Francisco [53]. Leake reported that Botsford had 3 good opportunities [54], but Kohl went instead to Eau de Clair, Wisconsin, to general practice, some anesthesia and lots of obstetrics [55]. She had a second baby in November, 1933 [56]. She disappeared from anesthesia directories after 1935. The 1940 AMA directory of physicians listed her as specializing in obstetrics and gynecology [57]. She was licensed in California in 1944, practicing general medicine [58] and divorced her husband in 1945 [56].

A 1942 letter, gave Waters' impression of Kohl:

"…during her service I was considerably disappointed in Leake (for his recommendation). She is good-looking and has brains and is capable, but she proved to be extremely nervous and easily upset…She, however, did a fairly good year's work in

Fig. 16.5 Female and total residents in various specialties at the University of Wisconsin Medical School from 1927 through 1949

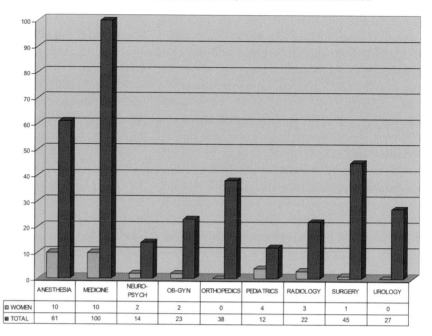

FEMALE AND TOTAL RESIDENTS 1927-1949, U. OF WISCONSIN MEDICAL SCHOOL

	ANESTHESIA	MEDICINE	NEURO-PSYCH	OB-GYN	ORTHOPEDICS	PEDIATRICS	RADIOLOGY	SURGERY	UROLOGY
WOMEN	10	10	2	2	0	4	3	1	0
TOTAL	61	100	14	23	38	12	22	45	27

spite of physical handicaps…the last time I saw her, she said her husband was in the military service and the care of the children was pretty much up to her…" He also noted she was found to have "some disturbance of the internal secretions and got better with treatment." [55]

Speaking of Kohl again, Waters revealed his aversion to women, including competent women:

"I have a woman resident who has been with me a year and a half who, as women go, is as good as any. Neither you nor I like women, so I presume you would not consider her. She knows, however, inhalation anesthesia in all its phases…with the possible exception of endotracheal work. She can however, do endo and work reasonably well. She can take care of major blocks, has done hundreds of spinals and a significant number of transacrals. She likes to teach, and I think is a good teacher. The only serious objection I have to her is that she is a woman…." [59]

These first 3 female residents were an inauspicious start for the Wisconsin department, failing to elevate Waters' attitude towards medical women. In a letter to Guedel, he wrote "…M.D. ladies…are useless in the profession. I am through with them. Ladies are nice socially but not (as) professionals [60]." Another 5 years passed before a fourth woman trainee came to Madison. Fortunately, she was outstanding.

Virginia Apgar

Virginia Apgar (1909–1974), a unique, charming and charismatic character became America's best-known anesthesiologist, male or female (Fig. 16.6). A 1933 graduate of Columbia University's medical school, she wanted to be a

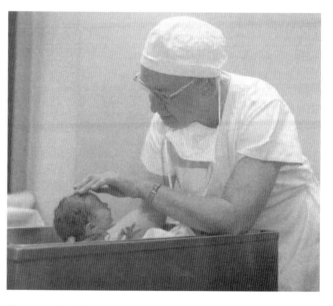

Fig. 16.6 Anesthesiologist Virginia Apgar attends one of her patients. Her Score ("the Apgar"), published in 1953, easily identified which newborns needed resuscitation. (From National Library of Medicine, http://profiles.nlm.nih.gov/ps/retrieve/Narrative/CP/p-visuals/true)

surgeon. But Alan Whipple, chair of surgery at Columbia wanted medical anesthesia at Columbia (only nurse anesthetists gave anesthesia at Columbia then). He saw Apgar as the best candidate to accomplish this, and persuaded her of the wisdom of that course. Apgar wrote to Francis McMechan (1879–1939) (then organizing national and regional anesthesia societies), asking about places to train [61]. McMechan wrote to Waters: "She seems to be an unusually ambitious person and might prove to be an excellent find for the specialty irrespective of her sex. Do what you can for her [62]." She stayed at Columbia, working with nurse anesthetists during the 2 ½ years it took her to find anesthesia training. She finally came to the University of Wisconsin as a "visitor," arriving on January 2, 1937 [63]. ("Visitors" were common then; only a few 3-year "resident" positions with room and board were available because of limited state budgets caused by the Great Depression).

Apgar faced the usual problem of housing for women physicians. House staff were poorly paid (Eger remembers getting $25 per month as an intern in 1955), and free room and board made survival possible. Lack of housing was used to explain the rejection of women house staff, although plenty of housing seemed available for nurses. Apgar initially slept in Waters' office for 2 weeks and, after moving several times, found a room in the maids' quarters. She recorded in her diary of being excluded from dinners after anesthesia meetings: "Stag dinner—MAD!" [61] Botsford also recorded her anger at exclusion from similar events.

In September 1937, Apgar returned to New York City as a resident in the new Bellevue program under Emery Rovenstine (1895–1960). At this time, Waters sent his partially trained staff to Rovenstine, to help Rovenstine succeed in a difficult situation. Rovenstine, a Waters' trainee and former UW faculty member, had rejected Apgar for a training position in April 1936 [64]. Her training with Waters must have made her acceptable this time around. Apgar wrote to Waters as she ended her time at Bellevue, "Did a small bird tell me you are risking two positions on women this next year? I hope you will not be disappointed…please don't expect anything less of them and make them work like the devil, for there is nothing worse than a poor woman anesthetist [65]." Another woman physician, Mary Lou Byrd (later Cowan, 1911–1994), started residency at Bellevue as Apgar left, so Apgar's performance must have been satisfactory.

On 1 January 1938, Apgar became Director of the Division of Anesthesia, and Attending Anesthetist at Columbia. Beginning the difficult job of developing academic anesthesia, she followed Waters' plan, focusing first on medical student teaching, then clinical care, and lastly research. World War II imposed enormous difficulties. In spite of these, she attracted residents, wrote papers, and did research, some with surgeons [61].

Her first 3 residents were men, for she did not immediately want women, writing to Waters in 1938: "If you have any applications for residencies which you cannot use (not women yet) maybe they would like to get a breath of Madison in NYC [66]." She sought advice from Waters for years on the problems she faced as a prominent woman in this developing specialty [67].

Waters probably instigated Apgar's 1940 selection as treasurer of the American Society of Anesthetists (later the American Society of Anesthesiologists, or ASA), a position held from 1929 by the powerful but then ailing ASA founder, Paul Wood (1894–1963). Apgar contributed greatly to the stabilization of the fledgling ASA. The organization's finances were poorly managed; there was no budget, a non-standard method was used for accounting, dues collection was erratic, and the launch of the journal *Anesthesiology* threatened to financially overwhelm the organization. Despite conflicts with Paul Wood, Apgar solved these problems, placing the ASA and the journal on a sound financial basis. Although it was clear that she had done a good job as Treasurer, she was the last woman officer to hold a significant ASA position for 27 years [27].

In the mid-1940s, a crisis arose concerning the state of anesthesia research at Columbia. As at other institutions, clinical demands exceeded the capacities of the available staff, precluding a sustained research focus. Apgar searched for a vice-chair for research, but there were few suitable candidates who wanted to be only a vice-chair. Ultimately, Emanuel Papper (1915–2002) came from Bellevue in 1949 as chief of the division. He became chair of a free-standing department at Columbia in 1952. After a year's sabbatical leave and now freed from the burdens of administration, Apgar moved laterally into obstetric anesthesia, a neglected area in which she had always been interested [61].

A medical student asked the question at a casual breakfast in the hospital cafeteria: How do you evaluate a newborn baby? "Easy," Apgar said, and in a moment, wrote down the "Apgar Score". After testing for validity, it was published in 1953, becoming the world-wide method to evaluate how well newborns made the transition to extra-uterine life. The beauty and power of the Apgar Score was its simplicity; it could be determined easily and quickly, and required no fancy apparatus. She and her team documented that, contrary to previous thought, hypoxia and acidosis were abnormal after birth and should be treated. Low Apgar Scores meant hypoxia and acidosis and indicated a need for prompt resuscitation. Using the Apgar Score and other measures, they found that maternal and neonatal outcomes improved when regional rather than general anesthesia was used for delivery. Thus they began the move to regional anesthesia for obstetrics, incidentally comparing various methods of neonatal resuscitation [68].

In 1959, Apgar became director of the National Foundation's (previously the March of Dimes) new effort to decrease the incidence of birth defects, later becoming Vice President for Research at the Foundation [61]. Because of her work on newborns, many thought she was an obstetrician or pediatrician, not suspecting that she was an anesthesiologist. Efforts led by the American Academy of Pediatrics and its Neonatal Section resulted in release of a US postage stamp in her honor in 1994, a fitting acknowledgement because Apgar was a dedicated stamp collector [69]. Since 1975, the section has maintained an annual Virginia Apgar Award in Perinatal

Pediatrics. The ASA's Distinguished Service Award, its highest honor, was awarded to Apgar, the first woman to receive it, in 1961 [70].

Another Successful Woman of the 1930s, Gertie Marx

A new source of US women physicians appeared in the 1930s: Jews fleeing Nazi Germany. Anesthesia training positions were available, and many of these immigrants found anesthesia to be their only opportunity. This small group included another notable woman, Gertie (Gesti in German) Marx (1912–2004), the "Mother of Obstetric Anesthesia." At the University of Frankfurt in Germany in 1931, nearly 40% of her medical school classmates were women, however anti-democratic legislation in 1933 prohibited the graduation of Jews. She completed the final semester for her MD at the University of Bern in 1936, and moved to the US in 1937. She had trouble finding an internship because of the so-called housing problem for women physicians. She found a rotating internship at Beth Israel in New York City when a male intern candidate withdrew and a room then magically opened for her in the student nurses' quarters. Her first rotation was surgery, but this tiny person was too weak to hold retractors. She was instead assigned to anesthesia for the next 4 months, and loved it. Anesthesia became her life's work.

Her long career (she practiced until age 85) focused on obstetric anesthesia. She reintroduced spinal anesthesia for obstetrics, documented the problems and treatments of aorto-caval compression in pregnant patients, advocated epidural analgesia for labor, and in 1969 co-founded the Society for Obstetric Anesthesia and Perinatology [71]. She received the ASA Distinguished Service Award in 1988 [85], and is remembered with great affection as a terrifyingly effective teacher who, Eger says, could skewer you with a question.

Women Chairs End for a While

Apgar and Marx established themselves just as the early women physician anesthetist leaders finished their careers. Botsford retired in 1932 and died in 1939. Herb retired in 1941 and died in 1943. Francis McMechan, the pivotal leader of the AAA, who had strongly supported women physicians in anesthesia, died in 1939. These deaths marked the end of that early era of professional anesthesia. There were still remnants however, women chairs of anesthesia departments, such as they were at the time. In 1940, 4 women chairs were in place: Isabella Herb at Rush, Dorothy Wood (1894–1963) at UCSF (soon to be replaced by Waters-trained Hugh Hathaway), Huberta Livingstone (1905–1980), another Herb trainee, at the University of

Chicago and Virginia Apgar at Columbia. This was down from 5 in 1932: Herb at Rush, Botsford at UCSF, Palmer at Stanford, Livingstone at the University of Chicago and Diamond at Iowa. Julia Arrowood (later Mason, 1900–1984) would be appointed Acting Chair at the Massachusetts General Hospital (MGH) from 1943–45, replacing Henry Beecher (1904–1984), who left for war service [72]. Hers was a difficult position, as MGH epitomized the white male establishment hostile to women. Harvard admitted no female medical students until 1945, and MGH only rarely employed female faculty and interns.

One might argue that these women did not chair freestanding departments, separate from the surgery department, but that was the usual situation then. All but one or two early departments were divisions or sections in surgery. As late as 1965, 40% of US anesthesia "departments" were sections of a surgery department [73]. All the divisions/sections-departments headed by women were organized for didactic and clinical teaching of students, interns and, in some cases, residents. Men replaced the women chairs just before or during World War II, leaving only Apgar at Columbia until 1949, Huberta Livingstone at the University of Chicago until 1952, and Alice McNeal (1897–1964), another Herb trainee, at the University of Alabama at Birmingham from 1948 to 1961. Then there would be none until 1974, when Dola Thompson became chair at the University of Arkansas. A 1949 University of Arkansas medical graduate, she interned with her surgeon-husband at CHSF [74].

World War II

Despite the anticipated need for more anesthesiologists as World War II approached, many anesthesia residencies perversely excluded women. Residency lists by specialty published in the AMA's annual *Directory of Physicians* did not note exclusion by gender until 1940. That year, 33 hospitals were approved for an anesthesia residency, and only half accepted women applicants. New York City, a major center for academic anesthesia, had 8 approved residencies, but only 3 accepted women. All 3 approved California hospitals accepted women, likely reflecting Botsford's legacy. Women headed 3 residency programs (Stanford, the University of Chicago and Columbia) [75].

In preparation for war, the Army began ordering male medical officers to anesthesia training programs [76]. A Subcommittee on Anesthesia of the National Defense Council was formed in 1940, enlisting prominent male chairmen and ASA leaders. It developed short training courses and the necessary didactic material. In July 1942, the Surgeon General appointed Ralph Tovell as consultant in anesthesia for the European Theater [77]. As in World War I, base hospitals were organized at major hospitals, and these units planned to include their usual female physician anesthetists, for example Apgar at Columbia (Base Hospital No. 2) and Alice McNeal at Rush-Presbyterian in Chicago (Base Hospital No. 13). (McNeal was a 1921 Rush medical graduate working in Herb's department [78]) And, again as in World War I, women physicians would not be commissioned officers, only less-prestigious and less-paid contract surgeons. Surgeon General James Magee proclaimed in 1942 that "Women should not belong [31]."

Medical women fought back, their argument focusing on the importance of women physicians in anesthesia. Writing to Magee on February 18, 1942, Emily Barringer, president of the American Medical Women's Association (AMWA), used women physicians' status as anesthetists as the main reason to commission medical women:

> "The field of anaesthesia is one in which women physicians have excelled and a field where many of the objections to a woman physician do not apply. At the present moment there are two anaesthetists who have applied to your office for permission to serve in the Unit from the Hospital to which they are attached. I refer to Dr. Alice McNeal of Chicago and Dr. Virginia Apgar of New York City. And I am asking you to please be willing to change your mind and appoint these two women in the Medical Reserve Corps, and let them go forward with their Units...By appointing these two outstanding women you will hearten all the women physicians of America...." [79]

Magee resisted, and the units left without their physician anesthetists. The *New York Times* and *Time* magazine reported McNeal's situation to the public [80]. (It is not clear why Apgar's situation was not also publicized.) A nation-wide lobbying campaign for commissions for medical women, especially anesthetists, drew support from unions and charitable organizations. Success came on April 16, 1943, when President Roosevelt signed the Sparkman-Johnson Bill, allowing women physicians to serve in the Army and Navy Medical Corps [2].

However, only 4 women physicians became Army anesthesiologists in World War II, out of 76 women commissioned as medical officers. Two of the 4 attended the new war-time short courses in anesthesia at Bellevue and Walter Reed. The Navy commissioned 57 female physicians, but only 2 were anesthesiologists. Only 1 of the 6 women, Bernice Walters, continued in anesthesia after the war, becoming a career Navy medical officer. She was the first woman physician assigned to a Navy ship in war time, during the Korean War [31]. Another woman doctor, Louise DeVore, was in Honolulu visiting her sister when Pearl Harbor was bombed. She rushed to Tripler Army Hospital to help, and gave anesthesia there for the next nine months as a "United States civil service worker attached to military service." Despite requests from her commanding officer, she was never commissioned [81].

In contrast to World War I, the military did not recruit female anesthesiologists for World War II. Although the numbers of soldiers and sailors serving in the armed forces in World War II exceeded those in World War I by 4 to 5-fold, only 6 female anesthesiologists served in World War II, in contrast to 16 in World War I. One went overseas (to England), compared to 11 in World War I, when women were placed in front-line situations.

The war-time shortage of men increased medical school, internship and residency opportunities for the available women. In addition to filling slots in established residencies, women became the first residents in new anesthesia programs that were to develop modern, post-war anesthesiology. Margo Deming (1914–1998) was the first resident at the University of Pennsylvania (HUP), beginning in October, 1942 [82]. In 1946 she became the first chief of anesthesia at Children's Hospital of Philadelphia and was a pioneer in pediatric anesthesia. Later she was chief of anesthesia at Philadelphia General Hospital. She was never acknowledged by the department as the first HUP resident [83]. Three women became the first residents at Charity Hospital, New Orleans, in 1941 when John Adriani became chair [84].

World War II changed American anesthesiology to a recognized, prestigious, more affluent and desirable specialty [77]—that left women behind. Many of the men trained in anesthesia by the armed services sought further anesthesia training after the war and filled positions previously held by women. And, the aging, earlier generation of women physician anesthetists was not replaced because fewer women became medical students and physicians. As noted above, men moved into anesthesia after World War II because they had been pressed into service as anesthetists and discovered that they liked the specialty. In addition, the war prompted employers to provide health insurance (wage controls meant they could not attract workers with increased wages). Anesthesiologists got paid just like the professionals they were—he/she sent a large bill. And, the insurance company, not the patient, paid the bill.

1950–2000

The civil rights movement and the Vietnam War began in the mid-1950s and both escalated in the 1960s, affecting many areas of American society, particularly medicine. Laws and legal actions increased the flow of women into medical schools. They included: The Civil Rights Act of 1964 (banning discrimination on the basis of color, religion or national origin), a sex-discrimination law suit against every medical school in the country in 1970, an amendment to the Public Health Service Act (banning employment discrimination in medical and other health professional schools), and in 1972, passage of Title IX of the Higher Education Act (banning discrimination in admissions and salaries in institutions receiving federal funds). Within two years after Title IX passed, women's applications to medical schools tripled. The number of women accepted to medical schools increased from 824 in 1964–5, to 1,295 in 1970–71 and to 3,392 in 1974–75 [30].

In 1964, the year the Civil Rights Act passed, Apgar described women's status in anesthesiology in a pamphlet published by the American Medical Women's Association for women medical students. It documented the situation for women in anesthesiology as the 1960s began. The final section, "Anesthesiology as a Career for Women," revealed what today might be considered patronizing and sexist stereotypes:

> "women were ideally fitted for this specialty because tact and diplomacy are part of their nature (with a few exceptions). Team work comes easily. Manual dexterity is a by-product of those who are expert at sewing or knitting." Apgar discussed the potential problems for women of her time, especially those with children: "Married women anesthesiologists with children are not, in general, popular as members of a group practice. They are, of necessity, less dependable than men."

She noted that women did much of the low-prestige medical student and intern teaching and held few of the higher prestige administrative positions. She ended with statistics: Women constituted 11% of the ASA membership in 1963, but comprised only 6% of the physician population [85], implying that anesthesiology continued to be an attractive specialty for women.

Women medical students and graduates progressively increased in numbers without a parallel increase in acceptance. Ten years after Apgar's pamphlet, Mary Howell, the first woman serving as a dean at Harvard Medical School, wrote a pivotal article, "What medical schools teach about women [86]", on what was happening in medical schools and residencies. The article profoundly influenced women physicians, especially older ones. They realized, many for the first time, that the issues they faced did not have to happen. Memoirs by two women anesthesiologists documented the situation in anesthesiology from the 1960s [87, 88].

As the number of women medical graduates increased, the total number of women in anesthesiology residencies and practice increased, in part a "mass effect" from the increased total numbers of female physicians. From the time of Apgar's observation to the present, the percentage of anesthesiologists who were women has progressively increased (Fig. 16.7). However, on a percent basis (percent of total women physicians who are in anesthesia), entry of women into anesthesia has actually fallen [89]. To many, it seemed that there were no problems for women in anesthesiology, but that was not quite the case.

In the 1980s and 1990s, women anesthesiologists worked to correct the limited presence of women leaders in the organizations that represent anesthesiologists. In 1983, Anne Barlow, then medical director at Abbott Laboratories and president of the American Medical Women's Association

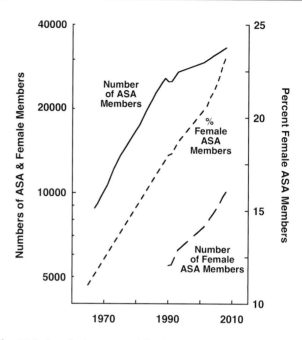

Fig. 16.7 Anesthesia as a specialty in the US grew progressively in the last half of the 20th century. Women anesthetists vigorously participated in this growth, females contributing an increasing percentage of the membership of the American Society of Anesthesiologists. (Data from ASA archives generously supplied by Karen Bieterman, MLIS, Manager of the Wood Library-Museum of Anesthesia, Park Ridge, IL.)

(AMWA), convened a group of 20 women anesthesiologist leaders during an ASA meeting. All agreed that a committee on women's issues was needed in the ASA and that male-specific organizational bylaws were a concern.

The next year, Caryl Guth of California surveyed other specialty organizations which were represented in the American Medical Association's House of Delegates and which were the same size as the ASA (then 18,000). All seven had committees on women's issues and had revised their bylaws to be gender neutral. The ASA had neither committees on women's issues nor gender neutral bylaws. Guth wrote to the ASA president-elect in 1986, requesting formation of an ad hoc committee on women and that the ASA sponsor a panel each year on women's issues at the ASA meeting. (Two informal sessions had already been held.) Both requests were denied [90].

In 1986, Wilkinson and Linde published the first analysis of women in academic anesthesiology [91]. This documented the lower academic advancement of women compared to men, and the lower board-certification rate. As Apgar noted 20 years earlier, women were more involved in teaching and patient care, with fewer research and administrative duties. There were 3 women academic chairs, less than there were in 1940.

At the 1986 House of Delegates meeting during the ASA meeting, Texan Betty Stephenson (1927–2006), presented a resolution to degender the language of the ASA's Bylaws.

ASA's Executive Secretary said it would be too burdensome to undertake, and the issue was referred to the bylaws committee (all male), asking, "Do the bylaws need to be degendered?" The answer was "no," reasoning that a footnote on page 1 of the bylaws stated that all masculine pronouns were to be considered gender-neutral. Stephenson became ASA president in 1991, the first and only woman ASA president. Other unsuccessful attempts were made, and the issue festered until ASA President Peter McDermott acted:

> "In October 1992, I became ASA president and issued an order degendering the language of ASA bylaws and other documents. It would have been embarrassing to have the issue debated by old white men. I also selected the first woman Rovenstine lecturer—Betty Bamforth—and established the women's forum at the ASA annual meeting that morphed into the Committee on Professional Diversity. My first partner, Kay Belton, sensitized me to gender discrimination, and my three daughters take no prisoners when it comes to asserting the importance of women." (Private communication to S. Calmes and E. Eger, July 28, 2010).

At the 1993 ASA meeting, the California delegation to the House of Delegates proposed formation of an ad hoc committee on women's issues, and it passed. The committee was formed in 1994 as the Committee on Women's Issues [90], renamed the Committee on Professional Diversity in 1996 [92]. It now focuses on all issues of diversity. No other committee or activity in the organization focuses on women.

2000 to the Present

A 2004 survey [27] found that 5 of the 7 major specialty organizations (not anesthesia) had a woman president that year. Two had women immediate past-presidents, and 1 had a woman president-elect. Only the American College of Surgeons had not had a woman president by 2004, but did in 2005–6 [93], and in 2011 has a second woman president [94]. The ASA's single woman president served in 1991, 20 years ago. However, Jane Fitch is the President-Elect for the ASA in 2013. As in Guth's 1984 survey, female contributions to ASA governance differed from that of other equivalent size specialty organizations, making the ASA unique among medical specialty organizations.

A 2008 article on the situation for women in academic anesthesiology [95], the second on this subject, compared 2006 data (the most recent available at that time) to 1985 data, and reported a mixed picture. The percentage of women anesthesiologists progressively increased (Fig. 16.7). Other areas of improvement included the number of female chairs (a 100 % increase in a decade) [96], an increased presence of female American Board of Anesthesiology examiners, and an increase in women serving in leadership positions in the increased number of subspecialty anesthesia organizations. These new subspecialty areas led to more opportunities for

women to be leaders. For example, women anesthesiologists have been important leaders in the move to out-patient surgery. Nine of the 22 presidents of the Society for Ambulatory Anesthesia, founded in 1974, have been women [97].

Women first joined editorial boards of the modern anesthesia journals in 1978 (*Anaesthesia and Intensive Care*), in 1980 (*Anesthesia & Analgesia*), and in 1987 (*Anesthesiology*). By 2011, 4 women were editors at Anesthesia and Analgesia and 2 at Anesthesiology. Nonetheless, a study of the gender of specialty and editorial boards reported found anesthesia was 1 of 6 specialties, out of 21, in which women were significantly under-represented compared to the number of women in the specialty [98].

Of female anesthesiology faculty in 2006, 6.5 % were full professors, compared with 17.7 % of male faculty. This had not changed significantly since 1986. No other specialty had a lower percentage of women full professors [95]. On the other hand, in 2010 women occupied many prestigious chairs in anesthesia, including those at the Massachusetts General Hospital (Harvard), University of Washington (becoming Dean at the University of Iowa in 2012), Columbia, UCLA, Yale, and SUNY Upstate Medical Center, as well as the University of Arkansas, University of Texas at Houston, Syracuse, Northwestern, University of Nebraska, University of Oklahoma, and New York Medical College. And in 2000, 27 % of residents were females; this increased to 38 % in 2010.

Contributions by Women Outside the US

The striking differences among countries in opportunities for women in medicine and the differences in the development of professional anesthesia among countries make a world-wide view of this subject difficult. Several consultants outside the US supplied their assessment of the leadership roles women have assumed outside the US. Information was difficult to collect, and some major countries, such as Japan and India, did not contribute. But the numbers in such roles appear to have been limited. As one consultant put it, "…considering the number of women practising anaesthesia in Europe at the present time, there have been very few women of note in the history of anaesthesia outside of the USA." To describe those who have made contributions, we have taken an exemplar approach, citing the contributions and when they were made.

1950–1980

Australia–New Zealand In 1935, Mary Burnell (Fig. 24.9; 1907–1996) became the first female member of the Australian Society of Anaesthetists. In 1953, she was elected president of the Society, the first woman attaining that position.

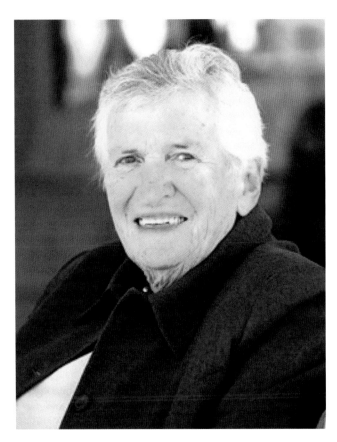

Fig. 16.8 Pat Mackay was a founding member of the Australian Patient Safety Foundation and President of the Australian Society of Anaesthetists from 1966–1968. She was Chairman of the Victorian Consultative Council on Anaesthetic Morbidity and Mortality from 1991 to 2005, and named 2001 Woman Doctor of the Year. (Courtesy of Dr. Patricia Macay, OAM)

She served as Dean of the Faculty of Anaesthetists, Royal Australasian College of Surgeons in 1966–67, the first female Dean of the Faculty. She had a sense of humor as indicated in a story told by Gwen Wilson: On one occasion,

> "after an hour's fruitless argument and nit-picking over a minor issue, a firm voice said, 'Mr Chairman, I've had a lot of committee experience and I know this committee is both tired and hungry. I propose we go to lunch'. The meeting broke up laughing, and on return after lunch, the matter was settled in less than five minutes."

Professor Tess Cramond (née Brophy) (1926 -) was the first female Fellow of the Australian Medical Association (AMA). She formed the Pain Clinic at the Royal Brisbane Hospital in 1967 where she directed the Multidisciplinary Pain Centre, now the Professor Tess Cramond Multidisciplinary Pain Centre. She was Dean of the Faculty of Anaesthetists of the Royal Australian College of Surgeons from 1972–3. From 1978 to 1993, she was Professor of Anaesthetics at the University of Queensland, the first female professor of anaesthesia in Australia. Accolades include an Order of the

British Empire (OBE) in 1977, the Gold Medal of the Faculty of Anaesthetists of the Royal Australian College of Surgeons in 1982, an Advance Australia Award in 1986, Officer of the Order of Australia (AO) in 1991, a Red Cross Long Service Award 1994, and the AMA Women in Medicine Award.

Neridah Dilworth established paediatric anaesthesia in Western Australia. She became the first Director of Anaesthetics at Princess Margaret Hospital for Children in December 1960, remaining Director until her retirement in 1992. With Peter Brine, she started the first ICU in Perth. "Physicians and the medical superintendent, who were unable to accept that anaesthetists could care appropriately for critically ill patients" opposed their efforts. The Australian Society of Anesthesiologists Western Australian Section named an award in her honour in 1988. She was awarded a Member of the Order of Australia (AM) in 1993, for services to medicine, particularly in paediatric anaesthesia, subsequently receiving the Australian Society of Anesthesiologists Medal.

While in London in the 1930s, Margaret (Greta) McClelland (1905–1990) documented the adverse interaction between trichlorethylene and soda lime. She returned to Melbourne in 1946, and became the first director of paediatric anaesthesia at the Royal Children's Hospital. She was President of the Australian Society of Anaesthetists in 1964, and received the OBE in 1975.

Patricia Mackay (nee Wilson; Fig. 16.8) was a founding member of the Australian Patient Safety Foundation. She was Secretary, then Treasurer of the Australian Society of Anaesthetists, becoming President from 1966 to 1968. In 1984, she was appointed Chairman and Head of the Department of Anaesthesia at the Royal Melbourne Hospital, a position she held until 1992. She established the first acute pain management unit in Victoria. She received the Order of Australia Medal (OAM) in the Queen's Birthday Honours on 9 June 2008, after serving as Chairman of the Victorian Consultative Council on Anaesthetic Mortality and Morbidity (VC-CAMM) from 1991 until 2005. As Chairman of VCCAMM she authored the 5th, 6th, 7th and 8th Reports of the Council (in 1993, 1996, 2000 and 2004). In 2000, she was awarded the Australian and New Zealand College of Anaesthetists Medal and shortly later received an award as the Woman Doctor of the Year by the Australian Medical Association.

Gwen Wilson (1916–1998) was one of the first female physicians to specialize in anesthesia in Australia. She has fame as a historian, having authored two books, one on the Australian Society of Anaesthetists, and another on anesthesia in Australia-New Zealand, "One Grand Chain". She was the first Laureate of the History of Anesthesia awarded by the Wood Library Museum [99].

Israel Florella Magora contributed to the development of intrathecal opioids for the management of pain, being a

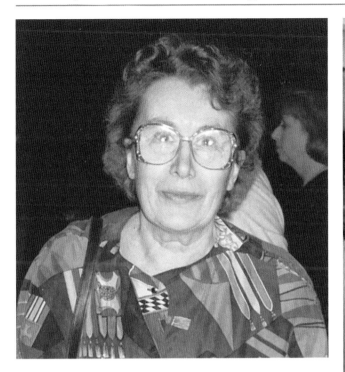

Fig. 16.9 Elena Damir was appointed chair of one of the first Russian departments of anesthesiology in 1959. She trained more than 15,000 students in the "Damir School" and was a member of the WFSA Executive for more than 20 years. (Courtesy of Kester Brown.)

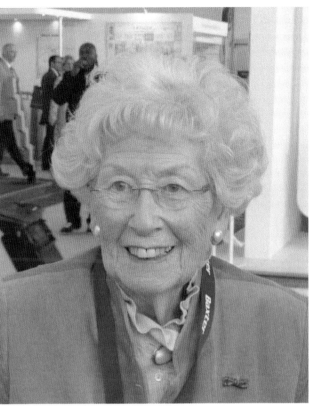

Fig. 16.10 Doreen Vermuelen-Cranch was appointed Professor of Anesthesiology in 1958 at Amersterdam's University Hospital, the first chair of anesthesiology on the Continent, and the first ever held by a woman in anesthesiology in Europe. (Courtesy of Dr. Christine Ball.)

co-author of the first report of epidural opioid for the management of postoperative pain [6].

The Netherlands Affectionately known as "The Missus," Doreen Vermeulen-Cranch (Fig. 16.10; 1915–2011; Amsterdam) trained in the UK during World War II at University Hospital, London, with experience with chest cases at the Brompton Hospital. She was asked to improve anesthesia at Amersterdam's University Hospital. She was the first trained anesthetist in the Netherlands, convinced the surgeons of the need for professional anesthesia, especially for chest cases, and was appointed Professor of Anesthesiology in 1958. This was the first chair of anesthesiology on the Continent, and the first ever held by a woman in anesthesiology in Europe [100].

Russia Elena Damir (Fig. 16.9) was one of three leaders of Russian anesthesia during the 1950s to 80s, the only prominent woman known at the beginning of Russian anesthesiology. After anesthesia training in Moscow, she went to Copenhagen for the World Health Organization training course. She chaired the Dept of Anesthesia at Botkin Hospital in Moscow from 1959–1998 and was active in the World Federation of Societies of Anesthesiology (WFSA).

United Kingdom Margaret Manford (1914–2007) focused on pediatric anesthesia at St Helier Children's Hospital in the 1950s and 60s, doing so when this was not a time of specialization in anesthesia. She had numerous trainees and published a variety of papers with them. She had an affection for the underserved, doing work in the late 1960s in Vietnam and Bangladesh, and after retirement she worked with disadvantaged families in Kent.

1980–Present

Australia–New Zealand Kate Leslie (1962-), Associate Professor at the Royal Melbourne Hospital at the University of Melbourne, is known for her collaborative work on awareness during anaesthesia. She was President of the Australia-New Zealand College of Anaesthetists from 2010 to 2012.

Jeanette Thirlwell (author of this book's essay on the History of Anesthesia Journals) has been the backbone of the journal, Anaesthesia and Intensive Care, since it began under the first editor, Ben Barry, in 1972. She was appointed as Assistant Editor in 1978, and remains as the executive editor, supervising all printing and publication.

There is a notable prominence of women a leaders in anesthesia organizations. In 2013, the incumbent president of the Australian and New Zealand College of Anaesthetists is the third woman in a row to hold the position (a two year term), with the current Vice-President (and likely next President), also a woman.

China Ailun Luo, was elected President of the Chinese Society of Anesthesiologists in 1997, She was subsequently elected as a fellow of the Royal College of Anesthetists.

Greece Helena Askitopolou from Heraklion in Crete, is active as a historian of early Greek contributions to anesthesia [101].

Mexico Estella Melman is Professor and Chair; Dept of Anesthesia, Hospital Infantil de Mexico, Mexico, D.F. She has played a prominent role in pediatric and regional anesthesia since the 1970s and authored one of the essays in this book.

United Kingdom Aileen Adams (1923-), an early neuroanesthetist, worked at Cambridge and made several political contributions. She was Dean of the Faculty of Anaesthetists, Royal College of Surgeons of England from 1985–1988. She also was President of the Section of Anaesthetics in the Royal Society of Medicine from 1985–1986 and President of the Section of the History of Medicine from 1994–1995. She was President of the History of Anaesthesia Society from 1990–1992 and the British Society for the History of Medicine from 2003–2005.

Griselda Cooper was recently Vice-President of the Royal College of Anaesthetists (RCA). She was awarded an OBE recently for services to obstetric anaesthesia.

Jean Horton (1924-) is a neuroanesthetist, who worked at Addenbrooke's Hospital, Cambridge. Her teaching in Hong Kong and Lagos improved anesthesia care in those areas. She was a founding member of the History of Anaesthesia Society and was President in 1997–1999.

Judith Hulf, on the faculty at Middlesex Hospital and University College Hospital, London, recently completed her term as President of the RCA.

Jennifer Hunter is currently Professor of Anaesthesia, University of Liverpool where she studied the pharmacodynamics and pharmacokinetics of neuromuscular blocking drugs in health and disease, especially in critically ill patients, and in patients with chronic renal failure and liver disease. She was Editor-in-Chief of the British Journal of Anaesthesia from 1997–2005 and subsequently was made Honorary Chairman of the Board of the Journal.

Jean Lumley at Hammersmith Hospital, London, is presently Vice-President of the RCA.

Reflections on the History of Women Anesthesiologists Outside of the US

These exemplars suggest that female anesthesiologists have made greater progress in the United Kingdom and Australia than in other countries. We cannot say whether this reflects differences in interest or opportunity. It does correlate with the origins of anesthesia and, perhaps with an earlier acceptance of anesthesia as a specialty in the countries of origin. If so, the increasing worldwide acceptance of anesthesia as a specialty suggests that the worldwide prominence of female anesthesiologists will increase in the future.

Concluding Thoughts

In the first few decades of the 20th century, women physicians contributed definitively to anesthesiology in the US, and in some parts of the country women physician anesthetists flourished. In part, this resulted from the efforts and vision of two physicians, Mary Botsford and Isabella Herb. In part, it resulted from a perception by surgeons that anesthesia was well-served by the psychic makeup of women. In part, it resulted from an unfavorable view of anesthesia, a specialty not worthy of a male physician's attention.

But there were concurrent opposing factors. Changes in medical education, the decline of women's medical institutions, and increasing technology (adding interest) contributed to the end of anesthesia as "women physicians' work." So did the increased interest in anesthesia by male physicians, exemplified by the great Ralph Waters, who despite his greatness failed to understand the potential of women physician anesthetists. Perhaps that should be surprising. Botsford and Herb had views in the 1900s and 1910s and 1920s that antedated but paralleled those expressed by Waters in the 1930s and 1940s on the development of anesthesiology. All emphasized clinical care, teaching, research, and the development of professional organizations. Botsford and Herb were committed to, and convincingly espoused the critical issues for anesthesia of the time. They were important leaders who were comfortable in their roles as leaders at a time when women were not leaders in any other medical specialty. The two women published articles describing complications, recorded clinical effects of various anesthetic techniques, and analyzed how care might be improved. Both advocated preoperative visits by physician anesthetists and got surgeons to agree. They argued that an understanding and observation of the operation should guide the conduct of anesthesia. Both were charismatic teachers who had medical school faculty appointments (the first ones for anesthesia in their schools), and they educated medical students, interns and residents. Their recruitment of women physicians into anesthesia attests to their ability and charisma.

World War II produced changes that further shifted dominance in anesthesia towards men. Male, but not female, physicians were drafted into the armed services and forced to become anesthetists, like it or not. Many did like it, and they swelled the numbers of male physician anesthetists. The war made anesthesia financially rewarding by providing workers with health insurance benefits that allowed payment to anesthesiologists, and, insult to injury, women physicians couldn't enlist and be trained at no charge as anesthetists, as commissioned officers, until the end of the war. Too late! Most women couldn't benefit from (didn't have a chance to earn) the GI Bill of Rights. Thus male physician anesthetists increasingly dominated anesthesia in the 1940s and 1950s, despite the great contributions of a few women physician anesthetists such as Virginia Apgar.

Then came the 1960s and the 1970s and the confrontation of bigotry. There was and is a good side to bigotry. The anger, sometimes rage, that it generates, the sense of injustice, prompts women and men to civil disobedience and other acts that have transformed the world, a transformation that continues to this day. The primary vehicles of transformation in the US were the 1960s civil rights movement and the feminist movement. These changed the face of anesthesia in the last third of the 20th century and into the 21st century. Some changes are obvious. Women now equal, sometimes exceed, men in medical school admissions (well, they are smarter, and they get better grades, don't they?) As anesthesiologists, they still lag although they've gained ground. Perhaps anesthesiology is less sought after by women, or perhaps until recently there were fewer role models. But that is changing now that women hold the chairs at some of the most prestigious departments in America.

Anesthesiology today differs qualitatively and quantitatively from that developed by Botsford and Herb in the early 1900s. These women from an earlier, simpler time left a legacy that influences today's vastly different specialty which still, however, focuses on teaching, clinical care, and research. It wouldn't hurt to remember that Herb and Botsford led the way a century ago.

References

1. Elizabeth H. Thomson. Elizabeth Blackwell. Notable American Women, 1607–1950: A Biographical Dictionary. Vol 1. In: James ET, James JW, Boyer PS, Editors. Cambridge: Belknap Press of Harvard University; 1971. pp. 161–5.
2. Walsh MR. Doctors wanted: no women need apply. Sexual barriers in the medical profession, 1835–1975. New Haven: Yale University Press; 1977.
3. Bonner TN. To the ends of the earth: women's search for education in medicine. Cambridge; Harvard University Press; 1992. pp. 6–30.
4. Calmes SH. The women physician anesthetists of San Francisco, 1897–1940: the legacy of Dr. Mary Botsford (1865–1939), The history of anaesthesia. In: Atkinson RS, Boulton TB, Editors. London: The Royal Society of Medicine Services; 1989. pp. 547–50.
5. Waters RM. Why the professional anesthetist? J-Lancet (Minn). 1919;39:32–7.
6. Oschner AJ. Surgical diagnosis and treatment by American authors vol I. New York: Lea and Febiger; 1920. p. 97.
7. Ravitch MM. A century of surgery, the history of the American Surgical Association, vol 1. Philadelphia: JB Lippincott; 1981. pp. 646, 648
8. No author. University of California Graduates, 1864–1905. Berkley: University of California; 1905. pp. 134–5.
9. No author. List of visiting and resident physicians and interns who have served in the hospital. 1903 Annual report, Hospital for Children and Training School for Nurses. Children's Hospital San Francisco 1875–1988 Collection (hereafter CHSF collection). The Bancroft Library, University of California, Berkeley.
10. 1898 Annual Report, Children's Hospital and Training School for Nurses. San Francisco: no publisher; 1898. p. 5. (CHSF collection, The Bancroft Library).
11. Strickland RA. Isabella Coler Herb, MD: an early leader in anesthesiology. Anesth Analg. 1995;80:600–5.
12. Doyle HM. A child went forth. New York: Gotham House; 1934. p. 307.
13. No author. Minutes, board of trustees CHSF 1903. CHSF collection, The Bancroft Library.
14. The California Board of Medical Examiners Directories list her as having afternoon office hours.
15. The 1920 and 1930 censuses record the niece and grand-niece living at the same address as Botsford, who was listed as head of the household. The niece had no occupation so probably kept house for Botsford, supporting Botsford's work as a professional woman.
16. No author. Augustana Hospital, history of medicine and surgery and physicians and surgeons of Chicago. No editor. Chicago: The Biographical Publishing Corporation; 1922. pp. 275–6.
17. Herb IC. Observations on one thousand consecutive cases of anesthesia in the service of Dr A.J. Oschner, Augustana Hospital. Chicago Med Recorder. 1898;15:397–403.
18. No author. Announcements Medical Department of the University of California, 1910–1911, vol I, p. 24. San Francisco: UCSF Archives and Special Collections.
19. Others often noted her expertise, and she presented papers and wrote articles on this. Most striking was her advocacy for nitrous oxide in children in Botsford ME: Nitrous oxid-oxygen anesthesia in children. Anes Analg. 1923;2:193–6. (This technique was thought to be contraindicated for children at the time).
20. Botsford ME. Nitrous oxid-oxygen anesthesia. Am J Surg Anes Supp. 1916;30:44–6.
21. Dutton AC. History of the anesthetic department at Lane Stanford University Hospital in San Francisco. Ca and Western Med. 1940;53:70–2.
22. No author. More honors richly deserved. Am J Surg Anes Supp. 1924;38:89–90.
23. Kress GH. A history of the medical profession in Southern California. Los Angeles: Times-Mirror Printing and Binding House; 1910. p. 183.
24. No author. Anesthetists organize. JAMA. 1919;72:1776.
25. Seymour E. The present state of anesthesiology and the anesthetist. Ca State J Med. 1920;18:355–8.
26. Ralph Milton Waters (hereafter RMW) to Arthur E. Guedel (hereafter AEG) Nov 12, 1928. Guedel papers, Guedel Memorial Center, San Francisco (hereafter GMC).
27. References for this section are in Calmes SH. Women anesthesiologists in the American Society of Anesthesiologists, The American Society of Anesthesiologists: a century of challenges and progress. Edited by Bacon DR, McGoldrick KE, Lema MJ. Park Ridge IL: Wood Library Museum; 2005. pp. 193–204.
28. Vedin A. Six months work in anesthesia. Am J Surg (Anes Supp). 1917;31:30–1.

29. AAA membership, both male and female, was counted from No author. American Medical Association (hereafter AMA) Directory of Physicians 1914. Chicago, American Medical Association, pp 122–7 and No author: AMA Directory of Physicians 1916. Chicago: American Medical Association, pp. 123–35.

30. More ES. Restoring the balance: women physicians and the profession of medicine 1850–1995. Cambridge: Harvard University Press; 1999. p. 98.

31. Bellafaire J, Graf MH. Women doctors in war. College Station: Texas A & M University Press; 2009. p. 38.

32. Sarnecky MT. A history of the Army Nurse Corps. Philadelphia: University of Pennsylvania Press; 1999. pp. 80–3.

33. Courington FW, Calverley RK. Anesthesia on the Western Front: the Anglo-American experience of World War I. Anesth. 1986;65:642–53.

34. No author (signature not readable). Circular of information. Employment of women physicians as contract surgeons. No date. Papers of Rose Alexander Bowers: US Army contract surgeon. History and Special Collections, Louise M. Darling Biomedical Library, UCLA.

35. No author. Frances Edith Haines, History of Medicine and Surgery and Physicians and Surgeons of Chicago. Chicago: The Biographical Publishing Corporation; 1922. p. 553.

36. MS-50 1.1 Frances Edith Haines, Women in Military Service Memorial Foundation, Arlington, VA. Memorial Register no. 218489.

37. Haines FS. Ether analgesia by inhalation for minor operations. Am J Surg Anes Supp. 1919;38:107–9.

38. Hocker EVC. The personal experience of a contract surgeon in the United States Army. Med Wom J. 1942;49:9–11.

39. Statement of Dr. Ollie Josephine Prescott Baird-Bennett, Washington D.C. Hearings before Subcommittee No. 3 of the Committee on Military Affairs House of Representatives Seventy-Eighth Congress First Session on H.R. 824 and H.R. 1857 March 10, 11 and 18th, 1943.

40. Haines FE. Economic problems in anesthesia: presidential address, Mid-Western Association of Anesthetists, 1926. Anes Anal. 1927;6:25–8.

41. WBBM-TV script for January 21, 1964. Sotir M. Woman doctor seeks equal pay for war. Chicago Tribune, July 12, 1964. Frances E. Haines biographic file, American Society of Anesthesiologists, Park Ridge: IL

42. Telegram. Harris (no initials) to Botsford ME October 16, 1918. Botsford papers, The Bancroft Library: University of California, Berkeley.

43. Papers of Rose Alexander Bowers. US Army contract surgeon. History and Special Collections, Louise M. Darling Biomedical Library, UCLA.

44. Morantz-Sanchez RM. Sympathy and science, women physicians in American medicine. New York: Oxford University Press; 1985. pp. 320–9.

45. Directory of Anesthetists. Am J Surg Anes Supp. 1920;34:61–4 (A copy published separately, at the WLM, has slightly different figures).

46. Davis DA, Moyers J. Harding of Iowa. Historical vignettes of anesthesia. In: Davis DA, Editor. Philadelphia: FA Davis Company; 1968. pp. 68–76.

47. Dorothy Sara Dimond, Application to the Board of Medical Examiners State of California, January 20, 1923.

48. Data for this statement was hand-counted from resident lists in Clark PF. The University of Wisconsin Medical School: a chronicle, 1848–1948. Madison: U Wisconsin Press; 1967. pp. 134, 140, 147, 152–5, 163–4, 165, 169–70, 173, 176–7, 177, 182, 185, 191–2.

49. Calmes SH. Women in the first academic department of anesthesiology. Proceedings of the Fifth International Symposium on the History of Anesthesia, Santiago de Compostela, Spain. In: Diz JC, Franco A, Bacon DR, Rupreht J, Alvarez J, Editors. New York: Elsevier; 2002. pp. 263–7.

50. Leake CD (hereafter CDL) to RMW. December 30, 1930. Leake Papers, San Francisco: UCSF Archives.

51. Wheaton N to Calmes SH. October 31, 2006. Letter in author's possession.

52. Kohl M to RMW, December 1, 1930. Application materials (complete), Waters papers, UW archives.

53. RMW to CDL, June 3, 1932. UCSF Leake papers.

54. CDL to RMW June 10, 1932. UCSF Leake papers

55. RMW to WA Munn, July 20, 1942. Box 2, Anesthetists Wanted, #39–42. Waters Papers, UW.

56. Martha Kohl family tree. http://trees.ancestry.com/tree/13851563/person/3400265. Accessed: 23 May 2010.

57. AMA Directory of Physicians 1940. p. 1850.

58. California Directory of Physicians 1944. p. 866.

59. RMW to CN Chipman June 10, 1933. Waters correspondence GMC.

60. RMW to AEG Febraru 16, 1932. Waters Correspondence, GMC.

61. Calmes SH. Virginia Apgar: A woman physician's career in a developing specialty. JAMWA 1984;39:184–8.

62. FH McMechan to RMW August 18, 1934. AEG Correspondence, GMC.

63. RMW to AEG, July 15, 1932. AEG Correspondence, GMC.

64. Emery A. Rovenstine to RMW April 8, 1936. Box 14, Waters correspondence, Box 14. Waters archives, UW.

65. V Apgar to RMW, November 13, 1937. Apgar Papers, Williston Memorial Library, Mt Holyoke College, Mt. Holyoke, MA (hereafter Mt. Holyoke).

66. V Apgar to RMW October 4, 1938. Apgar Papers, Mt Holyoke.

67. Calmes SH, Dr. Virginia Apgar. The effect of Dr. Ralph Waters on her career. Ralph Milton Waters MD: Mentor to a Profession. In: Morris LE, Schroeder ME, Warner ME, Editors. Wood Library Museum, Park Ridge, IL, 2004, pp 94–9.

68. Calmes SH. Virginia Apgar, MD: at the forefront of obstetric anesthesia. ASA Newsletter. 1992;56:9–12.

69. Calmes SH. Stamp to be released honoring Dr. Virginia Apgar. AHA Newsletter. 1994;12:4–5.

70. Schaner PJ. A history of the Distinguished Service Award. ASA Newsletter, Centennial Edition, no page. Available at http://www.asahq.org/Newsletters/2005/Centennial/schaner100.html.

71. Kean C. Gertie Marx called the "Mother of Obstetric Anesthesia." Anesthesiology News 2001 (Jan) 27; 48–49. Pearce J: Dr. Gertie F. Marx, 91, a pioneer in her specialty. New York Times, January 29, 2004. Kritchman MS: Gertie Marx, MD: Role Model Extraordinaire. ASA Newsletter. 2001;1992 56:13–5.

72. No author. Henry Knowles Beecher: Pioneer in anesthesiology and medical ethics, "This is no Humbug." Reminiscences of the Department of Anesthesia at the Massachusetts General Hospital. Edited by Kitz RJ. Boston, Massachusetts General Hospital Anesthesia and Critical Care, 2003, pp 108.

73. Keown KK. Status of anesthesiology 1965. JAMA. 1966;195:141–3.

74. No author. Dola Searcy Thompson, MD, has served the College of Medicine for six decades. University of Arkansas Medicine, spring-summer 2009. pp. 22–3. Available at http://www.uams.edu/com/Mag/summer-2009.pdf. Accessed: 18 May 2010..

75. Approved Residencies and Fellowships. AMA Directory of Physicians 1940. pp. 114, 134.

76. Tynes AL, Nichol WW, Wiggin SC. Anesthesia for military needs. War Med. 1941;1:789–98.

77. Waisel DB. The role of World War II and the European Theater of Operations in the development of anesthesiology as a physician specialty in the USA. Anesth. 2001;94:907–14.

78. Alice McNeil. Directory of Medical Specialists vol IV. Chicago: A.N. Marquis Co.; 1949. p. 583.

79. E Barringer to JC Magee Feb 18, 1942. AMWA Archives, Drexel University College of Medicine, Philadelphia.

80. No author. Woman physician barred by Army is urged to refuse inferior rating with the WAACS. New York Times, July 30, 1942. No author. Equality for women doctors. Time. April. 1943;41:46.

81. No author. Dr. DeVore served in Hawaii. News notes. The Med Woman's J. 1942;49:322.

82. Eckenhoff JE. Anesthesia from Colonial Times: a history of Anesthesia at the University of Pennsylvania. Philadelphia: JP Lippincott Co; 1966. p. 154.

83. Calmes SH. The first anesthesiologist at America's first children's hospital: Margo Deming, MD, (1914–1998), and the Children's Hospital of Philadelphia. ASA Newsletter. 1998;62:22–4.

84. Zepernick RG, Hyde EG, Naraghi MA John Adriani, The genesis of contemporary anesthesiology. In: Volpitto PP, Vandam LD, Editors. Springfield: Charles C. Thomas Publisher; 1982. p. 137.

85. Apgar V. Careers in anesthesiology. JAMWA. 1964:19;675–80.

86. Howell MC. What medical schools teach about women. NEJM. 1974;291:304–7.

87. Calmes SH. Anesthesiology from the far side, 1966–1996. Careers in anesthesiology, autobiographical memoirs. vol 2. In: Fink RB, Editor. Park Ridge: IL, WLM; 1998. pp. 3–33.

88. Kraft M. Women in the DACC: A personal story, "This is no humbug." Reminiscences of the Department of Anesthesia at the Massachusetts General Hospital. Edited by Kitz RJ. Boston, Massachusetts General Hospital Anesthesia and Critical Care. 2003, pp. 251–67.

89. Calmes SH. Anesthesia demographics: women physicians changing specialty choices and implications for anesthesiology's workforce shortage. ASA Newsletter. 1995;59:26–9.

90. Guth CJ A committee whose time has come. ASA Newsletter.1995;59:26–9.

91. Wilkinson CJ, Linde HW. Status of women in academic anesthesiology. Anesthesiology. 1986;64:496–500.

92. Kerr GE. Diversity…why? ASA Newsletter. 2009;73:48–9.

93. List of presidents of the American College of Surgeons is available at http://www.facs.org/archives/presidentslist.html. Kathryn D. Anderson of Children's Hospital of Los Angeles was ACS president in 2005–2006. Accessed: 26 May 2011.

94. Walker EP ACS president resigns over controversial editorial. April 18, 2011. Available at http://www.medpagetoday.com/anesthesiology/generalsurgery/25997. Accessed: 26. May 2011.

95. Wong CA, Stock MC. The status of women in academic anesthesiology: a progress report. Anes Analg. 2008;107:178–84.

96. Email communication CA Wong to SH Calmes, May 22, 2010.

97. SAMBA past presidents Available at http://www.sambahq.org/index.php?src=gendocs&refs=PastPresdients&category=Professional. (Note misspelling in this address.) Accessed: 2 June 2011.

98. Morton MJ, Sonnad SS. Women on professional society and journal editorial boards. J Natl Med Assoc. 2007;99:764–71.

99. Cooper MG. A Woman of History. Gwenifer Wilson 1916–1998. Obituary. Anaesth Intensive Care. 1999;27:110–1.

100. Vermeulen-Cranch DME. From open ether to open hearts. In: Rupreht J, van Lieburg MJ, Lee JA, Erdmann W, Editors. Anaesthesia: essays on its history. New York: Springer-Verlag; 1985. pp. 265–70.

101. Astyrakaki E, Papaioannou A, Askitopoulou H. References to anesthesia, pain, and analgesia in the Hippocratic collection. Anesth Analg. 2010;110:188–94.

Anesthesia, Anesthesiologists and Modern Medical Ethics

Stephen H. Jackson and Gail Van Norman

Summary

Historically, anesthesiologists have played pivotal roles in medical ethics by developing and applying technology that posed ethical dilemmas, and by their leadership in answering ethical questions and posing new ones. In 1853, Queen Victoria's demand for chloroform for her labor undermined the religious demand that women must suffer the pains of childbirth. In the 1950s, Pope Pius XII consulted with anesthesiologists concerning humane and ethical pursuits centered in anesthesia. In 1957, the Pope supported the treatment of pathologic pain, even though such treatment might shorten life (the "double effect"). In 1973, John Bonica proposed that relief of pain is a basic human right.

Horrific abuses by Nazi physicians during World War II attacked the moral traditions of medicine and medical research. These and subtler unethical actions of honorable researchers led anesthesiologist Henry Beecher in the 1960s to support the development of institutional review boards and informed consent protections for human subjects of research. In 1968, Beecher again advanced medical ethics when his Harvard-based committee defined death in permanently unconscious patients. Robert Truog and other anesthesiologists continue to opine about ethical repercussions of the practice of anesthesiology by the dead donor rule, organ donation after cardiac death, and terminal sedation/anesthesia.

Dutch anesthesiologist Pieter Admiraal has made an ethical case for physician assisted suicide and euthanasia since the 1980s. In 1982, an anesthesiologist recommended what soon became the preferred lethal drug recipe for state-sponsored executions. However, in 2006 the American Society of Anesthesiologists (ASA) condemned physician participation in execution as unethical, and in 2010 the American Board of Anesthesiology threatened rescission of board certification for such unethical behavior.

Throughout the last 25 years, the ASA Committee on Ethics has advanced the cause of ethical medical care by anesthesiologists, particularly through its 1995 *Guidelines for the Ethical Practice of Anesthesiology*. The 1993 *Ethical Guidelines for the Patient with Do-Not-Resuscitate (DNR) Orders or Other Directives That Limit Care* argued for the routinely-neglected ethical right of a surgical patient with an existing DNR directive to refuse resuscitation should a cardiac arrest occur under anesthesia. Other specialties (e.g. the American College of Surgeons) used these documents to develop their ethical guidelines.

In the first decade of this century, a cluster of notorious cases of research and publication fraud by anesthesiologists prompted a coordinated response from the specialty to rectify these unethical breaches.

In their reach across specialty boundaries (pain medicine, critical care, and transplantation) anesthesiologists have contributed to the evolution of medical ethics in the US and abroad, in anesthesia in particular, and medicine in general.

S. H. Jackson (✉)
Department of Anesthesiology, Good Samaritan Hospital of San Jose, San Jose, CA, USA
e-mail: hojacks@gmail.com

G. V. Norman
Department of Anesthesiology and Pain Medicine, Department of Biomedical Ethics, University of Washington Medical Center, Seattle, WA, USA
e-mail: lbsparrow@yahoo.com

Introduction

The School of Hippocrates [1] advised that the relationship of physicians with their patients should be gentle and pleasant, comforting and discreet. The traditional Hippocratic Oath also suggested the obligations of physicians to their patients—benefit the sick and do them no harm; keep confidences; refrain from exploitation; and show concern and caring—even at a cost to the physician's health and wealth. Then and now, physicians must justify their worthiness of social trust and demonstrate that they deserve so-

E. I Eger II et al. (eds.), *The Wondrous Story of Anesthesia,* DOI 10.1007/978-1-4614-8441-7_17, © Edmond I Eger, MD 2014

cial authority and reward. Societies expect that a physician's primary concern is that of their patients' well being. These three themes—personal character, interpersonal duty and social responsibility—are recurrent topics of ethical reflection, and they constitute the threads that bind medicine and morality, what has become known as medical ethics.

This chapter examines some of the ethical dilemmas unique to anesthesia and considers contributions that anesthesia and anesthesiologists made to the advancement of modern medical ethics as a whole. Because of the specialty's broad scope, with connections to most aspects of medicine, anesthesiologists have played critical roles in the major ethical issues of our age: Should pain be relieved even if treatment may hasten or cause death? Is it ethical to relieve the pain of childbirth? Should anesthesiologists participate in legal executions? How should ethical research be carried out on human subjects?

Anesthesiologists and the Ethics of Birth, Pain, and Death

The ethical history of anesthesiology goes beyond the responses of anesthesiologists to the shifting moral and ethical demands of society, to how they produced and promoted moral change. One example is the role of anesthesia and anesthesiologists in changing Western attitudes towards the pain of childbirth, and the implications of that change for the role of women in society. Another addresses the question of whether relieving pain by administering potentially fatal doses of medication is morally acceptable. A third considers patients who want to forgo life-sustaining medical interventions and the evolving definition of the principle of 'beneficence'[1] in biomedical ethics. These examples touch on fundamental problems: where does life begin and end; when does a person cease to be a person; and is it moral to withdraw life-sustaining therapies at the end-of-life?

Moral Questions About Pain Relief

Labor Analgesia

Traditional stories blame Woman (Eve) for introducing knowledge (sin) into the Garden of Eden. The pain of childbirth served as eternal punishment for this: [2]

Genesis 3:16 Unto the woman He said, "I will greatly multiply thy sorrow and thy conception. In pain[2] thou shalt bring forth children; and thy desire shall be to thy husband, and he shall rule over thee." [3]

Western culture used these passages to justify the subjugation of women (as the originators of sin) and to rationalize suffering during childbirth. To relieve labor pain neutralized God's justice and repudiated God's dictum that women should be subordinate to men.

Violations of this concept in Western society could have capital consequences. Although efforts to relieve the pain of labor date to the dawn of historic times in Egypt and Persia, [4] in Christian-dominated society, those acting to relieve pain for laboring women might lose their lives. Even requesting labor analgesia could be heresy. In the 16th century CE, Euphemia McCalyean and Agnes Sampson were burned at the stake because Euphemia asked Agnes for something to relieve her labor pains [5, 6].

Fast forward to 1847, a momentous year in a quiet revolution for women. On 19 January, James Simpson, Professor of Midwifery at the University of Edinburgh, became the first physician to use ether to relieve labor pain in the UK [7]. Less than a year later, Simpson discovered the anesthetic property of chloroform and, having determined it to be a superior anesthetic agent, immediately employed it in his obstetric practice. The parents of the first baby he delivered under chloroform, in gratitude, baptized the child 'Anaesthesia.' Some representatives of the clergy criticized this practice as against the will of God. Simpson responded by famously quoting Biblical text supporting anesthesia as a divine invention:

Genesis 2:21 So the Lord God caused the man to fall into a deep sleep and while he was sleeping, He took one of the man's ribs and closed up the place with flesh [3].

The bold actions of three famous families on both sides of the Atlantic Ocean quickly followed Simpson's treatment. On 7 April 1847, Fanny Longfellow, wife of Henry Wadsworth Longfellow, received ether administered by her physician, Nathan Keep, to relieve the pain of labor [8]. The belief that relief of labor pain was against God's will was prominent in rural America in the 19th Century [7], but there was a reason why Fanny would defy Christian edicts. The Longfellows belonged to a precursor of the modern Unitarian Church, which did not believe in original sin, did not believe that relief of labor pain opposed God's will, and held enlightened views of the role of women in society. This would become the leading edge of women's rights in the US, and an early step in a movement that would reach beyond the labor suite.

[1] Beneficence is a moral obligation to act to benefit the patient, to promote the patient's best interests. Originally interpreted to mean "preservation of life," from the late 20th century onward, this obligation was interpreted to mean promoting a 'good quality of life,' and acting with the patient's desires and goals in mind.

[2] Many theologians argue that this translation of the Hebrew text is incorrect, and that the proper word in the second sentence is 'sorrow,' and not 'pain,' as it was originally phrased in the King James Version of the Bible.

In July of the same year, Charles Darwin administered chloroform to his wife, Emma (who also held Unitarian beliefs) [9] for the birth of their seventh child, Elizabeth [10]. And on 7 April 1853, Queen Victoria received chloroform from John Snow for the birth of Prince Leopold [11]. The acceptance of labor analgesia by the monarch, who was also the head of the Church of England, promoted the widespread acceptance of labor analgesia in England and beyond.

Anesthesia arose in an age of evolving liberal views, and obstetrical anesthesia appeared at a time ripe for liberalization of society's view of women. The development of anesthesia and labor analgesia not only resulted from—but also fostered the growth of—enlightened ideas regarding humanism, compassion, and the worth of human life [7]. In 1956, the Pope of the Catholic Church accepted that Christian women could seek pain relief for childbirth, although they should not do so "with exaggerated haste." [12]

The Moral Acceptability of Pain Relief, and the Principle of Double Effect

The religious imagery of global cultures, including Western civilization, accepts pain as divine punishment. Eastern faiths such as Hinduism describe pain as the result of wickedness in previous lives, and the Abrahamic religions (Judaism, Islam, and Christianity) draw direct relationships between pain and punishment.

Medieval Christian theology glorified martyrdom and man's obligation to accept suffering imposed by God. Was induction of unconsciousness in the pursuit of pain relief a sin against God? And was it morally acceptable to seek to relieve pain if the treatments intended to accomplish relief also risked an unintended shortening of life—the principle of 'double effect'? At the 1957 Congress of the Italian Society of the Science of Anesthetics, the president, Piero Mazzoni, posed these questions to Pope Pius XII [13]. The Pope affirmed that Christians legitimately used pain treatments, "in accordance with the Creator" to bring suffering under man's control. The Pope agreed that producing unconsciousness for surgery was acceptable, but enjoined that deprivation of consciousness (sedation) in a dying patient for reasons other than to relieve pain was not morally acceptable.

Pain Relief as a Human Right

As advances of modern medicine prolonged lifespan, chronic pain and its attendant suffering became a key factor in determining the quality of life, particularly in the developing world which has less capacity to control pain. The medical profession experienced a heightened ethical impetus to treat pain and suffering, "to develop those dimensions of practice that seek to heal what cannot be cured … the physician is both a therapeutic and moral agent, given that any (if not all) clinical decisions affect the vulnerability of the patient, reflecting the asymmetries of knowledge and power between physician and patient, and (thus) impact trust within the medical relationship." [14]

The founding father of the field of pain medicine, and the driving force in establishing the International Association for the Study of Pain (IASP) in 1973, was John Bonica, professor and chair of the Department of Anesthesiology at the University of Washington (1960–1978) [15]. This visionary figure achieved recognition of the importance of pain as a fundamental element of human suffering, and established the specialty of pain medicine as an international, multidisciplinary scientific effort. His preeminent contribution to medical ethics lay in his championing of pain relief as a human right. In 2004, with the support of the World Health Organization, the IASP issued the first international call for pain relief as a human right, and not merely as a medical issue [16]. Alex Cahana continued carrying Bonica's torch, by advocating at both a national and international level for the consideration of pain as a distinct phenomenon, and not a symptomatic byproduct of disease. He has advocated for the appropriate, measurement-based and safe administration of opioids for chronic pain, and for an enhanced appreciation for the impact that psychosocial elements of pain have on patient outcomes [17, 18].

Ethical Issues at End-of-Life

Forgoing Life-sustaining Medical Interventions

The rapid advances of anesthesia and intensive care in the mid-20th century prompted a succession of moral questions. War and plague contributed to advancements in medical care and ethics. The development of open-chest cardiac massage in World War II (with subsequent modification to closed chest massage and cardiopulmonary resuscitation—CPR), and the need for long-term ventilation of patients suffering from respiratory paralysis brought about by polio, led to further medical and theological dialogues—this time between the World Congress of Anesthesiologists and Pope Pius XII.

Mechanical ventilation had existed before the polio epidemics of the 1940s and 1950s. "Iron lungs" (tank respirators) were intermittent negative pressure chambers in which the patient was placed with their head outside the chamber. The negative pressure expanded the chest, passively drawing gas into the lungs. Long-term therapy was possible—as of 2008, approximately 30 patients still depended on iron lung therapy, one having lived this way for more than 60 years [19]. However, such therapy was expensive, and the limited access to the patient hindered their care.

A crushing polio epidemic struck Copenhagen in 1952, when hundreds of patients succumbed from respiratory paralysis, spurring a search for a new therapy. Anesthesiologist Björn Ibsen suggested supplying manual positive pressure ventilation via tracheal tubes placed through tracheotomies, and delivered by diverse personnel [20]. Over two hundred medical students (backed up by anesthesiologists and dental students) provided "hand ventilation" around the clock to support as many as 75 patients at any one time [21]. The success of their efforts encouraged the development of positive pressure ventilators and intensive care units.

CPR and artificial respiration raised potential moral implications. Were patients or physicians obliged to institute or continue such therapy in hopeless situations? Should such therapy be withdrawn if the family of the patient wished to discontinue it? And when, exactly, was an unconscious patient dead: when they were unable to breath on their own, or when their heart had stopped beating? Bruno Haid, chief of anesthesia at the surgical clinic of the University of Innsbruck Hospital, posed these questions to Pope Pius II, on behalf of the World Congress of Anesthesiologists in 1957. The Pope's response acknowledged the broad role of anesthesiologists in medicine, in the relief of pain, and in end-of-life care. In answer to the specific questions, he stated:

> "The doctor has no separate or independent right where the patient is concerned. In general he can take action only if the patient explicitly or implicitly, directly or indirectly, gives him permission." [22]

Further, he said that doctors were not obliged to use modern artificial respiration apparatus, and that the family could morally act only in accordance with the known will of an unconscious patient who is 'of age.' He stated that a definition of death "could not be deduced from any religious and moral principle" and "does not fall within the competence of the Church … It remains for the doctor, and especially the anesthesiologist, to give a clear and precise definition of death …" [22]

Out of this dialogue would come discussions of how to define death, socially and medically. Henry Beecher, first chair of Anesthesiology at the Harvard School of Medicine would lead these discussions.

Defining Death

In 1968, Beecher received permission to use the Harvard Standing Committee on Human Studies, to examine the issue of declaring death in the permanently unconscious patient. Within a year, his committee published their definition of death in terms of a neurologic standard, in the "Report of the Ad Hoc Committee of the Harvard Medical School to Examine the Definition of Brain Death." [23] The sole refer-

ence listed in this Committee's original report was a speech by Pope Pius XII. This Ad Hoc Committee's Report cited two primary purposes for defining irreversible coma, with no discernible central nervous system activity as a new criterion for death:

> "1) Improvements in resuscitative and supportive measures have led to increased efforts to save those who are desperately injured. Sometimes these efforts have only partial success so that the result is an individual whose heart continues to beat but whose brain is irreversibly damaged. The burden is great on patients who suffer permanent loss of intellect, on their families, on the hospitals, and on those in need of hospital beds already occupied by these comatose patients. 2) Obsolete criteria for the definition of death can lead to controversy in obtaining organs for transplantation." [23]

Beecher had to repeatedly dispute allegations that securing a better supply of organs for transplantation had provided the primary motivation for his committee [24]. His emphasis was antithetical to this contention; instead it developed stringent objective criteria to determine that the patient had died, thus enabling the physician to pronounce a patient dead. While the criteria for brain death promulgated by Beecher's committee would be modified over the next fifty years, these guidelines have remained the bulwark of the present day's definition of death.

Physician-Assisted Suicide and Euthanasia

After World War II, physician involvement in euthanasia[3] was closely scrutinized because of abuses of prisoners and vulnerable patients by physicians employed by the Third Reich. Expanding medical technology in the latter half of the 20th century also forced a medical profession that had previously been dedicated to preservation of life, at almost any cost, to confront the ethics of end-of-life care. The seemingly endless new means of prolonging life raised ethical and

---

[3] "Euthanasia" refers to another party ending a patient's life at the patient's request. Currently, it is only legal if it occurs at the patient's request. It differs from withdrawal of life-supportive therapy or refusal of life-supportive therapy, in that it is active (not passive). "Physician-assisted suicide" (PAS) refers to the use of powers and privileges restricted to physicians and a few other health-related professions (for example, prescriptive privileges) to provide a patient with the means by which they may, at a time of their choosing, end their life. Distinguishing between the two partly relies on asking which party "acted" last. If the physician acts last to inject a lethal substance, then they have committed euthanasia. If the patient acts last to voluntarily ingest a lethal substance, then they have committed suicide. A physician who uses common powers not related to health care (for example, a physician might purchase a gun with which a patient then uses to commit suicide) to assist a suicide is not providing PAS, but merely "assisted suicide." The differences are significant in that PAS raises questions related to the ethics of the physician's role in suicide, while assisted suicide does not.

legal debate about patient rights to forgo life-saving medical therapies, and about the role of physicians in end-of-life management. "Euthanasia", the active ending of a life at the request of the patient, became an issue because unregulated physicians in many Western countries were, quietly and compassionately, actively assisting patients to die.

The Netherlands became one of the first countries to accept the practices of euthanasia and physician-assisted suicide (PAS), ironically so because among occupied countries during World War II, it alone refused to participate in the Nazi euthanasia program [25]. However, by the 1980s, Dutch physicians, like those of many other countries, undertook covert euthanasia in patients who were suffering from incurable disease, and who requested it. The first official study of the Dutch practice of euthanasia—the 1991 Remmelink Report [26]—indicated that PAS and "voluntary euthanasia" (where the patient requests euthanasia) had occurred in about 2,700 patients during the previous year, and "involuntary euthanasia" (where the physician ended a patient's life without their request) had occurred in 1,300 patients during the same time. Another 8,100 patients died of narcotic overdose that physicians intended to hasten death. All in all, in 1990, physicians deliberately assisted about 9.1 % of deaths in the Netherlands.

A prominent Dutch anesthesiologist, Pieter Admiraal, became the major international advocate for euthanasia and PAS, as he pioneered the field of voluntary euthanasia [27, 28]. He was President of the Dutch Society of Anesthesiology, the first president of the Dutch Society for the Study of Pain, and a member of the Committee of Pain and Committee of Euthanasia of the Dutch Health Council. In 1994, he received the royal decoration, Officer Oranje Nassau, and in 2000 he was awarded the Janet Good Memorial Award from the US Hemlock Society. In 2000, partly as a result of his advocacy, the Dutch Parliament legalized euthanasia and PAS under strict conditions, becoming the first Western country to legalize both. Belgium, Lichtenstein and several other countries have since followed suit, and liberalization of laws in Britain, Germany and France is being debated. As in many countries, physicians in the US, such as anesthesiologist Lawrence Egbert, often pushed the legal boundaries to actively assist patients in dying [29].

The Ethics of Research and Publication

Rights of Human Research Subjects; Obligations of Human Subject Researchers

Following revelations of experimentation by Nazi physicians in German prison camps, the world rebelled against abuses in human experimentation. The physicians were tried and convicted at Nuremberg, and the Nuremberg Code

[30] was created, emphasizing the importance of informed consent and voluntariness of human subjects of experiments. The Code forcefully addressed the need to protect human safety, to not experiment frivolously, and to only allow experimentation by qualified researchers. Indeed, the influence of the Code marked "a new beginning in the moral traditions of medicine, a beginning that would become bioethics." [21] These regulations primarily addressed "physician-researchers" who were not in a therapeutic relationship with their subjects, and therefore, were to be distinguished from "physician friends." Interestingly, the Nuremberg Code had, over the next decade, little effective influence on American investigators performing research upon human subjects [31].

In the 1950s and early 1960s, US funded research was initiated in earnest, and included both 'volunteer' subjects and 'subject-patients'. Not being patients, volunteers failed to qualify for the fiduciary responsibilities traditionally provided by physicians, and subject-patients risked being harmed by their well-meaning physician's experiments. Thus, again, the awareness of a distinction between the moral quality of the researcher-physician, and the treating-physician arose [32]. Was the good will of the investigator sufficient to safeguard the rights and welfare of all experimental subjects?

Henry Beecher's interest in the ethics of human experimentation dated from 1947, when he requested information about Nazi medical experimentation from the Office of the Surgeon General at the War Department [33]. In 1959, Beecher prepared an essay that appeared in the *Journal of the American Medical Association* (JAMA) [34] and broadly distinguished the motives and practices of research from those of therapy, but it received little attention and stirred minimal controversy. He continued to write on informed consent and ethics in human investigations in 1962 and 1963 [35–37].

In 1964, James Shannon, the Director of the National Institutes of Health (which over two decades, had increased the funds available for research by over 600-fold to nearly half a billion dollars yearly) [38], appointed a committee to review the ethics of human experimentation. It concluded that "the judgment of the investigator is not sufficient as a basis for reaching a conclusion concerning the ethical and moral set of questions in that relationship," thus repudiating a traditional, century-long view. Shannon then declared that the researcher's judgment must be subject to prior peer review to ensure an independent determination of risks and benefits [39].

In 1966 in a paper published in the *New England Journal of Medicine* (after its rejection by the JAMA), Beecher described examples of abuse in human experimentation [40]. This landmark article contained 22 anonymous but concrete examples of what he considered to be unethical experimentation, many by leading investigators at respected academic institutions (including his own). He did not specifically cite the examples "for the condemnation of individuals," but rather with the hope that "calling attention to (the examples) will help to correct abuses present." [33, 37] While he stated that "thoughtlessness and carelessness, not a willful disregard of the patient's rights, accounted for most of the cases encountered," his article nonetheless shocked the medical community by offering an unfavorable exposure of the practice of human experimentation. The fact that this ethical indictment came from such a renowned scientist, and was published strategically in perhaps the most respected medical journal of its time, testified to Beecher's extraordinary "courage" [31]. In fact, Beecher's report had a great impact, and without that report,

> "*the movement to set new rules for human experimentation would have proceeded on a much slower track. Few others had the scientific knowledge and ethical sensibilities to call into question, researcher's ethics.*" [31]

Because of Beecher's publication, and others, a Presidential Commission was formed to examine the behavior of US medical researchers, and the rights of human subjects. The resulting Belmont Report reiterated the rights of human subjects and proposed formal independent oversight of research, giving birth to the concept of Investigational Review Boards (IRBs) [41]. In 1966, the National Advisory Council of the NIH issued a policy requiring reviews of research proposals by IRBs, a mandate that presently must be followed in all institutions conducting human research.

Beecher kick-started a transition from an insulated research community with minimal internal or external oversight to a medical community requiring informed consent and public oversight of both standard and research medical procedures. His report ultimately overthrew a naïve conception that placed ethical decision-making in the purview of an insular research profession, whose paternalistic practitioners made moral decisions based on their professional training and personal integrity, but not necessarily based on a formal understanding of rules governing morality. However, Beecher believed that the best interests of patients involved in research investigations was served, not necessarily by a code of ethics—or even informed consent (which he thought was an absolute necessity)—but rather by "the presence of an intelligent, informed, conscientious, compassionate investigator." [40]

The Oaths of Hippocrates and Lasagna

After obtaining his medical degree from Columbia University, Louis Lasagna became a research fellow and then an associate in Beecher's anesthesia laboratory at the Massachusetts General Hospital. Later acknowledged as the father of clinical pharmacology, Lasagna worked with Beecher in

the early 1950s, on the placebo effects of medications, including the study of the psychotomimetic (not psychedelic) effects of lysergic acid diethylamide (LSD), at that time a legal drug, to investigate subjective responses [42]. This and other army-sponsored research that Beecher, in retrospect, believed to have been unethical, may have prompted his advocacy for the ethical treatment of human research subjects [43, 44]. Lasagna authored the popular Oath of Lasagna, commonly referred to as the contemporary version of the Oath of Hippocrates, and first presented in 1964 [45] while he was at Johns Hopkins. This holistic and humanistic oath had no prohibition against abortion, nor a promise of the physician to abide by the ethical principle of nonmaleficence,[4] nor an admonition against prescribing a "lethal medicine." It includes:

> "*avoiding those twin traps of overtreatment and therapeutic nihilism ... that warmth, sympathy, and understanding may outweigh the surgeon's knife or the chemist's drug ... if it is given me to save a life, all thanks. But it may also be within my power to take a life; this awesome responsibility must be faced with great humbleness and awareness of my own frailty ... I do not treat a fever chart, a cancerous growth, but a sick human being, whose illness may affect the person's family and economic stability.*" [45]

Beecher's thoughts, ideas, and opinions were complex, and occasionally seemingly contradictory and enigmatic, yet inevitably open to his own reconsideration and public deliberation, while participating in the groundbreaking work that was integral to the foundation of clinical ethics. As already noted, he advocated the ethical treatment of human subjects, but he had engaged in potentially unethical work on hallucinogens. Perhaps he was led to champion the ethical treatment of human subjects because of such personal experiences. Another enigma: Beecher knew of the Nazis' forced experimentation with psychoactive drugs, but in 1959 he opposed the application of the Nuremberg Code to American medical experimentation, and even at that juncture he questioned the concept of informed consent [34]. Yet, nearly a decade later, his evolving bioethical perspective supported a more stringent view of ethical violations in human experimentation, one that ultimately produced IRBs and applied informed consent. Nonetheless, he continued to adhere to the belief that the ethical obligation of scientists might better serve society if it rested with investigators rather than their institutions or standardized regulations.

---

[4]Abstaining from whatever is deleterious; primum non nocere (Latin: "first do no harm"). In modern times beneficence coupled with nonmaleficence are considered to be maximizing ethical principles—not simply doing good and avoiding harm, but providing the greatest good and the least amount of harm for the patient.

Research and Publication Fraud

Physicians have a social contract with the public that they serve—a contract that includes the spirit of sacrifice and service to society. They are expected to collectively and individually exercise moral integrity, this behavior fostering the public trust and serving as a structurally stabilizing and protective force. We are aghast and angry when they fail us. In return, physicians retain considerable authority and privilege to control key aspects of the practice of medicine. The medical profession has an obligation to expel those physicians who fail to maintain technical and intellectual competence and the ethical norms of professional integrity. Fraudulent research and publication practices divert and undermine the search for truth, corrupt the scientific literature, and damage the image of scientific investigation as a noble enterprise. Publication of scientific research serves the medical profession's ethical obligation to advance knowledge that benefits patients (beneficence), and discredits harmful or ineffective treatments (nonmalfeasance) . Falsification and fabrication of data increases the potential for delivery of ineffective or even harmful treatments, and the loss of beneficial treatments. False information can divert other researchers from productive paths of inquiry.

Sadly, in the last decade, several anesthesiology researchers provided some of the largest individual acts of research fraud and misconduct ever detected in the medical literature. An audit in 2008, revealed fraudulent research by American anesthesiologist Scott Reuben, promoting the routine use of postoperative pain medications with theoretically detrimental effects on bone healing in orthopedic patients [46]. After the Baystate Medical Center in Springfield Massachusetts, (the institution in which the fraud had been conducted) announced the fabrication, Steven Shafer, editor-in-chief of *Anesthesia and Analgesia*, listed 21 journal articles (ten from *Anesthesia and Analgesia*, three from *Anesthesiology*) that had been based on that data, and then correctly predicted the retraction of most if not all of them [47]. Reuben was fined and imprisoned.

German anesthesiologist, Joachim Boldt misrepresented key aspects of a published study, including probable fabricated data, on the use of hydroxyethyl starch as a priming solution for cardiopulmonary bypass [48]. The article contained other egregious ethical transgressions, such as failure to gain IRB approval and to obtain informed consent. In an unprecedented international collaboration, the editors of sixteen journals published a collective letter acknowledging that 89 (now corrected to 88) of 102 studies by Boldt had not received IRB approval [49]. Subsequently, the hospital at Ludwigschafen announced its findings in August of 2012 [50], adding that no evidence indicated patient harm consequent to the research. However, of 91 articles examined, study files were incomplete or missing in most; nearly all

had not received IRB approval; and most had no record of informed consent. False data were published in at least 10 of the 91 studies. Boldt was stripped of his professorship, and faces both fines and potential imprisonment, under direction by the State Medical Association of Rhineland-Pfalz which has jurisdiction over such physician misconduct in Germany [51].

More recently, in what may be a record number (approximately 172) of fraudulent publications by a single investigator [52], retractions were announced of virtually all research published by Japanese anesthesiologist, Yoshitaka Fujii. Whereas questions were initially raised about the integrity of his research in 2001 [53], serious investigation did not commence until approximately 2010 [54]. Allegations included lack of IRB approval, failure to follow ethical standards for research, and questions about the veracity of data presented in the papers. Moreover, in some cases, listed co-authors were unaware of being listed, and it is alleged that submission letters to journals contained forged signatures. Once again, a bevy of respected editors from prominent anesthesiology journals, including Shafer, Steven Yentis (*Anaesthesia*) and Donald Miller (*Canadian Journal of Anesthesia*), successfully pursued appropriate investigation at the host institutions, as well as correction in the published literature. Fujii was dismissed from Toho University and almost all of his research retracted. Indeed, the international community of editors for anesthesiology journals is "completely engaged with the process of coordinating our efforts to identify and reduce research fraud. … It is a team effort. … Everyone is on board." [55–57] Importantly, anesthesiologists introduced statistical methodology as a novel tool to identify unnatural patterns of categorical and continual variables in order to identify fabricated data [58, 59]. This expands the armamentarium of editors to detect research and publication fraud far beyond acts of plagiarism [60].

Ultimately, as Beecher stated, the integrity of medical knowledge and advancement of patient care relies on the honest pursuit of ethically designed research, and therefore on the integrity of individual researchers [40].

Anesthesiologists and the State

Lethal Injection

Physicians receive financial benefits and social as well as professional prestige for their skills and their adherence to rules that prevent them from taking advantage of vulnerable persons or using their skills in immoral ways. For most of the history of medicine, the physician has had a role similar to that of a priest or shaman, and hallowed tenets of the medical profession forbid the use of a physician's skills for personal or political purposes or gains.

Use of a physician's expertise for non-medical, state-sponsored activities such as torture, medical incarceration, or executions is forbidden. Physicians may swear ancient oaths to "keep patients from harm or injustice." [1] From ancient times, individual physicians have ignored these principles, and governing states have employed execution for the most serious of human crimes. Ritualistic, even "religious" overtones of executions unite a community in virtue, and separate the condemned from society. Until recently, protracted torture was also a common element of executions that exacted retribution.

Execution methods have evolved to ensure that society's laws and punishments are humane (not 'cruel or unusual'), to prevent prisoners' suffering during the execution process. Physicians have contributed to the development of many modern methods, such as the guillotine (Antoine Louis and Joseph Ignace-Gillotin), hanging (Samuel Haughton) and the gas chamber (Allen McLean Hamilton).

When macabre aspects of many modern execution methods rendered them repugnant to the public, Jay Chapman, a medical examiner, and Stanley Deutsch, an anesthesiologist at the University of Oklahoma, introduced a recipe for a lethal intravenous injection—combining a hypnotic (e.g., thiopental or pentobarbital), a paralyzing agent, and potassium—for the execution of prisoners [61]. This formula was first used in 1982, and became the preferred method of execution in most of the US. It continues to be the subject of ongoing, acrimonious debate among the public, and among physicians in the US.

Participation of individual physicians in state executions is debated as an issue of beneficence (providing a 'humane death' for the prisoner) versus a violation of the principle of nonmaleficence, and an erosion of the physician's professional ethic. However, social action in pursuit of social justice in other Western countries has demonized and eliminated the death penalty. In fact, such actions have reached beyond individual country boundaries. When a shortage of the hypnotic thiopental occurred in the US in 2009, Hospira Inc. exited the market for barbiturates, under pressure from death penalty abolitionists in the European countries where the company's manufacturing plants were sited [62]. An initial attempt by the US to obtain the drug from DreamPharma in the UK, was thwarted when Great Britain banned the export of thiopental for use in lethal injections [63]. More recently, prisons have turned to the use of pentobarbital, a drug also used in veterinary euthanasia [64].

In 2006 anesthesiologists were drawn into the national debate on lethal injection. In California, death row inmate Michael Morales successfully argued that lethal injection might go awry and be cruel, leading Justice Jeremy Fogel to rule that a physician had to be present at all executions to prevent mistakes [65]. Two anesthesiologists, Robert Singler and another identified subsequently as "Anesthesiologist 2," initially volunteered [66], thinking that they would only monitor the prisoner and declare death. They both withdrew when they learned that, in the event of a mishap, they might have to administer drugs to execute the prisoner. Both claimed that, in contrast with their feelings about declaring death, 'active' participation in the execution itself violated their medical ethical principles. In that same year, a federal judge in Missouri ordered that a board-certified anesthesiologist be present at all lethal injections [67]. The then President of the American Society of Anesthesiologists (ASA), Orin Guidry, declared that:

> "*Clearly, an anesthesiologist complying with the Missouri ruling—and despite the court's position on ethical obligations—would be violating the AMA position which ASA has adopted. It is my belief that the court cannot modify physicians' ethical principles to meet its needs.*" [68]

This reflected the ASA's Committee on Ethics statement that executions were not medical activities, that execution by lethal injection is not the practice of medicine (particularly anesthesiology) [69], and that participation in executions would constitute a violation of the ASA's ethical code. Later that year, the mandate for an anesthesiologist's presence at executions in Missouri was reversed, although in 2008, an anesthesiologist who demanded anonymity joined the Missouri execution team, thus violating the ethical guidelines of the ASA [70]. It is not known whether that anesthesiologist is even a member of the ASA. In any case, no disciplinary action could be pursued by the ASA, presumably because the identity of the physician was never released.

Years before the California and Missouri cases, the ASA adopted principles upheld by the American Medical Association [71], which were expounded by Robert Truog's article in the *New England Journal of Medicine* [72]—indicating that participation in lethal injection, including prescribing tranquilizers, monitoring consciousness or vital signs, attending or observing the execution, rendering technical advice or assistance, selecting injection sites, starting IV infusions, preparing the drugs, supervising the injection of lethal drugs, inspecting or maintaining equipment used in the execution, and consulting with or supervising execution personnel, was unethical and violated foundational medical ethical principles. In fact, all medical professional organizations in the US hold that physician participation in state executions is unethical, although as of 2010, no US physician organization had outlined punitive action against any member for providing the means for—or carrying out—state executions.

In 2010, the American Board of Anesthesiologists (ABA) made the historic announcement that not only was participation in lethal injection unethical, but doing so by a board-certified anesthesiologist would be investigated, and that punitive action could result, which might include rescission of board certification [73]. In so declaring, the ABA became the first physician organization to indicate that it would actually punish physician members who violated its ethical code regarding physician involvement in executions.

Despite a steady opposition by professional medical societies, and anesthesiologist-ethicists, to physician participation in the death penalty [74, 75], some anesthesiologist-ethicists have questioned the ABA edict. David Waisel argues that, whether physicians support the death penalty or not, perhaps anesthesiologists are best positioned to provide humane 'euthanasia' and should be permitted to do so under specific circumstances. Waisel argued further that humane euthanasia should be available to any individual, regardless of whether or not death is ordered by the state [76, 77].

The future of lethal injection, and of executions in general in the US, is uncertain: for the first time in history less than half of Americans favor capital punishment if life-long incarceration is assured for certain crimes [78]. Whatever the ultimate outcome of the debate, anesthesiologists will continue to have a major role in the debate regarding physician participation in executions—from formulating methods of execution, to potentially being the first specialty to punish its members should they participate.

The American Society of Anesthesiologists Committee on Ethics

The history of the Committee on Ethics of the American Society of Anesthesiologists (ASA) is best understood by reviewing the content of the original "*Guidelines to the Ethical Practice of Anesthesiology*," dating to the 1960s. These guidelines appropriately included an anesthesiologist's responsibilities to patients, other physicians, hospitals and nurse anesthetists. It also addressed financial aspects of anesthesia practice, such as fee-for-service rules, billing, and hospital contracts [79]. Credibly, those guidelines, also ruled against exploitation of patients, healthcare personnel and other anesthesiologists; warned against inappropriate prevention of qualified anesthesiologists from securing staff appointments; and promoted billing of reasonable fees, only for services personally rendered. These "ethical" guidelines notwithstanding, in 1977, the Federal Trade Commission (FTC) issued a proposed complaint against the ASA, alleging that the provision in its "ethical guidelines" that prohibited ASA membership by most employed physicians (i.e., those not practicing on a fee-for-service basis) impaired competition and thus violated antitrust laws. In truth, aspects of these guidelines, *at least* in part, were intended both to prevent exploitation of anesthesiologists by institutions, and to protect the best interests of patients from institutional economic interests. The ASA was forced to abandon that so-called "ethical" standard [80].

In the 1960s, the ASA had no committee on ethics, and its *Guidelines to the Ethical Practice of Anesthesiology* received no input from ethicists. In the late 1980s, some anesthesiologists and medical ethicists declared as unethical the common practice of automatically suspending existing Do-Not-Resuscitate (DNR) orders of surgical patients coming to the operating room. The need for the ASA to resolve this issue of not honoring a *patient's informed refusal* for resuscitation, as well as to decide upon other ethical matters (both past and into the future) led the ASA, in 1992, to establish a formal Committee on Ethics, chaired by Robert Stoelting. The following year and for the next decade, Stephen Jackson assumed the chairmanship, and he was succeeded, chronologically, by Susan Palmer, Gail Van Norman and Jeffrey Jacobs. The Committee on Ethics, a distinguished group of anesthesiologist-ethicists, has over a period of two decades, contributed to medical ethics well beyond its reconstruction and expansion of the ASA's ethical guidelines for anesthesiologists.

ASA Guidelines for the Ethical Practice of Anesthesiology

The 1992 formal Committee on Ethics re-wrote the ASA *Guidelines for the Ethical Practice of Anesthesiology* [81] to reflect ethical, rather than economic, issues. Guided by the American Medical Association's Principles of Medical Ethics and by ethical guidelines of other medical as well as non-medical professional organizations, Susan Palmer led the committee in composing guidelines that recognized physician responsibilities to patients, to colleagues, to health care facilities, to themselves and to the community. In so doing, the Committee empowered the ASA to be among the first medical organizations to declare such obligations to include the duty to provide health care to patients regardless of their ability to pay, to advise colleagues whose ability to provide care had become impaired to cease practice, to assist in the rehabilitation (when possible) of impaired colleagues to return to work, and to modify or cease practice if the anesthesiologist's physical health or ability to practice was in doubt [82].

ASA Ethical Guidelines for Patients with Do-Not-Resuscitate (DNR) Orders or Other Directives that Limit Care

The passage in the US Congress of the Patient Self-Determination Act of 1990 [83] responded to public concerns regarding the lingering authoritarianism and paternalism in the medical profession for decisions about life-sustaining therapies. The law stated that patients have the right to consent to *and to refuse* medical therapy, that health care institutions accepting government funding must both recognize those rights and inform patients of them, that institutions cannot then discriminate against patients because they have executed advance directives, and that the institutions must then see that such advance directives *are implemented to the extent permissible under state law*. This important Federal Law focused on a patient's right to refuse medical therapy, including life-sustaining therapy, tacitly recognizing that, without informed refusal, there cannot be *informed consent*.

Federal legislation to the contrary, until the early 1990s, the routine and essentially noncontroversial exception to this covenant was the surgical patient with preoperative DNR orders. As a universal institutional culture, pre-existing DNR orders were automatically suspended upon the patient's entrance into the operating room. Both bioethicists and patient-rights advocates vehemently challenged this violation of patient autonomy, and a flock of commentaries virtually unanimously declared that automatic suspension of DNR orders could not be ethically justified [84–95].

An early task for the newly established ASA Committee on Ethics, therefore, was to develop opinion and guidelines relevant to DNR orders. Led by Perry Fine and Joseph Layon, a task force of the committee created the *Ethical Guidelines for the Anesthesia Care of Patients with Do-Not-Resuscitate Orders or Other Directives that Limit Treatment* [96] that the 1993 ASA House of Delegates adopted, including:

> "*policies automatically suspending DNR orders ... may not sufficiently address a patient's rights to self-determination in a responsible and ethical manner. Such policies ... should be reviewed and revised.*" [96]

These guidelines required reconsideration and renegotiation of the DNR order [97, 98].

At the ASA's prompting, the American College of Surgeons [99] and the Association of Operating Room Nurses [100] soon followed suit with documents that paralleled the ASA's guidelines, advocating for the fundamental right of competent patients to define and limit what treatment would be provided to them in the operating room.

Whereas the original "DNR-in-OR" guidelines detailed specific procedures to avoid in the operating room, in 1998, the ASA Committee on Ethics revised the guidelines to incorporate a goals- and values-directed approach, in which the patient's goals would be outlined, and the anesthesiologist would be allowed more procedural flexibility. The revised guidelines recognized that the context of a cardiac arrest would play a larger role in determining the clinical response that it generates [101–103]. These efforts have gone a long way to draw the anesthesiologist into understanding the autonomous rights of patients in the operating room, but questions remain as to whether the quest for honoring patient autonomy is best served by a goals-directed process that may

introduce, rather than eliminate, ambiguities in decisions about therapeutic interventions [102].

The ASA's "DNR-in-OR" ethical guidelines also considered the moral views of individual physicians, and a means of resolving conflicts that might arise from conscientious objections [96, 104] of the physician to aspects of patient care. Indeed, in order for these guidelines to be ethically whole, anesthesiologists, surgeons and nurses must agree about how to manage ethically and emotionally perplexing scenarios.

Unequivocal enthusiasm did not greet the early efforts by the ASA Committee on Ethics to establish ethical, rather than economic, guidelines for physician behavior. The first proposal of the *Guidelines for Ethical Practice of Anesthesiology* was met with skepticism and at least one comment that the committee 'Must be made of West-Coast tree-huggers' (although only 3 of the 13 members of that committee hailed from west of the Rockies) and 'moon-beamers' (referring to a past—and present—governor of California).[5] After publication of the *Ethical Guidelines for the Anesthesia Care of Patients with DNR or other Directives that Limit Treatment*, a proposal was put forth to rescind the guidelines after the question of a lawsuit was raised against an anesthesiologist-member, who had resuscitated a patient against their will.[6] Despite these political hurdles, both guidelines remain cornerstones of the Committee's work. To this day, the only formal criterion for potential expulsion from ASA membership is failure to observe the guidelines of the Committee on Ethics. This growing role of medical ethics in shaping the specialty of anesthesiology was underscored by the 1999 ASA Annual Rovenstine lecture delivered by anesthesiologist-intensivist-ethicist Carl Hug Jr entitled 'Patient Values, Hippocrates, Science and Technology." [105]

Ethics of Medical Tests

The ethical implications of medical tests, such as genetic testing, have been widely discussed in the literature. However, until recently, professional societies have not formally addressed the ethical implications of routine testing despite the ethical dimensions—those of beneficence and nonmaleficence as well as implications for patient autonomy, privacy, and social justice.[7] [106]. Preoperative testing for pregnancy,

---

[5] Personal communication to the then chair of the ASA Committee on Ethics, Stephen Jackson.

[6] Letter of protest to the ASA Committee on Ethics.

[7] Social justice is the distribution of the limited resources made available by society for health care such that the burdens and benefits are borne fairly by others in society. In contradistinction to an individual patient's autonomous medical choices (self determination), distributive justice does not require serving the immediate good of the patient (beneficence). Thus it underscores a physician's obligation to society as well as to the individual.

HIV and hepatitis can introduce complex social implications and potential harms [107, 108]. The ethics of medical testing became of particular concern to the ASA Committee on Ethics when, despite the absence of supportive scientific evidence, the ASA published a Practice Advisory on Pre-anesthetic Evaluation in 2002 that buttressed the practice of unconsented routine pregnancy testing. Citing issues ranging from women's rights to women's autonomy and privacy, and the lack of evidence of medical benefit accruing from routine mandatory pregnancy testing, the ASA Committee on Ethics objected to this unsubstantiated advisory, finding that routine mandatory pregnancy testing may be unethical. The ensuing discussion between the *clinical practice* and the *ethical* arms of the ASA led to an amended Practice Advisory that recommended *offering* pregnancy testing with informed consent [109]. The change reflected both the limited existent scientific information and the ethical considerations involved with preoperative pregnancy testing [107]. In so doing, the ASA took an ethical leadership role that both questioned and limited a heretofore-paternalistic approach in routine medical care.

Council of Medical Specialty Societies' Contemporary Ethic of the Practice of Medicine

The Council of Medical Specialty Societies (CMSS) was created in 1965 to provide an independent, yet collaborative forum for the discussion by medical specialists of issues of national interest and mutual concern. In 1996, as an organization of then 17 (currently 39) national specialty societies, the CMSS established a Task Force to examine the traditional professional ethic of medicine—the attitudes and behaviors of physicians as ethical professionals—in modern healthcare delivery. This effort responded to the question of whether the traditional ethic should be abandoned, or adapted to fit the current realities of health care that, while having become more scientifically deciphered, also had fallen siege to potentially corrupting influences of the profession by public and commercial entities. Moreover, whereas the traditional ethic was rooted in the relationship between physician and patient, contemporary pressures had begun to shift physician responsibility from individual patients to patient populations (and only secondarily to individual patients), and thereby produce the greater good for the greater number of people. As with every ethic, this was likely to overlap with moral guidelines and the law.

It was envisioned that statements or concepts representing a consensus framework for ethical medical practice could be developed for consideration by each specialty society, and serve as a direction and stimulus for further initiatives, as well as a reference for practicing physicians. As the ASA's representative of that Task Force, Stephen Jackson intro-

duced the Task Force to the ASA's recently adopted *Guidelines for the Ethical Practice of Anesthesiology* [81]. The ASA Guidelines became the framework for the consensus statement that the CMSS adopted in 1999 [110][8]. This document, as with the ASA guidelines upon which it was built, acknowledged that it introduced only some of the values and principles governing the relationship between physicians and their patients, colleagues, organizations/institutions, and the larger society in which they practice. It remains to be determined whether one consensus ethic could guide the entire health care enterprise, as it did in the past, and whether any contemporary ethic based on the physician-patient relationship, would be sufficiently sensitive to the ethical demands of the greatly modified contemporary work environment.

Ethics and Anesthesiologists and the Shape of Things to Come

Anesthesiologists continue to be engaged in the evolving field of medical ethics. Robert Truog has challenged the dead donor rule (DDR), guiding principles in the transplantation of vital organs from one patient to another. He has also raised questions surrounding established practice concerning brain death and the declaration of death in patients providing organ donation after cardiac death (DCD) [111–115] He brings us, once again, back to Beecher's work [23] on revising the definition of death such that some patients with devastating neurologic injury become ethically and legally suitable for transplantation of their organs under the DDR. Indeed, individuals diagnosed as brain dead "maintain an extensive range of biological functioning of the organism as a whole." [116–118] Maintaining that the DDR has necessitated "unnecessary and unsupportable revisions of the definition of death," Truog also opines that the arguments supporting why these patients should be considered dead have never been "ethically convincing." Indeed, DCD challenges the reliance on the DDR because DCD patients are not brain dead, but rather undergo an orchestrated withdrawal of life support that leads to a cardiac asystole, for which a decision has been made to *not* attempt resuscitation. As the cardiac definition of death incorporates the irreversible cessation of cardiac function, that irreversibility is the consequence of a choice to *not* reverse, and indeed, these patients' hearts have been successfully transplanted. Truog does conclude that "characterizing the ethical requirements of organ donation in terms of valid informed consent [from patients or surrogates] under the limited conditions of devastating neurologic injury is ethically sound," and even that it is ethical to retrieve vital organs *before* death in such patients, provided that anesthesia is administered." [119]

---

[8] Steve Jackson's personal observation.

The prominent French bioethicist, Sadek Beloucif, has focused on ethics in informed consent for procedures with special societal implications—such as psychosurgery (e.g., lobotomy) and electoconvulsive therapy [120]—as well as patient rights with regard to pain relief, organ transplantation, and issues of self-determination at end-of-life. Beloucif has explored the preeminent ethical issues relating to psychosurgery: their scientific validity, the unique ethical intricacies of the process of informed consent for such interventions, and the potential conflict between the interests of the patient and those of society, particularly for violent individuals. He emphasizes that human dignity is deeply embedded in the concept of free will, as he advocates for ethical safeguards to protect the rights of mentally afflicted patients who present for psychosurgical techniques and functional psychiatric interventions.

The first textbooks of ethics for anesthesiologists, published in 2003 and 2011 [121, 122], addressed topics beyond anesthesiology, and they have relevance to "the domain of other physicians and surgeons," [123] reflecting the broad reach of the specialty. As one surgeon wrote,

"Although there is room for discussion and disagreement about how truly distinct the ethics of anesthesiology should be from, for example, the ethics of surgery [or any other medical discipline], there should be no disagreement over the importance of addressing ethical issues from the perspective of specific disciplines ... the field of clinical medical ethics requires attention from all specialties in medical practice." [124]

The specialty of anesthesiology touches on issues from birth to death involving clinical care and research, and even human rights. Medical ethics continues to evolve, shaping the nature of medical care and the kind of practitioners who will care for us in the years to come. Anesthesiologists will continue to shape debate about the intersection of medical science and moral obligations.

References

1. Edelstein L. The hippocratic oath: text, translation and interpretation. Ancient Medicine: selected papers of Ludwig Edelstein. In Temkin O, Temkin CL. Baltimore, Johns Hopkins Press, 1967. pp. 3–63.
2. Cohen J. After office hours. Doctor James Young Simpson, Rabbi Abraham De Sola, and Genesis Chapter 3, verse 16. Obst Gyn. 1996;88:895–8.
3. Holy Bible. New King James Version.
4. Takrouri MSM. Basis of obstetric analgesia and anaesthesia during childbirth. Internet J Health. 2009;9.
5. Defalque RJ, Wright AJ. In the name of God: why Agnes Sampson and Eufame McCalyean were burned at the stake. Bull Anesth History. 2004;22.
6. Lurie S. Euphemia McLean, Agnes Sampson, and pain relief during labour in 16th Century Edinburgh. Anaesthesia. 2004;59:834–5.
7. Snow S. Blessed days of anaesthesia: how anesthetics changed the world. Oxford:Oxford University Press; 2008.
8. Calhoun CC. Longfellow: a rediscovered life. Boston: Beacon Press; 2004. p. 189.
9. Darwin Correspondence Project. Cambridge University Library. West Road, Cambridge UK. http://darwinproject.ac.uk/what-did-darwin-believe-article. Accessed: 15 Aug. 2012.
10. Robinson A. Taking the Pain Away. Oxford: Oxford University Press; 2008. p. 226.
11. Ellis Richard H, Editor. The case books of Dr. John Snow, Medical History, Suppl No. 14. London: Wellcome Institute for the History of Medicine; 1994. p. 271.
12. Sanghavi D. The mother lode of pain. The Boston Globe, July 23, 2006.
13. Address by Pope Pius XII to the Ninth National Congress of the Italian Society for the Science of Anesthetics. Feb. 24, 1957.
14. Giordano J, Hover G. Conjoining interventional pain management and palliative care: considerations for practice, ethics and policy. In: Van Norman G, Jackson S, Rosenbaum S, Palmer S, Editors. Clinical Ethics in Anesthesiology. Cambridge: Cambridge University Press; 2011. pp. 143–7.
15. Benedetti C, Chapman CR, John J. Bonica: a biography. Minerva Anestesiol. 2005;71. 7–8, 391–6.
16. International Association for the Study of Pain. Global year against pain. http://www.iasp-pain.org/Content/NavigationMenu/GlobalYearAgainstPain/20042005RighttoPainRelief/default.htm. Accessed: 15 Aug. 2012.
17. Cahana A. Testimony before the Untied States Senate Finance Subcommittee on Health. March 22, 2012.
18. Cahana A. Pain and philosophy of the mind. Pain Clin Updates. 2007;15:1–4.
19. Fox M. Martha Mason, who wrote a book about her decades in an Iron Lung, dies at 71. The New York Times. May 9, 2009.
20. Ibsen B. The anaesthetist's viewpoint on the treatment of respiratory complications in poliomyelitis during the epidemic in Copenhagen, 1952. Proc Royal Soc Med. 1954;47:72–4.
21. Jonsen AR. The Birth of Bioethics. Oxford: Oxford University Press; 1998. pp. 133–40, 236–8.
22. Pope Pius XII. Address to the International Congress of Anesthesiologists. November 24, 1957, L'Osservatore Romano. Nov. 25–26, 1957.
23. A definition of irreversible coma. Report of the Ad Hoc Committee of the Harvard Medical School to Examine the Definition of Brain Death. JAMA. 1968;205:337–40.
24. Lowenstein E. Defining brain death: motivations and future directions. Int Anes Clin. 2007;45:121–3.
25. Leo Alexander. Medical science under dictatorship. NEJM. 1949;241:45.
26. Medical Decisions About the End of Life. I. Report of the Committee to Study the Medical Practice Concerning Euthanasia. II. The Study for the Committee on Medical Practice Concerning Euthanasia (2 vol.). The Hague, September 19, 1991.
27. Admiraal P. Justifiable euthanasia. Issues Law Med. 1988;3:361–70.
28. Admiraal P. Listening and helping to die: the Dutch way.In: Kuhse H, Singer P, Editors. Bioethics: an anthology. 2nd edn. Oxford: Blackwell Publishing; 2006. pp. 391–8.
29. Egbert L. Death with dignity: what is the role of the physician? Tex Med. 1991;93:57–9.
30. Shuster E. Fifty years later: the significance of the Nuremberg Code. NEJM. 1997;337:1436–40.
31. Rothman D. Strangers at the bedside: a history of how law and bioethics transformed medical decision making. New York: Basic Books; 1991. Pp. 62–3, 85–94.
32. Guttentag O. The problem of experimentation in humans. Science. 1953;117:205–14.
33. Freidenfelds L. Recruiting allies for reform. Int Anes Clin. 2007;45:79–103.
34. Beecher HK. Experimentation in man. JAMA. 1959;169:461–78.

35. Beecher HK. Some fallacies and errors in the application of the principle of consent in human experimentation. Clin Pharmacol Ther. 1962;3:141–6.

36. Beecher HK. Ethics and experimental therapy. JAMA. 1963;186:858–9.

37. Gaw A. Exposing unethical human research: the transatlantic correspondence of Beecher and Pappworth. Ann Int Med. 2012;156:150–5.

38. National Institute of Health Almanac. Appropriations. http://www.nih.gov/about/almanac/appropriations/index.htm. Accessed: 10 Aug. 2012.

39. Silverman WA. Bad science and the role of institutional review boards. Arch Ped Adolesc Med. 2000;154:1183–4.

40. Beecher HK. Ethics and clinical research. NEJM. 1966;274:1354–60.

41. Belmont Report. United States Department of Health and Human Services, April 18, 1979. US DHHS, 200 Independence Ave SW, Washington DC 20201. http://www.hhs.gov/ohrp/humansubjects/guidance/belmont.html. Accessed: 10 Aug2012.

42. Von Felsinger J, Lasagna L, Beecher H. The response of normal men to lysergic acid derivatives. J Clin Exp Psychopathol. 1956;17:414–28.

43. Mashour G. From LSD to the IRB: Henry Beecher's psychedelic research and the foundation of clinical ethics. Int Anes Clin. 2007;45:105–11.

44. Moreno J. Bioethics and the national security state. J Law Med Ethics. 2004;198–208.

45. Lasagna L. "Hippocratic Oath—Modern Version". From: The Hippocratic Oath Today by Peter Tyson, NOVA. 1964. http://www.pbs.org/wgbh/nova/body/hippocratic-oath-today.html. Accessed: 10 Aug 2012.

46. Borrell B. A medical Madoff: anesthesiologist faked data in 21 studies. Scientific American, March 10, 2009. http://www.scientificamerican.com/article.cfm?id=a-medical-madoff-anesthestesiologist-faked-data.

47. White PF, Carl R. Shafer S. The Scott Reuben saga: one last retraction. Anesth Analg. 2011;112:512–5.

48. Retractions Watch. http://retractionwatch.wordpress.com/2011/02/28/22-papers-by-joachim-boldt-retracted-and-67-likely-on-the-way/. Accessed: 10 Aug 2012.

49. Yentis SM. Lies, damn lies, and statistics. Anaesthesia. 2012;67:455–6.

50. Kompetent leistungsstark innovativ partnershaft lich umsorgen. http://www.klilu.de/content/aktuelles_presse/pressearchiv/2012/hospital_presents_results_of_final_report_committee_completes_investigation_in_the_case_of_dr_boldt/index_ger.html. Accessed: 15 Aug. 2012.

51. Wagner E. Who is responsible for investigating suspected research misconduct? Anaesthesia. 2012;67:462–6.

52. Normile D. "A New Record for Retractions?", Science Insider (American Association for the Advancement of Science). 2 July 2012.

53. Kranke P, Apfel CC, Roewer N. Reported data on granisetron and postoperative nausea and vomiting by Fujii et al. are incredibly nice! Anesth Analg. 2000;90:1004–7.

54. Moore RA, Derry S, McQuay HJ. Fraud or flawed: adverse impact of fabricated or poor quality research. Anaesthesia. 2010;65:327–30.

55. Shafer S. Anesthesia and Analgesia policy on institutional review board approval and informed consent for research. Anesth Analg. 2011;112:494–5.

56. Yentis S. Research, audit, and journal policies. Anes Analg. 2011;112:496–7.

57. Shafer S. Personal communication to Stephen Jackson. Nov. 1, 2012.

58. Carlisle JB. The analysis of 168 randomised controlled trials to test data integrity. Anaesthesia. 2012;67:521–37.

59. Pandit JJ. On statistical methods to test if sampling in trials is genuinely random. Anaesthesia. 2012;67:456–62.

60. Shafer S. You will be caught. Anesth Analg. 2011;112:491–3.

61. Human Rights Watch. So long as they die. 2006;18(1).

62. Hospira Statement Regarding Penthothal (sodium thiopental) market exit. Hospira. Lake Forest, Ill. Jan 21, 2011. http://phx.corporate-ir.net/phoenix.zhtml?c=175550&p=irol-newsArticle&ID=1518610&highlight=Pentothal. Accessed: 15 Aug 2012.

63. Casciani D. US lethal injection drug faces UK export restriction. BBCnews, UK. Nov 29, 2010. http://www.bbc.co.uk/news/uk-11865881. Accessed: 15 Aug. 2012.

64. Lohr K. New lethal injection drug raises concerns. Jan 29, 2011. National Public Radio. http://www.npr.org/2011/01/29/133302950/new-lethal-injection-drug-raises-concerns. Accessed: 16 Aug. 2012.

65. Morales MA, Hickman RQ. Secretary of the California Dept of Corrections and Rehabilitation. US District Court N. Calif. Case 5:06-cv-00219-JF. http://www.deathpenaltyinfo.org/Calif.leth.inj.Order.pdf. Accessed: 15 Aug. 2012.

66. Smith S. Doctor leaves prison to avoid participating in Morales' execution. Recordnet.com Sept 29, 2006. http://www.recordnet.com/apps/pbcs.dll/article?AID=/20060929/NEWS01/609290328. Accessed: 15 Aug. 2012.

67. Weinstein H. Showdown looming over lethal injection in Missouri. The Seattle Times. July 17, 2006. http://seattletimes.nwsource.com/html/nationworld/2003131722_execute17.html. Accessed: 15 Aug. 2012.

68. Guidry OF. Message from the president: observations regarding lethal injection. June 30, 2006. American Society of Anesthesiologists. Park Ridge, Il. http://asatest.asahq.org/news/asanews063006.htm. Accessed: 15 Aug. 2012.

69. American Society of Anesthesiologists Committee on Ethics. Statement on physician non-participation in legally authorized executions. Approved by the ASA House of Delegates on October 18, 2006; reaffirmed on October 19, 2011. www.asahq.org.

70. Associated Press. Anesthesiologist joins Missouri's execution team. Missourian, May 25, 2008. http://www.columbiamissourian.com/stories/2008/05/25/anesthesiologist-joins-missouris-execution-team/. Accessed: 15 Aug. 2012.

71. Opinion 2.06. Capital punishment. American Medical Association Code of Medical Ethics. Issued July 1980. http://www.ama-assn.org/ama/pub/physician-resources/medical-ethics/code-medical-ethics/opinion206.page. Accessed: 15 Aug. 2012.

72. Truog R, Brennan T. Participation of physicians in capital punishment. NEJM. 1993;329:1346–50.

73. Anesthesiologists and Capital Punishment. Professional Standing. A statement of the American Board of Anesthesiology, Park Ridge, Il. Issued February 2010. http://www.theaba.org/Home/notices#punishment. Accessed: 15 Aug. 2012.

74. Truog R. Are there some things doctors just shouldn't do? Hastings Center Rep. 2011;41:3.

75. Lanier WL, Berge KH. Physician involvement in capital punishment: simplifying a complex calculus. Mayo Clin Proc. 2007;82:1043–6.

76. Waisel D. Physician participation in capital punishment. Mayo Clin Proc. 2007;82:1073–80.

77. Gawande A, Denno D, Truog R, Waisel D. Perspective: physicians and execution – highlights from a discussion of lethal injection. NEJM. 2008;358:448–51.

78. Newport F. In U.S. 64% support death penalty in case of murder. Nov 8, 2010. Gallup Inc. 2010. http://www.gallup.com/poll/144284/Support-Death-Penalty-Cases-Murder.aspx. Accessed: 15 Aug. 2011.

79. American Society of Anesthesiologists. Guidelines for the ethical practice of anesthesiology. Directory of members. 33rd Edn. ASA: Park Ridge, IL; 1968.

80. Scott M. 1979 adventures in antitrust: some justice here, some FTC there. ASA Newsletter. 2004;68:18–9.

81. American Society of Anesthesiologists Committee on Ethics. Guidelines for the ethical practice of anesthesiology. Approved by the ASA House of Delegates, October 15, 2003. Last amended, October 19, 2011. www.asahq.org.

82. Specht T, Ward C, Jackson S. The impaired anesthesiologist—addiction. In: Van Norman G, Jackson S, Rosenbaum S, Palmer S, Editors. Clinical Ethics in Anesthesiology. Cambridge: Cambridge University Press; 2011. pp. 219–23.

83. H.R. 4449 IH—Patient Self Determination Act of 1990. (101st Congress, 1989–1990) http://thomas.loc.gov/cgi-bin/query/z?c101:H.R.4449.IH:. Accessed: 15 Aug. 2012.

84. Truog R. "Do-not-resuscitate" orders during anesthesia and surgery. Anesthesiology. 1991;74:606–8.

85. Lees D. Do not resuscitate orders and the anesthesiologist. ASA Newsletter. 1991;55:19–21.

86. Steer P. Do not resuscitate orders: considerations for the anesthesiologist. Anesthesiol Rev. 1992;19:12–6.

87. Martin R, Soifer B, Stevens W. Ethical issues in anesthesia: management of the do-not-resuscitate patient. Anesth Analg. 1991;73:221–5.

88. Youngner S, Cascorbi H, Shuck J. DNR in the operating room: not really a paradox. JAMA. 1991;266:2433–4.

89. Walker R. DNR in the OR. JAMA. 1991;266:2407–12.

90. Franklin C, Rothenberg D. DNR in the OR. JAMA. 1992;267:1465.

91. Truog R, Rockoff M, Brustowicz R. DNR in the OR. JAMA. 1992;267:1466.

92. Cohen C, Cohen P. Do-not-resuscitate orders in the operating room. NEJM. 1991;325:1879–82.

93. Keffer M, Keffer H. Do-not-resuscitate in the operating room: moral obligations of anesthesiologists. Anes Analg. 1992;74:901–5.

94. Clemency M, Thompson N. Do not resuscitate orders and the anesthesiologist: a survey. Anesth Analg. 1993;76:394–401.

95. Rothenberg D. Ethical issues in the operating room. Clinical Anesthesia Updates. 1993;4:1–11.

96. American Society of Anesthesiologists. Ethical guidelines for the anesthesia care of patients with do-not-resuscitate orders or other directives that limit treatment. 2012. www.asahq.org.

97. Waisel D, Jackson S, Fine P. Should do-not-resuscitate orders be suspended for surgical cases? Cur Opin Anes. 2003;16:209–13.

98. Fine P, Jackson S. Do not resuscitate in the operating room: more than rights and wrongs. Am J Anes. 1995;22:45–51.

99. American College of Surgeons. [ST-19] Statement on advance directives by patients: do not resuscitate in the operating room. Bull Amer Coll Surg. 1994;79:29.

100. Association of Operating Room Nurses (AORN—currently titled Association of Perioperative Registered Nurses). Position statement: perioperative care of patients with do-not-resuscitate or allow-natural-death orders. AORN. Approved by the House of Delegates, March, 1995. http://www.aorn.org/search.aspx?searchtext=DNR#axzz23p9HidZl. Accessed: 15 Aug. 2012.

101. Truog R, Waisel D, Burns J. DNR in the OR: a goal-directed approach. Anesthesiology. 1999;90:289–95.

102. Jackson S, Van Norman G. Goals- and values-directed approach to informed consent in the "DNR" patient presenting for surgery: more demanding of the anesthesiologist? Anesthesiology. 1999;90:3–6.

103. Waisel D, Truog R. Informed consent for the patient with an existing DNR order. ASA Newsletter. 2001;65:13–4.

104. Morgenweck C, Jackson S. Physician conscientious objection in anesthesiology practice. In: Van Norman G, Jackson S, Rosenbaum S, Palmer S, Editors. Clinical ethics in anesthesiology. Cambridge: Cambridge University Press; 2011. pp. 257–60.

105. Hug C Jr. Rovenstine lecture: patient values, hippocrates, science, and technology: what we (physicians) can do versus what we should do for the patient. Anesthesiology. 2000;93:556–64.

106. Van Norman G. Ethical challenges of routine preoperative tests. ASA Newsletter. 2012;76:42–3.

107. Van Norman G. Informed consent for preoperative testing: pregnancy testing and other tests involving sensitive patient issues. In: Van Norman G, Jackson S, Rosenbaum S, Palmer S, Editors. Clinical Ethics in Anesthesiology. Cambridge: Cambridge University Press; 2011. pp. 79–84.

108. Rosenbaum S, Jackson S. Ethics and the HIV/AIDS epidemic. ASA Newsletter 1996; 60:16-9

109. American Society of Anesthesiologists Task Force on Preanesthesia Evaluation: Practice advisory for preanesthesia evaluation: an updated report. Anesthesiology 116:522–538, 2012.

110. Council of Medical Specialty Societies. Ethics statement. November 1999. www.cmss.org. Accessed: July 15, 2012.

111. Truog R, Capmbell M, Curtis JR, Haas C, Luce J, Rubenfeld G, Rushton C, Kaufman DC. Recommendations for end-of-life care in the intensive care unit: a consensus statement by the American college of critical care medicine. Crit Care Med. 2008;36:953–63.

112. Truog R, Brett A, Frader A. The problem with futility. NEJM. 1992;326:1560–4.

113. Truog R. End-of-life decision-making in the United States. Eur J Anaesth. 2008;25 (Suppl 42):43–50.

114. Truog R. Is it always wrong to perform futile CPR? NEJM. 2010;362:477–9.

115. Truog R. Tackling medical futility in Texas. NEJM. 2007;357:1–3.

116. Truog R. Brain death—too flawed to endure, too ingrained to abandon. J Law Med Ethics. 2007;35:273–81.

117. Truog R, Miller F. Are donors after circulatory death really dead, and does it matter? No and not really. Chest. 2010;138:16–8.

118. Truog R, Miller F. The dead donor rule and organ transplantation. NEJM. 2008;359:674–5.

119. Truog D, Brock D, White D. Should patients receive general anesthesia prior to extubation at the end of life? Crit Care Med. 2012;40:631–3.

120. Beloucif S. Consent for anesthesia for procedures with special society implications: psychosurgery and electroconvulsive therapy. In: Van Norman G, Jackson S, Rosenbaum S, Palmer S, Editors. Clinical ethics in anesthesiology. Cambridge: Cambridge University Press; 2011. pp. 55–60.

121. Draper H, Scott W. Ethics in anaesthesia and intensive care. Edinburgh: Elsevier. 2003.

122. Van Norman G, Jackson S, Rosenbaum S, Palmer S. Clinical ethics in anesthesiology: a case-based textbook. Cambridge:Cambridge University Press; 2011.

123. Dauber M. Book review of clinical ethics in anesthesiology: a case-based textbook. JAMA. 2011;306:1603–4.

124. Angelos P. Book review of clinical ethics in anesthesiology: a case-based textbook. Anesthesiology. 2012;117:222–4.

A History of Drug Addiction in Anesthesia

Christopher D. Kent and Karen B. Domino

Summary

Heroes from the early history of anesthesia, Davy, Wells, Glover, and Halsted, all displayed a sometimes fatal addiction to inhaled anesthetics, cocaine, or opioids. Even before the 1900s, society debated whether addiction was a disease or an immoral weakness of will. In the 1890s, states (but not the Federal US government) passed anti-morphine laws to stem addiction. Observations at this time indicated that physicians might be at increased risk of addiction. In 1906, the Federal Pure Food and Drug Act banned importation of potentially harmful drugs, and the 1914 Harrison Narcotic Tax Act required the Treasury Department to enforce the law. In the 1930s, the US Public Health Service established drug addiction treatment hospitals having features consistent with a view of addiction as both disease and vice.

In his 1955 treatise on drug addiction among physicians, Marks estimated that roughly "…one out of every hundred physicians in the United States has been, or is, addicted to narcotics…", and several (but not all) observers considered that anesthesiologists were at greater risk than other physicians. In 1975, the Georgia Medical Association funded an Impaired Physician Program to treat impaired physicians. In 1983, it found that anesthesiologists comprised 9.6% of its first 507 patients but made up only 4% of the physicians in the US. Studies from 1983 and 1984 corroborated the Georgia data. Surveys in the 2000s revealed that anesthesiologists frequently abused synthetic opioids, with propofol also emerging as a drug of abuse.

In the 1980s and 1990s, the anesthesia community responded to the addiction "epidemic" with tools for preventing drug abuse, for early detection of abuse, and for assisting in recovery. No study has shown that these tools are effective.

A retrospective survey of anesthesiology program directors in 1983 found a large incidence of relapse with death in anesthesiology residents using parenteral opioids, concluding that such residents should be redirected to an alternative career. However, a 1984 review of addiction among anesthesiologists by Spiegelman and colleagues suggested that 60–80% of addicted physicians sustained recovery after a return to practice, with the same recovery success as that of other physicians. Estimates from treatment programs in the 1990s suggested that up to 70% of addicted health care professionals successfully returned to medical practice, with a sustained recovery among anesthesiologists similar to that of physicians working in other areas. Independent reviews in 1994 and 2005 did not reveal that any patient injury resulted from errors made by impaired anesthesiologists.

The problem of addiction in anesthesia is real and substantial. Although much of the discussion applies to anesthesiologists, parallel problems and solutions appear for nurse anesthetists. For both groups, the history of addiction's causes and management indicates that it is a soluble problem.

Introduction

"It's a poor sort of memory that only works backwards."
—Lewis Carroll from *Through the Looking Glass and What Alice Found There*

Despite what Jefferson Airplane may have implied in their song *White Rabbit*, no evidence indicates that drug use inspired the fantastic scenes from Lewis Carroll's stories. This introductory quotation merely reminds us that we need to project what we learn from our memories and history onto the future.

Discoveries and innovations in anesthesia and patient care are largely triumphs of hard work and celebrations of brilliant insights. But much might be learned from darker stories. The history of drug addiction in anesthesia reveals few triumphs, but does provide opportunities for insight, and perhaps redemption, in the stories of the lives affected and sometimes ended by this occupational hazard. Our burden of this disease has made us leaders in the struggle against it. By facing the problem of addiction in our profession, we better

C. D. Kent (✉) · K. B. Domino
Department of Anesthesiology and Pain Medicine,
University of Washington, 1959 NE Pacific Street, Seattle,
WA 98195-6540, USA
e-mail: Kentc02@u.washington.edu

insure that our patients do not become additional victims of the disease.

Perhaps no other story in the history of anesthesia evokes such powerful emotional responses from anesthetists. At its heart are fundamental human questions; what are the limits of free will and of responsibility for choices affected by environment and genetics. It raises questions specific to our role as self-regulating professionals. How should we respond to the violation of professional trust? How do we simultaneously protect our patients while assisting and providing a safe second chance for each colleague in recovery? This chapter reviews the history of addiction, particularly as it broadens our understanding of the history of addiction among anesthetists. The review focuses on the medications used in daily anesthetic practice, those to which anesthetists have direct and sometimes unique access. We examine the stages of our recognition, as a specialty, of our problem with addiction, and the history of our evolving response to it.

Some terms we use require clarification. Drug addiction, drug abuse, and chemical and controlled substance misuse can be found in source materials on this topic but are not synonymous. Aside from alcohol, the substances most abused and the primary focus of addictions among anesthetists are opioids, so we frequently employ the terms opioid abuse and opioid addiction. The term narcotic originally meant any drug that produces narcosis or sleep, but now this term refers to substances whose use is legally restricted and includes activating substances such as cocaine, so the term is avoided except in direct quotation.

Finally, we note that the problem of addiction extends to all of the anesthesia community. The present chapter focuses on the problem in physicians. Nurse anesthetists and organizations such as the American Association of Nurse Anesthetists have confronted the same problem (see Chapter 22).

Pioneers in Discovery and Addiction

The story of addiction and anesthesia coincides with the discovery of inhalational anesthesia. In 1795, building on the work of Joseph Priestley, Humphry Davy isolated, contained and inhaled nitrous oxide. He briefly noted nitrous oxide's potential as an anesthetic agent, but as the center of a group of creative luminaries such as the potter Josiah Wedgwood, and the poets Samuel Coleridge and William Wordsworth, Davy focused much of his attention on its recreational use. From 1798 to 1800, Davy inhaled nitrous oxide compulsively, providing evidence for an addiction in this description; "I ought to have observed that a desire to breathe the gas is always awakened in me by the sight of a person breathing, or even by that of an air-bag or an air-holder." Although he eventually controlled his use of the drug and went on to unparalleled success as a chemist (e.g., he discovered the

element sodium), Davy seems to have suffered short term health consequences from its use and the consequent inactivation of methionine synthase from prolonged exposure to nitrous oxide: "increased sensibility of touch: my fingers were pained by anything rough, and the tooth-edge produced from slighter causes than usual. I was certainly more irritable and felt more acutely from trifling circumstances [1]."

Fifty years later, Horace Wells in the U.S. and Robert Glover in the U.K. were not as fortunate as Davy. They lived out parallel stories of thwarted recognition and addiction that led to their deaths. Wells considered himself to be the discoverer of inhalational anesthesia. He provided a proof of concept with nitrous oxide use in his dental practice, and a partially successful demonstration with nitrous oxide in 1845 at the Massachusetts General Hospital. But William Morton's triumph at the same site eclipsed Wells' efforts on what became known as Ether Day in 1846 [2]. The perception that Wells' anesthetic was "humbug" while Morton's was a miraculous success plagued Wells, as he vied, largely unsuccessfully with Morton and Charles Jackson, for recognition as the discoverer of anesthesia. Similarly, Glover felt cheated by James Simpson from the recognition of his (Glover's) discovery of chloroform's anesthetic potential. Glover had published the results of his studies with chloroform in animals 5 years before Simpson's reports of chloroform anesthesia in humans [3].

The greatest tragedy in the lives of Wells and Glover was not the lack of recognition of their roles in the discovery of anesthesia, but their lack of recognition of the consequences of self-experimentation with chloroform. Wells was among the first practitioners to use it in the US but failed to appreciate the hazards that might result from its frequent use. Upon moving to New York City in 1848, Wells advertised his arrival in the *Herald*:

> H. Wells, Surgeon Dentist, who is known as the discoverer of the wonderful effect of ether and various stimulating gases in annulling pain, would inform the citizens of New York that he has moved to this city, and will for the present attend personally to those who may require his professional services. It is now over three years since he first made this valuable discovery, and from that time to the present, not one of his patients has experienced the slightest ill effects from it; the sensation is highly pleasurable [2].

Wells asserted that breathing chloroform was "highly pleasurable", a view arising from his frequent personal use of the anesthetic. What may have started as "scientific" experimentation to master the use of chloroform changed to something more sinister. Wells turned from its use as an anesthetic to its use for pleasure.

In an incident in the days leading up to his death, Wells recounted helping a male acquaintance obtain revenge upon a woman by providing sulfuric acid used subsequently to attack her. Three days later, after a prolonged chloroform binge, Wells apparently went on his own sulfuric acid rampage. Allegedly, he threw acid on two women. He claimed his chloroform-induced delirium impaired his memory of what happened. Wells was arrested and imprisoned. He was tortured by guilt over the effect that his actions would have on his personal and professional reputation, and the reputation of his family. He was escorted to his home to obtain toiletries for his stay in prison, and while there surreptitiously obtained chloroform and a razor. After returning to his cell, Wells wrote to his wife and others outlining his actions and remorse over the events of the preceding days. Then in the desperate isolation of his cell, Wells soaked a handkerchief with chloroform, secured it in his mouth, and slashed an artery in his left thigh. His death was reported as "suicide while under temporary insanity."

Confounding our ability to make sense of the circumstances surrounding Wells' death is the contemporaneous report of a police officer who could not find evidence of any women injured in an attack with acid. Nor could the officer find anyone who corroborated the initial testimony of the accusers appearing in court when Wells was arrested [1]. Did Wells die in part as a result of the guilt and shame over hallucinatory experiences produced by chloroform intoxication? Wells' death tragically parallels the deaths of others who desperately thought that they were trapped by the consequences of their drug use.

Glover's equally tragic death from addiction was less dramatic and more protracted. He appears to be the first physician with documented poly-substance abuse. He became addicted to both opium and chloroform after treating himself for symptoms associated with dysentery acquired during the Crimean War in 1856. His death followed a slow decline over the next three years from heavy chloroform and opium use and was ruled an "accidental death by overdose of chloroform ingested to produce intoxication."

William Halsted: Addiction to Cocaine and Morphine

In the first century after the introduction of ether, few physicians dedicated their practice to the delivery of anesthesia. Many who practiced anesthesia were surgeons like William Halsted. While he was a faculty member at Columbia University, Halsted experimented with the use of cocaine as a local anesthetic, demonstrating its capacity to block superficial nerves [4]. He produced plexus anesthesia by direct application of cocaine to the nerves after open dissection and exposure, a lengthy process that should put in perspective present complaints by surgeons about delays associated with peripheral nerve blocks. While developing this expertise, Halsted became addicted to cocaine. The severity of his addiction prompted his closest friend and fellow physician,

William Welch, to take Halsted on a long sea voyage to attempt a cure [5]. Halsted demonstrated the depth of his addiction first by sneaking a stash of cocaine on board and then by breaking into the Captain's locked medicine chest when his supply ran out.

Following this unsuccessful treatment, Halsted checked into a psychiatric hospital where in addition to the holistic treatments of "seclusion, fresh air, exercise, a healthful diet, and a gradual withdrawal from cocaine" he received morphine to treat the symptoms of cocaine withdrawal—thereby starting his lifelong addiction to morphine. In the first two years of his battle with morphine addiction, he re-entered the treatment facility and struggled to re-establish his reputation as a physician. Despite signs that he secretly used morphine and possibly cocaine for the rest of his life, Halsted became the Chief Surgeon at Johns Hopkins, recognized as both a great surgeon and pioneer in patient safety. In a diary unsealed in 1969, William Osler recounted having seen Halsted suffering from extreme chills. His conversation with Halsted on this subject led Osler to write, "[Halsted] has never been able to reduce the amount to less than three grains [of morphine] daily, on this he could do his work comfortably and maintain his excellent physical vigor…. I do not think that anyone suspected him… [6]." An entry in a letter from Halsted to Osler illustrates Halsted's good fortune relative to some other colleagues, "Poor Hall and two other assistants of mine acquired the cocaine habit in the course of our experiments on ourselves—injecting nerves. They all died without recovering from the habit [7]."

Addiction: Moral Failure or Disease?

Halstead acquired his first addiction—to cocaine—through self-experimentation with a substance unrecognized as addictive, and his second addiction—to morphine—as treatment for the first. His life-long secrecy on the matter suggests that neither his accidental path to addiction nor the fact that opioids were widely and legally available in patent medicines could mitigate his shame in this matter. The recreational use of opioids in the US in the 19th century was primarily thought to be confined to opium smoking, a practice symbolically associated with Chinese immigrants. The most common path to opioid addiction, however, was through prescription and non-prescription medical use. Opium and its derivatives were used to treat acute and chronic pain, stress, insomnia, and menstrual pain [8].

Although 19th century control over opioid importation and distribution was limited, addiction to opioids appears to have been stigmatized. Some medical literature characterized opioid addiction as a loss of "moral will" or a problem that affected susceptible, weak individuals in the lower social classes [8, 9]. In a brief chapter on the "Morphia Habit" in his textbook of 1892, Osler wrote, "Persons addicted to morphia are inveterate liars, and no reliance whatever can be placed upon their statements. In many instances this is not confined to matters relating to the vice [10]." Osler's words have a moralizing tone absent from those used by his contemporary JB Mattison, the medical director of a home in Brooklyn for treatment of opiate addiction. Mattison wrote in 1894, "it is easy to moralize on the weak will—as many, mistakenly, are wont to put it … but talk about weak will as a reason why strong men succumb to morphia …is twaddle [11]."

The idea that addiction, starting with alcohol and later encompassing other drugs, is a disease rather than a sign of moral intemperance is more than 2000 years old. References to chronic drunkenness as a sickness of the body and soul, and the existence of specialized roles to care for people suffering from "drink madness" appear in writings from ancient Egypt and Greece [12]. Benjamin Rush (1745–1813), a prominent American physician, advanced this idea, asserting that alcoholism was a disease in which alcohol is the causal agent, loss of control over drinking behavior the characteristic symptom, and total abstinence the only effective cure [13]. Since the 1930s, the successful treatment approaches used by Alcoholics Anonymous and Narcotics Anonymous incorporate the idea that addiction is a disease requiring multi-faceted treatment [14, 15].

In contrast, many societies and individuals, including physicians, held and continue to hold conflicting views as to the idea of addiction as disease. Physicians surveyed by the Treasury Committee's 1919 report *Traffic in Narcotic Drugs* were almost evenly divided on whether drug addiction was a disease or a vice [16]. This idea of addiction as something other than disease has persisted, as apparent in this statement from a 1962 review article by a psychiatrist purportedly specializing in addiction: "Addiction is caused far more by human weakness than the drugs themselves and from the psychiatric point of view is essentially a symptom of personality maladjustment [17]." Even recently, psychologists and psychiatrists expressed dissenting opinions in response to the Recognizing Addiction as a Disease Act of 2007. This act was intended to change the name of the National Institute on Drug Abuse to the National Institute on Diseases of Addiction and the name of the National Institute on Alcohol Abuse and Alcoholism to the National Institute on Alcohol Disorders and Health. Some may consider this an empty battle over semantics, but therapists resisting the change assert that the disease terminology is bad for the public's "mental health literacy" and is excessively fatalistic and disempowering, implying that users cannot fully free themselves of their drug or alcohol problems [18].

These opposing viewpoints underlie the conflicting responses to societal and individual problems associated with opioid addiction in US governmental policies, policies that have sometimes focused on the restriction of access to opioids and enforcement of legal penalties for abuse, while at other times centered on treating a disease. In the 1890s, although no federal laws restricted opioid distribution, various states began to pass anti-morphine laws, ostensibly to stem the rapidly increasing numbers of addicted individuals [8]. Federal regulation of narcotics started with the passage of the Pure Food and Drug Act of 1906 which banned importation of any drug that could be considered harmful to the health of the people [8]. But no practical means of regulating narcotic distribution existed before the 1914 Harrison Narcotic Tax Act that made the Treasury Department responsible for enforcement of the law. This required that physicians, pharmacists, dentists and veterinarians register to dispense certain opioids and cocaine. It made possession of these drugs illegal without a license or a prescription from a licensed professional. Initially, the Supreme Court ruled that the Harrison Act regulated a vice, and that professionals could not dispense opioids solely for the maintenance of an opioid addiction in the absence of another reason such as chronic pain [8].

Although there is a long history of private hospitals, retreats, and homes in the U.S. for the treatment of drug addiction, treatment at the federal level started in the 1930s with establishment of drug addiction treatment hospitals by the US Public Health Service in Fort Worth, Texas and Lexington, Kentucky. Having features of hospitals and prisons, these facilities manifested the divided view of drug addiction as both vice and disease. Drug-addicted individuals convicted of other crimes could be remanded involuntarily for treatment while persons without a criminal record but with a drug addiction could also apply for treatment [8].

Addiction as an Occupational Hazard for Anesthesia Providers

The stigma attached to drug abuse and addiction may compromise our ability to measure the incidence of addiction, particularly among health care professionals. In 1892, Osler noted that physicians who used morphine via hypodermic injection to control pain had a greater incidence of morphine addiction, perhaps the first suggestion of a physician-occupation risk for addiction to opioids [10]. In 1894, Mattison reported that 70% of the morphine-addicted patients in his Home for Habitues were physicians [11]. Of the male morphine addicts treated between 1883 and 1900 in an Ontario treatment center, 35% were physicians [19]. In 1955, Jan Marks published *Doctor Purgatory*, a treatise on the problem of drug addiction among physicians. He provided what appears to be the first estimate of the incidence of addiction among physicians: "It is estimated roughly that one out of every hundred physicians in the United States has been, or is, addicted to narcotics… [20]." In the United Kingdom, the Home Office recorded the proportion of its citizens known to be drug addicts, in part to establish eligibility for maintenance treatment. According to its records, 21 % of the addicts in 1947 were physicians [21], and in 1956 this figure was 23 % [22], both figures far exceeding the proportion of physicians in the population. Despite these data, some authors writing more recently have concluded that the incidence of drug addiction among physicians remains unknown [23, 24], while others suggest that the prevalence is similar to that in the general public [25].

Some "circumstantial" evidence from the 1990s suggests that anesthesiologists are at greater risk for addiction and abuse than other physicians. This evidence comes from surveys of anesthesiologists, reports from chairs of anesthesia departments, and records from treatment centers, particularly those specializing in treating drug abuse and addiction among physicians. Problems with the surveys include the likelihood of underreporting by affected physicians, and the possibility that the memories of anesthesia chairs may be biased. In contrast, at least one report indicates that resident anesthesiologists do not have a greater incidence of drug abuse than residents in other specialties [26]. The apparent overrepresentation of anesthesiologists in treatment may not be related to an increased prevalence of addiction in the specialty, but to the choice of abused substance [27]. The incidence of deaths related to drug abuse in anesthesia may be greater than in other specialties because the drug of choice, an opioid, has a high addictive risk and low therapeutic index. These factors lead to a relative risk of drug-use-related death of 2.79 in anesthesiologists when compared to a cohort of matched internists, with the greatest frequency of deaths occurring in the first 5 years after graduation from medical school [28].

If anesthesiologists do have a higher risk of addiction, why might that be? Theories include the stress of a demanding career, easy access to addictive substances, and a sense of invincibility stemming from an innate sense of control over our destinies or an exaggerated sense of personal control over potent substances as a result of working with them every day [29]. A 1988 report from providers in treatment programs suggested that individuals predisposed to drug abuse by previous experience and exposure may select anesthesiology for the access to drugs that it provides [30]. Some investigators in the 2000s suggested that exposure to potent opioids through aerosolization and subsequent inhalation primes craving in the anesthesia provider and thereby leads to abuse [31]. Vaporized fentanyl in parts per billion may exist in the air surrounding an anesthetized patient's head [32]. That such a concentration could exert a subtle but significant long-term priming effect in susceptible individuals seems fantastical; we might equally blame the release of endorphins.

With regard to the written history of drug abuse and addiction specifically among anesthetists, nothing appears to have been published from the time of Halsted's story in 1884 (we count Halsted as an anesthesiologist as well as a surgeon), until an article by Bloomquist in 1959 [33]. Bloomquist focused on the problems associated with providing anesthesia for patients with addiction. He also raised concerns about the addiction potential of anesthesia medications, opining that "anesthesiologists are advised to refrain from sampling anesthetic drugs for any reason." He particularly advised against teaching anesthesia trainees to smell anesthetic gases to check their concentration and content, asserting that this might bring on addiction in susceptible individuals. He reported what might be the first case of a patient harmed by an anesthesia provider's addiction: a 2 ½ year old child who died while under the care of an anesthesiologist impaired by the inhalation of nitrous oxide and halothane [34].

In 1962, at the request of the American Association of Nurse Anesthetists, John Lundy, an anesthesiologist, and Florence McQuillen, a nurse anesthetist, wrote a review acknowledging (1) the hazards of addiction in the anesthesia work environment; (2) the lack of published information on the topic; and (3) the then reliance on anecdotal reports [35]. The authors surveyed the experience of the American Association of Nurse Anesthetists regarding drug abuse among perioperative personnel. There was a low rate of return on their questionnaires, limiting their value as a comprehensive review of the problem. Notwithstanding this limitation, the survey identified 25 individuals with drug abuse problems: 6 nurse anesthetists, 2 physician anesthesiologists, and 17 other allied health professionals. The most frequently abused medication was meperidine. This corroborated the reported use of meperidine as an abused drug among health professionals from the Lexington Public Health Hospital: 50 % of the patients at Lexington addicted to meperidine between 1955 and 1958 were either physicians or allied health professionals. In the Lundy-McQuillen survey, neither of the two addicted physician anesthesiologists and only one of the nurse anesthetists remained in the workplace.

Although problems with addiction among anesthetists surely occurred in the 1960s and 1970s, there is little or no published recognition of its impact. In 1975, the Georgia Medical Association (GMA) pioneered treatment for drug-addicted physicians, funding an Impaired Physician Program (IPP) for the treatment of impaired physicians throughout the country. In a 1983 editorial, Talbott and Farley noted that 9.6 % of the first 507 patients in the GMA IPP were anesthesiologists [36], but anesthesiologists comprised only 4 % of the physicians in the US [37]. In the same journal, Gravenstein et al. published the results of anonymous surveys sent to the chairs and clinical personnel in 31 academic anesthesia departments [38]. The chairs reported that 1–2 % of anesthesia providers abused drugs, with at least 47 drug-abuse-related deaths between 1974 and 1979. Despite the availability of synthetic opioids, there were still anesthesia providers addicted to inhalational agents (shades of Glover and Wells).

In 1983, Ward et al. [39] surveyed all anesthesia training programs in the US regarding their experience with resident and attending physician drug abuse. Seventy four percent of programs reported at least one incident of drug abuse among the residents or attending physicians during the 10 years under study. Their extrapolation from the number of attendings and residents in the programs surveyed indicated that the incidence of drug abuse among anesthesia providers was 1%. The most frequently abused drugs were meperidine, fentanyl, and morphine. Interestingly, droperidol made the list of abused substances despite reports that it could produce severe dysphoria. Perhaps this abuse was of Innovar, a combination of droperidol and fentanyl. Most impaired physicians in this study were referred for psychiatric care, with few needing detoxification. Detailed follow-up was available for about 40% of the reported incidents; 71 practitioners were offered a return to their original employment; tragically, 30 died of drug overdose.

Two other studies of physician drug addiction treatment programs from 1983 and 1984 corroborated the Georgia data on disproportionate numbers of anesthesiologists in treatment: 13.8% of physicians in the California Diversion Program [40] and 13% in the Depaul Rehabilitation Treatment Program [41]. In 1984, Spiegelman and colleagues published a comprehensive review of addiction among anesthesiologists suggesting that 60–80% of addicted physicians remained successfully in recovery after a return to practice [41]. Based on their personal communications with addiction treatment specialists, Spiegelman et al. suggested that despite their particular work environment, anesthesiologists had the same recovery success as other physicians. This review also provided the strongest statement to date on the impact of drug addiction on the specialty: "The 1979 survey [42] of the causes of death of anesthesiologists concludes that the high mortality rate for suicide appears to be the only major health problem among American anesthesiologists. In fact, it may be more accurate to say that the major health problem associated with the practice of anesthesia is chemical dependency."

In a landmark study published in JAMA in 1987, updated data from the GMA IPP for the first 1000 patients in the program indicated that the trend first noted in their treatment program had continued—although anesthesiologists comprised only 4% of physicians, they again represented 13% of the physicians in the treatment program [43]. More remarkable were the data for residents in treatment: anesthesia residents constituted 4.6% of all residents, but 45% of the residents in treatment.

The published data on the incidence of drug problems among anesthesiology trainees and attending physicians has remained consistent in recent years. Menk et al. [44] and

Booth et al. [45] reported on the results of their surveys sent to academic anesthesia programs, finding that the incidence of residents with known drug abuse was 2% and 1.6% respectively. Booth also surveyed attending anesthesiologists and once again estimated the incidence of abuse to be 1%. Fentanyl was the most frequently abused substance, but other opioids, benzodiazepines, propofol, thiopental, and inhalational agents were also misused. Ominously, in Booth's study 18% of the persons abusing drugs were identified by a drug overdose producing death or a near-death event.

Atypical, Emerging, and Reemerging Substances of Abuse

From surveys of anonymous practicing anesthesiologists and from reports of those in treatment, the most frequently abused substances are consistently opioids, especially synthetic opioids. Fentanyl surpassed meperidine as the most frequently abused drug in the 1980s. The history of drug abuse in anesthesia contains stories of abuse that are novel and perhaps surprising in both the manner of abuse and some of the substances involved, e.g., an individual in a motor vehicle accident who was driving while under the influence of enflurane inhaled from a soaked rag [46].

In 18% of departments recently surveyed, propofol emerged as a drug of abuse. This generates an incidence estimate of 10 per 10,000 anesthesia providers per decade [47], a fivefold increase from earlier surveys [39, 45]. Of 25 individuals reported to abuse propofol, 7 died as a result of the abuse, 6 of whom were residents. Volatile agents and propofol are especially problematic in that there is little or no provision for regulating and monitoring the diversion of these substances. Results of a 1993 study suggested the potential for the misuse of propofol, with 50% of the study participants reporting liking the drug [48]. In 2010, the federal government responded to the perception of a growing problem with propofol abuse by proposing to place it in Schedule IV of the Controlled Substances Act [49].

The Response from the Anesthesia Community; Tools for Enhancing Prevention, Early Detection of Drug Abuse, and Recovery

Efforts to prevent drug abuse and detect it before addiction becomes a career- and life-destroying force include provider education, enhanced controlled-substance dispensing systems, and improved drug testing. In 1986, Lecky and colleagues at the University of Pennsylvania developed and published a departmental policy aimed at increasing general awareness and directing actions effectively when dealing with physician impairment [50]. The policy outlined the importance of education and specified that incoming residents receive an introductory lecture on the hazards of substance abuse. These efforts anticipated the mandatory requirement for formal education regarding drug abuse, instituted by the American College of Graduate Medical Education (ACGME) for all residency training programs. In 1993, a group led by Tom Hornbein, then Chair of the University of Washington Department of Anesthesia, supported the production of the video *Wearing Masks* (produced and directed by Dirk Wales), an emotionally powerful tool for increasing awareness of the problem of drug abuse among anesthesia providers and their spouses and partners. The Coalition for the Prevention of Substance Abuse in Anesthesia has continued this work, having produced the *Wearing Masks Series,* a collection of videos that addresses many aspects of the problem, including the issue of the recovering anesthesia provider returning to practice [51].

Lecky's protocol and the Hornbein-Wales films provide excellent and sometimes dramatic illustrations of attempts by the anesthesia community to decrease the numbers of addicted anesthetists and thereby, the number of associated deaths. We do not know, however, whether either is effective. No controlled study has examined whether the protocol or films decrease abuse or death. It is not enough to say that their application should or might be effective. We have had half a century or more to determine whether we can affect the problem of abuse and death. We have not yet done that.

Historically, one of the obstacles to effective intervention was the lack of a urine drug test for the most frequently abused [52] and arguably the most dangerous drugs of abuse for anesthesiologists: fentanyl and sufentanil. The American Society of Anesthesiologists funded the development of a urine drug screen for the detection of fentanyl. In addition, programs using statistical analysis of providers' drug acquisition from dispensing systems have been developed to improve the detection of unusual patterns that might indicate the diversion of controlled substances [53].

In the 1990s, the predominant belief was that the high rate of relapse with death in anesthesiology residents using parenteral opioids indicated that they should be redirected to an alternative career. This belief was based upon results from a highly publicized retrospective survey of anesthesiology program directors describing a poor success rate of reentry, with a high death rate for residents using parenteral opioids [40]. Treatment protocols and monitoring methods have changed markedly over the past 2 decades and now include frequent contact for behavioral assessment, random urine testing with observed micturition, and workplace surveillance [43, 55]. Treatment programs now estimate that up to 70 % of health care professionals successfully return to medical practice [56], with similar rates of success among anesthesiologists to other physicians, despite their more widespread use of parenteral opioids [56, 57]. A family history of substance use disorder and a co-existing psychiatric disorder, such as depression or a personality disorder increase the risk of relapse [54]. The use of a major opioid only increased the risk of relapse in the presence of a coexisting psychiatric disorder, but not in its absence. These observations should be considered in the decision regarding return to anesthesiology practice of anesthesiologists with substance use disorders.

The concern regarding anesthesia providers in recovery returning to anesthesiology practice also extends to concerns over patient safety. Two separate reviews utilizing different types of databases did not reveal any incidents of patient injury resulting from lapses in vigilance or errors made by impaired anesthesiologists [58, 59]. A controversial article in Men's Health Magazine, and the online correspondence following the article, highlighted incidents of severe patient injury attributed to impaired anesthesiologists [60]. However, the problems described were not related to anesthesiologists with a known substance abuse problem in recovery and in a monitored work environment. Hence, there is little evidence to support the assertion that monitored anesthetists in recovery pose a danger to their patients.

Controversy over Returning Recovering Anesthesiologists to Practice

The issue of a return to anesthesia practice for practitioners in recovery has elicited strong opinions and focused discussion. Opponents of the "one strike and you are out" approach suggest that this might discourage affected individuals from seeking early help. Other opponents suggest that the Americans with Disabilities Act mandates an opportunity to return to work with reasonable accommodation [54]. In the middle ground, between the extremes of return to work for all or none, are those investigators looking for predictors and optimization of monitoring and treatment programs to allow an individualized approach.

Conclusion

Addiction has been the dark shadow companion of anesthesia since the earliest days of the discovery of the remarkable effects of its central actions. The recognition of the dangers that anesthetic medications pose to anesthetists has slowly developed, with accelerated growth in recent years. Although anesthetists have taken many steps to identify, prevent and treat addiction among the members of the profession, the stigma attached to addiction has added to the complex challenges associated with broadening and deepening our understanding of it. The evaluation of the effectiveness of treatment and monitoring programs for addicted practitioners is limited at best and may, by nature of the problems faced, always be imperfect. The vigilance that anesthetists apply to their patient care must also include vigilance regarding the possibility of addiction among their colleagues to ensure that more anesthetists do not suffer the tragic fates of some pioneers in the profession.

References

1. Cartwright FF. Humphry Davy's contribution to anaesthesia. Proc R Soc Med. 1950;43:571–8.
2. Fenster JM. Ether day: the strange tale of America's greatest medical discovery and the haunted men who made it. New York: Harper Collins; 2001. p. 178–83.
3. Defalque RJ. Wright AJ: The short, tragic life of Robert M. Glover. Anaesthesia. 2004;59:394–400.
4. Olch PD, William S. Halsted and local anesthesia: contributions and complications. Anesthesiology. 1975;42:479–86.
5. Markel H. The accidental addict. New Engl J Med. 2005;352:966–8.
6. Osler W, Bates DG, Bensley EH. The inner history of the Johns Hopkins Hospital. Johns Hopkins Med J. 1969;125:184–94.
7. Penfield W. Halsted of Johns Hopkins. JAMA. 1969;210:2214–8.
8. Musto DF. The American disease: origins of narcotic control. New York: Oxford University Press; 1987. p. 1.
9. Terry CE, Pellens M. The opium problem. New York: Committee on Drug Addictions; 1928.
10. Osler W. The principles and practice of medicine. New York: D Appleton and Company; 1892. p. 1006.
11. Mattison JB. Morphinism in medical men. JAMA. 1894;23:186–8.
12. White W. Addiction as a disease: birth of a concept. Counselor. 2000;1:46–51, 73.
13. Meyer RE. The disease called addiction: emerging evidence in a 200-year debate. Lancet. 1996;347:162–6.
14. Gossop M, Stewart D. Marsden J: Attendance at Narcotics Anonymous and Alcoholics Anonymous meetings, frequency of attendance and substance use outcomes after residential treatment for drug dependence: a 5-year follow-up study. Addiction. 2008;103:119–25.
15. Kaskutas LA. Alcoholics Anonymous effectiveness: faith meets science. J Addict Dis. 2009;28:145–57.
16. Musto DF. The American disease: origins of narcotic control. New York: Oxford University Press; 1987. p. 137.
17. Harrington J: Drug addiction. J Forensic Sci Soc. 1962;3:37–42.
18. Newsweek Interactive Satel S, Lilienfeld S. Medical misnomer: addiction isn't a brain disease. Congress. Slate: Washington Post Co. http://www.slate.com/id/2171131/pagenum/all/Â. Accessed 15 Feb 2010.
19. Krasnick CL. The aristocratic vice: the medical treatment of drug addiction at the Homewood Retreat, 1883–1900. Ont Hist. 1983;75:403–27.
20. Marks J: Doctor Purgatory. New York: Citadel; 1959.
21. East WN. The British Government report to the United Nations on the traffic in opium and other dangerous drugs. Br J Addict. 1949;46:38–9.
22. Anonymous. United Kingdom: Drug addiction. JAMA. 1957;165:181.
23. Brewster JM. Prevalence of alcohol and other drug problems among physicians. JAMA. 1986;255:1913–20.
24. Matsumura JS, Berry AJ. Addicted anesthesiology residents: recommendations after treatment. Anesth Analg. 2006;103:513–5.
25. Hughes PH, Brandenburg N, Baldwin DC, et al. Prevalence of substance use among US physicians. JAMA. 1992;267:2333–9.
26. Hughes PH, Baldwin DC Jr, Sheehan DV, et al. Resident physician substance use, by specialty. Am J Psychiatry. 1992;149:1348–54.

27. McGovern MP, Angres DH, Leon S. Characteristics of physicians presenting for assessment at a behavioral health center. J Addict Dis. 2000;19:59–73.
28. Alexander BH, Checkoway H, Nagahama SI, Domino KB. Cause-specific mortality risks of anesthesiologists. Anesthesiology. 2000;93:922–30.
29. Gold MS, Byars JA, Frost-Pineda K. Occupational exposure and addictions for physicians: case studies and theoretical implications. Psychiatr Clin North Am. 2004;27:745–53.
30. Gallegos KV, Browne CH, Veit FW, Talbott GD. Addiction in anesthesiologists: drug access and patterns of substance abuse. QRB Qual Rev Bull. 1988;14:116–22.
31. Gold MS, Melker RJ, Dennis DM, et al. Fentanyl abuse and dependence: further evidence for second hand exposure hypothesis. J Addict Dis. 2006;25:15–21.
32. Gold MS, Melker RJ, Pomm R, et al. Anesthesiologists are exposed to fentanyl in the operating room: addiction may be due to sensitization. Int J Neuropsychopharmacol. 2004;7(S1):p01.023
33. Bloomquist ER. Addiction, addicting drugs, and the anesthesiologist. J Am Med Assoc. 1959;171:518–23.
34. Anesthetist Jailed. Foreign Letters. J Am Med Assoc. 1959;169:235.
35. Lundy JS, McQuillen FA. Narcotics and the anesthetist: professional hazards. J Am Assoc Nurs Anesth. 1962;30:147–76.
36. Farley WJ, Talbott GD. Anesthesiology and addiction. Anesth Analg. 1983;62:465–6.
37. Roback G, Mead D, Randolph L. Physician Characteristics and Distribution in the US. Chicago: American Medical Association; 1989.
38. Gravenstein JS, Kory WP, Marks RG. Drug abuse by anesthesia personnel. Anesth Analg. 1983;62:467–72.
39. Ward CF, Ward GC, Saidman LJ. Drug abuse in anesthesia training programs. A survey: 1970 through 1980. JAMA. 1983;250:922–5.
40. Gualtieri AC, Consentino JP, Becker JS. The California experience with a diversion program for impaired physicians. JAMA. 1983;249:226–9.
41. Spiegelman WG, Saunders L, Mazze RI. Addiction and anesthesiology. Anesthesiology. 1984;60:335–41.
42. Lew EA. Mortality experience among anesthesiologists 1954–1976. Anesthesiology. 1979;51:195–9.
43. Talbott GD, Gallegos KV, Wilson PO, Porter TL. The Medical Association of Georgia's Impaired Physicians Program. Review of the first 1000 physicians: analysis of specialty. JAMA. 1987;257:2927–30.
44. Menk EJ, Baumgarten RK, Kingsley CP, et al. Success of reentry into anesthesiology training programs by residents with a history of substance abuse. JAMA. 1990;263:3060–2.
45. Booth JV, Grossman D, Moore J, et al. Substance abuse among physicians: a survey of academic anesthesiology programs. Anesth Analg. 2002;95:1024–30.
46. Musshoff F, Junker H, Madea B. An unusual case of driving under the influence of enflurane. Forensic Sci Int 2002;128:187–9.
47. Wischmeyer PE, Johnson BR, Wilson JE et al. A survey of propofol abuse in academic anesthesia programs. Anesth Analg. 2007;105:1066–71.
48. Zacny JP, Lichtor JL, Zaragoza JG, et al. Assessing the behavioral effects and abuse potential of propofol bolus injections in healthy volunteers. Drug Alcohol Depend. 1993;32:45–57.
49. http://www.federalregister.gov/articles/2010/10/27/2010–27193/schedules-of-controlled-substances-placement-of-propofol-into-schedule-iv. Accessed 27 March 2011.
50. Lecky JH, Aukburg SJ, Conahan TJ 3rd, et al. A departmental policy addressing chemical substance abuse. Anesthesiology. 1986;65:414–7.
51. Wearing Masks Programs… the potential for drug addiction in anesthesia. http://www.allanesthesia.com/Wearing_Masks_Programs.html. Accessed 11 March 2010.
52. Bryson EO, Silverstein JH. Addiction and substance abuse in anesthesiology. Anesthesiology. 2008;109:905–17.

53. Epstein RH, Gratch DM, Grunwald Z. Development of a scheduled drug diversion surveillance system based on an analysis of atypical drug transactions. Anesth Analg. 2007;105:1053–60.
54. Oreskovich MR, Caldeiro RM. Anesthesiologists recovering from chemical dependency: can they safely return to the operating room? Mayo Clin Proc. 2009;84:576–80.
55. Leshner AI. Science-based views of drug addiction and its treatment. JAMA. 1999;282:1314–16.
56. Pelton C, Ikeda RM. The California Physicians Diversion Program's experience with recovering anesthesiologists. J Psychoactive Drugs. 1991;23:427–31.
57. Paris RT, Canavan DI. Physician substance abuse impairment: anesthesiologists vs other specialties. J Addict Dis. 1999;18:1–7.
58. Sivarajan M, Posner KL, Caplan RA, et al. Substance abuse among anesthesiologists [letter]. Anesthesiology. 1994;80:704.
59. Domino KB, Hornbein TF, Polissar NL, et al. Risk factors for relapse in health care professionals with substance use disorders. JAMA. 2005;293(12):1453–60.
60. The Junkie in the O.R. Men's Health. http://www.menshealth.com/men/health/doctors-hospitals/the-junkie-in-the-o-r/article/d7a4dfaa4d41e010vgnvcm20000012281eac/4. Accessed 11 March 2010.

The American Society of Anesthesiologists' Contributions to the Development of Anesthesiology

Peter L. McDermott

Summary

Eight Brooklyn physicians and a medical student founded the Long Island Society of Anesthetists (LISA) on 6 October 1905. LISA became the New York Society of Anesthetists (NYSA), and in 1936, in pursuit of AMA recognition, became the American Society of Anesthetists (ASA). The AMA rejected the ASA's effort. Two highly respected anesthesia leaders, John Lundy and Ralph Waters, asked the American Board of Surgery (ABS) to recognize the American Board of Anesthesia (ABA) as a sub-board. The ABA gained recognition in 1937 and the Advisory Board for Medical Specialties approved this action in 1938.

In 1940, the ASA established the journal *Anesthesiology*. In 1943, the ASA Committee on Fellowship revived the Fellowship process and in 1947, developed the American College of Anesthesiologists. In 1945, the ASA became the American Society of Anesthesiologists. Membership quadrupled between 1940 and 1960. In 1949, Paul Wood's collection of historical materials became the Wood Library-Museum (WLM), with a permanent home at the new ASA offices in 1963.

In 1950, with AMA support, the ASA threatened to deny membership to any salaried physician who allowed a corporation (e.g., a hospital) to offer their services for a fee. However, in 1978, the Federal Trade Commission required that the ASA sign a Consent Decree, agreeing "that an anesthesiologist is free to choose whatever arrangement he prefers for compensation of his professional services."

In 1962, the ASA House of Delegates authorized the ASA Medical Student Preceptorship Program, placing thousands of medical students with practicing anesthesiologists, until the program ended in 1983.

In the mid 1970s, malpractice claims increased and professional liability insurance premiums rose sharply. In 1984, the ASA began studies of closed claims—resolved litigated cases—to learn what underlay adverse outcomes and define solutions to those outcomes. By 1985, Ellison Pierce, ASA Immediate Past President, proposed the creation of The Anesthesia Patient Safety Foundation (APSF), a foundation dedicated to eliminating harm from anesthesia.

In 1985, the ASA established an ad hoc Committee on Industry Relations, to encourage anesthesia-related industries to support ASA activities. This led to the establishment of the ASA Foundation for Anesthesia Education and Research (FAER). In the 1980s, the ASA's Committee on Occupational Health of Operating Room Personnel developed programs for monitoring, education, and intervention that would protect patients and rehabilitate drug-impaired physicians.

Founding of the Society

The world's first anesthesia society, the London Society of Anaesthetists, was founded in 1893. A dozen years later, on the evening of October 6, 1905, eight young Brooklyn doctors and a medical student met to form the second—the Long Island Society of Anesthetists, LISA [1]. Adolph Erdmann (Fig. 19.1) was the driving force behind an American association dedicated to placing "the science of anesthesia upon its proper plane with the other cognate sciences whose aim is to make man well [1]." From this beginning, through name changes and vast expansions of membership, arose the American Society of Anesthesiologists.

Erdmann was not the first to believe that safe and effective administration of anesthetic agents required knowledge of physical science and medicine, careful calculation of drug dosages and techniques of administration, and the development of equipment for airway management and drug delivery. John Snow had made similar observations a half century earlier but had not acted to form a society, because there were few anesthesiologists. Before LISA's inaugural meeting, Erdmann and his colleagues had concluded that conditions for successful surgery and improved patient

P. L. McDermott (✉)
Camarillo, CA, USA
e-mail: PMcVane@juno.com

E. I Eger II et al. (eds.), *The Wondrous Story of Anesthesia*, DOI 10.1007/978-1-4614-8441-7_19, © Edmond I Eger, MD 2014

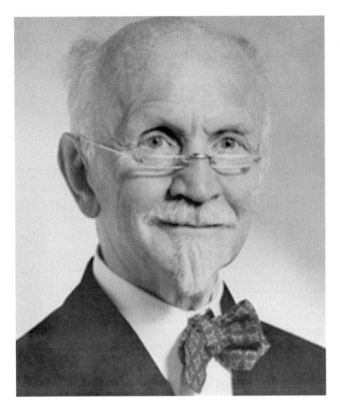

Fig. 19.1 Adolph Erdmann, founder of the Long Island Society of Anesthetists (LISA). (From the Wood Memorial Library-Museum of Anesthesiology, Park Ridge, IL)

No doubt, Erdmann and his colleagues dedicated themselves to promoting "the art and science of anesthesia"[3], but we need not accept this statement as explanation in full. A cynic of today, condescending to the past might ask—what art and what science? But there were techniques and tricks and a knowledge of physics and chemistry that could be shared. The same cynic might ask if Erdmann and his colleagues were driven by greed (money) and hunger for power, or unearned status or respectability? The historical record does not overflow with admissions of self-interest. We do know that physicians were modestly paid, their annual income averaging $750 according to AMA surveys [2]. The profession lacked control over the practice of individual physicians, the respective states controlling the profession through licensure and review boards. Whatever interests physicians shared, whatever their competing loyalties, they were, perhaps unconsciously, discovering a new identity. E. P. Thompson, in his *The Making of the English Working Class,* describes the way in which awareness of belonging to a class or group follows the struggle to clarify relationships in terms of values and moral agency:

> Class happens when some men, as a result of common experiences (inherited or shared), feel and articulate the identity of their interests as between themselves, and as against other men whose interests are different from (and usually opposed to) theirs [4].

outcomes demanded improved education and training of those who administered anesthetics.

There may have been further motivations to form a society. Historians are wedded to context. In 1905, in America, surgeons directed anesthetic administration by diverse personnel, including nurses, medical students, janitors, secretaries, interns, orderlies – and sometimes physicians. Equipment generally consisted of a vaporizer made from a towel, gauze, or a rag [1]. The administrator's eye, ear, nose, and fingertips served as monitoring devices. The anesthetist performed a task but hardly practiced medicine. Physicians practicing anesthesia might have wished to separate themselves from those less educated, and to establish qualifications for education and practice, but medical education in the US at the turn of the 20th century was unregulated, patchy, and sometimes almost fictitious. The American Medical Association (AMA) had little influence, and primarily existed during its annual meeting. In 1900, with 8,000 members out of approximately 120,000 physicians in the US, the AMA was an annual occasion rather than an institution. Remarkably however, in 1904, it established the Council on Medical Education which initiated the process of assessing medical schools and their curricula, leading to the revolutionary 1910 Flexner Report on medical education [2]. With support from the Carnegie Foundation, and publication nationally, Flexner's report radically improved medical education.

LISA established its identity in the February 1907 issue of the *Long Island Medical Journal,* with eight articles on anesthesia practices and techniques, as revealed in the Table of Contents:

1. Spinal Anesthesia
2. The Techniques of Tubation of the Pharynx to Facilitate Administration of Anesthetics
3. Major Surgery with Minor Anesthesia
4. Conditions Governing the Selection of General Anesthesia
5. Nitrous Oxide and Gas-Ether Sequence for Inducing Anesthesia, with Special Reference to the Bennett Apparatus
6. The Chloroform and Ether Solution for Anesthesia
7. Ethyl Chloride and the Newer Anesthetics, Some Personal Experiences
8. Ethyl Chloride in Oral Surgery

As a final consideration concerning the circumstance of this newly created medical society: US courts had recently shifted in their interpretation of medical malpractice and standards of care. According to Paul Starr,

> "physicians came increasingly to rely on each other's good will for their access to patients and facilities. I have already alluded to the instrumental role of the rise of hospitals and specialization in creating greater interdependence among doctors. Physicians also depended more on their colleagues for defense against malpractice suits, which were increasing in frequency. The courts, in working out the rules of liability for medical malpractice in the late nineteenth century, had set as the standard of care that of the local community where the physician practiced [2]."

Such an argument provided an impetus for defining the practice of medicine, specifically the practice of anesthesia, by standards agreed upon by local practitioners.

A fire destroyed the early records of the society in 1911, the same year that the society changed its name to the New York Society of Anesthetists (NYSA) [1]. The charter of the new society proclaimed its commitment to the "science and art of anesthesia [3]." Erdmann became the first president of the new society and James Gwathmey succeeded him in 1912. In that year, Gwathmey reported that in the US "mortality rates for anesthesia were one death in 5,623 anesthetics, three-fold greater than in the United Kingdom where physician anesthetists by then were on duty in almost all major hospitals [5]." Gwathmey attributed this to the minimal training of US physicians in anesthesia and the use of nurses as anesthesia providers [5].

Other Societies Arose

During the next two decades, a spate of anesthesia societies sprang up in the US: the American Association of Anesthetists (1912), the Interstate Association of Anesthetists (1915), the American Society of Regional Anesthesia (1923), and the International Anesthesia Research Society (1925). These and a multitude of local and regional societies sought to define the education and practices of this developing medical specialty, and to create some certifying system for practitioners [6]. But such fragmentation or "Balkanization of anesthesia into fiefdoms and principalities" delayed agreement on LISA/NYSA's goals of establishing criteria for qualification as a proficient anesthetist [6].

Physician vs. Nurse Anesthesia

During the 1930s, battle lines were drawn over the relationship between physicians and nurse anesthetists, and whether the NYSA should continue to seek recognition by the AMA. At the same time, a concurrent reality needed to be addressed. Profits were to be made by the administration of anesthetics, and hospitals, surgeons, and nurses competed with physician anesthetists for the rewards. In 1926, the NYSA supported legislation in the New York legislature that would have increased the number of physicians providing anesthesia while limiting the anesthesia practice of others. This unrealistic proposal, which would have created a serious shortage of anesthesia providers, engendered the opposition of surgeons, nurses, and hospital associations. It was not enacted but left bitter feelings against physician anesthetists [7].

As Douglas Bacon wrote:

"Because administration of an anesthetic was a profit center for surgeons and hospitals, physician specialists were struggling.

Surgeons could hire a nurse, or other individual, and have that person give the anesthetic. The surgeon charged an anesthetic fee, and the money collected was in excess of the salary paid to the 'anesthetist.' Hospitals likewise hired a nurse to give anesthetics and collected a fee that more than paid the nurse's salary. Finally, general practitioners (GPs) often would refer surgical cases to surgeons who would in turn use the GP as an anesthetist, and by administering the occasional anesthetic the GP increased his/her income [7]."

Multiple forces drove the aspirations of physician anesthetists in the mid-1930s:
1. Formal recognition of anesthetist's work as the practice of medicine (which would provide status and financial leverage);
2. Establishment of quality practice through education, performance standards, examinations, and certification by a recognized American accrediting authority;
3. Professional independence from the influence of others on clinical decision-making;
4. Freedom from economic exploitation by surgeons and hospitals.

Certification and Specialty Recognition

In 1930, the NYSA established a committee to revisit the issue of member certification. As I recorded:

"Simultaneously, the Associated Anesthetists of the United States and Canada (AAUSC), under Francis Hoeffer McMechan, recognized the need for a national certification.... As is generally the case with intelligent people who find themselves with a problem, the AAUSC created another committee. As is often the case when intelligent people find themselves in a committee, they failed to agree, leading to another two years of delay and indecision [6]."

During the 1930s, the NYSA began anew, the efforts to achieve specialty recognition from the AMA. That route was unproductive when, in 1912, Gwathmey requested and was refused AMA recognition for a section on anesthesia [7]. By 1935, the Fellowship Committee of the NYSA had established a certification process consisting of oral and written examinations, and a practical demonstration of clinical competence. Physicians from twenty-three states requested applications, but to obtain recognition by the AMA, would require a national organization "in name as well as in fact". Thus, in February 1936, the NYSA Executive Committee recommended approval of a name change to the American Society of Anesthetists (ASA) [8]. In order to establish some mechanism for awarding fellowship status to qualified physicians, representatives of the ASA, the Surgical Section of the AMA, and the American Regional Society of Anesthetists, met in October 1936 to discuss formation of an American Board of Anesthesia.

In December 1936, the NYSA, having received membership applications from nine other states, officially changed its name to the American Society of Anesthetists by action of its House of Delegates, meeting the AMA's requirement for a nationwide organization, at least in name. The ASA now had 487 members [9]. They sent John Lundy, head of anesthesia at the Mayo Clinic and a long-time consultant to the AMA, to meet with the Guiding Committee of the AMA and the Advisory Board of Medical Specialties [9]. Although these groups would not agree to a separate Board or Section for anesthesia, a "side-door for entrance into organized medicine" opened.

Erwin Schmidt, Chief of Surgery at the University of Wisconsin in Madison, and a friend of Ralph Waters, proposed an affiliate status for anesthesiologists within the American Board of Surgery (ABS). On January 10, 1937, two representatives of the ASA, Waters and Paul Wood, successfully argued for this proposal before the ABS [10]. In June 1937, the ABS officially recognized the American Board of Anesthesia (ABA). In February 1938, the Advisory Board for Medical Specialties approved this affiliation, thus officially recognizing anesthesia as a medical specialty [3].

While the ASA pursued board status, it concurrently sought recognition as a medical specialty within the family of medicine. In June 1937, in its pursuit of recognition by the AMA through the creation of a Section on Anesthesia, the ASA limited its membership to physicians who were members of the AMA. This removed dentists, scientists, and foreigners from membership [3].

The 1939 World's Fair in New York provided an opportunity for the ASA, through the Winthrop Corporation, to promote the specialty of anesthesia to the general public (Fig. 19.2). With the theme "The Physician Anesthetist of Tomorrow," an ambitious display was assembled including a simulated patient and operating theatre. Just how many of the 45 million visitors to the Fair took in the ASA display is unknown—it competed with over 60 foreign government exhibits, 300 priceless works of art from the galleries of Europe, an original copy of the Magna Carta, and an amusement section with a 10,000 seat amphitheatre.

State associations of anesthesiologists in California, Connecticut, and Indiana had established sections on anesthesia within their state medical societies, and offered educational programs and scientific displays. In May 1939, at the annual AMA meeting in St. Louis, the ASA presented a session on anesthesia, and leaders of the AMA increasingly supported recognition of anesthesia as a specialty [3]. Members of the Council on Scientific Assembly of the AMA, at their meeting in December 1939, recommended establishment of a Section on Anesthesia within the AMA. This recommendation was submitted to the AMA House of Delegates Annual Meeting in June 1940, and was approved unanimously. Anesthesiology was now recognized as a medical specialty by the AMA.

Publication of the ASA Journal, *Anesthesiology*

The process of legitimizing the specialty also required establishment of organs of communication. First came a monthly *Newsletter,* begun in April 1938, which reported items of interest to anesthetists, appointments, meetings, and activities [7]. Next came the journal *Anesthesiology,* in July 1940. Development of *Anesthesiology* had been suspended out of respect for Francis McMechan and his dedication to *Current Researches in Anesthesia and Analgesia. Anesthesiology* commenced publication shortly after McMechan's death in 1939. It thrived, becoming the pre-eminent journal for anesthesia-related articles.

On February 16, 1941, the ABA gained independent status. The process of organizing anesthetists, developing a corporate identity, defining standards of practice and education, and incorporating these activities within those of other physicians was complete. Anesthesia had arrived as a medical specialty.

World War II Accelerates ASA Growth

The entry of the US into World War II, late in 1941, profoundly changed progress in anesthesia. The expectation of great numbers of casualties and the unfortunate experience of World War I battlefield anesthesia by episodically supervised and diverse anesthetists (corpsmen, nurses, secretaries, and the occasional physician), caused the National Research Foundation to ask eminent anesthesiologists how to manage the anticipated demand. Ralph Waters headed this group of ASA leaders, including Emery Rovenstine, John Lundy, Henry Ruth, Henry Beecher, Paul Wood, Ralph Tovell, and Lewis Booth [10]. They developed an anesthesia training program for physicians that joined the educational and training potential of American anesthesiologists to the emergent demand. Hundreds of physicians received an accelerated program of instruction, at class 'A' medical schools with established departments of anesthesia having a chairman who was certified by the ABA. Certain military hospitals handling a large volume of surgical cases with adequate staff were also included, as well as the Mayo Clinic and similar institutions [10].

This program, supported by ASA, contributed to the rapid growth of the specialty after the war. To accommodate the credentialing demands of this new population of partially trained physicians practicing anesthesiology, the Committee on Fellowship of the ASA revived the Fellowship process in 1943, and by 1947, it expanded into the American College of Anesthesiologists. For returning physicians who did not qualify for ABA certification, or who practiced anesthesia part-time, fellowship offered an opportunity to certify skills

Fig. 19.2 This postcard (front and back) pictured the ASA/Winthrop Corporation's effort to inform the public, to convince them of the considerable advantages offered by the skills of the anesthesiologist

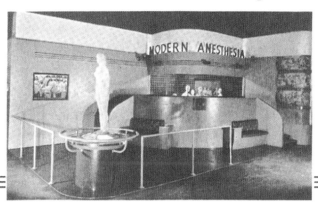

Visit New York World's Fair

SEE WINTHROP'S ANESTHESIA EXHIBIT
The *"Hit Show"* in
Medicine and Public Health Building

10-39 (6000)

ANESTHESIA AT THE WORLD'S FAIR

"MODERN ANESTHESIA", the *hit show* in the Medicine and Public Health Building of the New York World's Fair, was conceived by a committee of prominent American anesthetists under the sponsorship of Winthrop Chemical Company, Inc.

The purpose of Winthrop's exhibit on modern anesthesia is to inform the public that anesthesia is a fully developed and important specialty of medicine. By means of a demonstration of inhalation anesthesia with life size models in a typical operating room, the spectators are given the indelible impression that the training, skill and resourcefulness of the anesthetist of today render modern anesthesia wonderfully efficient and remarkably safe.

WINTHROP CHEMICAL COMPANY, INC.
Manufacturers of
AVERTIN • EVIPAL SOLUBLE • PONTOCAINE • NOVOCAIN

and knowledge of the practice of anesthesiology [6]. The post-war expansion in the number of residencies and positions indicates the accelerated growth of anesthesiology: in 1940 there were 37 residency programs with 108 positions, in 1950 there were 216 residency programs with more than 700 positions [11].

The ASA Changes its Name

In 1945, the total membership of ASA was 1,977. Of those, 739 (37%) served in the military [3]. As the war drew to a close, the ASA changed its name to the American Society of Anesthesiologists and held the first of its Annual Sessions.

Paul Wood, the 1945 first recipient of the ASA Distinguished Service Award, had made the suggestion for a name change the year before, citing correspondence from MJ Seifert of Illinois:

> "In 1902, while teaching at the University of Illinois, I coined the word 'anesthesiology' and defined it as follows: The science that treats of the means and methods of producing various degrees of insensibility to pain with or without hypnosis. An Anesthetist is a technician and an Anesthesiologist is the scientific authority on anesthesia and anesthetics. I cannot understand why you do not term yourself the American Society of Anesthesiologists?"

Apparently the term anesthesiologist predated the society itself.

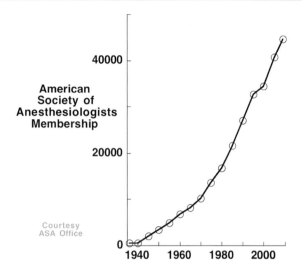

Fig. 19.3 World War II spurred the growth in ASA membership. Growth accelerated further starting at approximately 1970, in part perhaps because of ASA efforts to educate medical students concerning the important role played by anesthesiologists in the care of surgical patients

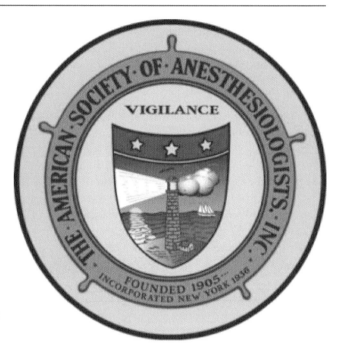

Fig. 19.4 In 1932, Paul Wood presented the ASA with the pictured seal of his design that became the Great Seal of the ASA. Bacon wrote [35] that this consisted of "… the pilot wheel, perfect circle, shield, stars, clouds, moon, ship, sea and lighthouse.…The patient is represented as the ship sailing the troubled sea with clouds of doubt, waves of terror, being guided by the skillful pilot (the anesthetist) with constant and eternal (*stars*) vigilance (*motto*) by his dependable (*lighthouse*) knowledge of the art of sleep (*moon*) to a safe and happy outcome of his voyage through the realm of the unknown. The perfect circle denotes unity of a closed group (the Society)* Quoting Wood, Bacon added that "the three dots after the founding date of 1905 were put there… to symbolize the name changes of the Society, from the original Long Island Society of Anesthetists, to the New York Society of Anesthetists, to the American Society of Anesthetists, and then the name under which the Society was incorporated, the American Society of Anesthesiologists." [36, 37] (Courtesy of the American Society of Anesthesiologists)

A Move to Chicago

In 1946, the ASA celebrated the centenary of the discovery of anesthesia, at its annual meeting in Boston, featuring the Morton Centennial Commemoration and the Ether Centenary celebration. It addressed part of the growing needs of the present and expanding membership, by hiring its first Executive Secretary, John Hunt, who was followed by John Andes in 1960. Need for more space and a more central location within the US prompted the movement of ASA offices to Chicago in 1947. Responding to the maturation of this new specialty, the ASA changed its constitution and bylaws [3]. The new governance structure created component societies at the state or regional level, a Board of Directors, a House of Delegates, and an Executive Committee. This model survives to this day. The House of Delegates first met in St. Louis in 1948. Refresher Courses, instituted at the 1950 Annual Session, continue to be offered today.

The 1940s saw an increase in membership from 538 to 3,393, and by 1960 it had increased to 6,785 [9]. Figure 19.3 indicates three phases of this growth: Slow before World War II: a steeper rise promoted by the war through 1970: and a still steeper increase thereafter, an increase that has yet to abate.

Founding of the Wood Library-Museum and Other ASA Foundations

In 1949, Paul Wood's collection of materials related to the history of anesthesia, officially became the Wood Library-Museum (WLM). George Bause admirably tells the

development and travels of this unique collection [12]. After being shuffled around New York for three decades, it found a permanent home at the new ASA offices in Park Ridge, Illinois in 1963. It now resides at the enlarged facility built there in 1993. This is the world's greatest collection of documents, letters, publications, memorabilia, and equipment related to anesthesia.

Wood gave the ASA something else. In 1932, he presented the ASA with a seal that became the Great Seal of the ASA (Fig. 19.4) [3]. Emblazoned on the shield is the patient as a ship on clouded troubled seas steered by the anesthetist (using the pilot wheel, a perfect circle suggesting the unity of the ASA) with stars and a lighthouse to guide the way, and a moon to reflect sleep. The three dots after "Founded 1905" symbolize the three successive societies – the Long Island Society of Anesthetists, the New York Society of Anesthetists, and the ASA. And above the shield lies the word "Vigilance", the motto of the ASA.

The WLM later achieved foundation status, but was not the first of the ASA's four foundations. First was the Anesthesia Memorial Foundation (AMF) established in 1956 to honor the passing of several prominent anesthesiologists who died that year—R. Charles Adams, Rolland Whitacre, Brian Sword, Robert Hammond, Henry Ruth, and Arthur Guedel. This foundation aimed "to loan or give money to deserving persons and to assist them in becoming specialists in anesthesia, or for research and study in the field of anesthesia and related fields." In 1984, its name was changed to The Anesthesia Foundation (AF). Over the years its effectiveness has grown. It provides loans to residents, as many as 60 per year, in amounts up to $6,000. It assisted in resident relief after hurricane Katrina hit New Orleans in 2005. Through its Anesthesia Foundation/Wellness Initiative Advisory Committee, it expanded its efforts to assist practicing physicians who experience hardship. Its assets exceed $1,250,000, all of it "committed to individuals in the form of loans [13–15]."

The ASA Opposes the Corporate Practice of Anesthesiology

The 1950s were notable for more than organizational changes of the ASA. Increasingly, hospitals sought to control the practice of anesthesia, largely to generate revenue. The growth of health insurance companies in the 30s and 40s, and the provision of insurance coverage as an employee benefit during World War II, coupled with the increased power of the hospital industry, put pressure on anesthesiologists to become salaried employees of hospitals. The ASA needed to craft effective responses to this challenge. Since the 1940s, the ASA had issued statements asserting the professional nature of anesthesiologists' services to the patient, as opposed to the institutional services supplied by hospitals and their employees. Having required its members to maintain membership in the AMA (and the ABA having required that its candidates be members of the ASA), the ASA now sought AMA support against profit-based hospitals and their exploitation of physician anesthesiologists [16].

In 1950, the Committee on Corporate Practice of Medicine of the AMA, working with members of the ASA, produced a report on the corporate practice of medicine that was adopted by the AMA House of Delegates. The report included the statement:

"that the overall policy of the American Medical Association shall be that it is illegal… and unethical for any lay corporation to practice medicine and to furnish medical services for a professional fee which shall be so divided as to produce profit for a lay employer, either individual or institutional, including hospital and medical schools… The licensed physician is the only person legally qualified at the present time to render any individual medical service [16]."

The ASA quickly followed with a Statement of Policy threatening denial of membership through its component society system, to anyone working for a salary and allowing another entity to offer his services for a fee. It was rumored that residencies would be disapproved if their directors did not comply with this policy [16]. The intended consequence of this effort was to align the specialty with the private practice of medicine. The private practice of medicine was based economically upon fee for service payment. Over the next dozen years, the percentage of anesthesiologists practicing under salary from an institution, decreased from 25.7% to 8.8% [16].

Academic anesthesiologists, as salaried faculty in medical schools, increasingly feared that the ASA wrongly connected salary source and ethical behavior. Between 1950 and 1953, several prominent academic anesthesiologists formed the Association of University Anesthetists, later the Association of University Anesthesiologists (AUA), in part to challenge this connection. The division was real and deep, and threatened the corporate identity that anesthesiologists had obtained with such difficulty in creating the ASA. Despite ASA opposition, 37 academicians (all ASA members) formed the AUA, held their first meeting in 1953, and contemplated a life in opposition to the ASA [16]. Eventually, cordial and respectful relations developed between the ASA and the AUA, and as a multiplicity of special interest associations arose, the ASA pitched larger tents, made accommodations, and held together the specialty whose identity continued to evolve.

Founding of the WFSA

In 1955, 28 societies from around the world founded the World Federation of Societies of Anaesthesiologists (WFSA). The US, the post-war global super power, had just passed through a virulent communist scare and was engaged in the Cold War. The ASA was the largest and most prosperous anesthesia organization on earth and initially considered that the WFSA offered little benefit to ASA members. If becoming a member required the ASA to relinquish any of its hard won authority, caution was necessary before contemplating membership. Thus, initially, the ASA elected to remain an "observer". Ultimately the ASA decided that WFSA membership had more advantages than disadvantages, and, perhaps that it had an obligation to the larger development of anesthesia implied by membership. In 1960, the ASA became a member of the federation that now has 116 member organizations [16].

Birth of the Relative Value Guide

The 1960s saw an economic revolution in medical care and government involvement in the production, delivery, and reimbursement for health care services. Even before the enactment of Medicare in 1965, medical associations sought to devise some system to quantify the value of medical services. California led the way in 1953, with the creation of a Relative Value System. It was not a fee schedule, but a formula for calculating the relative value of specific medical services. From this, a dollar amount could be derived by application of a conversion factor. Joseph Failing developed a Relative Value Guide (RVG) specific to operative anesthesia services, and saw to its passage by the California Medical Association and the California Society of Anesthesiologists [17]. It was based upon the type of surgical procedure (e.g., gall bladder removal), pre-existing risk factors (e.g., heart disease and the extent of heart disease), modifying units for use of complicated modalities (e.g., hypothermia, extracorporeal circulation), and actual time for anesthesia services. The ASA adopted this RVG in 1962, which was therefore in place when Medicare came into effect [18]. Because the conversion factor varied with the prevailing cost of living and practice, it was not considered a fee schedule or a method of fixing prices. Despite legal challenges, the ASA-RVG survived and continued in use [18, 19].

Formation of the ASA Medical Student Preceptor Program

In 1962, the ASA House of Delegates authorized a systematic analysis of the practice of anesthesiology beginning with a survey of practice, research, and teaching [20]. Using the resources of a professional consultant, the ASA identified several areas deserving special attention. Medical student attitudes regarding the specialty led the ASA to include them in focused educational experiences—meetings, curriculum modifications, and the ASA Medical Student Preceptorship program. The last of these placed hundreds of medical students in direct contact with practicing anesthesiologists each year. Over the sixteen years before the program ended in 1983, thousands of medical students experienced the practice of anesthesiology first hand. Some then chose it as a specialty and many viewed it with increased favor [21]. Such recruitment to anesthesiology may explain a portion of the increase in numbers of anesthesia residents/anesthesiologists at this time (Fig. 19.3).

Support Programs for ASA Members Grow

Appointed in 1966, the ASA Council on Education developed guidelines for the inclusion of anesthesia education for interns, in the curriculum established by the AMA [20]. In addition, a heightened public education program was developed, including brochures, films directed at medical students, and similar materials directed at patients or the general public. Anesthesiology became a separate section in the AMA, thereby increasing its status in the eyes of other physicians [20]. The recognition and respect that the ASA and its members desired from the public in general, required public education beyond that described above. Specifically, anesthesiologists wanted the general public to appreciate the distinctions between physicians administering anesthetics, and other anesthetic providers. To this end, the ASA called attention to the academic aspects of anesthesiology and mounted a public relations campaign. The emphasis on science focused on research funding and the assessment tools for continuing competence. The latter prompted the American College of Anesthesiologists (ACA) to develop the Self Education and Evaluation (SEE) program. Thus began periodic verification of practice competence, and assessment of the currency of member education, ultimately resulting in an ABA recertification mechanism. The ACA, in response to information gleaned from the SEE program, developed educational programs, regional refresher courses, and publication of the ASA Regional Refresher Courses—for many years the best selling publication of the specialty [6].

During the 1970s, the ASA developed further programs and support systems for its members. It established Ambulatory Surgery Guidelines in 1973 [18]. That same year the ASA, in conjunction with the ABA, mandated a resident in-training examination. In 1975, the ASA began assisting recovery room nurses in forming their own organizations, regionally and nationally. This resulted in the 1982 formation of the American Society of Post-Anesthesia Care Nurses (ASPAN) [19].

The ASA and the Federal Trade Commission

It would be wonderful to say that the ASA devoted all its resources and energies to the art and science of anesthesiology, but the 1965 Medicare and Medicaid legislation unleashed governmental agencies seeking economies in reimbursements that had overrun their predictive models. Membership in the ASA had been restricted to those who adhered to the ASA's approved methods of reimbursement. Punitive sanctions were pursued against those who deviated from the prescribed economic and ethical imperatives of the ASA.

> "In September 1975, the Department of Justice filed an antitrust suit against ASA charging that 'the *Relative Value Guide* promulgated by the Association (sic).... which sets values on particular procedures...are used by the Association (sic) members to determine what fee to charge… (and) have the effect of raising, fixing, stabilizing, and maintaining fees.'" [18]

Two years later, the Federal Trade Commission (FTC) began an investigation of the ASA and its Guidelines to the Ethical

Practice of Anesthesia [22]. The Guidelines stated that "financial return from the private practice of anesthesia should be on a fee for service basis… Physicians should bill their own patients for the services and only the services they perform personally [18]." This, thereby restricted membership to those who demanded a fee for service. Whereas the ASA successfully defended its *Relative Value Guide* against the Department of Justice, it had to retreat on its Ethical Guidelines, accepting a consent decree with the FTC that agreed to stop "importuning or engaging in threats or actions of reprisal, coercion, or intimidation with purpose or effect of restraining or impeding anesthesiologists individually or as a class of practitioners from engaging in the practice of anesthesiology other than on a fee for service basis [18]." In the same year, 1975, the ASA established an advocacy presence in Washington D.C. [18] That presence continues today and enables advocacy on behalf of members and their patients with the federal government.

In August 1979, the FTC launched another investigation into allegations of anti-competitive practices, by anesthesiologists against nurse anesthetists. This matter was resolved within a year in favor of the ASA, but the FTC continued to threaten further action over the next decade [19]. The ASA faced more than legal challenges from the federal government. Bureaucracies instituted several regulatory activities in the early 1980s that threatened development of the specialty. The ASA began a series of activities to prepare anesthesiologists for some of the new realities of practicing in a highly regulatory environment. "Legislative Workshops" were begun—first in Chicago and then in Washington D.C. The Annual Legislative Workshop continues as a resource to component society leaders and their counsels [19]. In 1980, the ASA instituted a program on governmental affairs at its Annual Meeting, and through a *Key Contact* program, ASA members were encouraged to form personal relationships with legislators at both state and federal levels, in order to present concerns over pending legislation and regulatory rules. Establishment of a political action committee (PAC) was considered, but not pursued at that time.

The ASA Establishes a Full-Time Presence in Washington

In the early 1980s, the US Bureau of Health Manpower formed a Graduate Medical Education National Advisory Committee (GMENAC), to advise the Secretary of Health, Education, and Welfare on the proper number of physicians in each specialty. The GMENAC advocated increased numbers of primary care physicians and fewer positions in anesthesia residencies – despite studies indicating a shortage of anesthesiologists. By 1984, it became clear that a full-time presence in Washington was necessary: the Office of Gov-

ernmental Affairs (OGA) was opened with full-time staff, lobbying consultants, and legal counsel. In the following year, the ASA sponsored Grass Roots Political Education Seminars in five locations around the country. Recognizing that precedents could be set at a local level that affected the laws and regulations in other states, it became imperative that the broad range of possible threats to the specialty be communicated to component societies [19, 23].

It is numbing to relate the multitude of skirmishes and challenges that the ASA faced from the 1982 Tax Equity and Fiscal Responsibility Act (TEFRA). They included the congressionally mandated Prospective Payment System (PPS), the schedule of Diagnostic Related Groups (DRGs), the Physician Payment Review Commission (PPRC), efforts to bundle physician services with those of the hospital, or proposals to separate radiologists, anesthesiologists, and pathologists (RAPs) and their reimbursement from that of other physicians. Two critical contests were afoot: 1) the professional nature of the practice of anesthesiology, particularly its autonomy from institutional control; and 2) the economic survival of residency teaching programs. The ASA, in conjunction with the AUA, the Society of Academic Anesthesia Chairmen (SAAC), and the Association of American Medical Colleges (AAMC) *defined* reimbursable services for an attending physician who was concurrently directing two residents or interns [19]. As the government exercised increasing control over reimbursement for medical services, new problems arose. What is the value of the physician component of medical services when supervising nurse anesthetists? How many nurses could reasonably or safely be supervised at one time—two? four? eleven? How and when is the input of the physician in medical care appropriate? And, as a bottom-line, what is the service worth?

Other problems required consideration: What are the ethical implications of exclusive contracts between anesthesiologists and hospitals? Are they designed to maintain quality care or to keep out competition? Are clinical decisions influenced by the one who pays the bill? Is the exclusion of qualified practitioners from access to hospital facilities morally justifiable? As far as economic credentialing is concerned, should a medical staff or hospital administration grant exclusive privileges to practice based upon cost rather than quality of care? These issues have yet to be resolved as the quality of anesthesia services and the value of those services are considered in the broader arena of health care reform.

Establishment of the APSF and FAER

During the mid 1970s, professional liability insurance premiums rose alarmingly as malpractice claims increased. The crisis presented an opportunity, an ASA mandate to reduce harm to the patient. In 1984, the ASA began a study of closed claims—litigated cases that had been resolved—in order to analyze problems with management decisions, practice methods, and their relationship with adverse outcomes. The Closed Claims Study eventually included thousands of cases. The ASA acted upon the information to focus educational programs on safety. The ASA also demanded better technologies, pharmaceutical agents and packaging, and developed guidelines and standards of care, peer review programs, and quality assurance programs for medical staff [19]. By 1985, Ellison Pierce, ASA Immediate Past President, had inspired creation of The Anesthesia Patient Safety Foundation (APSF), a foundation dedicated to a simple purpose—that no patient be harmed by anesthesia. Rather than focus on tort reform, it extended its hand to a coalition that included anesthesiologists, nurse anesthetists, nurses, pharmaceutical and equipment manufacturers, regulators, insurers, attorneys, and hospital representatives [24]. Actions of the foundation, together with the work of ASA committees on safety and standards, profoundly influenced the practice of anesthesia through development of standards for monitoring, promotion of alarm systems, use of simulators for training personnel, education in risk management, and information management and sharing [24, 25]. The result was that patient safety dramatically increased—and malpractice costs dramatically decreased. Sometimes good is rewarded.

At the same time the APSF was created in 1985, the ASA established an ad hoc Committee on Industry Relations, whose purpose was to obtain funding from anesthesia related industries to support ASA activities. This is called non-dues income, and, while priding itself on its frugality and efficiency in meeting its members' needs while keeping dues low, the ASA imagined treasure flowing into its general revenue account. The Committee, having reviewed the economic, ethical, public relations, and professional implications associated with multiple commercial marriages, identified two areas in which the ASA and industry shared respectable goals and interests—research and education. The committee then proposed the establishment of the ASA's fourth and last foundation, the Foundation for Anesthesia Education and Research (FAER), declared a victory, and vanished [26]. FAER has grown and fulfilled the expectations of its founders. King and Hug found that by 1998, "234 of the 296 FAER grant recipients then surveyed had received more than $100 million in subsequent grant funding, from an initial FAER investment of just over $5 million. I challenge you to find a better example of return on investment anywhere [27]." The emphasis on supporting post residency fellows and junior faculty also aided in the retention of academic faculty. FAER currently has assets of over $20 million, awards grants in excess of $2 million annually, and has organized an Academy of Mentors to encourage the exchange between senior academicians and those in the early stages of their research careers [28].

Substance Abuse

In the 1980s, the ASA addressed another significant problem: the plight of the impaired physician. Anesthesiologists used and abused addictive substances, including alcohol and other substances, more than did other specialists. This problem presented a need for investigation and intervention. The ASA's Committee on Occupational Health of Operating Room Personnel was charged with the responsibility for developing the programs of monitoring, education, and intervention needed to protect patients, and to rehabilitate physicians who could be rescued [19]. During the next three decades, other medical associations joined the effort to solve the problem. Did these and the ASA's activities produce remediation of physician impairment? There is no unequivocal answer, but hospital personnel with whom I've spoken seem confident that the problem is less severe than it had been. On the other hand, James Arens wrote (personal communication) that "Unfortunately there has been little to no change in the incidence of substance abuse in anesthesia residents." Thus, despite three decades of effort, we do not know whether remediation has occurred and, if it has, what specific efforts produced the remediation.

Public Relations

The ASA's forays into public relations programs dwindled after the 1960s. By the 1980s, the complex practice of anesthesiology had become sub-specialized and in need of renewed public understanding. The ASA Committee on Communications developed a program of Public Education, with a press information kit, spokesperson training, media tours, renewed medical student recruitment efforts, and video releases for television [19]. However, subsequent studies of the effectiveness of public education efforts indicated that the effort and funds expended on the program minimally affected the general public's appreciation of the role and importance of the anesthesiologist [19].

Bluntly speaking, no one was interested until they were about to have surgery. The ASA decided it was more effective to educate the decision-makers in government, the media, and other health care professionals. The ASA enhanced its presence at the AMA, developed stronger connections with other medical associations, and established annual media awards, presented to honorees at its Annual House of Delegates Meeting. The education of those in government was motivated by more than the economic interests of ASA members. Its efforts to limit the scope of practice of less qualified practitioners, and its determination to educate legislators and regulators on the consequences of their decisions cannot be reduced to mere lobbying. Lobbying, historically, signifies the pressure of self-interested groups on those in government. The ASA has certainly represented the economic concerns of its members, but it has also been an advocate for the care of patients.

Subspecialization

As the 1990s began, sub-specialization within the practice of anesthesiology needed to be addressed: was the ASA to passively observe the fragmentation of the specialty or proactively adopt a supportive role? The Executive Office offered administrative support for the subspecialties as it had for the Foundations. Specifically, the ASA headquarters office helped with communications, membership services, meetings, and many of the needs of the new societies. By 1990, the House of Delegates had amended the ASA Bylaws to allow voting status to representatives from the American Society of Critical Care Anesthesiologists (ASCCA), the Society for Obstetric Anesthesia and Perinatology (SOAP), the Society of Cardiovascular Anesthesiologists (SCA), the Society for Pediatric Anesthesia (SPA), the Society for Ambulatory Anesthesia (SAMBA), the American Society of Regional Anesthesia and Pain Management (ASRA), and the Society for Neurosurgical Anesthesia and Critical Care (SNACC) [19].

Nicholas Greene had long been a volunteer with the overseas medical missionary project *Hope*. At his urging, in 1990, the ASA began an Overseas Teaching Program (OTP) in support of volunteer ASA members who would train anesthesia personnel in safe practices. In the past two decades the ASA-OTP has enlisted more than 100 volunteers for temporary teaching posts in Uganda, Zambia, Tanzania, and Kenya [29]. In 2009, it changed its name and mission. The new ASA Committee on Global Humanitarian Outreach (GHO) coordinates its activities with other organizations and specialties such as the WFSA, the World Health Organization (WHO), Health Volunteers Overseas, and the American College of Surgeons (ACS) [29].

Primary Care Growth Transiently Forces a Retreat

In 1991, the ASA, responding to the need for more effective representation of the political and economic interests of its members, approved the formation of a political action committee (ASAPAC). Some in the ASA had been reluctant to separate their representation at the federal level, from that of the AMA and its political action committee [23]. A gap had developed however, between the interests of the ASA and the AMA. There had been growing pressures on the AMA to represent the interests of primary care physicians and, within a short time, a federal Council on Graduate Medical Education (COGME), recommended an increase in

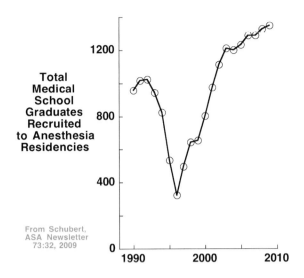

Fig. 19.5 This summary of match results for recruitment to first year positions in residency programs from 1980–2009 shows the considerable impact of the attempt of the Clinton Health Initiative in the early 1990s, to divert physicians from specialty to family care practice. The impact was large but relatively short-lived. (From Armin Schubert essay in the ASA newsletter 73, p 32, 2009)

the number of primary care physicians at the expense of specialty education. Specifically, anesthesiology residency positions would be reduced by 40% [30]. Such measures, combined with reaction to the Clinton health care initiative, the growth of managed care, the increase in exclusive contracts between hospitals and closed panels of anesthesiologists, and concerns over the numbers and qualifications of future anesthesia providers, dramatically decreased recruitment into anesthesia (Fig. 19.5). ASAPAC activities and increased programs to recruit medical students into anesthesia ensued, and recruitment into anesthesia residencies recovered. The sub-specialization in anesthesia and the expansion of clinical opportunities for general anesthesiologists, restored the demand and the specialty grew again. Subspecialties grew in number and membership, and the ASA responded by supporting them administratively and by incorporating them into the political structure of the ASA. In 1990, membership was 27,034. By 2010, it had grown to 44,599 [31]. The ASA's annual budget is approximately $36 million.

Activities in the 2000s

As the century drew to a close, the ASA began another process of self-examination like that of the 1960s. In 1992, the ASA leadership convened a retreat/workshop consisting of the Administrative Council and other key leaders. Task forces were appointed to study and report upon the ASA's research and education efforts and the extent to which they responded to identified needs, set goals and priorities, and measured outcomes. Another taskforce studied the structure and function of the society—leadership, governance, and administrative support systems. Others reviewed member services, economics and governance as they affected the strength of the society, and potential changes in the role of the anesthesiologist in the future. This process of planning and goal setting has continued, using facilitators, consultants, and other professional resources. Some results include an expansion of the Board of Directors to include representatives of all the component societies, representatives from subspecialty societies, related foundations, and academic organizations. The ASA House of Delegates continues to meet annually, and has expanded its membership to nearly 400. It has a reference committee format for handling reports and resolutions, a consent calendar for managing action and information, and a parliamentary structure for meetings.

The growing number of women entering the medical profession prompted an ASA workshop on women's issues in 1993, that evolved into a standing committee on diversity that addresses concerns of underrepresented sectors of the specialty and the particular interests that they might have. These sectors include medical students and residents, young physicians, uniformed services and veterans, anesthesia assistants, and anesthesia care team members. The ASA also established ongoing projects dealing with geriatrics, ethics, and practice management. The Annual Session added a subsection on history with panels, posters, and papers.

Formed in the mid 1980s, the Committee on Standards of Care produced a series of standards on monitoring, practice guidelines, and algorithms useful in dealing with special procedures. Practice parameters have been written based upon evidence or consensus. To date, the ASA has approved twenty evidence-based parameters [32]. They deal with such matters as preoperative evaluation, the prevention of intraoperative and postoperative complications, pain management, transfusion therapy, and postoperative care. The ASA has supported the development of anesthesia simulators, both in training and in maintaining proficiency in anesthesia practice. Concern for physician wellness, beginning as an awareness of the problem of substance abuse, has expanded to include active involvement in impairments of other kinds, including those related to aging, distraction, and unhealthy lifestyles. Other medical organizations and most medical staffs have embraced the ASA's concern, and instituted measures of detection and intervention to identify impaired physicians, and guide them toward recovery.

In response to an era of almost instant information dissemination, the ASA and its foundations and subspecialties have developed web sites and electronic alerts and bulletins, knitting the various anesthesia communities and their interests together. *Advocacy* has become a fashionable term, describing the duty of organizations to their members. To speak for ones members' interests is a laudable goal of an organization. When that organization is a professional society however, it must behave as more than a trade association. Whatever member interests are advocated, they must also represent the best interests of the patients they serve and the collective good of society. The ASA has become the voice of most anesthesiologists in the US, representing them before the public, the government, industries, and the world. Despite diverse interests, anesthesiologists find common ground in socio-economic, public relations, scope of practice issues, and the improvement of patient care, as stated in the ASA's current Mission Statement:

> The American Society of Anesthesiologists is an organization of physicians and other professionals dedicated to serving the best interests of its members and their patients. ASA supports patient safety by promoting improved quality, ethical behavior, discovery of new knowledge, and involvement of an anesthesiologist with every patient receiving anesthesia services, including perioperative care, pain management, and critical care [33].

One might argue that these goals cannot be realized, given the existence of dentists, veterinarians, and others doing their best to care for patients where anesthesia is required, but where there is no anesthesiologist. One might also argue that in some ways anesthesiology has become a victim of its own success. Improvements in practice have enabled application of more complicated and riskier procedures to sicker patients, but as a practice approaches fail-safe status, the virtuosity of the provider becomes a given. How relevant to or proportional to the outcome of the medical experience, is the investment in education and training of the provider? To answer this question, the ASA has established an Anesthesia Quality Institute, gathering data in preparation for the creation of a National Anesthesia Clinical Outcomes Registry [34].

The Specialty has Matured

In summary, over the past century, the ASA has developed a sustaining culture of shared values and assumptions that have advanced the progress of anesthesiology as a medical specialty. Its four foundations, jewels in the crown of the ASA, have shaped the development of the specialty. The ASA's educational efforts—meetings, communications, the most prestigious journal in anesthesiology—have informed and enriched generations of anesthesiologists. Awards and eponymous lectureships and scholarships have directed attention to the accomplishments of those whose contributions to the specialty have been noteworthy. The communities of anesthesiologists and those associated with the specialty rely upon a network of relationships, values, and communications; the ASA has provided these. The ASA can claim credit for creating an environment in which knowledge is shared and valued through education and research, and in which safe patient care is the primary consideration.

References

1. Erickson JC. In the beginning: Adolph Frederick Erdmann and the long island society of anesthetists. American Society of Anesthesiologists: a century of challenges and progress. In: Bacon DR, McGoldrick KE, Lema MJ Editors. The Wood Library Museum. Park Ridge; 2005. pp. 1–8.
2. Starr P. The social transformation of American medicine: the rise of a sovereign profession and the making of a vast industry. Basic Books; 1983. pp. 92–111.
3. Betcher AM, Ciliberti BJ, Wood PM, Wright LH. The jubilee year of organized anesthesia. Anesthesiol. 1956;17:229–67.
4. Thompson EP. The making of the english working class. Harmondsworth: Penguin; 1968. p. 9.
5. Smith BE. ASA newsletter 64. The genesis of the American Society of Anesthesiologists; Sept 2000; pp. 5–7.
6. McDermott PL. The American college of anesthesiologists: the ghost in the basement. American Society of Anesthesiologists: a century of challenges and progress. In: Bacon DR, McGoldrick KE, Lema MJ Editors. The Wood Library Museum. Park Ridge; 2005. pp. 137–57.
7. Bacon DR. The New York society of anesthetists: building the foundation. American Society of Anesthesiologists: a century of challenges and progress. In: Bacon DR, McGoldrick KE, Lema MJ. The Wood Library Museum. Park Ridge; 2005. pp. 9–18.
8. Wood PM. Cited in Betcher et al. The jubilee year of organized anesthesia. anesthesiol. 1956;17:229–67.
9. Little DM, Betcher AM. The diamond jubilee. ASA annual meeting. 1980.
10. Bacon DR. The creation of the American Society of Anesthesiologists: an intriguing decade. American Society of Anesthesiologists: a century of challenges and progress. In: Bacon DR, McGoldrick KE, Lema MJ Editors. The Wood Library Museum. Park Ridge; 2005. pp. 19–34.
11. Curry TB, Berger I, Tandy CC. The post-world war II era. American Society of Anesthesiologists: a century of challenges and progress. In: Bacon DR, McGoldrick KE, Lema MJ. The Wood Library Museum. Park Ridge; 2005. pp. 43–54.
12. Bause GS. The nine lives of paul wood's collection: the wood library-museum of anesthesiology. American Society of Anesthesiologists: a century of challenges and progress. In: Bacon DR, McGoldrick KE, Lema MJ Editors. The Wood Library Museum. Park Ridge; 2005. pp. 55–73.
13. Owens WD. ASA newsletter special commemorative issue 2005. The Anesthesia Foundation. 2005; pp. 23–24.
14. Warfield CA. ASA newsletter 73. Aug 2009; pp. 24–5.
15. Sessler AD. ASA newsletter 68. The 4 Foundations: jewels in the ASA Crown. Sept 2004; pp. 9–11.
16. Curry TB, Tandy CC. The 1950s: a Decade of turmoil. American Society of Anesthesiologists: a century of challenges and progress. In: Bacon DR, McGoldrick KE, Lema MJ Editors. The Wood Library Museum. Park Ridge; 2005. pp. 75–84.
17. Ogunnaike BO, Giesecke AH. ASA newsletter 68. Nov 2004; pp. 13–5.
18. The GAW 1970s: a decade of crisis. American Society of Anesthesiologists: a century of challenges and progress. In: Bacon DR, McGoldrick KE, Lema MJ Editors. The Wood Library Museum. Park Ridge; 2005. Pp. 147–57.
19. The SBE 1980s: a decade of change. American Society of Anesthesiologists: a century of challenges and progress. In: Bacon DR, McGoldrick KE, Lema MJ Editors. The Wood Library Museum. Park Ridge; 2005. pp. 173–91.
20. Ogunnaike BO, Giesecke AH. The 1960s: the ASA comes of age. American Society of Anesthesiologists: a century of challenges and progress. In: Bacon DR, McGoldrick KE, Lema MJ Editors. The Wood Library Museum. Park Ridge; 2005. pp. 103–21.
21. Morrow JG, Steinhaus JE. The anesthesia survey and the medical student preceptorship. American Society of Anesthesiologists: a century of challenges and progress. In: Bacon DR, McGoldrick KE, Lema MJ Editors. The Wood Library Museum. Park Ridge; 2005. pp. 123–36.
22. Weiss JB. ASA newsletter 64. Sep 2000; pp. 21–2.
23. Hattox JS. Personal communication.
24. Stoelting RK. www.apsf.org.
25. Stoelting RK. ASA newsletter 73. Anesthesia patient safety foundation update. June 2009; pp. 38–9.
26. McDermott PL. Personal communication.
27. Todd MM. ASA newsletter 73. Why you should donate your hard-earned dollars to FAER-funded research. June 2009; pp. 54–5.
28. Gelman S. ASA newsletter 70. Nov 2006; pp. 35–6.
29. Bridenbaugh DH, Bridenbaugh PO. ASA newsletter 73. Overseas Teaching Program Goes Global! July 2009; pp. 42–3.
30. The JGW 1990s: growing pains. American Society of Anesthesiologists: a century of challenges and progress. In: Bacon DR, McGoldrick KE, Lema MJ Editors. The Wood Library Museum. Park Ridge; 2005. pp. 205–12.
31. Sim P. Personal communication.
32. Arens JF. ASA newsletter 73. Practice Parameters—2009 Update. Mar 2009; pp. 43, 51.
33. Http://www.asahq.org/aboutAsa/StrategicPlanRevisedAC120608.pdf.
34. Http:///www.AQIHQ.org.
35. Bacon DR. Iconography in anesthesiology. The importance of society seals in the. and 30s. Anesthesiol 1996. 1920s;85:414–9.
36. Minutes of Meeting of the New York Society of Anesthetists, April 13,1932. Collected Papers and Minutes of the Long Island, New York and American Society of Anesthetists (1905–1945). The Wood Library-Museum Collection. Park Ridge; Illinois.
37. Letter from Paul Wood to Winthrop Hall, June 5, 1961. The Collected Papers of Paul Wood, MD, The Wood Library-Museum Collection. Park Ridge; Illinois.

The Role of the International Anesthesia Research Society in the History of Anesthesia

Douglas Craig, Michael Cahalan, Davy C. H. Cheng, Colleen G. Koch and Robert N. Sladen

Summary

The 10-decade old, 14,000-member International Anesthesia Research Society (IARS) was born and grew through the efforts of Francis McMechan (1879–1939) and his wife Laurette McMechan (1878–1970). By 1911, severe rheumatoid arthritis prevented McMechan from continuing his medical practice, and he turned his skills to the development of anesthesia organizations. In 1914, McMechan became editor of the *Quarterly Supplement of Anesthesia and Analgesia*. In 1919, he established the National Anesthesia Research Society (NARS) which in 1922, initiated publication of *Current Researches in Anesthesia and Analgesia*. The IARS succeeded the NARS in 1925. In 1957, the Journal became *Anesthesia and Analgesia...Current Researches*, and in 1979 it became *Anesthesia & Analgesia*.

Laurette acted as Assistant Editor, assuming greater responsibilities as illness increasingly disabled McMechan in the 1930s, leading to his death in 1939. In 1940, Howard Dittrick (Laurette's gynecologist) was appointed Directing Editor and Laurette continued as Assistant Executive-Secretary-Editor. Dittrick died in 1954 and Harry Seldon became Editor-in-Chief (1954–1976).

The fourth Editor-in-Chief (1976–1990), Nicholas Greene, improved scientific content, expanded circulation, and increased profitability, enabling the IARS research awards program. Greene was succeeded by Ronald Miller (1991–2006), who created a "journal within the Journal" for subspecialty societies, including the Society of Cardiovascular Anesthesiologists. Miller also appointed international editors, and inaugurated the Chinese Language Edition.

The sixth Editor-in-Chief, Steven Shafer (2006–), continued development of the electronic edition enhancing interactivity and facilitating continuing medical education and links to OpenAnesthesia.org. He led the charge in identifying and combating plagiarism and fraud in anesthesia publication.

The IARS provided logistical and financial assistance in the establishment of the World Federation of Societies of Anaesthesiologists (WFSA), which in 1955 elected Harold Griffith (Chair of the Board of Trustees of the IARS) as the first WFSA President.

IARS founders envisioned support of research and education as primary objectives, and from 1983 to the present, the IARS provided more than $ 12,000,000 to support research. In 2009, responding to growing concerns that anesthetics may impair mental development in young animals, the FDA and the IARS launched a public-private partnership (SmartTots), to raise $ 30,000,000 to support research needed to determine the safest sedatives and anesthetics for young patients. Finally, from 1997 to 2012, the IARS gave 21 anesthesiologists Teaching Recognition Awards totaling $ 220,000.

D. Craig (✉)
Department of Anesthesia, University of Manitoba, 66 Chancellors Cir, MB R3T 2N2, Winnipeg, Canada
e-mail: doug.craig@bell.net

M. Cahalan
Department of Anesthesiology, University of Utah, 30 N 1900 E, Room 3C444, Salt Lake City, UT 84132-2501, USA
e-mail: Michael.cahalan@hsc.utah.edu

D. C. H. Cheng
Department of Anesthesia & Perioperative Medicine, University of Western Ontario, London Health Science Centre & St Joseph's Health Care, 339 Windermere Road, C3-172, London, ON N6A 5A5, Canada
e-mail: davy.cheng@LHSC.ON.CA

Introduction

The International Anesthesia Research Society (IARS) arose concurrently with the accelerating development of anesthesiology that marked the beginning of modern anesthesia. Where other new anesthetic societies failed, the IARS succeeded, principally through the efforts of an extraordinary man, Francis McMechan (Fig. 20.1). He had a vision for an international society of specialists in anesthesia that would support research, organize meetings as venues to present research results, publish a journal, and provide a mechanism for specialty certification [1]. This

E. I Eger II et al. (eds.), *The Wondrous Story of Anesthesia*, DOI 10.1007/978-1-4614-8441-7_20, © Edmond I Eger, MD 2014

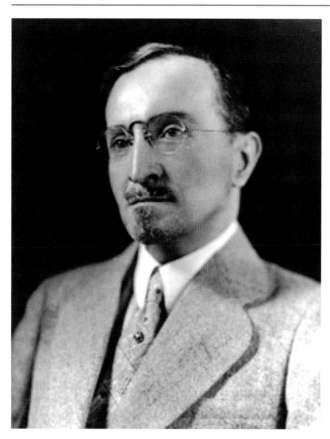

Fig. 20.1 Francis McMechan. (Courtesy of the Wood Library-Museum of Anesthesiology, Park Ridge, IL.)

chapter describes his role in the creation of the IARS, and the continuing contributions of that society to the advancement of anesthesiology.

The McMechans

McMechan's grandfather and father were physicians. While in college, McMechan (1879–1939) won gold medals for oratory and essay writing. He was attracted to dramatics and music. Too young to enter medical school after graduation from college, he worked for 3 years as a playwright, as the Director of the Shuster-Martin School of Acting in Cincin-

C. G. Koch
Department of Cardiothoracic Anesthesia (J-4), Cleveland Clinic
Lerner College of Medicine of Case Western Reserve University,
9500 Euclid Avenue, Cleveland, OH 44195, USA
e-mail: kochc@ccf.org

R. N. Sladen
Division of Critical Care, Department of Anesthesiology, PH 527-B,
College of Physicians & Surgeons of Columbia University, 630 West
168th St, New York, NY 10027, USA
e-mail: rs543@columbia.edu

nati [2], and as a reporter for the Cincinnati Post. In 1900, he entered the College of Medicine at the University of Cincinnati. After graduating in 1903, he joined his father's general practice in Cincinnati. An interest in anesthesia led McMechan to approach surgeons known to his father and ask if he could administer anesthetics for them. They soon appreciated that McMechan possessed unusual skills as an anesthetist, and although he began his career as a general practitioner in Cincinnati, he established a successful anesthetic practice, evolving into one of the first full-time anesthesiologists in the United States [3].

Laurette van Varseveld McMechan (1878–1970) claimed to be a descendant of Baron Larrey, Napoleon's Surgeon in Chief. While detailed analysis of historic records does not support this claim, there is no doubt that Laurette had a major positive role in the development of the specialty of anesthesiology, earning the affectionate title "Mother of Anesthetists" [4]. She was a student at the Shuster-Martin School, displaying an interest that coincided with McMechan's [3]. They married in 1909.

Unfortunately, Francis McMechan developed rapidly progressing rheumatoid arthritis and by the age of 32, his skeletal deformities were so debilitating that he could not continue his medical practice. The disease eventually forced him to sleep while seated and to rely on assistance from others, particularly Laurette. Unable to practice medicine, a tenacious McMechan applied his considerable skills as physician, reporter, playwright and amateur actor, to written communications within the fledgling specialty, and to the development of its organizations. McMechan was the Editor and Executive Secretary of the IARS and had similar appointments in several affiliated organizations. Laurette became his assistant, increasingly assuming responsibilities for the conduct of these organizations as McMechan's health failed during the late 1930s. She continued with these responsibilities after his death. McMechan spent most of his adult life in a wheelchair, "a device which contained but never confined him" [5]. With the support of his wife and colleagues at the IARS, he remained productive until the late 1930s, traveling throughout the world on behalf of anesthesiology. The following provides the details of his story and the associated history of the IARS.

Formation of the International Anesthesia Research Society (IARS)

The London Society of Anaesthetists (1893), the Long Island Society of Anesthetists (1905) and its successor, the New York Society of Anesthetists (1911) constituted the world of formal organizations in anesthesia at the start of the 20th Century. Formal anesthesia training programs had

Fig. 20.2 A graphic depiction of the societies McMechan helped create and their approximate creation dates. (From Seldon TH: Anesthesia and analgesia—50 years of publication. Anesth Analg 1971; 50: 571–7, with permission.)

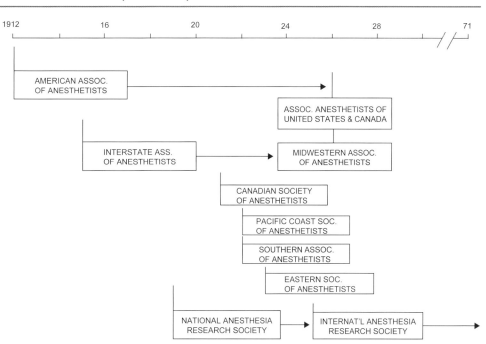

not been established for physicians[1], and no process existed to certify anesthetic practitioners. The specialty was truly in its infancy.

Two parallel streams of anesthesia organizations emerged in the United States. First, the New York Society became the American Society of Anesthetists (1936), to be renamed the American Society of Anesthesiologists (ASA) in 1945. Although the ASA initially included Canadian provinces as components, and one Canadian (Wesley Bourne) served as the ASA President in 1942, this arrangement lapsed and full ASA membership was then restricted to US residents.

Second, McMechan developed competing organizations in the US and Canada, some with international membership categories (Fig. 20.2). The American Association of Anesthetists (AAA, 1912), was linked initially with the American Medical Association, but through McMechan's influence, soon became fully independent. Additions to the AAA, included state and regional anesthesia societies within the US, and the Canadian Society of Anesthetists. A North American society (Associated Anesthetists of the United States and Canada) succeeded the AAA in 1926. McMechan led the establishment of the National Anesthesia Research Society (NARS) in late 1919. The announcement of the launching of NARS formed part of a report of the 8th Annual Meeting of the American Association of Anesthetists in New Orleans, April 26–27, 1920 [6]. NARS had a mandate to promote

research in anesthesiology and to communicate the results of this research, a mandate consistent with McMechan's vision of the importance of research for the future of anesthesia, and the need to link research with clinical practice. Members included both medical practitioners and industry representatives. However, the inclusion of members from industry prompted controversy and led to the decision to change both the society name and membership eligibility in 1925.

The IARS officially began on the 8th February 1925, by resolution of the "Professional Board of Governors (pro tem)" of the IARS, as the successor of the NARS. The IARS adopted the mission of the NARS, changing only the society name and society membership criteria (by excluding industry representatives). The IARS concurrently became the Publisher of *Current Researches in Anesthesia and Analgesia*, the first major anesthesia medical journal in the world, a journal started by the NARS in 1922 (Fig. 20.3). The 1925 Constitution and By-Laws of the IARS noted that the Society "…shall have the following Objects: 1) To initiate and foster research in all phases of anesthesia; 2) To establish and maintain the International Research Foundation; and 3) To extend the publication of the literature of anesthesia in so far as its resources may permit and its governing powers may direct" [7]. IARS membership was restricted to physicians, dentists and researchers with advanced degrees. The name change from NARS to IARS followed McMechan's belief that 'his' societies could and should have an international role, as evidenced by the IARS constitution listing its roles as the "official research and publications society of the International Federation of Anesthetists".

The Federation appears, from the limited information now available, to have been an entity under the IARS umbrella

---

[1] Agnes McGee established a school for nurse anesthesia at St. Vincent's Hospital in Portland Oregon in 1909. Agatha Hodgins and George Crile founded a school for nurse anesthesia at the Lakeside Hospital in Cleveland (part of the Cleveland Clinic) in 1915. (see Chapters 22 and 36 on the evolution of nurse anesthesia.)

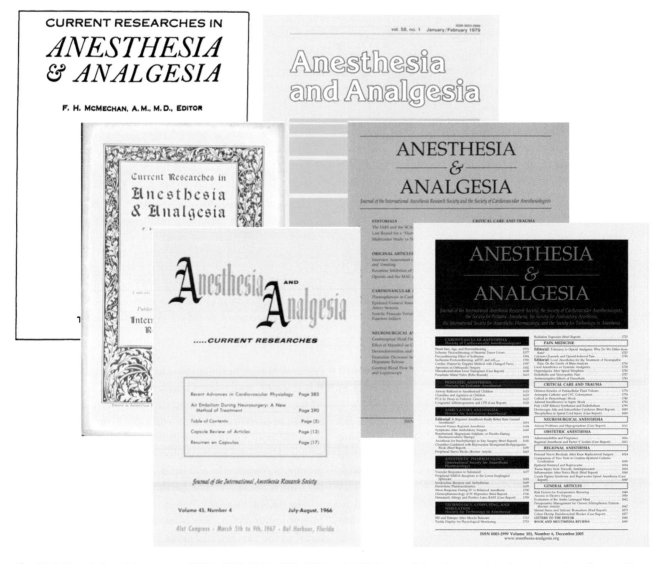

Fig. 20.3 From left to right, covers of 1922, 1926, 1966, 1979, 1994 and 2005 issues of *Anesthesia and Analgesia* in various flavors. (From *Anesthesia and Analgesia*, with permission.)

which, at various points in time, included anesthesia societies in the United States, Canada and the United Kingdom. For example, the 1930 Directory of Anesthetists (accessed in the Wood Library-Museum of Anesthesiology) lists first the Associated Anesthetists of the United States and Canada, followed by the IARS and eight other societies based in the United States, plus one in Canada and three in the United Kingdom.

McMechan conceived the Federation as an organization that would certify specialists in anesthesia in the United States, Canada and the United Kingdom. However, when the certification process for anesthesia specialists was implemented, it was the International College of Anesthetists (not the Federation) that was the certifying entity. Medical and dental anesthesia specialists received the designation FICA—Fellow of the International College of Anesthetists. The IARS Board of Governors served as the review

committee of applications for certification. The 1941 certification requirements included 14 elements, ranging from professional qualifications through clinical anesthesia experience (minimum 2000 cases over 5 years), to IARS membership, and a pledge "to the ethical practice to the specialty of anesthesia". Applicants were required to "present themselves to the Certification Board for questioning and for receiving certification" [8].

McMechan's position on certification, as well as his condemnation of non-physician anesthetic practitioners, and those who taught them or worked with them, in part separated his organizations from ASA organizations. When invited in the late 1930s to join the ASA's collaborative efforts with the AMA in the formation of the American Board of Anesthesiology (ABA), the IARS declined, responding that they already provided certification and that it should be "entirely separate from any other larger medical or surgical organization and free from its domination or control" [9]. Thus, the IARS missed its chance to play a role in the formation of the ABA, and once the ABA was formed, the IARS certification gradually became irrelevant [10]. Newly developed specialty certification processes in Canada and the United Kingdom made the F.I.C.A. qualification irrelevant in those countries as well.

One historical discrepancy remains unresolved. The announcement in the April 1925 issue of *Anesthesia and Analgesia, Current Researches,* clearly states 1925 as the official start date for the IARS, succeeding the NARS. However, 1922 (the year of the first journal issue) is the date on the IARS seal. The seal was designed by, or under the authority of, the IARS Board of Governors, so the use of the year 1922 appears deliberate. The records now available do not further explain the seeming discrepancy. The year 1922 continues to be used as the official IARS start date.

Creation and Development of an Independent IARS Journal

McMechan recognized the importance of written communications to the development of anesthesiology. By 1914 he had convinced Joseph MacDonald, Managing Editor of the *American Journal of Surgery*, to publish a *Quarterly Supplement of Anesthesia and Analgesia*, with McMechan as editor. The Supplement continued until 1926, despite commencement of publication of *Current Researches in Anesthesia and Analgesia* in 1922 by NARS, with McMechan as editor. The latter publication coincided with the year in which MacDonald died.[2] The Editorial Foreword [11] of the first issue of *Current Researches in Anesthesia and Analgesia,* in August 1922, included the modest statement: "With this issue the former Bulletin becomes a regular Journal to carry on the organization and educational campaign of the National Anesthesia Research Society. As in the past, the Journal will print papers from the Transactions of the several Associations of Anesthetists, special and selected articles of pertinent interest, as well as abstracts from the current literature of anesthesia and analgesia." A one-year subscription to the journal cost $ 3.00, and single copies 50 cents.

With formation of the IARS in 1925, the Board of Governors of the IARS became the owners and governing body of the journal. McMechan continued as the Journal's first editor until his death in 1939. His death precipitated a crisis for the IARS and its Journal, for the IARS Board of Governors had not prepared a succession plan. On 1 July 1939 the Board appointed Board member Emanuel Klaus to the acting positions of Executive Secretary and Editor, and Laurette

McMechan as Assistant Executive-Secretary-Editor, the positions she had held before her husband's death. She continued in these roles until she retired in 1956. Thereafter, she was appointed Honorary Assistant Editor, a position she held until her death in 1970. A published summary of its 24 September 1939 meeting, noted that the Board had considered suggestions that the IARS should "amalgamate with other societies" [12]. In response, the Board approved an amendment to the IARS Constitution and Bylaws, requiring consultation with the membership via a mail vote for any proposal to change the status of the IARS as an organization. A change of IARS status required a two-thirds affirmative vote from at least two-thirds of the members. The IARS Board participated in initial discussions with an ASA committee but then withdrew, ultimately maintaining two societies, two journals (*Anesthesiology* was not launched until 1940), and two annual meetings [13].

In a further step toward editorial independence for the Journal, unlike two of three prior editors (McMechan and Seldon), Nicholas Greene, appointed as the fourth Editor-in-Chief of *Anesthesia & Analgesia* in 1977, declined to serve on the IARS Board of Trustees. This separation of the IARS governing board and the Journal editorial leadership, endured until 2012 when the IARS Board of Trustees (BOT) voted to invite Steven Shafer to participate in all BOT meetings (with certain exceptions) as a guest. This arrangement strengthened the communication between the IARS BOT and the Journal Editor-in-Chief, while maintaining the editorial independence of *Anesthesia & Analgesia*.

The history of the Journal, which became *Anesthesia and Analgesia...Current Researches* in 1957, and *Anesthesia & Analgesia* in 1979, may best be appreciated by a review of the contributions of the six Editors who have led it since 1922. In 1971, Seldon chronicled the Journal's first 50 years [14], and in 1997, Craig and Martin reflected on the first 75 years [5]. We summarize those reviews below and add vignettes for Ronald Miller and Steven Shafer to bring us to 2013.

Francis McMechan (Editor from 1922–1939)

McMechan dominated the early years of the NARS/IARS and of the Journal (Fig. 20.1). As noted above, he had edited the *Quarterly Supplement of Anesthesia and Analgesia* of the *American Journal of Surgery*, from 1914 to 1926. As a former newspaper reporter and playwright he brought effective communication skills to these tasks. Through written communications, in an era when communication tools were basic by modern standards, and by extensive travel during which he promoted the specialty of anesthesiology and "his" societies, McMechan attracted authors, society members and journal subscribers. The Journal was successful and became a vehicle not only for scientific communication, but also for

---

[2] The British Medical Journal of 18 Feb 1922 reported MacDonald's death on p 22.

NARS/IARS announcements. Some of these appear in the indexed pages of the Journal while others are 'hidden away' in the annual index, and are not highlighted on the index itself. Commercial advertising was introduced, with a note that "for permanent binding the advertising pages may be withdrawn, without discarding any of the content." Laurette McMechan held an active position as Assistant Editor and influenced the operations of both the Journal and the various societies. During the 1930s, when chronic illness frequently disabled McMechan, Laurette increasingly assumed governance of Journal operations. This experience proved valuable following McMechan's death in June 1939. Laurette's contributions to anesthesia worldwide, including her recognition as the "Mother of Anaesthetists", were included in tributes published following her death [15].

In 1937 Francis and Laurette were jointly recognized for their many achievements with the presentation of a loving cup trophy with the following inscriptions: "To F. Hoeffer McMechan, M.A., M.D., F.I.C.A. Editor, Secretary-General and Laurette van Varseveld McMechan Associate Editor, Secretary and hostess. In loving appreciation of devoted services and splendid achievements for the organization, economics, research, practice, teaching, journalism and fellowship of the specialty of anesthesia. For the world conquest of human pain in behalf of suffering humanity. Presented by the International Anesthesia Research Society and International College of Anesthetists. Sixteenth annual Congress of Anesthetists. 1937" [16].

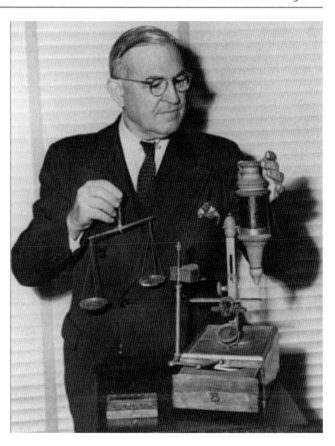

Fig. 20.4 Howard Dittrick, second editor of *Current Researches in Anesthesia and Analgesia* shows one of the many surgical artifacts he collected. (From the Case Western Reserve Dittrick Medical History Center, Cleveland, OH.)

Howard Dittrick (1940–1954)

As outlined earlier, the IARS did not have a succession plan ready when McMechan died in 1939. Assisted by Laurette McMechan and the IARS Governors, Emanuel Klaus, a member of the IARS Board of Governors, assumed editorial responsibility for the final three issues of 1939. The January–February 1940 issue announced Dittrick's appointment as Directing Editor, reporting to the IARS Board (Fig. 20.4) [17]. Dittrick (1877–1954), a gynecologist, had a background in medical editing (Editor of the *Bulletin of the Cleveland Academy of Medicine*) and medical history. His appointment is thought to have been as a result of the IARS Board's positive view of his academic credentials and international recognition, as well as Dittrick's longstanding friendships with Klaus and both McMechans [18]. The first Journal issue for 1940 also confirmed the continuing role of Laurette McMechan as Assistant Editor and continued the IARS Board of Governors as the Editorial Board.

The 1940s were difficult years for the Journal. Dittrick functioned more as a copy editor than an Editor-in-Chief, and had a limited ability to recruit reports for the struggling Journal. Commencing in July 1940, the publication

of *Anesthesiology* by the American Society of Anesthetists (becoming the American Society of Anesthesiologists in 1945) provided stiff competition for *Current Researches in Anesthesia and Analgesia*. The difficulties created by World War II, including the suspension of the IARS Congresses from 1942 to 1945 (a major source of papers published in the Journal), were also a negative factor. To the credit of the editorial team, the Journal continued bimonthly publication throughout the 1940s, but the numbers of society members and subscribers declined. Dittrick continued as Directing Editor until his death at age 77 early in 1954.

T. Harry Seldon (1954–1976)

After Dittrick's death, Thomas Harry Seldon, (always addressed as Harry), a member of the IARS Board, assumed the Editor-in-Chief position, in addition to his full time clinical practice as an anesthesiologist at the Mayo Clinic (Fig. 20.5). Laurette McMechan's appointment as Assistant Editor continued, as did the role of the IARS Board as the Editorial Board of the Journal. Seldon (1905–1991) recognized that the competition provided by *Anesthesiology* re-

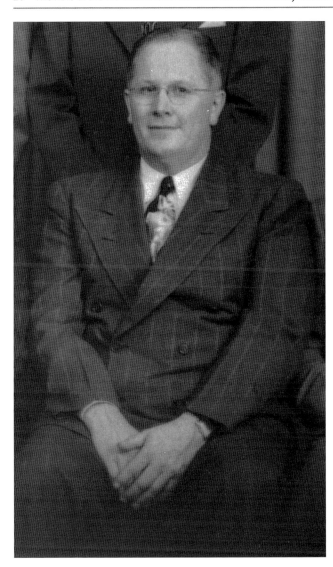

Fig. 20.5 Thomas Harry Seldon. (Photo courtesy of Mayo Foundation for Medical Education and Research. Used with Permission.)

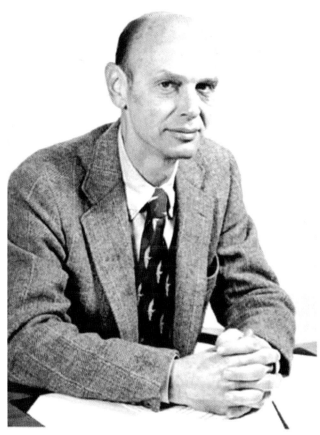

Fig. 20.6 Nicholas M. Greene. (From Medicine at Yale website.)

Nicholas Greene (1976–1990)

The appointment of Nicholas Greene (1922–2004) as Editor-in-Chief began a new phase for the Journal (Fig. 20.6). He had served for 18 years as the Chair of the Department of Anesthesiology at Yale University, and had just completed a term as Editor-in-Chief of *Anesthesiology*. Greene offered a wealth of knowledge, experience and credibility as an editor and academician [20]. Tellingly, Greene declined an invitation to become an IARS Trustee. The Editorial Board was expanded, with most Editors not simultaneously acting as Trustees on the IARS Board. Thus, although the Journal was still responsible to the IARS Board, it gained increasing editorial independence. Another redesign was introduced in 1979 (Fig. 20.3), the Journal was renamed *Anesthesia & Analgesia*, and the following year it became a monthly publication.

Greene's authoritative approach to the scientific review process, and his kind but firm communications with authors had a salutary effect on the reputation of *Anesthesia & Analgesia* and the IARS, and the number of quality manuscripts increased. Elsevier Science Publishing (New York) was engaged as Publisher, replacing a complex set of in-house management steps that could be traced back to 1922.

quired major changes to the Journal. The official title of the journal was changed in 1957 to *Anesthesia and Analgesia… Current Researches*. The appearance of the journal changed (Fig. 20.3). The page size was increased, color highlights were added, and new content features were introduced, all to make the Journal more interesting for the reader. These included short notes about new drugs and equipment, historical vignettes and the inclusion of photographs and biographical sketches of first authors. More significant was Seldon's legendary kindness and patience in helping first authors create publishable articles, through the revision and editing process. The Editorial Board was expanded to include non-IARS Board of Trustee members, a step with symbolic and practical importance. Credited to Harry Seldon, the decline in the status of the Journal was arrested, confidence in it increased [19] and *Anesthesia and Analgesia…Current Researches* was ready for the next phase.

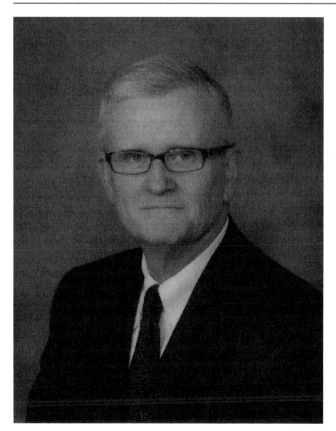

Fig. 20.7 Ronald Miller. (From UCSF physician website.)

A crucial Miller legacy was his accomplishment of a "Journal within the Journal", a publishing home for several anesthesiology subspecialty societies [21]. In 1993, the IARS changed publishers from Elsevier to Lippincott Williams & Wilkins (LWW), and in 1994, the Society of Cardiovascular Anesthesiologists (SCA) became the first and largest subspecialty society to adopt *Anesthesia and Analgesia* as its official journal. The IARS agreed to appoint an Associate Editor-in-Chief for Cardiovascular Anesthesiology, nominated by the SCA. This agreement strengthened the Journal by increasing its subscriber base and the number of manuscripts available for potential publication Subsequently, Miller succeeded in negotiating with four more societies to affiliate with *Anesthesia & Analgesia* as their official journal:the Society for Pediatric Anesthesia (SPA) and the Society for Ambulatory Anesthesia (SAMBA) in 1996, the international Society for Anaesthetic Pharmacology (ISAP) in 2000, and the Society for Technology in Anesthesia in 2001. With the exception of SCA, affiliate society members were not required to subscribe to the Journal or join the IARS.

Miller advanced the worldwide influence of the Journal by appointing several international members to the Editorial Board, by creating the on-line edition of the Journal, and by inaugurating the Chinese Language Edition, published and distributed in China. The appearance of the printed Journal changed twice during his 15-year tenure (Fig. 20.3).

The enhanced scientific content and more efficient management process expanded circulation and increased profitability, which in turn supported the establishment of the IARS Research Awards program. When he stepped down as Editor-in-Chief in 1990, Greene left a legacy of a vibrant, scientifically based Journal, and a society that could now actively support anesthesiology research.

Ronald Miller (1991–2006)

Ronald Miller was a successful editor and academician before assuming the role of Editor-in-Chief of *Anesthesia & Analgesia* (Fig. 20.7). His textbook, *Anesthesia*, was in its third edition and was regarded as among the definitive textbooks in anesthesiology. Miller was Chair of the Department of Anesthesiology at the University of California San Francisco. While Editor-in-Chief, he was elected to the Institute of Medicine of the United States National Academy of Sciences. Miller moved the Journal Editorial Office to San Francisco, where it functioned relatively independently from the IARS Office in Cleveland, Ohio. The relationship between the Editor-in-Chief and the IARS Board of Trustees was similarly independent, with the interaction primarily that of regular reportage.

Steven Shafer (2006–Present)

In 2006, after an extensive and competitive search by the IARS Board of Trustees, Steven Shafer was selected as Editor-in-Chief (Fig. 20.8). Shafer is an academic anesthesiologist whose research focus is pharmacokinetics and pharmacodynamics. Shafer created a new look for the Journal in its printed and on-line versions. The covers of the printed versions contain original artwork: sometimes humorous, sometimes puzzling, but always arresting (Fig. 20.9). He further expanded the editorial content and correspondence sections of the Journal to amplify the significance of its content, and support subsequent debate. Dr. Shafer enhanced the interactivity of the on-line Journal using a multimedia approach, creating and encouraging links to innovative sites such as OpenAnesthesia.org. During Shafer's tenure the impact factor of *Anesthesia & Analgesia* increased from to 2.1 in 2006 to 3.4 in 2012, placing it in the top tier of anesthesiology journals. In 2013, the Journal stopped publishing Case Reports, instead creating a new online journal, *Anesthesia & Analgesia Case Reports,* naming Lawrence Saidman as Editor-in-Chief.

Shafer continued the recruitment of subspecialty societies and expansion of the editorial board. The Anesthesia Patient Safety Foundation (APSF) became affiliated with the Jour-

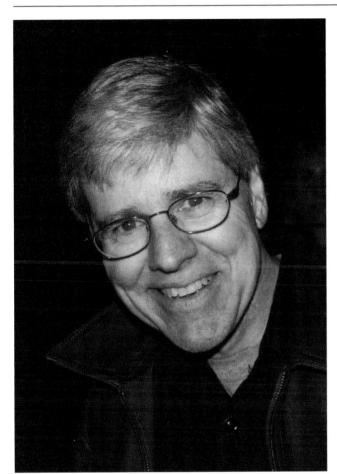

Fig. 20.8 Steven Shafer. (Courtesy of Dr. Pamela Flood.)

nal in 2007. In 2008, *Anesthesiology* decided to divest itself of subspecialty society affiliations. Shafer made a new home for the Society for Obstetric Anesthesia and Perinatology (SOAP), and the American Society for Critical Care Anesthesiology (ASCCA)—now called the Society of Critical Care Anesthesiologists (SOCCA).

A sad topical reflection on academic anesthesiology (and the scientific community as a whole) has been the increasing revelations of plagiarism and fraud in scientific publications. Shafer had to deal with three major such events in his first term, and many other minor ones. In every case he met the challenge head-on, with resolve, persistence and editorials (Fig. 20.9) [22–24]. Through his leadership, he brought together several national and international scientific journal editors to take joint action against academic fraud.

An important aspect of Shafer's role as Editor-in-Chief of *Anesthesia & Analgesia,* has been his active and ongoing dialog with the IARS Board of Trustees. He has engaged with the Board of Trustees in strategic planning, and has increased the exchange of ideas between the Board of Trustees and the Editorial Board. The move of the IARS Head Office to San Francisco and its amalgamation with the

Editorial Office (see below) further enhanced this relationship. Shafer was appointed to a second five-year term by the IARS Board of Trustees in 2011, and in 2012, he was invited to participate in BOT meetings (with certain exceptions) as a guest.

Creation and Evolution of the IARS Congress

McMechan initially convened his several societies as an annual "Congress of Anesthetists" at various locations in the United States and Canada. The first American Association of Anesthetists Congress took place in 1913. As new societies were formed, they participated in the Annual Congress, although with some inconsistency in sponsorships and inclusion—even the ASA co-sponsored the Congress for a short time. The first NARS Congress was held in Columbus, Ohio in 1922.

Since its formation in 1925, a major activity of the IARS has been its Annual Congress, renamed the Annual Meeting in 2009. Through this time the IARS has conducted 85 meetings, omitting only those coinciding with World War II (1942–1945) and the first WFSA meeting in 1955. Most meetings have been held in the United States (with a tradition of a meeting in Hawaii every five years), but other venues have included Puerto Rico, the Bahamas, Canada and England.

For many years two Trustees working with the IARS Head Office essentially ran the Annual Congress. This model devolved into an Annual Meeting Committee, still led by two Trustees, but which reached outside the Board of Directors for new energy and ideas.

Rather than trying to compete directly with the ASA meeting, the IARS has positioned its Annual Meeting as a much smaller (1,000 attendees), interactive international forum with direct and easy access between faculty and registrants. The attractiveness of the Annual Meeting has been enhanced by innovations such as a half to full day thematic scientific symposium, and replacing the formal industrial exhibition by an interactive 'table top' gathering of sponsors and anesthesia expert opinion leaders. As a consequence, the IARS Annual Meeting continues to fulfill a unique, valuable role in enhancing the missions of the Society.

The IARS and the World Federation of Societies of Anaesthesiologists

The IARS played critical roles in the establishment of the World Federation of Societies of Anaesthesiologists (WFSA) and in the first World Congress, in Scheveningen, The Netherlands in 1955 [25]. Continuing the tradition of international cooperation established by McMechan decades

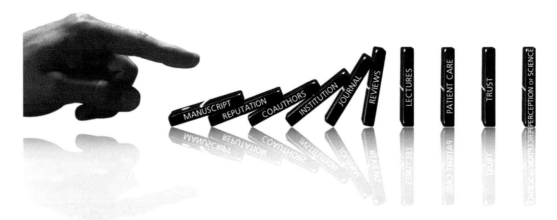

www.anesthesia-analgesia.org

March 2011 • Volume 112 • Number 3

ANESTHESIA & ANALGESIA®

MISCONDUCT

IARS International Anesthesia Research Society

Fig. 20.9 Cover of March 2011 issue of *Anesthesia and Analgesia*

earlier, the IARS held its 1951 Congress in London, in joint session with the Association of Anaesthetists of Great Britain and Ireland. This meeting was followed by another international anesthesia congress in Paris, attended by IARS officers, during which the creation of a new world-wide anesthesia organization was proposed. Harold Griffith (at the time Chair of the Board of Trustees of the IARS) chaired the committee established to explore the issue. After soliciting reports about the numbers of anesthesiologists throughout the world, the committee met again in June 1953. The national organizations representing the specialty reported that there were about 7,000 practicing anesthesiologists and also confirmed interest in the development of a new international organization. The IARS represented the US on the planning committee since the ASA elected to remain an "Official Observer" rather than become involved at that point. Steps to establish the WFSA began, as did planning for the 1955 Congress. The IARS provided secretarial support and financial assistance for the Society and Congress planning processes, and later paid the full costs for the preparation and printing of the proceedings of the 1955 Congress, which were mailed to all IARS members and the 2,000 attendees. Griffith chaired the World Congress and was elected as the first WFSA President.

The WFSA Constitution, which was legally registered in the Netherlands in 1956, described the aim of the Federation as: "To make available the highest standard of anaesthesia to all peoples of the world". McMechan's vision of an international organization of anesthesiologists had been fulfilled, 15 years after his death [26].

By the time of the second World Congress in Toronto, Canada in 1960, the WFSA society membership criteria had been established, with each component national society required to be representative of all anesthetic practitioners in its own country. The IARS Board recognized and accepted that in the United States this role belonged to the ASA, not the IARS. The ASA, after its initial reluctance to become involved in 1955, became a strong and loyal supporter of the WFSA.

More recent IARS support for WFSA programs included the provision of 200 copies of the printed annual IARS Review Course book, from 1983 to 2007 (the last print edition) as well as major support for the costs of the Harold R. Griffith Symposium at the WFSA 9th World Congress in Washington, DC, in 1988.

IARS Governance

The Board of Governors of the NARS (1919–1924) and then the IARS (from 1925) included physicians, dentists, and scientists. These individuals ran the society, conducted the congresses, and starting in 1922, served as the editorial board of

the journal under the direction of McMechan. This unincorporated arrangement continued until 1952, when the IARS incorporated as a not-for-profit organization in the state of Ohio, to "foster progress and research in all phases of anesthesia." The articles of incorporation charged the IARS Board of Trustees with all the responsibilities and authorities of the Society, including the management of its Journal. The title of the IARS Board members changed with incorporation from Governor to Trustee. A listing of all IARS Board members is available on the IARS website (IARS.org).

Initially, Board members were appointed without term limits. Later, the limit was set at 24 and then 18 years. Finally, in 1999, Stephen Thomas stepped down after twelve years, in an effort to push the Board of Trustees toward the twelve-year term, which has been in place since then. This term appears to have achieved the right balance between experience and innovation in the Board of Trustees. The Board has also become increasingly representative of women and minorities, as well as more international in character.

The listing of the IARS Board of Governors and the Honorary Officers and Advisory Board, in the 1930 Directory of Anesthetists (IARS Archives, Wood Library-Museum), reveals the international reach of the IARS, under McMechan's influence. While 7 of 8 Governors were from the US, and one from Canada, the honorary officers were from (order and spelling as in Directory): United States, Germany, France, Holland, Sweden, Brazil, Cuba, England, Czecho-Slovakia, Scotland, Australia, Russia, New Zealand, and the Irish Free State—further evidence of McMechan's international vision!

Except for the years 1962 to 1973, there has been at least one Board member from Canada. In 1999, the first European Trustee was elected to the Board of Trustees, followed in 2001 by the first Asian Trustee from Japan. These two seats have remained "international".

The relationship between the IARS Board of Trustees and the Editor and Editorial Board of *Anesthesia & Analgesia* has undergone a continuous evolution. At its inception, the Board of Trustees essentially directed activities of the Journal. Greene's decision to not become a Trustee initiated establishment of the editorial independence of the Editor-in-Chief and the Editorial Board, which developed further over the next three decades. Greene and Miller organized and directed the activities of the Journal through the Editorial Board and the Editorial Office, which moved to San Francisco during Miller's tenure. The IARS Head Office remained in Cleveland, Ohio, with a local staff and limited interaction with the Editorial Office on the West Coast. The Editor-in-Chief had a largely reporting relationship to the Board of Trustees, which had little input into the day-to-day running of the Journal.

After the appointment of Shafer in 2006, this distant relationship started to reverse. Shafer brought new ideas for discussion with the Board of Trustees. In 2007 the Board of Trustees hired a new Executive Director, Tom Cooper. In 2009, the IARS moved its office from Cleveland, Ohio to San Francisco, California, where it amalgamated with the Editorial Office with a new staff (save for Ms. Laura Kuhar, who has been with the IARS for 32 years!). The centralized office facilitated the productive integration of all the operational activities of the IARS—*Anesthesia & Analgesia*, the Annual Scientific Meeting, and support of research and education in anesthesiology and perioperative medicine. This development is consistent with the strategic missions of the IARS, and has enhanced teamwork between the editorial and IARS staff, increased operational efficiency and realized substantial cost savings.

Indicative of the enhanced interaction between the IARS Office and the Editorial Office, was the 2010 appointment of a Director of Publishing and Strategic Partnerships. In 2009, a Journal Strategic Planning Committee (JSPC) was formed that included the Editor-in-Chief, the Chair of the Board of Trustees, the IARS Executive Director, the Director of Publishing and Strategic Partnerships and a senior BOT member as Journal Liaison. This Committee has met twice a year to discuss financial issues of importance to both the Journal and the BOT, and steered the recent renewal of the Journal contract with Lippincott Williams & Wilkins. The JSPC also promoted the development and close association of the IARS and the Journal with OpenAnesthesia.org, an exciting on-line interface with great appeal to residents and younger anesthesiologists, as well as an iPad version of *Anesthesia & Analgesia*.

IARS Affiliation with Specialty Societies

In 1994, the IARS and the Society of Cardiovascular Anesthesiologists (SCA) reached an affiliation agreement in which the SCA made *Anesthesia & Analgesia* its official journal to be received by all its members. The IARS agreed to provide a "Journal within the Journal" for cardiothoracic and vascular related articles selected by the existing editorial process. In addition, the IARS agreed to appoint an Associate Editor-in-Chief for Cardiovascular Anesthesiology nominated by the SCA. This agreement strengthened the journal by increasing its subscriber base and the number of manuscripts available for potential publication. Subsequently, seven other societies, as listed in the section on Editors, established joint publishing relationships with the IARS and selected *Anesthesia & Analgesia* as their official journal. The subsequent affiliations strengthened the Journal, but the SCA affiliation remains the only agreement that required its members to subscribe to *Anesthesia & Analgesia*. In mid 2013, *Anesthesia & Analgesia* had 14,000 IARS member subscribers and 3,567 institutional subscribers.

IARS Support of Research and Teaching

Although the founders of the IARS envisioned support of research as a primary objective, a formal and sustained research awards program was not established until 1983. Before that time, the IARS recognized outstanding research by presentation of a "Scroll of Recognition for Meritorious Research in Anesthesia and Analgesia." The IARS presented the first such award to Dennis Jackson in 1924. C McKesson (President), W Jones (Vice President) and F McMechan (Editor—Executive Secretary) signed the scroll. The IARS awarded two scrolls in 1925. It was not until decades later that the IARS contributed funds to support research: a $ 10,000 donation to the ASA in 1976 and a $ 5,000 donation to the Canadian Anesthesiologists' Society in 1985, the latter in recognition of the many years of service of Canadian Trustees on the Board of the IARS.

In 1983, the IARS began its systematic support of research, establishing the BB Sankey Anesthesia Advancement Award ($ 25,000) in recognition of Sankey's long service to the IARS as Executive Secretary (1965–1983). The IARS Board of Trustees served as the review committee for these applications and subsequent awards noted below—with one exception. Applicants had to be IARS members and to submit formal research proposals. From 1983 to 1993, the IARS granted 45 Sankey awards, totaling $ 1,078,495. From 1993 to 2004, the IARS provided seven individuals with $ 143,237 (total) as the Ben Covino Research Awards, in honor of Covino's pioneering work in regional anesthesia.

In 1988, the IARS Board determined that the financial success of *Anesthesia & Analgesia* permitted expansion of the IARS Research Awards Program. The Board reached two conclusions. First, it decided that the specialty needed larger awards (initially $ 50,000, later $ 80,000) focused on clinical research. To address this need, the Board created the IARS Clinical Scholar Research Award (CSRA) replacing the smaller Sankey award, a change made with Sankey's consent. From 1994 to 2011, 62 individuals received Clinical Scholar Research Awards, including researchers from seven different nations (US, Canada, Germany, Israel, Netherlands, Switzerland, and the UK), totaling $ 4,696,613. In 2012 the CSRA was replaced by the $ 150,000 IARS Mentored Research Award, with four awards made in 2013.

Second, the Board concluded that anesthesiology needed a major award (initially $ 500,000, currently $ 750,000) to "foster innovation and creativity in anesthesia research by an individual researcher." To address this need, the Board created the IARS Frontiers in Anesthesia Research Award. The Board appointed expert panels of scientists to review applications. From 1995 to 2012, this award has been granted nine times to researchers in four different countries (US, Canada, Germany, and Switzerland), totaling $ 4,750,000. In 2009, in partnership with the Society of Cardiovascular Anesthesiologists (SCA), the IARS pledgcd $ 1,000,000 over five years to the SCA Foundation in support of cardiothoracic and vascular anesthesia research projects. To date the IARS has provided over $ 12,000,000 of support for research, including $ 250,000 for the SmartTots Initiative discussed below.

In addition to research awards, the IARS provided recognition of excellence in education. From 1997 to 2012, 21 anesthesiologists have received Teaching Recognition Awards. Academic departments nominate and document the work of their outstanding teacher. The IARS Board selects the recipients and presents the awards at the IARS Annual meeting. Currently there are two awards ($ 17,000 total), one recognizing Innovation in Education, the other, Achievement in Education. In total, the IARS has awarded $ 220,000 in recognition of teaching excellence. A listing of all IARS awardees since 1983 is available on the IARS web site[3].

The IARS-FDA SmartTots Initiative

In 2008 the US Food and Drug Administration (FDA) approached the IARS with a proposal to launch a private-public partnership to study the safety of anesthetics and sedatives in young children. This initiative was developed in response to a growing concern that anesthetics and sedatives may impair mental development in young animals. The FDA chose the IARS for this partnership because it considered the Society to be apolitical, independent and capable of garnering the scientific and financial resources required for this unique project.

After considerable discussion and planning, the partnership was unveiled in 2009 as SmartTots (Strategies for Mitigating Anesthesia Related neuro-Toxicity in Tots). (The program was introduced as SafeKids, but the title was changed when it was discovered that another entity was already using this name).

(http://www.fda.gov/NewsEvents/Newsroom/PressAnnouncements/ucm149543.htm).

Guided by a joint IARS-FDA Steering Committee, a multidisciplinary Scientific Advisory Board was formed to provide oversight for research strategy and proposal review as well as an Executive Board to lead fundraising. SmartTots appointed as its Executive Board Chair, Michael Roizen, a noted academic anesthesiologist, a well-known health advocate having a particular interest in the issue of neurotoxicity in the very young, and a proven expertise in gathering funds for such a major enterprise.

More than 250 physicians and scientists attended the SmartTots inaugural scientific symposium that took place at the 2010 IARS Annual Meeting in Honolulu. Guided by Roizen and his Executive Board, SmartTots (www.Smart-

Tots.org) seeks to raise $ 30,000,000 from private sources, to support the research needed to determine the safest agents to be used for the youngest patients requiring sedation or anesthesia. The IARS has donated $ 250,000 to SmartTots thus far, and is leading the charge in soliciting donations from the anesthesiology community and the general public.

Conclusions

The IARS is a unique organization, now in its tenth decade as an apolitical, international medical society with a voluntary membership of 14,000 worldwide. The IARS has provided more than $ 12,000,000 to support research, and many millions of dollars more to publish *Anesthesia & Analgesia*, the first major journal devoted to the profession of anesthesiology. Eight specialty societies have adopted *Anesthesia & Analgesia* as their official "Journal within a Journal." Over the lifetime of meetings organized by the IARS, approximately 50,000 professionals have attended an annual IARS meeting to participate in the presentation of research findings and educational sessions. Today, the IARS is pioneering discovery and improved patient care through its SmartTots partnership with the United States Food and Drug Administration. As it approaches completion of a century of activity, the IARS continues to fulfill its trifold mission to support research investigation and education in anesthesiology, and disseminate new information through its prestigious Journals and its Annual Meeting.

Acknowledgments The authors wish to thank Laura Kuhar of the IARS staff and the Wood Library-Museum of Anesthesiology for their help in providing material for this review.

References

1. Bacon DR. Special article: Francis Hoeffer McMechan, MD: Creator of Modern Anesthesiology? Anesth Analg. 2012;115:1393–400.
2. Martin JT (JTM). Vignettes about Francis Hoeffer McMechan, MD. IARS Archives, WLM, Park Ridge Illinois; undated.
3. Atkinson RS. Francis Hoeffer McMechan—1879–1939. Hist Anaesth Soc Proc. 1995;18:53–5.
4. Calmes SH. Special article: Laurette McMechan (1878–1970): "Mother of Anesthetists". Anesth Analg. 2012;115:1401–9.
5. Craig DB, Martin JT. Anesthesia & analgesia: seventy-five years of publication. Anesth Analg. 1997;85:237–47.
6. Archives of the International Anesthesia Research Society and its predecessors. Wood Library-Museum of Anesthesiology, Park Ridge, Illinois.
7. International Anesthesia Research Society constitution and by-laws. Curr Res Anesth Analg. 1925 April;3:66; 126–7.
8. New requirements for medical certification in the International College of Anesthetists. Curr Res Anesth Analg. 1941;20:March suppl, p 32.
9. Part of a letter from McMechan as recorded in the Minutes of a March 2, 1936 meeting of the New York Society of Anesthetists.

---

3 http://www.iars.org/awards

10. Betcher AM, Ciliberti BJ, Wood PM, Wright LH. The jubilee year of organized anesthesia. Anesthesiology. 1956;17:226–64.

11. McMechan FH. Editorial Foreword. Curr Res Anesth Analg. 1922;1:1.

12. Report of Dr. E. Klaus, Acting Executive Secretary-Editor. Proceedings of the Board of Governors' Meeting of July 1st, 1939. Curr Res Anesth Analg. 1940;19:7–12.

13. Bacon DR. The promise of one great anesthesia society. The 1939–1940 proposed merger of the American Society of Anesthetists and the International Anesthesia Research Society. Anesthesiology. 1994;80:929–35.

14. Seldon TH. Anesthesia and Analgesia–50 years of publication. Anesth Analg. 1971;50:571–7.

15. Daly HJ, Kaye G. Tributes to Mrs. Laurette McMechan. Anesth Analg. 1970;49:655.

16. Bause GS. Special article: recovering the long-lost trophy awarded in 1937 to the founders McMechan by the International Anesthesia Research Society. Anesth Analg. 2012;115:1433–6.

17. Editorial. The Board of Governors has the honor to present Howard Dittrick, M.B., M.D. Curr Res Anesth Analg. 1940;19:1.

18. Bause GS, Edmonson JM. Special article: Howard Dittrick: curator to the McMechans' legacy journal. Anesth Analg. 2012;115:1410–5.

19. Southorn P, Rehder K, Sessler AD. Special article: T. H. Seldon (1905–1991). Anesth Analg. 2012;115:1416–22.

20. McGoldrick KE. Special article: Nicholas M. Greene: visionary educator, clinician, editor, and humanitarian. Anesth Analg. 2012;115:1423-30.

21. Tuman KJ. Special article: Ronald D. Miller: tribute to a past editor-in-chief. Anesth Analg. 2012;115:1431–2.

22. Shafer SL. Tattered threads. Anesth Analg. 2009;108:1361–3.

23. Shafer SL. You will be caught. Anesth Analg. 2011;112:491–3.

24. Shafer SL. Shadow of doubt. Anesth Analg. 2011;112:498–500.

25. Griffith HR. A history of the World Federation of Anesthesiologists. Anesth Analg. 1963;42:389–97.

26. Bacon DR. The World Federation of Societies of Anesthesiologists: McMechan's final legacy? Anesth Analg. 1997;84:1130–5.

Francis P. Hughes, and Myer H. Rosenthal

Summary

The NY Society of Anesthetists (NYSA) established a Committee on Fellowships in 1931, incorporating as the "American Board of Anesthesiology" (ABA) in 1935. The ABA certified only local practitioners, excluding recognition by the nationally-based American Medical Association (AMA). In 1936, the NYSA renamed itself the American Society of Anesthetists (ASA). Waters and Wood presented the need for formal recognition of credentialing by the ASA to the American Board of Surgery (ABS). The ABS instructed the ASA to form an examining board as a sub-board of the ABS. In 1938, the Advisory (later American) Board of Medical Specialties (ABMS) approved the ABA as a sub-board of the ABS. In 1939 the ABA awarded its first certificate. In 1941, the ABMS approved the ABA as a primary board with standing equal to that of other boards.

In the 1940s, the ABA evaluated each anesthesia residency training program application submitted to the AMA Council of Medical Education (AMACME). This became too burdensome for the 11 Board Directors, leading the AMACME to establish the Residency Review Committee (RRC) for anesthesiology in 1957. Similarly, the ABA abandoned the use of practical examinations and surveys of practice to define clinical competence in the 1940s, substituting yearly reports of competence by residency directors or preceptors, in 1946.

In 1940, the ABA defined two pathways for entry to its examination system: Two years of approved post-internship training followed by 3 years of 100% anesthesia practice, or 5 years of 100% anesthesia practice. In 1944, the ABA made two years of approved anesthesia training mandatory. From 1937 to 1947, the ABA allowed graduates of AMA-approved foreign medical schools to enter its examination system. In 1969, the ABA admitted Fellows of English, Irish, South African, Australasian and Canadian Colleges (of anesthesia) to its examinations, but the Faculty of Anesthetists of the Royal College of Surgeons of England barred US trained anesthesiologists from their examination system because their training demanded more years than did the US. The ABA mandated an increase in residency from 3 to 4 years in 1976, implementing the increase in 1984. In 1993, the ABA withdrew recognition of residency training in any foreign country except Canada.

In 1985, the ABMS authorized the granting of certification in Anesthesia Critical Care Medicine, with the first examination in 1986. In 1991, the ABMS authorized certification in Pain Management, with the first examination in 1993.

In 1994 and 1995, the ABA declared its intent to issue 10-year time-limited certificates for its primary certificate and for all current and future subspecialty certificates, to commence for all certificates awarded after January 2000. Pain Management certification was granted with a 10-year time limit at its inception in 1993. In 2009, a program for Maintenance of Certification in Anesthesiology (MOCA) replaced the recertification program in place since 2000.

Background[1]

[1] Unless specifically referenced, quotations and material came from minutes and reports from committees and Boards or from Booklets of Information dating from the beginning of this history.

M. H. Rosenthal (✉)
Medicine and Surgery, Stanford University School of Medicine, 783 Tolman Drive, Stanford, CA 94305, USA
e-mail: mhr@stanford.edu

F. P. Hughes
12097 Markridge Loop, The Villages, FL 32162, USA
e-mail: fph3242@yahoo.com

The first US medical organization focused on anesthesiology was the Long Island Society of Anesthetists (LISA), established in 1905. T Drysdale Buchanan, later the first President of the American Board of Anesthesiology (ABA) and recipient of ABA certificate #1, graduated from the New York Homeopathic Hospital in 1897 and in 1898 became the first anesthetist appointed to the Flower Hospital Staff in New York City. In 1904, he became the first professor and head of the Department of Anesthesia at the New York Homeopathic Hospital (later the New York Medical College and Flower Hospital.) In 1912, the LISA combined with anesthetists from Manhattan, to become the New York Society of Anesthetists (NYSA). The NYSA established the Committee on

Fig. 21.1 Members of the New York Society of Anesthesiologists' Committee on Fellowships. (Courtesy of the New York State Society of Anesthesiologists, New York, NY.)

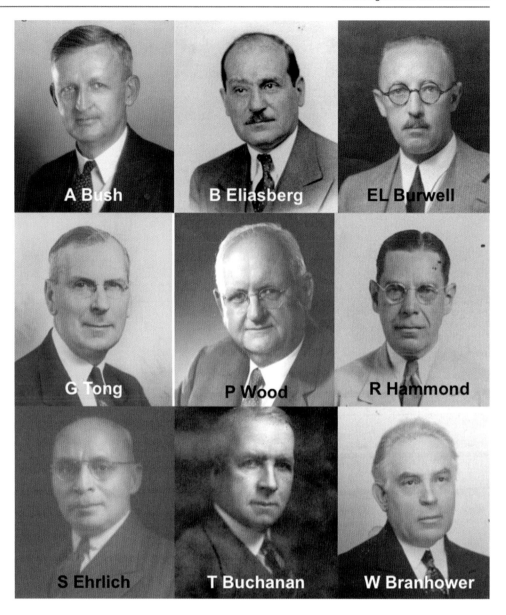

Fellowships in 1931 (Fig. 21.1), beginning a 9-year effort to develop a certification process for anesthesiologists.

Francis McMechan established the International Anesthesia Research Society (IARS) in 1922, and the International College of Anesthetists (ICA—which awarded the first certificate in anesthesiology in 1935), but circumstances militated against his efforts to establish a US based certification.

ICA certification required:

1. Documentation of graduation from medical school and type of anesthesia practice
2. Documentation of the candidate's practice for the previous 3 years, meetings attended, and papers published
3. Submission of 10 complete records including preoperative evaluation, with a discourse on that which was learned from each case.

McMechan, crippled with rheumatoid arthritis, would not tolerate dissent and rarely sought compromise. His adamant opposition to anesthesia practiced by nurses, placed him in direct opposition to surgeons and the American Medical Association (AMA) who favored non-physician anesthesia, demonstrating their allegiance to the nurses providing anesthesia in support of their surgeries. McMechan, an internationalist, married to a French woman, favored international over a more limited US certification. The AMA, the NYSA, and the ABMS established in 1933 by the AMA, opposed such an approach. McMechan's internationalism came at a time of increasing isolationist views in America. Having suffered over a million casualties, beginning with the Revolutionary War and continuing through the Great War (World War I), American society had turned inward, giving a deaf-ear to McMechan's proposals. His uncompromising persona precluded reconciliation.

Paralleling McMechan, the Committee on Fellowships of the NYSA, with Buchanan as Chair and Paul Wood, (an Obstetrical Anesthesiologist at the 5th Avenue Hospital in New York City who famously created the Library-Museum bearing his name) as secretary, began developing its own certification process, a process that eventually established the ABA. The Committee formally incorporated in 1935 "under and by virtue of the laws of the State of New York, (and) the name…shall be the Examining Board, Committee of Fellowship, American Society of Anesthetists or American Board of Anesthesiology." Initial Committee members were Buchanan, Wood, and William Branhower, E Leslie Burwell, Archer Bush, Simon Ehrlich, Bernard Eliasberg, Robert Hammond, and George Tong.

On 23 July 1935, approximately 1 year after McMechan's ICA awarded its first certificates, the Committee met for the first time. In 1936, Fellowships were granted to 88 members of the NYSA, "certifying on record only". The Committee's intent for establishing specific certification for anesthesiologists was that "the basic science for anesthesiology must, of course, stress pharmacology and physiology which, apparently, are less important to the operating surgeon".

In 1927, at the University of Wisconsin, Ralph Waters created the first academic Department of Anesthesiology. His protégés subsequently developed parallel anesthesia programs that enlarged the recognition of anesthesiology as a physician-led, independent specialty and thereby prompted the formation of a certification processes. One protégé, Emery Rovenstine, established the Department of Anesthesia at the Bellevue Hospital at New York University College of Medicine, in 1935. Rovenstine, Buchanan, Wood and Waters would join the first Board of Trustees of the new Examining Board.

Restriction of the certification by the Fellowship Committee of the NYSA to locally trained practitioners precluded support by the nationally-based AMA. In 1935, the NYSA extended membership outside New York, accepting anesthetists from 17 other states. Further to the national focus of the AMA, on December 10, 1936, the NYSA incorporated in New York as the American Society of Anesthetists (ASA). Reflecting McMechan's concerns regarding non-physician practitioners, the ASA by-laws stated that the purpose of the Committee on Fellowships was "to protect the public against irresponsible and unqualified practitioners who profess to be specialists in anesthesiology."

The ABMS rebuffed early ASA attempts to establish a primary certification process. The ABMS and the AMA considered anesthetists as "surgeons specializing in anesthesia". This hostile climate led the Committee on Fellowships to seek other options, leading to a discourse with the American Board of Surgery (ABS) which was organized on 1 Janu-

ary 1937. On 10 January 1937, Waters and Wood presented the ASA position to the ABS. The ABS instructed the ASA to form an "examining board in anesthesiology" as a sub-board of the ABS. A formal affiliation was established on 2 June 1937. The initial examining board consisted of 3 members nominated by the ASA, 3 by the ABS and 3 by the Section of Surgery of the AMA. A 10th member would be a representative from the ABS. The initial articles of incorporation specified that the Examining Board would establish criteria of fitness to practice anesthesia, and arrange, control and conduct examinations to determine the qualifications, and grant certificates to those who voluntarily apply and meet these required standards.

The initial Board of Trustees, as it was called, included the then giants of anesthesia (Fig. 21.2): Buchanan (NYC), Arthur Guedel (Los Angeles), John Lundy (Rochester, Minnesota), Rovenstine (NYC), Henry Ruth (Philadelphia), Ralph Tovell (Hartford, Connecticut), Waters (Madison, Wisconsin), Wood (NYC), and Philip Woodbridge (Boston). The surgical representative from the ABS was Arthur Elting from Albany, New York. Buchanan was designated Chair with Ruth as Vice-Chair and Wood as Secretary-Treasurer.

The Examining Board established criteria for entering the examination process:
1. Medical school graduation
2. Completion of internship
3. 2 years of training, including 18 months of practical training in anesthesia
4. 2 years in the sole practice of anesthesia
5. Membership in the AMA or a comparable approved national medical society (a change from the original criteria that required NYSA membership)

The Board developed categories for the first candidates for certification:
I. Founders: Professors and Associate Professors previously elected to Fellowship in the ASA were to be certified without examination
II. Group A: Those having practiced for 15 or more years were to appear before the Board and could be certified without examination
III. Group B: Those practicing for 7.5 years or more or having administered anesthesia in at least 1500 major procedures could be certified following only an oral examination
IV. Group C: Those who met the 5 "criteria for entering the examination process" listed above and submitted 150 of their cases for evaluation were allowed to enter the full examination system

Finally, certification required a positive vote of two-thirds of the Board of Trustees of the Examining Board and approval by the ABS.

Arthur Guedel did not fall under any of the group designations, and he was removed as a Trustee and replaced by

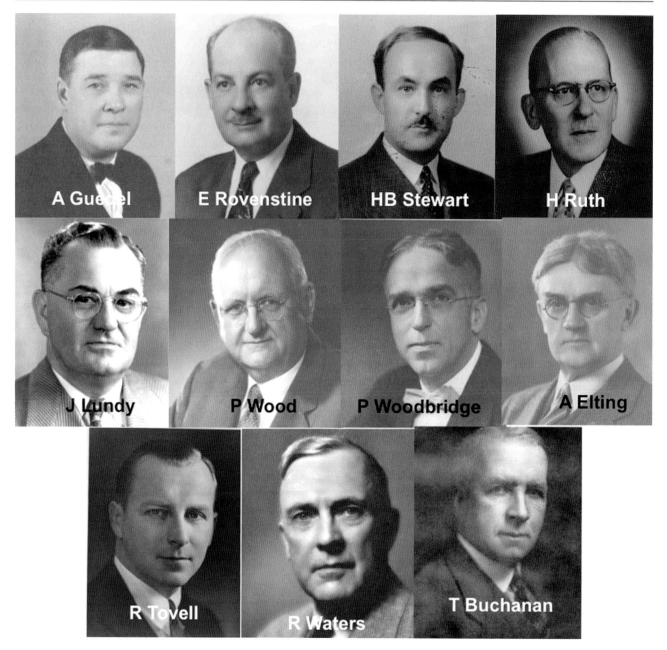

Fig. 21.2 The initial Board of Trustees of the American Board of Anesthesiology. (Courtesy of the American Board of Anesthesiology, Inc., Raleigh, NC.)

H. Boyd Stewart of Tulsa, Oklahoma. In 1943, recognizing Guedel's enormous contributions to anesthesiology, the Board of Directors of the ABA approved his certification without examination. Guedel said, "thank you".

The AMA initially resisted certification of the Founder's group of 40 anesthetists and suggested placing this group in Group A. The ABS rejected this proposal as it would have eliminated 95% of the candidates including Rovenstine, Wood, and Tovell. On 1 January 1939, the ABA awarded certificates to the Founders and 6 candidates from Group A (Fig. 21.3).

The ASA Trustees next sought independent recognition by the ABMS, and thus the medical establishment, for anesthesiology. In February 1938, the ABMS approved the ABA as a sub-board of the ABS, and on 23 March 1938, this new Board was incorporated in the State of New York. The final articles of incorporation began the separation from the ABS, as desired by the ASA Trustees, by replacing the 3 nominations previously assigned to the ABS with 3 nominations from the American Society of Regional Anesthesia (ASRA). The role of the ASRA in the nominating process ended with its merger with the ASA in 1939. These articles also identified the former Trustees as Directors.

Fig. 21.3 The second certificate given by the American Board of Anesthesiology. (Courtesy of the American Board of Anesthesiology, Inc., Raleigh, NC.)

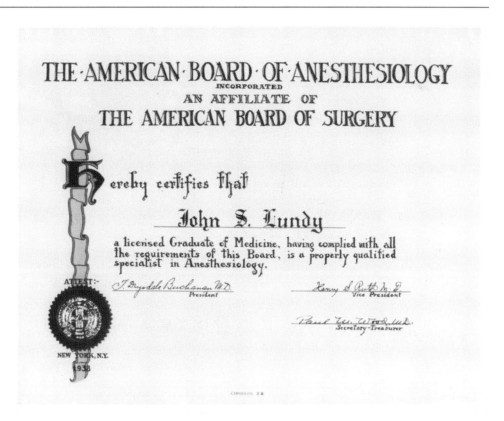

An early issue faced by the new sub-board of the ABS was the status of nurse anesthetists and "non-professional" practitioners. (This could be almost anyone, including a first-year medical student such as Eger, who with his first anesthetic nearly killed a patient [1].) The National Association of Nurse Anesthetists (NANA—later the American Association of Nurse Anesthetists or AANA) asked the ABS to protect the position of nurse anesthetists. The ABS requested a meeting between the NANA, the ABS and the ABA to examine the feasibility of having the ABA sanction a training curriculum and certification for nurse anesthetists. They met on 27 November 1938. The minutes of this meeting indicated that the NANA wanted to "compile a pattern curriculum which we expect to have taught in the various schools of anesthesia for nurse anesthetists. After this has been introduced we expect to have examinations for the students with eventual certification."

Discussions revealed mutual distrust and ABA apprehension concerning independent nurse anesthesia practice. Elting, the ABS representative to the ABA, attempted to encourage discussion, stating that "Just as the American Board of Surgery is perhaps in the relative position of the god-father of the American Board of Anesthesiology, so the American Board of Anesthesiology might perhaps be the god-father to the Association of Nurse Anesthetists or the nurse anesthetists of this country." The ABA continued the dialogue to avoid offending the ABS, but expressed little en-

thusiasm for involvement with nurse anesthesia. At an ABA meeting in May, 1939, Buchanan related a conversation with an ABS surgeon who cautioned, "To be frank with you I want to state that Dr. Graham, Dr. Elting and I are very concerned about the way you are handling this nurse anesthetist question … Frankly we feel that you are side-stepping it." At this May meeting, Buchanan reported that he had told Elting and Rodman that he "would not consent to the American Board of Anesthesiology being sponsors to any nurse anesthetists and they both agreed with me that I was right."

Thus the two protagonists—anesthesiologists and nurse anesthetists—missed an opportunity. Trained anesthetists—nurse and physician—were scarce, and the approaching World War indicated a great increase in the need for trained anesthetists. A formal teaching arrangement might have been established that would have benefited the nurse-physician relationship and the quality of care given to our patients. Anesthesiologists—especially those involved in certification—might have taken the opportunity to participate in nurse certification. The nurses asked for guidance and physicians rejected their overtures to the detriment of their relationship.

An October 1939 report to the ABA by John Lundy exemplifies the physician perception of nurse anesthetists: "The Committee has functioned perfectly. There have been many opportunities offered to the girls to come to us for advice on what would be the best books to read and the advice hasn't been sought." Several ABA discussions considered withdrawing or not certifying physicians who were involved in training nurse anesthetists. Furthermore, when in 1950, the ABA added membership in "good standing" in the ASA, as a criteria for candidacy for certification, the board stated that "If a man signs a nurse's training certificate he is not in good standing in the ASA". However, we cannot find that the ABA acted against any physician working with or training nurse anesthetists. In a statement in 1976, the ABA demonstrated an attempt at accommodation with nurse anesthesia, in proposing to become involved in and accept responsibility "for examination and certification of non-physician anesthesia personnel." Subsequently, the ABA refrained from involvement with nurse anesthetist certification, leaving such matters to the ASA as the representative of the practicing anesthesiologist. Anesthesiologists do contribute to nurse anesthetist education, participating importantly in training, but without the sanction of the ASA or the ABA.

The ABA relationship with its "god-father", the ABS, was sometimes contentious. In October, 1939, Lundy reported on a conversation with the ABS's Elting. Elting stated that "The first thing I want to tell you is that the American Board of Anesthesiology is not an independent Board. They cannot issue a certificate without our consent and while we haven't bourn [sic] down on them previously, we may have to." The ABA remained sensitive to their position as an affiliate of the ABS, and attempted to limit concerns raised by the ABS as evidenced by a Lundy statement at the October 1939 ABA meeting: "I too hope that this Board will keep those problems under their consideration and that they won't do the thing that will offend that Board [ABS] and make them think that we are unsympathetic as to the problem they have to face."

In March 1940, the ABMS with the support of the ABS, recommended ABA independence to the AMA. On 16 February 1941, the ABMS approved the ABA as a primary board with equal standing to others, including the ABS. Neither Buchanan nor McMechan lived to see this event. McMechan died on 26 June 1939, with some speculating that the AMA's decision to establish the Section on Anesthesiology in June 1940 was not just coincidental. Buchanan died suddenly on 22 March 1940 and was replaced as President by Ruth, and as Director by Charles McCuskey, from Glendale, California. In recognition of his contributions in establishing certification for anesthesiologists culminating in the acknowledgement of anesthesiology as a primary specialty, the ABA directors paid tribute to Buchanan.

The by-laws of the ABA as a primary ABMS Board listed the following objectives:

1. To elevate the standard of anesthesiology
2. To familiarize the public with its aims and ideals
3. To protect the public from irresponsible and unqualified practitioners
4. To examine and certify

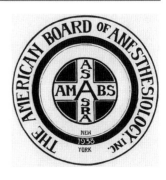

Fig. 21.4 The ABA seal (logo). (Courtesy of the American Board of Anesthesiology, Inc., Raleigh, NC.)

Organization of the ABA and its Directors

Achievement of a balanced national representation motivated selection of future directors. The merger of the ASRA and the ASA in 1939, eliminated the short-lived role of the ASRA in the nomination process. The seal (logo) of the ABA, designed in 1941 and still in use today, reflects this relationship of the ABA with the ASRA along with the AMA, ASA and ABS (Fig. 21.4). In 1942, the AMA provided four nominees (Lundy, McCuskey, Ruth, and Tovell), the ASA provided four (Rovenstine, Waters, Wood, and Woodbridge) and the Southern Medical Society provided one (Stewart). In 1944, the New England Society of Anesthesiology nominated a tenth (Meyer Saklad). Over the following decade, the ABA asserted increasing control over the selection process, assuming sole responsibility for the final selection of nominees, while expressing its desire for input from the nominating bodies. Notwithstanding that expression of desire, conflicts arose between the ABA and the nominating bodies. With Stewart's resignation in 1946, the Southern Medical Society nominated John Winter. Winter completed Stewart's term in 1949, by which time nominations by component societies (Southern and New England) had been assigned to the ASA. The ASA refused to re-nominate Winter, and instead nominated Harvey Slocum who was selected. When, in 1950, the ASA also refused to re-nominate Ruth and Lundy, expressing concern over their "heavy-handedness" and length of service, the ABA "in defiance of their wishes" re-elected the two and made it clear that if the ABA so desired, the AMA and ASA were compelled to nominate a specified candidate, thereby insuring the re-election of existing Directors and control by the ABA of its own makeup.

Differences between AMA and ABA continued into the 1950s. In 1955, the AMA refused to re-nominate Edward Touhy, appointed in 1951 to fill Ruth's unexpired term. The last founding Director, Lundy, retired in 1955 after 18 years of service. Albert Faulconer and Forrest Leffingwell replaced Ruth and Lundy.

The controversy over control of the nominating process was resolved when the ABA, AMA and ASA created a joint nominating committee, with 2 representatives from each organization. The ABA president served as the non-voting chair of the committee. The ABA gained the control it desired when it was agreed that each ASA and AMA representative would have 1 vote and each ABA representative would have 2 votes. The ABA could not be out-voted. Established in 1961, this Triple Committee would nominate 3 candidates for each position, and the ABA would elect its Directors from this slate. As the work of the ABA increased, the number of Directors increased from 10 to 11 in 1950, and to its current number of 12 in 1973. Director's terms as a member of the Board were initially 6 years without term limits. In 1950, this changed to a maximum of two 6-year terms, and in 1957 to three 4-year terms, requiring re-nomination and re-election at each interval. Gender was also considered as a factor in discussions related to Director nominations in 1938, when Huberta Livingstone was considered "… as the probable female member of the Board when it was organized….", but the first female Director, Judith Donegan, was not elected until 1983. Gender equality continued to evolve slowly so that as of October 2012, there are three female directors.

Notoriety came to Emery Rovenstine, one of the original Board Directors. He was the second professor and chair of an academic anesthesiology program (at NYU), Waters being the first in both categories. Rovenstine was President of the ASRA. In the fall of 1947, a series of articles appeared in the New Yorker Magazine that favorably described his contributions to this new specialty, anesthesiology. At this time the medical profession abhorred any advertisement of services. The articles describing Rovenstine and anesthesiology in the New York area led to investigation of his role in the publications, and the material was found to be "self-serving and self-promoting" and therefore inconsistent with the standards of a medical professional. Rovenstine was censured and suspended from membership by the New York State Society of Anesthesiologists. He resigned as a member of the ABA Board of Directors on 19 July 1948, and in support of his good friend and colleague, Wood also resigned. Rovenstine fell victim to pressures of the times, but his reputation as educator and clinician, did not suffer among his colleagues.

The expanding activity of the ABA mandated increasing administrative support. In 1950, an administrative leadership position of Executive Secretary was established and occupied by Charlotte Hickcox, sister of ABA Director Curtis Hickcox. She served until 1979. With Ms. Hickcox's retirement, a new Executive Secretary was hired whose performance was deemed unacceptable. Litigation followed and after settlement, in 1981, search for a replacement resumed. As it had in 1974, the ABA considered asking a physician/former Director to assume this position, a direction consistent with that of other ABMS Boards. But the ABA reasoned that appointment of a former Director could concentrate responsibility and decision making processes in a single individual, diminishing the role of the entire Board. Accordingly, the ABA selected Francis Hughes, PhD as Executive Secretary

in 1982, a title changed to Executive Vice-President in 1994, and to Executive Director in 2000. Duties of the Executive Director position altered in 2007 due to both an increasing role of Board executive directors in the governance of the ABMS, and Hughes' impending retirement.

In June, 2008, Mary Post, MBA was appointed Executive Director for Administrative Affairs while Hughes assumed the new position of Executive Director for Professional Affairs. In this position, Hughes continued his involvement in the governance of the ABMS, serving together with representatives from the other ABMS Boards. As most other board representatives were physicians, Hughes opined and the ABA determined, that physician representation provided more credibility to the views expressed at the ABMS by the ABA. Consistent with its earlier views regarding a physician executive director, the ABA chose to designate a new position of Executive Director for Professional Affairs without involvement in the administrative functions within the Board office. Initially that position was filled by the appointment of a Former Director, David Chestnut to represent the ABA at meetings of the ABMS Board of Directors. The ABA presently intends that the Executive Director for Professional Affairs will be a sitting Director, acting for a maximum of 2 consecutive 3 years terms.

The tenure of Frank Hughes as Executive Director and Executive Vice President coincided with the development of the current written examination and the increased emphasis on validated psychometric tools. Hughes' background as a psychometrician proved invaluable to these processes, and the credibility of the ABA certification process. The reader is referred to Chapter 35 regarding Hughes' crucial role in the development of the certifying examination.

Anesthesia Training and Program Accreditation

The ABA was created to establish a certification process that would eliminate "irresponsible" practitioners, and to guarantee the quality of the educational processes leading to certification. Thus, the ABA would both certify practitioners and accredit programs. The initial articles of incorporation stipulated that the ABA should "increase educational facilities in medical schools and hospitals, and furnish lists of these, together with lists of individual instructors who give adequate instruction and training in anesthesiology". ABA criteria for candidacy for certification included "2 years of training of which 18 months should be practical training in anesthesia." Thus, the ABA was tasked with evaluating each anesthesia residency training application that an institution submitted to the AMA Council of Medical Education for approval. Members of the ABA acted as program inspectors. By 1943, there were 45 approved training programs in anesthesiology, increasing to 213 by 1950. Desire for accreditation exceeded resident interest—in 1950, there were only 107 anesthesiology trainees. By comparison, in 2010, 132 accredited programs trained 5,556 residents.

The responsibility for evaluating and recommending programs became increasingly burdensome for the 11 Board Directors, leading to discussions with the AMA Council on Medical Education and the 1957 establishment of the Residency Review Committee (RRC) for anesthesiology. The RRC was composed of 3 ABA Directors and 3 appointees by the AMA who were recommended by the ABA. In 1981, the AMA, ABMS and the American Hospital Association (AHA) established the Accreditation Council for Graduate Medical Education (ACGME), retaining the RRC as an arm of the ACGME. The ACGME assumed responsibility for accrediting both internship and residency training programs. Concurrently, the ABA modified its requirements to include satisfactory completion of a residency in anesthesia at an ACGME accredited program. The ABA continues to nominate Directors to the RRC as does the Anesthesia Section of the AMA and more recently the ASA. These nominations are forwarded to the RRC/ACGME, who select the RRC members. Beginning in 1998, an anesthesia resident representative was (and still is) nominated by the ASA Resident Component Governing Council. With approval by the ASA Board of Directors, RRC and the ACGME, this resident becomes a member of the RRC. Survey and evaluation of programs by the RRC and accreditation by the ACGME eased the burden on the ABA. The ABA continued to determine the training necessary for admission to its examination and certification system, and therefore continued to influence the content and accreditation of training programs.

The Anesthesia Curriculum and Resident Evaluation

Since its formation, the ABA established education requirements, training curricula and evaluation procedures for certification of physicians in anesthesiology. These were guided by Committees on Education, Curricula, Residencies, Written Examinations, Oral Examinations, Practical Examinations, and Requirements and Credentials. The Committee on Education established "maximum and minimum suggestions for teaching purposes, undergraduate and post-graduate." The work of the Curricula Committee was eventually "blended" with that of a similar committee of the ASA. The ABA Committee on Curricula would be responsible for approving the curriculum assembled by the ASA. The ABA also believed that multiple curricula should be approved to avoid implying "that's all you have to know." In 1947, through a process of elimination and consolidation, the Board reduced its committee structure to a Finance and Executive Committee, a Committee on Credentials and Residency, an Examination Committee, and the Committee on the Administration of Anesthetics in the US.

In March 1972, the Board determined that the Continuum of Education in Anesthesiology consisted of three postdoctoral years; 24 months devoted to approved residency training in clinical anesthesia, and 12 months devoted to internships or any combination of such, approved for the individual by the training program director. The program director, in consultation with each candidate, determined when during the Continuum, the candidate received training in clinical anesthesia and clinical experience versus training in an area or areas other than clinical anesthesia, but the Board urged that at least part of the latter should occur early in the Continuum. The Board also determined that candidates who passed the written examination would have to complete two years of anesthesia practice or an Optional Year of training, before appearing for oral examination.

The increase in information and ideas in the last half of the twentieth century affected all aspects of medicine, including anesthesia, and mandated (at least in the eyes of the Board) an increased duration of training. In October 1976, the Board eliminated the "Optional Year of training" and required all candidates to complete a four-year continuum. Two options in lieu of a fourth (i.e., specialized) year of approved training were added to the required 12 months Clinical Base and 24 months Clinical Anesthesia training: (1) two years of practice or (2) a year of residency in other specialties, or a year of anesthesia related research. This change could be implemented without the RRC having to revise the "Essentials" because all programs had to offer three years of anesthesia training. In 1987, the essentials were changed to require a fourth year of training for all anesthesiology residents.

Subsequently, the ABA convened two meetings of anesthesiology program directors, to inform and obtain input about implementation of a mandated fourth year of training. The ABA announced the continuum, mandating a fourth year of training, at a meeting of Program Directors in April 1984. The Board described three possible tracks for the mandatory fourth (or CA-3) year—Advanced Clinical, Subspecialty Clinical, and Clinical Scientist. The ACGME subsequently mandated a fourth year of training and required that each program offer all three CA-3 tracks. Over the ensuing 15 years, most residents selected the Advanced Clinical Track, spending more than the minimum number of months in subspecialty training—or devoting time to research. Consistent with these dominant choices, the Subspecialty Clinical Track was eliminated and the Clinical Scientist Track (CST) was modified to define opportunities for academic investigators. The CST consisted of 2 options. Option A allowed the candidate to complete 6 months of research at any time during the 48 month continuum. Option B was designed for academic investigators and provided for 18 months of clinical or laboratory research at any time during a 60 month continuum, of which 12 months were devoted to clinical base training and 30 months to clinical anesthesia. In time, options for research during the residency replaced the Academic Investigator Track. These options required that the program director develop a plan with strict guidelines for research activity and "work product" oversight for resident's research activities exceeding 6 months. Scholarly activities had to generate a specific permanent "work product." A local Scholarship Oversight Committee assessed the trainee's progress, and verified the completion of a permanent work product.

With one exception, until recently, the ABA had not stipulated duration of time spent in anesthesiology subspecialties, nor had it mandated the number of cases in any particular area of anesthesia. The exception was Critical Care Medicine. In 1983, the Board required that 2 months be spent in Intensive Care, in 2008 increasing that to 4 months, 1 of which might be in the Clinical Base Year (internship). With input from the ABA, the RRC has now, however, provided definitive expectations regarding specific experiences in both subspecialties types of cases and experience in the entire scope of perioperative care.

More recently, after several meetings with other ABMS primary specialty boards and with approval of ABMS, the ABA has established combined training programs with Pediatrics beginning in 2010, and with Internal Medicine in 2013. Completion of a combined program will result in eligibility for certification in both specialties in less time than that needed to complete each residency separately.

The Clinical Competence Certificate

From its inception, the ABA defined competence with more than grades in the written and oral examinations. Initially, the ABA used a practical examination and surveys of practice, but these proved too burdensome for the small Board. Recognizing that those who trained the candidates might be best able to evaluate competence, in 1946, the ABA mandated yearly reports by residency directors or preceptors. In April 1973, the ABA proposed "a new method for determining competency" to address "long-standing problems of the ABA … related to judging the clinical competence of candidates desiring certification by the ABA." The Board subsequently required appraisal of "satisfactory achievement as assessed by an Evaluation Committee within the candidate's institution of training".

In October 1973, the Board mandated "that a Certificate of Clinical Competence (CCC) be a requirement in the process leading to certification for all candidates who complete their training …." In November 1973, Anesthesiology Training Program Directors were told

> "…that candidates for certification who complete the two years
> of Clinical Anesthesia subsequent to December 31, 1974, will

be required to have a CCC on file with the ABA attesting to their having achieved at least satisfactory clinical competence …." This did not eliminate any existing requirements. Program Directors had to "appoint a Clinical Competence Evaluation Committee… [that] is best chaired by someone other than the Program Director."

The new procedure required that the Committee formally evaluate "the candidate's performance in each of the categories," make a judgment of overall clinical competence, and forward the completed evaluations to the ABA during June and December of each year of Clinical Anesthesia training. "The evaluation of overall clinical competence by this committee during the final six months of the two years of Clinical Anesthesia training will be the evaluation used by the Board in its final determination of eligibility for certification." In time, the Board identified Essential Attributes in the semi-annual evaluation form and required that overall clinical competence be judged unsatisfactory if any "Essential Attribute" was judged unsatisfactory. By 2000, the Board required that programs extend Clinical Anesthesia training for residents receiving consecutive unsatisfactory evaluations of overall clinical competence.

Qualifications and Credentialing of Candidates

In its first Booklet of Information in 1937, the ABA identified the criteria for admission to the examination process.
1. Satisfactory ethical and moral standing
2. Membership in the AMA or other medical societies acceptable to the Council on Medical Education and Hospitals of the AMA
3. Practice limited to anesthesiology (as stipulated by the ABS)
4. Graduation from a Grade A medical school in the US or Canada recognized by the Council of Medical Education and Hospitals of the AMA or graduation from an approved foreign school
5. Satisfactory completion of 1 year or more of an approved internship
6. Duly licensed by law to practice medicine
Although in 1938, the ABS "stipulated" the requirement for practice to be limited to anesthesiology, ABA minutes of 1939 revealed that the ABS felt that the ABA was too strict in implementing this guideline. The ASA leadership expressed concern over the next two decades, regarding the rule limiting practice to anesthesiology. Failure to meet this requirement caused several Diplomates to lose certification. Non-anesthesia practice included general medical practice, surgery or other non-anesthetic specialty practice. The ASA represented many of these "part-time anesthesiologists" and brought pressure on the ABA to remove the 100% requirement. In response, a 1957 Board action removed the 100% requirement for those who already had certification but retained it as

a credentialing criterion for prospective candidates. In 1960, the Board eliminated the 100% practice requirement for certification, retaining it only during residency training.

The numbers of physicians entering the practice of anesthesia grew slowly in the 1930s, and this may have influenced the view of what constituted adequate training in anesthesiology. The approach of World War II and the potential need for greatly increased numbers of trained anesthetists may also have influenced that view. In June 1940, the ABA identified 2 entrance pathways for its examination system

1. Two years of approved post-internship training, followed by 3 years of 100% anesthesia practice or
2. 5 years of 100% anesthesia practice

The 2 years of training could be either in an approved program, or under the supervision of an ABA approved preceptor. In 1944, the ABA eliminated Groups A, B and C categories for certification identified at its creation in 1937. Pathway 2 above, the full practice option, was eliminated in 1945, thus making two years of approved anesthesia training mandatory—except that the Board allowed credit for military anesthesia practice: "In exceptional instances the Board may, in its discretion, accept for examination, candidates who have met all the preliminary requirements, and have clearly demonstrated their identity as an anesthetist over a period of years, but whose formal training does not comply with the full requirements to be exacted in the future." In 1950, the Board again modified their requirements, allowing candidates to take the written board examination (the first examination phase for certification) following the second year of practice, however, final certification would still not take place until after 3 years of practice.

In its 1937 Booklet of Information, the ABA stated that effective from 1 January 1944, requirements for entrance to the examination system would be 3 years of post-internship anesthesia training plus 3 years of anesthesia practice. Although the Directors favored such a plan, it was not implemented. Again in 1957, the ABA voted to increase training to 3 years post-internship, beginning on 1 July 1963, and to only admit those with this option after 1 July 1965. Furthermore, the ABA indicated its plans to withdraw recognition of any training program that did not offer the 3 years after 1 July 1964. However, program directors and the ASA criticized this decision. Led by John Dillon and Robert Virtue, this opposition caused the ABA to hold a special meeting with program directors on 8 December 1959 and again on 5 October 1960. Subsequently, the ABA again rescinded its plans for the required 3 years of residency. As an alternative it created the "optional 3rd year".

In 1962, the ABA announced two pathways to certification beginning 1 July 1966:

1. Two years of clinical anesthesia training post-internship plus a 3rd year spent in research in the basic or clinical sciences, pathology, internal medicine, surgery, advanced

anesthesia training or an anesthesia subspecialty. These 3 years would be followed by 1 year of practice
2. Two years of training post-internship of clinical anesthesia followed by 4 years of practice

In 1966, the Board granted credit for 2 years of the 4 year practice requirement in the second pathway, for 1 year of scientific work performed after completion of undergraduate training, 1 year of training in a medical specialty recognized by the ABMS, or pursuit of a PhD degree in a scientific field. In 1970, the ABA increased the credit for these activities to 3 of the 4 years of required practice.

Just as the ABA had accepted on-the-job expertise gained from military service during World War II, it accepted the value of anesthesia experiences during the Viet Nam conflict. Military personnel completing at least 6 months of formal anesthesia training could receive additional credit for military anesthesia experience on an individual basis evaluated by the ABA.

In 1973, the ABA revised its credentialing under the "optional 3rd year" program:

1. Clinical Base Year (CBY) plus 3 years of anesthesia training, or
2. CBY plus 2 years of anesthesia training and 2 years of practice

Credit towards the 2 years of practice in pathway 2 could include military experience, training in or practice of anesthesia in a foreign country, or any of those previously credited in 1966. In 1977, a candidate with a PhD in a related field or satisfactory completion of another ABMS specialty could apply for full credit for the third year in pathway 1.

In 1984, 47 years after first suggesting it, the ABA announced its decision to increase the required training to 3 years following the CBY. The Board identified the continuum of 4 years—CBY, CA-1, CA-2 and CA-3 (CA=clinical anesthesia). The new continuum was to be introduced for those beginning the CA-1 on 1 May 1986. Again the ABA met opposition but experiences with the optional third year supported the Board's decision, and implementation took place as planned.

International Medical Graduates

Foreign medical graduates (FMGs) or, as more recently designated, international medical graduates (IMGs), presented two concerns for the ABA: Would acceptance of IMGs affect standardization of training; and could the ABA identify acceptable programs including medical schools, internships and residencies satisfying criteria leading to approval by identifiable regulating agencies such as state licensing boards? The Board sought assurance that only IMGs educated comparably to US physicians be admitted to the certification process, an often impossible task. From 1937 to

1947, the ABA allowed graduates of AMA-approved foreign medical schools to enter its examination system. In 1947, the Board deleted direct reference to FMGs in its Booklet of Information, favoring a statement indicating acceptance of Diplomates of the National Board of Medical Examiners (NBME). In 1961, after introduction of the Educational Commission of Foreign Medical Graduates' Examination (ECFMG), the ABA announced that the only acceptable screening organizations were the NBME and the ECFMG. In 1972, the Board added the Federal Licensing Examination (FLEX), and included in its Booklet of Information, the words "or any recognized licensing body".

The ABA first adopted a formal policy regarding IMGs in April 1969, after conducting a 2-year investigation of certification requirements of English, Irish, South African, Australasian and Canadian Colleges or Faculties (of anesthesia) that revealed them to be comparable to those of the ABA. The ABA subsequently admitted holders of the Fellowships of these Colleges or Faculties to its examinations if all other entrance requirements (except for training in an ACGME accredited program) were satisfied. The Board stated that "… dual certification was neither necessary nor desirable." Furthermore it discouraged the need for ABA certification for those with Fellowship status in the above Colleges, a position that had significant future implications when the ABA deleted reference to "equal and comparable" regarding the Colleges and the ABA's certification.

In 1969, the Faculty of Anesthetists of the Royal College of Surgeons of England indicated their appreciation for the equivalency statement by the ABA, however, adding that they would not admit US trained anesthesiologists to their examination system, because British anesthesia training required more years than in the US. The Canadian College sent similar correspondence. Over the next 14 years, the ABA continued to refine the acceptance qualifications for entrance to its certifying examinations for holders of these Fellowships in 1977, adding the requirement for 1 year of practice or training in the US. In 1982, all Fellows except for those from Canada were required to have a year of training in an ACGME accredited anesthesia training program. In 1986, the requirement was added for Fellows from Canada. The refusal of the various foreign Colleges to admit US residency graduates to their examinations certainly contributed to these policies.

In 1993, the ABA withdrew recognition of residency training in any foreign country except for the CBY from Canadian institutions affiliated with medical schools approved by the Liaison Committee on Medical Education (LCME). This change arose from the realization that the ABA could not objectively verify the comparability of any other organizations' certification nor could it verify the equality of training programs certified outside the US not controlled by the ACGME. The removal led to complaints from those with Fellowship certificates, who, because of the ABA's language

regarding "equality" in the past, elected not to take the examination. Sympathetic to this dilemma, the ABA allowed IMG holders of the Royal College Fellowships to apply through an alternative pathway, expiring in 1997, for entrance to the examination with either 1 year of US training or 2 years of practice in the US with the second year between 1 January 1992 and 31 December 1995.

The ABA continued to examine these policies, and review of their minutes indicates that consideration is ongoing regarding IMGs practicing in the US, with special emphasis on faculty in US academic training programs. A trial program limited to 2 faculty members from a given ACGME approved academic program, is currently in place. The program permits IMGs to eventually qualify to take the ABA certifying examinations. Subsequent evaluation of this trial program will determine future ABA policies for IMG anesthesia practitioners.

Doctors of Osteopathy

Initially, the ABA denied osteopathic physicians entry into the examination process. However, the decision by the California State Legislature to recognize doctors of osteopathy (DOs) as medical doctors, changed the ABA stance, and the ABA subsequently treated MDs and DOs equally. In 1981, the ABA accepted the clinical base year from a program approved by the American Osteopathic Association (AOA). Thus, the Board required all candidates to have satisfactorily completed residency training in an anesthesia program accredited by the ACGME, with the exception of those completing their CBY in either a Canadian institution affiliated with a medical school approved by the LCME, or an osteopathic program approved by the AOA.

The ABA and Anesthesia Subspecialty Certification

When initially confronted with the issue of subspecialty certification, the Board reacted negatively. In the early 1970s, referring to Critical Care Medicine (CCM) certification, the ABA indicated that it would not allow its credentialing policies to be used to limit the ability of its Diplomates to practice in certain subspecialties: "We cannot condone economic credentialing". Undeterred, in 1977, the Society of Critical Care Medicine (SCCM) initiated discussions with the ABMS Boards of Internal Medicine, Pediatrics, Surgery and Anesthesiology. These foundered on disagreements over guidelines and duration of training, but prompted ABA reconsideration. Recognizing the possibility of hindering the practice of ABA Diplomates in CCM if other Boards individually allowed certification, the ABA submitted an application to the ABMS for authorization to grant certification in Anesthesia CCM. The ABA application was approved on 21 March 1985, with the first written examination on 27 September 1986. Recognition of Pain Management (PM) as a multi-disciplinary subspecialty, caused the ABA to request authorization to certify PM from the ABMS. Authorization was granted on 26 September 1991, with the first written examination on 11 September 1993.

In the early 1990s the ABA decided not to object to ACGME accreditation of subspecialties, if requested by their respective organizations. At that time, however, the ABA was still not favorably disposed to approve certification for subspecialties where patient care was restricted to anesthesiologists. Most recently in 2009, the ABA decided to begin the process to offer subspecialty certification in Pediatric Anesthesiology, and the first certification examination is scheduled for 2013. Furthermore, ABA subspecialty certification is now a reality for Hospice and Palliative Medicine with the first examination in 2008, and for Sleep Medicine in 2011. Recognition of these latter two subspecialties with certification available to anesthesiologists, was done in conjunction with several other ABMS primary boards and reflects, as with Pain Medicine and Critical Care Medicine, the ABA's efforts to protect its Diplomates practicing in areas recognized by other specialty Boards. Other subspecialties including cardiac anesthesia remain under consideration. The implications for intra-disciplinary competition, and the potential inability of rural hospitals to provide care in the absence of board certified anesthesia sub-specialists, remain unresolved.

Continuing Medical Education, Recertification and Time-Limited Certificates

In 1994, and again in 1995, the ABA declared its intent to issue 10-year time-limited certificates for its primary certificate, and for all certificates awarded after 1 January 2000. Pain Management certification was granted with a 10-year time limit at its inception in 1993.

Why had it taken so long? A 1932 report of the Commission on Medical Education noted that "The time may come when every physician may be required in the public interest to take continuation courses to insure that his practice will be kept abreast of current methods of diagnosis, treatment and prevention." In 1940, the Advisory Board of the AMA stated, "…as the certifying boards become better established and as they complete the examination of a large group of physicians already practicing the specialties, they may find it desirable to issue certificates that are valid for a stated period only." Thus, the seeds for CME and recertification were planted before the ABA existed. CME became increasingly popular with the advent of local, regional, national and in-

ternational meetings offering a plethora of reviews, updates and presentations. State licensing departments soon required continuing education as a condition of continued licensure. New Mexico became the first state (in 1971) to require CME for medical license renewal. While agreeing with the need for currency, the ABA determined that the responsibility for CME belonged to the ASA rather than the ABA. In 1949, the ABA recommended that the ASA establish a Refresher Course Program, a program offered first in 1950 and annually ever since. The ABA maintained that education is the purview of the ASA and its components, while certification is that of the ABA. However, the ABA proactively works with the ASA and others to promote educational opportunities in support of its certification examinations and the currency of its Diplomates.

In 1973, the ABMS called for all boards to adopt voluntary recertification, asking that a "… reasonable deadline [be established] when voluntary, periodic recertification of medical specialists will have become a standard policy of all medical boards." Thus began the ABA's prolonged assessment of recertification for its Diplomates. The first ABA proposal came in 1977 with adoption of a plan for voluntary recertification to be implemented in 1984. Although proposed to ensure public trust, maintain a high standard of practice, motivate CME and comply with the ABMS resolution of 1973, the ABA felt continuing concern over numerous issues, particularly the best tool for reassessment, and lack of evidence on how long it took to degrade knowledge and skill. Perhaps most importantly, the ABA believed it lacked proof of the validity of the initial certification certificate! As stated by one director "Board certifying procedures do not test clinical competence", a crucial concern since the maintenance of clinical competence underlay the enthusiasm for recertification.

Given increasing lack of confidence that the goals of recertification might not be met, the ABA reversed course in 1980 and rescinded its proposal for the 1984 implementation of voluntary recertification. Over the following 13 years the ABA continued to assess both the climate for recertification and evidence of its worth. Pressure from the ABMS and from government, both state and federal mounted, with most ABMS Boards implementing recertification procedures. State licensing agencies considered mandating recertification as either a requirement or an alternative pathway for licensure renewal, and the federal government began considering legislation to require recertification. Representative Pete Stark from California introduced proposals in Congress, calling for recertification of physicians, one of which appeared in the 100th Congress on 7 August 1987 as an amendment to the Social Security Act as the "Medicare Physician Competency Certification Act of 1987". It would "…require periodic competency certification of physicians as a condition of participation under the Medicare program."

Pressure built for the ABA to join other ABMS Boards in offering recertification. Publications began to appear, including those of Silber and Slogoff in the 1990s, validating certification as a means to predict and assess satisfactory clinical care [2, 3]. Experiences of other boards suggested the value of reassessing knowledge and performance. During that period a joint committee of the ABA and ASA met to define the best way to proceed with recertification. The Committee recommended both a credentialing process and examination to provide Continued Demonstration of Qualifications (CDQ). The ABA adopted this proposal, with implementation in 1993. Having taken the first major step in recertification, the remainder of that decade witnessed the continued maturing of recertification, renaming CDQ to simply Recertification in 1996. As a final step, the ABA proposed to the ABMS, with acceptance on 21 March 1998, the issuance of only time-limited certificates, beginning on 1 January 2000. Consistent with the policies of several ABMS Boards, the ABA "grandfathered" all those with non-time-limited certificates. Such holders would remain certified without requiring recertification except that all Associate Examiners and Board Directors of the ABA had to be recertified within 10 years of their original certificate, and every 10 years thereafter.

From 2000 to the present, the ABA continued to emphasize education and credentialing beyond that provided in its written examination. This philosophy led the ABA and the ASA to develop an educational based approach to recertification which "includes a commitment to continuing education, an assessment of the quality of practice in the local environment, and an evaluation of knowledge." In 2009 the recertification program in place since 2000 was replaced by a program for Maintenance of Certification in Anesthesiology (MOCA). MOCA originated from a concept of maintenance of certification (MOC) approved by the ABMS in 2000, and endorsed by the 24 ABMS Member Boards. The ABA also plans to complete the transition from its current subspecialty recertification examinations to a MOCA-SUBS process in 2017. The 2010 ABA Booklet of Information describes MOCA as "a 10-year program of ongoing self-assessment and lifelong learning, continual professional standing assessment, periodic self-directed assessments of practice performance and quality improvement, and an examination of cognitive expertise." The program begins immediately following the awarding of an ABA certificate.

Although it took the ABA what many may have thought an inordinately long time to recognize the appropriateness of its final decision regarding recertification and time-limited certification, the Board believed that the depth and resulting duration of its assessment was appropriate. The ABA recognized that such a major philosophical change with significant impact on its Diplomates required a cautious and thoughtful approach. Having issued 49,877 primary certificates, 1,616 for Critical Care Medicine 4,739 for Pain Medicine, 59 for Hospice and Palliative Medicine, and 5 for Sleep Medicine as of 30 November 2012, the ABA continues to examine several complex issues. These include subspecialty certification, recertification and the role of simulation, the relationship to IMGs practicing in the US, modification to the anesthesia curriculum and its existing examinations to ensure currency, the appropriate emphasis on research, and scholarly activity, as part of the continuum.

At the time of preparation of this chapter the ABA has served as the specialty's primary certification board for 70 years. During that period the Board has met its responsibilities to the public, the specialty and its Diplomates in its decisions impacting the education, training and continued excellence in clinical care. Whether it was duration of training, components of the anesthesia curriculum, certification for subspecialists, or more recently, recertification, the ABA has persisted in rigorous evaluation and reevaluation prior to implementation. The ABA's demonstrated capacity to establish educational standards, to certify trainees and their training programs, and to work productively with other anesthesia societies and organizations will be essential to the continued growth of physician led anesthesia.

References

1. Eger EI II. After you, please: the second Annual John W. Severinghaus Lecture on Translational Science. Anesthesiology. 2010;112:786–93.
2. Silber JH, Williams SV, Krakauer H, Schwartz JS. Hospital and patient characteristics associated with death after surgery. A study of adverse occurrence and failure to rescue. Med Care. 1992;30:615–29.
3. Slogoff S, Hughes FP, Hug CC Jr, Longnecker DE, Saidman LJ. A demonstration of validity for certification by the American Board of Anesthesiology. Acad Med. 1994;69:740–6.

The Evolution of Nurse Anesthesia in the United States

Bruce Evan Koch

Summary

From 1870–1890, many US surgeons asked nurses to provide anesthesia. The Mayo brothers trained Alice Magaw and Florence Henderson, who perfected smooth and safe anesthesia with ether. In 1909, Agnes McGee opened the first school of nurse anesthesia in Portland Oregon. In 1915, supported by surgeon George Crile, Agatha Hodgins opened a more influential school at Lakeside Hospital (later the Cleveland Clinic), spawning 54 schools by 1950.

In the early 1900s, legislative efforts and lawsuits unsuccessfully sought to preclude nurse anesthesia, arguing that it allowed nurses to practice medicine. Subsequent state statutes legalized nurse anesthesia practice but specified physician supervision of nurse anesthetists. The second Bush administration modified a federal corollary to these statutes, allowing states to "opt out" of the supervision requirement. By 2011, 17 of 31 eligible states had opted out.

Hodgins, Helen Lamb, and Gertrude Fife saw the need to protect nurse anesthesia through a formal organization that would certify competence of its members, leading in 1931, to the American Association of Nurse Anesthetists (AANA). The first AANA qualifying examination was administered in 1945, leading in 1956, to the Certified Registered Nurse Anesthetist (CRNA). The AANA implemented recertification in 1978. By the end of the twentieth century, nurse anesthesia training had increased to >2 years and will increase to 3 or more years after 2015.

In 1955, the Dept. of Health, Education and Welfare recognized the AANA as the accrediting agency for nurse anesthesia educational programs. In 1974, the US Office of Education (USOE) required that an independent organization supply accreditation and the AANA proposed establishment of an autonomous Council on Accreditation of Nurse Anesthesia Educational Programs (COA) composed of CRNAs, anesthesiologists and members of the public. In 1976, the USOE granted the COA the authority to accredit nurse anesthesia training programs.

In 1978, Swiss nurse anesthetist Hermi Löhnert discussed the potential for international cooperation with AANA President Ron Caulk. In June 1989, representatives from 11 countries founded the International Federation of Nurse Anesthetists. Nurse anesthetists are an essential part of world health. A 2011 survey of 107 countries found that nurse anesthetists usually delivered 70 to 89 % of the anesthetics.

In the past 20 years, volunteer nurse anesthetists have increased access to anesthesia care in underdeveloped countries and began to formalize nurse anesthesia education. Also in the past 20 years, the AANA has faced up to the epidemic of drug abuse and addiction among nurse anesthetists.

Social Factors and Anesthetic Delivery Between 1850 and 1900

Three revolutions changed the status of women in the eighteenth and nineteenth centuries. The American and French Revolutions caused women to believe that they were entitled to the rights enjoyed by men [1]. The Industrial Revolution forced women to seek work outside the home. Because medical schools would not accept them, many women entered nursing. Florence Nightingale (1820–1910) elevated nursing from custodial care to a profession, based on hygiene and nutrition [2]. During the Civil War (1861–65), surgeons used nurses to meet the need for anesthesia care, [3, 4] generating the first US group of nurses to practice anesthesia.

In the second half of the nineteenth century, the US economy expanded rapidly westward. Small Midwestern towns accumulated wealth, established hospitals, and attracted physicians eager to operate on patients anesthetized with ether or chloroform. For half a century or more after Morton's 1846 demonstration of ether anesthesia, "midwives, first-year medical students, husbands, chauffeurs, and inexperienced general practitioners were all pressed into service" [5] to provide anesthesia. Deaths inevitably resulted from the poor care that they provided. According to Gunn and Thatcher,

B. E. Koch (✉)
Clinical Nurse Anesthetist, Kootenai Medical Center, 30899 North
Nautical Loop, Spirit Lake, Coeur d'Alene, Idaho 83869, USA
e-mail: Evan_Koch2000@yahoo.com

[3, 6] anesthesia came to be regarded as a "failed promise" [6] or "not an unmixed blessing" and Thatcher (pp. 49–52) [3] and Bankert (pp. 21–24) [7] reported that descriptions of late nineteenth century anesthesia contained words like "barbaric," "reckless," and "dangerous."

The experience of Harvey Cushing (later the father of neurosurgery), giving anesthesia in 1894 as a student at Harvard, illustrates the problem. He reported, that in the course of his administration of ether anesthesia to an older man with a strangulated hernia, the patient vomited, aspirated the vomit, and died. An orderly had directed Cushing's administration of the ether, and this was Cushing's first administration of anesthesia. "To my perfect amazement, I was told it was nothing at all, that I had nothing to do with the man's death, that he had a strangulated hernia and had been vomiting all night anyway, and that sort of thing happened frequently …." [8].

Referring to nineteenth century anesthesia, Helen Clapesattle, the historian of the Mayo family of physicians, wrote that "only the most courageous patients would submit to it" [9]. Concern for their patients and professional standing led surgeons to seek skilled inexpensive anesthetists who would remain attentive. Both Thatcher (p. 53) [7] and Bankert (p. 16) [3] wrote that the job required intelligence and acceptance of a subordinate role that would not compete with that of the surgeon.

Then Matters Improved

In 1877, some Midwest surgeons turned to nurses, particularly Catholic Sisters, for anesthesia service (p. 54). [3] First taught by surgeons, they added intuitive skill to the delivery of anesthesia. Sister Secundina Mindrup

"devised her own method for judging when more ether or chloroform or an alcohol-chloroform-ether mixture should be given—a decade of prayers on the rosary and it was time to give a little more. In an apron with two split pockets she carried everything that anyone in the hospital might want, and in one of the pockets she secreted a bottle of chloroform. This she quietly and judiciously used to supplement the ether anesthesia when the surgeon required more relaxation" (Thatcher, p. 55). [3]

Sister Secundina embodied a change from most previous anesthetists. She added anesthesia to her other duties, yet was innovative (e.g., devising her own means of knowing when to re-dose), and proficient with three anesthetics.

By the late 1880s, Catholic hospitals throughout the Midwest turned to sisters/nurses like Sister Secundina for anesthesia. Thatcher documented over 90 by name (p. 285–6) [3]. The practice spread to other hospitals. Between 1884 and 1888, the Missouri Pacific Railroad established hospitals for its employees in Illinois, Indiana, and Missouri, and Thatcher noted (p. 54) [3] that the Hospital Sisters of St. Francis provided the nursing and the anesthesia.

Records describing the earliest nurse anesthetists are scant, but what began in Catholic Hospitals spread to other institutions. The earliest example was the Augustana Hospital in Chicago where Lotta Frejd, the Matron: "acted as cook, laundress, anesthetist, janitress, and carried patients up and down stairs" [10].

These pioneer nurses advanced anesthesia, in part by mastering the difficult and sometimes perilous inhalation induction of anesthesia. The difficulty and danger arose in the phase from wakefulness to deep sleep. In this phase, inhibitions and the ability to swallow are diminished, but involuntary movements can result in struggling, coughing, vomiting and aspiration (recall Cushing's patient). The phase could last several minutes, or longer in unskilled hands.

Magaw and Henderson Advance Anesthesia Beyond the Mayo Clinic

The employment of nurses as anesthetists developed at St. Mary's Hospital (The Mayo Clinic) in Rochester, Minnesota. Clapesattle wrote [9] that "The Mayos had given the job to Miss (Edith) Graham and then to Miss (Alice) Magaw in the first place through necessity; they had no interns. And when the interns came, the brothers decided that a nurse was better suited to the task because she was more likely to keep her mind on it, whereas the intern was naturally more interested in what the surgeon was doing." Magaw and her star student, Florence Henderson, perfected the induction of anesthesia with ether in the 1890s. Magaw and those she taught used an Esmarch mask covered with two layers of gauze. They administered ether continuously, drop by drop, onto the gauze. They initially held the mask a short distance from the face and gradually lowered it, applying the ether slowly at first and then faster as the patient accepted the smell. This graded approach minimized the sense of suffocation and limited the struggling [9]. The anesthetist would observe the face for flushing (vasodilation) and sought evidence of relaxation, both changes denoting the onset of anesthesia. Support of the lower jaw and turning the head helped maintain an open airway. Turning the head might also facilitate the discharge of regurgitated gastric contents and thus lessen the likelihood of aspiration. These techniques resulted from an awareness of the importance of upper airway management [11]. The pioneer surgeon William Mayo praised Magaw as "The Mother of Anesthesia" [12].

Magaw and Henderson applied different techniques to gain a patient's confidence and cooperation. Magaw wrote that "one must be quick to notice the temperament, and decide which mode of suggestion will be the most effective in the particular case: the abrupt, crude, and very firm; or the reasonable, sensible, and natural" [11]. Harris and Dean wrote (p. 11) [13] that Henderson was gentle, and made patients feel they were in control of the anesthetic.

Magaw and Henderson applied other measures to improve the patient's experience, including inducing anesthesia within the operating room, and warming the patient. To decrease stimulation and suggest sleep during the induction, they enforced silence. At all times they displayed self confidence. Henderson wrote that: "If the administrator is nervous or loses the confidence in her ability to secure a rapid narcosis, it invariably affects the patient." Writing of her work between 1899 and 1906, Magaw described her experiences in over 14,000 cases, all "without an accident, the need for artificial respiration, or the occurrence of pneumonia or any serious results" [11, 14] Testimonials by physicians visiting the Mayo Clinic reflect the esteem that Magaw and Henderson enjoyed. Henry Munro observed that: [13]

> "… it is quite the common occurrence for an anesthetist who does not understand the use of suggestion to use from ten to twenty times the amount of ether in anesthetizing a patient that is used by Alice Magaw and Miss Henderson, who make use of suggestion in every possible way in a given operation." And "there is no period of excitement, no struggling of the patient that demands restraint, comparatively little stertorous breathing, no feeling of the pulse, and no hypodermics administered in the course of the operation, and more yet, an unbroken record of approximately seventeen thousand cases of anesthesia without a single death from the anesthetic."

First the Midwest, and then larger regions adopted the methods developed and refined by Magaw and Henderson. Nurses came to St. Mary's from hospitals in New York, Philadelphia, Seattle, New Orleans, and Denver, returning to teach others. And those who learned, passed the word to hospitals in Illinois, Oregon, Maryland, Iowa, Upstate New York, California, Michigan, Virginia and Minnesota. According to Thatcher (p. 77), [3] by the second decade of the twentieth century, a wide spectrum of institutions in the US had "capitulated to nurse anesthesia."

Nurses Introduce Nitrous-Oxide/Oxygen Anesthesia in World War I

World War I Opens a Door and Hodgins Walks Through

The contributions of US nurse anesthetists during World War I were important in numbers and in the introduction of new techniques. In Europe, nurse anesthetists provided anesthesia in the American field hospitals for almost three years before the 1917 entry of the US into the war. The hospitals, known as "ambulances" (from the French), were shipped in their entirety from the US.

One of these was led by the surgeon George Crile (Fig. 22.1) from Lakeside Hospital (associated with the Cleveland Clinic), assisted by nurse anesthetist Agatha Hodgins (Fig. 22.2). Crile had learned the use of nitrous

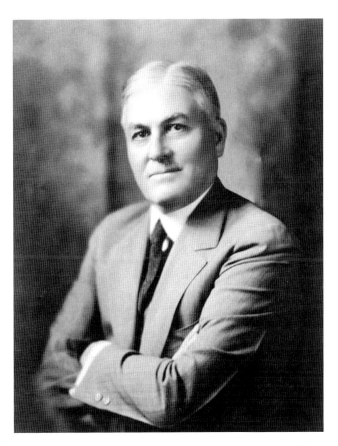

Fig. 22.1 George Crile Sr. who was of one of the founders of Cleveland Clinic. (Courtesy of the American Association of Nurse Anesthetists Archives.)

oxide-oxygen ("gas-oxygen") from the dentists John Stephan and Charles Teter. With Hodgins' help, Crile conducted experiments on animals, determining that nitrous oxide produced less cardiovascular depression than chloroform or ether, and from that surmised that nitrous oxide might be better suited to wartime trauma surgery.

Hodgins described her work as a nurse anesthetist in the early war years (Bankert, pp. 44–5): [7]

> "The unit…in the charge of Dr Crile, left in December, 1914, for service in the American Ambulance in Neuilly, Paris, France. Attached to this unit were three anesthetists—the writer and two members of her staff. The assignment of this anesthesia unit was to introduce gas-oxygen in war surgery, from that base hospital. The fortunate result was that of being able to successfully accomplish this assignment both on this special unit, and later, on the French surgical division of the American Ambulance Hospital."

Nitrous Oxide/Oxygen for Trauma Victims

In 1915, Hodgins returned to the US to direct one of the earliest formal nurse anesthesia educational programs. Other

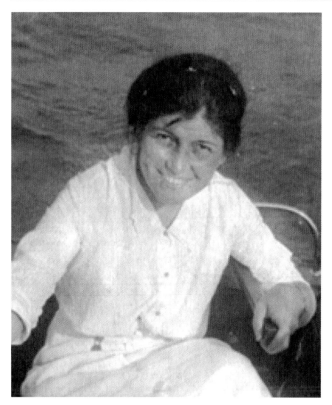

Fig. 22.2 Agatha Hodgins. (Courtesy of the American Association of Nurse Anesthetists Archives.)

American nurse anesthetists continued to provide nitrous-oxide/oxygen anesthesia until the armistice in 1918. Crile and Hodgins added pre-operative injections of scopolamine or atropine and morphine prior to nitrous-oxide and oxygen administration. The combination produced a "dissociated" mental state that Crile termed anoci-association, a state in which patients did not perceive pain. This was a forerunner of balanced anesthesia. Anoci-association, but particularly the administration of nitrous oxide with limited concentrations of oxygen and no oxygen monitor, required special skills.

Alice Hunt, a nurse anesthetist on the Yale faculty, described her approach.

> "The technique calls for careful attention to detail in several ways, as follows: (1) an endeavor to gain the patient's confidence and cooperation and to allay apprehension; (2) adequate narcotic premedication for relief of pain; (3) rinsing out of all diluting air from the lungs and tissues of the body; (4) avoidance of painful manipulation during the induction period; and (5) gentle surgical handling of the body tissues throughout the operation-a strong plea for this anesthesia, for it is a well-recognized fact that an important contributing cause of surgical shock is trauma to the tissues." [15]

Crile also knew that the technique demanded observant care.

> "Oxygen is a pilot light to keep the flame of life burning safely. If the light burns too high, the patient immediately comes out

from the anesthesia, if too low, the patient is too deeply submerged; if it is turned out, the patient dies. Yet with a steady flow of gas under constant pressure, the patient is carried easily through the narrow zone of anesthesia. Miss Hodgins made an outstanding anesthetist for she had to a marked degree both the intelligence and the gift." [16]

Personal accounts reveal some unusual stresses of wartime experiences. Sophie Winton (1887–1989), who worked with James Gwathmey wrote that she averaged twenty-five to thirty anesthetics a day. "As soon as they were through operating on one patient, I would have the next patient anesthetized....Many a night I had to pour ether or chloroform on my finger to determine the amount I was giving, because we had no lights except the surgeon had a searchlight for his work, so the only sign I had to go by was respiration" [17].

From "The History of the Pennsylvania Hospital Unit":

> "Throughout the British Army, anesthetics had hitherto only been administered by doctors and when shortly after our arrival our women began their work they (the British) were greatly astonished. The skill and care which was displayed soon caused their amazement to yield to admiration. The idea was soon adopted by the British authorities, and in the early spring of 1918, classes were formed of British nurses who received instruction at our hospital and at several others, and before the end of the war a number of British nursing sisters were performing the duties of anesthetists in various hospitals throughout the British Expeditionary Forces...." [18]. In 1936, Crile reflected that: "if the Great War had gone on another year, the British army would have adopted the nurse anesthetists right in the middle of the war." [19]

Accolades accrued to Winton and her colleagues: "All the nurses in Winton's unit were awarded the Croix de Guerre. Bankert reported (p. 48) [7] that Winton herself was also awarded six overseas service bars as well as honors from the Overseas Nurses Association, the American Legion, and the Veterans of Foreign Wars." They were paid $ 60 per month. But as they were associated with the Red Cross nurses, they "did not receive full military rank, nor the pay and allowances equal to male military personnel. Veterans' compensation was also denied them" [20].

Thatcher (p. 97) [3] traced two other changes to World War I. The Army and Navy both began to formally train nurses for duty as anesthetists for war service, a practice that continues to this day. The other change stemmed from the increased popularity of nitrous oxide: a "booming demand" after the war for trained nurse anesthetists" familiar with the technique of nitrous oxide anesthesia.

Success Triggers Opposition

The success of nurse anesthetists during World War I and afterwards, triggered opposition among the growing number of physicians entering anesthesia. According to Thatcher

(p. 108) [3]. "The rapid growth of postgraduate schools of anesthesia in which nurses were trained, as well as the increasing enthusiasm for the trained nurse anesthetist during and after World War I, did not escape the attention of physician specialists in anesthesia, and during the 1920s resentment against the nurse anesthetist culminated in attempts to legislate her out of existence."

The movement began in New York as early as 1912 with an article by attorney Lawrence Irwell entitled "The Case Against the Nurse-Anaesthetist". "The moment that a nurse of her own volition, in consequence of symptoms observed by her, increases or decreases the amount of an anesthetic, which is being given to man, woman or child, she unquestionably and beyond doubt practices medicine in the legal sense of the words and violates the law of New York, Ohio, or Illinois, as the case may be." He snidely concluded his article urging: "self respecting nurses to turn their attention to other matters—perhaps urinalysis" [21].

Bankert considered that Frank McMechan, the founder of the Interstate Association of Anesthetists, was "probably the most virulent" opponent to nurse anesthetists. In an editorial in the American Journal of Surgery, [22] he inveighed: "The nurse anesthetist must go, because she is unlicensed, and because her employment is as much an economic crime against the profession and public as *fee splitting* (emphasis original)." McMechan threatened: "to bring an end to the administration of anesthetics by unlicensed persons in every state in the middle West in which such can be secured" [22].

In 1916, McMechan attempted to close the Lakeside School, a high profile source of nurse anesthetists. Through the Interstate Association of Anesthetists, McMechan petitioned the Ohio Medical Board to adopt a resolution that stated in part, "it has been charged by many well-known and reputable physicians, that the law regarding the administration of anesthetics by others (sic) than licensed physicians has been systematically violated by Lakeside Hospital, Cleveland, Ohio, and that courses in anesthetics are given nurses in Lakeside Hospital." Thatcher wrote (p. 113) [3] that together with physicians Albert Freiberg and J Baldwin, McMechan: "denounced in no uncertain terms the administration of anesthetics by nurses."

More subtle opposition came from giants in anesthesia. Ralph Waters, the father of academic anesthesiology, held nurse anesthetists in low esteem:

"I hear that some surgeon in this state is using a nurse or an office girl—I'm not sure which—to administer anesthetics to his patients. Do you know why? The only honorable reason he could give is because he believes that she can give an anesthetic better than any practitioner of medicine available in his community. Surgeons with this handicap can be found in many communities in the United States today." He believed that: "A nurse's training is not sufficient foundation for becoming an anesthetist of value to both patient and surgeon."(Bankert, p. 56). [7]

Program closures occurred or were threatened. A program had been established at the Johns Hopkins Hospital in 1917. In 1931, Olive Berger became its director, and in 1941 the pioneer thoracic surgeon Alfred Blalock, became the Chief of Surgery. According to Bankert (p. 199), [7] Berger:

"managed the anesthesia department, administered anesthesia, and trained at least four nurse anesthesia students a year. She administered the anesthesia for the first total pneumonectomy at John Hopkins and, with Helen Lamb, developed an endotracheal technique for intrathoracic surgery. She was the first nurse anesthetist to administer anesthesia to infants for tetralogy of Fallot."

In 1941, Blalock invited Austin Lamont, an alumnus of Ralph Waters, to open a residency at Hopkins. "Lamont's concept of an anesthesia department that included physician anesthesia, residency training and a resident research program was forged by the model presented in both Wisconsin and New York" [23]. But Lamont and Blalock "came to a parting of the ways". Lamont wrote that his resignation was "due to Blalock's opposition to my wish to increase the number of physician anesthetists and decrease the number of anesthetic nurses" [23]. The Johns Hopkins program survived until 1985, a time when numerous programs closed (see below).

Attempts to Outlaw Nurse Anesthesia

During the first half of the twentieth century, two lawsuits unsuccessfully argued that nurse anesthesia practice was illegal. In Frank v. South (Kentucky, 1917), surgeon Louis Frank, together with nurse anesthetist Margaret Hatfield, sued the Kentucky State Board of Health to test the contention that Hatfield was practicing medicine. The court ruled that both nurses and physicians could practice anesthesia without breaking the law (Bankert, p. 116) [3].

In Chalmers-Francis v. Nelson (California, 1936), the Los Angeles County Medical Association and its Anesthesia Section sued nurse anesthetist Dagmar Nelson for allegedly practicing medicine. Nelson however, with support from surgeon Verne Hunt, convinced the court:

"(1) (that) the giving of drugs upon the direct or understood instruction of a physician was a recognized practice and within the limits of the definition of nursing, (2) that the recognition and the reporting of changes in a patient's condition and acting accordingly under the direct or understood supervision of a physician was within the province of nursing, (3) that nursing education as accepted by law gave instruction in the administration of anesthetics and the recognition of the signs and stages of anesthesia and (4) that it was an established practice within the law for registered nurses to give anesthetics as a nursing duty" (Bankert, p. 146). [3]

Acting with the backing of these two rulings, nurse anesthetists sought legislation in some state legislatures to legalize their work. "A number of states adopted statutes recognizing the practice of nurse anesthetists. Typically, these statutes followed the formulation in Frank v. South, and provided that nurse anesthetists were to work under the 'supervision' or 'direction' of a physician" [24]. Stoll wrote (p. 86) [25] that "Any nurse anesthetist would have been convicted of practicing medicine without such direction and supervision." Ultimately, twenty-three states enacted a supervision requirement either in their medical practice act, nursing practice act, or hospital licensing requirements [26].

Attempts to Control Nurse Anesthesia

Decades later, the concept of required supervision would be turned against nurse anesthetists. In 1985, H Ketcham Morrell, president of the American Society of Anesthesiologists (ASA) wrote: "…the operating surgeon or obstetrician who purports to provide medical direction of the nurse, in the absence of an anesthesiologist, carries a high risk of exposure, on a variety of legal theories, for the acts of the nurse" [24].

Additionally, two federal (Medicare) payment schemes, the Tax Equity and Fiscal Responsibility Act (TEFRA-1982), and the Prospective Payment System (PPS-1983), disadvantaged Certified Registered Nurse Anesthetists (CRNAs). TEFRA and PPS were accountability measures meant to ensure that an anesthesiologist oversaw no more than 4 CRNAs at once, and personally performed certain services as part of a given anesthetic, to qualify for payment. However, the PPS inadequately compensated the physician/nurse team. Rita Rupp, a policy expert who was Special Assistant to the Executive Director at the AANA, concluded that: "Simply put CRNA services were, for all practical purposes, non-reimbursable" [11] The PPS and TEFRA rules were misconstrued as a standard of care, despite the government's caution that they were not (Bruton-Maree and Rupp, pp. 361–3) [27].

CRNAs sought legislative and then regulatory relief. Medicare rules were the logical place to request removal of the supervision requirement, because they impacted all the states where *state* laws did not impose supervision (p. 408) [24]. Efforts by the AANA and the ASA to renegotiate TEFRA ended after "the ASA had second thoughts" about agreed upon revisions (Bruton-Maree and Rupp, p. 363) [27]. The Clinton administration removed the other supervision requirement. This was overturned by the GW Bush administration, with a proviso that states could "opt out" of supervision if the governor so chose. To date, Governors in 17 of the 31 eligible states have done so (Table 22.1).

Other activities pertinent to education included ostracism of anesthesiologists participating in training programs,

Table 22.1 States in which the governor has opted out of the federal CRNA supervision requirement, and the date

State	Date of opting out
Iowa	2001
Nebraska	2002
Idaho	2002
Minnesota	2002
New Hampshire	2002
New Mexico	2002
Kansas	2003
North Dakota	2003
Washington	2003
Alaska	2003
Oregon	2003
Montana	2004
South Dakota	2005
Wisconsin	2005
California	2009
Colorado	2010
Kentucky	2012

Data from http://www.aana.com/Advocacy.aspx?id=2573

(see for example, John Adriani below; Bankert, p. 154) [7] and an attempt to control school accreditation (also discussed below) [28]. Like the preceding lawsuits and attempts to legislate restrictions, both of these efforts failed.

What prompted the opposition to nurse anesthesia? Bankert argued (p. 57) [7] that economic factors were key. She cited C McCauley, a colleague of Ralph Waters: "I think the main reason that we are having nurses give anesthetics, at least up in this country, is the question of money." Thatcher wrote (p. 135): [3] "Undoubtedly, it was the economic pinch of the depression that led the California physician anesthetists to renew their attack against nurse anesthesia in October, 1933, leading to the trial of Dagmar Nelson…" Stoll, citing (p. 200) [25] Hodgins (1935) wrote that opposition was greatest against nurse anesthetists who worked on a fee for service basis, at a lesser price than anesthesiologists.

Bankert added (p. 62 and p. 95) [7] that surgeons like Louis Frank and Verne Hunt, recognized the limited resources of nurse anesthetists, and financially supported the pursuit of their claims or defense. Attempts to control the activities of nurse anesthetists prompted them to form state associations for self protection (e.g., Ohio in 1931, New York in 1933, and California in 1935 and others) (Thatcher p. 162) [3] Closer ties developed between the AANA and other nursing organizations (Stoll, p. 200) [25]. Finally, efforts to improve education, which lagged between the mid 1950s and the 1970s, were reignited when anesthesiologists moved to control the accreditation of nurse anesthesia schools (Stoll, pp. 128–38) [25].

Nurse Anesthesia Education

Teaching the Art of Anesthesia

Surgeons taught nurses to administer anesthesia in the 1870s and 1880s. By the mid to late 1890s, nurses began to train other nurses. As noted earlier, the first formal training in anesthesia took place in the 1890s at St. Mary's Hospital (the Mayo Clinic) with Magaw and Henderson doing most of the teaching. Initially they learned from surgeons, adding education by trial and error, supplemented with keen observation. They knew little pharmacology or physiology, and offered no theories, but they understood how to deliver chloroform and ether effectively and safely. They gave their students guidance, plenty of time, and individual oversight. Thatcher wrote (p. 62) [3] that "Sometimes the nurses (students) stayed for 2 or 3 months and learned to give ether under supervision." Education was tailored to the learning style of each student, and respectful of the need for oversight for patient protection. Such early nurse education in anesthesia differed from most education of anesthetists, which historian AJ Wright described (p. 15) [5] as: "on the spot training of any person available."

From Technical Training to Professional Education

As the twentieth century began, Thatcher described (p. 93) [3] the training of nurses in anesthesia as taking three forms:

"(1) that given by graduate nurses in a hospital in which they were to be employed as anesthetists;
(2) that provided gratuitously to visitors-physicians and nurses-who went to a hospital to observe and sometimes give anesthetics under supervision; and
(3) that given by the manufacturers and the demonstrators of gas machines, who often traveled round the country to sell and teach the operation of machines to anyone who would buy."

Although better than training by trial and error, these methods lacked uniformity or a didactic component. They were technical and only addressed the need to cover service requirements.

The recognition of the importance of asepsis in the 1890s, underlay the expansion of surgery, and this, in turn increased the need for safer, better, more consistent anesthesia. According to Thatcher (p. 48) [3] "The new (aseptic) surgery, combined with the new knowledge of other practical aspects of bacteriology, stimulated organized efforts to set standards of education and service in all phases of medical care."

In 1910, Medical Education Changed, and Nurse Education Followed

Publication of the Flexner Report in 1910, contributed to the closure of many inadequate medical schools. Medical education became university based, science-driven and research oriented [29]. Nursing education needed to change to keep pace.

"Early on, before anesthesia education was regulated, there were a lot of substandard schools. They needed to be improved or closed to ensure *safe patient care*. Our profession took on that responsibility." (April 2011 personal communication, Betty Horton, AANA Education Director from 1990–2002,)

The First Schools of Nurse Anesthesia

Agnes McGee graduated in 1907, from St. Joseph's Hospital School of Nursing in Chicago, and received anesthesia training in Heidelberg, Germany, before settling in Portland, Oregon. In 1908–09, Good Samaritan and St. Vincent's hospitals in Portland used interns to deliver anesthesia, but the interns rebelled, resolving that 'they were not going to spend their internship giving anesthetics.' Their revolt opened the way for McGee, and in 1909, at St. Vincent's Hospital; she opened the first school of nurse anesthesia in the US. [30–31]

According to Brown, the school "expanded and flourished under McGee's leadership" [31]. The initial course occupied four months. It was extended to one year in 1939. The students studied the "anatomy and physiology of the respiratory tract, pharmacology of anesthetic agents and techniques of administration of anesthesia" [31]. St. Vincent's curriculum was the first to contain both didactic and clinical components. The program continued until 1956, training 142 students over its life span. Other programs followed at St John's Hospital, Springfield, Illinois (1912); the New York Post-Graduate Hospital, New York City (1912); and the Long Island College Hospital, Brooklyn (1914). For her pioneering work, McGee received the AANA Award of Appreciation in 1953.

A second pivotal event for nurse anesthesia education took place in 1909: the twelfth annual convention of the Nurse's Associated Alumni of the US, in Minneapolis. The meeting was to feature a presentation on the nurse as anesthetist by Henderson, and a response by Hodgins. Instead, nurses in attendance took over the agenda, and expressed their desire for formal specialty training programs in anesthesia. Thatcher wrote (p. 91) [3] that Hodgins was said to have gone home: "with a bee in her bonnet", perhaps remembering J Baldy's

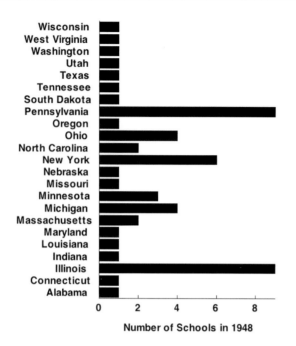

Fig. 22.3 Distribution of the 54 schools of nurse anesthesia listed by the AANA, that produced graduates qualified to take the certifying examination in 1948

declaration the year before, that: "At present there is no place to my knowledge where a nurse or anyone else could apply for a training in anesthesia." Hodgins and Crile began their school at the Lakeside Hospital in Cleveland, thinking their program was the first. Regardless, the meeting in Minneapolis produced the Lakeside program, a program from which 54 other institutions developed six-month-long postgraduate training programs—modeled on the one at Lakeside. Hodgins and Crile trained nurses, doctors, and dentists in the administration of nitrous-oxide-oxygen anesthesia. Founded in 1915, the school became known for this anesthetic approach, just as the Mayo Clinic had evolved as a center for teaching ether anesthesia. In 1916, 11 nurses, 6 physicians, and 2 dentists graduated. In 1917, the Lakeside school was closed by the challenge from the Ohio Medical Board described above. Thatcher reported (p. 106) [3] that it reopened in 1918, and by 1919, 54 nurses and 2 physicians had graduated.

The Lakeside School was housed within the anesthesia department. From 1915–1933, Hodgins directed and was the driving force behind both. As reported by Thatcher (p. 76) [3] "One now famous surgeon, who as a student went to Cleveland to learn the technic (nitrous oxide-oxygen anesthesia), was admonished by his chief: 'George (Crile, the surgeon) will talk a lot, but you watch Agatha'." The curriculum lasted six months, tuition was charged, and a diploma was granted. Hodgins gave the classroom instruction (added in 1918), and she had up to three assistants to help supervise the students. To widen clinical experience, students rotated to operating rooms in hospitals around Cleveland (Thatcher, p. 106) [3].

The Lakeside School had considerable influence. In her 1948 presentation of a posthumous award to George Crile, for his support of nurse anesthesia education, AANA President Lucy Richards noted: "Living memorials to him are the 54 formal schools for the training of nurse anesthetists in registered hospitals in this country. Because of his vision and his confidence, the anesthesia service in over 75 per cent of the nation's registered hospitals is being conducted by nurse anesthetists educated in schools patterned after the one of which he was the founder" [32]. Three-quarters of the 54 schools established by 1948 were centered in the mid-west (39%) and Northeast (35%) (Fig. 22.3).

Anesthesia education improved during this era. Classroom instruction began to supplement on-the-job training. But as Thatcher described (p. 96), [3] "while these pioneer educational ventures started a shift of emphasis from service to education, the service requirements of hospitals remained paramount in the majority of the training programs that sprang up during World War I and the postwar period. All other considerations were secondary to that of turning out anesthetists who had technical proficiency."

Assuring Quality in Anesthesia Education

Between 1931 and 1955, Hodgins, Helen Lamb, and Gertrude Fife changed anesthesia education by organizing a national nurse anesthetists' association, promulgating educational standards and agitating for their acceptance. These pioneers fought to accredit schools, determine curriculum standards, certify graduates by examination, educate educators, and initiate continuing education for practicing nurse anesthetists.

In 1931, many programs were deficient. Requirements for opening a school were lax, consisting "merely of obtaining the consent of the hospital and the surgeons and a willingness on the part of the instructor to impart knowledge and techniques to the student apprentice."(p. 103) Some schools did not keep pace with scientific and technical advances. Thatcher reported (p. 96) [3] that "the courses represented all shades of adequacy depending on the native intelligence and the teaching ability, experience and education of the instructor." Certification was needed to ensure that graduate nurse anesthetists met an acceptable standard. Hodgins appreciated that achieving this goal required a coordinated nationwide effort.

Birth of the American Association of Nurse Anesthetists (AANA) and Education Standards

The National Association of Nurse Anesthetists (NANA—changing its name to the American Association of Nurse Anesthetists, or AANA, in 1939) was born in 1931, at a meeting convened by Hodgins, of members of the Lakeside Alumnae Association. The organization was the culmination of her life's work, and became a singular force for bettering anesthesia education [3, 33] Membership was to be contingent upon certifying that the applicant's practice and capabilities met set standards. Applicants for membership either had to have practiced anesthesia more than 3 years, or graduated from a program of nurse anesthesia that met standards set by the AANA. Certification of a nurse anesthetist or a school by the AANA would signify quality in education. Thatcher wrote (p. 209) [3] that the accomplishment of these intended goals would "place the association in the position of a pioneer among nurse specialty groups."

An Education Committee was formed to define and achieve these goals. Its work became "the main plot development in the story of the national organization," and Lamb chaired the Education Committee. After training at the Lakeside School under Hodgins, Lamb had been recruited by Evarts Graham to the Barnes Hospital in St. Louis. There, she founded a program of nurse anesthesia in 1929, remaining as its director until retiring in 1951. With Graham, Lamb pioneered endotracheal anesthesia, and collaborated with the engineer Richard von Foregger on the design of anesthesia equipment. She administered anesthesia for the world's first pneumonectomy (Thatcher, p. 158, and Bankart, p. 202) [7]. She was an exacting teacher, and is today remembered annually by an award in her name, bestowed by the AANA upon an outstanding nurse anesthesia educator.

Lamb "could size people up very quickly (Kelly JW: personal communication, 2011)," "and looked into the future with sharper vision than had anyone else up to that point" (Thatcher, p. 189) [3]. Her career overlapped those of Mc-Mechan who opposed nurse anesthesia, [23] and Waters who resisted the presence of nurse anesthetists in academic centers [34]. Observing these men and their actions, Lamb probably suspected that nurse anesthesia would be threatened if it failed to keep up with the progress made by physicians.

The Education Committee first surveyed existing schools to determine the current state of anesthesia education. From the survey results, the Committee published minimum curriculum standards for schools in 1933, making these increasingly stringent in 1935, 1936 and 1948 (Fig. 22.4). The Committee then established and maintained a list of "accredited" schools that met those standards. These were the first universal standards in nurse anesthesia education.

Defining adequate schools was only one of the AANA's educational goals. Beginning in 1933, the Association published a journal; it has subsequently been in print continuously. The Education Committee also established a certifying examination that all graduates would have to pass to obtain AANA membership (see also Chapter 36). World War II delayed implementation of the examination by several years. In the interim, the AANA established an Education Department in 1935, with Lamb as its first director.

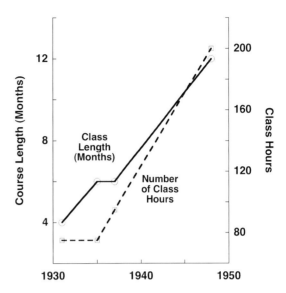

Fig. 22.4 Course requirements for nurse anesthesia programs markedly increased between 1931 and 1948. (Data from Stoll DA: The emerging role of the nurse anesthetist in medical practice (dissertation). Evanston, IL, Northwestern University, 1988)

In her 1934 address at the annual meeting in Memphis, Fife articulated the AANA's intention to become the sole authority on nurse anesthesia education: "The Association will serve as a pace-maker for the better schools and will influence the poorer schools to meet the required standards. The Association will secure for (accredited) schools on its list a recognition throughout the United States such as could not be secured in any other way, and will make possible the acceptance of guiding principles in matters pertaining to the education of the nurse anesthetist" (Thatcher, p. 210) [3].

Hodgins vs. Fife: How Should Certification Be Achieved?

To accomplish these goals, the Association had to arbitrate a dispute between Hodgins and Fife over how certification should be achieved. Hodgins favored state registration. Bankert wrote (p. 97) [3, 7] that "her reasons for doing so may have been the result of her conviction that the work fell under neither the category of medicine nor of nursing, and that nurse anesthetists needed the protection of a separate legal status. She may also have been affected by years of listening to the charge leveled by physician-anesthetists hostile to the existence of nurses in the field, that they were 'unlicensed' practitioners."

Fife took the position that national certification would be more practical.

"Furthermore, every anesthetist should be required to pass a National Board examinations (sic). I do not believe that state board registration for nurse anesthetists is either practical or possible. Quicker and more direct action can be obtained through a National Board, and more uniform methods of teaching will result from the establishment of universal rather than sectional standards" (Bankert, p. 211) [7].

This "contest of wills" ended only after Hodgins' death, with the eventual implementation of national certification.

Strengthening the AANA by Affiliation with Other Organizations

Other matters diverted attention from the move to establish standards. Organized physician groups filed law suits—the two discussed above and several in other states—challenging the right of nurses to practice anesthesia. To confront the lawsuits of organized physicians, maintain standards in the face of the government's wartime needs, and keep up with expanding marketplace needs was daunting. And the AANA was weak, having fewer than 1,000 members, each paying only $ 5 in annual dues. However, the AANA persevered.

Hodgins, Lamb, and Fife, and their fellow organizers affiliated the AANA with the American Hospital Association. Philosophical differences hindered attempts to work with other associations. Hodgins had written to the American Nurses Association (ANA) seeking affiliation as a subsection, prior to establishing the NANA: "Our reason for asking affiliation with the ANA, is simply recognition of the primary fact that we are registered, graduate nurses, qualified for and pursuing a special work" (Bankert, p. 70) [7]. The ANA stalled and finally rejected the request, creating a rift that would not be healed until the 1970s.

At the sixth annual meeting of the NANA, Lamb spoke of efforts to enlist support from the American Hospital Association: "The (Education) Committee's most important activity centers around the movement now under way to enlist the endorsement of the American Hospital Association…for the inspection of schools of anesthesia for nurse anesthetists; and upon the basis of inspection to eventually approve those schools whose curriculum proves to be the equivalent of the standard already adopted by our Association" [35].

Before settling on the American Hospital Association, the NANA held "numerous conferences" with other organizations. Thatcher listed (p. 233): [3] "a talk by Miss Lamb on the association's educational aims before the American Board of Surgery in St. Louis…a meeting of the entire Board of Trustees with members of the American Board of Surgery and the newly organized American Board of Anesthesiology in New York City on November 27, 1938, and subsequent conferences with representatives of the American Hospital Association and the American Board of Anesthesiology."

The specifics of those meetings are unknown. For the American Hospital Association (AHA) to contemplate imposing new standards on a school must have been politically delicate. Thatcher would conclude (p. 233): [3] "The conferences pointed to the facts that the AHA would be the most desirable sponsoring body, but that a more detailed plan should be prepared for formal submission to that organization and that the association could effect a raising of standards in schools of anesthesia by having definite rather than nonspecific requirements for admission to membership."

Liaison with the AHA was instrumental in this formative stage. As John Garde observed: "By 1933, the NANA had still not held its first national meeting, and suffered from general disarray organizationally" [36]. The AHA, recognizing the value of nurse anesthetists to their hospitals, invited the NANA to hold its first national meeting in conjunction with them [36]. The relationship was a success, and the AANA (renamed from the NANA in 1939) and the AHA held their annual conventions together for 43 years, from 1933 to 1976.

Other imperatives trumped the educational aims of the association. Stoll wrote (p. 6) [25] that "While it may be rationalized that the primary reason for the support from administrators and surgeons was based on the proven capabilities of nurse anesthetists, the reality of this support was the need for an inexpensive provider of anesthesia services. It is important to state that when serious challenges to nurse anesthetists' right to work began, these organizations and individuals provided the necessary peer and professional support required to ensure that nurse anesthetists remained in practice."

World War II Delays Educational Advancement

The demands for trained anesthesia personnel posed by World War II were a challenge. The need for nurse anesthetists was so great that the Army pressed them into service after as little as three months training, some within "earshot of battle." This compounded a severe shortage of civilian nurse anesthetists. The AANA wisely (it would turn out) did not resist the accelerated training programs, although these emergencies delayed implementing the leaders' plans for a national certifying examination and a school accreditation program. Fife articulated the AANA's position, including its attempt to maintain minimum standards of competence, in a recruiting brochure published in 1942:

> "The need for nurse anesthetists both in civilian and Army hospitals is becoming increasingly urgent. In order to meet the situation many Schools of Anesthesia have increased the student body. The degree of expansion is limited, however, because in order to qualify for membership in the AANA, each anesthetist must have administered a certain number of anesthetics during her training. The AANA has been opposed to lowering the standards by allowing the student to be graduated with less clinical experience than necessary to prepare her properly for work in active surgical clinics" [37]. Instead of resisting the accelerated training, Bankert wrote (p. 124) [7] that the AANA: "encouraged the establishment of schools in hospitals equipped to offer training in this field."

With the war's end, the AANA renewed its education program. Bankert reported (pp. 130–5) [7] that opposition from anesthesiology organizations reappeared as threats of sanctions against anesthesiologists who were involved in training nurse anesthetists. John Adriani directed a major school of nurse anesthesia at Charity Hospital, in New Orleans. In 1947, the Board of Directors of the American Society of Anesthesiologists "adopted a statement in its bylaws to the effect that it was unethical for an anesthesiologist to participate in the training of nurses" and "precluded giving lectures at the annual meeting for the AANA." "In addition, Adriani was personally informed by Dr. Paul Wood, secretary of the American Board of Anesthesiology, that the board was 'seriously considering' the revocation of certification of any anesthesiologist who trained nurse anesthetists." "Promising to respond with a federal lawsuit to any revocation of his certification, Adriani heard no more and continued his work." The bylaw was not rescinded until 1964. Its effect on other anesthesiologists cooperating with nurse anesthesia education was never assessed.

The first qualifying examination was administered in 1945. The wartime contributions of trained nurse anesthetists indirectly sped the move to accreditation of schools of nurse anesthesia. In 1947, the Education Consultant for the Army Nurse Corps, Lt. Col Katherine Balz, explained that "World War II conclusively demonstrated the need for nurses trained in anesthesia, both for battle-front duty and for service in Army hospitals caring for military personnel. The very fact that the Army has founded schools for the training of nurses in anesthesia is confirmatory evidence of the value of the nurse anesthetist to the armed forces" [38]. Balz next observed that the Army planned training programs at five hospitals, ensuring that "upon completion of the course, the Army nurse will be prepared to take the qualifying examination and become a member of the Association" [38]. The endorsement of civilian hospitals followed the Army's acceptance of the AANA plan, and the accreditation of programs and certification of graduates became universal after the Korean conflict.

The aftermath of the war in Korea added to the pressure to accredit programs. Federal education benefits for military personnel could not be obtained for training at unaccredited schools. In 1955, the AANA successfully appealed to the United States Office of Education to recognize the AANA as the accrediting agency for nurse anesthesia educational programs (Bankert, p. 138) [7]. Unaccredited programs then gradually disappeared, but were more than replaced by accredited programs (Fig. 22.5).

Between 1953 and 54, just before the accreditation mechanism was approved (1955), the number of programs nearly doubled within one year. Stoll explained (p. 98) [25] that "only the schools which adhered to AANA educational guidelines were counted prior to 1952, and after the United

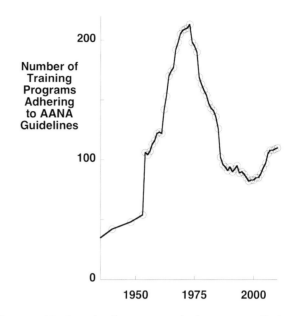

Fig. 22.5 Number of active nurse anesthesia programs adhering to AANA guidelines from the 1940s

States Office of Education approval, those non-recognized programs that met requirements, received accreditation status, and were added to the approved list."

A continuing expansion ended with a peak of 213 programs in 1973, and an equally rapid descent between 1978 and 1988. Half the programs closed, and graduates decreased by one third [39]. Concurrently, "the number of anesthesiology residents nearly doubled" [39]. Sandra Maree-Ouellette, a former AANA President recalled: "As a profession we thought we were dying on the vine" (personal communication July 2011).

DePaolis-Lutzo suggested diverse reasons for the striking decrease in the number of programs, with the main problems being funding, cost, competition from anesthesiology residents (subsidized by the US government), and the lack of anesthesiologist support within joint departments [40]. Similarly, Denise Martin-Sheridan attributed closures to: "lack of financial support from the hospital, university, and anesthesiologists; changes in state and federal reimbursement, and reconfiguration of the delivery of healthcare services under managed care systems...." [41] Jeffrey Beutler contrasted third-party payment policies for anesthesiologists teaching residents, and CRNAs teaching student nurse anesthetists, finding that they "burden CRNAs and nurse anesthesia students with financial disincentives and payment exclusions...." [42].

By 1989, fears for professional survival prompted AANA President Richard Oullette to appoint a 17-person commission of nurse anesthetists, anesthesiologists, and administrators of educational institutions and health systems, to study school closures and recommend what should be done. Sandra Maree was the chair.

The commission reached several conclusions. Program closures had caused a CRNA shortage, ranging geographically from 10–20%. Access to anesthesia had become limited in rural areas where CRNAs practiced alone. Anesthesia had grown more expensive as demand outstripped the supply of providers, and where anesthesiologists had displaced CRNAs. Quality was compromised because untrained (non-anesthesia) providers were substituted to administer intravenous sedation. Resolution of these problems would require the training of 25,000 additional CRNAs by 2010 [43].

Where nurse anesthesia educational programs shared facilities with anesthesiology residencies, the lack of sufficient cases posed a major obstacle to training more CRNAs. Nurse anesthesia programs resolved this problem by diversifying. Some developed relationships with community hospitals. Additional remedies separated nurse anesthesia training programs from other training (residencies), or even from schools of nursing [44]. Some nurse anesthesia training programs affiliated with allied health departments, and some found ways to co-exist happily within schools of nursing [45–53]. Horton and Brunner described how programs became more numerous and complex between 1992 and 1997, a period in which the number of clinical sites rose from 266 to 577 and the number of graduates recovered from 669 in 1990, to almost 1100 in 1996 [54]. These efforts restored the independence and vitality of nurse anesthesia as shown by the stabilization of the number of accredited training programs in the late 1980s (Fig. 22.5). In the end: "Almost a third of the nation's 6,000 hospitals participated in the education of nurse anesthetists" (personal communication Sandra Maree-Oullette July 2011. Sandra Maree and Richard Ouellette married in 1994).

Will We Soon Call a Nurse *Doctor*?

In 2004, the American Association of Colleges of Nursing (AACN) recommended that by 2015, all advanced practice nurses earn a doctoral degree. A 2006 AANA task force explored the consequences and concluded that: "it is essential to support doctoral education…" [55]. But a 2015 deadline would deprive existing programs of sufficient time to prepare. Consequently, the task force proposed delaying the doctoral requirement to 2025, and the AACN (which accredits colleges of nursing, some of which contain anesthesia educational programs) has not objected.

For differing reasons and for some time, doctoral education has been a goal of nurses. According to Sandra Edwardson, Professor and Director of the Doctor of Nursing Practice Program at the University of Minnesota: "From the beginning, the primary reason for wanting doctoral preparation in nursing was to develop the knowledge necessary for practice and to gain credibility within the academy" [56].

The AACN, referring to a National Academy of Sciences recommendation, says: "the growing complexity of the healthcare environment, coupled with the rapid expansion of knowledge required for practice" demand higher degreed nurses (http://www.aacn.nche.edu/media-relations/fact-sheets/dnp). Phelps and Gerbasi examined why 14 health care professions adopted doctoral education. Most pointed to: "changes in the scope of practice relating to increasing responsibility and/or independence of practice…" [57]. Doctoral education has become a trend.

But what type of doctoral degree should student nurse anesthetists earn? Phelps and Gerbasi compared accreditation requirements of doctoral programs in clinical laboratory sciences, dentistry, medicine, nursing, nurse anesthesia, osteopathic medicine, pharmacy, physical therapy, podiatry, and psychology [57]. They found a swing away from universal educational standards, which are considered by many administrators as "unnecessarily prescriptive." Instead, almost all accrediting agencies identify essential competencies that graduates should obtain.

Thus, the AANA did not prescribe a type of doctoral degree, allowing nurse anesthesia educational programs to offer research-based or practice-based degrees. The doctor of philosophy (PhD), doctor of education (EdD), doctor of nursing science (DNSc or DNS) are research-based. The doctor of nursing practice (DNP or DrNP), doctor of nurse anesthesia practice (DNAP), and doctor of management practice in nurse anesthesia (DMPNA) are practice-based [58].

However between the degrees there are: "subtle although uncertain distinctions" [56]. One distinction is the requirement for a thesis. Mary Marienau who is Program Director at the Mayo Clinic Nurse Anesthesia Educational Program, and Chair of the Council on Accreditation of Nurse Anesthesia Educational Programs, noted that: "Just like other professional (practice-oriented) degrees, including the MD degree, a thesis is not a requirement." Instead; "A capstone project is an expectation, which still requires a rigorous in-depth investigation into a research question, but it does not necessarily need to be a thesis" (personal email communication, October 2011).

Eight essentials for a practice doctorate in nursing have been identified: 1) Nursing Science & Theory: Scientific Underpinnings of Practice; 2) Systems Thinking, Healthcare Organizations, & the Advanced Nurse Practitioner; 3) Clinical Scholarship and Evidenced Based Practice; 4) Information Systems/Technology Systems, and Patient Care; 5) Health Care Policy for Advocacy in Patient Care; 6) Interprofessional Collaboration for Improving Patient and Population Health; 7) Clinical Prevention and Population Health for Improving a Nation's Health; and 8) Ethics [59].

The minimum time required to earn a doctoral degree has also been assessed. Upon graduation, a nurse anesthetist with a DNP degree will have spent a minimum of 8 years in training (4 undergraduate, 1 ICU, and 3 graduate years). Mary Marienau, explained that: "Four years of baccalaureate (nursing) education, plus one year of ICU experience (as a nurse), plus three years of doctoral education is comparable to other doctoral degrees....Possibly we should be calling the ICU experience an RN-ICU Internship so that it equilibrates to the MD model of internship time."

However, even with the postponement of implementation to 2025, and near universal support, the transition to doctoral education may prove difficult. The diluting affect of nursing "essentials" on the anesthesia component within the curriculum will be assessed. Mary Marienau noted that some within the AACN would like to see more classroom time devoted to non-anesthesia topics—but that the Council on Accreditation will fight "tooth and nail" to retain and in fact expand the time devoted to anesthesia. It is too soon to predict if doctoral preparation will increase nursing's presence within the academy, but AANA Executive Director Wanda Wilson recently reiterated Helen Lamb's hope (noted below) that: "nurse anesthetists with doctoral degrees could participate more fully in university life" (personal communication, June 2011). Finally, no one has ventured to predict whether doctoral education leads to better or more cost effective anesthesia.

Support for the Safety of Nurse Anesthesia

The increasing complexity of surgery and anesthesia in the 1950s did not diminish the role of nurse anesthesia. Training and numbers of nurse anesthetists increased (Figs. 22.4 and 22.5). "There had been a constant market for nurse anesthesia services, and surgeons had provided them with support and acclaim. There were no major indicators demonstrating any significant problems, although there was little question that studies demonstrating accountability in terms of patient outcomes were on the horizon" [6].

In 1954, Beecher and Todd [60] published the first major multi-institutional study assessing anesthesia outcomes among anesthesia providers. Their study showed that in patients at comparable risk: "although the physician specialist anesthetizes only half as many patients as the nurse, he is charged with an equal number of anesthesia deaths." The authors speculated that this finding was due to the "complexities of the situation" and the "common observation" that the physician "cares for the patient faced with the more trying and difficult operation…" Without citing evidence they concluded that: "to deny the greater difficulty of the physician specialists' cases is to reduce the matter to an absurdity where one would be obliged to argue that the physician's learning was a dangerous thing." Perhaps the nurses' learning had also amounted to something.

This issue resurfaced in the 1990s. Between 1992 and 2003, anesthesiologists published five studies [61–65] that the AANA critiqued. Four supported the view that "CRNAs should be anesthesiologist-supervised, and that such supervision improves anesthesia outcomes." The fifth found that: "office surgery may not be as safe when an anesthesiologist is not present." The AANA review concluded that "Anesthesia-related accidents are infrequent; those that do occur tend to result from lack of vigilance rather than the level of education of the provider.... Studies to date have not demonstrated statistically significant differences in the safety of anesthesia care provided by CRNAs working alone, CRNAs working with anesthesiologists, or anesthesiologists providing care alone" [66].

Increasing Educational Demands on Nurse Anesthesia Increase University Affiliations

It was anticipated that an increased number of nurse anesthesia faculty with academic degrees, would promote college and university affiliations for nurse anesthesia programs [67]. In 1936, Lamb pointed to the desirability of this evolution towards university based education: "The School of Anesthesia should strive to secure the benefits which Universities have extended to other professional groups. Such University recognition and affiliation should eventually result in broadened facilities, both practical and cultural" [68].

But what Lamb urged took half a century to achieve. Stoll explained (p. 66) [25] the delay by noting that early nurse anesthetists "…had enough to do in beginning this organization (the AANA) and fighting to keep it viable that they could not address the issue of university affiliation which was beginning to consume the leaders of nursing". CRNAs also resisted the imposition of greater educational requirements. Hudson reports (p. 15) [69] that John Garde recalled "…CRNA faculty standing up in 1975 stating: 'if you think you are going to get CRNAs to have a bachelor's degree to be a program director, you are not going to have any anesthetists in this country. We will be replaced by technicians because these people cannot teach, work all day and get baccalaureate degrees'". Horton argued that advancing anesthesia education "could not have been done without" the "deliberate actions" of nurse anesthesia leaders. These included setting educational standards, approving curricula, inspecting schools, and developing an accreditation process [70].

In the last half of the twentieth century, advances in anesthesia education were accomplished, but not linearly. Until 1980, nurse anesthesia training concluded with possession of a certificate or a bachelor's degree. Masters' degree programs emerged in the 1980s. A bachelor's degree became the minimum requirement in 1990, and in 1998 the requirement universally increased to a masters degree. As noted above, a clinical doctorate will be fully implemented in 2025 [70].

Assuring an Absence of Conflict of Interest in Accreditation

In 1974, the US Office of Education (USOE) revised its standards for accrediting organizations. Of particular importance was "Standard 7. Avoidance of Possible Conflicts of Interest such as the separation of the decision making body responsible for the accreditation of educational programs and that body responsible for the certification of graduates of those programs." In order for students (Korean War veterans) to be eligible for federal education dollars, the AANA would have to meet Standard 7. After decades as a de facto accrediting agency, the AANA would have to end its involvement in the accreditation process.

An ad hoc group of CRNA educators, led by Ira Gunn and Ruth Satterfield, pioneering educators who had developed anesthesia programs for the US Army, organized the changes that would be required to meet the new USOE requirements. Both Gunn (p. 11) [6] and Hudson wrote (p. 9) [69] that "it would be necessary to change the organizational structure of the AANA to assure the degree of autonomy for the accrediting element to maintain continued recognition as the accreditor of nurse anesthesia education." They proposed an independent organization, to be called the Council on Accreditation of Nurse Anesthesia Programs, to undertake the work. It would be composed of CRNAs, anesthesiologists and members of the public, representing a 'community of interest' in anesthesia.

Anesthesiologists Compete for Control of Nurse Anesthesia Education

In 1975, anesthesiologists proposed a competing accrediting organization, the Faculty of Nurse Anesthesia Schools (FNAS). All existing nurse anesthesia faculty were invited to join. Hudson wrote (p. 2) [69] that if authorized by the USOE, the FNAS would "effectively (cede) control of nurse anesthesia education to anesthesiologists".

At the same time, the ASA brought a 1972 manpower study to the USOE which the ASA claimed had support from the AANA (it did not; Bankert, pp. 156–8) [7]. The study concluded that the best interests of patient care would be served by: "more direct involvement of the anesthesiologists in establishment of policy relative to accreditation, curriculum, certification, and quality assurance for the nurse

involved in anesthetic care" [71]. Nurse anesthetists saw this initiative as a threat to the control of their profession.

Bankert (pp. 156–62) and Hudson (p. 11) [69] reported that concern increased further in 1976 when, in confidence, three leading anesthesiologists filed "letters of complaint against the AANA's accreditation program with the USOE…", questioning the competence, adequacy, composition, and autonomy of the Council proposed by the AANA. The AANA petitioned the USOE for copies of those letters, and the USOE mistakenly sent the AANA a letter meant for the physicians who had complained about the Council. Ira Gunn explained to Hudson (p. 21) [69] that John Profit (head of the Accreditation Unit at USOE) wrote to the three anesthesiologists indicating "that they probably didn't need to worry (regarding the AANA petition) because they didn't expect the AANA to come into compliance with the new criteria…Mr. Profit's secretary at the USOE furnished us with that letter rather than the three complaints, and there is no question that prompted a strong willingness for the AANA to get involved."

Disclosure of these letters to the AANA provoked outrage. Hudson noted (pp. 11–12) [69] that President Bernice Baum wrote that the letters contained "innuendo, misrepresentation, and out-of-context quotations to discredit the AANA accreditation program." Baum observed that "While some of the allegations expressed may stem from sincere concerns about the anesthesia care in the United States, there can be little question that the real issues are: control, power, and economics…."

The USOE decision to recognize the Council on Accreditation or the FNAS was delayed, pending resolution of the complaints. In September 1976, in Washington DC, the AANA's Council on Accreditation, the ASA and the FNAS presented their views to the USOE (Hudson p. 18) [69]. The AANA argued that "Individual professions must assume primary responsibility for quality assurance mechanisms relative to their membership while providing adequate input from the community of interest and the public…. The FNAS is neither representative of historical precedence, professional tradition, nor recognized by the USOE and has no experience in the accreditation of nurse anesthesia educational programs and certification of nurse anesthetists." [72] The USOE sided with the AANA and granted the authorization to the Council on Accreditation.

"An Impetus to Formalize Nurse Anesthesia Education"

To Hudson (p. 9), [69] "the newly mandated standards gave the AANA an impetus to formalize nurse anesthesia education." Gunn agreed, saying that as a result of this ordeal "It also became apparent that this would be the best time to implement new standards not only incorporating USOE criteria but those which would also set the stage for movement of nurse anesthesia education in university frameworks" [73].

Other related education reforms took place concurrently. Standards of Practice were written in 1974, with subsequent periodic revisions. Mandatory continuing education was initiated in 1977, and recertification was implemented in 1978. Recertification required that for every two year period, nurse anesthetists must possess an active unrestricted license, earn forty hours of continuing education, and document that they remain "substantially engaged in the practice of nurse anesthesia" [73].

Global Improvements in Anesthesia Education

A dream and a conversation lead to international cooperation One day in August 1978, a Swiss nurse anesthetist travelled to Detroit carrying a dream. Hermi Löhnert had come to attend the AANA Annual Meeting. He shared this dream with President Ron Caulk. Might the AANA "be interested in co-sponsoring (with the Swiss Association of Nurse Anesthetists) an international symposium in Switzerland?"(p. 5) [74]. Caulk, who would become an enthusiastic co-founder of the symposium, learned much later "that the Swiss had not formed their (own national) organization yet."

> For Löhnert (p. 5), [74] attending the AANA Annual Meeting was a "tremendous experience…One take home message I will never forget: 'be professional!' I received all the support needed to strengthen and improve the situation of our Swiss Association of Nurse Anesthetists. The many discussions with nurse anesthetists at the congress triggered my interest for international cooperation."

Achieving international cooperation was easier dreamed than done. Löhnert, together with Caulk, pursued it for eleven years. Under the auspices of the American and Swiss Associations, they sponsored two international symposiums (Lucerne 1985 and Amsterdam 1988) and numerous organizing meetings. The symposiums contained educational presentations, but were better remembered for overcoming provincialism. Pascal Rod, of France, recalled (p. 11): [74] "It was amazing how much each country was promoting its own education and practice as being the only one available." Ron Caulk recalled (p. 9) [74] that being 'more open' entailed a "major adjustment"…in Finland "when we discussed business in the sauna…nude!"

On June 10th 1989, representatives from Austria, Finland, France, Germany, Iceland, Norway, Slovenia, South Korea, Sweden, Switzerland, and the USA signed a charter in St. Gallen Switzerland, and the International Federation of Nurse Anesthetists was born [75]. From the outset, the IFNA

faced problems that recalled the early years of the AANA. Pascal Rod recalled that advanced practice nursing was opposed in many nations, and not just by physicians. Nursing organizations looked at nurse anesthetists as "only technicians doing medical tasks." Just as in the 1930s, nursing and medicine denied nurse anesthetists a home [74].

But the IFNA was anxious to announce its presence. The newly elected officers, Löhnert as President, Caulk as Vice President, Hanna Birgitsdottir of Iceland as Secretary, and Svein Olaussen of Norway as Treasurer, reached out to the International Council of Nurses, the World Federation of Societies of Anesthesiologists, and the World Health Organization. New member countries were recruited, especially from Africa and Asia. The officers vowed to convene a World Congress of Nurse Anesthetists every two to three years, which they did in Oslo (1991), Paris (1994), Vienna (1997), and Chicago (2000) [75] Today, preparations are underway for the 11th World Congress in Tunis in 2014.

They then tried to "find their colleagues." No one, including the chief nurse scientist at the World Health Organization, knew the world-wide extent of nurse anesthesia. Sandra Maree-Ouellette reported: "When meeting with her (the chief nurse scientist) she said 'why should we take nurses to do technicians work.' The answer we gave her was: because nurses are administering anesthesia all over the world. She said 'show me!' And we did." (email communication July 2011)

McAuliffe and Henry found that nurse anesthetists are an essential part of world health. They surveyed the education, practice and regulation of nurse anesthetists worldwide, reporting in 1996 that nurses administered anesthesia in 107 countries—the majority of member states of the World Health Organization [76]. Nurse anesthetists from 96 countries subsequently completed questionnaires about their practice, education and regulation. Respondents from 62 countries reported that educational programs to prepare nurses to give anesthesia existed within their countries. Of these, 81% indicated they had classroom instruction in anatomy and physiology, 87% in pharmacology including anesthetic agents and adjunctive drugs, 65% in chemistry and physics of anesthesia, and 91% in basic principles of anesthesia practice.77–78 However, the duration of anesthesia training varied, ranging from 12 months or less to over 22 months, and clinical training varied from 5 months or less to more than 22 months. Only half of the respondents reported access to continuing nurse anesthesia education after completing their entry level education. McAuliffe further wrote that: "The data were reconfirmed with data collected over a (sic) 10 years, including repeat mailings of surveys to original study participants, recruitment of additional participants from international educational meetings, and in depth interviews of nurse anesthesia leaders throughout the world." (Personal email communication Maura McAuliffe, 6 October 2011).

Though groundbreaking, McAuliffe's survey is but a pilot study that provides an incomplete view. Data were gathered from little more than half the countries of the world, and from only a minor fraction of the anesthesia providers. Given the potential importance of nurse anesthesia to the health of the world and given the apparently unequal distribution, contribution and education of nurse anesthetists, this survey bears repeating with greater control and in greater depth.

Notwithstanding the limitations of McAuliffe's findings, they anticipated IFNAs' next big endeavor: establish a committee to set international standards for nurse anesthesia education. Sandra Maree Ouellette chaired this Education Committee, and like the original Education Committee chaired by Helen Lamb, this one had to define what it means to be a nurse anesthetist. Between 1989 and 2001, the committee wrote (and the IFNA adopted) Educational Standards for Preparing Nurse Anesthetists, Standards of Practice, a Code of Ethics, and Patient Monitoring Guidelines. [75]

The IFNA grew. As many as 4200 registrants from 35 member countries attended its tri-annual World Congress meetings. Proceedings, which were translated into several languages, covered scientific, clinical, and educational topics. There were poster sessions and, of course, much socializing.

A forum for teachers of anesthesia began at the 1991 World Congress in Norway. Although it was "put together at the last minute, the room was filled to capacity, and the response to the presentation of educational issues was enthusiastically received." An expanded forum is now a permanent part of the World Congress [74].

The IFNA has begun to "globalize" nurse anesthesia. Ouellette and Horton counted the ways: IFNA developed international professional standards; IFNA interacted with appropriate regional and international organizations and professions; IFNA examined and recorded the range of nurse anesthesia and its contributions to progress in anesthesia; and IFNA has developed a worldwide quality assurance program for educational programs [79].

The quality assurance program, known as the anesthesia program approval process or APAP, is the first international accrediting program for educational programs in nurse anesthesia. Starting in the early 2000s, it evolved through "a pilot project, a call for public comments, feedback from internal and external parties, and final approval of the documents and process by IFNA decision-making bodies in 2010." [79] Ultimately, three increasingly stringent, but voluntary categories of approval were devised. Each acknowledged: "1. The diversity of nurse anesthesia programs throughout the world, 2. The economic stage of development of a country, 3. The resources available to individual programs, and 4. A commitment of diverse programs to a common standard of educational quality" [79].

Today, anesthesia programs officially recognized by the IFNA can be found in: The Netherlands, US, Iceland, France, and Sweden. They and the details of the APAP program can be found at: (http://ifna-int.org/ifna/news.php, accessed July 16, 2011) Herme Lohnert's dream has largely been realized.

Nurse Anesthetists from the US Contribute to World Health

With 80,000 licensed anesthesia providers (nurses and physicians) in the US, there may be a sufficient number to meet the country's needs. Developing nations present a different picture. Richard Henker, the Program Coordinator of a nurse anesthesia training program in Bhutan, reported in 2011 (personal email communication February 2011), that 18 nurse anesthetists and 4 anesthesiologists serve that nation's population of 700,000 people, a proportion roughly one-tenth of that found in the US. Similar situations exist in some countries of Africa, Southeast Asia, and Latin America [75].

CRNAs have provided assistance in developing nations for decades. Ruby Hills volunteered for physician Tom Dooley in Viet Nam in the 1950s [80]. Hundreds of volunteer CRNAs followed in Ruby's footsteps. Sponsored by religious, military, or non-governmental organizations, they traveled as part of surgical teams to remote locations to establish temporary operating rooms, gave many anesthetics in a relatively short time, and returned home.

Such care was of limited value. Only surgeries requiring minimal postoperative care could be performed, and, because of the brevity of involvement, no local nurses received an education in anesthesia, and the host countries remained dependent on outsiders for anesthesia. (Personal communication: Suzanne Brown 2011).

How it Began

At the 1989 AANA Annual Meeting, an educational session on "Third World Anesthesia" drew a standing room only crowd. The strong interest among CRNAs prompted AANA support of volunteerism. However, overseas work demanded greater resources than the AANA could provide, leading in 1992 to affiliation of the AANA with Health Volunteers Overseas (HVO). (Personal communication: Clyde Tempel, 2010) HVO is a private non-profit organization headquartered in Washington, DC, coordinating activities of sponsors from various surgical specialties. Most importantly, HVO

Table 22.2 Teaching programs established by nurse anesthesia overseas (NAO)

Country	Year initiated	CRNA volunteers	SRNAs	MDs
Uganda	1993	9	20	0
Guyana	1994	28	6	0
Belize	2001	40	15	0
Cambodia	2003	17	7	0
Eritrea	2005	7	14	0
Bhutan	2009	17	8	3
Ethiopia	2010	7	13	0

Source: NAO 2011

facilitates training and education of local health care providers [81]. In 1992, CRNAs established a new organization within HVO, Nurse Anesthesia Overseas (NAO).

According to Suzanne Brown, a principle CRNA at NAO, teaching anesthesia to local nurses began with a few realizations. American standards might not always be attainable in foreign settings, but some set of standards would be needed if a program were to have legitimacy. A physical plant, a clinical setting, and legal recognition of graduates would also be required. NAO looked to the International Federation of Nurse Anesthetists (IFNA) for educational standards and recruited a local "champion" within each host country who could overcome cultural and legal barriers. (Personal communication: Suzanne Brown 2010) The IFNA had developed Educational Standards in 1994, that served as the cornerstone of the education plan.

An Example

Since 1994, teaching programs have been established in seven countries (Table 22.2). A representative example is the one developed in Belize, home to 300,000 people, and before 2001, dependent on transient foreigners for anesthesia. At the request of the Belize Ministry of Health, in 2001, 40 volunteer American CRNAs opened a school of anesthesia in Belize City, making numerous trips at their own expense. One volunteer described her experience as the greatest gift she could give another person and herself. The 2-year program conformed to curriculum standards established by the IFNA. Working through NAO and Belizean health authorities, the CRNAs selected top performing nurses for education as nurse anesthetists. Students spent seven months completing 73 didactic assignments in anatomy and physiology, biochemistry, physics, advanced pharmacology, and anesthesia case management. Frequent examinations kept them on track to succeed in the accelerated program. During the remaining 17 months, students devoted 1,000 hours to clinical rotations in Belize City hospitals, each student anesthetizing at least 450 patients. Students had to be trained to work alone since small rural hospitals serve most of the country. The program

taught more than clinical anesthesia. Students were trained to lead continuing education classes, administer tests, and obtain information from the internet that was not locally available.

The program aroused strong feelings. One student was "petrified on the first day," and another expressed her devotion to the region she came from because "I have to go home and take care of my people." In the final week, a student said that the volunteers "did an excellent job of preparing us for what we would face." [82] These students became the first "generation" of CRNAs for their country. They made anesthesia available to more Belizeans.

Nancy Kelly MHS, the Executive Director of HVO believes that: "The Nurse Anesthesia Overseas program in Belize is an outstanding example of the HVO mission in action. (The) volunteers…transformed anesthesia care in Belize so that it is safer and more cost effective" [82].

Program descriptions and longevity vary from country to country. The program in Belize trained one generation of providers only. Similar, but ongoing, programs that train nurse anesthetists exist in Ethiopia and Cambodia. In Bhutan, the program focuses on continuing education of existing nurse anesthetists. The programs in Uganda, Guyana and Eritrea have completed their missions and closed.

CRNAs Combat Drug Abuse

A Tragedy Provokes Action

CRNA Jan Stewart had been the President of the AANA in 1999–2000. Her death at age 50, in 2002, caused CRNAs to confront drug misuse and addiction. Friends, loved ones, and colleagues believed she was happy, healthy and busy. Her daughter, teacher Sarah Gomes suspected otherwise. She knew her mom had been under a lot of stress, but believed she could handle it. Sarah learned too late that the medication Jan said she was taking for headaches was not Imitrex. In 2004, Sarah disclosed that her mom's death had been caused by an overdose of sufentanil. In a tribute, Sarah lamented that there are

> "…a lot of challenges facing nurse anesthetists, and nurses in general, who give so much of themselves… and often times forget to take care of themselves. It's really important that we are able to talk about this openly before, and after, someone dies. If we talk about it before hand maybe we can prevent the drug use from even starting. If we talk about it while someone is using drugs, perhaps we can get them help so that they do not die. And if we talk about it after they die, unfortunately like I'm doing, we can learn the realities of what drug abuse does to families, individuals, and how easily death comes" [83].

Jan's death and Sarah's admonition to 'talk more openly encouraged AANA leaders to alter the way addiction was handled. The AANA Board of Directors commissioned a "Blue Ribbon Panel" to explore establishment of a wellness initiative. The panel's recommendations led to the AANA Wellness Program.

Almost a Disease: 1846–1975

Drug misuse and addiction in anesthesia has a long history. Ether frolics and nitrous-oxide parties, the recreational use of these drugs, preceded the discovery of anesthesia. Addiction to chloroform contributed to the suicide of Horace Wells, one of several claimants to the discovery of anesthesia, in 1848. One newspaper obituary described his affliction as "amounting almost to disease" [84].

However, many considered drug abuse a moral failure rather than a disease. In 1910, Flexner likened alcohol and drug use to vice and moral turpitude. Congress and the states passed laws criminalizing drug use and depriving addicted physicians of licensure. Similar laws governing nurses followed. Some recognized the need for a different view. In 1962, anesthesiologist John Lundy and nurse anesthetist Florence McQuillan, described addiction as "an occupational hazard within the anesthesia community" deserving greater medical attention. [85] Still, few if any studies examined addiction among nurses before 1975.

Investigations of drug misuse among nurses revealed its considerable dimensions. State boards of nursing reported in 1984, that drug addiction among nurses was "significant and rising." Of all nurse disciplinary actions, 67% were drug-related. At that time, there were approximately 1,800,000 nurses in the US, [86] 20,000 (1.1%) of whom were CRNAs. But CRNAs accounted for an astonishing 75% of drug abuse cases. Denial and self-delusion made meaningful data on incidence hard to obtain. Drug misuse by nurses was a secret epidemic. Addiction often resulted, and CRNAs were at greatest risk [87].

Enlightenment and Rehabilitation after 1975

To prevent negative publicity, hospitals might discharge addicted CRNAs. Databases, like the National Practitioner Data Bank kept the names of those discharged, so it might be difficult for a recovered CRNA to find work. The 1980s produced more enlightened attitudes toward addiction. It received a new name, chemical dependency, and was designated as a psychiatric disorder in the Diagnostic and Statistical Manual of Diseases. Essentially all states decriminalized addiction for doctors, but only 30 states did so for nurses. The American Nurses Association passed a resolution advocating treatment before discipline. Self help support networks and rehabilitation hospitals emerged. CRNAs led by

Diana Quinlan, Rusty Ratliffe, and Art Zwerling brought an "alternative-to-discipline" program to nurse anesthesia, Quinlan spearheading these efforts for more than 20 years. She worked with a nationwide network of peer assistance advisors, and established education materials, resource lists, and guidelines. Peer assistance advisors served in every state to facilitate recovery of CRNAs suffering from addiction and their re-entry into the workplace [88].

The alternative-to-discipline approach appeared to decrease the problem. Addicted nurses were removed from work faster. They were helped to recover, to retain a nursing license, and in some cases to remain in or return to practice. In 1996, alternative programs were found to double the recovery rate relative to that found in discipline programs (68% versus 37%) [89]—although this assertion is difficult to evaluate because states with purely disciplinary programs were generally unwilling to share outcome data for fear "it would cast the program in a negative light" [90]. Because alternative-to-discipline programs removed impaired nurses from practice faster, they were said to improve patient safety. Quinlan attributed success to a 12-step program, support group attendance, random drug screening, and the use of recovering CRNAs to serve as mentors/sponsors for other recovering CRNAs [91]. However, none of the studies cited above pertained specifically to CRNAs.

Causes and Epidemiology: Drug Abuse as a Gender Problem

In the 1990s, the first publications by CRNAs, about CRNAs, suggested causes for drug misuse. John McDonough found that student nurse anesthetists have "excitement seeking" traits that place them at greater risk of developing addiction disorders than other graduate nursing students. McDonough urged anesthesia educators to prepare students for this danger [92]. He also echoed what others had stated: CRNAs are at greater risk of addiction due to easy access to addictive drugs and time spent alone. In 1995, Quinlan suggested a link between job-related stress and the risk of addiction among CRNAs [93]. In her 1996 review, Quinlan pointed out that addiction remained a criminal offense for nurses in 20 states. Substance abuse was a greater occupational hazard than either hepatitis B or HIV infection [94].

In 1999, Donald Bell et al. [95] surveyed 10% of CRNAs, finding that 9.8% of respondents reported "anesthesia drug misuse" of inhaled anesthetics, narcotics, sedatives, and other drugs. Sixty-two percent of those misusing drugs were male, consistent with Quinlan's 2001 observation that: "Although men account for more than 40% of the CRNA population, they represent about 80% of the callers (to the AANA peer assistance hotline) with addiction…" (pp. 431–2) [87]. Bell's 9.8% prevalence matched results from a similar study of anesthesiologists, [96] but because it was self-reported, the incidence may have been artificially low. Bell also found that CRNAs were more likely to misuse drugs ten years after graduation.

The Wellness Program Attacks Stress

These studies shed light on the problem, but did nothing to mitigate it. The AANA Wellness Program had as its premise the possibility that some people resort to drugs in response to stress. Tony Chipas, a nurse anesthesia education program director, said: "It's not just about addiction; It's about reducing stress…Practicing anesthesia is stressful. Sources of stress include: the expectation of perfect outcomes, long work hours, disrupted sleep patterns, emotional exhaustion, and the lack of control over the workplace." (Personal communication March 2011). Bell concurred: "Benjamin Rush called alcoholism a disease almost 250 years ago. Yet, today we are still trying to find a means of derailing the disease without fully understanding its biological basis. We hope that by addressing stress as an environmental precursor, we can reduce the overall incidence of chemical dependency and abuse" (Personal communication March 2011). Finally, CRNA Sandra Tunajek, who led the Wellness Program for six years, wrote: "CRNAs recognized the detrimental effect that stress plays in their lives." [97]

The AANA Wellness Program began by subsuming and building on existing peer assistance activities. An annual lecture named for Jan Stewart was begun at the AANA Annual Meeting in 2004. Topics have included aging, stress management, substance abuse and workplace issues. Subsequently other elements were created. A variety of resources are housed on the internet, at http://www.aana.com/Resources.aspx?id=6088&linkidentifier=id&itemid=6088.

A monthly column in the AANA News Bulletin entitled "Wellness Milestones" began in 2005. Written by Sandra Tunajek, it addressed topics not usually found in professional journals. Some were intangible like harmony, compassion, fatigue, and spiritual dimensions of wellness. In 2011, the effect of stress on learning formed part of revised nurse anesthesia curriculum standards. It had been recognized that stress threatens learning. Twenty learning modules, all evidence based, were developed. They are to be implemented in 2012.

Have Good Intentions Succeeded?

Considerable effort has gone into the several studies and programs attempting to address the problem and the tragedies caused by addiction, but we have little evidence, yet, of their success. Alternative-to-discipline treatment did not appear

to decrease diversion, addiction, or mortality. Bell found that in 2006, abuse rates and death rates among CRNAs had not changed since his 1999 study (Unpublished manuscript, Personal communication, 2011). Measuring outcomes from the Wellness Program has not yet happened. Sandra Tunajek recently said: "Evidence to support conclusions is not there. It's very difficult to measure the ability of people to cope with or manage the pressures of anesthesia practice (personal communication 2011)." It remains to be seen if drug misuse and its adverse results can be reduced, and if stress is a major factor leading to misuse. Thus far, the plausible notion that stress may contribute to the problem of addiction, is just that. Eger is fond of quoting from a poster that was in the laboratory of his hero, John Severinghaus: "For every question there is an answer: neat, plausible, and wrong." (personal communication to EK, 31 Oct 12).

Conclusions

Nurses provided the earliest substantial numbers of professional anesthesia practitioners in the US. They paid attention to details of anesthetic administration and used positive suggestion to lead the patient smoothly through the induction process. They made anesthesia safe, and facilitated the evolution of the "Golden Age" of surgery. Nurses provided the first formal training programs and the first formal educational programs in anesthesia. They progressively increased the quality of education by accrediting schools. They assured quality practitioners by certifying graduates. Nurses established education for anesthesia educators, and mandated continuing education for practicing CRNAs. They supported surgery for the trauma imposed during World War I and played crucial roles in every war thereafter. Nurse anesthetists helped improve anesthesia globally by writing standards through the IFNA, volunteering in developing nations, and establishing volunteer run training programs. Finally, nurse anesthetists have established a wellness program with the hope of combating substance abuse and other stress related diseases that affect CRNAs. Taken together, these contributions define what nurses contribute to the care of patients under anesthesia.

Acknowledgments I wish to thank Sandra Maree-Ouellette and Rita Rupp for fact checking. I'm also grateful to Edmond Eger, Larry Saidman, and Rod N. Westhorpe for editing, and to Kathy Koch (no relation) for help with the reference list. And finally, I thank my wife, Loree Peery, who did everything else while I composed this paper.

References

1. Stansell C. The feminist promise: 1792 to the present. New York, Modern Library; 2010. p. 3–26.

2. Roberts JI, Group TM. Awake ye women awake, nursing and feminism: an historical perspective on power, status, and political activism in the nursing profession. In: Robert JI, Group TM. Westport, CT, Praeger Publishers;1995. p. 1.

3. Thatcher VS. History of anesthesia with emphasis on the nurse specialist. Philadelphia, JB Lippincott; 1953

4. Lawrence CW. Sketch of life and labor of Miss Catherine S. Lawrence. Albany, NY, Amasa J. Parker, Receiver of the Weed, Parsons & Co.; 1893. p. 1–174.

5. Wright AJ. Appeals for physician anesthesia in the United States between 1880 and 1920, Ralph Milton Waters, MD: Mentor to a Profession. In: Morris LE, Schroeder ME, Warner ME. Park Ridge, IL, Wood Library-Museum of Anesthesiology; 2004. pp. 14–9.

6. Gunn IP. Nurse anesthesia: a history of challenge, nurse anesthesia, 3rd edition. In: Nagelhout J, Zaglaniczny K. Philadelphia, WB Saunders; 2005. pp. 1–29.

7. Bankert M. Watchful care: a history of America's nurse anesthetists. New York, Continuum; 1989. p. 234.

8. Cushing HW, Letter to FA Washburn, Anaesthesia Charts of 1895, Treadwell Library, Massachusetts General Hospital, Boston. Cited in Shephard DA: Harvery Cusing and anaesthesia. Can Anaesth Soc J. 1965;12:431–2.

9. Clapesattle HB. The doctors mayo. Rochester, MN, Mayo Foundation for Medical Education and Research; 1969. pp. 13, 256–7.

10. Schjolberg AO. A history of the Augustana hospital school of nursing, 1884–1938. Chicago, Alumnae Association of the Augustana Hospital School of Nursing, 1939. Available at the National Library of Medicine, call number WY 19 S337h 1939. p. 5.

11. Magaw A. A review of over fourteen thousand surgical anesthesias. Surg Gynecol Obstet. 1906;3:795–9.

12. Nelson J, Wilstead S: Alice Magaw (Kessel). Her life in and out of the operating room. AANA J 2009;77:12–6.

13. Harris N, Dean J. The art of Florence Henderson, pioneer nurse and anesthetist (master's thesis). Rochester, MN, Mayo School of Health Related Sciences; 2007. pp. 1–27.

14. Magaw A. Observations in anesthesia. Northwestern Lancet 1899;19:207–10.

15. Hunt AM. Anesthesia: principles and practice, a presentation for the nursing profession. New York, GB Putnam's Sons; 1949. p. 72.

16. Crile GW. George Crile: an autobiography. Philadelphia, JB Lippincott; 1947, p. 199.

17. The war years: Nurse anesthesia at the front lines, AANA News Bulletin November1984;38 suppl:6.

18. History of the Pennsylvania hospital unit, base hospital number 10, U.S.A in the Great War. New York, Hoeber; 1921. pp. 67, 93.

19. Crile GW. Greetings. Bull Am Assoc Nurse Anesth. 1936;4:182–4.

20. Harsch T. Nurse anesthetists in the US Army Nurse Corps in World War II (master's thesis). Peoria Illinois, Bradley University; 1993. p. 25.

21. Irwell L. The case against the nurse-anaesthetist. International Clinics 1912;2(Series 22):204–9.

22. McMechan F. Editorial. Anesthesia supplement, Am J Surg 1915;29:120.

23. Harmel M. Austin Lamont, MD (1905–1969), Ralph Milton Waters MD: mentor to a profession. In: Morris L, Schroeder M, Warner M. Park Ridge, IL, Wood Library-Museum of Anesthesiology; 2004. pp. 107–11.

24. Blumenreich GA. Supervision. AANA J 2000;68:404–8.

25. Stoll DA. The emerging role of the nurse anesthetist in medical practice (dissertation). Evanston, IL, Northwestern University, 1988.

26. Koch BE. Nurse anesthesia: a history of challenge, Nurse Anesthesia, 4th edition. In: Nagelhout J, Plaus K. St. Louis, Saunders Elsevier; 2010. p. 19.

27. Bruton-Maree N, Rupp R. Federal healthcare policy: how AANA advocates for the profession, A Professional Study and Resource Guide for the CRNA. In: Foster S, Faut-Callahan M. Park Ridge, IL, AANA Publishing; 2001. pp. 357–79.

28. Gerbasi F, Horton BJ. Nurse anesthesia education in the United States, Nurse Anesthesia, 4th edition. In: Nagelhout J, Plaus K. St. Louis, Saunders Elsevier; 2010. pp. 34–9.

29. Starr P. The social transformation of American medicine. New York, Basic Books Inc.; 1982. pp. 116–27.

30. Klein R: The first 100 years, The History of Anesthesia in Oregon. Edited by Klein R, Kendrick A. Portland, OR, Oregon Trail Publishing, 2004. pp. 3–26.

31. Brown S. Nurse anesthesia in Oregon, The history of anesthesia in Oregon. In: Klein R, Kendrick A. Portland, OR, Oregon Trail Publishing, 2004. p. 53–87.

32. Second award of appreciation. J Am Assoc Nurs Anesth 1948;16:331–3.

33. Koch K. AANA's 75th anniversary: Agatha Hodgins, Lakeside Alumae Association, and the founding of the AANA. AANA J 2005;73:259–62.

34. Sykes K. How Ralph Waters influenced the development of anaesthesia in the British Commonwealth and in Europe, Ralph Waters MD: Mentor to a Profession. Park Ridge, IL, Wood Library-Museum of Anesthesiology; 2004. p. 198.

35. Report of the educational committee. Bull Nat Assoc Nurse Anesth. 1938;6:199–200.

36. Garde JF. The role of the professional organization, A Professional Study and Resource Guide for the CRNA. In: Foster S, Faut-Callahan, M. Park Ridge, IL, AANA Publishing; 2001. pp. 45.

37. Anesthesia: A career for the graduate nurse. Bull Am Assoc Nurse Anesth. 1942;10:97–104.

38. Balz KE. The value of special training in anesthesia for the Army nurse. J Am Assoc Nurse Anesth. 1947;15:138–40.

39. Rosenbach M, Cromwell J, Pope G, Butrica B, Pitcher J. Study of nurse anesthesia manpower needs. AANA J. 1991;59:233–40.

40. DePaolis-Lutzo M. Factors influencing nurse anesthesia educational programs: 1982–1987 (dissertation). University of Pittsburgh; 1987. p. 111

41. Martin-Sheridan D. Factors that influence six nurse anesthesia programs to close. AANA J. 1998;66:377–84.

42. Beutler JM. Federal legislative and regulatory impact on funding of nurse anesthesia educational programs: medicare reimbursement for nurse anesthesia education: Report of the National Commission on Nurse Anesthesia Education. AANA J. 1991;59:180–2.

43. Report of the National Commission on Nurse Anesthesia Education. Park Ridge, IL, American Association of Nurse Anesthetists; 1990. p. 5

44. Foster SD. Regionalized education and the accreditation process: report of the National Commission on Nurse Anesthesia Education. AANA J. 1991;59:62–4.

45. Booth MJ. Current and future perspectives regarding the framework for nurse anesthesia education: within the framework of allied health departments: Report of the National Commission on Nurse Anesthesia Education. AANA J. 1991;59:487–90.

46. Worth P. Current and future perspectives regarding the framework for nurse anesthesia education: nurse anesthesia curriculum in the College of Pharmacy and Allied Health Professions, Wayne State University: report of the National Commission on Nurse Anesthesia Education. AANA J. 1991;59:561–2.

47. Bullard WG. Current and future perspectives regarding the framework for nurse anesthesia education: military education of nurse anesthetists and the case for centralized academic programs with multiple clinical affiliates (USAF): Report of the National Commission on Nurse Anesthesia Education. AANA J. 1991;59:294–5.

48. Byrnes G. Current and future perspectives regarding the framework for nurse anesthesia education: Military education of nurse anesthetists and the case for centralized academic programs with multiple

clinical affiliates: US Navy: Report of the National Commission on Nurse Anesthesia Education. AANA J. 1991;59:490–1.

49. Masters F, Skidmore M, Thibodeaux B. US Army/Texas Wesleyan University program in anesthesia nursing: report of the National Commission on Nurse Anesthesia Education. AANA J 1991;59:480–1.

50. DePaolis-Lutzo MV. Current and future perspectives regarding the framework for nurse anesthesia education: nurse anesthesia education within the framework of nursing education: report of the National Commission on Nurse Anesthesia Education. AANA J. 1991;59:492–6.

51. Waugaman WR. Graduate nurse anesthesia education: the university based model: report of the National Commission on Nurse Anesthesia Education. AANA J. 1991;59:559–60.

52. Faut-Callahan M. Graduate education for nurse anesthetists: Masters versus clinical doctorate: report of the National Commission on Nurse Anesthesia Education. AANA J. 1992;60:98–103.

53. Lebeck LL. The need for alternative educational pathways in nurse anesthesia education: report of the National Commission on Nurse Anesthesia Education. AANA J. 1992;60:183–4.

54. Horton BJ, Brunner M. Nurse Anesthesia Education Programs, 1991–1997. AANA J. 1998;66:338–42.

55. American Association of Nurse Anesthetists. AANA Announces Support of Doctorate for Entry into Nurse Anesthesia Practice by 2025. September 20, 2007. http://www.aana.com/newsandjournal/News/Pages/092007-AANA-Announces-Support-of-Doctorate-for-Entry-into-Nurse-Anesthesia-Practice-by-2025.aspx.

56. Edwardson SR. Imagining the DNP role, The Doctor of Nursing Practice Essentials: a New Model for Advanced Practice Nursing. In: Zaccagnini M, White KW. Sudbury, MA, Jones and Bartlett; 2011. p. xvii–xxviii.

57. Phelps MR, Gerbasi F. Accreditation requirements for practice doctorates in 14 healthcare professions. AANA J. 2009;77:19–26.

58. Hawkins R, Nezat G. Doctoral education: which degree to pursue? AANA J. 2009;77: 92–6.

59. Zaccagnini M, White KW. The doctor of nursing practice essentials: a new model for advanced practice nursing. In: Zaccagnini M, White KW. Sudbury, MA, Jones and Bartlett; 2011.

60. Beecher HK, Todd DP. A study of the deaths associated with anesthesia and surgery: based on a study of 599,548 anesthesias in ten institutions 1948–1952, inclusive. Ann Surg. 1954;140:2–35.

61. Silber JH, Williams SV, Krakauer H, Schwartz JS. Hospital and patient characteristics associated with death after surgery: a study of averse outcomes and failure to rescue. Med Care. 1992;30:615–29.

62. Abenstein JP, Warner MA. Anesthesia providers, patient outcomes and costs. Anesth Analg. 1996;82:1273–83.

63. Wiklund RA, Rosenbaum SH. Anesthesiology (parts one and two). N Engl J Med. 1997;337:1132–41 and N Engl J Med. 1997;337:1215–9.

64. Silber JH, Kennedy SK, Even-Shoshan O, Chen W, Koziol LF, Showan AM, Longnecker DE. Anesthesiologist direction and patient outcomes. Anesthesiology. 2000;93:152–63.

65. Vila H Jr, Soto R, Cantor AB, Mackey D. Comparative outcomes analysis of procedures performed in physician offices and ambulatory surgery centers. Arch Surg. 2003;138:991–9.

66. Quality of Care in Anesthesia: synopsis of published information comparing certified registered nurse Anesthetist and Anesthesiologist Patient Outcomes. Park Ridge, IL, American association of nurse anesthetists, 2009, available at: http://www.aana.com/resources2/professionalpractice/Documents/Quality%20of%20Care%20in%20Anesthesia%2012102009.pdf. Accessed February 21, 2012.

67. Horton BJ. Upgrading nurse anesthesia educational requirements (1992–2006)–Part 2: Curriculum, faculty and students. AANA J. 2007;75:247–51.

68. Lamb H, Berger O, Cameron M, Hard M, Muller M. Report of the Educational Committee. Bull Natl Assoc Nurse Anesth. 1936;4:57–65.

69. Hudson J. Autonomy in nurse anesthesia education: the creation of American Association of Nurse Anesthetists Council on Accreditation. 1995, Available from Oakland California, Samuel Merritt College Program of Nurse Anesthesia. Unpublished manuscript, p. 15.

70. Horton BJ. Upgrading nurse anesthesia educational requirements (1933–2006)–Part I: Setting standards. AANA J. 2007;75:167–70.

71. Stephens C. Nurses in Anesthesia. American Society of Anesthesiology Manpower Report. Washington, D.C., United States Department of Health Education and Welfare, 1969.

72. AANA Reaffirms Its Position on Credentialing: views formation of FNAS with concern. AANA NewsBulletin, January 1976; 30:1, 36 [Editors: this publication begins numbering at page in each issue, so I included the month].

73. National Board for the Certification and Recertification of Nurse Anesthetists: 2011 Criteria for recertification of nurse anesthetists. Park Ridge, IL, NBCRNA, 2011, p. 6. Also available at: http://www.nbcrna.com/recert/Documents/2011%20COR%20Criteria%20for%20Recertification%20Brochure.pdf. Accessed 21. Feb. 2012.

74. International Federation of Nurse Anesthetists: the very beginning: the History of the International Federation of Nurse Anesthetists 1989–2009. Paris, International Federation of Nurse Anesthetists; 2009. pp. 1–103, Available from the AANA Archives, WY 11.1 I6154 2010.

75. Caulk RF, Ouellette SM. The International Federation of Nurse Anesthetists, A Professional Study and Resource Guide for the CRNA. In: Foster S, Faut-Callahan M. Park Ridge, IL, AANA Publishing; 2001. pp. 381–403.

76. McAuliffe M. Countries where anesthesia is administered by nurses. AANA J. 1996;64:469–79.

77. McAuliffe, M Henry B. Survey of nurse anesthesia practice, education, and regulation in 96 countries. AANA J. 1998;66:273–86.

78. Henry B, McAuliffe M. Practice and education of nurse anesthetists. Bull World Health Organ. 1999;77:267–70.

79. Ouellette SM, Horton BJ. Towards globalization of a profession. AANA J. 2001;79:12–4.

80. Brown S. Oral history with Ruby Hills, CRNA [DVD], Portland, Oregon Association of Nurse Anesthetists, 2010.

81. Health Volunteers Overseas: a lasting impact: 2009 Annual Report. Washington, D.C., Health Volunteers Overseas; 2009. p. 1.

82. Teaching the Healers: the story of health volunteers overseas [DVD]. Washington D.C., Treehouse Productions, 2005. Available from Health Volunteers Overseas

83. About Wellness [DVD # 318]. Park Ridge IL, American Association of Nurse Anesthetists, 2010. Available from American Association of Nurse Anesthetists.

84. Fenster JM. Ether day: the strange tale of America's Greatest Medical Discovery and the Haunted Men Who Made It. New York, Harper Collins; 2001. p. 186.

85. Lundy J, McQuillen FA. Narcotics and the anesthetist: Professional hazards. J Am Assoc Nurse Anesth. 1962;30:147–75.

86. Health Resources and Services Administration: the Registered Nurse Population: finding from the National Sample Survey of Registered Nurses. http://bhpr.hrsa.gov/healthworkforce/rnsurvey04/2.htm, accessed April 25, 2011.

87. Quinlan D. Peer Assistance–Part 1, A Professional Study and Resource Guide for the CRNA. In: Foster S, Faut-Callahan M. Park Ridge, IL, AANA Publishing; 2001. pp. 425–51.

88. Quinlan D. Peer assistance reaches its 25th year. AANA J. 2009;77:254:254–8.

89. Yocom C, Haack: Interim Report. A Comparison of Two Regulatory Approaches to the Management of the Chemically Dependent Nurse. Chicago, National Council of State Boards of Nursing; 1996.

90. Monroe T, Pearson F, Kenaga H. Procedures for handling cases of substance abuse among nurses: a comparison of disciplinary and alternative programs. J Addict Nurs. 2008;19:156–61.

91. Wilson H, Compton M. Reentry of the addicted Certified Registered Nurse Anesthetist: a review of the literature. J Addict Nurs. 2009;20:177–84.

92. McDonough JP. Personality, addiction and anesthesia. AANA J. 1990;58:193–200.

93. Quinlan D: The impaired anesthesia provider: the manager's role. AANA J 1995;63:485–91.

94. Quinlan D. Peer assistance: an historical perspective. AANA News-Bulletin, January 1996;50:14–5.

95. Bell D, McDonough J, Ellison J, Fitzhugh E. Controlled drug misuse among Certified Registered Nurse Anesthetists. AANA J. 1999;67;133–40.

96. Farley E, Talbott G. Anesthesiology and addiction. Anesthesiology 1983;62:465–6.

97. Tunajek S. Why wellness? AANA News Bull, September 2009;63:24.

Eugene P. Steffey

Summary

The Royal Veterinary College, London, adopted anesthesia soon after Morton's 1846 demonstration. However, reports of accidents and deaths hindered widespread veterinarian acceptance of anesthesia, especially with large animals. In the late 1800s, anesthesia was used more to restrain than to alleviate pain. In 1875, Humbert described the oral, rectal and intraperitoneal administration of chloral hydrate to horses, usually as an adjunct to local or inhalation anesthesia. Later studies in Western Europe supported intravenous chloral hydrate in horses. In 1915, Hobday published the first English textbook devoted to veterinary anesthesia. In 1919, the British Parliament enacted an Anaesthetics Bill for Animals, specifying that anesthesia must "...prevent the animal feeling pain".

In his first edition of Veterinary Anaesthesia in 1941, Wright laid the foundations of *modern* veterinary anesthesia. The 1950s saw the first veterinarians who exclusively practiced anesthesia. From 1960–1979, the number of faculty and trainees in university-based programs increased in both Europe and the US. Alphaxalone, azaperone, droperidol, fentanyl, halothane, enflurane, ketamine, and xylazine appeared, and their effects were defined in species of interest to veterinarians. Growth of new university-based programs in the US and UK paralleled the growth in numbers of veterinary anesthesiologists. By the early 1980s, 25 faculty positions were assigned to teaching and research programs in the US, with 2 in Canada.

Established in 1964, the Association of Veterinary Anaesthetists of Great Britain and Ireland (reduced to AVA in 1991) awarded its first Diploma of Veterinary Anaesthesia (DVA) in 1967. The European College of Veterinary Anaesthesia and Analgesia (ECVAA) incorporated in 1995, and was registered in the Netherlands in 1997. The ECVAA Diploma became the primary certification as a specialist in veterinary anesthesia in Europe, and the DVA was phased out.

Founded in 1970, the American Society of Veterinary Anesthesiology (ASVA) was immediately recognized by the American Veterinary Medical Association (AVMA). In 1971, the ASVA facilitated establishment of the American College of Veterinary Anesthesiologists (ACVA), to credential specialists in veterinary anesthesiology. The AVMA recognized the ACVA in 1975. Two organizations were not needed, and the ASVA was dissolved in 1981. Presently, there are 222 ACVA diplomats, with 16 approved residency programs of veterinary anesthesia in the US, and 4 in Canada.

The International Congress of Veterinary Anesthesia was established in 1985 "...to promote veterinary anaesthesiology within the international community of veterinarians, through...triennial World Congresses of Veterinary Anaesthesiology".

Introduction

The reviews of Hall [1], Smithcors [2, 3], Stevenson [4], Wright [5], Westhues & Fritsch [6], Weaver [7], and Jones [8], provided material for the present discourse. I will briefly describe the early years of veterinary anesthesia, focusing more attention on events occurring during my lifetime, a period that most impacted clinical practice and fostered the evolution of veterinary anesthesia as an organized discipline of veterinary medicine. I choose this tack because information from the last half century is incomplete or unpublished, yet is known to me from personal experiences in teaching, research and clinical practice.

The Early Development of Veterinary Anesthesia

"...the history of anesthesia is a disturbing account of 'what might have been'...." [3]

Why was the use of anesthesia to relieve the pain of surgery in animals delayed? Despite knowledge of the discovery of

E. P. Steffey (✉)
Department of Surgical and Radiological Sciences, School of Veterinary Medicine, University of California Davis, Davis, CA, USA
e-mail: epsteffey@ucdavis.edu

E. I Eger II et al. (eds.), *The Wondrous Story of Anesthesia,* DOI 10.1007/978-1-4614-8441-7_23, © Edmond I Eger, MD 2014

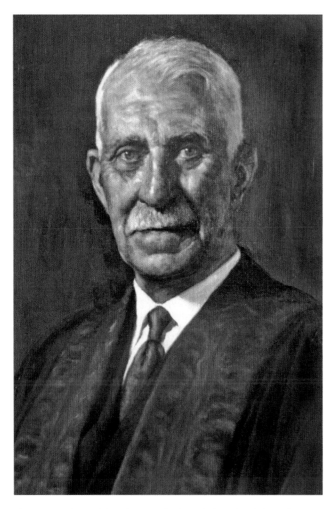

Fig. 23.1 John Wright (Photograph of a painting of Wright; painter unknown. Photo taken by Robert Pearson and sent to EPS by Ron Jones)

anesthesia, progress in veterinary anesthesia lagged behind that in humans, and reliance on mechanical restraint persisted [1, 3, 9].

Mid-1800s

The use of nitrous oxide, ether, chloroform, and even carbon dioxide in laboratory animals, antedated William Morton's 1846 public demonstration of ether as a general anesthetic, at the Massachusetts General Hospital [3]. An absence of a veterinary journal published by a veterinary anesthesia association hinders a determination of anesthesia's first clinical use. Several historians cite Charles Jackson's 1853 account of his experiences with "Etherization of Animals" [10], as one of the earliest (if not the first) published accounts of general anesthesia in animals [2–4]. Even this might be questioned as this shameless self promoter also claimed to have invented the telegraph. John Wright (Fig. 23.1) noted that, "Almost immediately after publication of Morton's use of [ether] in

human surgery (1846), it was adopted in the Royal Veterinary College, London [5]".

In 1847, Edward Mayhew reported in the Veterinarian[1] on the use of ether for "minor surgery" in cats and dogs [2, 3]. Despite the absence of evident pain, the excitatory stage of the anesthesia disturbed him:

"The results of these trials are not calculated to inspire any very sanguine hopes. We cannot tell whether the cries emitted are evidence of pain or not; but they are suggestive of agony to the listener, and, without testimony to the contrary, must be regarded as indicative of suffering. The process, therefore, is not calculated to attain the object for which in veterinary practice it would be most generally employed, namely, to relieve the owner from the impression that his animal was subject to torture…" [2]

In response to Mayhew's perception that the animals' cries reflected pain, Percivall, an editor of the journal with credentials as both a physician and veterinarian published a contrary view:

"… after perusing Mr. Mayhew's interesting cases, we … augur more favourably of the inferences deducible from them than he would seem to. To us it appears questionable whether the cries emitted by the animals during experiments are … 'evidence of pain'" [2]

This in turn prompted Mayhew to test his convictions, by convincing his dentist to 'etherize' him multiple times over the next 2 days, to have a *dens sapienta* extracted. Although he noted that the inhalation of ether was pleasant, he apparently was completely unaware of his excitatory state—and that each administration resulted in unsuccessful attempts at the extraction he had requested. After multiple attempts on the first day and another attempt the following day, the dentist and his assistant refused to continue. Nonetheless Mayhew "… concluded that ether did have a place in veterinary surgery, but warned, 'We should be cautious lest we become cruel under a mistaken endeavor to be kind' [2]" Smithcors described as unfortunate, Mayhew's suggestion that the principle use of anesthesia in veterinary practice would be to relieve the owner's perception of pain. Consideration for the patient's suffering appears to have arisen later [4, 11].

Chloroform's use in the horse in the UK quickly followed Simpson's discovery of chloroform anesthesia in humans [5]. WJ Goodwin, veterinary surgeon to Queen Victoria, administered chloroform to a horse at the Royal Mews for a neurectomy associated with navicular arthritis. Wright, in his review continues [5]:

---

[1] The 'Veterinarian' was a journal launched in 1828 by William Percivall in the UK. It conveyed information concerning veterinary medicine in general (i.e., it was not a specialty publication). It likely was the earliest such publication in veterinary medicine but was independent of any organized veterinary association. It ceased publication in 1902 probably because the Veterinary Record was launched in late 1888 by the British Veterinary Medical Association.

"In the same year, William Field reported (that) …'However satisfied I may feel about the power of chloroform over the horse as an anaesthetic agent, I cannot think of using it for casting in lieu of hobbles…the fall of the animal is too uncertain to admit of restraint or limitation and consequently violent injury may result in the struggles and staggerings preparatory to its fall, as well as in the fall itself.' "

Over the next few years, reports of accidents and deaths of animals subjected to anesthesia militated against veterinarian acceptance of anesthesia, especially with large animals. Only later in the nineteenth century and early in the twentieth century, when Frederick Hobday developed better techniques for agent delivery, did veterinarians accept anesthesia.

In the US, the physician George Dadd, was perhaps the first to use ether and chloroform for surgical procedures in animals. Dadd moved from human patients to veterinary practice soon after ether's introduction by Morton, and his familiarity with medical developments likely prompted his use of inhalation anesthesia in animals. In his 1854 book, *Modern Horse Doctor* [12] (beginning page 252):

"…we recommend that, in all operations of this kind, the subject be etherized, not only in view of preventing pain, but that we may, in the absence of all struggling on the part of our patient, perform the operation satisfactorily, and in much less time after etherization has taken place than otherwise. So soon as the patient is under the influence of that valuable agent, we have nothing to fear from his struggles, provided we have the assistance of one experienced to administer it. We generally use a mixture of chloroform and chloric ether in our operations, and consider it far preferable, so far as the life of the patient is concerned, to pure chloroform."

Thus, as in humans, this veterinarian recognized the greater safety of ether.

The Later 1800s

The difficulties accompanying inhalational anesthetic administration in large domestic animals, prompted a search for better anesthetics. Liebig discovered chloral hydrate in 1832, and after experimenting in animals, Pierre-Cyprien Oré used it intravenously to produce anesthesia in humans in 1872. Humbert described its use in horses in 1875, at doses of 30–70 gm. It was given by mouth or via the rectum, and occasionally by intraperitoneal injection, usually as an adjunct to local or inhalation anesthesia. The later intravenous use of chloral hydrate in full anesthetic doses in the horse is credited to experiments conducted in Western Europe. Degive, a prominent Belgian professor, described this method of administration in horses, in 1908. Degive wrote (as quoted by Wright [13]):

"Chloral hydrate injected into the jugular vein of the horse … produces in 1 to 2 minutes complete general anaesthesia without causing preliminary excitement in the animal [as commonly seen with chloroform]. The method is most valuable when prac-

ticed with full aseptic precautions but it has been followed by several accidents which have put its value into doubt."

Later, Wright wrote:

"It is a drug the value of which is continually being rediscovered. … Half a century later I … arrived at the same conclusion except to say that provided adequate technical care is exercised the doubt he [Degive] expresses becomes removed. In fact even today, with the great advances in our knowledge of anaesthesia and anaesthetics, it is my opinion that chloral hydrate by intravenous injections is the best method of inducing general anaesthesia in the horse …"

Organized veterinary medicine had but limited interest in anesthesia through much of the last quarter of the nineteenth century. In his review of the History of Veterinary Anesthesia [3], Smithcors notes:

"In the first volume of the 'American Veterinary Review' (1877), … there is but one reference to anesthetics, and none in volume 2….Early advocates of anesthesia, mainly Dadd and his colleagues, worked outside the pale of urbanized veterinary medicine. Perhaps one had to be a maverick to stray far from conventional practice."

And in his *Manual of Operative Veterinary Surgery* Alexandre Liautard wrote [14]:

"In veterinary surgery, the indication for anesthesia has not, to the same extent as in human, the avoidance of pain in the patient for its object, … the administration of anesthetic compounds aims principally to facilitate the performance of the operation for its own sake…."

1900–1939

In the 1915 edition of *The Principles of Veterinary Surgery*, Louis Merillat echoed the above sentiments but noted a trend to a use of anesthesia to relieve pain [11]:

"Anaesthesia in veterinary surgery today is a means of restraint and not an expedient to relieve pain. So long as an operation can be performed by forcible restraint without imminent danger to the technique, the operator or the animal, the thought of anaesthesia does not enter in the proposition. But, on the other hand, when a certain technique requires perfect repose of the surgical field, or when there is danger of personal injury or injury to the animal, it is **sometimes** (sic) administered, minority reports to the contrary notwithstanding."

"(However, it is a matter of fact that practitioners who once begin the practice of administering inhalation anaesthetics for their operations soon find it indispensable to the success of their work. As they become more and more confident in their ability as anaesthetists they resort to this in all kinds of operations, minor and major, and the result is always the enlargement of their scope of usefulness as surgeons.)"

Humanitarian concerns for animals led to legislation in Great Britain (Cruelty to Animals Act, 1876), to restrict the use of animals in experiments to those persons who were licensed and had Home Office permission for particular procedures (later succeeded by the Animals [Scientific Procedures] Act of 1986). In 1913, the British Parliament discussed and later enacted an Anaesthetics Bill for Animals [15],—the Animals (Anaesthetics) Act of 1919 (reproduced in the appendix of Wright's textbook [16]). It specified that general or local anesthetic must be used in specific surgical procedures in a horse, dog, cat or a bovine, and that the anesthetic must be "…of sufficient power to prevent the animal feeling pain". Any person subjecting, or causing, or procuring, or being the owner of the animal subjected "… to an operation contrary to the regulations … shall be guilty of an offence under this Act" and liable upon conviction, for a fine and/or imprisonment. Its focus on general anesthesia inhibited the development of regional anesthesia until 1954. The 1919 Act was a precursor to legislation of the present day Act, i.e., The Protection of Animals (Anaesthetics) Act of 1954 and 1964 [7]. The 1964 version allowed veterinary surgeons to choose the type of anesthetic as long as it produced "adequate anaesthesia" [8].

In 1915, Hobday published the first English textbook devoted exclusively to veterinary anesthesia, *Anaesthesia and Narcosis of Animals and Birds* [15]. In his Preface he wrote that "The progress of anaesthetics in veterinary surgery has not been as rapid as it ought to have been, and it is in the hope that a small textbook specially devoted to the subject may be helpful in his direction."

Wright laid the foundations of *modern* veterinary anesthesia. He qualified and spent the early part of his career as a veterinary surgeon in the Department of Surgery at the Beaumont Hospital of the Royal Veterinary College, London. He moved to the veterinary school at the University of Liverpool in 1941, where he established the Field Station. Like Hobday, Wright's interest in anesthesia lay in his desire as a surgeon to avoid pain, to provide a safe anesthetic, and to ensure a proper environment for the performance of surgery. He published his first edition of *Veterinary Anaesthesia* in 1941. In 1961, Wright and LW Hall (of Cambridge University) co-authored the 5th edition. In 1966, the 6th edition appeared as *Wright's Veterinary Anaesthesia and Analgesia*, with Hall as the single author. No textbook of veterinary anesthesia has been published for a longer time, and it recently reached its 10th edition (now authored by Hall, KW Clarke and C Trim).

Two major advances occurred in the decade before World War II [4]: the introduction of barbiturates and epidural anesthesia to clinical practice. In America, Kreutzer [17] reported the first use of pentobarbital (administered intraperitoneally; IP) in veterinary anesthesia. Two years later in Britain, Wright published his own experiences with IP pentobarbital in 100 dog and cat patients. Humans were given barbiturates intravenously, and this route was soon applied to animals [18]. Some veterinarians thought that this method, particu-

larly for anesthetic induction was "…infinitely superior to the accepted methods of inhalation anesthesia; in fact by its introduction canine surgery became revolutionized [19]." Shortly thereafter, thiopental and later thiamylal were found to be more satisfactory for many common needs of veterinary medicine, like short periods of deep sedation and anesthesia for minor surgery [20]. Following intravenous barbiturate anesthetic induction, the needle was maintained in situ in the vein, and the attached syringe taped to the (usually) patient's foreleg for ease of added drug dosing as needed.

Such a technique was common in a small animal-focused clinical practice, when I entered the profession in 1967. Until I purchased my first inhalation anesthetic machine (with in-circuit glass vaporizer) from a regional General Services Administration (federal agency disposing of obsolete/unwanted medical equipment) auction in 1968, most anesthetics I administered in general veterinary practice were barbiturates. The notable exception was the use of diethyl ether for short-term anesthetic management of cats undergoing routine castration or abscess incision and drainage. Why ether? Part of the problem was poorly socialized, especially rural and semi-rural cats. In addition, the re-used needles of that time had varying degrees of sharpness. Accordingly, it was easier for the veterinarian and cat to place the fasted cat into a top-hinged wooden box with glass panel. The lid was quickly closed after a few milliliters of diethyl ether were poured onto the box floor. If additional anesthetic time was needed, more ether was administered using an open-drop technique.

Short and ultrashort acting barbiturates which appeared in the 1930s remained two of the most widely used anesthetic drugs (as a sole agent) in both small and large animal practice until late in the twentieth century. Their use as a sole agent however, required large doses to eliminate movement in response to pain. Accordingly, recovery times were undesirably prolonged.

To deal with the prolonged recovery time, during the 1970s, the increasing use of halothane and the newly introduced enflurane supplanted pentobarbital. In the 1980s, the introduction of ketamine and isoflurane as primary agents, either alone or in various species-related anesthetic drug cocktails, and then propofol (especially in small animals), gradually replaced the ultra-short acting barbiturates. In the past decade, a few investigators have used desflurane to accelerate recovery from anesthesia in large and fractious animals. Sevoflurane has seen an expanded, but still small clinical application for companion animals and horses. Cost has limited a broader application of both anesthetics. Isoflurane remains, by far, the primary inhaled anesthetic in veterinary medicine.

The development of local and regional anesthetic techniques for human patients fostered similar developments in veterinary medicine. For example, since the late part of the nineteenth century, local anesthesia has been used to

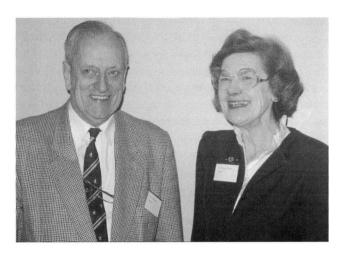

Fig. 23.2 Leslie Hall and Barbara Weaver. (EP Steffey photograph, 1994.)

assist diagnosis of the cause of lameness in horses. In the US, in 1924, Bemis and colleagues published a summary of regional nerve blocks in contemporary use with horses [21]. Regional anesthesia achieved only limited popularity in veterinary medicine because both local and regional anesthesia require a cooperative patient. Smithcors notes, "It remained for veterinarians Retzgen of Berlin [and also Pape and Pitzch] in 1925, and Franz Benesch of Austria in 1926, to demonstrate in horses and cattle respectively, that epidural anesthesia with the needle introduced distal to the spinal cord proper, was a safe technique. [3]" In 1940, Farquharson described paravertebral blocks of thoracic and lumbar nerves for abdominal operations (eg, rumenotomy and exploratory laporatomy) in standing cattle [22]. In 1953, Larson introduced the internal pudendal (pudic) nerve block for anesthesia of the penis and relaxation of the retractor penis muscle in bulls [23].

1940–1959

Veterinary anesthesiology did not exist as a discipline before 1950. Surgeons and general practitioners gave anesthesia as part of their care. The first veterinarians devoting their practice exclusively to anesthesia and its clinical development were Barbara Weaver and Leslie Hall (Fig. 23.2). Weaver qualified from the Royal Veterinary College (RVC) in 1949, and was appointed House Surgeon, then Lecturer at the RVC Beaumont Animals Hospital, London. Hall qualified in 1950, also from the RVC. After three months in general practice he was awarded a Veterinary Education Trust research training scholarship to work under E. Amoroso in the Physiology Department of the RVC. He was awarded a PhD degree from London University in 1957 for an investigation of the control of arterial blood pressure under general anesthesia.

Hall and Weaver's paths repeatedly crossed. They began meeting with medical anesthesiologists in 1951, meetings that facilitated the application of knowledge and skills of anesthetic management of humans to animals. Weaver wrote:

"In the 1950s when Leslie and I became interested in anaesthesia, realizing we were some 50 years behind the 'medics' we adapted human techniques for our patients in the Beaumont Animals Hospital, mainly dogs and cats and an early trial in the horse. We introduced 'Balanced Anaesthesia' with three phases, i.e., premedication, induction and maintenance. For maintenance, using semi closed systems without absorption, we maintained anaesthesia with nitrous oxide, oxygen and trichlorethylene (trilene). Endotracheal intubation was carried out and intermittent positive pressure ventilation was also carried out to assist or control ventilation as necessary. Muscle relaxant agents were used with care, facilitating the control of ventilation when necessary." (Weaver, personal communication, 2010)

In 1952, early in his PhD studies, Hall was appointed to a faculty surgery post in the new veterinary school at Cambridge University. He taught ophthalmology, gastrointestinal and thoracic surgery—and anaesthesia. Appointment of more teaching staff allowed him to focus on anesthesia teaching and research. After 8 years at the RVC, Weaver moved to the University of Bristol (5 November 1957) with a special remit to establish a division of anaesthesia within the Department of Veterinary Surgery. There she introduced balanced anaesthetic techniques in the management of small animals, and facilitated further development of inhalation equipment for anesthesia in adult horses and cattle [24, 25].

Weaver and Hall worked closely with physician and basic science colleagues (including William Weipers, William Mapleson, Brian Marshall, and Michael Halsey). Both were recognized by physicians for these interactions and their many contributions. For example, Hall was elected President of the East Anglian Society of Anaesthetists, and Weaver was elected President of the Society of Anaesthetists of the South Western Region. In 1977, Hall became the first veterinarian to be awarded the Faculty Medal of the Faculty of Anaesthetists of the Royal College of Surgeons of England, the highest award given by the Faculty. A few years later, Weaver was similarly honored, as Ronald Jones was still later, (discussed below), and all three were elected Fellows of the Royal College of Anaesthetists in 2001.

Veterinarians used and sometimes misused neuromuscular blocking agents, as a substitute for or as an adjunct to veterinary anesthesia. Wright credits William Sewell at the University of London, as the first person to experiment with curare as a remedy [13]. In 1935, Sewell used it to treat tetanus in a horse and a donkey, by implanting an arrow head coated with curare in the fleshy part of the afflicted equine shoulder, publishing accounts of this, years later. We aren't told of the results, but they were likely no better than those of similar trials in humans (see Chapter 50 on Neuromuscular Blockade by J Caldwell).

1960–1979

In the next two decades, the number of faculty and trainees in university based programs increased dramatically in both Europe and the US. Alphaxalone (Althesin, Saffan), azaperone, droperidol, fentanyl (or Innovar, a combination of droperidol and fentenyl), enflurane, ketamine, and xylazine appeared, and their effects were defined in species of interest to veterinary medicine. Anesthetic and monitoring equipment, developed for use in humans, subsequently entered veterinary practice.

Ronald Jones (Fig. 23.3) was the third academic veterinarian appointed in the U.K., and in 1962, became the first person designated as a lecturer in veterinary anesthesiology, in the veterinary faculty of the University of Liverpool. He became the first full professor in veterinary anaesthesia in the UK in 1990. At Liverpool he overlapped tenure with Wright (just before Wright's retirement), but spent most of his time in the medical school's department of anaesthesia in association with Cecil Gray, Jackson Rees, John Utting and Jennifer Hunter. Indeed, he was influenced by and in turn influenced the medical anesthesia community. He served as Chair of the medical school's Department of Anaesthesia (the only veterinarian to my knowledge to hold such an honor), and was a reviewer and later Assistant Editor (1993–2001) of the British Journal of Anaesthesia. Like Hall and Weaver, he mentored numerous trainees, many of whom contributed to veterinary anesthesia programs elsewhere.

As documented by the careers of Hall, Weaver and Jones, collaboration and encouragement by physician anesthesiologists facilitated the progress of veterinary anesthesia in Great Britain. Weaver recently wrote to Steffey (personal communication), "The 'medical' anaesthetists have been hugely supportive of what we were trying to do for veterinary anaesthesia. I found their support and encouragement indispensable and no doubt was a major contribution to my lasting interest in comparative anaesthesia studies."

A parallel growth, similarly facilitated by physician involvement, occurred in North America (Table 23.1). Most of these first generation academicians trained in medical school anesthesia residency/fellowship programs. Lawrence (Larry) Soma (Fig. 23.4) graduated from the University of Pennsylvania School of Veterinary Medicine in 1957. After an internship at the Animal Medical Center in New York City in 1958, he returned to the University of Pennsylvania in 1960, training for three years in human anesthesia under the direction of Robert Dripps.

Soma recounted to me, his start with Dripps. Immediately after receiving his VMD, Soma applied for a newly established fellowship in veterinary cardiology under David Detwiler at Penn (another example of the many clinical disciplines new to veterinary medicine gaining its start at Penn). However, before a decision on his application was made, Soma enlisted in the US Army veterinary corps, and

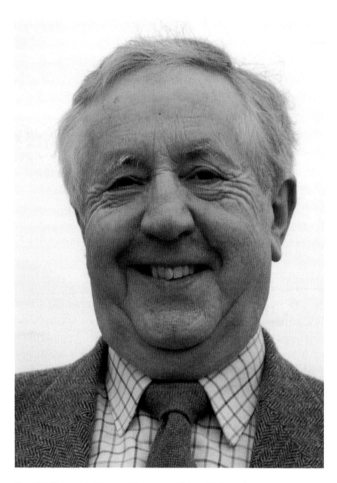

Fig. 23.3 Ronald Jones. (Courtesy of Ronald Jones.)

Clinical veterinary use of neuromuscular blocking drugs followed more than a decade after Griffith and Johnson's 1942 report of curare in the anesthetic management of human patients [26]. In 1954, Hall and Weaver introduced "balanced anesthesia", including curare, to the clinical management of dogs and cats [27]. Peculiarly, Weaver did not find the bronchospasm in dogs that had discouraged Stuart Cullen from extending his studies to humans: "I did not find bronchospasm a serious problem in dogs. I was aware that it was a concern and so was prepared for it." (personal communication to E Steffey) By the early 1970s, 3 major textbooks of veterinary anesthesia discussed muscle relaxant pharmacology and the clinical use of relaxants [28–30]. However, their application in veterinary medicine remained modest. For example, the use of neuromuscular blockade to facilitate atraumatic tracheal intubation or intermittent positive pressure ventilation, both common to the management of human patients, is unnecessary with most veterinary patients. Thus, current use is focused largely on particularly delicate and/or complicated surgeries in small companion animals and in horses, e.g., some ocular operations, open reductions of large bone fractures, and specialized cardiovascular or intracranial surgeries.

Table 23.1 First Generation US Veterinary Anesthesiologists

Year[a]	Veterinarian	Medical School Supporting Training	School Supporting Veterinarian's Appointment
1954	William Lumb	Surgeon with graduate training at University of Minnesota, School of Medicine (surgery)	Colorado State University
1954	E. Wynn Jones	Surgeon	Oklahoma State University
1963	Lawrence Soma	University of Pennsylvania	University of Pennsylvania
1965	J. R. Gillespie	University of California, San Francisco	University of California, Davis
1965	Charles Short	Baylor University	University of Missouri
1966	R. Bruce Heath	Ohio State University	Colorado State University
1969	John Thurmon	Baylor University College of Medicine & University of Illinois @ Chicago	University of Illinois, Urbana
1970	Wayne McDonnell	University of Toronto,	Ontario Veterinary College at Guelph
1970	Donald Sawyer	Colorado State University & University of California, San Francisco	Michigan State University
1971	James Heavner	University of Washington	University of Washington
1973	Eugene Steffey	University of California, San Francisco & University of California, Davis	University of California, Davis
1975	William Muir	Ohio State University	Ohio State University

[a] Year starting at indicated institution devoted to veterinary anesthesia as a member of the faculty

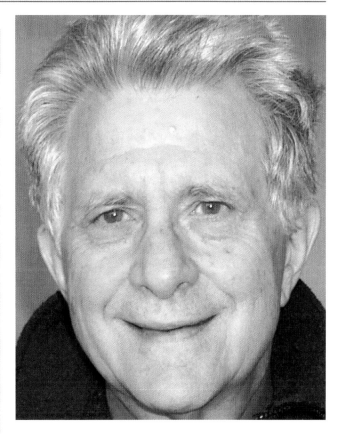

Fig. 23.4 Lawrence Soma. (Courtesy of Lawrence Soma.)

spent 2 years in research at Walter Reed Medical Center. During this time, a valuable racing thoroughbred at Penn's veterinary hospital required major surgery. The then Veterinary Medicine Dean, Mark Allam asked Dripps to consult on the anesthetic management of this horse. Dripps reportedly replied,

> "Thank you for inviting me but I can't do anything. You need a veterinarian trained in anesthesia! You select him and I'll train him."

In 1960, after completing his army service, Soma phoned Robert Marshak, then Chair of the Department of Clinical Studies, asking if he had any vacant positions. "Marshak replied, 'Go see Dripps'." Soma did, and the rest is history. Upon completion of training with Dripps, Soma joined the veterinary faculty at Penn with the charge by Allam to develop anesthesia as a distinct discipline in the veterinary

school; the first such program in the world. He published his *Textbook of Veterinary Anesthesia* in 1971, with contributions by Dripps and 11 other prominent anesthesiologists. Others quickly followed Soma's lead (Table 23.1).

Two of the earliest individuals helping to create veterinary anesthesiology as a discipline in North America, established their credentials in anesthesia to improve the quality of their results as surgeons. The first, William Lumb, was an established veterinary surgeon who directed a National Institutes of Health funded surgical training/research laboratory, at the veterinary school at Colorado State University, beginning in 1963. In 1963, he also published the first US veterinary anesthesia text, *Small Animal Anesthesia*, and then, with co-author E Wynn "Ginger" Jones, published a broader species based text, *Veterinary Anesthesia* in 1973. E. Wynn Jones qualified at the RVC in London and then came to Cornell University, for advanced clinical training in large animal surgery and completion of an anesthesia-related PhD dissertation. In 1954, he was offered and accepted a faculty post in large animal surgery in the veterinary college at Oklahoma State University. Research with disease-free swine at Oklahoma in the early 1970s involved him in early studies of the pathogenesis of malignant hyperthermia (MH), and subsequent development of a susceptible strain of swine for use as a model. Jones and Lumb are Charter Diplomates of both the American College of Veterinary Surgeons (est. 1967),

Table 23.2 First Generation Veterinary Anesthesiologists Outside the US

Year[a]	Veterinarian	Country	Institution
1951	Leslie Hall	UK	Royal Vet College & Cambridge U
1951	Barbara Weaver	UK	Royal Vet College, & Bristol U
1962	Ron Jones	UK	University of Liverpool
1969	Don Turner	Australia	University of Sydney.
1969	Mike Rex	New Zealand & Australia	Massey University,
1971	Urs Schatzmann	Switzerland	University of Berne
1971	Evert Lagerweij	Netherlands	University of Utrecht
1974	Ives Moens	Belgium,	University of Ghent,
1976	Flavio Massone	Brazil	UNESP, Campus of Botucatu
1977	Len Cullen	Australia	University of Perth
1979	Dimitris Raptopoulos	Greece	University of Thessaloniki
1988	F. Tendillo	Spain	Complutense University, Madrid
1988	I. Gomez de Segura	Spain	Complutense University, Madrid
1989	J. Curz Madorran	Spain	University of Zaragoza
1994	Carlos Valadao	Brazil	UNESP, Campus of Jaboticabal
1996	Firmino Marsico	Brazil	Fluminense Federal U (Rio de Janerio)

[a] Year (approximate) starting as faculty in veterinary anesthesiology at the indicated institution

and the American College of Veterinary Anesthesiologists (more on this below).

Some others during this time established credentials in other ways. Following his Comparative Pathology PhD program at the University of California, Davis (UCD), JR Gillespie completed a respiratory disease fellowship at the Cardiovascular Research Institute of the University of California, San Francisco. He then returned to UCD in 1965, to establish the first clinical teaching program in respiratory system physiology/pathophysiology, and the first pulmonary function laboratory in a school of veterinary medicine. He set the stage for the later anesthesia program at UCD. For approximately the first decade of his career after his postdoctoral training in neurosciences, Jim Heavner worked with Rudy DeJong at the University of Washington, investigating basic and clinical actions of local anesthetics.

At this time, individuals dedicated to veterinary anesthesia appeared in Western Europe and other parts of the world (Table 23.2).

1980–to Date

Growth of new university-based programs in the US and UK paralleled the growth in numbers of veterinary anesthesiolo-

gists. Before 1960 in North America, no veterinarians were recognized as anesthesiologists, and no academic anesthesia programs existed in veterinary medicine. Both Lumb and Jones were surgeons. However, by the beginning of 1980, 25 faculty positions were assigned to teaching and research programs in colleges and schools of veterinary medicine in the US, and there were 2 in Canada.

Veterinary schools now add courses in anesthesia to both core and elective curricula. For example, the DVM curriculum at the University of California at Davis mandates an introductory 15 hours of lectures, 2 laboratory sessions on principles of veterinary anesthesia at the end of the second year, and a laboratory course on applied techniques of anesthesia at the beginning of the third year. In the third year it also mandates at least one of 3 species-specific elective courses, and the fourth year requires a 2-week clinical rotation in anesthesia.

A parallel growth in postgraduate professional training in veterinary anesthesia occurred. For example, beginning in 1966 as a single 2-year residency position in anesthesia at the University of Pennsylvania (held by Alan Klide, with Soma as director), by the 1980s there were 16 positions throughout North America. Five of the then 11 postgraduate clinical training programs, progressed from 2 year to 3 year training programs. This timing did not include a pre-residency internship year requirement after obtaining the DVM/VMD degree. According to American College of Veterinary Anesthesiologists (ACVA; described below) records, in 2010 there are 46 individuals at various stages of training, within 20 residency programs in North America (16 in US and 4 in Canada).

Organizations of Veterinary Anesthesiology

The first formal society of veterinary anesthesia was the Association of Veterinary Anaesthetists (AVA; until 1991 it was the AVA of Great Britain and Ireland). The constitution of the AVA paralleled the Constitution of the Association of Anaesthetists of Great Britain and Ireland (AAGBI), and was written with the assistance of physician colleagues active in the AAGBI. The first general AVA meeting was held in 1964, and bi-annual meetings of the association followed with increasing national and international attendance. By 1968, there were 46 members of whom 9 were Corresponding Members including those from North America. Postgraduate specialist qualifications were subsequently established and recognized by the Royal College of Veterinary Surgeons, with particular enthusiasm and encouragement from William Weipers. The AVA awarded the first Diploma of Veterinary Anaesthesia (DVA) in 1967. Weaver has prepared a detailed account of the formative years of the AVA [31].

On January 1995, the European College of Veterinary Anaesthesia and Analgesia (ECVAA) was incorporated, and

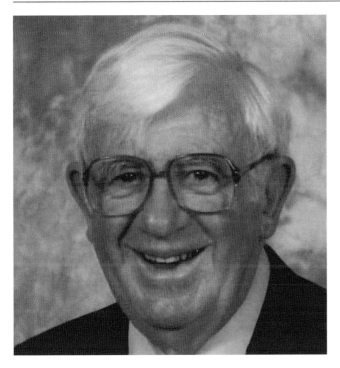

Fig. 23.5 Charles Short. (Courtesy of Charles Short.)

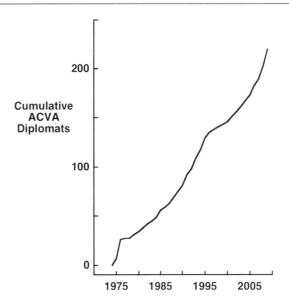

Fig. 23.6 ACVA Diplomate numbers progressively increased since the inception of the examination process

was registered in the Netherlands in May 1997. The ECVAA regulates the standards of specialization in veterinary anesthesia and certified specialists in Europe. The DVA was phased out because the Diploma of the ECVAA became the primary route for certification as a specialist in veterinary anesthesia. The AVA evolved into an organization focused on regional political issues, organized scientific meetings for the specialty, and supported educational opportunities.

The American Society of Veterinary Anesthesiology (ASVA), with Charles Short (Fig. 23.5) as first president, was founded in 1970, and was immediately recognized as a professional society by the American Veterinary Medical Association (AVMA). In 1971, President Larry Soma appointed an ad hoc committee to investigate the establishment of a specialist college, the American College of Veterinary Anesthesiologists (ACVA), that would credential specialists in veterinary anesthesiology. The AVMA Executive Board recognized the ACVA in 1975, with JC Thurmon serving as the College's inaugural 2-term president. Because two organizations were not sustainable at the time, the ASVA was dissolved in 1981. Seven Founding Charter Diplomates and 13 additional Charter Diplomates attended the first ACVA meeting. The number of awardees progressively increased (Fig. 23.6) [32]. To date there are 222 ACVA diplomates and 16 approved residency programs of veterinary anesthesiology in the US, and 4 approved in Canada. In 2010, in the US and Canada, 41 and 5 individuals respectively, are training in these graduate clinical programs.

The World Congress of Veterinary Anaesthesiology (WCVA), was established in 1985 (changed from the International Congress of Veterinary Anesthesia in 2004) "…to promote veterinary anaesthesiology within the international community of veterinarians, through…triennial World Congresses of Veterinary Anaesthesiology". Hall was the inaugural president. Nine World Congresses followed the first Congress in Cambridge, England, with 4 subsequently hosted in Europe, 3 in North America, and 1 each in Australia and South America.

Reprise

The history of veterinary anesthesia has paralleled but lagged behind that of anesthesia for human patients (Fig. 23.7). The two have been intimately intertwined, each contributing to the advancement of the other. The introduction of veterinary anesthesia was delayed by the misperception that the induction of anesthesia in animals was painful—and unnecessary—one needed but to hobble the animal. Fortunately this misperception gave way to reality, and led to the governmental demand for the application of anesthesia to relieve the pain of surgery in animals. The conduct of anesthesia in animals today, as does surgery in animals, is remarkably similar to that in humans, particularly in the US, Great Britain, and Europe.

Acknowledgments I particularly acknowledge S Allweiler, RB Heath, S Luna, I Segura, LR Soma, and BMQ Weaver who supplied their first hand knowledge of names, locations and activities for this essay. Special thanks to RS Jones for my repeated botherings, and Dennis Sylvain for timely and accurate library searches.

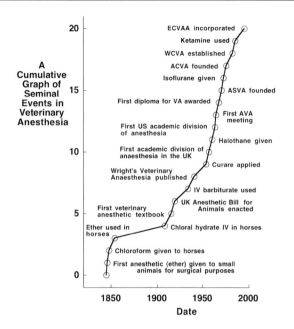

Fig. 23.7 A graphic representation of the history of veterinary anesthesia suggests immediate parallels to progress in anesthesia in humans

References

1. Hall LW. Anesthesiology. In: Brandly CA, Jungherr EL, Editors. Advances in Veterinary Science. 3. ed. Academic Press, New York, 1957. pp. 1–32.
2. Smithcors JF. The early use of anaesthesia in veterinary practice. Brit vet J. 1957;113:284–91.
3. Smithcors JF. History of veterinary anesthesia. In: Soma LR, Editor. Textbook of veterinary anesthesia. 1. ed. Williams & Wilkins, Baltimore, 1971. pp. 1–23.
4. Stevenson DE. The evolution of veterinary anaesthesia. Brit Vet J. 1963;119:477–83.
5. Wright JG. Anaesthesia in animals: a review. Vet Rec. 1964;76:710–3.
6. Westhues M, Fritsch R. Introduction: history of general anaesthesia. In: Westhues M, Fritsch R, Editors. Animal anaesthesia. 1st English ed. Lippincott, Philadelphia, 1965. pp. xiii–xxi.
7. Weaver BMQ. The history of veterinary anesthesia. Vet History. 1988;5:43–57.
8. Jones RS. A history of veterinary anaesthesia. An vet (Murcia). 2002;18:7–15.
9. Larsen LH. Recent advances in anaesthesia. Aust Vet J. 1952;28:323–32.
10. Jackson CT. Etherization of animals. Report of the Comissioner of Patents for the Year of 1853. 1853, 59. 1853. Washington, D.C., Beverly Tucker Senate Printer. Ref Type: Report.
11. Merillat LA. The principles of veterinary surgery. Chicago: Alexander Eger; 1915.
12. Dadd GH. The modern horse doctor. Boston: J.P. Jewett; 1854.
13. Wright JG. Anaesthesia and narcosis in the horse. Vet Rec. 1958;70:329–36.
14. Liautard A. Manual of operative veterinary surgery. New York: Sabiston & Murray; 1892.
15. Hobday FTG. Anaesthesia & narcosis of animals and birds. Chicago: Alexander Eger; 1915.
16. Wright JG. Veterinary anaesthesia. Chicago: Alexander Eger; 1941.
17. Kreutzer RH. The use of nembutal in small animal practice. Vet Med. 1931;26:524–5.
18. Wright JG, Oyler M. Nembutal anaesthesia in the dog. Vet Rec. 1934;14:1463–71.
19. Wright JG, Oyler M. Some aspects of general anaesthesia in animals. Vet Rec. 1935;15:1223–30.
20. Wright JG. The use of a new, short-acting barbiturate—pentothal sodium—as a general anesthetic in canine surgery. Vet Rec. 1937;49:27–9.
21. Bemis HE, Guard WF, Covault CH. Anesthesia, general and local. J Am Vet Med Assoc. 1924;64:413–39.
22. Farquharson J. Paravertebral lumbar anesthesia in the bovine species. J Am Vet Med Assoc. 1940;97:54.
23. Larson LL. The internal pudendal (pudic) nerve block for anesthesia of the penis and relaxation of the retractor penis muscle. J Am Vet Med Assoc. 1953;123:18–27.
24. Fisher EW, Jennings S. A closed circuit anaesthetic apparatus for adult cattle and for horses. Vet Rec. 1957;69:769–71.
25. Weaver BMQ. An apparatus for inhalation aneaesthesia in large animals. Vet Rec. 1960;72:1121–5.
26. Griffith HR, Johnson GE. The use of curare in general anesthesia. Anesthesiology. 1942;3:418.
27. Hall LW, Weaver BMQ. Some notes on balanced anaesthesia for the dog and cat. Vet Rec. 1954;66:289–93.
28. Soma LR. Textbook of veterinary anesthesia. Baltimore: Williams & Wilkins Co.; 1971.
29. Hall LW. Wright's veterinary anaesthesia and analgesia. London: Bailliére Tindall; 1971.
30. Lumb WV, Jones EW. Veterinary anesthesia. Philadelphia:Lea & Febiger; 1973.
31. Weaver BMQ, Hall LW. Origin of the association of veterinary anaesthetists—editorial. Vet Anaesth Analg. 2005;32:179–83.
32. Website, American College of Veterinary Anesthesiologists. The History of the American College of Veterinary Anesthesiologists. ACVA.org. Accessed: 17. Jun. 2009.

The History of Anaesthesia in Australia and New Zealand

Rod N. Westhorpe

Summary

Before Europeans arrived in Australia and New Zealand, neither of the indigenous peoples, aborigines or Maori, used any form of anaesthesia. The news of anaesthesia arrived in Britain's furthest colonies in May 1847. Australians William Pugh and John Belisario independently gave ether on 7 June 1847. In New Zealand, an instrument maker gave the first surgical anesthetic on 27 September 1847. Chloroform arrived in 1848. Portable and non-flammable, it was the ideal agent in a country of widely scattered rural communities. In the late 1870s, the risks inherent to chloroform became increasingly apparent and ether and nitrous oxide replaced chloroform.

By the end of the 19th century, physicians administered most anaesthetics. The lowly status of anaesthetists limited the attraction of young doctors to the specialty. Not until 1934, did Geoffrey Kaye convene a meeting in Hobart to found the Australian Society of Anaesthetists (ASA). Kaye assisted in the founding of the New Zealand Society in 1948.

Anaesthesia training until the1940s consisted largely of observing senior anaesthetists. In 1944, a diploma course began at Sydney University, followed by another at Melbourne University in 1946. 1946 also saw publication of "Anaesthetic Methods" the most important anaesthesia textbook in Australia and New Zealand.

In 1952, the Faculty of Anaesthetists, Royal Australasian College of Surgeons was inaugurated, and examinations began in 1956. Successful candidates became Fellows and could claim the specialist status accorded by the post-nominals FFARACS. The Faculty Fellowship soon replaced the diplomas as defining the position of the specialist anaesthetist. Over the next fifty years non-specialist anaesthetists gradually disappeared, except for remote rural communities. In 1994, the Faculty separated from the College of Surgeons, and became a College in its own right, the Australian and New Zealand College of Anaesthetists. In 2011, there were 4000 Fellows of the College.

The ASA initiated publication of Anaesthesia and Intensive Care in 1972. In ensuing years it became and presently continues as a major international journal. In 1996, the ASA hosted the largest medical congress ever held in the southern hemisphere, the World Congress of Anaesthesiologists, in Sydney. In Australia and New Zealand, doctors administer all anaesthetics. They have established a proud tradition of safety and quality care.

Pain Relief Before Anaesthesia

Excluding indigenous aborigines, the 1847 population of Australia was around 300,000. Most lived in New South Wales (NSW) or Tasmania, and consisted of settlers, convicts transported from Britain, and government and military personnel. No accurate record indicates the number of aborigines. Bringing diseases and weapons, the European pioneers had decimated the aborigines, and by 1847 the number of aborigines in NSW had declined from an estimated 50,000 to 20,000. In New Zealand, the indigenous Maori outnumbered the 14,000 settlers 5 to 1. The great gold rush had not yet begun.

Pain relief before European settlement was rudimentary. Neither the aborigines nor the Maori conducted surgery except for tribal rituals—circumcision, skin scarification and tattooing, all without pain relief. They did however, use some plant preparations for relief of toothache, arthritis (a common complaint), and other ailments. They also had access to a drug, "pituri", that produced mild euphoria, enabling them to endure strenuous activity for long periods.

Aboriginal medicine was closely linked to their culture and beliefs—the "dreamtime", and their knowledge of the land and its flora and fauna. Many aboriginal bush medicines contained pharmacologically active compounds, but none produced anaesthesia. There were no measured doses or specific times of treatment. Since most were applied externally, there was little danger of toxicity [1].

The most widely known aboriginal herbal preparation is "pituri". Joseph Banks, the botanist accompanying Cook

R. N. Westhorpe (✉)
Melbourne, Australia
e-mail: westhorpe@netspace.net.au

on his voyage of 1770 *"...observed that some, tho few, held constantly in their mouths, the leaves of an herb which they chewd as a European does tobacco or an East Indian Betele. What sort of plant it was, we had not an opportunity of learning...[2]."*

When the starving John King, only survivor of the ill-fated Burke and Wills expedition to central and northern Australia, was rescued in 1861, he had Wills' diary. It told how aborigines had fed them fish, bread and a

> *"stuff they call bedgery or pedgery; it has a highly intoxicating effect when chewed even in small quantities. It appears to be the dried stems and leaves of some shrub".* King described it as *"nasty dirty-looking balls of chewed grass (producing) much the same effect as two pretty stiff nobblers of brandy."* [2, 3]

Joseph Bancroft immigrated to Brisbane from England in 1864, becoming the first resident surgeon at Brisbane Hospital. He studied the use of native plants in medicine, introducing many into his practice *"thanks to the beneficent rule of this colony (Queensland), where no law prevents professional men from experimenting...."* He found that infusions of minute amounts of pituri caused respiratory arrest and death in frogs, rats, cats and dogs [3, 4].

Duboisia hopwoodii and species of *Nicotiniana* supplied the active ingredient of pituri, *d-nornicotine*. Its use was generally confined to adult men, and its preparation and source were jealously guarded. Only men whose beards were grey were taught the secret of preparation [5].

The then small and scattered population of Australia/New Zealand merited little surgery. William Bland, a former naval surgeon, had been sentenced to seven years penal servitude in Australia after killing a fellow naval officer in a duel. Arriving in Sydney in 1814, he was pardoned almost immediately by Governor Macquarie because of the urgent need for qualified doctors in the colony [6]. In 1832, Bland attempted to ligate a subclavian artery aneurysm on William Mullen, a convict. Mullen's wife had paid Bland the princely sum of 20 pounds. The patient died after 18 days, presumably from infection. Bland attempted another operation in 1837, the patient remaining on the operating table for five and a half hours [6].

The News of Anaesthesia Arrives

The news of Morton's 16 October 1846 demonstration spread to England within a few weeks of the momentous event, coming as a personal letter aboard the *Acadia*, which left Boston on December 2, arriving in Liverpool on December 16. From there, in 100 days, the news journeyed to Australia and New Zealand, arriving in March 1847. Ironically, in both Australia and New Zealand, reports of anaesthesia rated only minor mention in newspapers [7].

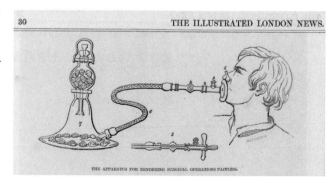

Fig. 24.1 Diagram from the 9 January 1847, issue of The Illustrated London News, showing the apparatus used for several anaesthetics in London during December, 1846. Both Belisario and Pugh are said to have copied their apparatus from this diagram. (Courtesy of R. Westhorpe.)

The news could have come directly to Sydney from Boston. The *Robert Pulsford* sailed from Boston on 21 October, just five days after Morton's demonstration, reaching Sydney on 5 February 1847. She carried the latest Boston newspapers, but no reports, either from them or by word of mouth from crew or passengers, appeared in local newspapers. The British admiralty regulated the transport of cargo to and from Australian ports under the English Navigation Laws of 1651, in order to keep out the Dutch. Non-British ships were unwelcome in Australian and New Zealand waters, and the *Robert Pulsford* was one of only two American ships to visit in 1847. No, the news had to come circuitously from Britain [7].

On 21 December 1846, Robert Liston performed painless surgery in London, and English Newspapers published news of Morton's discovery. The *Mount Stuart Elphinstone* left England on 23 December carrying Bell's Weekly Messenger of 21 December, describing anaesthesia. The ship reached Sydney Cove on 28 April 1847, afterwards proceeding to New Zealand. Sydney newspapers made no mention of anaesthesia, apparently sceptical or thinking little of the news. The Maitland Mercury in Stroud, 130 miles away, thought differently and published an account on 8 May [7].

More ships came with published articles, and from 17 May, major newspapers extracted details from various English publications. Taking from the *Lancet* of 2 January, the *Illustrated London News* of 9 January described the apparatus that Francis Boott used to supply ether (Fig. 24.1). This led to the first anaesthetics in Australia.

The "January Mail" for New Zealand reached Wellington on board the *Waterwitch*, on 4 July, 1847. On 7 July, the Wellington Independent reported *"It appears by the London papers that the use of Sulphuric Aether, inhaled by vapour, by patients about to undergo painful operations, has reduced them to a state of unconsciousness while the operations were performed. Cases are given in which the most serious operations were performed without causing pain to the patient".*

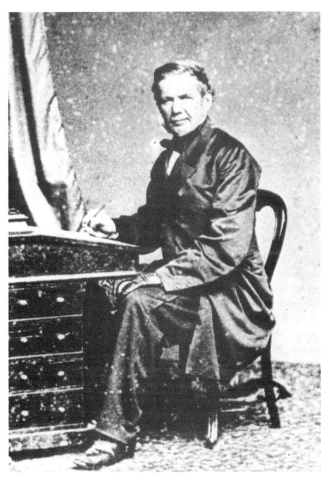

Fig. 24.2 William Pugh, general practitioner of Launceston, Tasmania, who administered ether for 2 surgical operations, on 7 June 1847. (Courtesy Geoffrey Kaye Museum of Anaesthetic History, Australian and New Zealand College of Anaesthetists, Melbourne.)

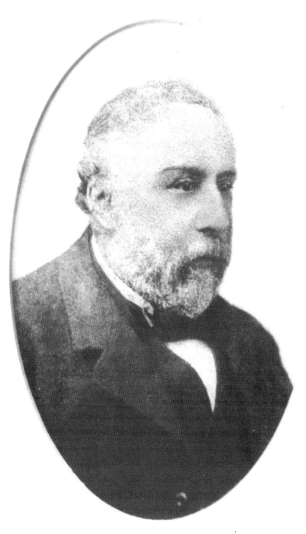

Fig. 24.3 John Belisario, dentist of Sydney, who used ether for dental extractions on 7 June 1847. (Courtesy Geoffrey Kaye Museum of Anaesthetic History, Australian and New Zealand College of Anaesthetists, Melbourne.)

The First Anaesthetics in Australia

On 7 June 1847, William Pugh (Fig. 24.2) administered ether for surgery in Launceston, Tasmania, and John Belisario (Fig. 24.3) gave ether for dentistry in Sydney. Both Pugh and Belisario based their apparatus on the sketch in the Illustrated London News. In the Sydney Morning Herald, 8 June, 1847, below a list of auction sales, there appeared: *"Painless Surgery—We had an opportunity yesterday of witnessing, at Mr Belisario's, the extraction of teeth from persons who had inhaled ether, and in two cases the effect was as described in recent papers from England, almost miraculous…."*

Further, on 16 June, the Herald published:

"…In the first case, a Mr Yarrow inhaled by means of a tube communicating with a vessel containing the ether, until from the entire relaxation of his whole frame, and the deathly expression of his physiognomy, we began to apprehend that the proceedings were taking a turn towards manslaughter, and that our curiosity was leading us into a scrape. As soon as Mr Yarrow was fairly off, as it was called; that is, as soon as his eyes closed,

his arms dropped and his body fell back as he sat…the tube was withdrawn from his mouth, and several persons in the room proceeded to satisfy their curiosity upon the patient, each in his own way. One pinched him in the arm, another in the leg, a third squeezed the top knuckle joints of the patient's hand violently together…but the patient gave no sign whatever of the sensation."

The report continues: *"….He concluded by asking like Oliver Twist 'for more', which however was not given to him, as another patient stepped in…"* This patient had two painful decayed stumps removed while under the influence of ether, and interestingly, *"he had on a previous occasion undergone…extraction under the ether application…."* When and where had this patient had his previous anaesthetic? Was it in Sydney, or in England—the mystery remains?

Pugh probably obtained the 'Illustrated London News' on 29 May via coach from Hobart where the *Lady How-*

den had berthed on 27 May. This gave him time to prepare the ether and apparatus, and plan the surgery. He also had willing patients who had previously undergone unsuccessful attempts at surgery. He proceeded to give two successful ether anaesthetics at St John's Hospital, in the presence of an audience that included the editor of the Launceston Examiner.

So, both Belisario and Pugh gave anaesthetics on 7 June 1847, but who was first? Belisario may have used ether previously, but no record has been discovered. He reportedly performed anaesthesia on 40 patients by 9th June, his successes leading him to advertise his services in the newspaper. David Thomas performed anaesthesia in Melbourne on 2 August, followed by Benjamin Kent in Adelaide on 30 September.

The First Anaesthetic in New Zealand

The first anaesthetic in New Zealand took place on 27 September 1847. That morning, Dr. John Fitzgerald and Mr. James Marriott went to the Wellington Gaol, *"where a prisoner was anxious to have a decayed tooth extracted"*. Marriott was an engraver with a talent for constructing mathematical and scientific instruments. He had constructed an inhaler for ether, although the particulars are not known [8]. Marriott administered the ether, and Fitzgerald extracted the tooth. That afternoon, Fitzgerald removed a fibromatous lesion of the shoulder from Hiangarere, a Maori chief, at the Colonial Hospital. Marriott was the anaesthetist, and several Maori tribesmen observed the operation [8].

Good News?

Was anaesthesia welcomed? Recall that the public in general and the medical profession in particular, considered that pain and surgery were inseparable partners.

On 7 June, Pugh wrote to the recently established *Australian Medical Journal* which published his letter on 18 June:

"As it may be of interest to your readers to receive local testimony in addition to the published reports of cases, in which surgical operations have been divested of the usual suffering attendant on such procedures by the use of ethereal inhalation, I beg to furnish you with the results of a trial of this novel discovery made at St John's Hospital today, the results which, although to a certain extent incomplete, were so far so satisfactory as to justify an opinion that large amount of suffering hitherto experienced by the patients may be superseded, and that many operations can be performed during the stage of unconsciousness which is so readily induced."

"I employed part of Nooth's apparatus in the manner delineated in the illustrated London News of the 9th (January) and I found it in every respect suited to the purpose."

The Journal responded with a long editorial that included: *"...we have no hesitation in predicting for this process a transient popularity. It will have its day, ultimately to be abandoned as useless and/or injurious...."*

The editor's stance mellowed modestly in the next issue:

"Since our last publication, accounts of the effects of the sulphuric ether inhalation have poured in upon us from all quarters; and loud have been the blowing of trumpets and great the jubilation and overwhelming the nonsense uttered and invited thereupon...it may for a time serve interested parties as a medium for puffing themselves and for mystifying the public by enveloping the matter in a cloud of pseudo-scientific balderdash; but the simple fact is, that to inhale the sulphuric ether is neither more nor less than a mode of getting drunk;"

"Do not let us be misunderstood. We do not say that it ought entirely to be eschewed; all we contend for is that it should be used not indiscriminately, but with caution; and only under the superintendence of medical practitioners, who, instead of allowing themselves to be run away with by the novelty of the process, should use it and investigate its effects coolly and philosophically, so that it may not, if calculated to be really useful, come as many other therapeutic means have come to a premature end through the discredit thrown upon it by its abuse...."

Chloroform or Ether?

Ether was the sole anaesthetic used in Australia, until chloroform arrived. On 31 March 1848, the Sydney Morning Herald reported:

"We have now to state that a new anaesthetic agent has been discovered by Professor Simpson of Edinburgh. It is a substance called chloroform. It is applied similarly to ether, that is to say, the patient is made to inhale it, and the advantages over ether are so great, that it is said the latter will be entirely superseded."

On 12 April, 1848, the following report was published:

"Chloroform. This new agent, for rendering the operations of surgery painless, was yesterday, in the presence of some visitors, most successfully tried by the Surgeons of the Sydney Infirmary. The subject, a little girl had to submit to a most tedious, difficult and hitherto excruciating operation. Dr McEwan operated, Mr Nathan administered the anaesthetic."

The Sydney Hospital surgeon who administered the anaesthetic was Charles Nathan, who had assisted Belisario in the first ether anaesthetics the previous year. Chloroform soon displaced ether as the agent of choice.

Gold was discovered in Victoria on 10 June 1851. By 1860, the non-indigenous population had more than doubled to exceed one million. Hundreds of the new settlers practiced medicine, many without qualifications. Most surgery was performed in makeshift surroundings, and chloroform was the most suitable anesthetic. Anesthesia required a dropper bottle, a handkerchief and a small volume of sweet smelling chloroform. And chloroform didn't catch fire, a particular advantage in a tent.

The first patient death under chloroform was reported just three months after its introduction to Australia [7]. It was not until the late 1870s, that ether challenged the dominance of chloroform, and until 1900, the word "chloroformist" was synonymous with "anaesthetist". Chloroform had other uses. An entry in the 20 September 1848 issue of the Sydney Morning Herald says "Chloroform is recommended as excellent for scolding wives. A husband who has tried it says— 'No family should be without it'".

William Purdie, one of Simpson's classmates, brought the benefits of chloroform to New Zealand. Purdie had been a regular attendee at meetings of the Obstetrical Society in Edinburgh, where he had commenced practice. Having arrived in New Zealand in late 1849, with a supply of chloroform, he set up practice in Dunedin [8].

Nitrous Oxide

Nitrous oxide emerged as an alternative, for dental surgery in particular, at about the same time as the re-emergence of ether. It must have been known in the early scientific circles of the colonies. In the Sydney Morning Herald of Monday, 21 July 1845, JS Norrie advertised his lecture on chemistry that evening on *"The simple substances and the metals. At the conclusion of the lecture the effect of the laughing gas will be exhibited."*

There is no further reference to the use of nitrous oxide until Colin Buchanan of Port Stephens, wrote in July 1847 of his administration of ether for the repair of a popliteal aneurysm. He wrote "...*not being aware of the kind of apparatus used for the inhalation of ether, I tried the simple bladder with mouthpiece, similar to what is used in the inhalation of nitrous oxide, or laughing gas, which answered the purpose admirably (I must tell you that I first tried it on myself, which convinced me as to its efficacy)."* We presume that Buchanan used nitrous oxide for recreational purposes [7].

Recreational use of nitrous oxide appears in a contribution to the NSW Medical Gazette, a letter perhaps stimulated by the introduction of nitrous oxide into dental practice around 1870:

"Gentlemen... perhaps it would interest some of your readers to know the effects (nitrous oxide) produced upon me when taken on two different occasions, several years back. I inhaled it first in Sydney, at the residence of one of my friends.

"I had breathed about three quarts when the landlady of the house entered the room, and looked in an angry manner at me, to reprove me for being so ridiculous as to have the opening of a bullock's bladder in my mouth, like the figures in an old fashioned caricature; this look and the gas together caused me to have a violent fit of laughing; I laughed in the chair that I was

sitting on, then I fell on the floor and rolled over and over on the ground still laughing, and this state lasted about five minutes. I then recovered perfectly without any unpleasant after-effects. I believe however, I made an enemy of my friend's landlady ever-afterwards as she never spoke to me again."

"I am, gentlemen, yours sincerely, A subscriber." Sydney August 20th 1870 [9]

In his *"History of Dentistry in South Australia 1836–1936"* Arthur Chapman writes that in the 1850s *"the introduction of laughing gas must have been greatly appreciated by those able to avail themselves of it* [10]*."* This presumably also refers to recreational use, because Chapman describes Lionel Blackmore, who arrived in Adelaide in 1870, as probably the first to use nitrous oxide for dental anaesthesia in Adelaide. The Sydney Morning Herald of 24 October 1870, reported that *"Mr E Reading, Dentist, 128 Phillip Street, administers the nitrous oxide gas on Tuesday, Wednesday, Thursday and Friday."* By the end of the 1870s, Chapman notes that *"we find gold, platinum and vulcanite in use for artificial denture bases, and nitrous oxide gas largely employed for extractions* [10]*."*

The Australian Medical Gazette was the first Australian journal to include an article on nitrous oxide anaesthesia, in 1870 reprinting a paper from the 1869 *Lancet* by Charles Fox, Dental Surgeon to the Dental Hospital in London. Having learnt techniques from Gardner Colton, his paper extolled the virtues of nitrous oxide anaesthesia, citing his experience of its administration to M. Blondin for *"extremely severe dental operations"* whereupon the patient *"performed all his most difficult feats on the high rope 430 feet long within three hours after I had given him the gas* [11]*."*

The NSW Medical Gazette of 1871 noted in the "Miscellanea" section, that nitrous oxide was likely to supersede chloroform for short operations [12]. However, for the remainder of the nineteenth century, medical journals scarcely mention nitrous oxide, although it continued to be used regularly by dentists (Fig. 24.4).

The Adelaide based FH Faulding and Company, a pharmaceutical company founded in 1845, published Faulding's Medical Journal.[1] The quasi-scientific journal of news and reviews of scientific papers included advertisements for dental anaesthesia such as the *"New York Dental Institute"* of Grenfell Street, Adelaide, offering in the May 1900 edition *"teeth extracted painlessly with Cocaine, Eucaine, Laughing Gas or Aether* [13]*."*

Evidence of the establishment of local manufacture appears in the British Journal of Dental Science in 1898:

"Australian Nitrous Oxide Gas—In addition to making their own dentists, Australia is beginning to make its own nitrous oxide, for an Australian Nitrous Oxide Gas Company has been

---

[1] FH Faulding and Company was taken over in 2010 by Mayne Group, and following a demerger in 2005, is now part of Symbion Pharmacy Services.

Fig. 24.4 Dental anaesthesia with nitrous oxide, in rural Australia (Colac) C 1900. (Courtesy of R. Westhorpe.)

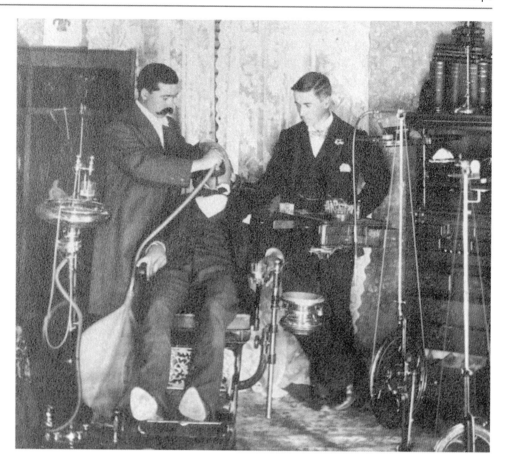

formed and a complete plant for the manufacture of the gas has been imported....The price will be lower than that of the imported gas, as the risk and expense of carriage as deck cargo is avoided, while the cylinders will be of uniform size. Advance Australia!" [14]

No record can be found of an Australian Nitrous Oxide Gas Company. If it was FH Faulding and Company, they didn't mention it in Fauldings' Medical Journal. Still, it is likely that they were manufacturing nitrous oxide by 1900, as they supplied apparatus and pre-filled cylinders according to advertisements in their journal.

Nitrous Oxide in New Zealand Before 1900

The story of nitrous oxide in New Zealand is similar to that in Australia. The December 1878 Napier newspaper reported: *"Our Dentist, Mr H C Wilson, is about to commence the use of nitrous oxide (laughing) gas for producing insensibility to pain during dental operations... we believe that Mr Wilson is the first dentist in the Colonies who has introduced the use of this anaesthetic into his practice: and we must add that we are glad to see Napier taking the initiative in this advance of science."* [15]

Septimus Solomon Arthur Wellington Daniel Myers registered as a Dentist in 1880, and is thought to have intro-

duced nitrous oxide in Invercargill. He then established a dental company in Dunedin, opening a Christchurch branch in 1888 [16].

An issue of stamps in 1893 with advertisements on the back indicates the expansion of nitrous oxide in New Zealand. Denominations ranged from one penny to one shilling, each stamp in a sheet bearing a different advertisement. The one advertising S Myers and Company noted that painless extractions are available using nitrous oxide gas. These stamps were withdrawn soon after issue due to a rumor that the ink, when licked, was injurious to health [16].

Deaths Under Chloroform

By 1870, the words anaesthesia and chloroform were virtually interchangeable. The deaths reported each year from 1848 had little influence on practice [17].

The July 1868 Australian Medical Journal, described a previously healthy 33 year old woman receiving chloroform at the Melbourne Hospital for surgery to her anal fistula and haemorrhoids. In the absence of the resident House Surgeon or Physician, the attending surgeon administered the chloroform. The patient struggled and died shortly thereafter. Although post mortem examination did not reveal the cause of death, kidney disease or impure chloroform was implicated.

It was recommended that the hospital appoint a full-time chloroformist. The proposal went unsupported [18].

In February 1891, the Australian Medical Journal reported another death in a patient receiving chloroform at the Melbourne Hospital with the City Coroner recommending *"...that there ought to be some specially qualified gentleman in the hospital for the administration and teaching of the use of chloroform."* The suggestion was put to the Medical Staff Committee who took no action [19].

In May 1891, a young man of 32 died during chloroform administration at the Melbourne Hospital. The "resuscitation" over 20 minutes included artificial respiration, hypodermic injections of ether, and intravenous ammonia. At inquest, the City Coroner declared that an expert should supervise chloroform administration. *"It appeared to him, that cases of death under chloroform occurred far too frequently at the Melbourne Hospital. Students were allowed to give chloroform without any supervision. The wonder was not that deaths should occasionally occur, but that they did not happen more frequently* [20, 21]."

In an editorial entitled *"Anaesthetics at the Melbourne Hospital"*, the Australian Medical Journal argued for the appointment of a specialist anaesthetist to administer chloroform and other anaesthetics, and to supervise and instruct residents in the practice of anaesthesia. The Melbourne Hospital Medical Staff dealt with the issue by passing motions of confidence in whoever administered the chloroform [22, 23].

At this time, physicians (internists) controlled most medical affairs, with surgeons not far behind and exerting increasing influence. Anaesthetists ranked poorly, anaesthesia being entrusted to junior staff or students. But when things went wrong, it was a problem with the patient or the chloroform, and not the administration or the administrator.

Non-Medical Anaesthetists

Non-medical anaesthetists gave many anaesthetics, particularly in rural Australia. The medical profession condemned such practices but did nothing to remove the problem by advancing the establishment of anaesthesia as a specialty.

In 1884, the Australasian Medical Gazette reported that a patient had died while receiving chloroform at Tamworth Hospital in central NSW. Mr Goodwin, a local chemist, had administered the chloroform. The journal asked why the surgeon, Eustace Pratt, did not use the anaesthetic services of another medical man. In the next issue, Pratt attacked the editor for his audacity, and chastised him for forwarding copies of his editorial to the local Tamworth papers and several prominent citizens. He described how *"hundreds of men, not legally qualified, have to give chloroform in the bush."* He described the Medical Gazette as a moribund and poverty stricken organ of a small clique of mutual admirers [24, 25].

Chloroform was easy to administer with a minimum of equipment. The status of the chloroformist was negligible, and surgeons regarded their anaesthetists as dependents rather than colleagues. Nonetheless, non-medical anaesthetists gradually disappeared, and by 1900, hospital residents or family doctors, gave virtually all anaesthetics. Until the mid-twentieth century, the family doctor who referred a patient to a surgeon would commonly provide the anaesthesia.

1900—The Beginnings of a Specialty

In 1901, the Legislative Council considered a Dental Act which would establish a Board registering Dentists with appropriate qualifications and would permit only those holding the Diploma of one of the American or British Dental Colleges to administer nitrous oxide. In November, Faulding's Medical Journal commented that

> *"it can hardly be claimed that (this) provision has been inserted for the benefit of the public, for it means that to less than one dozen dentists in South Australia is granted the sole right to administer this anaesthetic. The members of this privileged class are all with high class practices, who charge high fees. It is therefore obvious that the poorer classes will be practically denied the comfort and benefit of nitrous oxide when undergoing dental operations..."*

In 1909, four honorary anaesthetists were appointed to the Melbourne Hospital, to instruct and supervise residents. The resident doctors, who covered all disciplines during their work, had to view 20 anaesthetics before attempting one. Although this was a major step forward, the honoraries did not normally attend cases out of hours, when residents provided anaesthetics. This led to a furore after a death in September 1912.

An extremely ill 66-year-old man presented for surgery at 6am. The unfortunate duty resident administered ethyl chloride and ether, whereupon the patient immediately succumbed [26]. One of the honorary anaesthetists, Rupert Hornabrook (Australia's first full-time specialist anaesthetist, and an advocate for the ethyl chloride—ether sequence) made a personal representation to the Coroner, leading to a public enquiry. Hornabrook argued that residents should not have to deal with such cases, and that a senior anaesthetic resident should always be present. He proclaimed, *"Anaesthetic work should be more respected than it was."* The Coroner added fuel to the fire by stating *"there appeared to be a feeling among medical men that the anaesthetist's work was not as necessary as some might think."* The hospital was outraged, claiming that Hornabrook's action was disloyal to the hospital and to the residents [26–28].

In the March 1914 Australian Medical Journal, Hornabrook wrote *"The anaesthetist should be placed on the staffs of hospitals... on equal footing with other members of the staff. It is useless to expect good men to come forward unless they are given some status ."* [29]

But things didn't change. Physicians and surgeons controlled public hospitals. Surgeons depended on referrals from general practitioners in their private practices, and often engaged those practitioners as assistants or anaesthetists. Surgeons may have wanted anaesthetists to provide services, but they were not prepared to give them more than a passing acknowledgement. The traditional relationship between the surgeon and the "chloroformist" was hard to break, and the idea of the surgeon collecting the fee on behalf of the anaesthetist was firmly entrenched.

Thus, competing factors influenced the establishment of specialist anesthetists. There was tacit recognition of the desirability of specialisation, but difficulty in attracting doctors into anaesthesia because of low status and poor remuneration. Their paltry remuneration forced anaesthetists to rely on activities such as general practice to survive. They had no time for research, and they were not unified.

There were exceptions. Edward Embley championed the cause of anaesthetists. He had gained worldwide recognition for determining that the cause of death from chloroform was cardiac and not respiratory [30]. His suburban general practice supported his unpaid weekend research at Melbourne University.

Hornabrook, recognised for his enthusiasm in experimentation (Fig. 24.5) and in teaching anaesthesia, was an outspoken advocate for patients and anaesthetists, and saw the need for anaesthetists to unite. He suggested in the April 1913 Australian Medical Journal, that a Society of Anaesthetists be established [31], also noting that:

> *"....more consideration should be shown by some surgeons towards their patients and the anaesthetist. Some gentlemen seem to have no idea of punctuality—half or three quarters of an hour late in the time of starting an operation seems to be nothing to them, they never appear to think of what that extra half hour or so must mean to the patient, in may cases it must be perfect hell."*

He went on to say how the lateness impacts on staff and other hospital arrangements. His forthright approach is obvious:

> *"On one occasion, after waiting an hour for a well-known surgeon, I walked out of the operating theatre as he walked into it. He remarked that he was ready to start, and I told him that if he was, I was not, and that if he wanted the patient put under an anaesthetic he had better get someone else to do it... ."* [31]

In the May 1914 Australian Medical Journal, he wrote of

> *"Some of the difficulties the anaesthetist has to contend against... One of the greatest difficulties the teacher has to contend with is the inborn idea that any fool can administer an anaesthetic."* He related the remark of a senior Melbourne surgeon that *"a drayman could administer chloroform"* [30]

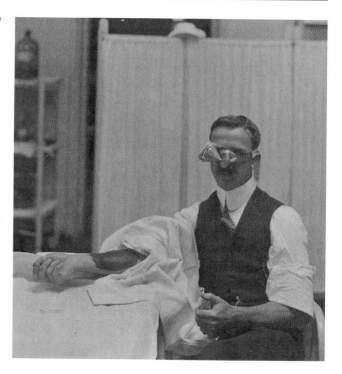

Fig. 24.5 Rupert Hornabrook, self administering ethyl chloride via a nasal inhaler, while submitting himself to an incision in his forearm, followed by suturing. He said pain only occurred during the suturing of the last half inch of the two inch wound, when he became diverted from anesthetic delivery by his conversation with the operator. (Courtesy Geoffrey Kaye Museum of Anaesthetic History, Australian and New Zealand College of Anaesthetists, Melbourne.)

It gets worse:

> *"A few years ago, I was stopped one morning and asked by a surgeon if I was not busy on the following day could I come to a certain private hospital and be present while he did a big abdominal operation. The patient was a lady who had been sent to him by Dr X. Dr X had sent him a case before, and on that occasion he had asked him to assist at the operation; that he had found Dr X to be such a fool at assisting that he had this time asked him to give the anaesthetic."*

> *"For the next few minutes the air was electric"* [30]

The situation did not improve for another 40 years. In 1927, a senior surgeon at the Alfred hospital told Geoffrey Kaye, when contemplating a career in anaesthesia, *"Why waste your opportunities"*. Kaye recalled that anaesthetics was poorly regarded as a specialty, the province of the physically handicapped or those who had failed in other branches of medicine. The surgeons of the day found that the best anaesthetists were the medical orderlies of the 1914 War, *"because those blokes did as they were told"*. [32]

This attitude was not peculiar to Australia and New Zealand. John Lundy recalled in 1946 that "There was a tendency for only those physicians who were incompetent in general practice or in other branches to limit themselves to the practice of anesthesia." [33]

Francis McMechan's Visit

In 1929, only Hornabrook and Fred Green in Melbourne, and Gilbert Brown in Adelaide, were full time anaesthetists. Notwithstanding their limited numbers, they, with several others and the young and enthusiastic Kaye persuaded the Australasian[2] Medical Congress to establish a section of anaesthetics in 1929. Accompanied by his wife, Laurette, Francis McMechan (Fig. 34.3) visited that Congress, having previously written to anaesthetists in Australia and New Zealand, encouraging them to convince the medical establishment to formally recognise anaesthesia. An editorial in the 1930 Australian Medical Journal stated: "The anaesthetist is a specialist in the truest sense. The time has come when he should be recognised as such". The suggestion fell on deaf ears.

Specialisation seemed similarly stalled in New Zealand, although formal instruction in anaesthesia began at the Dunedin School of Medicine in 1892. McMechan visited New Zealand after the 1929 Australasian Medical Congress in Sydney, and it is likely that he further encouraged anaesthetists to join forces. At the February 1930 BMA annual conference in Christchurch, there was a Section of Anaesthesia.[3] The Section of Anaesthesia met again at the 1932 Annual Conference in Auckland. A Society seemed to form but died without trace. In 1949 F Fullerton recalled: *"We elected a President, a Secretary and a Treasurer, and we handed over 5 shillings each as our modest contribution to expenses. Well, if you'll believe me, that was the last we ever heard of the Society. No further meeting was ever called...and I don't know what became of our 5 shillings."* [8]

The Influence of Geoffrey Kaye (1903–1986)

Australia had better luck, but it depended on the 26 year old Kaye, whose enthusiasm for anaesthesia research impressed McMechan. Kaye had a small private income enabling him to travel to England and Germany at the end of 1929, and McMechan convinced Kaye to visit North America. Kaye remembered McMechan's "quite electrifying" description of the American approach to anaesthetics: anaesthetists trained in basic sciences, keeping anaesthesia record charts, and looking after their patients [32].

So in late 1929, Kaye returned to London briefly, as an Honorary research worker at St Thomas' Hospital, before continuing on an extended tour of the US, Canada, and Germany. Prior to returning to Melbourne in early 1931, Kaye took several courses, including one with Elmer McKesson in Toledo, Ohio. McKesson, who trained as a physiologist and became an anaesthetist and manufacturer, advocated clinical measurements. McKesson's technique of rebreathing and secondary saturation after intentional hypoxia from 100% nitrous oxide impressed Kaye who, however, later recognized the dangers of this approach. McKesson induced in Kaye a lifelong interest in engineering and metalwork. Kaye studied regional anaesthesia with Gaston Labat in New York, and spent time with Paul Wood, John Lundy, Wesley Bourne, and Ralph Waters, who more than anyone else shaped and encouraged Kaye's development as a teacher and researcher. Kaye attended anaesthetic society meetings in Canada and the US, including the IARS meeting in New York in October 1930 [32].

On returning to Melbourne, Kaye assumed editorship of the first Australian textbook on anaesthesia. *Practical Anaesthesia* appeared in 1932, the collated work of several anaesthetists at the Alfred Hospital. McMechan wrote the introduction. Kaye joined in the organization of anaesthesia, becoming secretary of the Victorian State Section of Anaesthetics, under the auspices of the British Medical Association. He was instrumental in developing a Section meeting at the 1934 Australasian Medical Congress in Hobart, the venue of the second meeting after the eventful 1929 Sydney meeting. The 1934 Congress was to have been held in Perth in 1932, but the great depression delayed the meeting. With the advantage of his private income, Kaye devoted his energies to correspondence with several anaesthetists preceding the 1934 Congress. He convened a meeting of 6 prominent anaesthetists from various States, together with a local representative of the BMA, at Hadley's Hotel where, in January 1934, the Australian Society of Anaesthetists was born, with Gilbert Brown elected as President, and Kaye as secretary [34, 35].

The first years of the Society were difficult times. Non-anaesthetists did not appreciate the necessity of a separate society; the BMA did not take kindly to the establishment of a group "in opposition" to the State Sections of Anaesthetics; the members of the Executive were idealistic in their expectations of the Society; and the general members struggled to make a living. Nevertheless, Kaye's dogged efforts as secretary ensured that the Society survived.

From 1931 to 1939, while continuing to provide clinical anaesthesia (Fig. 24.6), Kaye published regular "memorandums" on new drugs and subjects of interest, and at least 16 scientific reports. One publication, for which he did not claim authorship, deserves particular mention. The June

---

[2] Australasia refers to Australia and New Zealand, as in the Royal Australasian College of Surgeons.

[3] Until 1962 in Australia, and 1967 in New Zealand, the local medical associations were branches of the British Medical Association.

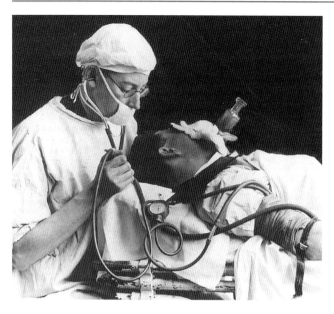

Fig. 24.6 Geoffrey Kaye administering ether, 1932. (Courtesy Geoffrey Kaye Museum of Anaesthetic History, Australian and New Zealand College of Anaesthetists, Melbourne.)

1938 "Anaesthetic Number" of the Medical Journal of Australia included the results of a survey of Anaesthetic fatalities presented at the 1937 Australasian Congress in Adelaide. Kay collated the data from nearly 400,000 anaesthetics at 14 hospitals from around the country, finding a mortality from anaesthesia of 1:1000 [36].

He also designed a demand flow anaesthetic machine, similar in principle to the McKesson. The DM machine was widely used in various forms for many years [37]. In 1938, Kaye again travelled overseas to Europe and America, this time because "it seemed inevitable that Europe was going to be shot up before long." [32]

He went via Canada and the USA, renewing his acquaintance with Waters. Believing he had a mission to complete in Australia, Kaye declined a thinly veiled invitation by Waters to stay in Wisconsin. Had he accepted, anaesthesia in Australia would have been critically altered. In Rochester, he met with Lundy who was jealous that he had visited Waters first. This was an unintentional slight—Kaye had timed his visit to coincide with the meeting of the Anaesthesia Travel Club at the Mayo Clinic.

He visited F Clement in Toledo, who then drove him 800 miles to the IARS Congress in New York where Kaye presented a paper comparing carbon dioxide absorption and positive pressure techniques of gas anaesthesia [32, 34]. McMechan also attended the Congress but was too ill to attend the programme. He summoned Kaye to his room. Kaye gave the following account.

> "He asked me if I knew why I had been so well received…on my previous visit to Europe and North America."

> "I said that I had possibly been a personable young man."

> "No", he said, that was not the reason: I was being "vetted" as his possible successor as Secretary General of the IARS. He indicated the requirements of the post, the incumbent had to be an anaesthetist, internationally known, capable of handling meetings and secretarial work, not at a loss in Congress ante-rooms or in private homes, and fluent in English, French and German."

> "But now", said McMechan, "it will not do. The world is sliding into war. When that war ends, the only country possessed of money will be the United States, and they will want an American Secretary General. Therefore, go back to Australia and do the best you can. If you survive the war, do your best to bring the anaesthetists of the world together again". [34]

World War II Intervenes

World War II deferred progress towards an organised specialist Society, and the ASA went into hibernation as did progress in New Zealand. At the 1946 BMA Conference, a proposal to establish a New Zealand Society revived the New Zealand BMA Section of Anaesthesia. Eric Anson, the director of anaesthesia at Auckland Hospital, led the movement and sought Kaye's advice on the process of establishment. Under the auspices of the BMA, The Society was formally established in 1948, with Anson as the first President [8].

Surgeons and patients appreciated the new intravenous barbiturates and more efficient apparatus developed by the 1940s, but these did not change their perception of the anaesthetist. And perhaps rightly so: There was no formal training or qualifying examination. "You simply followed around after senior anaesthetists and copied their tricks as best you could". [32]

In 1939, Kaye had tried unsuccessfully to convince the President of the Royal Australasian College of Surgeons, of the need for an Australian Diploma in Anaesthetics similar to the British Diploma. In 1943, after serving as advisor to the Australian Army during World War II, Kaye returned to the University of Melbourne University, where he pursued his plans for the establishment of formal training of specialist anaesthetists [34].

Diplomas in Anaesthesia

Kaye sought, and failed, to establish a Diploma conjointly awarded by the Royal Australasian College of Surgeons and the Royal Australian College of Physicians. In 1944 however, the University of Sydney established a DA, and in 1946, the University of Melbourne followed. Kaye wanted the DA to be based in Melbourne, and later claimed that he had really envisaged an inaugural College of Anaesthetists. It was

Fig. 24.7 Geoffrey Kaye lecturing to medical students at Melbourne University, C1950. The first display of his museum collection may be seen in the background. (Courtesy Geoffrey Kaye Museum of Anaesthetic History, Australian and New Zealand College of Anaesthetists, Melbourne.)

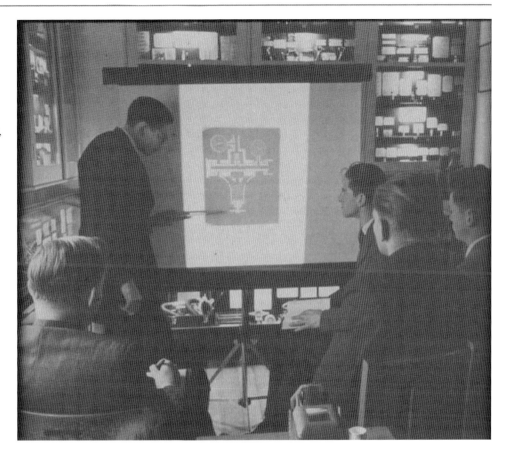

not to be. What eventuated were two DAs in the two major cities of Australia [34].

Kaye threw himself into his teaching responsibilities at the University, supported by newly allocated teaching space, and facilities for a library and museum (Fig. 24.7). On 16 October 1946, the Centenary of Morton's demonstration, Kaye led the celebration of the official opening of his new teaching "Centre" for anaesthesia, in the Physiology Department at the University of Melbourne. With the introduction of the DA in Melbourne, and having got the ASA on its feet, the 43 year-old Kaye resigned as secretary of the Society, believing it time for a "younger man". [34]

1946 also saw the publication of the second Australian textbook on anaesthesia. "Anaesthetic Methods", a popular practical guide for both the specialist and non-specialist anaesthetist was written by Kaye, Orton, and Douglas Renton, all from the Alfred Hospital. The book was dedicated to Waters.

Orton and Renton assumed the task of sorting out the chaos resulting from two different DAs, further complicated by the credentials of anaesthetists who had obtained an English DA or held the FRCS or FRCP [34]. In 1946, the ASA created the Education Subcommittee, which would play a major role in the establishment of the Faculty. Organization of two more subcommittees. International Relationships, and

Standards, quickly followed, and in 1948, the State Sections of the Society were established [34].

The Faculty of Anaesthetists—Early Negotiations

In 1947, as President of the Australian Society, Harry Daly again approached the Royal Australasian College of Surgeons and the Royal Australasian College of Physicians, seeking the creation of a Federal Diploma of Anaesthesia. To no avail. In the meantime, Daly was awarded a Fellowship of the English Faculty on the occasion of its inauguration in 1947. Wishing to accept this honour in person, he and his wife set off to London in 1949 via cargo ship. On returning, their ship docked in Adelaide, and the Dalys stayed for several days with Mary Burnell. A meeting at Burnell's home was arranged with Ivan Jose (later Sir Ivan), a member of the RACS Council. This meeting led to negotiations with the RACS—and ultimately to the establishment of the Australian Faculty of Anaesthetists [34].

In 1949, Kaye travelled to Scandinavia, Great Britain and North America to review anaesthesia training in these countries, and particularly to seek some parity between the Australian DA, or at least one of them, and the English DA. Like Daly, Kaye had been elected to Fellowship of the Faculty of

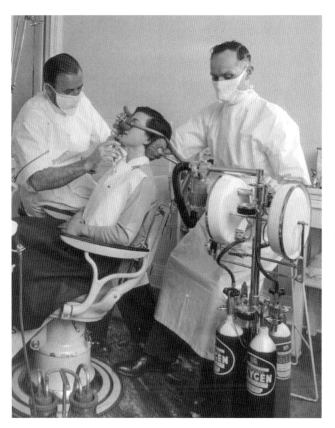

Fig. 24.8 The "DM" or "Dental Midwifery" machine in use, C1950. (Courtesy Geoffrey Kaye Museum of Anaesthetic History, Australian and New Zealand College of Anaesthetists, Melbourne.)

Anaesthetists of the Royal College of Surgeons (England) without examination, giving him some influence. Having sensed dissatisfaction among some members of the new Faculty of the RCS, he returned home with a plan [34].

Kaye's Experiment

Kaye considered that the US led the world in research and organisation, but Britain offered the best clinical anaesthesia. He also believed that the apparatus used in Australia equalled that found elsewhere (Fig. 24.8). [34]

He participated in the negotiations by the Society with the RACS to establish an Australasian Faculty. Renton and Orton, assisted by others on the ASA Executive continued their negotiations with the RACS. By mid 1950, Kaye again became Acting Secretary of the Society, owing to the illness of the incumbent, thrusting him again into the centre of the action. Kaye really wanted a College of Anaesthetists to be established in Melbourne. Behind the scenes he sought a suitable building to house his dream of a "centre" of anaesthesia. At the time, the membership of the Society stood at around 100.

In his retiring address as president of the ASA in 1949, Orton reflected on what would improve the status of anaes-

thesia in Australia: Anaesthetists should be properly trained, with higher qualifications required for senior appointments; and surgeons should be convinced of the advantages of modern anaesthesia. There was one unsaid factor: anaesthetists needed access to larger fees, and payment for public hospital work. Finally, Orton suggested that the anaesthetist should provide preoperative assessment and preparation, intravenous fluid therapy, and postoperative care [38].

The Faculty is Established

In October 1950, the College of Surgeons approved the establishment by the Society of an interim Board of Faculty that would become the Faculty of Anaesthetists. Concurrently, Kaye proposed a "Headquarters" of the Society, the establishment of his dream—a centre of excellence for Australian anaesthesia. Kaye was a man of vision—and incredible optimism. He purchased a substantial property in Melbourne and renovated it, converting the downstairs to include a meeting room, library, museum, laboratory and darkroom, and retaining the upstairs for his accommodation. Robert Macintosh officially opened the Centre in March 1951 [34, 35].

On 25 August1952, the Faculty of Anaesthetists of the Royal Australasian College of Surgeons was inaugurated—in the same week that the ASA held its Annual General Meeting in Kaye's mansion. All were impressed by what they saw, but did they appreciate what it meant? Kaye must have had an inkling that his "experiment" might not succeed: He inserted a clause in the five-year lease to the Society that its extension was at his discretion. Although he continued to arrange scientific meetings and invite overseas speakers, Kaye's mansion primarily became a venue for the monthly meeting of the Victorian Section of the Society. Kaye managed the library and museum, and single-handedly produced the Society newsletter. He wrote some 15 papers for the newsletter for distribution to all members, eg, explosions, oesophageal thermometry, and anaesthesia for snakes. He encouraged young anaesthetists to learn engineering skills, and had them help in the sectioning[4] of apparatus for teaching purposes [35].

The Experiment Fails

The experiment abruptly ended in 1955, when Kaye withdrew the lease. He lamented to his colleague Daly, *"our own members, who tread cigarette ends into the carpets, burn holes in the linoleum, ignore the washing up and generally*

[4] Sectioning refers to the use of a lathe and other engineering equipment to cut apparatus in different planes, so as to demonstrate their internal construction and operation.

leave the place a pigsty when they depart" [35]. He later wrote:

> *"In backing the experiment at "49" (49 Mathoura Road, Toorak), I was gambling in "anaesthesia futures" for heavy stakes. The premises, and their rebuilding for the Society's purposes, cost me £12,000, my entire fluid capital. The scientific equipment which I put into the pool was the collection of years, assembled for such a purpose. The upkeep of house and grounds has absorbed my surplus income for five years, abolishing all freedom of movement. Finally, the Society appeared to hold itself entitled to a blank cheque upon my physical energy".* [35]

Kaye was years ahead of his time, but did not comprehend the needs of the ordinary anaesthetist. The new specialists of the infant specialty in the immediate post war period had young families to support in a new environment. Their goals did not extend to scientific development. In contrast, Kaye, was unmarried and had an independent private income from his father. He "hated private practice". This may reflect his reputation as an anaesthetist, where he had a tendency to exasperate his surgical colleagues by always trying new things.

In 1955, Kaye sold "49" and severed his relationship with anaesthesia. The museum and library were gifted to the Faculty of Anaesthetists at the Royal Australasian College of Surgeons in Melbourne. Only reluctantly did he, in 1958, agree to have his name associated with the museum.

Kaye joined the Department of Electrical Engineering at Melbourne University, where he designed and developed electrometrical equipment. His most ambitious project was the construction of a "Patient Watching Machine" which might monitor multiple parameters, and was reputedly the size of a large refrigerator. In 1965, the university refused to continue funding the project and, despite having contributed $16,000 of his own money into it, he was forced to abandon it.

He shifted to his other passion, collecting objets d'art. However, his own financial status came under threat and he was forced to earn a salary. At the age of 62, he spent some five years working in the development section of Commonwealth Industrial Gases (CIG), the Australian equivalent of the British Oxygen Company (BOC). Once his finances improved, he resumed his passion, establishing a substantial collection of artwork, decorative arts, furniture and tableware.

He became an acknowledged expert on "Old English Glass", "Chinese Monochromes of the 18th Century", and "Antique English Silver". In 1984, at the age of 81, he gave an opening address at the fiftieth anniversary meeting of the Australian Society of Anaesthetists. He died in 1986.

Specialization and Recognition

The establishment of the Australian Society in 1934, the New Zealand Society in 1948; the offering of Diplomas in both Sydney and Melbourne, in 1944 and 1946; and the founding of the Australasian Faculty in 1952, laid foundations for a specialty with status in both Australia and New Zealand.

In the 1950s, despite many enlightened surgeons, especially those involved in the RACS, surgeons and anaesthetists were uneasy partners. Each needed the other, but neither used the benefits of the relationship to enhance the status of anaesthesia. There was a lot of tradition to overcome.

Stuart Marshall, President of the ASA in 1951–1952, and a member of the interim Board of Faculty 1951, wrote *"Problems which surgeons create for anaesthetists"* in the Australian Medical Journal in 1954 [39]. This appeared soon after the first Commonwealth Medical Benefits Schedule, where, as Orton might have predicted, the rebates for surgery services far exceeded those for anaesthesia. They were, of course, based on the fees commonly charged at the time.

> *"The outmoded idea that the anaesthetic is any fool's business still persists, not only in responsible medical circles, but also among hospital authorities, government officials and the public as well. Surgeons in general are apparently not averse to other perpetuation of these anomalies, and thus play a major part in creating serious economic problems for anaesthetists."*

> *"None can deny the enormous benefits of good anaesthesia, yet there are surgeons who seek to preserve a degraded status for anaesthetists; who decry their achievements; who ridicule their knowledge and skill..."*

In concluding the paper Marshall wrote *"Contrary to widespread surgical and lay belief, the acquisition of reasonably comprehensive knowledge and skill in specialised anaesthetics is not a matter of a few weeks training, but of at least two to three years' intensive postgraduate study and practical work. Fortunately many surgeons, both senior and junior, have a lively appreciation of the situation...The recent establishment of the faculty of Anaesthetists of the RACS marks a great step forward in this respect ."* [39] And it indeed it was!

Early Days of the Faculty

The RACS had established an eminent interim Board in January 1951, including Daly, Renton, Len Travers, and Gilbert Troup. Troup, Daly, and Renton had been Presidents of the ASA, Renton in the immediate period leading to the establishment of the faculty. Travers had been a respected surgeon, until a serious skin disorder of his hands ended his surgical career. He then became a skilled anaesthetist who retained a strong influence in surgical circles.

The interim Board, acting under the auspices of the College of Surgeons Council, admitted several Foundation Fellows, and asked for recommendations from each State section of the ASA, and the New Zealand Society. This process caused disquiet, as there were approximately 100 members of the ASA and 60 in the NZSA, but the College Secretary invited only 36 anaesthetists to join the 5 interim Board members as foundation Fellows of the new Faculty. They included Kaye, and Renton was elected as the first Dean.

Having established the list of foundation Fellows, the Board then sought applicants for Membership to the College. Fellows would be admitted by election, and Members by application. Both had to be practising anaesthetists, with a Diploma in Anaesthetics (or similar). There was liable to be disquiet again because of the potential for discrimination. Regulations were required! The Chairman of the Executive of the College of Surgeons, Henry Searby took this in hand, drafted the regulations, and presented them *fait accompli* to the Board.

Notable among the regulations were the following clauses:

> *"Subject always to the approval of the Council (of the College of Surgeons), the Board shall govern and control all of the business of the Faculty", and "...if it (the Faculty) does not accept what the College wants, then it ceases to exist"* [34]

A great start! Well, at least we knew who the boss was.

Sixty Members were invited to join the Faculty, ensuring an initial Faculty of 100 anaesthetists. Thereafter a maximum of five recommendations for election to Fellowship, and two applications for Membership would be considered per year. Not surprisingly, some anaesthetists were upset at not being grandfathered into the Faculty, straining relationships with the Society. Following inauguration, Fellowships were conferred by election, but once examinations were instituted, they were also gained by successful examination. A Fellowship gave the holder the entitlement to place the letters FFARACS (Fellow of the Faculty of Anaesthetists, Royal Australasian College of Surgeons) after their name. Memberships by application were discontinued in 1959, once the examination process was established.

Of the seven candidates taking the first Fellowship examination in 1956, four were women. Six of the seven passed, becoming the first Fellows (by examination) of the Faculty. The two part examination began in 1957, with the first Primary examination. The Diplomas became increasingly irrelevant, with the Sydney DA discontinued in 1974, followed by the Melbourne DA in 1985.

The 1950s, Time of Change

As the Faculty consolidated its role and began training new specialists, the ASA entered a turbulent time. Besides Kaye selling its headquarters, there were financial concerns. The Society disaffiliated from the BMA in 1951. The timing may have been unfortunate, as the Minister for Health in the recently elected Government introduced the "Commonwealth Medical Benefits Schedule"(CMBS).[5] Even the BMA had

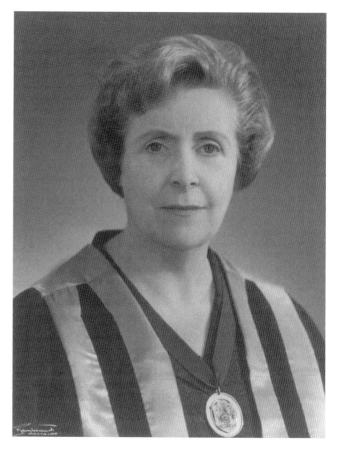

Fig. 24.9 Mary Burnell (1907–1996), the first woman member of the ASA (1935), the first woman President of the ASA (1953), and the first woman Dean of the Faculty of Anaesthetists, Royal Australasian College of Surgeons (1966). (Courtesy Geoffrey Kaye Museum of Anaesthetic History, Australian and New Zealand College of Anaesthetists, Melbourne.)

difficulty resolving issues with Government over anomalies in the schedule, and the Society's concerns fell on deaf ears. In 1959, the Minister responded to BMA requests for amendments to the Schedule, saying he would consider them "if they did not involve too much arithmetic". Anaesthetists remained the "poor relations" in the operating room, receiving an income less than that of surgeons for many years [34].

Mary Burnell (Fig. 24.9) became the first woman President (1953–54) of the ASA, and Patricia Mackay (nee Wilson) served as treasurer/secretary (1955–61), later becoming President (1966–68). This indicates the major role women played in the ASA from its inception. In 1966, Burnell became the first woman Dean of the Faculty

---

[5] The Commonwealth Medical Benefits Schedule (CMBS) is an indexed list of medical procedures and consultations to which the Commonwealth Government ascribes a "fee" that determines the basis of

reimbursement to patients of medical fees paid. All Australian citizens are entitled to a refund of 75 % of the CMBS "fee", and optional private health insurance can be taken to cover the remaining 25 %. The "fee" is indexed each year. However, indexation at minimal rates over the years has seriously eroded the value of the refunds paid, and in many cases, they now fall far short of medical fees actually charged. Nowhere has this been more evident than with anaesthesia fees.

The New Zealand Society arose in the 1950s, in the process becoming a voice for specialist anaesthetists, important because New Zealand specialists had minimal representation in the new Faculty. Not having an established home, the headquarters of the Society rotated every two years between the major cities, similar to the ASA's situation once Kaye sold 49 Mathoura Road. A regular newsletter was begun, and regular meetings held. Patricia Mackay became Secretary/Treasurer in 1954, before moving to Melbourne and fulfilling the same role for the Australian Society. Of great concern, few doctors entered the specialty because of the lack of suitable full-time and registrar posts in public hospitals, and private practice was poorly remunerated. The importance of anaesthetists charging patients directly (rather than via the surgeon) was raised with the College of Surgeons, and a scale of fees drawn up. A meeting called by the Director General of Health was attended by hospital superintendents, surgeons, and Society members, resulting in an increase in hospital posts, and ultimately, independence from surgeons in the setting of fees. This long preceded similar changes in Australia. By 1959, New Zealand, with a population of just over 2 million had 147 physician anaesthetists, quite an achievement [8].

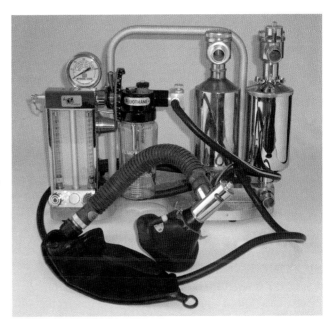

Fig. 24.10 Portable "Midget Anaesthetic Machine", typical of those used in Australia in the 1960s by anaesthetists in private practice. The anaesthetist carried this machine, as well as all drugs and other equipment, to each hospital. The hospital provided only oxygen. (Courtesy Geoffrey Kaye Museum of Anaesthetic History, Australian and New Zealand College of Anaesthetists, Melbourne.)

The 1960s

In Australia, the 1960s saw the aftermath of the introduction of the CMBS, and the gradual introduction of sessional payments for specialists in public hospitals. Under the old "honorary" system, specialists gave their time free of charge in the treatment of non-private patients in public hospitals, their income being derived entirely from their private practice. Such a system was fine for surgeons and other well established specialists, but anaesthetists received far less remuneration than their colleagues. It was not uncommon for the anaesthesia fee to be a quarter or less of the surgical fee, and the 1960s anaesthetist in private practice followed the surgeon to operating rooms in diverse small private hospitals, carrying their own apparatus and drugs, even nitrous oxide and halothane (Fig. 24.10).

At the end of the 1950s, academic anaesthesia had not recovered from the aftermath of World War II. No-one had taken up the initiative that Kaye had started. It was John Lowenthal, Professor of Surgery at the University of Sydney, who initiated establishment of an academic appointment. Driven in part by self-interest, his proposal would ensure the availability of specialist anaesthetists for his surgical practice, and for expansion of the Department of Surgery, In 1960, he proposed the appointment of an Associate Professor in the Department of Surgery, and sought financial assistance from the Nuffield Foundation [34].

The similarity of events, to those in Oxford some 22 years previously, was uncanny. Having obtained a grant of £ 20,000 from the Nuffield Foundation, the advertisement was placed, stipulating that "the successful applicant will work under the direction of the Professor of Surgery"! Harry Daly was having none of it! As inaugural Vice-Dean of the Faculty and former President of the ASA, the prominent Sydney anaesthetist prevailed upon his friend, Robert Macintosh, and sought a meeting with Lord Nuffield, who was visiting Sydney at the time. A polite exchange of letters followed, resulting in an increase in Nuffield's grant to £ 50,000, in order to fund a full academic chair in anaesthesia (similar to that of Nuffield's funding the first professorship in anaesthesia in Great Britain. See also Chapter 30) Douglas Joseph became Australia's first Professor in May, 1963 [34].

Opinions differed as to whether the ASA or the Faculty should represent anaesthetists on medico-political-economic matters. The argument began in the State of Victoria, prompted by the Government's establishment of a committee to determine salaries and conditions for doctors in public hospitals. The debate continued over several years, however Gwen Wilson recalled that if both organisations had looked closely at their history, constitutions, and previous legal judgements, the issue might have been resolved more quickly. At the height of the disquiet, in 1963, the Society had 460 members compared to the Faculty's 248 Fellows. The ASA affiliated with the Australian Medical Association in 1965, and ultimately, became recognised as representing anaesthetists on all matters related to fees and conditions of employment, while the Faculty concerned itself with training and standards of practice. This separation of roles has continued, and both bodies support education and research. A similar relationship exists in New Zealand [34].

Over the late 1950s and the 1960s, the ASA and the NZSA increasingly co-operated, particularly on matters of education and overseas aid. That relationship has continued, with each represented on the other's Board/Council meetings, and with joint support of congresses.

Low anaesthesia fees continued as an issue, with the Government schedule for anaesthesia fees priced at a fraction of the recommended surgical fee for the surgical procedure performed. After a visit to the US in 1970, Brian Pollard and Brian Dwyer introduced the "relative value" concept. After 30 years, and countless hours of lobbying by Pat Maplestone, Peter Hales, John Lodge, Greg Deacon and others, the Australian Government agreed to adopt the Relative Value Guide so that anaesthesia fees and rebates were determined by the anaesthesia service, and not by what the surgeon did [35].

The 1970s and Beyond

The 1970s also saw the first publication of *Anaesthesia and Intensive Care*. The proposal to publish a Society journal was raised in 1954, but interstate differences caused an 18-year delay. The first editor-in-chief was Ben Barry, and Neville Gibbs is now the fifth. Jeanette Thirlwell has been assistant and then executive editor of the journal since its beginning.

In 1970, the ASA established a permanent secretariat with a full time staff first housed in the offices of the private anaesthetic practice shared by several Sydney anaesthetists. In 1985, the Society moved to its current permanent headquarters in Sydney.

The 1970s and early 80s was a consolidation period for the specialty in Australia and New Zealand. Non-specialist, general practitioner anaesthetists diminished in numbers or vanished, as surgeons, hospitals, and eventually the public, increasingly appreciated the safety and quality of anaesthesia provided by trained specialists. Non-specialists were (and still are) required in remote rural parts of Australia. The Society and Faculty continue to support them with education and advocacy.

Over the 40 years from 1952, the Faculty grew in strength and numbers, as more doctors saw specialist anaesthesia as a fulfilling career. The relationship with the College of Surgeons was a necessary step at the time, and although Kaye dearly wanted an independent College established in 1951, the College of Surgeons provided the specialty with infrastructure and political clout that it would not have had as an indepen-

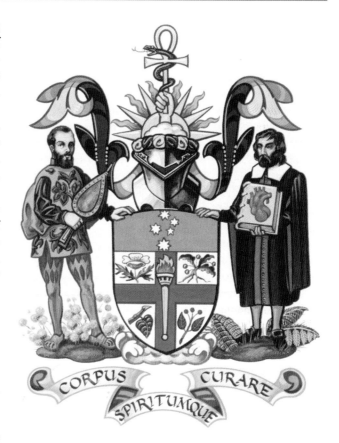

Fig. 24.11 Armorial Bearings of the Australian and New Zealand College of Anaesthetists, inaugurated in 1992. On the left, standing on wattle, the Australian national flower, is Vesalius with bellows signifying "ventilation". On the right, standing on the New Zealand silver fern, is William Harvey, who described the circulation of the blood. The Latin motto means "to care for the body and its breath of life". (Courtesy Geoffrey Kaye Museum of Anaesthetic History, Australian and New Zealand College of Anaesthetists, Melbourne.)

dent entity. Nevertheless, to many, the subordinate status of the Faculty sustained prejudices established over 100 years. Finally, in 1992, the Faculty separated from the surgeons to become the Australian and New Zealand College of Anaesthetists (ANZCA; Fig. 24.11). In 1994, the College moved to its current premises in Melbourne, a grand Victorian mansion now adjoined by a modern multi-story office building.

The Societies also prospered. They developed co-operative programs with the Faculty and with one another. The New Zealand Society began the first Conference of Anaesthetists of New Zealand (CANZ) in 1978, this becoming a major regular educational event. CANZ soon became a joint venture of the Society and the Faculty. In 1986, the Continuing Education Committee of Anaesthetists of New Zealand (CECANZ) was established as an educational arm of the Society, with a funded Director. CECANZ ultimately embraced the CANZ meeting and other educational meetings, refresher courses, and incident reporting. In 2004, CECANZ was replaced by NZAEC, the New Zealand Anaesthesia Education Committee, a formal joint educational program with the Australian and New Zealand College of Anaesthetists.

The NZSA and ANZCA acted to overturn a peculiar "medical manslaughter" law in New Zealand. Under this legal aberration, medical practitioners responsible for the death of a patient might be liable to criminal prosecution for manslaughter, regardless of whether or not the death had been due to negligence. A lengthy and enthusiastic representation finally resulted in passage of the Crimes Amendment Bill in 1997. No longer could doctors be charged with manslaughter after a medical error, unless gross negligence could be proven.

The NZSA has supported anaesthetists in the Pacific islands since the 1970s, and today the ASA is also closely involved. The ASA funded the establishment of the lecturer in anaesthesia at the University of the South Pacific in Fiji, and continues to fund the Pacific Fellowship.

Promulgation of Faculty policy documents was initiated in the 1980s, producing statements defining standards of facilities, training, assistance, and routine monitoring. These lay the basis for anaesthetists to argue for better conditions and facilities for the safe care of patients. Regularly reviewed and updated, such policies have become, by default, the standards by which hospitals and facilities are now judged. In 1987, Bill Runciman and colleagues established the Australian Patient Safety Foundation, placing Australian and New Zealand anaesthetists at the forefront in patient safety.(see History of Patient Safety in Anaesthesia-Chapter 41)

A landmark event for Australasian anaesthesia, was the 1996 staging of the World Congress of Anaesthesiologists in Sydney, hosted by the Australian Society of Anaesthetists. The largest medical congress held in the southern hemisphere up to that time, it attracted some 10,000 delegates.

Anaesthesia in Australia and New Zealand has made enormous strides in the last century. Anaesthetists now play significant roles in Australian and New Zealand health care. Intensive Care Medicine grew from the "hobby" of a few anaesthetists in the 1950s, to a joint specialty faculty of the College of Anaesthetists and the College of Physicians, now an independent College of Intensive Care Medicine. The Faculty of Pain Medicine was a world-first initiative in the training of specialists in chronic and cancer pain, and many hospitals now boast pain units for the management of postoperative and other pain.

Times have changed. In 1927, Kaye described the practice of anaesthesia.

"The care of patients was rudimentary in the extreme. Nobody ever dreamt of paying them a preoperative visit. Anaesthetists and patient met as strangers in the operating theatre. Nobody ever charted blood pressure, pulse or respiration during operations." [32]

As noted earlier, in 1936 Kaye determined that anaesthesia mortality was around 1:1000. Australian mortality reporting has been amongst the most comprehensive in the world. Although reporting criteria have changed over the years, later mortality reports suggest enormous progress. Holland reported anaesthesia related mortality in 1960 of 1:5,500, reducing to 1:10,250 by 1970. This coincided with many general practitioners voluntarily leaving anaesthesia practice, and junior and untrained medical staff no longer providing the backbone of anaesthetic service. In 1984, the published anaesthesia-related mortality was 1:26,000, and the most recent figures suggest an incidence of less than 1:50,000, including patients classified as "high risk". [40, 41] Australian and New Zealand anaesthetists take great pride in their achievements.

References

1. Devansen D. Traditional aboriginal medicine practice in the northern territory. International Symposium on Traditional Medicine, September 2000, WHO, Kobe, Japan.
2. Ratsch A, Steadman KJ, Bogossian F. The Pituri Story: a review of the historical literature surrounding traditional Australian aboriginal use of nicotine in central Australia. J Ethnobiol Ethnomed. 2010;6:26
3. Cribb A, Cribb J, Pearn J. Pituri, plants and physic. In: Pearn J, Powell L, Editors. The Bancroft Tradition. Brisbane: Amphion Press; 1991.
4. Foley P. *Duboisia myoporoides*: The medical career of a native Australian plant. Historical Records of Australian Science. 2006;17:31–9.
5. Stack E. Aboriginal Pharmacopeia. Northern territory Library Service, 1989; Darwin.
6. Dunlop N. Dr William Bland. J R Aust Hist Soc. 1926;11:321–51.
7. Wilson G. One grand chain—the history of anaesthesia in Australia 1846–1962 volume 1 1846–1934. Australian and New Zealand College of Anaesthetists. Melbourne; 1995.
8. Hutchinson BR, Gibbs JM, Newson AJ. Safety through knowledge—a fifty year history of the New Zealand Society of Anaesthetists. New Zealand Society of Anaesthetists. Auckland; 1998.
9. Chapman A, Editor. History of dentistry in South Australia 1836–1936. Australian Dental Association, South Australian Branch. Adelaide; 1937.
10. "A Subscriber" Laughing Gas (Letter to the Editor). NSW Med Gaz. 1870;25.
11. Fox CJ. Nitrous oxide gas as an anaesthetic. Aust Med Gaz. 1870;130–2.
12. "Miscellanea" Anaesthetics—Nitrous Oxide Gas. NSW Med Gaz. 1871;30.
13. Faulding's Medical Journal. May, 1900; p. 20.
14. Letter. Australian Nitrous Oxide Gas. Brit J Dental Sc. 1898;41:789.
15. Hutchinson BR. Early anaesthetics in New Zealand. NZ Med J. 1992;105:343.
16. Newson AJ. Nitrous Oxide Advertisements on New Zealand Postage Stamps. NZSA Newsletter 1972;19:161.
17. Cooper MG. The first reported death associated with anaesthesia in Australia. Anaes Int Care. 1991;19:265–6.
18. Rudall JT. A case of death under chloroform. Aust Med J. 1868;13:215–20.
19. "Local Subjects" Death under Chloroform at the Melbourne Hospital. Aust Med J. (New series) 1891;13:103–4.

20. "Local Subjects" Death under Chloroform. Aust Med J. (New series) 1891;13:327–8.
21. "Notices" Victoria. The Australasian Med Gazette. 1891;10:282.
22. Editorial. Anaesthetics at the Melbourne Hospital. Aust Med J. (New series) 1891;13:316–8.
23. "Hospital Intelligence" Melbourne Hospital. Aust Med J. (New series) 1891;13:321–2.
24. "Notices" The Australasian Med Gazette. 1884;3:131.
25. "Editorial" A Champion of Irregular Practice. The Australasian Med Gazette. 1884;3:157.
26. "Editorial" The Responsibility of Anaesthetists. The Australasian Med Gazette. 1912;31:391.
27. "Editorial" The Responsibility of Anaesthetists. The Australasian Med Gazette. 1912;31:420–1.
28. "Hornabrook RW" Letter to the Editor re: The responsibility of Anaesthetists. The Australasian Med Gazette. 1912;31:421.
29. Hornabrook RW. Some of the difficulties the anaesthetist has to contend against. Aus Med J. 1914;19:1559–72.
30. Embley EH. The causation of death during the administration of chloroform. Br Med J. 1902;1:817–821, 885–893, 951–61.
31. Hornabrook RW. A plea for the more considerate treatment of patient and anaesthetist by the surgeon. Aus Med J. 1913;18:1009–12.
32. Kaye G. Anaesthesia since 1927, people and ideas. Australian Society of Anaesthetists presentation 1962. Unpublished.
33. Lundy JS. Factors that influenced the development of anesthesiology. Anesth Analg. 1946; 25:38–43.
34. Wilson G, Kaye G, Phillips G, Baker AB. One grand chain—the history of anaesthesia in Australia vol. 2. 1934–1962. In: Thirlwell-Jones J, Editor. Australian and New Zealand College of Anaesthetists. Melbourne; 2004.
35. Wilson G. Fifty years—the Australian society of anaesthetists 1934–1984. Australian Society of Anaesthetists. Sydney; 1987.
36. Kaye G. Anaesthetic fatalities. Med J Australia. 1938;1:995–1031.
37. Westhorpe R. The D.M. anaesthetic machine. Anaes Int Care. 1989;17:128.
38. Orton RH. The surgeon-anaesthetist relationship. Med J Aust. 1949; 2:239–41.
39. Marshall SV. Problems which surgeons create for anaesthetists. Med J Aust. 1954;2:891–2.
40. Holland R. Anaesthetic Mortality in New South Wales. Br J Anaesth. 1987;59:834–41.
41. Gibbs N, Editor. Safety of Anaesthesia. A review of anaesthesia-related mortality reporting in Australia and New Zealand 2003–2005. Australian and New Zealand College of Anaesthetists. Melbourne; 2009.

History of Canadian Anesthesia

25

Douglas Craig, Diane Biehl, Robert Byrick and John G. Wade

Summary

The first reported anesthesia in a territory that would become part of Canada (in 1867) was in the British colonial province of New Brunswick, in January 1847. In the late 19th century, Canadian anesthesia was linked primarily with that in the UK, leading to a physician-based practice, which continues to the present. In the early 20th century, US influence increased. By the 1930s a true Canadian identity began to emerge and, in time, to dominate.

The Canadian Society of Anaesthetists formed in 1920, but lapsed in 1929 with the start of the Anaesthesia Section of the Canadian Medical Association. The Montreal Society of Anaesthetists, established in 1930, became the Canadian Anaesthetists' Society (CAS) in 1943. The CAS was renamed the Canadian Anesthesiologists' Society in 1993. The CAS began a medical journal in 1954, an international education fund in 1967, and a research foundation in 1979.

McGill University established the first Canadian academic Department of Anesthesia in 1945, with independent departments evolving in all sixteen Canadian universities over the next 25 years. Important for these departments was the Royal College of Physicians and Surgeons of Canada (RCPSC), established in 1929, which oversaw the education curriculum in all specialty training programs and offered specialty examinations. In 1972, the RCPSC mandated that all specialty training programs operate under the auspices of a university. The Association of Canadian University Departments of Anesthesia (ACUDA) formed in 1976 to support academic departments and research. Canadian anesthesia researchers have contributed to many areas of medicine.

In the 1970s the focus on patient safety became increasingly important, and led to the CAS publishing Guidelines for the Practice of Anesthesia. The CAS assisted in creating and implementing new anesthesia gas machines standards of the Canadian Standards Association.

Since 1972, the Canadian universal healthcare system has provided patients in all provinces with comprehensive health services, including physician services. This unique system allows anesthesiologists (specialist or family-practitioner) to provide anesthesia services for all patients, regardless of their ability to pay.

In the Beginning

Canadian anesthesia began before the four eastern provinces formally amalgamated as the Dominion of Canada on July 1, 1867. Physicians, drugs and techniques from the neighboring United States (US) and the United Kingdom (UK) strongly influenced medical care in the provinces that would become Canada. According to the 22 Jan edition of the Weekly Chronicle, St. John, New Brunswick, the first reported anesthetic was on 17 Jan 1847, three months fol-

lowing the successful demonstration of ether anesthesia by William Morton in Boston. A visiting dentist from Boston (Samuel Adams) administered a "vapor of a compound of which aether appeared to form the chief ingredient" to a man to produce "complete sleep and insensibility" for removal of a tumor on his arm [1]. The proximity of St. John to Boston by sea explains how the news spread quickly. Other newspaper reports of the use of ether in Canada in early 1847 have been reviewed, [2] but none antedated that in St. John. A surgeon, Edward Worthington, provided the first medical report of the use of ether in Canada, in Eaton Center, Quebec, on 11 March 1847, describing a below-knee amputation [3]. Worthington was also the first in Canada to report (4 November 1847) the use of chloroform, soon after its introduction into surgical practice by James Simpson in Edinburgh.

Despite the proximity of the US, Canadian medicine in general and anesthesia in particular, were linked primarily to the UK during the second half of the 19th century. Many physicians then in Canada had completed their medical training in the UK before immigrating to a country that was part of

D. Craig (✉) · D. Biehl
Department of Anesthesia, University of Manitoba,
Winnipeg, Canada
e-mail: doug.craig@bell.net

R. Byrick
Department of Anesthesia, University of Toronto,
St. Michael's Hospital, Toronto, Ontario, Canada

J. G. Wade
Faculty of Medicine, Department of Anesthesia,
University of Manitoba, Winnipeg, Canada

E. I Eger II et al. (eds.), *The Wondrous Story of Anesthesia*, DOI 10.1007/978-1-4614-8441-7_25, © Edmond I Eger, MD 2014

the British Empire. The pioneering anesthesia research in the UK by John Snow (1813–1858) also encouraged the long-term link between anesthesia in Canada and the UK. From the outset and continuing to the present, anesthetic practice in Canada has been physician-based, as in the UK. Although US influences on Canadian anesthesia became stronger by the early 20th century, a Canadian identity evolved and later dominated. This chapter charts the key steps in the development of that Canadian identity.

1899–1920: Origins of Anesthesia as a Specialty in Canada

From 1899 to 1920, anesthesia was performed as a 'craft', with a developing empirical base but little scientific evidence to guide its use [4]. Hospital appointments were an important step in recognizing anesthesia as a worthy profession. The appointment, in 1899, of William Hutton as an 'honorary anaesthetist' at the Winnipeg General Hospital in Manitoba, marks the beginning of the specialty in Canada [5]. Hutton graduated from the Manitoba Medical College in 1887 and was later appointed as Professor of Practical Chemistry and also Registrar of the College [6]. Other appointments soon followed, most notably William Webster (1865–1934) in Winnipeg, and Samuel Johnston (1869–1947) in Toronto [7]. Webster, born in Manchester, UK, came to Snowflake in rural Manitoba as a school teacher in 1888, then entered the Manitoba Medical College, graduating in 1895. After postgraduate training in Pathology in the UK, he returned to Winnipeg, working in both General Medicine and Pathology. Without further formal training, he began to include anesthesia in his practice, eventually on a full-time basis. In 1905, he was appointed Lecturer on Anesthesia at the Manitoba Medical College. He found that safe anesthesia relies on application of basic physiological and pharmacological principles [8]. His 1924 publication of *The Science and Art of Anaesthesia*, the only comprehensive anesthesia textbook written by a Canadian anesthetist, demonstrated his interests in teaching and research.

Johnston graduated from Trinity Medical College in Toronto in 1901. He began a general medical practice, but turned to full-time work in anesthesia. He later wrote: "I know I was the first physician in Canada to give up general practice and go into the specialty of anaesthesia." (Personal Communication: Edward Shorter, Hannah Professor of History, University of Toronto. 2012.) Johnston was invited to organize the Department of Anesthesia at Toronto General Hospital in 1904, where he instructed house officers in anesthesia. In 1907, he was appointed Lecturer in Anesthetics in the Faculty of Medicine, University of Toronto. He spent 1908–09 in the UK, acquiring further training before returning to Toronto to his career in anesthesia. He taught medical students about anesthesia and was probably the first anesthesiologist to do so in Canada. Canada's 'formal' teaching track record in anesthesia therefore goes back to 1910.

Charles LaRocque, at Hotel Dieu Hospital, and William Nagle, at the Royal Victoria Hospital, both in Montreal, Quebec, joined Webster and Johnston as the only doctors in Canada at that time devoting themselves solely to anesthesia [9]. General practitioners, or interns and residents supervised by surgeons (in some of the teaching hospitals), provided much of the clinical anesthesia in Canada. Of interest, Margaret McCallum Johnston (wife of Samuel Johnston) was appointed as the first Chief of Anesthesia at Women's College Hospital in Toronto in 1914, and is believed to be the first woman to practice anesthesia full-time in Canada.

Webster and Johnson travelled to the UK and the US to observe anesthetic practice, teaching, and the beginnings of anesthesia-related research. Although links to the UK had a greater influence on Canadian anesthesia in the first decade of the 20th century, influences from the US increased after 1910 because of mutual concerns about the quality of basic medical education resulting from Abraham Flexner's comprehensive report [10]. The report, entitled "Medical Education in the United States and Canada", transformed medical education in both countries. Academic-based training programs undertaken in Universities replaced the apprentice model, controlled by private practitioners.

Francis McMechan (1879–1939) of Cincinnati, Ohio probably created the most significant US link to Canada, from the late 1910s to the 1930s. Despite severe rheumatoid arthritis, which prevented him from continuing his anesthetic practice, he profoundly affected the organization of anesthesia in the US, Canada, and indeed worldwide. This included the creation of several anesthesia societies, which held annual scientific meetings, and his creation and editorships of both the Quarterly Supplement of Anesthesia and Analgesia of the American Journal of Surgery (1914–26), and Current Researches in Anesthesia and Analgesia, starting in 1922. Through his worldwide contacts with anesthetists, including Webster, Johnston and others in Canada, and Waters in the US, McMechan promoted academic anesthesia, with an emphasis on the link between the basic science laboratory and the clinical practice of anesthesia. Canadian anesthesia benefited greatly from McMechan's promotion of anesthesia as a valid specialty.

Leaders in the specialty from both countries met regularly, including as the "Anesthesia Travel Club", formed in 1929. Four of the 14 members at the initial meeting were Canadian—Easson Brown, Charles Robson, Harry Shields and John Blezard.

In 1933, Ralph Waters (1887–1979) was appointed Head of the first autonomous Department of Anesthesia, in Madison, Wisconsin. He created an academic department that provided exemplary patient care, undergraduate and postgraduate teaching, and quality research. Waters had a major impact on Canadian anesthesia, similar to his influence on American anesthesia.

In the subsequent decades, the scientific foundation for anesthetic practice established by Webster and Johnston, became the base for the evolution of anesthesia in Canada from that of a 'service-oriented craft', to a discipline recognized by others, and finally to a specialty based in science.

1920–1929: Canadian Society of Anaesthetists

The Canadian Society of Anaesthetists, Canada's first formal association of specialists, [11] was founded mainly through the efforts of Wesley Bourne of Montreal as Secretary, and Samuel Johnston as the first President. They were encouraged and assisted by McMechan, who had established several anesthesia societies in the US and who had developed links with anesthesia organizations outside North America. The first annual scientific meeting was held in 1921 at Niagara Falls, Ontario, in conjunction with the Interstate Association of Anesthetists (Ohio, Kentucky), and the New York Society of Anesthetists (the precursor of the American Society of Anesthesiologists). The scientific program included presentations from Canadian, American and British anesthetists. HEG Boyle of London was the Honorary Chairman of the meeting and the Official Representative of the Anaesthesia Section, Royal Society of Medicine. Boyle's participation demonstrated both McMechan's far-reaching influence, and the different maturity of anesthesia organizations in the UK and Canada. By 1926, the Canadian society had over 100 members, but in 1928 the society Executive decided to terminate the Canadian society, and transfer its role to the Section of Anaesthesia of the Canadian Medical Association, thereby muting the voice of anesthesia. Although consideration was given in the 1930s to reviving the Society, no action was taken [6].

1930–1943: Montreal Society of Anaesthetists

The Montreal Society of Anaesthetists was established to facilitate interactions between and support French and English-speaking Montreal anesthetists. Its national importance emerged in 1943. Five members of the Society, with the support of colleagues in Toronto, applied to have the Society formally converted into a national entity – the Canadian Anaesthetists' Society. The applicants were Wesley Bourne, Harold Griffith, M. Digby Leigh, Georges Cousineau, and Romeo Rochette.

1943: Canadian Anaesthetists' Society (CAS)

A Memorandum of Agreement of 27 May 1943, signed by the five anesthetists, established the objectives of the new society, objectives that remain in place today:

> *"To advance the art and science of Anaesthesia and to promote its interests in relation to Medicine with particular reference to the clinical, educational, ethical and economic aspects thereof, to associate together in one corporate body members in good standing of the Medical Profession who have specialized in this particular science, to promote the interest of its members, to maintain a Society Library and Bureau of Information, to edit and publish a journal of Anaesthesia, to acquire and own such property and real estate as may become necessary to effectively carry out the purposes of the Society, and to do all such lawful acts and things as may be incidental or conducive to the attainment of the above Objects."*

On 24 June 1943, the Office of the Registrar General of Canada signed the Letters Patent confirming registration of the CAS in Canada as a "Body Corporate and Politic". Canadian Anesthesia again had its own voice and this time had no intention of relinquishing it. The CAS office was initially sited in Montreal but moved to Toronto in 1946, where it remains. The CAS grew to its present size of 2000 members across Canada, with Divisions in each province. There are now 12 sub-specialty Sections within the CAS, reflecting expansion of modern anesthetic practice beyond the operating room, and advances in anesthesia for specialist surgical interventions. The Society name was changed to the Canadian Anesthesiologists' Society in 1993. Although never officially recognized as such, the adoption of the US term anesthesiologist and the elimination of the dipthong ('ae') indicate the shift away from the early primary links of Canadian anesthesia with the UK. While a full description of CAS activities exceeds the scope of this summary, three Society programs deserve note, as do CAS roles in the World Federation of Societies of Anaesthesiologists (WFSA).

1954—Canadian Anaesthetists' Society Journal

The Founders' vision in 1943, that the Society publish a "journal of Anaesthesia", was fulfilled in July 1954 with the first issue of the Canadian Anaesthetists' Society Journal. The quarterly publication was distributed to the 500 Society members and a small number of subscribers. The first editor, Roderick Gordon of Toronto, held that post for 28 years (1954–1982). While the content initially consisted of papers presented at national and regional meetings in Canada, the Journal soon attracted manuscripts and subscribers from outside Canada. By 1961, 25% of the content originated from the US. In time, an increased volume of submissions prompted the publication frequency to increase to bi-monthly and then monthly. The title change in 1987, to *Canadian Journal of Anaesthesia/Journal Canadien d'Anesthésie*, reflected the expanding international nature of submissions and readership. From the first issue, articles have been published in English or French, according to the language of submission. The inclusion of international Editorial Board members and Guest Editors also indicates the evolution of the Journal to a member of the international community of anesthesia journals.

Gordon (1911–1998) deserves recognition beyond his role as journal Editor. Within the CAS, he served as Secretary-Treasurer from 1946 to 1961, and President in 1963–64. He received the CAS Gold Medal in 1969. He was Professor and Head of the University of Toronto Department of Anesthesia from 1961 to 1977. The Dr. R.A. Gordon Research Award of the CAS continues to honor the man who influenced Canadian Anesthesia for decades.

1979: Canadian Anesthesia Research Foundation (CARF)

CARF was established as the Canadian Anaesthetists' Society Research Fund. The CAS Research Fund became the CARF in 1992, without changing its basic structure and mission. CARF is a Registered Charity in Canada and supports the Research Awards Program of the CAS. Led by a founding Trustee, Gordon Sellery of London, Ontario, CARF's resources grew until it could fund the first annual award in 1985, assisted by the CAS and its Journal. This award became a catalyst for additional awards in the CARF/CAS awards program, supported either by CARF or external sources. With total annual awards exceeding $200,000, the CARF/CAS Program has become the largest provider of funds for Canadian anesthesia research, increasing from one award in 1985, to 12 in 2005 [12]. CARF supported 3 of the 12 awards in 2005, the remainder being externally funded. The seed planted in 1979 with the start of CARF grew to a single tree in 1985—and a small forest by 2005! The review also noted the important role of CAS new-investigator awards, [12] as the first step in successful long-term research careers of Canadian anesthetists. By 2012, the cumulative number of awards from the CARF/CAS Program had increased to more than 200—with the Program being the primary source of funding for new anesthesia investigators in Canada.

1967: CAS International Education Fund (IEF)

The IEF was established as the CAS Anaesthesia Training and Relief Fund, a Registered Charity, in response to a 1964 challenge from the WFSA for national societies to make modern anesthesia available worldwide. The Fund, led by Rod Gordon, initially supported Canadian involvement with overseas training programs, principally in Nigeria, as well as supporting foreign trainees' short-term learning experiences in Canada. In 1993, the Fund was renamed and took on the mission of assisting anesthesia providers in developing countries to establish self-sustaining programs relevant to each country's needs. Canadians have helped Nepalese anesthesiologists, over a period of 15 years, to develop a training program in Katmandu. More recently, the main focus has been on a training program in Kigali, Rwanda. The Fund has also arranged visits by Canadian anesthesiologists to Ethiopia and Madagascar. The 1964 WFSA challenge continues to be recognized.

CAS and WFSA: 1955–2012

Harold Griffith of Montreal, the first CAS President (1943–1946) was elected in 1955, as the Founding President of the WFSA. (A fuller account of his WFSA roles can be found in Chapter 20). The second World Congress of Anaesthesiologists (WCA) was held in Toronto in 1960, and the 12th in Montreal in 2000. From the outset, Canadians have supported the WFSA through the CAS and through individual participation within the WFSA structure and at World Congresses. Angela Enright of Victoria, British Columbia, served as the WFSA President from 2008–2012, leading the WFSA component of the Lifebox pulse oximeter initiative. She was awarded the Order of Canada, the highest civilian honor, in 2010, and in 2012 was a recipient of the Queen Elizabeth II Diamond Jubilee Medal in Canada and the American Society of Anesthesiologists (ASA) Nicholas M. Greene Outstanding Humanitarian Award.

University Departments of Anesthesia (starting in 1945)

Anesthesia slowly became an autonomous academic specialty recognized by universities in Canada. Although Webster and Johnston were lecturers in anesthesia in Winnipeg (Webster) and Toronto (Johnston), their appointments were within the Department of Surgery (Webster) and Therapeutics (Johnston). The 1945 appointment of Wesley Bourne as Chair of the autonomous Department of Anaesthesia at McGill University was a key factor in the advancement of academic anesthesia in Canada. The McGill Department followed the creation of the first ever university anesthesia department in 1933, in Madison Wisconsin (Ralph Waters, Head), and the second in 1937 with the appointment of Robert Macintosh to the Nuffield Professorship of Anaesthetics at Oxford University. The founding of the McGill department deserves special recognition, both because it represented establishment of the first academic anesthesia department in Canada, and because it provides the opportunity to recognize three key members of the new department – Wesley Bourne, Harold Griffith, and Digby Leigh.

Bourne (1886–1965), the first Head at McGill, was nearing the end of a distinguished career. He had been an outstanding clinician, teacher, and investigator, holding an appointment in the McGill Department of Pharmacology. His honors included the first Henry Hill Hickman Medal of the Royal Society of Medicine, the first Gold Medal of the Canadian Anaesthetists' Society, and the 1942 Presidency of the American Society of Anesthetists (renamed the American Society of Anesthesiologists in 1945). Bourne was the only non-American ever to hold this position. An endowed Chair at McGill and the annual Dr. Wesley Bourne Lecture continue to honor this man.

Griffith (1894–1985) is best known for the first clinical use of curare in 1942, but his contributions to anesthesia at McGill (Head 1951–56), nationally and internationally, were broadly based and extraordinary [13]. An outstanding clinician and teacher, he made major contributions to the development of anesthesia organizations in Canada and beyond. He served as the first CAS President, as Chair of the Board of Trustees of the International Anesthesia Research Society (IARS), and as Founding President of the WFSA. Honors included the Hickman Medal, the 1959 Distinguished Service Award of the ASA, the CAS Gold Medal and appointment as an Officer of the Order of Canada. Griffith was also recognized in 1991 with a commemorative Canadian postage stamp bearing his image.

Leigh (1904–1975) was a University of British Columbia (UBC) undergraduate and a McGill medical graduate, who began training in surgery in Montreal, but was convinced by Bourne to change to anesthesia. He trained at the University of Wisconsin under Waters, returning to Montreal as a Research Fellow in Pharmacology, before becoming Head of Anesthesia at the Children's Hospital. He and Bourne established a two-year course in anesthesia at McGill, accepting candidates following a year of internship. Leigh elected to return to UBC, and later moved to Los Angeles Children's Hospital in California, where he developed a major pediatric anesthesia training program and remained as Chief for several years. In 1948, Leigh and Kathleen Belton authored *Pediatric Anesthesia* one of the first major pediatric anesthesia texts.

The University of Toronto Department became the second Canadian University Department in 1951. On 14 May 1951, in a letter to the President of the University, Dean MacFarlane of the Faculty of Medicine articulated the rationale for recommending an autonomous academic department of anesthesia: "anaesthesia has made considerable advances in the past 15 years" and "there is constantly a search for new methods of inducing anaesthesia which constitutes greater measures of safety in seriously ill and injured patients". The importance of establishing an independent body of knowledge as the basis for the specialty was recognized, and patient safety became a focus for the growth of anesthesia in other Canadian Universities. However, it took another 20 years to place independent departments in all 16 Canadian Faculties of Medicine.

The Royal College of Physicians and Surgeons of Canada (RCPSC)

Unlike other international colleges and boards, the RCPSC accredits training programs and examines candidates in all medical and surgical specialties. In addition, since 1974, the RCPSC has required all Canadian specialty training programs to be university-based and accredited by the RCPSC. Accreditors include anesthesiologists, who also review programs in Surgery, Internal Medicine, and the many sub-specialty programs. The RCPSC requirements have strengthened postgraduate medical educational programs across Canada.

The RCPSC was established in 1929 with a different mandate to that existing today. As originally designed, it provided a Fellowship diploma for physicians to confirm competence in special work. Initially, a limited number of these were conferred without examination, on physicians in academic posts. However, from 1931, the Fellowship has been awarded by examination. Regardless, from its inception, Fellows were expected to be grounded in basic sciences and in general medicine and surgery. The Fellowship, to quote, was "the hallmark of the academic man" and thus at that time was an academic qualification rather than a confirmation of specialist competence.

In the 1930s, about one third of Canadian physicians performed some form of specialist work, without holding a RCPSC Fellowship. Many physicians wanted recognition for their specialty, but not by means of the Fellowship. The RCPSC responded by creating an added RCPSC Certification program. Certification requirements were less rigorous than those for the Fellowship, but did confirm specialist status. Initially, Anesthesia was not one of the specialties recognized by Certification.

During the 1930s, anesthetists in Canada had other major issues to deal with. Many were salaried hospital employees while others were remunerated on a fee for service basis. Another concern was the emerging possibility of a National Health Insurance Program. These concerns, arising mainly in Montreal and Toronto, caused the Royal College to agree in 1942 to include Anesthesia in the Certification program.

However, the two-tier recognition of specialists, in all specialties, as either Fellows or Certificants, created further conflict within the College. A single standard of training and examination, leading to a single qualification resolved this issue in 1971. The new form of specialist certification opened the way for Fellowship to all successful candidates, leading therefore to full membership in the RCPSC. In particular, this meant that the status of anesthesia was now the same as that for other specialties in Canada. Anesthesia candidates are certified in the RCPSC Division of Internal Medicine, not Surgery. This recognized that anesthesia residencies (requiring four years of clinical training after completion of internship), include one year of internal medicine, with an emphasis on intensive care.

The RCPSC enhanced independent Canadian-based research at the graduate level, by recognizing a Clinician-Investigator training program (CIP) in 1995. This program gave all residents access to funding and encouragement to undertake graduate research training as part of their fellowship. Prior to this program, no funding was available to support such research training during residency, and most anesthetists seeking research experience went abroad after their residency. This vital part of postgraduate education now allows residents to develop research skills during their residency, helping them to become successful career clinician scientists.

1976: Association of Canadian University Departments of Anesthesia (ACUDA)

A 1975 meeting instigated by Stuart Vandewater, then Chair of Anesthesia at Queen's University in Kingston, Ontario greatly advanced Canadian academic anesthesia. Previously, anesthesia department heads had met only informally. The Kingston retreat included representatives from all university departments of anesthesia, the RCPSC, the Medical Research Council of Canada and the Canadian Anaesthetists' Society. This hallmark meeting led to the formation of ACUDA, in June 1976. ACUDA's bylaws/goals caused academic anesthetists in Canada:

- To affiliate in a single organization, representatives of all Canadian University Departments of Anesthesia.
- To develop and promote undergraduate, postgraduate and continuing education by Canadian University Departments of Anesthesia.
- To advise in the training of allied health personnel as it relates to anesthesia.
- To promote the development of research and scientific progress in anesthesia.
- To represent the academic departments of anesthesia and to promote their interest within professional and learned societies, advisory boards and councils to government or public service organizations.

- To promote exemplary patient care and advise responsible bodies on matters concerning the standards of anesthetic practice.
- To support the interests of the profession through the objectives of the Canadian Anesthesiologists' Society.

ACUDA differed from the previous conference of department heads, in that it comprised all elements of the academic departments, rather than just department heads. Standing committees considered issues in undergraduate and postgraduate education, research, and departmental management.

Throughout this period it was essential that ACUDA and the Canadian Anesthesiologists' Society had a consistent and cooperative partnership. Emerson Moffitt, Department Head at Dalhousie University, Halifax Nova Scotia noted: [14] "the Society has many aims and functions but the responsibility for survival and development of academic anesthesia ultimately rests with the 16 University departments". During the 1990s, ACUDA provided a forum for the specialty to address human resource needs specific to anesthesia in Canada. The planning model used, [15, 16] allowed the specialty to lobby the government and universities in promoting the case for more providers.

Patient Safety and Quality of Care

In the 1960s and 1970s, anesthesia-related mortality of perhaps 1 in 5000 attracted the highest Canadian Medical Protective Association (CMPA) liability fees of any specialty in Canada. Following publication by the Canadian Anesthesiologists' Society, of the "Guidelines for the Practice of Anesthesia" in 1977, [17] Canadian anesthesiologists performed outcome studies in many institutions across Canada [18]. Reviewed annually, expanded, and renamed, the Guidelines are now published in an accessible on-line format [19]. Mortality has decreased to approximately 1 in 200,000 and anesthesia now has among the lowest CMPA fees.

Canada became the first country to have a comprehensive standard for anesthetic machines. The Canadian Standards Association published this in 1978 as a preliminary standard, followed in 1980 by the definitive standard [20]. Preceding the preliminary standard by one year was the June 1977 "Advance Standards Information" bulletin, sent to all Canadian hospitals. The stimulus for the bulletin, and for the publication of the preliminary standard, was the simultaneous presence in Canada of anesthetic machines of UK origin (oxygen as the left side flowmeter) and US origin (oxygen as the right side flowmeter). The new Standard, in addition to a number of other safety enhancements, required 'oxygen right'. In time, all clinical anesthetic machines met the new standard.

The importance of a national Guideline for the Practice of Anesthesia was further established when pulse oximetry and capnography were introduced into clinical practice. The CAS-approved Guidelines made these monitors de facto standards. This document supported efforts by anesthesia leaders, mandating that hospitals purchase this equipment to provide safe care. Later, the Guidelines dealt not only with technical aspects of monitoring equipment, but also the professional qualifications of providers, and eventually the role of members of the anesthesia care team appropriate to ensure patient safety.

In 1995, anesthetists developed Canada's first high-fidelity simulation-based education facility at the University of Toronto and Sunnybrook Health Sciences Centre. This was the third such centre in North America (after Stanford and Harvard Universities). Anesthesiologists from both Harvard and Stanford contributed their time and experience to train Canadian anesthesiologists in this emerging educational tool, and collaborated in research projects.

Research

Canadian research in anesthesia began in the 1920s and 1930s. Bourne had a faculty appointment in Pharmacology at McGill and was one of the early anesthesiologists to teach and conduct research. In Toronto, practicing physician Easson Brown, worked with George Lucas and Velyien Henderson to develop cyclopropane as an anesthetic agent. Henderson volunteered to receive cyclopropane in Lucas and Henderson's laboratory at the University of Toronto. In a later demonstration in the same laboratory, attended by members of the local anesthetic community, [21] the volunteer was Frederick Banting (later Sir Frederick Banting), who along with John Macleod received the 1923 Nobel Prize in Medicine for their discovery of insulin. This auspicious history notwithstanding, several unfortunate anesthesia-related deaths in Toronto and a fear of explosive agents led Samuel Johnston to forbid the use of cyclopropane on patients in Toronto. International relationships proved important, and the agent was supplied to Waters who introduced it into clinical practice.

In January 1942, Harold Griffith, and anesthesia resident Enid Johnson introduced curare into clinical practice at the Homeopathic Hospital of Montreal, publishing their results in the July edition of Anesthesiology [22]. They reported the use of Intocostrin (Purified Extract of Curare, Squibb) during 25 general anesthetics for a range of procedures from minor (curettage of the uterus, hemorrhoidectomy) to major (laparotomy, nephrectomy). This demonstration that curare could be used "safely" (although no reversal of blockade was done) was a major step forward and clinical anesthesia was forever changed for the better. Johnson moved to Dalhou-

sie University in Halifax after completing her training, and eventually became a Professor in the Department of Physiology at Dalhousie.

Research by pharmacologist Werner Kalow, at the University of Toronto, provided the first evidence of the importance of pharmacogenetics in anesthesia, with the discovery of the genetic basis for atypical plasma cholinesterases [23]. Later, in collaboration with clinical anesthesiologist Beverly Britt, Kalow described the genetic basis for malignant hyperthermia [24].

However, until the late 1960s or early 1970s, less research took place in anesthesia than in other specialties, such as internal medicine. At the Vandewater meeting in 1975 in Kingston, the head of the Medical Research Council of Canada, Malcolm Brown, pointed out that if Canadian anesthesiology were to produce research, they would have to do what other specialties had done: institute 'practice plans' that would free up time, allowing faculty to do research (protected time), and support investigators' training after the RCPSC fellowship. This launched research in many Canadian departments, and created a career path for the graduates of Clinician-Scientist training programs into the future.

Considerable input into the development of anesthesia came from other University departments. For example, Mark Nickerson (Pharmacology) and Reuben Cherniak (Internal Medicine) in Manitoba, promoted a 1963 report on anesthesia [25] at the University of Manitoba by Robert Dripps of the University of Pennsylvania. Dripps recommended establishing a University Department of Anesthesia (done in 1967) and pointed to the potential for anesthetists to do clinical research, a point he had made many years earlier [26]. Also at that time, with the advent of cardiac surgery and the advances in respiratory medicine, some anesthesiologists began to work in critical care medicine. Barry Fairley (anesthesia) in Toronto, and Cherniak in Winnipeg, were instrumental in this. Fairley worked with a pulmonary physiologist, Charles Bryan, recruited to the Department of Anesthesia in Toronto, on a series of classic experiments on lung volumes (FRC) and positive end-expired pressure (PEEP). Many clinical anesthesiologists trained in research with "Charlie", and this experience led to the elucidation of many important concepts that are still fundamental to clinical practice – including diaphragmatic function during anesthesia, [27] and mechanical ventilation using high frequency oscillation [28].

Alan Conn (1925–2010), Chief of Anesthesia at the Toronto Hospital for Sick Children (1960–71), recognized the need for a pediatric intensive care unit with specifically trained anesthesiologists. Conn followed in the footsteps of Charles Robson [29] (1884–1969), recognized as the "Father of Pediatric Anesthesia" (see chapter 65 on Pediatric Anesthesia for details). From 1971 to 1981, Conn directed the Intensive Care Unit. He was committed to both education and research, and established the Dr. Alan W. Conn Lectureship in Pediatric Anesthesia and Critical Care in 1986.

At that time many young Canadian anesthesiologists went to the US for further research training at the University of California, San Francisco (UCSF), Boston, and the University of Washington. Their return stimulated research in many Canadian departments of anesthesia. Beverley Orser, who completed her PhD in neuroscience following her anesthesia fellowship, demonstrated benefits of training Canadian anesthesiologists as Clinician Scientists. Her studies in the basic molecular mechanisms of anesthesia were recognized in 1995, by the first "Frontiers of Anesthesia" research award ($500,000) from the International Anesthesia Research Society. She was the first anesthesiologist to receive a Canada Research Chair, in 2003, under a Government of Canada program recognizing research excellence. Her success demonstrated that anesthesia had become a specialty in Canada which could train Clinician Scientists at the highest level. Graduate programs which were recognized by the Royal College in their Clinical Investigator Program, were established within the university departments to support such graduate level training for anesthesiologists.

In the 1970s, recognizing a growing clinical need in obstetrical units, especially in large hospitals, several Canadian anesthesiologists pursued obstetrical anesthesia fellowships in the US. In 1979, following the lead of the Society of Obstetrical Anesthesiologists and Perinatologists (SOAP) established in the US in 1968, several obstetrical anesthesiologists in Canada convinced the CAS Executive to create an Obstetrical Anesthesia section, the first subspecialty Section within the CAS. The Section arranged an Obstetrical Anesthesia clinical session at each CAS Annual Meeting and assisted members in research strategies and ways to improve obstetrical anesthesia in their individual hospitals. Following on the creation of this section, other anesthesiologists formed sections devoted to the anesthesia care of cardiac, neurosurgical, and pediatric patients. Today there are 12 such sections, which help the CAS to provide an Annual Meeting with excellent research and sub-specialty educational activities.

Clinical Anesthesia Across Canada

Canada is the second largest country in the world (after Russia) with a land mass of 3.8 million square miles, but a population of only 34 million. This is roughly 10% of the US population and 40% of the UK population. Although most Canadians live within 100 km of the US border, many are in rural and remote areas, some accessible only by air. Delivery of health care, including anesthesia services, presents major challenges as a result. Canada's universal healthcare system (Medicare) has been in place in all provinces and territories

since 1972. The federal Canada Health Act (1984) provides the basic guidelines for the Canadian Medicare system (universality, comprehensiveness, accessibility, portability, public administration), but the actual delivery of healthcare is the responsibility of the ten Provinces and three Territories.

Because of the geographic challenges and the requirement for physician-based anesthetic delivery, specialist anesthesiologists (see RCPSC section) or Family Physicians (FPs) with advanced training in anesthesia, provide all anesthetic services. The training of FP anesthesiologists has evolved over the years. In 2002, the College of Family Physicians of Canada (CFPC) formally accredited anesthesia for a third year of family medicine training, with a specified training curriculum within any of the 16 university Anesthesia departments.

The university departments of anesthesia and the CAS provide programs for ongoing anesthesia education for all practitioners in Canada. Anesthesiologists have become major contributors to patient care outside the operating room. In common with other countries, many Canadian departments now include "Perioperative Medicine" in their official titles. Many obstetrical wards have had anesthesiologists in-house providing epidural analgesia during labor, as well as anesthesia for patients undergoing elective and emergency cesarean sections. In the past two decades, pre-operative assessment clinics have been widely established. Management of both acute post-operative pain and chronic pain has become a special area of expertise. In all these areas, nursing staff and more recently physician assistants have allowed anesthesiologists to assume a supervisory role, helping reduce physician manpower requirements.

The Canadian Anesthesia Identity

The combination of the physician-based provider model from the UK, and the university-based clinical training system originating with Waters in the US, has resulted in a uniquely Canadian entity, operating within Canada's universal Medicare system and adapting to the geographical and political health service delivery challenges of Canada. It led to the development of the Canadian identity.

The CAS 'Guidelines for the Practice of Anesthesia', first published in 1977 was many years ahead of those of other nations, and improved the outcomes of anesthesia, while decreasing liability insurance premiums.

Until the 1960s, some anesthesiologists worked as hospital employees, but with the introduction of universal Medicare in the late 1960s and early 1970s, anesthesiologists became independent contractors. Since healthcare was a provincial/territorial responsibility, fees were negotiated separately in each province or territory. Initially, fees were less than attractive, but with time, they increased to levels of appropriate remuneration. In many university departments, anesthesiologists organized into groups to provide opportunities for research, education and subspecialty clinical careers.

Reflecting the breadth of their clinical work, Canadian anesthesiologists accepted management positions in intensive care units, obstetrical care, pain clinics and other areas. Anesthesiologists became Vice Presidents of Medicine, Chiefs of Staff, and Chief Executives Officers of major health regions and hospitals, Deans of Faculties of Medicine, and Deputy Provincial Ministers of Health. Anesthesia has provided leaders in many of the medical associations at the Provincial and National level. They were instrumental in the 2003 formation of the Canadian Patient Safety Institute (CPSI), with John Wade of Winnipeg, Manitoba as the Founding Board Chair. Wade also had a major role in the early 1990s development of the Can Meds (Canadian Medical Education) system, by the RCPSC, which led to a revolution in the teaching of medicine at the undergraduate, postgraduate, and continuing education levels in Canada. Anesthetists have served as Registrars of provincial Colleges of Physicians and Surgeons, which regulate the medical profession, and as elected Presidents of the Colleges.

Over time, anesthesia emerged as a leading specialty in Canada and internationally, with leaders in research, education and patient care. The key factor in this evolutionary process was the development of a professional identity. Professionalism has been referred to as "the presence of individuals who have acquired knowledge by means of training and study and desire to pass on that knowledge to others" [30]. Combining the physician-based model from the UK with the positive influence of University-based departments of the US facilitated the development of the Canadian identity.

References

1. Shephard DAE, Turner KE. Preserving the heritage of Canadian anesthesiology. A panorama of people, ideas, techniques and events. Canadian Anesthesiologists' Society. 2004. http://www.cas.ca/English/Page/Files/74_Preserving%20the%20Heritage.pdf. Accessed:June 2012.
2. Steward DJ. The early history of anaesthesia in Canada: The introduction of ether to Upper Canada, 1847. Can Anaesth Soc J. 1977;24:153–61.
3. Jacques A. Anaesthesia in Canada, 1847–1967: I. The beginnings of anaesthesia in Canada. Can Anaesth Soc J. 1967;14:500–9.
4. Shephard D. From craft to specialty: a medical and social history of anesthesia and its changing role in health care. Thunder Bay: ON York Point Publishing, 2009.
5. Hutton_WAB. University of Manitoba Faculty of Medicine Archives.
6. Shephard DAE. History of Canadian Anaesthesia. The evolution of anaesthesia as a specialty in Canada. Can J Anaesth. 1990;37:134–42.

7. Griffith HR. Anaesthesia in Canada 1847–1967: II. The development of anaesthesia in Canada. Can Anaesth Soc J. 1967;14:510–8.
8. Carr I, Beamish RE. The Anaesthetists. In: Manitoba Medicine. A brief history. Winnipeg:The University of Manitoba;1999. pp 112–3.
9. Shields HJ. The history of anaesthesia in Canada. Can Anaesth Soc J. 1955;2:301–7.
10. Flexner A. Medical education in the United States and Canada: a report to the Carnegie Foundation for the Advancement of Teaching. New York: Carnegie Foundation for the Advancement of Teaching;1910.
11. Shephard DAE. The first century of anaesthesia in Canada 1847–1942. In: Watching closely those who sleep. A history of the Canadian Anaesthetists' Society. 1943–1993. Canadian Anesthesiologists' Society, Toronto;1993.
12. Miller DR, Wozny D. Research Awards Program of the Canadian Anesthesiologists' Society / Canadian Anesthesia Research Foundation: survey of past recipients. Can J Anesth 2007;54:314–9.
13. Harold Griffith. The evolution of modern anaesthesia. Bodman R, Gillies D, Editors. Toronto: Hannah Institute and Dundurn Press;1992.
14. Moffitt EA. Academic Anaesthesia Organizes (editorial). Can Anaesth Soc J. 1978;25:1–3.
15. Byrick RJ, Craig DB, Carli F. A physician workforce planning model applied to Canadian anesthesiology: assessment of needs. Can J Anesth. 2002;49:663–70.
16. Craig D, Byrick RJ, Carli F. A physician workforce planning model applied to Canadian anesthesiology: planning the future supply of anesthesiologists. Can J Anesth. 2002;49:671–7.
17. Minimum guidelines for the standards of practice of anaesthesia. Canadian Anaesthetists' Society. Toronto;1977
18. Cohen MM, Duncan PG, Pope WDB, Biehl D, Tweed WA, MacWilliam L, Merchant RN. The Canadian four-centre study of anaesthetic outcomes: II. Can outcomes be used to assess the quality of anaesthesia care? Can J Anesth. 1992;39:430–9.
19. Guidelines to the practice of anaesthesia. 2012 Edition. Can J Anesth. 2012;59:63–102.
20. Continuous flow inhalation anaesthetic apparatus (anaesthetic machines) for medical use. CSA Standard Z168.3-M1980. Rexdale:Canadian Standards Association;1980.
21. Lucas GHW. The discovery of cyclopropane. Anesth Analg. 1961;40:15–27.
22. Griffith HR, Johnson GE. The use of curare in general anesthesia. Anesthesiology. 1942;3:418–20.
23. Kalow W. Atypical plasma cholinesterase: a personal discovery story: a tale of three cities. Can J Anesth. 2004;51:206–11.
24. Britt BA, Kalow W, Gordon A, Humphrey JG, Rewcastle NB. Malignant Hyperthermia: an investigation of five patients. Can Anaesth Soc J. 1973;20:431–67.
25. Dripps RD. Confidential report to the Dean of Medicine, University of Manitoba. Archives, Faculty of Medicine;1963.
26. Dripps RD. Research and its relationship to clinical anesthesiology. Anesthesiology. 1949;10:690–5.
27. Froese AB, Bryan CB. Effects of anesthesia and paralysis on diaphragmatic mechanics in man. Anesthesiology. 1974;41:242–55.
28. Butler WJ, Bohn DJ, Bryan AC, Froese AB. Ventilation by high-frequency oscillation in humans. Anesth Analg. 1980;59:577–84.
29. Steward DJ. Historical vignette: Dr. Charles Robson. Pioneer Canadian pediatric anesthetist. Pediatric Anesthesia. 2012;22:275–7.
30. Vandam LR. Early American Anesthetists. The origins of professionalism in anesthesia. Anesthesiology. 1972;38:264–74.

The History of Anesthesia in Mexico, the Caribbean Islands, and Central America

Estela Melman

Summary

Mexico and Cuba rapidly adopted anesthesia following Morton's 1846 demonstration, and US and Mexican forces used ether in the Mexican-American war in 1847. Ether was used in Cuba and Guatemala in 1847, but not until 1861 in the Dominican Republic, 1875 in Panama, and 1889 or later in El Salvador, Nicaragua, and Costa Rica. Surgeons in Cuba used cocaine for topical and local anesthesia in 1884. Spinal anesthesia appeared from 1899 (Mexico first) to 1910 in Mexico, Cuba, Guatemala, El Salvador, Nicaragua and Panama. At the Hospital General de Mexico from 1905 to the mid-1920s, Vázquez found a mortality of approximately 1:1,500 with spinal anesthesia and 1:440 with chloroform. In 1946, Cuban, Manuel Curbelo, performed continuous lumbar epidural anesthesia. Vicente García Olivera created the first center for pain treatment in 1948, in Mexico. Keith Holder followed, in Panama in 1975. In 1956, Mexican anesthesiologists assumed responsibility for obstetric anesthesia.

Tracheal intubation arrived in the 1930s–1950s in Cuba, Mexico, El Salvador, and Panama. Short-acting barbiturates, were adopted in the 1930s in Mexico, Cuba, Guatemala, and El Salvador while curare and succinylcholine came into use in the 1940s–1950s in every country. After Michael Johnstone's 1956 demonstration (Mexico), halothane rapidly replaced ether and cyclopropane throughout the region. Sevoflurane, given in oxygen, displaced halothane and isoflurane in most Central American countries in the 1990s. Desflurane appeared in a few countries (e.g., Panama and Mexico) at this time.

The Society of Anesthetists of Mexico developed in 1934, and societies formed between 1950 and 1993 in the remaining countries. The Mexican Society published a journal in 1951 (the second in Latin America), but except for the Cuban Society (which developed a journal in 2001) other societies were too small to publish a bulletin or journal.

Institution of specialty training in anesthesia roughly paralleled the development of societies, beginning in Mexico in 1957. 1974 saw the creation of the Mexican Board of Anesthesia. Residencies currently last for 3–4 years. Of all the countries in this region, only Mexico and Panama have recertification programs (every five years).

Initially, surgeons administered most anesthesia in Central America, but the shortage of physicians dictated that nurses and technicians also performed this task. Increasing numbers of anesthesiologists appeared after 1950, leading some countries to limit delivery of anesthesia to physicians: Panama, in 1971; Cuba, after 1978; and Mexico, 1998. Dominican Republic anesthesiologists currently provide anesthesia in even the smallest villages. Technicians still give most anesthetics in Guatemala, Honduras, El Salvador, and Nicaragua.

A Historical Perspective

Before Europeans came to North and South America, Mexico and neighboring countries were home to advanced Meso-American cultures. From the 1519–1521 Spanish conquest to Mexico's independence in the early nineteenth century, this region was part of the Viceroyalty of New Spain, embracing Mexico, the Spanish Caribbean Islands and Central America as far South as Panama. A viceroy residing in Mexico City and appointed by the Spanish monarch administered the Viceroyalty.

Following the Mexican declaration of independence in 1810, protracted countrywide fighting erupted until independence was won in 1821. War left Mexico in disorder, but slowly Mexicans rebuilt the social and political infrastructure needed to support a republican government. The US invasion of Mexico in 1846 interrupted this process. Adding further to disorder and disarray, in 1848, Mexico was forced to cede California, Arizona, Nevada, New Mexico, Utah, Colorado, Wyoming and Texas to the US.

E. Melman (✉)
Department of Anesthesia, American British Cowdry Medical Center, Mexico City, Mexico
e-mail: bierzmel@prodigy.net.mx

E. I Eger II et al. (eds.), *The Wondrous Story of Anesthesia,* DOI 10.1007/978-1-4614-8441-7_26, © Edmond I Eger, MD 2014

While under Spanish rule, Central America was a colonial backwater and lagged economically and culturally behind Mexico. However, fortunately Central America was spared the bloody wars that characterized the independence movements of Mexico and Spanish South America, and in 1821, Costa Rica, El Salvador, Guatemala, Honduras and Nicaragua proclaimed their independence from the Spanish Crown. In 1823, these five countries transiently formed the United Provinces of Central America, dreaming that they might achieve a united and prosperous independent Central American nation. This dream ended in 1841 when the five countries split apart. In 1821, the Dominican Republic gained its independence from Spain. However, Cuba remained a Spanish territory until 1898 when the US defeated Spain in the Spanish-American War. Cuba gained its independence from the US on 20 May 1902.

Mexico

Anesthesia Begins in Mexico

Anesthesia began in Mexico during the Mexican-American war [1]. Edward Barton, a University of Pennsylvania graduate, and surgeon to the 3rd Dragoons Cavalry Brigade, Twiggs Division, wrote to Thomas Lawson, US Surgeon General, in December 1846, citing Morton's recent demonstration of ether anesthesia. He urged Lawson to use Morton's agent for the relief of surgical pain in wounded soldiers. At President Polk's request, Barton joined General Winfield Scott in Veracruz, in February 1847 during Scott's siege of the port city. On March 29, 1847, Barton administered the first ether anesthetic in Mexico. A German teamster had accidentally discharged his musket, shattering both of his legs. On March 28, one leg was amputated, but the patient cried so intensely that amputation of the other leg was postponed. The next day, Barton, assisted by doctors Harney, Porter, and Laub, used ether during the amputation, administered with an apparatus that Barton had brought from the US (probably similar to Morton's). Barton described it as a complete success [1]. The patient became insensitive to pain and "the limb was removed without the quiver of a muscle."

Barton taught his aides, including John Porter who chronicled medical aspects of the Mexican-American war, including how to administer ether anesthesia [2]. Porter in turn, taught ether anesthesia to his Mexican counterparts, including Pedro Van der Linden, surgeon in chief to the Mexican Army (Fig. 26.1). During the Cerro Gordo's battle (Jalapa, Mexico), Van der Linden gave ether anesthesia to wounded Mexican soldiers. "Occasionally the physicians on both sides engaged in actual fighting, but more often they were kept busy, first attending their own compatriots, then the

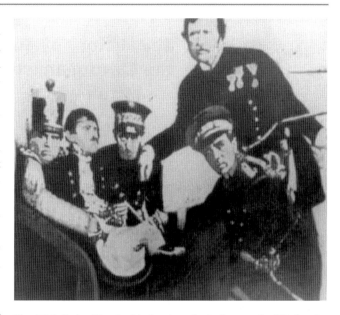

Fig. 26.1 Pedro Van der Linden (standing), Surgeon in Chief to the Mexican Army, after performing his first amputation in a patient anesthetized with ether. Two soldiers hold the wounded soldier, perhaps still asleep (second from left), and a third soldier holds the amputated limb. This daguerreotype copy was taken at the Battle of Cerro Gordo, 18 April 1847 from reference 3 with permission from the publisher. (Courtesy of Gaceta Médica de México)

wounded enemy. The rule, rather than the exception, was that gallant and noble gestures were displayed by physicians on both sides" [2, 3]. The use of ether spread to other cities. On June 15 1847, Jose Sansores used it successfully for an upper limb amputation in Merida, Yucatan [4].

Pablo Martinez del Rio introduced ether into Mexico in 1848 (for general and obstetrical surgery), and then introduced chloroform in 1849. Years later (1878), he reported his experiences with chloroform in obstetric anesthesia [5]. He supported the use of chloroform anesthesia during general surgery, but advised against it in obstetrics in order to avoid massive blood loss and death, particularly in uterine dystocia. He suggested that it should be used only to achieve analgesia: "More than one mishap could have been avoided if the parturient would not have been under the influence of chloroform."

Fernando López Sánchez, a surgeon and ophthalmologist in the armed forces, was trained in Paris. In 1886, he returned to Mexico and began using cocaine topically, for superficial ocular surgery. During the 1890s, to avoid the use of general anesthesia with chloroform, he described a technique in which he injected 1 % cocaine around the eyeball to perform enucleations and other major procedures [6].

In July 1900, in Oaxaca, Mexico, following a description published by Theodore Tuffier in 1899, Ramon Pardo used 15 mg cocaine hydrochloride injected at the 5th lumbar interspace to produce spinal anesthesia for amputation of a leg. He used a Pravaz syringe and a 9 cm long needle designed by

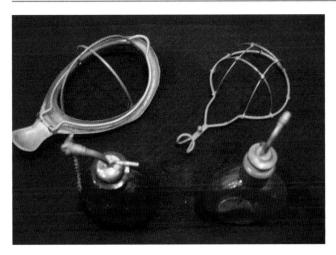

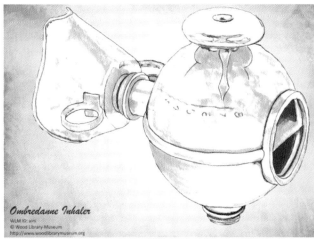

Fig. 26.2 Examples of the metal frames that were used to support the gauze onto which ether and chloroform were dropped. Two examples of the drip bottles used to deliver ether or chloroform also are shown. (Courtesy of Museo del Palacio de Medicina y de la Dirección General del Patrimonio Universitario, UNAM (DGPU/1239/2013), Mexico City, Mexico)

Fig. 26.3 The ether inhaler designed by Louis Ombrédanne in 1908. (Courtesy of the Wood Library-Museum of Anesthesiology, Park Ridge, IL)

Table 26.1 Anesthetics Given at the Hospital General de Mexico, 1905-mid-1920s

	Number of Cases	%
Spinal anesthesia with cocaine	9452	100.00
Spinals completed with chloroform	687	7.27
Failed spinals	661	6.99
Deaths related to spinal anesthesia	6	0.06
General anesthesia with chloroform	8372	100.00
Cardiac arrests during chloroform	18	0.19
Deaths related to chloroform	19	0.22
Mixed anesthetics	401	
General anesthesia with ether	307	
Anesthesia with ethyl chloride	80	

Tuffier to obtain cerebrospinal fluid and inject the cocaine, achieving excellent anesthesia without side effects [7–9].

Bandera reported [10] that in the early 1900s, the most common anesthetic techniques used by surgeons in Mexico were local/topical anesthesia with cocaine for ophthalmic surgery, ethyl chloride for incision and drainage of superficial abscesses, and chloroform or spinal anesthesia for general surgery. Ether was reserved for very sick patients only. The consensus among surgeons was that chloroform was a potent and "toxic" anesthetic that could kill the patient instantly, or in the immediate postoperative period, by producing profound depression leading to coma, anuria and death [11, 12]. They considered that ether was a "safer" anesthetic, and was better tolerated than chloroform by sick patients [12]. Induction was said to be more pleasant with chloroform, which explains its continued use. However, they concluded that "it is about time to discard chloroform, but unfortunately we are immersed in a

tight routine of spinal and chloroform for all patients...." Ether was available.

To deliver chloroform, a gauze mask was used. A similar mask could be used for ether, or alternatively, a Fowler, Clover or Allis's mask or inhaler (metal frame, covered with leather and containing a folded cloth to absorb the ether) [13]. A dropper (Fig. 26.2) was also required, together with a mouth opener, and forceps to hold the tongue in case of a sudden respiratory arrest. Caffeine and strychnine were used to treat cardiac depression manifested by bradycardia and "cerebral anemia" (loss of consciousness or profound depression), and adrenalin was used for accidents occurring during spinal anesthesia. A report of anesthetics given at the Hospital General de Mexico, shows the greater popularity of spinal anesthesia (Table 26.1) and its lower mortality (p < 0.0001– chi square analysis) [12].

In addition, the author compared the mortality occurring in the US at the time, with the same anesthetics: chloroform 1 death/2,500, ether 1/16,000 and nitrous oxide 1/200,000 cases [12].

In 1908, Louis Ombrédanne described an anesthetic apparatus for the simple delivery of ether anesthesia (Fig. 26.3), popularizing its use [14]. Nitrous oxide anesthesia, and carbon dioxide absorbers were introduced in the 1910s and 1920s respectively [10].

In 1932, Federico Vollbrechthausen, a trainee from the Mayo Clinic, came to Mexico to practice anesthesia, bringing ethylene, cyclopropane, and a closed circuit apparatus for their administration. He brought hexobarbital (later replaced by thiopental) for intravenous use, and procaine for spinal and local anesthesia. In 1941, an American thoracic surgeon, Leo Eloesser, and his anesthesiologist colleague William Neff, a former pupil of Ralph Waters, came to Mexico City to demonstrate thoracic surgery and anesthesia at the Hospital for Tuberculosis Diseases. Neff used tracheal intubation and controlled ventilation with a closed circuit apparatus [15]. Jorge Terrazas and Martin Maquívar then employed it, reporting in 1944 on the first "19 cases of anesthesia with controlled ventilation for thoracic anesthesia" [16]. The 1940s also saw the introduction of curare, and the monitoring of vital signs. Cyclopropane became as popular as ether due to its capacity to produce a rapid induction, its potency, and the wide margin between anesthetic and lethal concentrations.

In 1956, Michael Johnstone came to Mexico to demonstrate the use of halothane, which then largely replaced ether and cyclopropane over the next decade [17] A lesser proportion of the flammable anesthetics were replaced by methoxyflurane and enflurane. However, neither achieved great popularity. Their use was discontinued in 1980, with the arrival of isoflurane. Halothane continued in use until the 1990s, when Melman and Lozano introduced desflurane and sevoflurane into Mexico [18, 19]. The latter agents are those currently in use.

Regional Anesthesia in Mexico

As noted earlier, Ramón Pardo introduced spinal anesthesia in 1900 [7, 8]. Cocaine, amylocaine (Stovaine), and subsequently procaine hydrochloride were the commonly used local anesthetics, until displaced by tetracaíne and lidocaine. In 1923, Leopoldo Escobar gave the first caudal anesthesia to a patient suffering from sciatica. In 1939, in Monterrey, Mexico, Rodolfo Rodriguez performed the first lumbar epidural block.

For almost two decades, obstetricians/gynecologists administered anesthesia for obstetrics, either intravenously with a combination of meperidine 50–100 mg plus promethazine 50 mg and promazine 25 mg, or as a spinal anesthetic with tetracaíne. In 1938, surgeon Isidro Espinosa de los Reyes, used a catheter to achieve a continuous caudal epidural [20]. Two other surgeons (Mateos Fournier and Jose Rabago) [21] later introduced Robert Hingson's and Waldo Edwards's continuous caudal analgesia technique for obstetrics In 1956, anesthesiologists Vicente García Olivera [22], Guillermo Vasconcelos [23], Fernando Rodriguez de la Fuente [24], and Carlos Martínez Redding [25] took obstetric anesthesia from the hands of the surgeons at the hospitals of the Social Security Institute. They replaced spinal (because of hypotension) and caudal (because of catheter contamination) anesthesia with lumbar epidural anesthesia. This practice, with its benefits for the parturient and the newborn, rapidly spread to other hospitals. Currently, unless contraindicated, lumbar epidural block is applied in 95–98% of obstetric cases (Marrón M. Personal Communication. Ob/Gyn Anesthesiologist. Former Director Division of Postgrade and Continuous Education in Health. Secretaría de Salud, Mexico).

Epidural or subarachnoid anesthesia had not been used in children until Melman, Marrufo, and Penuelas, working at the Children's Hospital in Mexico City (Hospital Infantil de México), compared the effects of subarachnoid versus epidural block, and from studies in cadavers and patients, Melman, Tandazo and Arenas, determined the doses needed to reach different dermatomes [26, 27]. Surgeons initially opposed the use of these techniques, but the benefits quickly overcame their reservations. Currently, at the Children's Hospital, central neuraxial anesthesia is used in about 50% of cases and results in the earlier discharge of patients [28]. Epidural anesthesia in children is nowadays used throughout Mexico, having displaced spinal anesthesia because of the longer postoperative analgesia possible with continuous epidural anesthesia.

In 1945, Vicente García Olivera went to New York to train under E Rovenstine at the Bellevue Hospital in New York who had founded a Pain Clinic in 1936. García Olivera later attended a course at the Veterans Administration Pain Clinic in McKinney, Texas [29]. He was an enthusiast in regional anesthesia, in all its modalities, central neuraxial, sympathetic, and peripheral blocks. In 1948, he created the first center for pain treatment at the London Clinic, in Mexico City (Hospital Clínica Londres). In 1975 he organized the first Pain Clinic at the Hospital General de México. which in 1992 became the National Center for Training in Pain Therapy (Centro Nacional de Capacitación en Clínica y Terapia del Dolor) [29].

The Mexican Society of Anesthesiology

In 1934, led by physicians Emilio Varela, Federico Vollbrenthausen, Juan Morquecho, Francisco Fierro and Benjamín Bandera, the Surgical Society of the Hospital Juarez in Mexico City founded the Society of Anesthetists of Mexico (Sociedad de Anestesistas de Mexico), the first anesthesia society created in Latin America. In 1948, the Society changed its name to the Mexican Society of Anesthesiologists (MSA), appointing members from other Mexican states [30].

In 1946, the MSA organized its first National Congress of Anesthesia, holding subsequent congresses every two years until 1974, when annual meetings were instituted. The MSA participated in the founding of societies of anesthesia in other states of Mexico, such as the Society of Anesthesiology of Jalisco in 1948, and the Society of Anesthesiologists of Monterrey, in 1954. In 1960, the societies assembled into a Federation of Mexican Societies of Anesthesia (FSARM). In 1955, the MSA participated as Mexico's representative in the creation of the World Federation of Societies of Anesthesia (WFSA), and in 1962, in the Confederation of Latin American Societies of Anesthesia (CLASA). The MSA was appointed by the FSARM to be the main organizer of the 6th World Congress of Anesthesiology held in Mexico City in 1976. In 1994 the MSA changed its name to Colegio Mexicano de Anestesiología (COMEXANE) to more effectively represent its members before government authorities [31]. The former Federation of Societies (FSARM) is now called FMCA, AC (Federación Mexicana de Colegios de Anestesia, Asociación Civil). The Mexican College of Anesthesiology, in Mexico City, has 1500 members. The total number of anesthesiologists in Mexico is approximately 12,000, with 8,000 board certified as of September 2011.

Goals of the Mexican College of Anesthesiology (Formerly Society)

1. *To promote information about anesthesia.* Aspects of the specialty are presented and discussed in monthly meetings. An Annual Meeting has been held with the participation of foreign and national speakers and professors since 1974.
2. *To promote research in anesthesia.* To further this aim, the "Benjamín Bandera Foundation" was created in 1976. A Trust Fund established with the profits from the 6th World Congress of Anesthesia held in 1976 in Mexico City, was used to support the Foundation.
3. *To improve clinical care*: anesthesia courses and workshops are conducted in different hospitals.
4. *To promote the countrywide development of societies of anesthesia.*

In 1960, the Society supported the founding of the Federation of Mexican Societies of Anesthesia (FSARM). State societies of anesthesia, one or two for each state for a total of 60, combined to form FSARM [32]. The Society (now College), also supported the founding and organization of societies of different anesthesia subspecialties including pediatrics (SAP), obstetrics and gynecology (SMAGO), cardiothoracic anesthesia, and pain [33].

Residency Programs in Anesthesia

The establishment of several major medical institutions in Mexico City in the 1940s facilitated the development of anesthesia training programs. They included the Children's Hospital in 1943, the National Institute of Cardiology in 1944, the Institute for Medical Sciences and Nutritional Diseases (Instituto Nacional de Ciencias Médicas y Nutrición) in 1946, and the Hospitals in the Mexican Institute for Social Security. The training programs were supported initially by the Mexican Society of Anesthesiologists (MSA) and later by the National University of Mexico (UNAM) and the Mexican Board of Anesthesiology.

In 1957, the MSA organized the first postgraduate course in anesthesia, appointing members of the Society as professors. The 24-month course was held in Mexico City at the General Hospital (Hospital General de México). Physicians taking the course and training received a monthly salary enabling them to leave their former practice and devote their entire time to anesthesia. The MSA continued to organize these courses until 1962. The anesthesiologists thus trained, and others trained in Canada and the US, initiated residency programs in anesthesia in several Mexican hospitals.

In 1966, the MSA and the National University initiated a two-year residency program [19, 20]. A 3 year program was established in 1986 at the National University. This was achieved through the co-operation of the National Committee for Postgraduate Education, the Ministry of Health, the MSA's Academic Committee in Anesthesia and the Mexican Federation of Societies of Anesthesia [21, 22]. Acceptance for subspecialty training in pediatrics, neuro-anesthesia, cardiothoracic anesthesia, critical care, obstetrics/gynecology, or pain, currently requires that the appointee be certified by the Mexican Board of Anesthesia. Subspecialty credentialing demands a further 2 years of training in the designated subspecialty [33].

Mexican Board of Anesthesia

In 1974, members of the MSA, as advised by the National Academy of Medicine, created the Mexican Board of Anesthesia (Consejo Mexicano de Anestesiología; Archivo del Consejo Mexicano de Anestesiología 1974). Candidates were certified after 3 years of a residency program in one of the hospitals appointed as training hospitals, and after taking a written and oral examination. The Board was also responsible for approving and certifying the congresses and the courses held as part of the continuing medical education programs. The Board also determined recertification of all anesthesiologists every 5 years, granting the permit to continue to practice anesthesia. This process of accreditation and certification by the Anesthesia Board, was equivalent to the process that was carried out by the 47 specialty councils recognized by the National Committee for Medical Specialties (CONACEM).

Practice of Anesthesia

As in many parts of the world, surgeons were the first to administer anesthesia in Mexico. However, the shortage of physicians also dictated that nurses and technicians perform these tasks. Nurses and technicians received one year tutorial courses from trained anesthesiologists; these courses ceased in the early 1970s. Finally, after a long campaign conducted by Mexican anesthesiologists, the authorities and politicians in Mexico became convinced that anesthesia was a medical specialty, best administered by trained physicians. This was incorporated into Mexican law in 1998.[1]

Revista Mexicana de Anestesiología (Mexican Journal of Anesthesiology)

The founding members of the MSA published the first anesthesia articles as a supplement called "Anesthesia" in the "Journal of Surgery of the Hospital Juarez" from 1936 until 1939. Subsequent anesthesia articles were published in "Medicina" [10, 31].

In July 1951, the first issue of Revista Mexicana de Anestesiologia (RMA) was published, with Benjamín Bandera as the first director and Vicente García Olivera as editor [10]. It was the second anesthesia journal (after Argentina's) published in Latin America. Since its first publication, it has appeared every three months. It is abstracted or indexed by standard databases (16 databases including Scopus, but not Medline), and is distributed to all members of the Mexican Society. It is the main anesthesia journal published in Mexico, and is the official publication of the Mexican College of Anesthesiology, (COMEXANE). The journal promotes the publication of clinical and basic research in anesthesia and perioperative medicine, critical care, and pain. The Editorial Board accepts papers submitted for publication by Mexican and Spanish speaking Latin American anesthesiologists.

Since 2006, the Colegio Mexicano de Anestesiología also edits quarterly, the Mexican Clinics of Anesthesia, with Raul Carrillo Esper as the current editor-in-chief of both publications [34]. Another Mexican journal "Anestesia", edited by the Mexican Federation (FMCAAC), has had an irregular publication schedule; currently it is published online every 4 months.

Globalization has permitted the rapid spread of knowledge and technology. In Mexico the quality of medicine may now be comparable to that practiced in first world countries. The US Joint Commission on Health Care Accreditation, (JAHCO) has accredited several hospitals in Mexico City and other states in Mexico, as having standards comparable to those in the US (e.g., the American British Cowdray Medical Center).

Anesthesia in Caribbean Islands and Central America

Anesthesia developed unevenly in Caribbean Islands and Central American countries in the several decades after Morton's historic demonstration in 1846 (Tables 26.2 and 26.3). This remarkable observation makes one marvel at the diverse conditions that led to a virtual absence of anesthesia in some countries until the last quarter of the nineteenth century, whereas other countries benefited from anesthesia within a year of its discovery. Of course, some of the information may overestimate how long it took to incorporate anesthesia into practice, since for some drugs, little data are available, while for others (ether-chloroform) we have sufficient information. Although a good explanation for the late arrival of anesthesia in many countries is lacking, socio-cultural and economic factors probably underlie the variability in the delay, but as Sherlock Holmes said: "it is a capital mistake to theorize before one has data."

Cuba

Vicente de Castro used ether in Cuba on 11 March 1847, in a patient requiring surgical treatment of a bilateral hydrocele. Nicolas Gutierrez introduced chloroform in 1848 (It did not replace ether), and cocaine was first used for local anesthesia in ophthalmology in 1884. In 1900, Emilio Nuñez gave subarachnoid anesthesia with cocaine, later replaced with amylocaine by Gonzalez Mármol [35] (Personal Communication: Humberto Sainz Cabrera, Presidente Sociedad Cubana de Anestesia y Reanimación, 2011). Fourneau had introduced spinal anesthesia, and Gonzalez Marmol used it in 100 obstetrical cases, reporting uterine inertia in five.

Luis Hevia, a physician who practiced anesthesia full-time, is considered to be the "founder of the specialty" in Cuba. He introduced nitrous oxide in 1918, ethylene in 1926, and cyclopropane in 1934 [35]. In 1938, he was appointed as Honorary President of the Anesthesia Research Society and the International College of Anaesthetists during the joint meeting with the Associated Anesthetists of the United States and Canada held in New York [36]. In 1939, he described the use of ether in the tropics [36].

In the 1930s, intravenous sodium amytal, hexobarbital, and sodium thiopental were used in Cuba to induce anesthesia, the last having the greatest popularity and remaining in use until recent times. Tracheal intubation was also introduced during those years [35], (Personal Communication: Humberto Sainz Cabrera, Presidente Sociedad Cubana de Anestesia y Reanimación, 2011) and epidural anesthesia was initiated in 1937 by Ferro [37].

In 1946, Manuel Curbelo performed continuous lumbar epidural anesthesia via a ureteral catheter inserted through a

---

[1] It appears as **NOM # 170 for The Practice of Anesthesiology** (Norma Oficial Mexicana #170-SSA1-1998 para la Práctica de la Anestesiología), which has been replaced **by NOM006-SSA3-2011**.

Table 26.2 Initial Use of Anesthetics in Mexico, Caribbean Islands and Central America

Country	Ether	Chloroform	Nitrous Oxide	Curare	Cocaine	Spinal	Epidural
Mexico	1847	1849	1910s	1942	1890s	1899	1923
Cuba	1847	1848	1918	1950s	1886	1900	1937
Dominican Republic	1861	1861	1930s?	1953	—	1916	1957
Guatemala	1847	1859	1930?	1950	1901	1901	1935
Honduras	1900s	1900s	1960s	1960s	—	1950s	1966
El Salvador	1899	1870	1937	1949	1886	1902	1941
Nicaragua	1889	1891	1955	1956	1891	1900	1960
Costa Rica	1890s	1875	1952	1947	—	1909	1962
Panama	1875+	1875+	1910	1957	—	1910	1970

Table 26.3 Initiation of Societies, Residencies and Journals

Country	Society	Residency	Journal
Mexico	1934	1957	1951
Cuba	1950	1962	2001
Dominican Rep	1970	1976	None
Guatemala	1958	1958	None
Honduras	1960	1998	None
El Salvador	1967	1974	None
Nicaragua	1993	1982	None
Costa Rica	1991	1974	None
Panama	1964	1971	None

16 G Huber tipped Tuohy needle. He was invited to demonstrate his technique in New York. The international anesthesia community acknowledged his contributions, electing him in 1955, as the first vice-president of the World Federation of Societies of Anesthesiology (WFSA) (Personal Communication: Humberto Sainz Cabrera, Presidente Sociedad Cubana de Anestesia y Reanimación, 2011).

Alberto Fraga introduced curare, succinylcholine and halothane for clinical use in the 1950s. Halothane rapidly replaced all other inhaled anesthetics (ether, ethyl chloride and ethylene) soon after its introduction in the late 1950s.

The exodus of many physicians after the 1962 Cuban Revolution, prompted initiation of a two-year residency program in anesthesia preceded by a one year rotating internship. No residency program, only tutoring, had existed previously. Physicians had practiced anesthesia as a part time specialty, supplementing income from other practices. The shortage of physicians and anesthesiologists, and the need to provide anesthesia services throughout the country, prompted the development of a one year anesthesia training program for registered nurses and, subsequently, for technicians. For more than a decade, these personnel provided most anesthesia services. In 1978, Sergio del Valle, Health Secretary, became aware of the considerable morbidity and mortality related to anesthesia, and determined that only trained physicians should administer anesthesia. Accordingly, the number of anesthesiologists increased from a few hundred in the early 1980s, to 1300 in 2012 (Personal Communication: Humberto Sainz Cabrera, Presidente Sociedad

Cubana de Anestesia y Reanimación, 2011). In 1986, anesthesia training increased to 4 years. The anesthesia training program was nationally designed and implemented by the Schools of Medicine. Trainees completing the program were awarded the title of specialist in anesthesia by the Ministry for Advanced Education (Ministerio de Educación Superior) (Personal Communication: Humberto Sainz Cabrera, Presidente Sociedad Cubana de Anestesia y Reanimación, 2011).

The shortage of resources and foreign currency due to the economic blockade of Cuba following the revolution hindered technical and scientific advancement. After the year 2000, globalization and the internet increased access to medical knowledge and thereby ameliorated this situation.

The Cuban Society of Anesthesiology (Sociedad Cubana de Anestesiología) was created in 1950. In 2000, the society was renamed Sociedad Cubana de Anestesiología y Reanimación (SCAR). It became the medical advisor to the Cuban Government and established national protocols for anesthesia practice throughout the country. SCAR has been an active member of CLASA since 1975 (Confederation of Latin American Societies of Anesthesia) and WFSA since its creation in 1955. It is also a member of FESACAC (Federation of Anesthesia Societies of Central America and the Caribbean), Humbero Saínz Cabrera from Cuba is the current President. Since 2001, the Cuban Journal of Anesthesia has been published online every 4 months, an initiative of Idoris Cordero, the current editor (Personal Communication: Humberto Sainz Cabrera, Presidente Sociedad Cubana de Anestesia y Reanimación, 2011).

Dominican Republic

Chloroform and ether anesthesia were introduced between 1861 and 1870, but were rarely used due to "complications". "Aguardiente" (an anise-flavored liquor) was preferred. The first reports of the use of chloroform and ether appeared in the 1900s. Ether was initially used with Julliard´s mask, and later with Ombrédanne's apparatus. There is no information as to why there was such an apparently long delay for anesthesia to emerge.

Francisco Puello, a general surgeon, reported the first spinal anesthesia in 1916. In 1923, he published an article describing 100 cases using "steraine with glucose". He reported two deaths and sphincter paralysis, leading him to substitute procaine for the mixture thereafter.

Between 1947 and 1950, the first anesthesia apparatus, a Heidbrink machine, [g] was brought to the island. It had a carbon dioxide absorber and a circle rebreathing system for administration of nitrous oxide and ether via a face mask. Tracheal intubation was not used. In 1951, Octavio Marmolejos went to Argentina to learn anesthetic techniques including selective bronchial intubation and cardiovascular anesthesia. Following his return to Santo Domingo he organized anesthesia services in clinics and hospitals, equipping them with Foregger anesthesia machines [38]. In 1953, he and Humberto Hernández initiated the use of tubocurarine. In 1957 Marmolejos also introduced epidural anesthesia with the "hanging drop technique" or Gutierrez's method, which he had learned in Buenos Aires. (Personal communication provided by José Fanduiz the senior member of the SDA).

In 1970, Cosme Battle, founder of the Dominican Anesthesia Society, became its first president. In 1978, the Society created the first School of Anesthesia for physicians in the country. In 1993 CLASA incorporated the Sociedad Dominicana de Anestesiología (SDA) as one of its members, encouraging them to organize national and international anesthesia congresses, such as the XXV Latin American Congress of Anesthesia held in Santo Domingo in 1999. The SDA is also a founding member of the Federación de Sociedades de Anestesia de Centro América y el Caribe (FESACAC). The bylaws of the Society were updated, in 2006 [39].

In 1976, two anesthesia residency programs were created, one at the Salvador B Gautier Hospital of the Social Security system, and the other at the Hospital Dr. Darío Contreras, by the Health Ministry. Initially, residency programs lasted 2 years, but in 2009 they were extended to 4 years. Currently there are 12 residency programs in the country, two are in military hospitals, two in the Social Security Institute, one private and the remaining seven are with the Health Ministry. All are sponsored by the Universidad Autónoma de Santo Domingo (Autonomous University of Santo Domingo) (Lambertus Tomás E: Personal Comunication. Dr. Lambertus is the Current Medical Director of the Department of Anesthesia at the Hospital Dr. Darío Contreras in Santo Domingo, Dominican Republic).

All hospitals have postanesthesia care units (PACUs). ICUs are available in the large hospitals with active participation by anesthesiologists in most. Anesthesiologists currently provide most anesthesia even in the smallest villages. Malpractice concerns ended anesthesia practice by all but a handful of technicians, some of whom are still in practice, but decreasing in number (Lambertus Tomás E: Personal Comunication).

The Dominican Republic occupies almost two thirds of the territory of the Island of Hispaniola (48,442 km^2); Haiti occupies the other third. Approximately 600 anesthesiologists serve this country with a population of more than 9.3 million inhabitants (Lambertus Tomás E: Personal Comunication).

Guatemala

José Luna, a Guatemalan-born physician trained in Paris, used ether in November 1847, to anesthetize Urbano Paniagua in order to amputate his finger. A few days later, two medical students, Juan Cañas from Guatemala and Felipe Arana from El Salvador, volunteered to be anesthetized with ether by Luna in a public demonstration at the Hospital General "San Juan de Dios". During induction they became excited and cyanotic and the experiment was suspended. On the next day, Luna amputated Marcelino Martinez's right arm under ether anesthesia [40, 41].

Following these four experiences, chloroform, which permitted a smoother induction and emergence, replaced ether. Luna used it first on 21 February 1850 and thereafter for 50 years. He was probably afraid to use ether again [40].

In 1901, Juan Ortega, after training in Paris, used spinal anesthesia with cocaine (0.15 g) for a patient undergoing inguinal herniorrhaphy. He named this technique "raquio-cocainización". It was used for the next 45 years for abdominal surgery [40].

In May 1913, surgeon Mario Wunderlich bought an Ombrédanne apparatus, for ether administration in Guatemala's General Hospital. The associated decrease in morbidity and mortality, and the ease of the use of ether with the Ombrédanne led to the displacement of chloroform by ether [40, 41].

Ethyl chloride was first used in 1910, at the General Hospital. In 1926, Wunderlich used ethyl chloride combined with chloroform and ether as the Schleich mixture, for anesthesia in 100 cases.

In 1930, a Foregger "Gwathmey" model anesthesia apparatus was brought to Guatemala and used to administer ether for the first cholecystectomy in Guatemala performed under general anesthesia. The 40-bed American Hospital was opened, equipped with an Ombrédanne's apparatus and an induction room for anesthesia [40, 41].

From 1935–1940, Mariano Herrarte and Enrique Penedo gave dibucaine/5 % glucose (Nupercaine) intrathecally as "saddle anesthesia" This technique gained popularity for gynecological and urological surgery. Applying a technique developed by the Mexican anesthesiologist Efrén Fierro, Lopez Herrarte produced segmental spinal anesthesia for thyroidectomies and neck surgery (brave anesthesiologist; braver patient). Herrarte also used caudal anesthesia for labor. Ramiro

Gálvez gave caudal anesthesia for urological and rectal surgery, and paravertebral and regional blocks for abdominal surgery [40].

Wunderlich introduced sodium thiopental into practice in 1939. Pablo Fuchs performed the first tracheal intubation in 1945 for a thyroidectomy. He used a rubber rectal tube adapted to Ombrédanne's ether apparatus [40, 41].

In 1948, two Guatemalans trained in the United States: Gustavo Ordoñez at Chicago's Cook County Hospital and Roberto Perez at Yale University. In addition, Flaviano Velazquez trained at the Children's Hospital (Hospital Infantil) and the National Institute of Cardiology (Instituto Nacional de Cardiología) in Mexico City. These three returned to Guatemala and pioneered development and training in anesthesia. They created the first departments, and were soon followed by others trained abroad. In 1950, they created the Chair of Anesthesia at the University of San Carlos in Guatemala City [41].

In 1958, they also founded the Anesthesia Society of Guatemala, which in 1968 became a member of WFSA, and in 1969 of CLASA. The society has been renamed as "Asociación Guatemalteca de Anestesiología Reanimación y Tratamiento del Dolor" (AGARTD). Guatemala's Society was also a founding member of the Federation of Anesthesia Societies of Central America and the Caribbean (FESACAC) (Personal communication from Dr. Eilin Valenzuela de Mazariegos, President of AGARTD).

In 1958, Samayoa de León started the first residency program in anesthesia, consisting of a 4-year training period developed by the University of San Carlos, the Health Ministry, Universidad Mariano Galvez, and the Institute for Social Security. At the end of the program, trainees were certified as anesthesiologists and became members of the Medical College of the University. They had to complete 32 hours per year of continuing medical education to remain active members, and to maintain the right to practice (Personal communication from Dr. Eilin Valenzuela de Mazariegos, President of AGARTD).

Although technicians still provide anesthesia in many parts of the country, in 1970, anesthesia was recognized as a medical specialty by the Medical College of Guatemala. The specialty has expanded into other fields such as ventilation therapy, peri-operative medicine, pain management, intensive care and other subspecialties. The AGARTD does not publish a journal or bulletin (Personal communication from Dr. Eilin Valenzuela de Mazariegos, President of AGARTD).

Honduras

Ether and chloroform both were first used in the early 1900s [42]. Initially, surgeons supervised the provision of anesthesia by nuns, nurses or laypersons. In the 1930s, Sor Roswindis, a German nun, served as an anesthetist and taught local personnel for many years. She is remembered as one of the pioneers. No information indicates who introduced ether or chloroform.

Ether was administered with an Ombrédanne's apparatus from 1908 to the 1950s. Subsequently, modern anesthesia apparatus, vaporizers, anesthetics, ancillary drugs and techniques were slowly incorporated into the practice of anesthesia. Current practice in large government hospitals and in some smaller private ones, is comparable to that in many other countries in Latin America. However, small government centers may provide a lesser standard of care. Government institutions hire anesthesia technicians with high-school degrees (secondary level), and with limited training given in a government school, to provide unsupervised anesthesia services. They are hired in preference to graduate anesthesiologists. Honduras has approximately 300 technicians. In private hospitals, anesthesia is provided by anesthesiologists who have graduated from a residency program. [39] (Montes GN, Personal Communication. Dr. Montes was a former trainee at Hospital Infantil de México in Mexico City and is Executive.Director of Hospital "Dr. Mario Catarino Rivas" in San Pedro Sula, Honduras).

The government controls 28 hospitals, and there are about an equal number of private hospitals. Only half of public hospitals have PACUs whereas all private hospitals have PACUs. Only 4 large government hospitals located in major cities have ICUs: Tegucigalpa—the capital city, San Pedro Sula and La Ceiba (Montes GN, Personal Communication). One editor of this book (LS) along with his wife Arlene spent two weeks in 1998 as a volunteer with a group from Interplast providing care in La Ceiba to children requiring cleft lip and palate repair. Arlene also assisted as the interpreter in preoperative preparation and postoperative observation. She refused to return the next year citing inadequate training for the job.

The University of Honduras was founded in 1847, and initiated its Medical School in 1881. In 1882, the first hospital opened in Honduras, the Hospital General San Felipe. Since then it has been the training site for medical graduates, specialists and technicians. In 1959, the Instituto Hondureño de Seguridad Social was created, and with it new clinics and hospitals with newly organized anesthesia departments. A formal residency program in Anesthesia, Reanimation and Pain was initiated in 1998, by Francisco Samayoa, who continues to be its academic coordinator. The National Health Department, the Social Security Institute, and the Universidad Autónoma de Honduras through its Post-graduate Division have supported this program since its creation [42].

The first Society of Anesthesia was founded in November 1960 by Napoleon Alcerro Oliva, an ENT specialist and anesthesiologist (the first director of the Anesthesia Service at San Felipe´s General Hospital), along with Zulema Canales, René Cervantes, Armando Rivera and Alejo Lara, all of whom had trained abroad. From 1995 to 1997, new bylaws of the Society were adopted and the Society changed its name to "Sociedad Hondureña de Anestesiología Reanimación y Dolor" (SHARD). Currently approximately 175 trained anesthesiologists serve a country of 5,500,000 inhabitants [42].

In 1974, the Society joined CLASA, and in 1976 joined WFSA. In 1994, the Society acted as a founding member of the Federation of Anesthesia Societies of Central America and the Caribbean (FESACAC). In 2002, the fifth congress of FESACAC was held in Honduras and in 2005, CLASA's XXVIII Congress of Anesthesia, was successfully organized in Tegucigalpa, Honduras, by Francisco Samayoa, acting as President of the organizing committee. Carolina Haylock, from San Pedro Sula, is the current president of SHARD. SHARD does not publish a journal or bulletin [42].

El Salvador

In 1870, 23 years following Simpson's 1847 discovery of the anesthetic properties of chloroform, Carlos Bonilla gave the first chloroform anesthetic in El Salvador. Surgeon Carlos Emilio Alvarez and his followers, pioneers of surgery as a specialty in El Salvador, used chloroform anesthesia for their surgical procedures. In 1886, Alvarez introduced the local anesthetic, cocaine. In 1899, surgeon Tomas Palomo brought ether to El Salvador for use by inhalation or rectally. In 1901, on a trip to Europe, he bought an Ombrédanne's apparatus, using it to administer Schleich's mixture of chloroform, ether and ethyl chloride [43]. Schleich's mixture was commonly used until 1920, when a modified Ombrédanne apparatus that delivered ether and oxygen, was substituted for the former one. Chloroform, which many surgeons had used was finally abandoned due to its toxicity [43, 44].

In 1902, Palomo used cocaine for spinal anesthesia in 28 cases, describing the symptomatic treatment used for spinal headache [44].

Medical students, who were responsible for bringing along a mask, and dripping chloroform onto it, provided anesthesia during the early twentieth century [43]. They also brought a mouth opener and a forceps to pull out the tongue in case of a sudden respiratory arrest (or perhaps airway obstruction).

In 1934, Carlos Leiva administered intravenous sodium hexobarbital to his brother for anesthesia, and Raul García Prieto induced obstetric analgesia with rectal paraldehyde.

In 1937, Raúl Argüello Manning convinced the board of the Hospital Rosales, of the need to improve the quality of medical care, and particularly anesthesia delivery to patients,

recommending the acquisition of the first two anesthesia machines in El Salvador. Two "Heidbrink" machines, each costing $ 1,500 USD, were purchased. They could deliver nitrous oxide, cyclopropane, ethylene and oxygen. At the same time, Manning hired an American nurse anesthetist, from Chicago, Miss Doris Nuggett, to provide and teach anesthesia in El Salvador—and initiate the delivery of oxygen with nitrous oxide, cyclopropane, or ethylene. She stayed for two years, leaving one of her pupils, Mr. Joaquin Herrador Tejada, in charge when she left [44].

In 1941, Joaquín Herrador, working with the surgeon Carlos B González, used tracheal intubation and positive pressure anesthesia for a pulmonary lobectomy. Antonio Lazo Guerra and Roberto Cañas Rivas initiated the use of sodium thiopental and epidural anesthesia for obstetric and perineal surgery [43, 44].

In 1948, two US trained Salvadoran anesthesiologists (Joaquín Coto from the Mayo Foundation and University of Minnesota, and Armando Milla from the University of Chicago) returned to found the Anesthesia Service at the Hospital Rosales (the first public hospital). Other anesthesiologists who had trained abroad soon joined them. Tracheal intubation and muscle relaxants were introduced, and modern anesthesia began (Aguilar ME: Personal communication. Aguilar is a cardiovascular anesthesiologist and was the President of CLASA for 2009–2011).

Halothane and methoxyflurane were introduced in the 1960s, and the use of cyclopropane ceased in 1972, with ether finally disappearing in 1976. Enflurane was introduced in the last half of the 1970s, and isoflurane in 1983. Sevoflurane displaced all of these agents in the 1990s. Nitrous oxide has now been abandoned in favor of air-oxygen mixtures. (Aguilar ME: Personal communication).

In the 1950s, Joaquín Coto tutored 12 physicians in anesthesia. Some of them went to the US to continue formal training. Others trained nurses to become anesthetists. In 1977, Coto founded the School of Technicians in Anesthesia, which has graduated around 1000 technicians to provide anesthesia in different provinces. (Aguilar ME: Personal communication.)

In 1974, a 2-year anesthesia residency program was initiated at the Hospital Nacional Rosales. In 1987, the program increased to 3 years plus a year in surgery or medicine, or to 4 years of anesthesia. (Aguilar ME: Personal communication; Sandra Leal Aquino. Personal communication. Aquino is the current President of AMAES.)

Currently, about 100 anesthesiologists work in El Salvador (mainly in the capital city of San Salvador), a country with more than 5.7 million inhabitants. El Salvador has 32 hospitals (four with ICUs) and 8 hospitals supported by the Social Security Institute (four with ICUs). Anesthesiologists care for the patients in all of those units. All hospitals have PACUs. (Aguilar ME: Personal communication; Sandra Leal

Aquino. Personal communication.). Technicians/nurse anesthetists provide anesthesia in most provinces. The anesthesiologist to technician ratio is approximately 1:10. (Aguilar ME: Personal communication.)

The anesthesiologists returning to El Salvador in the 1950s founded the first Society of Anesthesia, but it disappeared after a short time. In 1967, Fernando Antonio Escobar re-established the former society and renamed it "Asociación de Médicos Anestesiólogos de El Salvador" (AMAES) which, in 1993, became a member of CLASA. In 2009, it was accepted by the WFSA as a member, finally ratified in 2012. It is a member of FESACAC (Federación de Sociedades de Anestesia de Centro América y el Caribe) and organized its 2nd congress in 1996. (Aguilar ME: Personal communication; Sandra Leal Aquino. Personal communication.) The Society has no journal or bulletin.

Nicaragua

There is no recorded description of anesthesia in Nicaragua before 1900. However, Juan José Martinez, a surgeon who trained for two years at the Bellevue Hospital in New York, probably introduced ether anesthesia when he returned to Nicaragua in September 1889. Although his autobiography [45] does not mention the use of anesthesia, he describes the surgeries he performed before 1900, probably done under ether anesthesia administered by nuns. He mentions his first surgery for removal of a cataract using local anesthesia with 5% cocaine in 1891, and his first spinal anesthesia with cocaine for a patient with an ankle fracture in 1900. He gave spinal anesthetics with cocaine in approximately 100 cases, mentioning that it caused a "horrible" headache. He therefore substituted amylocaine for cocaine, reporting its use in 500 additional cases. Later, he substituted procaine hydrochloride for amylocaine [45].

At the end of 1891, Luis H Debayle, a surgeon trained in Paris, arrived in Nicaragua. Since chloroform was commonly used for surgical procedures in France, Debayle probably introduced it into Nicaragua. No recorded description identified the year or the person responsible for introducing chloroform, although it is generally thought that chloroform was used before 1900 (Denis F. Nava. Personal Communication. Nava was the former National Director of Education in Anesthesiology and Past President of Asociación Nicaragüense de Anestesiología y Reanimación (ANARE)).

Lay providers continued to administer ether and chloroform anesthesia until 1956 when Cayetano Espinoza Valdés, an anesthesiologist trained in Chicago, returned to practice in Nicaragua. He organized the anesthesia department at the General Hospital in Managua, where he was joined by other anesthesiologists trained abroad. He introduced succinylcholine and halothane, thus ending the use of ether and chloroform. Between 1964 and 1972, methoxyflurane was introduced and used. Enflurane was used for a short period in the 1970s. Halothane was used until 2000, when it was replaced by sevoflurane. Nitrous oxide was used in the first half of the 20th century but is no longer used. Sevoflurane-oxygen is currently the dominant anesthetic. (Denis F. Nava. Personal Communication.)

In 1960, Denis Nava, who had been trained in Mexico City, introduced epidural anesthesia. In the 1980s, 25 cases of arachnoiditis were reported after spinal and epidural anesthesia, probably attributable to the detergents used to sterilize reusable glass syringes and needles. Heat sterilization was then adopted as advised by Armando Fortuna from Brazil (who was lecturing in Nicaragua at the time), and this unfortunate complication has not recurred in any of the 25 hospitals serving the country. Regional anesthesia is still a popular anesthesia technique. No disposable equipment is available. Lidocaine and bupivacaine are the common local anesthetics used, with or without opioids. (Denis F. Nava. Personal Communication.)

A new private hospital, "Hospital Metropolitano Vivian Pellas" was opened in 2005, and has a gas sterilizer. It has been recognized by the JAHCO and is the most expensive hospital in Nicaragua. (Denis F. Nava. Personal Communication.)

The Ministry of Health (MINSA), and the National University of Nicaragua established a 3 year residency program in anesthesiology in 1982. Currently in Managua, the Antonio Lenin Fonseca hospital, the Berta Calderón hospital, the Roberto Calderón hospital and the Manuel de Jesús Rivera (pediatric hospital) offer anesthesia residencies, as does the Oscar D Rosales hospital in León. By 1979, 44 trained anesthesiologists provided anesthesia in Nicaragua, but with the overthrow of Anastasio Somoza, most of them emigrated, leaving only 18. At present, 190 anesthesiologists serve a population of almost 6 million inhabitants, leaving many vacant shifts covered by technicians, particularly in small provinces.

In 1993, the anesthesia community founded the Asociación Nicaragüense de Anestesiología y Reanimación (ANARE), which has been a member of CLASA and WFSA for the last 10 years. ANARE was also a founding member of FESACAC. In November 2009, the XXX Latin American Congress of Anesthesia, organized by CLASA and the VIth Nicaraguan Congress of Anesthesia and Pain were held at the same time in Nicaragua. No journal or bulletin has been published (Denis F. Nava. Personal Communication.)

Costa Rica

Anesthesia began in Costa Rica in 1875, with Carlos Duran's arrival from Guy's Hospital in London, where he had graduated in medicine and surgery, supervised by Joseph Lister, Queen Victoria's private physician. At the Hospital

San Juan de Dios in San José, he performed surgery on patients anesthetized with chloroform, teaching other physicians the technique of its administration. He founded the School of Obstetrics, the School of Nursing, the Asylum for Insane Patients, and the Sanatorium for Patients with Tuberculosis–a remarkable man. Nuns ran the hospital and administered the anesthesia. Chloroform was dropped over 8 layers of gauze, 6 drops during the first minute, 12 during the second, 24 on the third and so on until they reached one drop per second [46, 47].

Physicians returning from medical studies in the US introduced ether in the late 1800s. To shorten the induction period they preceded ether administration with ethyl chloride administration. Ether continued in use until 1962. On 15 December 1909, surgeon Luis Paulino Jiménez used spinal anesthesia with amylocaine for the first time, in a 45 year old male with an inguinal hernia [47].

After many years of practicing both surgery and anesthesia, Ricardo Jimenez Núñez decided to devote his full attention to anesthesia. In 1940, he wrote a book in which he argued that "anesthesia should not be administered by nurses alone, they always have to work under the supervision of a medical doctor" [47]

Gonzalo Vargas Aguilar was the first trained anesthesiologist in Costa Rica. In 1941, he went to the Memorial Hospital in New York to train, returning in 1942. In 1947 he initiated the use of curare (Intocostrin, Squibb) for his cases. The introduction of anesthesia machines to Hospital San Juan de Dios, by Enrique Sotela in 1952, and their use by trained anesthesiologists, increased the popularity of neuromuscular blocking drugs, presumably because anesthetic machines allowed the support of ventilation [47]. In the 1950s, other physicians went to Mexico to train in anesthesia. On their return, they gave 9-month courses in anesthesia to nurses and technicians, who replaced a declining supply of nuns in the operating rooms. Such training continued for more than a decade, producing 130 technician anesthetists. The courses were suspended in 1981 [47]. Epidural anesthesia was introduced in 1962, by Luis Guillermo Hidalgo on his return from training in Denmark.

In 1974, there were 12 anesthesiologists in Costa Rica who had trained abroad. Supported by the University of Costa Rica, they initiated a two and a half year residency program, extended to 3 years in 1982. Physicians trained in residency programs have become the primary providers of anesthesia, and the few remaining technicians are used to monitor patients receiving intravenous sedation or to assist anesthesiologists. A subspecialty residency program in Pediatric Anesthesia is available at the Hospital Nacional de Niños "Dr. Carlos Saenz Herrera" (National Children's Hospital), and lasts one year. Other subspecialty training must be accomplished abroad. All hospitals have PACUs, and larger hospitals have ICUs (Celia Hofman: Personal Communica-

tion. Hofman is former Director of the Anesthesia Service at the Hospital Mexico, Past President of AMACR and is the Coordinator of the European Foundation for Education in Anesthesia for Central America). Currently 200 trained anesthesiologists serve a country of 4,301,712 inhabitants (2011 census).

In 1987, Costa Rica converted to a partial barter system with England: coffee from Costa Rica was exchanged for new and modern anesthesia equipment to supply the country's 57 hospitals.

In 1960, 8 anesthesiologists founded the first Anesthesia Society, but this ceased to exist after a few years. It was re-created in 1991 as "Asociación de Médicos Anestesiólogos de Costa Rica" (AMACR). It is a member of CLASA, WFSA, and FESACAC. In 1995, the Society promulgated Safety Standards for the Practice of Anesthesia based on international standards. These have been accepted by the Ministry of Health and are compulsory. In order to practice after finishing a residency program, regardless of the specialty, one must become a member of the Colegio de Médicos y Cirujanos de Costa Rica (College of Medical and Surgical Physicians) which acts as a board of certification and grants a permit to practice. AMACR has not developed a journal or bulletin (Celia Hofman: Personal Communication).

Panama

Geographically and historically, Panama was a part of Greater Colombia—from 28 Nov 1821 to 3 Nov 1903. After several insurrections, it became independent in 1903.

No precise record describes the development of anesthesia in Panama in the 1800s. In Colombia, ether and chloroform were widely used during the last quarter of the 1800s [48] In 1846, the US signed the Bidlack-Mallarino treaty with Colombia, granting the US rights to build railroads in Panama and to intervene militarily. In 1855, the world's first transcontinental railroad—across the Isthmus, from Colón at the Atlantic Ocean to Panama City at the Pacific Ocean—was completed. From 1880 to 1889, the French company that had built the Suez Canal, attempted to build a sea-level canal in Panama. They constructed dispensaries next to the railroad stations and large hospitals in the main cities to treat construction workers afflicted by accidents, yellow fever, malaria and cholera. French physicians, nurses and technicians served in these facilities. In September 1882, the 500 bed L'Hopital Notre Dame du Canal was established in Panama City, at a cost of 500 million francs [49, 50].

In 1904, during Theodore Roosevelt's presidency, the US bought the rights from the French to build the abandoned project in a deal that included hospitals and dispensaries. The Panama Canal was then constructed. American and French medicine strongly influenced the development of medicine in general and anesthesia in particular. There is no precise reference as to when or who introduced chloroform and ether, but both were widely used by French and American personnel who taught local personnel the art or technique of anesthesia [50]. (Solange de los Ríos, Personal communication: Former trainee at Hospital Infantil de Mexico, Mexico City. Jefe del Servicio de Anestesia, Hospital de Especialidades Pediátricas de la Caja del Seguro Social, Ciudad de Panamá, Panamá).

In the first half of the 20th century, surgeons provided spinal anesthesia while nurses cared for the patient during the surgery. Gabriel Sosa recalls that in 1938, amylocaine was used for spinals, and chloroform and ether were administered "open drop" by the nurses. Ramirez Duque bought an Ombrédanne apparatus ether inhaler from the US that "delivered ether more safely" (Solange de los Ríos, Personal communication) [49, 50].

In the 1950s, Augusto Ramos, an ENT specialist, traveled to Cuba to learn anesthesia, and tracheal intubation in particular. (Solange de los Ríos, Personal communication). In 1957, Rodrigo Bernal, the first anesthesiologist formally trained in Washington DC, arrived in Panama and was joined 2 years later by Dante Viggiano, who also trained in the US. Both worked at the Saint Thomas Hospital (Hospital Santo Tomás) supervising nurse anesthetists and administering anesthesia in more complex cases. Curare was introduced by Rodrigo Bernal in 1957 (Solange de los Ríos, Personal communication).

In 1962, the first anesthesia service was organized at the General Hospital of the Social Security (Caja del Seguro Social). Open drop ether and cyclopropane were the anesthetics used until 1975, when they were replaced successively by halothane, enflurane and isoflurane. In 1995, sevoflurane was introduced and two years later, desflurane appeared on the market (Solange de los Ríos, Personal communication).

Regional anesthesia has been widely used in adults and children. Rodrigo Bernal introduced epidural anesthesia in adults in 1970 (Solange de los Ríos, Personal communication). Central neuraxial anesthesia has been used in children since the 1980s when Solange de los Ríos, a trainee at the Children's Hospital in Mexico City, returned to Panama and taught the technique. Lidocaine, bupivacaine, and occasionally ropivacaine are the local anesthetics currently used in adults and children (Solange de los Ríos, Personal communication).

In 1975, neurosurgeon Keith Holder developed the first Pain Clinic, followed in 1991 by Luis Pretto, an anesthesiologist who specialized in Pain Medicine (Solange de los Ríos, Personal communication).

Since 1971, administration of anesthesia by nurses or non-medical practitioners has been forbidden by law. A 3 year residency program was initiated in that year, at the Social Security and Santo Tomás hospitals by the Univer-sity of Panama and the Ministry of Health. Training in subspecialties has been done abroad. Anesthesiologists work as generalists or as subspecialists in cardiovascular anesthesia, neuroanesthesia, intensive therapy, pediatrics, obstetrics, or pain. Presently, 300 anesthesiologists serve a population of more than 3.4 million inhabitants. The influence of American Medicine is still strong; it is the "raw model" to follow. Drugs not approved by the FDA in the US, are not allowed (Solange de los Ríos, Personal communication).

In 1964, Rodrigo Bernal and Dante Viggiano founded the Anesthesia Society, "Sociedad Panameña de Anestesiología, Reanimación y Algiología" (SPARA). In 1977, it became a member of CLASA, and in November 2011, staged the XXXI Latin American Congress and the XIV National Congress of Anesthesia. It has been a member of WFSA since 1984 and of FESACAC since its foundation in 1994. SPARA does not publish a journal or bulletin (Solange de los Ríos, Personal communication).

Reflections

The use of anesthesia in Mexico, Central America, Cuba and other Caribbean islands variably followed Morton's and Simpson's demonstrations, Mexico and Cuba often leading the way with delays of up to decades in some of the other countries. Similarly, anesthetic advances in this region, advances in equipment, drugs, training, and anesthetic societies lagged behind those in more developed countries. All countries in this region now have anesthetic societies. Gradually, full-time anesthesiologists, usually trained for three or four years, have increased in numbers, doing so to the point where in several countries in this region (and subspecialists in a few countries) they now are responsible for most of or all anesthetic delivery. However, in several other countries in this region, technicians still deliver a substantial portion of anesthetics.

References

1. Aldrete JA, Marron GM, Wright AJ. The first administration of anesthesia in military surgery: on occasion of the Mexican-American War. Anesthesiology. 1984;61:585–8.
2. Porter JB. Medical and surgical notes of campaigns in the war with Mexico during the years 1845, 1846, 1847, and 1848. Am J Med Sci. 1852;24:13–30.
3. Del Castillo F. ¿Cuándo y por quién se aplicó por primera vez en Mexico la Anestesia por inhalación?. Gac Med Mex. 1948;78:265–78.
4. Primera anestesia por inhalación en la Republica Mexicana. "El Noticioso de Yucatán". Mérida; 1847 (Junio 15).
5. Martinez del Rio JP. La Anestesia en la Práctica de la Obstetricia. Gac Med Mex. 1878;13:459–61.
6. López F. Técnica para obtener la analgesia por la cocaína en las operaciones mutilantes del globo ocular. Anales de Oftalmología. 1901;IV:65–8.

7. De Avila Cervantes A. La primera anestesia espinal en Mexico. Rev Mex Anest. 1960;51:323–8.
8. Pardo R. La cocainización lumbar por el método de Tuffier. Cron Med Mex. 1901; 1.(Tomo) lV:1
9. Vasconcelos PG. La primera anestesia raquídea en Mexico. Cron Med Mex. 1988;124:246–8.
10. Bandera B. Historia de la Anestesia en México. Evolución, desarrollo, futuro. Rev Mex Anest. 1960;38:83–94.
11. Nuñez T. Breves consideraciones sobre los accidentes a que puede dar lugar el cloroformo cuando se emplea para obtener la anestesia quirúrgica. Gac Med Mex. 1901;38:134–8.
12. Vázquez M. Breves Consideraciones Acerca de la Acción de los Anestésicos sobre el Organismo. Rev Mex Ciencias Médicas. 1927;2:6–16.
13. Macouzet R. Cién Eterizaciones. Gac Med Mex. 1901;38:139–40.
14. Plotz J. The ether inhaler of Louis Ombredanne. Remarks on his career outside France and his invention. Anaesthesist. 2001;50:605–11.
15. Melman E. La Anestesiología en México durante el Siglo XX. Gaceta Médica de México. 1988;124:251–3.
16. Maquívar M, Terrazas J. 19 casos de anestesia con respiración controlada. Sus posibilidades en la Anestesia de Torax. Memorias del 1er. Congreso de Tuberculosis y Silicosis. 1944.
17. Morales OA, Odor GA. Anestesia con Fluothane en Método Cerrado. Rev Mex Anest. 1957;6:153–4.
18. Melman E, Berrocal M. Seguridad y Eficacia del Desflurano durante la Anestesia General en el Paciente Pediátrico. Rev Mex Anest. 1998;21:75–81.
19. Lozano NR, Moreno MA, González MA, Galindo E. Valoración de la Seguridad del Desflurano en Anestesia General en Adultos. Rev Mex Anest. 1998;21:253–7.
20. Sandoval CA. Anestesia Obstétrica. Evolución Histórica. En: Gandera JA, Ayala FS, Editors. Anestesia Obstétrica y Perinatología, Temas Selectos. Edición Homenaje al Dr. Guillermo Vasconcelos Palacios. México; 1978. pp. 7–22.
21. Mateos-Fournier M. Un caso de Anestesia Caudal con Accidente. Gac Med Mex. 1944;74:146–54.
22. Garcia OV. Raquianalgesia y sus modalidades. Rev Mex Anest. 1958;7:91–100.
23. Vasconcelos PG. Consideraciones sobre Anestesia Obstétrica. Rev Mex Anest. 1958;7:302–6.
24. Rodrigues de la Fuente F. Anestesia en Obstetricia. Rev Mex Anest. 1962;11:484–93.
25. Martinez RC, Martinez OS, Vasconcelos PG, Rodrigues de la Fuente F. Bloqueo Peridural en Cirugía Obstétrica. Rev Mex Anest. 1962;11:67–73.
26. Melman E. Anestesia Regional en Pediatría. En: Moyao GD, Editors. Anestesia en Pediatría. PAC Anestesia -2. 1ª. Ed. México: Intersistemas S.A. de C.V.; 2000. pp. 50–6.
27. Melman E, Penuelas JA, Marrufo J. Regional anesthesia in children. Anesth Analg. 1975;54:387–90.
28. Moyao GD, Garza-Leyva M, Velazquez-Armenta EY, Nava-Ocampo AA. Caudal block with 4 mg × kg⁻¹ (1.6 ml × kg⁻¹) of bupivacaine 0.25% in children undergoing surgical correction of congenital pyloric stenosis. Paediatr Anaesth. 2002;12:404–10.
29. García OV. Anecdotario de un Anestesiólogo. Ed. Diana. México; 1996:13–228.
30. Moreno AC. Historia de la Sociedad Mexicana de Anestesiología. Rev Mex Anest. 1984;7:191–200 (Editorial).
31. Moreno AC. Los Colegios Médicos en México. Rev Mex Anest. 2007;30:55–60.
32. Acta Constitutiva de la Federación de Sociedades de Anestesia de la República Mexicana (FSARM). Rev Mex Anest. 1960;47:124–9.
33. Las Sociedades Anestesiológicas de Sub o Supraespecialidad. Rev Mex Anest. 1995;18:223–4.
34. Carrillo ER. Dos Años Después. Rev Mex Anest. 2005;28:123–4 (Editorial).
35. López SJ. Historia y Evolución del Uso de la Anestesia Quirúrgica en Cuba. Nicolás Gutierrez Academy. Finlay Medical Society. Finlay online www.cmw.sid.cu.
36. Hevia L. Ether as safest anesthetic in ordinary surgical work in the tropics. Anesth Analg Curr Res. 1939;18:241–51.
37. Ferro AH. Consideraciones sobre la Anestesia Epidural. Informaciones Médicas. La Habana. 1937;1:9–14.
38. Moscoso Puello FE. Apuntes para la Historia de la Medicina de la Isla de Santo Domingo. Editorial República Dominicana 1978.
39. Historia de la Anestesia en República Dominicana (1844–1997). www.sda.com.do.
40. Asturais F. Historia de la Medicina en Guatemala. Guatemala: Ed. Universitaria; 1959.
41. Rivas J. Historia de la Anestesia en Guatemala. Tesis de Graduación. Guatemala: Ed. Piedra Santa; 1970.
42. Samayoa F, Graugnard M. Historia de la Anestesiología en Honduras y de la Sociedad de Anestesiología, Reanimación y Dolor (SHARD). Tegucigalpa; 2012.
43. Infante Meyer C. e Infante Díaz S. División Diagnóstica y Servicios de Apoyo. En Hospital Rosales-Una Institución Centenaria "1902–2002". Colección Catelo. San Salvador: Ed. Laboratorios López; 2002. pp. 129–134.
44. Infante SD. La Anestesiología en El Salvador. En Salvador Díaz Infante, "Cáncer en El Salvador." San Salvador: Ed. Dirección de Publicaciones del Ministerio de Educación; 1964. pp. 93–98.
45. Martinez JJ. Autobiografía. Editorial Bolsa Médica, Managua, Nicaragua. No. 29 y 30; 1996.
46. Gonzalez Pacheco CE. Hospital San Juan de Dios, 150 años de Historia. San José: Editorial Nacional de Salud y Seguridad Social; 1995.
47. Enrique SJ. Reseña Histórica de la Anestesia en Costa Rica. San José: Editorial Nacional de Salud y Seguridad Social; 1997.
48. Pontón HJ. Historia de la Anestesia en Colombia. Rev Colom Anest 1974; 1:Art. 7.
49. de San Martin TM. Tesis Doctoral (en prensa) (Doctoral Thesis, in press). Anestesióloga del Instituto Oncológico Nacional, Cd. de Panamá, Panamá. 2012.
50. Panama. In Encyclopaedia Britannica, Inc. William & Helen Hemingway Benton, Publishers, Chicago, Ill. Macropaedia. 1978;13:940–7.

A History of Anesthesia in China

27

Xiaomei Feng, Buwei Yu, Xuerong Yu, Yuguang Huang, Guolin Wang and Jin Liu

Summary

Peter Parker introduced ether anesthesia into China on 4 October 1847, using an apparatus supplied by Charles Jackson. A year later, he used chloroform after reading a pamphlet written by James Simpson. Open-drop ether or chloroform, and local and spinal anesthesia were used in China up to the mid-20th century. Physicians, students, nurses, nuns, and technicians—but few professional anesthesiologists—delivered clinical anesthesia. The People's Republic of China was founded in 1949 after the devastation of World War II and the civil war. Jone Wu and Xingfang Li from Shanghai and Deyan Shang, Rong Xie and Huiying Tan from Beijing then returned from the US and Europe, bringing back modern ideas concerning anesthetic delivery. In 1953, Rong Xie organized the first training course in anesthesiology, sponsored by the Peking Union Medical College and Beijing Medical Universities. Development of anesthesiology as a specialty, and the establishment of training programs began in the 1950s, aided by publication of two books, *Clinical Anesthesiology* by Jone Wu, and *Anesthesiology* by Rong Xie.

During the Chinese Cultural Revolution (1966–1976), research and funding were interrupted, and patient care switched to acupuncture and traditional Chinese medicine. Although the above techniques were later abandoned because of their poor performance on their own, acupuncture continued in use as a supplement to anesthesia and analgesia. At the conclusion of the Cultural Revolution, a few pain management programs and post-anesthesia care units and intensive care units were established. In 1979, 44 anesthesiologists were elected as inaugural members of the Chinese Society of Anesthesiology (CSA). The *Chinese Journal of Anesthesiology* (1981), *Foreign Medical Sciences (Anesthesiology and Resuscitation; 1982), and The Journal of Clinical Anesthesiology* (1983) began their publication.

A College of Anesthesia was established in Xuzhou Medical School in 1987. In 1989, the Ministry of Public Health formally defined the essential facilities and professional scope of a department of anesthesiology, thereby establishing anesthesiology as a clinical specialty. Chinese editions *of Anesthesia & Analgesia* (2002)*, Anesthesiology* (2007)*,* and *Anaesthesia* (2007) began their publication.

Chinese medical schools currently have 8-, 7-, and 5-year options for training in anesthesiology. Anesthesia given by nurses has not been established in China. Data obtained by Shuren Li, Emeritus President of the CSA, said that in 2007, more than 80,000 anesthesiologists were available in mainland China.

X. Feng (✉) · B. Yu
Department of Anesthesiology, Shanghai Ruijin Hospital,
School of Medicine, Shanghai Jiaotong University, Shanghai, China
e-mail: leaflet1981@gmail.com

B. Yu
e-mail: yubuwei@yahoo.com.cn

X. Yu · Y. Huang
Department of Anesthesiology, Peking Union Medical College
Hospital, Dongcheng District, Beijing China
e-mail: yxr313@yahoo.com.cn

Y. Huang
e-mail: pumchhyg@yahoo.com.cn

G. Wang
Department of Anesthesiology, Tianjin Medical University
General Hospital, Tianjin, China
e-mail: wangguolin@tjmugh.com.cn

J. Liu
Department of Anesthesia and Critical Care, West China Hospital,
Sichuan University, Chengdu, Sichuan, China
e-mail: scujinliu@yahoo.com.cn

Anesthesia in Ancient China

Anesthesia in China dates back to 500 BCE, to the era of Bian Que (Fig. 27.1) the earliest known physician of ancient China. He and Hua Tuo are the most famous early Chinese physicians. Acupuncture, herbs and wine were used to provide anesthesia. Bian Que excelled in pulse taking and acupuncture therapy.

Documents from the Eastern Han Dynasty(25CE-220CE) and the Three Kingdoms (220CE-265CE) periods indicate that Hua Tuo (Fig. 27.2) was respected for his expertise in surgery, anesthesia, and acupuncture, and that he was the first person in China to apply anesthesia for surgery. His general anesthetic combined wine with herbs in a concoction called mafeisan ("boiled cannabis powder"). The Book of Sui Dynasty listed five books attributed to Hua and his disciples, but none survived and Hua's prescription for mafeisan has

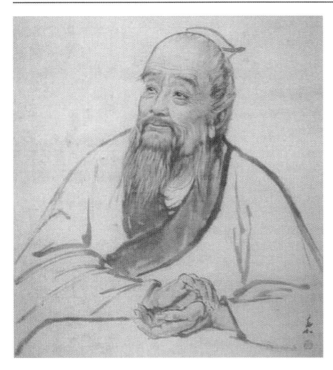

Fig. 27.1 Portrait of Bian Que. the earliest known physician of ancient China. (Courtesy of the Chinese Society of Anesthesiology, Beijing, China.)

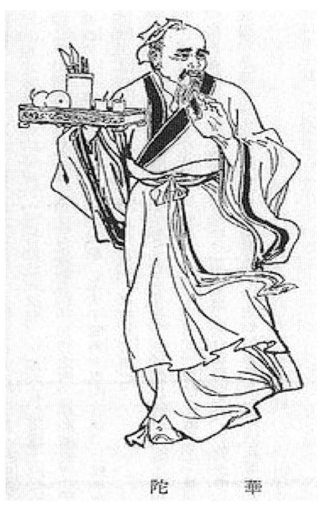

Fig. 27.2 Portrait of Hua Tuo from a Qing Dynasty print. He was the first person in China to apply anesthesia for surgery. (Courtesy of the Chinese Society of Anesthesiology, Beijing, China.)

been lost [1]. Hua was also considered the first surgeon in China. He has been compared to Jivaka of India, who lived at the time of Buddha (about 500 BCE.) and was also renowned for surgery and anesthesia. Hua had no significant successors until modern times, when surgery and anesthesia were reintroduced by Western physicians [2]. Biographical information about *Hua Tuo* appeared in English in three works: an article in the *Journal of Traditional Chinese Medicine*; [3] a monograph in Chen's *History of Chinese Medical Science*; [4] and a report in the *Advanced Textbook on Traditional Chinese Medicine and Pharmacology* [5].

The Introduction of Western Anesthesia into China (1847–1949)

News of the 1846 public demonstration of ether anesthesia for surgery in the US [6, 7] spread to London in December 1846 and Paris in January 1847. Peter Parker, who received degrees from both the divinity and medical schools at Yale, introduced ether anesthesia into China on 4 October 1847, using an apparatus received from Charles Jackson of Boston. He anesthetized a middle-aged farmer for the separation of the eyelid from the eyeball (symblepharon) in Canton Hospital, Guangzhou. A year later, Parker used chloroform in 8–10 cases, after reading a pamphlet written by James Simpson [8].

Anesthesia, as demonstrated by Morton and Simpson, was quickly introduced into large cities including Beijing,

Tianjin, Shanghai, and Guangzhou. Open-drop ether or chloroform, along with local and spinal anesthesia were used throughout the rest of the 19th century and up to the middle of the 20th century. During this time, physicians, students, nurses, nuns, and technicians might administer anesthesia. Although the anesthesia methods were simple, gastrectomy, cholecystectomy, and even some neurological surgeries were successfully completed. For example, in September 1938, a pituitary adenoma resection was completed in the Peking Union Medical College Hospital (PUMCH) using a combination of local anesthesia with procaine and rectal anesthesia with Avertin.

Modern anesthesiology in China developed formally with the founding of Peking Union Medical College (PUMC) in 1921, by the US Rockefeller Foundation. FC Mclean, a 28-year-old graduate of the University of Chicago, and professor of internal medicine, was appointed the Dean. PB Seam was assigned as the president of its subsidiary hospital, PUMCH. General surgery, orthopedics,

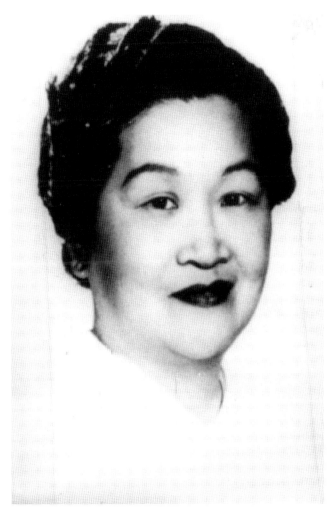

Fig. 27.3 Ma Yueqing, the first Chinese anesthesiologist in Beijing. (Courtesy of the author.)

urology, gynecology, ENT and other surgical departments were immediately established. Miss Helen Holland was in charge of anesthetic delivery. From 1938 to 1941, Yueqing Ma, a 1934 graduate from PUMC, worked in the department of anesthesia as the first Chinese anesthesiologist in Beijing [Fig. 27.3]. The PUMCH was equipped with US-made equipment. A Heidbrink anesthesia machine and a McKesson intermittent flow anesthesia apparatus, believed to have been used in the 1940s, were found in the storeroom of PUMCH in the 1950s,

Development of Anesthesiology in China (1949–1966)

World War II devastated China no less than Europe. The internal disruptions required to oppose the Japanese occupation were compounded by the Chinese civil war that followed. The Marshall Plan assisting reconstruction in Europe did not apply to China. Thus, anesthesiology, like all of

Chinese medicine, faced enormous economic and physical burdens. Anesthesiology as a clinical specialty and science had to begin at ground level, starting in the great cities and spreading from there.

Pioneers in Chinese Anesthesiology

Before World War II, anesthesiology in China strove to keep pace with that in America and Europe. Interns and junior surgical residents were trained to administer anesthesia, but no formal residency program existed, nor was there a professional society to promote the "art and science" of anesthesiology. There was neither a Chinese textbook of anesthesiology, nor a journal devoted to anesthesia.

After World War II, the Ministry of Education underwrote grants to send promising physicians to North America for training in anesthesia with the hope that these physicians would return with the knowledge and expertise to ensure the growth of the specialty in China. The following includes brief biograhical sketches of some of these pioneers in Chinese anesthesiology.

Jone Wu (Fig. 27.4), a 1938 graduate of the National Shanghai Medical College, had pursued a career as an instructor in pharmacology at his alma mater for almost a decade. In 1947, he won a Ministry of Education Scholarship to study anesthesiology in the US, and from 1947 until 1949, he studied at the University of Wisconsin in Madison. Wu returned to China in 1950, and founded the Department of Anesthesiology in Zhongshan Hospital of the National Shanghai Medical College, and established the first blood bank in China. By 1954, Wu founded an independent academic department of anesthesiology, to provide a clinical service to the six hospitals affiliated with the medical school. He also helped develop the first Chinese ventilator and anesthetic machine [9]. In 1954, Wu published the first Chinese-language anesthesia text, with a second, expanded edition appearing in 1959. He was instrumental in establishing postgraduate training in anesthesiology and personally trained more than 150 residents.

Deyan Shang (Fig. 27.5) completed a 5-yr medical program in Lanzhou University in 1942. After graduation, he served as a surgeon at his medical school, becoming chief resident surgeon in 1945. Because there was no anesthesia service in Lanzhou at that time, the chief executive officer of Lanzhou Central Hospital persuaded young surgeon Shang to pursue anesthesia training in America, and sent him to the anesthesiology residency program at the University of Illinois (Chicago) in 1948. Shang returned to China in 1949 and established the first Department of Anesthesiology in China in the National Lanzhou Hospital. He began a research program in cardiac physiology, critical care medicine, and resuscitation.

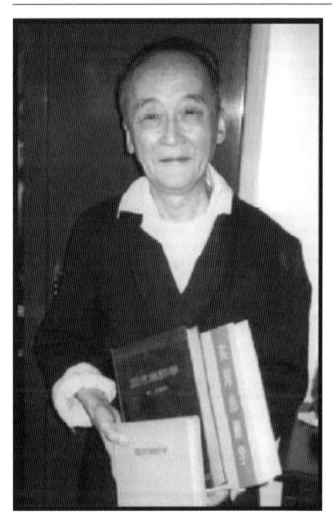

Fig. 27.4 A photograph of Jone Wu taken in February 1986 at his residence in Shanghai. He holds three books that he wrote on anesthesiology. The middle one is mentioned in the memorial tribute to him published in 1954 in Clinical Anesthesiology. (Courtesy of Joseph Rupreht, MD, PhD.)

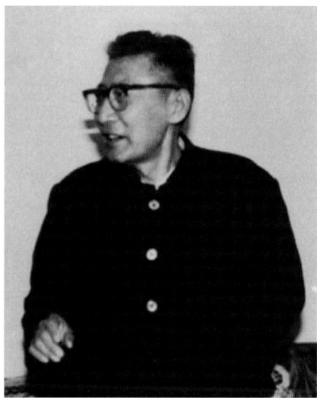

Fig. 27.5 Deyan Shang (1918–1985), the first president of Chinese Society of Anesthesiology. (Courtesy of the Chinese Society of Anesthesiology, Beijing, China.)

In 1956, he moved from Lanzhou to the Fu Wai hospital in Bejing, a major teaching affiliate of the PUMC, where his career blossomed. In 1957, he established the first animal research laboratory in China, investigating issues associated with invasive cardiothoracic anesthetic management, hypothermic anesthesia for cardiac surgery, and resuscitative studies. Shang helped found the Chinese Society of Anesthesiologists (CSA) in 1979, and became its first president. In addition, he helped establish the Chinese Journal of Anesthesiology in 1981.

Rong Xie (Yung Shieh) (Fig. 27.6) graduated from the Tong Ji University School of Medicine in 1946. He traveled to America, and received training at the Detroit Receiving Hospital in Michigan, affiliated with Wayne State University. He received additional training in Pittsburgh, Pennsylvania, before returning to China in 1950. He first traveled to his home province of Yunan to develop anesthesiology in the southwest region of China. In 1956, Xie started a collaborative relationship with Shang in Beijing. He was appointed associate professor at Peking Medical University in 1957, and succeeded Shang as the second president of the CSA, in 1984. He established the first Surgical Intensive Care Unit directed by an anesthesia department in China in 1985. He was also the founding editor-in-chief of the Chinese Journal of Anesthesiology.

Xingfang Li went to the US in 1947 for training in anesthesia. After returning to China in 1947, Li began work in the Renji Hospital at the Shanghai Second Medical School, establishing the Department of Anesthesiology there in 1954. Three years later, Li moved to the Ruijin Hospital, also affiliated with the Shanghai Second Medical School, where she established another Department of Anesthesiology following the anesthesia group established by the famous surgeon, Jixiang Shi. Li was an expert in hypothermia and cardiac anesthesia.

Huiying Tan graduated from Yunnan Medical School, and went to Europe in 1947, to study and work in the Department of Anesthesiology of the University of Paris. In 1956, she returned from France and pioneered "artificial hibernation

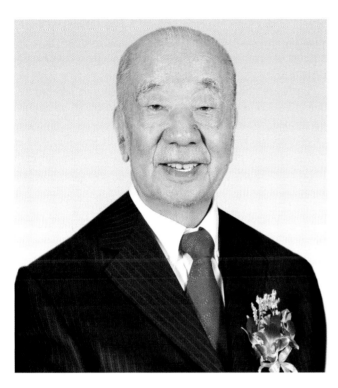

Fig. 27.6 Rong Xie (Yung Shieh), the second president of the CSA in 1984. He established the first SICU directed by an anesthesia department in China in 1985. He was also the founding editor-in-chief of the *Chinese Journal of Anesthesiology*. (Courtesy of the Chinese Society of Anesthesiology, Beijing, China.)

therapy", a state of deep sedation induced with pethidine and chlorpromazine (or promethazine).

These five pioneers are credited with elevating the national standard of anesthesia in clinical training, research, and education. They were instrumental in shaping Chinese anesthesia.

Progress in Anesthesia Methods and Machines

In the 1950s, most anesthesia practice consisted of open-drop ether inhalation, local infiltration anesthesia, and single-injection spinal anesthesia. Some anesthesia machines were in use, and nearly all equipment was imported, including Heidbrink machines from the US, Drager machines from Germany, and Boyle machines from the British Oxygen Company. Meanwhile, domestic manufacturers progressed from simple imitation of non-Chinese equipment to modification and improvement of machines built in China. Chinese brands included the Shanghai Tao Gen Ji (later the "Zhong Hua" brand, similar to the Heidbrink anesthesia machine); the Zhonghua compound anesthesia machine (with an attachment for pediatric anesthesia), a multi-functional anesthesia machine (with positive and negative pressure ven-

tilation), and the "103" closed circuit anesthesia machine. The first continuous-flow anesthetic machine was made in Shanghai in 1956, and the first artificial heart-lung machine was constructed, also in Shanghai, in 1957.

Most hospitals once used and are still using these products which combined quality and reasonable price. Chinese anesthesiologists were innovative and adaptive. If equipment was not ready-made, anesthesiologists used considerable ingenuity. For example, they might obtain smooth and slippery rubber tubing of appropriate diameter from grocery stores, and cut them into different lengths to make tracheal tubes. The distal end might be beveled and smoothed with sandpaper [10]. Meanwhile, other equipment was manufactured, including epidural and spinal needles, and laryngoscopes.

Anesthetic drugs, including ether, procaine, and succinylcholine were also manufactured in China, starting in the 1950s. Locally made procaine became available in 1955, and succinylcholine in 1964. During the 1950s and 1960s, epidural anesthesia, intravenous anesthesia with procaine, and nerve blocks became the most popular anesthesia techniques in China, largely because these techniques were simple and inexpensive.

Despite the problems of the times, major complicated surgery and related therapies by anesthesiologists were initiated in some major city hospitals. For example, the first mitral valvuloplasty was performed in 1954, in Shanghai, and the first interventricular septal defect repair using cardiopulmonary bypass, was performed successfully in 1958, in Xi'an. In 1958, steel worker, Caikang Qiu, suffered extensive burns to 89% of his body, and was thought unlikely to survive. But the efforts of anesthesiologists, internists, surgeons, and nurses resulted in his successful treatment in Ruijin Hospital in Shanghai.

Yuanchang Wang (1922–1998) from Tianjin Medical College is the world's pioneer of external chest compression for cardiopulmonary resuscitation, providing what may be the first report of such therapy. In 1955, he used external chest compression successfully in 2 patients suffering cardiac arrest following epidural anesthesia. He published a report of "*Management of Complications in Epidural Anesthesia*", in the Chinese Journal of Surgery in 1957. In his paper, Wang described external chest compression and its advantages in detail, emphasizing the importance of immediate recognition of arrest and action to restore cardiac function [11]. The following gives a summary of the two cases and the resulting conclusions:

Case 4: "Although 25 mg ephedrine was injected intravenously two times, the patient's condition was not improved and cardiac arrest subsequently occurred. External chest compression was immediately performed. After one minute, powerful heartbeat reappeared and blood pressure returned to 140 mmHg."

Case 5: "Pulse and blood pressure were undetectable, and the heart sound was not audible. External chest compression was performed at once, and ephedrine and Nikethylamide were also given intravenously. Five minutes later, the first chest compression operator tired and was then replaced by another person to continue the external cardiac compression. Within half a minute, regular and powerful heartbeats returned. Blood pressure returned to 150/70 mmHg and pulse to 140 beats per minute."

In the Discussion, Wang wrote: "Cardiac massage should be immediately applied without any hesitation once heart beat stopped. Details of the methods are described in the literature. We performed external chest compression in two patients (cases 4, 5) in this paper. To do external chest compression, operator should stand on the left side of the patient, facing patients head. Palm with curved fingers is placed on the cardiac region of anterior chest wall, pressing the chest wall backwards like punching, about 70 to 90 times per minute. Such compression should be performed using the palm without moving fingers. External chest compression would not be effective if compression on the chest wall is not powerful.

The advantage of external chest compression is very simple, so that every health-care provider can do it. According to animal study, within one and half minutes of cardiac arrest, myocardium excitability and conductivity increase. Therefore, heart beat can easily return by cardiac massage during such period. External cardiac compression should be immediately applied when cardiac arrest occurs during epidural block. Because opening chest or abdomen is avoided, one may get precious time to save patient's life. In addition, bleeding and infection caused by opening the chest or abdomen are also avoided by using this external cardiac compression. So far we can not get a final conclusion on the effects of the method due to limited experiences from the only two cases in this paper. But, at all events, whenever cardiac arrest occurs during epidural block, we should try our best to use this method." [11]

Dexin Li, Chairman and professor of the Department of Anesthesiology, Nanjing General Hospital of Nanjing Military Command, led advances in brain resuscitation and blood gas analysis. In 1962, he combined selective head cooling with osmotic diuresis, to successfully resuscitate a patient who had been in cardiac arrest for more than 10 min. He also applied blood gas analysis to guide the monitoring and treatment of respiratory failure, and saved the lives of many patients with multiple organ failure.

Academic Development and Personnel Training

As indicated above, in the early 1950s, professional anesthesiology was established in the hospitals of major Chinese cities. At that time, Anesthesiology was a sub-discipline of surgery, and consistent with the expansion of surgery, the number of professional staff engaged in anesthesia gradually expanded.

Early anesthesia practice focused on surgical operations, and was limited by the number and types of operations performed. With the expansion and increasing complexity of clinical work in sometimes severely ill patients, greater demands were placed on anesthesiologists to expand both basic knowledge and expertise. Training and education assumed increasing importance. Thus, in July 1953, Rong Xie chaired the first training course in anesthesiology, a course organized through the joint efforts of PUMC and Beijing Medical University. Support of the course included compilation of a "Clinical Anesthesiology Lecture". The lecture systematically traced the development of modern anesthesia, including general anesthesia, spinal anesthesia, and blood transfusion. The course laid the foundation for future training and education [12].

Academic Activities in Anesthesiology

The earliest academic activities in Chinese anesthesiology were described in the first anesthesiology report to PUMC in 1951, by Rong Xie. Discussion included the significance and practical application of premedication, anesthetic techniques, and new anesthetics. After the Korean War (1950–1953), Deyan Shang trained many anesthesiologists for the army, significantly increasing their numbers. In February 1954, the Society of Surgery (Beijing Branch, Chinese Medical Association) organized a conference on epidural anesthesia at the PUMC. Dexin Li initiated the First National Conference on Anesthesia in Nanjing in 1964 (Fig. 27.7). The conference systematically reviewed the development and achievements of Chinese anesthesiology, including research on respiratory physiology, treatment of shock, cardiac arrest and resuscitation, and anesthetic management of heart and major vascular surgery. These early discussions lagged behind international standards for at least five years, but stimulated interest in technical development and scientific research. Gradually, academic activities became formalized under the imprimatur and name of the Chinese Society of Surgery—Anesthesiology Branch, and the Chinese Society of Anesthesiology. This support of academic activity has continued to increase [12].

Anesthesiology Books and Journals

Before the 1950s, there was no Chinese anesthesiology journal because Anesthesiology was a division of surgery rather than an independent specialty, and most research articles

Fig. 27.7 The First National Conference on Anesthesia was held in Nanjing in 1964 to systematically review the development and achievements of Anesthesiology. (Courtesy of the Chinese Society of Anesthesiology, Beijing, China.)

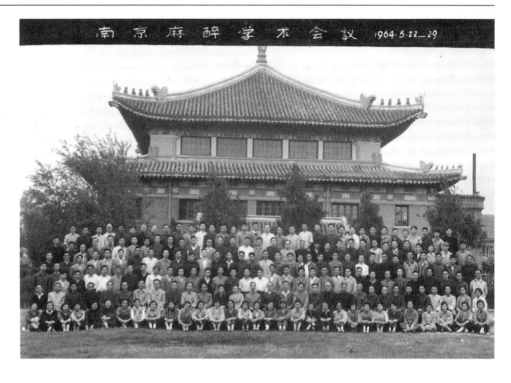

were published in surgical journals. Two books published in the 1950s played a major role in the development of Chinese anesthesiology and the training of practitioners. They were *Clinical Anesthesiology* by Jone Wu (Shanghai), and *Anesthesiology* by Rong Xie (Beijing). [12]

The Cultural Revolution and the Recovery Period

The Cultural Revolution in China (1966–1976) caused social, political and economic upheaval. Prominent intellectuals, especially professors, were persecuted, and this greatly impeded the development of anesthesiology and surgery. Scientific work either stopped or switched to acupuncture and Traditional Chinese Medicine. The limited research funding that existed was allocated solely to these two areas. Fortunately, China continued research on nerve growth factor and the endogenous opioid, endomorphin, as they were related to studies of acupuncture; and studies of the microcirculation were promoted. Only a few new drugs were developed, such as cissampelosime methiodide, for muscle relaxation. This drug was extracted from a Chinese Medicine called Herbacissampelotis. Its structure and purity are not known to the present authors. In addition, domestic ketamine, fentanyl and haloperidol were produced, thus enabling the development and use of dissociative and neurolept anesthesia and analgesia. Except for these few bright spots, the Cultural Revolution significantly and adversely affected the development of Anesthesiology in China.

Because ties between China and the outside world were severed during this period, development of Chinese anesthesiology missed the halothane epoch. Routine anesthesia applied intravenous procaine plus ether inhalation, along with epidural anesthesia. Because of the special status of the Chinese People's Liberation Army (PLA), the anesthesia and resuscitation group that existed within the PLA were not subjected to the same restrictions as others, and thus became an important force in Chinese anesthesiology.

In 1976, the Cultural Revolution officially ended, and all that had been left undone now awaited attention. Anesthesiology was among those scientific fields to be reconstructed. Inspired by the National Science Conference held in 1978, Anesthesiology resumed its advance.

Anesthesiology and Anesthesiology Societies Develop (1979–1989), and Anesthesiology Becomes an Independent Academic Discipline

The pioneers mentioned above established the specialty of anesthesiology in some hospitals affiliated with medical schools. These became the bases for clinical work, scientific research, and education and training in China. In the 1950s, daily clinical anesthetic work was the principal focus. As time progressed, further areas of activity were developed. In the 1960s, these included cardiopulmonary and cerebral resuscitation. In the 1970s, a small number of hospitals began to develop pain medicine, together with the establishment of post-anesthesia care units and intensive care units. In the 1980s, consistent with the world-wide development of new specialty areas within anesthesiology, the specialty achieved further recognition. However, anesthesiology was often viewed as a technical rather than a clinical department in domestic hospitals. In 1989, the Ministry of Public Health formally defined the facilities within the professional scope of a department of anesthesiology:

> "The department of anesthesiology should be a clinical department rather than a technical department. More emphasis should be showed on personnel training, instrument and equipment. The working level should be improved to meet the demands of medical development."

This established Chinese anesthesiology as a recognized clinical specialty, as opposed to a technical specialty in a supporting role for another clinical specialty, and therefore with a lower status [12].

As reform and open policies progressed, Chinese interchanges with the world increased. More advanced anesthesia equipment, anesthetic medications, and techniques were introduced from abroad. Anesthesia machines (Drager, Datex, Ohmeda) and modern volatile anesthetics, including isoflurane and enflurane, were eventually imported and employed in routine clinical practice.

The Chinese Society of Anesthesiology Is Founded In August 1979, the 2nd National Anesthesiology Annual Meeting of the Chinese Medical Association (CMA) was convened in Harbin, Heilongjiang Province. During the meeting, besides academic discussion and paper presentations, 44 anesthesiologists were elected as inaugural committee members of the Chinese Society of Anesthesiology (CSA) of the CMA. Deyan Shang, the chairman of the department of anesthesiology in Fuwai Hospital, Beijing, was elected as the first President. Rong Xie, Jone Wu, and Huiying Tan (from Beijing Soviet Red Cross Hospital, currently Beijing Friendship Hospital) were elected as vice-Presidents. In contrast to the order often followed in other countries, local Societies of Anesthesiology followed establishment of the National Society.

Following formation of the Society, international academic activities increased. In 1986, the Beijing International Conference on Anesthesia was successfully held. From that time, Chinese anesthesiologists began to communicate more with their international colleagues. At the first Sino-Japanese Clinical Anesthesia Symposium held in 1986, the CSA and the Japan Society for Clinical Anesthesia, represented respectively by Rong Xie and Kosaka Futomi, agreed to hold a symposium every 2 years. These symposiums promoted the modernization of Chinese Anesthesiology.

Journals Several journals were launched, including the *Chinese Journal of Anesthesiology* in Shijiazhuang in 1981, *Foreign Medical Sciences (Anesthesiology and Resuscitation)* in

Xuzhou in 1982, and *The Journal of Clinical Anesthesiology* in Nanjing in 1985.

Colleges of Anesthesia One of the most important indications of progress during this period was the 1987 establishment of the College of Anesthesia in Xuzhou Medical School by Yinming Zeng, who devoted his life to education in anesthesiology. This was the first College of Anesthesia founded in a medical school in China and represented a landmark in the history of Chinese anesthesiology. In effect, it was an enlarged anesthesia residency. Students underwent 5 years of study and training in anesthesiology, pain management, and critical care medicine to get their Medical Degree. This College of Anesthesia cultivated a greater knowledge and expertise in anesthesiology.

Many other Colleges of Anesthesia have been established, such as in Harbin Medical University, Hunan Medical University, and Tongji Medical University, all in 1988. By 2011, 54 medical universities had established Colleges of Anesthesia. This is a characteristically Chinese approach of anesthesia training. However, whether this approach should exist as an undergraduate major in medical school remains controversial.

The Rapid Development of Anesthesiology in China (1990-present)

The last 20 years have been exciting for Chinese anesthesia, largely because of the increasing opportunities that allowed the sharing of clinical and research experiences, making anesthetic practice safer and better than ever before. By 2007, China had 80,000 anesthesiologists (nurses do not provide anesthesia in China).

Advances in Anesthetic Equipment and Medications

More advanced anesthetic technology and medication were introduced into China from abroad. The manufacture of anesthetic instruments in China developed from imitation of foreign anesthetic machines and assembly of imported components, to the creation of original products. Improvements by anesthesiologists and technicians narrowed the gap between Chinese components and foreign ones in both quality and accuracy. In the 1990s, various anesthetic and adjuvant medications were available, and most new medications manufactured abroad were accessible in clinical practice. Indeed, some of our products now meet international standards.

During the last 20 years, Chinese anesthesiologists have advanced some innovative ideas and practices. The former president (2009–2012) of the CSA, Buwei Yu, has initiated the concept of "ideal anesthesia", which aims to monitor and control vital signs at predetermined "ideal" (normal) values, and achieve other desirable outcomes (e.g., minimizing postoperative nausea and vomiting). Hopefully, ideal anesthesia should provide patients with greater satisfaction and safety.

In addition, in the 2000s, Jin Liu from West China Hospital, Sichuan University completed a lot of animal studies and a phase I clinical trail on 130 human volunteers with emulsified isoflurane. These studies indicate that induction of and recovery from anesthesia with emulsified isoflurane is faster than with propofol, and provides stable hemodynamics. Therefore, it may be particularly suitable for rapid sequence induction and short and invasive examinations and therapies. In addition, it would reduce pollution (because may be equivalent to closed circuit anesthetic delivery), and is convenient to carry and use in the wild or on battlefields. As with inhaled potent anesthetics, emulsified isoflurane preconditioning has a protective effect against liver and lung injury, improves survival in hemorrhagic shock [13], and provides protection against cardiac ischemia reperfusion injury [14, 15].

The Chinese Society of Anesthesiology (CSA)

The CSA has built cooperative relationships with international associations, such as the American Society of Anesthesiologists, the International Anesthesia Research Society, and the Association of Anaesthetists of Great Britain and Ireland. Young Chinese scholars increasingly participate in major international meetings held in the US, Europe, Japan, and surrounding countries and regions. Famous professors from abroad (e.g., Ronald Miller and Edmond Eger) have visited China as keynote speakers. These activities enhance Chinese anesthesiologists' familiarity with and contribution to international achievements and developments in anesthesiology. In return, these efforts make Chinese anesthesiology known to the world, and provide a foundation for the future development and international communication of Chinese anesthesiology.

The CSA plays a vital role in the progress of Chinese anesthesiology, acting as the conduit for official connections with many developed and developing counties; publishing many guidelines and recommendations on clinical practice; supervising the Quality Control Centers for Clinical Anesthesia; and establishing refresher courses for anesthesiologists from undeveloped regions.

Anesthesia Training Reforms that followed the cultural revolution enabled many young anesthesiologists to go abroad to receive training. In Chinese medical universities, there are now several training programs, varying in their lengths of study. Many are 8-year training programs, initiated by famous medical schools at the end of the twentieth century. The first 8-year training program was established in PUMC, reflecting practice in the US (i.e., 4 years of medical school and 4 years of training devoted to anesthesia). There also are 7-year and 5-year programs. Most specialists in anesthesiology come from undergraduate and postgraduate programs. A system of nurse anesthesia training has not been established in China.

According to 2007 data from Shuren Li, Emeritus President of the CSA, more than 80,000 anesthesia professionals are available in mainland China which is a large number. However, the population in China is 1.3 billion, and at least 150,000 anesthesiologists are needed. In addition, economic and medical development has been uneven among regions. About 4000-to-5000 medical school graduates begin to study anesthesiology each year. However, no national standardized training system currently exists. Usually, anesthesia residents take 3 years for basic anesthesia training and 2 years for advanced sub-discipline anesthesia training, such as cardiovascular anesthesia, pediatric anesthesia, intensive care, and pain management. After these 5 years of training, they must pass a national examination before being certified as attending anesthesiologists.

Academic and Research Activities Since the 1990s, academic activities have been promoted both domestically and internationally. The National Conference on Anesthesia has been held annually since 2000, and symposiums attracting young scholars and specialists are held all over China throughout the year. In addition, international communications have been enhanced. Ailun Luo, after being elected President of CSA in 1997, advocated China's integration into the world anesthesia community. She was conferred an Honorary Fellowship of the Royal College of Anaesthetists of the United Kingdom.

From the 1990s until today, research in Chinese anesthesiology has moved as fast as the economy of China would permit. Many well-known journals including, *Anesthesia & Analgesia*, *Anesthesiology*, and *Anaesthesia*, have been published in Chinese editions from 2002, 2007 and 2007, respectively, extending their influence among Chinese professionals. These localized journals become the window for communication in anesthesiology between China and the world. Moreover, with the progress of Anesthesiology, the numbers and qualities of research funds have been increasing. Clinical and basic studies have been conducted and increasing numbers of papers from mainland China have been published in international academic journals. In *Anesthesiology*, there were no Chinese studies published in 1999, and 5 in 2009.; In *Anesthesia and Analgesia*, the number rose from 1 to 14, and in the *British Journal of Anaesthesia*, the number rose from 0 to 4.

Conclusions

Anesthesiology in China has met many obstacles and opportunities during modern times. Several generations have striven to catch up with western countries, having had to contend with poverty, civil war, and great societal upheaval from the Cultural Revolution. Anesthesia practice today is performed by well-educated anesthesiologists using increasingly advanced anesthetic technology and medications. Academic and research activities are developing rapidly, as are anesthesia training and international communication. Future Chinese anesthesiologists will play an increasing role in the international arena. A bright future lies ahead.

References

1. Wai FK. On Hua Tuo's position in the history of Chinese medicine. The Am J Chin Med. 2004;32:313–20.
2. Unschuld PU. Medicine in China: a history of ideas. Berkeley: University of California Press; 1985.
3. Zheng B. The miracle-working doctor. J Tradit Chin Med. 1985;5(4):311–2.
4. Hsu HY, Peacher WG. Chen's history of Chinese medical science. Taiwan: Modern Drug Publishers Co.; 1977.
5. State administration of traditional Chinese medicine, advanced textbook on traditional Chinese medicine and pharmacology. Beijing: New World Press; 1995.
6. Fenster J. Ether day: the strange tale of America's greatest medical discovery and the haunted men who made it. New York: HarperCollins; 2001.
7. Sykes W. Essays on the one hundred years of anesthesia. Edinburgh: Livingstone; 1960.
8. Hune EH. Peter Paker and the introduction of anesthesia into China. J History Med Allied Sci. 1946;1:671–3.
9. Sim P, Du B, Bacon RD. Pioneer Chinese anesthesiologists: American influences. Anesthesiology. 2000;93:256–64.
10. Zhao J. The path we explored. Anesthesia tribune. 1996;4:7–8, 11.
11. Wang Y. Management of complications in epidural anesthesia. Chin J Surg. 1957;5:828.
12. Zhao J. The path we explored. Anesth tribune. 1995;4:2–3.
13. Zhang L, Luo N, Liu J, Duan Z, Du G, Cheng J, Lin H, Li Z. Emulsified isoflurane preconditioning protects against liver and lung injury in rat model of hemorrhagic shock. J Surg Res. 2011;171:783–90.
14. Huang H, Zhang W, Liu S, Yanfang C, Li T, Liu J. Cardioprotection afforded by St Thomas solution is enhanced by emulsified isoflurane in an isolated heart ischemia reperfusion injury model in rats. J Cardiothorac Vasc Anesth. 2010;24:99–103.
15. Hu ZY, Luo NF, Liu J. The protective effects of emulsified isoflurane on myocardial ischemia and reperfusion injury in rats. Can J Anaesth. 2009;56:115–25.)

David Baker, Jean-Bernard Cazalaà and Marie-Thérèse Cousin

Summary

The first trial of ether in France antedated use of the agent in England. During the next few years, France's Académie des Sciences examined the claims for the discovery of anesthesia, finally according it jointly to Morton and Jackson. By 1848, chloroform displaced ether despite inexplicable fatalities associated with its use. In 1908, ether spectacularly returned with the introduction of the Ombrédanne inhaler, remaining popular in France to the 1960s.

As World War II began, doctors, pharmacists, dentists and medical orderlies might be briefly trained in anesthesia. Surgeons directed anesthesia, and article 45 of the 1947 code of practice gave the "*surgeon...the right to choose his operating assistants as well as the anaesthestist.*" Students completing a 6-week course, supervised by surgeons or physicians and supplemented by a 6-month hospital assignment, received a "Certificate of Anaesthesia". The institution of examinations in 1948 led to the award of the Diplôme d'Anesthésie-Réanimation (Diploma in Anesthesia and post-operative care)

In 1934, surgeon Monod founded the Société d'études sur l'anesthésie et l'analgésie (SEAA). The Society published a review (*Anesthésie et Analgésie*) since 1935. In 1938, the Society became the Société Française d'anesthésie et d'analgésie (SFAA), but went dormant during World War II, reviving in 1946 with 117 members, mostly surgeons but including 17 anesthetists.

Until 1947, only surgeons received fees, giving about 10% to "assistants". Anesthetists provided all supplies, promoting use of the least expensive approaches. From 1947, "Special anesthesia" by a qualified anesthetist warranted a separate fee. In 1958, a major reform of hospitals created full-time anesthesia posts and services. A 1960 Government decree recognized anesthesiology as a specialty, renamed in 1970 as Anesthésie-Réanimation, emphasizing the anesthetist's role in post-operative care. In 1979, the Conseil National de l'Ordre recognized anesthesiologists as medical specialists, independent of surgeons. From 1989, postgraduate medical education expanded to include anesthesia (previously restricted to older medical specialities), and 5 years of training led to the Diplôme d'études supérieures en anesthésié-réanimation (DESA). Concurrently, schools for nurse anesthetists opened, and examination led to the Certificat d'Aptitude aux Fonctions d'Aide Anesthésie. Like physicians, nurse anesthetists organized training programs and trade unions, and worked in accordance with statutes they devised. They competed with doctors, creating still unresolved antagonisms.

French anesthesiologists developed the prehospital emergency system, SAMU (Service d'Aide Médicale Urgente) in the 1970s, reasoning that in emergencies the hospital should go to the patient. In 1982, two previously disparate groups fused into la Société Française d'Anesthésie et Réanimation (SFAR), establishing the journal, Annales Françaises d'Anesthésie et de Réanimation (AFAR).

D. Baker (✉)
Hôpital Necker-Enfants Malades, Paris, Club de l'histoire de l'anesthésie et de la réanimation français, Souillac, France
e-mail: 113445.3600@wanadoo.fr

J.-B. Cazalaà
Hôpitaux de Paris, Club d'histoire de l'anesthésie et de la réanimation (CHAR) français, Paris, France
e-mail: jbcaz@noos.fr

M.-T. Cousin
Anesthésiologiste des Hôpitaux de Paris, Club de l'histoire de l'anesthésie et de la réanimation France, Buc, France
e-mail: mtcoucou@yahoo.fr

Introduction

Anesthesia in France initially developed in parallel with English speaking countries, but the details of that history are little known outside France. Nineteenth century French innovations reported in French often went unnoticed elsewhere. In addition, the development of anesthesiology as a speciality was slow. This chapter provides insights into the problems faced by anesthetists in France, from the middle of the 19th century to the end of the 1980s, when French anesthesia could be regarded as being again in step with the progress of the speciality in other parts of the world [1–4].

The Early Years of Surgical Anesthesia (1846–1850)

France Adjudicated the American Quarrel about Discovery

From January 1847, the use of ether spread in France, as it did in England and throughout the rest of continental Europe. Charles Jackson (1805–1880), William Morton (1819–1868) and then Horace Wells (1815–1848) battled for recognition as the discoverer of anesthesia. They appealed to France to adjudicate, since for them a valid opinion could only come from Paris, at that time the medical capital of the world.

At the meeting of the Académie des Sciences, [4] on 18 January 1847 (six days after the first French communication about anesthesia to the Academy of Medicine), Christophe Ducros (1808–1849) claimed the discovery of anesthesia, recalling his paper of 16 March 1846 on the effects of sulphuric ether. His experiments carried out in 1842 showed the hypnotic effects of ether rubbed into fowls, and also mentioned similar effects in man. Accordingly, he claimed to have invented anesthesia, before the American who had recently suggested that the ablation of consciousness using ether could be of value in patients undergoing surgery. At the meeting, Léonce Elie de Beaumont (1798–1874), a geologist and a friend of Jackson requested that a sealed envelope[1] which he had delivered to the meeting of 28 December 1846, be opened. This contained three letters from Jackson which were read to the Academy. The first was dated 13 November 1846, and the second, 1 December 1846. The following are extracts from the letters:

> 'I request permission to communicate to the Academy of Science through your intermediary a discovery which I have made which I believe to be important for the alleviation of human suffering and of great value for the art of surgery' (…) 'On learning that a local dentist was giving ether to patients requiring tooth extractions I asked him to go to the Massachusetts General Hospital and to give the vapour to a patient undergoing a painful surgical operation. The result was that the patient did not feel the slightest pain during the operation and was well afterwards.' The letters claimed responsibility for the discovery and maintained that Morton had been but a technician. He did not even mention the latter by name.

Elie de Beaumont supported Jackson's claim and his scientific credentials, and brought the discovery to the attention of the Academy. After this lecture, the surgeon Alfred Velpeau (1795–1867) noted that:

> 'The secret in question in the note which I have just read has not been a secret for long. The journals in America and England have revealed it since the month of November. I personally learned about it in a letter from Dr Warren in Boston over a month ago and Dr Willis Fisher, from the same town came to ask me to conduct a trial at the Charité (hospital) about the middle of last December'.

There followed a short narrative in which Velpeau cited the name of Morton, and related the results of his own experiments in anesthesia and those of others, about which he had learned in Paris.

At the 25 January 1847 meeting of the Académie des Sciences, Ducros again laid claim to the invention of anesthesia, but was ignored. For the moment, the French academics gave the credit for the discovery to Jackson.

Horace Wells, who had arrived in Paris at that time to start an engraving and painting business was welcomed by his friend and fellow Bostonian, Christopher Brewster (1799–1870), who practiced in Paris. Wells convinced Brewster that he was the inventor of anesthesia. Brewster introduced him to his circle of friends, and Wells lectured on nitrous oxide and ether. His presentation to the Société Médicale de Paris on the 17 February 1847 (*A history of the discovery of the application of nitrous oxide gas, ether and other vapors to surgical operations* [5]) propelled him to fame. He wrote to the Academy of Medicine (the meeting of the 23 February 1847) [4] and to the Academy of Science (the meeting of 8 March 1847) [4] to claim recognition for the discovery:

> 'Reasoning from analogy, I was led to believe that surgical operations might be performed without pain (…) By these facts I was led to enquire if the same result would not follow by the inhalation of exhilarating gas (…) I accordingly procured some nitrous oxide gas, resolving to make the first experiment on myself, by having a tooth extracted, which was done without any painful sensations (…) This discovery does not consist in the use of any one specific gas or vapour, for anything which will cause a certain degree of nervous excitement, is all that is required to render the system insensible to pain.(…).'

There followed a lively discussion in the Academy, not just about who made the discovery but also on the use of nitrous oxide, which was contested by Matéo Orfila (1787–1853) and Pierre Boullay (1777–1869), since the gas appeared to them to be dangerous. Nicolas Gérardin (1790–1868) recalled that a London surgeon had written a letter bringing this topic to the attention of the Academy 17 or 18 years previously, when only Baron Larrey (1766–1842) had defended the use of nitrous oxide. This letter from Henry-Hill Hickman (1800–1830), read to the Académie de Médecine on the 28 September 1828, developed the idea that '*by introducing certain gases into the lungs the ability to feel could be*

---

[1]A sealed envelope is a system whereby an inventor may guard his rights to an invention which are still uncertain. The latter is kept by the Academy and is not opened until requested by the depositor.

suspended'. This letter remained forgotten by the Academy of Medicine, and was finally lost.

The Academy of Science received a similar demand from Wells. The secretary added that this claim could not be considered until the documents proving the claims had been received. Jackson's friend, Elie de Beaumont, noted that the delays involved in examining the claim were unduly long and consequently diminished the value of the claim. He supported Jackson noting '*the true benefactor to humanity is the person who asked the dentist to pull a tooth from a person who was in a state induced by the inhalation of ether.*' Wells returned to Boston to collect documents proving his claims.

During the session of the Académie des Sciences [4] of 22 March 1847, Elie de Beaumont read a new, Machiavellian letter from Jackson, dated 28 February 1847. He noted a respiratory problem during an anesthetic given in Boston, and recommended the use of oxygen and precautions that should be taken before any anesthetic. This valuable scientific information brought honour on its author. In a second paragraph he justified the claim for a patent for anesthesia '*I was very opposed to the idea of taking out patents for anything that could reduce human suffering (...) but I decided to do so in order to establish my rights as author of the discovery and to be able to authorize others to use it*'. In a footnote he said that he had been obliged to include Morton in the patent since Morton had worked under his orders, but that he had been surprised to see him as sole owner of the rights six months later, although only for the US. These facts were proven to be false some months later, but the French Academies were not informed of this. The third paragraph contained an attack on Wells' requests. He finished with the final discovery he had made—dental cement—which confirmed his position as a man of science.

On the same boat that left Boston for Europe on 1 March 1847, Jackson sent copies of the Boston Advertiser of the 1st March 1847 to a hundred medical and other personalities. This contained the minutes of the meeting (written by him) of doctors in Boston where he had claimed his rights to the invention. In the minutes, he listed all the doctors and other persons who were present at the meeting. His carefully drafted text gives the impression that all present warmly favoured his claim. But the minutes are a fiction, since the meeting was not held until 2 March, after the departure of the mail boat for England! The honesty of Jackson had been placed in some doubt in Boston, but in Europe and particularly in Paris, the falsehood was accepted, and Jackson remained the discoverer of anesthesia.

Morton's response was to send a letter to the Académie des Sciences, which was received on 17 May, and a memorandum to the Académie de Médecine, mentioned in the Proceedings of 2 November 1847 under the title *Works received: 'Memorandum on the discovery of a new use of sulphuric ether by Morton'*.

Jackson continued to send legal documents supporting his claim to the Académie des Sciences (meetings were held on 5 May and 5 July 1847). The disregard of Morton's claim incensed the French consul in Boston. He wrote to the Ministère de l'instruction publique (Minister of Education), requesting him to kindly communicate the contents of his letter to the Academies. The letter was duly read to the Académie de Médecine on 21 September:

> '*I forward (some) publications sent by Mrs Gray and Warren (the son of John Collins Warren who had welcomed Morton) which put beyond doubt the fact that the honour for this discovery is due to Dr WTG Morton (following the receipt of the abstract of the brevet by Morton and the general attitude of Jackson). Jackson had so little confidence in the effectiveness of the 'ether' that he ceded all his rights to the discovery to Dr Morton for the sum of 500 dollars.*'

The Académie des Sciences did not mention this submission until the proceedings of 18 October. On 13 December 1847, and 27 March 1848, Elie de Beaumont sent further notes by Jackson and announced an emissary (Mr Peabody), to confirm his priority.

On 24 January 1848, in a state of despair, Horace Wells committed suicide in prison while awaiting trial. Several days following his burial, a letter arrived in Hartford, sent from Paris by Brewster: "*My dear Wells I have just returned from a meeting of Paris Medical Society, where they have voted that to Horace Wells of Hartford, Connecticut, USA, is due all the honour of having first discovered and successfully applied the use of vapours or gases whereby surgical operations could be performed without pain.*" [6] But the Association des Médecins in Paris was not the Academy, and Wells had only obtained this recognition from the Société Médicale de Paris. The announcement of Wells' death arrived in Paris after this honour had been granted. In 1910, a statue of Wells was erected in the Place des Etats-Unis in Paris (Fig. 28.1).

On 24 April 1848, Morton announced to the Académie des Sciences that documents had been sent, which proved his claim and cited Dr. Bigelow as a witness. The Academy did not however receive these documents in April, and would indeed never receive them. They were contained in six cases which had been mislaid during Customs clearance. When Morton was informed after a delay of six months, he asked to whom in Paris he might send them. He requested the dentist Brewster (the friend of Wells) to assist. Brewster managed to clear the cases from Customs using money sent by Morton, but then held onto them for two years without responding to Morton's queries.

The Commission that was charged with the task of establishing who had made the discovery, took its time. On 16 April 1849, the Ministère de l'Instruction Publique (Minister of Education) sent a copy of a letter from Jackson to the Academy of Sciences on the occasion of his being awarded the decoration of Chevalier de la Légion d'Honneur. In the

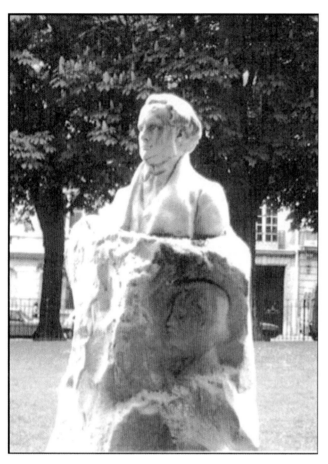

Fig. 28.1 Statue of Horace Wells in the Place des Etats–Unis in Paris, erected in 1910 by subscription by the members of the Franco—American Society of Dentists. On one face of the pedestal is a bas-relief of Paul Bert's bust. (Courtesy of MT Cousin)

letter, he expressed his gratitude to the Academy for the welcome he had received from it, following his discovery of ether anesthesia.

Morton re-sent a letter to the Académie des Sciences dated 16 March 1849, which was read at the 23 April 1849 meeting, concerning the question of ownership of the discovery. He reminded the Academy that the annual report of the Massachusetts General Hospital of 1848, formally accorded him the honour of having made the discovery. He added that, when the question was raised in the US Congress, the majority of the Congress reached the same decision.

The results of a Commission in charge of awarding a prize in Medicine and Surgery (the Prix Montyon), for the years 1847 and 1848, were announced by Dr Roux on 25 February 1850 [4]. '*A prize in the sum of 3000 francs[2] is awarded to Dr Jackson for his observations and experiments on the anesthetic effects produced by the inhalation of ether;' (...) and a further prize of a similar sum is given*

to Dr Morton for having introduced the method into surgical practice, following guidance from Dr Jackson. In the report concerning these prizes, read during the subsequent session (4 March 1850), [4] the Academy concluded that it could not determine who of the two, had made such a marvellous discovery. The prizes were duly reduced to 2500 francs.

The judgement was that of Solomon for some, but unfair for others. Jackson was unhappy to be associated with Morton, but still accepted the prize. For his part, Morton protested against the decision of the Academy and refused the prize. This caused a scandal in the Academy, since it was thought unacceptable that Morton had not received any reward because the Academy had received several documents favourable to his case over a period of time. After long discussions, the Commission decided to create a gold medal to the value of the prize. On one side of the medal was the Institut de France, surrounded by a Minerve (the Roman goddess of science and the official emblem of the Institut de France); and on the other side, the inscription 'Académie des Sciences, Montyon prize for medicine and surgery Concours of 1847 and 1848 WTG Morton 1850'. However the value of this medal was still less than that of the prize, so the Academy requested the maker to add a laurel wreath to make up the difference, All this enraged Jackson who had only a diploma, while the name of Morton appeared on the medal. Several years later, Morton had to sell the medal to provide for his family [6]. The fight between Jackson and Morton would continue in the US.

The Early Demise of Chloroform: A Clash of Two Personalities

The first death from chloroform in France occurred in 1848, several months after Hannah Greener died in England. The French Government ordered judicial and medical inquiries. The Academy of Medicine set up a special commission which arrived at contentious conclusions. The patient, a healthy 35-year-old woman, needed surgery for an abscess that had formed around a foreign body resulting from a riding accident. Within a minute of inhaling from a gauze pad onto which 20 drops of chloroform had been poured, she exclaimed '*I am choking*', turned pale and died despite two hours of attempted resuscitation (involving insufflation of air into the airways) [7]. Malgaigne, who had presented his studies on ether anesthesia to the Academy one year earlier, led the inquiry. The Commission included Antoine Jobert (de Lamballe) (who had given the first ether anesthetic in Paris on December 15 1846), Alfred Velpeau (an adept enthusiast of surgical anesthesia), and Frédéric Blandin (author of a lengthy academic study on the effects of ether in 1847). Of the 13 Commissioners 7 were surgeons and the remainder veterinarians, pharmacists and chemists.

---

[2] What corresponded to approximately one year of salary for a worker.

Fig. 28.2 Joseph-François Malgaigne and Jules Guérin. (Malgaigne image from http://www.biusante. parisdescartes.fr/histmed/ image?anmpx37x0163terb Guérin image from http://www.biusante. parisdescartes.fr/histmed/ image?anmpx05x0189)

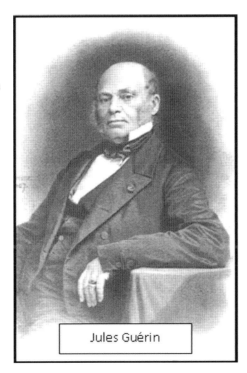

Jules Guérin

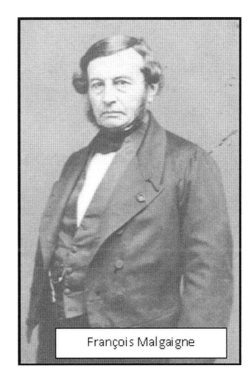

François Malgaigne

Malgaigne presented the Commission's findings to the Academy in October 1848. They questioned the details of the report written by the surgeon who had conducted the anesthesia and operation, focussing on the dose of chloroform and the delay to the moment of death. They noted that the woman said '*I am choking*', indicating in Malgaigne's view that the chloroform had not started to work. They suggested therefore that the sudden death was, without doubt, due to anxiety, or to a gas embolism (gas was found in the blood vessels at autopsy). Finally, the death was attributed to asphyxia (as Simpson had suggested for Hannah Greener). Other deaths occurred subsequently, but such cases were rare, being less than a dozen in one year out of several hundred chloroform anesthetics. Concerning the overall safety of chloroform, Malgaigne noted that '*one could not set up rules starting from exceptions. It was only necessary therefore to introduce certain precautions to avoid asphyxia*'.

This conclusion was not unanimously accepted, some members of the Commission noting that sudden deaths had occurred in animals as well as in humans. Blaming chloroform might mean abandoning general anesthesia itself, despite the successes with ether. Velpeau hoped that '*for the honour of chloroform*' the real cause of the deaths would be found. Jules Guérin (1801–1886) supplied the most virulent criticism, saying that to deny chloroform as the cause of death ran contrary to the facts and would render the Academy responsible for future accidents. He suggested a research program to establish the contributions of dose, setting, delay of action, and supply, through a program of animal experiments. This program had been preceded by intensive research

on many animals (mostly dogs, but also including rabbits, chickens, birds and frogs) conducted by chemists, veterinarians, and surgeons, including some members of the Commission. Guérin himself had studied the effects of chloroform on dogs, rabbits and frogs. However, Malgaigne remained content with clinical experience alone and thereby began a bitter dispute in which he denied the fact that Guérin had experimented on anesthetics. Further, he insinuated that Guerin had previously referred to '*non-existent results*', inferring that Guérin was a liar. Guerin made no immediate response to this accusation but went on the attack the following day.

The confrontation had nothing to do with the anesthetic question. The real reason was a quarrel beginning ten years earlier. Both were surgeons, members of the Academy, and directors of medical journals—and their dispute had only been resolved a few months previously. In his journal, Guérin had reported on tenotomies for correction of club foot and spinal deformations. Of 750 operations, he described 650 cures or improvements. Thinking these results to be too good to be true, Malgaigne had attacked Guérin who then sued Malgaigne for defamation. Guérin won this case, but Malgaigne, having pursued the matter legally, attracted public attention by his eloquence. Guérin then asked for, and won the right for a Commission to judge the results of his new cases occurring during the following 3 months. The Commission judged that the results were consistent with those that Guérin had previously reported, and the Commission noted '*Mr Guérin had brought honour to science and to humanity*'. (Fig. 28.2)

During the following days, Guérin threw down the gauntlet declaring '*In deference to all I had to refrain previously from rising to this provocation. However, now you will no doubt be ready to provide the satisfaction that is normal among persons of honour'.* Malgaigne refused the invitation to duel but also refused to withdraw his accusations.

The Academy, wishing to end this affair quickly, voted on 6 February 1849, to accept the conclusions of a new report about chloroform. The conclusions were identical to those of the first report, adding that rules could not be established 'on the basis of exceptions'. Chloroform was thus reinstated although, on 24 January 1849 in Lyon, another fatal accident was immediately reported in the journal, L'Union Médicale, with the objective of persuading the Commission to alter its conclusions.. After this latest accident, the surgeons of Lyon completely abandoned the use of chloroform, however they remained at odds with most other French surgeons who, as in England, used it successfully over much of the nineteenth century.

The Early Twentieth Century—The Ombrédanne Inhaler Reigns

Based on the work of Paul Bert (1833–1886), the use of nitrous oxide increased in the latter half of the nineteenth century, with ethyl chloride appearing at the end of the century. In 1908, the Parisian surgeon, Louis Ombrédanne (1871–1956) described his ether inhaler. It was a modification of Clover's inhaler, which he criticised "*….as these are not provided with means of admission of fresh air, they rapidly produce cyanosis if one does not constantly raise the mask from the face.*" Ombrédanne's ether inhaler allowed the regulated admission of fresh air, and soon became the most commonly used apparatus in France, displacing the use of chloroform. It also became the usual means of anesthesia in many countries around the world, particularly Latin America.

Several other developments took place. Intravenous anesthesia, first used by Cyprien Oré (1828–1889) with chloral hydrate in 1872, was adopted from 1935 with the arrival of barbiturate compounds from Germany. Henri Laborit (1914–1995) described '*re-inforced anesthesia*' using other compounds, notably neuroleptics, antihistamines and morphine-like compounds, which had the ability to 'produce anesthetic states without using anesthetics'. His work also included the discovery of gamma hydroxybutyrate and its anesthetic effects.

Local anesthesia was largely the surgeons' domain. It started with simple infiltration (Paul Reclus 1847–1914), followed by nerve trunk blocks introduced by Victor Pauchet (1869–1936) and his pupil Gaston Labat (1876–1934). Finally, Théodore Tuffier (1857–1929) followed in the path of the German August Bier (1851–1949), and popularised spinal block. This new technique appeared shortly before caudal epidural anesthesia, which was discovered independently

by Fernand Cathelin (1873–1945) and Jean Athanase Sicard (1872–1929) in1901.

In the late 1940s, Daniel Bovet (1907–1992) at the Institut Pasteur synthesized new muscle relaxants, used in clinical practice by Pierre Huguenard (1924–2006). Powerful opioids were discovered by the Belgian Paul Jansen (1926–2003) in 1961, and were tested by his fellow countryman Georges de Castro (1918–1990), who also worked in France.

The Slow Path to Professional Recognition in the Twentieth Century

Anesthesia in France was based almost entirely on the use of the Ombrédanne ether inhaler well into the twentieth century. The context of the times slowed professional progress. At the end of World War II, the French hospital system was essentially an antiquated nineteenth century structure. Doctors, surgeons and anesthetists were employed part-time, working on a voluntary basis in the mornings and earning their living in private practice in the afternoon. Surgeons reigned supreme and guarded their privileges.

In 1946, a dedicated anesthetist, Ernest Kern (who had obtained his Diploma in Anesthetics in England) reflected the stagnation pervading the medical services, in his book, *Mes Quatre Vies* [8]. He described several anecdotes that followed his return to France after the Libération:

> - After asking for some modern anesthetic equipment, the director of a clinic replied '*we have used the Ombrédanne inhaler in France for 100 years to everyone's satisfaction. I do not see why we should change now to expensive foreign techniques. If you want other equipment you just have to bring it in yourself*'.

> - For one anesthetic he recalled '*I did not have curare available at the time and so used cyclopropane (which was at that time very expensive). This achieved perfect muscle relaxation and the surgeon thought the anesthesia was excellent. With total disdain the operating theatre sister threw me two 100 franc coins (the sum usually given to the theatre porter for giving the anesthetic). But this anesthetic had cost me five times as much…*'

> - In 1946, Kern presented a lecture to the Société Française d'Anesthésie et d'Analgésie (SFAA) on controlled respiration during thiopental and curare anesthesia. Afterwards, the President, surgeon Pierre Fredet (1870–1946), observed '*God caused man to breathe and God alone has the right to take away breathing. I challenge any man and any anesthetist to have this right; that would be sacrilege*'.

First Step: Towards a Trade Union

Several anesthetists gathered together to defend their rights and establish a separate speciality. On 25 November 1941, Louis Amiot (1897–1978), Jacques Boureau (1909–2004), and Geneviève Delahaye (1906–1970) founded a 'co-operative of anesthetists' in Paris, made up of 19 Members (under the Vichy regime, trade unions were banned) with the approval of the recently-formed Ordre des Médecins. After the Libération, the 'co-operative of anesthetists' (now with 23 members) changed its name to the Syndicat des Anesthésistes Francais, and was officially recognised.

Second Step: Freedom from Surgical Domination

Professional Organization and Establishment of Qualifications (1947–1970) Other specialities saw anesthesia as a professional threat, resulting in confrontations with the Ordre des Médecins, hospitals, and universities—all organizations controlled by surgeons. Despite this, the scientific development of anesthesia progressed through congresses and publications. In 1947, the 'new doctors' who had arrived in the operating theatre, were controlled by an article of the code of ethics, (Code de Déontologie), written by the Ordre des Médecins, and officially published as a decree [9] stating that the '*surgeon had the right to choose his operating assistants as well as the anesthestist*'. In 1955, despite a revision of the code of ethics, this article (article 45, a pet hate of the anesthetists) was unchanged. Surgeons continued to control anesthesia, and the speciality could not financially support practitioners. Anesthesia was merely a 'competence' held by suitably qualified doctors with a university diploma (which did not yet exist) or who had passed a suitable hospital open examination (when they were indeed set up).

The situation changed gradually. Three Commissions to review qualifications were set up in 1950, with surgeons and anesthetists appointed by the Union and SFA, supervised by the surgeon Jean Baumann (1906–1981) and two anesthetists, Jacques Boureau and Louis Amiot. Little by little, the profession was recognised, which meant higher remuneration, better conditions and more consideration. On 18 November 1965, anesthesiology was added to the list of medical specialities, following a decree by the Minister of Health giving it official recognition. In 1970, the speciality became known as 'Anesthésie-Réanimation' instead of Anesthesiology, to recognize the role of the anesthetist in post-operative care. In 1979, when the Code was changed for the third time, the infamous article 45 was abandoned. The Conseil National de l'Ordre finally recognized the anesthesiologist as an independent medical specialist, no longer under the control of the surgeon.

The Problem of Fees

One major problem was the payment for providing anesthesia care. Before 1947, only surgeons received fees. Approximately 10% of these (at most!) were given to 'assistants', medical and non-medical. The anesthetist provided all drugs and equipment. Since doctors could not financially survive as anesthetists, most continued to work as part time general practitioners. This situation led to the term '*docteur 10%*'. Some pioneers, such as Kern, paid for the new drugs and apparatus, but most stayed with ether and the Ombrédanne inhaler.

From 1947 however, arrangements for payment for anesthetic services emerged. "Special anesthesia" given by a medically qualified anesthetist was paid for separately from the surgeon's fee, and the surgeon's fee was reduced, providing an incentive for surgeons to use anesthetic nurses. Whether the '*special anesthetic*' was determined by the state of the patient, or by the nature of the surgery, was a decision left to the health insurance companies. In 1953, the payment for anesthesia services improved slightly. Every patient, regardless of their condition, was thought to benefit from a modern anesthetic without the anesthetist having to justify it. Finally in 1960, anesthesia was separated completely from surgery with the understanding that it was given personally by a medical practitioner. At last, the fee for anesthesia was completely separated from that of the surgeon.

Hospital and University

Creation of the Union did not necessarily confer status on the new speciality. In 1939, a project to create funded posts for anesthetists went unrealized. An ambitious programme of recruitment set up by the Paris hospital service in 1947 envisaged a chief anesthetist with posts for part time assistants. The programme was not formalized, but a competitive application was instituted for the post of hospital assistant, for 15 posts in Paris. The application specified that the post did not carry any remuneration. The greatest names in French anesthesia entered into this system but continued to earn their living by providing anesthesia in private hospitals.

In 1958, a major reform of French hospitals occurred when Charles de Gaulle returned to government. It had been formulated during World War II by the "Conseil National de la Résistance" of which Robert Debré was a member. Its authors were driven by a 'generous mystic', according to Debré's word, who affirmed equality of all French people when faced with illness. When Debré's son, Michel Debré, became the First Minister of the de Gaulle Government, he facilitated the implementation of the reform. It was financed in part by the Government (French state finances improved with the ending of the Algerian War) and partly by the Sécurité Sociale [10] (whose funds came from the contributions of salaried employees). The new structures united hospitals and universities. It led to creation of full-time posts and to the definition of future anesthesia services, giving the Union a new opportunity. A Government decree in December 1958, created heads of departments, although it took two more years to include anesthetists as a recognized speciality. Anesthesia departments were instituted seven years later. Dual university and hospital appointments were created, and from that time specialists were trained, and posts created for them in large numbers.

Training in Anesthesia

Training in anesthesia in France, was formally organized after World War II. Until then, only a few private initiatives existed for training nurses. In 1939, at the outbreak of the war, training for doctors, pharmacists, dentists and medical orderlies was established to provide anesthetists for the Army.

In 1945, the surgeon Pierre Moulonguet (1890–1981), who held the newly created Chair of Surgical Techniques in Paris, assembled a formal training program for anesthetists, based upon modules used for teaching Army doctors and medical orderlies. The six week course started in 1947, and was supplemented by a six month hospital assignment supervised by members of the Société d'Etudes, either surgeons or internists. Students completing this course, received a 'Certificat d'anesthésie'. In 1948, a written examination was taken before entering the course, and a final examination led to the award of the Diplôme d'Anesthésie-Réanimation (Diploma in Anesthesia and post-operative care). Nurse anesthetists continued to receive the Certificate of Anesthesia, now awarded following a written examination. In 1951, doctors wishing certification had to be examined for the award of the Certificat d'Etudes Spéciales d'Anesthésie (CESA, the certificate of special studies in anesthesia). Faculties of medicine in major cities around the country organized the examinations, and the certificate became a national standard in 1956. By now the word 'réanimation' (post-operative care) had been dropped. However in 1966, CESA became CESAR with the addition of 'réanimation'. Holders of the CESAR could practice in both public and private hospitals, but not teach.

The growth in specialist medical anesthetists numbers was impressive. The 20 or so qualifications granted yearly between 1947 and 1951 increased tenfold, with a dozen city faculties introducing their own training. In 1966, there were 1000 trained anesthetists, and the number of trainees increased from 400 a year in the 60s and 70s, to 700 between 1970 and 1982. From 1989, anesthesia was included in immediate postgraduate medical education in Paris (the 'Internat'), previously restricted to the older medical specialities. However, the annual number of trainees in anesthesia was reduced by nearly 80 % due to a quota system for the 'internat'. Successful students received the exclusive new diploma (Diplôme d'études supérieures en anesthésié-réanimation, DESA) at the end of five years of anesthetic training.

Anesthesiologists and Intensive Care Physicians and Precedence

During conversations with one of the authors, Maurice Cara (1918–2009) said that he had always insisted that anesthesiologists were capable of looking after patients with respiratory impairment, either pathological or from neuromuscular blocking drugs. It was an anesthetist, Björn Ibsen (1915–2007), who had convinced Henry Lassen (1900–1974) in Copenhagen in 1952, that polio patients required artificial ventilation [11].

Cara was a thoracic physiologist, and later an anesthesiologist. He was part of a specialist group working on silicosis for the European Coal and Steel Community (a forerunner of the European Union). In this group he met other European lung specialists including Benjamin Baudraz, who alerted Cara to what was happening in Copenhagen. On hearing the news, Cara immediately put himself at Ibsen's disposal. He noted that the Engstrom ventilator had been able to replace medical students who been used to squeeze bags to keep patients with respiratory failure alive. Cara finally met Carl Engstrom (1912–1987) in Stockholm, and the latter was obliging enough to lend him one of his machines. Cara had the opportunity to study the device at the Hôpital Necker—Enfants Malades in Paris, and he bought several for the Paris hospital service.

He used the device when the polio epidemic struck France in 1954. The first patient given intermittent positive pressure artificial ventilation was a child admitted to the hospital with polio at the beginning of 1954. At this time, Pierre Mollaret (1898–1987) had treated numerous adults afflicted with polio using cabinet ventilators (the 'iron lung'). To convince Mollaret of the value of mechanical positive pressure ventilation, Cara and a biochemist colleague ventilated a dog for a week (although they noted that patients had already been treated in this way in Denmark for more than two years). Finally convinced, Mollaret bought several Engstrom ventilators and opened the first 'respiratory resuscitation' service for adults at the Claude-Bernard Hospital in Paris in September. Numerous other French centers' duplicated this because of the concern about polio.

In 1955, under the aegis of SFAA, Cara convened a meeting of those with practical experience using mechanical ventilation, including French and Swiss practitioners who were anesthesiologists, physiologists, biochemists and medical intensivists. Mollaret was, of course, invited but his antipathy (jealousy?) towards Cara was such that he actually forbade Cara to attend, even though Cara had organized the meeting! For this reason, Louis Amiot, the President of the SFAA at that time, read the introductory address, drafted by Cara. Cara seems to have accepted the "diktat" without complaint, but never forgot it.

The dispute between anesthesiologists and medical intensivists, about who should control postoperative, and even aspects of perioperative care, lingered. Surprisingly, anesthesiologists found allies in the surgeons who did not wish to see two doctors at the head of the operating table. Anesthesiologists increasingly realized that life support was important to their work. In 1957, not wishing to restrict their practice to the operating room, they asked authorities to increase training by 1 year (to a total of 3 years) devoted to 'reanimation' (post-operative and intensive care). They also modified the name of their society, to '*Société Française d'Analgésie d'Anesthésie et de Réanimation*', and also the name of their journal which became '*Anesthésie Analgésie Réanimation*'.

Medical and Nurse Anesthetists: An Unfortunate Confusion of Identity

In 1946, nurse anesthetists received, in Paris, the same Certificate of Anesthesia as did doctors. From 1948 to 1973, nurse-anesthetist training schools trained 1500 students. From 1960 almost all cities with universities had a nurse-anesthetists school, and an examination was devised leading to the *Certificat d'Aptitude aux Fonctions d'Aide Anesthésiste*. During this period (1947–1965), nurse anesthetists advanced their own ideas about training. The word 'anesthésiste' presented a problem. It was used equally to describe doctors, nurses or auxiliary personal (including nurses) who had undergone any training in anesthesia. However, a legal ruling obliged nurses who were giving anesthesia, to put the word 'Aide' in front of 'Anesthésiste' (literally to describe them as anesthetic assistants).

The first nurse anesthetists were pioneers. Like medical anesthetists, they purchased their own equipment and drugs, and were entirely self-supported, including going abroad for further training. Like physicians, they organized trade unions and worked in accordance with statutes that they devised. With the support of surgeons they obtained the right to practice from the Ministry of Health. Thanks to close relations with the then Prime Minister, they obtained the exclusive right to practice as nurse anesthetists (Infirmière Anesthésiste Diplomée d'Etat or IADE) provided they had completed an official training program that they themselves had inspired. They organized their training programs, and thereby excluded other paramedical staff from giving anesthesia.

Far from being mere anesthetic assistants, they competed with the doctors, resulting in an antagonism. Anesthesiologists could not see (and some still cannot today) that the IADE were skilled technicians (rather like paramedics) who followed "cookbook" like protocols. They gave the anesthetic under the direct and exclusive supervision of a medical anesthesiologist, who could intervene at any moment. This mirrored systems used in Sweden and other countries. They could not work independently as was (but no longer is in many states) the case in the US.

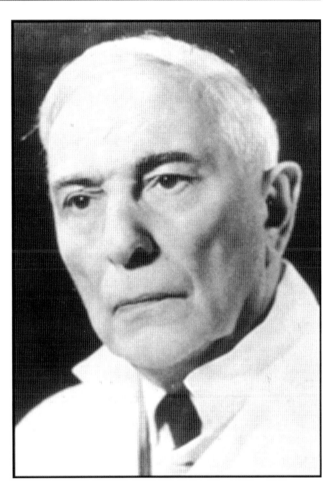

Fig. 28.3 Robert Monod, surgeon and founder of the Société d'études d'anesthésie et d'analgésie (1934). (From reference [1], pp 591, with permission)

The Successive French Societies of Anesthesiology

Société d'Études d'Anesthésie et d'Analgésie (SEAA)

In 1934, surgeon Robert Monod (Fig. 28.3) founded the Society for the study of anesthesia and analgesia (Société d'études sur l'anesthésie et l'analgésie SEAA), with surgeon Antonin Gosset (1872–1944) as President (already President of the Society of Surgery). At the first meeting of the Society, Monod stated that '*its objective was not to become a society of anesthetists*' (probably since surgeons held themselves superior to other physicians of the time) [12].

World War II and the Birth of a New Society

The society published a review (*Anesthésie et Analgésie*), with Monod as editor-in-chief, from 1935 until 1951. In

1934, the Society had 100 members from medical, physiological, pharmaceutical and veterinary disciplines, but only four anesthetic practitioners. In 1935, membership increased to 120. In 1938, the Society became the Société française d'anesthésie et d'analgésie (SFAA), but its activity and archives were suspended in 1939, following the outbreak of war. In 1946, the SFAA was reborn with 17 anesthetists out of a total of 117 members. The attraction of anesthetists towards the SFAA grew and was accompanied by the development of a trade union. As they were often anesthetists working with the surgeon-memberss of the SFAA, they were elected members of this society.

World War II had introduced modern anesthesia to France, but there would be a long battle to replace the Ombrédanne inhaler introduced in 1908. By 1948, anesthetic practice had progressed considerably from Fredet's notions. At a meeting of the general assembly on 15 January 1948, Monod (President of the society in 1947) [13] noted:

> '*We have been criticised, not without cause, for having created a society too much concerned with theory and research and not with practice. In this respect we have considerable work to do, since, despite the journal we publish, it is evident that anesthesia in France is not yet up to the standard found abroad, notably in America and Great Britain, a situation which is regrettable. I am speaking obviously as a surgeon and it has to be taken into account that really one of the reasons that surgery in this country is behind that of others is the fact that the practice of anesthesia is certainly not what it should be and does not have the degree of expertise it has achieved elsewhere*'.

While some surgeons agreed with Monod about the primitive nature of anesthesia practice, and the need to catch up with that in the US and the UK, others did not. In 1946, almost everything remained to be achieved. Formal teaching needed to be established, and anesthetists needed to be recognized by surgeons and the general public, by health insurance, by the *Ordre des Médecins*, and by hospitals and universities. With the new generation of anesthetists, the SFAA and the French anesthetists' Union, the battle to establish French anesthesia began. It would last more than 20 years.

The Founding of the World Federation of Societies of Anaesthesiologists

Before World War II, an international congress originally planned for 1942 was arranged by the SFAA President, Monod, and the Vice President of the International Anesthesia Research Society (IARS), Francis McMechan (1879–1939). In 1951, this project was revived and an international congress of anesthesia was organized under the auspices of the International Congress of Surgery. The congress was duly held in Paris, and 32 countries took part. Lectures were presented by Maurice Cara (on graphical recording of physiological functions during anesthesia) and Pierre Huguenard

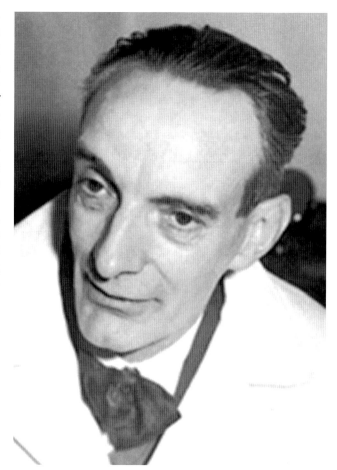

Fig. 28.4 Daniel Bovet, discoverer of synthetic muscle relaxants and winner of the Nobel Prize for Medicine. (From http://www.nobelprize.org/nobel_prizes/medicine/laureates/1957/)

(on the use of synthetic muscle relaxants). Daniel Bovet (1907–1992) (Fig. 28.4), a member of SFAA and a 1957 recipient of the Nobel Prize for medicine, reported on the chemistry of muscle relaxants.

The 1951 congress was a success, attracting great names from throughout the world of anesthesia, including Henry Beecher, Harold Griffith, Virginia Apgar, William Mushin and chemists and physicists such as Bovet and Robert Brinkmann. The idea of founding an international society linking the Société d'Etudes and the IARS of McMechan was considered. In March and May of 1951, Marcel Thalheimer, treasurer of the SFAA, set in motion the ideas for organization of such a society, and renewed them at the Congress of Anesthesia in London in September 1951. This British congress was held a week before the Paris meeting, bringing together English-speaking anesthetists and colleagues from the IARS in France. The participants debated whether it would be better to create a new society or to turn the IARS into an international society, not exclusively for research. The idea of a society open to several disciplines based on the model of the SFAA, was not popular with

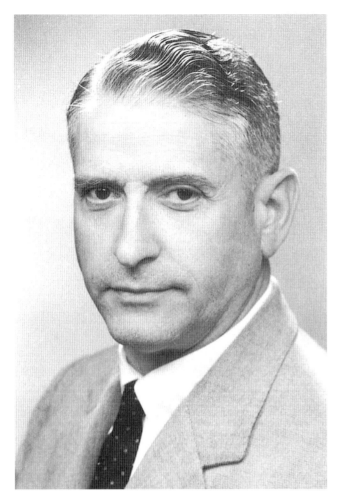

Fig. 28.5 Jacques Boureau (1909–2004) President SFAAR 1958–1961 and Vice President WFSA (1965). (From reference [1], pp 575, with permission)

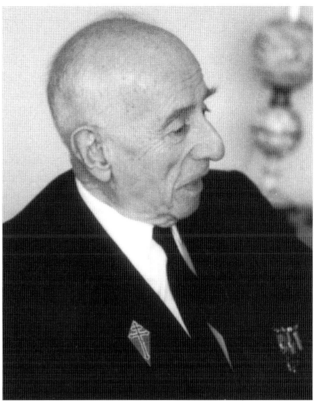

Fig. 28.6 Jean Lassner. (From www.histanestrea-france.org/SITE/Regards-sur-l-anesthesie-d-hi.)

ing skill, his overall knowledge, and his mastery of anesthetic techniques.

1960–1982: Division in French Anesthesia Societies

A controversy divided French anesthetists from 1960 to 1982. The problem lay with the concept of anesthesia. On one side was traditional anesthesia, dominated by inhalational anesthesia; quick and effective but often accompanied by untoward physiological reactions (e.g. nausea, hypotension). On the other side were the 'Laboritiens' who supported the views of Henri Laborit (1914–1995). He argued that the use of neuroleptic and other inhibitory agents protected the patient. The main actors in this drama were Jean Lassner (1913–2007; Fig. 28.6), Guy Vourch (1919–1988), and supporters of the English-speaking school of anesthesia on one side; and Pierre Huguenard (1924–2006) and other 'Laboritiens', mainly from Southern France (Louis Campan in Toulouse, Jean Bimar in Marseille and Jacques du Cailar in Montpellier), on the other.

The proposed election of a new member of the French Society of Anesthetists (SFAAR) started the division. The President, Jacques Boureau, following the rules of the parent

English-speaking anesthetists who had already founded a society of their own. Above all, they feared that the new society would be controlled by surgeons, as had occurred in France.

Representatives of the 32 societies present at the London conference elected an interim committee, charging the committee with the tasks of drafting statutes for a new international society, and organizing the next (1955) congress. Membership of the committee included Alexandre Goldblatt (Belgium), Torsten Gordh (Sweden), Harold Griffith (Canada), John Gillies (Scotland) and Jacques Boureau, (France) in his capacity as President of the French Anesthestists Union. There was also a representative of SFAA. Thus it was that the World Federation of Societies of Anaesthesiiologists was born. In 1959, Boureau (Fig. 28.5), President of the SFAA (now called 'Société Française d'Anesthésie, d'Analgésie et de Réanimation', SFAAR), became one of the Vice Presidents of the WFSA. His many qualities included his struggle to assert the independence of anesthetists, his bilingual negotiat-

society SEAA founded 25 years earlier, wished to elect a pharmacologist. Huguenard, then secretary of the SFAAR and Editor-in-Chief of its journal Anesthésie, Analgésie et Réanimation (AAR), opposed the election. Several years earlier, Lassner (and his English-influenced school) who had founded a new journal, Les *Cahiers d'Anesthésie*, thought that the editor of AAR was biased, favoring the Laboritiens. For his part, Huguenard thought the objectives of the *Cahiers* (whose motto was '*the method of giving an anesthetic was more important than what was given*') were too restrictive and blocked pharmacologic innovation. Huguenard left the SFAAR, and together with Bimar, founded l'Association des Anesthésistes Français (AAF) with its own journal, Les Annales de l'Anesthésie Française. Cara accepted the position of President, since he saw in the new society, a dynamism and capacity for innovation lacking in the old society. In fact, if the two journals are compared, new topics such as drugs, techniques and intensive care were more apparent in the AAF than the SFAAR journal. *Les Cahiers*, for its part, addressed more professional problems such as ethical questions, legislation, pain relief, and working relations with surgeons. The dispute continued until the end of the 1970s, when Lassner, in association with du Cailar, tried to bring the two societies together to form a united society, while Cara tried to reconcile the main protagonists of the two camps. However, anesthetist members remained distant from the discussions and still remained divided between the two societies.

The Société Française d'Anesthésie et de Réanimation (SFAR)

The divisions finally ended in 1982, with fusion of the two societies into a single organization (la Société Française d'Anesthésie et Réanimation (SFAR), with its journal, Annales Françaises d'Anesthésie et de Réanimation (AFAR). SFAR at present includes over 3500 doctors. The annual congress attracts more than 7000 participants making it the largest French-speaking congress in the world. The main activities of SFAR, then as now, concerned education, research, safety, ethics, professional life and relations with other specialities (including surgeons, intensivists, and nurse anesthetists).

In addition to training, central subjects for SFAR included the new organization of the national congress, editing successively professional guidelines from 1989, consensus conferences from 1993, meetings of experts from 1996 clinical standards from 1999, and an inquiry into postoperative pain from 2002. The training committee, created in 1992, became the Collège Français des Anesthésistes Réanimateurs (CFAR). This body linked all the key players in the profession including SFAR, the universities and the unions. In 1994, with Philippe Scherpereel as its first President, CFAR undertook control of continuing medical education and the upholding of standards in the profession.

In 1990, SFAR helped research by organizing joint meetings with the 'Institut national de la santé et de la recherche médicale (Inserm). In 2001, SFAR financed the conduct of anesthetic research and in 2007, introduced the prize for multicenter research in anesthesia. Safety during anesthesia became a priority for SFAR, with an enquiry into morbidity and mortality in 1981, and establishment of the safety committee from 1989. A mortality enquiry was established in 1999, and a risk assessment and management committee from 2000. This Committee developed standards for anesthetic ethical considerations and established the scientific support Committee from 1999.

The professional conduct committee was formed in 1992. This regulates all aspects of professional practice. In parallel, SFAR has contributed to specific professional enquiries, notably the practice of anesthesia from 1996 and demographics from 1997. Professional relations have been clarified with the surgeons, intensive care physicians (through the interface between SFAR and the French language resuscitation society SRLF), and nurse anesthetists. Finally, SFAR communicates through its web site [14] set up in 1998, and internal journals: La lettre de la SFAR (1992–1997), and Vigilance (since 2004). Thus, SFAR became the definitive partner, and scientific point of reference for concerns regarding anesthesia by ministers and agencies involved in the management of health in France.

From Craft to Profession (1970–2000)

The Painful Path to Safer Anesthesia

Death on the operating table is anathema to surgeons, anesthetists, and the general public. Such accidents make front-page news and lead to corrective measures. In France, three dramas attracted media and judicial attention, and influenced the development of safety in anesthesia.

The Anesthetist Shares Responsibility with the Surgeon

On 10 July 1967, in Montpellier, the 29 year-old author, Albertine Sarrazin, died during surgery for tuberculous pyelonephrosis. The non-medical, unqualified 'anesthetist' first met Sarrazin in the operating theatre and was unaware of her serious medical history. Although this was likely to be a bloody operation, no provision was made for transfusion. The hypovolemic patient suffered a cardiac arrest during a change in position. The first inquiry (December 1970) acquitted the practitioners involved. At appeal, only the anesthetist was held responsible. A later hearing (June 1972) referred the case to the court of appeal in Toulouse (April

1973) which condemned the ancsthctist for the superficial approach to the case, and the surgeon for not having realized the potential likelihood of major hemorrhage requiring transfusion. Both received a two month suspended sentence and a heavy fine. The separate responsibilities of the two practitioners were recognized for the first time.

Death Prompts a Study of Mortality from Anesthesia

On 11 July 1973, in Paris, a 20 year-old patient suffered a hypoxic-related cardiac arrest during a tonsillectomy. Recovery from anesthesia was improperly monitored, the patient returning directly from theatre to his hospital room. He died a few days later from the consequences of cerebral hypoxia. The anesthetist was deemed responsible, and the surgeon was acquitted at the initial hearing. At appeal, a higher court ruled that the surgeon was also responsible for improper patient observation postoperatively. Both practitioners left the hospital but resumed work elsewhere.

This accident prompted issuance of ministerial statements concerning anesthetic safety and procedures in the recovery room. In 1974, in a ministerial circular (a document without regulatory power) the Minister of Health recommended the establishment of recovery rooms, and specified the required equipment and personnel. However, the recommendations were ignored for reasons of cost. Two other circulars had equally little effect.

In 1976, the cumulative effect of the recommendations led to a major epidemiological enquiry into anesthetic deaths. At the request of the Society's president, Jean Lassner, Simone Veil, the Minister of Health, created a national commission on anesthesiology. This commission, chaired by Guy Vourc'h, organized the first epidemiological enquiry into anesthetic accidents, one similar to the Beecher-Todd report in 1954 [15]. The resulting INSERM inquiry (1978–82) [16] considered 200,000 anesthetics, finding a mortality of 1 in 13,000, and a greater incidence (60 % of deaths) in the immediate postoperative period, in patients who had a moderate risk of respiratory insufficiency.

A Death Produces New Safety Standards

On 10 October 1984, in Poitiers, Nicole Berneron, aged 35 years, died at the end of an ENT procedure, possibly from switched nitrous oxide and oxygen pipeline supply to the anesthetic machine. The following trial raised great media interest. The accused practitioners were found not guilty, and the public hospital concerned paid damages to the victim's family.

Immediate measures were taken concerning the safety of anesthetic equipment in operating theatres, starting with a ministerial circular of 10 October 1985 on medical gases. The report of the Committee of public health on anesthetic safety (Nov 1993) [17] led to a Ministerial decree on 5 December

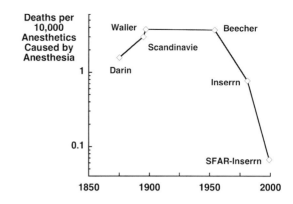

Fig. 28.7 Measures taken in the past few decades markedly decreased mortality from anesthesia in France. [15–20]

1994 (such a decree is the equivalent of a law in France). The decree established safety standards for anesthesia, including an obligatory preoperative anesthetic consultation more than 24 hours before elective surgery and to a final examination which had to take place the evening before or several hours before the start of anesthesia. This allowed verification of the pre-operative investigations, to find out whether there had been any change in medical condition since the consultation and to answer any further questions from the patient following the first consultation. Premedication was also prescribed at this time.

Conditions for the use of anesthesia equipment were also issued, and finally, the unbinding suggestions in the first ministerial circular of 1974 (i.e. 20 years before) were mandated. It was now an obligation that the patient be taken from the operating theatre to a recovery room. This revolution responded to several requests by anesthetists. All hospitals and clinics in France now had to be equipped according to these requirements, or risk being closed.

The recommendations of SFAR from 1989, meetings of experts, and risk management, changed anesthesia from a craft to a profession. A new study by SFAR and INSERM in 1999, showed the effectiveness of the measures. Anesthetic mortality had decreased to 1 death per 150,000 anesthetics (Fig. 28.7) [15–20].

French Research and International Recognition

Jean-Claude Otteni and Lassner, both German speakers, had special links with anesthetists in Germany, and frequently crossed the Rhine to give lectures, particularly after 1965. Other French anesthetists rarely visited Germany until 1977 (see next paragraph). Ernest Kern, Lassner, and Vourc'h created links with England and Canada, but these were essentially personal.

In 1977, Lassner created the European Academy of Anesthesiology (EAA) in Paris, sharing a common headquarters with the Société Française d'anesthésiologie. Its aim was to promote meetings between European anesthestists, and thereby exchange ideas, notably on teaching methods. Out of the Academy came the European Journal of Anaesthesiology (1984) whose first editor was Mike Vickers. From this organization John Zorab proposed the idea of a European Diploma of Anesthesiology.

The arrival of two new anesthetic department heads in Paris, Jean-Marie Desmonts at the Bichat hospital, and Pierre Viars at the Pitié—Salpêtrière, would open French anesthesia to influence from North America. Desmonts had learned the technique of gas chromatography at Stanford University in California. Several contacts in that institution spent sabbatical periods in his department. In 1978, he produced the first publication from France in Anesthesiology on the cardiovascular effects of naloxone. His assistant, Philippe Duvaldestin was a known specialist in the use of muscle relaxants.

As part of the EAA Desmonts had close contacts with Vickers, Rozen and Fries. His research team travelled regularly to the US for the American Society of Anesthesiologists (ASA) conferences where they presented their work. He also maintained his relationship with the WFSA and was a member of the executive committee from 1992–2000, and Vice-President between 2000 and 2004.

Pierre Viars (1930–1998) followed a different path. He was committed to the advancement of French anesthesia. He sent his assistant Francois Clergue, to contact US anesthetists, and he invited American experts to lecture at his annual postgraduate education conference (Journées d'enseignement post-universitaire de la Pitié-Salpêtrière, JEPU).

Concurrently Viars guided French anesthetists towards the laboratory, and encouraged them to present PhD theses in pharmacology, pneumonology and cardiology. Thus, with an approach different from that in other countries, including the US where anesthetists usually were recruited after completing a PhD, he succeeded in moving anesthetists from a clinical to an academic environment. This explains the particular nature of the anesthesia related research of many French physicians.

Viars, a pharmacologist by training, understood the role of industry in developing new medicines and the need for rigorous research. The work of his department was among the first accepted by the FDA in the US from a foreign source. He sponsored attendance of his colleagues (particularly his pupils) at international congresses, notably the American Society of Anesthesiologists (ASA) Annual Meeting. He insisted that they publish in English noting that this language had replaced Latin in the medical world. However, writing for an American journal was not simple. Among the first to overcome this obstacle were André Lienhart, Kamran Samii, Francois Clergue and Pierre Coriat. Many others including Bruno Riou and Jean jacques Rouby followed, and by 1988, more than 50% of communications to the ASA from outside

the US came from pupils of Viars. One of the editors of this book (LS) was Editor-in-Chief of Anesthesiology during this period (1986–96) and was impressed with the high quality of French research then submitted to and published in Anesthesiology.

Viars also co-founded the new European Society of Anesthesiology which, in 1991, brought together the EAA, the ESA and the European National Society of Anaesthesiology. Philippe Scherpereel from Lille, was initially an intensive care practicionner. He came to Paris as assistant in Viars's department to study anesthesia and later became chief of the anesthesiology department in Lille. With Johan Spierdijk from Leiden, he put in place the Foundations for European education in Anaesthesiology (FEEA) in 1986. From January 2009 this organization joined the European Society of Anaesthesiology. There still exists a joint initiative between the ESA and the WFSA for the operation of 110 training centres around the world.

Desmonts and Viars provided inspiration to anesthestists who followed them. French anesthetists now participate in all international activities and are recognized for the quality of their original research. The success of the world congress of the WFSA in Paris in 2004 was proof of this.

Following the work of the modern pioneers, French anesthesiology has developed into a speciality of perioperative care which covers all medical and surgical cases requiring special resuscitative care. Although in University hospitals there are medical and surgical special care units this is not the case in the smaller hospitals where resuscitation and intensive care are largely the responsibility of anesthetists.

Anesthetists Outside the Hospital: The Founding of SAMU

In the latter part of the 20th century, French anesthesiologists pioneered the development of the provision of prehospital emergency care. The French prehospital emergency system is known as SAMU (Service d'Aide Médicale Urgente) and is a medical and not a paramedical service. Anesthesiologists, Maurice Cara (Paris), Pierre Huguenard (Créteil), Louis Lareng (Toulouse) and Louis Serre (Montpellier) (Fig. 28.8) developed SAMU during the 1970s, reasoning that in emergencies the hospital should go to the patient and not the contrary. Consequently, medical teams (often including an anesthesiologist) go from hospitals in specially equipped ambulances to care for patients with life-threatening emergencies. Doctors dispatch and control the emergency response teams. Unlike many emergency medical services, SAMU is an extension of the hospital service itself.

Following the Algerian War in the 1960s, the health authorities asked anesthetists to organize emergency medicine and prehospital care in France. This urgent request was intended

Fig. 28.8 The early pioneers of the SAMU: Maurice Cara (Paris), Pierre Huguenard (Créteil), Louis Lareng (Toulouse) and Louis Serre (Montpellier) (from Archive of Char with permission)

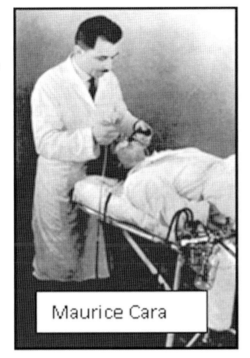

Maurice Cara

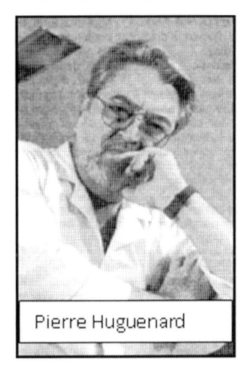

Pierre Huguenard

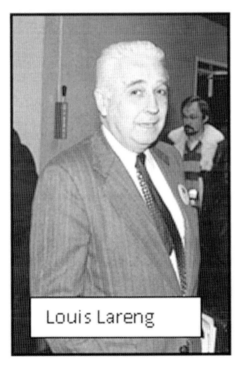

Louis Lareng

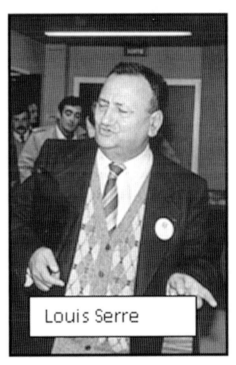

Louis Serre

to address the rising death rate from automobile related accidents, which had reached 13,000 per year and more than 290,500 injured, 90,150 of them seriously. The creation of mobile emergency units in the south (by Paul Bourret at Salon de Provence, and Louis Serre at Montpellier) began in 1957 and gradually grew. The first mobile medical emergency response units were created in 1965 (Service mobile d'urgence et de réanimation, SMUR). The treatment and transport of high-risk patients required the immediate provision of medical care, and its continuation through transport to hospital. This was achieved using specially trained and equipped medical teams who could perform resuscitation and emergency care in emergency ambulances, helicopters or fixed wing aircraft. In 2006, this service conducted 1,890,439 missions.

A 1986 French law [21] specified that SAMU should act as a dispatch and reception center for all medical emergency calls, 24 hours a day. SAMU now operates under Government control throughout France in over 100 regional subunits united in their training and equipment. Before the organization of SAMU, Fire Brigades (Sapeurs Pompiers) provided prehospital emergency medical care. This service still provides primary emergency care, especially in rural regions, and works alongside SAMU in large towns. The development of SAMU demonstrates the widening borders of anesthesiology, a speciality only relatively recently recognised in France. In 2006, SAMU received 15 million calls.

Epilogue

The discipline of anesthesia in France is now securely established. It has become reliable with a mortality rate approaching 1:150,000 to 1:300,000 for patients having an ASA Physical Status of 1–2. Qualifications of trained medical graduates in anesthesia equal those of other specialists, and the discrimination against anesthesia consultants present up to the 1990s has ended. At the end of training, the anesthetist can undertake research in the university in preparation for the Diplôme d'Etudes Approfondies (DEA), a qualification now essential for those wishing to hold a university chair.

As with all living organisms, anesthesiology continues to evolve. The struggle between anesthetists and medical resuscitators is over. The SFAR has woven links with the Société de Réanimation de Langue Française and the two are currently drafting the basis of ministerial decrees relating to the speciality. Anesthetists now provide preoperative assessment. Often in smaller hospitals, anesthetists also run the intensive care units, caring for a wide range of acutely ill patients. Anesthetists have taken charge of prehospital emergency medicine and created SAMU. Following the lead of Americans, they were the first in France to organize pain clinics.

But the path of anesthesiology is not always smooth. Sometimes it has lost control of structures it created such as SAMU and pain clinics. The demands of the 'internat qualifiant' examination has drastically reduced the number of practitioners, and uncertainty about the future weighs heavily on a profession which was the first speciality in France to make demographic projections. The risk at present, is the possibility of delegating specialist tasks to nonmedical personnel as was formerly the case, or relinquishing certain professional activities such as perioperative care to nonspecialists. To do so would be to negate what has been an intrinsic part of our profession and part of the specific character of French anesthesia.

References

1. Cousin M-Th. L'anesthésie-Réanimation en France des origines à 1965. Paris: L'Harmattan; 2005.
2. Cazalaà JB, Baker DJ, Cousin M-T. Apparatus for anaesthesia and intensive care. Paris: Editions Glyphe; 2005.
3. Zimmer M. Histoire de l'anesthésie Méthodes et techniques au XIXe siècle. Les Ulys: EDPS; 2008.
4. Website of CHAR (Society for the history of anaesthesia and intensive care in France): http://www.char-fr.net/SITE/index.php
5. Wells H. A history of the discovery of the application of nitrous oxide gas, ether and other vapors in surgical operations. Hartford: J Gaylord Wells; 1847.
6. Fülöp-Miller R. Triumph over pain. New York: Charter Books; 1938.
7. Gorré F. Observation d'un cas de mort causé par l'inhalation du chloroforme. B Acad Nat Med Paris. 1848;13:1144–60.
8. Kern E. Mes quatre vies. Paris: Arnette; 1971.
9. Code de déontologie médicale: introduction. Paris: Seuil; 1996.
10. Cousin MT. La création des départements d'anesthésiologie dans le cadre de la réforme hospitalo-universitaire. Cah Anesthésiol. 2002;50:447–52.
11. Ibsen B. The anaesthetist's viewpoint on the treatment of respiratory complications during the epidemic in Copenhagen 1952. Proc Roy Soc. 1953;47:72–4.
12. Monod R. But général et moyens d'action de la société. Anesth Analg Paris. 1935;1:61.
13. Monod R. Rapport du président à l'assembléée générale de la société d'anesthésie du 15 janvier 1948. Anesth Analg Paris. 1949;6:290–2.
14. Website of Société Française d'anesthésie et de réanimation http://www.sfar.org
15. Beecher HK, Todd DP. A study of the deaths associated with anesthesia and surgery. Ann Surg. 1954;140:2–34.
16. Hatton F, Tiret L, Maujol L, N'Doye P, Vourc'h G, Desmonts JM, Otteni JC, Scherpereel P. Enquête épidémiologique sur les accidents d'anesthésie. Premiers résultats. Ann Fr Anesth Réanim. 1983;2:331–86.
17. Rapport du Haut Comité de la santé publique sur la sécurité anesthésique. Ministère de la santé et de l'action humanitaire, Paris 1993. (In line to www.sfar.org).
18. Lienhart A, Auroy Y, Péquignot F, Benhamou D, Warszawski J, Bovet M, Jougla E. Survey of anesthesia-related mortality in France. Anesthesiology. 2006;105:1087–97.
19. Darin G. Sur les anesthésiques. Arch Physiol Norm Pathol. 1875;25:711–5.
20. Buxton DW, Report of the special chloroform committee. Br Med J. 1902;116–28.
21. Loi du 6 janvier 1986 relative à l'aide médicale urgente et aux transport sanitaires. Journal Officiel de la République Française 7 janvier 1986.

The Development of Anaesthesiology in German-Speaking Countries

29

Michael Goerig

Summary

Heyfelder administered the first ether anaesthetic on 24 January 1847. For the next century, surgeons gave anaesthesia or directed its administration by a nurse or a less experienced person. To the 1940s, most surgeons-anaesthetists dripped ether or chloroform onto Esmarch or Schimmelbusch masks. In 1902, Roth described an anaesthetic machine produced by the Dräger brothers using compressed gases and reducing valves. In 1907, Dräger added its Pulmotor, a ventilator. In 1903, Fischer and von Mering synthesized barbitone, the first of the barbiturates. In 1905, Kuhn advocated Macewen's technique of orotracheal intubation and until the 1950s, tracheal tubes were usually inserted under local anaesthesia and digital control. In 1908, Küppers patented the rotameter, subsequently used by Neu in 1910 to deliver anaesthetic gases from the Rotameter Company's new anaesthesia machine, and ultimately used to control gas flow for much of the next century. Pharmacologist Straub produced the first electrically driven roller pump in 1911 to accurately infuse intravenous fluids and drugs during anaesthesia, and surgeon Martin developed today's drip-chamber. Schmidt introduced the Codman-Cushing anaesthetic records into Germany at the end of the 1920s. In 1932, pharmacist Weese described a new, water-soluble, ultra-short acting barbiturate, hexobarbital. In 1953, Frey devised an electronic device for continuous analysis of volatile agents.

Koller's 1884 discovery of cocaine's anaesthetic properties introduced local and regional anaesthesia. German surgeons became regional anaesthesia advocates. In 1899, Bier gave the first spinal "block". Some surgeons rejected cocaine because of its side effects, inspiring Einhorn to synthesize procaine in 1904. Bier described intravenous regional anaesthesia, and obstetrician Sellheim described paravertebral blocks in 1908. In 1911, Hirschel invented the axillary approach to the brachial plexus, while Kulenkampff described the supraclavicular approach. In 1912, Perthes used electrical stimulation to locate peripheral nerves. In the early 1930s Capelle prescribed continuous subcutaneous abdominal injection of local anaesthetic to facilitate deep breathing and decrease the incidence of postoperative pneumonia.

In the early 1900s, Gauss suggested use of scopolamine-morphine to enable pain-free childbirth but its dangers led to its abandonment after only a few years. Surgeon Hercher used hypertonic solutions for fluid resuscitation during World War I, and Schück and Simenauer revived this concept in the 1930s. In 1943, Weese invented 4% polyvinyl pyrrolidone to manage hemodynamic instability.

Increasing complexity of surgery and use of new anesthetics and delivery apparatus in the 1920s revived interest in anaesthesia specialization. But influential surgeons rejected the idea, and World War II stopped the discussion. US and UK advances in anaesthesia rekindled discussion after World War II, and in 1953, the German Society of Anaesthesia was founded.

In the Beginning

Little time separated the successful demonstration of anaesthesia in Boston on October 1846, from the first ether administration in Germany. Johann Heyfelder (1798–1869) gave ether at the Erlangen University on 24 Jan 1847 to facilitate incision of a gluteal abscess [1]. Few advances followed in the next fifty years. Surgeons gave anaesthesia or directed a nurse or a less experienced assistant to drip ether or chloroform. Surgeons Esmarch and Schimmelbusch introduced apparatus and techniques, and their wire and gauze masks (see below). Medical, gynaecological or surgical journals reported observations on anaesthesia.

At the turn of the twentieth century, the first association of professional anaesthesiologists was formed in New York. Parallel developments in Germany might have occurred at the instigation of Carl-Ludwig Schleich (1859–1922; Fig. 29.1). He was among the first surgeons to condemn the existing state of anaesthesia, advocating specialization and

M. Goerig (✉)
Department Anesthesia and Intensive Care, University Hospital
Hamburg-Eppendorf, Hamburg, Germany
e-mail: goerig@uke.uni-hamburg.de

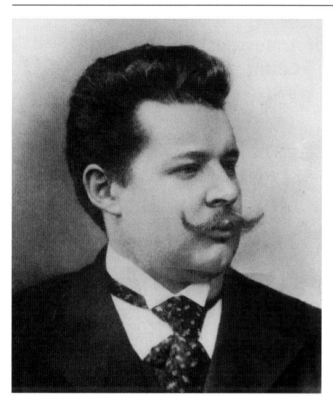

Fig. 29.1 Carl-Ludwig Schleich, father of infiltration anaesthesia, insisted that local anaesthesia could decrease or eliminate the need for general anaesthesia. He advocated training in anaesthesia. (The picture, taken around 1905, is from the collection of the author.)

training in anaesthesiology to improve quality and minimize risks. Schleich however, was "persona non grata" within the German Society of Surgery, and therefore (see below) his ideas went unheeded. Anaesthesia did not develop as a specialty in Germany until after World War II.

Nevertheless, many German surgeons, chemists and other physicians, produced anaesthetic innovations. These included the introduction of regional anaesthesia, development of the barbiturates, and invention of anaesthesia apparatus.

Local and Regional Anaesthesia

The 1884 discovery of cocaine's anaesthetic properties by the ophthalmologist Carl Koller (1857–1944) of Vienna, introduced local and regional anaesthesia [2]. The same concentrations of cocaine used for topical anaesthesia were then used for injection, and such high concentrations sometimes caused fatal complications, leading other investigators, including Schleich, to dilute the solutions to produce "infiltration anaesthesia".

Schleich described his techniques in a lecture to the 21st annual Congress of the German Surgical Society in 1891 in Berlin. After reviewing infiltration anaesthesia including indications, and the pros and cons, using humanistic,

legal and ethical arguments, Schleich denounced chloroform anaesthesia as dangerous, and denied the need for general anaesthesia for most surgical procedures. A tumult arose. Although the audience knew little about the new technique, nobody agreed with Schleich's arguments, and he left the congress without further discussion. Schleich continued to perform major surgical procedures including hernia repair, laparotomy, and limb amputation under infiltration anaesthesia, stating that general anaesthesia was not needed. The initial negative response eventually subsided, and his method was later considered a "great feat in the discipline of surgery in Germany" [3].

In 1894, Schleich again inflamed his fellow surgeons by arguing, in his textbook "Schmerzlose Operationen" (Painless Surgery), that only specially trained physicians should perform anaesthesia, and moreover that the specialist should teach younger colleagues. This was then a revolutionary concept in Germany [4].

Regional Anaesthesia: Further Developments

At the end of the nineteenth century, the side effects of cocaine inspired the German chemist Alfred Einhorn (1856–1917), to search for a better local anaesthetic. In 1904, Einhorn and his colleagues produced procaine (Novocaine), which until the 1940s discovery of lidocaine by Swedes Nils Löfgren (1913–1967) and Bengt Lundquist (1878–1922), was the prototypic local anaesthetic.

In 1903, Heinrich Braun (1862–1934) of Leipzig recommended adding adrenaline to cocaine to decrease the speed of absorption. This allowed the safe administration of larger amounts of cocaine and more extensive surgery. Braun also realized that the simultaneous use of adrenaline would minimize procaine's vasodilating properties, decrease the toxic side effects of procaine and prolong its anaesthetic properties. Not surprisingly, procaine became the most important local anaesthetic for decades, worldwide. In the 1920s, variants of procaine, such as isocaine and nirvanine were introduced, but failed to challenge procaine [5].

Specialized regional anaesthesia techniques including splanchnic, paravertebral, sacral-caudal and brachial plexus blocks, were developed subsequently and local anaesthesia increasingly displaced general anaesthesia. Braun described these new options in his famous textbook "Local Anaesthesia—Scientific Basis and Practical Use", first published in 1905, with several editions following until 1951 [6]. A 1914 translation popularized local anaesthetic techniques in the English-speaking world [7].

Arthur Läwen (1876–1958) trained with Braun, and in 1933 succeeded him as editor of the textbook. Läwen enthusiastically supported local and regional anaesthesia. He provided a clinical evaluation of a bicarbonated procaine solution, which he developed in collaboration with his pharma-

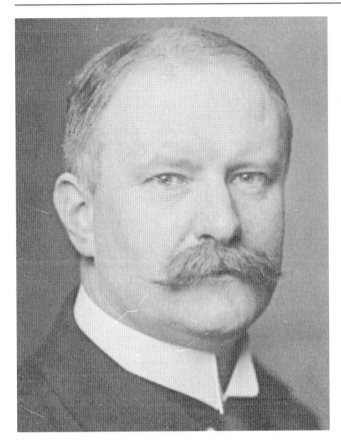

Fig. 29.2 August Bier gave the first spinal block and invented intravenous regional anaesthesia. (The picture, taken around 1910, is from the collection of the author.)

administered the first spinal or regional "block" to adult patients. Bier sought to "render a large part of the body insensitive to pain for surgical purposes." Using a fine hollow needle, as described by Heinrich Quincke (1842–1922), Bier performed a lumbar puncture with the patient in the lateral recumbent position. The puncture itself was made painless by local anaesthetic infiltration using Schleich's method. Bier then injected 0.10–0.15 mg of cocaine into the lumbar subarachnoid space. Following an initial enthusiasm, German surgeons rejected the new method because of reports of severe side effects [9].

Bier himself called for caution in applying the method. The problem of an excessively high spinal block with its attendant side effects represented a major challenge, and the means to prevent these adverse reactions were often inadequate. Side effects such as the unsolved problem of postoperative nausea and vomiting, post spinal headache, and hypotension caused Bier to call for restricted use of the brand-new technique. Moreover, the analgesic cocaine was far from the ideal anaesthetic [10]. Thus, most physicians contented themselves with local infiltration and inhalation anaesthesia and only a few enthusiasts persisted in administration of spinal anaesthesia [11]. In the mid 1920s, new atraumatic spinal needles and hypo- or hyperbaric anaesthetic solutions renewed interest in spinal anaesthesia [12]. A better knowledge of physiology and newly developed vasoconstrictive drugs like ephedrine, further augmented enthusiasm [13].

In the 1930s, the Hamburg surgeon Helmut Schmidt (1895–1979) popularized Pitkin's 20–22 gauge short bevel needle in Germany. This special needle, originally described by Georg Pitkin (1885–1943) of New Jersey in 1924, decreased the incidence of post-dural puncture headache (PDPH) to less than 5 % [14].

With wider use of spinal anaesthesia in German speaking countries in the mid 1970s, the call for less traumatic spinal needles increased. This prompted the Würzburg anaesthetist, Günther Sprotte (1947), to develop a spinal needle, with a "pencil point" tip and aperture positioned slightly back from the tip. The design minimized trauma during perforation of the dura, further decreasing the incidence of PDPH to less than 2%. Since then the "Sprotte needle" has found worldwide acceptance among anaesthesiologists [15].

Unlike surgeons, obstetricians and gynaecologists persisted in advocating the use of spinal anaesthesia. After the London surgeon, Arthur Barker (1850–1916), described hyperbaric and hypobaric solutions in 1907, Freiburg obstetrician Carl Gauss (1875–1957; Fig. 29.3), assessed the use of gravity as revealed by experiments in Great Britain with a glass model of the spinal canal, evaluating the potential of hyperbaric/hypobaric solutions to control intrathecal spread [16]. Gauss recommended hyper- or hypobaric solutions in spinal anaesthesia for patients undergoing operative gynae-

cological colleague Oskar Gross (1877–1947) from Leipzig. This preparation had a faster onset, longer duration of action, and less potential for toxicity [8].

New Conduction Anaesthesia Techniques are Established

In 1911, Georg Hirschel (1875–1963) invented the axillary approach to the brachial plexus while Diedrich Kulenkampff (1880–1963) described the supraclavicular approach. Hirschel also published a textbook of local anaesthesia which gained world-wide recognition due to its excellent illustrations and detailed descriptions. Several editions were published in Germany. Translations into English, French, Spanish and Russian popularized local anaesthetic techniques outside Germany [1].

Spinal Anaesthesia

In 1899, August Bier (1861–1949; Fig. 29.2), a colleague of the Kiel surgeon, Friedrich von Esmarch (1823–1908),

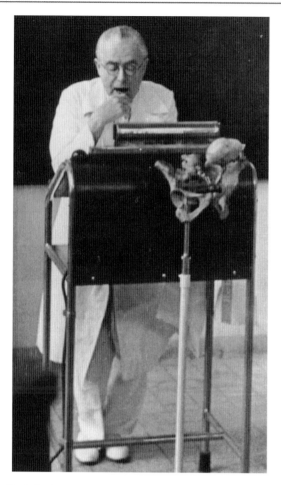

Fig. 29.3 Carl Gauss gives a lecture at the University of Würzburg. Gauss used baricity to control the level of spinal anaesthesia. He contributed to the invention of twilight sleep. (The picture, taken around 1938, is from the collection of the author.)

cology. However, his technique did not become popular until the mid 1930s [17]. In 1900, Oskar Kreis (1872–1958) of Basle used spinal anaesthesia to ameliorate labour pain, describing the parturients as remarkably alert compared with women receiving other forms of labour analgesia [18]. Later, spinal anaesthesia was often combined with a low dose of subcutaneously administered scopolamine for sedation, as recommended by the Austrian obstetrician Richard von Steinbüchel (1865–1952) in 1903 [19]. It was hoped that the scopolamine would also decrease the incidence of vomiting.

Paravertebral and Epidural Conduction Anaesthesia

Most regional anaesthetic procedures designed to avoid the adverse effects of spinal anaesthesia were developed during the early 1900s. Tübingen obstetrician Hugo Sell-heim (1871–1936), described paravertebral anaesthesia in 1908 [20], but surgeons did not become interested until Max Kappis (1881–1938), of Hanover, published articles on

it [21]. Kappis suggested applying it to differentiate indistinct types of abdominal pain, a method approved by Läwen [22]. Läwen also advanced the use of epidural anaesthesia, particularly "sacral anaesthesia", in urology and obstetrics [23, 24]. The initially inferior quality of epidural anaesthesia stimulated Läwen's efforts to improve the technique to one that allowed safe cholecystectomy, gastrectomy or nephrectomy [25]. To shorten the time of onset and to prolong the duration of anaesthesia, he used a new bicarbonated preparation of the local anaesthetic procaine [26]. He combined epidural and general anaesthesia in 1912 [27].

Safety First: Localization of Peripheral Nerves by Electricity

The increasing popularity of conduction anaesthesia in the twentieth century prompted development of techniques that located peripheral nerves using electrical stimulation. Georg Perthes (1869–1927) from Tübingen, described this method in 1912. Unfortunately his technique lay fallow until the 1960s, when it was rediscovered and became the "gold standard" until the twenty-first century when ultrasound became available for localization of peripheral nerves [28].

Quality Management in Regional Anaesthesia: Realized in 1910

In 1908, Bier described regional intravenous anaesthesia [29]. He injected up to 40 ml of 1 % procaine intravenously into a limb previouly made bloodless by an Esmarch bandage. Complete anaesthesia and motor paralysis could be achieved. Known as "Venenanästhesie" in German speaking countries, and "Intravenous Regional Anaesthesia" (IVRA) or "Bier's Block" in Anglo-American countries, the method achieved limited popularity. Fear of local anaesthetic overdose, or the cumbersomeness and limited duration of the block may have hindered its use [30]. IVRA also may not have competed with new conduction techniques for blocking peripheral nerves and plexuses percutaneously. Fear of intravenous overdose inspired Bier's colleague Fritz Momburg (1870–1939) to invent a double tourniquet, still applied today when IVRA is used [31]. Concerns regarding the side effects of IVRA prompted the development of a remarkable risk/benefit questionnaire [32] marking the beginning of quality control measurements in German anaesthesia.

Pain Therapy

The pioneers of local anaesthesia appreciated the adverse effect of acute and chronic pain upon daily life, and evaluated the possible role of local anaesthetics in pain management.

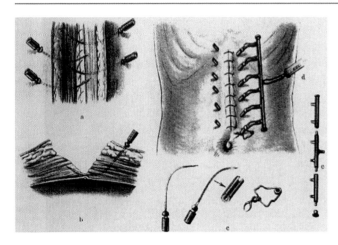

Fig. 29.4 This set of specially designed needles allowed the continuous application of local anaesthetics into the abdominal muscles for post-operative pain relief. (From Capelle W: Die Bedeutung des Wundschmerzes und seiner Ausschaltung bei Laparotomierten. Dtsch Zschr f Chir 1936; 246: 466–85.)

Surgeons Schleich, Braun, Läwen, Kappis and Kirschner explored various regional anaesthesia techniques in the management of chronic pain. A lesser known pioneer was the Berlin surgeon Walter Capelle (1881–1950), who in the early 1930s suggested continuous subcutaneous injection of local anaesthetic. Specially designed needles (Fig. 29.4) were inserted into the subcutaneous tissue of the abdominal wall surrounding the surgical incision. He hypothesized that pain relief would facilitate deep breathing and decrease the incidence of postoperative pneumonia [33]. His contemporaries did not appreciate the importance of this concept and it seems that only his surgical colleague Ewald Fulde (1899–1971) in 1933 praised Capelle's innovative concept [34].

Tübingen surgeon Martin Kirschner (1881–1942), introduced the modern treatment of trigeminal neuralgia [35]. In 1932, he used an electrocoagulating current to produce discrete lesions and to limit the spread of substances injected into the trigeminal nerve and Gasserian ganglion. Kirschner inserted the electrode through the foramen ovale into the ganglion. Decades previously, Georg Perthes had used a similar apparatus to localize peripheral nerves, and perhaps this stimulated Kirschner to invent a comparable device [36].

The Long Way to Painless Childbirth: The Medicated Birth

In the early twentieth century, childbirth moved from the home to hospital. Progress in anaesthesia, and the introduction of new anaesthetics, led women and their obstetricians to expect a painless birth through medication. Unlike surgeons, obstetricians and gynaecologists applied spinal anaesthesia widely from its beginning. By 1900, Gauss had suggested the use of combinations of scopolamine and mor-

phine to alleviate pain during childbirth. Although anaesthetic drugs affected the baby, physicians believed that the benefits of the combination outweighed the risks to mother and baby. Morphine relieved or dulled the pain, and scopolamine produced mental sedation and amnesia. There was the unproven perception that the drug combination enhanced the effectiveness of each single drug, thereby enabling a reduced dose of medication and a minimization of side effects. Labour might progress uninterruptedly without the pregnant woman being aware, or at least remembering, that she had suffered any discomfort. Gauss' concept, known as "twilight sleep" attained transient popularity world-wide but its dangers to the baby and mother [37] rapidly led to its abandonment.

Later, caudal anaesthesia was recommended as a substitute for spinal anaesthesia. By the 1950s, epidural blocks, often performed via a catheter, became popular. This allowed more precise control over the extent of sensory loss and enabled the mother to assist in pushing during labour [38].

Early Intravenous Anaesthesia—Beginning with Intravenous Ether

Rectal and intravenous alternatives to the inhalation route were tried soon after the 1846 discovery of the anaesthetic properties of ether. In 1847, the Russian surgeon Nicolai Pirogoff (1810–1881) described such experiments in his monograph [39]. Decades later, French physiologist Cyprien Oré (1828–1899) attempted to popularize the intravenous injection of chloral hydrate, but failed due to inadequate analgesia and side-effects. Intravenous anaesthesia was forgotten for another thirty years, and rediscovered by the Würzburg surgeon Ludwig Burkhardt (1872–1922).

In 1909, Burkhardt reported that intravenous infusion of 4% chloroform or ether in a warmed saline solution could produce unresponsiveness and could sustain anaesthesia. He thought that intravenous infusion should minimize pulmonary complications because evidence of respiratory irritation such as coughing, laryngeal spasm, and cyanosis was markedly decreased. There were the added benefits of little or no excitement during induction, and intra- and postoperative cardiovascular stability, probably a consequence of the infusion of several litres of fluid. Burkhardt suggested that IV-ether was indicated for patients undergoing surgery of the head, face and neck, and especially for cachectic and hypovolemic patients [40]. Hamburg surgeon Hermann Kümmel (1852–1937) praised IV-anaesthesia as an "ideal narcosis" and recommended it for oesophageal surgery, gastric resection, craniotomy, and hypophysectomy. Intravenous ether was used during World War I, especially in hypovolemic patients [41].

But IV-ether never became popular. In the writer's view, the technique died for two reasons: There was the problem of easily establishing reliable intravenous access; and few

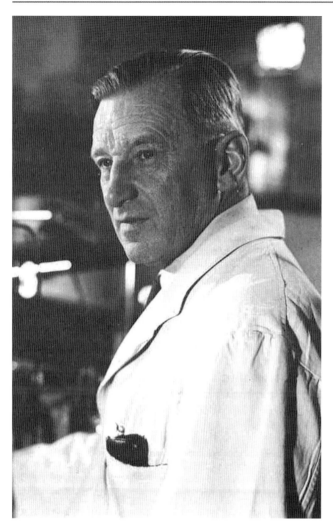

Fig. 29.5 Hellmuth Weese invented hexobarbital in 1932, and the plasma substitute, 4% polyvinyl pyrrolidone in 1943. (The picture, taken around 1950, is from the collection of the author.)

experienced persons knew how to use IV needles (i.e., to avoid the need for cut-down access). Nevertheless, until the late 1920s, notable German surgical journals and textbooks of surgery discussed the use of IV-ether, recommending it in selected cases and calling for further research. The introduction of the short acting barbiturates, cyclopropane, and intubation techniques, made IV ether superfluous by the early 1930s [42].

From Intravenous Ether Anaesthesia to Balanced Anaesthesia

In the early 1930s, oral barbiturates became widely used for premedication. Berlin chemist Emil Fischer (1852–1919) winner of the 1902 Nobel prize in chemistry in collaboration with Josef von Mering (1849–1908) synthesized barbitone (Veronal)®, the first effective sedative barbiturate, in 1903.

In the mid 1920s, others reported on water soluble preparations of limited value due to unwanted pharmacological properties [43]. Their pharmacological properties caused a deep sleep lasting for up to 24 hours. Moreover, respiratory and circulatory side effects were noted and often the patient's airway was compromised by the drug's action, producing life-threatening situations [44]. In 1932, Bayer pharmacist Hellmuth Weese (1897–1954; Fig. 29.5) reported his experiences with a new, water-soluble and ultra-short acting barbiturate that changed anaesthetic practice, Evipan® (hexobarbital) [45].

The pharmacological properties of hexobarbital created a breakthrough despite untoward effects, including life-threatening cardiovascular depression, induced respiratory depression with airway obstruction, local phlebitis and allergic reactions. IV hexobarbital anaesthesia offered considerable advantages, particularly a smooth induction which was then followed with an inhalational anaesthetic. Unlike ether, hexobarbital did not burn or explode with the use of cautery. Its portability recommended its application in war zones, if administered with caution, and as often suggested, "with an individual dosage" [46]. Cumbersome anaesthesia apparatus could be eliminated. These advantages plus changing surgical requirements led to the broad acceptance of hexobarbital.

Weese, Professor of Pharmacology at Dusseldorf and Director of Pharmacology at Bayer Wuppertal-Elberfeldt, was a major contributor to modern intravenous anaesthesia, illustrating a beneficial partnership between academia and industry [47]. In 1938, he was elected as an honorary member of the International Anesthesia Research Society, and became one of the first honorary members of the German Anaesthesia Society (DGA) on its founding in 1953 [48]. In the later 1930s, thiopental displaced hexobarbital. The Munich scientist, Alfred Doenicke (born in 1928), reported on a new hypnotic, etomidate, [marketed as Hypnomidate®] synthesized in 1971 and introduced in 1973. Its minimal depression of the circulation facilitated anaesthesia in hemodynamically compromised patients [49].

On the Way to Target-Controlled-Infusion (TCI)

In the 1960s and 1970s, pharmacokinetics and pharmacodynamics with new available hypnotics and analgesics became a topic of scientific interest in Germany [50].

The onset and elimination characteristics of drugs administered via precision infusions pumps were analysed. These tests identified dosages of the drugs for used for "target controlled infusion" (TCI). The invention of microprocessor controlled infusion pumps facilitated development of TCI. A group of anaesthetists guided by Horst Stoeckel (1930) in Bonn published the first paper on "closed–loop total

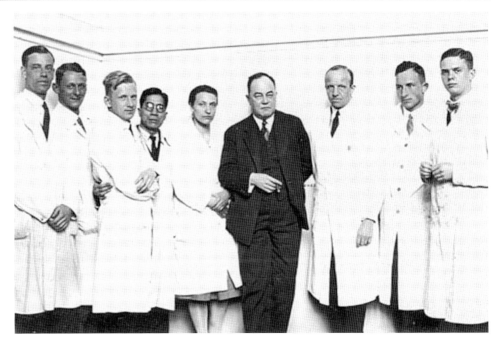

Fig. 29.6 Walter Straub (center and with cigar) produced the electrical roller pump for accurate infusion of liquids. Weese is third from left. (The picture, taken around 1930, is from the collection of the author.)

intravenous anaesthesia", using the EEG as the feedback variable in estimating pharmacokinetic and pharmacodynamic values [51]. Of note, closed loop delivery of inhaled ether anesthesia had already been realized by the US physiologist Reginald Bickford (1913–1998) with his so-called Servo-Anesthesizer for the EEG-controlled dosing of ether in the early 1950s [52].

Rectal Anaesthesia

Pioneering anaesthesiologists found that rectal administration of pure ether produced excellent narcosis but adversely affected local tissues. The method was abandoned, but was revived early in the twentieth century by the American anaesthetist James Gwathmey (1862–1944) whose mixture of ether with olive oil produced satisfactory narcosis without injuring tissues [53]. It enjoyed some popularity in the US, especially for obstetric analgesia. In Germany it never became popular. Similarly, rectally administered paraldehyde was used as a basal narcotic in Great Britain, but was rarely given in German speaking countries.

Paraldehyde's unpleasant odour, and the occasional violent restlessness associated with its use, caused German anaesthetists to prefer Avertin® (tri-bromoethanol), which became available in the mid 1920s. The surgeon Otto Butzengeiger (1885–1968) observed that convenience, a smooth induction, and ready acceptance by patients recommended the use of Avertin® [54], particularly where calmness during preparation for anaesthesia was desirable (e.g., in children and patients suffering from thyrotoxicosis). However, adverse local tissue reactions were described shortly after

Avertin's® introduction, leading to cautionary headlines in the lay-press and medical journals. With a revised dosage regimen, and administration restricted to selected patients, Avertin® remained in use until the middle of the 1960s.

Some Early Developments in Infusion Therapy

Experiences with IV anaesthetics stimulated the design of devices that administered precise volumes. In 1911, the pharmacologist Walter Straub (1874–1944; Fig. 29.6) produced the first electrically driven roller pump [55]. Straub suggested the use of his device to accurately infuse intravenous fluids, and drugs during anaesthesia, but only after the beginning of the 1950s were these pumps introduced into clinical practice. In German speaking countries, various models then became available, the most popular being the "Perfusor"®, designed by the Braun Company, Melsungen, in the early 1950s. (Fig. 29.7). Even today, the term "Perfusor"® is colloquial for an anaesthesia IV pump in German speaking regions, even if it is a microprocessor-controlled computerized model [56].

Synonymous with the use of an intravenous infusion needle is the term "Strauss-Kanüle", a needle made of steel and invented in the first decade of the twentieth century by the Berlin internist Strauss (1868–1944) [57]. A comparable model, made of polypropylene, became available in the mid 1950s. It was produced by the Braun Company, Melsungen, hence it is usually named "Braunüle"® [58].

The first appearance (in 1911) of today's ubiquitous drip-chamber may be credited to the Cologne surgeon Emil Martin (1865-?) [59].

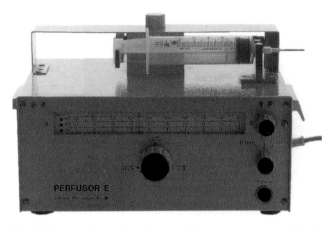

Fig. 29.7 An early model of Braun's infusion pump, named "Perfusor", used in clinical practice around 1955. (From the collection of the author.)

From Short-Acting Salt-Solutions to Volume Expanding Fluids

Early in the twentieth century, the importance of a sufficient intravascular fluid volume during anaesthesia became increasingly appreciated. Attempts were made to retain infused solutions within the intravascular space longer than normal saline by using a solution of gum acacia [60]. The research of the English physiologist Ernest Starling (1866–1927), suggested that a 3% solution might be best. His concept was correct, as shown by tests during World War I in wounded soldiers. But serious adverse effects such as allergic reactions, fever and even shock, led to tests of new approaches, such as the administration of hypertonic solutions [61]. Surgeon Friedrich Hercher (1881–1958) may have been the first to use such hypertonic solutions, giving them during World War I. He administered a "maximum of 50 ml of a 9% hypertonic solution" and praised its immediate cardiovascular stabilizing effects in several publications. Berlin surgeons Franz Schück (1888–1958) and Erich Simenauer (1901–1988) revived this concept in the 1930s. Schück noted the positive circulatory effects that appeared in 3–5 minutes. Why this revolutionary concept did not change clinical practice is unclear. One explanation is that both scientists were Jewish and emigrated to escape persecution. Their idea was temporarily forgotten, and rediscovered in the early 1980s. Today their concept is known world-wide as "small-volume resuscitation" [62].

A world-wide search for a solution with volume expanding properties proceeded in parallel to the studies of a concentrated saline or sugar solution. The lack of safe and effective blood-volume expanders became apparent during World War II. In Germany, Weese devised a non toxic, biocompatible solution with the desired blood-volume expanding properties, but without side-effects in 1943. This was Periston® (Polyvidone) [63], containing 4% polyvinyl pyrrolidone (PVP) with

an average molecular weight of 30,000. It was successfully tested as a plasma substitute in wounded soldiers, primarily during the campaign in France in 1940. Later it was not uncommon to administer Periston® into the sternal marrow of hypovolemic soldiers to manage hemodynamic instability. However it was generally infused intravenously during surgical procedures in anaesthetized patients. It was noticed that the pyrrolidone could bind with toxic substances like botulism and diphtheria toxins that were then renally excreted, thus being detoxified. Bayer subsequently developed a 6% preparation for this use, and this preparation was used to treat intoxication-hazards, such as barbiturate poisoning in suicide or in septic patients [64]. In the mid 1960s, pyrrolidone was withdrawn from the market, as better new synthetic colloids became available, especially modified fluid gelatins, dextrans and new preparations of starch solutions [65].

Around 1920, Straub developed an infusion of a "serum saline solution". Its use became widespread, since it could be prepared from hot water and a powder. A "Normosal-solution", manufactured at the "Sächsische Serum Werke" was available in ampoules by the middle of the 1920s. Some years later, other saline solutions, such as Tutofusin became available

Professional Developments in Surgical Pain Relief in Germany

Schleich's call to raise the quality of anaesthesia practice in the early part of the twentieth century fell on deaf ears. However the introduction of acetylene as an anaesthetic, the greater use of nitrous oxide, and the increased administration of intravenous or rectal anaesthetics in German speaking countries in the early 1920s, revived the idea of a specialty of anaesthesia. The development of complex apparatus for anaesthetic delivery, and more intricate operations increased the pressure for specialization. Physicians and state institutions favoured specialization, and the founding of a German Anaesthesia Society was discussed during the nineteeth Meeting of the German Natural Scientists and Physicians in Hamburg in 1928. But influential surgeons rejected the idea of anaesthesiologists. Most surgeons feared losing their place as the "captain of the ship" in the operating theatre. There was also an economic reason. Accepting the anaesthesiologist's important role in the treatment of patients during surgery would result in monetary requests to the patient, and this was not acceptable! In a popular textbook, Greifswald surgeon Friedrich Pels-Leusden (1866–1944) argued: "Fortunately, we do not have specialists in anaesthesiology like in the United States and hopefully they will never annoy us". Thus for decades, nurses experienced in the administration of anaesthetics were responsible for anaesthesia [66].

The enormous progress in anaesthesia in the US and UK during the 1930s and 1940s, rekindled discussion after

World War II. But major surgical circles continued to deny the need for specialization in anaesthesiology. Karl-Heinrich Bauer (1890–1978) argued: "For the training of anaesthesia physicians there is no urgent need; on the contrary, a better training of the anaesthesia nurses is more urgent" [67]. But the development of anaesthesiology as an independent branch of medicine could no longer be stopped. In 1953, the German Society of Anaesthesia (Deutsche Gesellschaft für Anaesthesie) was founded [68].

Because in Germany there was no educational program for nurses to specialize in anaesthesia, their role diminished as the medical specialty developed [69]. For decades, nurses have not been allowed to perform anaesthesia unless controlled (directed) by a physician [70]. In contrast to this situation in Germany and Austria, trained nurses in Switzerland are permitted to perform anaesthesia when an anaesthesiologist is nearby.

Journals and Textbooks Reflect the Increasing Importance of Anaesthesia

Publication of the first German anaesthesia-related journals "Der Schmerz" and "Narkose und Anaesthesie" in 1928, considerably preceded the founding of a professional specialty of anaesthesia. These journals merged to "Schmerz, Narkose und Anaesthesie" for economic reasons in 1929 and continued publication until 1944, interrupted then by the devastation of World War II. In the early 1950s, discussion by those working to form the German Anaesthesia Society led to publication of the journal "Der Anesthesist". Indeed, the first issue of "Der Anesthesist" appeared in 1952 when the Austrian and Swiss Societies were founded. It is noteworthy, that this happened before the founding of the German Society of Anaesthesia! Der Anesthesist subsequently became the official organ of the German, Swiss and Austrian Anaesthesia Societies. In the mid 1960s, additional anaesthesia related journals appeared: Anästhesiologie und Intensivmedizin (Anaesthesiology and Intensive Medicine), Anästhesiologie-Intensivmedizin-Notfallmedizin-Schmerztherapie (AINS; Anaesthesiology, Intensive Care Medicine, Emergency Medicine, Pain Therapy) and these are still published [71]. The official journal of the German Society and Intensive Therapy of the former German Democratic Republic (DDR) merged with AINS after West and East Germany reunified in the late 1990s. Presently, all publications are official organs of the German Anaesthesia Society [72].

An increasing demand for information concerning anaesthesia encouraged publication of new textbooks for both the novice and the experienced anaesthetist. In the first decade of the twentieth century, German speaking authors Fritz Dumont (1854–1932) from Bern, Switzerland, Benno-Wilhelm Müller (1873–1947) from Berlin, and Max von

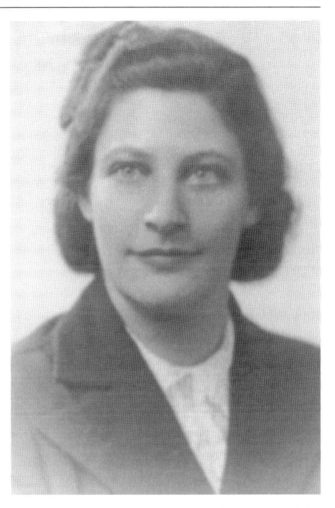

Fig. 29.8 Jean Henley at age 30. Reproduced from a photograph that accompanied her application for internship at Santa Barbara Cottage Hospital. In 1949, she wrote the first modern German textbook on anaesthesia. (From Zeitlin GK, Goerig M. An American contribution to German anesthesia. Anesthesiology 2003:99; 496–502, with permission)

Brunn (1875–1924) from Tübingen published anaesthesia related monographs. Dumont's textbook, "Handbuch der der allgemeinen und lokalen Anästhesie" [Textbook of general and local anaesthesia] appeared in 1903, Müller's monograph "Narkologie—Narkosen und Methoden der lokalen Anaesthesie" [General anaesthesia and methods of local anaesthesia] followed in 1908. Max von Brunn's monograph "Allgemeinnarkose" [General Anaesthesia] became available in 1913. In 1934, two monographs were published: Hans Killian's "Narkose für operative Zwecke" (General Anaesthesia for Operative Surgery) [73] and Ludwig Lendle's, Fritz Hesse's and Rudolf Schoen's "Allgemeinnarkose und örtliche Betäubung" (General Anaesthesia and Local Anaesthesia) [74].

After World War II, the American anaesthetist Jean Henley (1910–1993; Fig. 29.8) worked for several months at various hospitals in the American Sector of Germany. During the second half of 1949, she completed the first modern

German anaesthesia textbook, entitled "Einführung in die Praxis der modernen Inhalationsnarkose" (Introduction to the Practice of Modern Inhalation Anaesthesia) [75]. The textbook became a "best-seller" with more than 15,000 copies through 13 editions [76]. Henley's textbook helped popularize modern anaesthesia techniques and endotracheal intubation in German medicine. She initiated the recording of preoperative assessment and postoperative complications. In 1981, the German Society of Anaesthesiology and Intensive Care Medicine (DGAI) awarded Henley an honorary membership [77]. Other anaesthesia related monographs by German authors soon followed publication of Henley's book, reflecting the rise of anaesthesiology as a new German speciality. These publications underpinned the academic and scientific needs of the speciality.

Airway Management: from Tracheotomy to Endotracheal Anaesthesia

In 1869, Friedrich Trendelenburg (1844–1924) introduced a cannula surrounded by an inflatable cushion through a tracheotomy and delivered an inhaled anaesthetic through the cannula. In 1878, the Scot, William Macewen (1848–1924), pioneered tracheal intubation when he passed a tube by mouth into the trachea. His technique was initially unrecognized in its importance. Decades later the Kassel surgeon Franz Kuhn (1866–1929) "rediscovered" Macewen's technique and praised orotracheal intubation [78] in a 1911 monograph [79] detailing the technique and its indications in anaesthesia and emergency medicine. His work led to the general recognition in Germany of the importance of tracheal intubation [80].

Kuhn never wearied of promoting the advantages of tracheal intubation. He repeatedly drew attention to the importance of an adequate airway during anaesthesia and of the avoidance of hypoxia. He demonstrated that intubation allowed provision of an adequate intrapulmonary pressure that would prevent pulmonary collapse when the pleural cavity was opened. Most of his German surgical colleagues did not realize the immense importance of intubation, perhaps being prejudiced by the influential surgeon Ferdinand Sauerbruch (1875–1951) who described positive pressure ventilation as "unphysiological" [81]. Another reason for the lack of interest in the intubation technique was the concurrently increasing importance of local anaesthesia in clinical practice. Some surgeons performed 70% of procedures under local anaesthesia, because the use of chloroform was thought to be (and probably was) dangerous [82]. In 1905, Kuhn designed an inflatable pharyngeal airway (Fig. 29.9), perhaps anticipating the development of the laryngeal mask airway [83]. We do not know why he discontinued this research.

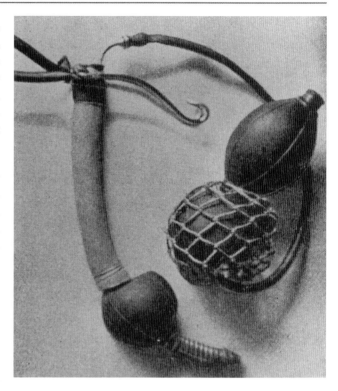

Fig. 29.9 Kuhn's inflatable pharyngeal airway (ca 1910) anticipated the laryngeal mask airway. (From Kuhn F: Perorale Tubage mit und ohne Druck. II. Teil Perorale Tubage mit Überdrucknarkose. Dtsch Zschr f Chir 1905; 76: 467–520.)

From "Autoscopia" to "Laryngoscopia"

Initially, tracheal tubes were inserted by digital guidance aided by topical cocaine-analgesia (Fig. 29.10) [84]. Later, the tube was passed orally under direct vision using a laryngoscope provided with distal illumination as described in 1895 by Berlin otolaryngologist Alfred Kirstein (1863–1922). Kirstein was among the first to develop a laryngoscope, but his intention was to visualize the larynx, trachea and oesophageal opening, and not tracheal intubation! Kirstein called his technique "autoscopia", and the instrument an "autoscope" (autos = self, copia = watch) [85]. His laryngoscope was rarely used by anaesthetists. Thus, up to the 1950s, tracheal tubes were still usually inserted under topical anaesthesia and digital control, as Kuhn suggested in 1910 [86]. With the clinical introduction of muscle-relaxants in the early 1950s, laryngoscopes became more widely used in Germany [87].

Origins of Premedication in Germany

In 1900, Eduard Schneiderlin (1875-?) of the Psychiatry Clinic in Emmendingen described the positive effects of scopolamine combined with morphine, terming the combination "new anaesthesia". He declared that he intended to prevent

in Germany. Patients now came to the operating theatre in a state of greater mental and physical tranquillity than before.

In addition to the purported sedative and anxiolytic effects of scopolamine-opioid medication, surgeons believed there was an antiemetic effect. Given the antiemetic effect of scopolamine on motion sickness, this had some basis. Moreover, they noticed a decreased incidence of post-operative pneumonia, attributed by Hermann Kümmell (1852–1937) of Hamburg, to decreased salivary secretions. Additionally, the course of anaesthesia became smoother with preoperative medication, and the amount of anaesthetic required could be reduced [90]. Leading pharmacologists suggested that morphine and scopolamine were mutually antagonistic in their effects on the human body, perhaps convincing physicians that side effects of each drug were lowered [91]. It became common practice to concurrently administer both drugs subcutaneously.

Schneiderlin's enthusiastic reports stimulated the Austrian obstetrician Richard von Steinbüchel (1862–1952) of Graz, to use morphine-scopolamine in his practice. The medication allowed the conduct of obstetric procedures such as perineal suture, dilatation of the cervix, or a delivery with forceps. He found that scopolamine-morphine premedication markedly decreased the requirement for inhalation anaesthesia [92, 93].

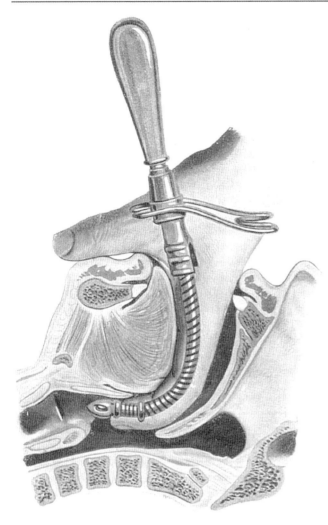

Fig. 29.10 Insertion of a tracheal tube under digit control. The index finger pulls the tongue and the epiglottis forward, as the tube equipped with an introducer is inserted along the index finger into the larynx, ca 1927. (From Kirschner M, A Schubert (Hrsg.) Allgemeine und spezielle chirurgische Operationslehre. Springer-Verlag. Berlin-Wien, 1927, p 130, with permission.)

"the act of anaesthesia (from) comprising painful sensations" and to "avoid events… that appear to be repulsive to a human being" [88]. Schneiderlin advised performing a trial injection of about 0.3 mg scopolamine and 10 mg morphine, and to repeat the dosage after an interval of up to two hours. As he recommended repeating the injection up to four times to achieve the desired effects, it is not surprising that side effects were also observed.

The Freiburg surgeon Bertholt Korff (1859–1918) appreciated the advantages of preoperatively administered scopolamine-morphine [89]. Unfortunately, the doses recommended by Schneiderlin were excessive, leading critics to question the advantages of the medication. Revised instructions for dosage, and the use of new agents such as Pantopon (a mixture of all the alkaloids in opium), reduced adverse events, and increased acceptance among surgeons

From Bottle Droppers to Complex Anaesthesia Machines

Resisting innovations in the design of inhalers and gas apparatus, most German surgeons continued to use the simple open drop method of anaesthesia administration in the first decade of the twentieth century. Special bottle droppers allowed the continuous application of controllable amounts of ether and chloroform [94].

The surgeon Oskar Witzel (1856–1925) reported this open-drop method of anaesthesia for the first time in 1895. His several publications made the technique popular in Germany and abroad. Continuously dripping ether or chloroform on a loosely fitting face mask, the concentration of the agent was progressively increased, thus minimizing side effects such as apnoea due to the sudden imposition of high concentrations of vapour. Moreover, Witzel was convinced that the use of his technique lowered the incidence of cardiovascular side effects and, in combination with the positioning of the patient's head in extension, minimized obstruction of the upper airway [95]. The broader use and acceptance of anaesthetic apparatus resulted from sequential advancements, including the production of pure oxygen, probably in the mid 1880s and the introduction of steel cylinders for storage of oxygen under high pressure in 1887.

Munich engineer Carl von Linde (1842–1934) liquefied oxygen in 1895. The storage and delivery of oxygen, and the manufacture of anaesthetic apparatus is closely connected with the name of the brothers Heinrich Dräger (1847–1917) and Bernhard Dräger (1870–1928), the founders of the Dräger-Company in Lübeck [96, 97].

In 1902, Lübeck surgeon Otto Roth (1863–1944) presented the first model of an anaesthetic apparatus, during the 31st Annual German Congress of Surgeons in Berlin. It was a sturdy oxygen-chloroform apparatus. Oxygen stored under high pressure was reduced in pressure and dispensed by a pressure reducing valve. Concurrently an injector drew liquid chloroform from a storage flask at a controlled rate that was allowed to vaporize in the oxygen stream. Roth detailed the improvements in anaesthetic control provided by the device:

"…We have now succeeded in making the falling drops of chloroform visible by using the suction effect of the oxygen stream and an especially made vessel; by virtue of this new construction the drops are always the same size so that about 50 drops always make one gram. An adjustable valve controls the number of drops and thus allows small or large amounts of chloroform on demand to fall into the oxygen stream, which is flowing at a known rate below the drip device, where they are able to evaporate. An indicator positioned above a scale of the valve gives details about the number of drops at any given time—and thus the chloroform dose in grams, which is evaporated per minute. In this way a true and accurate drip procedure is guaranteed which cannot be affected by the impatience of the operator." [98]

This new anaesthetic apparatus was a milestone in anaesthesia—the modern beginning of delivery of precisely controlled dosages of anaesthetic vapours [99].

Following the suggestion of the gynaecologist Bernhard Krönig (1863–1917) of Jena, in 1911, a second drip for ether was added. A later addition to the anaesthetic apparatus made artificial ventilation possible. An oxygen operated injector, independent of the anaesthetic components, alternately imposed positive and negative pressures to the tightly-fitting breathing mask. By virtue of their manufacture and development of such devices, Dräger became and continues as a leading manufacturer of anaesthetic apparatus in the world [100].

Another milestone was the incorporation of the Pulmotor into an anaesthetic apparatus to allow automatic ventilation of the lungs. Dräger built the first Pulmotor for rescue purposes in 1907. A clockwork motor controlled the flow of oxygen to positive and negative pressure Venturi tubes. A later model was oxygen powered. The apparatus continued in use to the beginning of the 1960s [100].

Concurrent with Witzel's open drop experiences at the end of the nineteenth century, Roth invented a completely metal, anaesthetic mask, which became the prototype for new models of anaesthetic masks. In contrast to the popular Schimmelbusch mask [96], Roth's model could be employed

with an anaesthetic apparatus and anticipated the face-mask used in modern anaesthesia apparatus [101]. Some models provided for carbon dioxide absorption. Kuhn tested the technique clinically in 1906, but did not pursue it beyond initial trials [102].

After World War I, Würzburg obstetrician Carl Gauss recommended administration of the strange smelling acetylene with the newly invented anaesthetic machines [103]. However, several explosions occurred, leading clinicians to abandon acetylene [104]. The Dräger Company developed a comparable machine for delivery of ether-nitrous-oxide-oxygen. Two Hamburg surgeons Helmut Schmidt (1895–1979) and Paul Sudeck (1866–1945) had initiated this development, and accordingly, the model was often called the "Sudeck-Schmidt" apparatus. A positive pressure attachment could be added to the model which might then be used for thoracotomies [105]. The apparatus helped popularize nitrous-oxide-oxygen anaesthesia in Germany. Obstetricians, in particular, applied it for pain relief during labour. In the mid 1940s, Gauss initiated the development of a device for the self-administration of nitrous oxide oxygen mixtures. The apparatus was introduced in 1949 as the "Dräger Spezial-Lachgas-Analgesie- und Narkoseapparat nach Prof. Dr. C. J. Gauss". A labouring parturient would inhale nitrous-oxide-oxygen via a tightly fitting mask as soon she felt contractions. The device could also deliver ether, allowing minor surgical procedures like suturing of the perineum or curettage to be done. This popular apparatus was also used in dentistry [100].

Monitoring and Documentation During Anaesthesia

At the turn of the twentieth century, heart rate, blood pressure and the amount of anaesthetic was sometimes noted in so-called "ether charts" [106]. This development was prompted by the American surgeon Harvey Cushing (1869–1930), and expanded despite rejection in the official statement of the Massachusetts General Hospital in 1903: "The adoption of blood-pressure measurement in surgical patients does not at present appear to be necessary as a routine measure" [107]. After Schmidt learned of the advantages of intraoperative documentation of vital parameters during a trip to the US at the end of the 1920s, he introduced the "anaesthesia protocol" into the Department of Surgery at the Eppendorf Hospital in Hamburg in 1929 where it continued to be used for decades [108].

Automated Measurement of Blood Pressure in Anaesthetized Patients

In 1932 the Siemens Company reported on the development of the "Autonograph", a sophisticated device for continu-

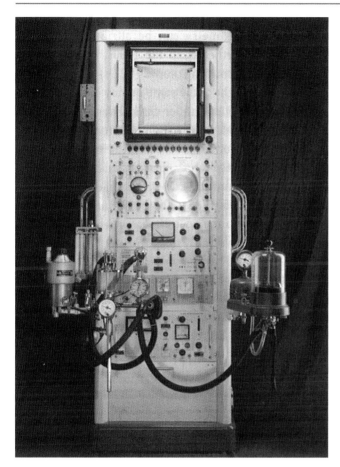

Fig. 29.11 Heinz Oehmig's anaesthesia "workstation" of the late 1950s with integrated sophisticated monitoring devices, comparable to those that we use today. (From Oehmig H: Sichere Narkose. Die Umschau in Wissenschaft und Technik 1962; 23:730–4, with permission.)

ous measurement of blood pressure. It provided a printout of its recordings and was recommended for safer anaesthesia: "The blood pressure data can be consulted at any time as evidence for 'flawless' monitoring of the anaesthesia should any lawsuits arise" [109]. A few years later, in 1937, another device, the "Kardiotron" was developed for the same purpose [110]. It allowed the surveillance of additional hemodynamic parameters. Facilitated by the invention of piezoelectronic crystals, even weak signals of heart rate or blood pressure could be transformed into acoustic and optical signals to alert the anaesthesiologist [111].

Monitoring and Recording Data from Patients after World War II

The importance of sophisticated monitoring was not appreciated immediately after World War II in Germany. The development of heart surgery in the mid 1950s changed this attitude. The anaesthetist Karl Oehmig (1919–2006) of Heidelberg, and later Cologne, was the most prominent Ger-

man advocate of comprehensive monitoring systems for use in the operating theatre. In the mid 1950s, he introduced a monitoring system similar to that which we use today. His sophisticated apparatus could continuously record blood pressure, heart rate, ECG, EEG, temperature, respiratory minute volume, exhaled carbon dioxide and the concentration of inspired air-oxygen mixture (Fig. 29.11). Later models also recorded the inspired and exhaled anaesthetic vapour concentrations [112].

Over decades, Oehmig sought to popularize such systems, but most anaesthetists felt little need for their use [113]. Problems associated with the new apparatus may explain part of their reluctance. For example, initially the ECG oscilloscopes provided a poor quality display subject to artifacts and interference, especially from diathermy. The use of needle electrodes or spiral-shaped stylus electrodes inserted into the skin also made the device less attractive [114].

On the Way to Inhaled Gas Control and Monitoring

The need to control the anaesthetic state stimulated the development of measurements of inhaled agents in anaesthetic circuits and in blood. Crucial to control was the measurement of the gas flow delivered from the anaesthetic machine. The engineer Karl Küppers (1874–1933) invented the rotameter to precisely measure the flow of gases, and his development was soon applied in anaesthetic apparatus. In 1908, Küppers obtained a patent for his invention, and in 1910, Heidelberg obstetrician Maximilian Neu (1877–1940) used rotameter flow meters to precisely control the delivery of different anaesthetic gas mixtures from a newly developed anaesthesia machine of the Rotameter Company, Aachen [115].

Cost initially limited the use of nitrous-oxide-oxygen anaesthesia in Germany. The anaesthetic had to be imported, making it expensive. Methods to minimize nitrous oxide consumption were sought, possibly leading to the reintroduction of rebreathing, a technology previously developed in an apparatus built by the Dräger Company in 1906. In 1925, rebreathing was revived in two models, the Gauss-Wieland apparatus for acetylene and the Dräger apparatus "Model A" for nitrous oxide [100]. These models also featured separate tubes for inhalation and exhalation, low-resistance micro foil valves, a carbon-dioxide absorber (as a single use cartridge, which could be shut off wholly or partly), and a breathing bag which allowed manual ventilation. A venting valve and an overpressure limiting valve were available extras [116].

The appeal of both rebreathing anaesthetic devices prompted new efforts to analyse the concentration of inhaled agents and carbon dioxide. Introduction of acetylene as a potent, expensive, and explosive inhaled anaesthetic was instrumental in the development of such a monitoring device in German speaking countries. In the early 1920s, the Dräger Company constructed a new anaesthetic apparatus that incorporated rebreathing to decrease the cost of this expensive anaesthetic, and limit exposure of operating room personnel to the strange smelling agent [100].

Despite these precautions, deaths from explosions limited the use of acetylene. Convinced that elevated concentrations of the anaesthetic gas inside the operating rooms caused this hazard, Hamburg physiologist and internist Wilhelm Knipping (1895–1982) recommended the use of a device to continuously monitor the exhaled concentration of acetylene [116]. By so doing, the anaesthetist could use closed-circuit anaesthesia, decreasing the concentrations in the operating room. Moreover, Knipping proposed that by using his device, the anaesthetist would know the concentration of gases within the circle system, thus minimizing the risk of administration of hypoxic mixtures, or awakening of the patient due to inadequate anaesthetic concentrations, anticipating in the mid-1920s modern concerns regarding the "awake" patient [117].

Monitors of Inhaled Gas Concentrations Become Available

As indicated above, the use of gas analysis during nitrous oxide anaesthesia would allow the anaesthetist to identify possible hypoxic mixtures [118]. But use of such an analytical device, manufactured by the Siemens Company, did not spread in the 1920s and 1930s despite being repeatedly mentioned in reports and in Hesse, Lendle and Schoen's textbook of anaesthesiology [74]. The device made use of the different thermal conductivity of different gases, measuring the effect of the gas on the rate of cooling of an electrically heated wire. The greater the thermal conductivity of the gas, the greater the cooling that resulted, measured quantitatively by the loss of resistance in the cooled wire [119].

After World War II, the Heidelberg anaesthetist Rudolf Frey reported his design of an electronic device that allowed continuous analysis of volatile agents. The apparatus, which became available in 1953, was similar to that which Knipping had constructed 20 years earlier. Frey repeated the arguments Knipping had advanced earlier [120]. Although Morris' Copper Kettle and the British variable bypass vaporizers appeared in the 1950s, many vaporizers (e.g., Boyles' vaporizer) provided uncalibrated concentrations of potent volatile agents like halothane or enflurane. The profound depression of circulation and respiration that these new anaesthetics could produce imposed a greater need for control over the anaesthetic state. Several new devices to measure

gas concentrations, like those developed by Helmut Vonderschmidt (1914–1998) or the already mentioned Karl Oehmig (Fig. 29.11), became available [121]. Since that time, such monitoring devices have become an integral part of all anaesthesia delivery systems. The Dräger company supplies the majority of anaesthesia equipment in Germany except for monitoring devices, where the influence of Anglo-American and Scandinavian companies has increased during recent times.

Anaesthetic Pollution—A Problem in the Operating Theatre?

Health risks to doctors and nurses by chronic occupational exposure to anaesthetic vapours, were repeatedly discussed in German journals of surgery. In the early 1920s, the Dresden surgeon Georg Kelling (1866–1945), called for decreases in such trace concentrations of inhaled agent [122]. His articles stimulated surgeons like Perthes (1869–1927) from Tübingen, and the Cologne obstetrician Josef Wieloch (1890–1944), to design devices for scavenging waste anaesthetic gases, designs similar to those used today [123].

Middle Twentieth Century Status of Physician and Nurse Anesthetists

Major deficiencies in the quality of anaesthesia in Germany were evident through the 1920s. Nevertheless, leading German surgeons opposed the development of an independent specialty of anaesthesiology. For decades all authors of German surgical textbooks stated that only experienced doctors, mostly attending surgeons in training, should administer anaesthetics in close cooperation with the operating and responsible surgeon. The trainee was part of the surgical team and this arrangement ensured that the surgeon controlled the doctors administering anaesthetics. The Ministry of Health played a passive role, and supporters of the development of an independent specialty of anaesthesiology were again rebuffed at the 43th Meeting of the Aerztetag in Bremen, in 1924 [124]. In 1937, another attempt was made to establish anaesthesiology as the 16th area of expertise among recognized medical specialities. Again, the attempt failed. After World War II, surgeons recognized the importance of the advances in modern anaesthesia that had occurred in the US and UK. Nevertheless the majority hesitated to support the idea of a speciality of anaesthesia, instead discussing legal issues concerning the training of nurses to become anaesthetists qualified for German operating rooms. "According to German law, the surgeon is still responsible for the whole surgical procedure and the anaesthesiologist is only an aide." [125] In the following years, surgeons realized that they had to accept that anaesthesia had become the responsibility of the anaesthesiologist instead of the surgeon or nurses.

Another consensus was achieved after World War II. Nurses were officially not allowed to perform any kind of anaesthesia in Germany, a position which is still current [126]. Nevertheless it must be conceded that even today the reality is different in daily anaesthetic practice, although in 1959, nursing authorities officially refused to perform "intravenous anaesthesia methods, intubation procedures, controlled ventilation or use of curare" [127]. In contrast to these "modern anaesthetic procedures", they did not object to performing traditional inhalational ether anaesthesia. By the 2000s, this limit was applied to Austria and Germany only [128] whereas in Switzerland, specialized trained nurses were officially still allowed to perform anaesthesia under the anaesthesiologist's surveillance [129].

Postgraduate Training in Anaesthesiology

When the German Society of Anaesthesia (DGA) became the 16th area of expertise among recognized medical specialties in 1953, the training time was set at 5 years. It was typical that the regulations for specialist physicians required only a minimum training period for individual specialties, without a formal curriculum. In 1953, for example, specialist physician training in anaesthesia required a postgraduate training period of 4 years, made up of:

- 1 year of surgery
- 2 years of anaesthesia
- 6 months of pharmacology or physiology
- 6 months of internal diseases

Agreement had to be reached on transitional regulations for those colleagues who had practiced as anaesthesiologists for a long time. For unclear reasons, in 1967 the professional training time was reduced to 4 years. New regulations governing accreditation of the specialty soon followed, demanding a revision of of the professional training curriculum. It was designed to be employed in surgery, but since the knowledge of an anaesthesiologist had to cover all areas of surgery, it was initially established only in anaesthesia related subjects.

The growing complexity of daily anaesthetic practice, especially during the 1960s and 1970s, increased the demand for qualified and well-trained anaesthesiologists. Specific training in thoracic, abdominal and obstetric anaesthesiology resulted in the neglect of other surgical disciplines, and led to the realisation that specific specialist education was required in anaesthesia itself. A new curriculum for the broader certification in anaesthesiology had to be established. In 1992, after several years of discussion, a 5 year education programme in anaesthesiology was restored. Finally, German anaesthesiology was on equal footing with other major European countries [130].

Training with the Anaesthesia Simulator

In the past 15 years, training on simulators has become widely accepted in Germany. Equipped with software allowing the display of a variety of physiological, pharmacological, respiratory and hemodynamic circumstances, these patient simulators allow an individualized sophisticated training commensurate with the participant's individual educational level. The various State Chambers of Physicians in Germany are now considering how to use simulators to validate certification. Such an application will encourage all university departments to purchase anaesthesia simulators for teaching [131].

Further Professional Training in Anaesthesiology

Reflecting the increasing sophistication and knowledge base in medicine and anaesthesiology, the Deutsche Akademie für Anästhesiologische Forschung (DAAD, German Academy of continuous Education in Anaesthesiology) was established by the DGAI and BDA (German Society of Anaesthesiology and Intensive Care Medicine and Professional Association of German Anaesthetists) in 1977. This institution oversees continuing medical education in the specialty. Since 2003, a uniform certificate, valid nationwide, has been established in Germany, but this may be replaced by the European diploma in the future [132].

A Reprise and Conclusion

German scientists have contributed to major aspects of the history of anaesthesia. In 1804, Sertürner isolated morphine from opium. And months after Morton's momentous 1846 demonstration, Heyfelder administered ether as an anaesthetic in Germany. Many advances followed, including the use of ethyl chloride anaesthesia (1848) in humans, the isolation (1853) and purification (1860) of cocaine, and the delivery of anaesthesia via a tracheotomy (1869). In 1884, Koller reported that cocaine had topical anaesthetic effects, opening the door to its application by numerous German-speaking physicians for infiltration and nerve blockade, and by Bier in 1898 for spinal anaesthesia. In 1890, Schimmelbusch invented his mask, used by Witzel in 1895 for continuous open drop anaesthesia.

In the early 1900s, the Dräger Company developed various anaesthetic machines, and new anaesthetic compounds were synthesized, including barbitone, the first useful sedative barbiturate (1903) and procaine (1904). In 1905, Kuhn invented an oro-pharyngeal airway, equipped with an inflatable cuff, the result anticipating by 80 years the development of laryngeal mask airways. By 1910, rotameters were invented and used in anaesthetic machines, and a decade later carbon dioxide absorbers were added. In 1912, Perthes described the localization of peripheral nerves by electrical stimulation. In 1925, Knipping developed a device to continuously monitor the exhaled concentration of respiratory and anaesthetic gases. Books and monographs were written, and in 1928, two anaesthesia related journals were published "Der Schmerz" and "Narkose und Anaesthesie". The 1930s saw the synthesis of hexobarbital (1932, and meperidine/pethidine (1939). Blood volume expanders were developed in the 1940s.

In 1950, Henley's German textbook "Introduction to the Practice of Modern Inhalation Anaesthesia" was published, followed by numerous texts written by German speaking anaesthesiologists. Several subsequent developments supported the advancement of anaesthesiology in German speaking countries, including publication of the journal "Der Anaesthesist" (1952), founding of the Austrian and Swiss Society of Anaesthesiology (1952) and the German Society of Anaesthesia (1953), and the establishment of increasing numbers of chairs in anaesthesiology (e.g., Innsbruck, Austria, 1959; Basle, Switzerland, 1963; Hamburg-Eppendorf, Germany, 1963). The "Berufsverband Deutscher Anästhesisten" (BDA; German Association of Anaesthetists) was founded in 1961. In 1971, Doenicke published the first report on the clinical use of etomidate.

In summary, German speaking scientists and physicians added to the development of anaesthesiology. Perhaps more than in other countries, surgeons and obstetricians led the way, doing so for a century. Only in the last half century has anaesthesiology developed as a specialty in its own right.

References

1. Wawersik J. History of anesthesia in Germany. J Clin Anesth. 1991;3:235–44.
2. Holubar K. Coca-Koller and his friends. On the 140th birthday of the Vienna Jewish trio: Carl Koller Sigmund Lustgarten and Sigmund Freud. Wien klin Wochenschr. 1997;14:170–5.
3. Seidel G. Ärzte ohne Nobelpreis, deren Entdeckungen Millionen Menschen geholfen haben. Genf: Ariston Verlag; 1974. pp. 24–32.
4. Schleich CL. Schmerzlose Operationen. Berlin: Julius Springer-Verlag; 1894.
5. Wulf H, Goerig M. Zur Geschichte der örtlichen Betäubung. In: Wulff H, van Aken H, Editors. Lokalanästhesie Regionalanästhesie Regionale Schmerztherapie. Stuttgart: Thieme Verlag; 2010. pp. 1–8.
6. Röse W. Heinrich Braun. Anaesth und Intensivmed. 2000;4:224–38.
7. Braun H. Local anesthesia—its scientific basis and practical use. Philadelphia: Lea & Febiger; 1914.
8. Wesemeier K. Arthur Läwen—Pionier der Anästhesiologie. Med Dissertation. Magdeburg: Otto von Guericke-Universität Magdeburg; 1993.
9. Bier A. Versuche über Cocainisirung des Rückenmarkes. Dtsch Zschr f Chir. 1899;51:361–9.
10. Bier A. Weitere Mitteilungen über Rückenmarksanästhesie. Verhandlungsbericht der Deutschen Gesellschaft für Chirurgie. Arch f klin Chir. 1901;64:236–59.
11. Goerig M, Agarwal K, Schulte am Esch J. Versatile August Bier (1861–1949)—father of spinal anesthesia. Clin Anesth. 2000;12:561–9.
12. Schmidt H. Lumbalanästhesie mit spezifisch leichter viscotischer Novocainlösung (Spinocain) und prophylaktischer Stabilisierung des Blutdrucks durch Ephedrin. Klin Wochenschr. 1930;16:748–56.
13. Ocherblad NF, Dillon TG. Use of epinephrine in spinal anesthesia—a preliminary report. JAMA. 1927;88:1135–6.
14. Wilhelm, et al. Postspinal headache—its prevention over the decades. In: Schulte am Esch J, Goerig M, Editors. Proceedings-the fourth international symposium on the history of anaesthesia. Lübeck: Draeger-Druck; 1998. pp. 631–34.
15. Ross BK, Chadwick HS, Mancuso JJ, Benedetti C. Sprotte needle for obstetric anesthesia: decreased incidence of post dural puncture headache. Reg Anesth. 1992;17:29–39.
16. Gauss CJ. Über den Ausbreitungsmodus des Anästhetikums bei der Lumbalanästhesie. Zbl f Gyn. 1909;33:1070–7.
17. Goerig M, Agarwal K. Iso- hypo- oder hyperbare Lokalanästhesielösung—das ist die Frage! Hauptstadtkongress HAI 2007. Berlin: Poster PO 3597.
18. Kreis O. Über Medullarnarkose bei Gebärenden. Cbl f Gyn. 1900;24:724–9.
19. Steinbüchel R von. Die Scopolamin-Morphium-Halbnarkose in der Geburtshilfe. Beiträge Geburtshilfe und Gynäkologie. 1903;1:294–326.
20. Sellheim H. Herabsetzung der Empfindlichkeit der Bauchdecken und des Peritoneums parietale durch perineurale Injektion anästhesierender Lösungen an die Stämme des N N intercostales subcostales des ileo-hypogastricus und ileo-inguinalis. Verhandlungen des 9. Deutschen Gynäkologenkongresses. Verhandlungen der Deutschen Gesellschaft für Gynäkologie. 1906. pp. 176–9.
21. Kappis M. Ueber Leitungsanästhesie am Bauch, Brust, Arm und Hals durch Injektionen am Foramen intervertebrale. Münch Med Wochenschr. 1912;13:224–38.
22. Kappis M, Gerlach F. Die differentialdiagnostische Bedeutung der paravertebralen Novokaineinspritzung. Med Klin. 1923;35:1184–7.
23. Läwen A. Fortschritte in der Sakralanästhesie. Zbl f Chir. 1924;51:1000–4.
24. Läwen A. Über Extraduralanästhesie für chirurgische Operationen. Dtsch Zsch f Chir. 1910;108:1–43.
25. Läwen A. Weitere Erfahrungen über paravertebrale Schmerzaufhebung zur Differentialdiagnose von Erkrankungen der Gallenblase, des Magens, der Niere und des Wurmfortsatzes sowie zur Behandlung postoperativer Lungenkomplikationen. Zbl f Chir. 1923;50:460–65.
26. Läwen A. Ueber die Verwendung des Novokains in Natriumbikarbonat-Kochsalzlösung zur lokalen Anästhesie. Münch Med Wochenschr. 1910;39:2044–6.
27. Läwen A. Ueber die Verbindung der Lokalanästhesie mit der Narkose, über hohe Extraduralanästhesie und epidurale Injektionen anästhesierender Lösungen bei tabischen Magenkrisen. Bruns Beitr f klin Chir. 1912;80:168–80.
28. Goerig M, Agarwal K. Georg Perthes—the man behind the technique of nerve tracer technology. Reg Anesth Pain Med. 2000;25:296–301.
29. Bier A. Ueber einen neuen Weg Lokalanästhesie an den Gliedmaassen zu erzeugen. Arch f klin Chir. 1908;86:1007–8.

30. van Zundert A, Helmstädter A, Goerig M, Motier E. Centennial of Intravenous Regional Anesthesia Bier's Block (1908–2008). Reg Anesth Pain Med. 2008;33:483–9.

31. Momburg F. Zur Venenanästhesie Biers. Zbl f Chir. 1909;41:1413–4.

32. Hayward E. Erfahrungen und Beobachtungen an 375 Fällen von Venenanästhesie. Arch f klin Chir. 1910;99:993–1019.

33. Capelle W. Die Bedeutung des Wundschmerzes und seiner Ausschaltung für den Ablauf der Atmung bei Laparotomierten. Dtsch Zschr f Chir. 1936;246:466–85.

34. Fulde E. Die örtliche Ausschaltung des Nachschmerzes Bauchoperierter. Langenbeck's Arch f klin Chir. 1933;237:637–49.

35. Kirschner M. Elektrokoagulation des Ganglion gasseri. Zbl f Chir. 1932;59:2841–2.

36. Goerig M, Beck H. Martin Kirschner—an outstanding surgeon and anesthetist. In: Fink BR, Morris LE, Stephen, CR, Editors. The history of anesthesia proceedings of the Third International Symposium Atlanta 1992. Wood Library-Museum of Anesthesiology Park Ridge. Illinois; 1992. pp. 233–40.

37. Caton DC. What a blessing—she had chloroform. The medical and social response to the pain of childbirth from 1800 to the present. New Haven and London: Yale University Press; 2000.

38. Gogarten W, Aken H van. A century of regional analgesia in obstetrics. Anesth Analg. 2000;91:773–5.

39. Pirogoff N. Researches Practique et Physiologique sur L'Ethérisation. Paris: St Petersbourg Chez Fd Bellizard et Co Librairies—Éditeurs; 1847. pp. 53–9.

40. Burkhardt J. Die intravenöse Narkose mit Aether und Chloroform. Münch Med Wochenschr. 1909;46:2365–9.

41. Kümmell H. Weitere Erfahrungen über intravenöse Aethernarkose. Bruns Beitr klin Chir. 1914;92:27–36.

42. Goerig M. Schulte am Esch J. Historical Remarks Regarding Intravenous Ether Anesthesia. Bull Anesth History. 1996;14:1–6.

43. Dundee JW. The history of barbiturates. Anesthesia. 1982;37:726–34.

44. Bumm R. Narkoseversuche mit intravenöser Darreichung von Barbitursäurederivaten. Dtsch Zschr f Chir. 1928;202:289–303.

45. Weese H, Scharpff W. Evipan—ein neuartiges Einschlafmittel. Dtsch Med Wochenschr. 1932;58:1205–7.

46. Lange K, v Wolffersdorf H. Über die Anwendung des Evipanatriums bei großen operativen Eingriffen und seine Gebrauchsfähigkeit im Kriege. Chirurg. 1939;11:681–4.

47. Goerig M, Schulte am Esch J. Hellmuth Weese—Der Versuch einer Würdigung seiner Bedeutung für die deutschsprachige Anästhesie. AINS. 1997;32:678–85.

48. Schulte Esch J, Goerig M. Die Anästhesie nach 1945. In: Schüttler J, Editor. 50 Jahre Deutsche Gesellschaft für Anästhesiologie und Intensivmedizin. Tradition & Innovation. Im Auftrag der Deutschen Gesellschaft für Anästhesiologie und Intensivmedizin unter Mitarbeit von M Goerig, H Petermann, J Schulte am Esch, W Schwarz. Berlin: Springer-Verlag; 2003. pp. 182–231.

49. Doenicke A. Hirnfunktion und Toleranzbreite nach Etomidate—einem neuen barbituratfreien iv-applizierbaren Hypnoticum. Anaesthesist. 1973;22:357–66.

50. Dost FH. Fundamental of Pharmacokinetics. Stuttgart: Thieme Verlag; 1968.

51. Schüttler J, Schwilden H, Stoeckel H. Pharmacokinetics as applied to total intravenous anesthesia, Practical implications. Anaesthesia. 1983;Suppl 38:53–6.

52. Bickford RG. Automatic encephalographic control of general anesthesia. Clin Neurophysiol. 1951;3:83–90.

53. Gwathmey JT. Obstetrical analgesia—a further study based on more than twenty thousand cases. Anesth Analg. 1931;10:190–5.

54. Goerig M. The Avertin-story. In: Fink BR, Morris LE, Stephen CR, Editors. The history of anesthesia proceedings of the Third International Symposium Atlanta 1992. Wood Library-Museum of Anesthesiology Park Ridge. Illinois; 1992. pp. 223–32.

55. Straub W. Zur Infusion von Flüssigkeiten unter konstanter Geschwindigkeit. Münch Med Wochenschr. 1911;28: 1514–1515

56. Schulte am Esch J, Goerig M. Anaesthetic equipment in the history of German anesthesia. Lübeck: DrägerDruck; 1997.

57. Strauss H. Zur Methodik der intravenösen Therapie. Dtsch Med Wochenschr. 1906;4:141–2.

58. Just OH, Dietzel W. Die historische Entwicklung der intravenösen Injektionstechnik und die heutige Verwendung der Plastikkanüle (Braunüle). Die Schwester. 1986;1:53–9.

59. Martin E. Die rektale kontinuierliche Kochsalzinfusion; der "Tröpfcheneinlauf" unter Kontrolle des Auges. Münch Med Wochenschr. 1911;18:949–52.

60. Bayliss WM. The action of gum acacia on the circulation. J Pharmacol Exper Ther. 1919;15:29–74.

61. Külz F. Zur Frage des Ersatzes von Blutverlusten durch Gummi-Kochsalzlösungen. Dtsch Med Wochenschr. 1921;49:1493–4.

62. Goerig M, Agarwal K. Small-Volume-Resuscitation—historical remarks. In: Diz JC et al. Editors. The history of anesthesia. Amsterdam: Elsevier Science BV; 2002. pp. 233–44.

63. Hecht G, Weese H. Periston ein neuer Flüssigkeitsersatz. Münch Med Wochenschr. 1943;1:11–5.

64. Schubert R. Die Anwendung von Periston N zur Serum- und Zellwäsche und ihre klinische Bedeutung. Dtsch Med Wochenschr. 1951;47:1487–92.

65. Przemeck M, Adams HA. Volumen—und Flüssigkeitsersatz. In: Kochs E, Adams HA, Spies, Editors. Anästhesiologie. Stuttgart: Thieme Verlag; 2008. pp. 153–64.

66. Goerig M, Schulte Esch J. Die Anästhesie in der ersten Hälfte des 20 Jahrhunderts. In: Schüttler J, Editor. 50 Jahre Deutsche Gesellschaft für Anästhesiologie und Intensivmedizin. Tradition & Innovation. Im Auftrag der Deutschen Gesellschaft für Anästhesiologie und Intensivmedizin unter Mitarbeit von M Goerig, H Petermann, J Schulte am Esch, W Schwarz. Berlin: Springer-Verlag; 2003. pp. 27–65.

67. Bräutigam KH. 40 Jahre "Facharzt für Anästhesie". Anaesth und Intensivmed. 1993;9:259–68.

68. Brandt L, Goerig M. Kurze Geschichte der Deutschen Gesellschaft für Anästhesie und Intensivmedizin. AINS. 2003;38:215–25.

69. Ahnefeld FW, Dick W. Das Berufsbild von Anästhesie und Intensivtherapie-Schwestern bzw. Pflegern. Anästh Inform. 1972;13:201.

70. Weissauer W. Die Entwicklung zum selbstständigen Fachgebiet. In: Schüttler J, Editor. 50 Jahre Deutsche Gesellschaft für Anästhesiologie und Intensivmedizin. Tradition & Innovation. Im Auftrag der Deutschen Gesellschaft für Anästhesiologie und Intensivmedizin unter Mitarbeit von M Goerig H Petermann J Schulte am Esch W Schwarz. Berlin: Springer-Verlag; 2003. pp. 68–78.

71. Taeger K, Schüttler J. Die Entwicklung der Fachzeitschriften: Die Zeitschriften Der Anaesthesist: eine lebendige wissenschaftliche und praxisbezogene Zeitschrift im Wandel der Zeit/1952–2003). In: Schüttler J, Editor. 50 Jahre Deutsche Gesellschaft für Anästhesiologie und Intensivmedizin. Tradition & Innovation. Im Auftrag der Deutschen Gesellschaft für Anästhesiologie und Intensivmedizin unter Mitarbeit von M Goerig, H Petermann, J Schulte am Esch W Schwarz. Berlin: Springer-Verlag; 2003. pp. 155–69.

72. Benad G. Die Entwicklung der Fachzeitschriften: Die Zeitschrift Anaesthesiologie und Reanimation. In: Schüttler J, Editor. 50 Jahre Deutsche Gesellschaft für Anästhesiologie und Intensivmedizin. Tradition & Innovation. Im Auftrag der Deutschen Gesellschaft für Anästhesiologie und Intensivmedizin unter Mitarbeit von M Goerig, H Petermann, J Schulte am Esch W Schwarz. Berlin: Springer-Verlag; 2003. pp. 169–74.

73. Killian H. Narkose zu operativen Zwecken. Berlin: Julius Springer-Verlag; 1934.

74. Hesse F, Lendle L, Schoen R. Allgemeinnarkose und örtliche Betäubung. Leipzig: Johann Ambrosius Barth; 1934.

75. Henley J. Einführung in die Praxis der modernen Inhalationsnarkose. Berlin: Walter de Gruyter & Co Verlag; 1950.

76. Zeitlin GL, Goerig M. An American contribution to German anesthesia. Anesthesiology. 2003;59:456–502.

77. Petermann H. Anglo-amerikanische Einflüsse bei der Etablierung der Anästhesie in der Bundesrepublik Deutschland im Zeitraum von 1949–1960. AINS. 2005;40:133–41.

78. Brandt L, Pokar H. Schütte S. 100 Jahre Intubationsnarkose. Anaesthesist. 1983;32:200–4.

79. Kuhn F. Die perorale Intubation. Berlin: S. Karger; 1911.

80. Goerig M, Schulte am Esch J. Franz Kuhn (1866–1929) zum 125 Geburtstag. AINS. 1991;8:416–24.

81. Klippe HJ. Zur historischen Entwicklung der endotrachealen Intubation. Schleswig-Holsteinisches Ärzteblatt. 1986;6:364–67 und 1986;7:425–27.

82. Braun H. Die Lokalanästhesie, ihre wissenschaftlichen Grundlagen und praktische Anwendung. Dritte, völlig umgearbeitete Auflage. Leipzig: Ambrosius Barth Verlag; 1913.

83. Kuhn F. Perorale Tubage mit und ohne Druck. II. Teil Perorale Tubage mit Überdrucknarkose. Dtsch Zschr f Chir. 1905;76:467–520.

84. Hirsch NPG, Smith P, Hirsch O. Alfred Kirstein pioneer of direct laryngoscopy. Anaesthesia. 1986;4:42–5.

85. Kirstein A. Autoskopie des Larynx und der Trachea (Laryngoscopia directa, Euthyskopie, Besichtigung ohne Spiegel). Berlin: Archiv für Laryngologie und Rhinologie Verlag von August Hirschwald; 1895. pp. 156–64.

86. Irmer W, Koss FH, Killian H. Die Endotrachealnarkose. In: Killian—Weese, Editor. Die Narkose—Ein Lehr- und Handbuch. Stuttgart: Georg-Thieme-Verlag; 1954. pp. 570–615.

87. Reinhardt M, Eberhardt E. Alfred Kirstein (1863–1922) Pionier der direkten Laryngoskopie. AINS. 1995;29:240–6.

88. Schneiderlin E. Eine neue Narkose. Aerztliche Mitteilungen aus und für Baden. 1900;10:101–3.

89. Korff B. Mitteilungen zur Morphin-Scopolamin-Narkose. Bln klin Wochenschr. 1906;51:1626–9.

90. Grimm W. Die mit Skopolamin-Morphium kombinierte Inhalationsnarkose und ihre günstige Beziehung zu den Pneumonien nach Bauchoperationen. Bruns Beitr klin Chir. 1907;55:1–8.

91. Von Brunn M. Die Allgemeinnarkose. Stuttgart: Enke Verlag; 1913.

92. Steinbüchel R von. Vorläufige Mitteilung über die Anwendung von Skopolamin-Morphium-Injektionen in der Geburtshilfe. Cbl f Gyn. 1902;26:1303–4.

93. Roth O. Kleinere Mittheilungen. Zur Sauerstoff-Chloroform-Narkose. Zbl f Chir. 1902;46:188–90.

94. Müller WB. Narkologie. Ein Handbuch der Wissenschaft über allgemeine und lokale Schmerzbetäubung (Narkosen und Methoden der lokalen Anästhesie). I. Band: Narkosiologie. Berlin: Trenkel Verlag; 1908.

95. Witzel O. Praktische Erfahrungen ueber das Operieren in der Narkose. Dtsch Med Wochenschr. 1895;30:605–8.

96. Reinhardt M, Eberhardt E. Curt Schimmelbusch (1860–1895)—Entwicklung einer Maske für Chloroform- und Äthernarkosen aus primär aseptischen Überlegungen. AINS. 1994;29:30–5.

97. Thompson PW. The house of Dräger. In: Atkinson RS, Boulton ThB, Editors. The history of anaesthesia. Royal Society of Medicine Service. London: The Parthenon Publishing Group; 1988. pp. 298–300.

98. Roth O. Kleinere Mittheilungen. Zur Sauerstoff-Chloroform-Narkose. Zbl f Chir. 1902;46:188–90.

99. Barns E. It began with the Pulmotor. One hundred years of Artificial ventilation. Lübeck: Dräger Medica; 2000.

100. Haupt J. Die Entwicklung der DRÄGER—Narkoseapparate. In: DRÄGER—Medizingeräte im Wandel der Zeiten Drägerwerk Lübeck Sonderdruck MT 1 aus dem Drägerheft Nr 280 281 282 Lübeck 1970 30–5.

101. Strätling M. Schmucker P. 100 Jahre Sauerstofftherapie (1902–2002)—Eine medizinhistorische Neubewertung. AINS. 2003;38:4–13.

102. Nemes C. Franz Kuhn (1866–1929)—Pionier der peroralen Tubage und der Überdrucknarkose. In: Stoeckel H, Editor. Deutsche Anästhesie-Pioniere der ersten 100 Jahre—1847 bis etwa 1950. DCS-Überlingen; 2011. pp. 95–111.

103. Gauss CJ. Die Narcylenbetäubung mit dem Kreisatmer. Zbl f Gyn. 1925;49:1218–26.

104. Oehlecker F. Die Explosionsgefahr bei der Narcylenbetäubung. Zbl f Chir. 1926;53:774–9.

105. Sudeck P, Schmidt H. Ein neues Modell eines möglichst druckkonstanten Überdruckapparates. Dtsch Zsch f Chir. 1926;1926:1–9.

106. Goerig M. Die Überwachung des narkotisierten Patienten. In: Brandt L, Editor. Illustrierte Geschichte der Anästhesie. Stuttgart: Wissenschaftliche Verlagsgesellschaft m b H Stuttgart; 1997. pp. 152–5.

107. Anonymus. Bulletin no 2 division of surgery. Massachusetts General Hospital 1902.

108. Schmidt H. Lumbalanästhesie mit spezifisch leichter viscotischer Novocainlösung (Spinocain) und prophylaktischer Stabilisierung des Blutdrucks durch Ephedrin. Klin.Wochenschr. 1930;16:748–56.

109. Anonymus. Werbeschrift der Firma Siemens-Reiniger für den Autonograph nach Dr. Lange zum fortlaufenden selbständigen Messen und Registrieren des menschlichen Blutdrucks. Berlin 1932.

110. Jaeger F. Die Blutdruck- und Pulskontrolle während der Operation. Schmerz-Narkose-Anaesthesie. 1937;1:44–7.

111. Lundy JS. Observations on Anesthesia in Europe in 1938. Proceedings of the Staff Meetings of the Mayo Clinic. 1938;13(29):447–50.

112. Oehmig H. Sichere Narkose. Die Umschau in Wissenschaft und Technik. 1962;23:730–4.

113. Kern ER. Gegensätzliche Strömungen der heutigen Anästhesiologie. Anaesthesist. 1964;13:277–9.

114. Herden N, Lawin P. Anästhesiefibel. Stuttgart: Thieme Verlag; 1973.

115. Foregger R. The rotameter and the waterwheel. Anaesthesist. 2001;50:701–8.

116. Dräger S. 111 Jahre: Dräger-Technik für das Leben—alles begann mit dem Oxygen-Automaten. In: Symposium, Editor. Deutsche Anästhesie-Pioniere der ersten 100 Jahre 1847 bis etwa 1950. DCS-Überlingen; 2011. pp. 95–106.

117. Knipping HW. Beitrag zur Acetylennarkose. Hoppe-Seyler's Zschr f Physiolog Chem. 1924;141:11–2.

118. Goerig M, Agarwal K. Hugo Wilhelm Knipping: a pioneer in continuous anesthetic gas monitoring during the administration of nitrous-oxide-oxygen based anesthesia. In: Diz JC et al. Editors. The history of anesthesia. Amsterdam: Elsevier Science BV; 2002. pp. 313–22.

119. Schmidt H. Dosierungsprinzipien bei der Gasnarkose. Narkose und Anaesthesie. 1929;1:65–80.

120. Frey R. H Göpfert. Kontrolle der Inhalationsnarkose durch fortlaufende elektrische Gasanalyse. Anaesthesist. 1953;3:99–101.

121. Vonderschmitt H, Gasteyer KH. Überwachung der Anästhesie durch fortlaufende Registrierung mit Vielfachschreibung. Anaesthesist. 1959;9:272–5.

122. Kelling G. Narkosemaske zur selbsttätigen Abführung der Chloroform- und Ätherdämpfe. Zbl f Chir. 1922;49:1064–6.

123. Wieloch J. Zur Beseitigung der Narkosedämpfe aus dem Operationssaal. Zbl f Gyn.1925;49:2768–70.

124. Anonymus. Der 43. Deutsche Aerztetag am 20. und 21. VI in Bremen. Dtsch Med Wochenschr. 1924;27:962–4.

125. Bauer KH. Zur geistigen Situation unseres Faches. Langenbecks Arch Klin Chir. 1952;273:9–14.

126. Hübner A. Standes- und Berufsfragen. Der Krankenhausarzt. 1952;9:92.
127. Anonymus. Fachnachrichten und Kongreßkalender. Anaesthesist. 1959;8:216.
128. Anonymus. Münsteraner Erklärung: Gemeinsame Stellungnahme des BDA und der DGAI zur Parallelnarkose. Anästh und Intensivmed. 2007;4:223–9.
129. Pasch T, Frei F. 50 Jahre Schweizerische Gesellschaft für Anästhesiologie und Reanimation. Anaesthesist. 2002;51:1015–19.
130. Lawin P, Opderbecke HW, Van Aken H. The Development of Intensive Care Medicine in the Framework of Anaesthesiology in the Federal Republic of Germany. In: Schüttler J Editor 55 Years German Society of Anaesthesiology and Intensive Care Medicine. Springer Verlag; 2012. pp. 147–74.
131. Schüttler J. DGAI-Projekt zur Optimierung der studentischen Lehre durch Anästhesie und Notfallsimulatoren erfolgreich angelaufen. Anästh Intensivmed. 2004;45:381.
132. Schulte am Esch, Goerig M, Agarwal K. Development of anaesthesia after 1945. In: Schüttler J, Editor. 55 Years German Society of Anaesthesiology and Intensive Care Medicine. Springer Verlag; 2012. pp. 116–46.

The Evolution of Anaesthesia in the British Isles

30

Cedric Prys-Roberts

Summary

In 1800, Davy suggested that nitrous oxide might be used to relieve pain during surgery, but no one acted on his suggestion. Morton's 16 Oct 1846 discovery led to ether anaesthesia in Scotland and London on 19 Dec 1846. Liston proclaimed *"This Yankee dodge beats mesmerism hollow"*. Simpson discovered and popularized chloroform anaesthesia in 1847. In the late 1840s, Snow developed an anaesthetic vaporiser and correlated anaesthetic dose and effect. In 1904, the General Medical Council (GMC), added anaesthetics as the 16th subject that every medical course and examination should contain.

The *British Journal of Anaesthesia,* and *Anaesthesia* began publishing in 1923 and 1946, respectively. Magill helped found the Association of Anaesthetists of Great Britain and Ireland (AAGBI) in 1932, and in 1935, the Anaesthetic Section of the Royal Society of Medicine awarded the Diploma in Anaesthesia. Lord Nuffield underwrote the Nuffield Department of Anaesthetics (NDA) at Oxford in 1937. Universities at Bristol (1946), Newcastle-upon-Tyne (1949), Cardiff (Welsh National School of Medicine; 1952) and Liverpool (1959) created Departments of Anaesthesia. In 1948, the Royal College of Surgeons established a Faculty of Anaesthetists, soon to introduce a Fellowship by examination (FFARCS). Parallel developments led to the Irish Faculty of Anaesthetists in 1959. Between 1960 and 1971, 15 new university departments headed by chairs of anaesthesia emerged in the UK.

In the early 1950s, ICI's Suckling and Raventós developed halothane which quickly became the world's anaesthetic, aided by the new calibrated vaporizer, the Fluotec. In 1967, Baird and Reid described the clinical use of pancuronium. JB Glen and colleagues at ICI discovered propofol in 1973, but formulation troubles delayed its release until the 1980s. In 1981, Wellcome Research Laboratories released atracurium, and in 1983, Brain introduced the laryngeal mask airway (LMA).

Established in 1988, the independent College of Anaesthetists (to gain Royal charter in 1992) participated in creating the Inter-Collegiate Faculty of Intensive Care Medicine in the late 2000s, and developed an independent Faculty of Pain Medicine. Similarly, in Ireland, a College of Anaesthetists (CAI) was created within the RCSI, becoming independent in 1998, and later creating an inter-Collegiate Faculty of Intensive Care Medicine, and its own Faculty of Pain Medicine.

In 2010, Pandit reported that only 6 of 23 UK universities sustained a departmental or divisional structure for anaesthesia. Will "anaesthesia" as "perioperative medicine"—encompassing anaesthesia, intensive care medicine, and pain medicine be a more attractive and effective format for the advancement of our specialties into the future?

Early British Medicine

In Britain and other European countries monks and priests, working as hospitallers, developed the science and art of healing. Two London hospitals, St Bartholomew's and St Thomas's, date from the 12th century. By the 15th century, many British physicians studied at Italian schools in Padua, Bologna, Pisa and Ferrara, and Protestant schools in Switzerland and Holland. These were the centres of the medi-

cal universe at the time [1]. Following a petition from the universities of Oxford and Cambridge in 1421, the English Parliament decreed that graduates of foreign universities should be granted the degree of Doctor of Medicine (DM Oxon, or MD Cambridge) to allow them, as well as graduates of Oxford or Cambridge, to practice medicine. Now, in the United Kingdom and in the Republic of Ireland, 'doctors' qualify with Bachelor's degrees in medicine and surgery (eg, MB, BS), whereas DM or MD are higher degrees based on research presented as theses or dissertations.

Thomas Linacre (1460–1524), a physician, scholar and humanist, studied at Padua for 12 years. With a group of distinguished physicians, he recognised the need for licensing physicians and apothecaries. Under charter from King Henry VIII, he founded the College of Physicians of London

C. Prys-Roberts (✉)
Past President, Royal College of Anaesthetists, Emeritus Professor, University of Bristol, Foxes Mead, Cleeve Hill Road, Cleeve, Bristol BS49 4PG, UK
e-mail: cedricpr@talktalk.net

in 1518 [1, 2]. The College licensed those qualified to prac-tice, and identified and allowed the law to punish unqualified practitioners and those engaged in malpractice. The College acquired the "Royal" prefix in 1674. Linacre also established lectureships at Oxford and Cambridge that later became the Regius Professorships of Medicine. Robert Sibbald and col-leagues founded a College of Physicians in Edinburgh and obtained a "Royal" charter from Charles II in 1681. Similar colleges had been established in Glasgow (1599), and in Ire-land (1654), both later acquiring the "Royal" prefix.

Surgery developed at a slower pace. In the 14th century, the Guild of Surgeons in London was in dispute with the Worshipful Company of Barbers, and in 1542, Henry VIII united the two groups to form the Company of Barber-Sur-geons. Unlike the physicians, they had no qualifications, let alone a medical degree. In 1745, the surgeons separated from the barbers to form the Company of Surgeons, and gained a royal charter in 1800 to become the Royal College of Sur-geons in London. In 1845, Queen Victoria granted them a further charter to become the Royal College of Surgeons of England [3], and the Royal College of Physicians concur-rently insisted that surgeons should acquire a medical degree before they could practise. Until then, surgeons could not prescribe medicines.

Surgeons in Glasgow functioned as a joint Faculty with physicians, becoming a Royal Faculty in 1909, and a Royal College of Physicians and Surgeons in 1962. Barber-surgeons in Edinburgh incorporated as a Craft Guild in 1505 and were granted a charter by George III to become the Royal College of Surgeons of the City of Edinburgh (1778) and finally the Royal College of Surgeons of Edinburgh (1851) [4].

The progress of surgery in Ireland was much more in-teresting. The Barber-Surgeons Guild of St Magdalene was incorporated in 1446 by King Henry VI, becoming the first such corporation in the British Isles. Limerick surgeon, Syl-vester O'Halloran, proposed a College of Surgeons modelled on the College de St Cosme in Paris, which had trained and regulated French surgeons since its receipt of a charter from Louis IX in 1255! However, this did not materialise and in 1785, George III chartered the Dublin Society of Surgeons as the Royal College of Surgeons in Ireland [5]. This col-lege is one of the five constituent Colleges of the National University of Ireland and, unlike all other Royal Colleges, has its own undergraduate medical school. Although Ireland became a republic in 1922, the Royal Colleges maintained their chartered names as they include both Northern Ireland and the Republic.

Until 1999, all British (and Irish) Royal Colleges, in ad-dition to their specialist training and regulatory functions, held examinations in medicine and surgery allowing them to license graduates to practise medicine. In 1993, the Society of Apothecaries, together with the five English and Scottish Colleges of Physicians and Surgeons, formed the United Examining Board (UEB) to conduct the non-university ex-amination for a registrable medical qualification. The UEB was dissolved in 2007, to conform to European Commission rules that allow only universities to grant qualifications in medicine. Other medical specialties, including anaesthesia, became chartered Royal Colleges after World War II.

Anaesthesia Develops as a Specialty in Great Britain

Humphry Davy (1778–1829) was neither an anaesthetist nor an academic, neither attending nor teaching at a university. At the age of 17, he was apprenticed to JP Borlase, a surgeon in Cornwall, and in that occupation he prepared and inhaled nitrous oxide, a gas discovered by Joseph Priestley (1733–1804). Priestley received the Copley medal of the Royal So-ciety for a paper entitled "*The Different Kinds of Air*". This paper stimulated Thomas Beddoes (1760–1808), an Oxford physician, to establish the Pneumatic Institution in Dowry Square, Bristol, ostensibly to treat pulmonary tuberculosis by the inhalation of these new airs. Beddoes met Humphry Davy during a holiday in Cornwall, and invited the 19 year old to become Superintendent of the Institution. There, Davy prepared nitrous oxide by heating ammonium nitrate as described by Berthollet in 1785, and studied the effects of breathing the gas, on himself and others. Some of Davy's experiments were conducted at a time when he suffered from inflammation of the gums. In 1800 he described his experi-ences: "*On the day when the inflammation was most trouble-some, I breathed three large doses of nitrous oxide. The pain always diminished after the first four or five respirations*". Based on this simple observation [6, 7], Davy concluded that as (nitrous oxide) "*appears capable of destroying physical pain, it may probably be used with advantage during surgical operations in which no great effusion of blood takes place*".

No power analysis, no randomised double-blind investi-gation but, nevertheless, a powerful prophesy. Davy went on to other great scientific discoveries, but missed his chance to provide the greatest advance in all of medicine. The discov-ery of anaesthesia was still 45 years away.

In 1823–4, Henry Hill Hickman (1800–1830), in Bir-mingham, experimented with inhaled carbon dioxide to cre-ate a state that he described as suspended animation, but his findings aroused little general or medical interest [8, 9].

News of the new paradigm called anaesthesia crossed the Atlantic Ocean on Samuel Cunard's ship the *Acadia,* in December 1846. William Fraser (1819–1863) was medical officer on board the Acadia and travelled on to Dumfries in Scotland. His personal report of Morton's public demonstra-tion of ether anaesthesia in Boston, resulted in the successful administration of ether at the Dumfries and Galloway Hospi-tal on 19 Dec 1846 [10].

A letter from Jacob Bigelow (the father of Henry Bigelow) to his friend Henry Boott in London, also travelled on the *Acadia*. Boott persuaded his neighbour in Gower Street, James Robinson, a dentist, to administer ether to a Miss Lonsdale for extraction of a molar tooth, also on 19 Dec 1846 [11], reported in the *Illustrated London News* on 9 January 1847. This early success led to the use of diethyl ether as an anaesthetic, when Robert Liston amputated the leg of Frederick Churchill on 21 December 1846, only four days after the news arrived in London. Liston proclaimed, "*This Yankee dodge beats mesmerism hollow*".

Three physicians, James Young Simpson (1811–1870), John Snow (1813–1858), and Joseph Thomas Clover (1825–1882) dominated the clinical and academic development of anaesthesia in Britain from 1847 to 1876.

Simpson, Professor of Midwifery at the University of Edinburgh and Doctor of Medicine, was primarily an obstetrician. He was persuaded by David Waldie, the chemist of the Apothecaries' Company of Liverpool, to test several volatile compounds, including chloroform, as potential anaesthetics to relieve the pain of labour (p24) [12]. Having inhaled these compounds, Simpson chose chloroform because it was effective, pleasant to breathe, and induced anaesthesia rapidly. In November 1847, Simpson presented a paper to the Edinburgh Medical and Chirurgical Society entitled "*Notice of a New Anaesthetic Agent as a Substitute for Sulphuric Ether in Surgery and Midwifery*".

John Snow was a remarkable man [13]. At age 14, he commenced studies as one of eight students attending the Medical School of Newcastle-upon-Tyne, at its inception in 1832. He left Newcastle in 1836 and walked 285 miles to London, where he attended lectures at the Westminster Hospital, and at the School of Anatomy founded by William Hunter, the elder brother of John Hunter. He qualified in medicine in 1838, as a Member of the Royal College of Surgeons. To prescribe medicines (which "Barber-Surgeons" were not allowed to do), he also passed the examinations at the Apothecaries Hall. In 1844 he became an MD in London University, and was appointed Lecturer in Forensic Medicine at the Aldersgate School of Medicine for 5 years.

Early in 1847, Snow attended an administration of ether by Robinson, who wrote "I again operated this morning with the most perfect success, in the presence of my friends—Mr Stocks, Mr Snow and Mr Fenney (p16) [12]. Anaesthesia caught Snow's imagination. He applied his mind to improving the administration of ether, soon developing an ether inhaler allowing production of constant saturated concentrations of ether vapour, thus increasing the safety of the procedure. Within the year, he had published "*On the Inhalation of the Vapour of Ether in Surgical Operations*" in which he described five degrees (today we might call them stages) of ether anaesthesia [14]. The anaesthetist might control the level—and safety—of anaesthesia by observing these degrees. Snow was appointed as anaesthetist to St George's Hospital. He also worked with Robert Liston at University College Hospital, and William Fergusson at King's College Hospital. He was the leading anaesthetist of his time, and probably of all time. He performed one of the earliest outcomes studies through a review of reports of deaths arising during anaesthesia, determining that chloroform might cause death by producing "cardiac syncopy". He investigated the effects of several vapours, including bromoform, ethyl bromide and amylene on himself and animals.

Snow developed a rebreathing system containing caustic potash (potassium hydroxide) for carbon dioxide absorption. Experimenting on himself, he showed that rebreathing chloroform present in the expired air prolonged anaesthesia. He found that the production of carbon dioxide during chloroform anaesthesia was decreased, suggesting that chloroform depressed metabolism [15].

By the time of his death in 1858, Snow had administered chloroform to more than 4000 patients with only one death potentially attributable to the agent. Snow administered chloroform to Queen Victoria during the births of Prince Leopold (1853) and Princess Beatrice (1857), deviating from his normal practice by dropping 15 minims (approximately 0.9 ml) of chloroform intermittently onto a handkerchief! Published posthumously in 1858, his book "*On Chloroform and other Anaesthetics*" was an extraordinary scientific treatise for that time [15]. He originated academic anaesthesia in Britain, perchance the world.

Snow had eclectic interests. He is considered the father of epidemiology, largely for his studies on cholera, his suppression of a cholera epidemic in London, and his 1849 book "*On the Mode of Communication of Cholera*" [16].

Clover succeeded Snow as the leading scientific and practical anaesthetist. Like Snow, Clover was primarily concerned with safety, and developed methods and apparatus for the delivery of precise concentrations of both chloroform and ether. In 1871, he claimed to have given 11,000 anaesthetics without a death, 7000 of them with chloroform. In the same year he showed that nitrous oxide's anaesthetic effect was not the result of asphyxia. In 1876, he introduced the nitrous oxide/ether sequence that evolved as the most widely used approach to anaesthesia for the next half-century [12].

By the last quarter of the century, formal appointments of anaesthetists were made in many teaching hospitals, but anaesthetics were largely administered by general medical practitioners. There were no official training programmes or specialised qualifications. Two more British anaesthetists emerged as successors to Snow and Clover. Sir Frederic Hewitt (1857–1916) was appointed Lecturer on anaesthetics at the London Hospital in 1886. He advocated instruction in anaesthesia to medical students, and persuaded the Government of the day to draft a Bill to prevent anaesthetic administration by unqualified people. In 1892, JFW Silk published a plea for anaesthesia to be an essential part of the medical curriculum [17].

We remember Dudley Buxton (1855–1931), anaesthetist at University College Hospital, for the first British textbook (1888) on "*Anaesthetics: their uses and administration*" [18], and for popularising the use of premedication with opiates, atropine or hyoscine, alone or in combination. However, his major academic contribution was to advocate for compulsory inclusion of the study of anaesthetics in the medical curriculum (1901) [19]. He argued that there should be a course of lectures during the final clinical year, and that every student should witness anaesthesia on at least 50 occasions, and have administered at least 12 anaesthetics before qualifying. Following representations to the Medico-Legal Society and the General Medical Council (GMC), *The Anaesthetics Bill* was proposed to the House of Commons. The first clause read that: "no person should be registered under the Medical Acts… unless he shall have produced evidence that he has received theoretical and practical instruction in the administration of anaesthetics" [20]. The *Anaesthetics Bill* never became law, but after another 3 years, the GMC added anaesthetics as the 16th subject that every medical course and examination should contain; not only for every university-based medical school, but also for the joint qualifications of the Royal Colleges of Physicians and Surgeons, and for that of the Society of Apothecaries. Up to 1922, the whole of Ireland was part of the United Kingdom, and thus these criteria also applied to Irish medical schools. At that time, almost every doctor might be required, as a house officer (intern), to administer anaesthetics.

The Twentieth Century

Surgeons and anaesthetists made innovations during the first thirty years of the twentieth century. Arthur Barker (1850–1916), Professor of the Principles and Practice of Surgery at University College Hospital, London, used beta-eucaine for infiltration analgesia in 1899; and pioneered spinal anaesthesia in Britain, controlling the level of blockade by using glucose to alter baricity. He used Stovaine (amylocaine), a synthetic local anaesthetic developed to avoid the toxic effects of cocaine, for spinal anaesthesia [21].

The introduction of continuous flow anaesthetic machines by Henry Boyle in the 1930s, popularized the co-administration of nitrous oxide and oxygen with ether or chloroform. Sir Ivan Magill (1888–1986; Fig. 30.1) and Stanley Rowbotham (1890–1979) worked with plastic surgeon Sir Harold Gillies, at Sidcup Hospital, treating servicemen injured during World War I. They developed tracheal insufflation of warm ether from a Shipway apparatus through one of two gum-elastic tubes (gas entering via one tube and exiting via the other) passed with the aid of laryngoscopy. Subsequently

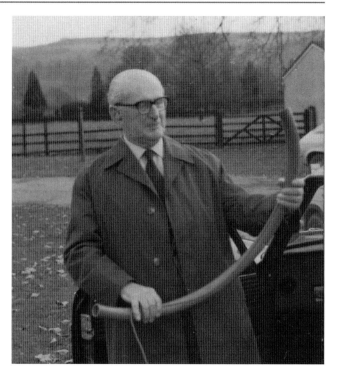

Fig. 30.1 Sir Ivan "Paddy" Magill (1888–1986) holding an equine version of his tracheal tube

Magill developed mineralised rubber tracheal tubes, and later endobronchial tubes and bronchus blockers to advance the feasibility and safety of thoracic surgery. Rowbotham developed the art of blind nasal-tracheal intubation.

Magill contributed to academic anaesthesia and the recognition of anaesthesia as a specialty through the founding of the Association of Anaesthetists of Great Britain and Ireland (AAGBI) in 1932, and through the inauguration of the Diploma in Anaesthesia (DA) in 1935, under the auspices of the Anaesthetic Section of the Royal Society of Medicine [12]. Other hospitals appointed specialist anaesthetists, but, even so, only 50 existed in the whole of the UK. Numerous hospitals employed general practitioners, many with limited training, as anaesthetists for general surgical procedures and for the administration of ethyl chloride or nitrous oxide for dental extractions.

Between 1901 and 1925, many universities established honorary or part-time anaesthetic appointments, mostly within surgical departments, to enable the teaching of undergraduates.

The Chair of Anaesthetics at the University of Oxford [22]

Oxford had no clinical medical school in the early 1930s. The then Minister of Health, Neville Chamberlain, (yes the same Neville Chamberlain who in September 1938 and as

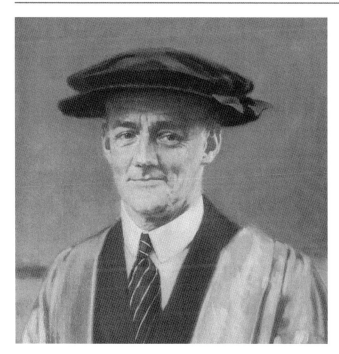

Fig. 30.2 Lord Nuffield (William Morris) (1877–1963), philanthropist and benefactor of anaesthesia, in academic regalia

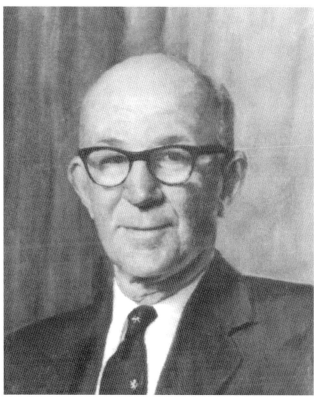

Fig. 30.3 Sir Robert Macintosh (1897–1989), the first Nuffield Department of Anaesthetics chair

Prime Minister returned from Munich stating "I believe it is peace for our time") consulted with the Regius Professor of Medicine, Farquhar Buzzard, about the desirability of setting up a postgraduate medical school. Douglas Veale, who had been Chamberlain's private secretary, moved to Oxford to become the University Registrar. Hugh Cairns, an Australian neurosurgeon who had trained with Harvey Cushing in Boston, was interested in this concept and wrote two extensive memoranda proposing a research-orientated medical school at Oxford. Buzzard, Veale and Cairns targeted Lord Nuffield for support. Nuffield, as William Morris, had developed a major automobile industry in Oxford and became one of Britain's great philanthropists. (Fig. 30.2) Nuffield initially offered the University £ 1.25 million to establish "*a school where professors and their assistants may pursue their research in clinical medicine unhampered by the claims of private practice or the routine teaching of students*" [22]. In a presidential address to the 104th Annual Meeting of the British Medical Association at Oxford in 1936, Buzzard stated that "*The task of the heads of medical research departments, who must all be recognized leaders in their field, would be to link observations at the bedside with those made in laboratories*" (translational research is not new!) [23].

Buzzard and Veale proposed that the grant be used to fund professors and departments of medicine, surgery, and obstetrics (and gynaecology). However, as a young man Nuffield had experienced problems following general anaesthesia for dental extractions, and was adamant that he wanted a Chair

of Anaesthetics as part of his endowment. In August 1936, Cairns wrote to Howard Florey (Professor of Pathology, representing pre-clinical disciplines) that a Department of Anaesthetics would be: "*quite feasible—to serve primarily as a training ground which could turn out all the young anaesthetists of the country at large, and probably many from the Dominions*". Meeting with Nuffield's secretary, Veale "*...wondered whether Nuffield really meant a Professorship, not a Readership, suggesting that anaesthetics might not be a subject of professorial status*" [22]. Veale also proposed allocating a lower salary for this position, £ 1500 compared with £ 2000 for the other professors. Nuffield increased his gift to £ 2 million provided that a Chair of Anaesthetics was included, and that Robert (later Sir Robert) Macintosh, a New Zealander, would be appointed to the chair (Fig. 30.3). The University reluctantly agreed to Nuffield's proposal, in doing so establishing anaesthesia as an academic subject, and creating the first Chair of Anaesthetics in Britain, the British Commonwealth, and Europe [22].

The Oxford hospitals created three major problems for the four new Nuffield professors, especially Macintosh. Who controlled a hospital service; who controlled fees from paying patients, and who controlled secondary costs to the hospital? After many discussions Macintosh won dominion in that " *... the Honorary Anaesthetists had no* *objection to Professor Macintosh being in general charge over the Department ...*" (p35) [22]. The Oxford hospitals insisted that the newly appointed Nuffield professors, and their medical assistants, would not undertake private practice, and the University introduced a £ 500 per annum bonus to a Nuffield Professor who did not accept fees from private patients. The third issue concerned the building of new departmental accommodations for the Nuffield professors. The Departments of Surgery (Hugh Cairns) and Obstetrics (Chassar Moir) controlled new wards and operating facilities, but Macintosh endured a prolonged battle for suitable accommodation. From the outset, and throughout the war years, Macintosh's department, now named the *Nuffield Department of Anaesthetics* (NDA) was housed in a temporary structure on the roof of another hospital building. The final purpose-built department came into being after Macintosh's retirement in 1965!

During the war years (1939–1945), the NDA had a heavy teaching commitment, training postgraduate specialists to achieve the new Diploma in Anaesthesia, and thereby supply the burgeoning demand for anaesthetists in the armed forces. Macintosh was an Air Commodore in the Royal Air Force and travelled widely to ensure that equipment for that service was up to standard. During the war years, the NDA developed a submarine escape apparatus using CO_2 absorption, and studied the physiological effects of flying at high altitude (up to 40,000 feet). A novel, but unsuccessful, study designed a system that would allow Winston Churchill to breathe oxygen at altitudes greater than 8000 feet while smoking the cigars to which he was habituated [22]. Edgar Pask (1912–1966) allowed himself to be anaesthetized and subject to ventilatory arrest by forced hyperventilation with 15 % ether in order to test the efficacy of various methods of resuscitation. To test the efficacy of 17 types of life-jackets, Pask allowed himself to be anaesthetized, have his trachea intubated, and then to be submerged under water on four separate occasions [22].

Macintosh's main contribution to research in anaesthesia was to develop, in co-operation with Hans Epstein, and Morris Motors (Nuffield's factory), an accurate portable draw-over vaporizer for ether (the Oxford vaporizer). The vaporizer allowed delivery of controllable ether vapour concentrations and thus safer anaesthesia, to be administered under field (armed forces) conditions, with or without added oxygen [24]. The principles of the Oxford vaporiser were later applied to the design, in 1956, of the EMO (Epstein, Macintosh, Oxford) vaporiser, and a subsequent miniature vaporizer, both robust and reliable devices. They formed the basis of future vaporizer designs. Macintosh also designed a laryngoscope blade that quickly gained worldwide acceptance.

Was Anaesthesia Safe?

In 1943, George Godber, Chief Medical Officer of Health (CMO), surveyed hospital services, finding that "virtually all the anaesthetists were also in general practice [25]. Unstated was the conclusion that the resulting occasional anaesthetist must compromise safety.

Immediately After World War II

Soon after World War II, four more universities created Departments of Anaesthesia. In 1946, the University of Bristol created a department headed by Ronald Woolmer (as a Senior Lecturer, later upgraded to Reader). In 1957, Woolmer was appointed Professor in the Research Department of Anaesthesia at the Royal College of Surgeons in London. Edgar Pask, became a Reader in the University of Newcastle-upon-Tyne in 1947, and full Professor in 1949. William Mushin (1910–1993), previously First Assistant in the NDA, was appointed Director of Anaesthesia to the Cardiff group of hospitals. In 1952 he was elected to a Chair of Anaesthesia in the Welsh National School of Medicine. T Cecil Gray (1913–2008) gained an MD in 1947, and was appointed Head of Department (Reader) in the University of Liverpool (Fig. 30.4). He was subsequently granted a Personal Chair in 1959. Gray and his Liverpool colleagues (Halton, G Jackson Rees, Utting, and Robinson) popularized the use of curare (d-tubocurarine) in British anaesthesia, and created the 'Liverpool technique' based on nitrous oxide anaesthesia, muscle relaxation induced by curare, and manually controlled ventilation [26]. Shafer, who argues that Gray's real innovation was that of balanced anaesthesia with a combination of drugs rather than a single inhalational agent, recently reviewed Gray's enormous contribution to modern anaesthetic practice [27].

Open cardiac surgery, mostly in adults, was made possible in 1952–1953 by pump-oxygenators (either the Melrose design developed at the Hammersmith Hospital, or the American Mayo-Gibbon machine), or profound hypothermia as pioneered at the Westminster Hospital. Induced hypotension techniques were developed to facilitate neurosurgery and plastic surgery. In the late 1940s, John Gillies (1895–1976) in Edinburgh, pioneered total spinal anaesthesia for the surgical treatment of hypertension by thoraco-lumbar sympathectomy, achieving drastic decreases in blood pressure (to less than 50 mm Hg) [28]. Subsequently, ganglion-blocking and adrenoceptor-blocking drugs combined with head-up tilt made the process potentially much safer [29].

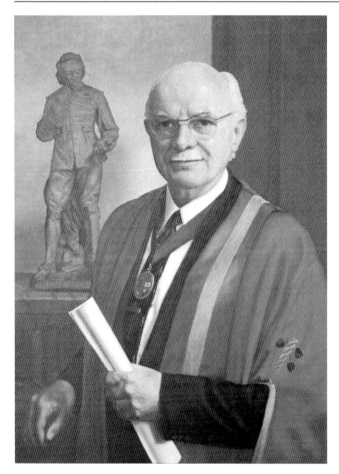

Fig. 30.4 T. Cecil Gray (1913–2008) in his robes as Dean of the Royal College of Anaesthetists

1948–1988

The Faculty of Anaesthetists of the Royal College of Surgeons of England

After World War II, academic aspects of anaesthesia progressed on several fronts. The Goodenough Committee proposed that medical schools should create clinical academic departments, and that universities should support whole-time staff [30]. Representations by the Association of Anaesthetists to the Spens Committee led to the recognition that anaesthetists should be accorded equal status (and thus pay) with other hospital-based specialists [31]. The inauguration of the National Health Service (NHS) in 1948, led to the recognition that the number of suitably qualified consultant (specialist) anaesthetists was too small to staff the major hospitals of the country. The specialty moved rapidly to upgrade the Diploma of Anaesthesia (DA), then organised jointly by the Royal Colleges of Physicians and Surgeons, to a two-part examination: Primary (basic sciences) and Final (clinical anaesthesia). The Association of Anaesthetists requested the Royal College of Surgeons to establish a Faculty

of Anaesthetists. The Board of the resulting new Faculty met on 23 March 1948 under its first Dean, Archibald Marston. It was considered that a proposed Fellowship (1952) of the new Faculty (FFARCS) "would greatly enhance the academic status of the Faculty as well as being a means to encourage anaesthetists to attain the highest distinction in their speciality". The GMC now considered anaesthesia to be a postgraduate subject, and consequently omitted the teaching of anaesthetics from the undergraduate curriculum in 1947, a regressive step that was corrected in the 1980s.

The training of specialist anaesthetists, which increasingly included intensive care, followed the pattern taken by other medical and surgical specialties. After internship, trainees occupied training posts in NHS hospitals, at senior house officer and then registrar status. The NHS assumed responsibility for trainee employment, while the Faculty (of Anaesthetists) controlled the setting and supervision of standards of training, and of examinations. After passing the final examination, trainees progressed to Senior Registrar posts for 3 to 5 years advanced training, after which they could apply for NHS consultant posts. Senior Registrars were encouraged to spend time abroad, expanding their research and clinical training, mostly in North America, Europe, Australia or New Zealand.

In the UK and the Republic of Ireland, unlike other countries in Europe, universities were not responsible for medical specialist training. The relevance of this statement will become evident later in this essay.

During its first forty years, the Faculty of Anaesthetists was accommodated in the Royal College of Surgeons, and the organization of its parent, the Royal College of Surgeons, largely determined the organization of the Faculty. Although the Faculty became financially independent, it enjoyed close support and good relations with its parent College. The Faculty had three major responsibilities: postgraduate (specialist) education, examination for the primary and final fellowship, and the setting of professional standards in anaesthesia, intensive care and, increasingly, treatment of severe and chronic pain.

The Faculty of Anaesthetists of the Royal College of Surgeons in Ireland, established in 1959, developed along almost identical lines, and until 1995 there was a reciprocal recognition of training standards and examinations between the two Faculties.

So, as the sixties began, academic anaesthesia was advancing well. Between 1960 and 1971, 15 new university departments headed by chairs of anaesthesia emerged. Britain differed from Germany and many other European countries, where a higher degree (doctorate, Habilitation) was an absolute requirement for advancement to an academic chair. John Nunn at Leeds (Fig. 30.5), and Alex Crampton Smith (Fig. 30.6) (as Macintosh's successor) at Oxford were the

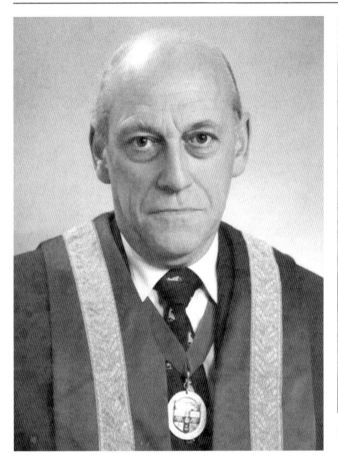

Fig. 30.5 John Nunn in his robes as Dean of the Royal College of Anaesthetists

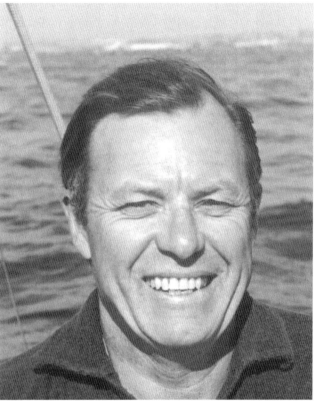

Fig. 30.6 Alex Crampton Smith (1917–2010) on the high seas

great facilitators of scientific research, and sought to raise the calibre of the specialty by promoting research doctorates (PhD and MD). NHS hospitals increasingly supported Intensive Care, and a few university anaesthesia departments (Leeds, Oxford, Glasgow, Royal Postgraduate Medical School—Hammersmith) concentrated research efforts on this new sub-specialty.

Anaesthetic Research Society and Publication of Research

The Anaesthetic Research Group began in 1958 as a discussion forum for research in progress, rather than completed work [32]. Initially some established professors (Macintosh, Gray, Mushin, and Pask) were not supportive, but by 1967, the group meetings attracted substantial pre-publication presentations of research from both university and NHS departments. The group was reformed as the Anaesthetic Research Society in 1968. Two anaesthesia journals, the *British Journal of Anaesthesia* (founded in 1923), and *Anaesthesia* (founded in 1946), contributed enormously to the development of clinical and research aspects of anaesthesia and in-

tensive care during this period, by supplying a distinguished print forum for the work of investigators in anaesthesia. The *Lancet* and BMJ only accepted articles of general interest to medical practitioners, and specialist journals such as the *Journal of Physiology, Journal of Applied Physiology,* and *Cardiovascular Research* were relevant to only a handful of researchers.

Drug Development

The success of the pharmaceutical industry in developing new drugs, greatly influenced four categories of progress in clinical anaesthesia: inhalational agents, opioid analgesics, intravenous anaesthetics, and muscle relaxants. Working at Imperial Chemical Industries (ICI), near Manchester, in the early 1950s, Suckling [33] and Raventós [34] developed halothane. Introduced into clinical practice in the late 1950s [35, 36], and delivered with a calibrated vaporizer, the Fluotec, halothane rapidly replaced the flammable anaesthetics, diethyl ether and cyclopropane. Although halothane caused hypotension, and indeed was used specifically for induced hypotension [29], this was widely considered to be safe because it had been described as a vasodilator [36]. However, studies in animals [37] and humans [38] showed that halothane produced a concentration-dependent depression of the myocardium.

In 1961, Tunstall [39] described the first use of a pre-mixed gas, nitrous oxide (50%) and oxygen (50%), for analgesia during childbirth. This development was to be of considerable benefit in obstetrics, and also in accident and emergency medicine.

Paul Janssen, in Belgium, developed a new series of synthetic opioids modelled on pethidine (meperidine). They were initially introduced in the UK in 1964, to add to the technique of neuroleptanalgesia [40], a technique combining an opioid (phenoperidine) with a neuroleptic drug (haloperidol) to produce a 'vegetative' state that could be augmented with nitrous oxide anaesthesia. Subsequently, fentanyl (1965), alfentanil (1976), sufentanil (1976) and remifentanil (1993) became widely used as the analgesic components to supplement 'balanced' inhalation anaesthesia and, from the mid-sixties onwards, of total intravenous anaesthesia.

Although thiopentone had been the standard induction agent, methohexitone and Althesin became popular in the UK and Ireland. Althesin, a combination of the steroids alphaxolone (the main effective anaesthetic) and alphadolone, solubilized in Cremophor EL, was developed by Glaxo Ltd (Uxbridge, Middlesex) in 1972. It was widely used as an induction agent and later as a continuous infusion [41, 42]. The rapid recovery from single or multiple doses of Althesin was a great advantage over thiopentone. The latter rapidly declined in popularity in the UK, whereas in the US it remained the main agent for induction of anaesthesia. Althesin was withdrawn from human use following reports of complement-mediated anaphylactoid reactions to Cremophor EL [43]. Glaxo Ltd subsequently developed a water soluble steroid anaesthetic, Minaxolone [44], but teratogenicity issues in animals caused it to be withdrawn. Finally, in 1980, Glen and colleagues at ICI Pharmaceuticals, near Manchester, developed a new intravenous anaesthetic: di-isopropyl phenol [45]. This lipid-soluble anaesthetic was also initially solubilized in Cremophor EL, but concerns that anaphylactic reactions might occur [46] led to its reformulation in a lipid emulsion [47]. Released in 1986, propofol, became the most popular agent world-wide for intravenous induction of anaesthesia, for the sedative component of total intravenous anaesthesia, and for continuous sedation in intensive care.

In 1967, Baird and Reid reported on the clinical use of pancuronium, a new muscle relaxant developed by Organon Laboratories, of Cambridge [48]. Pancuronium became widely used as a medium duration neuromuscular blocking agent (NMB), that had mild vagolytic effects on the cardiovascular system. In 1981, atracurium was released by the Wellcome Research Laboratories, of Beckenham, Kent, as a novel NMB that underwent spontaneous degradation by the Hofmann reaction [49, 50]. Cis-atracurium, a stereoisomer of atracurium, has largely superseded the parent drug.

The Eighties

Archie Brain designed, and in 1983 introduced, a remarkable advance in airway management, the laryngeal mask airway (LMA) [51]. This simple device evolved into the most widely used new airway since the introduction of the oral airway and tracheal tube. Although the main use of the mask has been in anaesthesia, it has also been applied in emergency medicine, in situations where manipulation of the head or neck is difficult because of potential cervical spine injury, or during rescue in confined spaces. Modifications include channels for gastric suction (LMA ProSeal™, LMA Supreme™), and for guiding endotracheal tubes into the larynx (ILMA—Intubating Laryngeal Mask Airway) and LMA-Fastrach™ [52].

A pilot study by Lunn and Mushin of mortality associated with anaesthesia [53] led to the initiation of a joint venture between anaesthetists and surgeons and the publication in 1987 of the first report of the Confidential Enquiry into Perioperative Deaths (CEPOD) [54]. This initial report quoted a mortality, within 30 days of surgery, of 0.7% in a cohort of half a million patients, with more than half the deaths in patients over 75 years old. The authors recommended that all anaesthetists and surgeons should audit their personal and departmental clinical practices, to enhance quality assurance for patient care; and that they should review consultants' supervision of trainees. NCEPOD (N for National) continued on an annual review basis, evaluating perioperative deaths in a range of patient age groups or surgical interventions. During the first 11 years, the number of deaths reported was fairly consistent (range: 18,132 to 20,442 deaths per annum), but the number of deaths attributed to anaesthesia decreased progressively and is now considered to be between 1 and 2 deaths per million anaesthetics. In 2004 the same acronym, NCEPOD, changed to mean National Confidential Enquiry into Patient Outcome and Death, thus expanding the objectives. A similar system had been established in 1952, as the Confidential Enquiry into Maternal Deaths (CEMD) and the Confidential Enquiries into Stillbirths and deaths in Infancy (CESDI) [55].

The most recent (2011) NCEPOD report [56] compared data on mortality for patients undergoing major non-cardiac surgery in the UK and US in comparable hospitals over the same time period. Applying the P-POSSUM (Portsmouth modified Physiological and Operative Severity Score for the enUmeration of Mortality and morbidity) index, the authors concluded that patients in the UK with a predicted 0–5% mortality risk had an actual mortality (2.5%) that was eight times higher than their counterparts in the US (0.3%). A critique of this report [57] pointed out that the US spends significantly more (15.3%) of its GDP on health care than does the UK (8.2%), and has nearly 6 times the number of intensive care beds than does the UK. Their conclusion that "…the NHS needs to invest in more critical care beds to improve outcomes in high risk surgical patients." was tempered in an accompanying editorial [58] which identified several strategies that could, with economy, improve outcomes.

Changes in Governance and Funding of Academia

From 1981 to 1985, Margaret Thatcher's Conservative government, driven by Keith Joseph, the Secretary of State for Education, greatly decreased funding of UK universities, a process previously regulated by the University Grants Committee (UGC) based on quinquennial estimates of financial needs from each university. Concurrently, Alex Jarratt, then chairman of the Committee of Vice-Chancellors and Principals, produced a report [59], responding to the growing demand from Thatcher for universities (and the NHS) to demonstrate efficiency, and accountability for public funds. Jarratt shocked many academics by his perception that universities should be seen as business enterprises in which students were customers. Academics were viewed as shop-floor deliverers of education, subject to performance indicators, rather than as a self-governing collegial group seeking to expand knowledge [60, 61]. The organizational functions of universities were viewed as requiring dedicated business managers, with a transfer of these roles from academics to such managers. The report thus laid the ground for the increase of "managerialism in the academy" [62] and it has become explicit government policy that university staff are paid to help their employers compete against sister institutions, rather than to serve the more traditional roles of university teachers. The adoption of the report led to the abolition of academic tenure.

In 1986, the government redistributed funding previously paid directly to universities. Funds were now directed to research councils, such as the Medical Research Council (MRC) and the Science Research Council (SRC), and University staff could then bid for grants from the research councils. Thus a substantial proportion of the funding of their university would depend on the quality of their grant applications. Another important consequence was the introduction in 1986, by the UGC, of the Research Assessment Exercise (RAE). Submissions from each subject area (or unit of assessment) were ranked by a subject specialist peer review panel. The rankings were used to inform the allocation of quality-weighted research funding that each higher education institution received from their national funding council. A decrease of one rank point (on a five point scale), by one or more small clinical academic departments, could decrease university funding by £ 1.5 million over a 4 year period. Most universities could only absorb such a loss by not reappointing academic staff.

For small clinical academic departments such as anaesthesia, these changes imposed major disadvantages. Firstly,

compared with their non-clinical colleagues, most clinical academics contracted to work 50 % of their time in the National Health Service (NHS), limiting the time assignable to research and the writing of grant applications. Secondly, for seemingly equivalent quality applications from academic anaesthetists versus those from other specialties, anaesthestists fared poorly in their applications to MRC or SRC, or the Wellcome Trust. In 1988 Professor Rosen, as the first President of the College of Anaesthetists, invited the MRC secretary, D Davies to explain why the MRC was so parsimonious in their support of anaesthesia research. To paraphrase his reply: heart disease, cancer, asthma, tuberculosis, malaria and AIDs kill millions of patients—anaesthesia may kill one in a million! Eight years later, the new Chief Executive of the MRC, George Radda, gave the Royal College of Anaesthetists much the same answer.

The Faculty of Anaesthetists Finds a New Home

During this period of academic upheaval, most anaesthetists believed that, despite excellent working relationships between the Faculty of Anaesthetists and their parent Royal College of Surgeons (RCS), the specialty needed independence and equal status with other specialities that had become, or were becoming, Royal Colleges. With the consent and support of the RCS, officers of the Faculty engaged with the Privy Council to seek a constitutional pathway to achieve their aims. The solution, of a College (of Anaesthetists) within a College (RCS), seemed to be a satisfactory arrangement that would allow the former to maintain its functional and geographical links with the surgeons. Thus the College of Anaesthetists came into being in 1988. However, further discussions with the Privy Council revealed that the concept of a 'Royal College within a Royal College' was not compatible with the charter of the RCS. It was therefore decided to petition the Privy Council to create a charter for an independent Royal College of Anaesthetists (RCoA).

The Nineties and Noughties (1990–2010)

The Royal College of Anaesthetists (RCoA) was granted its charter (Fig. 30.7) in 1992 and occupied premises in Russell Square, London until 2002 when the College acquired larger premises in Red Lion Square (Fig. 30.8). In 1996, the RCoA sought to create a Faculty of Intensive Care Medicine but found little support from the various Colleges of Physicians and Surgeons, and settled eventually for an Inter-Collegiate Board. Continuing discussions over the ensuing fourteen years led to creation of the Inter-Collegiate Faculty of Intensive Care Medicine [63]. The RCoA also established an independent Faculty of Pain Medicine.

Similarly, in Ireland, a College of Anaesthetists was initially created within the RCSI, but in 1998 the College

Fig. 30. 7 Charter of the Royal College of Anaesthetists (1992)

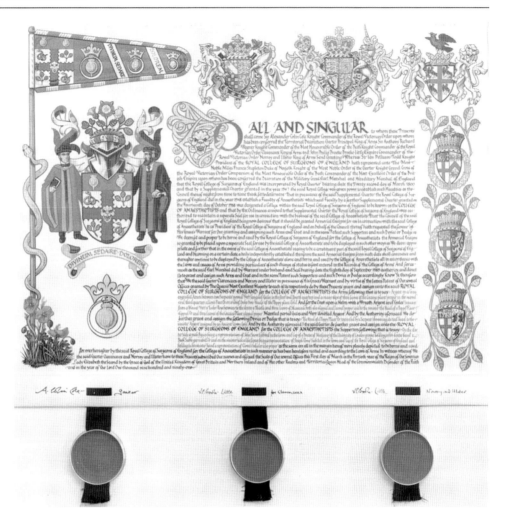

(CAI) became independent, and later also created an inter-Collegiate Faculty of Intensive Care Medicine, and its own Faculty of Pain Medicine.

Like other Colleges, during the 1990s, the RCoA had to respond to the directives of the Council of Europe. Firstly, changes were required in the way that anaesthesia in the UK recognised 'specialists' so as to conform to Council Directive 93/16/EEC 'to facilitate the free movement of doctors and the mutual recognition of their diplomas, certificates and other evidence of formal qualifications' [64]. In the UK and the Republic of Ireland, trainees had acquired the status of 'Consultant' as the final point of training, whereas in most other European countries, a doctor became a 'Specialist' after a shorter period of training. The European Specialist Medical Qualifications Order 1995; No 3208 [65] created a new system in which, at the end of a structured training programme overseen by the relevant Royal College, the Specialist Training Authority (STA) granted a Certificate of Completion of Specialist Training (CCST). The STA was a new regulatory body set up by, and responsible to, the government; as an expedient alternative to empowering the GMC for this purpose.

Secondly, the European Working Time Directive 93/104/EEC [64] required that by 2003, trainees should not work for more than 56 hours per week, and that by 2009, they should not work for more than 48 hours per week. This directive, initially promulgated in 1998, paralleled a general directive aimed at workers in many industries. It was perceived by the BMA and by the Royal Colleges to be incompatible with the traditional programme of training in which trainees spent a substantial number of hours each week 'on call', and profited from the experience. The Temple report [66] concluded that "… high quality training can be delivered in 48 hours per week, but not where trainees: have a major role in out-of-hours services; are poorly supervised; (and) have limited access to learning opportunities". In order to comply with these requirements, consultants in specialties such as surgery, obstetrics and anaesthesia, have had to take on night call duties in place of trainees. Consequently trainees have had their exposure to emergency anaesthesia substantially decreased. Nevertheless, a recent study [67] in a London teaching hospital concluded that "High quality anaesthetic training is still possible in the UK despite reductions in junior doctors' hours".

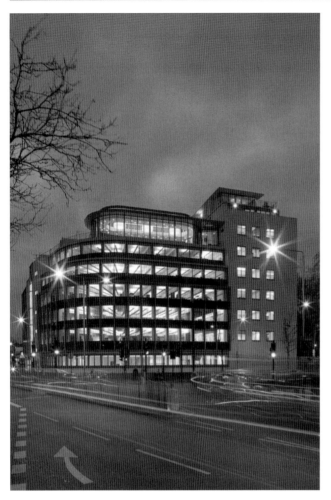

Fig. 30. 8 Present home to the Royal College of Anaesthetists, London

The Evolution of Specialist Training and Academia in Anaesthesia

As noted earlier, unlike the US, Canada and most of Europe, universities in the UK and Ireland have no direct responsibility for training specialist doctors; they exist primarily to teach undergraduates (including students preparing for first degrees in medicine, dentistry and veterinary medicine), and to prosecute research (including postgraduate research-orientated degrees such as MSc, PhD, and MD). University teachers in medical and dental subjects are appointed according to the importance of their specialist subject in the undergraduate curriculum, and their research profile. During the 1950s to 1970s, universities usually paid all grades of academic anaesthetists from UGC funds. However, with the growing importance of specialist training, some Regional Health Authorities, seeking to improve the quality of basic science education in certain specialties, funded university lectureships and chairs. In 1997, in preparing the inaugural Macintosh Lecture in Oxford, I consulted my British academic colleagues and found that 50% of professors and readers, and 75% of senior lecturers (all at NHS consultant equivalence) were paid by the NHS! Nunn produced similar data in his 1999 review

[68]. Fig. 30.9 shows the expansion of academic departments of anaesthesia headed by professors, from 1937 to 2000. These foregoing changes prompted many universities to distance themselves from their responsibilities for small clinical departments, using the savings to enhance non-medical subjects. All the while, the NHS demanded a greater role of clinical academics in the education of specialist trainees.

During the 1970s and onwards, the provision of specialist training was the responsibility of the NHS; co-ordinated for the Government by Postgraduate Deans, appointed by the Regional Health Authorities that were responsible for healthcare on a geographical basis. Universities initially played host to the Postgraduate Deans (often granting them personal professorships) and their Deanery offices, although the deans drew their salaries from the NHS (Department of Health) and not from the universities (Department for Education and Science). During the past ten years, there has been a functional and geographical detachment of most Postgraduate Deans and Deaneries from Universities, further undermining the health:education sector partnership. Medical Schools have played a decreasing role in postgraduate training, reflecting their emphasis on undergraduate education and research, the latter driven by the three-yearly RAE.

One problem bedevilling the relationships between successive governments (tasked with staffing the NHS) and the Royal Colleges (tasked with maintaining standards of training and clinical practice), has been the disparity between the number of doctors in training and the number required to provide clinical services on a 24-hour basis. In 2004, following national devolution (transfer of certain powers from the UK parliament to regional governments), the four UK Health Ministers (for England, Wales, Scotland and Northern Ireland) responded to a paper by the CMO, Liam Donaldson, entitled "*Unfinished business: Proposal for reform of the SHO grade*", by establishing a new system for specialist training [69]. The future shape of foundation, specialist and general training programmes was enshrined in the document "*Modernising Medical Careers (MMC)—The Next Steps*" [70]. The essence of MMC would be a two-year foundation training common to all specialties, followed by 5 to 7 year fixed-term specialist training appointments (FTSTAs) that were competency-based and 'run-through', (Fig. 30.10). The RCoA welcomed the changes and rapidly adapted their training programmes to the new outline.

Unfortunately, MMC was linked to MTAS (Medical Training Application Service), a computerised centralised admission system set up to enable recruitment into the first year of the new First Specialist Training year (ST1 in Fig. 30.10). This scheme was intended to be similar to the National Resident Matching Program in the USA. However, from early 2007 there were reports of technical problems with MTAS and evidence of unacceptable variation in the individuals selected for interview, together with evidence that doctors who previously would have been regarded

Fig. 30.9 Schematic of the expansion of departments of anaesthesia headed by professors in UK universities in decades from 1937 to 2000. Each small rectangle represents a professorial department. In the list of departments only the name of the initial professor is given, except where more than one professor was appointed (mainly for subjects, such as physics, related to anaesthesia). One academic department was merged with another within the University of Glasgow. Individual professors were funded either by HEFCE (Higher Education Funding Council for England and Wales)—open rectangles, or by the NHS through Regional Health Authorities

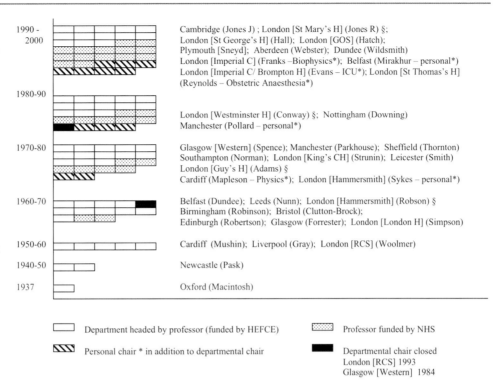

Fig. 30.10 Schematic of the process of specialist medical training since the introduction of "Modernising Medical Careers" in 2007. Letters A to E in circles represent the 5 policy instruments of MMC. The scheme differs from the previous process in that (1) F1 and F2 replace the single year of medical/surgical internship with a 2 year foundation programme for all doctors; and (2) Specialist Training (ST1 to ST 7) is now a run-through appointment that does not require periodic re-appointment in intermittent grades. The number of trainees in each specialty will be based on predicted manpower requirements for the relevant specialty as agreed between the Royal Colleges and the Department of Health.

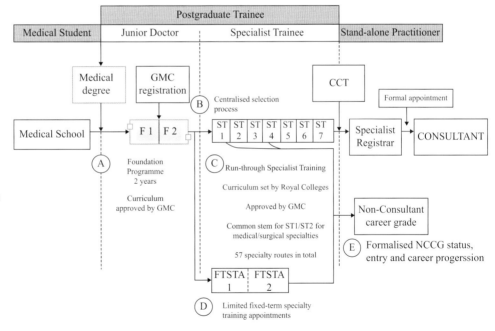

as first-class candidates were not being short-listed. That MTAS was a disaster became evident later in 2007, provoking the government to establish yet another inquiry led by John Tooke. The report—"Aspiring to Excellence" was scathing and recommended corrective action on eight major issues in MMC [71].

A sub-committee of MMC, chaired by Mark Walport, Chairman of the Wellcome Trust was tasked with reviewing what was described as "... *the perilous state of academ-*

ic medicine and dentistry in the UK.", and recommending processes for training clinical academics in line with the main MMC recommendations. The report [72] started by identifying three barriers for potential clinical academic trainees:

1. Lack of both a clear route of entry and a transparent career structure
2. Lack of flexibility in the balance of clinical and academic training
3. Shortage of properly structured and supported posts on completion of training.

The core proposal of the report was to ensure that:

> *"dedicated academic training programmes are developed in strong host environments, in partnerships between universities and local NHS Trusts and Deaneries"*, and that *"substantial efforts are made to develop academic training programmes in those specialties that have been subject to decline in their academic activity"*. Additionally, a National Institute of Health Research (NIHR) was created, *"in which the NHS supports outstanding individuals, working in world class facilities, conducting leading edge research focused on the needs of patients and the public. The NHS reputation for international excellence is growing as it gains recognition for being the preferred host for collaborative and multi-centred research in the public interest in partnership with and for industry."*[73]

In addition to increasing problems on the training front, the Academy of Medical Sciences perceived an impending crisis in academic medicine in general, especially in anaesthesia [74]. The RCoA commissioned a review by a strategist (J Pandit) who was appointed to work with the College's Academic & Research Committee chaired by JAW Wildsmith. A central tenet of Pandit's Strategy Report [75] was that *"… academic anaesthesia is an important and necessary activity: it includes not just research but also teaching, the development of new techniques for patient care, and professional leadership. As such, academic anaesthesia is essential for the future of the specialty as a scientific (and consultant-based) discipline"*. The report identified as the main cause of the crisis, the Research Assessment Exercise (RAE) and its effect on the policies of various universities on the staffing and structure of their medical schools. The report also pointed to the slow adaptation by the Royal Colleges to the changes imposed by government from 1986 onwards. A multidisciplinary campaign by the British Medical Association, the Academy of Medical Sciences, and others, sought to redress the harm done to clinical academic medicine. The Department for Education and Science responded with a consultation document *Reform of Higher Education Research Assessment and Funding* [76] in which they proposed to replace the RAE by 2010, with a simpler metrics-based system derived from various forms of research income other than QR (rather than the existing peer-review system). It is too early to assess the effects on academic anaesthesia of any proposed changes.

Seeking to redress potential damage to academic anaesthesia, and following the recommendations of the Pandit Report, the RCoA, together with the Association of Anaesthetists and the British Journal of Anaesthesia, established a National Institute of Academic Anaesthesia (NIAA). The College envisaged that the NIAA would engage with NIHR and other funding bodies to press the cause of academic anaesthesia. (However, it appears that the NIAA relates to individual researchers, in training or in career positions, rather than with universities or other employing agencies.) In its first report on the years 2008–11 the NIAA reported

that over £ 2million had been sourced and distributed as research grants, a very significant success story. Data in the Pandit report suggested that only six out of 23 UK universities sustained an independent departmental or divisional structure for anaesthesia. Between 2000 and 2012, twelve London medical schools have been merged within a new Collegiate structure (University College, King's College, Imperial College, and Queen Mary College), and there has been a consequent decrease in the number of chairs of anaesthesia compared with the number shown in Fig. 30.9. Despite the restructuring within universities, most Divisions of Anaesthesia have been able to sustain their identity and their clinical links. It is worthy of note that the NDA (now Nuffield Division of Anaesthetics) has been subsumed into a new Nuffield Department of Clinical Neurosciences, and that the current Nuffield Professor of Anaesthetic Science (Irene Tracey) is Director of the Oxford Centre for Magnetic Resonance Imaging of the Brain.

The quantity and quality of research publications can give an estimate of the productivity of academic departments. Feneck and colleagues surveyed the output of original research from British university departments from 1997 to 2006, concluding that there had been a severe progressive decline in research publications from the UK, compared with other parts of the world [77]. A parallel assessment used bibliometric data and indices, to conclude that from 2004 to 2008, UK anaesthetists published research on a par with their European and Canadian peers [78]. Of the 23 UK academic units assessed, four (Oxford, Cambridge, University College and Imperial College, London) contributed 51 % of all publications. A similar preponderance of research output in the US comes from a small fraction of the academic institutions there.

The Future

As the oarsman steers by his wake, we also rely on the history of our specialty to guide our progress into an uncertain future. The RCoA, the CAI and the AAGBI have collaborated to develop "perioperative medicine" as the focus of their activities, encompassing intensive care medicine and pain medicine. The training programmes and curricula developed by RCoA and CAI are now an integral component of the MMT process, and will undoubtedly ensure for the future, a steady supply of fully-trained anaesthetists, intensivists and pain specialists. The specialty of clinical anaesthesia is thriving in the UK and Ireland, and remains attractive to medical students as a springboard to specialist training.

The future of academic anaesthesia in the UK is less certain. Whereas academics, at all grades, were previously primarily anaesthetists, universities are now tending to appoint professors (and related staff) within groups of allied clinical and non-clinical scientists to form university departments with common purposes (for instance neurosciences, cardiovascular sciences and pharmacology). Thus there are greater opportunities to expand the other aspects of perioperative medicine, such as pain management, and intensive care medicine, linking these activities with research in allied areas such as immunology and sepsis. However, there is a danger that such developments may sequester the academicians both geographically and functionally from their clinical counterparts, making it more difficult to maintain a holistic environment for the academic and clinical education of trainees, and thus the future integrity of the specialty.

References

 1 Fulton JF. History of medical education. BMJ. 1953;ii:457–61

 2. Clark G. A history of the Royal College of Physicians vol 1. London: Royal College of Physicians; 1964.

 3. www.rcseng.ac.uk/about/history.

 4. www.rcsed.ac.uk/site/345/default.aspx.

 5. www.rcsi.ie/index.jsp?p=109 & n=156.

 6. Davy H. Researches, chemical and philosophical; Chiefly Concerning Nitrous Oxide. London: J.Johnson; 1800. (also facsimile reproduction, Butterworths, London, 1972).

 7. Smith WDA. A history of nitrous oxide and oxygen anaesthesia. Part II: Davy's researches in relation to inhalation anaesthesia. Br J Anaesth. 1965;37:871–82.

 8. Smith WDA. A history of nitrous oxide and oxygen anaesthesia. Part IV: Hickman and the "introduction of certain gases into the lungs". Br J Anaesth. 1966;38:58–72.

 9. Henry Hill Hickman by W.D.A. Smith.: A. Padfield, E. N. Armitage, F. E. Bennetts and P. M. E. Drury (editors). History of Anaesthesia Society, Sheffield, 2005.

10. Baillie TW. The first European trial of anaesthetic ether: the Dumfries Claim. Br J Anaesth. 1965;37:952–7.

11. Robinson J. A treatise on the inhalation of the vapour of ether. London: Webster; 1847. (Facsimile edition: Eastbourne, Baillière Tindall, 1983).

12. Rushman GB, Davies NJH, Atkinson RS. A short history of anaesthesia—the first 150 years. Oxford: Butterworth Heinemann; 1996. pp. 16, 26, 27, 96.

13. Shepard DAE. John Snow, anaesthetist to a queen and epidemiologist to a nation. A biography. Cornwall: York Point; 1995.

14. Snow J. On the inhalation of the vapour of ether in surgical operations. Reprinted in Br J Anaesth. 1953;25:53–67, 162–9, 253–67, 349–82.

15. Snow J. On chloroform and other anaesthetics. London: John Churchill; 1858.

16. Snow J. On the mode of communication of cholera. 2nd ed. London: John Churchill; 1855.

17. Silk JFW. Anaesthetics a necessary part of the curriculum. Lancet. 1892:1178–80.

18. Buxton DW. Anesthetics: their uses and administration. London: HK Lewis; 1888.

19. Buxton DW. On the advisability of the inclusion of the study of anaesthetics as compulsory subject in the medical curriculum. BMJ. 1901; i:1007–9.

20. Prys-Roberts C, Cooper GM, Hutton P. Anaesthesia in the undergraduate curriculum. Br J Anaesth. 1988;60:355–7.

21. Barker AE. A report on clinical experiences with spinal analgesia in 100 cases. BMJ. 1907;i:665–74.

22. Beinart J. A history of the Nuffield Department of Anaesthetics, Oxford 1937–1987. Oxford: Oxford University Press; 1987. pp. 24, 30, 35, 51, 52–4.

23. Buzzard EF. 'And the Future'. BMJ. 1936;ii:163–6.

24. Epstein HG, Macintosh R. An anaesthetic inhaler with automatic thermocompensation. Anaesthesia. 1956;11:83–8.

25. Godber G. 'The Domesday Book of British hospitals'. Bull Soc Hist Med. 1983;32:4–13.

26. Gray TC, Rees GJ. The role of apnoea in anaesthesia for major surgery BMJ. 1952;ii:891–2.

27. Shafer SL. From d-tubocurarine to sugammadex: the contribution of T. Cecil Gray to modern anaesthetic practice. Br J Anaesth. 2011;107:97–102.

28. Gillies J. Anaesthesia for the surgical treatment of hypertension. Proc Roy Soc Med. 1949;42:295–8.

29. Enderby GEH. Historical review of the practice of deliberate hypotension, Hypotensive anaesthesia. Enderby GEH, editor. London:Churchill Livingstone; 1985.

30. Goodenough W. Report of the Inter-departmental Committee on medical schools. London: HMSO; 1944.

31. Spens W. Report of inter-departmental committee on the remuneration of consultants and specialists. London: HMSO; 1948. (also BMJ 1948; i: 1146).

32. Nunn JF. The first meeting of the Anaesthetic Research Society. Br J Anaesth. 1988;61:639–41.

33. Suckling CW. Some chemical and physical factors in the development of fluothane. Br J Anaesth. 1957;29:466–72.

34. Raventós J. The action of fluothane; a new volatile anaesthetic. Br J Pharmacol. 1956;11:394–410.

35. Bryce-Smith R, O'Brien HD. Fluothane: a non-explosive volatile anaesthetic agent. BMJ. 1956;ii:969–72.

36. Johnstone M. The human cardiovascular response to fluothane anaesthesia. Br J Anaesth. 1956;28:392–410.

37 Prys-Roberts C, Gersh BJ, Baker AB, Reuben SR. The effects of halothane on the interaction between myocardial contractility, aortic impedance and left ventricular performance. I. Theoretical consideration and results. Br J Anaesth. 1972;44:634–49.

38 Prys-Roberts C, Lloyd JW, Fisher A, Kerr JH, Patterson TJS. Deliberate profound hypotension induced with halothane: studies of haemodynamics and pulmonary gas exchange. Br J Anaesth. 1974;46:105–16.

39. Tunstall ME. Obstetric analgesia. The use of a fixed nitrous oxide and oxygen mixture from one cylinder. Lancet. 1961;2:964. (single page article).

40. Edmonds-Seal J, Prys-Roberts C. The pharmacology of drugs used in neuroleptanalgesia. Br J Anaesth. 1970;42:207–16.

41. Sear JW, Prys-Roberts C. Plasma concentrations of alphaxolone during continuous infusion of Althesin. Br J Anaesth. 1979;51:861–5.

42. Sear JW, Prys-Roberts C. Dose-related haemodynamic effects of continuous infusions of Althesin in man. Br J Anaesth. 1979;51:867–73.

43. Watkins J, Appleyard TN, Thornton JA. Immune mediated reactions to Althesin (alphaxolone). Br J Anaesth. 1976;48:881–6.

44. Aveling W, Sear JW, Fitch W, Chang H, Waters A, Cooper GM, Simpson P, Savege TM, Prys-Roberts C, Campbell D. Early clinical evaluation of minaxolone; a new intravenous steroid anaesthetic agent. Lancet. 1979;ii:71–3.

45. Glen JB. Animal pharmacology of ICI 35,868, a new i.v. anaesthetics agent. Br J Anaesth. 1980;52:230P. (single page article).

46. Glen JB, Davies GE, Thomson DS et al. An animal model for the investigation of adverse responses to I.V. anaesthetic agents and their solvents. Br J Anaesth. 1979;51:819–27.

47. Glen JB, Hunter SC. Pharmacology of an emulsion formulation of ICI 35,868. Br J Anaesth. 1984;56:617–26.

48. Baird WLM, Reid AM. The neuromuscular blocking properties of a new steroid compound, pancuronium bromide. Br J Anaesth. 1967;39:775–80.

49. Hughes R, Chappell DJ. The pharmacology of atracurium: a new competitive neuromuscular blocking agent. Br J Anaesth. 1981;53:31–44.

50. Payne JP, Hughes R. Evaluation of atracurium in anaesthetized man. Br J Anaesth. 1981;53:45–54.

51. Brain AIJ. The laryngeal mask—a new concept in airway management. Br J Anaesth. 1983;55:801–5.

52. Baskett PJF, Parr MJA, Nolan JP. The intubating laryngeal mask. Results of a multicentre trial with experience of 500 cases. Anaesthesia. 1998;53:1174–9.

53. Lunn JN, Mushin WW. Mortality associated with anaesthesia. Oxford: Nuffield Provincial Hospitals Trust; 1982.

54. Buck N, Devlin HB, Lunn JN. The report of a confidential enquiry into perioperative deaths. London: The Nuffield Provincial Hospitals Trust and Kings Fund; 1987.

55. Cooper GM. Editorial II. Confidential enquiries into anaesthetic deaths. Br J Anaesth. 2007;99:606–8.

56. National Confidential Enquiry into Patient Outcome and Death. Knowing the Risk: a Review of the Perioperative Care of Surgical Patients. London, NCEPOD, 2011.

57. Wong DJN, Wickham AJ. The UK needs more critical care investment in order to improve peri-operative outcomes. Anaesthesia. 2012;67:541.

58. Goldhill DR, Waldmann CS, Soni N. 'The future ain't what it used to be'—reflections on the future of anaesthesia. Anaesthesia. 2012;67:470–3.

59. Jarratt A. Report of the steering committee for efficiency studies. London: CVCP; 1985.

60. McNay I. From the collegial academy to corporate enterprise: the changing cultures of universities, The Changing University. Schuller T, editor. Buckingham:Open University Press; 1995.

61. Tapper T, Palfreyman D: Oxford and the Decline of the Collegiate Tradition. London: Woburn; 2000.

62. Randle K, Brady N. Managerialism and professionalism in the 'Cinderella Service'. J Vocat Edu Train. 1997;49:121–39.

63. Nightingale P. Development of the faculty of intensive care medicine. Br J Anaesth. 2011;107:5–7.

64. http://europa.eu/legislation_summaries/about/index_en.htm.

65. http://www.legislation.gov.uk/uksi/1995/3208/.

66. Temple J. Time for training. A review of the impact of the European working time directive on the quality of training. London: HMSO; 2010.

67. Paul RG, Bunker N, Fauvel NJ, Cox M. The effect of the European working time directive on anaesthetic working patterns and training. Anaesthesia. 2012;67:951–6.

68. Nunn JF. Development of academic anaesthesia in the UK up to the end of 1998. Br J Anaesth. 1999;83:916–32.

69. http://www.publications.parliament.uk/pa/cm200708/cmselect/cmhealth/25/2505.htm

70. http://www.dh.gov.uk/publications.

71. http://www.mmcinquiry.org.uk/MMC_FINAL_REPORT_REVD_4jan.pdf.

72. http://www.mmc.nhs.uk.

73. http://www.nihr.ac.uk/.

74. Academy of Medical Sciences. Clinical academic medicine in jeopardy: recommendations for change. London: Academy of Medical Sciences; 2002.

75. Pandit JJ. A national strategy for academic anaesthesia. London: Royal College of Anaesthetists; 2005.

76. www.education.gov.uk/.../RAE%20response%20summary%20250107.doc.

77. Feneck RO, Natarajan N, Sebastian R, Naughton C. Decline in research publications from the United Kingdom in anaesthesia journals from 1997 to 2006. Anaesthesia. 2008;63:270–5.

78. Moppett IK, Hardman JG. Bibliometrics of anaesthesia researchers in the UK. Br J Anaesth. 2011;107:351–6.

Kunio Suwa

Summary

In 1804, Seishu Hanaoka performed breast surgery in women anesthetized with herbs producing unconsciousness for 8–24 hours. News of Morton's discovery arrived in Japan in 1850 with Seikei Sugita's translation of Schlesinger's German monograph. In 1855, Sugita gave the first ether anesthetic, and Genboku Ito gave chloroform in 1861. Nagayoshi Nagai discovered ephedrine in 1887. In what may have been the first use of intrathecal opioids, Otoziro Kitagawa injected two patients with 10 mg of morphine in 1901, relieving pain in both.

In 1934, the Nippon Dental Junior College established the first anesthesia department, but anesthesia remained relatively undeveloped until after World War II. Anesthesia usually consisted of open drop ether and spinal anesthesia, administered by the youngest member of the surgical team. In 1950, American Meyer Saklad lectured in Tokyo, attracting the interest of Japanese surgeons in tracheal intubation and artificial ventilation. Surgeon Kentaro Shimuzi, convinced a young surgeon, Hideo Yamamura, to concentrate on anesthesia. Following study in the US, in 1956 Yamamura became the Professor and Chief of the Department of Anesthesia at the University of Tokyo. The Japanese Society of Anesthesiologists initiated board examinations in 1963.

In 1972, Takuo Aoyagi of Nihon-Kohden invented and patented the basic principles of pulse oximetry. The Maruishi Drug Co obtained the rights for sevoflurane in 1983, and sevoflurane was approved for clinical use in Japan in 1990—and the rest of the world soon thereafter.

The Japanese Journal of Anesthesia, *Masui*, began publication in 1954. An English language journal, The Journal of Anesthesia began publication in 1987. Perhaps the event most increasing recognition of the specialty was Emperor Showa's (Hirohito) surgery in 1987. It increased the public appreciation of epidural anesthesia, the scope of the specialty, and the capabilities of anesthesiologists. As of 2009, more than 20,000 Japanese physicians were qualified to practice anesthesia.

History of Anesthesia in Japan During the Edo Era (1600–1867)

Between 1637 and 1853, Japan was closed to all Western countries except Holland. Contact was maintained with China and Korea. Medical concepts were principally governed by Chinese principles, adjusted and modified to Japanese needs, and supplemented by information from the few Dutch people residing in the Western part of Japan.

One record relates that in 1689, Tokumei Takamine (1653–1738) successfully repaired a cleft lip in Ryukyu while using mafutsu-san, which was considered at the time to be some form of general anesthesia. Ryukyu, now called Okinawa and located at the western end of Japan, was a semi-independent country at that time, ruled loosely by both Japan and China. Akitomo Matsuki, a medical historian and one of Japan's leading anesthesiologists, has studied the original record and concluded however, that mafutsu-san was not an anesthetic but rather was an ointment applied to dress the incision and surgical wound [1].

In 1804, Seishu Hanaoka (1760–1835; Fig. 31.1) performed the first successful surgical treatment of breast cancer under general anesthesia. Many claim that it was the first ever general anesthetic administered for a surgical procedure. Hanaoka performed surgery for many other kinds of surgical procedures in a total of 156 cases prior to his death in 1835 [2]. The "anesthetics" consisted of mixtures of various ingredients obtained from herbs and were given per mouth. The medication kept the patients unconscious for 8 to 24 hours. Detailed information is given in Matsuki's article [2]. Although Hanaoka taught this technique to his students, it was not widely publicized beyond his school, thereby limiting its application to a relatively small group of physicians and patients.

In 1850, Seikei Sugita (1817–1859) translated the Dutch version of J. Schlesinger's monograph on ether anesthesia (in German) into Japanese. He also coined the word "Masui",

K. Suwa (✉)
Department of Lifecare, Section of Medical Engineering,
Teikyo Junior College, Shibuya, Tokyo, Japan
e-mail: kunio.suwa@nifty.com

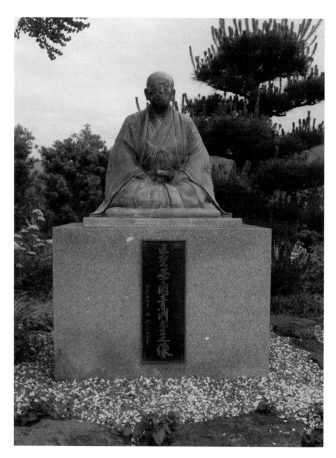

Fig. 31.1 Seishu Hanaoka. (Open source)

literally meaning "paralysis" plus "unconsciousness". In 1855, Sugita himself gave ether anesthesia, probably the first inhalational anesthetic given in Japan. The record indicates that he performed a mastectomy under ether anesthesia, but no additional details are available. There are also records describing Genboku Ito administering chloroform anesthesia for limb amputation in 1861, as taught by Franz von Siebold (1796–1866), who was a German physician and scientist. Chloroform was imported from Holland by a Dutch Navy doctor.

1868 to 1950

In 1853, Commodore Perry, a US naval officer commanding four battle-ships, forced Japan to open herself to various Western countries. In 1868, the Shogun officially resigned, starting the Meiji Era, and initiating aggressive efforts to obtain information from Western civilizations.

In 1878, cocaine was imported, but its use was not recorded until 1885, when it was administered for pain relief during tooth extraction. The route of administration is not known. In 1887, a pharmacist Nagayoshi Nagai discovered ephedrine, extracting it from a Chinese herb. This was reported

to a German journal, [3, 4] and mentioned by KK Chen and Carl Schmidt who rediscovered this agent in 1924 [5]. Before 1900, a few sporadic records described importation of nitrous oxide and the equipment required for its use.

In 1901, Otoziro Kitagawa performed spinal anesthesia for the first time in Japan using the local anesthetic "eucaine" ($C_{15}H_{21}NO_2$), an agent supplied as either alpha or beta eucaine (the latter known also as betacaine). This anesthesia was given to patients with intractable pain. It was used for some time around the turn of twentieth century because it was less toxic than cocaine, yet later abandoned because of its side-effects.

In two patients, Kitagawa injected 10 mg of morphine intrathecally. One patient was a 33-year-old man who was relieved of severe pain for several days, and the other was a 43-year-old woman who was relieved of pain in the lower back for two days. This may be the earliest description of narcotic use in the subarachnoid space [6]. Recognizing that this intrathecal dose of morphine might have been associated with profound respiratory depression, Matsuki comments that Kitagawa used a large needle, possibly enabling a leakage of CSF and preventing (of course, fortuitously) respiratory depression [6].

In 1912, surgeon Hakaru Hashimoto of Kyushu University reported four cases of an unusual type of thyroid disease, later known as "Hashimoto disease" or "Hashimoto' thyroiditis" [7]. In this report, he performed surgery in all four cases under "chloroform anesthesia".

1900 to 1930 saw the use of various techniques and instruments, including epidural anesthesia, intravenous alcohol administration, and tracheal tubes. In 1934, a Department of Dental Anesthesia was established at Nippon Dental Junior College (now the Nippon Dental College). This is believed to be the first Japanese academic department specializing in anesthesia, more than 20 years before any department in a Japanese medical school.

Beginning in 1936, Daisuke Nagae, an Army surgeon, spent two years at the Mayo Clinic in Rochester, Minnesota, observing the practice of medicine. Upon returning in 1938, he published a report entitled "Trends in Surgical Anesthesia at Mayo Clinic [8]." In retrospect, although this superb report clearly described various aspects of general anesthesia including tracheal intubation, it had little impact upon Japanese medicine because it was published in the Journal of Army Medicine, and access was not only difficult but was more or less deliberately kept secret. This period immediately preceded hostilities between Japan and the US, and Nagae, an Army Surgeon, could not officially report the superiority of American techniques, although he did publish the article.

In 1941, Japan attacked Pearl Harbor, and following the war, was occupied by the US until 1952. Despite his contributions to medicine and his sympathies towards the US,

Nagae was excluded from official or governmental positions because he was a high ranking official in the Army when the war ended, and was considered to have contributed to the war effort. He died in 1957 and his contributions to Japanese medicine became known only after his death, mainly due to the efforts of Matsuki [9].

There is little published information describing how anesthesia was practiced during this period. Anecdotal evidence suggests that the youngest member of the surgical team administered open drop ether and spinal anesthesia. There were no known formally trained anesthetists, although there might have been a few individuals who gave anesthesia routinely. There are records showing that Japan manufactured a small amount of anesthesia equipment. Tracheal tubes, if used at all, were probably inserted by dentists rather than by physicians, and even most thoracic surgery was done under local anesthesia. Clearly, Nagae's revolutionary report made little impact.

1950 to the Present: Various Academic Anesthesia Departments

The Impact of Meyer Saklad's Lecture on Japanese Medicine/Anesthesia

In August 1950, Meyer Saklad of Rhode Island Hospital attended the Japanese-American Joint Conference of Medical Educators, held in Tokyo. This meeting was a part of Unitarian Service Committee (USC) activities, American efforts aimed at the exchange of medical information and the establishment of close relationships between the American medical profession and members of the profession in post-war foreign countries.

This Conference had a major impact on Japanese surgeons (there were no anesthetists at that time) attending the meeting. They were particularly interested in tracheal intubation and maintenance of artificial respiration. Saklad's lecture was translated into Japanese by Kentaro Shimizu (Fig. 31.2), a leading surgeon of the University of Tokyo who had just returned from a visit to the US. Hideo Yamamura (Fig. 31.3), a 30 year old surgeon in Shimizu's department, attended the meeting only reluctantly to satisfy the request of Shimizu, but was soon attracted to anesthesia. (This story was told to me by Yamamura himself.) Recognizing Yamamura's interest, Shimizu suggested that Yamamura abandon surgery and concentrate on anesthesia. Yamamura agreed and in 1952, Shimizu established a small section of anesthesia in the department of surgery at the University Hospital, and then sent Yamamura to the US for further study.

Saklad's lecture attracted many other surgeons to this new field, particularly because of the delivery of anesthesia via tracheal tubes, resulting in an enormous increase in the

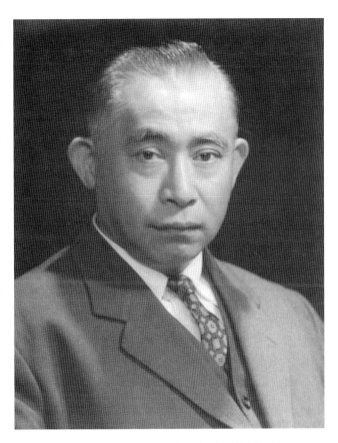

Fig. 31.2 Kentaro Shimizu. (From the author's collection.)

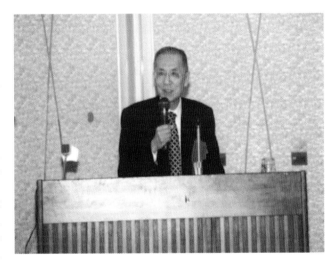

Fig. 31.3 Hideo Yamamura. (From the author's collection.)

number of anesthesia-related reports at surgical meetings. In 1954, Shimizu organized the first meeting of the Japanese Society of Anesthesiology (JSA). In the same year, publication of the Journal, *Masui* (The Japanese Journal of Anesthesiology) began. This journal was, and still is, published only in Japanese, yet it achieved semi-official status as the journal of JSA. On return from the US in 1956, Yamamura

Table 31.1 Each of these individuals became professors and chiefs of their departments

Names	Affiliation	Mentor and training site
Kenichi Iwatuki	Tohoku University	Benjamin Etsten, Boston University
Etsutaro Ikezono	Tokyo Medical and Dental University	Merel Harmel, Johns Hopkins University
Tohru Yamamoto*	Nihon University	Ferdinand Greifenstein, Wayne State University
Yoshio Kurosu*	Toho University	Leroy Vandam, Peter Bent Brigham, William Derrick, Arthur Keats, Baylor Medical College
Yu Miyake*	Tokyo Medical College	Meyer Saklad, Rhode Island Hospital
Tatsushi Fujita	Gumma University	Solomon Albert, George Washington University
Kunio Ichiyanagi*	NiigataUniversity	Robert Dripps, University of Pennsylvania
Seizo Iwai*	Kobe University	Digby Leigh, Los Angeles Children's Hospital
Tetsuji Furukawa*	Kyushu University	Ferdinand Greifenstein, Wayne State University
Tohru Morioka	Kumamoto University	Louis Orkin, Albert Einstein Medical School
Ryo Tanaka*	Kitasato University	Francis Foldes, Mercy Hospital Pittsburg
		Robert Virtue, University of Colorado
Mitsugu Fugimori	Osaka City University	Robert Dripps, University of Pennsylvania
Yusuke Itoh	Toyama University	Merel Harmel, Johns Hopkins University

* Deceased

became the Professor and Chief of the Department of Anesthesia at the University of Tokyo, the first such department in a Japanese Medical School. Yamamura retired from academic medicine in 1980 at age 60, and in 2010 at the age of 90, still practices medicine in his clinic. He does not smoke, drink, or take coffee. He ate little even when he was young. He is not active in any sport, but does play the piano, his only hobby besides studying, of which I am aware.

At this time, many young physicians went to the US for anesthesia training, adding to those already in the US who were training in other fields but switched to anesthesia. The information describing who studied in which institutions and when they were there, was mostly lost, but fortunately the "The Aqualumni Tree" by Lucien Morris, appearing in the September 2001 ASA Newsletter, prompted discussion and interest among Japanese anesthesiologists about this matter. The following list of those who were trained in 1950 resulted from that discussion (Table 31.1) [10]. Alas, I am certain that I must be missing many other names due to the difficulty in tracing them.

In the meantime, several companies began producing carbon-dioxide absorbents (Soda-lime: Wako Junyaku Co.),

thiopental (Tanabe Co., Now Tanabe-Mitsubishi Drug Co.) and nitrous oxide (Showa Denko Co.). Ether and chloroform were already available for inhalational anesthetic use. Anesthesia machines and equipment were originally imported, but were soon manufactured locally (Senkosha Co., Acoma Co, and AIKA Co.).

Establishment of the Specialty

Until recently, once qualified (holds a permanent medical license) a Japanese physician could practice any specialty. The names of these specialties were legally recognized, but as late as the middle of the 1950s, anesthesia was not included in the list of recognized specialties, because at the time the law was written, anesthesia as a specialty was unknown in Japan. As it became widely known, pressure increased, to include anesthesia as a legally recognized specialty. Subsequent discussion resulted in making anesthesia a "special" specialty which meant that unlike all other specialties, anesthesia could not be chosen (as could other specialties), without fulfilling one of two requirements: completion of two years of training, or experience administering general anesthesia to 300 patients using anesthesia equipment. In addition, a category for those not satisfying the above requirements that allowed the "choice" of anesthesia was extended to the "pioneers" trained in overseas programs.

This system was established in 1961 and still exists. It consists of a permanent qualification (i.e., medical license) that once obtained, remains in force indefinitely. According to the law, therefore, any physician of any specialty may practice anesthesia as long as he or she is qualified once, as described above.

Currently a debate exists as to whether this system should be maintained. In some respects, it is a stronger and more legitimate qualification than that required to practice any other specialty because the training requirements are written into law, and thus established officially. Qualification in other specialties is weaker because it is determined by individual private societies.

Recognizing that this system provided only a limited test of the quality of training in anesthesia, ten leading anesthesiologists decided to establish a specialty board using an American model—the first formal certification of and by a medical specialty in Japan. The Japanese Society of Anesthesiology conducted the first examination in 1963, and although the exact number of candidates is no longer known, 44 anesthesiologists qualified by passing the examination consisting of oral and written examinations, and the testing of skills. The JSA initiated certification of "Instructing Hospitals" (i.e., residency programs) in 1973, dictating minimum standards for the instructing staff and residency experience. In 1991, Renewal of Instructor and Instructing Hospital Certification became necessary every 5 years. In 2004, guidelines for certification and accreditation common to all specialties were established. To comply, the JSA certification mandated a three stage system: Certified Anesthesiologist, Certified Anesthesia Specialist, and Certified Anesthesia Instructor. Certification had to be renewed every 5 years, and was judged by document review.

The present specifics are as follows. Hospitals may post clinical services that they provide, including anesthesiology, when they have staff anesthesiologists who have been trained by JSA Certified Instructors for 2 years or more, or have been instructed by such Instructors in 300 cases or more at a Certified Instructing Hospital. Such staff anesthesiologists have been recognized by the Ministry of Health, Labor and Welfare (MHLW) with posting permits since 1960 and now total more than 20,000. The posting permit does not have to be renewed and the MHLW does not keep track of permits once issued. The number of postings does not define the number of anesthesiologists presently in practice. Today's physicians trained in anesthesiology might include four groups.

1. Some are non-anesthesiologists who had trained in anesthesiology (see previous paragraph) but who principally practice a discipline other than anesthesia.
2. As of 2012, approximately 2,500 physicians are Certified Anesthesiologists. These are senior residents or junior faculty who have had at least 2 years of training (not simply those who have given 300 cases or more under supervision), have gained a MHLW permit, and have joined the JSA. They would usually have had more than 3 years of postgraduate training. Through a review of documents, a JSA committee adjudges that they have reached this stage (no test is given).
3. Approximately an additional 3,000 physicians are Certified Anesthesia Specialists. These usually have faculty status at an academic hospital and have taken 4 or more years of training in anesthesia and 6 or more years of postgraduate training. They must pass a written, an oral, and, if deemed necessary, a skill test.
4. Approximately an additional 3,300 physicians are Certified Anesthesia Instructors. They have held the position of Certified Anesthesia Specialist for more than 4 years. A committee for adjudging instructor certification in the JSA has found them capable of training Anesthesia Specialists. During their fifth year as a Specialist they will apply for the title of Certified Anesthesia Instructor.

My Experience Taking the American Board of Anesthesiology Examination

Among Japanese physicians, anesthesiologists as a group are particularly fond of America. There are several reasons for this: anesthesiology was born and developed in America; most of us learned from American textbooks and journals;

and many, including me, received part or all of their training in America.

Between the 1950 and the 1970, America was considered so wealthy that, coming from Japan, a country still recovering from the devastation of World War II, it seemed like a paradise. In addition, I was impressed that such an affluent society was at the same time a "fair society", far fairer than I had expected.

I began residency training at the Massachusetts General Hospital in Boston in July 1963. At the end of the second year of training, I passed the written examination of the American Board of Anesthesiology. In my third year, I studied pulmonary gas exchange while also working in the OR (partly to earn my keep). Coincidentally at that time, the ABA changed the requirements for entrance into the Oral Exam from two years of clinical training and two years of practice time to three years of clinical training or two years of clinical training and one year of research. Taking into account the time required for completion of the application process, I was eligible to take the Oral Exam in the Spring of 1967.

I was a Fulbright scholar, and the scholarship covered travel expenses and allowed me to stay in the country for three years. However, even with extensions, the maximum was 3 years, 3 months and 2 weeks. It was before the era of the jumbo-jet, and international airfares were astronomical, especially for Japanese, because Japan had just begun her economic redevelopment and the currency exchange rate was 360 yen to a dollar (ah, how times have changed!) Had I been forced to return to Japan in 1966 upon completion of residency training, the cost of a return trip to America in 1967 to take the examination would have consumed my annual income.

However, the examination in October 1966 would be held just within the time-limit allowed by the Fulbright committee. In desperation, I wrote to the Board explaining the situation and pleading that I be allowed to sit for the examination for which I was, strictly speaking, not eligible. I thought that my chances were minimal because, after all, I was asking the ABA to break its own rule, but to my delight, the ABA allowed me to sit for the exam in October, cautioning me that I would know the result—success or failure—only after April 1967. I was jubilant. Not only could I take the exam, but the ABA had flexibly applied its rule without breaking its basic position. I learned later that the ABA ruling in my case was not only an expression of fairness, but resulted partly from the amusement of the ABA staff. I think they enjoyed both my letter, and giving me this opportunity. The oral exam held in the Broadmoor Hotel in beautiful Colorado Springs was an anticlimax. Overcoming the hurdles preceding the test gave me confidence that I would pass. In May 1967, I learned the good news. (Coincidentally, Lawrence J. Saidman, one of the editors of this book and later a Director of the ABA also took his Oral Exam in Colorado Springs at the same time and Ted

Eger, also an editor of this book was an examiner at that exam. It is a small world.)

For a few years, I was one of only a few Japanese certified by the ABA. Japanese members were Fellows of the American College of Anesthesiology (FACA). We held regular meetings. I remember attending one where I felt envied because I was both FACA and ABA accredited.

The History of Pulse Oximeters in Japan

Takuo Aoyagi of Nihon-Kohden invented and patented the basic principles of pulse oximetry in 1972. Only a month later, Akio Yamanishi of Minolta and others applied for similar patents but were rejected, because of the prior submission by Aoyagi. Although the latter request from Yamanishi of Minolta was rejected, Minolta did succeed in obtaining the patent internationally, including in the US and Britain, because Aoyagi or Nihon-Kohden failed to apply for international patent protection. Furthermore, while Nihon-Kohden produced only a few test models, Minolta produced a commercially viable version and began selling it. This Minolta model reached both William New at Stanford and the Biox Company in Colorado, and sparked the development of a more practical unit, both in the use of photodiodes and digital technology, including microprocessors. It was the Biox Company (now a part of Ohmeda) that incorporated most of the technical improvements. William New was trained as an anesthesiologist, but after spending a year in the Stanford Business School's Sloan Program, and realizing the usefulness of pulse oximeters in the OR, ICU and other hospital environments, he decided to leave academia and establish Nellcor.

As an aside, there is no evidence that Minolta imitated the Nihon-Kohden device. It appears that they simply pursued a similar idea by a different route. Minolta's initial model used a finger probe rather than the Nihon-Kohden earlobe probe, fixing the subsequent path of development of this instrument.

The Contribution of John Severinghaus

In addition to his great contributions to various fields in anesthesia and medicine, Severinghaus also clarified the history of pulse oximeters. While studying pulse oximeters and the history of blood gas measurement, Severinghaus became interested in who actually invented the pulse oximeter. Realizing that the pulse oximeter was invented in Japan, he consulted Yoshiyuki Honda, Professor of Physiology at Chiba University with whom he had been cooperating in research. Honda traced the discovery back to Aoyagi and supplied this information to Severinghaus. Severinghaus subsequently described the circumstances surrounding the discovery, in the *Journal of Clinical Monitoring*, giving Aoyagi priority as the discoverer of the principle of pulse

oximetry and the inventor of the instrument, a fact not known widely, even inside Japan. Severinghaus subsequently wrote a book on the History of blood gas measurement, further securing Aoyagi's seminal role in this discovery [11–13].

My Regrets and a Little Pride

In 1974 I attended the meeting in Osaka at which Aoyagi made the first public presentation of his work. It was a large meeting with many simultaneous sessions, and I did not attend the particular session at which Aoyogi presented his findings. The abstract had been sitting on my bookshelf, and I only found it many years later.

Sometime in 1976, I first came across the Minolta model of the pulse oximeter, immediately realizing its potential as well as its drawbacks. I then had young Masayuki Suzukawa with me, and asked him to study it. His resulting paper was published in Japanese in 1978 [14]. Mr. Nakamura (first name lost), a professional science writer, translated it into high quality English, but this English version was never submitted to an English language journal, probably because I thought it was after all, only a description of our experiences, and not an original paper. Suzukawa's paper, of which only the abstract was in English, has been quoted many times. Suzukawa was quite young at that time, and it was entirely my responsibility to decide whether and when to submit the paper. I greatly regret that I failed to make a little more effort to submit the English version.

Minolta's pulse oximeter was supplied to us for clinical trials and was the device Suzukawa studied. After successfully applying for funds from the Ministry of Education and Culture of the Japanese Government the following year, I bought a Minolta unit. I was later told that although the Minolta Company successfully patented the pulse oximeter outside Japan, they sold only 100 units or so before making major revisions using a combination of digital technology and optical diodes similar to Nellcor and Biox. I am glad that I had the sense to write about this Minolta instrument in one of my books on blood gases. So I take quiet pride in my early recognition of the instrument's potential [15].

In 1985, the chairman of a major anesthesiology department complained to me that during his sick-leave, his vice-chairman bought and installed pulse oximeter units in every OR in the hospital. This chairman then mentioned that we should not rely on such devices for knowing patient's oxygen levels. I responded, saying, "By taking sick-leave, you have done a great service to your patients and to the department. With the help of pulse oximeters, your patients will be much safer and do much better under anesthesia. Also, your residents will learn more quickly about the dynamics of oxygen during anesthesia." He might have taken this statement of mine as a joke, but I was serious. Indeed, we used a pulse oximeter when we anesthetized the Emperor (see below).

Introduction of Sevoflurane into Clinical Use (See also Chapter 46)

Sevoflurane was independently developed in the US by Ross Terrell at the Ohio Chemical Co, and by Richard Wallen at Baxter-Travenol Laboratories. After studies in the early 1970, both companies stopped further development because of sevoflurane's modest rate of metabolic degradation and its breakdown by soda-lime. The breakdown issue seemed especially important because isoflurane was being studied at about the same time and showed an extremely low degree of metabolism, more than an order of magnitude less than that of sevoflurane.

In 1983, the Maruishi Drug Co. obtained the rights for this agent from Travenol. Because Maruishi did not have an extensive knowledge of any inhalational agent, Kazuyuki Ikeda, Chairman of the Anesthesiology Department of Hamamatsu Medical School was consulted. Ikeda was chosen because he had worked closely with Maruishi on some sterilizing agents to be used in the OR. They concluded that while metabolism of sevoflurane is high, it was not enough to preclude sevoflurane's clinical use. Later Ikeda stated that he was impressed with both the reported low value of the blood-gas partition coefficient and with the ease of anesthetizing animals. He said that the ease of anesthetizing animals was so impressive that he thought, even if it failed as a clinical agent, it would be a superb agent in the laboratory.

Sevoflurane was approved for clinical use in 1990 in Japan, and its acceptance was immediate because of its low blood:gas partition coefficient and its minimal or absent pungency. Both induction and emergence proved to be fast and smooth. Currently, sevoflurane is used for more than 90 % of cases of inhalational anesthesia in Japan. It is the only inhalational anesthetic in which Japanese anesthesiologists played a major role in its clinical introduction. Ikeda recently retired and lives happily with his family. Tomiei Kazama, who played an active role during the development of sevoflurane, is now the Professor and Chairman of Anesthesiology of National Defense Medical College.

An English Language Japanese Journal: Journal of Anesthesia

As described above, the first Japanese academic departments were formed around 1952. A Specialty Journal originated at this time. *Masui* or the "Japanese Journal of Anesthesiology" was and is published in Japanese. Although it is indexed, many Japanese anesthesiologists wanted a journal published in English. Towards the end of the 1950s and into the early 1960s, several issues of the *Far-East Journal of Anesthesia* were published in cooperation with American anesthesiologists stationed in Japan. The journal failed to thrive, however.

The Japanese Society of Anesthesiologists prepared for, and finally published an English language journal, the *Journal of Anesthesia*, in 1987. It was published by Kokuseido originally, the same company publishing *Masui*, but its publication was transferred later to Springer. It too, is now included in Medline.

The Emperor's Surgery and its Effect on Anesthesia

Emperor Showa (HIROHITO) headed the Royal family from 1926 to 1989. In the Fall of 1987, at the age of 86 he developed signs of duodenal obstruction and surgery was performed on a semi-emergency basis in a small hospital inside the palace. The hospital was poorly staffed and poorly equipped, and major surgery was performed only a few times a year. Personnel from the University of Tokyo, including surgeons, two anesthesiologists (including me), and nurses were asked to participate.

Although we were not given the opportunity to see the patient before the planned surgery, we were allowed to check the OR and its equipment. An old anesthesia machine was available. It could only deliver nitrous oxide, oxygen, and halothane but appeared to function satisfactorily. The monitoring equipment consisted of a few manual blood pressure instruments. We asked the hospital personnel to obtain at least one EKG monitor. Originally they asked if it might be possible to use a regular paper-recording EKG instrument instead. We said "No" and they said "OK, we will get one. The Ministry of Finance won't be happy if we simply ask for a new instrument, but they would be willing to get one for the Emperor." We thought they were kidding, but they were serious.

The Word "Epidural" Becomes Famous

The emperor was in poor health, suffering from cardiac and kidney disease. Nevertheless, he tolerated 2 hours of surgery fairly well, including a gastro-jejunostomy. Anesthesia consisted of a combined epidural and general (halothane and nitrous oxide) anesthetic. We used a pulse oximeter and monitored CVP postoperatively.

One newspaper ran a headline "The Emperor had surgery done under general anesthesia". We immediately informed the journalists that it was not simply general anesthesia but was combined with epidural anesthesia. However the term "epidural" was not familiar and we had to explain it in detail—first to them, then to the public. Interestingly, this resulted in a fee increase in health insurance. Before this surgery, the fee was the same whether general anesthesia was given alone, or combined with an epidural. After the event, insurance regulators agreed that the reimbursement for combined general-epidural should be increased.

Although we had not intended it, this event turned out to be a great advertisement to the general public, about anesthesia and the role of the anesthesiologist. Few knew that specialists gave anesthesia, and the Emperor's surgery changed things dramatically. Patients now knew the word "epidural", and we anesthesiologists had no difficulty explaining its usefulness to our patients during the routine preoperative visit. In fact, our patients often asked to receive the anesthesia given to the Emperor. Several anesthesiologists, including me, wrote books for the general public explaining what anesthesia was, and the Japanese public now is far more aware of anesthesia and anesthesiologists than they had been prior to the "Emperor's anesthetic".

Similar transformations occurred in surgery. Previously, surgeons had difficulty persuading elderly patients to undergo surgery, simply because they thought they were too old. The fact that the old Emperor benefited from surgery done at 86, made elderly patients considerably less hesitant to have surgery.

The transfer of a pulse oximeter from the hospital to the palace provided an additional unintended consequence of "the surgery". At that time, we had only four units for our 14 operating theaters. After the surgery, the journalists wanted to know everything we had done to this patient. I mentioned the pulse oximeter after which I was asked to write an article describing the device for the newspaper's readers. This was probably the first time a pulse oximeter became known to the general public beyond the medical environment. I was quite aware of the possibility that such an article would help practicing anesthesiologists when asking their hospital administration to buy pulse oximeters for their operating rooms. Though not immediately, we obtained a good number of pulse oximeters for the entire OR suite. We also explained the use of pH and blood gases (the samples were taken to the University hospital and analyzed there), and the incentive spirometer for resolving atelectasis, each of which received considerable newspaper coverage. In the early 1990, JSA set the standards for monitoring in anesthesia, which included the use of pulse oximeters, but this was probably related to the standards already established in other countries, rather than the use of a pulse oximeter in caring for the Emperor.

In retrospect however, we made one mistake that fortunately did not cause any adverse outcome. The surgery was performed in a small, little-used hospital. Although these circumstances were for the most part out of our control, we were fortunate that nothing untoward resulted. Some fifteen years later, when the current Emperor (succeeding Showa Emperor) suffered from prostate disease, surgery was done in a University Hospital, a more logical and sensible solution.

The PC and the Software Contest Impacts Japanese Anesthesiology

Computer programming appeals to many Japanese including anesthesiologists. Indeed, Japanese found programming attractive before the PC appeared. The number of Japanese engaged in programming increased considerably when the PC was introduced. At the time of the introduction of the PC, commercially available software applications were expensive and of poor quality.

A group of anesthesiologists in JSA set up what we called a Software Contest within the JSA. Contestants presented their products to compete for the prize. If they won the prize, they were asked to make their product free to all. Usually, some 15 to 20 software applications were submitted annually, including some from foreign countries. This contest continued annually for fifteen years before being absorbed into the general session of the JSA [16].

One example coming from the contest was Hiroshi Hagihira's BSA (bispectral analyzer). When the BIS monitor appeared on the market, we wanted to know what and how it analyzed the EEG. Understandably, the Aspect Company (recently bought by Covidian) did not disclose the details of this proprietary analysis. But someone with knowledge and capacity should be able to write similar software, and that was what Hagihira did. Before it was reported to a highly cited journal like *Anesthesiology*, it was presented and discussed extensively among local anesthesiologists. Unlike the BIS, Hagihira's BSA was open and the source-code was freely available. Hagihira's software has not totally replaced the BIS, but it has been used in many ways in analyzing the EEG [17].

A Shortage of Anesthesiologists and the Lack of Group Practice

An important problem related to anesthetic practice in Japan, is that except for those anesthesiologists associated with academic institutions, (and who are interested in research and teaching) there are relatively few Japanese physicians practicing only anesthesiology. These academic physicians are paid a more or less fixed salary, and never create a group practice.

Institutions (e.g., medical schools) or hospitals employ nearly all anesthesiologists. Until recently, private practice in anesthesia—whether solo or as a group—was rare. The law does not prohibit private practice, but the insurance system and many other hurdles discourage it. I believe that this situation provides a major explanation for the limited supply of anesthesiologists.

An additional reason for the shortage of anesthesiologists is that the daily surgical schedule is unusually long. Whereas other specialties may manage their workload by controlling activity, anesthesiologists have little control over their workload and the ratio of surgeons to anesthesiologists often exceeds 10 to 1. Surgical patients come to the OR one after another, with too few anesthesiologists trying to cope with the load. As a consequence, anesthesiologists sense that they have failed and resign.

There are exceptions of course. A few anesthesia chiefs negotiate a reasonable ratio of procedures to anesthesiologists, or a hospital administrator wisely realizes the advantage of such a ratio. Then the size of the anesthesiology department may be expanded substantially, and incidentally, the status of the staff may increase. Unfortunately, these more favorable situations are the exception rather than the rule.

Since 2000, there have been several examples in which anesthesiologists, especially those from government institutions, and usually because the work load increased, have resigned as a group. This increased the workload of those remaining, resulting in both longer working hours and occasional "parallel anesthesia", or one anesthesiologist caring simultaneously for more than one patient at a time. Because these incidents occurred in leading institutions, such as the National Cancer Center Hospital in Tokyo and in the National Cerebral and Cardiovascular Center Hospital in Osaka, forcing a decrease in the number of surgeries, they were widely publicized on television and in the newspapers. However, it is unclear whether society really understood the problem and whether the journalists accurately portrayed the difficulties.

Some institutions solved the problem by increasing the number of positions. In others, group practices finally appeared. Groups successfully negotiated working conditions, including their income, with the hospital. Whether such group practice continues and thrives is difficult to predict.

Concluding Remarks

Japanese medicine has a long and honorable history, but anesthesiology began only after World War II and was largely influenced by those physicians studying in America. Academically, the specialty has been modestly successful, and its research and training systems are running smoothly. A major problem is the shortage of anesthesiologists resulting from the relatively low prestige of the specialty and the high workload. Group practice is increasing, but whether this will solve the problem is difficult to predict.

References

1. Matsuki A. New study on the history of anesthesiology–(5) and (6). Reevaluation of surgical achievements by Tokumei Takamine. (Article in Japanese). Masui. 2000;49:1285–9.
2. Matsuki A. Annals of anesthetic history. Seishu Hanaoka, a Japanese pioneer in anesthesia. Anesthesiology. 1970;32:446–50.
3. Miura K III. Aus der chirurgisch-ophthalmologishen Universitaetklinik in Tokio (Japan). Vorlaefige Mittheilung ueber Ephedrin, ein neues Mydriaticum. Berl klin Wochenschr. 1887;36:707.
4. Nagai N. Ephedrin (Fischer B. Ueber einige neuere Arzneimittel). Pharmazeutische Zeitung. 1887;32(98):700.
5. Chen KK, Schmidt CF. The action of ephedrine, the active principle of the Chinese drug, Ma Huang. J Pharm Exp Therap. 1924;24:339–57.
6. Matsuki A. Nothing new under the sun–a Japanese pioneer in the clinical use of intrathecal morphine. Anesthesiology. 1983;58:289–90.
7. Hashimoto H. Zur Kenntnis der lymphomatosen Veranderung der Schilddruse (Struma lymphomatosa). Archiv fur klinische Chirurgie. 1912;97:219–48.
8. Nagae D. Current trend in surgery in Mayo Clinic. Army Medical Journal 1938. (details unknown) (In Japanese)
9. Matsuki A. Tracks of Pioneers. Medi Science. 1990. (Book published in Japanese)
10. Morris LE, Ralph M. Waters' Legacy: The establishment of academic anesthesia centers by the 'Aqualumni' ASA Newsletter. 2001 Sept;65. Number 9.
11. Severinghaus JW, Honda Y. History of blood gas analysis. V. J Clin Monit. 1985;1:180–92.
12. Severinghaus JW, Honda Y. History of blood gas analysis. VII. J Clin Monit. 1987;3:135–8.
13. Severinghaus JW, Astrup PB. History of blood gas analysis. Boston: Little, Brown & Co; 1987.
14. Suzukawa M, Fujisawa M, Matsushita F, Suwa K, Yamamura H. Use of a pulse oximeter in anesthesia. Masui. 1978;27:600–5. (Abstract in English)
15. Suwa K. Blood gas training. Tokyo: Chugai Med. Pub.; 1983. (In Japanese)
16. Suwa K, Miyasaka K, Tanaka Y, Ozaki M, Mori T, Iwase Y, Nishi S. Report on the computer software contest at 38th Congress of the Japan Society of Anesthesiology. J Anesthesia. 1991;5:441–4.
17. Hagihira S, Takashina M, Mori T, Ueyama H, Mashimo T. Electroencephalographic bicoherence is sensitive to noxious stimuli during isoflurane or sevoflurane anesthesia. Anesthesiology. 2004;100:818–25.

A History of Nordic Anesthesia

32

Kjell Erik Stromskag, John G Brock-Utne, Jan Eklund
and Martin H:son Holmdahl

Summary

News of anesthesia's discovery came via Great Britain and France, and ether was given by February 1847. Chloroform quickly followed, but its lethality caused a reversion to ether by 1900. During the last half of the nineteenth Century, surgeons directed delivery of anesthesia by nurses and non-medical persons. Operations were few in number, and infections remained the dominant surgical risk. Surgeons introduced local and regional anesthesia after Koller's 1884 demonstration of the anesthetic effects of cocaine.

Until the 1930s, nurse anesthetists, directed by surgeons, continued to provide most anesthesia. Surgeons persuaded a few colleagues like Gordh (Sweden) to pursue a career in anesthesia. Gordh returned home in 1940 after 2 years training in the US. World War II delayed the training of other Nordic pioneers. Swedish scientists synthesized lidocaine, and Gordh clinically tested it in 1943. In 1950, Thesleff, and von Dardel in Sweden studied succinylcholine in patients.

In 1949, the World Health Organization established a one-year anesthetics course in Copenhagen for European and third world countries physicians. The course was repeated 23 times. After 1950, Nordic doctors needed 3 years of anesthesia training to become specialists in anesthesia. Besides the course in Copenhagen, each country developed its own annual postgraduate course.

In 1950–1952, polio epidemics struck Denmark and Sweden, and Ibsen applied long-term ventilation to decrease mortality, leading to the development of intensive care units (ICUs). In December 1952, Bauer opened the first ICU in Sweden, and in 1953 Ibsen did the same in Denmark. In the 1950s, Norwegian toy manufacturer Laerdal developed "Resusci-Anne". He supported Safar's 1961 first-ever meeting on closed chest cardiac massage.

Nordic anesthesia associations were founded in the mid-twentieth century. The first congress took place in Oslo in 1950. In 1957, the Association launched *Acta Anaesthesiologica Scandinavica*, with Eric Nilsson as the first editor.

From the 1960s onwards, Nordic anesthetic practice paralleled that in other developed countries. For example, the Swedish Society of Anesthesiologists increased from 180 members in 1966, to 400 in 1974, and 1400 in 2011. Within a department of anesthesia, teams of anesthesiologists and nurse anesthetists delivered anesthesia. Nordic anesthetists also provided prehospital acute care, intensive and postoperative care, and support for interhospital transportation.

J. G. Brock-Utne (✉)
Department of Anesthesia, Stanford University Medical Center,
300 Pasteur Drive, Stanford, CA 94305–5640, USA
e-mail: brockutn@stanford.edu

K. E. Stromskag
Department of Anesthesiology and Intensive Care, Molde Hospital,
Molde, Norway
e-mail: kjeer-st@online

J. Eklund
Department of Anesthesiology and Intensive Care, Karolinska Institute
and Hospital, Karolinska vägen, 171 76 Solna, Sweden
e-mail: jan.eklund@telia.com

M. H:son Holmdahl
Uppsala University, S:t Olofsgatan 10B, 753 12 Uppsala, Sweden
e-mail: martin.holmdahl@surgsci.uu.se

Introduction

Anesthesia is a young Nordic specialty. The first position for an anesthesiologist in Scandinavia and mainland Europe was established in 1940, at the Karolinska Hospital in Stockholm, Sweden. Why did anesthesiology take longer to develop in Nordic countries than in Great Britain (GB) and the United States (US)? Until the 1930s, Nordic medical practice followed that on the European mainland. Nordic students and young doctors traveled to Germany and France to further their education, and anesthesiology in these countries lagged behind that in GB and the US. While European surgeons needed modern anesthesia as much as did their British and American counterparts, they regarded this new 'technology' as another "surgical method" for nurses or technicians. Every young physician wanted to be THE surgeon. Besides, there were no paid hospital jobs for anesthesiologists.

The Early Days

The political geography of Scandinavian countries in 1846 differed from today. Finland was a part of the Russian Empire, albeit with considerable independence. Its cultural bonds were to Sweden of which it had been part for 400 years. Sweden and Norway were united in an unpopular union, created in 1814 after the Napoleonic wars. Norway had its own constitution (created in 1814) and longed for independence. Norway was also the Scandinavian country most closely connected with GB. As part of the large European peninsula, Denmark had always been more influenced by the south. Denmark also ruled Iceland until World War II, and shaped its development.

Health care provided to Nordic inhabitants before 1850 was limited to urban areas. Operative reports indicate that all surgeries were performed without anesthesia or systematic use of analgesics [1]. Operations included treatment of skull fractures, removal of the mandible, gastrotomy, and repair of inguinal hernias and cleft lips.

The Start in Scandinavia

News of ether anesthesia reached Scandinavia in February 1847. Swedish chemist Jöns Jacob Berzelius wrote a letter from France, describing the discovery, a letter read to the Swedish Society of Medicine on 2 February. One month later, Carl Ekströmer, head surgeon at the Karolinska Institute reported satisfactory anesthesia in young healthy colleagues who volunteered to receive ether [2].

The Finn, Carl von Haartman, had a son studying in Paris who heard of ether's effects. He wrote of these to his father who read the letter to the Finnish Medical Association on 13 February [3], leading to the first anesthetics in Finland at the beginning of March.

On 18 February, in Norway, a letter from the young physician Petter Winge describing anesthesia, was read to the Norwegian Medical Society. The first trials of ether anesthesia took place at the national hospital (Rikshospitalet) at the beginning of March [4].

How the news reached Denmark is uncertain, but the first anesthetic was given on 20 February, 1847 [5]. Medical practice in Iceland lagged behind that in Europe, the first hospital opening in 1866. A general practitioner, Jon Finsen, working in the small town of Akureyri on Iceland's north coast, gave the first anesthetic in 1855 [6].

1847–1900; Ether, Chloroform and Complications

As in mainland Europe, Nordic anesthetic practice developed slowly after 1847. Many surgeons, other doctors, and even lay members of society maintained a continuing skepticism concerning anesthesia. Eventually, the use of ether became accepted throughout Europe, but these European anesthetic experiences were seldom documented and no "champion anesthesiologist" (like John Snow in England) advanced the specialty. Different methods for the administration of ether were 'imported' or invented. A Swedish surgeon, EG Palmgren, designed an apparatus for ether vaporization within one month of the news of the discovery reaching Sweden [7].

Chloroform became popular in Scandinavia, soon after Simpson described its anesthetic properties. In Finland, Carl von Hartmann (the man who reported Morton's discovery), visited Simpson and became an enthusiastic chloroform champion, persuading Finns to use chloroform instead of ether for 4 decades [8]. For a time, chloroform was the most common anesthetic in all Nordic countries, but it gradually decreased in popularity as complications with its use became obvious. After 1880, ether again became the primary anesthetic with chloroform's use eliminated by the beginning of the twentieth century.

Although the incidence of complications related to anesthetics indicated that the work demanded significant professional skill, nurses or technicians provided part-time anesthesia care throughout continental Europe. As noted, part of physician disinterest in anesthesia lay in low pay and status. In addition, there was a shortage of doctors and especially surgeons in all Nordic countries. Denmark, with 1.9 million inhabitants, had only 80 doctors in 1857, and surgery had become a medical specialty only 15 years earlier [9]. The total number of operations remained small for nearly two decades after the introduction of anesthesia. Concern about the risk of postoperative infections and associated morbidity and mortality may have limited surgery. Only when antiseptic, and then, aseptic surgery were introduced, could the surgeon's world expand.

The relationships between anesthetic depth, inadequate ventilation, hypoxia and hypercarbia were poorly appreciated during the first decades after the discovery of anesthesia. Few anesthetists considered the implications of carbon dioxide accumulation, inadequate oxygen transport and cyanosis. Patients might breathe (and even re-breathe) hypoxic mixtures of air and ether or chloroform gas, in inadequate volumes, with partly obstructed airways, without assistance.

Few reports described Nordic anesthesia during the nineteenth century. In Denmark, Berthelsen found 24 anesthesia-related papers published in the decade after 1847 [9]. Most articles discussed techniques, complications, and comparisons distinguishing ether and chloroform. Few dealt with pharmacology and physiology. None considered the question of who should administer anesthetics.

At its first meeting (in Gothenburg), the Scandinavian Society of Surgeons (Nordisk kirurgisk forening) launched an inter-Nordic anesthetic survey for 1894–1895. In 11,047 open drop chloroform anesthetics, 5 patients died (one death per 2,209 cases), while no deaths occurred in 1,279 ether anesthetics. When chloroform was used only as the induction agent, preceding 2,122 ether anesthetics, no deaths occurred. The greater "chloroform mortality" was consistent with results from Germany, France and Great Britain [10].

Anesthetic Delivery

Technical improvements focused on anesthetic administration. Though open drop anesthesia was preferred, many physicians constructed versions of Morton's original 'inhaler'. In Europe, the most common 'ether inhaler' became the French Charrière model.

In Denmark, around 1880, surgeon Oskar Wancher introduced a curious and potentially dangerous method for the administration of ether. Wancher's bag was a rubber bag of unknown volume connected to a breathing mask. The anesthetist placed 50 ml of ether into the bag, forming a pool in the bottom of the bag which was then filled with the patient's exhaled air. The ether evaporated into this air. The decreased oxygen and increased carbon dioxide in the rebreathed gases stimulated ventilation and thereby accelerated induction of anesthesia. "Fresh air" was added by letting the patient occasionally breathe room air [11]. The influential Danish surgeon, Professor Thorkild Rovsing strongly recommended this method in 1901, and it remained in frequent use for 30–40 years! The associated mortality remains unknown.

The use of nitrous oxide is mentioned around 1860. The slow development of nitrous oxide anesthesia is not surprising given the absence of a good method of storage, difficulty in manufacture, absence of an ability to easily add oxygen, and the limited potency of nitrous oxide. In 1894, the Gothenburg dentist Hjalmar Carlsson rediscovered ethyl chloride as a general anesthetic, reporting his accidental observation that ethyl chloride acted as a general anesthetic if used for local anesthesia in the mouth [12]. It became popular for rapidly inducing anesthesia before maintenance of anesthesia with ether.

Norwegian surgeon Jacob Heiberg (1843–1888) became an expert on treating anesthetic-associated complications in the 1870s. When respiration and circulation deteriorated, he taught: "*Throw away your surgical instruments. Stop the operation and open all windows and bathe the patient in masses of cold water* [13]." Heiberg soon realized that airway obstruction (and not warm rooms) was the major cause of complications stemming from inhalational anesthesia. He invented the "jaw thrust" to open the airway, and published this in 1873 [13]. The jaw thrust saved thousands of lives. Five years later, Johan von Esmarch (1823–1908) a German (who introduced the tourniquet), described a similar technique, for a time known as the Esmarch-Heiberg technique, but later attributed only to von Esmarch [14].

In 1898, Ingjald Reichborn-Kjennerud (1865–1949) published the first comprehensive description of anesthesia practice in Norway: "Anesthesia and local anesthesia" (Narkose og local anestesi) [15]. In the introduction, he wrote: "The number of general anesthetics is so few that one can't get much experience with its use. Hence one is at a disadvantage compared to larger towns in Europe, with hundreds of patients to evaluate one's technique."

The development of anesthesia as a clinical and scientific specialty, in Sweden before 1900, was similar to that in Norway. Fritjof Lennmalm (a neurologist) described that history in a review presented to the Swedish Society of Medicine in 1908 [16]. Except for mention of the 1847 demonstration of ether anesthesia, Lennmalm found no additional references describing progress in anesthesia before 1908 [16]. He stated that from 1838–1858 "*the great time for the surgeons had not yet come*" and when he summarized the years 1879–1904 he described surgical progress with scarcely a mention of anesthesia. He did note that chloroform was the most commonly used anesthetic.

In the second half of the nineteenth century, Swedish physiologists immobilized experimental animals with curare and gave them artificial ventilation. In Stockholm where only a narrow street separated laboratories and operating theatres, the famous Finnish/Swedish physiologist Robert Tigerstedt (who discovered and named renin in 1898) used this technique [17]. In Uppsala, his colleague Frithjof Holmgren, proposed the use of curare and intermittent positive pressure ventilation (IPPV) in a patient with tetanus, intending to evaluate whether curare had any analgesic effects [18].

The Nordic Medical Society recognized the importance of anesthesia at the end of the nineteenth century. At the 1898 meeting of the Swedish Society of Medicine, John Berg, professor of surgery, gave an honorary lecture entitled "*the start, development and current status of surgical anesthesia*". His presentation seems to have produced no effect on anesthesia research or clinical development.

Specialization in Anesthesia

Rovsing, the Dane who recommended Wancher's bag, became professor of surgical techniques, including anesthesia, without facilitating the specialty's development. It would perhaps have been better if his colleague, Fritz Levy, had been given the opportunity to take the lead. At a 1904 meeting, Levy stated:

> "*To perform a good anesthetic is an art which has to be taught just as everything else in life. It is also a gift which not all have been given. Thus this task cannot be handed over at random to anyone in the surgical staff. On the contrary it is necessary to secure an adequate number of well trained anesthetists*" [19].

A Roth-Dräger's anesthesia machine came into use in Copenhagen in 1902–03. For the first time a Nordic anesthetist could administer chloroform in a controlled way and also give the patient "a surplus of oxygen".

Local Anesthetics

News of Karl Koller's demonstration of the local anesthetic effects of cocaine, in Vienna in 1884, traveled quickly to Scandinavia. In 1885, the Swedish laryngologist, K Malmsten, vividly described the application of this breakthrough. After relating how earlier trials with local application of morphine/chloroform had been unsuccessful, he stated that "in 6 months all earlier scientific quarrels stopped when cocaine came into use" [20]. The Dane, Ernest Schmiegelow, used it in 1886 for topical administration [21]. Shortly thereafter another Dane, Christian Paulsen, performed the first trials with infiltration of cocaine for local anesthesia

In Norway's Tromsoe hospital, still the most northern university hospital in Europe, a young surgeon, Kristian Igelsrud, performed a spinal anesthetic shortly after August Bier's 1898 report. He also gave cocaine for superficial and infiltration anesthesia. These techniques gave the lone surgeon a perceived safer method than general anesthesia, safer because the surgeon could establish a stable level of anesthesia before attending to the surgery [22]. In major centres, the spinal anesthetic was often placed by a junior doctor with little experience in anesthesia, and when it was seen to work, nurses or technicians took over observation of the ongoing effect of the anesthetic. Contemporaneous similar reports were published by H Munch-Pedersen in Denmark [23] and by G Nyström in Sweden [24].

1900–1920

Surgeons in Control

By the early 1900s, many doctors in England and the US had specialized in anesthesia, but in Nordic countries, surgeons were responsible for anesthetic delivery and remained so for another four decades. Nurses provided general anesthesia under the surgeon's supervision. Such approaches became increasingly used in all Nordic countries No scientific reports refer to general anesthesia in Scandinavia in this period. In the weekly journal Hospitaltidende, the co-editor, Aage Kiaer, stated in 1904: "As well as I don't want to be operated by anyone, I don't want to be anesthetized by anybody" [25]. His warning went unheeded. In 1916, the need to control the supply of ether and oxygen by an anesthetic machine was questioned (the equipment would be too expensive!) by a Danish professor of internal medicine.

Surgeons like Regional Anesthesia

Surgeons like Kristian Igelsrud in Norway, and Gunnar Nyström and his teacher KG Lennander in Sweden, brought regional anesthetic techniques to various hospitals. In 1904, Nyström, who later became professor of Surgery in Uppsala, published a comprehensive review of local anesthesia including the production of regional anesthesia by nerve blocks in the journal of the Swedish Society of Physicians [24]. In 1907, Lennander wrote a chapter about local and subarachnoid anesthesia in Keen's Surgery [26] in which he presented his results for spinal anesthetics, and described Cushing's method of anesthetizing the abdominal wall and the lower thoracic region with intercostal blocks, using cocaine.

Central Europe, rather than GB or the US, influenced anesthetic developments in Scandinavia during this period. A 1906 Swedish summary of a survey on spinal anesthesia, by the Austrian E Slajmer, recommended restricting the method to surgery below the umbilicus, using the thinnest needle possible, and applying pure alcohol for skin disinfection [27]. In 1909, Swedish surgeon G Bäärnhielm, reported on 100 spinal anesthetics with procaine [28]. Three years later Gustaf Petrén described his use of intravenous regional anesthesia with 0.5% procaine, as advocated by Bier. Procaine remained the standard local anesthetic until the introduction of lidocaine in the 1940s.

Much knowledge of this period comes from the research of the Dane, Preben Berthelsen. He describes a 1904 report of a trial with "Scopolamine/Morphine anesthesia for otologic surgery" [29],and a report on "Subcutaneous nutrition with dextrose and peptone."

Intermittent Positive Pressure Ventilation (IPPV)

In 1910, Holger Mollegaard, a young student working with Christian Bohr, constructed a ventilator providing continuous positive pressure [30]. A mixture of chloroform and air was used for ventilation in 17 operations involving the lung. The trial was stopped because the surgical technique was inadequate and severe postoperative infections ensued.

Swedish surgeon K Giertz used Sauerbruch's sustained negative pressure method, proving in dogs that IPPV was needed to guarantee carbon dioxide elimination. He unfortunately published his results only in Swedish [31]. Giertz' pupil Clarence Crafoord, used IPPV for thoracic surgery. In his thesis, "On pneumonectomies in Man", Crafoord describes anesthesia with cyclopropane, using tracheal intubation and mechanical IPPV [32]. The Swedish company AGA and Paul Frenckner (A Swedish ENT physician), had constructed the respirator (Spiropulsator). It was used in Sweden until the 1970s.

Except for Finland, Nordic countries were sheltered from the worst effects of World War I, suffering however from isolation, leading to shortages of medical supplies, and to a lack of information. In Finland, the 1917 civil war did not make things better.

In 1916, Norwegian Nils Backer Groendahl, published the first Nordic anesthesia textbook for nurses entitled: *Anesthesia and Care of Surgical Patients* [33]. In this book he stresses the importance of skill and knowledge. By 1920, anesthetic practice had improved. Experienced nurses gave most of the anesthetics.

1920–45

Anesthetic Practice

The Swedish pioneer in neurosurgery, Herbert Olivecrona, observed that

> '*usually the American neurosurgeons prefer ether anesthesia. This method is, however, very difficult and demands an anesthetist with long experience... For myself I have entirely changed to only use local anesthesia in brain surgery as long as the patient's mental condition permits it*' [34].

This reflected the situation in all Nordic countries. Surgeons wanted to expand their practice but were constrained by a lack of experienced anesthetists. In part, this was a problem of their own making; they were "in charge" and unable/unwilling to relinquish this power.

In the 1930s, new ultra short acting barbiturates (in Scandinavia the German compound hexobarbital, Evipan was practically the only one) attracted interest, but their introduction in Sweden was marred by scientific quarrels about their use and dangers. New equipment like the McKesson apparatus increased interest in nitrous oxide anesthesia. These developments pointed to a need for specialists in anesthesia. Prominent surgeons like P Nylander in Finland, E Husfeldt in Denmark, J Holst and C Semb in Norway, and C Crafoord, J Strömbeck and G Söderlund in Sweden became convinced that anesthesia should be established as a medical specialty. Young surgeons were approached but their enthusiasm was limited for reasons previously discussed.

Wars usually bring improvements in surgical care. World War I advanced thoracic and neurosurgery, but did little to improve the performance of anesthesia. World War II varied in its effect on Nordic countries. Denmark was mostly spared. Norway was less fortunate, especially northern Norway where in late 1944, Russian troops fought the Germans, who burned everything as they retreated, leaving a desolate countryside. Medical development in both Denmark and Norway suffered from 5 years of isolation and restrictions. Nazi deportations of medical doctors (not only Jews) caused great hardship. JGBU's father, a doctor, remembers the Germans taking a Dr. Bernstein while he was on ward rounds. He

never returned. The Allies occupied Iceland which was minimally affected by the war. In contrast, Finland fought two bitter wars against the Soviet Union, one in 1939, and the second in 1941–44. The Finns were obliged to pay a postwar indemnity to the Soviet Union, a huge financial burden for many years. Sweden remained neutral during the war, and thanks to Torsten Gordh's pioneering work, anesthesiology began to develop as a specialty.

Nordic Pioneers: Denmark

A Danish pharmacologist, Knud Moeller, believed that most surgeons had little interest in anesthesia. He began a campaign to develop anesthesiology as a specialty. In 1936, while participating as a member of a doctoral committee involving a candidate defending a doctoral thesis about lumbar anesthesia, he raised public awareness that the quality of Danish anesthesia was inferior to that in other countries [35].

The first Danish anesthetist for a patient undergoing pneumonectomy (1939) was Ole Lippmann, the young director of Simonsen & Weel (a Danish manufacturer of medical instruments). He was not a physician but had learned how to administer nitrous oxide anesthesia during a 3 month stay in Toledo, Ohio while attached to the McKesson factory [35]. Lippmann introduced the technique to Ernst Trier Mørch, who later became Denmark's first anesthesiologist [36].

The thoracic surgeon, Erik Husfeldt, had recruited Mørch to help with his operations. Between 1941 and 1949, Mørch acted as a freelance anesthetist in Copenhagen. In 1943, the Germans permitted him to have a 3 week sabbatical stay with Torsten Gordh in Stockholm, an experience that committed him to anesthesia. During the rest of the war he also contributed to the Danish resistance and took an active part in the smuggling of Jews to Sweden.

Immediately after the war, Mørch spent two years studying anesthesia in London and Oxford. Returning to Denmark, he taught anesthesia and established anesthesiology as a specialty there. He published the first Danish textbook on anesthesia in 1949. In 1949, he abruptly emigrated to the US, perhaps protesting against the government's failure to create a department of anesthesiology at the Rigshospitalet (the National Hospital). In the US he led departments of anesthesia at major hospitals in Kansas City and Chicago [36].

Nordic Pioneers: Finland

After visiting Crafoord, Per Nylander, a Finnish surgeon, brought a 'Spiropulsator' back home. Another surgeon, Aare Järvinen, went to Sweden to study new anesthetic techniques. Nylander, and pharmacologist Armas Vartiainen, persuaded two resident surgeons, Eero Turpeinen and Lauri Aro, to become anesthetists. Before the war Turpeinen had studied the effects of anesthetic gases on animals, work for which he earned a PhD. Aro began work as an anesthesiologist after 1944.

In 1941, Turpeinen planned to travel to the US. The war delayed this until 1945, when he spent three months in the US and another three in the UK. On returning home he proposed the establishment of a position for an anesthetist at the Surgical Hospital in Helsinki. When this was rejected, he specialized in surgery, but in 1950 he was appointed as an anesthetist at Maria Hospital in Helsinki. After this, Turpeinen played a central role in the development of the specialty in Finland, and in founding both the Finnish and the Scandinavian Societies of Anesthesiologists.

Lauri Aro began surgical training in 1943 but, encouraged by Nylander, he converted to anesthesia. In 1948, he spent half a year in the UK, training at the Brompton Chest and Westminster Hospitals. Returning home he became a full time anesthesiologist with a special emphasis on anesthesia for thoracic surgery. He played a prominent role in the development of the specialty in Finland. In 1953, a new anesthetic position was created for him in Helsinki University Hospital [37].

Nordic Pioneers: Iceland

Three of the first four anesthesiologists in Iceland trained in the US, reflecting the close contact with the 'occupants' during World War II. Although Elias Eyvindsson studied anesthesia at the Mayo Clinic from 1948 to 1950, he became a surgeon after working for a few years at Landspitalinn (Iceland's National Hospital). Torbjörg Magnusdottir became the real pioneer, returning home in 1952 after training in Copenhagen and Lund (Sweden). The other two anesthesiologists trained in the US, were Alma Torarinsson and Valtyr Bjarnason [38].

Nordic Pioneers: Norway

Otto Mollestad (1908–1973) became the first Norwegian anesthetist, having shown a special interest in anesthesia during his medical studies. He had become friends with the surgeon Semb, just before World War II. After the war, Semb, who had joined the Norwegian resistance in London, arranged a position for Mollestad as an assistant to Robert Macintosh in Oxford. In 1946, a position as an anesthesiologist was created for Mollestad in Rikshospitalet, in Oslo.

Another surgeon, Johan Holst, arranged a residency position for Ivar Lund (1911–1992), at the Massachusetts General Hospital, with Henry Beecher. Lund returned to fill the second position for anesthesia in Norway in 1947. By 1950, four Norwegian hospitals had salaried positions for anesthesiologists [39].

Nordic Pioneers: Sweden

In Sweden, Gustaf Söderlund, professor of surgery in Stockholm, and the British anesthesiologist, Michael Nosworthy, persuaded a 29 year-old surgeon, Torsten Gordh (1907–2010), to train with Ralph Waters' at the University of Wisconsin in 1938. The start of World War II shortened Gordh's stay with Waters to 18 months, but before returning home, Gordh made a 'grand tour' through the US, meeting American pioneers including Virginia Apgar and Emery Rovenstine, contacts that later proved valuable to the development of Nordic anesthesiology. Just before the German invasion of Denmark and Norway (April 1940), Gordh journeyed home to Sweden, bringing with him a Foregger anesthesia machine, laryngoscopes, tracheal tubes and two Waters soda lime canisters [40].

Gordh immediately (1940) took up the first anesthetist position created in Sweden (and mainland Europe), a position at the Karolinska university hospital in Stockholm, and worked independently from the start. In contrast to the evolution of anesthesia in other Nordic countries, Sweden's neutrality allowed Gordh to develop anesthesiology in (relative) peace, albeit with an enormous clinical workload. Not only did he direct anesthesia at the Karolinska, he also provided anesthesia for the neurosurgical department at the Seraphimer hospital, the original university hospital in the city centre.

His biggest problem was a shortage of medicines and instruments. Gordh had his Foregger machine, but further imports proved impossible. However, the Swedish company AGA, an enterprise founded at the end of the nineteenth century by the Nobel laureate Gustaf Dahlén, soon met the demand for anesthetic machines. AGA, manufacturer of the ingenious equipment for lighthouses and also the 'Spiropulsator', also provided oxygen, nitrous oxide and cyclopropane. Swedish manufacturers of surgical equipment started making laryngoscopes, and the pharmaceutical company Astra synthesized a new ultra short acting barbiturate (Narkotal). Other drugs and items remained scarce.

A remarkable pharmacological breakthrough occurred in Sweden during the early part of the war. The local anesthetic lidocaine, was synthesized and tested by two chemists, Löfgren and Lundqvist [41] Initially they had difficulty interesting the Swedish Pharmaceutical Industry in lidocaine. They even considered travelling to London for negotiations with the British pharmaceutical industry, but German air attacks made any flight too dangerous. In 1943, Astra acquired the rights to lidocaine. It became Astra's first 'golden' product. Sweden continued to play a major role in local anesthetic development. Pharmacologist Bo af Ekenstam, introduced mepivacaine and bupivacaine in the 1960s. Ropivacaine was introduced in 1995. All three drugs were tested in Swedish hospitals [42] (Table 32.1).

Doctors and nurses in Sweden and other Nordic countries recognized Gordh's great ability as a teacher, and came to train with him. Three additional anesthesia positions in Sweden were established in the 1940s, and given to doctors trained in GB or the US. In Stockholm, Olle Friberg was employed in 1943 at the Sabbatsberg's hospital, where Crafoord had his cardiothoracic center. In 1945, Eric Nilsson

Table 32.1 Some Nordic contributions to anesthesiology

Country	Date	Contribution	Contributor/manufacturer
Denmark	1950s	Gas analysis	P Astrup; O Siggaard Anderson
	1955	Ruben valve; Ambu bag	H Ruben
Sweden	1940s	Gordh-Olovsson needle	T Olovsson; T Gordh
	1940s	Lidocaine	N Löfgren, B Lundqvist
	1957	Mepivicaine	Bo af Ekenstam
	1965	Bupivicaine	Bo af Ekenstam
	1996	Ropivacaine	Bo af Ekenstam
	1952	Engström ventilator	CG Engström
	1971	Servo ventilator	B Jonsson, L Nordstrom; Elema-Schönander
	1958	Implanted pacemakers	Å Senning, R Elmqvist; Elema-Schönander
	1948	*Inkjet ECG printers*	R Elmqvist; Mingograph-Elema-Schönander
Norway	1870	Jaw thrust	J Heiberg
	1901	First open CPR	K Igelsrud
	1961	Resuscitation simulators	B Lind; Asmund Laerdal Industries

was appointed in Lund, and is remembered for his contributions to intensive care. At the Bispebjergs Hospital in Copenhagen, Nilsson, together with the director Carl Clemmesen, adapted basic anesthesiological principles (open and clear airways, physiotherapy, frequent changes of body positions and careful positioning of the patient; and, if necessary, artificial ventilation and circulatory support) to treat patients with barbiturate intoxication, thereby decreasing the mortality rate from 20 to 1 %. This 'Scandinavian method' continues as a cornerstone of the treatment of barbiturate intoxication and of intensive care [43].

In 1947, Olle Lundskog was appointed in Malmoe, and in 1949, Karl-Gustav Dhuner received the first position for an anesthetist in Gothenburg—Sweden's second largest city. Göran Haglund, the first pediatric anesthetist in Sweden and a pioneer in pediatric intensive care, was appointed in 1951. At Uppsala University, Martin Holmdahl, a PhD in physiology and trained in Great Britain, received an independent position in 1954. He developed a prominent research center and produced several academic scientists, including Ake Grenvik.

A Nordic Society

In 1949, Gordh, Mollestad, Turpeinen and Henning Poulsen (Denmark) met in Helsinki to form a Nordic Society (Nordisk Anaesthesiologisk Forening, NAF) and create a Nordic Anaesthesia journal. In 1950, the first congress was held in Oslo and the first bylaws were approved. Subsequently, these congresses have been held every second year, the venue rotating between countries. The president of the current congress also

serves as society chairman. A general secretary guarantees continuity.

Acta Anaesthesiologica Scandinavia (*AAS*) first appeared in 1957. Eric Nilsson in Lund, became the first editor-in-chief, and Poulsen played a pivotal role, acting as a member of the first Editorial board and taking responsibility for publishing the journal. For the first 15 years, the journal was printed in his home town in Denmark—Aarhus [44]. He also became the NAF's first Secretary General.

1945–60

An expanding surgical work load forced the few existing anesthesiologists to focus on clinical demands. Such pressures precluded research or teaching, and recruitment of doctors into anesthesia. Although the specialty had become indispensable, financial constraints limited the number of new anesthesiologist positions.. Despite these problems, Nordic anesthesiology developed rapidly.

While almost all of the first generation of Nordic anesthetists went to GB or the US for training, domestic centers slowly developed specialty training. Initially, importation of British and Irish colleagues was needed to fill new positions, and some of these doctors stayed and became valuable contributors to the specialty, particularly outside regional centers.

The initial creation of only one anesthesia position per hospital, required anesthesiologists to recruit anesthetic nursing staff to get the work done. But the nurses had worked under the surgeon's supervision, and both surgeons and nurses sometimes found it difficult to accept physician anesthesia-led departments. Eventually harmonious anesthetic departments were created with teams of nurses (with postgraduate specialty training) directed by anesthesiologists.

This team approach continues to the present. Although the number of doctors progressively increased, a shortage existed early in the history of the specialty, partly because anesthesiologists earned less than most other doctors (they received the same hospital salary but lacked the opportunity to gain income from private outpatients). Mollestad's successor, Jacob Stovner summarized the situation: *'At the end of the working day we biked homewards in the exhausts from the surgeons' limos'!*

Anesthesia from 1945–1960 paralleled that in the rest of the western world, a barbiturate induction and maintenance with nitrous oxide and ether. Cyclopropane was sometimes used for pediatric anesthetic induction. The introduction of muscle relaxants was enthusiastically accepted. Although Hunt and Traveau synthesized succinylcholine in Boston in 1906, the Swedes Thesleff, von Dardel, and Holmberg first tested it clinically in 1950 [45]. In the same year, the Swedish ENT surgeon Eric Carlens published experiences with the use of his invention, the double lumen tracheal-bronchial tube for separation of the lungs [46]. a prerequisite for pulmonary surgery.

A Gradual Expansion

Denmark is more densely populated than Finland, Iceland, Norway or Sweden, but all have metropolitan areas where a majority of the inhabitants live. In Iceland and Norway, the population is concentrated in coastal areas. These conditions led to differences in the development of anesthesiology. Hence separate descriptions are necessary for each country. We rely on the book *Scandinavian Anaesthesia during 150 years.* (Nordisk anestesiologisk forening), to describe these differences.

Denmark [47]

In Denmark, development after Lippmann and Mørch was slow. Willy Dam (1914–1990) assumed the first position as an anesthetist, created in 1944 at Bisbebjergs Hospital in Copenhagen (within the department of surgery). In 1948, Erik Andersen was employed at Gentofte hospital, where he provided anesthesia services to three different surgical departments. He was later given the first independent anesthetic position.

Poulsen and Ole Secher started their careers after the end of World War II. Secher worked at the major state hospital—Rigshospitalet—where in 1953, he received an academic position as a lecturer. Poulsen initially worked in Copenhagen, soon moving to Aarhus where he created a university department. As noted, in 1949, he started the Danish Society for Anaesthesiologists and was a founder of the Nordic association.

Around 1950, the state recognized anesthesiology as an independent specialty and anesthesia development expanded throughout Denmark. The World Health Organization started a one-year international course in anesthesiology (the Anesthesiology Centre) in Copenhagen, with the initial faculty including Henry Beecher, Harry Churchill-Davidson, Stuart Cullen, Francis Foldes, Emmanuel Papper, John Severinghaus and Jackson Rees. The course was repeated 23 times in the ensuing two decades. In 1953, the first independent anesthetic departments were created under Secher and Henning Ruben (famous for the development of the Ruben valve and the self filling ventilating bag, Table 32.1).

In 1952, a lethal poliomyelitis epidemic in Copenhagen led to the development of Intensive Care Units (ICUs). The epidemic prompted professor HCA Lassen to form an expert group charged with finding a strategy for treatment of cases with severe respiratory insufficiency. The free-lancing anesthetist, Bjørn Ibsen, (who had earlier spent a year in Boston with Beecher) with physiologist Poul Astrup, convinced this group that the patients had to receive intermittent positive pressure ventilation (IPPV). Physiologist Poul Astrup helped guide the ventilation by pioneering a new method of blood:gas analysis. Volunteer doctors, nurses and students performed this radical treatment, manually squeezing reservoir bags attached to tracheotomy tubes. Mortality decreased from 87 to 37 per cent, a remarkable achievement. Ibsen established a permanent ICU in the city hospital (Kommunehospitalet), in April 1954. Two Danish anesthesiologists, Henrik Bendixen and Henning Pontoppidan, emigrated to the US in the 1950s, becoming pioneers of ICU medicine at the Massachusetts General Hospital.

Finland [48]

Immediately after World War II, severe shortages of medical equipment, and the absence of positions for anesthesiologists, hindered development of anesthesia. Some conservative surgeons claimed that "*ether anesthesia administered by a nurse was quite sufficient*" (a well-known point of view). The first positions were created in the county hospital in Lahti in 1950, for Sakkari Pelttari and Jorma Airaksinen. As mentioned before, the pioneers Turpeinen and Aro had to wait until 1950 and 1953 before obtaining positions. Turpeinen, Aro and their colleagues worked diligently to establish the specialty. Turpeinen was one of the 1949 founding fathers of the Nordic Society. In 1952, he and three colleagues founded a national society, promoting the spread of the specialty in Finland. The Society focused on the need for education and training of doctors in anesthesia, and the creation of independent departments and positions for specialists.

The WHO anesthesiology centre in Copenhagen provided an important educational resource, attended by 22 Finnish anesthetists between 1950 and 1967. Others gained training in the UK. A domestic training program began in 1957–1958, requiring three years of anesthesiology, and one year of surgery, internal medicine, otology or basic sciences. The Society proposed establishment of university departments in Helsinki and Turku (Åbo), a dream realized in 1969–1970.

During this period, the Finnish Society of Anesthesiologists successfully negotiated for new positions and salaries. However, recruitment remained difficult and several measures were taken to improve the situation. A three-month compulsory training course in anesthesia for all surgical residents was implemented, and at their own request medical students were approached by the Society regarding careers in anesthesiology at several meetings. How much these measures affected recruitment is unclear, but the number of specialist members in the Finnish Society of Anesthesiologists steadily increased to reach 300 in 1980.

Iceland [49]

Jon Sigurdson observed that

> "*In Iceland as in all neighboring countries the development from 1950 was gigantic... When the specialty anesthesiology*

took its first steps it was not highly valued by other specialists. Less experienced colleagues, medical students, nurses and even unqualified staff members were entrusted to perform anesthetics. Anyone could do it!"

After Magnusdottir, came Alma Torarinsson and Valtyr Barnason, both having studied in the US. Thereafter, most anesthesiologists were educated in Nordic countries. The number of specialists increased from 11 in 1975 to 67 in 1999, for an Iceland population of 300,000 (i.e., by 1999 the same ratio as in the US). Several of these doctors pursued research in and outside Iceland.

Norway [50]

The first anesthesiologists worked in Oslo; Mollestad at the central State hospital (Rikshospitalet), and Ivar Lund at Ullevål's hospital (the major city hospital). Both faced a lack of support and understanding of what anesthesia could provide. Upon retirement, Mollestad noted that he started without a chair to sit on. The challenges were a general lack of doctors and low salaries for anesthesiologists, but an advantage that half of the specialists in Norway were women. The Norwegian pioneers worked to establish a professorship, finally succeeding in 1973, when Jakob Stovner was appointed at Rikshospitalet.

Norway/Scandinavia Contributed to Cardiopulmonary Resuscitation (CPR)

In 1901, Igelsrud performed the world's first successful open CPR (i.e., where an incision is made in the chest to allow resuscitation by directly squeezing the heart in a rhythmical manner), at the Tromsoe Amtsykehus (Hospltal) where he was the only doctor. Igelsrud has not received proper acknowledgement for this crucial first step in CPR. The description of this first resuscitation was published in 1904 in Therapia Gazette, by an American doctor WW Keen from Philadelphia, who was visiting Igelsrud.

In the late 1950s, in cooperation with Peter Safar and Åsmund Lærdal of Laerdal Industries, Norwegian anesthesiologists further contributed to the field of resuscitation. Bjørn Lind, at the hospital in Stavanger, pioneered the development of Resusci-Anne (Fig. 32.1). Laerdal's support facilitated the first meeting on the new management of cardiovascular collapse, "Symposium on Emergency Resuscitation-Rescue Breathing and Closed Chest Cardiac Massage" in Stavanger Norway from 21–25 August 1961 [51]. Since then Laerdal Industries have achieved international prominence, producing Resusci-Anne and her followers and also developing sophisticated equipment for simulators (Table 32.1).

In 2000, doctors at Tromsoe Hospital were again in the news, saving a victim of severe accidental hypothermia (13.7 °C), a world record [52]. While skiing, the victim fell head first through a hole in thick ice. Rushing water filled

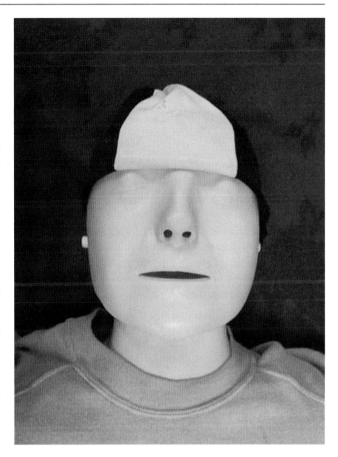

Fig. 32.1 Resusci Anne's face was supposedly based on "the death mask of an unidentified young woman reputedly drowned in the Seine River around the late 1880s." (Courtesy of Phil Parker, Leamington Spa, UK)

her clothes, wedging her in place. But she managed to turn her face sufficiently to breathe air beneath the ice. After 40 min, she ceased to move. When the rescue team arrived they declared her clinically dead. But they started Basic CPR because she was so cold. Within 2 hours cardiopulmonary bypass was initiated, and she was slowly warmed. She made a remarkable recovery, returning to work as a physician. What would Igelsrud have said about this achievement?

Sweden [53]

From 1945 to 1960, hospitals outside the major cities recruited increasing numbers of anesthetists. By 1960, almost all hospitals had anesthetic departments. However, as stated before, usually only one doctor was initially appointed. The anesthetist could not do all the cases and needed help from nurses who had previously performed anesthesia. This reflected the typical development of doctor–nurse teams in operating wards in all Nordic countries.

Surgeons in the central hospital in Borås (a regional centre in Southwest Sweden), convinced the board of directors in 1951, that it was necessary to engage an anesthesiologist. Eric Nilsson suggested Åke Bauer who accepted the offer with three conditions. (1) He should finish his specialty training. (2) He should be allowed to travel to GB and Germany to visit the postoperative wards of some major military hospitals. (3) An ICU should be established in Borås. All proposals were accepted, and on 1 June 1952, a properly equipped ICU was opened. For a few months it was only open during the daytime, but from December 1952, it was open 24 hours a day, caring for both surgical and medical cases. Bauer created nursing routines and even ethical guidelines for intensive care. He is regarded as one of the world's pioneers in intensive care [54].

A few years earlier, using the van Slyke method for gas analysis, Carl-Gunnar Engström at the Stockholm Hospital for Infectious Diseases, found that the available external methods for artificial ventilation (e.g., iron lungs) did not adequately ventilate the lungs of patients with severe poliomyelitis. He had been working with Crafoord and the 'spiropulsator', and realized that the problem could be solved by IPPV via a tracheotomy. At first this was done manually, but soon Engström and the engineer Paul Herzog constructed the ventilator thereafter named for Engström. The ventilator soon came into use in Stockholm, and in the 1952 polio epidemic in Copenhagen [54, 55].

1960–1980

During this period, anesthetic developments in Nordic countries converged. All hospitals established departments as the specialty's importance to medical care became obvious. Domestic specialist training and the number of specialists increased, although the number of positions lagged. For example, the Swedish Society of Anesthesiologists in 1966 had around 180 members; in 1974, 400 members; and in 2011, 1400 members. 'Sub-specialization' arose early in pediatric, cardiothoracic and neurosurgical sectors, and in intensive care medicine.

ICUs were gradually established, mostly as the province of departments of anesthesiology. Separate units also arose in some departments of cardiothoracic and neurological surgery. In smaller hospitals, postanesthesia care units (PICUs) might care for trauma and septic cases, drug overdoses, and severe internal medical emergencies. Most of these smaller units evolved to include intensive care. Before the development of coronary care units, PICUs might care for medical patients with cardiac dysfunction. Demand for care in ICUs was greater in larger hospitals. The severity of illness was greater and the criteria for admission stricter. In these hospitals, doctors increasingly specialized in ICU medicine, leading to a new subspecialty.

After 1975, Nordic anesthesiology developed in line with the rest of the western world—with some stylistic differences. Kjell Eric Strömskag described these in the context of a Specialty on Four Pillars—(1) Anesthesia, (2) Intensive Care Medicine, (3) Prehospital Emergency Care and Transportation and (4) Pain treatment [51].

Regarding anesthesia, the close cooperation between anesthesiologist and nurse anesthetists is a typical Scandinavian feature, without which early development would have been difficult. This cooperation has resulted in mature organizations with well-defined roles. Another feature is the small size of the private sector. The public sector runs most hospitals and is financed by taxation.

ICU Medicine. The early bonds created between anesthesia and ICU medicine remain close. Departments of anesthesiology run most ICUs, and the directors are anesthesiologists. Patients' primary care physicians and the director jointly decide treatment, but the director decides who is admitted.

Prehospital acute care and transportation. Scandinavian anesthetists have taken responsibility for prehospital acute care and interhospital transportation, particularly in Norway. Norway's long and jagged coastline hinders emergency access, and a good helicopter service is imperative. Anesthetists are responsible for the organization and medical protocols applied in this service. An anesthetist or ICU nurse usually accompanies the patient in the helicopter. Similarly, an anesthetic nurse is almost always in the crew of an ordinary ambulance service.

Another condition necessitating a special transportation organization is that patients in need of specialized care must often be transported to a tertiary hospital some 300 to 600 kilometers away. This has created a need for special expertise both in smaller and large hospitals. Some of the large centers have a special organization for these transports.

Treatment of pain. Nordic anesthesiologists have always participated in the development of pain treatment, beginning with consultations in terminal cases. Special pain units were formed in the 1970s, and the need for close cooperation with other specialties has resulted in the present multidisciplinary pain-clinics.

Nordic Organizations

Since its inauguration in 1951, congresses of the Nordisk Anestesiologisk Forening have been held every other year, alternating among the five countries. Before 1999, the president of the coming congress also acted as the chairman of the Society during the 2 year interval. However, the elected Secretary General in reality guaranteed the continuity of the administration. As the activities grew, the way of working with alternating presidents became inadequate. In 1997, the NAF General Assembly agreed on a change. Now a board and an executive president are elected for four years. The Society acts as an umbrella organization for the 5 national societies. This organization became the Scandinavian Society for Anesthesiology and Intensive Care (SSAI). The SSAI has assumed responsibility for education, quality of care, and research in anesthesiology in the original five countries and in the three Baltic countries. The national Societies continue their work both as unions and as organizations for education and research [56].

From its first issue, the journal *Acta Anaesthesiologica Scandinavica* (AAS) was published in English, intending to have an international presence. The first editor-in-chief was Eric Nilsson from Lund, Sweden, with Ibsen and Poulsen as Co-editors. Initially, four issues totaling approximately 250 printed pages were published each year. The number of pages increased progressively and several supplements were published.

In 1972, Olof Norlander succeeded Nilsson as Editor-in-Chief. Viggo Dyrberg from Gentofte, Denmark and Jan Eklund joined the board. Munksgaards became the publisher, and the characteristic red cover appeared. Under the editorship of Norlander and his successors Eklund and Sven E Gisvold (Trondheim, Norway), AAS has become a truly international, peer reviewed journal, which in 2010, published ten issues containing approximately 1300 printed pages [57].

Conclusions

Outside influence prompted the initial development of anesthesia practices in Nordic countries. Subsequently, Nordic physicians have made key contributions to anesthesia, intensive care medicine, pain therapy, airway management, blood-gas analysis, ventilatory care, the development of PACUs and ICUs, resuscitation, and simulations (Resusci-Ann), They have played an important part in making anesthesia and perioperative care what it is today—safer.

Acknowledgments Substantial parts of this text originate from the book: 150 År med Nordisk Anestesiologi (Scandinavian Anesthesia during 150 years, SA 150 yrs) which was published by the Nordic Society of Anesthesiologists, (Stockholm 1999). The contributing authors who are frequently cited in this text were: Preben G. Berthelsen, Denmark, Lena Janhunen, Finland, Jon Sigurdson, Iceland, and Per H. Rosenberg, Finland for the Society. We thank them all for valuable insights.

References

1. Nicolaysen J. Kirugien i Norge i det 19de århundrede [supplement]. Oslo (NO): Tidskrift for den norske laegeforening; 1933 (in Norwegian).
2. Gordh T. The development of anesthesiology in Sweden. Acta Anaesthesiol Scand. 1975;19:344–8.
3. Railo JO. Eeräs narkoosi. Medisiinari. 1955;XIX(9):13–4 (in Finnish).
4. Faye FC, editor. Forhandlinger I Lægeforeningen I Christiania I aaret 1847. Norsk Magazin for Lægevidenskapen; 1847. pp. 511–534 (issue 2) (in Norwegian).
5. Brandes LI. (Minutes from) Philiatriens Forhandlinger 1847. Mödet d. 23 Februar (in Danish).
6. Magnúsdóttir T. The development of anaesthesiology in Iceland. Acta Anaesthesiol Scand. 1975;19:336–40.
7. Palmgren EG. En ny bedöfningsapparat. In: Lindorm E, editor. Ny Svensk Historia; 1942, Part 2. p. 263 (in Swedish).
8. Jahunen L. Development of anaesthesiology in Finland. In: Eklund J, editor. Scandinavian anaesthesia during 150 years. Stockholm: Nordisk anaesthesiologisk forening; 1999. p. 58.
9. Berthelsen PG. Anaesthesiens 150-årige historie i Danmark. In: Eklund J, editor. Scandinavian anaesthesia during 150 years. Stockholm: Nordisk anaesthesiologisk forening; 1999. pp. 10–2 (in Danish).
10. Lindh A. Sammanställning af narkosstatistiken från de nordiska länderna för året 1 mars 1894 till 1 mars 1895. Nordiskt Medicinskt Ark. 1895;23:1–27 (in Swedish).
11. Wancher O. Aether versus Kloroform. Nordiskt Medicinskt Ark. 1898;29:1–8 (in Danish).
12. Gordh T. Anestesiologins utveckling I Sverige. Sv Läkartidningen. 1974;71:477 (in Swedish).
13. Faye FC, editor. Forhandlinger I Lægeforeningen I Christiania I aaret 1873. Norsk Magazin for Lægevidenskapen; 1873 (no. 4).
14. Strömskag KE. Norsk anestesis historie. In: Eklund J, editor. Scandinavian anaesthesia during 150 years. Stockholm:Nordisk anaesthesiologisk forening; 1999. pp. 99–134 (in Norwegian).
15. Reichborn-Kjennerud I. Narkose og lokal anestesi. Tidsskrift for Den norske Lægeforening; 1898. pp. 238-249 (no. 11) (in Norwegian).
16. Lennmalm F. Svenska Läkaresällskapets Historia 1808–1908. Stockholm: Svenska Läkaresällskapet; 1908. p. 302 (in Swedish).
17. Gordh T. The development of anesthesiology in Sweden. Acta Anesthesiol Scand. 1975;19:344.
18. Holmgren F. Om smärtförnimelse vid curareförgiftning. Upsala läkarförenings förhandlingar. 1880–81. p 557.
19. Levy F, editor. 10de Möde I Medicinsk Selskab. Bibl for Laeger. 1898;41:703–12 (in Danish).
20. Eklund J. Historien om Svensk anestesiologi ur ett NAF-perspektiv. In: Eklund J, editor. Scandinavian anaesthesia during 150 years. Stockholm: Nordisk anestesiologisk forening; 1999. p. 138 (in Swedish).
21. Schmiegelow E. Lidt om anvendelsen af Kokain ved Sygdomme I Struben, Svaelget, Naesen och Örene. Hospitalstidene. 1885;3RBIII:57–60 (in Danish).
22. Igelsrud K. Om kokain-anaesthesi af rygmarven. Tidskrift for Norges Laegeforening. 1905;11:389–97 (in Norwegian).
23. Munch-Petersen H. Rygmargsanaestesi ved Cocain. Hospitaltidende. 1902;45:289–93 (in Danish).
24. Nyström G. Lokal och regional anestesi med kokain och kokain-adrenalin. Läkartidningen. 1904;1:594 (in Swedish).
25. Editorial KA. Hospitaltidende. 1904;4RB12:510–1 (in Danish).
26. Lennander KG, Zachrisson LJF. Local and subarachnoid (Spinal) anestesia. In: Keen WW, DaCosta JC, editors. Surgery, its principles and practice. Philadelphia: WB Saunders; 1909. pp. 1045–100.
27. Forssner M. Report of: Slajmer E: Erfahrungen über Lumbalanästhesie mit Tropakokain in 1200 fällen. Sv Läkartidningen. 1906;3:492–4 (in Swedish).
28. Bäärnhielm G. Redogörelse för 100 fall av lumbalanästesi. Sv Läkartidningen. 1909;6:209–14 (in Swedish).
29. Saxtorph-Stein V. Mastoidaloperationer I Skopolamin-Morfin Narkose. Hospitaltidende. 1904;4RB12:1065–83 (in Danish).
30. Möllgaard H Teknisk redegörelse for et nyt 2 till overtrycksrespiration. Hospitalstidende. 1910;5RB3:569–80 (in Danish).
31. Giertz KH. Studies on pressure-difference respiration according to Sauerbruch and on artificial respiration (rhytmic insufflations of air)

[academic dissertation]. Uppsala (SE): University of Uppsala; 1916 (in Swedish).

32. Crafoord C. On pneumonectomies in man [academic dissertation]. Stockholm (SE): Karolinska Institute Medical University (Acta Chirurgica Scand); 1938 (suppl 65).

33. Backer-Grøndahl N. Narkose og pleie av operasjonspasienter. Oslo; 1920 (in Norwegian).

34. Olivecrona H. Några erfarenheter från 1925 om operativa ingrepp I bakre skallgropen. Läkartidningen. 1925;22:689–96 (in Swedish).

35. Moeller KO. Anestesiologiens udvikling I Danmark fra 1915, delvist beskrevet på grundlag af egne oplevelser. Medicinsk Forum. 1958;11:97–118 (in Danish).

36. Rosenberg M, Axelrod JK. Ernst Trier Mørch: inventor, medical pioneer, heroic freedom fighter. Anesth Analg. 2000;90:218–21.

37. Janhunen L. Development of anaesthesiology in Finland. In: Eklund J, editor. Scandinavian anaesthesia during 150 years. Stockholm: Nordisk anaestesiologisk Forening; 1999. pp. 57–63.

38. Sigurdsson J. Anaestesi i Island. In: Eklund J, editor. Scandinavian anaesthesia during 150 years. Stockholm: Nordisk anaestesiologisk forening; 1999. pp. 79–97 (in Scandinavian).

39. Strömskag KE. Norsk anestesis historie. In: Eklund J, editor. Scandinavian anaesthesia during 150 years. Stockholm: Nordisk anaesthesiologisk forening; 1999. pp. 99–134 (in Norwegian).

40. Gordh T. The development of anaesthesiology in Sweden. Acta Anaesthesiol Scand. 1975;19:344–8.

41. Löfgren N. Studies on local anesthetics: xylocaine a new synthetic drug [doctoreal dissertation]. Stockholm (SE): University of Stockholm; 1948.

42. Dahlgren N. Snille och tur har format svensk regionalanalgesi. Sv läkartidningen. 2011;108:739–41 (in Swedish).

43. Clemmesen C, Nilsson E. Therapeutic trends in the treatment of barbiturate poisoning. The Scandinavian method. Clin. Pharmacol Ther. 1961;2:220–29.

44. Poulsen H. The Scandinavian society of anaesthesiologists 1950–1975. Acta Anaesthesiol Scand. 1975;19:317–23.

45. Dardel O von, Thesleff S. Clinical experience with succinylcholine iodide, a new muscular relaxant. Curr Res Anesth Analg. 1952;31:250–7.

46. Carlens E. A new flexible double-lumen catheter for bronchospirometry. J Thorac Surg. 1949;18:742–6.

47. Berthelsen PG. Anaesthesiens 150-årige historie i Danmark. In: Eklund J, editor. Scandinavian anaesthesia during 150 years. Stockholm: Nordisk anaestesiologisk forening; 1999. pp. 9–56.

48. Janhunen L. Development of anaesthesiology in Finland. In: Eklund J, editor. Scandinavian anaesthesia during 150 years. Stockholm: Nordisk anaestesiologisk forening; 1999. pp. 57–78.

49. Sigurdsson J. Anaestesi i Island. In: Eklund J, editor. Scandinavian anaesthesia during 150 years. Stockholm: Nordisk anaestesiologisk forening; 1999. pp. 79–98 (In Scandinavian).

50. Strömskag KE. Norsk anestesis historie. In: Eklund J, editor. Scandinavian anaesthesia during 150 years. Stockholm: Nordisk anaesthesiologisk forening; 1999. pp. 99–134 (in Norwegian).

51. Strömskag KE. Et fag på søyler, anestesiens historie i Norge. Oslo: Tano Aschehoug; 1999 (in Norwegian).

52. Gilbert M, Busund R, Skagseth A, Nilsen P, Solbø JP. Resuscitation from accidental hypothermia of 13·7 °C with circulatory arrest. Lancet. 2000;355(9201):375–6.

53. Eklund J. Historien om svensk anestesiologi – ur ett NAF-perspektiv. In: Eklund J, editor. Scandinavian anaesthesia during 150 years. Stockholm:Nordisk anaestesiologisk forening; 1999. pp. 135–78 (in Swedish).

54. Wåhlin Å. Anestesi- och intensivvårdsläkarens roll i 1900-talets akutsjukvård. Sv Läkartidningen. 2004;101:2091–4 (in Swedish).

55. Engström CG. Treatment of severe cases of respiratory paralysis by the Engström universal respirator. Br Med J. 1954;2:666–9.

56. Rosenberg PH. The Scandinavian society of anaesthesiologists—50 years from the minutes. In: Eklund J, editor. Scandinavian anaesthesia during 150 years. Stockholm: Nordisk anaesthesiologisk forening; 1999. pp. 179–208.

57. Eklund J. Acta Anaesthesiologica Scandinavica—the journal. In: Eklund J, editor. Scandinavian anaesthesia during 150 years. Stockholm: Nordisk anaestesiologisk forening; 1999. pp. 209–27 (in Swedish).

A History of Anesthesia in South America

33

Adolfo Héctor Venturini

Summary

Before the discovery of anesthesia, clergy and shamans used opium, herbal extracts, and alcohol to diminish surgical pain. Infection and mortality were great. By 1847, ether anesthesia was used in Peru, Uruguay, Brazil, Argentina, and Venezuela, and in 1848, in Chile. By 1850, chloroform displaced ether. Surgeons gave or directed anesthetic delivery by colleagues, nurses, medical students, orderlies, midwives, priests or sisters. Chloroform use continued until the late 1800s when reports of cardiac arrest and liver damage decreased its appeal. French surgeon Ombrédanne invented an ether inhaler in 1908 that became the preferred method of anesthetic delivery in the first half of the 1900s. Waters' 1930s experiences with cyclopropane prompted its use until fatalities from explosions occurred in Chile and Peru. Various barbiturates were given in the 1920s and 1930s, with thiopental becoming the preferred induction agent throughout Latin America. Curare was used by the early-mid 1940s in Brazil, Venezuela, Argentina, and Uruguay. Many Latin American countries took up anesthesia with the inexpensive combination of procaine and thiopental, after its description in Argentina in 1949. Halothane replaced ether in the 1960s.

Soon after Bier's demonstration in 1899, most Latin American countries adopted spinal blocks with cocaine. In 1910, Peruvian Odriozola described paracervical block. Epidural blocks were reported in most Latin American countries between 1915 and 1939.

In 1939, Chilean anesthesiologist Meneses designed the "*Chilean Midget*" portable anesthetic machine that the Foregger company manufactured. In 1951–1952, Brazilian anesthesiologist Takaoka developed the Takaoka Respirator, and subsequently the Takaoka Universal Vaporizer which delivered various volatile anesthetics.

In 1921, Argentine surgeon Arce founded a "*School of Anesthesia Specialists*" in Buenos Aires. Aspects of training in anesthesia were offered in 1934, expanding to the first Brazilian specialty school in 1941. In 1947, Marín founded the first "*School of Anesthesia*" for Columbian physicians. In 1948, the University La Plata, Argentina, created the first University Graduate Course in Anesthesiology. Residencies arose in the 1950s in Brazil, Colombia, and Uruguay, and in Peru and Bolivia in the 1960s. In 1967, the Postgraduate Course of Anesthesia in the University Hospital of Caracas became the first International Training Center of Anesthesiologists of the World Federation of Societies of Anaesthesiologists (WFSA). The Latin American Confederation of Societies of Anesthesiologists was founded in Lima, Peru in October 1962, and in October 1987 became a Regional Chapter of the WFSA. The South American Federation of Anesthesiology was established in Paysandú, Uruguay, in 1987.

The first Spanish language journal, "*Revista Argentina de Anestesia y Analgesia*" (today "*Revista Argentina de Anestesiología*"), began publication in Buenos Aires in 1939. Currently, anesthesia societies in Argentina, Bolivia, Brazil, Colombia, Chile, Ecuador, Peru, Uruguay, and Venezuela publish journals.

Introduction

Ether and chloroform were used in South America only a few months after their first administration by Morton in Boston, and Simpson in Edinburgh. South America has subsequently been home to political and scientific events that influenced the history of anesthesia.

The Nineteenth Century

Pre-anesthesia Period

Before anesthesia came to South America, common surgical operations included exploration, draining and suturing of wounds, setting of fractures and dislocations, opening and

A. H. Venturini (✉)
Faculty of Medicine, University of Buenos Aires, Nueva York 2563, 1419 Buenos Aires, Argentina
e-mail: aventurini@anestesiologo.org

E. I Eger II et al. (eds.), *The Wondrous Story of Anesthesia*, DOI 10.1007/978-1-4614-8441-7_33, © Edmond I Eger, MD 2014

draining of boils and abscesses, excision of external tumors, and amputation followed by cautery with a hot iron [1]—procedures that could be rapidly accomplished. Operations were performed in homes or hospitals. Infection, erysipelas, septicemia, tetanus and gas gangrene were common and mortality was great, even for simple operations. Chest and abdominal wounds were invariably fatal.

Various practitioners provided treatment [2]. Physicians and Surgeons were "*Latinos*" and "*Romancistas*", classifications deriving from the Spanish. The Latin surgeon, equivalent to the current surgeon, was called a medical surgeon. Those setting fractures were "*ensalmadores*", "*calculistas*" and "*algebristas*", while "*flebótomos*" or "*sangradores*" (bleeders) performed bleeding, applied leeches and cupping glasses, and used tourniquets to stop bleeding. Midwives conducted home deliveries. Apothecaries prepared and dispensed medicines, and as in other parts of the world, members of religious communities, including Jesuits, Bethels, Dominicans and Franciscans provided medical care. Self-taught religious sisters and nuns living in hospitals, assisted in surgery. There were no schools of nursing.

Opium, Herbs, and Alcohol

As elsewhere in the world before the advent of anesthesia, the substances used to "alleviate" surgical pain [3] included opium, herbal extracts and alcohol. Pain killing confections ("*electuario*") such as "henbane opiate" might offer anise, fennel, myrrh, henbane seeds, opium, cinnamon, saffron and chamomile flowers, with honey as a carrier. Alcohol, including wine, sugar-cane liquor, beer, gin and rum were also used. In Argentina's Province of Mendoza "*analgesia was achieved through alcohol intoxication and opium, but these methods were not very effective to relieve pain during operations*" [4]. In Chile, according to Bulnes [5], "*the only anesthetic used, when mercy called for it, was alcohol*", which was given "*in the form of rum, wine, beer or ale, until the patient was drunk*". Jaime Pontón [6] wrote that in Colombia, it was common to use "*large doses of alcoholic beverages or preparations based on mandrake, Indian hemp and opium; the patient was strapped to a pallet or table and held by as many assistants as possible*".

Surprise, Deceit, and Restraint

In the absence of analgesic substances, the methods applied might include surprise, deceit and restraint. All ancient societies applied restraint. Pontón [6] wrote that in 1844, José Quevedo performed the first caesarean section "*without anesthesia*", in Medellín, Columbia. In 1838, in Montevideo, Uruguay, Spanish surgeon Cayetano Garviso [7] operated on a patient with an iliac artery aneurysm. He applied a peritoneal ligature to the left common iliac artery "*without anesthesia*", in twelve minutes.

The First Administration of Anesthesia with Ether

The news of Morton's demonstration of ether anesthesia on 16 October 1846 in Boston reached South America within months, and during 1847 and 1848, ether anesthesia was administered for surgery in several South American countries. The adoption of chloroform anesthesia decreased the use of ether (Table 33.1).

Peru

Higgins Guerra and Hernández de la Haza [8] wrote that Julián Bravo gave the first ether anesthetic on April 29, 1847, in Lima, adding that a headline in the local newspaper "*El Comercio*" announced: "*First test on etherization in this Capital City*". However, Zaldívar Sobrado [9] wrote:

> "*In Peru, the first anesthesia with ether was applied in 1848 by the great surgeon Dr. J. Sandoval at Remy Apothecary on a young man who had fractures in the right humerus at the neck and its lower third. Anesthesia came from a bottle at the bottom of which there was a sponge soaked with sulfuric ether and two tubes, one of which was for gas inhalation. A few minutes later, while already intoxicated, the fractures were set and a plaster bandage applied*".

The author concluded that the patient awoke without pain.

Uruguay

In early April 1847, the Montevideo newspaper "*Comercio del Plata*" reported the discovery of ether anesthesia [10]. In late April, the surgeon Adolfo Brunel tested the effect of ether by inhaling it himself. On 2 May, in the "*Charity Hospital*" of Montevideo, Brunel amputated the lower right arm of a soldier, accidentally shot when handling a cannon, the soldier being under ether anesthesia. Patricio Ramos, an Argentine physician born in Buenos Aires, administered the ether using an animal bladder (loaded with an ounce of ether) attached to a long tube that ended with a nozzle inserted into the patient's nose. The operation lasted four minutes, and the patient said he had felt little pain. During the ensuing months, Brunel as surgeon and Ramos as anesthetist, performed twelve operations with some untoward results, including restlessness, excessive saliva, coughing, and inadequate analgesia.

Brazil

In Rio de Janeiro on 20 May 1847, Roberto Lobo [11] and Domingo Marinho de Azevedo anesthetized Francisco Leme, a medical student. A descripton of this experiment was later published: "*As experiencias insensibilizantes do éter*". On 16 July, Leslie Curtis and Borges Monteiro used ether for surgical anesthesia in the "*Court of Military Hospital*", in Rio de Janeiro [12].

Table 33.1 First Administrations of Ether and Chloroform in Latin America

Date	Country	City	Anesthesia	Surgery	Anesthetist
11 Mar 1847	Cuba	La Habana	Ether	Hydrocele	V de Castro
29 Mar 1847	Mexico	Velacruz	Ether	Wound repair	E Barton
29 Apr 1847	Peru	Lima	Ether	Fractured humerus	J Sandoval Bravo
2 May 1847	Uruguay	Montevideo	Ether	Arm amputation	P Ramos
20 May 1847	Brazil	Rio de Janeiro	Ether	Experiment	RH Lobo
Aug 1847	Argentina	Buenos Aires	Ether	Strabismus	J Tewksbury
30 Nov 1847	Guatemala	Guatemala City	Ether	Finger amputation	J Luna
1847	Venezuela	Maracaibo	Ether	–	B Valbuena
Feb 1848	Uruguay	Montevideo	Chloroform	Phimosis	F Ferreira
Feb 1849	Cuba	La Habana	Chloroform	Breast tumor	N Gutierrez
July 1848	Argentina	Buenos Aires	Chloroform	Osteoclasia	J Mackenna
23 Oct 1848	Chile	Valparaiso	Chloroform	Arm amputation	F Villaneuva
1848	Brazil	Rio de Janeiro	Chloroform	Delivery	R de Bivar
1849	Columbia	Bogota	Chloroform	Breast tumor	A Reyes
1860	El Salvador	–	Chloroform	–	E Alvarez
1864	Paraguay	–	Chloroform	War injuries	–
1873	Ecuador	Quito	Chloroform	–	D Domec

"–" indicates absence of data

Argentina

Assisted by Teodoro Aubain (1814–1896), Jacob Tewksbury (1814–1877 operated on a male for correction of convergent strabismus, in Tewksbury's house, in Buenos Aires, without anesthetic or surgical complications. A report was published in the "*British Packet and Argentine News*", in Buenos Aires, on Saturday, 4 September 1847: "*A few days ago, we saw a correction of strabismus in a patient who was under the narcotic influence of ether vapor.*" In 1849, Tewksbury married Emilia Sutton, an Argentine, and returned with her to San Francisco, California, where he gained fame and wealth, thanks to the discovery of gold, but not ether [13].

Venezuela

Francis Ramírez [14] reported that "*according to the information obtained from the Revista Venezolana de Anestesiología, some historians argue that Dr. Blas Valbuena witnessed*" the anesthesia procedure performed by Morton on 16 October 1846, "*and that he took to Maracaibo a round glass instrument with two holes, similar to that used by Morton*", where he put a male patient to sleep with ether in 1847. No mention is made of the day or month.

Chile

While visiting the "*Hospital San Juan*" of Santiago, Chile on 13 April 1848, the historian Arnold Greene [15] wrote that "*Ether is now used here to perform operations*".

Colombia

There is no precise record of the first time anesthesia with ether was used in Colombia., Referring to the early years of the second half of the nineteenth century, Herrera Pontón wrote that "*ether and chloroform had probably arrived in Bogotá by that time*" [6].

The First Administrations of Anesthesia with Chloroform

In November 1847, Edinburgh obstetrician and surgeon, James Young Simpson used chloroform to ease the pain of childbirth. As in Great Britain, chloroform soon competed for acceptance with ether, initially tending to displace ether because of the faster and smoother induction found with chloroform. There was also the belief (without proof) that in abdominal operations it might cause greater muscle relaxation. Chloroform thus became widely used. However concerns arose regarding cardiac arrest associated with chloroform (white syncope) especially during induction, and chloroform ultimately fell into disuse.

Uruguay

"*Comercio del Plata*" [16] of Montevideo reported Simpson's successful use of chloroform. The French pharmacist Francisco Thibalier in Montevideo then distilled ethyl alcohol over calcium chloride to obtain chloroform. On 11 February 1848, in the "*Charity Hospital*" of Montevideo, Fermín Ferreira applied a sponge soaked with this chloroform to Jose Silva, and then operated to correct his phimosis. On 17 February, using chloroform for anesthesia, Bartolomé Odiccini operated on two soldiers. Subsequently, Brunel, with the same anesthetic, repaired a strangulated hernia in a 52 year old patient, and reported no complications.

It seems likely that the substance prepared by Thibalier was, in fact, chloroform, but this is not certain. In 1853, pharmacy student Mario Isola, at a meeting in the Society of Medicine of Montevideo, introduced chloroform prepared according to the standards set by "*Codex Medicamentorum Gallicus*", edition 1851.

Argentina

In 1848, John Mackenna in the "*British Medical Dispensary*" (from 1853 called the *British Hospital of Buenos Aires*) operated on a female patient for osteoclasia of the femur anesthetized with chloroform. On Saturday, 8 July 1848 the "*British Packet and Argentine News*" [17] in Buenos Aires, reported the event without referring to the day or the month of the surgical procedure.

Chile

In Valparaiso, in October 1848, Francisco Javier Villanueva administered chloroform for an upper limb amputation. The 23 October issue of "*El Mercurio*"[18] of Valparaiso, reported:

> "*Brilliant success of chloroform...A 90 year old woman had been taken to the hospital with a shattered arm caused by a fall. Dr. Villanueva decided to make the amputation of the arm with the aid of chloroform, which took effect without the patient feeling any pain; today, 15 days later, she is almost fully recovered.*"

Brazil

Chloroform was used on a recently delivered mother by Rodrigo de Bivar [11] in Rio de Janeiro in 1848. There is no reference as to the day or month.

Colombia

In 1849, Antonio Reyes successfully resected a breast tumor with the patient anesthetized with chloroform [19]. In Bogotá, in 1864, chloroform was used to perform the first resection of an ovary, while in Medellín, it was first used in 1880.

Venezuela

Eliseo Acosta [14] used chloroform in Caracas in 1848, and Guillermo Michelena subsequently enhanced its popularity. In 1856, Carlos du Villards bought the first apparatus for administration of chloroform (an accurate description of the apparatus is not available).

Paraguay

Chloroform was used during the War of the Triple Alliance (1864–1870, Argentina, Brazil and Uruguay against Paraguay). Sanabria Ortiz wrote that "*Anesthesia, that had already begun to be used during the War of the Triple Alliance, was popularized*". Apparently, chloroform came late to Paraguay.

Ecuador

Ettine Gayraud and Dominique Domec wrote in 1873 about "*the professionalism of surgical procedures in Quito since the early usage of chloroform anesthesia. In those years, alcohol (liquor) and exotic weeds were used for surgery*" [20]. Domec, an anesthesiologist from "*San Eloy Hospital*" of Montpellier, appointed as Professor of Anatomy and Anesthesia, introduced chloroform in 1873, at the "*Hospital San Juan de Dios*" in Quito, applying it with a handkerchief or dressing.

Ether or Chloroform?

In South America, chloroform was initially used more than ether because induction was faster and quieter, without salivation or coughing. It was easier to use in obese patients. There was the perception that greater relaxation was obtained during abdominal surgery and that patients awoke more rapidly. In the late nineteenth century, its use decreased because of reports of liver damage.

In 1848, Brunel (see above) said: "*Judging by the first times I used chloroform, it seems to have more advantages than ether; with the new chemical preparation, the patient does not cough, does not have muscle contractions and the effect is both more secure and faster*".

Argentine surgeon and historian Oscar Vaccarezza [15], commented on the thesis by Leopoldo Montes de Oca "*Notes on surgical clinic in Buenos Aires in 1852, 1853, 1854*", writing that Montes de Oca "*widely used chloroform anesthesia, which by then had displaced ether in the rest of the world and here in Buenos Aires*". In Argentina, during the second half of the nineteenth century, eight doctoral theses were presented at the School of Medicine of Buenos Aires, all concerning chloroform administration: L Montes de Oca (1854), J Clara (1857), R Gutiérrez (1868), W Taylor (1880), E de Elía (1881), CR Seguí (1888), E Pittaluga (1888), and DI Rapela (1897). And Ricardo Gutierrez' thesis "*Elimination of childbearing pain by means of chloroform*", indicates that he was one of the first Argentine anesthetists ("*cloroformista*") to treat pain in obstetric patients.

In Colombia, during the last quarter of the nineteenth century, according to Herrera Pontón [6], "*ether and chloroform were widely used, but it seems that the latter was the anesthetic product on the rise*". Doctoral theses at the University of Colombia indicate that chloroform "*was mostly used*". In 1891, Teodoro Castrillón suggested that the lower partial pressures of oxygen in the highlands of Bogotá contraindicated the use of chloroform and recommended that oxygen be added to devices used to vaporize chloroform. José Joaquín Azula's 1895 thesis entitled "*General anesthesia*" is exclusively dedicated to chloroform. He argued that anesthesia procedures should be performed by physicians.

During the Pacific War (1879–1884), when Chile fought Bolivia and Peru, Huete Lira [21] wrote that chloroform "*was simpler to use than ether, and it was not explosive, which was very important when operations were performed under the light of candles or gas lamps*".

In Brazil from 1896, ether acquired a greater popularity thanks to Daniel d'Almeida, a pioneer of Brazilian anesthesia who wrote "*Do éter como anestésico em cirurgia*". Nevertheless, the Rio de Janeiro surgeon, Álvaro Ramos separated conjoint twins, Maria and Rosalina in 1899. The "narcotizers" Fajardo and Pereira (Maria) and Couto and Leal (Rosalina) used chloroform [22].

In Venezuela, chloroform was most popular until the early twentieth century.

Who Administered Ether and Chloroform?

Initially, surgeons administered anesthesia, but soon the task was delegated to internal medicine physicians, medical students, nurses, orderlies, midwives, priests and sisters, and, according to Herrera Pontón, hospital porters [19]. The surgeon directed the "*cloroformista*", "*cloroformizador*" or "*eterizador*", the people who administered chloroform or ether.

Administration Technique: The First Inhalers

The first South American anesthetists dropped ether or chloroform onto dressings, tissues, sponges and towels applied to the nose and mouth of the patient. In Buenos Aires [15], in 1852, anesthetists used a paper bag stuffed with fabric or lint (the precursors of gauze) obtained by fraying old sheets. The lips and nasal mucous membranes were smeared with substances such as cerate (white wax and olive oil) or sweet almond oil to protect them.

A Scottish physician, John Alston, performed the first ovarian resection in Argentina in 1870, administering chloroform with Snow's Apparatus [15]. In 1877, Ignacio Pirovano, the most prestigious Argentine surgeon of the nineteenth century, also resected an ovary with the patient anesthetized with chloroform given via a Junker's Inhaler [15]. Physicians praised the method because it produced "*the surgical anesthetic effect quickly without generating a period of excitement*".

Sites of Anesthesia and Surgical Procedures

As mentioned above, surgery might be performed in hospitals or patients' homes. In Montevideo [23], surgery was also performed in local inns, where a guest room, bare of furniture, became an operating room. The table used for lunch and dinner became the operating table. The patient recovered in his usual bedroom. After Lister's work was publicized in 1867, the "operating" room was sprayed with carbolic acid.

Nitrous Oxide

The high cost of storing and transporting nitrous oxide restricted its use in Latin America during the nineteenth century. It did attract interest because of its non-pungency, nonflammability, rapid action, and absence of circulatory depressant effects. However, the use of pure nitrous oxide by inexpert anesthetists sometimes led to hypoxia and cardiac arrest. Coadministration of oxygen would circumvent this problem, but added to the storage and transportation costs. Most use in the nineteenth century was as brief administrations in dental operatories. Ecuador, Argentina, Colombia and Chile did use it in the nineteenth century, while other Latin American countries introduced it in the twentieth century. Its use became popular in the 1950s when it was locally manufactured.

Ecuador
In 1870, Alejandro Shibbeye, a Swedish national, used "*the nitrous oxide anesthetic, as advised by its discoverer*" [24], in Quito. The identity of the "discoverer" is unclear, but the author of the reference (Oswaldo Pinto) studied under Rovenstine in 1960–2.

Argentina
The dental surgeon, Louis Ernest [15], introduced nitrous oxide on 16 June 1871 in Buenos Aires, performing practical demonstrations of dental extractions before prestigious physicians. Ernest volunteered to take "*laughing gas*" (*sic*) administered by his colleague, Winkelman, a surgeon in the War of Paraguay. On 18 May 1874, the "*Buenos Aires Medical Surgical Journal*" called attention to deaths from the use of 100 % "*laughing gas*" in dental extractions.

In 1905, Nicasio Etchepareborda spoke on "*Short general anesthesia*" at the School of Medicine of Buenos Aires, saying that nitrous oxide "*is the safest of all anesthetics*" according to statistics published in the US and England, and that accidents occurred in Argentina because the gas was "*handled by incompetent hands*". He also suggested the addition of "*small amounts of oxygen.*"

Colombia
Lázaro Restrepo [6] used nitrous oxide in 1885, in the city of Antioquía.

Chile
According to Aureliano Oyarzún [18], some American dentists used "*nitrous oxide or laughing gas*" in Chile before 1890.

Uruguay

Nitrous oxide use began in the early twentieth century, although only in rare cases. Pedro Cantonet, José Bado and Manuel Herrera performed the first documented anesthesia procedures with it in 1926.

Paraguay

In Paraguay, nitrous oxide use was sporadic in the early twentieth century.

Venezuela

Beltrán Hurtado [14] delivered nitrous oxide in 1917 at the "*Hospital Vargas*" de Caracas.

Peru

In 1918, Novoa presented his doctoral thesis "*The N₂O narcosis*". The author wrote that Graña administered most of the anesthetics, using an apparatus that delivered nitrous oxide, oxygen and ether. He said that nitrous oxide use should be reserved for short operations.

Brazil

Using Desmarest's device, Leonido Ribeiro introduced nitrous oxide anesthesia in Rio de Janeiro in 1926, and then in Sao Paulo. In 1930, Pedro Netto of Sao Paulo presented his doctoral thesis "*Anestesia Geral pelo Protóxido de Azoto*", the thesis becoming the first paper on anesthesia to be awarded a prize in Brazil.

August Bier was a Rural Physician in Argentina

The German physician August Bier (1861–1949) pioneered spinal analgesia in surgical procedures. After graduating in 1896, he served for a short time as a doctor in the rural city of Lincoln [15] in Buenos Aires province, 320 km from the city of Buenos Aires. He returned to Germany, where his further career is well known. Bier's best quote is: "Medical scientists are nice people, but you should not let them treat you!"

Twentieth Century

Spinal Blocks

The first spinal anesthetics were performed in the late nineteenth century, in Brazil and Uruguay, but only in the twentieth century was this method fine-tuned and accepted worldwide. August Bier performed the first spinal anesthetic, anesthetizing his graduate student on 16 Aug 1898, in Kiel, Germany, injecting 3 ml of 0.5 % cocaine. Bier should have received the first "spinal", but after introducing the needle,

and while spinal fluid gushed forth, the graduate student found that the syringe containing cocaine didn't fit the hub of the needle. Bier got a spinal headache, and the graduate student got the spinal anesthetic. Spinal anesthesia quickly spread throughout South America. Favoring its application were its low cost and the flexibility it permitted the surgeon who could (sequentially) give the anesthetic and perform the surgery. Spinal anesthesia also did not impose some of the dangers of general anesthesia, such as hypoxia and hepatotoxicity.

Brazil

Paes Lemes performed spinal anesthesia in the "*Santa Casa de Misericordia*" of Rio de Janeiro in 1898 (no reference as to day or month). Starting in 1901, Daniel de Almeida [11] promoted the "*spinal*" in Brazil.

Uruguay

In 1899, Alfredo Navarro [25] used spinal anesthesia in the "*Hospital Maciel*" with 0.5 % cocaine for amputation of a gangrenous leg. In 1921, Alberto Roldán [26] published a paper in the "*Annals of the School of Medicine*" on "*spinal anesthesia*", using procaine in 165 patients at the "*Hospital Galán y Rocha*" of the town of Paysandú.

Venezuela

On 17 July 1900, Pablo Ortiz [14] used spinal anesthesia with cocaine, at the "*Hospital Vargas*" of Caracas. In that hospital on 18 August 1908, a medical student, Eudoro González, used stovaine for spinal anesthesia.

Argentina

In 1900, José Sabatini, in the "*Hospital Rawson*" in Buenos Aires, graduated from the School of Medicine of Buenos Aires. His thesis was: "*Analgesia with spinal injection of cocaine*" [15]. In another doctoral thesis, "*Cocaine injections in the lumbar arachnoid*", Bartolomé Podestá [15] wrote that he had performed 195 spinal anesthetics under the surgery service of Aguilar, in "*Hospital San Roque*" of Buenos Aires, without complications. In 1905, surgeons Heinrich Braun (1862–1934) in Germany and José Arce [15] (1881–1968) in "*Hospital Alvear*" in Buenos Aires (where he was Chief of Surgery) used procaine for spinal anesthesia.

In the 1920s, Arce, as Director of the Institute of Surgery Clinic of the "*Hospital Clínicas*" in Buenos Aires, devoted his efforts to improving anesthesia in Argentina. In 1921, he founded a school for anesthesia specialists, and established a course "*Anesthesia for all practical physicians*" where he taught spinal anesthesia techniques and the use of Ombrédanne's apparatus. In a 1931 paper presented at the Fourth National Congress of Medicine held in Buenos Aires, Arce and Braulio Pérez wrote: "*We believe that over 80 % of operations can be performed with local or spinal anesthesia and in this way, the patient will benefit, because we avoid the serious poisoning threat that general anesthesia represents".*

Ecuador

Barzallo Sacoto [27] claimed that spinal anesthesia was introduced in 1901 in the city of Quito. However Moran Pinto [24] said that *"in 1903 in Guayaquil, Dr. Miguel Achig Alcívar applied the first spinal anesthesia procedure".*

Peru

In 1902, at the *"Hospital Dos de Mayo"*, Barton gave a spinal anesthetic with cocaine for the resection of a testicle [8]. In the same year, two doctoral theses were presented: E Muñoz graduated with *"Spinal anesthesia with cocaine at birth"*, and V Diez Canseco with *"Spinal surgery"*, both physicians injecting 3 ml of 0.5 % cocaine.

Colombia

In 1905, Lisandro Leyva at *"Hospital San José"* in Bogotá, performed the first spinal anesthetic [6] in Colombia. In 1913, Juan Montoya y Flores presented a paper at the Second National Medical Congress, on spinal anesthesia with cocaine and stovaine.

Chile

Vargas Salcedo [18] performed the first spinal anesthetic in 1905, according to a paper he presented in October 1923, at the *"Chilean Medical Society"*.

Headaches Due to *Dura Mater* Puncture

In 1963, Edgar Aguirre de Caracas [28] reported headache relief after a *dura mater* puncture, obtained by placing a "blood patch" in the epidural space. In 1967, José Usubiaga, Lilia Usubiaga and Jaime Wikinski [29] of Buenos Aires, addressed the same complication, by administering 60 ml of saline solution.

Paracervical Block

In 1910, the Peruvian doctor, E Febres Odriozola [30] presented the first description of the paracervical block, specifying the indications and contraindications that are still recognized today.

Ombrédanne's Apparatus

The French surgeon, Louis Ombrédanne (1871–1956) created a hand-held inhaler for the administration of ether in

1908: *"Un appareil pour l'anesthésie par l'éther"* [31]. It was subsequently widely used in Europe, especially in France and Germany, and in Latin America, when ether started to prevail over chloroform. Ombrédanne's inhaler found minimal acceptance in English-speaking countries, but was the most popular *"anesthesia machine"* in the first half of the twentieth century in many hospitals in Latin America, largely because of its safety and simplicity.

Ether was administered in increasing concentrations from Ombrédanne's inhaler by moving a pointer that went from zero to eight. The device precluded spillage of liquid ether onto the patient's face. A source of oxygen could be placed under the mask of the device. Practitioners, medical students, nurses and nuns used Ombrédanne's inhaler.

Uruguay

In 1910, Enrique Pouey brought an Ombrédanne's inhaler from Paris. The use of this apparatus greatly expanded the popularity of ether.

Argentina

Argentine surgeon, Pedro Chutro [32], introduced Ombrédanne's inhaler in 1911. Until the mid 1950s, hospital interns in municipal hospitals in Buenos Aires were charged with its use in emergency operations. The intern who arrived late to the Emergency Service of *"Hospital Juan A. Fernández"* was punished by having to use Ombrédanne's apparatus (author's personal experience). The seat reserved for the anesthesiologist had a small drawer underneath that contained Heister's mouth opener, a metal airway, Lucas Championnière's tongue forceps and a Schimmelbusch mask.

Venezuela

Ombrédanne's apparatus arrived in 1912, according to F Ramírez [14], and ether *"displaced the use of chloroform almost completely".*

Chile

In October 1912, Zegers presented a paper on the use of Ombrédanne's apparatus at the *"Chilean Medical Society"* [18]. The apparatus continued to be a mainstay of anesthetic practice in Chile for the next 50 years. In 1925, González Ginouvés [33] said: Ombrédanne's apparatus was *"the responsibility of an intern who, upon arrival, received nervous brief instructions from another intern who was finishing his shift. In infra-umbilical conditions, spinal anesthesia is preferred".* In 1927, Ombrédanne himself, visited the Pediatric Surgery Department at *"Hospital Infantil Manuel Arriarán"* in Santiago de Chile [34]. In 1960, the *"Plan of Anesthesiology Education"* at the School of Medicine, University of Chile, by Raúl Jería, included a *"hands-on learning approach"* using Ombrédanne's apparatus [35].

Peru

In 1914, L de la Puente described the first ether anesthesia using Ombrédanne's apparatus, administered by the intern R Ugaz [8].

Ecuador

Ombrédanne's inhaler was used after 1917, together with Ricard's apparatus [24].

Colombia

In the "*Hospital Municipal*" of the town of Manizales "*in the beginning, anesthetics were administered by an emergency nurse, or some young ladies, or a surgeon using ether with Ombrédanne's apparatus*". In 1932, Juan Marín, an important Columbian anesthetist of the time, gave ether anesthesia using Ombrédanne's apparatus [6].

Bolivia

According to Crespo Villegas [36] of the Medical Institute in the city of Sucre "*in Bolivia, there is no information on its* (Ombrédanne's apparatus) *use*".

Cyclopropane

After its first clinical administration in 1930, and the publication of Ralph Waters' experiences in 1934, cyclopropane use became widespread in South America—until explosions claimed several lives. Manufacture and use of cyclopropane then ceased.

Paraguay

In 1928, Roberto Olmedo, an orthopedic surgeon, returned from the US. Using a Foregger anesthetic machine, he was the first to give cyclopropane.

Venezuela

In the 1930s, Roberto Baptista [14] gave cyclopropane using a Foregger anesthetic machine.

Argentina

The first to use cyclopropane in Buenos Aires, was Roberto Elder [36], in 1935.

Brazil

Álvaro de Aquino Salles used cyclopropane in 1936, and in 1940 presented his paper "*Anestesia gaseosa em ginecología y obstetricia*".

Uruguay

In 1936, Eduardo Palma [37] administered cyclopropane to obstetric patients.

Colombia

Herrera Pontón wrote that cyclopropane was first used in 1938 by Juan Martínez, in the "*Clínica de Marly*" in Bogota [6].

Chile: Lethal Explosions with Cyclopropane

In April 1945, an assistant was transferring oxygen from a large cylinder at high pressure to a small cylinder of cyclopropane [38]. An explosion resulted, killing the assistant.

On 6 May 1963, in Santiago "*Hospital de Niños Manuel Arriarán*", a cyclopropane cylinder exploded, causing, in turn, the explosion of another cylinder on an adjacent anesthesia machine [39]. A fire ensued. Four doctors (two anesthesiologists and two surgeons) and two patients, both children, died. Two other physicians were seriously injured, and 12 assistants suffered injuries of various severity, two requiring amputation of the leg. The use of cyclopropane was then banned throughout the country.

Peru: Lethal Explosions with Cyclopropane

A uterine curettage was scheduled in July 1971, at a clinic in Lima [40, 41]. A portable lamp with a loose electric cable was switched on while near a leaking cylinder of cyclopropane. The resulting explosion killed an anesthesia resident and a nurse assistant.

Epidural Blocks

Peru

To produce obstetrical analgesia in 1915, F Ferreyra [42] used caudal epidural blocks (via the sacral hiatus), injecting 3 ml of 0.3 % procaine. Patients were sedated with morphine and scopolamine subcutaneously.

Chile

In March 1920, Basilio Muñoz [18] published a paper on "*epidural anesthesia*".

Brazil

In 1926, Francisco Linz wrote on "*lumbar-sacrum epidural anesthesia*" as did Enio Mondatori in 1938. In 1940, Pedro Netto and Nicolau Manzini, published "*Contribution to the study of epidural anesthesia*" in "*Revista Argentina de Anestesiologia*".

Venezuela

At the Medical Congress of Venezuela held in 1926, in Maracay, A Van Tienhoven [14] of Caracas, presented cases of caudal epidural anesthesia.

Argentina and the "Hanging drop sign of Gutiérrez"

Alberto Gutiérrez (1892–1945), Professor and Chief of surgery at the "*Spanish. Hospital*" in Buenos Aires, founded the magazine "*Revista Argentina de Anestesia y Analgesia*" in 1939. In 1933, while performing an epidural needle insertion using the "loss of resistance" method (sign of Dogliotti,), he found considerable resistance when reaching the ligamentum flavum (yellow ligament). On detaching the syringe, he noted a drop of anesthetic solution (1 % procaine) hanging from the needle hub. He decided not to reattach the syringe, but slowly advanced the needle. Moments later, the drop disappeared into the needle, and he decided to inject 5 ml of procaine, repeating four boluses sparingly, and thus achieved successful analgesia. That year, Gutiérrez announced the finding in the Buenos Aires publications "*El Día Médico*" [43] and "*Revista de Cirugía*" [44]. Gutiérrez' technique has gained international acceptance.

Ecuador

Barzallo Sacoto [27] wrote that he performed the first epidural in 1937, but Moran Pintos [23] claims it was 1938, and that it was performed by Elias Andas.

Uruguay

With Alonso and Pérez Fontana, Eduardo Palma [24] spoke on "*Segmental epidural anesthesia*" at the 22 November 1939 meeting of the Society of Surgery. After visiting Alberto Gutiérrez, Palma used 1 % procaine.

Invention of Apparatus and Instruments

In 1934, José Delorme (Buenos Aires, 1903–1986), an important pioneer, a member of the National Academy of Medicine, and an advocate of anesthesiology in Argentina, created a machine for the delivery of anesthesia, particularly ethyl chloride, ether and chloroform. Delorme was a founding member and first president of the Argentine Association of Anesthesiology in 1945 [45, 46].

In 1939, Argentines Juan Miranda and Roberto Goyenechea, both anesthesiologists from the Institute of Surgery Clinic of the "*Hospital de Clínicas*" of Buenos Aires, devised a portable anesthesia machine called ADELIC (Institute of Surgery Apparatus). It worked with the "to and fro" system created by Ralph Waters, and could administer ether and cyclopropane. This device was taken to Montevideo by the Uruguayan, Ignacio Villar [47].

In 1939, the Foregger company in New York built a portable anesthesia apparatus, designed by the Chilean anesthesiologist Ernesto Meneses. The unit was called the "Chilean Midget" [48]. It was equipped with four cylinders (two oxygen, one cyclopropane, and one nitrous oxide), a flowmeter for each of the gases, and a vaporizer for ether. Meneses was a founding member of the Chilean Society of Anesthesiology, and President from 1957–1958.

In 1943, E de Souza [49] from Rio de Janeiro, Brazil, invented an apparatus comprising a balloon indicator, to confirm the correct location of an epidural needle. Robert Macintosh described this device in 1950, and introduced it into the anesthesia market.

In 1949, Argentine anesthesiologist and inventor Osmán Yanzón [50] created a device called "*Resucitador de Yanzón*" for newborns with respiratory problems. The device delivered oxygen during resuscitation and enabled aspiration of secretions. Yanzón was a founder, in 1945, of the Argentine Association of Anesthesiology.

In 1951–1952, Brazilian anesthesiologist and manufacturer Kentaro Takaoka developed a portable ventilator (Takaoka Respirator) for controlled artificial ventilation, cycling with a fixed delivered pressure [51]. In 1955, he conducted the first clinical trials. Subsequently, Takaoka designed and manufactured a small vaporizer (Takaoka Universal Vaporizer) [52] allowing the use of any of the available volatile anesthetics: ether, chloroform, trichlorethylene, halothane, or methoxyflurane.

In 1988, Alberto Torrieri of Buenos Aires, with the help of J Antonio Aldrete, introduced a needle for combined spinal-epidural block (First global communication) [53].

Intravenous Anesthetics: Somnifene—Pernocton—Eunarcon—Hexobarbital—Thiopental

Several barbiturates played small roles in anesthesia in South America in the early 1900s, including Somnifene® (a combination of barbital and diallylbarbituric acid), Eunarcón, Evipan, and hexobarbital. These vanished from clinical use after the arrival in the 1930s of the ultra-short-acting thiopental.

Uruguay

In 1925, A Langón [54] published his experiences with Somnifene® (first used intravenously in 1924) for obstetric analgesia (nine cases), caesarean section (one case), and hernia surgery (one case). In 1934, MB López, A Stábile, M Albo and P Martincich, presented their experiences with hexobarbital. No reports indicate the commercial introduction of thiopental [55].

Venezuela

Leopoldo Aguerrevere gave Pernoctón® (the first barbiturate used frequently to provide intravenous general anesthesia) in 1933, at the Maternity "*Hospital Vargas*" of Caracas. The first to use hexobarbital in Venezuela were P Gásperi, A Castillo and L Santana. Santana [14] also was the first to administer thiopental, giving it in 1942.

Argentina

In 1934, Germán Wernicke introduced hexobarbital for short-term anesthesia. In 1939, two anesthesiologists from the "*British Hospital*" of Buenos Aires, Leslie Cooper and Alberto Daniel, conducted the first trials with thiopental sodium, writing that "*The turbulent induction caused by inhalants has been left behind us*" [46].

Peru

In 1934, P Nagaró [8] presented his thesis "*Anesthesia of sodium Evipan*" (hexabarbital), and N Pareja wrote "*Sodium Evipan in short-term obstetric interventions*". In 1940, commenting on the current status of anesthesia in Peru, R Rubatto said that general anesthesia was widely accepted, but its delivery lacked anesthesiologists. He then stated that adoption of gas anesthesia had failed while intravenous general anesthesia had been widely accepted. In 1943, M Falvi presented his doctoral thesis "*About childbearing analgesia with sodium pentothal*", a trial performed at the "*Maternity Hospital*" of Lima. In the 1950s, the use of thiopental became widespread.

Colombia

An advertisement, printed by Abbott Laboratories de Colombia in 1934, suggests that thiopental was introduced as an anesthetic agent in 1934. According to Herrera Pontón [6], the first anesthesia procedures using cyclopropane and thiopental were performed in 1938.

Ecuador

In 1938, hexobarbital was first used in Riobamba [24].

Muscle Relaxants

As in the rest of the world, the arrival of the first muscle relaxant (Intocostrin®) to South America, fundamentally changed anesthesia and surgery. This was literally a drug that had come home. The obvious advantages of paralysis on demand were balanced by the less obvious drawbacks of this first neuromuscular blocking drug (e.g., histamine release, arterial hypotension, bronchospasm, and, most importantly, residual paralysis after anesthesia). These effects stimulated the search for safer synthetic compounds.

Brazil

In 1942, Oswaldo Vital extracted alkaloids from the *Strychnos* plant, which had a relaxing effect on striated muscle. Purified, this substance became *chondodendrum platyphyll*, and was marketed in 1945 as "*Condrocurare*"®. This drug was marketed only in Brazil, and had the merit of having been discovered by a Brazilian.

Venezuela

Pascual Scannone [14] trained in the US and introduced the use of curare in Latin America in 1942, performing the first tracheal intubation at the "*Hospital del Algodonal*" in Caracas, in a patient paralyzed with curare.

Argentina

Roberto Elder (1904–1969), was a founder of the Argentine Association of Anesthesiology. In 1945, he published an article in "*La Semana Medica*" [56] "*The use of curare in surgery and anesthesia*", noting the importance of "*highly experienced anesthesiologists with a perfect notion of directed ventilation and equipped with a suitable anesthesia machine to do it*".

Uruguay

Walter Oría, Juan Scasso and Antonio Cañellas administered the muscle relaxant Intocostrin®, the first commercial curare extract, in 1945 [57].

Colombia

Herrera Pontón [6] wrote that cyclopropane was first used in 1938, adding that curare was later incorporated, but not specifying the date.

Ecuador

In 1950, in Guayaquil, Rafael Comte performed naso-tracheal and oro-tracheal intubations after injecting muscle relaxants.

Peru

In the 1950s, Peter Safar visited Peru, promoting tracheal intubation and the use of muscle relaxants.

Specialization in Anesthesiology

Argentina

In 1921, Arce founded a "*School of Anesthesia Specialists*" at the "*Hospital de Clínicas*" in Buenos Aires, the first in Latin America. He taught "*Anesthesia for all practical physicians*". The thirty attendees learned spinal anesthetic techniques with procaine, and the use of ether with Ombrédanne's apparatus.

In 1936, Arce with Oscar Ivanissevich organized the second course in "*Anesthesia for all practical physicians*". Mexican Federico Vollbrechthausen, who had trained at the Mayo Clinic, taught the course. It was also held at the "*Hospital de Clínicas*". Attendees learned to intubate, and to use Foregger's anesthetic machine with an open, semi-open, or closed circuit, using mixtures of cyclopropane, ethylene, and nitrous oxide with ether.

In 1961, in Buenos Aires, Roberto Elder introduced a "*Graduate Course*" of two years duration, the beginning of a residency in anesthesiology. Later, the School of Medicine of the University of Buenos Aires agreed to the development of a four-year program leading to award of the "*Degree of Medical Specialist in Anesthesiology*". In 2008, the course was extended to five years.

Brazil

Mario d'Almeida, Oscar Ribeiro and Ivo Thiago, established some aspects of training in anesthesia, in 1934 in Rio de Janeiro. They expanded this to the first Brazilian specialty school in 1941. After 1955, "*Centros de Ensino e Trein-amento*" opened in major Brazilian states to train qualified specialists. These centers were key to the development of anesthesia in Brazil.

Colombia

In 1947, Juan Marín [6] founded the first "*School of Anesthesia*" for physicians in the "*Hospital de San José*". In 1948, supported by the School of Medicine in Antioquía, Iván Sánchez organized a course on anesthesia. The first residency began in 1958.

Uruguay

Teaching in the clinical practice of anesthesiology began in 1947. In 1954, Alfredo Pernin established the first course for graduate anesthetists at the School of Medicine of Montevideo. In 1976, he created the Chair of Anesthesiology at the Medical School [58]. In 1981, Pernin and Dardo Vega authored the book, the History of Anesthesiology in Uruguay.

Venezuela

In 1950, José Mazziotta taught the first official postgraduate course in anesthesia at the "*Hospital Central*" in Valencia, marking the first official academic recognition of anesthesiology.

In 1959, Argentine anesthesiologist, Juan Nesi (1909–2001) from Buenos Aires, and Venezuelan Carlos Larrazábal (1924–1988) (both founding members of their societies) established the Postgraduate Course in Anesthesia at the University Hospital of Caracas. In 1962, Nesi and Larrazábal created the Chair of Anesthesiology in the School of Medicine of the Universidad Central de Venezuela. In 1966, the Postgraduate Course became the Latin American Center of Anesthesiology [59] and in the following year, the first International Training Center of Anesthesiologists of the World Federation of Societies of Anaesthesiologists (WFSA).

Peru

In 1964, a university level Anesthesiology Residency (Postgraduate training) was established in the Hospital of the "Universidad Nacional Mayor de San Marcos", Lima [8].

Bolivia

In 1968, Carlos Castaños [60] established an anesthesia residency in the University Hospital in La Paz.

Ecuador

In 1971, a Chair of Anesthesiology was created at the School of Medical Sciences in Quito.

General Anesthesia with Intravenous Procaine: An Argentine Invention

During the Second Argentine Congress of Anesthesiology and First Latin American Congress, in 1949 in Buenos Aires, Gregorio Aranés and Ivar Castellanos gave a paper on "*Brief observations on anesthesia with Pentothal Sodium and Procaine*" [61]. They noted that Fraser and Hamilton had combined thiopental and intravenous procaine (as an analgesic agent), with continuous spinal analgesia or other anesthetics (cyclopropane, ethylene or nitrous oxide) and muscle relaxants to supply anesthesia. They then described their experiments at the Institute of Surgery in Haedo, Buenos Aires, using thiopental-procaine as a general anesthetic, adding a muscle relaxant in some cases. The authors concluded that: "*We believe that procaine, as an anesthetic agent, deserves dedication and studying from all anesthesiologists in the world*".

Several things recommended this technique to South American anesthesiologists. First, the technique was effective, supplying smooth anesthesia with analgesia that extended into the postoperative period. Second, the ingredients were inexpensive and easy to deliver. Third, the material needed for delivery of anesthesia was compact and therefore easily transported and stored. Thus, with several variations, use of intravenous procaine became widespread in South American countries, including Argentina, Uruguay, Bolivia, Chile, Peru and Paraguay.

For several subsequent decades, anesthesiologists studied intravenous procaine, presenting papers at conferences and in international journals. For example, Jaime Wikinski, José Usubiaga, and others presented "*Clinical evaluation of procaine as a general anesthetic*" at the Third World Congress of Anaesthesiologists, in 1964 in Sao Paulo, Brazil. The Peruvian anesthesiologist, Hernández de la Haya [8] wrote, "*intravenous procaine technique was widely accepted. It is highly used in Argentina and Uruguay and broadly accepted in our field, especially in health hospitals*".

The First Latin American University Professor of Anesthesiology

In 1948, the School of Medicine of the University La Plata, Argentina, created the first university course in anesthesiology for graduates, appointing Gregorio Aranés (1908–1996) as Professor and Course Director [46].

The first Latin American Anesthesiologist Appointed as Professor of Anesthesiology and Pharmacology in the United States

Jose Usubiaga (1931–1970) was born in Buenos Aires, earning his degree in medicine in 1953. In 1964, after publishing outstanding work—116 papers in his lifetime—he settled in the US with his wife, Lilia Usubiaga, also an anesthesiologist. In 1967, he was appointed Associate Professor of Anesthesiology and Pharmacology, at the School of Medicine of the University of Miami and, in 1970, he was appointed Professor [62, 63]. Sadly, he died a few months after this appointment. LJS, one of the editors of this book was a faculty colleague of "Dr Jose" at the University of Miami and comments that he was "highly respected not only for his scientific accomplishments but also for the remarkable kindness and obvious respect showed to all with whom he worked".

Corporate and Scientific Activities

Founding of Anesthesiology Societies in South America
Most Latin American Societies in individual countries arose immediately after World War II (Fig. 33.1)

Founding of the Latin American Confederation of Societies of Anesthesiologists (CLASA)
CLASA was founded at the VI Latin American Congress of Anesthesiology, held in Lima, Peru, in October 1962, and was primarily the result of the efforts of Argentine anesthesiologist José Delorme [18]. Founder countries were Argentina, Bolivia, Brazil, Colombia, Chile, Ecuador, Peru, Uruguay and Venezuela [64]. In October 1987, the Confederation became a Regional Chapter of the WFSA.

Participation in the Founding of the World Federation of Societies of Anaesthesiologists (WFSA)
The WFSA was founded in 1955 in Scheveningen, the Netherlands, during the First World Congress of Anaesthesiology. Founders were the Societies from 28 countries, including five from South America: Argentina, Brazil, Colombia, Chile and Uruguay. The Brazilian representative, Olegario Laranjeiras, was named Vice President for Latin America. From 1984–1988, Brazilian anesthesiologist, Carlos Parsloe (1919–2009; Fig. 33.2) was President of the WFSA. According to Almiro dos Reis Júnior, Parsloe was *"the most important and popular Brazilian anesthesiologist, and the one with the highest global impact"*. His career spanned all of modern anesthesia, starting in the 1940s and continuing to his death. He was a student, teacher, politician

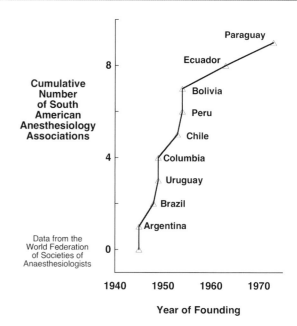

Fig. 33.1 Most Latin American Societies formed in the decade immediately following World War II. (Data kindly supplied by the World Federation of Societies of Anaesthesiology.)

(in the best sense of that word), and traveler all his life, a kind humane man with a consummate interest in worldwide anesthesiology [65].

In 1964, Brazil hosted the World Congress of Anaesthesiologists in Sao Paolo. The 2012 Congress was held in Buenos Aries.

South American Federation of Anesthesiology (FASA)
FASA was established in Paysandú, Uruguay, in 1987, by delegates from Argentina, Brazil, Paraguay and Uruguay. Bolivia, Chile, and Colombia subsequently became members.

Latin American Congress of Anesthesiology
During the Second Argentine Congress of Anesthesiology in Buenos Aires, in October 1949, Argentine José Delorme suggested that the event should become the first Latin American Congress of Anesthesiology, a suggestion unanimously approved by the representatives of those Latin American Societies present [66]—Argentina, Brazil, Colombia, Cuba, Chile, Mexico, Uruguay and Venezuela. Thus, the Latin American Congress antedated the First World Congress of Anesthesiology, held in 1955 in Holland. The First Latin American Congress took place in 1949, in Buenos Aires, and the Second in 1954, in Sao Paulo, Brazil.

Anesthesiology Journals Published in South America
The first Spanish language journal, *"Revista Argentina de Anestesia y Analgesia"* (today *"Revista Argentina de Anes-*

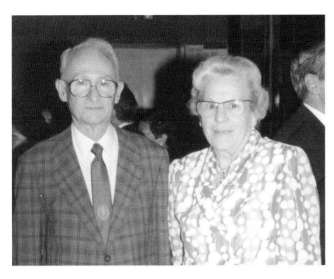

Fig. 33.2 A photograph of Carlos Parsloe and his wife, Edith. Both are remembered with affection by all who knew them, including the three editors of this book. (Courtesy Dr. Kester Brown.)

tesiología"), was founded in Buenos Aires by Argentine, Alberto Gutiérrez [67] in 1939, preceding the launch of "Anesthesiology" (1940) and "Anaesthesia" (1946). Daniel D'Almeida started publication of the oldest specialty newsletter in Latin America, the Portuguese language newsletter, "*Boletim de Anestesia*", in 1903. Currently, anesthesia societies in Argentina, Bolivia, Brazil, Colombia, Chile, Ecuador, Peru, Uruguay, and Venezuela, all publish journals.

Emblems of the CLASA and the WFSA
The Sixth General Assembly of the CLASA, held in 1971 in Rio de Janeiro, Brazil, adopted the emblem of CLASA suggested by Juan Marín, pioneer from Colombia. That year, Francis Foldes, President of the WFSA, proposed that Marin's emblem should also be adopted as the Presidential Medallion of the World Federation, a suggestion accepted during the Fifth World Congress of Anaesthesiologists held in Kyoto, Japan in 1972. The then elected President, Otto Mayrhofer from Austria, was first to wear the new medallion.

References

1. Venturini AH. Tratamiento del dolor quirúrgico en Buenos Aires durante la primera mitad del siglo XIX. Rev Arg Anest. 2008;(66)5:458–63.
2. Venturini AH. Cómo se aliviaba el dolor quirúrgico en 1810. Revista Con Anestesia, Buenos Aires. 2010;182:20–1.
3. Venturini AH. Historia de la Anestesia en la Argentina: La primera mitad del siglo XXº. Actas digitales del 37º Congreso Argentino de Anestesiología, Buenos Aires, 2008. Biblioteca de la Asociación de Anestesia, Analgesia y Reanimación de Bs. Aires. 2008.
4. Cassone E. Historia de la cirugía en Mendoza. Actas del Vº Congreso de Historia de la Medicina Argentina, Mendoza. 1983;69–78.
5. Bulnes A. Epistolario 1855–1881. Edit. Andrés Bello, Santiago de Chile. 1967;19.
6. Herrera Pontón J. Historia de la Anestesia en Colombia. Rev Colomb Anest. 1974;1:7.
7. Praderi RC, Bergalli L. Notas para una Historia de la Cirugía Uruguaya. Historia de la Cirugía Uruguaya, Montevideo. 1981;5.
8. Hernández de la Haza C. en Salaverry García O, Delgado Matallana G. Historia de la Medicina Peruana en el siglo XX, Tomo 1º. Universidad Nacional Mayor de San Marcos, Lima. 2000;273–288.
9. Zaldívar Sobrado C. Historia de la Ortopedia y Traumatología en el Perú. Universid. Nacional de San Marcos, Lima. 2002;22.
10. Higgins Guerra LF. Cronohistoriografía de la Anestesiología. www.anestesia.com.mx/histor2.html. (Accessed August, 2013)
11. Bezerra do Vale N. Sesquicentenario da Anestesia Obstetrica. Rev Bras Anest. 1998;(48)5424–440.
12. Pernín A, Vega DE. Historia de la Anestesia en el Uruguay. Roche, Montevideo. 1981;3.
13. Periódico British Packet and Argentine News, 4 Septiembre 1847: 1. Hemeroteca de la Biblioteca Nacional, Bs. Aires. 1847:1.
14. Ramírez F. Historia de la Anestesiología en Venezuela. VITAE Academia Biomédica Digital, Facultad de Medicina, Universidad Central de Venezuela, Nº 25, Octubre-Diciembre 2005. 2005.
15. Vaccarezza OA. Apuntes para la historia porteña de la anestesia quirúrgica en el siglo XIX. Actas del Primer Congreso Nacional de Historia de la Medicina Argentina, Buenos Aires. 1968;225–238.
16. Pernín A, Vega DE. Historia de la Anestesia en el Uruguay. Roche, Montevideo. 1981;2.
17. Periódico British Packet and Argentine News, 8 de Julio de 1848: 1–3. Hemeroteca de la Biblioteca Nacional, Bs. Aires. 1848:1–3.
18. Muñoz E, et al. Los orígenes de la Anestesia en Chile, Revisión histórica. Rev Chil Cir. 2000;(52)3:305–312.
19. Herrera Pontón J. Historia de la Anestesia en Colombia. SCARE, Bogotá. 1999;65.
20. Diario "El Comercio", Serie M, Quito, 13 de febrero de 2000.
21. Huete Lira I. La medicina militar chilena durante la guerra del Pacífico (1879–1884). Revista Ars Médica, Universidad Católica de Chile. 2002; Vol. 4, Nº 4.
22. Meira DG. Origens e evolugáo da anestesiología brasileira. Rio de Janeiro: Arte Moderno. 1968.
23. Pernín A. Maestros de la cirugía uruguaya: Prof. Luis Mondino. Rev Cir Urug. 1966;36:91–3.
24. Morán Pinto O. En busca de mitigar el dolor. Revista Cambios, Vol.II, Nº 4, Julio-Diciembre. 2003:327.
25. Silva JM. Para la divulgación de la raquianestesia. Anales de la Facultad de Medicina. Montevideo. 1925;10:909.
26. Roldán A. Raquianestesia. Anales de la Facultad de Medicina. Montevideo. 1921;6:758–65.
27. Barzallo Sacoto J. Historia de la Anestesiología, Universidad de Cuenca. rai.ucuenca.edu.ec/facultades/ciencias_medicas. (last accessed October 2012)
28. Martínez Aguirre E. Epidural blood match. Pub. Centro Médico de Caracas. 1963;2:81–3.
29. Usubiaga JE et al. Intermittent saline solution inyections lumbar epidural catéter. Anesth Analg. 1967;46:293–6.
30. Febres E. De l'anesthésie locale de l'utérus: "metro-cacainisation". Bull Soc Obst Paris. 1910;13:432–4.
31. Ombrédanne L. Un Appareil pour l'anesthésie par l'éther. Gaz des Hôpitaux. 1908;81:1095.
32. Venturini AH, González Varela A. Aparato de Ombrédanne. Revista Con Anestesia, Buenos Aires. 1985;84:26–27.
33. González Ginouvés I. Discurso de aceptación del título de Maestro de la Cirugía Chilena. Arch Soc Cirug Chilena. 1972;24:328–35.
34. Artigas R. Algunos aspectos históricos de la evolución de la cirugía pediátrica chilena. Revista Jornadas de la Historia de la Medicina, Edit. Universitaria, Santiago. 1989.
35. Mena Jería R. Plan de Enseñanza de Anestesiología, Hospital Clínico de la Universidad de Chile, Santiago Chile. 1960:85.

36. Crespo Villegas Z. Historia de la Anestesia: Louis Ombrédanne. Revista Historia de la Medicina, Instituto Médico Sucre. www.inmedsuc.8m.com/131/historia2.htm. (last accessed October 2012)

37. Delorme J. Elogio al Dr. Roberto O. Elder. Rev Arg Anest. 1971;31:15–7.

38. Palma EC. Analgesia obstétrica con ciclopropano. Archivos Uruguayos de Medicina, Cirugía y Especialid. 1936;9:185–190.

39. Barros S. Explosión por ciclopropano. Santa Casa da Misericordia, Santos, Brasil, Edición N° 11, mayo de 2003.

40. Artigas Nambrard R. Historia del Servicio de Cirugía Infantil, Ortopedia y Traumatología del Hospital Manuel Arriarán Rev Chilena Cirugía. 1998;(50)11:24–127.

41. Hernández de la Haya C. en Salaverry García O, Delgado Matallana G. Historia de la Medicina Peruana en el siglo XX, Tomo I, Universidad Nacional Mayor de San Marcos, Lima. 2000;284.

42. Hernández de la Haza C. en Salaverry García O, Delgado Matallana G. Historia de la Medicina Peruana en el siglo XX, Tomo I. Universidad Nacional Mayor de San Marcos, Lima. 2000;277.

43. Gutiérrez A. El valor de la aspiración líquida en el espacio peridural en la anestesia peridural. El Día Médico. 1933, 27 de marzo. 1933.

44. Gutiérrez A. Valor de la aspiración líquida en el espacio peridural, en la anestesia peridural. Rev Cirugía, Buenos Aires. 1933;12:225–7.

45. Delorme JC. Aparato universal para anestesias por inhalación. Asociación Argent. Cirugía, Actas Sesión, 26 octubre 1934. 1934.

46. Venturini AH, Fuentes OA. Historia de la Anestesiología en la República Argentina. Rev Arg Anest. 1979;37:139–54.

47. Arce J ADELIC, Aparato de anestesia en circuito cerrado con ciclopropano. Boletín Instituto Clínica Quirúrgica, Buenos Aires. 1941;17:107–14.

48. Aparato Chilean Midget. Revista Con Anestesia, Asociación de Anestesiología de Buenos Aires. 2001;94:14–15.

49. De Souza E. Puncao extradural. tecnica de un novo sinal. Rev Bras Circ. 1943;12:120.

50. Yanzón O. El resucitador-aspirador de Yanzón. Entrevista personal, año 2001. 2001.

51. Dobkin AB. Takaoka respirator for automatic ventilation of the lungs. Canad Anaesth Soc Jour. 1961;8:556.

52. Amaral RG. Emprégo do fluotano com o vaporizador de Takaoka em cirurgia torácica. Rev Brasil Anest. 1964:14:9.

53. Torrieri A, Aldrete JA. The T-A pair leedle (setter). Acta Anaesth Belg. 1988;39:65–6.

54. Langón AB. El Somnifeno como anestésico en Obstetricia y Cirugía. Anales Facult Med Montevideo. 1925;10:464–8.

55. Pernín A, Vega DE. Historia de la Anestesia en el Uruguay. Roche, Montevideo. 1981:25.

56. Elder RO. El uso del curare en cirugía y anestesia. La Semana Médica. 1945;3:831.

57. Fernández OW, Scasso JC, Cañellas A. Curare en cirugía general. Bol Soc Cir. 1947;18:298–307.

58. Pernín A, Vega DE. Historia de la Anestesia en el Uruguay. Roche, Montevideo. 1981:31.

59. Herrera García L. Carlos Rivas Larrazábal y la Anestesiología Venezolana. Fac. Medicina U.C.V., Caracas. 1995:67–70.

60. Ríos Dalénz J. Historia de la Residencia Médica en Boloivia. Archivos Bolivianos de Historia de la Medicina, La Paz, Vol. 1, N° 2, Julio-Diciembre. 1995:185–186.

61. Aranés GM, Bluske Castellanos I. Breves consideraciones sobre anestesia con Pentothal sódico y Procaína. Actas II° Congr. Arg. Anest. y I° Latinoamericano, Buenos Aires. 1979:566–570.

62. Venturini AH. XX Congresos después: recordando a un Maestro de la Anestesiología Argentina. Rev Con Anestesia, agosto-septiembre. 2002:26.

63. Wikinski J. En memoria de José E. Usubiaga. Rev Arg Anest. 1970;29:9–10.

64. Ocampo Trujillo B. Historia de la Confederación Latinoamericana de Sociedades de Anestesiología (CLASA) durante 50 años. Rev Col Anest. 2007;35:3.

65. dos Reis Junior A. Carlos Parsloe (1919–2009) in memoriam. Rev Bras Anest. 2009;59:4.

66. Libro de Actas. Asociación Argentina de Anestesiología. Libro I°, Acta N° 53, p. 91. Secretaría de la Asociación de Anestesia, Analgesia y Reanimación de Buenos Aires 1949.

67. Gutiérrez A. Revista Argentina de Anestesia y Analgesia, 1939, Año I, N° 1, Biblioteca de la Asociación de Anestesia, Analgesia y Reanimación de Buenos Aires. 1939.

A History of Anaesthesia Journals

Jeanette Thirlwell

Summary

The *Lancet* first appeared in 1823. The Boston Medical and Surgical Journal (later the New England Journal of Medicine) followed in 1828. These were the principal journals describing medical discoveries, particularly ether's anaesthetic properties. The Lancet in 1838 called Elliotson's performance of operations under mesmerism "humbug". Undeterred, Elliotson published '*The Zoist: A Journal of Cerebral Physiology and Mesmerism, and their Applications to Human Welfare*' from 1843 to 1855.

Were '*Current Researches in Anesthesia and Analgesia*' (1922) and the '*British Journal of Anaesthesia*' (1923) the first anaesthesia journals? In 1891, US dentist Samuel Hayes published '*Dental and Surgical Microcosm*', arguing for the provision of oxygen to avoid 'asphyxial (nitrous oxide) anaesthesia'. Hayes and Microcosm died in 1897.

From 1914, Francis McMechan edited a 'Quarterly Supplement' '*Anesthesia and Analgesia*' for the 'American Journal of Surgery'. In 1922, he founded the National Anaesthesia Research Society with the supplement as the Society's journal. He renamed it '*Current Researches in Anesthesia and Analgesia*' in 1925 when the Society became the International Anaesthesia Research Society.

Hyman Cohen soldiered in the US Army, married a Manchester girl in 1904, and became a full-time anaesthetist after completing medical school at St Bartholomew's Hospital. *The British Journal of Anaesthesia* was first published in 1923 with Cohen as the editor. He introduced the journal as a publication "devoted entirely to the interests of anaesthesia and its practitioners".

German surgeons edited '*Schmerz, Narkose und Anesthesie*' which appeared from 1928 to 1943. The '*AANA Journal*' was published in 1933, as a report of the first annual meeting of the National Association of Nurse Anesthetists. In 1935, the French Society of Anaesthesia and Analgesia launched '*Anesthésie et Analgésie*'. Perhaps the first multinational anaesthesia journal, '*Revista Argentina de Anestesia y Analgesia*', was published in 1939. Out of respect for McMechan, the American Society of Anesthesiologists refrained from publishing its own journal until McMechan died in 1939. '*Anesthesiology*' appeared in 1940. More journals in various languages appeared after World War II, reflecting the establishment of anaesthetic societies or specialist societies. That is, the rise of subspecialties and associated journals, beginning with 'Pain' in 1975, mirrors the continuing growth of anaesthesiology. The successive contents pages of journals reveal the chronological development of anaesthesia.

Assisted by Roger Eltringham, Iain Wilson founded and edited the on-line journal '*Update*' in 1992 to support the safe scientific practice of anaesthesia in the developing world. The WFSA adopted '*Update*' as its official journal.

Ethical misconduct in medical publishing has recently received great publicity. Three cases of spectacular deliberate deceit were uncovered, one resulting in prison for fraud. More plagiarism has been detected and eradicated by use of electronic software that can compare submissions to texts in huge databases.

An Overview

Scientific journals allow communication among individuals in all fields of learning, be they general and popular sciences, pure sciences such as mathematics, or pursuits as diverse as astrology, psychology or linguistics. New ideas, discoveries, and inventions are documented, theories proposed and phenomena documented. Details of experimentation and their results and applications are offered for discussion among peers, furthering collaboration and progress. Specialty journals such as those for anaesthesia and its many subspecialties have a more singular focus than those serving broader fields. There follows a history—the stories—of the evolution of some of the more important journals devoted to anaesthesia.

J. Thirlwell (✉)
Executive Editor, *Anaesthesia and Intensive Care,*
Australian Society of Anaesthetists, Sydney, Australia
e-mail: jeanette@thirlwell.com.au

E. I Eger II et al. (eds.), *The Wondrous Story of Anesthesia,* DOI 10.1007/978-1-4614-8441-7_34, © Edmond I Eger, MD 2014

The Early Anaesthesia Journals

Modern anaesthesia began with the 1840s introduction of nitrous oxide, ether, and chloroform. At that time, newspapers or early medical journals such as the Lancet (first appearing on October 5, 1823) disseminated written communications of discoveries which could produce analgesia with or without unconsciousness. In Lancet's first issue, the editor Thomas Wakley wrote of his aims: "A Lancet can be an arched window to let in the light or it can be a sharp surgical instrument to cut out the dross, and I intend to use it in both senses" [1].

But the story begins earlier. In the late eighteenth century, the Austrian physician Anton Mesmer, introduced and popularised mesmerism, or hypnotism with his 1779 monograph, "Mémoire sur la Découverte du Magnétisme Animale" [2]. After marrying a wealthy young French widow, Mesmer lived comfortably in Parisian society. His monograph argued, in less than idiomatic French, that his technique might provide adequate analgesia for even radical surgery. Mesmer's publication, a forerunner of a journal, and word of mouth, spread his views from France to England and Scotland. James Esdaile and James Braid, both Scottish surgeons excised tumours and amputated limbs under this early form of "anaesthesia", publishing books documenting their operative cases.

John Elliotson was first an Assistant Physician at St Thomas's Hospital, London in the 1830s, then at the University College Hospital. He performed operations under mesmerism, but not without challenge and criticism. In the Lancet in 1838, Wakley, true to his aim to "cut out the dross", famously pronounced mesmerism as "humbug", prompting John C. Warren, the surgeon at Morton's 1846 demonstration of ether anaesthesia in Boston, to declare "Gentlemen, this is no humbug!" [3].

However, Wakley's rebuke did not stop Elliotson in his practice of mesmerism, and with a considerable cult following, Elliotson began a journal titled 'The Zoist: A Journal of Cerebral Physiology and Mesmerism, and their Applications to Human Welfare'. Publication extended from April 1843 to December 1855, with complete volumes annually for thirteen years. An international journal, it was published by Bailliere in London and Paris and by Weigel in Leipzig. It reported on mesmerism as used for chronic aches and pains, psychological and psychiatric disorders, superficial tumour excisions and major surgical procedures such as leg amputations [4]. Was this the first anaesthesia journal?

The First "True" Anaesthesia Journals

Until recently it was generally believed that the first anaesthesia journals were published in the early 1920s, with Volume 1 of 'Current Researches in Anaesthesia and Analgesia'

appearing in August 1922, closely followed by Volume 1 of the 'British Journal of Anaesthesia' in 1923–4. But the Reverend Samuel Hayes, a Pittsburgh Pennsylvania dentist and former preacher in the Church of the United Brethren of Christ, published the first true anaesthesia journal in 1891. Hayes, like many dentists of the time, practised nitrous oxide analgesia for his patients. He criticized the technique used by some of his colleagues, preaching against their 'asphyxial anaesthesia'. Hayes argued for the provision of oxygen with nitrous oxide (or any other inhaled anaesthetic) in the administration of anaesthesia. In 1881 he therefore devised a foot-operated bellows to 'aerate' the gas delivered via the bubble-through vaporisers which he had also invented for ether and chloroform.

As a dentist, Hayes knew of a handbook published by the SS White Dental Manufacturing Company (SSW-DMC) of Philadelphia. From the 1880s the company published its proprietary journal, 'Dental Cosmos'. Hayes decided to confront Cosmos with his own quarterly, titled, with tongue-in-cheek, 'Dental and Surgical Microcosm' (DSM; Fig. 34.1). Hayes was 'Proprietor and Controlling Editor' of this challenging new volume. George Bause noted that "Hayes prided himself on defining 'anaesthesia' as distinct from 'asphyxia'" [4].

In 'Microcosm', Hayes publicised various design modifications of his "generators" (vaporisers), with thermoregulation to control the rate of vaporisation of chloroform and therefore the dosage received by the patient. Hayes died of tuberculosis in 1897 and with his demise, his journal ceased publication.

Anesthesia and Analgesia

'Current Researches in Anaesthesia and Analgesia Research Society Inc.' was first published bimonthly by the National Anaesthesia Research Society Inc., with Francis McMechan (Fig. 34.2) its instigator and editor. Though wheelchair-bound by rheumatoid arthritis, McMechan was a dynamic and enthusiastic advocate for the advancement of anaesthesia practice and research. Described as one of "the most militant figures of the history of the speciality" [5], he realised the need for a journal that would promote the specialty and disseminate the results of research. McMechan's involvement in editing and publishing began with his appointment by Managing Editor, Joseph McDonald, in 1914 as editor of a 'Quarterly Supplement' ('Anesthesia and Analgesia') to the 'American Journal of Surgery'. McMechan recruited the transactions of meetings of anaesthetists worldwide to publish in his Supplement. In the process he became known to medical researchers and leaders in the development and manufacturing of anaesthetic agents and commercial design of equipment.

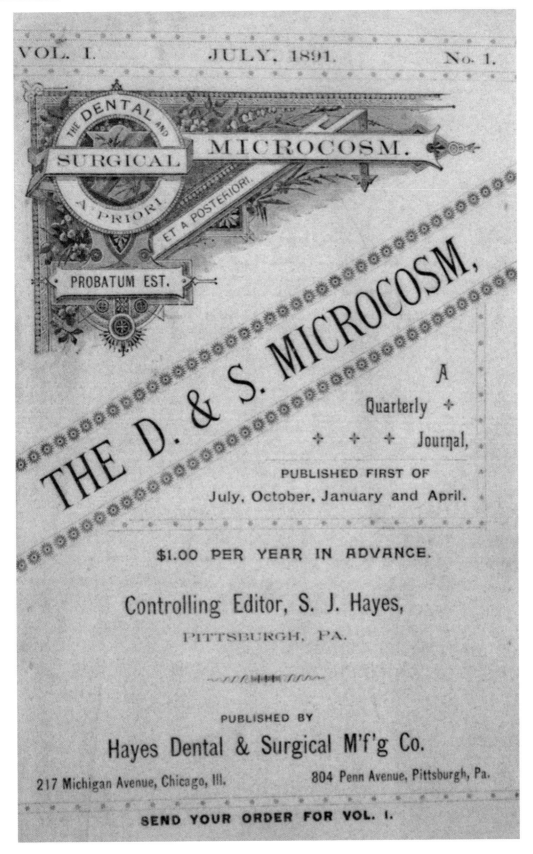

Fig. 34.1 The cover of the summer quarter, 1891, issue of the *Dental & Surgical Microcosm* issue, published and edited by SJ Hayes of the Hayes Dental and Surgical Manufacturing Co. (Courtesy of George S Bause, MD, MPH, Case Western Reserve University, Cleveland, OH.)

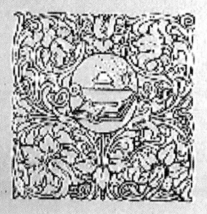

CURRENT RESEARCHES IN

ANESTHESIA

& ANALGESIA

F. H. MCMECHAN, A. M., M. D., EDITOR

1923

Published Bi-Monthly by
The National Anesthesia Research Society, Inc.

Fig. 34.2 The cover of a 1923 issue of *Current Researches in Anesthesia & Analggesia*, edited by Francis H McMechan, MD, published by the National Anesthesia Research Society, predecessor of the international Anesthesia Research Society

With McDonald's death in 1922, McMechan campaigned to establish a formal anaesthesia research organisation to continue the activities of the supplement. Thus in August of that year McMechan founded the National Anaesthesia Research Society which then published its own journal. McMechan was justifiably proud of this journal, actively discouraging the establishment of an alternative. Anesthesiology's first edition in 1940, had to await McMechan's death, as mentioned below.

The second page of Volume 1, Number 1 of 'Anaesthesia and Analgesia' lists the members of the Board of Convenors of the National Anesthesia Research Society and the research committee. It contains many notable names such as McKesson and Guedel. The journal's title changed in 1925 when the National Anesthesia Research became the International Anesthesia Research Society.

In 1909 McMechan married actress Laurette van Varsveld (Fig. 34.3), who assumed the role of constant carer/companion of her husband. McMechan, with Laurette at his side, travelled nationally and internationally to Canada, England, and the European continent. In his travels, McMechan met a young Australian, Geoffrey Kaye. On McMechan's strong recommendations, in 1934 Kaye became the principal instigator and founder of the Australian Society of Anaesthetists, initiating the long path to establishing the Australian Journal, 'Anaesthesia and Intensive Care', in 1972. McMechan inspired similar actions by others in Canada. Laurette, in the 1920s and 30s, became widely known and highly regarded for her contribution to her husband's journal, so much so that after his death in June 1939, she was appointed Assistant Editor and continued in that role until her death in 1970.

There were relatively few editors-in-chief of 'Anesthesia and Analgesia' over its almost 90 years of existence, promoting continuity of style. Its second editor, Howard Dittrick was succeeded by Thomas Seldon (1959–1976), then Nicholas Greene (1976–1990), Ronald Miller (1990–2006), and currently, Steven Shafer.

The 1940 November–December issue of 'Anesthesia and Analgesia' published a eulogy to McMechan by Omar Ranney, followed by tributes from Kaye, the then Secretary of the Australian Society of Anaesthetists. McMechan was more than founder of Anesthesia and Analgesia. As Kaye wrote to Laurette McMechan:

"He was an inspiration. We admired his courage, which rose superior to every physical disability. We admired his amazing knowledge of anaesthesia. We recognised in him a man of culture, with the wide and tolerant outlook which was capable of converting a national into an international endeavour…Above all, I think we admired his vision and the ideal to which it led him. He was not the parent of American anaesthesia, although he was, more that any man, its co-or-

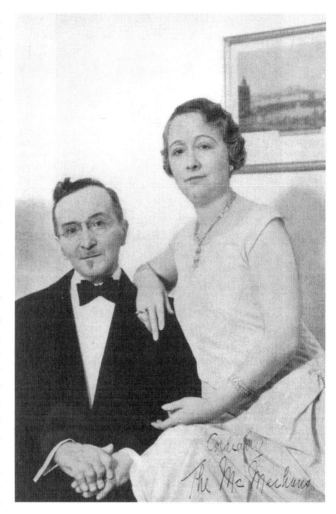

Fig. 34.3 Francis and Laurette McMechan. (Courtesy of the Geoffrey Kaye Museum of Anaesthetic History, Australian and New Zealand College of Anaesthetists.)

dinator. Of international anaesthesia, however, he was both co-ordinator and parent" [6, 7].

Other journals appeared between the first issues of 'Current Researches in Anaesthesia and Analgesia' in 1922 and its rival 'Anesthesiology' in 1940. In 1923–4 the 'British Journal of Anaesthesia' arrived, followed in 1935 by the French journal, 'Anesthesie et Analgesie' and the Argentinean journal 'Revista Argentina de Anestesia y Analgesia'.

British Journal of Anaesthesia

The 'British Journal of Anaesthesia' was the second major English language journal. It was first published in July 1923 and edited by Hyman Cohen until 1928. Initially a soldier in the United States Army, Cohen married a Manchester girl in 1904, then entered medical training at St Bartholomew's Hospital in London. He graduated in 1916 and became a full-time anaesthetist. He introduced his journal as a publication "devoted entirely to the interests of anaesthesia and its practitioners", saying that the journal "anticipates acting, not only as the mouthpiece for those who desire to give public expression to the results of their research and experience, but to place before its readers, an account of what is being done generally in the anaesthetic world" [8].

In 2002, J Norman of Southampton, UK published a paper entitled "The British Journal of Anaesthesia—An Informal History Of The First Twenty-Five Years", listing the pioneer founders in this developing medical specialty as SR Wilson and HEG Boyle, of the University of Manchester, F Shipway, J Bloomfield, DW Buxton from London, HB Fairlie from Glasgow and AJ O'Leary from Liverpool [9]. Although of necessity reducing publication from quarterly to twice a year for most of World War II, this journal flourished thereafter, rising high in the ranks of anaesthesia journals.

Anesthésie et Analgésie

In 1935, 'Anesthésie et Analgésie', the official publication of the French Society of Anaesthesia and Analgesia was launched. In the first issue, the chief editor, Robert Monod explained that the Society aimed to create a "review of anaesthesia in the French language" [10], and that, like anaesthesia journals established before and after, it sought to document research in the laboratory and in clinical practice, impartially and without bias.

Revista Argentina de Anestesia y Analgesia

Volumes 1 and 2 of 'Revista Argentina de Anestesia y Analgesia' were published in 1939–40 (Fig. 34.4). Articles came mostly from Argentina, but also included one paper each from France and Italy, making 'Revista Argentina de Anestesia y Analgesia' possibly the first journal with an international list of contributors. In his introductory editorial, Emilio Forgue, a Member of the Academy of Surgery and a Corresponding Member of the Institute of France, noted the widely differing techniques of anaesthesia used in different countries in the late 1930s, the choices varying according to the medical school and hospital traditions and the results of their research. He argued that the safest anaesthesia is "the one with which the anaesthetist has most experience" [11]. He acknowledged the originality and leadership of Americans at the time in the use of inhalational agents, while anaesthetists in Germany led the way in the use of regional techniques. Forgue was a protagonist of regional anaesthesic techniques. In contrast, in France he noted that particularly in Lyon, preference was given to intravenous induction.

Antonio Gutierrez, a Member of the National Academy of Medicine and Honorary professor of the Faculty of Medicine in Buenos Aires, wrote an editorial in the second issue of 'Revista Argentina de Anestesia y Analgesia', May–August 1939 titled, 'What is a Surgical Operation from the physical-biological point of view?' In answer, he described the 'offence, injury and aggression' inflicted, and the subsequent responsibility of the anaesthetist to support the patient [12]. Both editorials were forthright and apposite, applying equally well in the present day.

Anesthesiology

In March 1935, John Lundy approached Maurice Fishbein, editor of the 'Journal of The American Medical Association', to suggest establishing a second American anaesthesia journal under the auspices of the American Medical Association (AMA). Lundy was keen to increase the quality and quantity of scientific papers published in the field of anaesthesia. He believed that his anaesthetic colleagues would back this venture, and wrote to fifty-five of the most prominent of these to gather their support. The response was mixed. Although agreeing that another American anaesthesia journal would be an otherwise appropriate venture, Arthur Guedel expressed concern that establishing a second journal might offend McMechan. In contrast, Guedel's friend, Ralph Waters, then professor of the world's first academic Department of Anesthesiology at Madison, Wisconsin, agreed with Lundy that a second journal would be an "excellent idea" and that contributions from his department would support the venture. Other responses were less positive, so the project was temporarily shelved. Lundy suspected that McMechan had negatively influenced some of those surveyed [13].

After McMechan died in June 1939, plans quickly proceeded for establishment of 'Anesthesiology'. On November 4, the Journal Committee and the Publishing Committee of the American Society of Anesthesiologists met, appointing Henry Ruth as first Editor in Chief with Ralph Tovell and E.A. Rovenstine as Associate Editors and Paul Wood as Managing Editor. An Editorial Board was then appointed with four Contributing Editors and nine Consulting Editors. An Editorial Policy Committee was then established to act as a steering Committee to determine editorial policy. The first issue opened with an unusual essay by Howard Haggard, Director of the Laboratory of Applied Physiology at Yale University. His article entitled "The Place of the Anesthetist in American Medicine" was a transcript of a paper presented at a meeting of the Society of Anesthetists at the New York World Fair, New York City on October 12, 1940. This was a newly established Section on Anesthesiology of the AMA, held during its ninety-first annual session in New York City,

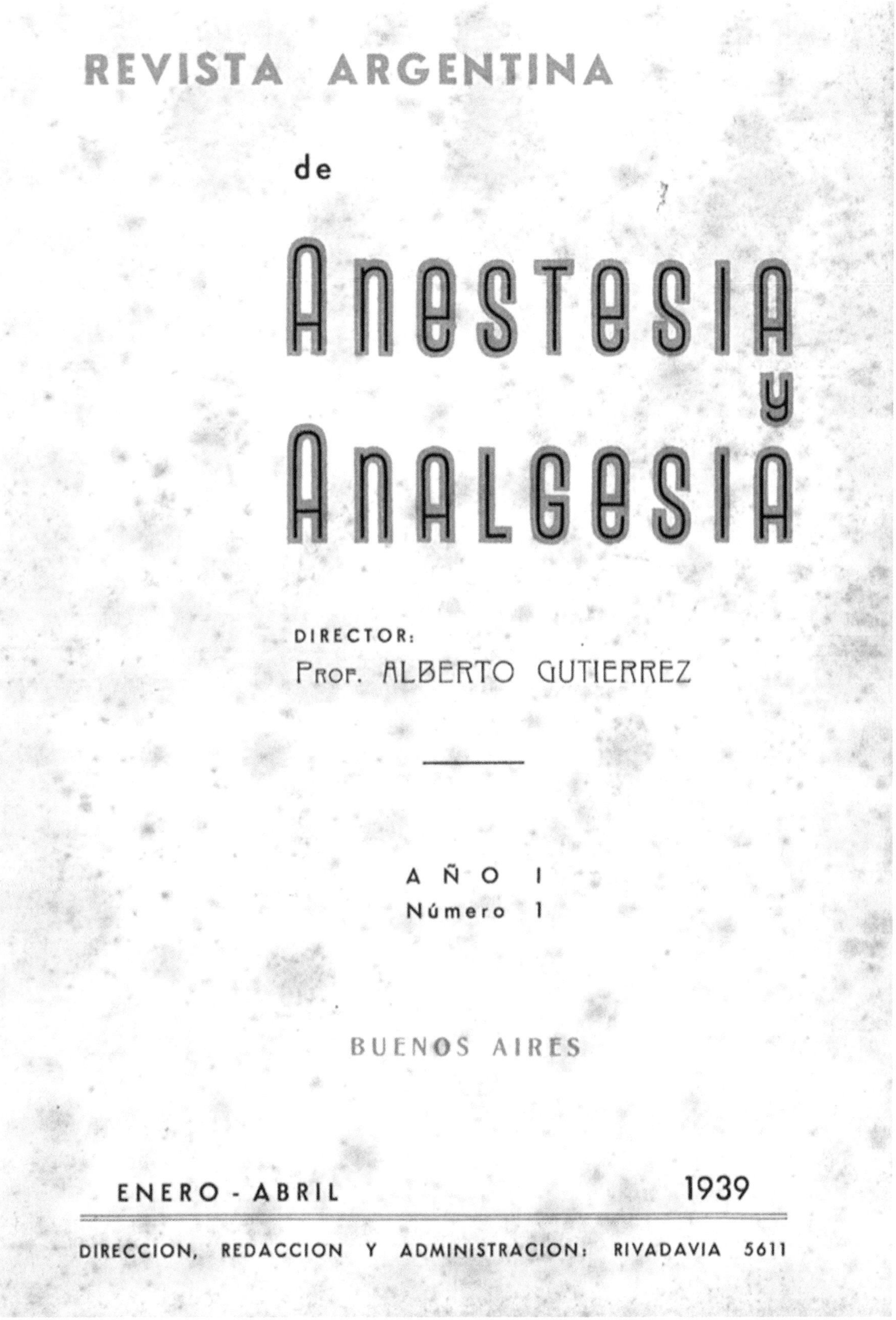

REVISTA ARGENTINA

de

Anestesia
y
Analgesia

DIRECTOR:
Prof. ALBERTO GUTIERREZ

———

A Ñ O I
Número 1

BUENOS AIRES

ENERO - ABRIL   1939

DIRECCION, REDACCION Y ADMINISTRACION: RIVADAVIA 5611

Fig. 34.4 A picture of the Volume 1, April, 1939 issue of *Revista Argentina de Anestesia y Analgesia.* (Courtesy of the Geoffrey Kaye Museum of Anaesthetic History, Australian and New Zealand College of Anaesthetists.)

October 10–14, 1940. Haggard's essay neither praised nor faulted anaesthesiologists [14]. His intent was to impress on the listener/reader that public opinion and an appreciation of the practice of anaesthesia as a professional skill were crucial to the development of the specialty. He maintained that the anaesthetist must shape public acceptance of the specialty of anaesthesia by the achievements of the anaesthetist in education, training and scientific development in physiology, pathology, biochemistry and general scientific endeavours. Haggard believed that good practical skills and professional personal presentations of anaesthetists to their patients were essential to the acceptance of the specialty of anaesthesia in its own right [14].

Volume 1, Number 1 continued with Guedel's review of his use of cyclopropane over the previous eight years in more than eight thousand cases, discussing controlled respiration, the production of abdominal relaxation, the presence of cardiac arrhythmias and techniques of administration. A readable, uncontrolled study of practice by one of the "great" anesthesiologists of the day [15].

Anaesthesia

'Anaesthesia', the Journal of the Association of Great Britain and Ireland, was established in 1946, remarkably soon after World War II. Its Editor was Cecil Hewer and Sub-Editor R. Blair Gould, with J.F. Gillies representing Scotland. Alfred Webb Johnson, President of the Royal College of Surgeons of England provided an introduction to this inaugural issue [16].

"I am grateful for the invitation to write a Foreword to this first number of the Quarterly Journal 'Anaesthesia', for it not only gives me the opportunity to wish the Journal every success, but also to say how pleased I am that the Association of Anaesthetists of Great Britain and Ireland has decided to launch a periodical publication on this important subject.

> "The year of the celebration of the centenary of the first operation under general anaesthesia in this country is a most opportune time for the institution of a Journal which will make British teaching and records of discovery and achievement available to the medical profession throughout the world. It is very fitting that the country which made such valuable contributions in the early days of anaesthesia by the pioneer work of Hickman, Simpson, Snow and Clover should be represented in the medical literature of the subject."

Hewer's editorial followed in the same vein, justifying the establishment of this new publication: "…the rapid advance in all types of anaesthetic and analgesic technique requires fuller and quicker expression than can be provided in the overloaded columns of the general medical press. The full and accurate presentation of observations, theories, new methods etc., is essential if true advance is to be maintained and if unprofitable detours are to be avoided."

Henry Featherstone, the first President of the Association of Anaesthetists, wrote of the "Inception and…Purpose" of the Association and its aims, objectives and formulated rules as set out at its establishment in 1930, and the subsequent successful introduction of a Diploma of Anaesthesia. This first issue also included a nine-page article by President AD Marsten on the "Centenary of Anaesthesia in Great Britain" in 1946, chronicling the events preceding the launch of "Anaesthesia" [17].

Thereafter followed twenty pages of dissertations on curarisation, local anaesthesia for abdominal operations, and an assessment by Noel Gillespie from Canada of the effect that World War II had on the "Position of the American Anaesthetist". The journal also included a case report, a review, abstracts and Association news. A small volume descriptive of anaesthetic interests of the time, 'Anaesthesia' quickly grew in stature and physical dimensions, from a small A5 quarterly booklet, half the size of its currently conventional A4 format, now issued monthly.

However, with the establishment of 'Anaesthesia' with such self-confidence it would be wrong to assume there was no rivalry between the long-established British Journal of Anaesthesia and this newcomer to the scene of anaesthesia journals. It was as if an unfair advantage of opportunity was being taken to rise above the British Journal of Anaesthesia which had suffered badly as a consequence of World War II because of a severe lack of papers offered for publication and a shortage of paper for printing of many medical journals at the time. It is fair to say that not all representatives of the Association of Great Britain and Ireland were in agreement with this proposal. This rivalry that the commencement of a second British journal aroused is clearly set out in a work by Thomas B. Boulton, titled 'The Association of Anaesthetists of Great Britain and Ireland 1932–1992, and the Development of the Specialty of Anaesthesia'. Ultimately the British Journal recovered from the ravages of wartime, while Anaesthesia maintained popularity as a more clinically orientated publication [17].

'Revista Brasiliera de Anestesiologica'

'Revista Brasiliera de Anestesiologica', the official publication of the Brazilian Society of Anaesthesiology, commenced publication in 1951, its first editor being Oscar Ribeiro. Ribeiro's introductory editorial was in Portuguese, while the second, by Ralph M. Waters, was in English. In nine pages, Waters congratulated his Brazilian colleagues for their inauguration of the first journal of anaesthesiology in a Portuguese-speaking country and the second in Latin

America. Waters gave a broad overview of the development of the specialty of anaesthesia from the latter part of the nineteenth century when, in the US, the administration of anaesthesia was largely entrusted to the temporarily idle medical student, intern, general practitioner, nurse or any individual who happened to be nearby. He then described the development of the specialty of anaesthesia through the 1940s, listing in detail the obligations of service, teaching and research. He also described the qualities of the "Good Anesthesiologist", citing the physical strength needed to practise well, moral obligations to the patient, the obligation to display a spirit of friendly cooperation with those with whom he works, and how he must "serve as the balance wheel which governs the smooth running of the machine of which he is a part. In short, he can make or break the success of the surgical team His pronouncement is as true today as it was some sixty years ago [18].

'Masui' (The Japanese Journal of Anesthesiology)

From 1951 to 1960, a profusion of anaesthesia journals emerged in Europe, the Middle East and the Far East. In April 1952, the first issue of the Japanese Journal of Anesthesiology was published. There were five Editors of this first issue; Shichiron Isikawa, Myoshi Urabe, Kingo Shinoi, Tikashi Suzuki and Shinobu Myamoto. In his Foreword, Tamotsu Fukuda, Professor of Surgery at Juntendo University in Tokyo, stated that several factors increasingly allowed surgeons to successfully perform major surgery, attributing their growing success to the development and availability of antibiotics including penicillin, and to "aggressive" pre- and postoperative management of their patients. He observed that regional anaesthesia had in the past, been the preferred technique, with reasonable results, but emphasised that it was now time for his anaesthesia colleagues to emulate anaesthesiologists in Europe and the United States, to allay not only the intraoperative pain of surgery but to continue their management of the patient as a whole, through surgery and the postoperative period. Generally known as 'Masui', the 'Japanese Journal of Anaesthesiology' is a Japanese language journal and is still in regular production [19].

The Japanese word 'masui' has an interesting story in itself. The news of the administration of successful anaesthesia in 1846 and the developments which followed spread quickly around the world with the publication of books such as Schlesinger's German book on ether anaesthesia. By 1848, six copies of the Dutch edition of this book had reached Japan and a Japanese edition was published in 1850. Seikei Sugita, an official translator of the Shogunate, executed the translation, coining the Japanese word 'masui', meaning 'paralysis and unconsciousness'.

Journal of Anaesthesia

The 'Journal of Anaesthesia', the journal of the Japanese Society of Anaesthesiologists is published in English. This journal made its debut in March 1987, its first Editor-in-Chief being Keisuke Amaha, with Kenjiro Mori (Kyoto University), Takesuke Mateki (Kurume University) Ryo Ogana (Nippon), Reiji Shimizu (Jichi) and Jurichi Yoshitake (Kyushu University) as co-founding editors. Indexed from Volume 17 in 2003, it achieved citation status in 2010. In parallel with other well-known journals, it has increased its publication from an initial two issues a year through four and now six issues per year.

In June 2010 at the Asian Australasian Congress of Anaesthesiologists in Fukuoka, Japan, Professor Akitomo Matsuki of the Department of Anesthesiology, Postgraduate School of Medicine of Hirosaki University, presented a paper entitled, 'Seshu Hanaoka's Philosophy of "Safety and Challenge"'. Hanaoka was a highly regarded Japanese surgeon in the late 18th and early nineteenth centuries. In 1804 he performed one of the earliest reported general anaesthesias, using an extract of Datura stramonium in an oral preparation, enabling him to excise an advanced tumour of the left breast. The patient, Kan Arya, expressed feeling no pain during the procedure, but died four and a half months later from dissemination of the original pathology. The successful anaesthesia and surgery which resulted is celebrated in the adoption of the flower of Datura, as the basis of the logo of the Japanese Society of Anaesthesia, appearing on the front cover of all issues of their 'Journal of Anesthaesia' since its inception. Datura has been used in South America, the Middle East and Far East in particular, for its 'medicinal' properties, and while it is not an anaesthetic, it is a known hallucinogen and is also known to alter the appreciation or memory of pain. The plant is recognized as containing scopolamine, hyoscine and atropine.

'Schmerz, Narkose und Anesthesie'

The first German language journal of anaesthesiology, 'Schmerz, Narkose und Anesthesie' (Pain, Narcosis and Anaesthesia) was published from 1928 to 1943. The title emphasised pain, anticipating the later development of pain as an anaesthesia subspecialty. The chaos of World War II ended publication of this journal.

Der Anaesthesist

In 1952/1953, Volume 1 of 'Der Anaesthesist' appeared, the journal of the Austrian Society for Anaesthesiology, its three editors being R. Frey of Heidelberg, W. Hugen of

Basel and O. Mayrhofer of Vienna. In 1953, it developed into the first multi-national society journal, in that with its Volume 2, Issue 3 it became the journal of the German Society for Anaesthesiology, while in Issue 4, it also became the journal of the Swiss Society for Anaesthesiology. Thus, 'Der Anaesthesist' has served the German-speaking fraternity of Europe while promoting co-operation with central European countries as well.

In 1979, Der Anaesthesist added a twenty-page journal-within-a-journal. Appearing every three to four months, this supplement, 'Regionale Anaesthese' supported the sub-specialist field of regional anaesthesia. Subsequent supplements commemorated pioneers of 'Regional Anaesthesia' such as Karl Koller, the discoverer of the local anaesthetic effects of cocaine, then Carl Schleich who developed infiltration anaesthesia, and August Bier, the champion of spinal anaesthesia. Many editors of 'Der Anaesthesist' and its included journal, 'Regionale Anaesthesie', have written editorials and articles on the history of both journals, and the importance of developments in regional anaesthesia as a peculiarly German-based subspecialty.

Canadian Anaesthetists Society Journal

The 'Canadian Anaesthetists Society Journal' was established in July 1954. An introductory page listed the executive officers and council of that society, including the president, Russell Fraser. The founding editor, Roderick Gordon, headed a three-member editorial board: Alan Noble, Louis Lamoureux and Ted Gain. The journal was printed in Toronto and published by the Society itself. An accompanying editorial described the evolution of the journal from the Society's newsletter, which had published papers presented at previous meetings [20]. The journal evolved over time from a quarterly to a monthly publication in 1993 and grew in international prominence within the specialty. In 1987, the name of the journal was changed to the Canadian Journal of Anesthesia. Reflecting the two official languages of Canada, articles in the Canadian Journal of Anesthesia are printed either in English or in French, according to the language of submission. In early 2012 the Journal's circulation was just under 6000, two-thirds external to Canada—from a modest beginning, as the successor to an anaesthesia society newsletter, it had grown to become a mainstream international journal.

Acta Anaesthesiologica Scandinavica

In 1940, a young anaesthetist, Torsten Gordh, returned to Sweden from training in the US, where his tutor Ralph Waters advised him to establish a Nordic Society of Anaesthe-

siologists. It took nine years to evolve, but in 1949, Gordh, Otto Mollestad (Norway), Henning Poulsen (Denmark) and Eero Turpeinen (Finland) founded, in Helsinki, the 'Nordisk Anesthesiologisk Forening' (NAF), that is, the Nordic Society of Anaesthesiologists [21].

Establishment of a journal was the next step, but this required interminable discussion to clarify the journal's aims. In 1950, after the Society's first congress in Oslo, approaches were made to various publishers with however, no general agreement on the proposed publication by the time of the General Assembly of the Society in 1952. There was still dissention concerning the nature of the contents and the scientific standard to be achieved. Finally, in 1956, at the General Assembly in Helsinki, a decision was made to proceed, with Bjorn Ibsen and Henning Poulsen as Editors, and Eric Nilsson (Sweden) as Editor-in-Chief. The name chosen for the Journal, 'Acta Anaesthesiologica Scandinavica' (AAS), conforms to the usual Latin style of other Scandinavian medical journals. Four issues appeared in 1958, with Olaf Norlander then added as Associate Editor for Sweden. The first issue was small, an A5 format, with a conservative creamy-coloured cover.

By 1971 it was noted that two-thirds of subscribers were non-Scandinavian, Acta Anaesthesiologica having effortlessly become an international journal. As with many journals in their first years, the editors did much of the editing and preparation of papers, while A. Ronsing, a lecturer in English at Ahrrus in Denmark, and Armstrong Davison of Newcastle-upon-Tyne, UK translated submissions in Scandinavian languages into English, and Otto Mayrhofer of Vienna translated abstracts into German.

Jan Eklund, Editor-in-Chief from 1985 to 1993, has described the history of this journal in a dissertation, 'Acta Anaesthesiologica Scandinavica—The First Fifty Years (From Lead to Electrons)'. Sven Gisvold followed Eklund as Editor-in-Chief in 1993, and in 2008, he was succeeded by Lars Rasmussen [21, 22].

In December 1971, when the AAS had grown sufficiently, Munksgaards became the publisher on contract to the Scandinavian Society. The journal format changed to the more conventional American A4, and a bright orange-red colour cover made it immediately identifiable. Each journal has a unique and readily identifiable cover, as well as a registered name and ISSN, but the individual appearance helps recognition on a library rack of journals side by side.

Middle East Journal of Anaesthesiology

Bernard Brandstater, an Australian graduate who was Professor at the American University of Beirut Medical Centre, pioneered the 'Middle East Journal of Anaesthesiology' in 1966. This journal was included in Index Medicus in 1976.

Brandstater, the first Editor-in-Chief, drew from Hamlet, Act III, Scene II for the journal's motto, "Some must watch and some must sleep". On the home page of its website, Brandstater also chose its symbol, the poppy flower (Papaver somniferum), first cultivated in the Middle East, a flower that has given unique service to suffering mankind for thousands of years. This journal is published three times a year, its consultant editors representing various Middle Eastern countries. Each volume consists of six issues and is therefore the sum of two years' publications. The journal is dedicated to promoting research and education in anaesthesia in these countries.

Anaesthesia and Intensive Care

In 'Fifty Years, The Australian Society of Anaesthetists 1934–1984', Gwen Wilson presented the history of the establishment of 'Anaesthesia and Intensive Care', the Journal of the Australian Society of Anaesthetists [23]. In 1934, Geoffrey Kaye, of Melbourne, acting on McMechan's recommendation, gathered six like-minded colleagues to found the Australian Society of Anaesthetists. One stated aim of the Society was to establish a journal. However, the long distances between cities and towns in a vast and thinly populated continent limited growth of the Society in those Depression years. Kaye first established a series of 'Anaesthetic Numbers' in the Medical Journal of Australia, and later wrote infrequent memoranda which developed into the Newsletter of the Society. The Newsletter contained some articles of a scientific nature, almost all written by Kaye himself, a demanding ongoing project. Most other Australian anaesthetists of that time sought greater exposure and recognition, sending their scientific articles to established overseas journals. The Newsletter was rightly regarded as a carrier of society news rather than a vehicle for scientific communication.

During World War II, many Australian medical graduates, including Kaye, were deployed overseas in the defence forces. Communications within the Society virtually ceased, and no scientific congresses were held in those years. At the Annual General Meeting of the Society in Perth, Western Australia in April 1954, the question of an Australian Journal of Anaesthetics, as it was referred to then, was raised again. However, a postal referendum by the Victorians revealed a consensus that the project was premature, and the proposal was abandoned.

In 1969, Ben Barry was appointed Honorary Federal Secretary of the Society. Barry favoured the establishment of a journal and quietly laid much of the groundwork, promoting the idea among members and accurately assessing costs with quotes from publishers. A motion to publish a journal was put to the Executive Committee in May 1971 and passed unanimously. Barry was appointed founding Editor, with an editorial board of twelve members. 'Anaesthesia and Intensive Care' was established, after four decades from its first consideration, with Volume 1 Number 1 appearing in August 1972. Barry continued as its editor for ten years. He was followed by B Horan, then J Roberts, A Duncan, and in 2007, N Gibbs. Barry continued to take a keen interest in the publication, opening each new issue and immediately calculating the income from advertisements contained within its pages to assess its continuing viability. Now in its fortieth year, 'Anaesthesia and Intensive Care' continues to be published in-house at the Australian Society's headquarters, employing a printer for the hard copy production only. It enjoys the official support of the Australian and New Zealand Intensive Care Society and the New Zealand Society of Anaesthetists (Fig. 34.5).

Since 1984, when the Australian Society of Anaesthetists celebrated its fiftieth year, an aspect of the history of anaesthesia has been featured as a cover photo, with a short informative covernote in the prepages. From 1984 to 1988, they were prepared by Gwen Wilson, followed by Rod N. Westhorpe and Christine Ball who have continued to provide the covernotes to this day. (Fig. 34.5) Other journals have also given prominence to history. 'Anesthesiology' has included a series of historical vignettes contributed by George Bause, curator of the Wood Library-Museum, Douglas Bacon and others. 'Anesthesia and Analgesia' recently included the cover image and story "The Amazing Nitrous Oxide", written by Naveen Nathan. For many years, the Newsletter of the Association of Anaesthetists of Great Britain and Ireland has included a "History Page."

Journals in Anaesthesia-Related Fields

Pain

In 1973, John Bonica was instrumental in organising the first International Symposium on Pain, held in Issaquash, Washington, US. Bonica's interest in pain began in the late 1930s and 1940s, during World War II, with his involvement as Chief of the Anesthesia and Operating Section of Madigan Army Hospital, Fort Lewis, Tacoma, Washington, where he was primarily involved in the treatment of pulmonary conditions and severe pain caused by war wounds. There, he taught himself regional anaesthetic techniques, and after the War initiated a training program in anaesthetics, first at Tacoma General Hospital in Tacoma Washington and then at the University of Washington.

Along with like-minded colleagues, Bonica established the International Association for the Study of Pain (IASP) in May 1974. At its first meeting in Washington DC, Bonica proposed the establishment of the journal, 'Pain'. Elsevier published the first issue of this quarterly journal in 1975 with Patrick Wall as its first Editor-in-Chief, while Bonica headed

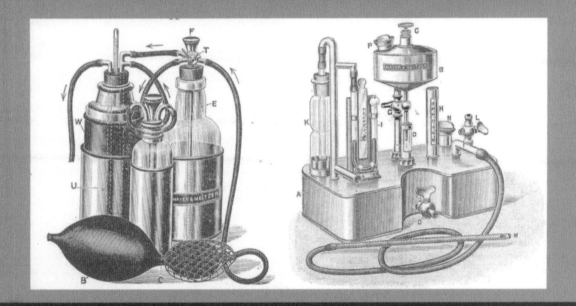

VOLUME 41 • NUMBER 3 • MAY 2013

Anaesthesia
and Intensive Care

- Australian Society of Anaesthetists
- Australia and New Zealand Intensive Care Society
- New Zealand Society of Anaesthetists

Visit *Anaesthesia and Intensive Care* online
www.aaic.net.au

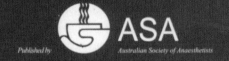

Fig. 34.5 *Anaesthesia and Intensive Care*, May 2013. Coverphoto: Shipway's warmed ether apparatus. (Reproduced with permission of the Executive Editor.)

the list of the Editorial Board. Definitions of pain were established and published in 1979 in 'Pain'. Publication expanded from a quarterly to a monthly in 1982. The IASP widened its base over the past 40 years to involve neurologists, neurosurgeons and other medical specialties, reflected by the increasingly range of articles published in the journal. It has become an interdisciplinary journal. In 2011, 'Pain' had an Impact Factor of 5.371(the highest of all journals classified as related to anaesthesia by ISI) and a 5-year Impact Factor of 6.125 [24].

Other notable journals specialist fields are 'Critical Care Medicine', established in 1972 'Regional Anesthesia and Pain Management' established in 1975.

'Thoracic and Cardiovascular Anesthesia', 1986, 'Journal of Neurosurgical Anesthesiology' 1989 and the 'International Journal of Obstetric Anesthesia', 1991 have also been established, following on closely since the original pioneering publications in new subspecialties.

Other Established Journals

These include the 'Indian Journal of Anaesthesia' which recently celebrated its fiftieth year of publication, having commenced in 1956, while the 'Romanian Journal of Anaesthesia and Intensive Care' was established in 1994.

Reasons for Writing

The British Medical Journal of 9 October 1965 contained a report of the nineteenth General Assembly of the World Medical Association held in London in that year. This session was in fact a conference of medical editors. Russell Brain made the first presentation. Brain was a British neurologist, principal author of Brain's 'Diseases of the Nervous System', and for many years, Editor of the journal, 'Brain'. His address, discussed the shortcomings of the presentations of scientific papers, pointing to poor construction of hypotheses and faulty reasoning, leading to erroneous deductions [25]. Austin Bradford-Hill followed with another paper, this in a more constructive vein, titled, "The Reasons for Writing" [26]. Bradford-Hill, or Hill as he called himself and preferred to be known, commenced by posing the question, "Why does the scientific worker write at all?" After dismissing examples of "authors who write to gain notoriety or to climb another rung or two on the ladder", he stated that the object of a scientific worker was to communicate to other workers in the field, just two things: "what was it the worker thought he had found out and how did he find it out". Hill was reacting to the loose and long-winded presentations of many papers published at the time. He declared that papers should have four sections which clearly answered the ques-

tions, 'Why did you start, what did you do, what answer did you get, and what does it mean anyway?' He argued that 'this seems to be a logical order of a scientific paper'. These four questions of Hill's, to be answered in the structure of the paper, constitute our now universally accepted format of Aims, Methods, Results and Discussion. Hill's basic guide to good scientific writing is clear and authoritative and continues to be quoted in "how-to" manuals such as the popular 'How to Write a Scientific Paper' by George Hall, the most recent edition being reprinted in 1999 [26].

'Update', Journal of the World Federation of Societies of Anaesthesiologists

The published reports in anaesthesia journals indicate the globalisation of the understanding and practice of anaesthesia. The spread of the English language as the language of science has facilitated communication of knowledge and ideas, of the results of drug trials, of new techniques and new equipment to facilitate the practice of these techniques. The prize for the journal published most broadly in geography and languages surely must go to 'Update', the Journal of the World Federation of Societies of Anaesthesiologists (WFSA). This Federation was formed in 1955 and its first World Congress held in 1957 in Scheveningen in The Netherlands. The World Congress of Anaesthesiologists has since been held at four-yearly intervals in cities worldwide. The original funding for the production of an international journal was given by the World Federation of Societies of Anaesthesiologists in 1992. UK aid from the Overseas Development Administration then added 16,000 Pounds Sterling over four years. 'Update' was launched, founded and edited by Iain Wilson in England, generously assisted by Roger Eltringham. The journal was then adopted by the WFSA as its official journal.

Since its beginning, this journal has aimed to spread the knowledge of the science and safe practice of anaesthesia throughout the developing world, its editors now being the Members of the Publications Committee of the WFSA, and its current Editor-in-Chief Bruce McCormick. This small band of volunteers from UK, US, Australia, Argentina, France, China and Togo edit all copy and translate the contents of every issue, resulting in its publication not only in English, but also Spanish (web), Russian (web and hard copy), Mandarin (hard copy) and French. At the time of writing, Portuguese and Persian editions are underway. Now fully funded by the WFSA, this journal is distributed in various countries where medical libraries and the Internet are not readily accessible or are prohibitively expensive, and has from the start, been available via the internet for free download. The journal reaches many anaesthetists, anaesthetic technicians and nurses in remote parts of South American countries, in sub-Saharan Africa, and in China, Southeast Asia and Mongolia and many other places where facilities for clinical practice and educational development are scarce, and textbooks and journals few or out of date. In terms of the populations they serve, collectively these countries are better termed 'the real world'. The aim of the WFSA and its committees is altruistic, supported by membership fees and donations of the individual societies of the WFSA.

Support and Survival

Why did some Anaesthesia Journals evolve as they did? Why, for instance, did 'Anesthesiology' eclipse 'Anesthesia and Analgesia'? Part of the answer may well lie in the economic and scientific dominance of the US after World War II. Relatively unscathed and growing economically, the US drew ahead in many aspects of science and its support, including that for anaesthesiology. NIH support increased markedly in the 1950s and 1960s. As part of this general development, the science of anaesthesia developed more in the US than in other countries, and perhaps being vulnerable to provincialism, researchers in the US submitted the results of their work to American journals. But probably most significant was that all members of the American Society received 'Anesthesiology' as part of their membership and the membership of the ASA quickly surpassed that of the IARS. The excellence of the selection of the editors-in-chief and editorial staff added greatly to Anesthesiology's prestige, and it became the journal of choice for research reports. Anesthesia and Analgesia was pejoratively referred to as the 'Yellow Peril' until its standards were raised by editors such as Nicholas Greene and those who followed.

Ethics of Publication—Plagiarism and Fraud

Regrettably we can't believe everything we read. Newspapers publish untruths which can result from inaccurate reporting, or deliberate misrepresentation of the facts for political or publicity purposes. Similarly in medical publications, be they in general articles or specialist fields of reporting or original research such as anaesthesia, there may be instances of either genuine mistakes or deliberate modifications of a study's results, to gloss over a defect in the collection of data or to prove a point that the author had as the original aim of the study. Unfortunately, it falls to the editor's lot or that of the reviewer to identify fraud before acceptance for publication. This is not an easy task, and inevitably some papers slip through the net.

Plagiarism is a well-recognised transgression in publication. Most journals request assignment of copyright by the authors on acceptance of the submission by that journal. Any part of another paper may be quoted as long as acknowledgement of the source is included. But the exact copy of text without

acknowledgement of the source and permission being granted by the copyright holder is plainly illegal. Self-plagiarism is certainly not unknown, where an author repeats verbatim his or her own already published text, whether it be originally in a journal or a paragraph in a major work such as a textbook.

A sharp-eyed and well-read editor or reviewer may recognise phrases or whole sentences in familiar subject matter that alerts him or her to the possibility or probability of plagiarism. More recently with the development of electronic software, such a submission may be scanned and compared to texts in the huge databases available such as Pubmed. Examples of software are eTblast, Deja-vu, DocCop and Turnitin, the last mentioned of these being in regular use in universities and schools when assessing students' examinations and 'original' essays. However, these electronic programs are helpful but not perfect; they assist in identifying closely similar text but must ultimately be used with caution. At best, they are useful tools, and editorial boards of anaesthesia journals are rapidly adopting the practice of scanning all submissions before acceptance for publication.

In the 1990s, various editorials were published on double publication and self-plagiarism to draw authors' and readers' attention to the serious nature of the problem. 'Anesthesia and Analgesia' and 'Anaesthesia and Intensive Care' have used these editorials to expose the practice, by instancing several cases within their own pages. In the 'British Journal of Anaesthesia' in April 1991, G Smith, R Miller, LJ Saidman and M Morgan published an editorial titled "Ethics in Publishing", which was closely followed by another in the same vein by JG Roberts in 'Anaesthesia and Intensive Care' the following month, the latter titled " Publishing in our Journals: Ethics and Honesty" [27, 28]. Similar editorials were published around the same time in Anesthesiology, Anaesthesia and the Canadian Journal of Anesthesia when it appeared that there was emerging an "epidemic" of double or multiple publication of data from a single study, and an increasing awareness of lack of ethics approval (of informed consent). As a result of this widely recognised and unacceptable incidence, the International Committee of Medical Journal Editors revised their document of 'Uniform Requirements'

Editors of journals in the same specialty fields communicate freely with one another when suspicion about the originality of a paper arises or when fraud is suspected; for instance, when no registration of a trial or clinical study is documented. For most journals, documented registration of a study or clinical trial is obligatory before acceptance for publication. An editorial by Martin Tramèr in the 'European Journal of Anaesthesiology' in 2011 describes a series of 88 clinical trials which were published in various medical journals from 1999 to 2011, all by the same author, Joachim Boldt [29]. Originally the total number of articles was 102, but at least 12 of these could be verified as approved by the Institutional Review Board (IRB) of the State Medical Association of Rheinland-Platz, Germany, where Boldt conducted his research. However, 88 remained without IRB approval, the research consequently could not be verified and to date is plainly unacceptable for publication. In his Editorial, Tramèr describes how the authors of the eighteen well-known medical journals have signed an "Editors-in-Chief Statement Regarding Published Clinical Trials conducted without IRB Approval by Joachim Boldt".

But to return to the beginning, Joachim Boldt, a German anaesthesiologist and former Head of the Department of Anaesthesiology at the Klinikum Ludwigshafen, a hospital which is not university-affiliated, published his 102 articles in various journals including the 'European Journal of Anaesthesiology' and 'Anesthesia and Analgesia'. Of these 102 articles, 12 were verified as having been approved by the IRB. The remaining 88 articles in question had no ethics committee approval as there was no ethics committee or IRB at this non-university-affiliated hospital at the time, and any claim published in these papers that the authors had such approval was plainly false. In another four articles in this series of 102, Boldt and his co-workers positively claimed that these studies had the approval of the IRB of the hospital, but no such committee has ever existed. However, there was in place until 2001, an arrangement whereby an author wishing to gain permission to proceed with some planned research could apply to the Landesartzkammer Rheinland-Pfalz, with a letter of approval from an ethics committee (IRB) together with patients' signed consent forms.

Scott Reuben graduated from the State University of New York Medical School at Buffalo in 1985 and trained in anesthesiology at Mount Sinai Medical Center in New York. In 2009 he held the position of Professor of Anesthesiology and Pain Medicine at Baystate Medical Center in Springfield, Massachusetts. Suspicion of fraudulent publication first occurred in 2008 when it was discovered that he had not submitted an application for IRB approval for two pieces of research which he planned to present at an in-hospital research week. In 2009, it was revealed by a staff member at Baystate that Reuben had admitted to failing to subject his proposed trials to an IRB, fabricating the results of trials and never even conducting the trials he wrote about in 21 articles he published in journals.

Reuben's first paper in a series of 21 clinical trials of doubtful validity appeared in 1996. Reuben fabricated some of the listed patients, no doubt wishing to add weight to the clinical "proof". He also listed co-researchers, some of whom knew nothing about the trials and had their signatures forged on submitted documents.

In 2009 Reuben also admitted to a member of staff that he had fabricated volunteers for his research and therefore the data in the results of his research in trials of various pain-killer preparations and an antidepressant drug for which Pfizer had made major grants for Reuben to perform the studies. The editors of the journals which had published Reuben's studies were obliged to retract these 21 articles. In 2010, Reuben was

charged and sentenced for health care fraud. He was relieved of his professorship at Baystate and sentenced to six months in gaol to be followed by supervised release for three years. He was also fined heavily and ordered to provide an enormous amount of monetary restitution [30]. According to Steven Shafer, Editor of 'Anesthesia and Analgesia', doctors had been applying his findings in their clinical practice, and thereby likely putting their patients at risk of serious and undocumented effects of the drugs. Shafer described Reuben's publications as "the biggest case of fraud in the history of Anesthesiology".

Some institutions such as the colleges of the medical specialties have their own systems to assist in the management of cases of plagiarism or fraud. One such is the General Medical Council of the United Kingdom. The recently established Committee on Publication Ethics (with the neat acronym of COPE) welcomes medical journal editors to join its international membership and to enjoy the full benefits it offers, assisting editors dealing with apparently insoluble issues with difficult authors and other problems of noncompliance with instructions [30].

But the history of this organisation is interesting in itself. In 1997 Michael Farthing, at that time Professor of Gastroenterology at St Bartholomew's Hospital in London, was appointed Editor of 'Gut, International Journal of Gastroenterology and Hepatology'. Within his first year as Editor, Farthing was surprised to encounter four cases of misconduct among the submissions received. This prompted some informal meetings of editors who were similarly concerned, where cases were discussed behind closed doors. In November of that year, a formal meeting of like-minded editors where anonymised cases were discussed, and the Committee on Publication Ethics was thus established. In his first annual report of the group meeting in May 1998, Farthing stated that "COPE is an experiment", adding that he would be delighted if the international response to research into misconduct significantly reduced its incidence. By the year 2000 COPE had a constitution, elected officers and a council. COPE is now a fully established organisation which has not only issued its 'Guidelines on Good Publication Practice', but assists individual editors personally and through its flowcharts (algorithms or guidelines), thereby directing editors in sorting out their problems with difficult and non-compliant authors. COPE's membership is currently around 350 editors worldwide, with a Code of Conduct and a quarterly newsletter.

Development of an Organization of Journal Editors

The International Committee of Medical Journal Editors (ICMJE) is a group of general medical journal editors worldwide. Originally known as the Vancouver Group after its first meeting in 1979 in Vancouver, British Columbia in Canada, the group now meets annually to discuss such items as recommendations for Instructions for Authors, a guide which all journals publish either once a year or regularly in each issue. These clearly set out the obligations which authors should observe for ready acceptability of their submissions. The committee also advises on such matters as registration of clinical trials and conformity.

Accessibility of Journals—HINARI

Lack of access to scientific journals has been recognised as a major hurdle to improvement in world health. After much deliberation and planning, in the year 2000 the World Health Organisation and the United Nations organisation agreed to co-operatively fund a program "Research for Life". One of the three programs under this banner is the Health Internet Access to Research Initiative, "HINARI". Under the HINARI banner, publishers who agree to allow their journals to contribute to this initiative donate one online subscription to the organisation. Microsoft Ireland provides free password-controlled access for approved institutions in low- and middle-income developing countries. This gesture is aimed at improving standards of health care and is already providing guidance to researchers in these countries as demonstrated at a combined meeting of General Partners, (the publishers) and recipients in London in July 2011.

All anaesthesia journals contribute to the distribution of the latest advances in the specialty, thus serving the needs of their readerships. But because of the wide range of their focus and differing readerships, direct comparisons and comparisons over the history of our specialty are inappropriate. As Nicholas Greene, a former Editor of 'Anesthesiology' indicated in a cautionary note in 1992: "Measuring something as subjective as the quality of the written word is as fraught with dangers as attempting to measure beauty" [31].

Publications as Measures of Progress

Each anaesthesia journal in its sequential issues reflects the development and progress of anaesthesia in a chronological order. By reading the contents pages of each issue of a journal, the titles of articles being very brief summaries, we can follow the chronological development of anaesthesia and form an accurate picture of trends and progress over the years. This is a different, but valid, way of looking at the history of anaesthesia.

Acknowledgments My thanks are due to Dr George S. Bause MD, MPH, Clinical Associate Professor, Case Western Reserve University, Cleveland, Ohio, USA, for his own photograph of the cover of the first issue of "Microcosm" and for the information relating to this journal; to Dr Gustavo Elena, Associate Professor of Anaesthesiolgy, Universidad Nacional di Rosario, Totoras, Argentina, for his translations of editorials; to Dr Shingi Sasaki, for also arranging translations; and to Ms Tereza Jiminez and Ms Karen Bieterman, Librarians at the Wood Library-Museum of the American Society of Anesthesiologists, Park Ridge, IL, USA, without whose generous assistance this small chapter would not have eventuated.

References

1. Rosen G. Mesmerism and surgery. A strange chapter in the history of anesthesia. J Hist Med Allied Sci (Henry Schumann, NY) 1946;1(4):527–50.
2. Mesmer A. Mémoire sur la Découverte du Magnetisme Animale. NY: Didot le Jeune; 1779.
3. Nuland SB. The origins of anaesthesia. Classics of medicine library. Birmingham, AL: Leslie B Adams, Gryphen Editions Ltd.; 1983;8:70.
4. Bause GS. America's first patented series of bubble-through anesthetic vaporisers. Anesthesiology. 2009;110:12–21.
5. Craig DB, Martin JT. Anesthesia and analgesia: seventy-five years of publication. Anesth Analg. 1997;85:237–47.
6. Ranney O. Francis McMechan (Tribute). Curr Res Anesth Analg. 1940; Nov–Dec (pp. not numbered in publication).
7. Kaye G. Francis McMechan (Tribute). Curr Res Anesth Analg. 1940; Nov–Dec (pp. not numbered in publication).
8. Cohen HM. Foreword. Br J Anaesth. 1923;1.
9. Norman J. The British journal of anaesthesia—an informal history of the first twenty-five years. Br J Anaesth. 2002;88(3):445–50.
10. Monod R. Introduction. Anesthesie et Analgesie. 1935;1–3.
11. Forgue E. Editorial. Revista Argentina de Anesthesia y Analgesia. 1939–1940;1:1
12. Gutierrez A. Introductory editorial. Revista Argentina de Anesthesia y Analgesia. 1939–40;1:3–6.
13. Bacon DR. The creation of anesthesiology. In: Bacon DR, McGoldrick KE, Lema MJ, editors. The American Society of Anesthesiologists—a century of challenges and progress. Park Ridge: Wood Library-Museum of Anesthesiology; 2005. pp. 35–42.
14. Haggard HW. The place of the anaesthetist in American Medicine. Anesthesiology. 1940;1:1–12.
15. Guedel AE. Cyclopropane anesthesia. Anesthesiology. 1940;2:13–25.
16. Webb JA. Foreword. Anaesthesia. 1946;1:3.
17. Langton HC. Editorial. Anaesthesia. 1946;1:4.
18. Waters RM. Editorial. Progress in anaesthesia in the western hemisphere. Revista Brasiliera de Anesthesiologica. 1951;1:3–12.
19. Fukuda T. Foreword. Masui. 1952; 1.
20. Gordon RA. Editorial. Can J Anaesth Soc J. 1954;1:1.
21. Eklund J. Acta Anaesthesiologica Scandinavica—the first fifty years (from lead to electrons). Acta Anaesth Scand. 2007;51:968–74.
22. Gisvold SE. There is much to learn from history. Editorial. Acta Anaesth Scand. 2007;51:965.
23. Wilson G. Fifty years—the Australian Society of Anaesthetists 1934–1984. Australian Society of Anaesthetists; 1984.
24. Kam P. Impact Factor; Overrated and Misused? Anaesth Intensive Care. 2005;33(5):567–70.
25. Brain R. Structure of a scientific paper. Br Med J. 1965 Oct 9; 868–9.
26. Bradford Hill A. The reasons for writing. Br Med J. 1965; 870–2.
27. Smith G, Miller R, Saidman LJ, Morgan M. Ethics in publishing. Br J Anaesth. 1991;66:421–2.
28. Roberts JG. Publishing in our journals: ethics and honesty. Editorial. Anaesth Intensive Care. 1991;18:163–4.
29. Tramèr MR. The boldt debacle. Editorial. Eur J Anaesth. 2011;28:393–5.
30. History of COPE. Committee on Publication Ethics. http://publicationethics.org/about/history.
31. Greene NM. Anesthesiology journals, 1992. Anesth Analg. 1992 Jan;74(1):116–20.

A History of the American Board of Anesthesiology Certifying Examinations

35

Stephen Slogoff

Summary

The American Board of Anesthesiology (ABA) incorporated as a sub-board of the American Board of Surgery, held its first written examination in 1938, and certified 9 diplomates by examination in 1939. In 1941, the ABA became a primary board. Its first written essay-style examination tested anatomy, pathology, pharmacology, physics and chemistry, and physiology. The unstructured oral examination aimed to test a candidate's clinical proficiency. A practical examination, held at the candidate's hospital, was used for 15 years—until growth in the candidate pool made it impractical. As a substitute, in 1975, the ABA required that a faculty clinical competence committee prepare an annual Certificate of Clinical Competence (CCC) for each resident in training.

In 1944, Saklad questioned the reliability of essay examinations, and after 1947 the written examination consisted of multiple choice questions. Other suggestions by Saklad, and later by Slocum, increased the reliability of the examination. In 1955, the ABA employed the Educational Testing Service (ETS) to provide psychometric support. Discussions between the ASA's American College of Anesthesiology (ACA) and the ABA, led to creation of an in-training examination for all residents in 1975. The 1979 introduction of the Rasch Model for grading examinations, permitted the Board to apply an ability-based standard rather than percent correct or a normative pass rate (i.e., the same level of knowledge was required each year to pass the written examination). In 1982, the ABA hired Francis Hughes as Executive Director. Hughes participated in every important decision concerning the Board's examination system until he retired in 2009.

In 1940, oral examiners chose the questions asked. In 1961, Adriani became chair of the Examinations Committee and in 1964 prepared a landmark guide for oral examiners. Paralleling one of Adriani's ideas, in 1969, Keats proposed using "suggested topics", forcing all test candidates to discuss the same subject. The resulting structured examination was first administered in 1970.

In 1995, the ABA sought the help of psychometrician Mary Lunz, to deal with concerns (first expressed in the mid 1980s) about how to control for reliability of individual guided questions, examiner grading, and the impact of new examiners giving their first examinations. In 2003, the ABA implemented multifactorial analysis scoring for its oral examination, to correct for question difficulty and examiner grading severity. During the 1980s and 1990s, the Board developed and refined certification in Critical Care and Pain Medicine subspecialties, and recertification for its primary (now Maintenance of Certification in Anesthesiology) and subspecialty certificates.

Over the course of 70 years, the ABA has provided increasingly objective certification of candidates in anesthesiology. The scoring system is now as objective as present methods and human frailty allow.

Introduction

The 1930s saw a sustained appeal to the American Medical Association (AMA) and its Advisory Board of Medical Specialties, to establish a certifying process for anesthesiology specialists. Advocates for this goal included Ralph

Waters, who founded the first university-based residency in anesthesiology at the University of Wisconsin in 1927, Paul Wood of the New York Medical College, and John Lundy of the Mayo Clinic (Lundy also lobbied successfully for the creation of the Section of Anesthesiology within the AMA). Complex motives prompted these men and those whom they represented. They believed that certification would bring legitimacy to this new medical specialty. Perhaps of equal importance, they believed that the recognition implied by certification would limit the intrusion of nurse anesthetists and minimally trained family physicians into the medical

S. Slogoff (✉)
Department of Anesthesiology, Stritch School of Medicine, Loyola University, Chicago, IL, USA
e-mail: sslogof@lumc.edu

Table 35.1 First Directors of the American Board of Anesthesiology (1938)

T Drysdale Buchanan, MD	New York, New York
John S Lundy, MD	Rochester, Minnesota
EA Rovenstine, MD	New York, New York
Henry S Ruth, MD	Philadelphia, Pennsylvania
H Boyd Stewart, MD	Tulsa, Oklahoma
Ralph M Tovell, MD	Hartford, Connecticut
Ralph M Waters, MD	Madison, Wisconsin
Paul M Wood, MD	New York, New York
Philip D Woodbridge, MD	Boston, Massachusetts

practice of anesthesia. Through their efforts, the American Board of Anesthesiology (ABA) was incorporated in 1938 as a sub-board of the American Board of Surgery.

The ABA acted quickly, giving its first written examination in 1938, and certifying nine diplomates by examination in 1939. Certificate #41, (the first to be awarded by examination), went to Rolland Hastreiter from University Hospital in Augusta, GA. He was certified on 3 Feb 1939. Certificate #1 (not by examination) went to T Drysdale Buchanan. Paul Wood became the first secretary of the Board and chair of the Examinations Committee. His considerable organizational and leadership skills qualified him for both positions. The Board modeled its process on that of the American Board of Surgery: written and oral examinations followed by a practical examination at the home site of the candidate. Based on national recognition of their expertise, 40 "Founders," including all the directors (Table 35.1) of the first ABA, were certified without examination. No further diplomates were certified in that manner. Those participating in the first oral examination included the ABA Directors and some of the other Founders.

In 1941, the ABA became a primary board, no longer a sub-board of the American Board of Surgery. Then, as now, the Board existed primarily to credential (confirm their suitability to enter the certification process) and certify candidates. In the past two decades, the ABA assumed certification of practitioners in two subspecialties within anesthesiology (Critical Care and Pain Medicine). It developed recertification for its primary and subspecialty certificates and, most recently, the conversion of recertification to maintenance of certification in anesthesiology (MOCA). Notwithstanding these diverse activities, certification remains its primary business.

This essay will describe the evolution of the examination process for the primary certificate through to approximately 2005, the date where my direct source material ended. This process has radically changed from the first examinations in 1938 and 1939. Logistics have changed because of the dramatic growth of anesthesiology and the consequent enrollment of increasing numbers of candidates for examination. A sustained commitment of the ABA to fairness in the evolution of the process, provided an underlying platform.

Fairness requires that every candidate is treated equally, but how could that be done for oral examinations by examiners with diverse qualities—some more demanding, some less demanding? How could that be done if the questions asked by different examiners differed? How does one factor into the process, the experience of the examiner or the time of day of the examination? And do the written and oral examinations test relevant knowledge and skills? This history of the ABA describes the struggle to answer these questions, and to achieve the best, if imperfect, answers.

Early Examinations

The ABA modeled the examination process on the written, oral, and practical components of the American Board of Surgery examination. Thus, the original Directors created a written essay-style examination with five basic science components: anatomy, pathology, pharmacology, physics and chemistry, and physiology [1]. In turn, each component consisted of five questions. Candidates had to answer three of the five questions in each component, within 45 minutes. Three directors on the Examinations Committee: the first ABA president Thomas Buchanan, Wood, and Emory Rovenstine, the fabled chair at Bellevue Hospital and a disciple of Ralph Waters, graded all examinations. All lived in the New York area and shuttled papers among themselves to complete the grading. As is the case today, in that first examination, graders were blinded to the name, personal information and location of the candidate. As the candidate pool grew, restricting grading to a small committee of directors became impossible, but at least one ABA director read every examination and retained final say over grading. Within a few years, Ralph Tovell and Lundy, both original directors, noted that teaching programs had obtained examination questions, and in response had changed their curricula. Some critics complained that the ABA gave the hardest basic science test of all specialties; Waters and Kenneth Woodbridge, the first Anesthesia Chair at Temple University accepted that as a compliment.

Initially, oral examinations were intended to test the candidate's proficiency in clinical anesthesiology, but were unstructured—examiners could ask questions about any area of anesthesia they chose. Unlike the written examination, examiners reviewed the candidate's application and list of publications before the test, and often asked the candidate "what he thought he did best." Not surprisingly, examination content varied widely. Each candidate was tested for 10 minutes in each of three rooms with two examiners in each room. ABA directors gave the first sets of examinations, but other "Founders" soon came to help, although only the directors graded the content. Then and subsequently, no one with personal knowledge of a candidate could examine that candidate.

After satisfactory completion of the written and oral examinations, a director or Founder went to the candidate's hospital, watched him/her provide anesthesia care, observed their interactions with patients and surgical colleagues, and even investigated whether they worked for a fee or were salaried by a hospital—salaried anesthesiologists were then considered to be acting unethically because all other physicians billed fee-for-service. On completion of the practical examination, the Board voted to award or not award a certificate to the candidate. By 1940, the ABA was already wavering on the feasibility of continuing the practicum phase of the certification process. Discussion in the ABA minutes focused on the impracticality of the exercise, particularly after the influx of candidates from World War II. There was no official end to the practical examination, nor was there mention of the last candidate so examined.

Rather than describe the evolution of all three components of the examination process simultaneously, the narrative now will follow each separately.

The Written Examination

The enormous surgical demands imposed by World War II, mandated drafting many young physicians into anesthesiology. Most of these became on-the-job trainees. For those few who were formally trained and eligible for examination after credentialing, the ABA initially provided written and oral examinations in Europe and the Far East, but that practice soon became unworkable.

In 1944, Meyer Saklad (Fig. 35.1), one of the first nine diplomates, and one of the creators of the original American Society of Anesthesiology's Physical Status Classification, became a director of the Board and the Board's first innovator. He questioned the reliability (the likelihood that the same candidate would get the same grade if taking a similar test at a different sitting) of essay-type examinations, arguing that the questions were too open-ended and responses too broad to establish true knowledge. Regardless, the horde of returning military anesthesiologists made the grading of essay examinations impractical. With little fanfare, the 1948 written examination of the ABA morphed into 125 multiple choice questions, and the next year into 300 questions, divided equally among the original five areas. The passing (the cut) score was arbitrarily set at 67% correct.

In 1950, administration of the written examination was decreased from twice to once a year. The multiple choice format was now firmly entrenched, although ABA minutes described the directors agonizing about teaching programs gearing their didactic material to passing such tests. When Fred Haugen of the University of Oregon succeeded Saklad as chair of the Examinations Committee, he opted to add more questions requiring reason and logic, rather than just

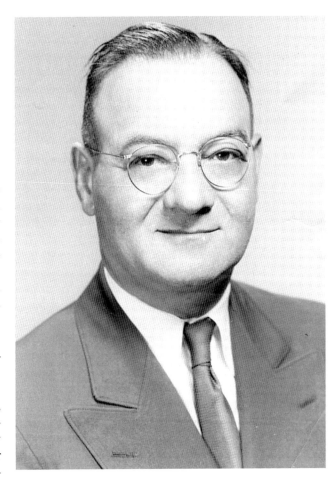

Fig. 35.1 Meyer Saklad. (Courtesy of the Wood Library-Museum of Anesthesiology, Park Ridge, IL.)

memory. By now, the written examination had a normative passing score, i.e., a certain percentage of candidates would pass independent of an arbitrary percent correct. In 1955, Saklad questioned this approach and suggested the imposition of a minimum pass score, regardless of the success rate. Saklad challenged the Examinations Committee to evaluate the test questions, to decide which should be answered correctly by a passing candidate, but little happened with this proposal. Prompted by such controversies, the ABA contracted with the Educational Testing Service (ETS) in Princeton to provide psychometric support. Two years later, ETS recommended eliminating the rigid five content sections, and reducing the length of the test from 300 to 180 items.

A "reliability index" provides a statistical assessment of the consistency or precision of a test; i.e., the likelihood that the same candidates taking a parallel, but different examination at another time would generate the same score. It ranges from zero (no reliability) to 1.0 (perfect reliability.) The changes instituted by Saklad and ETS dramatically increased the reliability index from 0.70 in 1956, to greater than 0.90 in 1957. However, "validity" (does the test examine what you hope it does) was a more elusive goal to assess, and had to be based on "content validity." This psychometric assessment, content validity, is based on the examination having a clearly defined content outline as the basis of its creation, and that test takers who are qualified in that domain perform better than those who are less well prepared in the content domain.

In 1960, Harvey Slocum, chair of Anesthesiology at the University of Texas Medical Branch in Galveston, became chair of the Examinations Committee. He enacted major changes in the written examination. First, the test would include 50 previously used questions from the 1957 and 1958 examinations for equating purposes. Equating would permit comparison of performance of examinees from different years on the same questions, and thereby allow psychometric conclusions about new items. Second, to allow reproducible analyses, statistical evaluations would only be made for data from first-time takers. With the benefit of these changes, the ABA went from a normative scoring system, in which a predetermined pass rate was used, to a criterion-based scoring system in which a predetermined cut score was used, resulting in a pass rate of 84 % the first time it was used. But these low failure rates produced discomfort for the Board and two years later the Board returned to normative scoring.

In 1965, the examination included more equating questions and increased to 210 items to prevent dilution by previously used questions. One year later, the ABA switched from ETS to the National Board of Medical Examiners (NBME) for psychometric support. The NBME distrusted equating, causing removal of all previously used items. The cut score was again now normative with a pass rate set arbitrarily at 75 % for first-time takers. Despite such arbitrariness, considerable data suggested that the written examination was performing well. The reliability index (see above) equaled 0.94 and director James Matthews noted that the current examination had never had a reliability index less than 0.86, a success level not yet achieved by any other specialty board. In that year, the "discrimination index" (comparing performance on items in aggregate by those who passed and failed the test) was 0.37; a good score is considered anything greater than 0.25. The Board was increasingly satisfied with the state of the written examination.

In 1967, two seemingly minor events changed the Board forever. An ad hoc committee of delegates from the Association of University Anesthetists, the American Society of Anesthesiologists (ASA), the AMA section on Anesthesiology, the Academy of Anesthesiology, and the ABA met to consider the possibility of an in-service examination for all US anesthesiology residents. David Little, secretary of the ABA, was the Board's delegate. Nothing came of the effort initially, but the seed for this concept was planted. The other event was election to the Board of the then chair of anesthesiology at Baylor Medical College, Arthur Keats (Fig. 35.2). Over the next twelve years, Keats changed the

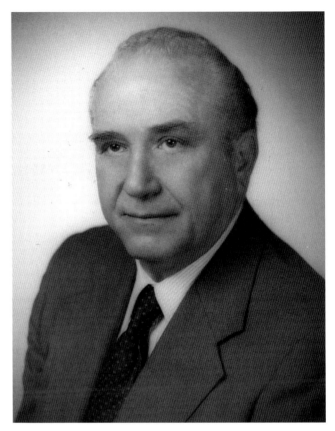

Fig. 35.2 Arthur Keats. (Wood Library-Museum of Anesthesiology, Park Ridge, IL.)

Board's written and oral examination more that any director before or since. No challenge was too great, no detail too small.

Keats became chair of the Examinations Committee in 1971, the same year that he became editor-in-chief of the journal, *Anesthesiology*. The committee immediately started discussions of computer-based examinations. He opined that such technology would not be appropriate for the primary examination, but "if recertification (an idea he and the rest of the Board opposed) ever came to pass, a computer-based examination might be ideal." He accurately foresaw the future.

Also in 1971, a second discussion of an in-service examination for all US anesthesiology residents was initiated between representatives of the ASA's American College of Anesthesiology (ACA) and the Board. For decades, the College had run a shadow certification process for anesthesiologists. Both the ACA and the ABA certified many practitioners, but the ACA also certified many who the ABA considered unqualified by training or who had failed the Board's examination. These competing certificates were a source of confusion to hospitals and their credentialing committees. Keats and Little represented the ABA and proposed that leadership of any in-service examination for all US anesthesiology residents must remain in the hands of the ABA, that the examination should be administered annually, and that participation would be a certification requirement of the ABA. At the next ABA meeting (1972), this enormously controversial proposal was discussed. First, the ABA had reservations about creating examinations with outsiders from the ASA and, secondly, they recognized the enormity of the undertaking. Albert Betcher declared opposition to the plan if the ACA continued its certification. Keats assured the Board that if the proposed plan were enacted, the ACA would cease awarding certificates, which it did a few years later.

In 1973, an ABA/ACA Liaison Committee for In-Training Examinations was formed. Membership from the ASA included Harry Bird, Charles Coakley and William Eggers. William Hamilton, Robert Patrick, and Keats as chair represented the ABA. Note the change in title from "in-service" to "in-training," a distinction that persists between surgery and anesthesiology to this day (surgical residents are in "servitude" and anesthesia residents are in "training"). The committee was charged with creating an examination that could be administered to all residents by 1975. Ultimately the ABA planned to use a subset of that examination as the written ABA examination. The challenge was so enormous that both organizations prepared their own examinations to use if creation of the in-training examination failed.

A key challenge for the committee was that a written certifying examination needs to test only a sample of knowledge from the field to be valid; but a useful in-training examination must be comprehensive; i.e., truly examine the total content of the domain of knowledge. No one had previously focused on the scope of the specialty. The liaison committee immediately went to work on creating a content outline (grid) that defined the entire contemporary scope of anesthesiology. Concurrently, Keats asked the NBME to help him create a new metric to assess whether the examination would test what was actually learned during residency training, as opposed to other educational experiences.

In the spring of 1975, amazingly on schedule, 1700 residents at multiple centers across the U.S. took the first in-training examination. The test had 350 questions, 140 from old ABA and ACA examinations, and 210 generated by writers solicited by Keats from US program directors. Performance on that examination would serve as the comparator for future examinations. In that year, the ad-hoc committee petitioned its two parents to change its status to a permanent council. The ABA-ASA Council on In-Training Examinations resulted. Keats (chair), Bird, Benson and Slogoff represented the ABA. Eggers, Howard Zauder, Coakley and Alan Sessler represented the ASA. As part of its charter and as a requirement of the ABA, the chair of the Council would always reside in the Board.

In the early days of the In Training Examination (ITE) Council, all examination questions were reviewed and edited by the 8 Council members. Disagreement about which of the five choices for the answer was correct, was not atypical. It then usually went like this. Keats, as chair, would let the discussion go on for several minutes during which one distinguished member would argue for answer "A," another for answer "C," and another for "D." After 10 minutes, Keats would say, "Time's up. The answer is 'E'. Let's move on."

The second examination in May 1976, was also given to all Canadian residents and was equally successful. Several enhancements were added. First, the "grid" was formalized as the "Content Outline of Anesthesiology," a description of the scope and breadth of the specialty, a document updated every several years with the appointment of a new Council chair, and provided to every anesthesia training department and resident.

Second, the Council debated over the feedback to departments and residents. In a qualifying test, only a score is required, but to have educational value, feedback had to be more meaningful. Options ranged from no feedback to providing the entire examination with answers. The latter was rejected for two reasons: all of the questions would be lost for future use and, more importantly, giving the questions and answers would suggest that those 350 items reflect all that you have to know about the domain, a flawed conclusion. The Council settled on a "keyword" feedback. The resident would receive a keyword phrase describing the essence rather than the point of the question, for each item they had answered incorrectly. This directed attention to an area of study rather than the more circumscribed correct answer to a specific question. An example might be a question dealing with drugs that do and don't cross the placenta with the correct answer being a muscle relaxant. The "keyword" phrase might be "placental transfer of relaxants." To avoid overwhelming junior residents with too many keyword phrases, feedback was limited to questions answered correctly by at least half of the graduating (CA3) residents. Keywords were created in advance, but could be modified if the responses to the question suggested a deficiency in knowledge different than expected. Program directors could therefore easily see what proportion of their residents incorrectly answered a question related to a specific keyword phrase, and draw conclusions about deficits in their departmental curriculum.

Third, the examination performed wonderfully by psychometric standards: reliability and discrimination indices (see above) were high.

The Council soon grew to 14 members, too unwieldy to review questions as a full group, so Keats divided us into three groups led by him, me (SS) and Phil Larson. Arthur always took the most opinionated people in his group. At the end of the first day of meeting in groups, we spilled out of the small rooms into our great room, and I noticed that a distinguished chair of a New England program emerged looking ashen. I asked him what was wrong. He said "for the past eight hours, Arthur splained (sic) anesthesia to us!"

And the new metric that Keats had requested of the NBME, the PGY (post graduate year of training) Index, demonstrated enormous utility. This index did not measure discrimination between high and low scorers, but between CA-3 residents and incoming residents. A high PGY Index suggested that the material tested was actually learned "in training" and a low or negative PGY Index suggested that the material was well known to residents just leaving medical school and/or not reinforced during training. A question about the Krebs cycle supplies an example that would contribute to a negative PGY Index. Such questions were dropped from the examination. A large corps of question writers and editors helped the Council prepare first-rate questions. At every Council meeting, Keats reminded us that every question should be answered correctly by a "good, not great resident graduating from a good, not great program." Keats also saw to it that there were no "PQ" (one paper-one question) questions and no "PAP" (piss-ass picayune [sic]) questions.

In 1977, the In-Training Examination moved from the spring to the second Saturday in July. This facilitated the ABA using a subset (about 250 questions) of the in-training examination for the written portion of its certification process after full completion of residency training, while still collecting data on the performance of the graduating CA3 residents on the entire ITE. (The examinations were administered together until 2008, when the ABA started computerized testing for its candidates and the ITE remained a pencil and paper examination.). The ABA applied two criteria for the subset: each question had to be clinically relevant and non-controversial. The change in date to July also provided baseline examination data from residents with no training.

Feedback concerning the In-Training Examination to departments, and the regularly updated Content Outline have likely improved training, and by extension advanced the specialty. The examination results prompted curricular changes, and books have been written based on the keyword phrases. Scores of question writers have become part of the Board's oral examination system based on their efforts for the Council. By 1980, the chair of the Council met regularly with all directors of the nation's residency programs at the annual meeting of the Society of Academic Anesthesia Chairs/Association of Anesthesia Program Directors, to review the examination and its performance and to describe widespread misinformation detected by the examination that might "surprise" these educators. Residents and their teachers received feedback indicating where those residents stood in their knowledge base, compared to their nationwide peers.

In 1979, the ABA reintroduced a criterion-based cut score for the written examination, which had become a subset of the In-Training Examination. The introduction of the Rasch Model [2] for grading examinations, a model that could

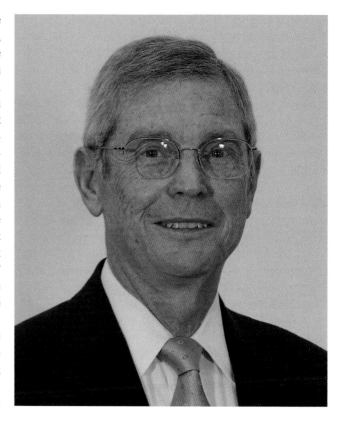

Fig. 35.3 Frank Hughes. (From the author's collection)

separate candidate ability from item difficulty, facilitated application of a truly defensible criterion-based cut score. It again required a pool of equating questions be included in each test from previous examinations, questions for which the difficulty was already known. The model measures difficulty and ability on a logit scale. A logit is a number without dimensions or boundaries and is an exponential transformation (a log scale) derived from the percent correct score of a test item. Using a cut score on the logit scale, permitted the Board to set a standard, arbitrary as it was, based on actual ability rather than percent correct or some normative pass rate. While understanding the Rasch Model is a challenge for even the most sophisticated examination committee, its usefulness is critical to objective scoring of examinations. With its use, the same level of knowledge is required to pass the Board's written examination from year to year, regardless of the actual pass rate.

At its winter meeting in January 1982, the ABA decided to hire an Executive Director to manage its administrative functions. The list of candidates numbered one. Francis Hughes (Fig. 35.3), a psychometrician at the NBME, had been the ITC (The In-Training Council) and ABA liaison for several years. His personal style and characteristics seemed to perfectly fit the administrative requirements of the job, and his psychometric skills and insight into the Board's examination system were a monumental plus. He was ready

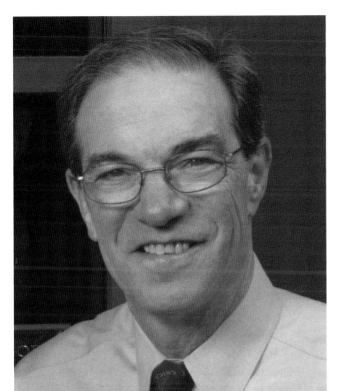

Fig. 35.4 Stephen Slogoff. (From the author's collection)

for a change and the rest was, as is said, history. Hughes became instrumental in every important decision concerning the Board's examination system, until he retired in 2009. Frank has been a close friend of this author since 1978 and I rarely remember anything funny about him, except when Harry Bird, in reference to Frank's obsessive compulsive behavior about details observed, "Frank is Catholic with both a capital C and a small c."

In 1982, I (Fig. 35.4) became a Board director and immediately migrated to full involvement in the examination process. A year later, Hughes and I "validated" the standard (cut score) for the written examination. To do so, we created the "borderline candidate" standard [3]. Each Board director received a 100 item sample of identical A-type (five choice) questions from the ABA subset, with varying, but known difficulties and was asked to assign a value to each item based on their expectations for the candidate who would just barely pass the examination, rather than the one who would excel. Correct answers were not provided. If they believed this imaginary borderline candidate would surely get it right, a value of one would be assigned. If they believed the borderline candidate would fail, then a score of 0.20 (a pure guess) was assigned. If they believed the candidate could narrow the choices to two, three or four possibilities (an educated guess)

then respective scores of 0.5, 0.33 or 0.25 were assigned. Scores for the 100 items were summed and then averaged for the 12 directors. The resultant score was converted to a logit level of ability based on the known difficulty of the 100 items and became the cut-score for the Board's written examination. Interestingly, this score was almost identical to the arbitrary score put in place a few years earlier. This standard was first used in the 1988 test. Over the ensuing decades, the Board repeated the "borderline candidate" exercise several times as it fine tuned and refreshed the standard for the written examination. In 1986, I became the chair of the Examinations Committee and the In-Training Council.

Originally, the ITC reported a standard score, placing the test takers along a continuum of success compared to their peers at training level. Starting in 1990, it reported a scaled score, a logit value of ability independent of the cohort taking the test. Since logits actually range narrowly above and below the number zero to several decimal points, and are hard even for those who understand them to conceptualize, the logit value was converted to a linear scale from 1-61 to make understanding easier for the trainee and program director. Henceforward, residents could track their own ability as training progressed, independent of cohort ability or test difficulty. By being able to track growth in knowledge of their residents individually and in aggregate, independent of these variables, educators have used these data to evaluate their residents and the effectiveness of their didactic programs.

In 1990, the Board and ITC administered the first non-standard examination to comply with the Americans with Disabilities Act. Examples of such disabilities might be dyslexia for the written examination or severe stuttering for the oral examination; each one requiring a longer test period. Every year since, a handful of candidates receive disability-specific non-standard written and oral examinations.

The Oral Examination

Although a grid of more than 100 suggested topics for the oral examination was created in 1940, the examiners had complete discretion in their choice of the actual questions asked. Two Board members in each of four rooms examined the candidates and assigned a grade from 0 to 100. The examiners then met to review the grades. By the mid-1940s, the ABA relied on an increasing pool of associates needed to administer the oral examination.

In 1945, Saklad questioned the validity of the oral examination, stating that he "frequently wasn't sure what the questions meant and what a correct answer was." In 1947, he became the first chair of the combined written and oral Examinations Committee. That fall, for the first time, grades of associate examiners were included in the final score, although they counted less than those of the

Directors. At that session, 29 candidates passed, 15 failed and 2 "conditioned," i.e., had to retest in one or more sections. The ABA began populating its examiner pool with a corps of "national" examiners, rather than local volunteers. Diplomates were only invited if they were expected to be effective examiners, and only re-invited if they demonstrated the requisite skills. The ABA believed that this change enhanced reliability, i.e., the likelihood that a candidate taking the examination at another time with different examiners would get the same grade.

Starting in 1950, four associate examiners and two directors examined each candidate, and all grades counted equally. For the first time, associate examiners were divided into "senior" and "junior", based on experience. Senior examiners were specifically expected to ensure the proper conduct of the examination. Saklad prepared a written outline of what the Board expected of a passing candidate, and introduced 3" × 5" question cards to facilitate inter-room reliability, provide a progression of easier to harder questions, and encourage examiners to stay on topic. However, use of these cards was not mandatory. After three years on the Board, Stuart Cullen, chair of Anesthesiology at the University of California San Francisco, said the Board should stop worrying about the questions, but focus on the issue that we "are examining physicians, not technicians and we need more than a safe anesthetist." He was demanding that questions focus more on the theoretical basis of clinical anesthesiology, rather than on issues of safe administration of anesthetics, an expectation that is consistent with the current examination. Midway through the decade, Frederick Haugen, the then chair of the Examinations Committee, began meeting with the associate examiners to describe what the ABA expected of the process and of a successful candidate, an important first step in standardizing expectations for a successful candidate. In 1956, the Board ruled that each examiner had to record the candidate's grade, independent of their co-examiner and before any discussion of the examination could occur, a policy that persists today.

As with the written examination, a cut score defined the difference between pass and fail for the oral examination. The Board agonized over whether the passing grade should be 75, or a little higher or lower. In 1957, ETS recommended recording grades in multiples of five from 65 to 85, and that the passing grade should be 75. In 1958, Forrest Leffingwell moved that the grade of 75 not be used, thus avoiding fence sitting by an examiner. Further, a director in the examination room would audit the performance of all associate examiners. It was suggested but not pursued, that case histories should be provided to examiners (shades of the coming structured examination). However, the only resulting change was that henceforward, examiners would list all topics discussed in the first examinations on a yellow sheet of paper,

to be taken by the candidate to subsequent rooms to ensure that topics were covered only once.

In 1961, the oral examination format was decreased to two rooms with two examiners in each, its current form. The grading system became 70, 73, 77, or 80 (i.e., low fail, fail, pass and high pass, respectively) with fence sitting (75) still not an option. The cut score settled at greater than 75 (e.g., 77, 77, 77, and 70 representing the lowest passing score of 75.25), the Board believing that no candidate should pass the examination having received failing grades from two of the four examiners.

During his tenure as chair of the Examinations Committee (1961-2), Robert Dripps refined the training and auditing of new, junior and senior examiners. Quality control was of prime importance to the Board, which didn't hesitate to terminate an underperforming examiner.

John Adriani became chair of the Examinations Committee in 1964, and prepared a landmark guide for oral examiners entitled "The Oral Examination of the American Board of Anesthesiology" [4]. He described (1) what characteristics an ABA diplomate should possess, (2) the requisites of a good examiner and (3) the type of questions an examiner should ask. A good examiner must have an adequate knowledge base, a clear understanding of what he/she expects from a diplomate, and the ability to elicit gradable information from the candidate. Questions should be easier at the beginning of the examination, should be modified by the style of the candidate's responsiveness, and should sometimes focus on depth and at other times on breadth of knowledge. Adriani's document, culled from observations by Board members, could serve as the basis for instructions to examiners today. However, Adriani was noted for opening his examination by handing the candidate a piece of paper and asking for the formula for atropine. I suppose that in the 1960s, he thought that was an easy question.

Ted Eger, one of the editors of this book remembers:

"Adriani was one of my Board examiners in the early 1960s. The other examiner was Bernard Briggs who asked me why the Ohio Chemical Co. had brought out the anesthetic fluroxene. Adriani quickly asked Briggs if he didn't mean halothane (but that couldn't be because halothane was produced by Imperial Chemical Industries.) No, Briggs insisted, he meant fluroxene. And I was caught in the middle with my mind frozen on the only reasonable answer: To make money—which was the answer I finally gave. It got a frosty reception from Briggs who elaborated that he wanted to know what qualities fluroxene had that recommended it. Oh, those. They passed me anyway [5]."

In 1966, Robert Patrick—a brilliant and gentle man who was a professor at the Mayo Clinic—suggested that a candidate could question the validity of their examination and request a repeat examination at the end of the day. Such a request would void the results of the first test; only the grades from the second examination would count. Few availed themselves of the opportunity and the opportunity lasted but one year.

Forrest Leffingwell—chair of Anesthesiology at Loma Linda University and president of the ASA in 1962 had "a great sense of humor, but came across as formal and thus highly respected but not feared [6]." In the 1968 ABA minutes, he opined that "It is apparent that the validity of the written examination is based on a good scientific foundation. It is equally apparent that the validity of the oral examination is based on quicksand." While the Board has persisted in its belief that the oral examination has a unique value, much remained to do to challenge Leffingwell's perception. In 1969, the ABA tested the correlation between results on the two different examinations and found a coefficient (r^2) of 0.45. That analysis suggested, but didn't prove, that the two examinations tested different attributes.

In 1969, Keats observed that Board directors and associate examiners never had an opportunity to mingle socially, since the Board met every day after the examinations. His suggestion that there be a formal reception for associate examiners and their spouses on the Sunday evening before the examinations started was unanimously adopted. That same year, Keats noted that the examiner pool lacked African-Americans, a rapidly corrected oversight.

In 1969, Keats was asked to standardize the oral examination. He "suggested topics" for each examination period so that all test candidates and examiners would discuss the same subject, albeit with the actual questions left to the individual examiners. This paralleled Adriani's suggestion and represented a revolutionary change. The first structured examination was administered in 1970, and in 1972, the first actual guided question was used. Before entering the examination room, each candidate received for review a brief summary describing the patient, the planned procedure, relevant medical problems and possibly some laboratory data. The examination focused on the preoperative, intraoperative, and postoperative issues of that case. This author took his oral examination in that year and was asked to deal with the anesthetic management of a child with a full stomach who had aspirated a peanut and required bronchoscopy for its removal. I was sure I had failed, but didn't.

Keats continued his assault on the examination process. He recommended redefining of the four grades (70, 73, 77, 80): 70 and 80 would represent a definite fail or pass, respectively, regardless of how poorly or well the candidate performed. 73 and 77 was to be used only when the examiner was uncertain. Fence sitting (75) was still not allowed. The lowest passing score remained 75.25 (e.g., 77, 77, 77, 70). No longer was there a concept of "high pass" or "low fail." Such inability to reward exemplary performance dissatisfied many examiners. This scoring system continued until the Board eliminated grading of the entire examination by the examiners in 2003 (see below). In 1972, examiners were instructed to grade candidates on five attributes: facts, application, judgment, adaptability, and organization and clarity of response. "Facts" were later removed as a grading issue, since the written examination covered these, and the stress associated with the oral examination could cause facts to be forgotten even though the candidate had an excellent grasp of important concepts.

In 1976, the Board introduced "Suggested Topics," (later called "Additional Topics" to reflect their mandatory use), which dealt with anesthetic issues not covered in the guided question. These brief vignettes were to follow the guided question to provide real topical breadth when all of the questions in the two examining rooms were combined. In an early use of these suggested topics, Jim Arens, a director from Galveston, was examining a poorly prepared candidate and got onto the subject of electrical safety in the operating room. He asked the candidate what he would do if the isolation monitor in the operating room turned from "green" to "red." Expecting the candidate to say that he would start unplugging pieces of electrical equipment to determine which one had a potentially dangerous ground fault, he was amazed when the candidate replied, "I will take my shoes off." Flustered, Arens replied, "I'm not worried about you, I'm worried about the patient!" The candidate quickly responded, "Don't worry about the patient, he already has his shoes off."

In the same year, a library of guided questions and suggested topics was initiated for use in future examinations. Also in 1976, the Board stopped discussing candidates at the end of the examination day; the grades generated were the final score. By then a rigorous system had been created to ensure that a candidate was never examined by someone who knew or had previously examined him/her. Occasionally the system failed, but a candidate could always be assigned a new examiner if, on entering the room, either the candidate or one of the examiner recognized the other in a way that could compromise the integrity of the process.

To ensure that every resident in the country had access to adequate oral examination preparation, the ABA, in 1982, started inviting faculty from programs not represented in the associate examiner pool, to training sessions and observation opportunities at real examinations, a program that continues today.

In 1983, the Board began examining reliability of individual guided questions, examiner "agreement" in grading, and the impact of "dubious" grades by new examiners giving their first examinations. Regarding the last of these issues, inspection of test results indicated that even if the new examiners' grades differed significantly from those of the other examiners, as long as a candidate was examined by only one new examiner out of the four, the impact was nil. Scratch that concern. Over the next five years, the Board, guided by Hughes, studied the psychometric reliability of the oral examination (i.e., assessed whether candidates would get the same grade if they took the examination with a different set of examiners or with a different pair of guided questions.)

These efforts by the ABA reflected its concern for any potential unfairness in the system: guided questions of differing complexity and difficulty, administration by better or poorer examiners and variability of grading among examiners.

For the next several years, these issues drove the Board to investigate numerous modifications in examination content, as well as examiner training and auditing, to ensure fairness in a process that was becoming increasingly important and less voluntary for practicing physicians. It would still be several years until true objectivity was achieved (see below).

Around 1975, external forces increasingly demanded that specialty boards not only certify diplomates, but also periodically recertify them. Some boards almost immediately acquiesced to this demand. The ABA resisted, not because it was opposed to the concept of recertification, but because it felt it still needed to better validate its primary certification before demanding recertification. "Validation" refers to whether the process of certification—credentialing, written and then oral examinations—meant that a diplomate was a better specialist than those who failed in the certification process or never attempted it. This was a major problem for most specialty boards. Recertification was also a threat to those anesthesiologists practicing without certification, but that consideration was never an issue or deterrent for the ABA. Wendell Stevens, the gentle, soft-spoken chair of anesthesiology at the University of Oregon and a new director, was assigned the unenviable task of stonewalling the external organizations, including the ABMS, pressuring for recertification.

Several years later, the Board published the results of an investigation that took over five years to complete, examining whether certification correlated with better skills and practice [7]. In each residency program, a faculty member familiar with the clinical attributes of all the residents, completed a questionnaire detailing the qualitative competence of their residents independent of their knowledge base and Certificate of Clinical Competence (which only documented minimally acceptable criteria; see below). The participating faculty member was blinded to the purpose of the questionnaire. Those residents were followed through the examination process over the next several years. The study was repeated with the next year's class as well. Success in the Board's oral examination clearly and significantly correlated with the earlier assignment of higher competence by the candidates' faculty. This appears to be the only validation of any specialty board's primary certification process.

However, the correlation is imperfect. That is, the oral examination does not reveal all the factors important to clinical excellence. Thus, these data, while statistically significant, are "soft". They reflect subjective data, collected from over 120 sources in more than 120 different programs. The only reproducible thing is the examination process. Consider-

ing all of these factors, the data and their implications are powerful. And, again, nobody else has attempted such a validation or come close.

With this study complete, and external pressure mounting, the ABA initiated its recertification process. One of the last holdouts, Robert Stoelting, chair at the University of Indiana, opined that "at least recertification will finally get people to read again after they passed their boards."

Attempts to strengthen and increase the fairness of the oral examination continued. In 1988, the Board declared that all programs should offer practice oral examinations to their residents. A parallel was added for new examiners. For the first few examinations in each week's cycle of the real thing, two directors served as the formal examiners, while new examiners observed these "real pros" before they started examining. While the Board continued to audit all examiners regularly, it also recognized that auditing examining style and content was different from evaluation of grading. The inherent differences in expectations of different examiners did affect candidate success. To deal with this concern, in June 1995, the ABA asked a psychometric consultant, Mary Lunz, to apply the Rasch model to the oral examinations with some common examiners over two examination cycles. Although candidate ability was the most powerful determinant of outcome, she identified four factors that influenced outcome: difficulty of the guided question, grading severity of the examiners, session of the day or week, and candidate ability. She recommended considering a Rasch model for the oral examination to control for those variables, a decision that would place the standard in the Board's hands, rather than the examiners.

A year later, led by Myer (Mike) Rosenthal of Stanford University, chair of the Examinations Committee, the ABA changed the format of the examination to emphasize the perioperative medicine nature of the practice, a name and focus anticipated by Saidman's 1994 Rovenstine Lecture, published a year later [8]. Time in each of the two rooms was extended to 35 minutes, and while intraoperative care was still stressed in the guided questions in both rooms (10 minutes in one and 15 minutes in the other), 10 minutes in one was devoted to preoperative evaluation and, in the other, 15 minutes was devoted to postoperative and intensive care. The new format was introduced in April 1997. The change included a requirement that each examiner had to provide scores for the individual components of each examination as well as the final, overall holistic grade.

In 1998, the Board started to explore the use of modular grading to replace the holistic grade. One year later, led by Jane Matjasko, chair at the University of Maryland, and by Hughes, the ABA began development of a plan for grading of the oral examination that used the Rasch model and considered three components: question difficulty, examiner severity (i.e., the harshness or leniency of grading), and candidate ability. A criterion-based passing score could then be derived by scoring the evaluation on each module of the examination. The new scoring system changed the thought process for grading from holistically and non-linear (see Keats' definition of score above), to grading on a ranked scale of performance. Examiners now graded each module as one in which a candidate (1) rarely, (2) sometimes, (3) often, and (4) almost always, demonstrates attributes of a board certified anesthesiologist. After three practice years with the multifactorial analysis, the ABA implemented multifactorial analysis scoring for its oral examination in 2003. The cut score was set at 3.0 ("often demonstrates attributes of a Board certified anesthesiologist") minus the standard error of the mean. Subtracting the standard error of the mean gave the benefit of doubt to the candidate. For the first time since its inception, grading of the certifying examination of the ABA corrected for the difficulty of the questions and the severity of the examiners. At least some of the objectivity that Leffingwell couldn't find in 1968 had now been realized.

The Practical Examination

From 1940 on, the ABA viewed the practical examination with ambivalence. On the one hand, the directors believed that they needed evidence that the potential diplomate was a good practitioner as well as a good test taker. They also recognized the impracticality of the task with an increasingly large candidate pool. Between 1945 and 1949, many candidates were certified without a practical examination if their practices were "well known" to a director of the Board, a practice necessitated by the large numbers of as yet uncertified anesthesiologists returning from WWII. By 1949, diplomates rather than directors performed practical examinations, and failed candidates could appeal for a second examination by a director.

By 1950, a "survey" of practice and references by a committee of certified anesthesiologists who lived and worked in the vicinity of the candidate, rapidly replaced the practical examination. Three years later, only one candidate underwent a practical examination. Less than five years later, a candidate-generated form describing what they had done since residency training and a list of diplomate references, replaced the survey. In 1957, practical examinations were formally discontinued and the survey committees were disbanded. Part of the credentialing process, the candidate-generated form of practice activity and references remained in place for the next two decades.

In 1975, the ABA required an annual Certificate of Clinical Competence (CCC) for each resident in training. The CCC, prepared by a knowledgeable faculty member and signed by the chair and resident, replaced all other sources that documented the candidate's clinical skills, personal characteristics, professional behavior and integrity. The CCC for the final six months of training became the primary credentialing tool for entering the examination system, and the candidate-generated form and list of references were retired.

Conclusions

Over the course of 70 years, the Board has moved towards an ever more objective and fair means of certifying candidates in anesthesiology. During the last decade, the Board developed and refined certification in its two subspecialties, Critical Care and Pain Medicine, and added recertification for its primary (now Maintenance of Certification in Anesthesiology) and subspecialty certificates. The primary examination process has never been better. The perfect examination remains the Board's (desired but unattainable) goal, and both the written and oral examinations continue to undergo refinement.

The scoring system is now as objective as present methods and human frailty allow, and standards for both examinations are criterion-referenced with solid evidence indicating the appropriateness of both cut scores. In the near future, the Board is likely to pursue further advances in the written and oral examinations with the use of computers and simulators.

While every Board director contributed to the examination process, I believe three people had the greatest impact: Meyer Saklad in the 1940s and 1950s repeatedly challenged the status quo and did something about it; Arthur Keats from the middle 1960s through to the 1970s led sea changes in both examinations; and Frank Hughes from his days with NBME until his retirement in 2009, guided the board through the complex task of creating defensible and valid criterion-referenced cut scores for both examinations. With the help of many Board directors, these three men contributed to making anesthesiology's certification process one of the fairest and most psychometrically defensible systems in organized medicine. I base this conclusion on numerous discussions with members of multiple specialty boards and am personally convinced that few, if any, boards have achieved the degree of fairness attained by the ABA.

Acknowledgments I thank the current directors of the American Board of Anesthesiology who gave me complete access to all of the minutes of that organization. Thanks also to Mary Post, the Executive Director of Administrative Affairs for the ABA, and Shirline Fuller, her Executive Assistant, who facilitated that access. I greatly appreciate the support of the late Patrick Sim and Felicia Reilly of the Wood Library Museum. I am also most grateful to the many former directors of the Board who gave me wonderful insights into the history and people described, as well as for critically reviewing this manuscript.

References

1. Bacon DR, Lema MJ. To define a specialty: a brief history of The American Board of Anesthesiology's first written examination. J Clin Anesth. 1992;4:489–97.
2. Embretson SE, Reise SP. Item response theory for psychologists. New Jersey: L. Earlbaum Associate, Inc.; 1997. p. 44–9.
3. Slogoff S, Hughes FP, Hug CC Jr. Development of the knowledge-based standard for the written certification examination of the American Board of Anesthesiology. Acad Med. 1992;67:124–6.
4. Broussard DM, Rossiter K. The influence of Dr. John Adriani on the American Board of Anesthesiology Oral Examination. J LA State Med Soc. 2008;160:225–30.
5. Eger EI. Personal Communication.
6. Siker ES. Personal Communication.
7. Slogoff S, Hughes FP, Hug CC Jr, et al. A demonstration of validity for certification by the American Board of Anesthesiology. Acad Med. 1994;69:740–6.
8. Saidman LJ. The 33rd Rovenstine Lecture. What I have learned from 9 years and 9,000 papers. Anesthesiology. 1995;83:191–7.

Other Sources

1. Minutes of the American Board of Anesthesiology business meetings. 1938–2005.
2. Rosenthal MH, Hughes FP. A history of the American Board of Anesthesiology, 1938–2003. Raleigh: The American Board of Anesthesiology Publisher; 2003.

Development of the Certification Examination by the American Association of Nurse Anesthetists (1933–2012)

Susan S. Caulk and Karen Plaus

Summary

The first US nurse anesthetists appeared in the 1870s. First directed by surgeons, these Catholic sisters later adding their own education and techniques. In 1908, surgeon Crile at Cleveland's Lakeside Hospital (later Cleveland Clinic) asked Agatha Hodgins to become his personal anesthetist. Hodgins developed a school of nurse anesthesia and promoted formation of the Lakeside Alumni in 1923, leading in 1931 to organization of the National Association of Nurse Anesthetists (NANA), In 1933, NANA president Fife proposed establishing a national board examination for nurse anesthetists, a proposal furthered in 1934 by appointment of an Education Committee to study establishment of the examination, and set standards for schools of nurse anesthesia. In 1939, the NANA became the American Association of Nurse Anesthetists (AANA). In 1941, Shupp suggested that passage of a certifying examination could define eligibility for AANA membership, and by mid 1940s new AANA members had to be certified by examination. The number of AANA-approved schools of nurse anesthesia progressively increased in the 1940s, but World War II delayed implementation of the qualifying examination until 1945. The title Certified Registered Nurse Anesthetist (CRNA), came into use in 1956.

To obtain GI benefits for training in nurse anesthesia, returning Korean War veterans had to apply to accredited schools. The AANA petitioned the Department of Health, Education and Welfare (HEW) for recognition as the accrediting agency for schools, receiving formal recognition from HEW Commissioner Brownell in 1955. In 1974, the HEW Office of Education required 12 new criteria to recognize AANA accreditation policies and procedures. By 1975, the AANA responded successfully to these mandates.

In 1978, the AANA adopted by-law amendments, establishing an independent Council on Recertification (COR), separating the AANA from certification and recertification processes, and separating membership from certification. In 1982, the "Qualifying Examination" became the *Certification Examination for Nurse Anesthetists,* because passing the examination certified an individual for entry into practice, not for AANA membership.

In the 1980s, attention focused on increasing the objectivity and quality of the examination process. Content validation procedures were documented through a 1987 analysis, with subsequent professional practice analyses in 1992, 1996, 2000, and 2007. Also beginning in 1987, examination scores were reported as scaled rather than raw scores, ensuring neither an advantage nor a disadvantage to taking the Certification Examination at a particular time.

In the mid 1990s, the Council on Certification of Nurse Anesthetists (CCNA) moved from paper and pencil test administration to a computer format, thereby allowing computer adaptive testing (CAT). This process objectively assessed the difficulty level that each examinee could pass.

S. S. Caulk (✉)
(Retired) Director of Continuing Education, Certification, Recertification, American Association of Nurse Anesthetists, 222 South Prospect Ave., Park Ridge, IL, 60068 USA
e-mail: scaulk@aana.com

K. Plaus
National Board on Certification and Recertification of Nurse Anesthetists (NBCRNA), 8725 West Higgins Road, Chicago, IL 60631 USA
e-mail: kplaus@NBCRNA.com

Introduction

Delivery of anesthesia increased rapidly after Morton's demonstration of the effectiveness of ether as an anesthetic, at the Massachusetts General Hospital in 1846. Lacking qualified anesthesia personnel, delivery of anesthesia passed to whomever was available, leading to considerable morbidity and mortality in Europe and the US. American surgeons believed that use of the untutored "part-time anesthetist"

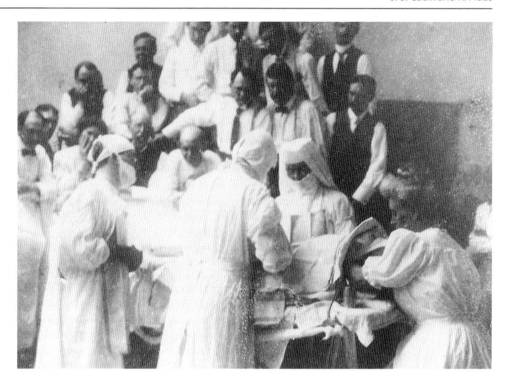

Fig. 36.1 Magaw at the head of the table, giving what appears to be ether anesthesia. (Courtesy of the American Association of Nurse Anesthetists Archive.)

explained the untoward effects. Surgeons wanted clinicians dedicated to the delivery of anesthesia, and nurses eagerly answered the call [1].

Virginia Thatcher's *History of Anesthesia with Emphasis on the Nurse Specialist* suggests that surgeons turned to nurses because they

> "wanted a person who would: (1) be satisfied with the subordinate role that the work required, (2) make anesthesia their one absorbing interest, (3) not look on the situation of anesthetist as one that put them in a position to watch and learn from the surgeon's technique, (4) accept relatively low pay, and (5) have the natural aptitude and intelligence to develop a high level of skill in providing the smooth anesthesia and relaxation that the surgeon demanded [1, 2]".

The earliest known nurse anesthetist was Sister Mary Bernard (1860–1924), a Catholic nun who administered anesthesia at St. Vincent's Hospital in Erie, PA, in 1877. By 1889, nine sisters of the Third Order of the Hospital Sisters of St. Francis had become nurse anesthetists [1].

The Sisters of St. Francis established St. Mary's Hospital in Rochester, Minnesota, in 1889, with the understanding that William Mayo (1819–1911) believed nurses would make fine anesthetists and that he would undertake their instruction. His sons, surgeons William (1861–1939) and Charles Mayo (1865–1939), "decided that a nurse was better suited to the task because she was more likely to keep her mind strictly on it, whereas the intern was naturally more interested in what the surgeon was doing [3]." Two sisters, Edith (1871–1943) and Dinah Graham (1860–1947), were the first nurse anesthetists at the Mayo Clinic.

In 1893, Alice Magaw (1860–1928, Fig. 36.1), the most famous nurse anesthetist of the nineteenth century, replaced the Graham sisters at Mayo Clinic. In her biography of the Mayo brothers, Helen Clapsattle noted that Magaw "won more widespread notice than that of any other member of the Rochester group apart from the brothers [3]." She earned international respect, and Charles Mayo dubbed her "the mother of Anesthesia" for her outstanding contributions [3]. She was the first nurse anesthetist to publish articles on anesthetic practice, beginning with "Observations on 1092 Cases of Anesthesia from Jan. 1, 1899 to Jan. 1, 1900," in the *St. Paul Medical Journal* [4].

In the article, Magaw said:

> I gave in a brief way our method of administering ether and chloroform. This is a method we have found, after several years' experience, to be the most satisfactory. I shall only report the cases on whom this method was used during this last year. I can report that out of this number, 1092 cases, we have not had an accident; we have not had occasion to use artificial respiration once; not one case of ether pneumonia; neither have we had any serious renal results.

Magaw also wrote, "That it is believed that if ether is given with plenty of air and the drop method, there are few, if any, bad results…the mortality can be much diminished by the careful selection of the anesthetic [4]."

Magaw reported administering open-drop chloroform and ether without a fatality attributable to the anesthesia, a considerable feat given a death rate due to anesthesia of perhaps 1:2000 in later years. Surgeons sent nurses to observe and learn from Magaw [4]. In December 1906, she published a review of her work in *Surgery, Gynecology, and Obstetrics*:

> "At St. Mary's Hospital our preference has always been ether. In 14,380 anaesthetics given by me, I have yet to see a death directly from the anaesthetic, but, no doubt, have had my share

of trouble in its administration, although artificial respiration with us is almost unheard of. In my series of cases, the 'open Method' has been the method of choice. We have tried almost all methods advocated that seemed at all reasonable, such as nitrous oxide gas, as a preliminary to ether (this method was used in 1,000 cases), a mixture of scopolamine and morphine as a preliminary to ether in 73 cases, also chloroform and ether, and have found them to be very unsatisfactory, if not harmful, and have returned to ether 'drop method' each time, which method we have used for over ten years. [5]"

In 1908, surgeon George Crile (1864–1943), at Lakeside Hospital in Cleveland, subsequently the teaching hospital for Case Western Reserve University, asked Agatha Hodgins (1877–1945) to become his personal anesthetist. Hodgins perfected administration of nitrous oxide-oxygen anesthesia, and Crile recalled,

"In 1909 I was able to report before the Southern Surgical and Gynecological Association that Miss Hodgins had administered nitrous oxide in 575 major operations, and in August 1911, I reported before the American Surgical Association, 10,787 surgical operations performed by me under either ether, or nitrous oxide supplemented by ether, with no anesthetic death. I reported also the use of morphine and scopolamine as adjuncts to ether or nitrous oxide anesthesia in over three thousand operations. [2]"

Between 1909 and 1915, local and visiting surgeons at Lakeside Hospital were sufficiently impressed by Hodgins' talent that they sent their nurses to be trained by her. She thus became a major participant in the education of physicians and nurse anesthetists at Lakeside Hospital [6, 7].

The contributions of America's nurse anesthetists to care in surgical units and hospitals during World War I increased the demand for nurse anesthetists after the war. The war prompted the first US military effort to train anesthetists. Nurses were taught anesthesia in 6-month on-the-job training programs, at four formal educational centers: St. Vincent's Hospital, Portland, OR (1909); St. John's Hospital, Springfield, IL (1912); The New York Post-Graduate Hospital, New York City, NY (1912); and Long Island College Hospital, Brooklyn, NY (1914). A diploma was issued upon completion, but there was no mention of an assessment or graduation examination.

After World War I, new nurse anesthesia educational programs moved into university hospitals and major community hospitals [1]: Johns Hopkins, Baltimore, MD (1917); the University of Michigan, Ann Arbor, MI (1919); Charity Hospital, New Orleans, LA (1917); Barnes Hospital, St. Louis, MO (1917), Presbyterian Hospital, Chicago, IL; Grace Hospital, Detroit, MI (1918); Grady Memorial Hospital, Atlanta, GA (1918); St. Joseph's Hospital, Tacoma, WA; St. Mary's Hospital, Minneapolis, MN; and Lakeside Hospital, Cleveland, OH (1915). The programs took 3 to 6 months, and there were no certification examinations upon completion.

The 6-month training programs initiated by the Armed Forces in World War II, and the subsequent 3- to 6-month civilian programs noted in the preceding paragraph established

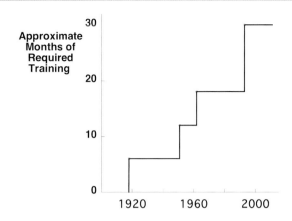

Fig. 36.2 Beginning with World War I, the required duration of training for nurse anesthetists was approximately 6 months, growing in roughly 6-month increments consistent with the need for progressively greater knowledge and skills

the minimum duration of required training (Fig. 36.2). In 1951, the requirement increased to a minimum of 1 year, and in 1962 became 18 months. This trend continued to the 1990s, at which time programs required a master's degree that demanded 24 to 36 months of training [8].

In 1930, at the biennial American Nurses Association (ANA) convention, Agatha Hodgins asked the ANA for recognition of nurse anesthetists as a subgroup within the organization. The ANA declined, as the ANA organizational structure did not envision such a possibility. Hodgins then led in the formation of a national professional organization for nurse anesthetists. The process began with the formation of the Lakeside Alumni in 1923. At the first Alumni meeting, Hodgins presented a plan for a national organization of nurse anesthetists. A tentative constitution and bylaws were drawn up, but not until 17 June 1931, in the Department of Anesthesia at University-Lakeside Hospital in Cleveland, was the organizational meeting for the proposed association held. A motion was proposed that a national association be formed, and the motion passed to form the National Association of Nurse Anesthetists (NANA). The NANA became, thereby, the oldest specialty nursing organization in the US. The early aims of the NANA were to place qualified anesthetists, supply continuing education, and provide professional recognition [1].

The 1930s

Because Hodgins became ill, Gertrude Fife (1902–1980), assistant director of the School of Anesthesia at University Hospitals in Cleveland, assumed a leadership role in the newly formed NANA. As president of the NANA at its first meeting in September 1933, Fife spoke on "The Future of the Nurse Anesthetist." She called for "establishment of a national board of examination for nurse anesthetists, arguing that such an examination would certify to surgeons that nurse anesthetists' knowledge in their field met the approval of an examining board – a board chosen and functioning to safeguard the interests of surgeons, hospitals, and the public [9]." At this first convention, the trustees established minimum standards for schools of anesthesia, specifically: duration of course, 4 months; number of cases of clinical experience, 250; and hours of class instruction, 75.

The second annual NANA meeting, in 1934, saw the appointment of an Education Committee to study the feasibility of establishing a national examination for nurse anesthetists, and standards for schools of nurse anesthesia. Fife observed that:

> "We must find a way whereby the hospitals and surgeons who employ nurse anesthetists can be assured that they have received the proper training, and are qualified to do the work" [10]. "An examining board should be chosen and every applicant applying for membership in the organization should be required to pass an examination. The examining board would be responsible for the preparation of the examination – the arrangements whereby the examination would be taken within the State – and responsible for the final decision which would allow the National Association to issue to the individual who successfully passes the examination a certificate signifying that the individual is sanctioned by this organization." [10]

Although state board registration could have accomplished this end, Fife reasoned that such registration was impractical; a national solution was needed. The national examining board she envisioned would (1) prepare the examination, (2) arrange for examination locations in each state, and (3) award certificates to successful candidates [10].

At the fourth annual meeting, in 1936, the NANA Education Committee continued to pursue its goal of establishing a national board of examiners, one that would be recognized by organizations that depended on nurse anesthetists. The Committee's report emphasized that a national examination and certification of nurse anesthetists should be compatible with professional trends in associated branches of medicine, including the newly created American Board of Surgery and the Council on Dental Education. Both organizations had been established in part for certification purposes [11]. The Education Committee's discussions with members of the American Board of Surgery and the American Hospital Association (AHA) suggested that those organizations would endorse the proposed examination for nurse anesthetists, and the inspection and accreditation of schools in anesthesia, as well as an examination and/or certification of currently active nurse anesthetists [12].

By the sixth annual meeting, in 1938, the Education Committee had (1) compiled a list of schools offering training in anesthesia to graduate nurses; and (2) obtained AHA endorsement of NANA plans for the inspection of schools of anesthesia for nurse anesthetists. On the basis of that inspection, the NANA foresaw that the AHA would approve those schools having curricula equivalent to the standard already adopted by the AHA [13].

In 1939, interest in nurse anesthesia as a career received a major endorsement in "Anesthesia – a Career," in the August issue of *RN Magazine.* The article drew 400 inquiries [14]. That year also saw formalization of a vital aspect of the anesthesia curriculum: Training in anesthesia programs had to be at least 6 months, and a NANA Curriculum Committee was formed to evaluate and present a curriculum in keeping with progressive education. Finally, in that year, the NANA resolved to change its name to the American Association of Nurse Anesthetists (AANA) [15].

From 1933 through the 1940s, the AANA studied ways to ensure the quality of the programs offered by schools of nurse anesthesia. In cooperation with the American Hospital Association, education committees of the AANA initiated efforts to establish a program for the inspection of schools. In 1945, the AHA's Council on Professional Practice proposed to put the program into operation. Representatives of the AANA and the AHA met in 1946, and recommended that the AANA, rather than any other agency, initiate the program. To undertake this action, the AANA board of trustees appointed an Approval Committee (to certify the quality of each school). Workshop conferences and the preparation of questionnaires preceded initiation of the program of school inspections. For the initial inspection of schools, the AANA board of trustees would appoint advisors from the field of adult education, and these advisors, with a nurse anesthetist, would visit each school of anesthesia to recommend accreditation. As originally envisioned, schools would be revisited at three-year intervals. This program of school evaluation was put into effect in the 1950s [8].

The 1940s

In 1940, AANA president Miriam Shupp (1901–1988), noted that a national examination of applicants could be used to measure their eligibility for AANA membership. "We have," she said, "arrived at that period in our development when this project can and should be put into effect to assure the members of AANA and those who employ nurse anesthetists that only properly qualified people are being admitted to membership [16]." Such a requirement had immediate appeal. It would motivate schools of anesthesia to improve their instructional programs, and the success of their graduates on the national examination would provide a measure of each school's quality [16].

At the ninth annual meeting, in 1941, AANA president Helen Lamb (1899–1973), envisioned development and operation of a national examination program by early 1943. The Education Committee laid the groundwork by requesting question sets from schools of anesthesia for use in the examination. Selection of the actual questions for the examination would be the responsibility of the yet-to-be-named examining board [17].

The AANA board of trustees appointed a Certification Program Committee, to plan for the examination of association members. A potentially contentious plan was to test anesthetists who had extensive experience in administering anesthetics but were not graduates of an approved school of anesthesia [18]. A 1942 resolution by the Certification Program Committee avoided this controversy, and was adopted by the AANA. The resolution required all AANA members to be certified by examination, except that the examination requirement would be waived for currently active members [19].

World War II, A Turning Point

World War II accelerated the coming of age of all anesthesia providers, nurses and physicians alike. Because the war drained the country of such providers, hospitals all over the US scrambled to fill the void, coping with the shortage in diverse ways. Some looked to the AANA's standards as criteria for training their students. However, because the AANA had no control over the quality of instruction, it was deeply concerned that those standards might not be met. How could the AANA ensure that these variously trained practitioners possess the skills required to safely provide anesthesia? [20]

Until the Examination Program came into being, the AANA knew little about the anesthesia programs being offered by schools around the country. What knowledge the AANA did have, was pieced together from questionnaires completed by program directors, information on applications for membership, and a fledgling school-visit program that the war had curtailed. There was great uncertainty about the adequacy of graduates applying for membership, because of doubts about the quality of training received in newly organized and older courses, and because of the lack of standards for approval of courses and schools. World events now added urgency to fulfillment of plans for a national board of examinations, plans that had been under discussion since 1933 [20].

The plan for the Certification Program, approved at the 1942 AANA meeting, was submitted to the Council on Professional Practice of the AHA. The AHA voiced reservations about what it saw as a conflict between the goal of raising the quality of service provided by nurse anesthetists and the exemption of those who were practicing. The AHA was also concerned that waiving the certification requirement for currently active members might weaken the program by including unqualified anesthetists. Finally, because the certification examination would only test theoretical knowledge, the AHA remained skeptical of the examination's ability to

test the practical skills of the candidates [21]. Some AANA members also objected to paying a fee for an examination that gave successful candidates no advantages over anesthetists who remained uncertified.

The examination program was approved at the 1944 AANA meeting, and the bylaws were amended to make successful completion of the qualifying examination a requirement for AANA membership. A Committee on Examinations was established, consisting of five members appointed by the board of trustees. The Committee's charge was to prepare a master set of questions for each examination, to prepare instructions for test-takers, and to grade the examinations [21]. The revised bylaws also established the Committee on Credentials, which replaced the Membership Committee. This new committee would accept or reject the qualifications of each applicant for the examination [21].

As 1944 drew to a close, the AANA invited 34 schools of anesthesia to participate in creating the examination. Thirty-four were selected perhaps on the basis of being better known to the educators, and perhaps because 34 was a workable number for construction of examination questions. Twenty-four schools submitted examination questions; all but two sent essay-type questions. The examination questions were drawn from these submissions. The Certification Program Committee then worked jointly with the Committee on Examinations, to prepare application forms for AANA membership, to create a transcript for each student, to refine the logistics of the program and examination, to prepare revisions of bylaws, and to develop test questions and a study outline [22].

Therefore, 12 years after it was proposed, the first qualifying examination was administered on June 4, 1945. A passing grade was a prerequisite for AANA membership, thus justifying the term "qualifying examination." This one aspect of eligibility set it apart from a state board examination or a certification examination [23].

Overseen by examination proctors chosen by the chairman of the Committee on Examinations and AANA's executive secretary, the examinees tackled the 38-page examination, which included true-false, fill-in, essay, and multiple-choice questions. There was no oral or practical component. The examination consisted of five parts: I, anatomy and physiology; II, anesthetic agents and medications; III, clinical aspects; IV, principles and techniques in administration of therapeutic cases; and V, miscellany, which included history, ethics, terminology, organization and management of an anesthesia and gas therapy department, and explosion hazards and safeguards [20, 24]. It consisted of true-false, short essay, and fill-in-the-blank questions about the uses (including those beyond anesthetic administration) of helium, carbon dioxide, nitrogen, oxygen therapy, and cyclopropane. The five content areas carried equal weight, and passing or failing the test was based on the average score [20, 24].

The grades for the first group of examinees were not revealed to them or their schools. However, after the second examination, the AANA provided percentile ranking reports to each anesthesia school [24].

Ninety-two nurse anesthetists from 39 hospitals in 28 states and Hawaii took the first examination. Eighty-nine passed with a grade of 70 % or more. One was disqualified for not having been authorized to sit for the test [24].

At last, 12 years after it was first proposed, the nurse anesthesia profession had established criteria enabling the AANA to "raise the standards of membership and the educational standards of schools of anesthesia, as well as increase the excellence of the services individual nurse anesthetists provided to patients, surgeons and society [20]." Comments from some of those taking the first examination reveal the diverse impact of this test on these new professionals [20]:

> JH, Charity Hospital, New Orleans: "We had been well prepared by our instructors at Charity Hospital, so I did not find the questions overly difficult. I did not take anesthesia lightly. I worked and studied very hard…the examination was a definite step forward."

> EC, Grace Hospital, Detroit: "I thought the examination was a good idea…Nurse anesthesia was a very hard job. I started at $250 a month and was on call every day and every other weekend…The examination was hard, too, considering the 9-month course I had taken in anesthesia. It took me all day to write it." (Note: Course length was a minimum of six months, but each program could impose a longer, but not shorter time.)

> MD, Mercy Hospital, Chicago: "That examination was so difficult that I remember thinking if I ever took another one it would be for a medical degree…Nevertheless, it was a good idea."

> BM, Grace Hospital, Detroit: "I can't recall a single question. Although the limited academic training I had received was not helpful in the examination, my hands-on experience served me well, not only on the examination but throughout the 35 years I practiced."

> AM, Charity Hospital, New Orleans: "I had just finished my anesthesia course the year before, so many of the answers to the questions were fresh in my mind…I was afraid that if I didn't pass I would lose my job."

The qualifying examination was administered subsequently in November and May, for the next 30 years. In 1976, administration of the examination was changed to June and December.

After the third administration of the qualifying examination in 1946, Adam Gilliland (d.1952), professor of psychology at Northwestern University, Evanston, IL, was appointed as an educational consultant to the AANA. Two key changes resulted from his consultation: (1) objectivity increased, because of the use of recognition-type test items rather than recall; and (2) examinees were not penalized for incorrect responses in multiple-choice test items [25].

Scoring and statistical analysis of the examination was now done by clerical workers under Gilliland's supervision.

This change hastened analysis of the results. Each program director received complete statistical reports on the performance of each graduate of the school. The reports included the name of each examinee, the percentile rank on each part of the examination, and the percentile rank on the total examination and on the General Information Test (GIT; see below). This information allowed school directors to correlate the successes of students while at the school with their performance on the qualifying examination [24].

The AANA now used percentiles to report grades on the qualifying examination. This method diminished problems resulting from questions that were too difficult or too easy, and it eliminated the differences in the grades reported by strict versus lenient examiners. The board of examiners determined the passing score for each examination in relation to the difficulty of questions and the quality of the group of applicants [26, 27].

In 1947, Gilliland suggested adding administration of a standardized general information test (GIT) to the qualifying examination, in order to establish the validity and reliability of the qualifying examinations. Since the duration for the fourth qualifying examination (November 11, 1946) had already been allotted, a short GIT was selected. Scores from this test correlated poorly with those from the fourth qualifying examination. Gilliland thought that the brevity of the GIT may have contributed to the low correlation, and at his suggestion, a longer GIT was used with the fifth qualifying examination. The correlation between the scores on the fifth examination seemed sufficiently high to serve as a fair basis for evaluating the examination [28, 29].

Next, Gilliland recommended administering the Bennett Mechanical Comprehension Test (BMCT), to determine whether a test could indicate manual skill in manipulating anesthetic equipment and in administering anesthetics. A questionnaire was sent to the director of each school of anesthesia asking for an estimate of the manual skill of each candidate from the school taking the ninth examination (May 1949). The information gathered from these questionnaires was compared with the results of the mechanical comprehension test [29, 30]. The BMCT was used with the next two examinations (November 1949 and May 1950.) Another questionnaire was sent to the directors of schools of anesthesia, asking for estimates of the manual skills of the candidates [30, 31]. It appears that the correlation with the BMTC results was insufficient, and the minutes and yearly reports do not mention the use of the BMCT after 1951.

The 1940s began a progressive increase in the number of schools of nurse anesthesia approved by the AANA (Fig. 36.3), reflecting the progressively increasing attractiveness of nurse anesthesia as a profession. The development of the examination and a certifying process could not have hurt the reputation and desirability of a career in nurse anesthesia.

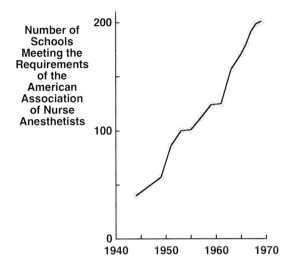

Fig. 36.3 By the 1920s, there were fewer than 20 schools training nurse anesthetists. However, starting in the 1940s, the numbers grew progressively in successive decades. Nurse anesthesia may have become increasingly attractive because of the aura of official approval conferred by the examination and certification process developed in the 1940s

The 1950s

The use of machine-scored answer sheets changed the content of the exams. Beginning with the fifth qualifying examination in May 1947, exam items were constructed to have only one possible correct answer. This allowed members of the committee to prepare a scoring key for each part. This was sent to the educational consultant, Gilliland, who oversaw the scoring and statistical analysis of the examinations. An important consideration in using machine-scored answer sheets was that effectiveness and validity of the test could be evaluated by statistical procedures that are largely inapplicable to essay tests. The machine-scored tests facilitated comparison of the scores of groups, and objective and precise evaluation of individual scores [32].

The Personnel Research Institute from Western Reserve University, developed a job description for the work of an anesthetist. This became a basis for the test outline and was used to test validity of the examination. The job description was constructed from interviews with anesthetists and observation of their work in hospitals in Cleveland and nearby Detroit and Cincinnati. An outline of major subject areas was prepared from the job description [33].

In 1951, in order to increase security of the test, testing agencies in cities throughout the country and abroad were employed. Because most of these agencies were connected to colleges and universities, the day of test administration was changed from Monday to Saturday. Candidates could now select any of the test cities, whereas previous candidates had been assigned to a test city near their place of residence [34].

In January 1952, the AANA adopted the first set of standards for accrediting schools of nurse anesthesia, and the program of accreditation went into effect. Subsequently, the standards were subjected to major and minor revisions. The compliance of schools with the standards is the basis for accreditation decisions made by the AANA Council.

Members attending the 1953 AANA annual meeting adopted an amendment that allowed experienced nurse anesthetists who did not have formal training, but were working in a recognized school of anesthesia, to take the qualifying examination after completing a specific refresher course. Only nonmembers of the AANA could take the refresher course [35]. The amendment also required that any candidate graduating from any recognized school more than five years before the date of application, had to present evidence of current clinical ability for evaluation by the credentials committee. This requirement was included so that a person who had administered only one type of anesthesia (e.g., for dentistry or obstetrics) could not qualify for membership [35].

In 1955, a bylaw was adopted in response to the misperception that membership in the AANA licensed an anesthetist to administer anesthesia. The bylaw sought to ensure compliance of all AANA members with the laws of the state in which they worked as nurse anesthetists. Through this bylaw, the AANA took thc stand that administration of anesthesia was a practice of nursing, and that all AANA members should maintain active registration as professional nurses in the state in which they worked [36].

Because each state had its own Veterans Administration policy concerning so-called "accredited schools," veterans returning from the Korean War faced problems obtaining GI benefits for training in schools of nurse anesthesia. The AANA applied to the Department of Health, Education, and Welfare (HEW) for recognition as the proper agency for accrediting these schools. On 20 November 1955, commissioner Brownell of HEW formally recognized the AANA as the accrediting agency for schools of anesthesia for nurses, thereby facilitating receipt of veterans' benefits [37].

In 1956, the initials CRNA, standing for certified registered nurse anesthetist, came into use. This title now signified to employers and the public that an individual nurse anesthetist had met the standards required for AANA membership [38].

The 1970s

From 1955, the AANA had been the recognized accrediting agency for schools of anesthesia. On August 20, 1974, the HEW Office of Education announced a change in the criteria for accreditation agencies [39]. The AANA formed a task force to assess and meet the requirements for compliance needed to successfully petition for continued recognition as the accrediting agency for nurse anesthesia educational programs. HEW mandated that 12 new criteria become part of the AANA accreditation policies and procedures. Three of the more important mandates included: (1) construction of due process mechanisms for students and faculty, including a mechanism for resolving grievances; (2) avoidance of possible conflicts of interest by separation of the decision-making body responsible for the accreditation of educational programs from the body responsible for the certification of graduates of those programs; and (3) public accountability to include representatives of the public and the community of interest in decision-making bodies, both at program and accrediting agency levels. New requirements also were imposed to ensure quality education [39].

In response to these mandates, the AANA made major revisions to its organizational structure to ensure absence of conflict of interest, autonomy in decision-making for the accreditation and certification bodies, and due process. The revisions supported the inclusion of public members of the community of interest on selected decision-making bodies [39]. The AANA acquired support for their petition from the American Nurses Association, the American College of Nurse Midwives, the Association of Operating Room Nurses, the Federation of Nursing Specialty Organizations, the National League for Nursing, and the US Public Health Service. Many individual anesthesiologists, surgeons, and hospital administrators also supported the AANA's endeavors [39].

In August of 1975, AANA members adopted a restructuring that included the formation of three councils within the corporate structure of the AANA—councils on accreditation, certification, and practice. These official groups affirmed AANA's compliance with the criteria mandated by HEW's Office of Education [40].

Autonomy of the Council on Accreditation (COA) eliminated the possible conflict of interest between the accrediting authority for educational programs, and the credentialing authority concerned with the initial certification of graduates. The Council on Certification would act independently in the initial certification of nurse anesthetists, and would be responsive to public interest. The Council on Practice would act as the appellate body for both the Council on Accreditation and the Council on Certification.

The Council on Accreditation assumed responsibility for establishing the standards and policies for nurse anesthesia educational programs, subject to consideration by its communities of interest. The standards addressed administrative policies and procedures, institutional support, curriculum and instruction, faculty, evaluation, and ethics. Thus, the COA (1) established standards, guidelines, procedures, and criteria for the accreditation of nurse anesthesia educational programs; and (2) accredited entry into nurse anesthesia practice educational programs. The Council's scope of accreditation applied to institutions and programs of nurse anesthesia at all levels of education—the post-master's degree certificate, the master's degree, and the doctoral degree [41].

Accreditation of an established program was based on self-evaluation by the program, and a site visit by a team of two or three reviewers. The process was repeated at intervals of up to 10 years, and might be supplemented by progress reports. A summary report of the review and the program's response to the report were presented to the Council for an accreditation decision. Accreditation signified that programs had completed the accreditation process successfully. Accreditation might be awarded for periods of from 2 to 10 years [41].

Responsibility for program accreditation by the AANA has been maintained without interruption since 1955. Today the Council for Higher Education Accreditation and the US Department of Education continue to recognize the Council on Accreditation as the accrediting agency of nurse anesthesia educational programs.

In September 1975, The Psychological Corporation in New York City assumed responsibility for the qualifying examination, including selection of testing centers, scoring and processing of test results, and consultation for examination development. The "bank" of examination questions remained the property of the Council on Certification, but was maintained by the testing agency.

The Council on Certification of Nurse Anesthetists (CCNA) first met on September 8–10, 1975. Over the next several years, it made several changes:

1. Candidates whose religious beliefs precluded taking an examination on a Saturday, took Sunday examinations;
2. Dates of the test administration changed to the second Saturday and Sunday in June and December;
3. New qualifying examination application forms and new transcripts were prepared;
4. The examination fee increased from $20 to $125;
5. An individual could apply for eligibility to take the qualifying examination regardless of the number of previous failures (previously, the candidate could not apply after failing three times);
6. Students enrolled in a program that had been placed on probation or had its accreditation status revoked, could apply for eligibility to take the Council's qualifying examination; but
7. Students admitted to a program that was on probation or had its accreditation status revoked, could not apply for such eligibility.

At the AANA annual meeting in 1978, the membership adopted the bylaw amendments that restructured the AANA. An independent Council on Recertification of Nurse Anesthetists (COR) was established, officially separating the AANA from the certification and recertification processes. The existing autonomous Council on Certification assumed responsibility for the initial certification of nurse anesthetists. Previously, after a graduate had passed the qualifying examination, he or she was certified, could become an AANA member, and could use the CRNA designation. No voluntary membership was available. The new bylaw separating membership from certification made voluntary membership available. An individual could be certified, and could use the CRNA designation, without becoming a member of the AANA [42].

Establishment of the Council on Recertification eliminated the need for external agencies (specifically, the US Office of Education, the Council on Postsecondary Accreditation, and the American Society of Anesthesiologists) to address the question of requiring AANA membership and recertification. Independence of the COR also allowed the AANA to increase political, economic, and government relations (lobbying) activities, and to engage a labor relations consultant to assist members and states. It separated evaluation of professional competence from association activities. It made AANA membership voluntary and no longer tied to initial certification or recertification [42].

The 1980s

On March 26–27, 1982, the "qualifying examination" became the "certification examination for nurse anesthetists," because formation of the Council on Certification eliminated the need to pass the certification examination in order to qualify for AANA membership. An individual passing the examination was certified by the Council on Certification for entry into practice, not for membership in the AANA [43].

In conjunction with the testing agency, the Council updated the nurse anesthesia examination process, and built a job-related examination. Nurse anesthesia programs had evolved from on-the-job training programs, to established hospital and university programs meeting the criteria of the Council on Accreditation for Accreditation of Nurse Anesthesia Programs Standards and Guidelines. Although differences in academic and clinical experiences existed among programs, standards and guidelines now identified the minimum requirements for nurse anesthesia educational programs.

Content validity refers to the degree to which examination content represents the area of work. A high degree of validity means that the questions on the examination accurately reflect requirements and expectations of the actual job, and that scores on the examination accurately indicate the examinee's mastery of those requirements. Content validation studies assess whether questions on an examination adequately represent a performance domain. Content validation procedures for the certification examination were documented through an analysis in 1987, and through subsequent professional practice analyses (PPAs) in 1992, 1996, 2000, 2007 and 2011 [44, 45].

For example, following the 1992 PPA, the Council revised the content outline and percentages of questions in each area to reflect current entry-level nurse anesthesia practice. These changes were justified by the consistency in the responses of the practitioners surveyed, in the major domains of knowledge and skills identified in the PPA. Knowledge was divided into five major areas related to anesthesia practice: basic sciences (30%); equipment (5%); basic principles of anesthesia (31%); advanced principles of anesthesia (30%); and professional issues (4%). The examination committee would use the new content outline to develop new questions for the certification examination as well as reclassify those currently in the repository of questions to meet the new specifications [45]. The examination content and percentages changed modestly after analysis of the results of the 2007 PPA: basic sciences (25%); equipment (10%); basic principles of anesthesia (30%); advanced principles of anesthesia (30%); and professional issues (5%) [46].

In April 1986, the Council accepted the Angoff method for "cut-score" determination, scaling, and equating of the certification examination. Psychometrically sound standards were used to set the passing score [44, 45].

Beginning with the December 1987 certification examination, scores were no longer reported as raw scores but as scaled scores. The use of a scaled score facilitated the equating of examination scores to ensure that candidates had no advantage or disadvantage based on having taken the test at a particular time [47].

In response to requirements of employers and states, that nurse anesthetists be certified in order to work, the Council implemented a certification-eligible status for applicants waiting to take the certification examination. As long as the certification-eligible status could be verified through the Council, the applicant could be employed [47].

The 1990s

The June 1990 certification examination included questions using graphs, diagrams, and electrocardiogram (ECG) strips. These questions facilitated testing of clinical knowledge and skills. The Examination Committee and the Council on Certification of Nurse Anesthetists worked collaboratively to ensure that the certification examination assessed the entry-level knowledge and skills necessary to perform the tasks identified in the on-going job analyses. Ongoing reassessment of the tasks, knowledge, and skills demanded by the test items, was a vital part of the process [44]. Graduates were increasingly pressured to pass the certification examination. States now required certification in order to be licensed as an advanced practice nurse, and Medicare required certification/recertification for reimbursement.

In 1993, suspected cheating prompted the Council to implement new policies ensuring the integrity of the certification examination:

> If the Council determines that there is reason to believe that one or more applicants have engaged in cheating or other improper behavior, or otherwise violated the security of the examination,

the Council may, at its discretion, (1) order one or more of those applications to retake the Certification Examination at a time and place to be determined by the Council, or (2) refuse to release the scores of one or more of those applications and thereby, deny their applications for certification [48].

The protection afforded by copyright was inserted into all levels of the instructions received by the candidates, forbidding the dissemination of copies of the examination by "review courses" claiming to prepare students for the examination using actual questions from the examination. The CCNA determined that all current council and committee members must sign a Work for Hire Statement, and that former examination and committee members must sign an Assignment of Copyright statement [48]. Candidates were warned that violation of the copyright not only subjected them to possible legal action but also endangered their credentialing.

In 1992, the CCNA considered changing its current paper-and-pencil test format to a computer format. The Council project manager, Karen Plaus, provided Council with information from the National League for Nursing regarding a new testing technology. It had recently been adopted by the National Council of State Board of Nursing, and was known as computer adaptive testing (CAT). CAT is based on the psychometric framework of the Item Response Theory (IRT) developed at the University of Minnesota in the 1960s. IRT is used to determine the difficulty of test questions and to estimate the ability of candidates [49]. Plaus advised Council of the advantages of this new technology – namely, more flexibility in test administration dates, the immediate availability of results, increased test security, and the possibility of self-paced administration of the test. By 1994, after meeting with experts in testing and with individuals from professional associations who used the computer for certification and licensure testing, Council began preparations for the transition [49, 50]. Implementation of CAT was approved in June 1996. Implementation required the development of educational materials for students and program directors, including three item-writing workshops and related lectures on CAT and IRT [49, 50].

Several advantages accrued from using the CAT format rather than the traditional paper-and-pencil format. The National Certification Examination (NCE) would be individualized for each candidate. The candidate would be examined individually at test administration sites, sitting at individual stations and taking the test at his or her own pace. The NCE would be offered up to four times a year, enabling a year-round test administration schedule. Candidates could schedule their own date, time, and test location. This advantage was more than simply a convenience, as many states required certification to practice. Because candidates could be promptly notified of their certification status, this flexibility accelerated their entrance into the workforce. Most important, the competence of candidates would be more accurately and fairly measured than before [49, 50].

How does CAT work? Each test is individualized and assembled interactively as the candidate is tested. Test questions are stored in a large item bank and are classified by content category and level of difficulty. After the candidate answers a question, the computer calculates an estimate of competency and chooses for the next question an item of appropriate content and difficulty. This process is repeated for each question, thus creating an examination that is both tailored to each individual's knowledge and skills, and fulfills the CCNA test plan requirements. The CAT NCE is fair to all candidates and conforms to the CCNA NCE outline content areas of basic sciences, basic and advanced principles of anesthesia, equipment, instrumentation and technology, and professional aspects. The passing score is identical for all candidates, ensuring a consistent difficulty level necessary to pass the NCE for all examinees [49].

The features for the CAT differed from those for the previous certification examination administered since 1945. (1) The test varied in length, with a minimum number of scored questions of 70 and a maximum of 140. Twenty pretest questions were not included with the minimum 70 that were scored. (2) The maximum length was three hours. (3) There were no options for review of previous answers. (4) The scores were reported as pass/fail [49].

On December 9, 1995, the last paper-and-pencil examination was administered to 820 individuals as the 102nd Certification Examination. On 15 April 1996, the first CAT was offered at the Sylvan Technology Centers. Student applicants now selected the date and location for their examination. Twice yearly administrations and the assembling of eligible candidates at university test centers on a Saturday were a thing of the past, incidentally eliminating the possibility of a cancellation due to a snowstorm.

Students and prospective employers pressured the Council to release results directly to the student upon completion of the examination. The Council rejected this request for three reasons. (1) The test agency first needed to verify all test results. (2) Each applicant needed to confirm that all criteria for certification criteria had been met. (3) Test center security required verification that the computer functioned properly, that the integrity of the data was maintained, and that the test session occurred under controlled conditions.

A New Century Arrives

By the twenty-first century, computer use affected most aspects of daily living. Every student had a computer, and nurse anesthesia programs placed many of their internal documents on such devices. Accordingly, the Council sought to make most documents available to students and program directors via the Web, including portable document format (pdf) files for transcript forms and examination information. By 2003, 55 % of all CCNA candidates registered on-line.

By 2004, all CCNA forms, including the official CCNA transcript and candidate handbook, were available as interactive pdf files.

The new systems for examination came none too soon. With the arrival of the new millennium, the popularity of nurse anesthesia as a profession continued to increase, with the number of graduates and clinical sites more than doubling in the years 2000 to 2009 (Fig. 36.4).

The Test Today

AANA bylaws originally stated that the examination should include written, oral, and practical portions. According to Thatcher, the difficulty of conducting more than a written examination led to the elimination of the oral and practical portions of the examination [6, 51], leaving only the written examination.

From its inception in 1945 to 2012, 68,784 students have taken the certification examination. The test evolved from a five-part, 38-page paper-and-pencil examination that used true-false, fill-in, essay, and multiple-choice questions, to a streamlined computer-format test having a maximum of 140 questions. The evolution resulted from concerns regarding the adequacy of the test instrument, and the equality and fairness of its application to all candidates.

Today diverse test designs, such as multiple correct responses, calculation, "drag-and-drop" and "hotspot" questions, enable a better test of issues difficult to pose in the traditional multiple-choice question format. Candidates now receive a preliminary pass/fail report as they leave the test center. This preliminary report is validated, and the National Board of Certification and Recertification for Nurse Anesthetists (NBCRNA) sends the official results within 2 to 4 weeks after the test (as opposed to the 3 months after the old paper-and-pencil test). Applicants now select the day, the time of examination, and the test site location. They register online. Some students say that one of the greatest benefits is that they are able to join the ranks of the employed more quickly.

What About the Future?

The NBCRNA continues to consider the use of simulation and other testing modalities. Looking into the future, by 2025, doctoral education for nurse anesthetists will become a requirement for entry into nurse anesthesia practice. With today's changing healthcare environment, providers must continue to expand their knowledge and skills. To position nurse anesthetists to meet this ongoing challenge, the AANA and NBCRNA support doctoral education as one way to incorporate technological and pharmaceutical advances, informatics, evidence-based practice, systems approaches to quality

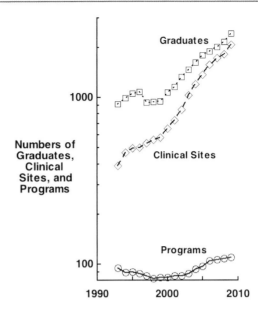

Fig. 36.4 The number of nurse anesthetist graduates and clinical sites for training more than doubled in the first decade of the new millennium. Computerization of examinations facilitated such rapid growth. (Data courtesy of the American Association of Nurse Anesthetists.)

improvement, healthcare business models, teamwork, and public relations. These are all subjects that will shape the future for anesthesia providers and their patients [52].

In 2011, the NBCRNA introduced the Continued Professional Certification (CPC) program that embraces lifelong learning for nurse anesthetists. Following initial certification, each nurse anesthetist will be required to complete continuing education and core competency modules every four years. A recertification examination is required every eight years.

References

1. Garde J. The nurse anesthesia profession: A past, present, and future perspective. Nurs Clin North Am. 1996;31:567–80.
2. Bankert M: Watchful Care: A History of America's Nurse Anesthetists. New York, Continuum, 1989, pp 1–58.
3. [Historical vignette] Nurse anesthetists. The dawn of a specialty. Milestones in Anesthesia. 1993;2:10–1.
4. Magaw A: Observations on 1092 cases of anesthesia from Jan. 1, 1899 to Jan.1, 1900. St. Paul Medical Journal 1900;2:306–11.
5. Magaw A. A review of over fourteen thousand surgical anesthesias. Surg Gynecol Obstet. 1906;3:795–6.
6. Thatcher V: History of Anesthesia with Emphasis on the Nurse Specialist. Philadelphia, J. B. Lippincott, 1953, pp 1–78.
7. [Historical vignette] Nurse anesthetists. The dawn of a specialty, part II. Milestones in Anesthesia. 1993;3:10–1.
8. O'Day E: Notes on the History and Organization of the American Association of Nurse Anesthetists. Planning Committee. Chicago, IL, American Association of Nurse Anesthetists, 1969, pp 1–74.
9. Fife G. Address of the president. Bull Natl Assoc Nurse Anesth. 1933;1:15–8.
10. Fife G. Address of the president. Bull Natl Assoc Nurse Anesth. 1935;3:5–7.

11. Salomon H. President's report. Bull Natl Assoc Nurse Anesth. 1936;4:185–7.
12. Lamb H. Report of the Educational Committee, National Association of Nurse Anesthetists. Bull Natl Assoc Nurse Anesth. 1936;4:190–1.
13. Lamb H. Report of the Educational Committee, National Association of Nurse Anesthetists. Bull Natl Assoc Nurse Anesth. 1938;6:199–200.
14. Lamb H. Report of the Educational Committee, National Association of Nurse Anesthetists. Bull Natl Assoc Nurse Anesth. 1939;7:266–7.
15. By-laws. National Association of Nurse Anesthetists. Bull Natl Assoc Nurse Anesth 1939;7:273–88.
16. Shupp M. President's report. Bull Natl Assoc Nurse Anesth. 1940;8:238–42.
17. Lamb H. Report of the president. Bull Natl Assoc Nurse Anesth. 1941;9:284–7.
18. Hodgins A. Report of Committee on Education. Bull Natl Assoc Nurse Anesth. 1941;9:297–8.
19. Amendments to the AANA by-laws. American Association of Nurse Anesthetists. Bull Natl Assoc Nurse Anesth. 1941;9:260.
20. Caulk S: 1st Qualifying Examination. A Developmental Historical Perspective of the Qualifying Examination First Administered in 1945. Park Ridge, IL, American Association of Nurse Anesthetists, 1994.
21. Shupp M. Report of the Certification Program Committee. Bull Natl Assoc Nurse Anesth. 1943;11:259–60.
22. Lamb H. Report of the Committee on Education. Bull Natl Assoc Nurse Anesth. 1944;12:254–5.
23. Campbell A: Second examination program scheduled for November: Membership requirements explained. Bull Natl Assoc Nurse Anesth 1945;13:35–7.
24. Shupp M. Annual report of the Committee on Examinations. J Am Assoc Nurse Anesth. 1946;5:52–4.
25. Shupp M: Minutes. Committee on Examinations. Chicago, IL, American Association of Nurse Anesthetists, June 9, 1946.
26. Shupp M. Report on qualifying examinations. J Am Assoc Nurse Anesth February. 1947;1:35–40.
27. Gilliland A: Percentile scores as a method of reporting grades. Bull Natl Assoc Nurse Anesth 1947;1:2.
28. McMahon J: Report. Committee on Examinations to the Board of Trustees. Chicago, IL, American Association of Nurse Anesthetists, February 11, 1947.
29. Gilliland A. Testing and general information tests. J Am Assoc Nurse Anesth. 1947;1:22–34.
30. McMahon J: Annual Report. Examination Committee. Chicago, IL, American Association of Nurse Anesthetists, September 1950.
31. McMahon J. Examination Committee report. Bull Natl Assoc Nurse Anesth. 1949;3:10.
32. Letter to F. McQuillen [executive director, American Association of Nurse Anesthetists, Chicago, IL], from the Professional Examination Service [New York, NY], November 8, 1951.
33. McMahon J: Annual Report of the Examination Committee. Bull Natl Assoc Nurse Anesth 1950;4:7.
34. McMahon J. Annual Report of the Examination Committee. Bull Natl Assoc Nurse Anesth. 1951;5:10–2.
35. Annual reports. Bull Natl Assoc Nurse Anesth 1953;7:1–10.
36. Vote to adopt revisions to by-laws. Bull Natl Assoc Nurse Anesth 1955;9:14.
37. Report of officers and committee chairmen of the American Association of Nurse Anesthetists. Bull Natl Assoc Nurse Anesth 1956;10:44–50.
38. Director emeritus report. Bull Natl Assoc Nurse Anesth 1970;24:15–16.
39. Gunn I. Annual report of the project director. Bull Natl Assoc Nurse Anesth. 1975;29:20–2.
40. Fevold N. Annual report of the acting executive director. Bull Natl Assoc Nurse Anesth. 1976;30:12–3.
41. Foster SC, Faut-Callahan M: A professional study and resource guide for the CRNA. Park Ridge, IL, AANA Publishing Inc., 2001, pp 51–2.
42. Caulk R. Annual report of the president 1977–1978. Bull Natl Assoc Nurse Anesth. 1978;32:28–32.
43. Minutes. Council on Certification of Nurse Anesthetists, American Association of Nurse Anesthetists. Park Ridge, IL, American Association of Nurse Anesthetists, March 26–27, 1982.
44. Zaglaniczny K: [Guest editorial] Development of the current certification examination. J Am Assoc Nurse Anesth. 1990;58:1;5–7.
45. Zaglaniczny K. Council on Certification Professional Practice Analysis. Council on Certification. J Am Assoc Nurse Anesth. 1993;61:241–55.
46. Muckle T. A report on the CCNA 2007 Professional Practice Analysis. A guest editorial. J Am Assoc Nurse Anesth. 2009;77:181–9.
47. Minutes. Council on Certification of Nurse Anesthetists, American Association of Nurse Anesthetists. Park Ridge, IL, American Association of Nurse Anesthetists, April 4–5, 1987.
48. Annual Council Reports. Bull Natl Assoc Nurse Anesth 1993;47:15.
49. Bergstrom B. Computerized adaptive testing for the National Certification Examination. Computer Adaptive Technologies, Inc. Bull Natl Assoc Nurse Anesth. 1996;50:119–24.
50. Zaglaniczny K. [Guest editorial] The transition of the National Certification Examination from paper and pencil to computer adaptive testing. J Am Assoc Nurse Anesth. 1996;64:9–14.
51. Shupp M: 2nd Annual Report, Committee on Examinations. Chicago, IL, American Association of Nurse Anesthetists, September 27, 1946.
52. Press release. Park Ridge, IL, American Association of Nurse Anesthetists, September 20, 2007.

The Development of Education in Anesthesia in the United States

Manuel Pardo

Summary

In 1850, four years after Morton's demonstration, Surgeon Warren described adequate anesthesia care: Have a dedicated person continuously deliver anesthesia to a fasting supine patient; administer anesthesia sufficient to produce relaxation; beware of obstructing breathing; and don't set fire to the operating room. Between 1847 and 1858, Snow documented how to safely give and assess ether and chloroform anesthesia. From 1860 to 1900, no formal training programs in anesthesiology existed. Surgeons, interns, medical students, nurses, and orderlies gave anesthetics. In 1916, surgeon Gatch, President of the American Association of Anesthetists, advocated training medical students and interns in anesthesia. In the 1910s–1920s, a few physician anesthetists, such as Botsford and Herb, established teaching programs.

In 1927, Ralph Waters became chairman of the world's first academic department of anesthesia. He created a 3-year post-graduate residency program: 2 years of clinical training and 1 of research. Because his graduating residents served as leaders, his vision for academic anesthesia influenced the country and world.

The American Board of Anesthesiology (ABA) conducted its first written examination in 1939. Three years of post-graduate training, 3 years in practice, and passage of written, oral, and practical examinations were required to become diplomates.

During World War II (1941–1945), many physicians were drafted into anesthesia after a few months of training. Finding that they liked what they were asked to do, along with improved remuneration, they found anesthesiology to be attractive. The number of US anesthesia residency programs grew five-fold in the decade after the war, and the number of residents increased.

In 1945, the American Society of Anesthesiologists created a "Committee on Postgraduate Education." A half decade later, the Committee recommended at least 2 years in residency training, increasing to 3 years (plus internship) in 1984. Created in 1972, the Liaison Committee on Graduate Medical Education began formal accreditation of graduate medical education programs in 1975, after reviewing the recommendations of individual Residency Review Committees.

Believing that an organization of teachers could improve education in anesthesia, junior anesthesia faculty in the US founded the Society for Education in Anesthesia (SEA) in the early 1980s. From the late 1990s to 2010, training and recertification with computerized simulators grew rapidly despite limited evidence of sustained efficacy. Since the 1990s, the most notable changes in anesthesia education have been the increase in specialty operating room experiences and non-operating room clinical experiences. In 2000, the ABA established time limited certification.

The Early Nineteenth Century

The US had four medical schools in 1800: University of Pennsylvania, Harvard University, Dartmouth College, and King's College (subsequently Columbia University). Twenty-six more schools were added by 1840. The curriculum typically occupied two four-month blocks, covering seven courses: anatomy; physiology and pathology; materia medica, therapeutics and pharmacy; chemistry and medical jurisprudence; theory and practice of medicine; principles and practice of surgery; and obstetrics and diseases of women and children [1]. Six to eight hours of didactic lectures occupied each day, lectures focused on practical rather than scientific concerns. Few effective therapies were available.

This mid-nineteenth century medical education had many deficiencies. Except for a few schools teaching anatomy with dissection, none offered laboratory instruction. Students were generally illiterate (even at Harvard), and few had a college degree. A brief and informal oral examination

M. Pardo (✉)
Department of Anesthesia and Perioperative Care, UCSF,
513 Parnassus, San Francisco, CA 94143–0427, USA
e-mail: pardom@anesthesia.ucsf.edu

E. I Eger II et al. (eds.), *The Wondrous Story of Anesthesia,* DOI 10.1007/978-1-4614-8441-7_37, © Edmond I Eger, MD 2014

qualified the student for graduation; there was no written examination. The medical school diploma was the sole document required to practice medicine; no state or national licensing procedures existed. Most medical schools were independent, "proprietary" institutions without any affiliation with a hospital or university. Most existed to make money, and the ability to pay entrance fees was the major criteria for admission.

Some physicians supplemented their training with apprenticeships, but the quality of instruction was generally poor, and many apprentices merely performed household chores. Nonetheless, starting in the early 1800s, the "house pupil" experience became an increasingly popular feature of American medical education. A few physicians or medical students spent a year in a hospital, rotating through all the hospital wards, helping staff physicians provide bedside care of patients. The terms "house pupil," "intern," and "resident" were used to describe these postings. The increasing number of surgeries performed after the introduction of anesthesia in 1846, significantly enlarged the work of the house pupil.

At this time, European medical training was considered the finest in the world. In the first half of the nineteenth century, Americans who could afford it chose Paris as a place for postgraduate medical study. What was special about French medicine at this time? French clinicians developed many approaches that became widely accepted, including modern approaches to pathology, physical diagnosis, and the use of statistics in clinical research. They placed the hospital at the center of medical teaching and research [1]. Their strength was astute clinical observation, eschewing speculative theories such as humorism that had crippled medicine. According to humorism, the human body was composed of four humors: black bile, yellow bile, phlegm, and blood. In health, the humors were balanced. Deficiency or excess of one of the humors explained all disease. Treatment could include bleeding (to reduce a surplus of blood) or applying a hot cup to a patient's skin, called "cupping" (to reduce a surplus of bile). French clinicians of this era did have a weakness: a distrust of experimental laboratory investigation [1]. By the mid-nineteenth century, German medical scientists had embraced experimental methods and subsequently made major discoveries such as cell theory, which eventually ended humorism's grasp on medical thinking. In the second half of the nineteenth century, Americans desiring additional medical training began to choose Germany instead of France, because of strengths in new clinical subspecialties (such as dermatology, ophthalmology, laryngology) as well as in the laboratory.

Good Advice

At the Massachusetts General Hospital, on 16 October 1846, William Morton publically demonstrated the capacity of diethyl ether to provide surgical anesthesia. John Warren presided as the operating surgeon. Four years later, Warren addressed the American Medical Association, reviewing the progress of surgery during the previous fifty years with a particular focus on how to administer ether safely [2].

"…I am in constant apprehension of some serious occurrence; and I would therefore venture to give a solemn warning to all surgeons who may have an occasion to use ether, not to omit any possible attention calculated to prevent a mischievous or dangerous accident. Our mode of application for the Hospital is very simple. First, The patient is not allowed to eat freely within three of four hours before an operation. Second, He is placed, if possible, in the horizontal posture. Third, If the operation is to be bloodless, the patient should be bled from the arm before it begins. Fourth, The pulse, respiration, and countenance should be carefully watched by an assistant, whose special duty it is to perform this office. Fifth, A large sponge, of a conical form, is filled with ether, and applied over the nostrils of the patient, but not in such a way as to prevent him from getting a quantity of atmospheric air into the lungs. Sixth, The application should not be too severely pressed upon the patient; and, if he coughs or exhibits symptoms of distress, the sponge should be raised for a moment, and then re-applied. Seventh, A perfect relaxation of the muscles is the test of full etherization, such as is required in every important surgical operation. Eighth, We generally continue the ether, with slight intermissions, till the operation is terminated, unless there is some reason for the contrary practice. Ninth, We avoid approaching the patient, during the administration of ether, with a light, the actual cautery, or any thing capable of setting fire to the vaporized ether."

Sensible observations: Have a dedicated person continuously deliver anesthesia to a fasting supine patient. Administer anesthesia sufficient to produce relaxation (no movement?). Beware of obstructing breathing; and don't set fire to the operating room. Education for the budding anesthetist.

1847–1858

John Snow, the first and arguably the greatest anesthesiologist, witnessed the use of ether for dental extraction in London on 28 December 1846 [3]. Over the next nine months, he designed a vaporizer that stabilized the temperature of the liquid ether and thus delivered a near constant (albeit high) concentration that he could crudely dilute by admitting more or less air to the inspired mixture. He developed an active ether administration practice, and published a monograph, *On the Inhalation of the Vapour of Ether in Surgical Operations,* that served as a comprehensive guide to the clinical use of ether anesthesia. In particular he described the "degrees" of anesthesia, a prerequisite to the control of the extent of anesthesia. He next applied his technical, clinical and educational skills to chloroform [4]. Reference works such as these were rare. The medical world learned the latest medical events through lectures, medical society meetings, journals, and newspapers.

1860–1900

Formal training programs in anesthesiology did not exist in the nineteenth century. Personnel with little or no experience, including medical students, interns, and ward nurses provided anesthesia. Occasional editorials in medical journals advocated teaching anesthesia to medical students. In 1900, one such editorial in *The Lancet* [5] noted that "Since the examining bodies apparently think little of the importance of the administration of anaesthetics, the medical schools, which naturally take their cue from these bodies, cannot insist upon much attention to the subject." The editorial mused on the importance of that omission: "A student may attend all the lectures available and read all the books, but until he has himself given an anaesthetic he can never become a safe anaesthetist." An understatement, indeed.

A 1900 editorial in The Philadelphia Medical Journal remarked [6]:

> "The faculties of our medical schools should recognize the tremendous responsibility of the anesthetist and the fact that all graduates are likely to be called upon to use anesthetics and in most cases quite frequently. Lack of knowledge or skill may jeopardize the patient's life and frustrate the surgeon's skillful endeavors. The facilities for teaching this subject should be increased; it should be made compulsory and the opportunity for hospital training should be given. In this way the students of the future will graduate much better equipped in a very important requisite than their predecessors have been."

Because medical schools did not attend to the training of anesthetists, the door was open for nurses to fill the gap. Indeed, at the Mayo Clinic in Rochester, Minnesota, surgeons William (1861–1939) and Charles Mayo (1865–1939) "decided that a nurse was better suited to the task because she was more likely to keep her mind strictly on it, whereas the intern was naturally more interested in what the surgeon was doing [7]." Edith (1871–1943) and Dinah Graham (1860–1947) became the first nurse anesthetists at the Mayo clinic. Their successor, Alice Magaw (1860–1928) is regarded as the most famous nurse anesthetist of the nineteenth century. Surgeons sent nurses to observe her practice and learn what they could.

1910: The Flexner Report

The American Medical Association (AMA) was founded in 1847, and in 1904, the Association formed the Council on Medical Education. Although the AMA was a practitioner-based organization, academic physicians advocating higher educational standards dominated the council [1]. In 1906, the council surveyed US medical schools, but never published the unflattering results of the survey, thinking it politically unwise for a medical organization dominated by practitioners to publicly criticize the nation's medical schools. Instead, the council invited the Carnegie Foundation for the Advancement of Teaching, to survey US medical schools. Abraham Flexner (1866–1959), an obscure educator at the Carnegie Foundation, led this survey. From 1908 to 1910, he visited every medical school in the US and Canada. His famous and widely distributed 1910 report, *Medical Education in the United States and Canada*, described the shortcomings of North American medical education compared to European education [8]. Describing each school's laboratory and clinical facilities, Flexner's observations were vivid and often critical. For example, he remarked on the laboratory facilities of the Kansas Medical College in Topeka:

> "The school occupies a three-story building, on the upper floor of which there have been improvised laboratories for pathology and bacteriology. They contain the necessary equipment for routine teaching, but are poorly kept…The dissecting-room is indescribably filthy; it contained, in addition to the necessary tables, a single, badly hacked cadaver, and was simultaneously used as a chicken yard."

The descriptions of individual facilities made for interesting reading—unless your school was criticized. The report contained much more than gaudy descriptions. Flexner first discussed principles underlying modern medical education. He then provided a detailed description of entrance requirements, attendance, teaching staff, resources for maintenance, laboratory facilities and clinical facilities available in each medical school. He advanced several tenets essential to medical education: 1) the medical student should be prepared by at least two years of college, including coursework in biology, chemistry and physics; 2) scientists rather than practitioners should teach basic sciences; 3) research should play a central role in the medical school; 4) medical schools needed financial resources to decrease their dependence on student fees; and 5) the schools needed ready access to hospitals for teaching purposes. While European schools possessed many of these elements, few American schools did. To Flexner, the model system of medical education was Johns Hopkins Medical School, and his report extolled its virtues repeatedly [8]. The Flexner report changed medical education over the next 10 years, leading to elimination of approximately one-third of US medical schools.

World War I (1914–1918)

There were few developments in anesthesia education during World War I. One outstanding example was Arthur Guedel (1883–1956), who served as an anesthesiologist with the

American Expeditionary Forces in France [9]. Because he was the only anesthesiologist in the region, he had to quickly train nurses, orderlies, and others to administer ether. Based on his observations from a decade of anesthesia practice, Guedel developed a chart describing stages of ether anesthesia based on patterns of respiration and the appearance of the patient's eyes (see Fig. 39.2). His trainees used this chart as they worked independently. Guedel was known for visiting his trainees at various hospitals using a motorcycle to navigate the muddy battlefields. This earned him the moniker "the motorcycle anesthetist of World War I." After the war, Guedel published the chart, which became widely used. Many modern anesthesia textbooks reproduced the chart as an example of the utility of clinical observations in evaluating depth of anesthesia.

1916

Although anesthesia continued to be taught in an unstructured manner, seeds of change had been sown. Anesthesia organizations in the US, including the American Association of Anesthetists, the predecessor to the American Society of Anesthesiologists (ASA), gained footing. In 1916, Willis Gatch, Professor of Surgery at the University of Indiana Medical Department, was elected president of the American Association of Anesthetists. In his presidential address, "Instruction of Medical Students and Hospital Internes [sic] in Anesthesia [10]" he remarked that

> "Nothing can do more to improve your standing as specialists than to educate physicians generally in this subject, and the best place to begin this course of instruction is with the medical student. Unless our leading medical schools give instruction in anesthesia not described in their catalogues, the training of students in this subject must be either entirely lacking or very inadequate…I am convinced that in most of our medical schools the student receives practically no instruction in anesthesia and that the instruction therein of internes [sic] in our hospitals is usually haphazard and frequently resented by its recipients." In his plan for supervision of interns, Gatch proposed "… that the duties of the anesthetist should not be limited to the actual conduct of the anesthesia, but should cover also the preliminary examination and preparation of the patient and his immediate post operative care."

1920

Gatch's address may have prompted the American Association of Anesthetists to form a committee to investigate the teaching of anesthesia in medical schools, and to develop plans for advancing anesthesia teaching and establishing a standard approach to training hospital interns in anesthesia. Isabella Herb (1863–1943), was on the committee, as one of the few individuals in the US with an academic appointment

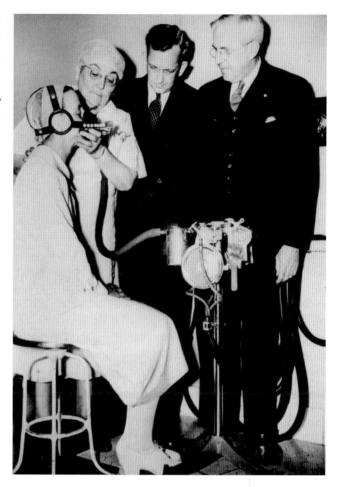

Fig. 37.1 Isabella Herb administers ethylene anesthesia while the discoverers of ethylene as an anesthetic, J. Bailey Carter and Arno Luckhardt, observe. (From [12]. Photo provided by Dr. John B. Stetson. Reprinted with permission)

in anesthesia. She was Assistant Professor of Surgery (Anesthetics) at Rush Medical College, and Chief Anesthetist at Presbyterian Hospital in Chicago (Fig. 37.1). Herb presented her teaching method at the annual meeting of the Interstate Association of Anesthetists, held in October 1920 in Pittsburgh, PA: "Anesthesia in Relation to Medical Schools and Hospitals [11]." She noted that "instruction in the art and practice of anesthesia is altogether absent from the curriculum of the majority of medical schools, or totally or inadequately dealt with…Nothing can improve the status of anesthesia, or bring about the proper recognition of anesthetics as a specialty, as the education of physicians and surgeons generally in this branch of medicine, and the proper place to begin instruction is in the medical schools when, true to the Arabian proverb 'A man knows not and knows that he knows not.'" Herb outlined her approach for teaching medical students at Rush Medical College and the Presbyterian Hospital in Chicago. Physiology, and the chemistry and pharmacology of anesthetic agents were taught during the first two years of medical school. During the senior year, a required didactic course in anesthetics was given, along with demonstrations and supervised administration of anesthesia. Her course topics resembled many of those that might be taught today. She began with the history of anesthesia and ended with legal matters. Between these bookends, she discussed the pharmacology of and the basis for the selection of the then used anesthetics (e.g., ether, chloroform, nitrous oxide). She continued with descriptions of the implications of patient pathophysiology, premedication with alkaloids, optimum patient position, resuscitation, how to deal with untoward events, and pulmonary complications following anesthesia.

Regarding interns and their training, she only admitted graduates of Rush Medical College, who thus had the anesthetic training outlined above. They became preceptees, with gradually increasing responsibilities. Herb noted "it is an exceedingly rare thing to find an interne [sic] who is not interested in this phase of his hospital work, in fact there is frequently considerable rivalry, in the desire to be considered the best anesthetist among the internes [11]."

Herb was among the first women physicians to specialize in anesthesia [12]. Beginning in 1899, she served as the first "physician anesthetist" at the Mayo Clinic in Rochester, working directly with Charles Mayo. Until that time, the Mayo Clinic used nurses or surgical residents to administer anesthesia. Herb also served as a pathologist at Mayo Clinic, in charge of the Section on Pathology. She left in 1904 for further study in Europe, and then returned to Chicago a year later to perform infectious disease research. In 1909, she became the chief anesthetist at Presbyterian Hospital in Chicago, a position she held until her retirement in 1941. She had a distinguished anesthesia career, reaching the rank of Professor of Surgery (Anesthesia) at Rush Medical College, and serving in many leadership positions in the specialty. She was the tenth president of the American Association of Anesthetists.

Mary Botsford (1865–1939) was another woman physician who specialized in anesthesia. Just as Herb was the first physician anesthetist at the Mayo Clinic, Botsford was the first physician anesthetist at the University of California Medical School in San Francisco, appointed in 1910 [13]. Botsford's anesthesia skills were self-taught, and Botsford herself was a charismatic and inspiring teacher. She educated women physicians, and many became interested in anesthesia practice. Indeed, in Botsford's time, the group of physician anesthetists at the University of California was composed entirely of women, reaching a peak of five from 1921 to 1928.

1921–1930

The 1910 Flexner report focused on medical student education because the prevailing view held that four years of medical school provided adequate preparation for the practice of medicine. That view changed as medical practice evolved

in the years after World War I. Long available but few in number, internships had no consistent format. An increasing recognition of the importance of post-graduate training prompted growth in the number of internship positions and the development of common internship structures, including the addition of formal didactic elements such as conferences, teaching rounds and lectures. The AMA Council on Medical Education, which had underwritten the Flexner report, and subsequently examined and approved medical schools, now extended this role to internships [14]. Reflecting the importance of the hospital setting to the internship, the council changed its name to "Council on Medical Education and Hospitals." While many internships lasted one year, others lasted two or even three years. Inconsistency in the internship experience was common, as interns were a source of service to the hospital as much as they were trainees learning to care for patients. Also, there was disagreement amongst medical educators about the role of the internship; some thought of internship as the end of medical school whereas others believed it was the start of post-graduate training. The AMA Council authorized three internship structures: rotating, straight, and mixed [15]. The rotating internship, considered the best overall training, allowed experience in the major specialties of medicine, surgery, obstetrics, and pediatrics, as well as some training in anesthesiology, radiology, and pathology. The straight internship, consisting of experience in only one major clinical area (e.g., medicine, surgery, pediatrics, radiology, or pathology), was considered more limited in scope, but was typically conducted in medical school teaching hospitals with increased access to educational activities [15]. The mixed internship offered experience in more than one clinical area, but in fewer disciplines than the rotating internship.

The term "residency" denoted training after the internship in a specific field of medicine. At that time, the residency was for the elite trainee, and programs only accepted the best students and interns [14]. Most had a pyramid structure, with more junior residents than senior residents, and only one achieving the position of "chief resident". In 1927, the list of hospitals with residency programs, under the AMA Council on Medical Education and Hospitals, contained 270 hospitals and 1699 residency positions. Of those, 15 hospitals offered anesthesia programs, with 19 residency positions in total [16].

1927—Waters Comes to Madison

In 1927, Ralph Waters joined the University of Wisconsin as the chairman of the world's first department of anesthesia. He sought to create an academic department that had four pillars: optimum patient care, education of medical students and interns, post-graduate education, and research into the scientific foundations of anesthesia [17]. While Herb and Botsford's programs taught medical students and interns, there was no provision for extended post-graduate anesthesia education in a university setting. Waters created a 3-year post-graduate residency program, with the first and third years dedicated to clinical training, and the second year to laboratory research. Reflecting on his career, Waters wrote:

"When I quit Kansas City to come here I had one idea in mind. That was that Anesthesia's great need was recognition by, and teaching in medical schools so that all M.D.'s would know what every doctor ought to know about it. So the residencies here came to be at least three years in duration…. [18]"

The choice of three years as the duration of his anesthesia residency may have reflected the duration of other specialty training. In 1923, three years of graduate medical education was required in general surgery, orthopedic surgery, obstetrics and gynecology, pediatrics, medicine, and neuropsychiatry. Specialties requiring only two years of graduate medical education at that time included ophthalmology, otolaryngology, and dermatology.

Waters started twice weekly departmental meetings: one reviewed the week's cases (at first such sessions were called M&M or Morbidity and Mortality Conferences; later they became more elaborate, morphing into Grand Rounds), and another reviewed current medical literature. Resident responsibilities included patient care, research, literature reviews, and teaching and supervision of medical students and interns. Waters acted to expand his vision for academic anesthesia across the country, expecting his graduating residents to serve as leaders. In a letter to Lincoln Sise (anesthesiologist at the Lahey Clinic in Boston), he wrote "my ambition is for the men who spend some time with me here to get eventually in teaching positions in other universities because I think that is the only way we can hope to improve the specialty in the future. It has therefore been a disappointment to me each time that one of my boys has gone to private practice [19]." Several of his graduates, and in turn, graduates of their programs, established most of North America's academic programs using Waters' approach. These included Emery Rovenstine, Robert Dripps, Stuart Cullen, and Emanuel Papper, each of whom spawned academic anesthesiologists and chairs. The University of Wisconsin residency program also served as a model for early programs in the United Kingdom and Canada [20].

1930–1940s

1937—Rovenstine's Address

Rovenstine's 1937 presidential address to the Associated Anesthetists of the US and Canada was titled "Anesthesia:

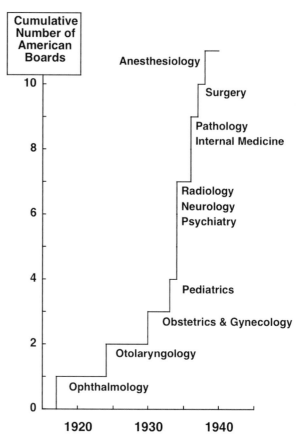

Fig. 37.2 Formation of many of the major examining boards took place in the 1930s, culminating with the formation of the American Board of Anesthesiology in 1938

Organization for Teaching." He advocated elements underlying contemporary anesthesia training programs, namely supervised clinical instruction in the operating room, didactic sessions, anatomy laboratory teaching for regional anesthesia, case conferences to review results and complications, and discussions of the current anesthesia literature. Further, he argued that "A teaching institution will not fulfill the spirit of service by the mere dissemination of knowledge but must accept as an integral part of its assignment, the accumulation of new knowledge…The attention of those responsible for postgraduate instruction must also be directed toward the preparation of students for teaching, administration, and organization."

1938–1939

Specialty board organizations demanded increased standardization in specialty training in the 1930s. The American Board of Ophthalmology and the American Board of Otolaryngology, were founded in 1917 and 1924, respectively. Several additional boards followed in the 1930s (Fig. 37.2) [14]. The American Board of Anesthesiology was established in 1938 as a board subordinate to the American Board

Table 37.1 Sample essay questions in the first written examination of the American Board of Anesthesiology, March 1939. (From [23], with permission)

Field	Essay question
Pharmacology	Define the term "secondary saturation" and give your opinion of its importance in the administration of nitrous oxide
Anatomy	Describe a method for producing block anesthesia for a surgical procedure involving a bunion
Physics and Chemistry	What safeguards do you advise against the hazard of explosion when inflammable anesthetic agents are being employed?
Pathology	If you had a patient suffering from marked cirrhosis of the liver and an intra-abdominal operation were necessary, what anesthetic agents would you avoid for this patient?
Physiology	Outline the protective mechanism which is called into place when acute hemorrhage occurs

of Surgery, becoming an independent board in 1939. An umbrella organization, the Advisory Board for Medical Specialties guided these specialty boards.

The boards required at least three years of post-graduate training, a few years in practice, and the successful completion of an examination (written, oral, and practical) to achieve diplomate status. Thus, while medical schools and teaching hospitals controlled the undergraduate educational experience, the professions themselves greatly influenced graduate medical education. In 1937, the Advisory Board for Medical Specialties created the Commission on Graduate Medical Education, with a mandate to "formulate the educational problems and principles involved in the continuation of medical training for a period of years after graduation and the adequate training of specialists, and to make recommendations for methods whereby those in practice, general and limited, may keep abreast of new developments in diagnosis, treatment and prevention [21]." The distinguished composition of the commission (albeit without a single anesthesiologist) strengthened the influence of its report. The report summarized what it believed were the basic principles of a residency:

"1. The residency should be the most satisfactory method of graduate training for specialized fields of practice.
2. The residency should be organized as a real educational experience provided by qualified teachers who are willing to assume responsibility for adequate instruction.
3. The residency should provide preparation in the sciences basic to the specialty as well as sufficient clinical experience, under supervision, to ensure real competence.
4. The residency should be a joint responsibility of medical schools and of those hospitals able to provide residencies of a satisfactory educational character [21]."

In 1939, 30 approved anesthesia residency programs in the US trained a total of 58 residents [22]. The American Board of Anesthesiology's 1937 Booklet of Information specified a requirement for three years of training after internship (like the other specialty boards), but this did not become mandatory until 1986. Eligibility for board certification also included a four-year period of practice limited to anesthesiology.

The first written examination conducted by the American Board of Anesthesiology, took place on 28 March 1939 [23]. It consisted of sections on pharmacology, anatomy, physics and chemistry, pathology, and physiology. Each section contained five essay questions, and the candidate selected three questions to answer (Table 37.1). Three directors of the American Board of Anesthesiology graded each examination, but the logistics of grading would grow in proportion to the number of candidates and the practicalities of duplicating and tracking the essays. The large number of post-World War II military anesthesiologists seeking ABA certification put an end to the essay examination, and the 1948 written examination changed from an essay to 125 multiple choice questions [24].

1941–1957

World War II changed attitudes toward medical specialization. Military physicians with specialty training received increased recognition, compensation, and responsibility. Anesthesiology in particular, benefited from the urgent need to enlarge the then small pool of anesthesiologists, to manage great numbers of casualties. A "crash" program to train many anesthesiologists (and non-physicians) resulted. Stevens Martin conducted the first armed forces anesthesiology didactic courses. These were offered to officers of station or general hospitals, officers of evacuation hospitals, and enlisted men of the Medical Corps on mobile auxiliary surgical teams [25]. The brief courses led students through the requisite basic sciences, anesthetic techniques and recognition of the stages of anesthesia (after all, they would be using ether!), how to recognize and treat cardiorespiratory complications, and the avoidance of fires and explosions (ether, again). The nitty-gritty of everyday anesthesia.

Daily lectures were given for 2–6 weeks, complemented by demonstrations of techniques, and practical instruction given as a preceptorship. Trainees were given unstructured assignments to an operative schedule, and were to undertake preoperative and postoperative rounds. Those assigned to evacuation hospitals learned techniques in inhalation anesthesia, intravenous anesthesia, some regional anesthesia, and tracheal intubation. Enlisted men only learned to deliver open drop ether anesthesia. The objective for all personnel was to learn enough to manage the technical demands of safe

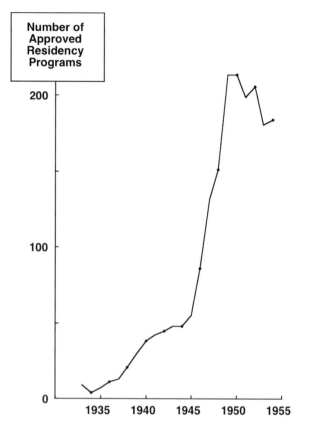

Fig. 37.3 The number of approved residency programs increased from the mid-1930s to the mid-1940s, consistent with the rising interest in a career in anesthesia. That interest was magnified by the enforced recruitment of physicians to anesthesia during World War II and the development of the means to pay anesthesiologists well. (Data taken from [27])

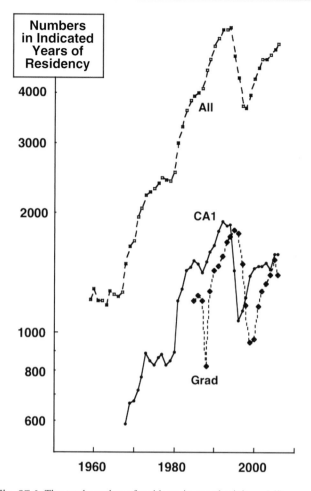

Fig. 37.4 The total number of residents in anesthesiology (all) more than quadrupled in the period from 1959 to 2006. The graph also presents the numbers in the CA1 year and the numbers graduating in a given year (grad; from data provided by [26])

anesthetic delivery. The academic veneer was necessarily thin. By the war's end, many physicians had perforce learned the trade we call anesthesia, learned it well, and learned that they liked the requirements placed on them.

After World War II, increasing demands for medical specialization led to a growth in specialty residents at teaching hospitals [14], and the number of US anesthesia residency programs increased almost five-fold over a decade (Fig. 37.3). As would be expected, the numbers of physicians subsequently recruited as residents, reflected this rapidly expanding interest in anesthesiology (Fig. 37.4) [26]. The total number of residents in training in a given year increased more than 4-fold between 1959 and 2006. There was however, a transient decrease in the early to mid 1990s, a dip reflecting a temporary focus on primary care rather than specialty training.

In 1945, the ASA created a "Committee on Postgraduate Education" (chaired by Stevens Martin) whose purpose was "to conduct a thorough study of the possibilities for postgraduate education in anesthesiology [28]". It was designed primarily to serve two groups: 1) returning veterans seek-

ing further training in anesthesiology, and 2) new initiates into the field. Approximately half a decade later, the Committee issued "Recommendations for a Curriculum in Anesthesiology [29]". The committee recommended two types of training: post-graduate refresher courses, or residencies and fellowships in anesthesiology. The term "fellow" was the most variable of the post-graduate training positions during the two decades after World War II, as the fellow could be assigned to one division or even one faculty member in a given department [14]. At some teaching hospitals, the resident was referred to as a "fellow" or "graduate fellow [14]".

The groups served by postgraduate refresher courses included World War II veterans seeking further training. The courses lasted three months or more, and covered general anesthesia, all forms of regional anesthesia, or a combination of both. The courses provided lectures, demonstrations, and group discussions on basic anatomy, physiology, pharmacology, physics, and chemistry. They were supplemented with weekly conferences to discuss "interesting cases and current literature" (M&M plus journal club). Perhaps most importantly, the participants were preceptees providing supervised anesthetic management of diverse cases. These courses were not a requirement for entrance to the ABA written examination, since the ABA began to require two years of post-internship training, starting in 1945. Instead, these "short courses" were part of the growing recognition that medical knowledge was progressing rapidly, and were designed to help physicians keep up with the latest developments in one's field [30]. As medical specialties (including anesthesiology) began to develop more rigorous residency training models, these short courses were eliminated as a means of learning a new specialty.

In contrast to the Postgraduate Refresher Courses, recommendations for residency or fellowship prescribed a minimum of 2 years spent in training for candidates with no prior instruction. Diplomates or Fellows in Anesthesiology would supply instruction. Candidates anticipating a position in a university or large institution, were urged to spend 3–4 years in residency or fellowship training.

The committee provided a 96 line "master and all-inclusive" list of subjects in outline form, that had four major headings: Introduction, General Anesthesia, Regional Anesthesia, and Related Subjects. The Related Subjects included topics contained in twenty-first century subject outlines, such as resuscitation, obstetric analgesia, and patient positioning. One subject, "psychology: surgeon–patient–anesthesiologist relationships" is notably absent in present-day subject outlines.

The Committee recommended a minimum case volume of "750 anesthesias per year under direct or indirect supervision, using all established agents and techniques for general and regional anesthesia performed for (all ordinary operations). They should be thoroughly familiar with the principles and practice of preoperative medication, postoperative rounds, bronchoscopy, fluid and inhalation therapy, diagnostic and therapeutic nerve blocks. A maximum of 14 days vacation per year should be given to each resident or fellow in Anesthesiology." Finally, the committee also encouraged all residents and fellows in anesthesiology to do original laboratory or clinical research, or write a thesis. It is not clear whether the encouragement had any impact, although subspecialty fellowships, in general, provided a greater opportunity for scholarly activities than residencies, which were clinically oriented by nature.

Who might review and regulate residencies? Return to 1940, when representatives of the American Medical Association's Council on Medical Education and Hospitals, and the American College of Physicians, formed the Conference Committee on Graduate Training in Internal Medicine. This Conference Committee appraised residency programs in internal medicine [31].

During World War II, members of the American Board of Internal Medicine also participated in these reviews. In June 1948, representatives of the three organizations met to reactivate the Conference Committee on Graduate Training in Internal Medicine. The Committee was charged with the establishment of standards for internal medicine residencies and the evaluation of internal medicine residencies. In May 1950, a parallel organization for surgeons arose. Representatives of the AMA, the American College of Surgeons, and the American Board of Surgery met to discuss a procedure for coordinated approval of surgical residency programs. They sought to, 1) encourage the adoption of uniform standards for residency training in surgery, 2) sponsor an "inspection service" for hospitals offering surgery training, and 3) approve and publish a list of acceptable surgical residency programs. The joint committee was called the Conference Committee on Graduate Training in Surgery. In 1953, the Conference Committee on Graduate Training in Internal Medicine officially changed its name to the Residency Review Committee (RRC) in Internal Medicine, in order to better describe its activities [31].

These experiences prompted the establishment of RRCs in other specialties. The AMA Council on Medical Education and Hospitals proposed that each RRC consist of representatives of the Council and the specific specialty board ("bipartite groups"). A few tripartite RRCs were established, similar to medicine and surgery, by incorporating a specialty society as a third sponsor. By 1957, all but a few of the established specialties had formed RRCs with the goal of formalizing accreditation in graduate medical education [31]. The RRC in Anesthesiology was formed in 1957, with three members representing the AMA Council on Medical Education and Hospitals, three members representing the American Board of Anesthesiology (ABA), and a Secretary who was a member of the Council staff. Residencies were surveyed by Council field staff or Diplomates of the ABA, who represented the RRC. In later years, the ASA sponsored committee members, thus making anesthesiology a tripartite RRC.

1957–1967

In 1962, the Anesthesiology RRC allowed residency programs to be approved for three years of training instead of two. The program had to offer research approved by the program director, subspecialty training in clinical anesthesia more advanced than the "usual" experience, or study in another clinical discipline. There was a benefit to participating in a three year program—the candidate was eligible to take the ABA written examination immediately after completion of training. Candidates who completed two years of anesthesia training were required to submit proof of four years of anesthesia practice over and above residency or fellowship training, prior to taking the written examination.

1966—The Citizen's Commission

In 1962, the Board of Trustees of the AMA appointed a Citizen's Commission on Graduate Medical Education, to study the problems in the graduate education of physicians. In 1966, the Commission, led by John Millis, president of Western Reserve University, issued its report. Five issues of paramount importance were highlighted [32]:

1. Discontinuity of the educational process
2. Persistence of apprenticeship in the process of education and training
3. Ineffectiveness and inadequacy in the organization of existing institutions of medical education
4. Failure to decide the role of the university in graduate medical education
5. Unsatisfactory balance between generalization and specialization

Accreditation of internships by the Internship Review Committee of the AMA, and accreditation of residencies by a separate RRC for each specialty, was cited as an example of discontinuity in the educational process. The Citizen's Commission also recommended that a new Commission on Graduate Medical Education be established, to review and approve standards for graduate medical education. Although the recommendation was never applied, this illustrated an early attempt to demonstrate accountability in the training of physicians.

1972—Birth of the Accreditation Council for Graduate Medical Education

In 1972, discussions between the AMA, the Association of American Medical Colleges, the American Board of Medical Specialties, the American Hospital Association, and the Council on Medical Specialty Societies, led to the creation of two new accrediting bodies in medical education [33]. The Liaison Committee on Graduate Medical Education (LCGME) was established to serve as the official accrediting body for graduate medical education, and the Coordinating Council on Medical Education (CCME) was established to consider policy matters for both undergraduate and graduate medical education. In 1980, the CCME was disbanded after years of disagreements among the five parent organizations.

The LCGME first met in December 1972, and was charged with the responsibility for accrediting graduate medical education programs, after reviewing the recommendations of individual RRCs. In 1975, the LCGME began to formally accredit programs. In 1981, the LCGME adopted a new name, the Accreditation Council for Graduate Medical Education (ACGME) [33]. The number of residency programs grew over the intervening years. In the academic year 2008–2009, there were 8,734 ACGME-accredited residency programs in 130 specialties and subspecialties. The number of active full-time and part-time residents for the academic year 2008–2009 was 109,482 [34].

1980s—Society for Education in Anesthesia

Believing that a broadly based organization of teachers of anesthesiology could improve education in anesthesia, a group of junior anesthesia faculty in the US founded the Society for Education in Anesthesia (SEA), in the early 1980s. Philip Liu, an anesthesiologist at the Massachusetts General Hospital, was "chairman pro tempore" of the fledgling organization. In the first SEA newsletter in February 1984, he expressed his hope that "members of this Society will develop a genuine sense of fellowship, so that individuals with an interest and vocation in the teaching of anesthesiology will find a network of support and a resource for communication." The first annual meeting and workshop of the SEA was held in October 1985, in San Francisco, with a meeting theme of "Training Residents for Competence." Over time, the SEA has served as an organization promoting the teaching of anesthesiology to medical students and residents. While individual members of SEA have served on the Anesthesiology RRC, the SEA has not asserted itself as an influential organization with respect to oversight or direction of anesthesia education.

The Duty Hours Era—1980s to Present

Training demanded extreme amounts of interns' and residents' time. For many years, it was common for an intern or resident to take "call" (staying in the hospital to admit and care for patients) every other night. On the post-call day, the intern or resident would remain in the hospital until the evening in order to tend to patient care needs. In this manner, over 120 hours of a possible 168 hours per week might be spent at work. While the culture of dedication to patients and one's professional work had its advantages, there was no doubt about the associated fatigue, and eventually about the limitations of performance that accompanied sleep deprivation. In the 1950s and 1960s, psychologists defined some of the effects of sleep deprivation, including reduced vigilance and cognition. A 1971 study showed that sleep-deprived interns (0 to 4 hours of sleep, mean of 1.8 hours) were twice as likely as a rested intern (7 hours sleep) to miss cardiac arrhythmias on an electrocardiogram [35].

However, it was the 1984 death of college student Libby Zion that brought resident duty hours to the national spotlight [35]. Zion was admitted to New York Hospital with fever, tremors and disorientation. She was diagnosed with a "viral syndrome", i.e., effects of a viral infection, and given intravenous hydration. She also received the painkiller and sedative mcpcridine, which likely caused a drug reaction with an antidepressant drug that she was taking, phenelzine. She developed extreme fever (107 degrees) and died of a cardiac arrest. Zion's father was Sidney Zion, an influential journalist with the New York Daily News. After learning more about his daughter's care, he became convinced that her death was the result of poor staffing at the hospital, including residents working too many hours, and covering too many patients with inadequate supervision [36]. A Manhattan grand jury investigation criticized the 36 hour duty periods worked by the residents, and the inadequate supervision by attending physicians [36, 37]. The New York Health Commissioner formed a committee that became known as the Bell Commission, led by primary care physician Bertrand Bell, a long-time critic of the lack of supervision of interns and residents [36]. The Bell Commission's 1987 report recommended an 80-hour per week limit on resident duty hours, a maximum of 24 consecutive hours on duty, and the requirement for senior physicians to be present in the hospital [37]. These recommendations were incorporated into the New York State Health Code in 1989, making New York the first (and so far, only) state that has adopted regulations for resident duty hours [36, 37].

The ACGME and the AAMC also formed task forces, and provided position statements on duty hours. However, progress was slow. In 1992, the ACGME approved requirements that all programs require one 24-hour period per week without patient care responsibilities, with call limited to every third night. While the 1992 ACGME rules did not specify hourly limits on resident duty hours, many individual specialty RRCs imposed such limits, including internal medicine, dermatology, ophthalmology, and emergency medicine. Most of these RRCs chose 80 hours as the weekly limit, with emergency medicine setting a limit of 72 hours [37]. The pressure mounted, however, when a 2001 petition requested that the Occupational Safety and Health Administration (OSHA) regulate duty hours of residents because of its potential role as a workplace health hazard. Also in 2001, the US Congress considered legislation to limit resident work hours [37]. Finally, in 2003, the ACGME set a maximum limit on the duty hours of residents in all specialties, of 80 hours per week. They also set a maximum of 24 hours of continuous duty, plus 6 hours for continuity and transfer of care.

Were patients safer as a result of these changes? The answer is not clear, given the many factors that impact on patient outcomes, and the complexity of the modern health care system. The Institute of Medicine (IOM), the health arm of the National Academy of Sciences, is an independent organization that advises the public and national decision makers, both private and governmental. Congress requested that the IOM study the relationship between resident duty hours and patient safety. In 2008, the IOM released a report titled "Resident Duty Hours: Enhancing Sleep, Supervision, and

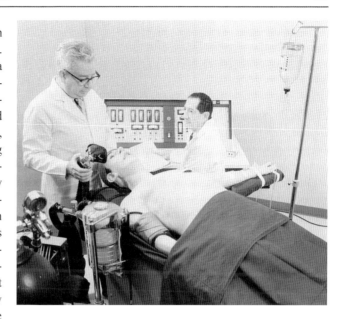

Fig. 37.5 Sim One, the first computer-controlled patient simulator lies on the table, attended by Judson Denson (*left*) and Stephen Abrahamson in the 1960s at the University of Southern California. (From [41]. Copyright (c) 1969 American Medical Association. All rights reserved)

Safety." The report "asserts that revisions to medical residents' workloads and duty hours are necessary to better protect patients against fatigue-related errors and to enhance the learning environment for doctors in training. The report recommends that residency programs provide regular opportunities for sleep each day and each week during resident training [38]." Subsequently, the ACGME revised its common program requirements to include additional restrictions on duty hours, the most notable being a reduction of continuous duty for interns to 16 hours maximum. However, the ACGME also addressed other aspects of patient safety, including new standards for supervision, teamwork, transitions of care, fitness for duty, alertness management, and fatigue mitigation [39].

Late 1980s—The Simulation Era

In the mid 1960s, the first computer-controlled mannequin simulator was created at the University of Southern California. Underlying its development was the question "how can computers be used in medical education?" Anesthesiologist Judson Denson and engineer Stephen Abrahamson received a \$272,000 grant from the US Office of Education, and created the simulator (nicknamed "Sim One") in collaboration with Aerojet General Corporation and Sierra Engineering (Fig. 37.5) [40, 41]. Lifelike features of the simulator included a chest wall that moved with respiration, blinking eyelids, anatomically correct airway structures, and palpable carotid and temporal pulses.

Sim One was used for an educational study of tracheal intubation skill acquisition, by new anesthesia residents. In the study, the investigators trained ten new anesthesia residents in how to check their anesthesia equipment, provide oxygen to a patient, induce anesthesia, intubate the patient's trachea, and stabilize anesthesia after intubation. Five residents were trained with Sim One, and the other five were trained in the operating room with real patients. A checklist of required actions was used to give the resident feedback on the relevant steps in the process. Once training was complete, the investigators determined the number of days until a resident completed nine consecutive successful tracheal intubations. Simulator-trained residents took 46 days on average, while conventionally trained residents took 77 days [41]. In other words, the simulator-trained group took less time to achieve the same performance benchmark. Because of limitations in computer technology at the time, Sim One was never commercialized.

Fast-forward to the 1980s. David Gaba at Stanford University Medical School created the Comprehensive Anesthesia Simulation Environment (CASE), to investigate human performance in anesthesia [42]. Michael Good and JS Gravenstein at the University of Florida developed the Gainesville Anesthesia Simulator (GAS) to help teach basic clinical skills to anesthesia residents [40]. The two groups were also influenced by the desire to improve patient safety in anesthesia. Over the next decade, these two simulators were produced commercially. The CASE system ownership changed repeatedly, eventually being sold to Medsim Ltd in Israel. GAS was licensed to Loral Data Systems, Inc, and a new company called Medical Education Technologies Inc (METI) in Sarasota, Florida. The CASE system was used by Gaba to create a training curriculum called Anesthesia Crisis Resource Management (ACRM), which was based on the aviation model of crew resource management [43]. The initial description was even published in an aviation journal.

From the late 1990s through to 2010, training with computerized simulators grew rapidly despite limited evidence of sustained efficacy. In the year 2000, there were less than 200 of these simulators in the world, but by 2011, the METI company reported that over 7000 institutions use its simulation products worldwide [44]. During this time, the cost of a computerized mannequin simulator decreased from $250,000 to $30,000. In 2009, the American Board of Anesthesiology required simulation training as part of its Maintenance of Certification in Anesthesiology (MOCA) recertification process. In 2010, the Anesthesiology RRC instituted a requirement of at least one simulated clinical experience per year.

Several factors led to the widespread adoption of simulators for training. Trainees generally reacted positively to this form of teaching, and many studies showed that learning objectives could be achieved at least as effectively as with traditional teaching methods. In addition, management of rare events such as malignant hyperthermia could be "practiced" repeatedly in a controlled setting. However, no large-scale randomized trial of simulator-trained clinicians versus non-simulator trained clinicians has examined the impact on patient outcomes. Because of the low morbidity rate attributable to anesthesia, such a study would involve large numbers of patients. To this criticism, Gaba has argued that "no industry in which human lives depend on the skilled performance of responsible operators has waited for unequivocal proof of the benefits of simulation before embracing it. In my opinion, neither should anesthesiology [45]."

The costs of developing a simulation education program are substantial. A typical budget would include the acquisition cost of the simulator, clinical equipment to promote realism, audiovisual equipment to facilitate video-based debriefing techniques, and personnel to teach and administer the simulation courses. While simulation programs are clearly part of the fabric of modern anesthesia training, the cost/benefit ratio may be quite high.

1990s–2010—The Development of Subspecialty Anesthesia

Since the 1990s, the most notable changes in anesthesia education have been the increase in sub-specialty and non-operating room clinical experiences. Beginning in the 1980s, the ABA required subspecialty anesthesia training, including obstetric anesthesia, pediatric anesthesia, cardiothoracic anesthesia, neuroanesthesia, anesthesia for outpatient surgery, recovery room care, regional anesthesia, pain management, and critical care medicine. Initially, the required duration of each experience was not specified by the ABA or the RRC, except for critical care, which had a 2 month minimum [46]. In 1985, the ABA began to issue certificates in critical care medicine to candidates completing one year of specialized training, the first subspecialty in anesthesia to receive such recognition [46]. In 1991, the ABA began issuing certificates in pain management. The recognition of these two subspecialties was indicative of the increased attention to subspecialty training in anesthesia, which occurred at both residency and fellowship levels. It was also a reflection of the ever-increasing complexity and specialization of medicine in general.

In the course of residency, the RRC now requires two month-long rotations in obstetric anesthesia, pediatric anesthesia, neuroanesthesia, and cardiac anesthesia. Non-OR required rotations include critical care medicine (four months), post-anesthesia care unit (2 weeks), preoperative medicine (one month), and pain medicine (one month each of acute, chronic, and regional). The increase in non-OR rotations, combined with the increased complexity of the specialty OR rotations, has resulted in the need for fellowship training to properly prepare for certain anesthesia subspecialties. Fellowships have become much more rigorous, especially if they must conform to the requirements of the ACGME. Currently, the ACGME accredits one-year fellowships in several anesthesia subspecialties: critical care medicine, pain medicine, pediatric anesthesia, cardiothoracic anesthesia, and obstetric anesthesia. In addition, some departments offer non-ACGME fellowships in areas such as obstetric anesthesia, regional anesthesia (including ultrasound), liver transplant anesthesia, and operating room management.

What does this mean for anesthesiology training in the twenty-first century? The "general" anesthesiologist, capable of caring for patients in any subspecialty will be a relic of the past. Increasingly, anesthesiologists will focus their practice in one or more subspecialties, and if a particular subspecialty is governed by an ACGME fellowship, then the fellowship will be the only path for training.

References

1. Ludmerer KM. Learning to heal: the development of American medical education. New York:Basic Books; 1985.
2. Warren JC. Address before the American Medical Association. Boston: John Wilson; 1850. pp. 52–3.
3. Vinten-Johansen P, Brody H, Paneth N, Rachman S, Rip M. Cholera, chloroform and the science of medicine: A life of John Snow. New York: Oxford University Press; 2003. p. 111.
4. Snow J. On chloroform and other anaesthetics: Their action and administration. London: John Churchill; 1858. pp. 1–443.
5. Anesthesia and the medical student. The Lancet. 1900 Oct 27;156(4026):1215.
6. The Teaching of Anesthesia. Phila Med J. 1900 Dec 29.
7. Historical Vignette. Nurse Anesthetists: The Dawn of a Specialty. Milestones in Anesthesia. 1993;2:10–1.
8. Flexner A. Medical education in the United States and Canada: A report to the Carnegie Foundation for the Advancement of Teaching. New York: Carnegie Foundation for the Advancement of Teaching; 1910.
9. Calmes SH. Arthur Guedel, M.D., and the eye signs of snesthesia. ASA Newsl. 2002 Sept;66(9):17–9
10. Gatch WD. Instruction of medical students and hospital interns in anesthesia. Am J Surg. 1916;30:98–9.
11. Herb IC. Anesthesia in relation to medical schools and hospitals. Am J Surg. 1921;35:50–1.
12. Strickland RA, Herb IC. An early leader in anesthesiology. Anesth Analg. 1995;80:600–5.
13. Calmes SH. Early MD anesthesia at the University of California: self-trained Mary Botsford to Waters-trained Hubert Hathaway. Anesthesiology. 2003; 99:A1273.
14. Ludmerer KM. Time to heal: American medical education from the turn of the century to the era of managed care. New York: Oxford University Press; 1999. pp. 80–3.
15. Leveroos EH, Albus WR, Corbett WW, Southard WW. Approved internships and residencies in the United States. JAMA. 1950;142(15):1145–8.
16. Council on Medical Education Hospitals. Hospital service in the United States. JAMA. 1927;88(11):789–839.
17. Bacon DR. Ament R: Ralph Waters and the beginnings of academic anesthesiology in the United States: the Wisconsin template. J Clin Anesth. 1995;7:534–43.
18. Waters RM. Letter from Ralph Waters MD to Paul Wood MD, February 23, 1948. The Collected Papers of Ralph Waters MD. Steenbock Library Collection. University of Wisconsin. Madison, Wisconsin.
19. Waters RM. Letter from Ralph Waters MD to Lincoln Sise MD, May 5, 1933. The Collected Papers of Ralph Waters MD. Steenbock Library Collection. University of Wisconsin. Madison, Wisconsin.
20. Prusinkiewicz CA, Maltby JR. The development of formal anesthesia training in Canada, the United States of America and the United Kingdom. Int Congr Ser. 2002;1242:385–91.
21. The Commission on Graduate Medical Education. Report of the Commission on graduate medical education. Chicago:University of Chicago Press; 1940.
22. Approved Residencies And Fellowships. JAMA. 1939;113:842–60.
23. Bacon DR. Lema MJ. To define a specialty: a brief history of the American Board of Anesthesiology's first written examination. J Clin Anes. 1992;4:489–97.
24. Slogoff S. A History of the American Board of Anesthesiology Certifying Examinations. Chapter 35 in Eger EI, Saidman LJ, Westhorpe RN (editors), The Wondrous Story of Anesthesia. Springer, New York, 2014.
25. Martin SJ. The teaching of anesthesiology in the Army. JAMA. 1942;119:1245–7.
26. Grogono AW. Resident numbers and graduation rates from residencies 2006. ASA Newsl. 2006 Nov. (Also accessible at http://www.grogono.com/nrmp/2006/Residencies06.pdf).
27. Betcher AM, Ciliberti BJ, Wood PM, Wright LH. The jubilee year of organized anesthesia. Anesthesiology. 1956;17:226–64.
28. New Committee of the American Society of Anesthesiologists, Inc. Anesthesiology. 1945;6:579.
29. Martin SJ. Recommendations for a curriculum in anesthesiology. Committee on postgraduate education, American Society of Anesthesiologists. Undated document from Wood Library-Museum of Anesthesiology. Estimated date 1951–1953.
30. The Commission on Graduate Medical Education: Report of the Commission on Graduate Medical Education. Chicago: University of Chicago Press; 1940. pp. 167–71.
31. Turner EL. Background and development of residency review and conference committees. JAMA. 1957;165:60–4.
32. Millis JS. Issues in graduate medical education. JAMA. 1966;197:989–91.
33. Council on Medical Education. Future directions for medical education. Chicago: American Medical Association; 1982. pp. 86–8.
34. Web site ACGME. http://www.acgme.org/acWebsite/newsRoom/newsRm_acGlance.asp. Accessed: 2010 Aug 17.
35. Friedman RC, Bigger JT, Kornfeld DS. The intern and sleep loss. N Engl J Med. 1971;285:201–3.
36. Lermer BH. A case that shook medicine—how one man's rage over his daughter's death sped reform of doctor training. The Washington Post. 2006 Nov 28.
37. Philibert I, Taradejna C. A brief history of duty hours and resident education. In: The ACGME. Duty hour standards: enhancing quality of care, supervision, and resident professional development. Chicago: Accreditation Council for Graduate Medical Education; 2011
38. Ulmer C, Wolman DM, Johns ME, editors. Resident duty hours: enhancing sleep, supervision, and safety. Washington, DC: National Academies Press (Institute of Medicine); 2009.

39. The ACGME. Duty hour standards: enhancing quality of care, supervision, and resident professional development. Chicago: Accreditation Council for Graduate Medical Education; 2011.

40. Cooper JB, Taqueti VR. A brief history of the development of mannequin simulators for clinical education and training. Qual Saf Health Care. 2004;13:i11–8.

41. Denson JS. Abrahamson S: A computer-controlled patient simulator. JAMA. 1969;208:504–8.

42. Gaba DM. DeAnda A: A comprehensive anesthesia simulation environment: re-creating the operating room for research and training. Anesthesiology. 1988;69:387–94.

43. Howard SK, Gaba DM, Fish KJ, Yang G. Sarnquist FH: Anesthesia crisis resource management training: teaching anesthesiologists to handle critical incidents. Aviat Space Environ Med. 1992;63:763–70.

44. Meti Company website. http://www.meti.com/about_family.htm. Accessed: 2011 Aug 8.

45. Gaba DM. Improving anesthesiologists' performance by simulating reality. Anesthesiology. 1992;76:491–4.

46. American Board of Anesthesiology Booklet of Information. January 1988.

Evolution of Education in Anesthesia in Europe

Thomas Pasch and Peter Simpson

Summary

In 1932, the Association of Anaesthetists of Great Britain and Ireland (AAGBI) was founded. Shortly thereafter, anesthesia societies arose in France and Italy. In 1935, the AAGBI established a Diploma in Anaesthetics (DA) and in 1940, Torsten Gordh introduced instruction in anesthesia in Sweden. World War II isolated Europe from anesthetic advances in the US and UK. However training programs began in many European countries soon after 1945, and European countries increasingly recognized anesthesia as a medical specialty.

In 1957, six countries signed the Treaty of Rome, creating the European Economic Community (EEC) that grew into today's European Union (EU) with 27 member states. Increasing mutual recognition of medical qualifications and harmonization of medical education accompanied this political process. In 1958, the European Union of Medical Specialists (UEMS) was founded, and in 1962 Specialist Sections were created, including one for Anaesthesiology. In 1963, the UEMS stipulated a minimum of 3 years training in anesthesia, increasing to 4 years in 1969. By 1973, training varied between 3 and 7 years in EEC countries and 2 and 6 years in non-EEC countries.

Before 1960, relatively few European anesthesiologists existed, nurse anesthetists giving most anesthetics (under a surgeon's direction). From 1960 to 1970, France, Sweden, Finland, Germany, Norway, the Netherlands, and Switzerland established formal educational programs for nurse anesthetists. From 1970 to 1990, growing numbers of anesthesiologists allowed increasing supervision of all non-physician anesthetists.

Beginning in the 1960s, national anesthesia training programs gradually incorporated intensive care, emergency medicine, and pain management, with variations among countries in duration and design of curricula. Founded in 1982, the European Society of Intensive Care Medicine (ESICM) created the European Diploma in Intensive Care (EDIC) in 1988.

Founded in 1978, the European Academy of Anaesthesiology (EAA) established the European Diploma in Anaesthesiology and Intensive Care (EDA) in 1984, with a two part, multi-lingual Diploma examination. In 1993, the Specialist Sections of the UEMS formed educational Boards, leading to the European Board of Anaesthesiology (EBA) which became the specialty's monitoring authority within the EU. The EBA developed guidelines for training anesthesiologists, coordinating activities with the EAA until 2005, and with EAA's successor, the European Society of Anesthesiology (ESA), since 2006. Established in 1986, the Foundation for European Education in Anaesthesiology (FEEA) promoted Continuing Medical Education (CME). Since 1990, recertification required evidence of annual CME in about 60 % of European countries.

Growing demands for and on anesthesiologists may lead to relative shortages in Europe. With increasing cost constraints and the EU Directive decreasing working hours, this may increase reliance on nurse anesthetists.

The Development of Anesthesia as a Specialty in Europe

Marked variations among European countries characterized the development of educational programs in anesthesia, before and after 1945. In the 1930s, a few dedicated physicians directed their professional activities towards anesthesia. In the UK, general practitioner anesthetists, junior hospital doctors, or medical students gave most anesthetics. General practitioner anesthetists received no fee for their work in "voluntary" hospitals and relied on general practice to earn

T. Pasch (✉)
Anaesthesiology, University Hospital Zurich,
Zurich, Switzerland
e-mail: thomas.pasch@t-online.de

P. Simpson
Royal College of Anaesthetists
London, UK

E. I Eger II et al. (eds.), *The Wondrous Story of Anesthesia*, DOI 10.1007/978-1-4614-8441-7_38, © Edmond I Eger, MD 2014

their living. Founded in 1932, the Association of Anaesthetists of Great Britain and Ireland instigated an examination for a Diploma in Anaesthetics in 1935, and trained full-time anesthetists during World War II. These Diplomates were already in place when anesthesia was recognized as a medical specialty in 1948.

In France and Italy, anesthesia societies were founded and instruction in anesthesia sporadically organized in the mid 1930s, on the personal initiative of surgeons dedicated to anesthesia. In Germany, demands for independent professional recognition of anesthesia were made in 1928 and again in 1939, but failed due to the opposition of surgeons, the dominant force in the operating room. Most powerful was Ferdinand Sauerbruch from Berlin, who rejected modern anesthetic techniques like endotracheal intubation and opposed initiatives to remove anesthesia from the surgeon's control. His influence extended beyond Germany to much of continental Europe. In addition, medicine in Europe was cut off from the advances in anesthesia occurring in the USA and UK during World War II. These circumstances delayed the recognition of anesthesia as an independent specialty, and the introduction of training programs in continental Europe, except in Scandinavia where specialists were already practicing and teaching anesthesia by the first half of the 1940s.

In the first postwar decade, virtually all European countries established training programs in anesthesia, the duration of training varying between 1 to 3 years. The curriculum included specialties like surgery, internal medicine and/or basic sciences because these were, and are, considered important for the practice of anesthesia. Over the ensuing 3 decades, the length of training in anesthesia increased, equalling that in other specialties such as surgery and internal medicine (Table 38.1 and Fig. 38.1). The following paragraphs describe examples of these developments in selected European countries.

United Kingdom

From its founding in 1932, a primary objective of the Association of Anaesthetists of Great Britain and Ireland (AAGBI) was the provision of a Diploma in Anaesthetics (DA). Since only a registered examining body could certify such a Diploma, the Diploma was placed under the Conjoint Examining Board of the Royal Colleges of Physicians and Surgeons. Candidate diplomates had to provide evidence of qualifications in medicine, surgery or midwifery, resident appointments in recognized hospitals for at least 12 months, including 6 months as a resident anesthetist, and delivery of at least 1000 anesthetics. The first examination took place in November 1935 [1, 2]. During World War II, the UK Armed Forces created Field Surgical Teams with surgeons, anesthetists, and supporting staff. The AAGBI oversaw their train-

ing and assessment, fortunately ensuring that by the end of the War, there were sufficient physician anesthetists to meet the needs of the nascent National Health Service (NHS) in 1948 [3, 4]. To ensure the independent eligibility of anesthetists for full consultant status, the President of the AAGBI approached the Royal College of Surgeons, requesting the formation of a Faculty of Anaesthetists. The Council of the College approved this request in February 1948 [1, 2, 4, 5]. The DA was quickly upgraded to a Fellowship Diploma with a two-part examination, a Primary in basic sciences and a Final in clinical anesthesia, medicine and surgery. Medical graduates could apply for Part I after completing 6 months as a House Physician or House Surgeon; Part II could be sat 2 years after passing Part I and after completing at least 12 months of specialty training in anesthesia. In 1953, the new DA became the Diploma of the Fellowship of the Faculty of Anaesthetists of the Royal College of Surgeons (FFARCS).

The Royal College of Surgeons retained responsibility for the FFARCS until 1983, when it passed to the Faculty of Anaesthetists. In 1988, the Faculty of Anaesthetists became the College of Anaesthetists, still based at the Royal College of Surgeons. In 1992 the College received Royal status, thereby achieving independence as The Royal College of Anaesthetists (RCoA) [4, 5].

Since 1992, the training leading to a Certificate of Completion of Training (CCT) in Anaesthetics has had a duration of 7 years. A trainee must follow a competency based program covering basic, intermediate, higher and advanced training in anesthesia, pain medicine and intensive care medicine (ICM). Basic, intermediate and higher training each normally last 2 years, followed by advanced training, normally lasting 1 year. Trainees are expected to pass the Primary FRCA examination during the basic, and the Final during the intermediate levels of training. Those who pass are inducted as Fellows of the College and can use the letters FRCA after their name.

France

In the 1930s, French surgeons and anesthetists sporadically organized training in anesthesia. Anesthesia became an independent medical specialty after World War II [6]. In 1946, two anesthetists, Ernest Kern and Nadia du Bouchet, who had trained during wartime in England and the US, held the first course in anesthesia in Paris. In 1947, surgeons Pierre Moulonguet and Jean Baumann, with anesthetists Louis Amiot, Geneviève Delahaye-Plouvier, du Bouchet and Kern, organized a formal, one-year, university-based course of training and theoretical study. A Diploma of Anesthesia was granted after success in an examination.

In 1948, the Ministry of National Education created a Certificate of Specialized Studies in Anesthesia (CES, Certificat

Table 38.1 A summary of the evolution of anesthesia training in Europe

Country	Training program introduced		Updates of training program						Current training program	
	Year	Duration: T/A/I/O; yr*	Year	Duration: T/A/I/O; yr*	Year	Duration: T/A/I/O; yr*	Year	Duration: T/A/l/O:yr*	Start year	Duration: T/A/I/O; yr*
Austria	1952	6/3/-/3	1981	6/3.5/0.5/2					1994	6/3/2/1
Belgium	1948	1/1/-/-	1954	2/2/-/-	1964	3/3/P/-	1974	4/4/P/-	1979	5/4.5/0.5/-/-
Bulgaria	1958	2.5/2/0.5/-	1969	3/2.5/0.5/-					1986	4/3/1/-
Croatia†	1954	2/1.5/-/0.5	1959	3/2/-/1	1974	4/3/0.5/0.5	2000	4.5/3/1/0.5	2009	5/3.5/1/0.5
Czech Republic¢	1954	6/3/-/3	1971	I°: 3/3/P/P II°: 3/3/P/-	2004	5/4.5/0.5/-			2009	5/4/1/-
Denmark	1950	5.5/3/-/2.5	1975	6/4/-/2					2004	5/3.5/1/0.5
Estonia‡	1961	2–6mo/2–6mo/-/-	1971	1/1/P/-	1993	2/1.5/0.5/-			2002	4/2.5/1.5/-
Finland	1958	4/3/-/1	1979	5/4/P/1					1999	6/4/0.75/1.25
France	1947	1/1/-/-	1948	2/2/-/-	1966	3/3/P/-	1984	4/3/1/-	2002	5/3/2/-
Germany^	1953	5/2/-/3	1968	4/4/-/-	1987	4/3.5/0.5/-			1992	5/4/1/-
Greece	1953	2/1/-/1	~1976	3/2/-/1					1994	5/4/0.5/0.5
Hungary	1961	4/2/-/2	1978	4/2/2/-					1993	5/3/2/-
Italy	1948	2/2/-/-	1968	3/3/P/-	1989	4/4/P/-			2008	5/3/2/-
Latvia‡	1962	10 mo/10 mo/P/-	1965	I°: 10mo/10mo/ P/-II°:2/2/P/-	1991	4/2.5/0.5/1			2004	5/2/2/1
Lithuania‡	1964	2.5–6mo/2.5–6mo/-/-	1969	10mo/10mo/-/-	1991	4/2/1/1	2003	5/2.5/1.5/1	2010	4/2.5/1.5/-
Netherlands	1947	3/2/-/1	1969	3.5/3/-/0.5	1978	4.5/3.5/ 0.5/0.5	1989	5/4.5/0.5/-	1996	5/4/1/-
Norway	1949	3/2/-/1	1952	4/3/-/1	1964	4.5/3/- /1.5	1978	5/4/-/1	2000	5/4/0.5/0.5
Poland	1952	3/3/-/-	1972	4/3/1/-	1983	5/3/2/-			1998	6/4/2/-
Romania	1951	2mo/2mo/-/-	1957	1/1/-/-	1959	3/P/-/-	1993	5/3/1/1	2007	5/4/1/-
Serbia†	1947	2/1/-/1	1953	3/2/-/1	1991	4/2.65/0.6/0.75			2010	5/3.25/1/0.75
Slovakia¢	1954	6/3/-/3	1971	I°: 3/3/P/P II°: 3/3/P/-					2005	5/3.5/1.5/-
Slovenia†	1947	3/2.2/-/0.8	1970	4/2.3/1/0.7	2000	6/3.5/2/0.5			2011	5/3.3/1.5/0.2
Spain	1955	1.5/1.5/-/-	1969	2/2/-/-	1972	3/2.75/ 0.25/-	1976	4/2.75/0.25/1	1996	4/3/0.5/0.5
Sweden	1958	4/3/-/1	1963	4/3/-/1	1967	5/4/-/1			1974	6.5/4/1/1.5
Switzerland	1954	4/2/-/2	1969	3/3/P/-	1982	5/3.75/0.25/1	1991	5/3.75/0.25/1	2001	6/4.5/0.5/1
Turkey	1955	4/-/-/-	1969	3/3/P/-	1982	4/4/P/-	2001	4/2.3/1/0.7	2010	4/2.7/1/0.3
United Kingdom	1935	1/0.5/-/0.5	1948	2.5/1/-/1.5	1958	5/5/-/-	1970	6/5/0.5/-	1985	7/6/1/-

T total; A = anesthesia (including emergency and pain medicine in most countries); I = intensive care medicine; O = others (e.g. internship, basic sciences, surgery, internal and general medicine); P part of anesthesia training but duration not specified; I° first level of training, including ICM and other specialties, but without specified duration; II° second (optional) level of training including ICM, but without specified duration
* indicated in mo = months where appropriate
† Part of Yugoslavia prior to 1991
¢ Part of Czechoslovakia prior to 1993
‡ Part of the Soviet Union prior to 1991
^ 1955–1969 two years and 1970–1976 one year of internship had to precede the specialist training program (not included in this table)

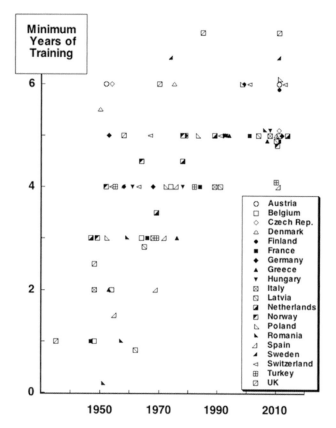

requirements specific to his/her specialty, and must present a thesis to a regional jury to receive the final Diploma (DES). A supplementary Diploma (DESC, Diplôme d'études spécialisées complémentaires) in non-surgical ICM, emergency medicine, pain and palliative medicine, hemobiology and transfusion, or clinical pharmacology may be obtained with 2–3 years of additional training.

Sweden

In Nordic countries, anesthesiology emerged earlier than in the large countries of continental Europe. One of the most influential pioneers was Torsten Gordh, who trained in Ralph Waters' Department in Madison, Wisconsin in 1938, and in 1940 became the first full-time anesthesiologist (at Stockholm's newly opened Karolinska Hospital) – not only in Sweden, but also in continental Europe. He immediately introduced training programs for doctors, students and nurses [7]. The National Medical Association recognized anesthesiology as a separate specialty in 1953. In 1960, the National Board of Health and Welfare officially followed suit. Initially, 3 years of anesthesia training were required to be included as a specialist on the register of "License to Practice". In the early 1970s, this changed to 5 years and included 6 months training in both a medical and surgical specialty, as well as 6 courses in basic sciences. The National Board of Health and Welfare determined the general rules for education of specialists, but the Swedish Society of Anaesthesiology and Intensive Care Medicine determined the details [8]. The European Diploma in Anaesthesiology and Intensive Care (EDA) examination, though voluntary, has been regarded as the national examination since 1989 [9].

Denmark

In Denmark the first doctor to undertake specialist training in anesthesiology was Trier Mørch, in 1940 [10]. Willy Dam filled the first anesthesiologist appointment, established in 1944 at Bispebjerg Hospital in Copenhagen. The National Health Service recognized anesthesiology as an independent specialty in 1950. Training requirements included 2 years of anesthesiology, 1.5 years of surgery, 1 year of internal medicine, and a 1 year course at the WHO Anaesthesiology Centre in Copenhagen (see below), followed by an examination. Training in pharmacology, physiology or biochemistry could replace 6 months of internal medicine. The requirements changed on several occasions. In 1975 they were: 4 years of training in anesthesiology, consisting of 2 years of theoretical training, and 2 years of training common to all specialties [11]. In 2004, the Danish Society of Anaesthesiology and

d'études spéciales d'anesthésie) to be granted by the Faculties of Medicine. Training lasted for at least 2 years and included 70 lessons, hospital training and a final examination. In 1966, mandated training increased to 3 years. In 1988, the Diploma of Specialized Studies (DES, Diplôme d'études spécialisées) replaced the CES. Admission to this new postgraduate specialist training program (now called "internat qualifiant"), required doctors graduating after 1984 to take a competitive entry examination common to all specialties, the specialty that candidates could ultimately choose being dependent on their ranking success. In 2002, the required duration of postgraduate training in anesthesia increased to 5 years. Trainees receive theoretical training (basic sciences 60 h, anesthesia-pain 150 h, intensive care and emergency medicine 150 h), while pursuing practical training (3 years anesthesia and 2 years ICM; 1 year of which can be replaced by a specialty related to anesthesia).

Admission of medical students to a specialist educational program, after their 6th year, now requires passage of a national classifying examination (introduced in 2004) in lieu of the examination for the "internat". Based on the test results, the student may select a specialty for training. After 5 years of training, a trainee must submit proof of having met the

Intensive Care Medicine's Postgraduate Training Manual prescribed 5 years of training, including 13 months in Intensive Care Medicine (ICM), 3 months in pain therapy, and 3 months in emergency medicine and trauma care. No compulsory specialist examination has existed since 1971. Since 2000, a performance-based assessment developed in detail for the first years of training has increasingly replaced the end-of-training examination [12]. A national hospital visiting program was introduced concurrently, to ensure that all centers fulfilled the conditions needed to provide adequate training.

The early 1950s saw development of two important events in anesthesiology in Copenhagen. First, a training center in anesthesiology was established in response to a request by the World Health Organization (WHO) to the Faculty of Medicine of the University of Copenhagen. The Centre organized 23 one-year courses, the first commencing 1 May 1950. Foreign instructors included Ralph Waters and Stuart Cullen, followed by Robert Macintosh, Henry Beecher, Jack Moyers, Leroy Vandam, Francis Foldes, and Torsten Gordh. From 1952 to 1974, 220 Danish and 205 European trainees, and 218 trainees from outside Europe, attended the courses [11, 13]. The second event was the 1952 poliomyelitis epidemic in Denmark. Led by Danish anesthesiologist Bjørn Ibsen, patients with life-threatening poliomyelitis were concentrated in one area and treated with controlled ventilation. These actions markedly decreased deaths, and their imitation led to the establishment of the first intensive care unit one year later [14].

Norway

The Norwegian pioneers were Otto Mollestad, who trained and qualified in Oxford with Macintosh, and Ivar Lund, who trained in Boston with Henry Beecher. Mollestad took the first anesthesiologist appointment at Rikshospitalet in Oslo in December 1946, and Lund joined the Ulleval Hospital one month later. Anesthesiology was recognized as a separate specialty in 1949. Training requirements for qualification as a specialist developed in parallel to those in other Scandinavian countries [8, 15]. Currently, education is based on a curriculum of 5 years including 6 months in ICM and 6 months served in any specialty other than anesthesiology, preferably internal medicine or pediatrics, or in research. There are 260 mandatory course hours in specific topics. As in Denmark and Sweden, the Norwegian Medical Association has not adopted examinations although the Norwegian Society of Anaesthesiology voted for a national examination in the early 1980s. A hospital visiting program introduced in the early 1980s evaluates the adequacy of training programs.

Finland

In 1940, Eero Turpeinen studied new methods of anesthesia with Torsten Gordh in Stockholm, but World War II cut short his stay. In 1945, he completed his anesthesia training in the US, and in 1948 he became the first Finnish specialist in anesthesia. From 1950 to 1967, most Finnish training in anesthesia occurred at the WHO courses in Copenhagen. The first dedicated residency posts in anesthesiology were founded during 1952 to 1955, and the post of chief anesthesiologist at Turku University was established in 1954. Criteria for training and accreditation were devised in 1955, based on a proposal by the Finnish Society of Anaesthesiologists. Anesthesiology was officially recognized as a separate specialty and a training program started in 1958 [4, 16]. Today the duration of training is 6 years, including 15 months in general practice and supporting disciplines, 4 years in anesthesiology, and 9 months in ICM. Of the 4 years in anesthesiology, a maximum of 3 years may be spent in a university hospital. The EDA examination can replace a written examination at the end of training, but no hospital visiting program exists.

Germany

Pressure in Germany for an independent professional identity for anesthesia arose in 1928 and again in 1939, but failed due to opposition from surgeons. World War II separated German medicine from the outside world [17, 18]. Soon after the War, many surgeons realized that anesthesia had enabled enormous advances in surgery, and consequently began sending young doctors to anesthesiology centers in the US, UK, Scandinavia, France and Switzerland [19]. Conversely, foreign anesthetists like Jean Henley (New York) and Karl Mülly (Zurich) visited German hospitals and taught modern anesthesia [20, 21]. In September 1953, the German Medical Assembly voted to include anesthesia as an independent discipline in the official list of medical specialties. The German Society of Anaesthesia had been founded just five months earlier. The duration of training was set at 5 years: 1 year of general medicine (as for every specialty at that time), 1 year of surgery, 6 months of internal medicine, 6 months physiology or pharmacology, and 2 years of anesthesia. In 1968, adapting to the widening responsibilities of anesthesiology, the duration of training specifically devoted to anesthesia increased to 4 years. Training in physiology, pharmacology, internal medicine, a lung function laboratory or a blood bank could replace 6 months of the 4 years. Trainees had to document the successful administration of 1200 anesthetics, and experience in ICM including artificial ventilation. Between 1955 and 1969, graduates from medical schools had to serve 2 years as an intern before being entitled to enter a specialist training program. This period was shortened to 1 year in 1970 and after 1976, the internship requirement ceased.

In 1987, training in ICM was set at 6 months and the minimum number of anesthetics was increased to 1800, including 100 regional blocks. In 1992, the duration of training continued to be 5 years: 4 years anesthesia and 1 year anesthesiology based ICM. An anesthesia-related specialty could replace 1 year of anesthesia training [18]. A final oral examination was introduced in 1978, organized by the State Chambers of Physicians (Landesärztekammern), which are officially responsible for both postgraduate medical training and continuing medical education. They also govern the recognition of training centers.

Austria

In the summer of 1947, the non-profit Unitarian Service Committee, sought to assist European refugees subjected to Nazi persecution, and sent a group of American anesthesiologists to Austria. They visited the Faculties of Medicine, gave lectures and demonstrated modern anesthetic techniques. This prompted some visionary surgeons to send assistants to the US and the UK [22]. In 1951, the Austrian Society of Anaesthesiology was founded, and in June 1952, the Federal Ministry of Social Administration recognized anesthesiology as an independent medical specialty. Training lasted 6 years, and consisted of 3 years of general medicine and 3 years of anesthesia, including basic sciences. Training in anesthesia increased to 4 years in 1981, and to 5 years in 1994, including 2 years of ICM. In addition, 6 months of surgery and 6 months internal medicine were required, resulting in a total duration of 6 years. At this time, the specialty was renamed "Anesthesiology and Intensive Care Medicine" [22]. A compulsory examination was introduced in 2002, and candidates could replace about half of the final examination with the Part I Examination for the EDA [23]. Since June 2010, all candidates have had to take the EDA Part I. If they pass, the number of oral examinations they must take during the final examination decreases from 8 to 4. In addition, the EDA Part II examination can be taken instead of the final national examination.

Switzerland

After World War II, the Swiss Academy of Medical Sciences recognized the need to adopt new developments in medicine in general, and anesthesiology in particular. It granted a clinical fellowship to Werner Hügin (Basel), who trained in Beecher's Department in 1947–1948. Others followed, and in 1952 they formed the Swiss Society of Anaesthesiology. They successfully petitioned the Swiss Medical Association to recognize anesthesiology as a specialty in January

1954. Training lasted 4 years, including 2 years in anesthesia (18 months in Switzerland and, until 1962, 6 months in a foreign training center). After 1961, training in anesthesia could be entirely undertaken in Swiss anesthetic departments. In 1963, training in anesthesia increased to 3 years at the expense of non-anesthetic training, and in 1967, to 4 years resulting in a total duration of 5 years (4 years in anesthesia and one year in non-anesthesia training). In 1991, 3 months of ICM became mandatory, increasing to 6 months in 2001 with a total duration of training of 6 years [24]. By 2013, the one year non-anesthesia training will be cancelled upon request of the Federal Government and the total duration of training will again be 5 years. The Swiss Society of Anaesthesiology and Reanimation (SSAR) introduced an optional examination in 1979. The SSAR persuaded the Swiss Medical Association to make the examination compulsory in 1986. One year later, the Part I EDA examination was adopted as the national written examination. Part II was organized as a national oral examination by the SSAR from the outset [25].

The Netherlands

Doreen Vermeulen-Cranch, from University College Hospital in London provided the first formal teaching in anesthesia, doing so in Amsterdam in January 1947. The first national training curriculum was proposed and accepted in 1947, with 2 years' training in anesthesia following 6 months in each of basic internal medicine and basic surgery. The Netherlands Society of Anaesthesiology (NSA) was founded in January 1948, and anesthesia was recognized as a medical specialty in that year. Training duration in 1954, 1969 and 1974 stepwise increased to 4.5 years and included training in basic sciences, ICM (6 months) and pain medicine (3 months) [26]. A five-year training program was established in 1989. Training guidelines were revised in 1996 and again in 2004, with the addition of specific learning goals. Examinations were offered from the beginning, but met with resistance. In 1989, a basic written and a final oral examination became mandatory. These examinations evolved into annual examinations A, B and C for training years 1, 2 and 3, with a final oral examination on three clinical cases. With the installation of new training guidelines in January 2011, competency based training in modules was implemented and changes to the EDA examination are planned. A delegation of the Board of Accreditation of the NSA inspects all medical specialist training institutions, at least once every five years.

Belgium

Belgian pioneers William De Weerdt and Jan Van de Walle, both trained in Macintosh's Department in Oxford. They established anesthesia services in the two University Hospitals of Leuven in 1947 and 1948 respectively, and began training courses in 1948. Two years training and conduct of a scientific project entitled trainees to the Diploma of Specialist in Anaesthesiology. In 1951, Van de Walle's division became an independent Department, and regular payment of anesthetists was introduced. Admission Boards for medical specialties were established in 1958 [27]. Anesthesia was officially recognized as an independent specialty in 1964. Postgraduate training in anesthesia existed in University Hospitals. The curriculum lasted 4 years, but a Diploma was not essential for specialist recognition. A Decree of the Federal Minister of Health issued in September 1979, prescribed the requirements of training centers, setting the duration of training in anesthesiology at 5 years. If post-anesthesia training included 12 months of training in ICM, anesthesiologists could be accredited as anesthesiologists specializing in ICM. Anesthesiologists and other specialists could obtain a supplementary certificate of competence in emergency medicine after an additional training of 1 to 2 years. This option was replaced by the creation of 2 new separate specialties, acute medicine and emergency medicine, in 2005.

Italy

Italian anesthesia evolved from 1947 to 1950 when open-minded surgeons encouraged young assistants to learn modern anesthetic techniques, some in the US, and some in the UK. "Schools of spezialization" in anesthesiology formed within medical schools. The first, in Torino in 1948, offered a postgraduate training program of 2 years. A parliamentary bill in July 1954, created independent anesthesia services in hospitals, thereby granting the specialty formal recognition [28]. The duration of training increased to 3 years in 1968, and to 4 years in 1989. Anesthesia services became strongly connected with ICUs, and in 1979, the Italian Society of Anaesthesia changed its name to the Italian Society of Anaesthesia, Analgesia, Reanimation and Intensive Therapy. In 2008, anesthesia training was harmonized with that of the European Board of Anaesthesiology, and the duration of training increased to 5 years, including training in basic sciences. The specialty now officially became Anaesthesia, Reanimation and Intensive Care Medicine. Trainee assessment relied on annual oral examinations in each of the training centers, and the evaluation of skills by the responsible tutors.

Spain

Civil War (1936–1939) and World War II markedly delayed the development of anesthesia in Spain. After 1945, some physicians trained as anesthesiologists in the UK, especially in Oxford, and in the US. In 1952, the Spanish Army recognized the position of specialist in anesthesia, establishing regulations for training. In the same year, the public health system (Seguridad Social) called for the establishment of the first positions for specialists in "anaesthesiology and reanimation". "Anaesthesiology and reanimation" first appeared as a medical speciality in the Official Bulletin of the Government (Boletín Oficial del Estado) in July 1955. In 1969, the Universities of Granada, Valencia and Barcelona opened the "University Schools for Professional Education of Anaesthesiologists" (Escuelas Profesionales de Anestesiología). Diplomas of anesthesiology were given after programs lasting 2 years.

In 1972, an official postgraduate program called MIR, "Médicos internos y residents" defined training in anesthesiology and reanimation, as well as all other specialties [29]. Many public hospitals then offered positions for residents in anesthesiology with a training duration of 3 years. 1976 saw the first 4 year residency program in the MIR system, and the 1996 guidelines for training in anaesthesiology and reanimation mandated 4 years of training. While there is an annual entry examination for every specialty, no final examination is required to obtain the relevant specialist diploma. With the inception of the MIR system, ICM was recognized as an independent specialty. Until then however, anesthesiologists or cardiologists directed ICUs, and the separate specialist recognition of ICM is considered a major problem for anesthesia. Spanish anesthesia trainees still devote at least 6 months of their training to ICM, and are legally allowed to work in the ICU.

Poland

Many Polish surgeons and anesthetists trained in the UK during World War II, returning to Poland when the war ended. They petitioned health care organizers to encourage the development of anesthesiology. In 1951, Mieczysław Justyna, Assistant Professor, was appointed as the national consultant for anaesthesiology and devised a program for specialization in anesthesiology. Based on this program, the Ministry of Health mandated 3 years training in anesthesia, of which 5 months would be spent in internal medicine and 11 months in surgery. In 1973, training increased to 4 years. In 1978, the name of the specialty became Anaesthesiology and Resuscitation and, in 1983, changed to Anaesthesiology and Intensive Care. Between 1983 and 1998, training in anesthesia and intensive care took 5 years, 3 years in the former and 2 years in the latter. In 1998, training increased to 6 years: anesthesia for 4 years and ICM for 2 years. From 1978 to 2008, the national examination comprised three parts: written, practical and oral. In autumn 2008, the EDA Part I examination replaced the written part of the National Specialization Examination [30, 31].

Table 38.2 Evolution of Anesthesia Training in the USSR (until 1991) and the Russian Federation (after 1991)

Year	Description	Duration of training			
		Total	Anesthesia	ICM	Public health and basic sciences
1956	Primary specialization ("pervichnaya spezializatija")	2 months	2 months	–	–
1958 to date	Primary specialization ("pervichnaya spezializatija") Now: professional re-training	5 months or 10 months	approx. 80%	approx. 20%	–
1960–1993	Clinical residency ("klinicheskaya ordinatura")	2 years	approx. 70%	approx. 30%	–
1982 to date	Internship ("internatura")	1 year	approx. 35%	approx. 35%	approx. 30%
1993 to date	Clinical residency (optional: additional 3 years)	2 years (+3 years)	approx. 40%	approx. 40%	approx. 20%

USSR and the Russian Federation

World War II probably devastated the USSR (Soviet Union) more than any country in Europe, greatly delaying progress in medicine in general and anesthesia in particular. The introduction of modern techniques such as endotracheal anesthesia began in 1946. In 1956–1957, leading surgical departments began training anesthesiologists, with training lasting 2 months. The first academic department and chair of anesthesia was established at the SM Kirov Military Medical Academy in St. Petersburg, in 1958. In that year, courses for primary specialization of 5 or 10 months duration were introduced and still exist today. In 1960, a so-called residency, i.e., 2-year training in anesthesia, was established as a second route, which since 1993, could be optionally extended to 5 years. The option of extending the residency from 2 to 5 years is virtually never taken up. In 1982, a one year-training program was introduced as a third alternative and called an internship (Table 38.2). Remarkably, these variants are equal from a legal point of view. Although the Professors, Chairs and the All-Union Society of Anesthesiologists played a consulting role, the Ministry of Health independently issued regulations for training and practical work of anesthesiologists. In 1986, the last decree of the former USSR made departments of anesthesiology and intensive therapy mandatory for every hospital. Today, there is no national examination. Efforts continue to persuade the Government to increase the duration of clinical training from 2 to 3 years, with the aim of eventually reaching the European standards of 5–6 years.

The system of parallel methods of qualification in anesthesia was also established in several former satellite states for a period following World War II. Countries which became independent after dissolution of the Warsaw Pact and the Soviet Union in the years 1989–1991, and who subsequently became members of the EU (Baltic States, Czechoslovakia, Hungary, Romania, Bulgaria) abandoned the parallel programs, instead assuming programs consistent with those in the EU.

The Evolution of Educational Components of Anesthesiology

In the 1950s and 1960s, anesthetists progressively expanded their expertise in the emerging fields of intensive care, emergency medicine, and pain medicine. Increasingly, these became constituent elements of education and clinical practice in anesthesiology, but anesthesiology was not the only base specialty through which these fields could be approached and certification obtained.

Intensive Care Medicine (ICM)

The 1952 poliomyelitis epidemic in Copenhagen and the initiatives instituted there by Ibsen [3, 4, 14], led to the establishment of one of the world's first ICUs in December 1953, under Ibsen's direction. Less well known, the anesthetist Åke Bauer had established an ICU in Borås (Sweden) at the same time. Anesthetists increasingly led the treatment of patients suffering from respiratory failure from all causes, and also the care of patients with compromised vital functions. These roles made anesthetists the leaders of ICM in many European countries, ensuring that ICM became a significant part of training in anesthesia. In the following decades, all European countries developed structures and regulations for education and training in ICM, but with significant differences identified in an international survey of 37 training programs within 28 European countries [32]:

> Supra-specialty model: Multidisciplinary access to a single common training program leading to dual specialist certification in a base specialty and ICM was the most frequent type of training (15 countries), e.g. Netherlands, UK, France, Belgium, Finland, Portugal.

> Multiple sub-specialty model: ICM training provided by multiple parent specialties, each with their own training programs provided dual certification or base specialty certification, including ICM (Austria and Germany).

Single sub-specialty model: Single parent specialty without multidisciplinary access provided ICM training. Dual certification or base specialty certification, including ICM (13 countries), e.g. Scandinavia, Italy, Poland, Czech Republic, Slovakia.

Primary specialty: Base specialty with access directly after graduation from medical school, leading to specialist certification (Spain and Switzerland).

At present, the duration of training usually ranges between 12 and 24 months, but is at least 36 months in Spain and Switzerland [33]. Some typical training programs will be briefly described.

United Kingdom

In 1992, the Royal Colleges of Anaesthetists, Physicians, and Surgeons formed the Joint Advisory Committee for Intensive Therapy which became the Intercollegiate Board for Training in Intensive Care Medicine (IBTICM). The RCoA was designated as the lead college. In 1999, the Specialist Medical Order was modified to include ICM as a joint Certificate of Completion of Training (CCT) with a base specialty. The IBTICM evolved into the Faculty of Intensive Care Medicine of the RCoA at the end of 2010. At the request of the General Medical Council, a primary specialty program for ICM was developed by January 2011, and runs in parallel with dual certification [34]. Another option for advanced training is pediatric ICM. In the UK, 80% of consultants leading adult ICUs are anesthetists by primary training [2]. The standard curriculum for anesthesia incorporates basic and intermediate training in ICM.

France

The first French ICUs opened in 1954, rapidly following the lead taken by Denmark. In the 1950s, ICM (réanimation) also became part of the practice of, and education in, anesthesia. Today, the training program for anesthesia-ICM includes 18 months practical training in ICM. Anesthetists, surgeons, internists, cardiologists, and neurologists can obtain an additional certificate (DESC) in non-surgical ICM (réanimation médicale). This requires 3 years of training beyond that for the base specialty.

Scandinavia

As seen in Table 38.1, Scandinavian training programs in anesthesiology include ICM training of 6-12-months duration [8]. In addition, the Scandinavian Society of Anaesthesiology and Intensive Care Medicine (SSAI) initiated a 2-year Scandinavian training program in ICM, in 1998.

Germany

The anesthesiology curriculum has included training and experience in ICM since 1968. A minimum training period of 6 months was introduced in 1979. In 1992 this increased to

12 months, and a multidisciplinary approach to ICM was officially established, i.e. supplementary training in specialty-related ICM was introduced for anesthesiology, surgery and its branches, internal medicine, pediatrics, neurosurgery and neurology. Training lasted 24 months, of which 12 months (anesthesiology) or 6 months (other specialties) could be set against training time in the base specialty [35].

Emergency Medicine

In the 1960s, many European anesthesiologists increasingly focused on emergency medicine. They took leading roles in cardiopulmonary resuscitation and formed physician-equipped ambulances providing a pre-hospital rescue service for critically ill patients – emergency medical services (EMS). Consequently, the German, Swiss and Austrian Societies of Anaesthesiology added "Reanimation" to their names in 1965, 1967 and 1972, respectively (in German, reanimation denotes resuscitation whereas it stands for ICM in the Romance languages). In the 1980s and later, several countries introduced supra-specialty qualifications. In 1984, a Certificate of Qualification in EMS in Germany could be acquired even before completion of specialization. The requirements were 12 months (later 18 months) of clinical training, 80 h of theoretical courses and 10 practical pre-hospital experiences as a supervised EMS physician. From 2003, mandated training increased to 24 months, and the number of pre-hospital supervised experiences to 50. The diploma became the Certificate in Emergency Medicine [36, 37]. In 2000, the Swiss Medical Association introduced a Certificate as an Emergency Physician, and a Certificate in Clinical Emergency Medicine was added in 2009 [25]. In France, an additional certificate (DESC) in emergency medicine could be obtained by anesthetists, surgeons, internists, and pediatricians. It required 2 years of training beyond that for the base specialty [38]. These specialists control both the pre-hospital EMS (SMUR, Service Mobile d'Urgence et de Réanimation) and the emergency departments in hospitals. Belgian anesthesiologists and other specialists could obtain a supplementary certificate in emergency medicine after an additional training of 1 to 2 years. A separate specialty status replaced this in 2005. For Scandinavian anesthesiologists, the Scandinavian Society of Anaesthesiology and Intensive Care Medicine (SSAI) offers a two-year masters course in advanced emergency medicine [8].

In the UK, a new specialty, Accident and Emergency Medicine, developed from casualty surgery in the 1970s, but never became part of anesthesia training. In 1991, an Intercollegiate Board in Accident and Emergency Medicine was established with representation from 8 Colleges and the British Association for Accident & Emergency Medicine [38].

Before this, a training program was available to those who had completed their specialization and the additional training lasted for 3 to 4 years. In 1993, the Board became the Intercollegiate Faculty and, in 2006, the College of Emergency Medicine. The minimum duration of specialist training in emergency medicine is now 6 years.

Pain Medicine

From the early 1970s, their expertise in treating acute postoperative pain drew anesthetists into pain therapy, and most European countries incorporated pain therapy into the core curriculum in anesthesiology [39]. Some countries established 1 to 2 year training programs in pain medicine, as a multidisciplinary supra-specialty. In Switzerland, an applicant must attend a given set of lectures and courses and perform a minimum number of interventions under supervision. In 2001, the SSAI opened a Nordic Education in Advanced Pain Medicine to its members, with training lasting 2 years [8, 40]. In the UK, the RCoA defines pain management as a special interest area for advanced training. Trainees in anesthesia may apply for a 6 to 12 month advanced training course in pain management. Within the RCoA, the Faculty of Pain Medicine was established in April 2007, replacing the previous Pain Management Committee. Doctors starting their Advanced Pain Training (APT) from 2011, are required to take the Fellowship of the Faculty of Pain Medicine of the RCoA examination, in addition to achieving the competencies of their APT.

Subspecialties of Anesthesia

Formal training programs in subspecialties such as cardiac/thoracic, pediatric, obstetric or neurosurgical anesthesia, are uncommon in Europe. The core curriculum includes these as it does acute pain therapy, management of chronic and malignant pain, emergency medicine and trauma care, ACLS training, and last but not least, ICM. Scandinavian anesthesiologists who recently obtained their specialist diploma in anesthesiology and intensive care can apply for the advanced Inter-Nordic education program in Paediatric Anaesthesia and Intensive Care, which is coordinated by the SSAI and lasts 12 months [8, 41]. In the curriculum organized and supervised by the RCoA, cardiac/thoracic, obstetric, pediatric anesthesia and neuroanesthesia are defined as special interest areas for advanced training, each lasting 6-12 months. However, the opportunity for trainees to gain such expertise depends on the availability of training posts in teaching hospitals, and the perceived demand for consultants trained in these fields.

Undergraduate Teaching

In most European countries, education of medical students in anesthesia began in the 1950s, when anesthetists first obtained posts as specialists and developed Anesthesia Divisions in University Departments of Surgery. In subsequent decades, university anesthesiologists increasingly committed themselves to the education and examination of students. Whether a student's surgical training included anesthesiology or whether anesthesiology was separated from surgical training varied, and still does, among European countries. National societies and their leading members increasingly appreciated the correlation of the quality of undergraduate teaching and the choice of anesthesiology as a professional career [8, 42, 43]. Some National Societies took special measures to familiarize medical students with anesthesiology and its various facets, e.g. the German Professional Association of Anaesthetists set up a website and a summer school for students and a "road show" at teaching hospitals. Based on the experience that courses in advanced life support using full-scale simulators proved particularly attractive to students if given by anesthesiologists, the German Society of Anaesthesiology and Intensive Care Medicine enabled 30 University Departments in 2003 to purchase full-scale anesthesia simulators for use in undergraduate teaching [44].

Continuing Medical Education (CME)

CME in anesthesiology developed simultaneously in most European countries and in some, evolved into Continuing Professional Development (CPD). Since 1990, about 60 % of European countries require a given number of annual credits as a prerequisite for recertification. In most countries, national Medical Associations and national Societies of Anesthesiology jointly organize and control CME activities. In the UK, the RCoA developed guidelines for CPD based on a so-called CPD matrix, specifying the knowledge and skill areas needed for revalidation (recertification). In France, the CME concept recently evolved into an evaluation of professional practices (EPP), integrated into a compulsory CPD system for all healthcare workers. For this purpose, in 1994, the scientific and professional associations of anesthesia formed the French College of Anaesthetists and Intensive Care Providers (CFAR, Collège Français des Anesthésistes Réanimateurs).

Harmonizing Education in Europe

The diverse systems of European medical education reflect European heterogeneity in history, language, political, legal, economic, and medical systems. In 1957, six countries signed the Treaty of Rome, creating the European Economic Community (EEC), which subsequently developed into today's European Union (EU) with 27 member states out of 47 European countries. The protracted and continuing process of harmonizing medical education will be described below, beginning with a description of the professional bodies guiding this development.

The European Union of Medical Specialists (UEMS) and the European Board of Anaesthesiology (EBA)

One year after the signing of the Treaty of Rome, medical specialists from the six member countries formed the UEMS (Union Européenne des Médecins Spécialistes) to serve as a source of discussion and consultation for EEC legislation [45–47]. Today the UEMS is the umbrella organization of the national associations of medical specialists of the 27 EU member states, together with 2 non-member states, Norway and Switzerland. Non-EU states can join as observers (Fig. 38.2). In 1962, the UEMS created the first Specialist Sections to offer expert advice to the EEC Commission. Representatives from the six initial member countries constituting the Section of Anaesthesiology, held their first meeting in September 1962. At that time, training in anesthesiology in these six countries ranged from 2 to 7 years. In 1963, the Section stipulated 3 years as the minimum period of training. In 1969, a re-assessment of training requirements for all EEC countries, including those about to join, again showed that training varied from 3 to 7 years. In 1969, the Section agreed on a minimum training period of 4 years, and in 1980 proposed a 5 year minimum period [48, 49]. In 1973, the periods of training still varied between 3 and 7 years in EEC countries, and between 2 and 6 years in non-EEC countries [47].

The Specialist Sections of the UEMS acted to harmonize specialist training, and proposed criteria that might allow the mutual recognition of specialists. These were established by "Doctors Directives" 75/362/EEC and 75/363/EEC in 1975, and were updated in 1993 by Directive 93/16/EC, which included requirements for recognizing training institutions and a minimum duration of training. In Directives 2005/36/EC and 2006/100/EC regulating the recognition of professional qualifications, anesthetics is named as one of the medical specialties with a minimum period of training of only 3 years, contrary to the proposal made by the Section of Anaesthesiology and endorsed by the Council of the UEMS.

Chapter 6 of the 1993 UEMS Charter on the Training of Medical Specialists stipulated individual input from each specialty. Accordingly, the Sections formed educational boards. Initially a separate European Board of Anaesthesiology (EBA) was formed. The Section and Board soon coalesced, with Section members normally also being Board members [46]. Two delegates represented each country in

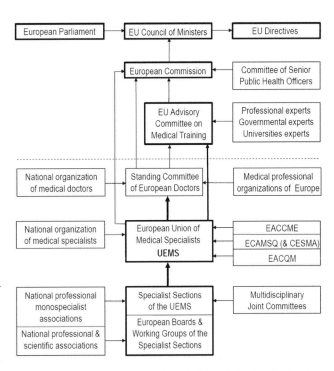

Fig. 38.2 The European Union of Medical Specialists (UEMS) and associated organizations are separated from the governing European political and professional structures (upper boxes) by the broken horizontal line. EU = European Union; EACCME = European Accreditation Council for Continuing Medical Education; ECAMSQ = European Council for Accreditation of Medical Specialist Qualification; CESMA = Council for European Specialist Assessment; EACQM = European Advisory Council for Quality Management of Specialist Medical Practice

the Section and on the Board. In 1993, the Section adopted requirements for the Specialty of Anaesthesiology and incorporated these in Chapter 6 of the Charter in May 1995. The Charter defined the tasks of the Board and confirmed it as the EU monitoring authority of the specialty [46].

The principal aims of the EBA, and procedures undertaken to achieve these were:

The publication of training guidelines in anesthesia, in booklet form in 1996, with revisions in 2001, 2008 and 2011 [50–52]. These produced changes, moving training programs in European countries, particularly in Eastern Europe, towards harmonization. In all versions, 5 years was recommended as the minimum duration of training.

Three guidelines were published in 2007: Directions for a core curriculum in emergency medicine integrated in the specialty of anesthesiology [53]; Guidelines for anesthesiologist specialist training in pain medicine [54]; and Guidelines for safety and quality of anesthesia practice in the European Union [55].

EBA endorsement of the examination for the European Diploma in Anaesthesiology and Intensive Care Medicine (EDA) of the European Academy of Anaesthesiology (EAA). In an editorial published in 2010, recommendations were made for trainee evaluation and assessment in Europe [56].

The Joint Hospital Visiting and Accreditation Programme of the EBA and EAA.

Medical specialties failing to fulfill given criteria were not listed as independent in the EU Directives on the recognition of professional qualifications (2005/36/EC and 2006/100/EC). They therefore could not form UEMS Specialist Sections and Boards. To overcome this problem, the Council of the UEMS was permitted to ask one or more Sections to create a Multidisciplinary Joint Committee (MJC) for defining competences or spheres of activity associated with several specialties. MJCs with active participation of the Section of Anaesthesiology were created for Intensive Care Medicine (MJCICM), Emergency Medicine (MJCEM), and Pain Medicine (MJCPM).

Based on its 1994 Charter on CME, in 1998 the UEMS Council developed a system for the exchange of CME credits at European level for countries recognizing credit points. For this purpose, the European Accreditation Council for CME (EACCME) was created one year later, becoming operational in 2000. UEMS/EACCME and several national accreditation authorities as well as the American Medical Association signed agreements on mutual recognition of credits. The EBA published guidelines on CME/CPD in 2007 [57].

To harmonize the assessment process in Europe, 11 Sections already conducting a European examination convened in 2007, and founded a Council for European Specialist Assessment (CESMA) with active participation of the Section of Anaesthesiology. They proposed the "Glasgow Declaration" on the significance and conditions of European Board Examinations.

A major challenge to the UEMS will be the revision of the EU Directive on Mutual Recognition of Professional Qualifications (Directive 2005/36/EC), which is expected in 2013. This revision will do the following:

Update the list of specialties recognized in the EU.

Update the content and length of training. This is of utmost importance for anesthesiology since in the Directive 2005/36/EC currently in force, the minimum duration of training is still 3 years despite the minimum of 5 years recommended in the 1996–2011 EBA guidelines [50–52].

Introduce the concept of "Particular Competencies" in intensive care and other specialties instead of defining them as independent specialties [58].

The European Academy of Anaesthesiology (EAA)

The EAA was founded in Paris in September 1978. Its main educational activities were to grant the European Diploma in Anaesthesiology and Intensive Care (EDA) and support the EAA/EBA Joint Hospital Visiting Programme (HVP). The latter role was to ensure that academic institutions met the criteria for teaching and training anesthesiologists in Europe, expressed in the training guidelines of the EBA [49, 59]. The

EDA was established in 1984 as an annual two part multi-lingual postgraduate (end-of-training) Diploma examination. Part I was a written multiple choice examination which European medical graduates could take even before training in anesthesia commenced. Eligibility for the Part II (final) examination required that candidates pass the Part I examination, complete 6 years of medical practice, including 4 years of training in anesthesia. They had to be eligible for specialist registration in a European country. The latter criterion was later modified insofar as candidates had to be certified anesthesiologists in any country, or trainees in the final year of training in anesthesiology in a European member state of the WHO. Part II consisted of four 30-minute oral examinations, each with a different pair of examiners. Successful candidates became Diplomates of the European Academy of Anaesthesiology (DEAA). Initially, this title was not officially recognized and was simply one of distinction. The Diploma neither replaced national specialist accreditation nor conferred the right to practice in another country.

In Switzerland, the EDA Part I examination became mandatory for all trainees in 1987, but the final (oral) examination remained in the hands of the National Society (SSAR). Malta accepted the European Diploma as a criterion for specialist status. From 1990, in a reciprocal agreement with the RCoA, those holding the EDA were exempt from passing the Primary FRCA when applying for the Final FRCA and those holding the FRCA were exempt from sitting the Part I EDA. In addition to the EDA examination, the EAA introduced an In-Training Assessment (ITA), which took place simultaneously and used the same multiple choice questions as the Part I Diploma examination. The ITA could be held in every European training centre accredited by the EEA examination committee [9].

In 1989, the EAA created a voluntary Hospital Recognition Programme. Although not accepted by the UEMS, it was supported and recommended by the Specialist Section of Anaesthesiology [49]. In 1996, it became the Hospital Visiting Programme (HVP) administered by a permanent Joint Committee of the EBA and the EAA. This program was mainly intended for training centers in countries without a national hospital visiting and accreditation program [59].

The European Society of Anaesthesiology (ESA)

The EAA limited the number of its members and was frequently regarded as a "closed" organization. To provide a broader forum, the European Society of Anaesthesiologists was formed in 1992, and was open to all practicing anesthesiologists. A parallel organization, the Confederation of European National Societies of Anaesthesiology (CENSA), evolved from the former European Regional Section of the World Federation of Societies of Anaesthesiologists. The

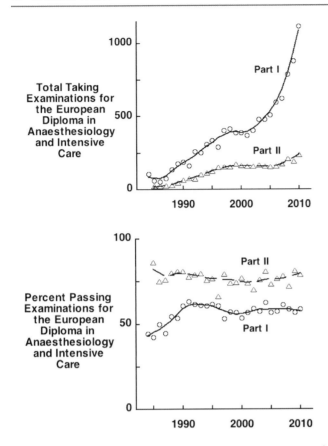

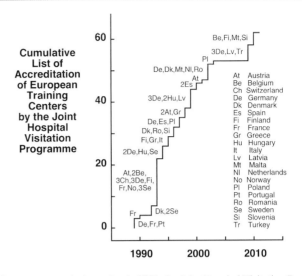

Fig. 38.4 From its inception in 1989, the Joint Hospital Visitation Program has accredited 62 European training centers

Fig. 38.3 Annual number of candidates sitting for Part I (written) and Part II (oral) Examinations for the European Diploma in Anaesthesiology and Intensive Care Medicine increased from 1984 to 2010 (*upper* graphs), whilst the percent passing each examination remained roughly constant at 60 % for Part I and 75 % for Part II (*lower* graphs)

complementary and partially overlapping nature of these three bodies led to an amalgamation which was realized in January 2005, by the formation of the "new" European Society of Anaesthesiology (ESA). CENSA became the National Anaesthesia Societies Committee (NASC) of the ESA. All activities of the combined organizations continued in the "new" ESA.

The Examinations Committee of the ESA governs the conduct of the EDA examination. New and past Diplomas have equal value. The title of Diplomate changed from DEAA to DESA. Candidates sitting the Part I and II examinations have steadily increased in numbers (Fig. 38.3). The Glasgow Declaration of the CESMA was approved by the Board of Directors and Examination Committee of the ESA and supported by the EBA. Article 6 of this document makes candidates of any nationality, i.e. also non-European nationals, eligible to sit European Board Examinations, and the EDA eligibility criteria had to be adapted accordingly. Article 7 allows candidates who pass a European Board Examination and who are certified specialists, to call themselves Fellows of the respective Board. This complies with a request made by the Section and Board of Anaesthesiology to the Council

of the UEMS in 2002 [60]. The EBA, with support of the ESA, prepared criteria for Membership and Fellowship that included more than just being a Diplomate: candidates must have been admitted to the Specialist Anesthesiology Register of a European member state, have been in clinical practice for 5 years, and have fulfilled the national or future European requirements for CME/CPD in the preceding 5 years. Implementation is scheduled for 2013. In 2007, Hungary joined Switzerland, in making the EDA Part I examination mandatory. In 2008, Romania and Poland followed suit [31], as did Slovenia and Turkey in 2009, and Austria in 2010. In February 2009, the Austrian Medical Chamber recognized the EDA Part II examination as equivalent to the Austrian national final examination in Anaesthesiology.

The Joint Hospital Visiting Programme of the EBA and EAA continued as the Hospital Visiting and Training Accreditation Programme (HVTAP), organized and supervised by a Joint Committee of EBA and ESA. It is offered on a voluntary basis to academic departments of anesthesia that apply for teaching accreditation, in accordance with European training guidelines. Figure 38.4 shows the cumulative number of training centers accredited since the program's inception.

In 1986, Johan Spierdijk (Netherlands), Philippe Scherpereel (France), George Rolly, Guillaume Hanegreefs and Maurice Lamy (all Belgium) founded the Foundation for European Education in Anaesthesiology (FEEA, Fondation Européenne d'Enseignement en Anesthésiologie). Initially, the FEEA aimed to provide CME in anesthesiology within the European Community by organizing refresher courses. Growth in the number of member countries progressively extended the area of activity of the FEEA, especially into Eastern Europe [61]. Since 1995, the FEEA also established educational centers outside Europe. In

January 2009, the ESA formally assumed the FEEA's activities with the creation of the CEEA (Committee for European Education in Anaesthesiology). The CME program of CEEA is based upon a cycle of six courses, and is accredited in Europe by the national systems of accreditation and the EACCME [62].

Subspecialties of Anesthesiology from the European Perspective

In most European countries, ICM, emergency medicine both inside and outside hospital, acute and chronic pain treatment, and palliative care, are considered special and essential areas of expertise in anesthesiology [8]. Note however, that ICM, critical care and pain medicine are not sub-specialties attainable exclusively by anesthesiologists, rather they are supra-specialties accessible from different base specialties including anesthesiology, surgery, and internal medicine.

Intensive Care Medicine

The European Society of Intensive Care Medicine (ESICM) was founded in March 1982, and created the European Diploma in Intensive Care (EDIC) in 1988. This became widely accepted and, according to a web-based survey published in 2009, was used by 10 European countries, with a mandatory exit examination [58]. The CoBaTrICE (*Competency-Based Training in Intensive Care medicinE*) collaboration was formed by the ESICM in 2003 to develop an internationally acceptable competency-based training program in ICM, and harmonize training standards across national borders [58].

As a multidisciplinary medical specialty, ICM could not be represented in the UEMS by a specialist section. Therefore a Multidisciplinary Joint Committee of Intensive Care Medicine (MJCICM) was established within the UEMS in 1999, with representation by delegates from 9 Sections, including anesthesiology. Delegates without voting rights represented the ESICM and the European Society of Paediatric and Neonatal Intensive Care. The MJCICM endorsed the EDIC, created an Intensive Care Unit Accreditation Visiting Programme in 2001, and published guidelines on structure, organization and training in 2002 [63]. To harmonize ICM training across Europe, the UEMS created a specialty Board for ICM (EBICM) in 2006, with representatives drawn equally from the MJCICM and from the ESICM, thus ensuring representation for the various national models of training. In April 2008, the Council of the UEMS supported the proposals made by the Chairmen of the MJCICM and EBICM, that ICM should be included in the revised version of Directive 2005/36/EC on the recognition of professional qualifications, as a particular medical competence/qualification. The

Council advised that the training content should be defined and managed through CoBaTrICE collaboration and monitored by the EBICM [33, 58].

Emergency Medicine

Currently, 15 members of the European Union (nine listed in EU Directive 2005/36/EC) recognize emergency medicine as an independent specialty. It is not yet a Specialist Section of the UEMS but, like ICM, it has been represented by a Multidisciplinary Joint Committee (MJCEM) since 2005. The MJCEM adopted a comprehensive Core Curriculum in Emergency Medicine, which the UEMS Council formally endorsed in April 2010. EU Directive 2005/36/EC sets European specialty training in emergency medicine at a minimum of 5 years of full-time training as a primary medical specialty. Within the 5 years, at least 3 must be spent in an Emergency Department accredited for training [64]. In October 2010, the Council of the UEMS agreed that the MJCEM and the European Society for Emergency Medicine should jointly form a European Board of Emergency Medicine.

Pain Medicine

Established in 1993, the European Federation of IASP Chapters (EFIC) is a multidisciplinary professional organization in the field of pain science and medicine, composed of the 30 European Chapters of the International Association for the Study of Pain (IASP). The EFIC aims to create a framework for European training and certification standards in pain medicine, including a core curriculum and subspecialty training. The typical duration of such a training program would be 2 years. At UEMS level, a MJC on Pain Medicine was established in April 2012.

Additional Competencies

The Federation of European Associations of Paediatric Anaesthesia (FEAPA) has developed guidelines for training, including the recommendation that all anesthetic trainees complete a minimum of 3 months of continuous training in pediatric anesthesia, regardless of their intended specialization [65].

Certification in transesophageal echocardiography (TEE) is a joint initiative, begun in 2005, between the European Association of Cardiothoracic Anaesthesiologists (EACTA) and the European Association of Echocardiography (EAE).

In 2006, the European Society of Regional Anaesthesia & Pain Therapy (ESRA) launched the European Diploma in Regional Anaesthesia & Pain Therapy, which certifies clinicians involved in regional anesthesia who achieve a uniformly high standard of knowledge. The Diploma is awarded to candidates who have passed a two-part examination.

Non-physician Anesthesia Team Members; Workload and Working Time

In Europe, responsibility for anesthetic services lies with trained physician anesthesiologists who may delegate anesthesia delivery to non-physician members of the anesthesia team. The degree of delegation varies enormously among countries, but independent delivery of anesthesia by nurse anesthetists is not allowed in any European country. Basic education, training, certification, roles, tasks and responsibilities of non-physician anesthetists differ due to the diversity in the historical development of health care systems in general, and anesthesia services in particular [66]. A recent study identified 4 models of non-physician anesthesia personnel: nurse anesthetists, circulating nurses, anesthesia technicians, and anesthesia physician assistants [67]. This paper describes the ways in which nationally certified nurse anesthetists can work alongside and under the responsibility of anesthesiologists. In most countries, they assist the anesthesiologist in giving anesthesia. In Denmark, France, Netherlands, Norway, Sweden, and Switzerland, nurse anesthetists perform both nursing and a delegated anesthesia practice. The number of nurse anesthetists equals 100 to 160 % of the number of anesthesiologists including residents, or between 105 % and 205 % without residents [67]. These numbers differ to some extent from those reported in a paper published 3 years earlier (45 to 230 % when residents are included and 50 to 320 % when they are not) [68]. Either way, nurse anesthetists clearly contribute substantially to patient care.

Reliable data on the contribution of each group to the provision of anesthesia in the decades after World War II are not available. Since few anesthesiologists practiced in European countries in the 1950s and 1960s, it is reasonable to assume that during that period nurses gave far more anesthetics than did doctors, the former nominally working under the supervision of the surgeon. Formal educational programs for nurse anesthetists were established after 1960 (1960 in France, 1962 in Sweden, 1963 in Finland, 1964 in Germany, 1965 in Norway, 1966 in The Netherlands, 1969 in Switzerland). From 1970 to 1990, the number of anesthesiologists increased to such an extent that virtually all non-physician anesthesia providers worked under the supervision of a certified anesthesiologist [66].

Although standardization of training and practice of nurse anesthetists or other anesthesia team members in Europe do not currently exist, such standards are becoming increasingly likely and necessary, given the existing or impending shortfall in numbers of anesthesiologists [69]. Escalating eco-

nomic constraints, increasing workload, growing demand for anesthetic care, demographic factors and inappropriate political decisions (e.g. too few places to study medicine or too few training positions in anesthesiology) underlie the likelihood of this impending shortfall [8, 68, 70−72]. However, it must not be taken for granted that sufficient numbers of nurse anesthetists will be available to compensate for a shortfall in anesthesiologists, because a lack of young doctors as well as nursing personnel, is becoming apparent in many countries.

Directive 2000/34/EC of the European Parliament and of the Council of June 2000, the so-called European Working Time Directive (EWTD) increases the need to train sufficient numbers of competent anesthesiologists. This limited the average working time for each 7-day period, including overtime, to 48 h (with a transitional period of 5 years from August 2004, for doctors in training). The effect of the EWTD on length and quality of training is not yet clear [73−75], but decreasing working time of trainees is a driving factor behind the replacement of the classical experience-based education of anesthesiologists by competency-based training programs [52, 56, 58].

Conclusion

Before 1945, anesthesia was not recognized as an independent medical specialty in Europe, due to the opposition from surgeons and the isolation of Europe during World War II. Influenced by developments in the US and the UK, modern anesthetic practice began in Europe after World War II ended. The growth of training programs between 1947 and 1958 supplied the basis for de facto or official recognition of anesthesiology as a separate, independent medical specialty. Not surprisingly, countries differed markedly in the clinical responsibilities of anesthesiologists and the content, quality and length of training. The principles of free movement of people, goods, services and capital underlying today's European Union of 27 Member States, stimulated efforts to harmonize the quality of anesthetic care and education. In the past 2 decades, this has enabled the mutual recognition of medical qualifications. The quality and uniformity of anesthesiology care and education has increased in Europe, not by lowering high standards, but by raising low ones, at first in the countries of Western Europe and then, following the dissolution of the Eastern bloc and the Soviet Union in 1989–1991, in most of the newly independent states of Eastern Europe.

Acknowledgments Large parts of this article could not be obtained from published literature and are based on information and support that we gratefully received from physician colleagues, including Iurie Acalovschi (Romania), Seppo Alahuhta (Finland), Helen Askitopoulou (Greece), Armen Bunatian (Russia), Lennart Christiansson (Sweden),

Karl Cvachovec (Czech Republic), Leon Drobnik (Poland), Sylvia Fitzal (Austria), Fernando Gilsanz (Spain), Slobodan Gligorijevic (Switzerland), Carmen Gomar (Spain), Jean-Pierre Haberer (France), Juozas Ivaskevicius (Lithuania), Hans Knape (The Netherlands), Krzysztof Kusza (Poland), Konstantin Lebedinskiy (Russia), Werner List (Austria), Jannicke Mellin-Olsen (Norway), Miodrag Milenovic (Serbia), Vesna Novak-Jankovič (Slovenia), Klaus Olkkola (Finland), Jean-Claude Otteni (France), Flavia Petrini (Italy), Indrek Rätsep (Estonia), Şükran Şahin (Turkey), Philippe Scherpereel (France), Olav Sellevold (Norway), Ivan Smilov (Bulgaria), Antonina Sondore (Latvia), Alan Šustić (Croatia), Stefan Trenkler (Slovakia), Hugo Van Aken (Germany), Elisabeth van Gessel (Switzerland), Eugene Vandermeersch (Belgium), Jørgen Viby-Mogensen (Denmark), Lars Wiklund (Sweden) and David Wilkinson (UK).

References[1]

1. Atkinson RS. Faculty of Anaesthetists, Royal College of Surgeons of England. The History of Anaesthesia. Edited by Atkinson RS, Boulton TB. London New York, Royal Society of Medicine Services, 1989, pp 162–3.
2. Boulton TB. The Association of Anaesthetists of Great Britain and Ireland 1942–1992 and The Development of the Specialty of Anaesthesia. London, The Association of Anaesthetists of Great Britain and Ireland, 1999.
3. Sykes K, Bunker J. Anaesthesia and the Practice of Medicine: Historical Perspectives. London, Royal Society of Medicine Press, 2007, pp 53, 87–8, 160–80.
4. Zuck D. The development of professional organizations in anaesthesia. Curr Anaesth Crit Care. 2000;11:141–9.
5. Adams AK. The foundation of the Faculty of Anaesthetists of the Royal College of Surgeons of England, The History of Anesthesia. Edited by Fink BR, Morris LE, Stephen CR. Park Ridge, Wood Library-Museum of Anesthesiology, 1992, pp 1–4.
6. Cousin MT. L'anesthésie-réanimation en France. Des origines à 1965. Tome I : Anesthésie. Tome II : Réanimation. Les nouveaux professionnels. Paris:L'Harmattan, 2005.
7. Gordh T Sr. How anaesthesiology came to Sweden. Acta Anaesthesiol Scand. 1998;42(Suppl 113):34–8.
8. Søreide E, Kalman S, Åneman A, Nørregaard O, Pere P, Mellin-Olsen J. Shaping the future of Scandinavian anaesthesiology: a position paper by the SSAI. Acta Anaesthesiol Scand. 2010;54:1062–70.
9. Zorab JS. The European Diploma in Anaesthesiology and Intensive Care of the European Academy of Anaesthesiology. Acta Anaesthesiol Scand 1995;39:579–81.
10. Rosenberg H, Axelrod JK. Ernst Trier Mørch: inventor, medical pioneer, heroic freedom fighter. Anesth Analg 2000;90:218–21
11. Haxholdt BF, Secher O. The twenty-fifth anniversary of the Danish Society of Anaesthesiology. Acta Anaesthesiol Scand. 1975;19:324–9.
12. Ringsted C, Østergaard D, van der Vleuten CP. Implementation of a formal in-training assessment programme in anaesthesiology and preliminary results of acceptability. Acta Anaesthesiol Scand. 2003;47:1196–203.
13. Secher O. Anaesthesiology Centre Copenhagen, Anaesthesia – Essays on Its History. Edited by Rupreht J, van Lieburg MJ, Lee JA, Ermann W. Berlin, Springer, 1985, pp 321–34.
14. Berthelsen PG, Cronqvist M. The first intensive care unit in the world: Copenhagen 1953. Acta Anaesthesiol Scand. 2003;47:1190–5.
15. Jørgensen B. The Norwegian Association of Anaesthesiologists—25 years. Acta Anaesthesiol Scand. 1975;19:341–3.
16. Jahunen L. On the activities of the Finnish Society of Anaesthesiologists 1952–1974. Acta Anaesthesiol Scand. 1975;19:330–5.
17. Rügheimer E, Schwarz W. Anesthesia training in West Germany. J Clin Anesth. 1991;3:249–52.
18. Brandt L, Goerig M. A short history of the German Society of Anaesthesiology and Intensive Care Medicine (DGAI). Anästhesiol Intensivmed Notfallmed Schmerzther. 2003;38:215–25 (German).
19. Petermann H. American influences on the development of anesthesiology in the Federal Republic of Germany between 1949 and 1960. Anästhesiol Intensivmed Notfallmed Schmerzther. 2005;40:133–41 (German).
20. Zeitlin GL, Goerig M. An American contribution to German anesthesia. Anesthesiology. 2003;99:496–502.
21. Schulte am Esch J, Goerig M, Agarwal K. Development of anaesthesia after 1945, 55 Years German Society of Anaesthesiology and Intensive Care Medicine. Edited by Schüttler J. Berlin, Springer, 2012, pp 116–46.
22. Fitzal S, Mayrhofer-Krammel O. A short history of the Austrian Society of Anaesthesiology, Resuscitation and Intensive Care Medicine (ÖGARI). Anästhesiol Intensivmed Notfallmed Schmerzther. 2003;38:226–30 (German).
23. Fitzal S. The Austrian specialist examination for anaesthesiology and intensive care medicine. Basic structure and experiences. Anaesthesist. 2005;54:808–15 (German).
24. Pasch T, Hossli G. A short history of the Swiss Society of Anaesthesiology and Resuscitation (SGAR). Anästhesiol Intensivmed Notfallmed Schmerzther. 2003;38:231–6 (German).
25. Pasch T, Zalunardo MP, Orlow P, Siegrist M, Giger M. Postgraduate specialist training in anaesthesiology in Switzerland. Anästh Intensivmed. 2008;49:270–80 (German).
26. Crul JF. The role of anesthesiology in the health care system of the Netherlands. J Clin Anesth. 1994;6:342–8.
27. Reinhold H. Anaesthesia in Belgium. J Roy Soc Med. 1978;71:770.
28. Pantaleoni M. The development of modern anaesthesia in Italy, Anaesthesia—Essays on Its History. Edited by Rupreht J, van Lieburg MJ, Lee JA, Ermann W. Berlin, Springer, 1985, pp. 242–52.
29. Lagunilla J, Diz JC, Franco A, Alvarez J. Changes in the social position of anaesthesiologists in the 19th and 20th centuries, The History of Anesthesia. Edited by Diz JC, Franco A, Bacon DR, Rupreht J, Alvarez J. Amsterdam, Elsevier, 2002, pp. 337–42.
30. Drobnik L. Looking beyond the own backyard – experiences with postgraduate education in Europe: anaesthesiology in Poland. Anästh Intensivmed. 2008;49:32–7 (German).
31. Kusza K, Goldik Z. Adoption of the European Diploma in Anaesthesiology as the National Board examination in anaesthesiology and intensive care: 2 year of experience in Poland. Br J Anaesth. 2011;106:148–9.
32. Barrett H, Bion JF. An international survey of training in adult intensive care medicine. Intensive Care Med. 2005;31:553–61.
33. Van Aken H, Mellin-Olsen J, Pelosi P. Intensive care medicine: a multidisciplinary approach. Eur J Anaesthesiol. 2011;28:313–5.
34. Nightingale P. Development of the faculty of intensive care medicine. Br J Anaesth. 2011;107:5–7.
35. Burchardi H. Regulations of education and training of intensive care medicine in Germany and their structural consequences. Intensive Care Med. 2005;31:589–90.
36. Dick W. Anglo-American vs. Franco-German emergency medical services systems. Prehosp Disast Med. 2003;18:29–37.
37. Reifferscheid F, Harding U, Dörges V, Knacke P, Wirtz S. Implementation of a specialist qualification in emergency medicine – do we have uniform requirements in Germany? Anästh Intensivmed. 2010;51:82–9 (German).
38. Yates DW. Education in emergency medicine. Ballière's Clin Anaesthesiol. 1992;6(1):161–75.

---

[1] The reader is also directed to the websites maintained by the national and European associations and societies mentioned in this article.

39. Breivik H. The future role of the anaesthesiologist in pain management. Acta Anaesthesiol Scand. 2005;49:922–6.

40. Breivik H, Lindahl SGE. Training programme in advanced pain medicine for Nordic anaesthesiologists. Acta Anaesthesiol Scand. 2001;45:1191–2.

41. Hansen TG. Specialist training in pediatric anesthesia – the Scandinavian approach. Pediatr Anesth. 2009;19:428–33.

42. Chaulier K, Ber CE, Allaouchiche B, Rimmelé T. Does the second cycle of French medical studies prepare students to be future anesthesiologists and intensivists? Ann Fr Anesth Reanim. 2010;29:536–42 (French).

43. Welker A, Baumgart A, Baja J, Schröpl K, Schleppers A. Professional profile of the anaesthetist—A qualitative and quantitative poll among students on the attractiveness of our specialty. Anästh Intensivmed. 2010;51:318–27 (German).

44. Schüttler J. Successful start of the DGAI project of optimizing undergraduate teaching by means of anaesthesia and emergency simulators. Anästh Intensivmed. 2004;45:381 (German).

45. Scherpereel P. The European Union of Medical Specialists (U.E.M.S.) and the European Board of Anaesthesiologists (E.B.A.). Acta Anaesthesiol Scand. 1995;39:438–9.

46. De Lange S. The European Union of Medical Specialists and speciality training. Eur J Anaesthesiol. 2001;18:561–2.

47. Hovat DDC. The European scene. The European Economic Community (EEC). Anaesthesia. 1974;29:211–21.

48. Howat DDC, Reinhold H. The Section of Anaesthesia and Intensive Care of the European Union of Medical Specialists and its contribution to the professional status of anaesthesiology in the European Economic Community, Anaesthesia – Essays on Its History. Edited by Rupreht J, van Lieburg MJ, Lee JA, Erdmann W. Berlin, Springer, 1985, pp 335–9.

49. Zorab JSM, Vickers MD. The European Academy of Anaesthesiology—and beyond. J Roy Soc Med. 1991. 1992;84:704–8.

50. European Board of Anaesthesiology. Training guidelines in anaesthesia of the European Board of Anaesthesiology Reanimation and Intensive Care. Eur J Anaesthesiol. 2001;18:563–71.

51. Carlsson C, Keld D, Gessel E van, Fee JPH, Van Aken H, Simpson P. Education and training in anaesthesia—revised guidelines by the European Board of Anaesthesiology, Reanimation and Intensive Care. Eur J Anaesthesiol. 2008;25:528–30.

52. Van Gessel E, Mellin-Olsen J, Østergaard HT, Niemi-Murola L, for the Education and Training Standing Committee of the European Board of Anaesthesiology, Reanimation and Intensive Care. Postgraduate training in anaesthesiology, pain and intensive care: the new European competence-based guidelines. Eur J Anaesthesiol. 2012;29:165–8.

53. De Robertis E, McAdoo J, Pagni R, Knape JTA. Core curriculum in emergency medicine integrated in the specialty of anaesthesiology. Eur J Anaesthesiol. 2007;24:987–90.

54. Cunningham AJ, Knape JTA, Adriaensen H, Blunnie WP, Buchser E, Goldik Z, Ilias W, Parver-Erzen V. Guidelines for anaesthesiologist specialist training in pain medicine. Eur J Anaesthesiol. 2007;24:568–70.

55. Mellin-Olsen J, Sullivan EO, Balogh D, Drobnik L, Knape JTA, Petrini F, Vimlati L. Guidelines for safety and quality in anaesthesia practice in the European Union. Eur J Anaesthesiol. 2007;24:479–82.

56. Van Gessel E, Goldik Z, Mellin-Olsen J, for the Education, Training Standing Committee of the European Board of Anaesthesiology, Reanimation, Intensive Care. Postgraduate training in anaesthesiology, resuscitation and intensive care: state-of-the-art for trainee evaluation and assessment in Europe. Eur J Anaesthesiol. 2010;27:673–5.

57. Alahuhta S, Mellin-Olsen J, Blunnie WP, Knape JTA. Charter on continuing medical education/continuing professional development approved by the UEMS Specialist Section and the European Board of Anaesthesiology. Eur J Anaesthesiol. 2007;24:483–5.

58. The CoBaTrICE Collaboration. The educational environment for training in intensive care medicine: structures, processes, outcomes and challenges in the European region. Intensive Care Med. 2009;35:1575–83.

59. Dick WF, Zorab JSM, Otteni JC. The assessment of European Departments of Anaesthesiology involved in teaching and training. Eur J Anaesthesiol. 1991;8:455–8.

60. Simpson P. Training, assessment and accreditation in anaesthesiology and the implications for the European Union. Eur J Anaesthesiol. 2003;20:679–81.

61. Scherpereel P. Foundation for European Education in Anaesthesiology. Fondation Européenne d'Enseignement en Anesthésiologie (FEEA). Eur J Anaesthesiol. 2000;17:75–6.

62. Mellin-Olsen J. Varieties of teaching programs matched to country needs. Int Anesthesiol Clin. 2010;48(2):9–21.

63. De Lange S, Van Aken H, Burchardi H. European Society of Intensive Care Medicine statement: intensive care medicine in Europe—structure, organisation and training guidelines of the Multidisciplinary Joint Committee of Intensive Care Medicine (MJCICM) of the European Union of Medical Specialists (UEMS). Intensive Care Med. 2002;28:1505–11.

64. Petrino R, Bodiwala G, Meulemans A, Plunkett P, Williams D. European Society for Emergency Medicine (EuSEM). EuSEM core curriculum for emergency medicine. Eur J Emerg Med. 2002;9:308–14.

65. Federation of European Associations of Paediatric Anaesthesia. European Guidelines for training in paediatric anaesthesia. Anästh Intensivmed. 2007; 48:S105–6.

66. Meeusen V, Van Zundert A, Gatt S, Knape H The history of nurse anaesthetists – a global perspective. The progress of non-medical professionals in anaesthesia, Risk factors for job turnover among Dutch nurse anaesthetists. By Meeusen VCH. University of Utrecht, doctoral thesis, 2010, pp 26–56.

67. Meeusen V, Zundert A van, Hoekman J, Kumar C, Rawal N, Knape H. Composition of the anesthesia team: a European survey. Eur J. Anaesthesiol. 2010;27:773–9.

68. Egger Halbeis CB, Cvachovec K, Scherpereel P, Mellin-Olsen J, Drobnik L, Sondore A. Anaesthesia workforce in Europe. Eur J Anaesthesiol. 2007;24:991–1007.

69. Clergue F. Time to consider nonphysician anaesthesia providers in Europe? Eur J Anaesthesiol. 2010;27:761–2.

70. Rolly G, McRae WR, Blunnie WP, Dupont M, Scherpereel P. Anaesthesiological manpower in Europe. Eur J Anaesthesiol. 1996;13:325–32.

71. Knichwitz G, Wenning M. Is Germany running out of anaesthesiologists? Anästh Intensivmed. 2009;50:276–82 (German).

72. Pontone S, Brouard N. Despite corrective measures, will there still be a lack of anaesthetists and intensive care physicians in France by 2020? Ann Fr Anesth Reanim. 2010;29:862–7 (French).

73. Waurick R, Weber T, Bröking K. Van Aken H. The European working time directive: effect on education and clinical care. Curr Opin Anaesthesiol. 2007;20:576–9.

74. Searle RD, Lyons G. Vanishing experience in training for obstetric general anaesthesia: an observational study. Int J Obstet Anesth. 2008;17:233–7.

75. Fernandez E, Williams DG. Training and the European working time directive: a 7 year review of paediatric anaesthetic trainee caseload data. Br J Anaesth. 2009;103:566–9.

Edmond I Eger II

Summary

Research in anesthesia has taken several forms. Other essays in this book supply detailed histories of those specific researches, including the discovery of new anesthetics and anesthetic adjuvant drugs, advances in anesthetic delivery and monitoring, measurement and codification of anesthetic pharmacodynamics and kinetics, and the development of vehicles for the exchange of information on research (societies, books and journals). We refer the reader to these chapters for details of the histories of specific researches. The present chapter supplies an overview, a summary of the progress in anesthesia research.

Research in anesthesia evolved from need and curiosity. Consider eight themes. Theme 1: The discovery of anesthetics and anesthetic adjuvants occupied the minds of anesthetists from the inception. Theme 2: The application of anesthetics demanded an immediate need to define and control the anesthetic state. The second theme demanded Theme 3: What did the body do to anesthetics (pharmacokinetics) and what did anesthetics normally do to the body—to breathing, circulation, indeed to all parts of the body (pharmacodynamics)? And what the anesthetics did to the body also led to Theme 4, outcomes. Sometimes these marvelous drugs did bad things, destroying the liver or brain and more; and sometimes they did good things, protecting the brain and the liver and more. Theme 5: How do anesthetics and anesthetic adjuvants accomplish their magic? The initial musings on mechanisms were far off the mark. I remember reading many books in my residency a half century ago. The one that excited me the most was The Mode of Action of Anaesthetics by TAB Harris published in 1951. It told how things worked and I was enthralled with the ideas, (almost) all wrong. In the past several decades that darkness seems to have lifted—but I wonder if a future reader will also say "all wrong." Theme 6: Scratch an anesthetist and you'll find a gadgeteer. Most anesthetists I know love gadgets and many have tried their hand at developing new ones. And Theme 7: who supplies support for research? Funding comes from many sources, but most comes from industry with lesser amounts coming from the NIH, anesthetic organizations (e.g., the ASA and IARS), and local sources (e.g., departmental and personal). Theme 8 makes use of the above seven themes: Translational research. How do laboratory discoveries move to the clinic—and vice versa?

Theme 1: New Drugs for Anesthesia

The discovery of new drugs began the history of anesthesia, and continues to the present. Figure 39.1 illustrates the chronology of the major drug discoveries. Some drugs are more equal than others, and the game changers are given in larger, bold type. For example, nitrous oxide, ether and halothane each moved anesthesia in giant steps. Although enflurane, isoflurane, and then sevoflurane and desflurane replaced halothane, they contributed much smaller steps.

The discovery/development of new drugs, and especially increasingly better anesthetic and adjuvant drugs, has often resulted from a collaborative effort between industry and academicians. Early on, such discoveries were often made by intellectuals. In 1774, Unitarian minister and genius Joseph

Priestley (1733–1804) synthesized nitrous oxide. Precocious Humphrey Davy (1778–1829) studied it, in 1800 noting that it might be used for surgery, and dentist Horace Wells (1815–1848) unsuccessfully attempted a public demonstration of its use as an anesthetic in 1845. Valerius Cordus (1515–1554) synthesized ether in 1540, and three centuries later, on 16 Oct 1846 (ether day) Morton (decidedly not an intellectual) used ether to publically demonstrate its anesthetic effect. Some additions arrived by trial and error (wild guesswork). Soubeiran, von Liebig, and Guthrie independently discovered chloroform in 1831, and Jean-Baptiste Dumas named and chemically characterized it in 1834. The obstetrician, Sir James Simpson discovered its anesthetic properties in 1847 by experimenting first on himself and then on his patients.

Ether, nitrous oxide, and chloroform supplied most of the needs for general anesthesia (some would add ethyl chloride) for the better part of a century, and the search for a better inhaled anesthetic was delayed. Discovery went elsewhere. In 1884, Carl Koller, (1857–1944) demonstrated that cocaine produced conjunctival anesthesia and within the year,

E. I Eger II (✉)
Department of Anesthesia and Perioperative Care, University of California, San Francisco, CA, USA
e-mail: egere@anesthesia.ucsf.edu

E. I Eger II et al. (eds.), *The Wondrous Story of Anesthesia,* DOI 10.1007/978-1-4614-8441-7_39, © Edmond I Eger, MD 2014

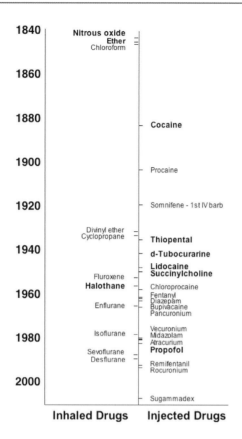

Fig. 39.1 The chronology of the major anesthesia drug discoveries began in 1844 with nitrous oxide. Some drugs were more equal than others, and the game changers are given in larger, *bold* type

cocaine was widely used for topical, infiltration and regional anesthesia. However, the toxicity of cocaine prompted a search for a better local anesthetic, leading to the synthesis of procaine by Einhorn in 1904.

The search for a better inhaled anesthetic was revived in the 1920s. Ethylene was discovered to put carnations to sleep and when given to animals put them to sleep, too. In 1923, Luckhardt and Carter introduced ethylene as an inhaled anesthetic at Presbyterian Hospital in Chicago [1]. Some discoveries had the insight of genius; simple things like Prof. Chauncey Leake's (1896–1978) suggestion to produce an ether with two ethylenes, to obtain the advantageous properties of both ethylene and diethyl ether. This led to divinyl ether in the early 1930s.

August Freund discovered cyclopropane in 1881, and cleverly proposed the correct cyclic structure. George Lucas and Velyien Henderson in Toronto discovered its anesthetic properties in the late 1920s. Henderson was the first human subject anesthetized with the gas. Waters demonstrated its anesthetic properties in patients in the early 1930s, using it in a rebreathing system.

And parallel to the expanding interest in inhaled anesthetics, Weese and Scharpff synthesized the short-acting

barbiturate, hexobarbital, in 1932 [2]. It was widely used in Europe. In the early 1930s, Ernest Volwiler (1893–1992) and Donalee Tabern (1900–1974), working for Abbott laboratories, discovered thiopental (Pentothal®). In 1934, Waters gave thiopental to a patient, inducing anesthesia without the unpleasant, sometimes terrifying, suffocating sensation associated with an induction of anesthesia with ether. Thiopental allowed a quick and pleasant transformation from wakefulness to sleep. "Count backwards, please, from 100…." Sleep came before 90.

One problem surgeons faced in the first half of the twentieth century was that, under ordinary circumstances, muscle relaxation was not sufficient to allow certain forms of surgery. Relaxation could be produced with the anesthetics at hand, but only by imposing deeper levels of anesthesia, levels that increased the risk of anesthesia. We knew of Ecuadorian Indians who painted the tips of darts with a substance called *woorari* ('poison' in the Carib language of the Macusi Indians of Guyana), now called d-tubocurarine ("curare"). An animal pricked by such a dart would become paralyzed, would die, and would be served for dinner. In 1780, Abbe Felix Fontana found that curare's action was not on the nerves and heart but on the ability of voluntary muscles to respond to stimuli. In the Nineteenth century, Claude Bernard demonstrated that paralysis resulted from an action on a small portion of the muscle, the so-called myoneural junction [3]. In 1811–1812, Benjamin Brodie (1783–1862) showed that curare does not kill by a direct effect, and that recovery eventually occurs if breathing is maintained artificially. In 1934, Henry Dale (1875–1968) showed that acetylcholine is the messenger mediating neuromuscular transmission, and that curare blocks such transmission.

Of course, one would not wish to permanently paralyze a patient, but what if the dose of curare were adjusted to produce just enough relaxation to facilitate surgery, a dose producing but a temporary paralysis? Stuart Cullen sought to test this possibility, injecting curare into dogs that promptly developed asthma-like symptoms. He abandoned curare. The credit for the discovery of the clinical usefulness of curare goes to the fearless Griffith and Johnson, who bypassed studies in animals, showing in 1942, that the bronchospasm found in dogs rarely applied in humans [4]. A new age had come to anesthesia, and curare was soon widely applied. Although it seemed safe, subsequent events suggested that the dangers implied by the deadly hunters of Ecuador might have some subtle application to humans (see below).

Cocaine and procaine had enabled topical, infiltration, and regional anesthesia, but neither was perfect. In the 1940s, local anesthesia was materially advanced by the introduction of the questionably safer, faster-acting amide, lidocaine. Lidocaine was synthesized by Nils Löfgren (1913–1967) and Bengt Lundqvist, and released for clinical use in 1948 [5].

It took World War II and advances in fluorine chemistry needed to enrich uranium isotopes, to give us modern inhaled anesthetics. The first successful modern anesthetic was halothane, synthesized by the British chemist Charles Suckling (b. 1920) for Imperial Chemical Industries. An inspired guess involved placing three fluorine atoms on one end of a two-carbon ethane, and adding a bromine and a chlorine atom on the other carbon. He thought the fluorine atoms would lend stability to and decrease toxicity of the molecule, and so they did. The bromine and the chlorine were probably included to secure a greater potency. In 1956, Michael Johnstone gave the first halothane anesthetic to a human [6]. Halothane quickly became popular because, unlike ether, the lack of pungency allowed a smooth, rapid, nonirritating induction of anesthesia.

And unlike chloroform—at least in the first years of its use—halothane did not seem to injure the liver. However, in 1958, a case of death in association with halothane use was reported, and more followed, leading to the National Halothane Study (see below). Enter Ross Terrell, a genius of a fluorine chemist, who was employed by the Ohio Chemical Company to find a replacement for halothane that would not injure the liver. He did that and more, synthesizing over 700 compounds in a search for the ideal anesthetic [7, 8]. First came enflurane, replacing halothane in the 1970s, particularly in the litigious US. Terrell's next anesthetic was isoflurane which replaced enflurane in the 1980s, and then he gave us desflurane in the 1990s. In parallel with Terrell, Bernard Regan, at Travenol Laboratories, synthesized sevoflurane [9]. This progression gave us and our patients increasingly safe and controllable anesthetics, nonflammable anesthetics with lesser blood solubilities allowing increasingly rapid awakening from anesthesia, with far less nausea than that from ether.

Further new drugs used in anesthesia resulted from the efforts of diverse clinicians, academicians and industry investigators. These included the muscle relaxants that replaced curare, increasingly safer and more controllable muscle relaxants. These newer muscle relaxants were made ever safer by better techniques for determining and eliminating any residual postoperative effects of such useful but potentially deadly drugs. Most recently we have, or nearly have, the reversal agent sugammadex, a drug eliminating the effects of particular relaxants by "hiding them from the muscle".

The new drugs included propofol, an intravenous induction agent largely replacing thiopental through greater controllability, secondary to metabolism an order of magnitude greater than that of thiopental. Propofol had some problems at its birth. Being poorly soluble in water, it had to be dissolved ("formulated") in an organic solvent. The solvent was initially cremaphor EL, and this combination was employed in 1977 in clinical trials. However, we soon learned that cremaphor might produce anaphylactoid (allergic-like) reactions that could be life threatening. Oops! Try again in 1986, using an emulsion of soy lipids to dissolve the propofol. Success!

1846–1920: Theme 2—Defining and Controlling Anesthetic Delivery

The discovery of anesthesia mandated research to address a simple question—how to conduct the patient safely through the operative procedure, and how to satisfy surgical requirements without injuring or killing the patient? We needed a clinically relevant assessment of what we came to call depth of anesthesia, we needed a controllable way to deliver anesthesia to achieve the "correct" depth, and we needed it right away. John Snow gave it to us. Golly, he was good. He invented the notion of depth of anesthesia, and he expressed that as five "degrees":

> "I shall divide the effects of ether into five stages or degrees; premising, however, that the division is, in some measure, arbitrary…In the first degree of etherization I shall include the various changes of feeling that a person may experience, whilst he still retains a correct consciousness of where he is, and what is occurring around him, and a capacity to direct his voluntary movements. In…the second degree, mental functions may be exercised, and voluntary actions performed, but in a disordered manner. In the third degree, there is no evidence of any mental function being exercised, and consequently no voluntary motions occur; but muscular contractions, in addition to those concerned in respiration, may sometimes take place as the effect of the ether, or of external impressions. In the fourth degree, no movements are seen except those of respiration, and they are incapable of being influenced by external impressions. In the fifth degree…the respiratory movements are more or less paralysed (sic), and become difficult, feeble, or irregular." (pp 1–2) [10]

Snow described how to achieve these degrees in his two books on delivery of the anesthetics of the day, diethyl ether [10] and chloroform [11]. We spent a century tinkering with the basic notions, Arthur Guedel being the greatest tinkerer. In World War I, he gave us not five degrees, but four stages, the third (surgical anesthesia; roughly equivalent to Snow's fourth degree) containing four planes (Fig. 39.2) [12]. Along the way, in 1895, Cushing (a neurosurgeon) and Codman added measurement of blood pressure and heart rate, and the anesthetic record [13].

1950–1980: Theme 3—Phenomenology: Pharmacokinetics

What Snow, Cushing, and Guedel taught us required attention to the patient's response to the anesthetic. What we saw in the patient, things such as the character of breathing, or the

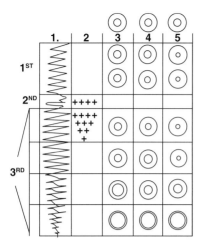

Fig. 39.2 The figure shows what constituted most of the characteristics of the first three of four stages (denoted at the furthest *left*) of anesthesia that Guedel devised. Four, successively deeper planes lay within the third stage. Stages and planes go from lightest level (*topmost*) to deepest level of anesthesia. *Column 1* characterizes inspiratory and expiratory movements, the depth and smoothness. *Column 2* indicates the activeness of movement of the eye in the second stage and the first plane of the third stage. *Columns 3, 4,* and *5* display the size of the pupil (*innermost circle*) and the iris (distance between the *innermost* and *outermost circles*) without (*column 3*) and with (*columns 4* and *5*) application of light to the eye. (From Guedel AE: Inhalation anesthesia: A fundamental guide. New York, Macmillan Co, 1937 pp 1-172)

size and responsiveness of the pupils to light, or changes in blood pressure, guided administration of more or less anesthetic or dictated cessation of anesthetic administration. Our observations had an enormous subjective element, meaning that delivery of anesthesia was as much an art as a science. This changed with our increased knowledge of anesthetic phenomenology in the 1950s, and the ability to deliver a precisely known amount of anesthetic that, additionally, we could directly measure.

In the mid-1900s we knew little about what we came to call anesthetic pharmacokinetics. We were ignorant about factors governing movement of anesthetics within the body (and thus we were hindered in our understanding of how to control and make use of such limits). Snow knew it was important, but could do little about it. In 1924, Howard Haggard explored the absorption, distribution and elimination of di-ethyl ether in dogs, dividing the distribution into that which went to the brain, and that which went elsewhere [14, 15]. In 1950, Seymour Kety (1915–2000) provided the first kinetic models, unintelligible for most mortals, and wrong in details (it failed, for example, to recognize the importance of differential distribution of the delivery of blood to different tissues) [16].

In 1954, John Severinghaus (b. 1922) started us properly down the pharmacokinetic road with his seminal study of nitrous oxide, the first investigation of uptake of an inhaled anesthetic in humans [17]. His investigation led to a more general, but empirical, description of uptake known as the square root of time rule, a rule stating that anesthetic uptake decreases as a function of the square root of time. It applied to anesthetics other than nitrous oxide [18]. Hal Price improved on the concepts of tissue distribution of intravenous anesthetics, noting that tissue bulk and blood flow had to be accounted for in our thinking of the redistribution of an anesthetic like thiopental (Pentothal®) [19]. His concepts led the way with thiopental and injected anesthetics, and prompted a broader view, one applicable to the inhaled anesthetics. In parallel with Price, Eger (b. 1930) studied inhaled anesthetic kinetics, doing so with a vengeance, measuring solubilities and uptake of all clinically-used and many experimental anesthetics [20]. In the late 1950s, he developed an iterative mathematical model explaining how inhaled anesthetics move into and throughout the body [21], a model that with a few modifications applies to all inhaled anesthetics used today. Other investigators used analog models to accomplish a similar explanation [22, 23], but these could not describe the effect of the inspired anesthetic concentration on pharmacokinetics.

1960–1980: Theme 3 Continued—Phenomenology, Pharmacodynamics

In 1963, we got a measure of anesthetic potency, a measure that would provide a standard that allowed a comparison among anesthetic effects. The measure of potency was MAC, the minimum alveolar concentration of an inhaled anesthetic producing immobility in 50 % of subjects given a stimulus such as a surgical incision [24, 25]. Three decades later, we got the equivalent of MAC for injected drugs such as propofol [26]. MAC allowed the comparative measurement of effects of inhaled anesthetics, everything from cardiorespiratory effects to what anesthetics did to brain and muscle and kidney and liver and pregnant ladies and infants and obese people and old people and… [27]. These phenomenology studies ("what does X do to Y?") poured out and dominated research through the 1970s and 1980s. Such studies continue to the present.

1950-Present: Theme 4: Outcome Studies

For the most part, important outcome studies appeared in the second half of the 20th century. But we must acknowledge earlier work, for example, Snow's careful dissection of the causes of death associated with chloroform anesthesia [11]. He repeatedly refers to a "sudden paralysis of the heart", possibly ventricular fibrillation or possibly severe myocardial depression. A less successful outcome study with the same theme was the work of the Hyderabad commission [28]. In 1902, echoing Snow's observations, Edward Embley provided support for the view that chloroform might cause sudden death by cardiac depression, believing that this resulted from a direct depressant effect of the vapor or by vagal irritability [29–31].

In 1954, at about the same time as we began to understand inhaled anesthetic pharmacokinetics, we got the first of the great outcomes studies, the work of Henry Beecher (1904–1976) and Donald Todd [32]. These investigators directed a consortium of 10 University hospitals in an investigation of the factors associated with death after anesthesia. Despite an absence of computers (after all, it was the early 1950s) they collected data on 599,548 patients coming to the astonishing conclusion that if a patient undergoing major surgery received curare, that patient was approximately 6 times more likely to die. The finding raised a ruckus, especially since it was published in a surgical journal and surgeons subsequently ordered anesthetists to stop using curare. No one likes being told what to do. Of course, the main problem was that apparently American anesthetists didn't understand that curare was apt to leave a residual paralysis that required reversal of the neuromuscular blockade [33]; the anesthetist did not recognize that although the patient might be breathing and appear grossly normal, he was still at risk from a remaining weakness, at risk of inadequate ventilation or an inability to react properly to vomiting—with vomit going into the lungs. You'd think we anesthetists would learn, but half a century later, another outcomes study again found that inadequate reversal of the effects of muscle relaxants grossly increased mortality [34].

Introduction of the inhaled anesthetic halothane, in the 1950s, was a smashing success. It quickly replaced all other potent inhaled anesthetics, including chloroform, cyclopropane and ether (halothane didn't explode but ether and cyclopropane did, and halothane had the added advantage of being less pungent than ether). Halothane also displaced the now infrequently used chloroform because chloroform injured the liver and halothane didn't seem to do so. Then in the late 1950s and early 1960s, sporadic cases of severe liver injury appeared after anesthesia with halothane, and we anesthetists feared that we might lose this new friend. The result was the National Halothane Study [35], a study of more than 800,000 patients given various anesthetics. The results suggested a rare, but believable connection between halothane and severe liver injury and death, a connection with signs and symptoms indicating that injury might be a consequence of an allergic response of the liver to halothane (or its metabolites).

The number of studies of outcomes, consequent to the activities of anesthetists, has increased dramatically. Outcome studies differ from phenomenology studies in that the outcomes intend to connect an action (of an anesthetic or a manipulation of some sort such as body temperature [36], oxygen concentration [37], or administration of beta blockers [38]) to either an adverse or beneficial outcome. In contrast, phenomenology studies connect an activity to a change where the change is neither inherently good nor bad. Sometimes outcome studies require data collection from large numbers of patients, as in the Beecher-Todd study or in the National Halothane Study, but more recent outcome studies might include just tens, hundreds, or a few thousand patients. Such small numbers were needed to demonstrate in the 1990s, that beta adrenergic blockage might provide long-term protection against postoperative myocardial injury [38].

One dramatic outcome study in the 1950s, was inadvertently conducted on patients suffering from tetanus [39]. These patients were given nitrous oxide to breathe, in order to decrease the pain of the muscle spasms produced by tetanus. The pain decreased, but after a few days, the number of white blood cells decreased and the patients began to die. The connection to nitrous oxide was clear, although the reason was not. The use of nitrous oxide continued in ordinary surgical patients because it appeared that the problem was only from prolonged breathing of the nitrous oxide. Anesthetists debated whether a more subtle noxiousness of this most ancient of anesthetics resulted from shorter exposures, with a consensus that the case was not proven, and the anesthetic had a long record of benefit and safety [40]. In 2007, an outcomes study of 2000 patients, given or not given nitrous oxide, suggested that nitrous oxide increased morbidity [41], possibly doing so for reasons related to the unique capacity of nitrous oxide to slowly inactivate a vital enzyme, methionine synthase [42]. However, not all recent outcome studies, even of 1000 patients, reveal an adverse effect of nitrous oxide [43]. The noxious effect of nitrous oxide continues to be debated, but the concerns over such noxiousness, including increased postoperative nausea and vomiting, have decreased the use of nitrous oxide in clinical practice.

The numbers of outcome studies are already large and will increase further. They will increase because of the need to supply better patient care, and to provide "evidence-based medicine." Their application may not only increase patient well-being, but will likely decrease the cost of patient care by causing us to discard ineffective remedies that often have the additional disadvantage of being expensive. This latter issue also concerns research on the comparative effectiveness of medical treatments and whether the incremental benefit of more effective treatments justifies the added costs.

1980-Present: Theme 5—Finally, Studies of Mechanisms

As indicated above, the major anesthesia research in the 2–3 decades following World War II was phenomenological, plus an increasing, somewhat later interest in outcomes. The 1970s and 1980s saw the start of a third major focus: how did anesthetics and anesthetic adjuvants work? A few such inquiries had been made earlier. In 1846, Claude Bernard (1813–1878) demonstrated that curare acted by interfering with the transmission of nervous impulses to muscle, at what is called the motor end-plate, the juncture of nerve and muscle [3]. Around 1900, Meyer [44] and Overton [45] connected anesthetic potency to an affinity for fatty substances, implying that anesthetics acted by doing something to the lipid parts of neurons, perhaps something to the lipid bilayers that encircle all cells, including the cells of the brain.

But only sporadic discoveries were made until the 1980s, when we began to make use of the great advances in our understanding of receptors, and in genetic engineering. Nick Franks and Bill Lieb deserve credit for shifting our attention away from thinking that anesthetics, especially inhaled anesthetics, must work by some action on lipids in membrane bilayers. As noted above, Meyer and Overton had focused on the correlation of anesthetic potency with affinity to lipid. In 1984, Franks and Lieb demonstrated that an equally good correlation could be made with an effect on a protein [46]. Then the floodgates opened, with many investigators showing that anesthetics affected numerous and specific receptors (proteins) in ways that plausibly explained the actions of anesthetics and anesthetic adjuvants, such as opioids and muscle relaxants.

Some phenotypic results (i.e., specific anesthetic effects such as the production of immobility in the face of noxious stimulation) of injected anesthetics such as propofol or etomidate clearly result from an action on a specific receptor. An important study in 2003 demonstrated that for propofol and etomidate, the action was on the gamma amino butyric acid (GABA) receptor, an inhibitory receptor [47]. Etomidate and propofol enhanced this inhibition, doing so by increasing the response of the GABA receptor to normally released GABA. In another important study, genetic engineering made a mouse with a specific GABA receptor that responded normally to GABA but no longer responded to the presence of etomidate or propofol—the enhancement was muted or gone. The bioengineered mouse did not display the usual phenotypic response to etomidate; the response was also muted or gone [47]. This brilliant experiment showed that the GABA receptor mediates at least part of etomidate's and propofol's effects. Future studies must deal with a more difficult question: what is the mechanism(s) by which etomidate and propofol affect the receptor to enhance inhibition?

Propofol and etomidate affect only the GABA receptor. In contrast, the inhaled anesthetics affect nearly all receptors or other proteins that allow nerves to function, usually by opening channels and thereby allowing the passage of ions (charged particles). Most of these effects could plausibly cause anesthesia, but in fact, none can explain more than a small part of the capacity of inhaled anesthetics to produce anesthesia [48]. For example, as with propofol and etomidate, inhaled anesthetics enhance the response of GABA receptors to GABA, but the results of several studies suggested that the GABA receptor does not mediate at least some of the effects of inhaled anesthetics, like immobility [49]. We made magical mice, mice like those telling us so much about etomidate and propofol, mice in which one particular type of GABA receptor no longer responded to isoflurane, but the isoflurane MAC for those mice wasn't changed [50].

Theme 6: Gadgets

Ancient Times

Research developing gadgets is part of the history of anesthesia. There was the initial scramble to produce delivery systems allowing the anesthetist to control the anesthetic state. Again, Snow led the way, the greatest anesthetist who ever lived. He saw the need to provide better control over the concentration of anesthetic delivered, and he developed a vaporizer to meet that need [10, 11]. Despite its imperfections, his work anticipated much of what evolved into our present vaporizers.

However, most anesthetists ignored his insights. The curmudgeon, Simpson, thought Snow foolish. A handkerchief and a bottle of chloroform were all that was needed. And thus anesthesia was given with primitive devices delivering an unknowable concentration of anesthetic. Anesthetic sprinkled on gauze or a handkerchief. Both I (EIE) and one of my co-editors (LJS) vividly remember the horror of being anesthetized (twice) by an anesthetist placing a gauze mask on our respective faces and dropping liquid ether on that mask until our world disappeared. I think it took four strong men to hold me down.

So, with exceptions, we learned how to give anesthesia safely if not pleasantly, guided by our observations of the patient's response to what we gave. We slowly added improvements prompted by suggestions of people such as Edmund Andrews who noted that nitrous oxide might be given for more than a few moments if oxygen were added [51]. Implementing that observation required the development of iron tanks to hold large amounts of (compressed) nitrous oxide and oxygen. Such tanks promoted construction of anesthetic machines, and onto these were grafted vaporizers that, while crude, allowed delivery of graded concentrations of potent inhaled anesthetics. Parallel developments were made in anesthetic delivery systems (to-and-fro and anesthetic circle systems), devices that accepted the gases and vapors made by the anesthetic machines, devices that enabled presentation of the gases and vapors to the patient to breathe and rebreathe—care being taken to remove the carbon dioxide from the rebreathed gases. Along the way in these developments, Cushing, after he killed a patient, led us to blood pressure monitoring and the recording of pulse rate and blood pressure in the 1890s [13].

Modern Times: So, for a century after the discovery of anesthesia, we made incremental improvements in anesthetic delivery systems and monitoring. World War II gave us the atomic bomb, and that invention required advances in fluorine chemistry—which, by the way, gave us Teflon® and modern (fluorinated) inhaled anesthetics. It also became crucial to better control the concentration of these powerful, potentially lethal, anesthetics. In the early 1950s, Lucien Morris invented the Copper Kettle, the first vaporizer intended to deliver a precisely known concentration of any volatile vapor, at any flow rate [52]. Control! Morris' approach was copied by other manufacturers (e.g., the Vernitrol produced by the Ohio Chemical Company.)

In a strange way, the atom bomb also gave us blood gas electrodes, devices allowing the measurement of oxygen and carbon dioxide partial pressures and acidity in small volumes of blood. John Severinghaus had begun a career in physics when the bomb exploded. His sense of the immorality of this device caused him to abandon physics and turn to a career in medicine and eventually anesthesiology. In the 1950s, this led to his invention of the carbon dioxide electrode and a device into which oxygen, pH and his newly invented carbon dioxide electrode could be placed allowing easy measurement of blood gases [53]. Severinghaus says he was given far more credit for the invention of the carbon dioxide electrode than was due. The real credit, he says should go to Richard Stow who thought of the basic idea (a slight pun), but couldn't make it work stably. Severinghaus supplied the additional thought needed to produce a functional electrode—Stow's electrode was simply a pH electrode covered with a latex film with distilled water separating the latex and the pH electrode. Carbon dioxide diffused across the latex and was read as a pH change. Severinghaus suggested adding sodium bicarbonate to the distilled water to ensure stability, and that worked like a charm. "The joke here is that I got the credit for inventing the CO_2 electrode but all I did was add soda."

At this time, we saw the development of analyzers of the gases that our patients breathed; anesthetic vapors and gases, oxygen and carbon dioxide. Because they absorbed infrared light (and thus were greenhouse gases—but I digress), the anesthetic gases and carbon dioxide could be analyzed by their absorption of infrared light at particular wavelength frequencies (the different frequencies allowed one gas to be distinguished from another). The German, Luft, had invented the device that used this principle right before World War II [54]. This analysis could be done on a breath-by-breath basis, and the results for the gas concentrations in the gases at the end of each breath closely correlated with the gases measured in arterial blood, using the blood gas analyzer. Thus, with each breath one could tell the concentration of these gases in the lungs and thus in the blood. Given a bit of time for equilibration, the concentrations in blood reflected the concentrations in tissues such as the brain. Such devices invited the determination of the anesthetic concentrations required to produce specific anesthetic phenotypes (i.e., the capacity of an anesthetic to produce a certain characteristic such as immobility or blockage of memory); as noted above, they facilitated the invention of MAC.

The realization that one could control the effects of inhaled anesthetics on vital functions such as breathing and blood pressure by controlling alveolar concentrations, in turn prompted an increasing demand for a clinical availability of monitors for respiratory (carbon dioxide and oxygen) and anesthetic gases. In the late 1970s, Severinghaus and Ozanne gave us such monitoring using a multiplexed mass spectrometer [55, 56]. (By now, dear reader, it should be clear that Severinghaus is the gadgeteer without peer [57]). Monitoring with the multiplexed analyzer usually worked well and was economical (it could serve a dozen rooms "simultaneously"), but the occasional breakdown of a system to which many anesthetists became addicted was unacceptable, and the multiplexed analyzer gave way in the late 1980s to the presently ubiquitous stand-alone infrared analyzers.

Not only could we now control the delivery, especially of inhaled anesthetics, we could measure and control what we did with those and other drugs. We controlled delivery in part by controlling ventilation. It sounds simple. When I (EIE) was a resident I usually controlled ventilation by squeezing a bag connected to the circuit which, in turn, was connected to the patient: when I squeezed, the patient got a breath. Because I was a graduate of much schooling, I (and every like anesthetist) was considered to have an "educated hand" that could precisely deliver the correct amount of breathing. Others decided that I was less educated than I thought [58, 59]. The educated hand wasn't. That, and a great interest in ventilating the lungs of patients suffering from polio in the 1950s, gave us ventilators, devices that continued to evolve, and gave us a precision over ventilation to the patient's great benefit. It also freed a hand that would otherwise be tethered to a bag.

And what about the heart? We could depress it with our drugs or stimulate it with other drugs. Increasingly, we measured various consequences of such depression and stimulation. As we've repeatedly noted, Cushing and Codman in the 1890s taught us to measure the blood pressure of patients indirectly, using the Riva-Roca method familiar to us in our doctor's office. But that didn't give us the pressure produced by every beat of the heart, and increasingly we applied the pressure transducer [the strain gauge invented by Edward Simmons (1911–2004) and Arthur Ruge (1905–2000) in 1938] that investigators used in animals, an application that is commonplace today.

Perhaps the most fascinating development was that of transesophageal echocardiography, the use of ultrasound to supply beat-by-beat images of the heart, images that tell the anesthetist how well the heart is doing its job [60]. First developed as a crude instrument by Oka in the late 1970s [60], it evolved from producing a one-dimensional to a two dimensional image. Today, it tells the anesthetist how well and where blood is flowing in the heart—right and wrong. A second application of ultrasound, one still developing, now tells the anesthetist just where to place the tip of a needle when performing regional anesthesia—or when trying to cannulate an artery or a vein.

Finally, consider today's ubiquitous pulse oximeter, a device that measures the amount of oxygen carried by the hemoglobin in blood, doing so with each beat of the heart and announcing the content with a beep whose pitch indicates the amount (percent). Severinghaus tells this rich story in Chapter 55. Many contributed to the history. Glen Millikan devised a working model in 1941 and coined the term "oximeter" [61]. Earl Wood supplied a key control in the late 1940s [62]. But the person who put it all together, and is credited with the discovery of pulse oximetry, is Takuo Aoyagi, a most modest Japanese bioengineer who was driven to his invention by the serendipitous observation of artifacts he saw in his studies of cardiac dye dilution with an earpiece densitometer. He reported on his invention on 26 April 1974, "Improvement of the Earpiece Oximeter," to the Japanese Society of Medical Electronics and Biological Engineering. The first report of Aoyagi's device was by the surgeon S Nakajima, in 1975 [63]. Anesthetists in all developed and many less developed countries use pulse oximeters, and many credit the device for decreasing the mortality associated with modern anesthesia. Curiously, attempts to prove this relationship have failed [64].

There are more inventions, gadgets devised by anesthetists, many trivial or potentially harmful (e.g., see my first publication) [65]. Some had considerable importance (e.g., transcutaneous measures of the partial pressure of carbon dioxide or oxygen). The reader is referred to Chapter 55.

1960-Present: Theme 7—Who Pays for Anesthesia Research?

For the era preceding WWII, the answer to the title question was "no one." Little research was done except for that supported by industry or occasionally the well-endowed institution, or the curious individual who took money from his pocket.

The major support for research in anesthesia has always come from industry. Industry underwrote the research into new drugs (see above) and advances in equipment (see "gadgets", also above). This relationship between industry and faculty investigators was symbiotic—industry got the data it needed to test and to gain approval for its' products. The investigators received support and the products required for clinical studies, and the subsequent academic recognition required for promotion, and the specialty gained access to marvelous (usually) new drugs. Most drug and equipment inventions were industry-inspired, but university investigators and practitioners often joined with industry in the evaluation of new products. Both developmental research and industry-investigator collaboration have decreased in the past two decades, as the cost of developing new drugs has increased and the perceived need for new products has decreased (as anesthesia as a specialty has matured). Rarely did industry support basic research in anesthesia, research into "how things worked". This fell to the National Institutes of Health (NIH) in the US and similar institutions in other countries, and to various foundations

In the US, the first named National Institute of Health was born in 1930. The (pleural, now) National Institutes of Health grew dramatically after World War II, but little in the way of funding went towards research in anesthesia until the 1960s. In the 1960s, Emanuel Papper (1915–2002), the chair of the first Department of Anesthesiology at Columbia University, contributed to several NIH committees and in 1965–6 acted as a principal consultant in the establishment of the National Institute of General Medical Sciences, an Institute serving as a primary source of support for research in anesthesia from that time to the present. He played a major role in freeing more NIH dollars for research in anesthesia. In terms of increasing dollars in support of research for anesthesiology, the NIH has been generous (Fig. 39.3) [66]. NIH support for anesthetic research appears to have exceeded (by an order of magnitude) and be more consistent that that supplied by the UK from its Medical Research Council (MRC) (Fig. 39.4), differences that have persisted for the past two decades.

A crucial but small source of research support in the US increasingly came from professional anesthesia organizations. This support was crucial because it supplied seed money. In 1987, the American Society of Anesthesiologists (ASA) organized FAER (Foundation for Anesthesia Education and Research).

"From 1988 to 2009, FAER awarded grants of over $24 million with another $1.4 million committed for disbursement in 2010 and 2011. Most of this was underwritten by the ASA and private industry which has given FAER a total of $24.9 million. The pace of donations and grants has increased in recent years. From 2005–2009, the ASA contributed $8.8 million and FAER gave $11.3 million in grants." (personal communication from Dr. Denham Ward to EIE.)

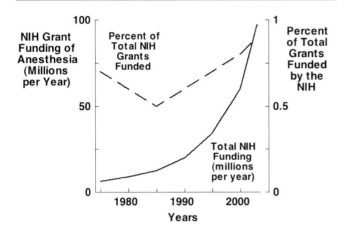

Fig. 39.3 From 1975 to 2003, NIH support for anesthesiology grew by 1600%, to nearly $100,000,000. This largely reflected increasing support of research in general, rather than acquisition of an increasing share of the research support pie by anesthesia researchers, which remained at less than 1% of the total grants funded by the NIH. (Data from Table 1 in Schwinn DA, Balser JR: Anesthesiology physician scientists in academic medicine: a wake-up call. Anesthesiology 2006; 104: 170–8)

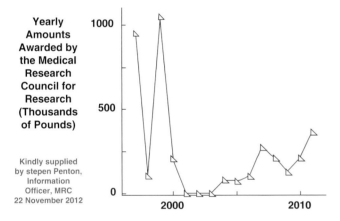

Fig. 39.4 The Medical Research Council in the UK also supports "anaesthesia research". As the graph indicates, support has been uneven in the past two decades, ranging from zero to over 1 million pounds per year. Support in the past decade appears to be on the ascent. (Data kindly provided as a communication from Stephen Penton, Information Officer, Medical Research Council, 22 Nov 2012, to EIE)

The International Anesthesia Research Society has similarly contributed to the support of research, providing more than $14,000,000 in support of research grants and fellowship training.

Conclusion: Theme 8

In greatest part, the seven themes exist to enhance clinical care. We have come to call this translational research, and the ASA has seen fit to emphasize its importance with an eponymous lecture named after one of the greatest contribu-

tors to such research, John Severinghaus—who was the first lecturer [57]. Such research does more than enhance clinical care. Not only does it move from bench to patient, but issues raised in the clinical care of patients lead back to laboratory work. Translational research is the eighth, and perhaps the most important, theme. Much of such research is described in great detail in Chapters 41–43, but I would argue that it appears in various guises in most of the chapters of this book.

Acknowledgment I thank Dr. John W. Severinghaus for his several suggestions.

References

1. Adriani J. The pharmacology of anesthetic drugs. Springfield: Charles C Thomas; 1952.
2. Weese H, Scharpff W. Evipan, cin neuartiges Einschlafmittel. Deut Med Wochenschr. 1932;58:1205–7.
3. Bernard C. Etudes phsiologiques sue quelques poisons americains. Revue des Deux Mondes 1864;53:164–90.
4. Griffith HR, Johnson E. The use of curare in general anesthesia. Anesthesiology. 1942;3:418–20.
5. Holmdahl MH. Xylocain (lidocaine, lignocaine), its discovery and Gordh's contribution to its clinical use. Acta Anaesthesiol Scand Suppl. 1998;113:8–12.
6. Johnstone M. Halothane: the first five years. Anesthesiology. 1961;22:591–614.
7. Vitcha JF. A history of Forane®. Anesthesiology. 1971;35:4–7.
8. Terrell RC. The invention and development of enflurane, isoflurane, sevoflurane, and desflurane. Anesthesiology. 2008;108:531–3.
9. Wallin RF, Regan BM, Napoli MD, Stern IJ. Sevoflurane: A new inhalational anesthetic agent. Anesth Analg. 1975;54:758–65.
10. Snow J. On the inhalation of the vapour of ether in surgical operations: containing a description of the various stages of etherization, and a statement of the result of nearly eighty operations in which ether has been employed in St. George's and University College Hospitals. London: John Churchill; 1847. pp 1–88.
11. Snow J. On chloroform and other anaesthetics: their action and administration. John Churchill, New Burlington Street. London 1858. pp 1–443.
12. Guedel AE. Inhalation anesthesia: a fundamental guide. New York, Macmillan; 1937. pp 1–172.
13. Cushing HW. Anaesthesia charts of 1895. Letter to F.A. Washburn. Treadwell Library, Massachusetts General Hospital, Boston, MA.
14. Haggard AW. The absorption, distribution and elimination of ethyl ether. II. Analysis of the mechanism of absorption and elimination of such a gas or vapor as ethyl ether. J Biol Chem. 1924;59:753–96.
15. Haggard AW. The absorption, distribution and elimination of ethyl ether. III. The relation of the concentration of ether, or any similar volatile substance in the central nervous system to the concentration in the arterial blood and the buffer action of the body. J Biol Chem. 1924;59:797–832.
16. Kety SS. Theory and application of exchange of inert gas at the lungs and tissues. Pharmacol Rev. 1951;3:1–41.
17. Severinghaus JW. The rate of uptake of nitrous oxide in man. J Clin Invest. 1954;33:1183–9.
18. Lowe HJ, Ernst EA. The quantitative practice of anesthesia. Use of closed circuit. Baltimore, Williams & Wilkins; 1981. pp 1–234.
19. Price HL. A dynamic concept of the distribution of thiopental in the human body. Anesthesiology. 1960;21:40–5.
20. Eger EI II. Anesthetic uptake and action. Baltimore, Williams & Wilkins; 1974. pp 1–371.

21. Eger EI II. A mathematical model of uptake and distribution. In: Papper EM, Kitz RJ, Editors. Uptake and distribution of anesthetic agents. New York, McGraw-Hill; 1963, pp 72–87.
22. Severinghaus JW. Role of lung factors. In: Papper EM, Kitz RJ, Editors. Uptake and distribution of anesthetic agents. New York, McGraw-Hill; 1963.
23. Mapleson WW. Quantitative prediction of anesthetic concentrations. In: Papper EM, Kitz RJ, Editors. Uptake and distribution of anesthetic agents. New York, McGraw-Hill; 1963, pp 104–19.
24. Merkel G, Eger EI II. A comparative study of halothane and halopropane anesthesia. Including a method for determining equipotency. Anesthesiology. 1963;24:346–57.
25. Saidman LJ, Eger EI II. Effect of nitrous oxide and of narcotic premedication on the alveolar concentration of halothane required for anesthesia. Anesthesiology. 1964;25:302–6.
26. Andrews DT, Leslie K, Sessler DI, Bjorksten AR. The arterial blood propofol concentration preventing movement in 50% of healthy women after skin incision. Anesth Analg. 1997;85:414–9.
27. Eger EI II, Eisenkraft JB, Weiskopf RB. The pharmacology of inhaled anesthetics. Chicago: Healthcare Press; 2002. pp 1–327.
28. Lawrie E. The Hyderbad chloroform commission. Lancet. 1889;1:952–3.
29. Embley EH. The causation of death during the administration of chloroform. Br Med J. 1902;2(2153):817–21.
30. Embley EH. The causation of death during the administration of chloroform. Br Med J. 1902;2(2154):885–93.
31. Embley EH. The causation of death during the administration of chloroform. Br Med J. 1902;1(2155):951–61.
32. Beecher HK, Todd DP. A study of the deaths associated with anesthesia and surgery: based on a study of 599, 548 anesthesias in ten institutions 1948–1952, inclusive. Ann Surg. 1954;140:2–35.
33. Prescott F, Organe G, Rowbotham S. Tubocurarine as an adjunct to anaesthesia. Lancet. 1946;2:80–4.
34. Arbous MS, Meursing AE, Kleef JW van, Lange JJ de, Spoormans HH, Touw P, Werner FM, Grobbee DE. Impact of anesthesia management characteristics on severe morbidity and mortality. Anesthesiology. 2005;102:257–68.
35. Summary of the National Halothane Study. Possible association between halothane anesthesia and postoperative hepatic necrosis. Report by Subcommittee on the National Halothane Study of the Committee on Anesthesia, National Academy of Science. JAMA. 1966;197:775–88.
36. Kurz A, Sessler DI, Lenhardt R. Perioperative normothermia to reduce the incidence of surgical-wound infection and shorten hospitalization. Study of Wound Infection and Temperature Group. N Engl J Med. 1996;334:1209–15.
37. Hopf HW, Hunt TK, West JM, Blomquist P, Goodson WH 3rd, Jensen JA, Jonsson K, Paty PB, Rabkin JM, Upton RA, Smitten K von, Whitney JD. Wound tissue oxygen tension predicts the risk of wound infection in surgical patients. Arch Surg. 1997;132:997–1004. (discussion 1005).
38. Wallace A, Layug B, Tateo I, Li J, Hollenberg M, Browner W, Miller D, Mangano D. Prophylactic atenolol reduces postoperative myocardial ischemia. McSPI Research Group. Anesthesiology. 1998;88:7–17.
39. Lassen HCA, Henriksen E, Neukirch F, Kristensen HS. Treatment of tetanus. Severe bone-marrow depression after prolonged nitrous-oxide anaesthesia. Lancet. 1956;1:527–30.
40. Eger EI II, Editor. Nitrous Oxide/N2O. New York: Elsevier; 1985. pp 1–357.
41. Myles PS, Leslie K, Chan MT, Forbes A, Paech MJ, Peyton P, Silbert BS, Pascoe E. Avoidance of nitrous oxide for patients undergoing major surgery: a randomized controlled trial. Anesthesiology. 2007;107:221–31.
42. Myles PS, Chan MT, Leslie K, Peyton P, Paech M, Forbes A. Effect of nitrous oxide on plasma homocysteine and folate in patients undergoing major surgery. Br J Anaesth. 2008;100:780–6.
43. McGregor DG, Lanier WL, Pasternak JJ, Rusy DA, Hogan K, Samra S, Hindman B, Todd MM, Schroeder DR, Bayman EO, Clarke W, Torner J, Weeks J. Effect of nitrous oxide on neurologic and neuropsychological function after intracranial aneurysm surgery. Anesthesiology. 2008;108:568–79.
44. Meyer HH. Theorie der Alkoholnarkose. Arch Exptl Pathol Pharmakol. 1899;42:109–18.
45. Overton E. Ueber die allgemeinen osmotischen Eigenschaften der Zelle, ihre vermutliche Ursachen und ihre Bedeutung fur die Physiologie. Vierteljahrschr Naturforsch Ges Zurich. 1899;44:88–114.
46. Franks NP, Lieb WR. Do general anaesthetics act by competitive binding to specific receptors? Nature. 1984;310:599–601.
47. Jurd R, Arras M, Lambert S, Drexler B, Siegwart R, Crestani F, Zaugg M, Vogt KE, Ledermann B, Antkowiak B, Rudolph U. General anesthetic actions in vivo strongly attenuated by a point mutation in the GABA(A) receptor beta3 subunit. FASEB J. 2003;17:250–2.
48. Eger EI, II, Raines DE, Shafer SL, Hemmings HC Jr, Sonner JM. Is a new paradigm needed to explain how inhaled anesthetics produce immobility? Anesth Analg. 2008;107:832–48.
49. Zhang Y, Sonner JM, Eger EI II, Stabernack CR, Laster MJ, Raines DE, Harris RA. GABAA receptors do not mediate the immobility produced by inhaled anesthetics. Anesth Analg. 2004;99:85–90.
50. Sonner JM, Werner DF, Elsen FP, Xing Y, Liao M, Harris RA, Harrison NL, Fanselow MS, Eger EI, 2nd, Homanics GE. Effect of isoflurane and other potent inhaled anesthetics on minimum alveolar concentration, learning, and the righting reflex in mice engineered to express alpha1 gamma-aminobutyric acid type A receptors unresponsive to isoflurane. Anesthesiology. 2007;106:107–13.
51. Lichtenstein ME, Method H. Edmund Andrews, M.D., a biographical sketch with historical notes concerning nitrous oxide anesthesia. Q Bull Northwest Univ Med Sch. 1953;27(4):337–52.
52. Morris LE. A new vaporizer for liquid anesthetic agents. Anesthesiology. 1952;13:587–93.
53. Severinghaus JW, Bradley AF. Electrodes for blood pO2 and pCO2 determination. J Appl Physiol. 1958;13:515–20.
54. Luft K. Über eine neue Methode der registrierenden Gasanalyse mit Hilfe der Absorption ultraroter Strahlen ohne spektrale Zerlegung. Ztschrf Techn Phys. 1943;24:97–104.
55. Severinghaus JW. Ozanne G: Multioperating room monitoring with one mass spectrometer. Acta Anaesthesiol Scand Suppl. 1978;70:186–7.
56. Ozanne GM, Young WG, Mazzei WJ, Severinghaus JW. Multipatient anesthetic mass spectrometry: rapid analysis of data stored in long catheters. Anesthesiology. 1981;55:62–70.
57. Severinghaus JW. Gadgeteering for health care: the John W. Severinghaus lecture on translational science. Anesthesiology. 2009;110:721–8.
58. Spears RS Jr, Yeh A, Fisher DM, Zwass MS. The "educated hand". Can anesthesiologists assess changes in neonatal pulmonary compliance manually? Anesthesiology. 1991;75:693–6.
59. Egbert LD, Bisno D. The educated hand of the anesthesiologist. A study of professional skill. Anesth Analg. 1967;46:195–200.
60. Oka Y. The evolution of intraoperative transesophageal echocardiography. Mt Sinai J Med. 2002;69:18–20.
61. Millikan GA. The oximeter: an instrument for measuring continuously oxygen saturation of arterial blood in man. Rev Sci Instr. 1942;13:434–44.
62. Wood EH, Geraci JE. Photoelectric determination of arterial oxygen saturation in man. J Lab Clin Med. 1949;34:387–401.
63. Nakajima S, Hirai Y, Takase H. Performances of new pulse wave earpiece oximeter. Respir Circ. 1975;23:41–5.
64. Moller JT, Pedersen T, Rasmussen LS, Jensen PF, Pedersen BD, Ravlo O, Rasmussen NH, Espersen K, Johannessen NW, Cooper JB, et al. Randomized evaluation of pulse oximetry in 20,802 patients: I. Design, demography, pulse oximetry failure rate, and overall complication rate. Anesthesiology. 1993;78:436–44.
65. Eger EI II, Hamilton WK. Positive-negative pressure ventilation with a modified Ayre's T-piece. Anesthesiology. 1958;19:611–8.
66. Schwinn DA, Balser JR. Anesthesiology physician scientists in academic medicine: a wake-up call. Anesthesiology. 2006;104:170–8.

Pharmacokinetic and Pharmacodynamic Modeling in Anesthesia

40

Dennis M. Fisher and Steven L. Shafer

Summary

Before 1950, we little understood what drugs did to patients (pharmacodynamics) or what patients did to drugs (pharmacokinetics). In 1949, Faulconer et al correlated the EEG with the sedative/anesthetic effects of nitrous oxide. In 1960, Price simulated thiopental pharmacokinetics. In 1963, Eger extended the simulation to inhaled anesthetics and invented MAC. From 1972 to 1997, Sheiner and Rosenberg used computer models to predict pharmacokinetics in individuals, leading to the population principle.

In 1978, Hull used the effect site concept to understand the time course of pancuronium's effect. From 1978 to 1986, Sheiner and Beal defined methods for estimating the parameters controlling drug behavior, developing NONMEM to estimate population pharmacokinetics. In the 1980s, Schwilden published models allowing control of anesthetic concentrations. With Stoeckel, he devised a target controlled infusion (TCI) system that could maintain a target drug concentration.

During 1983 to 1995, Rampil related his EEG "spectral edge" to response to noxious stimulation. Shafer developed algorithms to target plasma and effect site concentrations, measure the performance of TCI devices, and estimate pharmacokinetics. During 1990 to 1998, the Stanford group used TCI to study pharmacodynamics in a "pseudo-steady state", assessing the effects of constant brain concentrations of thiopental, midazolam, flumazenil, and propofol. In 1991, Hughes et al defined the time for a 50% decrease in plasma concentration, as the "context-sensitive half-time."

During 1992–2001, Glass and Sebel used TCIs to study fentanyl interactions with other anesthetic drugs. The Stanford group applied Sheiner and Beal's concepts to produce the "Minto" kinetic-dynamic model of remifentanil, now used for TCI of remifentanil. Fisher et al used the differential effects of muscle relaxants on adductor pollicis and respiratory muscles to create a dose-effect model that did not require measurement of plasma concentrations.

From 1996 to 2007, Sheiner used the population principle to show that population pharmacokinetic analysis does not require complete data. He proposed that a single clinical trial plus causal evidence of effectiveness can merit drug approval. Stanski in 2005 called this "Getting the Dose Right."

From 1989 to 1999, the Stanford group developed a pharmacokinetic—pharmacodynamic model of propofol incorporating age and gender as covariates, and yielding the "Schnider" model. With Glass et al. they developed TCI for sedating critically ill patients with propofol, midazolam, and lorazepam. From 1998 to 2004, Minto and the Stanford team initiated response surface methods to characterize drug interactions, including context-dependent time courses. From 1994 to 2005, Henthorn, Avram, and Krejcie demonstrated that accurate initial drug dosing required use of "front end" pharmacokinetics.

Prologue

Nearly four decades ago, Dennis Fisher and Steve Shafer independently encountered remarkable people changing the course of pharmacokinetic and pharmacodynamic modeling. This chapter reflects their admiration of those individuals, and adds their personal experiences during an era transforming anesthetic clinical pharmacology and altering our understanding of and clinical practice with the drugs we use every day.

In the Beginning

Fisher spent the 1970s at the University of Pennsylvania in pediatric and anesthesia residencies, followed by a fellowship in critical care. His mentors, Ted Smith and Henry Rosenberg, introduced him to the prolific neuromuscular

D. M. Fisher (✉)
P Less Than, 218 Castenada Avenue, San Francisco, CA 94116, USA
e-mail: fisher@plessthan.com

S. L. Shafer
School of Medicine, Stanford University, 300 Pasteur Drive, MC-5640, Stanford, CA 94305-5640, USA
e-mail: steven.shafer@stanford.edu

E. I Eger II et al. (eds.), *The Wondrous Story of Anesthesia,* DOI 10.1007/978-1-4614-8441-7_40, © Edmond I Eger, MD 2014

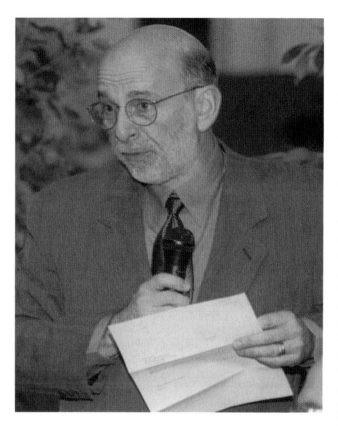

Fig. 40.1 Lewis Sheiner—Visionary Pharmacologist (1940–2004)

research coming from Ron Miller's group at the University of California, San Francisco (UCSF). Following residency Fisher applied to Miller for a fellowship, primarily drawn to UCSF by the opportunity to work with Lewis Sheiner (Fig. 40.1), the god of pharmacokinetics and pharmacodynamics. Many years of NIH support followed.

Shafer started closer to San Francisco, enrolling in Stanford Medical School in 1978. In his last year at Stanford, Shafer worked with Stanski, a previous Sheiner fellow, who was building a program in anesthetic pharmacology. Here are the stories of people—exemplars—who changed the world of anesthetic-related pharmacokinetics and pharmacodynamics.

Sheiner trained in internal medicine but never did much clinical work. Following his residency he went to the NIH to study Clinical Pharmacology, focusing on computer programs to individualize the dosing of warfarin [1]. In the late 1960s, computers were expensive, and programs were tediously assembled with punched cards that the computer could read. Applying this cumbersome technology to individualize dosing was a radical concept: it seemed too expensive and difficult to be practical. It was but one of Sheiner's visions.

Soon after arriving at UCSF, Sheiner developed a collaboration with Barr Rosenberg, economics professor at Berkeley and the entrepreneur founding Rosenberg mutual funds. Rosenberg told Sheiner that the econometrics community used sophisticated techniques to address problems inherent in issues such as warfarin dosing. Sheiner, Rosenberg and Ken Melmon (one of the founders of clinical pharmacology) proposed a general mathematical framework for optimizing drug dosage [2]. Sheiner's mother encountered problems with regular digoxin overdosing or underdosing, prompting his early study of computer aided digoxin delivery [3].

The "Population Principle"

Such modeling led to Sheiner's most important contribution, application of the "population principle" to pharmacology. According to the population principle, the behavior of drugs in individuals can be accurately predicted based on knowledge about how drugs behave in a population of patients with similar characteristics. The population principle defined drug behavior using "mixed effect" models combining the roles of "fixed effects" (e.g., dose, weight, height, age, gender), and the roles of "random effects" (things like the unexplained person-to-person differences in clearance, volume of distribution, or sensitivity to a drug) to explain drug behavior (pharmacodynamics). Further, the population principle separated the components of variability into those between individuals (interindividual variability, such as differences in clearance, which account for individual response to drugs) and those within an individual (intraindividual variability, such as assay noise). The aim was to predict drug effect as precisely as possible, taking known variables such as weight, height, gender, age, and other patient factors (e.g., genetics), to accurately predict the pharmacokinetic and pharmacodynamic factors controlling the response to a drug, factors such as clearance, volume of distribution, and potency. Thus, measurement of the right fixed effects should allow prediction of the response to a drug accurately, reducing the previously unexplained subject-to-subject variability. Reduction of residual inter-individual variability, things like assay noise, would require more precise measurements and perhaps refinement of models to more accurately describe the underlying biology.

Sheiner described the population principle in 1977 [4]. One of his insights was that pharmacokinetics in a population of patients could be estimated from routine clinical data. Sheiner's methods allowed the design of more efficient and informative clinical trials, optimizing dosing recommendations, and, via empirical Bayesian methods, optimizing individual therapy. The work transformed clinical pharmacology [5], the pharmaceutical industry [6, 7], and drug regulation [8].

A Fortuitous Bus Ride

Sheiner needed a statistician to develop his ideas, and a programmer to create software that would convert his concepts into research tools. In 1976, while riding on the UCSF

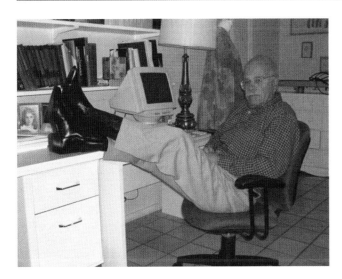

Fig. 40.2 Stuart Beal—Creator of NONMEM (1941–2006)

commuter bus to Marin County, he fortuitously sat next to Stuart Beal (Fig. 40.2), an aspiring statistician recently recruited to UCSF. Sheiner explained his ideas, piquing Beal's interest. A friendship and collaboration began that day and lasted a lifetime.

Beal expanded on Rosenberg's concepts for dose individualization [9], leading to his developing the statistical basis for mixed-effects modeling. Beal also wrote the program NONMEM, an acronym for non-linear mixed effects modeling. It is arguably the greatest intellectual advance in the history of clinical pharmacology. NONMEM's methodology opened the "population principle" of drug behavior to clinical pharmacologists, and became the standard modeling technique for the pharmaceutical industry. In the 1980s, Sheiner and Beal validated NONMEM against other popular approaches [10–12]. NONMEM outperformed those approaches.

In 1989, Ted Grasela approached Sheiner with a problem. Someone had sampled blood to determine theophylline concentration in neonates given theophylline to prevent apnea of prematurity. Each patient supplied a few samples. Grasela asked if a pharmacokinetic analysis could be done with such sparse sampling (compared to the standard of 10 samples or more). Sheiner realized that mixed-effects methods could be applied to Grasela's problem: the pharmacokinetic characteristics could be determined with a sufficient number of subjects (i.e., trading fewer samples per subjects for more subjects). The analysis succeeded [13], spawning a new approach to assessing population pharmacokinetics: study many subjects (thereby learning more about the population) but obtain few samples per patient (still learning about individual characteristics because of the large number of samples). This approach is known as sparse sampling coupled with population (mixed-effects) methods.

The "Effect Compartment"

Another novel Sheiner concept was mathematical modeling of the "effect compartment" in the context of a pharmacokinetic model. Clinicians have always known that a delay exists between drug dosing and drug effect. In 1960, Price described the time delay between thiopental concentration and drug effect [14]. Eger also provided insight into this delay or "hysteresis" for inhaled anesthetics [15]. However, this work did not link the delay to a pharmacokinetic model of the plasma drug concentration.

Stanski came to UCSF from his anesthesia residency at Massachusetts General Hospital. He wanted to develop a model explaining the delay between administration of a muscle relaxant and the resulting muscle paralysis. Immediately after receipt of a bolus dose, the plasma concentration of the muscle relaxant is at its highest concentration, but there is no drug effect. Over time the plasma concentration steadily decreases, and the level of muscle relaxation ("twitch depression") rises, reaches a maximum, and then recedes. This leads to the curious situation where there are two different plasma concentrations associated with the same twitch: one observed while the drug effect was increasing, and the other while the effect was decreasing. How could markedly different concentrations produce the same twitch depression?

Sheiner argued that the relevant concentration is the one at the neuromuscular junction (Sheiner chose the general term "effect site"). He linked it to the plasma concentration by simple "first order" diffusion down the concentration gradient. Sheiner and Stanski introduced the concept of the effect site" in a manuscript describing the time course of d-tubocurarine [16]. It became Stanski's most cited manuscript. Interestingly, using the same principle of first order diffusion down the concentration gradient, Chris Hull, a British anesthesiologist in Newcastle, UK, developed an effect compartment model for pancuronium [17]. Although Hull's publication preceded Sheiner's, Hull did little to popularize his work, and the Sheiner-Stanski contribution is considered pivotal.

Sheiner's Legacies

Sheiner pursued other issues: nonparametric approaches making minimal assumptions [18], therapeutic drug monitoring [19], how to handle missing dose data [20], and modeling drug compliance [21, 22]. He was a formidable intellect engaging anyone having interesting questions. He loved data. He was never just the visionary. Sheiner formatted the data, wrote NONMEM control streams, fitted the data to models, created the graphs, and analyzed the outputs. Fisher or Shafer would call Sheiner with a question, and his answer was often "Let me see the data, and I'll get back to you." He rarely looked anything up in books. It might be faster, but if he forced himself to do the derivation, he would then understand it better. Besides, it was more fun.

Sheiner mentored more than a generation of investigators and clinical pharmacologists. Most clinical pharmacology papers continue to reflect his work. He mentored Carl Peck, former Director of the FDA Center for Drug Evaluation and Research which incorporated Sheiner's concepts into FDA work. Sheiner was Stanski's mentor and greatest friend. He mentored Fisher whose papers in the 1990s benefited from Sheiner's insights.

Beal's education at UCLA included a BA degree in mathematics with a minor in Logic and Fine Arts, and MS and PhD degrees in biostatistics. He started at UCSF in 1973 as a Senior Statistician in the Office of Information Systems, joining the faculty in 1976, the year of his bus ride with Sheiner.

Sheiner was the front man—meeting people, giving lectures, looking for good questions and informative data, and raising new ideas. Beal was the implementer, the developer of statistics, translating Sheiner's grand ideas into NONMEM. NONMEM was Beal's life. He created new methods in NONMEM to handle the challenges raised by Sheiner and others. NONMEM came to encompass all of statistics to Beal.

In 2001, Shafer asked Beal how to perform a repeated measures ANOVA. Not trained as a statistician, Shafer had no idea about the "right" way to approach it, but had coded the problem using NONMEM. Beal laughed. Like Shafer, he could perform a repeated measures ANOVA using NONMEM, but had forgotten how to do it with conventional approaches. Indeed, Beal used NONMEM for t-tests. That conversation speaks volumes about NONMEM's versatility. Why use anything else, if NONMEM can provide any statistical test?

Beal and Sheiner offered NONMEM for a modest user fee to colleagues in academia and industry. If you didn't renew your license, then Beal (yes, the same Beal who developed the code) would personally call and ask you to return your magnetic tape or, once that was obsolete, the floppy disks. A week later you got another call, again from Beal.

Sheiner's colleague, Malcolm Rowland, thought that making NONMEM available inexpensively was a terrible idea: if Sheiner and Beal didn't make NONMEM profitable, then there would be no posthumous support structure for NONMEM. Eventually Sheiner and Beal accepted Rowland's wisdom and turned over NONMEM distribution to Globomax (now ICON Development Systems). Rowland's suggestion proved prescient. Despite Sheiner's and Beal's premature deaths, NONMEM has grown in popularity, usability, and statistical power.

Beal and Shafer—A Relationship Built on Questioning

Although many found Beal to be distant and reserved, he and Shafer were unusually close. Their friendship grew from a 1990s disagreement about modeling. Shafer, whose research was in target controlled drug delivery, had numerous reser-

vations about NONMEM. NONMEM could not be used for TCI, which required changing infusion rate every 10 seconds. Shafer had modeled all patients' responses simultaneously, ignoring inter-subject variability [23]. Beal dismissed the approach as "naïve" but allowed Shafer to deluge him with data, graphs, and analyses. Eventually Beal agreed that the naïve approach had merits, and was sometimes powerful. In the process, Beal showed Shafer how data settle scientific debates. Beal's patient mentorship led to Shafer's interest in the role of data in evidential reasoning [24]. Their relationship is evident in a letter Shafer sent to Beal in January, 1995:

> "I'm a physician with no formal training in mathematics or statistics. My role in clinical pharmacology is to bring the tools developed by your group to bear on questions important to me as a clinician. Your mentoring has allowed me to perform my work at a more sophisticated level than would otherwise be possible.

> "Mentoring takes time and patience, and God knows I've sorely tested your store of each. You have been patient with me, careful in your explanations, and considerate of my lack of formal training in mathematics and statistics. With your permission, I'll continue to pester you with problems, bother you with bugs, quiz you with questions, and irritate you with irreverent e-mail."

Epilogue to Lewis Sheiner and Stuart Beal

In 2004, Sheiner had a heart attack on a train from Basel Switzerland. He had just received the Rawls Palmer award at the American Society of Clinical Pharmacology and Therapeutics meeting. He was resuscitated but never regained consciousness, dying several days later.

Two years later, without his friend, collaborator, and soul mate, Beal completed his testing and validation of NONMEM VI. He sent it to Globomax with the enigmatic comment that it was nearly done, and that it could be released even without a final OK. A few days later he died.

Sheiner and Beal invented concepts, methodologies, and tools that changed how we understand therapeutics. Every drug is dosed a little better because of their work.

Dennis Fisher and the UCSF group

Fisher (Fig. 40.3) arrived in San Francisco in 1980, his interests quickly attracting him to Sheiner's circle. A pediatric anesthesiologist, Fisher initially studied pharmacokinetics and pharmacodynamics of muscle relaxants and intravenous anesthetic drugs in children, infants, and neonates. He developed a model describing the kinetics of drugs like atracurium that were degraded in plasma [25]. Burroughs Wellcome (now GSK) repeatedly challenged the model without explaining their rationale. Their stance galled Fisher because they adopted a similar model for cisatracurium, and claimed that they developed the model [26].

Francois Donati obtained simultaneous measurements of twitch depression at the thumb (adductor pollicis) and the laryngeal muscles, leading Fisher to a remarkable insight:

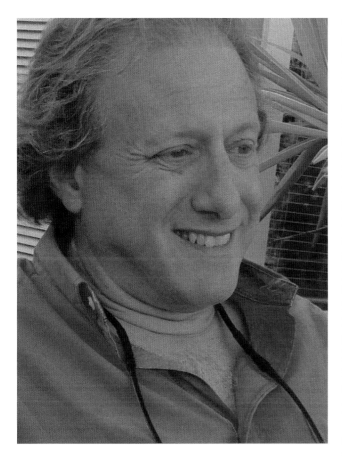

Fig. 40.3 Dennis Fisher. (Courtesy of the author)

with two different rates of onset, both driven by the same plasma drug concentrations, he could estimate the relative potency of the two drugs, and the rate of plasma-effect site equilibration for each with no measurement of plasma concentrations. The manuscript [27] prompted a suggestion by "an anonymous reviewer" (Shafer) to validate the model by repeating the study with plasma sampling and computing the outcome with and without those data. Fisher did, the results confirming his thesis [28].

Fisher presently evaluates many new drugs, most having nothing to do with anesthesia. His software, PLT Tools (in which Shafer also has a commercial interest) provides a powerful environment for harnessing NONMEM. Fisher and Shafer have now taught several hundred pharmaceutical scientists how to model their data with NONMEM. Through his teaching, and development of PLT Tools, Fisher continues the tradition of teaching, innovation, and service to pharmaceutical development that characterized Lew Sheiner.

Anesthesia and Brainwave Pioneers

The EEG has long been used to measure anesthetic effect. In 1875, Caton observed electrical activity in the scalp of rabbits, and found that the currents on one side of the head were influenced by light stimulation of the contralateral retina, suggesting the brain as a site of action [29]. Fifteen years later, Fleischl von Marxow demonstrated that chloroform extinguished the scalp electrical activity that Caton reported [30], confirming that the brain itself was the source of this activity. In the early 1930s, advances in amplification and recording allowed Berger to quantify EEG responses to chloroform-induced changes in consciousness [31]. In 1937, Gibbs observed that anesthetics changed the EEG from a low-voltage high-frequency pattern to a high-voltage, low frequency pattern, suggesting that the EEG could be used to measure the state of anesthesia [32]. In the late 1940s, Bickford at the Mayo clinic demonstrated the EEG effects of nitrous oxide [33]. In 1952, Faulconer correlated the arterial blood concentration of diethyl ether with specific EEG patterns, showing that the EEG responded predictably to a specific anesthetic [34]. Then as today, the finding was controversial. For example Galla and colleagues examined raw EEG signals for 43 patients and found a discrepancy between the clinical signs of anesthetic depth and the concurrent EEG [35]. Martin, Faulkoner, and Bickford, later demonstrated the classic biphasic response of the EEG to sedative/anesthetic drugs [36]. Bickford continued his work for nearly 50 years, publishing his last paper in 1992.

The microcomputer revolution of the 1970s allowed numerous investigators to attempt to link the EEG with anesthesia effect. For example, Levy and colleagues tried to correlate anesthesia drug concentrations with EEG at 50% (median frequency) or 95% (spectral edge) of wave activity, and concluded that the behavior of the EEG prevented any single number from describing the anesthetic state [37, 38]. What wise men! Drummond and colleagues calculated median frequency, spectral edge frequency, a frequency band power ratio, total power, and dominance shift during states of patient arousal during anesthesia [39], and concluded that none of these descriptors reliably predicted imminent arousal. But Long and coworkers undertook a similar analysis, and found that an abrupt decrease in delta EEG power always presaged arousal [40]. Dwyer and colleagues found no difference in the EEG power spectrum between patients anesthetized with isoflurane who moved on incision and those who didn't move [41]. What these investigators did not appreciate is that different drugs used to produce the anesthetic state produce different effects on the EEG. Stanski sorted out that riddle.

Don Stanski

After Stanski (Fig. 40.4) completed his fellowship training with Sheiner, Phil Larson recruited him to Stanford University to continue Stanford's program in clinical pharmacology, a program founded by William Forrest, Ellis Cohen, and Ty Smith. With Ed Meathe, Stanski used EEG algorithms de-

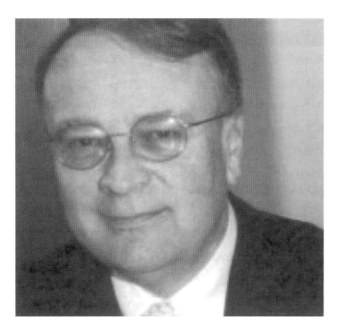

Fig. 40.4 Donald Stanski

veloped by Ira Rampil [42] to calculate the "spectral edge" [43] of the EEG response to thiopental. Stanski sent his EEG recordings following thiopental administration to engineer Meathe at UCSD, who calculated the spectral edge using Rampil's algorithm and returned the results to Stanski [44]. Stanski linked the EEG response to the effect site, the concept he developed at UCSF, to provide an integrated pharmacokinetic-pharmacodynamic model of thiopental [45]. His work disproved Dundee's 1950s claim that there was acute tolerance to thiopental [46] and showed that elderly brains are more sensitive to thiopental because of a change in pharmacokinetics, not because of a greater sensitivity to thiopental [47].

Stanski's success with the 95% spectral edge as a measure of thiopental drug effect was essential to his goal of creating integrated pharmacokinetic/pharmacodynamic models of intravenous anesthetic drugs. However, relying on UCSD to analyze his EEG recordings presented a significant logistical bottleneck. Shafer met Stanski in 1982, a year before Shafer completed medical school. Stanski needed a local programmer, and with help from Stanford Research Institute, Shafer wrote Fortran programs to digitize analog EEG data and calculate the 95% Spectral Edge. Stanski moved the EEG analysis to Stanford, and used Shafer's software for his subsequent studies on thiopental, benzodiazepines, and intravenous opioids. Stanski paid Shafer the munificent sum of US$ 1,000 at the end of the year for his contribution.

Stanford and "Ratsicles"

Stanski's work eventually provided integrated pharmacokinetic/pharmacodynamic models for thiopental [48, 49], fentanyl and alfentanil [50, 51], sufentanil [52], etomidate

[53], ketamine [54], and midazolam [55, 56]. Stanski's papers "hit" while Shafer pursued his residency (1984–1986) at the University of Pennsylvania. The papers garnered attention and befuddlement. Shafer was asked: "Do you know Stanski? Do you understand this effect site stuff?" Shafer answered "Yes" and "Maybe". Stanski recruited Shafer back to Stanford after residency, seducing him with visions of an academic career in computerized delivery of intravenous anesthetics.

Over the next six years, Stanski's laboratory became a center for clinical pharmacology in anesthesia. Stanski thought that defining the flow of drug to individual tissues could provide insights into the physical processes underlying common empiric pharmacokinetic models. He injected thiopental into rats, injected microspheres to identify regional blood flow then dropped the rats into liquid nitrogen. He dissected the tissues, counted microspheres, and assayed tissue concentrations of thiopental in twelve tissues from the frozen "ratsicle". From these he constructed detailed physiologic models of drug behavior [57]. It was a colossal effort with a small return on investment. These mathematically complex, detailed models did not provide more insight than simple empiric models consisting of 2 or 3 compartments linked by first-order drug transfer [58].

G187084B Becomes Remifentanil

Stanski's vision, partly implemented by Shafer, was that modeling and simulation could change drug development. In 1992, fortunate coincidences led Stanski, with Shafer in tow, to a paradigm changing experiment. Glaxo Pharmaceuticals had a new "ultra-fast" opioid, GI87084B, later known as remifentanil. They recruited one of Sheiner's former fellows, Keith Muir, to lead the remifentanil development program. Muir was well versed in pharmacokinetic and pharmacodynamic modeling. In preparing for his job interview, Muir read a paper by Shafer and Varvel summarizing the pharmacokinetic and pharmacodynamic parameters determined by Stanski for fentanyl, alfentanil, and sufentanil [59]. Muir took the modeling and data from the paper, and proposed to Glaxo that they use the EEG to guide the clinical development program for GI87084B. Fortunately, the FDA assigned Dan Spyker as the medical reviewer for GI87084B. Spyker was a toxicologist, but his PhD in electrical engineering probably drove his abiding interest in pharmacokinetic and pharmacodynamic modeling. He had formed a business, Cedar Systems, in the 1980s to develop software to model drug behavior. Spyker was convinced that Muir's concept was sound. He also thought it was a revolutionary paradigm change. Muir then contacted Stanski and Shafer with a proposal: use the fentanyl, alfentanil, and sufentanil work as a template for studies of remifentanil, And use those results to simulate how the drug should be used clinically. Stanski and Shafer jumped at the opportunity.

Three Stanford fellows were assigned to the project: Talmage Egan, Charles Minto, and Thomas Schnider. Together they produced the highest resolution pharmacokinetic/pharmacodynamic model that had been created for an intravenous anesthetic [60, 61]. They then applied the pharmacokinetics in simulations showing what to expect clinically with remifentanil [62]. These simulations reproduced the concentrations associated with different opioid effects, and provided precise guidance for clinical use.

The experiment worked. There were no failed clinical trials in the remifentanil development program, because the doses, based on simulation, were correct in every trial. The FDA approved the drug a mere 4 years after the patent was granted, a record for a drug not on a fast track (e.g., HIV therapy). And, most critically, it set an example of how modeling and simulation could create a "fingerprint" of a new pharmaceutical [63], resulting in safer, faster, and less expensive clinical development. It was the first demonstration of Sheiner's vision.

In retrospect, remifentanil was an "easy" demonstration. Remifentanil followed fentanyl, alfentanil, and sufentanil. For each of those opioids the EEG, a surrogate marker of effect, had already been mapped to clinical concentrations. Few other drug classes have such a clear relationship between a surrogate effect (EEG) readily measured in volunteers and the clinical effects.

Stanski Applies Sheiner's Vision

Stanski wanted to see if Sheiner's concepts could be more broadly applied. He left Stanford in late 1998 to work at Pharsight Corporation. Pharsight was founded to improve drug development using modeling. Stanski, Shafer, Fisher, and Sheiner were all involved in its early evolution. At Pharsight, Stanski directed a team applying modeling and simulation to drug development. Pharsight made some inroads in the area, but biological challenges (the difficulty of finding useful surrogate effects) combined with decreased FDA enthusiasm for modeling and simulation limited the implementation of Sheiner's vision. Stanski then went to the Commissioner's Office at the FDA to help them apply the kinetic/dynamic modeling skills developed at Stanford. In 2005 Stanski left the FDA for a position at Novartis Corporation where he built a team of approximately 80 clinical pharmacologists and modeling scientists. The concepts of quantitative drug development initially advanced by Sheiner and Beal, and refined for nearly 20 years at Stanford by Stanski, are being used today to develop new pharmaceuticals for human diseases. This is the wholesale application of Sheiner's vision to drug development: multiple programs, ranging from pre-clinical to post-approval, all guided by mathematical models of pharmacokinetics and pharmacodynamics, with specific incorporation of patient covariates and models of intersubject and intrasubject vari-

ability. The whole shebang. And it works! In 2011, Stanski was awarded the first Sheiner-Beal Pharmacometrics Award by the American Society of Clinical Pharmacology and Therapeutics.

Stanski is not a mathematician, statistician, modeler, or computer programmer. He has no intuition with equations. Basic statistical concepts do not come naturally. He never programmed a computer or wrote an Excel macro, although he did run an early version of NONMEM using punch cards. Stanski is a visionary. He knows what the tools do, and can match the tools to important questions. He doesn't need to model drug data. There are propeller heads like Shafer for that. Sheiner said it best, when introducing Stanski for the Rawls Palmer award in 1998: "I would rather hear a good question from Don, than a good answer from anyone else."

Stanski was Shafer's primary mentor, a lifetime relationship beginning nearly 30 years ago. Although Stanski is widely recognized for his scientific achievements, Shafer regards mentorship as Stanski's greatest talent. Stanski mentored dozens of fellows, most having gone on to academic and scientific careers. Shafer regularly gives talks on mentorship. They are always dedicated to Stanski.

Helmut Schwilden and Colleagues

It is easy to compute the infusion rate required to maintain a constant concentration for drugs described by one compartment models: it is the target concentration times the clearance. However, by the late 1960s it was clear that one compartment models describe few, if any, drugs. Distribution of drugs between central and peripheral compartments influences the accumulation of drug in the peripheral compartment and thereby affects the infusion rate required to sustain a constant effect. In 1968, Krüger-Thiemer described the mathematics required to maintain a steady drug concentration for drugs described by more than one compartment [64]. However, the calculations were intractably difficult, and in 1968 nobody envisioned microprocessors. More than a decade passed before implementation of Krüger-Thiemer's methodology.

Helmut Schwilden (Fig. 40.5) was a physicist who became an anesthesiologist. In the late 1970s, while Sheiner developed mixed-effects modeling and Stanski, modeled plasma-effect site relationships, Schwilden applied mathematics to instantly achieve and then maintain a constant drug concentration in the plasma.

The Beginnings of TCI

Schwilden published his *tour du force* in 1981 [65]. To implement the Krüger-Thiemer equations required a bolus injection of drug to nearly instantly achieve the desired plasma concentration, followed by an infusion that changed in rate

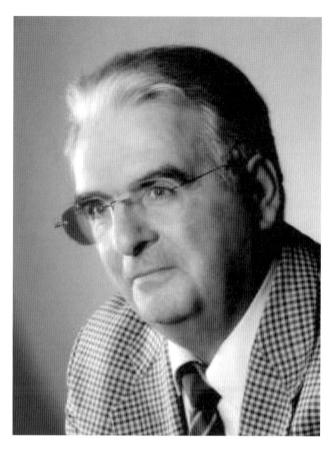

Fig. 40.5 Helmut Schwilden

every few seconds to maintain a constant concentration by replacing the drug that left the plasma. Schwilden's team built CATIA, Computer Assisted Titration of Intravenous Anesthesia [66], the first "Target Controlled Infusion" or "TCI" device. In the 30 years since TCI has become a standard technique to administer intravenous anesthetics worldwide, except in the US.

In the early 1980s, Max Ausems, a junior member of the faculty at Leiden University, created a new implementation of CATIA, "Titration of Intravenous Agents by Computer" or "TIAC" [67]. Ausems proved the accuracy of TIAC delivery of alfentanil [68] in human trials. He then used TIAC to "lock" the plasma alfentanil at a target concentration, and measured the effect of various alfentanil concentrations, thereby establishing concentration vs. response curves in the presence of various stimuli, and for spontaneous ventilation [69]. This pioneering work led to the development of TCI as a method of rapidly achieving a titratable steady state for understanding concentration vs. response relationships for intravenous drugs. It also led to a host of other "home-grown" TCI systems, only two of which are still in use: STANPUMP, developed by Shafer, and RUGLOOP (which was derived from STANPUMP), developed by Struys and De Smet [70].

The EEG and Feedback Control

Schwilden believed that such devices incompletely achieved the correct concentration in each patient. Adding the EEG would supply a continuous measure of drug effect that could be used to fine-tune drug delivery. Of course, there was precedent for this work. Bickford had implemented an EEG based closed loop system for anesthesia in 1950 [71], and Bellville followed suit in 1957 [72]. In 1962, Eger produced a constant EEG anesthetic level (burst suppression) in patients by adjusting and measuring the rate of an intravenous infusion of a 5 % solution of ether [73]. Thus he combined a servo (human) titration of the level of anesthesia (pharmacodynamics) with an assessment of uptake (pharmacokinetics).

Schwilden improved on these pioneering efforts, concluding that the median frequency contained the information needed to control an infusion pump [74]. In 1987, he developed a pioneering closed-loop feedback system, using the EEG to titrate methohexital [75]. While many question whether the EEG means anything during clinical anesthesia, two decades ago Helmut Schwilden demonstrated that the EEG alone could be used to successfully guide methohexital anesthesia, convincingly answering the question.

Schwilden was not only a visionary, he was an international ambassador for using mathematics (i.e., computers) to control the delivery of anesthetic drugs. Schwilden ushered in the field in 1981, built the first devices, and demonstrated that they worked. He gave brilliant, insightful, and stimulating lectures. But he showed frustration at the pace of development. He had developed and implemented the mathematical framework for fundamental principles of anesthetic drug delivery. However, it was not until 1995, that TCI became commercially available in Europe. It is now popular worldwide, although it remains unavailable in the US. But the capacity of the EEG to guide anesthesia remains controversial, and closed-loop intravenous anesthesia delivery systems may never appear despite Schwilden's demonstration in the 1980s, and the pioneering demonstrations by Bickford [66] and Bellville [67] more than 50 years ago.

Paul White

While Don Stanski mentored Steve Shafer, Paul White mentored Shafer's wife, Audrey Shafer. Following residency, the Shafer's returned to Stanford as post-doctoral fellows. In her fellowship years with White, Audrey Shafer studied a novel drug, propofol, that ICI Pharmaceuticals thought would be a suitable replacement for thiopental. ICI sought FDA approval for induction of anesthesia, but White had other ideas. In his view, propofol should also be infused to maintain anesthesia. ICI begrudgingly supported this research, which Audrey Shafer assumed as her fellowship project. Her resulting paper on the pharmacokinetics and pharmacodynamics of propofol [76] was the first definitive manuscript on propofol pharmacology.

Three Laboratories

Laboratories, like individuals, have a trajectory and a lifespan. To illustrate the history we provide an admittedly parochial description of three US laboratories contributing mightily to our understanding of the pharmacokinetics and pharmacodynamics of intravenous drugs. These three laboratories were populated by groups that we knew personally, and their selection does not mean that teams of investigators from other institutions (e.g., Emory University, Harvard University, University of Bonn, and the University of Leiden) made lesser contributions.

The Stanford Group

In the 1980s Stanski recruited fellows and investigators to characterize the clinical pharmacology of intravenous anesthetics. By 1986, Shafer, Pierre Maitre and Michael Buhrer from Switzerland, and Bill Ebling, a PhD from Buffalo, New York had joined the laboratory. Maitre was an "expert" in NONMEM by virtue of getting the program to run [77], a superhuman task in 1987. Buhrer studied benzodiazepine effects on the EEG [51, 52].

Stanski had a pleasant surprise for Shafer upon his arrival in 1986. While at the University of Alabama, Jerry Reves developed "computer assisted continuous infusion" or "CACI" [78]. Now at Duke University, Reves had joined with a young engineer, Jim Jacobs, to create CACI II [79]. Reves sent Stanski the software and Shafer was directed to test the CACI II device on patients. However, uncertain about the workings of the program, Shafer first tested the CACI II software. The resulting report [80] described numerous problems in the CACI II software, and Shafer was apprehensive about submitting such a critical manuscript for publication. Larry Saidman, Editor-in-Chief of *Anesthesiology*, asked Reves to review the submission. Reves was understandably annoyed by Shafer's criticisms but supported publication, feeling that development of computer controlled anesthetic delivery demanded rigorous evaluation of software. In a rapprochement, Reves, Peter Glass (then a fellow at Duke), and Jacobs spent two days with the Stanford team in Palo Alto. Fellowship mixed with rigorous science, and Shafer found lasting soul mates in Jacobs (someone who loved programming and mathematics), and Glass (an avid clinical investigator).

Mathematical Simulation vs. Empirical Pharmacology

The difficulties with CACI (later fixed by Jacobs) prompted Shafer to write STANPUMP ("STANford PUMP") to provide a competing platform, which he mostly completed from 1986–1990. Shafer noted that alfentanil, the drug with purportedly "rapid" pharmacokinetics, didn't seem to work as promoted. Ebling, the resident genius, suggested that Janssen Pharmaceuticals had not positioned fentanyl, alfentanil, and sufentanil correctly: "Janssen says you should use alfentanil for short cases, but I don't think it makes sense to use it for short cases. The drugs will look the same. The drug with the shortest half-life only makes sense for long cases, because there the rapid (terminal) half-life may pay off." Shafer wrote software to simulate TCI infusions, and with John Varvel (his first fellow) demonstrated that Janssen Pharmaceuticals had not understood the clinical implications of the multicompartment pharmacokinetics of fentanyl, alfentanil, and sufentanil [55]. Jansson had not done the necessary simulations to see if the pharmacokinetics of alfentanil predicted unusually rapid recovery (they don't). Shafer believed that pharmacokinetics might be widely misunderstood if a multibillion dollar pharmaceutical company had incorrectly positioned their product in the market. The paper provided a new framework to relate the time course of recovery to dose duration, (unknowingly having followed Eger's work with inhaled anesthetics) [81] and subsequently given the name "context-sensitive half-time" by Glass and Jacobs [82].

In the early 1990s a series of novel opioids were in development. Shafer created a table of clinical and EEG potencies with the explicit intent of guiding the development of novel opioids. When Muir read the paper the following year, he immediately understood the implications for the development of GI87084B. He did not realize that Shafer planted the table in the paper for exactly that purpose.

It was a time of innovation. Orlando Hung dissected thiopental concentration vs. response relationships using TCI methodology [83]. Varvel developed metrics to measure TCI performance [84]. Shafer produced TCI algorithms to control effect site concentrations with TCI [85], and pharmacometric methods to estimate kinetics from TCI studies [23]. Keith Gregg, a statistician, developed a novel EEG based measure optimized for opioid drug effect [86].

At Work and Play

Shafer wrote of the personal relationships fostered by their work: "At home Audrey and I looked after Thomas, who was born in the middle of our fellowship year. John and Liz Varvel had two young children, and Jeanette and Orlando Hung had a son, Christopher, who was Thomas' age and rapidly became his closest friend. We lived at each other's houses, the kids entertaining themselves while we played

Pictionary—men against women. Liz, Jeanette, and Audrey were superior artists and skilled guessers. John, Orlando and I only won by inventing increasingly elaborate cheating schemes."

New Kids on the Block Continue the Sheiner Legacy

In the mid 1990s a second influx of fellows initiated another productive period. Pedro Gambus (Spain), focused on a high-resolution study of intravenous dynorphin [87]. Valerie Billard (France) investigated plasma-effect site equilibration for propofol [88]. Thomas Schnider (Switzerland) undertook a high-resolution study of propofol pharmacokinetics [89] and pharmacodynamics [90] producing the standard propofol model for TCI. The work of Egan, Minto, and Schnider on remifentanil has been mentioned. Juliana Barr (Stanford), Jacques Somma (Canada), and Katie Zomorodi (UK) performed pharmacokinetic studies of propofol, midazolam, and lorazepam for ICU sedation [91–93], informing the dosing guidelines in the FDA package insert for propofol and midazolam sedation. In a 6 week mini-sabbatical, Tim Short (New Zealand) created a model [94] that became the standard for describing anesthetic drug interactions. Minto demonstrated that one could "observe" effect site equilibration from the time to peak effect [95], providing a means to directly validate the equilibration between the plasma and the site of anesthetic drug effect proposed by Sheiner and Stanski decades earlier [16].

In 1997 Thomas Bouillon became the last fellow to join Shafer's PK/PD research team at Stanford. The pharmacokinetic/pharmacodynamic underpinning of the potential of remifentanil or propofol to depress ventilation and produce apnea had not been modeled. Bouillon created a model relating the dose of these drugs to ventilatory drive in patients breathing room air under non-steady state conditions. Bouillon directed the most complex human studies conducted by the Stanford team. It took 10 people to measure a volunteer's CO_2—ventilatory response via a rebreathing circuit; set up and manage TCIs of propofol or remifentanil; provide graded stimuli to assess pharmacodynamics; and gather blood samples and arterial blood gases every minute. At the day's end, Bouillon always took the crew and the volunteer out for beer. Three papers published in *Anesthesiology* [96, 97, 98] years after Bouillon's fellowship ended described his seminal work.

By 1999, clinical pharmacology no longer seemed sexy to Shafer. His VA Merit Review grant ran out after 11 years of funding, and he did not seek renewal. Stanski left for Pharsight. The fellows had gone. No new anesthetic drugs appeared. The research had achieved its goals. In two decades, Stanski, and then Shafer, had produced models characterizing the pharmacokinetics and pharmacodynamics of intravenous hypnotics and opioids. Shafer went to Pharsight for a sabbatical. Other investigators maintained a clinical pharma-

cology programs at Stanford, but since 1999, Shafer has not had a research laboratory.

The Duke Group

In the early 1980s Reves brought TCI technology from Schwilden and Ausems to the US, developing the first incarnation of CACI at the University of Alabama. Reves was evangelical about TCI, believing it would transform intravenous anesthesia. He had a particular interest in using CACI in cardiac surgery, believing TCI would improve patient safety [99]. He found that aging increased sensitivity to midazolam [100].

Reves recruited Glass from South Africa, to help him with this project, initially performing clinical evaluations with TCI [101]. Like Reves, Glass increasingly used TCI as a tool to characterize hypnotic—opioid interactions [102, 103]. In the 1990s Glass also became interested in the processed EEG as a measure of drug effect, with a specific focus on the bispectral index (oddly called "BIS" rather than "BSI") developed by Aspect Medical Systems. Glass collaborated with Carl Rosow (Harvard) and Peter Sebel (Emory) in multicenter studies examining the clinical utility of BIS monitoring [104–106].

Reves brought Jacobs from the University of Alabama to develop and maintain CACI. Jacobs also provided pioneering work in TCI algorithms, insights into the "context-sensitive half-time" [82, 107], and novel pharmacokinetic models [108].

Some interests of the Duke laboratory mirrored those of the Stanford team, including TCI, novel drugs (propofol, remifentanil), modeling, and simulation. The personal friendships formed at their meeting in Palo Alto fostered an environment of ongoing collaboration. However, the Duke laboratory had a different focus. The Stanford team pursued fundamental pharmacokinetics and theoretical development. Most Stanford studies were in healthy volunteers. The Duke group used TCI to characterize the clinical potency (called the "effective concentration" or "EC_{50}") of anesthetic drugs in the tradition of Ausems. Nearly all of their studies were in patients. As at Stanford, a dearth of new drugs, and the departure of Reves, Glass, and Jacobs reduced the Duke team. Duke still has an active clinical pharmacology program, but one no longer focused on pharmacokinetics and pharmacodynamics.

The Northwestern Group

Three contemporaries of Fisher and Shafer created a laboratory in clinical pharmacology at the Northwestern University: Thomas Henthorn (the tallest of the group, and hence the presumed leader), Mike Avram (the pharmacologist), and

Tom Krejcie (the implementer). Classical pharmacokinetics characterized the disposition of drugs over many hours. However, in the mid 1980s, Henthorn, Avram, and Krejcie became obsessed with what happened seconds after an intravenous bolus injection. The classical model assumed that the concentration at zero minutes after bolus injection is the dose divided by the central compartment volume. That's the supposed peak, and it drops from there. But that's not how it works. Right after giving a slug of, say, propofol, the arterial concentration is 0, because it takes 30–60 seconds for drug to flow through the heart and lungs and reach the radial artery. After this initial delay the concentration abruptly shoots up as the main wave of drug passes down the radial artery. After the peak the concentration rapidly drops, but oscillates from the rapid return of a small amount of drug taken up by the heart and lung vasculature in the first pass. The oscillations subside in a minute or two, after which the concentration follows the smooth polyexponential decay described by classic models.

Like Price a generation earlier [109], Henthorn, Avram, and Krejcie focused on these "front end" pharmacokinetics, and gathered arterial blood samples during the initial moments after bolus injection. Shafer thought they were nuts. If the model is off for minute or two, but then works OK, that's good enough. Shafer didn't see a value in precise models for the first 2–3 minutes.

In the 1990s Henthorn, Avram, and Krejcie argued that plasma-effect site equilibration could not be properly modeled after bolus injection unless the model correctly defined the "front end" pharmacokinetics, particularly arguing that misspecification of the concentrations in the first 30–60 seconds drastically affected the equilibration occurring in the ensuing 2–5 minutes. They prevailed intellectually, but the Stanford group never incorporated "front end" pharmacokinetics into their PK models. The focus continued to be the "long term" pharmacokinetics for anesthetic drugs. Experimentally, the Stanford group sidestepped the issue (and greatly decreased the error) by using 10 minute infusions rather than bolus injections.

Henthorn, Avram, and Krejcie were right about the importance of front end pharmacokinetics [110]. Multiple investigators with slightly different research methodologies developed different estimates of the plasma-effect site equilibration rate (k_{e0}) for propofol because of inaccurate assumptions about drug behavior in the first 2 minutes after bolus injection. Indeed, Shafer published 4 different propofol k_{e0} estimates, because studies with slightly different arterial sampling schemes gave different results. These "dueling k_{e0}" values created a nightmare for companies developing effect-site target controlled infusion algorithms for propofol. The approach of Henthorn, Avram, and Krejcie would have prevented this confusion.

Henthorn, Avram, and Krejcie have a nickname. In 1996 Shafer chaired a site visit for a T32 training grant in Clinical Pharmacology submitted by the Northwestern University. As part of the review process, Henthorn, Avram, and Krejcie described the hours of early morning preparation each investigator contributed to the arterial blood sampling every 5 seconds after drug administration. Impressed by the effort and coordination required, Shafer asked "at what ungodly hour does your SWAT Team arrive to make this happen?" The name stuck. The outside world knows these investigators as Henthorn, Avram, and Krejcie. However, to their academic colleagues, they are "the SWAT Team".

The Industry Link

New drugs and devices benefit from the research conducted at Universities, but all products are eventually introduced by companies. Sometimes businessmen/scientists at these companies made significant contributions, as in the following two examples.

David Goodale

Dentist David Goodale was the propofol product manager in the US. for nearly 20 years, beginning in 1988. Goodale had pursued research before joining Stuart Pharmaceutics. Throughout the 1990s Goodale worked with Shafer to characterize the fundamental pharmacokinetics and pharmacodynamics of propofol. In the early 1990s, Goodale asked Shafer to help ICI (previously Stuart, later Astra Zeneca) analyze the existing clinical database to provide dosing guidelines for propofol for sedation. Elderly patients had died because the wrong dose of midazolam was prescribed, and the FDA wanted to avoid similar problems with propofol. Goodale believed this could be accomplished with a thorough pharmacokinetic/pharmacodynamic characterization. After several months of modeling Shafer provided ICI with doses for MAC sedation, the adjustment in dose required for elderly patients, and the scientific basis of the dosing guidelines. Those doses are still in the package insert, affirming Goodale's belief that modeling would develop dosing guidelines that would withstand the test of time. Similarly, Goodale enabled Schnider's high-resolution pharmacokinetic/pharmacodynamic model of propofol for use in general surgery patients [89, 90]. and Barr's pharmacokinetic/pharmacodynamic model of propofol for use in the intensive care unit [91]. Much of this work was directly translated into the dosing recommendations in the propofol package insert—and every one has stood the test of time.

Nassib Chamoun

Around 1990, Nassib Chamoun, founder of Aspect Medical Systems, approached Stanski to discuss an improved method of EEG analysis. Virtually all prior EEG analyses had ignored the "phase" relationships in the signal, mostly because nobody had any idea what to do with them. Chamoun thought there was gold in the phase information, believing that the EEG consisted of multiple interlocking frequencies, and the phase information revealed which frequencies were interlocked. Sleep or anesthesia would decrease synchrony between interlocked frequencies, because the sedated brain could not sustain the connections. Stanski was intrigued, and introduced Shafer to Chamoun. Shafer agreed to share his EEG tapes so that Chamoun could test his algorithm.

Aspect Medical Systems recruited bright engineers and found investors to pay for the expensive research and development that Chamoun believed were needed to validate his bispectral analysis—BIS—as a measure of anesthetic effect. Based on promising results from the data provided by Stanski [111] and similar results from other investigators, Chamoun underwrote an ambitious series of clinical trials. Indeed, an enormous amount of what we know about the potency of anesthetic drugs, the pharmacodynamic interaction of anesthetic drugs, and the relationship of individual drugs to the EEG stems from the hundreds of millions of dollars that Aspect Medical Systems invested in research. Other vendors subsequently introduced processed EEG monitors to assess drug effect and "anesthetic depth", but Chamoun did the heavy lifting, funding hundreds of clinical studies so that the use of BIS would be based on data.

The End of An Era

From the early 1970s through the end of the 20th Century our exemplars and their colleagues mathematically described the clinical pharmacology of most intravenous anesthetic drugs. All are older than 50 years. Few young investigators in anesthesia have arrived to replace them. Perhaps the paucity of drug development in anesthesia explains this drought. The excellence of drugs available to anesthesiologists (e.g., propofol, rocuronium, desflurane, sevoflurane) diminishes the incentive for pharmaceutical industry to develop new drugs. We may get sugammadex, but what then? Or perhaps all the important ideas have been offered? Is a lack of mentors the problem? Stanski moved to industry more than a decade ago. Shafer shifted his focus to his job as Editor-in-Chief of *Anesthesia and Analgesia*. Fisher left anesthesia to devote his efforts to early-stage drug development in other therapeutic areas. Henthorn, Glass, Schüttler, and Schnider became chairmen, an effective way to kill research careers. Schwilden, Reves, and White have retired. A few are still

active: Krejcie and Avram at Northwestern, Egan in Utah. However, perhaps it is the deaths of Sheiner and Beal, fountains of creative energy, that closed the era.

The era of innovation in pharmacokinetic/pharmacodynamic modeling in anesthesia peaked a decade or two ago. It was great fun while it lasted.

References

1. Sheiner LB. Computer-aided long-term anticoagulation therapy. Comput Biomed Res. 1969;2:507–18.
2. Sheiner LB, Rosenberg B, Melmon KL. Modelling of individual pharmacokinetics for computer-aided drug dosage. Comput Biomed Res. 1972;5:411–59.
3. Peck CC, Sheiner LB, Martin CM, Combs DT, Melmon KL. Computer-assisted digoxin therapy. N Engl J Med. 1973;289:441–6.
4. Sheiner LB, Rosenberg B, Marathe VV. Estimation of population characteristics of pharmacokinetic parameters from routine clinical data. J Pharmacokinet Biopharm. 1977;5:445–79.
5. Sheiner LB, Steimer JL. Pharmacokinetic/pharmacodynamic modeling in drug development. Annu Rev Pharmacol Toxicol. 2000;40:67–95.
6. Sheiner LB. Learning versus confirming in clinical drug development. Clin Pharmacol Ther. 1997;61:275–91.
7. Stanski DR, Rowland M, Sheiner LB. Getting the dose right: report from the Tenth European Federation of Pharmaceutical Sciences (EUFEPS) conference on optimizing drug development. J Pharmacokinet Pharmacodyn. 2005;32:199–211.
8. Peck CC, Rubin DB, Sheiner LB. Hypothesis: a single clinical trial plus causal evidence of effectiveness is sufficient for drug approval. Clin Pharmacol Ther. 2003;73:481-90.
9. Sheiner LB, Beal S, Rosenberg B, Marathe VV. Forecasting individual pharmacokinetics. Clin Pharmacol Ther. 1979;26:294–305.
10. Sheiner LB, Beal SL. Evaluation of methods for estimating population pharmacokinetics parameters. I. Michaelis-Menten model: routine clinical pharmacokinetic data. J Pharmacokinet Biopharm. 1980;8:553–71.
11. Sheiner LB. Analysis of pharmacokinetic data using parametric models. II. Point estimates of an individual's parameters. J Pharmacokinet Biopharm. 1985;13:515–40.
12. Sheiner LB, Beal SL. Evaluation of methods for estimating population pharmacokinetic parameters. III. Monoexponential model: routine clinical pharmacokinetic data. J Pharmacokinet Biopharm. 1983;11:303–19.
13. Grasela TH, Sheiner LB, Rambeck B, Boenigk HE, Dunlop A, Mullen PW, Wadsworth J, Richens A, Ishizaki T, Chiba K et al. Steady-state pharmacokinetics of phenytoin from routinely collected patient data. Clin Pharmacokinet. 1983;8:355–64.
14. Price HL. A dynamic concept of the distribution of thiopental in the human body. Anesthesiology. 1960;21:40–5.
15. Eger EI. II: Application of a mathematical model of gas uptake. In: Papper EM, Kitz RJ editor. Uptake and distribution of anesthetic agents. New York, McGraw-Hill; 1963. pp. 88–103.
16. Sheiner LB, Stanski DR, Vozeh S, Miller RD, Ham J. Simultaneous modeling of pharmacokinetics and pharmacodynamics: application to d-tubocurarine. Clin Pharmacol Ther. 1979;25:358–71.
17. Hull CJ, Van Beem HB, McLeod K et al. A pharmacodynamic model for pancuronium. Br J Anaesth. 1978;50:1113–23.
18. Verotta D, Sheiner LB. Simultaneous modeling of pharmacokinetics and pharmacodynamics: an improved algorithm. Comput Appl Biosci. 1987;3:345-9.
19. Sheiner LB. The use of serum concentrations of digitalis for quantitative therapeutic decisions. Cardiovasc Clin. 1974;6:141–51.

20. Soy D, Beal SL, Sheiner LB. Population one-compartment pharmacokinetic analysis with missing dosage data. Clin Pharmacol Ther. 2004;76:441–51.

21. Girard P, Sheiner LB, Kastrissios H, Blaschke TF. Do we need full compliance data for population pharmacokinetic analysis? J Pharmacokinet Biopharm. 1996;24:265–82.

22. Kshirsagar SA, Blaschke TF, Sheiner LB, Krygowski M, Acosta EP, Verotta D. Improving data reliability using a non-compliance detection method versus using pharmacokinetic criteria. J Pharmacokinet Pharmacodyn. 2007;34:35–55.

23. Shafer SL, Varvel JR, Aziz N, Scott JC. The pharmacokinetics of fentanyl administered by computer controlled infusion pump. Anesthesiology. 1990;73:1091–102.

24. Shafer SL. Critical thinking in anesthesia: eighth Honorary FAER Research Lecture. Anesthesiology. 2009;110:729–37.

25. Fisher DM, Canfell PC, Fahey MR, Rosen JI, Rupp SM, Sheiner LB, Miller RD. Elimination of atracurium in humans: contribution of Hofmann elimination and ester hydrolysis versus organ-based elimination. Anesthesiology. 1986;65:6–12.

26. Kisor DF, Schmith VD, Wargin WA, Lien CA, Ornstein E, Cook DR. Importance of the organ-independent elimination of cisatracurium. Anesth Analg. 1996;83:1065–71.

27. Bragg P, Fisher DM, Shi J, Donati F, Meistelman C, Lau M, Sheiner LB. Comparison of twitch depression of the adductor pollicis and the respiratory muscles. Pharmacodynamic modeling without plasma concentrations. Anesthesiology. 1994;80:310–9.

28. Fisher DM, Wright PM. Are plasma concentration values necessary for pharmacodynamic modeling of muscle relaxants? Anesthesiology. 1997;86:567–75.

29. Caton R. The electrical currents of the brain (abstract). BMJ 1875;2:278.

30. Fleischl von Marxow E. Mittheilung betreffend die Physiologie der Hirnrinde. Zentralbl Physiol. 1890;4:537–540.

31. Berger H. Uber das Elektrenkaphalogramm des Menschen. Arch Psychiatry. 1933;101:452.

32. Gibbs FA, Gibbs EL, Lennox WG. Effect on the electro-encephalogram of certain drugs which influence nervous activity. Arch Intern Med. 1937;60:154.

33. Faulconer A, Pender JW, Bickford RG. The influence of partial pressure of nitrous oxide on the depth of anesthesia and the electroencephalogram in man. Anesthesiology. 1949;10:601–9.

34. Faulconer A Jr. Correlation of concentrations of ether in arterial blood with electro-encephalographic patterns occurring during ether-oxygen and during nitrous oxide, oxygen and ether anesthesia of human surgical patients. Anesthesiology. 1952;13:361.

35. Galla SJ, Rocco AG, Vandam LD. Evaluation of the traditional signs and stages of anesthesia: an electroencephalographic and clinical study. Anesthesiology. 1958;19(361):328–38.

36. Martin JT, Faulconer A Jr, Bickford RG. Electroencephalography in anesthesiology. Anesthesiology. 1959;20:359–76.

37. Levy WJ, Shapiro HM, Maruchak G, et al. Automated EEG processing for intraoperative monitoring: a comparison of techniques. Anesthesiology. 1980;53:223.

38. Rampil IJ. What every neuroanesthesiologist should know about electroencephalograms and computerized monitors. Anesthesiol Clin North Am. 1992;10:683.

39. Drummond JC, Brann CA, Perkins DE, et al. A comparison of median frequency, spectral edge frequency, a frequency band power ratio, total power and dominance shift in the determination of depth of anesthesia. Acta Anaesthesiol Scand 1991;35:693.

40. Long CW, Shah NK, Loughlin C, et al. A comparison of EEG determinants of near awakening from isoflurane and fentanyl anesthesia. Anesth Analg. 1989;69:169.

41. Dwyer RC, Rampil IJ, Eger EI, et al. The electroencephalogram does not predict depth of isoflurane anesthesia. Anesthesiology. 1994;81:403.

42. Rampil IJ, Holzer JA, Quest DO, Rosenbaum SH. Correll JW: Prognostic value of computerized EEG analysis during carotid endarterectomy. Anesth Analg. 1983;62:186–92.

43. Rampil IJ, Matteo RS. Changes in EEG spectral edge frequency correlate with the hemodynamic response to laryngoscopy and intubation. Anesthesiology. 1987;67:139–42.

44. Hudson RJ, Stanski DR, Saidman LJ, Meathe E. A model for studying depth of anesthesia and acute tolerance to thiopental. Anesthesiology. 1983;59:301–8.

45. Stanski DR, Hudson RJ, Homer TD, Saidman LJ, Meathe E. Pharmacodynamic modeling of thiopental anesthesia. J Pharmacokinet Biopharm. 1984;12:223–40.

46. Dripps RD, Dundee JW, Price HL. Acute tolerance to thiopentone in man. Br J Anaesth. 1956;28:344–52.

47. Homer TD, Stanski DR. The effect of increasing age on thiopental disposition and anesthetic requirement. Anesthesiology. 1985;62:714–24.

48. Bührer M, Maitre PO, Hung OR, Ebling WF, Shafer SL, Stanski DR. Thiopental pharmacodynamics. I. Defining the pseudo-steady-state serum concentration-EEG effect relationship. Anesthesiology. 1992;77:226–36.

49. Hung OR, Varvel JR, Shafer SL, Stanski DR. Thiopental pharmacodynamics. II. Quantitation of clinical and electroencephalographic depth of anesthesia. Anesthesiology. 1992;77:237–44.

50. Scott JC, Stanski DR. Decreased fentanyl and alfentanil dose requirements with age. A simultaneous pharmacokinetic and pharmacodynamic evaluation. J Pharmacol Exp Ther. 1987;240:159–66.

51. Scott JC, Ponganis KV, Stanski DR. EEG quantitation of narcotic effect: the comparative pharmacodynamics of fentanyl and alfentanil. Anesthesiology. 1985;62:234–41.

52. Scott JC, Cooke JE, Stanski DR. Electroencephalographic quantitation of opioid effect: comparative pharmacodynamics of fentanyl and sufentanil. Anesthesiology. 1991;74:34–42.

53. Arden JR, Holley FO, Stanski DR. Increased sensitivity to etomidate in the elderly: initial distribution versus altered brain response. Anesthesiology. 1986;65:19–27.

54. Schüttler J, Stanski DR, White PF, Trevor AJ, Horai Y, Verotta D, Sheiner LB. Pharmacodynamic modeling of the EEG effects of ketamine and its enantiomers in man. J Pharmacokinet Biopharm. 1987;15:241–53.

55. Bührer M, Maitre PO, Hung O, Stanski DR. Electroencephalographic effects of benzodiazepines. I. Choosing an electroencephalographic parameter to measure the effect of midazolam on the central nervous system. Clin Pharmacol Ther. 1990;48:544–54.

56. Bührer M, Maitre PO, Crevoisier C, Stanski DR. Electroencephalographic effects of benzodiazepines. II. Pharmacodynamic modeling of the electroencephalographic effects of midazolam and diazepam. Clin Pharmacol Ther. 1990;48:555–67.

57. Ebling WF, Wada DR, Stanski DR. From piecewise to full physiologic pharmacokinetic modeling: applied to thiopental disposition in the rat. J Pharmacokinet Biopharm. 1994;22:259–92.

58. Björkman S, Wada DR, Stanski DR, Ebling WF. Comparative physiological pharmacokinetics of fentanyl and alfentanil in rats and humans based on parametric single-tissue models. J Pharmacokinet Biopharm. 1994;22:381–410.

59. Shafer SL, Varvel JR. Pharmacokinetics, pharmacodynamics, and rational opioid selection. Anesthesiology. 1991;74:53–63.

60. Egan TD, Lemmens HJ, Fiset P, Hermann DJ, Muir KT, Stanski DR, Shafer SL. The pharmacokinetics of the new short-acting opioid remifentanil (GI87084B) in healthy adult male volunteers. Anesthesiology. 1993;79:881–92.

61. Minto CF, Schnider TW, Egan TD, Youngs E, Lemmens HJ, Gambus PL, Billard V, Hoke JF, Moore KH, Hermann DJ, Muir KT, Mandema JW, Shafer SL. Influence of age and gender on the pharmacokinetics and pharmacodynamics of remifentanil. I. Model development. Anesthesiology. 1997;86:10–23.

62. Minto CF, Schnider TW, Shafer SL. The influence of age and gender on the pharmacokinetics and pharmacodynamics of remifentanil. II. Model application. Anesthesiology. 1997;86:24–33.

63. Egan TD, Muir KT, Hermann DJ, Stanski DR, Shafer SL. The electroencephalogram (EEG) and clinical measure of opioid potency: defining the EEG-clinical potency relationship ("fingerprint") with application to remifentanil. Int J Pharm Med. 2001;15:1–9.

64. Krüger-Thiemer E. Continuous intravenous infusion and multicompartment accumulation. Eur J Clin Pharmacol. 1968;4:317–24.

65. Schwilden H. A general method for calculating the dosage scheme in linear pharmacokinetics. Eur J Clin Pharmacol. 1981;20:379–86.

66. Lauven PM, Stoeckel H, Schwilden H. A microprocessor controlled infusion scheme for midazolam to achieve constant plasma levels. Anaesthesist. 1982;31:15–20 (German).

67. Ausems ME, Hug CC Jr, Lange S de. Variable rate infusion of alfentanil as a supplement to nitrous oxide anesthesia for general surgery. Anesth Analg. 1983;62:982–6.

68. Ausems ME, Stanski DR, Hug CC. An evaluation of the accuracy of pharmacokinetic data for the computer assisted infusion of alfentanil. Br J Anaesth. 1985;57:1217–25.

69. Ausems ME, Hug CC Jr, Stanski DR et al. Plasma concentrations of alfentanil required to supplement nitrous oxide anesthesia for general surgery. Anesthesiology. 1986;65:362–373.

70. Available from www.opentci.org, last accessed June 20, 2011

71. Bickford RG. Automated electroencephalographic control of general anesthesia. J EEG and Clin Neurophysiol. 1950;2:93–96.

72. Bellville JW, Attura GM. Servo control of general anesthesia. Science. 1957;126:827–830.

73. Eger EI II, Johnson EA, Larson CP Jr, Severinghaus JW The uptake and distribution of intravenous ether Anesthesiology. 1962;23:647–50.

74. Schwilden H, Schüttler J, Stoeckel H. Quantitation of the EEG and pharmacodynamic modelling of hypnotic drugs: etomidate as an example. Eur J Anaesthesiol. 1985;2:121–31.

75. Schwilden H, Schüttler J, Stoeckel H. Closed-loop feedback control of methohexital anesthesia by quantitative EEG analysis in humans. Anesthesiology. 1987;67:341–7.

76. Shafer A, Doze VA, Shafer SL, White PF. Pharmacokinetics and pharmacodynamics of propofol infusions during general anesthesia. Anesthesiology. 1988;69:348–56.

77. Maitre PO, Vozeh S, Heykants J, Thomson DA. Stanski DR: Population pharmacokinetics of alfentanil: the average dose-plasma concentration relationship and interindividual variability in patients. Anesthesiology. 1987;66:3–12.

78. Alvis JM, Reves JG, Spain JA. Sheppard LC: Computer-assisted continuous infusion of the intravenous analgesic fentanyl during general anesthesia-an interactive system. IEEE Trans Biomed Eng. 1985;32:323–9.

79. Reves JG, Glass P, Jacobs JR. Alfentanil and midazolam: new anesthetic drugs for continuous infusion and an automated method of administration. Mt Sinai J Med. 1989;56:99–107.

80. Shafer SL, Siegel LC, Cooke JE, Scott JC. Testing computer controlled infusion pumps by simulation. Anesthesiology. 1988;68:261–6.

81. Eger EI II. Anesthetic uptake and action. Williams and Wilkins; 1974. pp. 240–2.

82. Hughes MA, Glass PS, Jacobs JR. Context-sensitive half-time in multicompartment pharmacokinetic models for intravenous anesthetic drugs. Anesthesiology. 1992;76:334–41.

83. Hung OR, Varvel JR, Shafer SL, Stanski DR. Thiopental pharmacodynamics: II. Quantitation of clinical and EEG depth of anesthesia. Anesthesiology. 1992;77:237–44.

84. Varvel JR, Donoho DL, Shafer SL. Measuring the predictive performance of computer controlled infusion pumps. J Pharmacokinet Biopharm. 1992;20:63–94.

85. Shafer SL, Gregg KM. Algorithms to rapidly achieve and maintain stable drug concentrations at the site of drug effect with a computer controlled infusion pump. J Pharmacokinet Biopharm. 1992;20:147–69.

86. Gregg K, Varvel JR, Shafer SL. Application of semilinear canonical correlation to the measurement of opioid drug effect. J Pharmacokinet Biopharm. 1992;20:611–635.

87. Gambús PL, Schnider TW, Minto CF, Youngs EJ, Billard V, Brose WG, Hochhaus G, Shafer SL. The pharmacokinetics of i.v. dynorphin a(1–13) in opioid naive and opioid treated human volunteers. Clin Pharmacol Therapeut. 1998;64:27–38.

88. Billard V, Gambus PL, Chamoun N, Stanski DR, Shafer SL. A comparison of spectral edge, delta power, and bispectral index as EEG measures of alfentanil, propofol, and midazolam drug effect. Clin Pharmacol Therapeut. 1997;61:45–58.

89. Schnider TW, Minto CF, Gambus PL, Andresen C, Goodale DB, Shafer SL, Youngs EJ. The influence of method of administration and covariates on the pharmacokinetics of propofol in adult volunteers. Anesthesiology. 1998;88:1170–1182.

90. Schnider TW, Minto CF, Shafer SL, Gambus PL, Andresen C, Goodale DB, Youngs EJ. The Influence of age on propofol pharmacodynamics. Anesthesiology. 1999;90:1502–16.

91. Barr J, Egan TD, Sandoval NF, Zomorodi K, Cohane C, Gambus PL, Shafer SL. Propofol dosing regimens for ICU sedation based upon an integrated pharmacokinetic-pharmacodynamic model. Anesthesiology.2001;95:324–33.

92. Zomorodi K, Donner A, Jacques S, Barr J, Sladen R, Ramsay J, Geller E, Shafer SL. Population pharmacokinetics of midazolam administered by target controlled infusion for sedation following coronary artery bypass grafting. Anesthesiology. 1998;89:1418–29.

93. Somma J, Donner A, Zomorodi K, Sladen R, Ramsay J, Geller E, Shafer SL. Population pharmacodynamics of midazolam administered by target controlled Infusion in SICU patients after CABG surgery. Anesthesiology. 1998;89:1430–43.

94. Minto CF, Schnider TW, Short TG, Gregg KM, Gentilini A. Shafer SL. response surface model for anesthetic drug interactions. Anesthesiology. 2000;92:1603–816.

95. Minto CF, Schnider TW, Gregg KM, Henthorn TK, Shafer SL. Using the time of maximum effect-site concentration to combine pharmacokinetics and pharmacodynamics. Anesthesiology. 2003;99:324–33.

96. Bouillon T, Bruhn J, Radu-Radulescu L, Andresen C, Cohane C, Shafer SL. A model of the ventilatory depressant potency of remifentanil in the non steady state. Anesthesiology. 2003;99:779–87.

97. Bouillon T, Bruhn J, Radu-Radulescu L, Andresen C, Cohane C, Shafer SL. Mixed-effects modeling of the intrinsic ventilatory depressant potency of propofol in the non-steady state. Anesthesiology. 2004;100:240–50.

98. Bouillon TW, Bruhn J, Radulescu L, Andresen C, Shafer TJ, Cohane C, Shafer SL. Pharmacodynamic Interaction between propofol and remifentanil regarding hypnosis, tolerance of laryngoscopy, bispectral index and electroencephalographic approximate entropy. Anesthesiology. 2004;100:1353–72.

99. Theil DR, Stanley TE 3rd, White WD, Goodman DK, Glass PS, Bai SA, Jacobs JR, Reves JG. Midazolam and fentanyl continuous infusion anesthesia for cardiac surgery: a comparison of computer-assisted versus manual infusion systems. J Cardiothorac Vasc Anesth. 1993;7:300–6.

100. Jacobs JR, Reves JG, Marty J et al. Aging increases pharmacodynamic sensitivity to the hypnotic effects of midazolam. Anesth Analg. 1995;80:143–8.

101. Glass PS, Jacobs JR, Smith LR, Ginsberg B, Quill TJ, Bai SA, Reves JG. Pharmacokinetic model-driven infusion of fentanyl: assessment of accuracy. Anesthesiology. 1990;73:1082–90.

102. Sebel PS, Glass PS, Fletcher JE, Murphy MR, Gallagher C, Quill T. Reduction of the MAC of desflurane with fentanyl. Anesthesiology. 1992;76:52–9.
103. McEwan AI, Smith C, Dyar O, Goodman D, Smith LR, Glass PS. Isoflurane minimum alveolar concentration reduction by fentanyl. Anesthesiology. 1993;78:864–9.
104. Sebel PS, Lang E, Rampil IJ, White PF, Cork R, Jopling M, Smith NT, Glass PS, Manberg P. A multicenter study of bispectral electroencephalogram analysis for monitoring anesthetic effect. Anesth Analg. 1997;84:891–9.
105. Gan TJ, Glass PS, Windsor A, Payne F, Rosow C, Sebel P, Manberg P. Bispectral index monitoring allows faster emergence and improved recovery from propofol, alfentanil, and nitrous oxide anesthesia. BIS Utility Study Group. Anesthesiology. 1997;87:808–15.
106. Glass PS, Bloom M, Kearse L, Rosow C, Sebel P, Manberg P. Bispectral analysis measures sedation and memory effects of propofol, midazolam, isoflurane, and alfentanil in healthy volunteers. Anesthesiology. 1997;86:836–47.
107. Kapila A, Glass PS, Jacobs JR, Muir KT, Hermann DJ, Shiraishi M, Howell S, Smith RL. Measured context-sensitive half-times of remifentanil and alfentanil. Anesthesiology. 1995;83:968–75.
108. Jacobs JR, Shafer SL, Larsen JL. Hawkins ED: Two equally valid interpretations of the linear multi-compartmental mammillary pharmacokinetic model. J Pharm Sci. 1990;79:331–3.
109. Price HA. Dynamic concept of the distribution of thiopentalthe human body. Anesthesiology.1960;21:40–5.
110. Krejcie TC, Avram MJ, Gentry WB, Niemann CU, Janowski MP, Henthorn TK. A recirculatory model of the pulmonary uptake and pharmacokinetics of lidocaine based on analysis of arterial and mixed venous data from dogs. J Pharmacokinet Biopharm. 1997;25:169–90.
111. Billard V, Gambus PL, Chamoun N, Stanski DR, Shafer SL. A comparison of spectral edge, delta power, and bispectral index as EEG measures of alfentanil, propofol, and midazolam drug effect. Clin Pharmacol Ther. 1997;61:45–58.

A Brief History of the Patient Safety Movement in Anaesthesia

William B. Runciman and Alan F. Merry

Summary

Approaches to safety began slowly. It took a century for ether to be fully accepted as a safer choice to chloroform and for PIN indexing for gas cylinders to be introduced as a safety design.

In the 1960s, Ross Holland in Australia and Gai Harrison in South Africa initiated longitudinal studies of mortality caused by anaesthesia, showing progressive declines over the next decades in first world countries.

In 1974, Cooper suggested applying the critical incident technique to identify the contribution of human behaviour to harm from anaesthesia, and in 1978 produced his seminal essay on preventable anaesthesia mishaps.

The medical indemnity crisis prompted the 1984 International Committee for Prevention of Anaesthesia Mortality and Morbidity (ICPAMM) meeting in Boston, at which Pierce conceived the Anesthesia Patient Safety Foundation, formed in 1985.

Cheney and others collected anecdotes from US "closed" malpractice claims, focussing attention on common errors, thereby pointing the way to their correction. A 1990 closed claims report found that respiratory events underlay 35 % of total claims, largely preventable with better monitoring. Parallel approaches included Lunn and Devlin's 1988 launch of the National Confidential Enquiry into Perioperative Deaths in the UK, the Runciman-led formation of the Australian Patient Safety Foundation, and the Australian Incident Monitoring Study.

In 1985, the 9 Harvard hospitals implemented monitoring standards, standards that other institutions then adopted. Similar movements arose in Australia, and the UK. The International Task Force of Anaesthesia Safety led to international standards adopted by the World Federation of Societies of Anaesthesiologists in 1992. In 1999, an Institute of Medicine report ("To Err Is Human") found that anaesthesia-related mortality had decreased from 2 deaths per 10,000 anaesthetics in the 1980s to about 1 death per 200,000 for fit patients. The WFSA Global Oximetry initiative, begun in 2004, led to The Lifebox Foundation, making pulse oximetry available to every anaesthetised patient.

In 1988, Gaba described mannequin-based anaesthesia simulation at Stanford University. In 1991, he convened a conference focussed on human error in anaesthesia, and the organisational theory of safety in healthcare. This work led to the introduction of crisis management algorithms and checklists.

Retrospective medical record reviews by the 1991 Harvard Medical Practice study (and by a similar Australian study in 1995), prompted the development of a comprehensive classification of things that go wrong. Runciman developed a 12,000 category classification subsequently enlarged to the 20,000 category "Generic Reference Model". With input from 250 international experts, this formed the basis for the International Classification for Patient Safety.

Arguably, improving the training and status of anaesthesia providers plays the key role in improving patient safety in anaesthesia.

Preface

Individual anaesthetists and others have advanced the safety of anaesthesia by improving drugs, devices, infrastructure, training, and techniques. These contributions have been supported by the strengthening of human factors such as teamwork, and the introduction of checklists, protocols and algorithms. To describe key elements of this story, we provide sketches of some key players, outline advances made by a few more, and mention and cite selected publications of some others. Our sketch relates only to clinical anaesthesia and largely to a few English-speaking countries. We apolo-

W. B. Runciman (✉)
School of Psychology, Social Work and Social Policy,
Sleep Research Centre, University of South Australia City
East Campus, North Terrace, Adelaide, SA, Australia
e-mail: william.runciman@unisa.edu.au

A. F. Merry
Department of Anaesthesiology, University of Auckland,
Auckland, New Zealand
e-mail: a.merry@auckland.ac.nz

E. I Eger II et al. (eds.), *The Wondrous Story of Anesthesia*, DOI 10.1007/978-1-4614-8441-7_41, © Edmond I Eger, MD 2014

gise to the many who made important contributions not mentioned in our brief account.

The Past—A Framework of the History of Patient Safety in Anaesthesia

The potentially lethal effects of anaesthesia became known shortly after Morton's historic demonstration [1]. Ann Parkinson, of Spittlegate, Lincolnshire, died during ether anaesthesia in early 1847. The coronial inquest, reported in the Times of London, sparked a lively debate on the risks of etherisation [2]. Within three months of chloroform's introduction, Hannah Greener died suddenly whilst inhaling it for a minor procedure [3, 4]. This young girl had painful bilateral ingrown toenails. One had been successfully removed under ether, but she had been nauseated postoperatively and feared the second anaesthetic, 'crying continually and wishing she was dead rather than submit to it' [5]. Although chloroform had advantages over ether, its safe use required greater skill. Only a few practitioners (e.g., John Snow and Joseph Clover) possessed such skill, and deaths associated with chloroform dominated mortality from anaesthesia for the next 50 years, attracting considerable media attention. The use, and perforce the deaths from use, of chloroform, waned and then virtually ceased after a further 50 years [5].

The risks of anaesthesia soon after its discovery did not concern most patients. Pain consequent on disease or injury was commonplace, and patients remembered the horrors of operations without anaesthesia. Furthermore, the hazards of surgery eclipsed those of anaesthesia; before the 1860s advent of antisepsis, amputation carried a mortality of 30 % and Caesarean section a mortality exceeding 80 % [5].

Stories like those of Anne Parkinson and Hannah Greener powerfully influenced human behavior. Such reports provided the first of five parallel approaches to improving safety in anaesthesia.

Approaches to Improving Safety in Anaesthesia

1. Telling stories
2. Counting the dead (or injured)
3. Trying to understand what went wrong, and why
4. Developing preventive and corrective strategies
5. Evaluating the interventions

Progress in each of these occurred over three periods:

- The first century (1846–1945) after the discovery of anesthesia, ending with the advances during World War II.
- The post war years (1946–1978), ending with Jeff Cooper's seminal paper on anaesthesia incidents [6].
- The recent years (1978–2012).

Table 41.1 A sample of the causes of death during the first 100 years of anaesthesia, selected to illustrate the diversity of causation

Uncalibrated chloroform dilution reservoir bag leading to overdose
Phosgene poisoning from chloroform decomposition with open gas lights
Misconnection of tubes leading to inhalation of liquid chloroform
Chloroform inhalers which when tilted, deliver liquid chloroform
Explosion with ether from open flames, electrical sparks, static
Explosions in patients' mouths or airways associated with ether
Ignition and burning of cuff of tracheal tube
Vomit forced into lungs by attempted resuscitation
Carbon dioxide instead of oxygen in a wrongly marked cylinder
Nitrous oxide instead of oxygen in a wrongly marked cylinder
Wrong volatile agent in bottle—no consistent colour coding
Toxic metabolites (phosgene) of trichloroethylene with sodalime
Percaine (nupercaine) confused with procaine (10-fold potency difference)
Ten times dose error because decimal point missed
Symbol for drachm (dram; 4.4 g) confused with symbol for ounce (28.3 g)
Death from infected anaesthetic agent for spinal anaesthesia
Air embolism during high pressure intravenous infusion
Cardiac arrest from combination of chloroform and adrenalin
Asphyxiation from poor positioning of patient with a lung abscess
Blocked tracheal tube
Airway obstruction due to impacting the epiglottis into the larynx with a gag
Electrocution by an ECG machine

From Sykes WS. Thirty seven little things which have all caused death. In Essays on the First Hundred Years of Anaesthesia. Volume 2, Chapter 1 (pp. 1–23), 1960. E & S Livingstone Ltd, London with permission

The pursuit of safety in anaesthesia is a work in progress: David Gaba argues that anaesthetic practice has yet to adopt many risk-reducing approaches accepted in other high risk environments (e.g., commercial aviation, mining and the nuclear power industry) [7].

Approach 1. Story Telling

Stanley Sykes collected anecdotes of lethal anaesthetic-associated errors during the first century of anaesthesia [5]. Table 41.1 documents the diversity of errors. Similarly, stories or 'cautionary tales' reported to medical indemnity organisations have been collected and published [8, 9]. They allow large numbers of practitioners to benefit from the experiences of an unfortunate few. This approach remains relevant today.

Approach 2. Counting the Dead

Death is a clear and objective endpoint, but several problems hinder attempts to monitor improvements in safety from the study of deaths nominally due to anaesthesia [10]:

- How much do surgery or pre-existing patient-related problems contribute?
- Are all deaths reasonably attributed to anaesthesia (i.e., the numerator) identified, recorded and reported?
- Has the total number of anaesthetics given (i.e., the denominator) been determined [11]?
- Does anaesthesia include sedation, analgesia or the use of other potent drugs, particularly when used by practitioners other than anaesthetists, or when not recorded as anaesthetics in emergencies and remote or unusual locations [12]?
- What time period between anaesthesia and death must be exceeded to exclude anaesthesia as a causal or associated factor? The number used has varied from a few hours to thirty days or longer [13].

A further confounder affects mortality rate comparisons at different points in history. Early studies of "anaesthetic deaths" typically examined deaths occurring in fit people having minor procedures. Increasingly, deaths included those in association with more complex and invasive procedures carried out in sicker patients, some at the extremes of age.

Several investigators counted deaths associated with anaesthesia in the first 100 years. John Snow collected 50 cases of chloroform associated deaths [5].

Sykes recorded that, in the early days, chloroform caused at least 1 death for every 3000 cases, whereas ether seemed to be associated with less than 1 in 12,000. An 1871 report cites a zero mortality from nitrous oxide, a rate of 1 in 2,723 for chloroform and a rate of 1 in 23,704 for ether [14].

After World War II and with the adoption of curare, more complex surgery was undertaken in increasingly sicker patients. Over a dozen studies of anaesthesia mortality were reported, and two important longitudinal studies commenced [12, 13]. In 1959, Ross Holland approached the Director-General of Health of the state of New South Wales, Australia, seeking and receiving ministerial support to obtain statutory immunity for a study of deaths associated with anaesthesia. With Douglas Joseph, he established The Special Committee Investigating Deaths Under Anaesthesia (SCIDUA), which began in 1960. This work continues to this day under the overall auspices of the Australian and New Zealand College of Anaesthetists (ANZCA) and the current chairmanship of Neville Gibbs. Since 1997, data has been garnered from each state and from New Zealand, providing the best longitudinal information on anaesthetic mortality in the world. Holland reported a mortality rate in the 1960s of around 2 deaths per 10,000 cases. This fell to 1 per 25,000 by the end of 1980, and is today thought to be about 1 in 50,000 overall, and perhaps 1 in 200 000 (approximately) for fit patients having minor procedures [15–20].

Gainsford ("Gai") Harrison in South Africa recorded comparable figures from a 30-year longitudinal study [21–23]. Mortality decreased from 1:1,000 in 1958 to 1:10,000 in 1986.

These results indicate that anaesthesia mortality has fallen progressively in high income countries, notwithstanding increasingly complex surgery in sicker and older people. Concurring with these observations, the 1999 report of the Institute of Medicine, "To Err Is Human", stated that anaesthesia-related mortality had fallen from 2 deaths per 10,000 anaesthetics in the 1980s to about 1 death per 200,000 or even 300,000 [24].

Not everyone agrees that this reflects the overall picture. Robert Lagasse's recent review calculated an overall rate of 2 deaths per 10,000 anaesthetics. A prospective study in The Netherlands found an overall rate of 1 death per 13,000 anaesthetics [10–25]. This is far better than the 15–40 times greater (0.3 %) overall healthcare-associated mortality associated with admission to an acute care hospital [26, 27]. Of course, healthy patients having minor procedures have very low hospital- and anaesthesia-related mortality in high income countries today, and estimates of an overall rate are of limited value without some indication of casemix. Clearly, older people with serious co-morbidities undergoing major surgery have a higher risk of dying, but estimates of how much higher vary substantially, depending on factors including the reliability of denominator data, the time period included in the assessment, and the process of attribution of causality. Few would dispute the claim that anaesthesia is, in general, much safer today than it was a few decades ago, but two facts should counter any complacency. First, potentially avoidable deaths continue to occur, even in healthy young patients [19, 28]. Second, some low-income countries have anaesthesia mortality rates 100 times those cited here [29, 30].

The pioneering work in Togo, by Aboudoul-Fataou Maman, is anaesthesia patient safety history in the making. As a medical student, Maman found that, because of deficiencies in anaesthetic standards, many patients died after surgery in the hospital in which he trained, and so decided on a career in anaesthesia. He went on to initiate a classic quality improvement programme. With colleagues, he documented the very high rate of perioperative mortality in his institution, identified factors contributing to this [30] and introduced corrective strategies. These included preoperative evaluation by medical staff, protocols for nurses, triage of difficult cases to specialists, the promotion of local and regional anaesthesia, the creation of recovery rooms, and the training of nurses in the use of morphine. His data have made an important contribution to the World Health Organization's Safe Surgery Saves Lives initiative [31] and the Global Oximetry Project [32] (now Lifebox: see www.lifebox.org).

In 1991, Pedro Ibarra was instrumental in seeing landmark legislation passed by the Colombian Congress (Ley 6 de 1991–Sixth Law of 1991) that, for the first time, defined a medical specialty (anaesthesia) in law. This set the stage for the introduction of minimal standards in Colombia in 1992 and, later, in the rest of South America (promoting, amongst other things, the widespread option of pulse oximetry) The impact of these minimal standards is evidenced by a drop in malpractice claims in Colombia where anesthesia is now ranked 12th among medical specialties.

Approach 3. Understanding What Goes Wrong and Why

Anaesthetic agents, techniques, equipment—"the system"—or humans may underlie things going wrong. How do we identify the problems?

Implicating Drugs

For a century after chloroform's introduction, its inherent toxicity was debated, especially in relation to lightly anesthetised patients receiving noxious stimuli [5]. The landmark 1954 publication by Henry Beecher and Donald Todd supported the notion of the inherent toxicity of anaesthetic agents [33]. This report examined outcomes after 600,000 anaesthetics administered over five years in ten university hospitals, finding that the data "strongly suggests an inherent toxicity" for neuromuscular blocking drugs, particularly curare. A furore followed. Sixteen distinguished anaesthesiologists sought to refute the suggestion [34], and from a study of 33,000 cases, Dripps concluded that neuromuscular blockers did not increase risk [11]. It became clear that the use of curare without reversal by neostigmine placed patients at risk of fatal respiratory failure.

Halothane was introduced in the mid 1950s, and soon replaced all other potent inhaled anaesthetics. Although its hepatotoxicity was rare, it led to halothane's replacement in the 1970s and 1980s by enflurane and isoflurane. In the 1960s and 1970s, volatile inhaled anaesthetics and succinylcholine were found to trigger malignant hyperthermia in susceptible individuals. In 1975, Harrison reported that dantrolene was an effective specific antidote and mortality fell from 80 % to virtually nil [35]. It is now appreciated that the drugs used in anaesthesia today rarely contribute directly to mortality, provided they are used with adequate skill and care.

Implicating Equipment

As Sykes noted, inadequate equipment was identified early as a major cause of mortality and morbidity (Table 41.1) [5]. Understanding equipment became fundamental to safety in anaesthesia, with contributions from many anaesthetists, notably Jerry and Susan Dorsch in the USA [36] and John Russell in Australia [37], whose books have become established

as readily understandable references in this field. Equipment for anaesthesia has become more complicated, and the increasing incorporation of electronics and computers within anaesthesia devices creates new risks. There are particular challenges in providing equipment for low income regions of the world that is affordable, appropriate, and simple to maintain. Mike Dobson and Phoebe Mainland, working through the World Federation of Societies of Anaesthesiologists (WFSA), have advanced the case with the International Standards Organization (ISO), for standards that address these needs.

Implicating Techniques, Training and the System

Early academic leaders recognized that an environment conducive to safe anaesthesia required proper training, infrastructure and support. Robert Macintosh forcibly expressed the importance of proper training in 1949 [38]. These points were articulated in the 1993 International Standards for a Safe Practice of Anaesthesia [39], and repeated when these standards were subsequently revised [40]. Greater understanding has developed about techniques for airway management, patient positioning, ventilatory support, cardiopulmonary bypass, and crisis management.

Implicating People

In a lengthy, fascinating, and at times vitriolic paper (already cited above), MacIntosh argued in 1949 that there should be no deaths due to anaesthetics, and that those that did occur were mostly (if not all) attributable to failures on the part of the anaesthetist, rather than any inherent dangers in the drugs used or any underlying pathology that the patients might have [38].

Debate about the legitimacy of "anaesthetic death" as a default diagnosis for all otherwise unexplained perioperative deaths continued through the 1950s, 1960s and 1970s. Longitudinal studies by Holland [15, 16] and Harrison [22, 23] considerably increased our understanding of why things go wrong. In 1979, Arthur Keats published an important paper in which he criticised Macintosh's 1949 article. He accepted that a proportion of anaesthetic deaths are attributable to error but suggested that this proportion might be about 10 %. He argued that many of the drugs and techniques used in anaesthesia are inherently hazardous (citing malignant hyperthermia and succinylcholine-induced hyperkalemia as examples) although he agreed that attribution of deaths to anaesthetic drugs was unacceptable, without demonstration of a cause-effect relationship [41]. In 1979, William Hamilton, a friend and hunting companion of Keats, followed with a very balanced editorial [42], accepting many of Keats' points but suggesting that the proportion of deaths attributable to error might be closer to 90 %. Clearly a better conceptual framework was needed to sort out the relative contributions of drugs, equipment, the "system", patients, and anaesthetists themselves.

Incident Reporting, Mortality Committees and Human Factors

The earliest statement on the importance of critical incidents probably came from RH Todd, anaesthetist to the Prince Alfred Hospital in Sydney, who wrote the following in 1889: "An accident may be defined as any event in the course of the administration which interferes with the simple process of inducing and maintaining a state of surgical anaesthesia. Some of these accidents are of slight importance in themselves, but in as much as small accidents are often the forerunners of greater ones, successful results may depend on a readiness in anticipating, and failing this, a promptitude in remedying small accidents." [43] He then went on to classify accidents as impediments to free respiration, and those in which cardiac failure occurs, with lists of causes.

In 1974, Jeffrey Cooper was a bioengineer at the Massachusetts General Hospital (MGH). Whilst helping carve a pumpkin at a Halloween party, he struck up a conversation which led to an invitation to speak on human factors in healthcare. The resulting lecture, 'The anaesthesia machine: An accident waiting to happen', led a listener to suggest that he use the critical incident technique pioneered by Flanagan in World War II. This led to the study which resulted in his landmark first paper on anaesthetist-reported incidents, demonstrating the multifactorial cause of most problems and the important contribution of human behaviour to things that go wrong [6].

In 1987, David Gaba introduced the concepts of "Normal Accident Theory" to the anaesthesia literature [44]. Gaba, Cooper [45], and then others, advanced the principles of a systems-based (rather than a person-based) response to error. At about the turn of the century, Alan Merry and Alexander McCall Smith (who was then Professor of Law in Edinburgh) extended these ideas into the debate about the most appropriate legal and regulatory response to human error [46].

Cooper's seminal publication coincided with a medical indemnity crisis that had begun in the mid 1970s, characterised by increased litigation and steep rises in insurance premiums [47, 48]. These factors and others led Cooper, with Ellison (Jeep) Pierce—(then President of the American Society of Anesthesiologists) and Dick Kitz (then Chairman of Anesthesiology at Harvard), to organise the first meeting of the International Committee on Anaesthesia Mortality and Morbidity (ICPAMM) in Boston in 1984 [48, 49]. This focused attention on how anaesthesia-related adverse events happened, and how they might be prevented. During the meeting, Pierce conceived the idea of the Anesthesia Patient Safety Foundation (APSF). With Cooper and others, Pierce formed the APSF in 1985 with the motto "to ensure that no patient should be harmed by anesthesia" [50]. The APSF became a potent advocate for preventing harm rather than cleaning up the mess after an (often tragic) event.

The Closed Claims Study

The Closed Claims Study also arose from the 1984 ICPAMM meeting, where preliminary findings were presented on "closed" malpractice claims [51]. Fred Cheney, then Chairman of the ASA Committee on Professional Liability, saw the value of such a study. He formed a team including Robert Caplan, Karen Posner and Karen Domino, and pursued the cooperation of medical indemnity organisations. Limitations notwithstanding [52], this approach produced an influential series of papers (from ICPAMM to the present) including a 1990 report showing that adverse respiratory events underlay the largest single class of injury (35% of the total), and an even larger percent of payouts [53]. It showed that better monitoring would prevent 75% of these injuries. Another landmark study showed the tendency of human beings to display "outcome bias"—the strong human tendency to find fault if there has been a bad outcome – even when there was no question of conciliation or compensation [54].

The ASA used the Closed Claims data to develop practice standards, guidelines and advisories which have increased safety. The Closed Claims Study now possesses the findings for 8,000 malpractice cases, from 34 insurance organisations that insure nearly 15,000 anesthesiologists.

A decrease in the cost of malpractice insurance for anaesthetists has been evident world wide. It is difficult to say how much of this is the direct result of the outcomes of Closed Claim Studies, or how much is due to improved training, newer and better monitoring, new drugs, crisis management algorithms etc.

The National Confidential Enquiry into Perioperative Deaths (NCEPOD)

John Lunn and Brendan Devlin launched NCEPOD in 1988, following a report on surgical and anaesthetic practice during 1985–86 in three UK regions. The report compared patients who had died in hospital within thirty days of a surgical procedure, with "index" (control) cases, using information from those who had cared for these patients [55]. Although frequencies could not be calculated, because of the voluntary nature of the data source and low response rates, NCEPOD reports led to substantial improvements in the availability of resources, supervision of junior staff, appropriateness of surgery and access to critical care facilities [55, 56].

The Australian Patient Safety Foundation

Inspired by developments in the US, William Runciman called a meeting in Australia of 65 influential anaesthetists in 1987. The group comprised department heads and academic leaders, together with past and current deans of the Faculty of Anaesthetists. Standards for anaesthesia monitoring were proposed, and the group decided to form the Australian Patient Safety Foundation (Aus.PSF) to promote patient safety in anaesthesia and, more ambitiously, throughout healthcare

[57]. An early initiative developed a voluntary national incident reporting system for anaesthesia – the Australian Incident Monitoring System (AIMS). In 1993, 30 publications resulted from analysis of the first 2,000 incidents [58]. This, with the US Closed Claims Study, established the utility of oximetry and capnography in anaesthesia, and influenced the promulgation of the International Standards for a Safe Practice of Anaesthesia, which were endorsed by the General Assembly of the WFSA in 1994 [59].

The International Classification for Patient Safety

Unexplained disparate results between retrospective medical record reviews by the Harvard Medical Practice study in 1991 [60], and by a similar Australian study in 1995 [61, 62], prompted the development of a comprehensive classification of things that go wrong in health care. This showed that there were, effectively, no qualitative or quantitative differences between adverse events in Australia and the US, but also confirmed how safe anaesthesia had become. Anaesthesia-related adverse events contributed less than 2 % of the total events, compared with nearly 50 % for surgery [61]. Anaesthesia related events were also, on average, less severe. Following this study, Runciman developed a 12,000 category classification (the Generic Occurrence Classification), subsequently expanded into "the Generic Reference Model", with 20,000 categories [63]. With input from 250 international experts, this formed the basis for the new International Classification for Patient Safety (ICPS) [64]. The Australian team led by Runciman, now has responsibility for populating the ICPS framework with concepts and preferred terms on behalf of the World Health Organisation (from 2006 onwards). This is being done in collaboration with the "Common Formats" project for reporting to Patient Safety organisations in the US. To this end, Runciman was a member of the National Quality Forum—the group in the US which oversaw this project.

Several other anaesthesia patient safety experts have promoted patient safety across all of healthcare [65]. For example, Cooper participated in the Institute of Medicine report "To err is human.…"; and was a key player in the formation of the National Patient Safety Foundation of the American Medical Association. In 2010, Alan Merry was appointed to chair the Board set up to establish the New Zealand Health Quality and Safety Commission.

Approach 4: Developing and Implementing Preventive and Corrective Strategies

As problems have been identified and understood, so preventive and corrective strategies have been developed and applied. Many problems listed in Table 41.1 were amenable to solution and were solved in the first century of anaesthe-

sia. Some, such as the correct identification of drugs with look-alike and sound-alike names, "decimal point" confusion, and problems with airway management continue to this day. Possible solutions to some of the causes of drug administration error have been developed and evaluated, but not yet widely implemented [66].

Improving the System Through Engineering

If it is possible to eliminate a problem by design, then this should be done. In the post war years, problems with equipment, particularly equipment used to deliver gases and vapours, were common [67–69]. In 1940, two patients died because carbon dioxide cylinders were substituted for oxygen cylinders, having had their green colour painted over with black [69]. The introduction of PIN indexing for gas cylinders in 1954 [69] is a classic example of an engineering solution to remove a latent factor [70] in the system that sets people up to make mistakes. Other examples include breathing circuits that can only be assembled in the correct manner [71, 72],and modifications to gas flowmeter systems of anaesthesia machines that prevent the administration of hypoxic gas mixtures.

Monitoring and Standards

By the mid 1980s, it became evident that some problems could not easily be "designed out" (inadvertent oesophageal intubation, breathing circuit disconnections, and adverse reactions to drugs or surgical stimuli), but more effective management was possible if they could be rapidly detected. Equipment monitors (the Ritchie Whistle was an early example of an alarm to warn of oxygen supply failure [73]) and highly effective patient monitors set the scene for the widespread promulgation of standards of care. These included pulse oximeters providing beat-to-beat measurements of arterial blood saturation (invented in 1972 by a bioengineer, Takuo Aoyagi and first used on patients by a surgeon, Susumu Nakajima, in1975 [74, 75]) and capnographs providing breath-by-breath measurements of carbon dioxide concentrations (the modern infrared capnograph was developed in 1937 by Karl Luft [76]) In 1986, the nine Harvard hospitals initiated the Harvard Monitoring Standards as a standard of care, thereby beginning a wider adoption of monitoring; John Eichhorn and Jeff Cooper played major roles in this process [77]. Monitoring devices became de facto standards across the US and prompted the setting of standards in Australia, UK, and the rest of the world. Eichhorn was the organiser of the International Task Force of Anaesthesia Safety that led to the original 1993 international standards for safe practice of anaesthesia [39], and a major contributor to the revision of these standards in 2008 [40]. Anaesthesia safety standards were proposed for Australia during the 1987 meeting that gave birth to the Australian Patient Safety Foundation [58]. The 1980s Closed Claims Study and the 1990s AIMS, indicated that half of all incidents could be detected by monitors, and that up to 90% of these would be detected by capnography and oximetry [53, 59]. These monitors have become the standard of care in high income regions of the world, but many operating rooms internationally are without them. In 2008, the revised International Standards for a Safe Practice of Anaesthesia [40] effectively elevated the use of pulse oximetry to a mandatory requirement for elective anaesthesia, in concert with the aims of the Global Oximetry project [32] (see below). National anaesthesia societies and the WFSA have endorsed these initiatives to enhance the safety of anaesthesia

Crisis Management.

It had long been recognised in the aviation industry, that if a cockpit crisis occurred, it was not managed effectively if dealt with through deductive reasoning. By the time a solution was found in increasingly complex aircraft control systems, it was invariably too late. Instead, pre-compiled responses, the basic steps of which could be learned by rote, were instituted. These algorithms enabled pilots to respond to crises in an ordered manner, and were designed to reach a management solution, with or without determining an immediate cause. In the early 1990s in the US, David Gaba spearheaded advances in the use of pre-compiled algorithms for the management of crises during anaesthesia [78]. This was followed in Australia by the development of a specific set of crisis management algorithms for anaesthesia, tested against 4,000 incidents [27]. The development of courses to pioneer the systematic management of crises in anaesthesia (including the use of algorithms when appropriate) was pioneered in the US, Australia and New Zealand [79].

The need to monitor things that might go wrong will persist. Each new initiative or technological advance contains new ways of making mistakes. An early example might be the introduction of the laryngoscope, that facilitated safe insertion of an endotracheal tube, but potentially damaged the patient's teeth. Unintended consequences, or "revenge effects", can have major implications [80].

A Just Culture-Speaking Out

In responding to accidents in healthcare, the focus has shifted from one on individual culpability, through one in which no blame is attributed, except in egregious circumstances, to a current view which emphasises a just culture [46]. There are times when "whistle blowing" is called for. Steve Bolsin exemplifies the importance of speaking up when things persistently go wrong. He is famous as the "whistle blower" whose actions changed the mortality of paediatric surgery at the Bristol Royal Infirmary from 30 to 5%. He conducted the Cardiothoracic Anaesthesia Audit in the UK from 1990, when he came to realise the high mortality rate in his own

unit. When his efforts to address this were blocked, he took his concerns to the media with the result that a major enquiry ensued. Many lessons were learned [81] and changes followed both at Bristol and in the United Kingdom generally [82]. His actions also had the less salutary effect of leading to his unemployment in Britain. This proved to be a watershed in the patient safety movement in the UK [83].

Human Factors and Simulation

In 1991, Gaba convened a conference on Human Error in Anaesthesia. Sponsored by the APSF and the United States Food and Drug Administration, the meeting brought together 30 experts in the field of human factors in patient safety, including James Reason and Jens Rasmussen. Reason, a psychologist from Manchester, had just published his classic book, Human Error[70], in which he advanced the view of accident causation that has subsequently became famous as the "Swiss Cheese Model." [84] He distinguished the role of active and latent failures in producing an accident, emphasising that latent failures lie dormant in a complex system, until by confluence of one or more additional failures, often triggered by an active failure, an accident occurs. The meeting launched important developments in the understanding of the role of human error in anaesthesia, and in the organisational theory of safety in healthcare, in particular the idea of learning from high-risk environments like aviation and nuclear power [7, 85]. The meeting accelerated the uptake of simulation as a tool for teaching and research in anesthesia [86–89].

Engineer Stephen Abrahamson, and anaesthesiologist Judson Denson, in the mid-1960s, had created Sim One, the first anaesthetic simulator [90, 91]. Little came of this until 1986, when Gaba developed mannequin-based anaesthesia simulation at Stanford University and subsequently promoted its teaching and research potential. Soon after, Nik Gravenstein and Mike Good developed the Gainesville Anesthesia Simulator, along similar lines. Complex pathophysiological scenarios could be used in teaching human factors and crisis management [7]. Dan Raemer conceived of the Society of Simulation in Healthcare and chaired the "Board of Overseers" which established the Society in January 2004. *The Simulation in Healthcare Journal* began publication in January 2006, and the use of simulation for training, research and assessment in anaesthesia is now widespread.

Drug Administration Error in Anaesthesia

The "wrong drug" problem featured prominently in the 1993 AIMS reports [56], and has remained a recalcitrant problem in anaesthesia despite numerous case reports, high profile legal proceedings [92, 93] and calls for improvement [94, 95]. This probably reflects the fact that there is no simple solution to the problem, which is indeed multifaceted. In January 2008 and again in 2010, Bob Stoelting chaired APSF consensus conferences to develop new strategies for safe medication delivery. The latter conference developed a new paradigm to reduce medication errors, based on four key principles: Standardization, Technology, Pharmacy/Prefilled/Premixed (medication), and Culture (STPC) [96]. Between 1972 and 1983, the DAME system at Duke University used technology to ensure correctness of anaesthetic drugs at the point of administration, but technological challenges led to the demise of the system. Many automatic anaesthesia record keeping systems are in use today but few have focused on improving the safety of drug administration. Alan Merry has led a team in New Zealand investigating drug administration error in anaesthesia over the last decade. The primary focus of this work has been the elucidation of the principles likely to enhance the safety of drug administration in anaesthesia, and the results provide support for the concepts of STPC [66, 97–99]. The challenge from 2013 onwards is to promote widespread uptake of these principles.

The Role of Anaesthesia Societies, Colleges, and Academic Departments

Arguably, improving the training and status of anaesthesia providers has been the most important factor in improving patient safety in anaesthesia in high and middle income countries.

Clover demonstrated early that specialisation is important to safety. He gave up general practice to pursue anaesthesia, and administered 10,000 anaesthetics (more with chloroform than ether) before losing a patient under chloroform in 1874 [2].

Improved training has resulted from the activities of many anaesthetists through academic departments, societies, colleges and other organisations. Academic departments have been critically important in providing a focus and home for researchers and educationalists, for advancing the scientific basis of anaesthesia through research, and promoting the standing of anaesthetists. Ralph Waters was appointed to the University of Wisconsin in 1927, with the challenge of creating an academic department of anaesthesiology. He had four major objectives: to provide the best possible anaesthetic care to patients; to teach interns and residents the fundamentals of clinical anaesthesia; to educate postgraduate doctors in anaesthesia; and to continue research into the scientific foundations of anaesthesia [100]. He appreciated the importance of establishing similar academic departments across the country and famous anaesthetists who promulgated the "Wisconsin model" included Emery Rovenstine and Robert Dripps. Lord Nuffield established the first Chair of Anaesthesia in Europe at Oxford in 1936, and Robert Macintosh (who had visited Waters) was appointed to this position. He too advanced teaching and research in anaesthesia, and many leaders in anaesthesia,

including academic anaesthesia, trained under Macintosh in Oxford and the first and subsequent generations of "offspring" of Ralph Waters. The detailed stories of the development of education in anaesthesia are told in other chapters of this book.

Organisations such as the American Society of Anesthesiologists (ASA) in the US, the Australian and New Zealand College of Anaesthetists (ANZCA) in Australia and New Zealand, the Royal College of Anaesthetists (RCA) in the UK, and several national anaesthesia societies have promulgated standards and have furthered their application through education and advocacy. The WFSA has been particularly important in this regard, because it provides a forum for all anaesthesiologists (i.e., medically qualified anaesthetists) to collaborate. The WFSA evolved from discussions at the International Anaesthesia Congress in Paris in 1951, and was established in 1955 with 26 founding member societies (there are now well over 100). Its primary aim was "to make available the highest standard of anaesthesia to all the peoples throughout the world." The World Congress of Anaesthesiologists is arguably the premier international anaesthesia conference; it brings together anaesthesia providers from all over the world thereby advancing education and collegial support, both of which are critical for improving the standards, and therefore safety, of anaesthesia in low income countries of the world, if not everywhere. In particular, it provides a voice for many important contributors who might not otherwise be heard. The Education Committee of the WFSA, particularly under the leadership of Angela Enright has provided training and educational resources to thousands of anaesthesia providers, physicians and non-physicians, who would otherwise have had access to neither. Under Kester Brown's presidency, the Safety and Quality of Practice Committee was established. This Committee was elevated to the status of a Standing Committee in 2004; amongst its other contributions to patient safety it initiated the global oximetry project and oversaw the first four pilot projects. This established the concept of combining education with the provision of affordable and robust oximeters, as a viable and effective strategy in advancing the standards of safe anaesthesia [32].

Global Initiatives to Improve Safety in Anaesthesia and Surgery

Anaesthesia and surgery are inextricably linked. The recognition that the delivery of healthcare is itself a science, has been pivotal to advancing the safety of patients undergoing surgery, as has recognition of the importance of teamwork, communication and collaboration between the members of the perioperative team [101–104].

Perhaps the greatest contribution from an anaesthesiologist in this context has come from Peter Pronovost, an anaesthesiologist and intensive care physician at Johns Hopkins [105]. In 2001, he began to study healthcare acquired infections, and demonstrated that implementing a five item checklist protocol dramatically reduced central line associated bacteraemia (CLAB) [106]. He extended this work to the state of Michigan. The mean rate of CLAB per 1000 catheter-days decreased from 7.7 to 1.4 at 16 to 18 months of follow-up [107]. This approach has now been adopted in many countries, undoubtedly saving many thousands of lives and millions of dollars. Pronovost established the Quality and Safety Research Group at Hopkins, and has been very effective in promoting the importance of rigour in research into patient safety (see below).

A major influence in this area has been the WHO Safe Surgery Saves Lives initiative, led by Atul Gawande. This initiative was undertaken in response to the problems of iatrogenic harm associated with surgery globally (a great deal of which is attributable to inadequate anaesthesia services in low income regions [108]). It resulted, amongst other things, in the development of the Surgical Safety Checklist and the advancement of the Global Oximetry project (now the Lifebox project) [32]. Olaitan Soyanwo, Jeff Cooper, John Eichhorn, Iain Wilson and Alan Merry formed the safe anaesthesia working group in this major interdisciplinary safety initiative. A landmark multicentre international evaluation of the Checklist, published in 2009, provides compelling support for believing that the widespread adoption of the Checklist has reduced avoidable harm to patients and indeed saved many lives [101]. Gawande's books[109–111] and regular articles in the New Yorker have been powerful instruments in advancing patient safety to a wide readership, extending an awareness of the importance of safety in healthcare well beyond the limits of those directly involved with the provision of healthcare.

The Lifebox Foundation was established in 2011, as a charitable organisation to further the Global Oximetry initiative of the WFSA. This initiative began at the 2004 Congress in Paris. Its aim was to sustainably improve safety in low income countries by providing high standard, robust, affordable pulse oximeters, supported by education and advocacy where appropriate. Since 2009, the project has included the WHO Checklist. The WHO Checklist explicitly addresses risks related to anaesthesia, and is designed to promote communication and teamwork within the operating room [101–104]. The inclusion of pulse oximetry within the checklist was intentional, to emphasise that its use during elective cases is viewed as mandatory (in line with the revised International Standards for a Safe Practice of Anaesthesia) [40]. Beneath this is a powerful message – that anaesthesia needs adequate resources, both in respect of its providers and their level of training, and the necessary equipment. In 2010, the global gap in pulse oximetry was estimated as 77,700 (95 % confidence limits 63,195 and 95,533) [112]. By mid 2012, the gap has been reduced to 75,000 [113]. This very

substantial ongoing project has depended on close teamwork between many people, including in particular Gavin Thoms, Iain Wilson, Angela Enright, Isabeau Walker, Ellen O'Sullivan, Florian Nuevo, Alan Merry, and Atul Gawande [32, 114].

Approach 5: Assessing Preventive and Corrective Strategies

Measuring the effectiveness of preventive and corrective strategies in patient safety for anaesthesia is difficult because things go wrong so infrequently, making conventional prospective quantitative research costly, and/or a logistical nightmare [115]. Compounding the problem, anaesthesia-related "signals" tend to be lost amongst the "noise" produced by complex procedures and patient-comorbidities.

Nevertheless, measurement is integral to quality improvement (and safety is integral to quality in healthcare) [116]. Donabedian introduced the framework of structure, process and outcome for measuring quality in healthcare [117, 118]. In 2009, for the first time, as an interesting output from the WHO Safe Surgery Saves lives project, some basic metrics were defined to assist in estimating the quality of surgical services in a particular country. They included the number of operating rooms, number of operations, number of accredited surgeons, number of accredited anaesthesia professionals, day-of-surgery death ratio, and postoperative in-hospital death ratio [119, 120]. It is reflective of the challenge in improving the standards of anaesthesia globally, that to meet the definition for their respective structural measures, a surgeon has to be a physician, but an anaesthetist does not.

The difficulties in measuring outcomes in anaesthesia have been touched upon in Approach 2, above, in relation to studies of anaesthetic mortality. Nevertheless, indirect evidence suggests that progress has been made. In 1989, Eichhorn reviewed one million anaesthetics provided to ASA 1 and 2 patients at Harvard University hospitals between 1976 and 1985, finding eleven major intra-operative accidents, of which seven resulted from unrecognised lack of ventilation [121].This finding prompted the introduction of the Harvard Monitoring Standards in 1985.

Indirect evidence from Australia supports the efficacy of introducing oximetry and capnography in the early 1990s. In 2005, Runciman noted that a five year study of medico-legal files, and an analysis of the last 2,000 incidents reported to AIMS had not revealed a single case of inadequate ventilation or undetected oesophageal intubation, although there had been several such problems resulting in brain damage or death each year before 1990 [27].

In Cooper's 1978 study on adverse events in anaesthesia, human errors in drug administration accounted for 19 % of events, equalling ventilation and breathing circuit errors at 19.5%. As noted, today's ventilation and circuit problems are passably low, but harm from drug administration error continues.

A major focus of the work by Merry's group into drug administration error (mentioned above) has been to quantify the extent of the problem. To this end they introduced a method of facilitated incident reporting in that a response is required after every anaesthetic, whether it be a simple negative reply or a more comprehensive account. This established, for the first time, realistic estimates of the likely rate of drug administration error in anaesthesia (about one error for every 130 anaesthetics) [98, 122]. This rate was orders of magnitude higher than most previous estimates, but is itself most likely to be an underestimate.

Amongst the many important contributions of Pronovost to advancing safety in healthcare are his recent contributions to articulating the importance of rigour in research in this field [123–125]. Lucian Leape, Donald Berwick and David Bates made an important point in 2002 [126]: they observed that safety in anaesthesia (as in aviation) had not been based on evidence but rather "by applying a whole host of changes that made sense, were based on an understanding of human factors principles, and had been demonstrated to be effective in other settings." This idea was further advanced the following year by a (now famous) ironical "systematic review" of randomized trials of parachutes as an intervention to manage "gravitational challenge."[127]

In 2011, Shekelle, Pronovost and their co-authors provided a more sophisticated analysis of these issues. They explain why randomized trials are clearly not needed for parachutes, but why rigorous empirical evidence (not necessarily from randomized controlled trials) might well be required for many of the interventions aimed at improving patient safety. Their key points are that an intervention to improve safety should be based on a sound theoretical construct; it should be sufficiently well described to be reproducible; desired outcomes should be clearly defined, the possibility of unintended consequences should not be overlooked; and the influence of context should be taken into account. This is really just a restatement of the essential elements of rigorous research into many other aspects of healthcare, but this important article underlines the point that there is no justification for abandoning rigour in research just because it happens to be in the field of patient safety.

This does not imply slavish subservience to artificial "hierarchies" of evidence [128]. Randomized trials certainly have a role but they are expensive, difficult to undertake, and may be difficult to interpret. Two examples of randomised controlled trials to investigate patient safety initiatives are the well known study by Moller and co-authors into pulse oximetry [129, 130] and a recent study in over 1000 patients by Merry's group investigating an intervention to

reduce error in the recording and administration of drugs in anaesthesia [66]. In their own ways each of these studies has provided insights into the challenges associated with evaluating safety initiatives. The negative result from the former study has contrasted with the almost universal perception of the value of pulse oximetry, and with other indirect evidence supporting its value. With the benefit of hindsight their result was predictable given that the outcomes for which the study was powered statistically would not be expected to be influenced by hypoxaemia [114]. In the latter study, the practical difficulty of getting compliance from a large number of participants in adhering to key elements of practice guidelines was well demonstrated.

If the randomized controlled trial is thought of as a hammer, not every problem is a nail. Research methods need to be appropriate to the questions to be answered, and to the context in which they are being considered [114, 128].

It is salutary to note that a number of recent, highly influential studies into checklists [101–104] and into the reduction of CLAB [107] have not been randomised trials. A very important incidental outcome from the Keystone project was some clarification, in the US context at least, of the distinction between quality improvement research and human-subject research involving novel interventions. There is a need for some pragmatism in regulatory requirements if the evaluation of large scale implementations of established best practice is to be affordable and practical [131].

Evaluation is fundamental to quality improvement, but uptake of best practices as evidence emerges is essential if gains in patient safety are to be realised. Despite the evidence supplied by studies such as those cited above, the adoption of initiatives supported by sound research to improve safety in healthcare has been patchy [132, 133], and anaesthesia has been no exception.

The Future

The history of the patient safety movement in anaesthesia is a proud one, with many fine achievements. Much progress notwithstanding, there remains much to be done. The biggest challenges lie in underfunded areas of the world but even in wealthy countries, preventable deaths continue to occur. The goal of the APSF, that "no patient shall be harmed by anaesthesia" has yet to be achieved.

Improving safety is an iterative process. At each iteration, the emphasis must be on identifying the most important of the residual problems, coming up with practical and affordable solutions, and implementing them. There is a place for pragmatism and for applying things simply because they make sense, but not for abandoning the commitment to the scientific foundations of anaesthesia that has been the hallmark of the contributions to patient safety of many of the anaesthesiologists discussed in this chapter. Ongoing commitment to this fundamental principle will provide powerful impetus in adding to the impressive advances that have justified this speciality's reputation for leading the pursuit of patient safety. The goal of the APSF may be aspirational, but it has served our patients well, and will continue to do so, well into the foreseeable future.

Notable Names

The following list gives a brief insight into the contributions to patient safety, of some of the individuals mentioned in the body of this chapter. The list is in order of appearance, and is by no means exhaustive. Limitations on space have determined that many deserving contributors are omitted, and some appear elsewhere in this book. The authors offer their apologies to those people.

David Gaba (1954-) graduated from Yale University School of Medicine, in 1980. He introduced human factors and the organisational theory of safety into anaesthesia and healthcare, first by Normal Accidents Theory and then by High Reliability Organisation Theory. He is credited with inventing modern mannequin-based immersion simulation, work he conducted from 1986 to 1992. He subsequently introduced Crew Resource Management into anaesthesia (Anesthesia Crisis Resource Management), and then to healthcare in general (Crisis Resource Management). His ongoing research on human performance, cognition and human factors using simulation as a tool has been a model for the scientific advancement of patient safety.

W Stanley Sykes (1894–1961) served as an anaesthetist before and during World War II, including while a prisoner of war, for which he was awarded an MBE. He returned to general practice, but remained fascinated by things that go wrong with anaesthesia, becoming a prolific writer of matters medical and a series of thrillers. His "Essays on the first 100 years of Anaesthesia" [5] provide a rich tapestry of background, trivia, contemporary accounts, and important milestones in the development of anaesthesia and the safety of anaesthesia for that early period.

Gainsford "Gai" Harrison (1926–2003), a graduate of the University of Cape Town, contributed to the safety of anaesthesia in three areas: He conducted a 30-year longitudinal study of anaesthetic mortality; he was a world authority on anaesthesia for patients with porphyria; and he was pivotal in introducing dantrolene to treat malignant hyperthermia.

Aboudoul-Fataou Ouro-Bang'na Maman (1974-) was born in Tchalo (Sokode) and graduated from the University of Lome, Togo in 2002. He obtained a Diploma in pain management ("Capacité d'Evaluation et de Traitement de la Douleur") from the University of Montpellier 2, in France,

in 2004, and a Diploma of anaesthesia from the Faculty of Health Science, Cotonou (Benin) in 2006. He worked in Togo, Martinique, and Guadeloupe. He translated the book "Safe Anesthesia" into French in collaboration with the WFSA publication committee.

Robert MacIntosh (1897–1989) was born in New Zealand and baptised with the Maori name Rewi Rawhiti. He pioneered the safety of anaesthesia in the English speaking world outside of the US. In World War I he served as a pilot in the Royal Flying Corps, was shot down in 1917, taken prisoner and escaped several times. After the war, he trained in medicine in London, and in 1937, became the first Professor of Anaesthesia outside the US. He was a proponent of "safe and simple' anaesthesia". In the 1940s, he argued that most "anaesthetic accidents" were preventable. With William Mushin, he tried to launch research on this topic in 1944. Despite initial opposition, in 1949, the Association of Anaesthetists appointed a committee to investigate anaesthesia-associated deaths, a committee that is still active.

Arthur Keats (1923–2007) graduated from the University of Pennsylvania in 1946. Henry Beecher mentored him during his residency at the Massachusetts General Hospital from 1948–1951. He was the first Chair of the Scientific Evaluation Committee of the Anesthesia Patient Safety Foundation (APSF). From 1970–1973 he was Editor in Chief of the journal Anesthesiology. He was also a member of the FDA's Respiratory and Anesthetic Drug Advisory Committee.

Jeffrey Cooper (1946-) was born and received his early schooling in Philadelphia, Pennsylvania. He received his BS in Chemical Engineering (1968), and an MS in Biomedical Engineering (1970) from Drexel University, and a PhD in Chemical Engineering at the University of Missouri (1972). He is a Professor of Anesthesiology at Harvard Medical School, and is the father of incident reporting in anaesthesia – indeed, in medicine. He received several honours for his work in patient safety, including the 2003 John M. Eisenberg Award for Lifetime Achievement in Patient Safety from the National Quality Forum and the Joint Commission and the 2004 Lifetime Achievement Award from the American Academy of Clinical Engineering. He has a particular talent for supporting and mentoring others, and both authors have cause for considerable gratitude in this respect.

Ellison (Jeep) Pierce (1929–2011) was President of the American Society of Anesthesiologists, founder of the APSF, and an elected Fellow of the Royal College of Anaesthestists. He received awards and citations from the Food and Drug Administration, the American Medical Association, the Royal Society of Medicine and the Russian Society of Anesthesiology. To quote from his obituary in the APSF Newsletter *"when the specialty was faced with a malpractice crisis at the start of the 1980s, Jeep thought about protecting* *patients first and doctors second. That was a risky political move, but he didn't hesitate. He just did the right thing."*

Frederick Cheney (1935-) completed his specialist training in 1964 and joined the Faculty at the University of Washington where, 30 years on, he became Chairman. As Chair of the American Society of Anesthesiology Committee on Professional Liability, he organised the Closed Claims Study. From 1989, he concentrated his research activities on the ASA Closed Claims Project. In 2007, he created an endowed Chair of Anesthesia Patient Safety in the name of his mother, Laura Cheney.

John Eichhorn (1947-) was born in Cleveland, Ohio, attended Princeton University, and graduated from Harvard Medical School in 1973. He was the creator and original Editor of the newsletter of the APSF. He was a member of the WHO Safe Anesthesia Working Group, and the Safe Surgery Saves Lives global initiative. In recognition of his seminal contributions he was awarded the 2010 John Eisenberg Award for Individual Achievement in Healthcare Quality and Safety from the Joint Commission of the National Quality Forum in the USA.

JS (Nik) Gravenstein (1925–2009) was born in Berlin. He graduated from the University of Bonn Medical School in 1951 and from Harvard Medical School in 1958. He contributed to the safety of anaesthesia as head of several departments of anaesthesia, as Editor of the International Journal of Clinical Monitoring, as author of a book "Clinical Monitoring Practice", and as a pioneer in high fidelity simulation. A founder of the APSF, he was a Board Member for ten years. He led a team at the University of Florida which developed the "Gainesville Anesthesia Simulator". He was a "calm and collected" mentor, and a gracious and generous host and teacher (to W.B.R. amongst many). On Gravenstein's retirement, Jeep Pierce stated "I have not met a greater gentleman who has contributed more to the specialty of anesthesia than Nik Gravenstein".

Dan Raemer (1950-) graduated in Electrical Engineering from the University of Massachusetts in 1972. He then studied BioMedical Engineering and received a Master of Science in 1975, gaining a PhD in Bioengineering from the University of Utah. In Vermont, he and others started a program providing clinical engineering services to hospitals throughout the State (this program continues today). In 1993 he joined the nascent Boston Anesthesia Simulation Program begun by Jeff Cooper. He streamlined the pilot courses that had been introduced into coherent curricular entities that could be applied to large cohorts of anesthesia trainees. He expanded simulation and crisis resource management into other fields such as emergency medicine, intensive care, medicine (codes), and air rescue and turned them into ongoing programs. His vision was responsible for the creation and success of the Society for Simulation in Healthcare.

Angela Enright (1947-) was born and raised in Ireland, graduating from University College Dublin. She interned at St Vincent's Hospital, Dublin, then moved to Canada, training in anaesthesia at the University of Calgary, Alberta. She was President of the Canadian Anesthesiologists Society in 1994–95, and chaired the Organizing Committee for the 12th World Congress of Anesthesiologists held in Montreal in 2000. She is known for her promotion of education around the world, particularly in low income areas, in many ways following in the footsteps of Kester Brown but adding her own mix of excellence, charm and inspiration. As the immediate past President of the World Federation of Societies of Anaesthesiologists she coordinated and largely undertook the development of extensive educational material – translated into several languages. She is a Founding Director of the Lifebox Foundation. She was awarded the Order of Canada in 2011.

T.C.K. (Kester) Brown (1935-) was born in Kenya. He became the Director of Anaesthesia at the Royal Children's Hospital in Melbourne, and developed a worldwide reputation for himself and his Department. He became a member of the WFSA Education Committee in 1984, and President of WFSA in 2000. He was dedicated to helping those with limited resources and opportunities. He encouraged others to share in this passion, and mentored both of the authors. He advanced patient safety through his teaching, advocacy and personal example.

Atul Gawande (1965-) was born in Brooklyn, New York. His parents, both doctors, were immigrants from India. He grew up in Athens, Ohio. He graduated from Stanford, and he majored in Philosophy, Politics and Economics at Balliol College, Oxford as a Rhodes Scholar. It may seem unusual to include a surgeon in a chapter on the history of the patient safety movement in anaesthesia, but Atul Gawande is no ordinary surgeon: his contribution to patient safety in anaesthesia has been exceptional and has not ended. He joined Al Gore's presidential campaign in 1988, worked closely with Bill Clinton during his 1992 campaign, and went on to become a senior advisor in the Department of Health and Human Services. He returned to school (Harvard), in 1993 completing his medical training and specialising in surgery. He has a Master of Public Health (from the Harvard School of Public Health). In 2007, he became director of the WHO Safe Surgery initiative, which has a strong emphasis on the importance of anaesthesia to the safety of patients worldwide.

Olaitan Soyannwo (1945-) was born at Ilisan-Remo, Ogun State, Nigeria. She went to Mayflower school, Ikenne and Queen's College, Yaba, Lagos and then the University of Ibadan Medical school, qualifying in 1971. She trained in anaesthesia in England and has been a Consultant in Anaesthesia and Intensive Care at the University College Hospital, Ibadan since 1981, serving as Professor and Head of Department of Anaesthesia and Dean of the Faculty of Clinical Sciences. She was a key member of the Anaesthesia Safety Group of the Safe Surgery Saves Lives Campaign, and her advocacy (in the face of external scepticism about the relevance of "expensive technology" to low income areas of the world) facilitated the decision to include pulse oximetry on the WHO Safe Surgery Checklist. She was a major contributor to the revision of the International Standards for a Safe Practice of Anaesthesia.

Iain Wilson (1936-) was born in the UK and graduated from Glasgow University. While training in anaesthesia he worked in the Royal Air Force (1979–85) and as a Lecturer at the University of Zambia (1986–8), where he co-authored the first perioperative outcome study in the region. He is internationally known for his contribution to training, and chairs the Publications Committee of the WFSA where he established Update in Anaesthesia, and Anaesthesia Tutorial of the Week, as freely available training and CPD resources. He is a co-editor of the Oxford Handbook of Anaesthesia. He was a member of the Anaesthesia Safety Group of the Safe Surgery Saves Lives Campaign and led the WFSA Global Oximetry project in Uganda (79). He was elected President of the Association of Anaesthetists of Great Britain and Ireland in September 2010, bringing the influence and resources of this organisation to the support of the Lifebox initiative.

References

1. Rushman G, Davies N, Atkinson R. A short history of anaesthesia. Oxford: Butterworth-Heinemann; 1996.
2. Sykes K. Personal Communication. "References to Anesthesia in 19th Centure British regional newspapers". March 19 1847 Times, 2011.
3. Sykes K. Personal Communication. "References to Anesthesia in 19th Centure British regional newspapers". February 3 1848 Times. 2011.
4. Knight PR 3rd, Bacon DR. An unexplained death: Hannah Greener and chloroform. Anesthesiology. 2002;96:1250–53.
5. Sykes W. Essays on the first hundred years of anaesthesia. London: William Clowes (Beccles); 1982.
6. Cooper JB, Newbower RS, Long CD, McPeek B. Preventable anesthesia mishaps: a study of human factors. Anesthesiology. 1978;49:399–406.
7. Gaba DM. Anaesthesiology as a model for patient safety in health care. BMJ. 2000;320:785–8.
8. Utting JE, Gray TC, Shelley FC. Human misadventure in anaesthesia. Can Anaesth Soc J. 1979;26:472–8.
9. Aders A, Aders H. Anaesthetic adverse incident reports: an Australian study of 1,231 outcomes. Anaesth Intens Care. 2005;33:336–44.
10. Lagasse RS. Anesthesia safety: model or myth? A review of the published literature and analysis of current original data. Anesthesiology. 2002;97:1609–17.
11. Dripps RD, Lamont A, Eckenhoff JE. The role of anesthesia in surgical mortality. JAMA. 1961;178:261–6.
12. Davies JM, Strunin L. Anesthesia in 1984: how safe is it? Can Med Assoc J. 1984;131:437–41.

13. Derrington MC, Smith G. A review of studies of anaesthetic risk, morbidity and mortality. Br J Anaesth. 1987;59:815–33.
14. Sykes K. Anaesthesia and the times. History of Anaesthesia Society Proceedings 2008;39:15–19 (paper given in York June 27th, 2008).
15. Holland R. Special committee investigating deaths under anaesthesia. Report on 745 classified cases, 1960–1968. Med J Aust. 1970;1:573–94.
16. Holland R. Anaesthetic mortality in New South Wales. Br J Anaesth. 1987;59:834–41.
17. Warden JC, Borton CL, Horan BF. Mortality associated with anaesthesia in New South Wales, 1984–1990. Med J Aust. 1994;161:585–93.
18. Gibbs N, Rodoreda P. Anaesthetic mortality rates in Western Australia 1980–2002. Anaesth Intens Care. 2005;33:616–22.
19. Gibbs N, Borton C. A review of anaesthesia related mortality 2000 to 2002. Melbourne: Australian and New Zealand College of Anaesthetists; 2006.
20. Gibbs NM. Milestones in anaesthesia-related mortality and morbidity reporting in Australia. Anaesth Intens Care. 2010;38:807–8.
21. Harrison GG. Anaesthetic contributory death—its incidence and causes. I. Incidence. S Afr Med J. 1968;42:514–8.
22. Harrison GG. Death attributable to anaesthesia. A 10-year survey (1967–1976). Br J Anaesth. 1978;50:1041–6.
23. Harrison GG. Death due to anaesthesia at Groote Schuur Hospital, Cape Town—1956–1987. Part I. Incidence. S Afr Med J. 1990;77:412–5.
24. Institute of Medicine. To err is human: building a safer health system. Washington DC: National Academies Press; 1999.
25. Arbous MS, Meursing AE, van Kleef JW, de Lange JJ, Spoormans HH, Touw P, Werner FM, Grobbee DE. Impact of anesthesia management characteristics on severe morbidity and mortality. Anesthesiology. 2005;102:257–68.
26. Hogan H, Healey F, Neale G, Thomson R, Vincent C, Black N. Preventable deaths due to problems in care in English acute hospitals: a retrospective case record review study. BMJ Qual Saf. 2012;21:737–45.
27. Runciman WB. Iatrogenic harm and anaesthesia in Australia. Anaesth Intens Care. 2005;33:297–300.
28. Greenland KB, Acott C, Segal R, Riley RH, Merry AF. Delayed airway compromise following extubation of adult patients who required surgical drainage of Ludwig's angina: comment on three coronial cases. Anaesth Intens Care. 2011;39:506–8.
29. Enright A, Merry A. The WFSA and patient safety in the perioperative setting. Can J Anaesth. 2009;56:8–13.
30. Ouro-Bang'na Maman AF, Tomta K, Ahouangbevi S, Chobli M. Deaths associated with anaesthesia in Togo, West Africa. Trop Doct. 2005;35:220–2.
31. WHO Safe Surgery Saves Lives. http://www.who.int/patientsafety/safesurgery/en/. Accessed 17 March 2010.
32. Walker IA, Merry AF, Wilson IH, McHugh GA, O'Sullivan E, Thoms GM, Nuevo F, Whitaker DK, teams GOP. Global oximetry: an international anaesthesia quality improvement project. Anaesthesia. 2009;64:1051–60.
33. Beecher HK, Todd DP. A study of the deaths associated with anesthesia and surgery. Ann Surg. 1954;140:2–34.
34. Abajian J, Arrowood JG, Barrett RH, Dwyer CS, Eversole UH, Fine JH, Hand LV, Howrie WC, Marcus PS, Martin SJ, Nicholson MJ, Saklad E, Saklad M, Sellman P, Smith RM, Woodbridge PD. Critique of "A Study of the Deaths Associated with Anesthesia and Surgery". Ann Surg. 1955;142:138–41.
35. Harrison GG. Control of the malignant hyperpyrexic syndrome in MHS swine by dantrolene sodium. Br J Anaesth. 1975;47:62–5.
36. Dorsch JA, Dorsch SE, Series Editor Gravlee GP. A practical approach to anesthesia equipment. Wolters Kluwer—Lippincott Williams and Wilkins, Philadelphia.; 2011.

37. Russell WJ. Equipment for anaesthesia and intensive care. Adelaide: W J Russell; 1997.
38. Macintosh RR. Deaths under anaesthetics. Br J Anaesth. 1949;21:107–36.
39. International Taskforce on Anaesthesia Safety. International standards for a safe practice of anaesthesia. Eur J Anaesthesiol. 1993;10 (Suppl 7):12–15; updated: http://anaesthesiologists.org/en/safety/2008-international-standards-for-a-safe-practice-of-anaesthesia.html. Accessed 17 March 10).
40. Merry AF, Cooper JB, Soyannwo O, Wilson IH, Eichhorn JH. International Standards for a Safe Practice of Anesthesia 2010. Can J Anaesth. 2010;57:1027–34.
41. Keats AS. What do we know about anesthetic mortality? Anesthesiology. 1979;50:387–92.
42. Hamilton WK. Unexpected deaths during anesthesia: wherein lies the cause? Anesthesiology. 1979;50:381–3.
43. Todd RH. On some points connected with the accidents of anaesthesia and their treatment. The Australasian Medical Gazette. 1889;9:38–42.
44. Gaba DM, Maxwell M, DeAnda A. Anesthetic mishaps: breaking the chain of accident evolution. Anesthesiology. 1987;66:670–76.
45. Cooper JB, Gaba DM. A strategy for preventing anesthesia accidents. Int Anesthesiol Clin. 1989;27:148–52.
46. Merry AF, McCall Smith A. Errors, Medicine and the Law. Cambridge: Cambridge University Press; 2001.
47. Holzer JF. Liability insurance issues in anesthesiology. Int Anesthesiol Clin. 1989;27:205–12.
48. Pierce EC Jr. The 34th Rovenstine Lecture. 40 years behind the mask: safety revisited. Anesthesiology. 1996;84:965–75.
49. Cooper J. Patient safety and biomedical engineering. In: Kitz R, editor. This is No Humbug: reminiscences of the Department of Anesthesia at the Massachusetts General Hospital. Boston: Department of Anesthesia and Critical Care, Massachusetts General Hospital; 2002. S. 377–420.
50. Eichhorn J. The APSF at 25: pioneering success in safety but challenges remain. APSF Newsletter 2010;25:1, 23–4, 35–9.
51. Solazzi RW, Ward RJ. Analysis of anesthetic mishaps. The spectrum of medical liability cases. Int Anesthesiol Clin. 1984;22:43–59.
52. Keats AS. The Closed Claims Study. Anesthesiology. 1990;73:199–201.
53. Caplan RA, Posner KL, Ward RJ, Cheney FW. Adverse respiratory events in anesthesia: a closed claims analysis. Anesthesiology. 1990;72:828–33.
54. Posner KL, Caplan RA, Cheney FW. Variation in expert opinion in medical malpractice review. Anesthesiology. 1996;85:1049–54.
55. Lunn JN, Devlin HB. Lessons from the confidential enquiry into perioperative deaths in three NHS regions. Lancet. 1987;2:1384–6.
56. Lunn JN. The history and achievements of the National Confidential Enquiry into Perioperative Deaths. J Qual Clin Pract. 1998;18:29–35.
57. Anaesthesia and Intensive Care Symposium—The Australian Incident Monitoring Study. Anaes Int Care. 1993;21.
58. Holland R, Hains J, Roberts JG, Runciman WB. Symposium—The Australian Incident Monitoring Study. Anaesth Intens Care. 1993;21:501–5.
59. Webb RK, van der Walt JH, Runciman WB, Williamson JA, Cockings J, Russell WJ, Helps S. The Australian Incident Monitoring Study. Which monitor? An analysis of 2000 incident reports. Anaesth Intens Care. 1993;21:529–42.
60. Brennan TA, Leape LL, Laird NM, Hebert L, Localio AR, Lawthers AG, Newhouse JP, Weiler PC, Hiatt HH. Incidence of adverse events and negligence 2 hospitalized patients. Results of the Harvard Medical Practice Study I. N Engl J Med. 1991;324:370–6.
61. Wilson RM, Runciman WB, Gibberd RW, Harrison BT, Newby L, Hamilton JD. The Quality in Australian Health Care Study. Med J Aust. 1995;163:458–71.
62. Runciman WB, Webb RK, Helps SC, Thomas EJ, Sexton EJ, Studdert DM, Brennan TA. A comparison of iatrogenic injury studies in Australia and the USA. II: reviewer behaviour and quality of care. Int J Qual Health Care. 2000;12:379–88.
63. Runciman WB, Williamson JA, Deakin A, Benveniste KA, Bannon K, Hibbert PD. An integrated framework for safety, quality and risk management: an information and incident management system based on a universal patient safety classification. Qual Saf Health Care. 2006;15 (Suppl 1):i82–90.
64. Sherman H, Castro G, Fletcher M, Hatlie M, Hibbert P, Jakob R, Koss R, Lewalle P, Loeb J, Perneger T, Runciman W, Thomson R, Van Der Schaaf T, Virtanen M. Towards an International Classification for Patient Safety: the conceptual framework. Int J Qual Health Care. 2009;21:2–8.
65. Cooper JB, Gaba DM, Liang B, Woods D, Blum LN. The National Patient Safety Foundation agenda for research and development in patient safety. MedGenMed. 2000;2:E38.
66. Merry AF, Webster CS, Hannam J, Mitchell SJ, Henderson R, Reid P, Edwards K-E, Jardim A, Pak N, Cooper J, Hopley L, Frampton C, Short TG. Multimodal system designed to reduce errors in recording and administration of drugs in anaesthesia: prospective randomised clinical evaluation. BMJ. 2011;343:d5543.
67. Meyer JA, Rendell-Baker L. Safety and performance of anesthesia and ventilatory equipment. Anesthesiology. 1970;32:473–4.
68. Rendell-Baker L. Some gas machine hazards and their elimination. Anesth Analg. 1976;55:26–33.
69. Pierce EC Jr. Analysis of anesthetic mishaps. Historical perspectives. Int Anesthesiol Clin. 1984;22:1–16.
70. Reason J. Human error. New York: Cambridge University Press; 1990.
71. Rendell-Baker L. Desirable performance characteristics of anesthetic machines. Int Anesthesiol Clin. 1974;12:1–24.
72. Rendell-Baker L. Standards for anesthetic and ventilatory equipment. Int. Anesthesiol Clin. 1982;20:171–203.
73. Ritchie JR. Letter: a simple and reliable warning device for failing oxygen pressure. Br J Anaesth. 1974;46:323.
74. Severinghaus JW, Honda Y. History of blood gas analysis. VII. Pulse oximetry. J Clin Monit. 1987;3:135–8.
75. Westhorpe RN, Ball C. The pulse oximeter. Anaesth Intens Care. 2008;36:767.
76. Westhorpe RN, Ball C. The history of capnography. Anaesth Intens Care. 2010;38:611.
77. Eichhorn JH, Cooper JB, Cullen DJ, Maier WR, Philip JH, Seeman RG. Standards for patient monitoring during anesthesia at Harvard Medical School. JAMA. 1986;256:1017–20.
78. Gaba D, Fish K, Howard S. Crisis management in anesthesiology. 1st ed. New York: Churchill Livingston; 1994.
79. Weller J, Morris R, Watterson L, Garden A, Flanagan B, Robinson B, Thompson W, Jones R. Effective management of anaesthetic crises: development and evaluation of a college-accredited simulation-based course for anaesthesia education in Australia and New Zealand. Simul Healthcar. 2006;1:209–14.
80. Tenner EW. Why things bite back—technology and the revenge of unintended consequences. New York: Vintage Books; 1997.
81. Treasure T. Lessons from the Bristol case. Br Med J. 1998;316:1685–86.
82. Smith R. All changed, changed utterly. British medicine will be transformed by the Bristol case. BMJ. 1998;316:1917–8.
83. Kennedy I. Learning from Bristol: The Report of the Public Inquiry into Children's Heart Surgery at the Bristol Royal Infirmary 1984–1995: CM 5207 (London: The Stationery Office). Available at: http://www.bristol-inquiry.org.uk/. Accessed 29 May 2006, 2001.
84. Reason J. Human error: models and management. Br Med J. 2000;320:768–70.

85. Gaba DM, Maxwell M, DeAnda A. Anesthetic mishaps: breaking the chain of accident evolution. Anesthesiology. 1987;66:670–6.

86. Denson JS, Abrahamson S. A computer-controlled patient simulator. JAMA. 1969;208:504–08.

87. Gaba DM, DeAnda A. A comprehensive anesthesia simulation environment: re-creating the operating room for research and training. Anesthesiology. 1988;69:387–94.

88. Schwid HA. A flight simulator for general anesthesia training. Comput Biomed Res. 1987;20:64–75.

89. Good ML, Gravenstein JS. Anesthesia simulators and training devices. Int Anesthesiol Clin. 1989;27:161–68.

90. Carter DF. Man-made man: anesthesiological medical human simulator. J Assoc Adv Med Instrum. 1969;3:80–6.

91. Cooper JB, Taqueti VR. A brief history of the development of mannequin simulators for clinical education and training. Qual Saf Health Care. 2004;13 (Suppl 1):i11–8.

92. Merry AF, Peck DJ. Anaesthetists, errors in drug administration and the law. N Z Med J. 1995;108:185–7.

93. Dyer C. Doctors suspended after injecting wrong drug into spine. Br Med J. 2001;322:257.

94. Orser BA, Byrick R. Anesthesia-related medication error: time to take action. Can J Anaesth. 2004;51:756–60.

95. Merry AF, Webster CS. Medication error in New Zealand—time to act. N Z Med J. 2008;121:6–9.

96. Eichhorn J. APSF hosts medication safety conference: consensus group defines challenges and opportunities for improved practice. APSF Newsletter. 2010;25:1–7.

97. Merry AF, Webster CS, Mathew DJ. A new, safety-oriented, integrated drug administration and automated anesthesia record system. Anesth Analg. 2001;93:385–90.

98. Webster CS, Larsson L, Frampton CM, Weller J, McKenzie A, Cumin D, Merry AF. Clinical assessment of a new anaesthetic drug administration system: a prospective, controlled, longitudinal incident monitoring study. Anaesthesia. 2010;65:490–9.

99. Jensen LS, Merry AF, Webster CS, Weller J, Larsson L. Evidence-based strategies for preventing drug administration errors during anaesthesia. Anaesthesia. 2004;59:493–504.

100. Bacon DR, Ament R. Ralph Waters and the beginnings of academic anesthesiology in the United States: the Wisconsin Template. J Clin Anesth. 1995;7:534–43.

101. Haynes AB, Weiser TG, Berry WR, Lipsitz SR, Breizat AH, Dellinger EP, Herbosa T, Joseph S, Kibatala PL, Lapitan MC, Merry AF, Moorthy K, Reznick RK, Taylor B, Gawande AA, Safe SSavesLStudyG. A surgical safety checklist to reduce morbidity and mortality in a global population. N Engl J Med. 2009;360:491–9.

102. de Vries EN, Prins HA, Crolla RMPH, den Outer AJ, van Andel G, van Helden SH, Schlack WS, van Putten MA, Gouma DJ, Dijkgraaf MGW, Smorenburg SM, Boermeester MA, Group SC. Effect of a comprehensive surgical safety system on patient outcomes. N Engl J Med. 2010;363:1928–37.

103. Neily J, Mills PD, Young-Xu Y, Carney BT, West P, Berger DH, Mazzia LM, Paull DE, Bagian JP. Association between implementation of a medical team training program and surgical mortality. JAMA. 2010;304:1693–700.

104. Birkmeyer JD. Strategies for improving surgical quality—checklists and beyond. N Engl J Med. 2010;363:1963–5.

105. The KK 2008 TIME 100. Time Magazine: Time Warner, 2009.

106. Berenholtz SM, Pronovost PJ, Lipsett PA, Hobson D, Earsing K, Farley JE, Milanovich S, Garrett-Mayer E, Winters BD, Rubin HR, Dorman T, Perl TM. Eliminating catheter-related bloodstream infections in the intensive care unit.[see comment]. Crit Care Med. 2004;32:2014–20.

107. Pronovost P, Needham D, Berenholtz S, Sinopoli D, Chu H, Cosgrove S, Sexton B, Hyzy R, Welsh R, Roth G, Bander J, Kepros J, Goeschel C. An intervention to decrease catheter-related bloodstream infections in the ICU. N Engl J Med. 2006;355:2725–32.

108. Walker IA, Wilson IH. Anaesthesia in developing countries-a risk for patients. Lancet. 2008;371:968–9.

109. Gawande A. Complications. New York: Henry Holt and Company; 2002.

110. Gawande A. Better. New York: Henry Holt and Company; 2007.

111. Gawande A. The checklist manifesto. New York: Metropolitan Books Henry Holt and Company; 2010.

112. Funk LM, Weiser TG, Berry WR, Lipsitz SR, Merry AF, Enright AC, Wilson IH, Dziekan G, Gawande AA. Global operating theatre distribution and pulse oximetry supply: an estimation from reported data. Lancet. 2010;376:1055–61.

113. Lifebox.

114. Merry AF, Eichhorn JH, Wilson IH. Extending the WHO 'Safe Surgery Saves Lives' project through Global Oximetry. Anaesthesia. 2009;64:1045–8.

115. Runciman WB, Baker GR, Michel P, Jauregui IL, Lilford RJ, Andermann A, Flin R, Weeks WB. The epistemology of patient safety research. Int J Evid Based Healthc. 2008;6:476–86.

116. Runciman B, Merry A, Walton M. Safety and ethics in healthcare: A guide to getting it right. Aldershot: Ashgate; 2007.

117. Donabedian A. The quality of care: how can it be assessed? JAMA. 1988;260:1743–48.

118. Donabedian A. An Introduction to quality assurance in health care. New York:Oxford University Press; 2003.

119. WHO Guidelines for Safe Surgery. Safe surgery saves lives. Geneva: WHO Press: World Health Organization, 2009.

120. Weiser TG, Makary MA, Haynes AB, Dziekan G, Berry WR, Gawande AA, Safe SSavesLM, Study GiM A. Standardised metrics for global surgical surveillance. Lancet. 2009;374:1113–7.

121. Eichhorn JH. Prevention of intraoperative anesthesia accidents and related severe injury through safety monitoring. Anesthesiology. 1989;70:572–7.

122. Webster CS, Merry AF, Larsson L, McGrath KA, Weller J. The frequency and nature of drug administration error during anaesthesia. Anaesth Intens Care. 2001;29:494–500.

123. Shekelle PG, Pronovost PJ, Wachter RM, Taylor SL, Dy SM, Foy R, Hempel S, McDonald KM, Ovretveit J, Rubenstein LV, Adams AS, Angood PB, Bates DW, Bickman L, Carayon P, Donaldson L, Duan N, Farley DO, Greenhalgh T, Haughom J, Lake ET, Lilford R, Lohr KN, Meyer GS, Miller MR, Neuhauser DV, Ryan G, Saint S, Shojania KG, Shortell SM, Stevens DP, Walshe K. Advancing the science of patient safety. Ann Intern Med. 2011;154:693–6.

124. Pronovost PJ, Lilford R. Analysis & commentary: a road map for improving the performance of performance measures. Health Aff (Millwood). 2011;30:569–73.

125. Pronovost PJ, Cardo DM, Goeschel CA, Berenholtz SM, Saint S, Jernigan JA. A research framework for reducing preventable patient harm. Clin Infect Dis. 2011;52:507–13.

126. Leape LL, Berwick DM, Bates DW. What practices will most improve safety? Evidence-based medicine meets patient safety. JAMA. 2002;288:501–7.

127. Smith GC, Pell JP. Parachute use to prevent death and major trauma related to gravitational challenge: systematic review of randomised controlled trials. Br Med J. 2003;327:1459–61.

128. Merry AF, Davies JM, Maltby JR. Qualitative research in health care. Br J Anaesth. 2000;84:552–55.

129. Moller JT, Pedersen T, Rasmussen LS, Jensen PF, Pedersen BD, Ravlo O, Rasmussen NH, Espersen K, Johannessen NW, Cooper JB, Gravestein JS, Chraemmer-Jorgensen B, Wiberg-Jorgensen F, Djernes M, Heslet L, Johansen SH. Randomized evaluation of pulse oximetry in 20,802 patients: I. Design, demography, pulse oximetry failure rate, and overall complication rate. Anesthesiology. 1993;78:436–44.

130. Moller JT, Johannessen NW, Espersen K, Ravlo O, Pedersen BD, Jensen PF, Rasmussen NH, Rasmussen LS, Pedersen T, Cooper JB. Randomized evaluation of pulse oximetry in 20,802 patients: II. Perioperative events and postoperative complications. Anesthesiology. 1993;78:445–53.

131. Savel RH, Goldstein EB, Gropper MA. Critical care checklists, the Keystone Project, and the Office for Human Research Protections: a case for streamlining the approval process in quality-improvement research.[see comment]. Crit Care Med. 2009;37:725–8.

132. McGlynn E, Asch S, Adams J, Keesey J, Hicks J, DeCristofaro A, Kerr E. The quality of health care delivered to adults in the United States. N Engl J Med. 2003;348:2635–45.

133. Runciman WB, Hunt TD, Hannaford NA, Hibbert PD, Westbrook JI, Coiera EW, Day RO, Hindmarsh DM, McGlynn EA, Braithwaite J. CareTrack: assessing the appropriateness of health care delivery in Australia. Med J Aust. 2012;197:100–5.

Where and How Does the Anesthetic Process Help or Hurt Patients Independent of Producing Anesthesia?

Harriet W. Hopf

Summary

This chapter provides exemplars of good and bad outcomes that can result from anesthesia and anesthetists. In the 1850s, Snow determined that chloroform could kill by "cardiac syncope." In the 1930s, Lundy guided the banking and administration of blood, and Lundy and Rovenstine established pain clinics. In the 1970s, Bonica established pain as a subspecialty.

Ibsen's response to the terrible 1952 Copenhagen polio epidemic, manual support of breathing, led to intensive care units, ventilator development, and the creation of modern blood-gas analysis by Astrup and Severinghaus. In 1953, Apgar devised her "score", a number describing the neonate's condition. In 1956, Lassen showed the lethality of prolonged nitrous oxide administration. Later investigators suggested health hazards to occupational exposure to nitrous oxide.

Beecher advocated the use of informed consent in volunteers and patients in 1959. In the 1960s, he argued for establishment of Institutional Review Boards to govern human experimentation, and he helped define brain death.

In the 1960s, surgeon Hunt demonstrated that surgical wounds often have low tissue oxygen levels that predisposed to infection and impaired healing. Hopf showed that surgical site infections correlated with low wound oxygen levels. In the 1970s, Huch, Lubbers and Severinghaus developed transcutaneous oximetry, later adding transcutaneous carbon dioxide measurements.

Studies in the 1980s showed that exposure to inhaled anesthetics protected the heart from subsequent ischemia. Also, in the 1980s, Cahalan led in the evaluation and application of transesophageal echocardiography.

In the 1980s and early 1990s, Hunt's group and Hartmann found that generous fluid administration benefited wound healing. In 1996, Kurz et al. reported that maintaining normal core temperature reduced wound infection rates, and Schmied et al. found that mild hypothermia increased intra-and postoperative blood loss. In the late 1990s, Weiskopf found that a hemoglobin of less than 7 g/dL impaired cerebral function in resting fit volunteers.

In 1985 and 1995, psychiatrist Langer and anesthesia colleagues demonstrated that deep anesthesia with isoflurane decreased patient suffering from mental depression. In the 2000s, Olney's group suggested that anesthetics could impair the developing brain of rats. This concern resulted in a presently ongoing multidisciplinary effort to determine whether similar effects occur in humans, particularly very young patients.

In the 1990s and 2000s, inhaled anesthetics were found to deplete the ozone layer (especially halothane) or act as greenhouse gases (especially desflurane). In the 2000s, the prolonged use of large tidal volumes was found to injure the lungs.

Introduction

Anesthesia offers amnesia and immobility, transporting patients painlessly through surgery and providing optimum conditions for surgeons. From the discovery of anesthesia to the present, anesthetists have accepted diverse challenges unrelated or only tangentially related to rendering patients unconscious and/or insensitive to the surgeon's knife. Some actions of anesthetists/anesthetics caused harm to patients (e.g., hepatitis, renal injury) or society (e.g., environmental pollution) while others had salutary effects (e.g., diminishing mental depression, increasing myocardial tolerance to ischemic injury).

We begin with a definition of outcomes research. Taking the two words at face value, any investigation defining good and bad outcomes might be considered outcomes research. But respected investigators may take a different view. Daniel Sessler (personal communication, 16 Sept 12) doubts that

H. W. Hopf (✉)
Department of Anesthesiology, University of Utah School
of Medicine, SOM 3C444, 30 N 1900 East, Salt Lake City,
UT 84132, USA
e-mail: harriet.hopf@hsc.utah.edu

we "should extend the term to include all important game-changing research. There are lots of small studies that are critically important, but aren't what most people consider to be outcomes research." Sessler would "reserve the term for large-scale clinical trials evaluating outcomes that are meaningful to patients."

Others, such as the editors of this book argue that large-scale outcomes trials are at one end of outcomes research—research that tells us about clinical outcomes, good and bad. The definition of large-scale itself is ambiguous. Such trials have to be large enough to reveal significant changes in outcome (if they exist), but the size needed depends on the incidence and consistency of the outcome. It might range from a few hundred to millions of subjects. Why should we not call the studies requiring only tens to a hundred or two hundred subjects to define a good or bad clinical outcome, outcomes research? Where one draws the line is arbitrary.

For the purposes of this book, we will take both views, assigning the stories of large-scale clinical trials to Chapter 43 written by the editors, with the invaluable assistance of Arthur Wallace, and usually assigning smaller trials to the present chapter. We draw a line at roughly two hundred subjects, and the present chapter will look at the history of studies of less than this "number" and Chapter 43 will look primarily at studies of more than this number, particularly (but not limited to) those involving cardiovascular studies. Using chronologies within themes, both chapters provide exemplars of good and untoward outcomes. Many contributions are covered in detail elsewhere in this history, and some will be dealt with but briefly in both chapters. Anesthetists and anesthesia contributed greatly to these advances and retreats, often leading these stories. Many others also contributed to what has been a collaborative effort shared with colleagues outside of anesthesia, all focusing on issues relevant to patients in the perioperative period. Finally, we acknowledge that there is insufficient space to tell all the fine stories that might be told.

1846–1860: William Morton and the Discovery of Anesthesia

Most would not think of Morton's grand discovery as outcomes research, unless one uses the broad definition suggested above. Morton's observations in patients repeatedly confirmed an outcome, the production of insensitivity to surgical pain—despite Morton barely knowing what he was doing. Morton did not need fancy statistics or large numbers to produce "anesthesia outcomes research" because his goal, "anesthesia", always occurred; anesthesia was produced 100 % of the time. If an outcome occurs 100 % of the time, small studies can readily document an end-point, an outcome.

1848–1854: John Snow Connects Chloroform and Cardiac Syncope

Unlike Morton, Snow knew what he was doing. He wrote books about anesthesia and recorded summaries of each of the thousands of anesthetics he administered [1, 2]. From observation, he defined the characteristics pertaining to increasing depth of anesthesia (called by Snow, degrees of anesthesia). An appreciation of these characteristics enabled Snow and others to deliver anesthesia safely, at least most of the time.

When the issue of death from chloroform arose, Snow referred to his case records and to experiments he had conducted in cats and frogs. Against this background, he provided a detailed, case-by-case examination of 50 published reports of deaths between 1848 and 1854, associated with chloroform administration throughout Europe, the US, and Jamaica [1]. Hannah Greener was the first of these deaths, and Snow opined "From the lips becoming suddenly blanched in the above case, there is every reason to conclude that the heart was suddenly paralysed." Snow considered several possible causes of death, concluding that

> "In all the cases in which the symptoms which occurred at the time of death are reported, there is every reason to conclude… that death took place by cardiac syncope, or arrest of the action of the heart. In forty of these cases, the symptoms of danger appeared to arise entirely from cardiac syncope and were not complicated by the over-action of the chloroform on the brain. It was only in four cases that the breathing appeared to be embarrassed…."

Thus Snow, applying his patient and research experiences (a large database) to bear on diverse reports, cleverly concluded that death resulted from sudden stoppage of the heart. We would add that the stoppage probably resulted from arrhythmias or excessive depression secondary to anesthetic overdose, something Snow had devised methods to avoid.

1850s: Treatment of the Spasms Induced by Tetanus

An arsenal of potent drugs may be given to patients with benefit in mind, but little understanding of the disease being treated or the mechanistic basis of the drugs' action. Lest we smile, beware, for our ignorance is greater than we can imagine. So in the 1850s, physicians thought to diminish the spasms from tetanus by administering curare. The patients died (e.g., see Sayres) [3]. Not until 1954, was curare applied to the management of tetanus in a more rational and beneficial manner when Lassen et al. [4] and Honey et al. [5] not only gave curare, but also ventilated the lungs of their patients, who then happily survived.

1930s–Present: Blood Banking/Transfusion Medicine

At the Mayo Clinic in 1933, surgeon Charlie Mayo set anesthesiologist John Lundy with the task of improving blood transfusion [6]. The expertise of anesthesiologists in obtaining venous access for transfusions made an anesthesiologist the logical choice for this role. By 1935, Lundy's successes indicated a need for a more dependable blood supply than donors giving blood directly to the patient. In 1935, he demonstrated that blood could safely be stored in an icebox for up to 14 days, thus establishing "the first blood bank in North America."

By the 1960s, transfusion of banked refrigerated blood had become routine, but administration of large volumes to hemorrhaging patients was noted to lead to cardiac arrest from hypothermia. Anesthesiologists Boyan and Howland devised a system to warm the blood by passing the intravenous tubing through a warm water bath before infusion into the patient [7]. By this means, they could increase the rate of blood administration while decreasing the incidence of cardiac arrest in massive transfusion from 21 of 36 patients, to 1 of 45 patients.

In the late 1960s, anesthesiologist Ron Miller was stationed at the US Naval Support Activity Hospital in Da Nang during the Vietnam War, giving him extensive experience with massive transfusion (defined by Miller as greater than 20 units of blood) [8]. Using his experiences he described the effects of massive transfusion on coagulation and acid-base balance. His observations helped define the best combination of blood products for managing the effects of massive hemorrhage on coagulation function.

Perioperative blood transfusion increases the risk of complications such as surgical site infection (SSI). Studies in the 2000s indicated that preoperative anemia predicted postoperative complications [9, 10]. Several studies focused on the acceptability of using 'old' (nearing the end of storage expiration date) blood for transfusions in surgical patients. Old blood may be a hazard in cardiac surgery and pediatric patients, but Weiskopf et al. did not find that it was a problem when only 1 or 2 units were transfused [11].

1930s–Present: Pain Management

Because they manage the pain otherwise associated with surgery, anesthetists are natural leaders in the management of pain outside the operating room. In the 1930s, anesthesiologists John Lundy at the Mayo Clinic and Emory Rovenstine at Bellevue Hospital, established regional block clinics in an attempt to manage pain [12]. Anesthesiologist John Bonica published his classic textbook "The Management of Pain" in 1953, and became Chair of Anesthesiology at the University of Washington in 1960, where he immediately created a multidisciplinary chronic pain program. Bonica helped demonstrate the key role that anesthesiologists play in the treatment of chronic pain [13]. In 1973, Bonica organized a meeting which resulted in founding of the International Association of the Study of Pain with its associated journal, Pain [14]. Anesthesiologists subsequently joined with other members of the medical community to collegially develop the field of pain management and pain clinics, but it began with Lundy, Rovenstine, and, most of all, with Bonica.

1940s–1960s: Beecher's Contributions to Ethics

Anesthesiologist, Henry Beecher, observed that the wounded at Anzio in 1944 had a remarkably decreased need for morphine to relieve pain [15]. Their wounds provided the means to exit from the horrors of war. This led Beecher to the thought that the mind could control perception, something plausibly explained by physiologists Melzak and Wall with their 1965 spinal gate theory [16]. Beecher emphasized how effective placebos were, making their inclusion in a blinded manner mandatory to provide a controlled experiment [17]. Beecher then questioned whether ethical practice demanded the application of informed consent. A series of publications by Beecher followed his first in 1959 on "Experimentation in man" [18]. These ultimately led to the present demand for informed consent and the authority of Institutional Review Boards to govern human research in all of medicine [19].

Beecher assisted in the birthing of transplantation which made use of organs harvested from the dead. But when were the dead really dead? Specifically, when was the patient's brain really dead? In 1968, Beecher led in the definition of brain death [20].

1950s: Status Asthmaticus and Status Epilepticus

Because volatile anesthetics relax bronchial smooth muscle, they (and even rectal ether) were used to treat patients with status asthmaticus in the 1950s and earlier [21]. This was effective during administration of the anesthetics but did nothing to treat the underlying problem, and required intensive monitoring and often hemodynamic support. Thus, this treatment of status asthmaticus was never widely adopted. Similarly, anesthesiologists and colleagues used volatile anesthetics as a last resort to treat status epilepticus [22] because of anesthesia's effect on electroencephalographic activity. Again, because the underlying disorder (rather than the

EEG) was not treated and hemodynamic support was usually required to achieve the degree of suppression required, the treatment never became routine.

1950s–Present: Training of Others in Resuscitation

Anesthesiologists have played a major role in treating and training others to treat victims of trauma and accident. This has extended to on-site management during major disasters and improved planning for such rare and catastrophic events.

Anesthesiologists pioneered instruction of members of the general public in emergency CPR in many countries. Peter Safar was one of these in the US. In Australia, the combination of readily accessible beaches and warm weather led to an alarming number of drownings, prompting Tess Cramond to begin teaching CPR in the early 1950s, in conjunction with Surf Life Saving Australia. She later taught CPR to the Ambulance Training School and other organizations, encouraging colleagues throughout the country to follow her example. She founded the Australian Resuscitation Council in 1976.

In the early 1990s, several anaesthesiologists were engaged in teaching primary resuscitation and anesthesia care in third world countries. In 1995, the WHO asked Douglas Wilkinson from Oxford, UK to write a review of trauma management for developing countries. Together with anesthesiologists Haydn Perndt, Marcus Skinner (both from Australia) and Michael Dobson of Oxford, he developed a Primary Trauma Care (PTC) course. Following several courses in Africa and the South Pacific, it became clear that there was a need for expansion of the courses, instruction programs, and educational materials.

With the assistance of the World Federation of Societies of Anaesthesiologists, the number of courses and the countries involved multiplied. Instructor courses took place first in Oxford, then expanding to countries around the world. In 2003, the PTC manual became a WHO official publication. By 2010, the manual had been translated into 14 languages and courses had been run in over 60 countries.

1950s–Present: The Anesthesiologist Goes to the Patient

In most parts of the world, the patient who suffers some disaster is transported to the nearest hospital for urgent care. But wartime experiences suggested that a more immediate application of therapy might provide a better outcome. In France, anesthesiologists acted to make this a reality. In the 1950s, French health authorities asked anesthesiologists to organize emergency medicine and prehospital care to deal

with the 13,000 yearly deaths on French roads. In the 1960s, the first mobile medical emergency response units (Service mobile d'urgence et de réanimation, SMUR) were developed. French anesthesiologists Maurice Cara (Paris), Pierre Huguenard (Créteil), Louis Lareng (Toulouse) and Louis Serre (Montpellier) expanded this into the prehospital emergency system known as SAMU (Service d'Aide Médicale Urgente). Medical teams (often including an anesthesiologist) went from hospitals in specially equipped ambulances, helicopters, or fixed wing planes to care for patients with life-threatening emergencies. A 1986 French law [23] specified that SAMU should act as a dispatch and reception center for all medical emergency calls, 24 hours a day. In 2006, this service conducted 1,890,439 missions, having received 15 million calls.

1952: Polio Leads to Artificial Ventilation, Monitoring and Intensive Care

Of the polio epidemics that moved through the world in the 1940s and 1950s, the one striking Copenhagen in 1952 was among the worst, with hundreds of patients requiring ventilatory support and driving development of intensive care medicine and the intensive care unit (ICU) [13]. Anesthesiologist Bjørn Ibsen, had spent a year as an assistant anesthetist at the Massachusetts General Hospital in 1949–50, becoming familiar with the use of intermittent positive pressure ventilation (IPPV). Despite Ibsen's youth, he convinced Lassen, the director of Blegdams Infectious Diseases Hospital in Copenhagen, to allow him to introduce IPPV via a tracheostomy to keep patients with respiratory failure alive (see Fig. 55.7) [24]. Hundreds of volunteer anesthetists and other medical personnel, including medical and dental students supplied the IPPV by manually ventilating the lungs of each patient. Their contribution was essential, since the supply of ventilators was virtually non-existent. Equally important was concentrating these terribly sick patients in one location where support, supplies and personnel could be focused. Polio had forced the development of the basic ingredients of ICU medicine.

An immediate need in this crisis was to assess the adequacy of ventilation by what IPPV did to individual patient blood gases. But the blood/gas machine had not been invented and the then known laboratory procedures were too cumbersome. Clinical chemist Poul Astrup took the first step towards modern carbon dioxide monitoring in blood [25], by supplying Ibsen's rag-tag team with much needed information about how well they were doing. The need for something more automated and more controllable to supply IPPV, also prompted the development of ventilators. And finally, the lessons Ibsen learned in the 1952 polio epidemic of 1) ventilatory support (including blood analysis) and 2) concentrating resources/personnel led him to organize the first ICU in 1953 [26].

1953: The Apgar Score

Anesthesiologist Virginia Apgar (1909–1974) was the first woman appointed as a full professor at the Columbia University College of Physicians and Surgeons (see Fig. 16.6). She sought to provide better care to newborns suffering from 'fetal anoxia' and requiring resuscitation. In 1950, she reported that oxygen levels in newborn blood might vary greatly immediately after delivery [27]. To assist in determining which newborns required a higher level of care, she developed the Apgar Score, a number between 0 (bad) and 10 (good) describing the neonate's condition. She published a description of the score in 1953 [28]. She later demonstrated that low Apgar scores correlated with low blood oxygen levels and pH. The "Apgar" remains as a cornerstone of newborn evaluation today.

1954–1958: Evolution of Blood-Gas Electrodes

Astrup had gone part way towards the rapid analysis of respiratory gases in the blood. Physical chemist Richard Stow introduced the carbon dioxide electrode at the 1954 meeting of the American Physiological Society [29]. His findings influenced anesthesiologist John Severinghaus, who tested and improved on Stow's ideas [30]. Leland Clark (similarly not an anesthesiologist, but who also influenced Severinghaus and other anesthesiologists interested in measuring blood gases) introduced the self-contained polarographic oxygen electrode in 1956 [31]. Severinghaus set to work adapting it to measure oxygen in the blood. In 1957, he combined a Stow-Severinghaus carbon dioxide electrode and a Clark electrode with a heated cuvette that stirred the blood sample, thus creating the first blood gas analysis system [32]. A year later, he added a pH electrode, creating the first blood gas machine, a device routinely used today (see Fig. 55.15) [33].

1956: Nitrous Oxide May Not Be Innocuous

In 1956, Lassen et al. administered nitrous oxide to diminish the pain from spasms produced by tetanus. The pain diminished, but after a few days of therapy with nitrous oxide, the patients developed severe bone marrow depression, and some died [34]. This is the same Lassen who appealed to Bjørn Ibsen to do something to save the Copenhagen patients suffering from polio in 1952.

Decades later, anesthesiologists and other investigators showed that this untoward effect probably resulted from the capacity of nitrous oxide to inactivate methionine synthase [35, 36], a vital enzyme responsible for synthesizing the essential amino acid, methionine, and producing folate, needed for formation of DNA.

Exposure to nitrous oxide as a patient or as a member of the operative team who may breathe the gas released from the anesthetic machine, may result in subtle or less than subtle injury because we are not created with an equal amount of methionine synthase. Even if we were, the production of methionine synthase requires absorption of vitamin B12. So the patient who is a vegetarian (with less access to B12) or is an alcoholic or is just old (with a decreased production of intrinsic factor—needed to absorb B12) may be more vulnerable to inactivation of methionine synthase and its consequences. Anesthesiologists and others showed that fatal consequences can result in patients with a rare deficiency in the capacity to manufacture methionine synthase, who breathe nitrous oxide even briefly (1–2 hours) [37].

1960s–1980s: Tissue Oxygen Levels, Infection, and Wound Healing

In the 1960s, surgeon Thomas Hunt demonstrated that surgical wounds commonly have tissue oxygen levels low enough to impair resistance to infection and healing capacity [38]. Hunt quickly recognized the value of collaborating with anesthesiologists, eventually spurring the creation of a major current area of investigation within anesthesia, specifically outcomes research related to wound healing.

In the 1970s and 1980s, Hunt and his collaborators developed minimally invasive methods, based on the Clark electrode, to continuously measure oxygen partial pressures in surgical wounds. They demonstrated that decreased PO_2 in wounds can impair white cell function. By the mid-1990s, anesthesiologist Harriet Hopf under Hunt's tutelage showed that surgical site infections (SSIs) correlated with low wound oxygen levels [39]. In that study, PO_2 in most surgical wounds was less than normal, often low enough to impair white cell function. In volunteer studies, infusion of epinephrine [a model of sympathetic nervous system (SNS) activation] decreased wound PO_2 levels substantially—as did hypovolemia. Hunt predicted that preventing perioperative cold exposure/hypothermia, hypovolemia, pain, and stress would lessen SNS activation, thus preventing peripheral vasoconstriction and maintaining wound oxygen levels close to normal. This would improve healing and resistance to infection. He also understood that anesthesiologists held the key to the SNS. Then a surgery resident working in his lab, I (HH) decided to switch to anesthesiology. This started a 25-year collaboration and provided a mechanism for recruiting other anesthesiologists to study wound outcomes, including Dan Sessler (Fig. 42.1), Andrea Kurz, Kate Leslie,

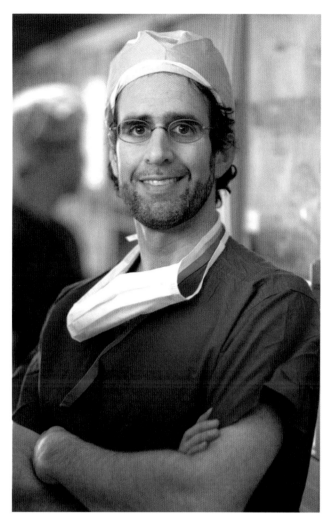

transcutaneous oximetry continues to be used for this purpose in neonatal ICUs. In older children and adults, measurement of transcutaneous oxygen partial pressures is less accurate, particularly at high PO_2 values. Transcutaneous oximetry did find new life, however, in the 1980s, when surgeons Hauser and Shoemaker demonstrated that transcutaneous oximetry could be used to quantify skin oxygen levels in ischemic limbs [45]. Transcutaneous oximetry is now used routinely in wound clinics to determine a patient's capacity to heal. Anesthesiologists have contributed to this field [46, 47].

1970s–Present: Anesthesiologists and Disasters

The involvement of anesthesiologists in on-site management of victims of major disasters came to the fore in the Moorgate Tube Train accident, in London in 1975. 43 people died and 72 required treatment in hospital. Prior planning, good communication, and the need for mobile medical teams to have emergency management experience, were all identified as key factors in the successful management of disaster victims. Anesthesiologists around the world subsequently became core members of local and national disaster planning processes.

In 1977, The Association of Anaesthetists of Great Britain and Ireland established the Pask Certificate of Honour. Named after Edgar Pask, anaesthetist and experimental physiologist in the Royal Air Force, the award honors the gallantry of a registrar anaesthetist in the Moorgate disaster. In 2010, the award was made to 113 anaesthetists who had served in the Armed Forces in Iraq from 2003 to 2009.

Successful completion of Fellowship training of anesthesiologists in Australia and New Zealand now requires accreditation in one of the following courses: Emergency Management of Severe Trauma (EMST), Advanced Trauma Life Support (ATLS) or Effective Management of Anaesthetic Crises (EMAC).

Fig. 42.1 Daniel Sessler. (From www.nlm.nih.gov/medlineplus/magazine/issues/summer07/articles/…)

Ozan Akca, Barbara Kabon, Elizabeth Fleischmann, and Paul Myles.

1970s–1980s: Transcutaneous Oxygen and Carbon Dioxide Measurement

The blood gas monitoring systems devised in the 1950s, could not be used to continuously monitor respiratory gases in the body. In the 1970s, Huch, Lubbers and Severinghaus developed transcutaneous oximetry to provide a nearly-continuous monitor of arterial oxygen [40–42]. In the late 1970s and early 1980s, Beran et al. and Severinghaus added transcutaneous analysis of carbon dioxide [43, 44]. The device heated the skin under the electrode, increasing cutaneous blood flow, thereby arterializing cutaneous gases and minimizing diffusion distances of oxygen and carbon dioxide to the electrode surface. Monitoring of both gases was found to accurately reflect arterial blood gas values in infants, and

1976: Volatile Anesthetics Can Predispose to Arrhythmias

Small studies are of limited or no use if they do not uncover a significant effect (they may be too small to reveal a significant difference). They are only useful if they reveal significant differences. For example, in 1976, Johnston et al. reported on the arrhythmias in 48 patients having transphenoidal removal of pituitary tumors after receiving submucosal injections of epinephrine in saline to minimize bleeding [48]. Of patients anesthetized with halothane, 50 % developed three or more premature ventricular contractions at a dose of 2.1 mg/kg epinephrine, a dose significantly less than the 6.7 mg/kg dose of epinephrine required to produce the same rate of PVCs during anesthesia with isoflurane. This small study in humans showed that the alkane, halothane, predisposed to ventricular arrhythmias far more than did the ether, isoflurane.

1980s: Potent Anesthetics May Decrease Myocardial Injury

In the 1980s, inhaled anesthetics were shown to have pre-conditioning effects mimicking ischemic preconditioning (a brief period of myocardial ischemia preceding a more prolonged period will protect the human heart from subsequent periods of ischemia [49] thereby reducing the impact of myocardial ischemia [50].) The protection was found to be long lasting (days) [51, 52], a change persisting in the absence of anesthesia, indicating that volatile anesthetics (all of them) can up-regulate and down-regulate genes. Perhaps this explains other phenomena such as the long-term remedy supplied by anesthesia to treat severe mental depression (see below).

1980s: The introduction of Trans-Esophageal Echocardiography

Studies examining survival of the heart in the face of stresses such as hypoxia make use of a now-ubiquitous device, transesophageal echocardiography. This noninvasive approach to evaluating the heart broke onto the scene in the early 1980s. Anesthesiologist Michael Cahalan was a leader of the evaluation and use of this device. His 1987 review article noted that echocardiography could be used to support the clinician (including the surgeon) and to further research [53].

1980s–2000s: Hypovolemia Increases Wound Infection

In the 1980s and early 1990s, Hunt's group examined the effect of hypovolemia on wounds, and found evidence for the benefit of generous fluid administration. Michael Hartmann, an anesthesiologist in Malmo, Sweden, demonstrated in 1992, that giving more fluid in response to low wound oxygen levels increased healing capacity (collagen deposition) in colon surgery patients [54]. This area of investigation was challenging. First, patients in the 1980s and 1990s were generally hypothermic. Hypothermia induced peripheral vasoconstriction and diuresis, thereby decreasing total blood volume by about 20% and limiting venous acceptance of additional fluid. A cold hypovolemic patient who received a fluid bolus might develop pulmonary edema, despite a low total blood volume. Second, heart rate, blood pressure, and

urine output frequently remained normal despite up to a 20% volume loss.

Optimum fluid volume management to prevent complications remains controversial [55]. Brandstrup's group in Copenhagen, demonstrated that giving about 2700 ml of colloid (large molecule) containing fluids improved wound outcomes more than giving 5000 ml of crystalloid (salt water). But Kabon and colleagues showed that giving high volumes of crystalloid intraoperatively led to higher wound oxygen levels than giving standard volumes (near the Brandstrup crystalloid value). Anesthesiologists, including TJ Gan, Markus Rehm, and Matthias Jacob, in addition to those already mentioned, continue this debate over fluid management. Current research is focused on so-called goal-directed therapy, in which transesophageal echocardiography, non-invasive cardiac output monitors, and other approaches are used to guide fluid therapy. Goal-directed therapy is promising, although formulation of guidelines must await completion of the large randomized trials that will provide the evidence.

In 2000 [56], anesthesiologists Greif and colleagues demonstrated that patients having colon surgery had less SSI (and an increase in wound oxygen) when given 80% oxygen during surgery. Several subsequent studies found similar results, but two found no benefit, leaving us with uncertainty about the value of high-inspired oxygen. Most agree that breathing high concentrations of oxygen for a few hours in the perioperative period is safe. A 2012 report by Meyhoff and colleagues found that mortality is not decreased by greater concentrations of oxygen for a subset of patients (those with cancer), and post-hoc analysis suggested the need to evaluate potential adverse effects of increased concentrations in patients undergoing surgery for cancer [57]. Ensuring the adequacy of perfusion by preventing activation of the SNS, appears to be a major determinant of success.

1985: Potent Anesthetics May Cure Mental Depression

Could volatile anesthetics be used to treat mental depression? Electro-convulsive therapy (ECT) (administered along with short acting hypnotics) is frequently and successfully used to treat major depression, but it is associated with prolonged memory loss. In 1985, psychiatrist Langer and anesthesia colleagues in Vienna reasoned that perhaps the therapeutic benefit of the convulsions might be associated with the electrical silence that follows seizures rather than the convulsion, itself. If so, perhaps the use of inhaled anesthetics to achieve electrical silence in such patients might be advantageous because there would not be a prolonged effect on memory. They demonstrated that deep anesthesia with isoflurane, inducing a period of 'electrocerebral silence,' reduced depression in 9 of 11 subjects [58]. These results were confirmed in 1995 [59].

In 1993, a separate group from Wurzburg also demonstrated that burst-suppression associated with a deep level of isoflurane anesthesia was as effective as ECT [60]. They noted that anesthesia required more time and monitoring than ECT, and therefore suggested it as a second level intervention. Use of isoflurane did not become routine, probably because psychiatrists make treatment decisions and the support for treatment with isoflurane came from small studies, only some of which were randomized and controlled.

Scott Tadler from the Dept. of Anesthesiology at the University of Utah revived the idea of treating depression in patients with concentrations of isoflurane sufficient to briefly cause burst suppression. First, using animal models of learned helplessness, he and colleagues demonstrated that isoflurane has an antidepressant-like effect (SC Tadler, A Light, R Hughen. (2009). Isoflurane Demonstrates Antidepressant-like Activity in a Mouse Model of Depression [Abstract]. *Anesthesia and Analgesia, 108*(S), 212.). The effect was comparable to that of desipramine, using the forced swim test in mice. Paul Shepard, a psychiatrist at the University of Maryland, picked up on these results and demonstrated an antidepressant like effect in rats for isoflurane, but not for halothane. These results imply antidepressant effects unique to isoflurane and perhaps a result of medication-induced cerebral isoelectricity (achieved by isoflurane but not halothane) These data suggest the need to explore the effects of other medications that cause isoelectricity. Next, in an open label pilot study, Tadler, Weeks and colleagues found that isoflurane effectively treated depression and caused less memory loss than traditional electroconvulsive therapy [61, 62]. Finally, preliminary results from a 2011 study indicate that ketamine acutely diminished depression in patients not responsive to ECT [63]. Whether this positive result would be sustained for more than a few hours is unknown but worth pursuing.

1990s: Post-Operative Cognitive Dysfunction

Anesthesia profoundly affects the central nervous system, but we assume that the alterations are transient, disappearing when anesthetic administration ceases. After all, the patient does awaken. Or are there persistent subtle effects that vex—or help—us? In the 1990s, Olney's group found that halothane could prevent MK-801 (a drug with properties similar to ketamine) from inducing neurotoxicity [64], later adding isoflurane and propofol [65]. However, in 2003, Olney's group suggested that midazolam, nitrous oxide and isoflurane given to the developing brain of rats caused cerebral apoptotic degeneration [66]. Injury to neurons in adult rat brains might be produced by nitrous oxide, with isoflurane acting to protect the brain [67].

Could similar effects produce postoperative cognitive dysfunction (POCD) in humans? In 1998, anesthesiologists Moller et al reported that patients older than 60 years were more likely to have POCD than unoperated peers, with operated patients still differing from controls 3 months after surgery [68]. But is this a consequence of the surgery, the anesthetic, being in a strange (hospital) environment or all of the above? In 2003, anesthesiologists Rasmussen et al. found that, yes, POCD occurred after surgery in patients aged 60 or greater, but that the extent of dysfunction after 3 months did not differ between patients given general versus regional anesthesia [69].

Finally, are children, particularly younger children, at risk of POCD? Considerable laboratory and epidemiological data have been gathered, with inconclusive evidence prompting concern. In 2011, this concern resulted in a presently ongoing multidisciplinary effort to determine whether such effects exist [70].

1990s: What Is Acceptable Anemia?

Renal transplantation and the AIDS epidemic transformed transfusion medicine, leading anesthesiologists to re-evaluate the management of anemia, blood loss, and transfusion. LT Goodnough championed approaches to reduce blood transfusion, acceptance of a lower transfusion threshold (7 g/dL hemoglobin rather than 10), and investigated the potential value of pre-donation of autologous blood and use of erythropoietin to increase red cell mass in patients scheduled for surgery potentially producing large blood loss. In the late 1990s, anesthesiologist Richard Weiskopf and his colleagues at UCSF, defined the physiologic responses to acute severe anemia in unanesthetized fit volunteers. Their findings supported the concept of a transfusion target of 7 g/dL [71].

1990s: Hypothermia, Oxygenation, and Infection

Sessler, at UCSF, defined how anesthesia leads routinely to hypothermia. In 1988, he and his colleagues found that anesthesia broadens the threshold to the body's response to hypothermia [72]. In the mid-1980s, Scott Augustine (a Navy anesthesiologist in San Diego) developed the forced air warmer (Bair Hugger), the first effective means of maintaining normal core temperature during anesthesia (aside from keeping the operating room too warm for the surgeons) [73]. Thus, by 1990, anesthesiologists were poised to examine whether preventing SNS activation by keeping patients warm during surgery would reduce SSI.

Based on Hunt and colleagues' demonstration that SNS-induced peripheral vasoconstriction caused wound hypoxia; on Sessler and his colleagues' demonstration of the mechanisms of anesthesia-induced hypothermia; and on Augustine's development of a successful method for preventing anesthesia-induced hypothermia (the forced air warming blanket), maintenance of intraoperative normothermia was investigated as a means of improving wound outcomes. The outcome trial that resulted was published in 1996 [74]. It demonstrated that maintaining normal core temperature (36.6 °C) while aggressively providing fluids and pain control reduced SSI by 67% in colon surgery patients, compared with a control group allowed to cool to 34.7 °C (the routine in clinical practice at the time). Schmied et al. in Sessler's group added further to the importance of maintaining normothermia [75]. They found that mild hypothermia (only a 1.6 °C decrease) increased intra-and postoperative blood loss.

The effect of these studies on practice was rapid and widespread. By 1999, Center for Disease Control (CDC) infection control guidelines incorporated maintenance of normal core temperature for patients undergoing colon surgery. Numerous devices are presently marketed to safely prevent and treat anesthesia-related hypothermia, including forced air warmers, resistive warmers, and conductive warmers. Of note, pre-warming the patient prevents much intraoperative hypothermia and should be considered for most patients [76].

1990s: Prevention of Deep Venous Thrombosis (DVT)

Venous thrombo-embolism significantly increases morbidity and mortality in patients undergoing surgery, and anesthesiologists have, along with surgeons, played a major role in instituting preventive measures. Pulmonary embolism is the third most common cause of preventable hospital related death, and commonly follows DVT in the lower limbs [77, 78]. Surgical patients are at significant risk of developing DVT, due to intraoperative venous stasis and changes in fibrinolytic activity, as well as low postoperative mobility. The simple technique of ensuring that occlusion of calf blood vessels is avoided during surgery, is the responsibility of the anesthesia care team. Additional measures have included intermittent calf compression with sequential compression devices, and the intra-operative use of low molecular weight dextrans [79]. Rapid post-operative mobilization is also a feature of modern surgery, and anesthesiologists have played a role by adopting drugs that are rapidly eliminated.

1990s–2000s: Inhaled Anesthetics Affect the Environment

Inhaled anesthetics can affect the environment in two ways. One is by depletion of the ozone layer. As proposed by chemists Frank Rowland and Mario Molina in 1973, breakdown of anesthetics containing bromine (halothane) or chlorine (chloroform, halothane, enflurane, isoflurane), releases the atomic halogen which, in turn, breaks down ozone [80]. Since ozone absorbs ultraviolet light, its loss would permit more ultraviolet light to reach the surface of the earth with potentially devastating effects. Rowland and Molina won the 1995 Nobel Prize for their work. The Montreal Protocol on Substances That Deplete the Ozone Layer was an international agreement limiting the release of such halogenated compounds into the environment and came into effect in the late 1980s [80], with subsequent improvement in the ozone layer. Release of inhaled anesthetics appears not to have been included in the Protocol. The anesthetics desflurane and sevoflurane in the 1990s, displaced the earlier chlorine- and bromine-containing anesthetics, and neither desflurane nor sevoflurane contain these halogens, being halogenated solely with fluorine (harmless to the ozone layer) [81].

However, inhaled anesthetics can affect the environment in a second way. All absorb infrared light. In 1937, Luft made use of this in his design of the infrared analyzer [82]. In 1991, Norwegian anesthesiologists noted the ability of nitrous oxide to act as a greenhouse gas and suggested use of lower inflow rates to minimize release into the atmosphere [83]. In 2010, anesthesiologist Susan Ryan, working with basic scientists, demonstrated that inhaled anesthetics are greenhouse gases, opening a new avenue for arguing about optimal anesthetic technique [84]. Not all anesthetics provided equal concern, desflurane having a several-fold greater potential environmental impact. However, "the overall contribution of inhalation anesthetics to greenhouse gas emission is miniscule…", [85] "approximately 0.01% of that of the CO_2 released from global fossil fuel combustion." [86] Even so, the anesthesia department at the University of Utah saved the equivalent greenhouse gas potential of driving 5.4 million miles over one year, by converting much of their anesthetic vapor use at their hospitals from desflurane to isoflurane. Ryan and Jodi Sherman from Yale addressed the wide range of environmental issues in anesthesia: [87] supply chain waste and contamination; disposal of unused drugs; entry of metabolized drugs into the water supply; greenhouse gas production; and disposable waste generation. The Stockholm County Council (http://www.janusinfo.se/In-English/) has compiled data that allows comparison of the environmental impact of various drugs based on persistence, bioaccumulation, toxicity, and expected concentration in the environment. Few anesthetic drugs have been classified in this way, but such data may ultimately guide anesthesiologists interested in providing the best anesthetic care with the lowest ecological footprint. For now, regional anesthesia appears to have the smallest footprint.

2000s: Prolonged Use of High Tidal Volumes May Cause Pulmonary Injury

A 2003 meta-analysis by anesthesiologists Petrucci and Iacovelli, found that using smaller tidal volumes in patients suffering from acute respiratory distress syndrome (ARDS) or acute lung injury (ALI) might decrease mortality [88]. In 2007, anesthesiologists Mascia et al. found that large tidal volumes per se produced lung injury in patients with severe brain injury [89]. In 2008, internists Meade et al. disputed the survival value of smaller tidal volumes in patients with ARDS or ALI [90]. However, Lellouche et al. reported in 2012 that large tidal volumes lead to organ failure and prolonged ICU stay in cardiac surgical patients [91].

2009–2012: Ethical Violations in Anesthesia

From 2009 to 2012, three anesthesiologists (Scott Reuben, Joachim Boldt, and Yoshitaka Fujii) and a cardiologist (Don Poldermans) engaged in anesthesia related research, admitted to research misconduct, ranging from ethics violations to fabrication of data. This worldwide misconduct, from the US to Europe to Japan, led to retraction of more than 100 articles, with at least 200 more in jeopardy. All four individuals were publishing research germane to the topic of this chapter; that is, in areas independent of producing anesthesia.

Does working outside the mainstream of traditional anesthesia related research make it easier to commit fraud? Is this a reflection of the degree to which anesthesia related research has come to be increasingly focused on topics outside of producing anesthesia? Are journals just getting better at identifying misconduct? Regardless, this is a concerning development!

2012: Uncertain Ethical Behavior in Anesthesia

Should anesthetists participate in the intravenous delivery of drugs deliberately intended to kill those sentenced to death? In 2012, the American Board of Anesthesiologists said no, indicating that they would revoke the certification of any anesthesiologist participating in such lethal injection, defending their action by pointing to the Hippocratic injunction that physicians do no harm. Those supporting lethal injection argued that anesthesiologists are best equipped to supply such injections humanely.

Reflections

The practice of anesthesiology touches patients managed by every surgical subspecialty and many medical ones, including radiology, cardiology, gastroenterology, and emergency medicine, prompting, as this chapter suggests, an awareness of the challenges within many disciplines and a collaboration with a broad range of colleagues. Thus it is appropriate that anesthesiologists have contributed to increased knowledge and improved practice in such disparate areas as blood banking, cardiac protection, infection prevention, critical care, pain management, patient safety, and patient comfort. They are likely to continue these contributions.

References

1. Snow J. On Chloroform and other anaesthetics: their action and administration. London: John Churchill; 1858. pp. 1–443.
2. Snow J. On the inhalation of the vapour of ether in surgical operations: containing a description of the various stages of etherization, and a statement of the result of nearly eighty operations in which ether has been employed in St. George's and University College Hospitals. London: John Churchill; 1847. pp. 1–88.
3. Sayres LA. Two cases of traumatic tetanus. New York J Med. 1858;4:250–3.
4. Lassen HC, Bjorneboe M, Ibsen B, Neukirch F. Treatment of tetanus with curarisation, general anaesthesia, and intratracheal positive-pressure ventilation. Lancet. 1954;267:1040–4.
5. Honey GE, Dwyer BE, Smith AC, Spalding JM. Tetanus treated with tubocurarine and intermittent positive-pressure respiration. Brit Med J. 1954;2:442–3.
6. Rabbitts JA, Bacon DR, Nuttall GA, Moore SB. Mayo Clinic and the origins of blood banking. Mayo Clin Proc. 2007;82:1117–8.
7. Boyan CP, Howland WS. Cardiac arrest and temperature of bank blood. JAMA. 1963;183:58–60.
8. Miller RD, Robbins TO, Tong MJ, Barton SL. Coagulation defects associated with massive blood transfusions. Ann Surg. 1971;174:794–801.
9. Koch CG, Li L, Duncan AI, Mihaljevic T, Loop FD, Starr NJ, Blackstone EH. Transfusion in coronary artery bypass grafting is associated with reduced long-term survival. Ann Thorac Surg. 2006;81:1650–7.
10. Wang D, Sun J, Solomon SB, Klein HG, Natanson C. Transfusion of older stored blood and risk of death: a meta-analysis. Transfusion. 2012;52:1184–95.
11. Weiskopf RB, Feiner J, Hopf H, Lieberman J, Finlay HE, Quah C, Kramer JH, Bostrom A, Toy P. Fresh blood and aged stored blood are equally efficacious in immediately reversing anemia-induced brain oxygenation deficits in humans. Anesthesiology. 2006;104:911–20.
12. Sen S, Martin DP, Bacon DR. Exploring origins: was John Bonica's model of modern-day pain management influenced by John Lundy's earlier work? Reg Anesth Pain Med. 2007;32:258–62.
13. Jacob AK, Kopp SL, Bacon DR, Smith HM. The history of anesthesia. In: Barash PG, Cullen BF, Stoelting RK, Cahalan M, Stock MC, editors. Clinical anesthesia. Philadelphia: Wolters Kluwer, Lippincott Williams & Wilkins. 2009. pp. 3–26.
14. Liebeskind JC, Meldrum ML, John JB. World champion of pain. In: Jensen TS, Turner JA, Wiesenfeld-Hallin Z, editors. Proceedings of the Eighth World Congress on Pain: Progress in pain research and management. Vol 8. Seattle: International Association for the Study of Pain Press; 1997. pp. 19–32.

15. Beecher HK. Pain in men wounded in battle. Ann Surg. 1946;123: 96–105.
16. Melzack R, Wall PD. Pain mechanisms: a new theory. Science. 1965;150:971–9.
17. Beecher HK. The powerful placebo. JAMA. 1955;159:1602–6.
18. Beecher HK. Experimentation in man. JAMA. 1959;169:461–78.
19. Kopp VJ. Henry Knowles Beecher and the development of informed consent in anesthesia research. Anesthesiology. 1999;90:1756–65.
20. A definition of irreversible coma. Report of the Ad Hoc Committee of the Harvard Medical School to examine the definition of brain death. JAMA. 1968;205:337–40.
21. Bentolila L. General anesthesia with cyclopropane for the treatment of status asthmaticus. Ann Allergy. 1951;9:519–21.
22. Kofke WA, Snider MT, Young RS, Ramer JC. Prolonged low flow isoflurane anesthesia for status epilepticus. Anesthesiology. 1985;62:653–6.
23. Loi du 6 janvier 1986 relative à l'aide médicale urgente et aux transport sanitaires. Journal Officiel de la République Française 7 janvier 1986.
24. West JB. The physiological challenges of the 1952 Copenhagen poliomyelitis epidemic and a renaissance in clinical respiratory physiology. J Appl Physiol. 2005;99:424–32.
25. Astrup P. A simple electrometric technique for the determination of carbon dioxide tension in blood and plasma, total content of carbon dioxide in plasma and bicarbonate content in "separated" plasma at a fixed carbon dioxide tension. Scand J Clin Lab Invest. 1956;8:33–44.
26. Berthelsen PG, Cronqvist M. The first intensive care unit in the world: Copenhagen 1953. Acta Anaesthesiol Scand. 2003;47:1190–5.
27. Apgar V. Oxygen as a supportive therapy in fetal anoxia. Bull N Y Acad Med. 1950;26:474–8.
28. Apgar V. A proposal for a new method of evaluation of the newborn infant. Curr Res Anesth Analg. 1953;32:260–7.
29. Stow RW, Randall BF. Electrical measurement of the PCO_2 of blood. Am J Physiol. 1954;179:678 (abstract).
30. Severinghaus JW. Gadgeteering for health care: the John W. Severinghaus lecture on translational science. Anesthesiology. 2009;110:721–8.
31. Clark LC. Monitor and control of blood and tissue O2 tensions. Trans Am Soc Artif Intern Organs. 1956;2:41–8.
32. Severinghaus JW, Bradley AF. Electrodes for blood pO2 and pCO2 determination. J Appl Physiol. 1958;13:515–20.
33. Severinghaus JW. Electrodes for blood and gas PCO2, PO2, and blood pH. Acta Anesth Scand Suppl. 1962;11:207–20.
34. Lassen HCA, Henriksen E, Neukirch F, Kristensen HS. Treatment of tetanus. Severe bone-marrow depression after prolonged nitrous-oxide anaesthesia. Lancet. 1956;1:527–30.
34. Banks RGS, Henderson RJ, Pratt JM. Reactions of gases in solution. III. Some reactions of nitrous oxide with transition-metal complexes. J Chem Soc Sec (A). 1968;3:2886–90.
36. Koblin DD, Watson JE, Deady JE, Stokstad ELR, Eger EII. Inactivation of methionine synthetase by nitrous oxide in mice. Anesthesiology. 1981;54:318–24.
37. Selzer RR, Rosenblatt DS, Laxova R, Hogan K. Adverse effect of nitrous oxide in a child with 5,10-methylenetetrahydrofolate reductase deficiency. N Engl J Med. 2003;349:45–50.
38. Hunt TK. A new method of determining tissue oxygen tension. Lancet. 1964;2:1370–1.
39. Hopf HW, Hunt TK, West JM, Blomquist P, Goodson WH 3rd, Jensen JA, Jonsson K, Paty PB, Rabkin JM, Upton RA, Smitten K von, Whitney JD. Wound tissue oxygen tension predicts the risk of wound infection in surgical patients. Arch Surg. 1997;132:997–1004; discussion 1005
40. Huch R, Huch A, Lubbers DW. Transcutaneous measurement of blood Po2 (tcPo2)—method and application in perinatal medicine. J Perinat Med. 1973;1:183–91.

41. Huch R, Lubbers DW, Huch A. Quantitative continuous measurement of partial oxygen pressure on the skin of adults and new-born babies. Pflugers Arch. 1972;337:185–98.
42. Severinghaus JW, Stafford M, Bradley AF. tcPCO2 electrode design, calibration and temperature gradient problems. Acta Anaesthesiol Scand Suppl. 1978;68:118–22.
43. Beran AV, Huxtable RF. Sperling DR: Electrochemical sensor for continuous transcutaneous PCO2 measurement. J Appl Physiol. 1976;41:442–7.
44. Severinghaus JW. A combined transcutaneous PO2-PCO2 electrode with electrochemical HCO3- stabilization. J Appl Physiol. 1981;51:1027–32.
45. Hauser CJ, Shoemaker WC. Use of a transcutaneous PO2 regional perfusion index to quantify tissue perfusion in peripheral vascular disease. Ann Surg. 1983;197:337–43.
46. Fife CE, Buyukcakir C, Otto GH, Sheffield PJ, Warriner RA, Love TL, Mader J. The predictive value of transcutaneous oxygen tension measurement in diabetic lower extremity ulcers treated with hyperbaric oxygen therapy: a retrospective analysis of 1,144 patients. Wound Repair Regen. 2002;10:198–207.
47. Fife CE, Smart DR, Sheffield PJ, Hopf HW, Hawkins G, Clarke D. Transcutaneous oximetry in clinical practice: consensus statements from an expert panel based on evidence. Undersea Hyperb Med. 2009;36:43–53.
48. Johnston RR, Eger EI II, Wilson C. A comparative interaction of epinephrine with enflurane, isoflurane, and halothane in man. Anesth Analg. 1976;55:709–12.
49. Deutsch E, Berger M, Kussmaul WG, Hirshfeld JW Jr, Herrmann HC, Laskey WK. Adaptation to ischemia during percutaneous transluminal coronary angioplasty: clinical, hemodynamic, and metabolic features. Circulation. 1990;82:2044–51.
50. Freedman BM, Hamm DP, Everson CT, Wechsler AS, Christian CM 2nd. Enflurane enhances postischemic functional recovery in the isolated rat heart. Anesthesiology. 1985;62:29–33.
51. Zaugg M, Lucchinetti E, Uecker M, Pasch T, Schaub MC. Anaesthetics and cardiac preconditioning. Part I. Signalling and cytoprotective mechanisms. Br J Anaesth. 2003;91:551–65.
52. Zaugg M, Lucchinetti E, Garcia C, Pasch T, Spahn DR, Schaub MC. Anaesthetics and cardiac preconditioning. Part II. Clinical implications. Br J Anaesth. 2003;91:566–76.
53. Cahalan MK, Litt L, Botvinick EH, Schiller NB. Advances in noninvasive cardiovascular imaging: implications for the anesthesiologist. Anesthesiology. 1987;66:356–72.
54. Hartmann M, Jonsson K, Zederfeldt B. Effect of tissue perfusion and oxygenation on accumulation of collagen in healing wounds. Randomized study in patients after major abdominal operations. Eur J Surg. 1992;158:521–6.
55. Chappell D, Jacob M, Hofmann-Kiefer K, Conzen P, Rehm M. A rational approach to perioperative fluid management. Anesthesiology. 2008;109:723–40.
56. Greif R, Akca O, Horn EP, Kurz A, Sessler DI. Supplemental perioperative oxygen to reduce the incidence of surgical-wound infection. Outcomes Research Group. N Engl J Med. 2000;342:161–7.
57. Meyhoff CS, Jorgensen LN, Wetterslev J, Christensen KB, Rasmussen LS. Increased long-term mortality after a high perioperative inspiratory oxygen fraction during abdominal surgery: follow-up of a randomized clinical trial. Anesth Analg. 2012;115:849–54.
58. Langer G, Neumark J, Koinig G, Graf M, Schoenbeck G. Rapid psychotherapeutic effects of anesthesia with isoflurane (ED narcotherapy) in treatment-refractory depressed patients. Neuropsychobiology. 1985;14:118–20.
59. Langer G, Karazman R, Neumark J, Saletu B, Schoenbeck G, Gruenberger J, Dittrich R, Petricek W, hoffmann P, Linzmayer L, Anderer P, Steinberger K. Isoflurane narcotherapy in depressive patients refractory to conventional antidepressant drug treatment.

A double-blind comparison with electroconvulsive treatment. Neuropsychobiology. 1995;31:182–94.

60. Engelhardt W, Carl G, Hartung E. Intra-individual open comparison of burst-suppression-isoflurane-anaesthesia versus electroconvulsive therapy in the treatment of severe depression. Eur J Anaesthesiol. 1993;10:113–8.

61. Tadler S, Weeks HR, Smith KW, Iacob E, Cahalan MK, Bushnell L, Sakata D, Light KC. Isoflurane treatment of depression. Anesthesiology. 2011;115:A002 (abstract).

62. Weeks HR III, Tadler SC, Smith KW, Iacob E, Saccoman M, et al. Neurocognitive effects of isoflurane anesthesia versus electroconvulsive therapy in refractory depression. PLos ONE 8:e69809. doi:10.1371/journal.pone.0069809

63. Ibrahim L, Diazgranados N, Luckenbaugh DA, Machado-Vieira R, Baumann J, Mallinger AG, Zarate CA Jr. Rapid decrease in depressive symptoms with an N-methyl-d-aspartate antagonist in ECT-resistant major depression. Prog Neuro-Psychopharm Biol Psych. 2011;35:1155–9.

64. Ishimaru M, Fukamauchi F, Olney JW. Halothane prevents MK-801 neurotoxicity in the rat cingulate cortex. Neurosci Lett. 1995;193:1–4.

65. Jevtovic-Todorovic V, Kirby CO, Olney JW. Isoflurane and propofol block neurotoxicity caused by MK-801 in the rat posterior cingulate/retrosplenial cortex. J Cerebral Bld Flow Metab. 1997;17:168–74.

66. Jevtovic-Todorovic V, Hartman RE, Izumi Y, Benshoff ND, Dikranian K, Zorumski CF, Olney JW, Wozniak DF. Early exposure to common anesthetic agents causes widespread neurodegeneration in the developing rat brain and persistent learning deficits. J Neurosci. 2003;23:876–82.

67. Jevtovic-Todorovic V, Beals J, Benshoff N, Olney JW. Prolonged exposure to inhalational anesthetic nitrous oxide kills neurons in adult rat brain. Neuroscience. 2003;122:609–16.

68. Moller JT, Cluitmans P, Rasmussen LS, Houx P, Rasmussen H, Canet J, Rabbitt P, Jolles J, Larsen K, Hanning CD, Langeron O, Johnson T, Lauven PM, Kristensen PA, Biedler A, Beem H van, Fraidakis O, Silverstein JH, Beneken JE, Gravenstein JS. Long-term postoperative cognitive dysfunction in the elderly ISPOCD1 study. ISPOCD investigators. International Study of Post-Operative Cognitive Dysfunction. Lancet. 1998;351:857–61.

69. Rasmussen LS, Johnson T, Kuipers HM, Kristensen D, Siersma VD, Vila P, Jolles J, Papaioannou A, Abildstrom H, Silverstein JH, Bonal JA, Raeder J, Nielsen IK, Korttila K, Munoz L, Dodds C, Hanning CD, Moller JT. Does anaesthesia cause postoperative cognitive dysfunction? A randomised study of regional versus general anaesthesia in 438 elderly patients. Acta Anaesthesiol Scand 2003;47:260–6.

70. Ramsay JG, Rappaport BA. SmartTots: a multidisciplinary effort to determine anesthetic safety in young children. Anesth Analg. 2011;113:963–4.

71. Weiskopf RB, Viele MK, Feiner J, Kelley S, Lieberman J, Noorani M, Leung JM, Fisher DM, Murray WR, Toy P, Moore MA. Human cardiovascular and metabolic response to acute, severe isovolemic anemia. JAMA. 1998;279:217–21.

72. Sessler DI, Olofsson CI, Rubinstein EH, Beebe JJ. The thermoregulatory threshold during halothane anesthesia in humans. Anesthesiology. 1988;68:836–42.

73. Augustine SD. The Bair Hugger patient warming system. J Post Anesth Nurs. 1991;6:2–4.

74. Kurz A, Sessler DI, Lenhardt R. Perioperative normothermia to reduce the incidence of surgical-wound infection and shorten hospitalization. Study of Wound Infection and Temperature Group. N Engl J Med. 1996;334:1209–15.

75. Schmied H, Kurz A, Sessler DI, Kozek S, Reiter A. Mild hypothermia increases blood loss and transfusion requirements during total hip arthroplasty. Lancet. 1996;347:289–92.

76. Sessler DI, Moayeri A. Skin-surface warming: heat flux and central temperature. Anesthesiology. 1990;73:218–24.

77. Lindblad B, Eriksson A, Bergqvist D. Autopsy-verified pulmonary embolism in a surgical department: analysis of the period from 1951 to 1988. Br J Surg. 1991;78:849–52.

78. Sandler DA, Martin JF. Autopsy proven pulmonary embolism in hospital patients: are we detecting enough deep vein thrombosis? J Roy Soc Med. 1989;82:203–5.

79. Anderson FA, Audet A-M. Best practices. Preventing deep vein thrombosis and pulmonary embolism. A practical guide to evaluation and improvement. University of Massachussets Medical School Centre for Outcomes Research. 1998. http://www.outcomes-umassmed.org/dvt/best_practice/.Last accessed 23 May 2012.

80. http://en.wikipedia.org/wiki/Montreal_Protocol. Accessed 23 May 2012.

81. Langbein T, Sonntag H, Trapp D, Hoffmann A, Malms W, Roth E-P, Mors V, Zellner R. Volatile anaesthetics and the atmosphere: atmospheric lifetimes and atmospheric effects of halothane, enflurane, isoflurane, desflurane and sevoflurane. Br J Anaesth. 1999;82:66–73.

82. Luft K. Über eine neue Methode der registrierenden Gasanalyse mit Hilfe der Absorption ultraroter Strahlen ohne spektrale Zerlegung. Ztschrf Techn Phys. 1943;24:97–104.

83. Dale O, Dale T. Anesthetic gases, the ozone layer and the greenhouse effect. How harmful are the anesthetic emissions for the global environment? Tidsskr Nor Laegeforen. 1991;111:2115–7.

84. Ryan SM, Nielsen CJ. Global warming potential of inhaled anesthetics: application to clinical use. Anesth Analg. 2010;111:92–8.

85. Ryan S, Sherman J. Sustainable anesthesia. Anesth Analg. 2012;114:921–3.

86. Andersen MP, Nielsen OJ, Wallington TJ, Karpichev B, Sander SP. Medical intelligence article: assessing the impact on global climate from general anesthetic gases. Anesth Analg. 2012;114:1081–5.

87. Sherman JD, Ryan S. Ecological responsibility in anesthesia practice. Int Anesthesiol Clin. 2010;48:139–51.

88. Petrucci N, Iacovelli W. Ventilation with lower tidal volumes versus traditional tidal volumes in adults for acute lung injury and acute respiratory distress syndrome. Cochrane database of systematic reviews 2003: CD003844.

89. Mascia L, Zavala E, Bosma K, Pasero D, Decaroli D, Andrews P, Isnardi D, Davi A, Arguis MJ, Berardino M, Ducati A. High tidal volume is associated with the development of acute lung injury after severe brain injury: an international observational study. Crit Care Med. 2007;35:1815–20.

90. Meade MO, Cook DJ, Guyatt GH, Slutsky AS, Arabi YM, Cooper DJ, Davies AR, Hand LE, Zhou Q, Thabane L, Austin P, Lapinsky S, Baxter A, Russell J, Skrobik Y, Ronco JJ, Stewart TE. Ventilation strategy using low tidal volumes, recruitment maneuvers, and high positive end-expiratory pressure for acute lung injury and acute respiratory distress syndrome: a randomized controlled trial. JAMA. 2008;299:637–45.

91. Lellouche F, Dionne S, Simard S, Bussieres J, Dagenais F. High tidal volumes in mechanically ventilated patients increase organ dysfunction after cardiac surgery. Anesthesiology. 2012;116:1072–82.

The History of Outcomes Research in Anesthesia

43

Rod N. Westhorpe, Lawrence J. Saidman and Edmond I Eger II

Summary

Anesthesia outcomes research as large-scale clinical trials, began at anesthesia's inception. Ether caused postoperative nausea and vomiting (PONV). By mid-twentieth century, many drugs were shown to decrease PONV. In 2004, Apfel reported that combining antiemetics with different actions enhanced efficacy.

Beecher and Todd's 1952 article on outcomes in 600,000 patients indicated that anesthesia killed 1 in 2000 patients, and that curare given without proper reversal increased the incidence 6-fold. The 1966 National Halothane Study of 856,515 patients, reported no increased mortality with halothane anesthesia but found rare cases of massive hepatic necrosis. Also in 1966, a 200-patient study connected methoxyflurane and renal injury, and in 1973 this was shown to be dose-related.

Notwithstanding the absence of quantitative numerators and denominators, 1980s-2000s' reviews of closed-claims data identified egregious anesthetic errors and prompted remedial measures. Similarly, in 1991, Rigler and Drasner found a cauda equina syndrome in 4 patients given 5 % lidocaine through a new spinal catheter that localized the injected lidocaine. This led to a 1998 study that found a more subtle injury from intrathecal lidocaine in 1,863 patients.

Slogoff and Keats' 1980s studies of patients having coronary artery bypass operations (CABG) showed that a greater heart rate correlated with postoperative myocardial infarction, independent of anesthetic choice. In 1989, Mangano, Leung and others initiated Studies of Perioperative Ischemia (SPI) which morphed into the Multicentered Study of Perioperative Ischemia (McSPI). These richly productive, prospective, expensive, outcomes researches in the 1990s-2000s showed: that surrogate evidence of ischemia (e.g., that obtained with TEE) predicted adverse clinical outcomes (e.g., myocardial infarction); that several drugs (e.g., acadesine, beta adrenergic blocking drugs, aspirin) might protect surgical patients at risk of myocardial injury from ischemia; and that aprotinin caused clotting of grafts and increased mortality. However, in 2012, critical re-analysis of earlier outcome studies supplied new information suggesting that perhaps aprotinin is useful after all. Wallace's inexpensive 2010 retrospective study of 38,779 electronic medical records of operations confirmed that perioperative beta blockade reduced perioperative mortality.

In the late 2000s, Pronovost led efforts to apply checklists to markedly decrease untoward consequences such as infection. Similarly, Loftus and Koff and colleagues at Dartmouth decreased hospital acquired infections by promoting hand hygiene by anesthesia providers in the operating room.

In conclusion, anesthesia outcomes research has led to evidence based outcomes, improved anesthesia care, and decreased perioperative risk.

R. N. Westhorpe (✉)
Melbourne, Australia
e-mail: westhorpe@netspace.net.au

L. J. Saidman
Department of Anesthesia, Stanford University,
Stanford, California, USA
e-mail: lsaidman@stanford.edu

E. I Eger II
University of California, San Francisco, CA 94143-0464, USA
e-mail: egere@anesthesia.ucsf.edu

Introduction

Assembling this history of outcomes research in anesthesia demanded decisions concerning what to include and exclude. By this apology, we note that we omitted important developments. The present essay follows the suggestion by Sessler (personal communication, 16 Sept 12) that outcomes research is "the term for large-scale clinical trials that evaluate outcomes that are meaningful to patients". A broader view might define outcomes research as research that tells us about clinical outcomes, good and bad, and includes small-scale as well as large-scale clinical trials. For the purposes of this book, Harriet Hopf provides (Chapter 42) a history of outcomes research in small-scale clinical trials, trials including as many as approximately 200 subjects (but we are liberal in our interpretation). The present chapter will focus on the large-scale trials with a particular emphasis on those investigating cardiovascular issues.

1846 to the 2000s and Apfel's Low Cost Study of Nausea and Vomiting

Starting with Morton's demonstration, postoperative nausea and vomiting (PONV) has been a problem of interest to anesthetists and patients. A 1936 survey of about 10,000 patients found that 40.6% vomited in the postoperative period [1]. The common anesthetics of the day—nitrous oxide, cyclopropane, and ether—are highly emetogenic, so the observation was not surprising.

Researchers sought drugs that might treat or prevent nausea and vomiting. Anti-histamine and anti-cholinergic drugs were introduced in the 1940s to prevent motion sickness, and made the first lasting impact on PONV. It seemed logical that drugs which worked against motion sickness might prevent PONV. In the early 1950s, two groups [2, 3] found that dimenhydrinate (Dramamine), introduced after World War II to decrease motion sickness, reduced PONV when given before induction of anesthesia. In 1955, anesthesiologists Dent, Ramachandra, and Stephen [4] showed that the antihistamine cyclizine (Marezine) given prophylatically, decreased PONV. This study of 3000 patients in the Post Anesthesia Care Unit also found that regional anesthesia produced less PONV than ether or cyclopropane. Sodium thiopental also produced less PONV than ether, but more than regional anesthesia. Head and neck surgeries had a higher rate of PONV than abdominal surgeries, although that may have been related to differences in anesthetic management. Interestingly, the group missed what is now recognized as one of the strongest predictors: female gender.

In 1960, anesthesiologists Bellville, Bross and Howland showed that phenothiazines protected against PONV [5, 6]. In this study of 3794 patients, they also found that 28% of females vomited vs. 9.3% of males. Larger total doses of anesthesia and intraoperative hypotension both predicted higher rates of PONV. Paul Janssen synthesized droperidol in 1961, and it was used in combination with fentanyl by the mid-1960s. It was one of a group of dopamine receptor antagonists useful for decreasing PONV. Developed by Glaxo in 1984, ondansetron, a 5-HT-3 (serotonin) antagonist, was released for use in the late 1980s and was quickly found to be effective against PONV [7]. In 1986, Doze et al. demonstrated that propofol was more effective than methohexital in decreasing PONV [8]. In 1994, McKenzie et al. found that adding dexamethasone to ondansetron further decreased PONV [9].

In 1961, Eger et al. reported that premedication could vastly influence PONV in children anesthetized with ether [10]. Premedication with the GABAergic drug pentobarbital, resulted in an incidence of vomiting of 18% in children. Omission of the barbiturate doubled the incidence of vomiting, while substitution of the opioids meperidine or morphine for pentobarbital, quadrupled the incidence compared with those receiving only an anticholinergic.

During the half century leading up to 2000, anesthesiologists applied diverse antiemetic drugs, including antihistaminics, anticholinergics, barbiturates, phenothiazines, dopamine receptor antagonists, serotonin receptor antagonists, dexamethasone, and propofol to minimize PONV. Each had merit but none was perfect. Each affected a different receptor, a clue that led to the next development. In 2004, Apfel reported an outcomes study in 5,199 patients at high risk for postoperative nausea and vomiting, in a randomized, controlled trial of factorial design to evaluate interactions among as many as three antiemetic interventions [11]. The primary outcome (nausea and vomiting within 24 hours after surgery), was evaluated blindly. The study found that combining antiemetic drugs, blocking different emesis-mediating receptors, decreased postoperative nausea and vomiting. The greater the number of different receptors blocked, the greater the prophylaxis. This 5,199 patient study was performed for $500,000 ($96/patient) by using a clever business model. German medical students needing to do research as part of their medical education, were recruited as study coordinators with the promise of being able to write manuscripts using the study database, and receiving credit toward their degree requirements. This special educational requirement allowed a large, inexpensive, outcomes study.

Understanding the Risks of Anesthesia

Anesthesia is inherently dangerous. Modern examples come to mind. In 2002, the Russian military conducted an unintended outcomes study involving 850 attendees held hostage by terrorists at the Moscow Opera House. It is speculated that both terrorists and attendees were anesthetized with an aerosolized version of fentanyl without benefit of anesthesia personnel: 129 (15%) died. "Studies" of the famous provide similar outcomes: John Belluchi, Chris Farley, Jimi Hendricks, Michael Jackson, Janice Joplin, Marilyn Monroe, Elvis Presley, Anna Nicole Smith, and Amy Winehouse to name a few. And we in anesthesia know of colleagues who, unattended, self-administered anesthesia with lethal results. Safe anesthesia demands the presence of the trained and vigilant anesthetist.

Many advances including improved equipment, education, better medications, and new or improved monitors, decreased anesthetic-induced mortality from the 15 % rate with no anesthetic care (the Moscow Opera House), to the miniscule rate associated with modern anesthesia. However, safety also resulted from the results of outcomes research, from large and small clinical trials.

1920s–1930s: Study Commissions to Improve Anesthesia Care

Anesthetic study commissions, supported by the American Medical Association (AMA), developed registries of case reports of anesthesia-associated deaths in the 1920s and 1930s. In April 1938, an editorial in the British Journal of Anaesthesia opined [12]:

> "If fault is to be found in the development of anesthetic practice, as it is seen today, that fault lies in our failure notably not to reduce the fatalities of anaesthesia. It should not be beyond the wit and skill of anaesthetists to secure safety without abandoning modern progress. The number of deaths on the table is not negligible, even when the patient is ordinarily fit and the operation not a grave one. The cure of this type of fatality is education and more education, for these fatalities do not occur, with the expert."

1946: Bishop Assembles Data

In a 1946 report, Harold Bishop considered the basis for "6 deaths which have occurred in the operating rooms of two hospitals with which we have been associated during the past four years. A total of 20,021 anesthetics have been administered during that time. Four of these patients had received an anesthetic; one patient died during the course of operation without anesthesia; one patient died during a therapeutic sympathetic nerve block [13]." Six deaths in 20,021 anesthetics indicated a mortality of 1:3,337. But anesthesia was not responsible for all of these (e.g., one patient died from a "fatal pulmonary embolism during manipulation of the hip under anesthesia" (embolism confirmed at autopsy), and thus the incidence was still less. On the other hand, Bishop's data did not include deaths from anesthesia that resulted after the conclusion of surgery, and thus his report probably underestimated mortality.

Bishop also discussed data for anesthetic-associated mortality from other reports, noting that in New York City for the years 1928 to 1936 there were 758 deaths in the operating room, and of this number, 412 were attributed to anesthesia. However, this collection of statistics lacked two dimensions: a complete numerator (the sum of all anesthetic-caused deaths, intraoperative and postoperative); and a denominator (the total population of anesthetized patients from which

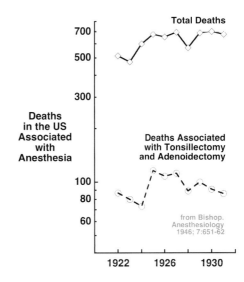

Fig. 43.1 From Bishop's report [13], we know that the total deaths, and deaths with tonsillectomy and adenoidectomy associated with anesthesia in the US, remained constant for a decade. We don't know how many anesthetics were given in each of these years, so we cannot tell whether matters were worse, better, or unchanged with time. (Data from Bishop [13])

these patients were drawn). Bishop also presented the number of deaths in the US associated with anesthesia, stating that "These figures would indicate that up until 1936, deaths under anesthesia were not decreasing". This conclusion can't really be made without an estimate of the number of operations per year. Bishop noted that one operation, tonsillectomy, supplied a substantial fraction (15 %) of the total deaths (Fig. 43.1), but failed to indicate what fraction of total surgery this procedure represented. Finally, Bishop cited the work of Gillespie for studies in the US, England, Australia and Canada for roughly the 1920s and 1930s, studies giving the deaths during anesthesia as 1 in 804 patients from a total number of cases of 227,546. Again, we didn't have a complete numerator (i.e., deaths after surgery were not considered). It was a beginning, but more was needed.

1949: Gregory also Wants a Commission

John Gregory's 1949 article, "The pathology of sudden and unexpected death under anesthesia" [14], reviewed the accepted causes of anesthesia-related mortality, criticized their lack of pathologic basis or validation, and called for a commission to:

Define detailed criteria for the study of sudden death under anesthesia.

- Be comprised of at least two physiologists, two pathologists, two pharmacologists, and two surgeons (but no anesthesiologist)
- Receive and study exhaustive data on all sudden deaths.

- Ensure that a postmortem examination was accomplished before a case could be considered for statistical purposes.

Gregory raised several important issues. Many reasons given for death had little pathophysiologic basis, and supplied no explanation (e.g., status lymphaticus). Several diagnoses were indistinguishable without an autopsy (e.g., acute coronary thrombosis and pulmonary embolism). Many blamed "the agent used or the ineptitude of the anesthesiologist." There also seemed to be a tension between blame assigned to the anesthesiologist and the surgeon. Gregory thought that the basis for

> "preventing deaths under anesthesia are the proper selection of agent and its mode of administration, and the management of the patient before and during anesthesia. The necessary knowledge of the normal and pathologic physiology and pharmacology of anesthesia is exceedingly large and complex. Not one surgeon in ten has been given such training or has the time or energy to acquire it. Thus, it is perfectly clear to me that the average surgeon should have little to do with anesthesiologic control. If an accident occurs the anesthesiologist is held accountable, either overtly or covertly. It is his duty to the patient and to medical science to demand the authority commensurate with his responsibility."

Gregory also noted an "apparent peculiar liability of the Negro to sudden death under anesthesia…The central commission should instigate, encourage and even direct these and other pertinent investigations [14]." Gregory identified socioeconomic differences and access to health care as causes of poor outcomes and the need for remediation of socioeconomic disparities in medical care. Aspects of this commission paralleled those of the American Society of Anesthesiology closed claims database that identified many issues essential to the improvement of anesthesia care [15–18].

1948–1952: The Beecher and Todd Study

At mid-century, Henry Beecher and Donald Todd took a giant step forward in anesthesia outcomes research [19]. They sought to determine the rate and etiologies of deaths attributable to anesthesia, and whether deaths were caused by the agent, technique, or misapplication. Finally, they attempted to assess the responsibility of the anesthetist. They believed that anesthesia caused an unnecessarily high death rate, that knowledge of what was dangerous was inadequate, and that directing attention to these issues would improve outcomes. Prospectively, they collected data on all deaths in 600,000 patients undergoing anesthesia at 10 major university hospitals, over a five-year period. A surgeon and the chief anesthetist of each institution, examined the record of every deceased patient and reported on anesthetic agents, techniques, type of surgical procedure, and causes and

classification of all deaths. Deaths were divided according to whether they resulted from patient disease, error in diagnosis, error in surgical judgment, error in surgical technique, or anesthesia. Residents, nurses, surgeons, anesthesia specialists, medical students, interns, and occasional physicians gave inhalation, intravenous, local, spinal, topical, regional, rectal, and caudal anesthetics. Although curare and curare-like drugs ("curares") were used in 44,100 cases, only 13,200 (4.3%) of all cases received controlled ventilation and 600 (0.2%) received assisted respiration. Deaths related to anesthesia when curares were not given (266) were 1:2,100, but were 1:370 (118) when curares were used. No discussion considered the possibility that the use of curares without supporting ventilation caused the 6-fold increased mortality, or that the lungs of patients receiving curares should be artificially ventilated, or that the residual effects of the curares should be reversed. They also identified increased mortality with thiopental, and with the use of tracheal tubes with inflatable cuffs—but just 2 cases: "one cuff got inflated with nasal oxygen, with fatal rupture, and the other broke during lobectomy for abscess and allowed the dependent lung to be suddenly flooded with detritus."

The discussion of the increased risk included power calculations, adjustments for case risk type, possible interactions with other agents, timing of deaths, surgical type, anesthetist experience, gender differences, gross misuse, and dose. Despite such sophisticated analyses, Beecher and Todd concluded that there must be some inherent toxicity of curare, and that the deaths were from circulatory collapse. Notwithstanding the failure to recognize partial paralysis from not reversing the effects of the curare as the probable cause of the curare-related deaths, this 600,000 patient study was a landmark in anesthesia outcomes research. An interview with Cecil Gray in 1996 [20] focused on the reason for the failure to reverse the residual effect of curare:

> "The Americans were frightened of prostigmine because of its effect on the heart. You give enough and the heart just stops. But atropine blocked that action but didn't block the action on the muscles, the reversal of the tubocurarine."

1966: A National Study Finds no Increased Risk with Halothane

Anesthetic molecules may be degraded by the alkali (bases) used to remove carbon dioxide, or may be metabolized by the patient's liver or kidney. The resulting degradation products may be injurious, sometimes highly injurious. In the late 1800s, deaths from hepatic injury were found to occur with chloroform use. Scholler showed in rats, that this noxious effect was due to the metabolism of chloroform to a noxious metabolite [21]. It was hoped that halothane, released for clinical use in 1957, would not share the hepatotoxicity possessed by chloroform. At first, as we all held our breaths, this seemed to be the case. But in the 1960s, rare cases of hepatic injury appeared, cases with a peculiar "syndrome" that had components suggesting that injury was based on an allergic mechanism [22]. The concern regarding halothane hepatotoxicity was intense. Halothane had largely replaced the older anesthetics, ether and cyclopropane. Few anesthetic converts to halothane wanted to return to the days of yesteryear, and again "drop" the flammable and irritating ether. But if ether were safer, well, then…. In December 1961, the Committee on Anesthesia of the National Academy of Sciences-National Research Council appointed a study group to report periodically on halothane anesthesia, with special attention to evidence of association with fatal postoperative hepatic necrosis. They found insufficient evidence to either establish or refute a causal relationship. Postoperative mortality at the time was 2%, and death attributable to massive hepatic necrosis appeared to be rare, perhaps one death in 10,000 operations. But in May 1963, the manufacturer issued a drug warning based on 12 cases of fatal hepatic necrosis following the use of halothane.

In response to the concern regarding hepatotoxicity, the National Halothane Study was initiated in June 1963, with funds provided by the National Institute of General Medical Sciences. It was appreciated that such a study would be large, difficult and costly, but the perceived great value of halothane justified the expense. Before the subcommittee completed its plans for a cooperative, randomized, prospective trial, several additional cases of hepatic necrosis were reported and several institutions severely restricted the use of halothane. Sensing some urgency, and after considering the feasibility, and cost of a prospective, randomized, clinical trial with sufficient power to identify a 1:10,000 risk, the subcommittee decided to survey the incidence of hepatotoxicity for the years before the issue of hepatotoxicity had been raised. Initially, 54 medical centers volunteered to participate in this collaborative retrospective study, but ultimately only 34 contributed data for the four-year study period from 1959 to 1962. This 37% drop-out of participants illustrates a difficulty of large-scale outcomes research.

The subcommittee sought to identify 0.1% differences in mortality rates, mandating a study of approximately one million patients. For all deaths thought to represent massive hepatic necrosis, a photocopy of the complete chart and sections of hepatic tissue were reviewed by a panel of six pathologists with a special interest in hepatic disorders. For the final 856,515 patients, 29.8% received halothane, 25.5% nitrous oxide-barbiturate, 17.2% cyclopropane, 11.9% ether, and 15.6% "other" agents [23, 24]. Massive hepatic necrosis per 10,000 patients was not increased for halothane (1.02), versus nitrous oxide-barbiturate (0.69), cyclopropane (1.7), ether (0.49), or other agents (0.82). Although mortality varied among the five anesthetic practices, mortality following

halothane (1.87%), was slightly less than the average for all anesthetics (1.93%). The study concluded that fatal postoperative hepatic necrosis was rare, and was usually associated with circulatory shock, sepsis, or previous hepatic disease. However, the possibility of halothane-induced hepatic necrosis following single or multiple administrations could not be excluded. There were unexpected large differences in postoperative mortality rates among participating institutions (halothane range 0.54 to 5.59%, nitrous oxide-barbiturate 0.17 to 6.55%, cyclopropane 0 to 21%, ether 0 to 13%, other 0.66 to 17.2%). Variations in measured criteria could not explain these differences.

The National Halothane Study resolved an important question using retrospective epidemiologic analysis. As such, it represented an important milestone in anesthesia outcomes research.

In the 1970s and 1980s, it was found that, as with halothane, the new inhaled anesthetics, enflurane and isoflurane, could produce hepatic injury. However, consistent with the lesser metabolism of enflurane and isoflurane, the incidence of hepatic injury with these anesthetics was much less. In the 1990s, desflurane and sevoflurane were released. It appeared that these anesthetics were still less injurious to the liver in that so few cases were reported after tens or hundreds of anesthetics have been given. For example, only a few cases of severe hepatic injury have been reported after desflurane anesthesia. One did appear to represent an allergic response to desflurane metabolism to an acetyl radical [25]. Another had nothing to do with the anesthesia, instead the hepatic injury resulted from a herpes virus infection coincident to anesthesia [26]. The minimal hepatotoxicity found with desflurane and sevoflurane in part may have resulted because neither contained chlorine, and in part because of low metabolism (especially desflurane)

1966: Nephrotoxicity Associated with Methoxyflurane Anesthesia

In the same year that the National Halothane Study determined halothane to be safe, Crandall, Papas, and Macdonald identified 16 cases (17% of patients) of high output renal failure after anesthesia with methoxyflurane, a significantly greater incidence than found in a comparison group of 100 patients given a different anesthetic [27]. They identified the pathology of the high output renal failure by fluid challenges, and the inability of ADH (Pitressin) injections to increase urine osmolality. Methoxyflurane was almost certainly the causal agent. But an editorial by Leroy Vandam concluded that more information was required before methoxyflurane could be indicted as a harmful drug, recommending its continued use until multiple, prospective, randomized, clinical trials were conducted [28].

Seven years passed until in 1973, Michael Cousins and Richard Mazze reported that subclinical toxicity occurred at 2.5–3 MAC-hours (i.e., administration of 1 MAC methoxyflurane for 2.5 to 3 hours) [29]. All patients exhibited clinical toxicity at dosages exceeding 5 MAC-hours. Cousins and Mazze cautiously suggested that methoxyflurane be used where it offered specific advantages, and where dosages of less than 2.5 MAC hours could be assured.

1978: Large, Prospective, Cardiology Outcomes Research

Modern perioperative cardiac outcomes research began with the 1978 publication *"Cardiac risk factors and complications in non-cardiac surgery"* by Lee Goldman et al. [30] Using multivariate regression analysis, these cardiologists demonstrated that postoperative cardiac death correlated significantly with (a) myocardial infarction in the previous 6 months; (b) third heart sound or jugular venous distention immediately preoperatively; (c) more than five premature ventricular contractions per minute, documented at any time preoperatively; (d) rhythm other than sinus, or premature atrial contractions on the preoperative electrocardiogram; (e) age over 70 years; (f) significant valvular aortic stenosis; (g) emergency operation; or (h) a 33% or greater decrease in systolic blood pressure for more than 10 min intraoperatively.

1980s–1990s: Prospective Anesthesiology Cardiac Outcome Research

Slogoff and Keats began the contribution by anesthesiologists to the modern era of cardiac outcomes, with their 1985 publication *"Does perioperative myocardial ischemia lead to postoperative myocardial infarction* [31]*?"* This study of 1,023 patients undergoing elective coronary artery bypass operations (CABG), found that postoperative myocardial infarction was unrelated to preoperative patient characteristics such as ejection fraction and left main coronary artery disease. Tachycardia, rather than patient selection, determined the frequency of infarction. This prospective study was sufficiently large to reasonably examine outcomes for both myocardial ischemia (a surrogate outcome), and postoperative myocardial infarction, showing a difference in infarction between those who had myocardial ischemia (6.9%), and those who did not (2.5%).

Slogoff and Keats extended this work in 1989 [32]. They prospectively randomized 1,012 patients to receive enflurane, halothane, isoflurane, or sufentanil. New ST segment depression (a surrogate outcome) appeared in 310 patients (30%), while the incidence of postoperative myocardial

infarction was 3.6–4.7%, and death was 1.2–2.4% (definitive clinical outcomes). The study demonstrated that preoperative myocardial ischemia was the strongest predictor of intraoperative ischemia. The authors concluded that approximately 90% of new myocardial ischemia observed during anesthesia reflected unrecognized preoperative ischemia, and only 10% arose from anesthetic management. They also concluded that, despite differences in the hemodynamic consequences of the study anesthetics, the choice of anesthetic did not influence outcome, and that the crucial role of the anesthesiologist is control of heart rate. Slogoff and Keats anticipated future cardiac risk reduction efforts when they stated "In the clinical situation studied here, the major role of the anesthesiologist in preventing PMI (perioperative myocardial infarction) remains limited to control of heart rate, primarily by beta-adrenergic blocking drugs [32]." A perhaps not surprising additional finding from their earlier study [31] was that the individual anesthesiologist could influence outcome: Their "anesthesiologist 7 had the highest incidence of intraoperative tachycardia, myocardial ischemia, and potoperative myocardial infarction."

1988: Use of Closed Legal Cases to Identify Risk

In the 1980s a new form of outcomes research began with the development of the American Society of Anesthesiologist's (ASA) closed claims database. Although providing important data, the limitation of this database was the lack of a denominator. Furthermore, the numerator was also limited since these cases represent only "closed" claims and not all such incidents. The ASA closed claims database has been used for analyses of cases wherein causation of complications and many factors including regional anesthesia [33], obstetric care [33], respiratory events [18], eye injuries [34], risk management issues [35], burns [36], awareness [37], difficult airway [38], pulse oximeters [39], capnography [39], pediatric anesthesia [40], regional anesthesia [41], drug errors [42], spinal cord injury [43], and chronic pain [44] might be inferred.

In 1988, anesthesiologist Robert Caplan and colleagues reported on the associations with unexpected cardiac arrest during spinal anesthesia in 14 patients, finding that ventilatory depression and sympathetic blockade with bradycardia played major roles [16]. One of the editors of this book (LJS) remembers a personal experience with such an event (fortunately not resulting in a significant adverse outcome or leading to legal action). He had given a spinal anesthetic to a surgical colleague and they were chatting as the operation, a urological procedure, began. Sudden profound bradycardia, cardiac arrest, and loss of consciousness ensued. The event was immediately noted and cardiopulmonary resuscitation (from the head of the OR table) initiated with rapid return of normal circulation. The patient opened his eyes, and upon seeing his shaken colleague said "Larry, you look terrible!"

In 1990, Caplan reported on adverse respiratory events occurring in 522 patients, finding that inadequate ventilation and intubation of the esophagus accounted for over half of the cases and much more than half of the settlement costs [15]. The "cure", in part, was an ASA-mandated use of capnography, a nearly perfect method of detecting when the tracheal tube was in the wrong place. Herein was an example of the value of this closed claims analysis in that establishing a standard (capnography) was associated with decreased liability insurance costs.

Closed claims analysis for detecting problems caused by anesthesia or anesthetists, and, sometimes, the cure of such problems continues to the present. These studies paralleled the earlier characterization of critical incidents in anesthesia [45, 46], incidents which led or *could have led* to patient injury. This process has in large part driven the developments in safe practice in anesthesia, including the promulgation of minimum monitoring standards, and crisis management algorithms. Other countries have taken up this approach to improving care, and the principles have been applied across a broad spectrum of health care practices, including other medical specialties and nurses [47, 48].

1989: Dennis Mangano, Jacqueline Leung, SPI and MCSPI

In 1989, Mangano (Fig. 43.2) assembled a group of investigators to form the Study of Perioperative Ischemia (SPI) that ultimately became The Multicenter Study of Perioperative Ischemia (McSPI). In 1989, Jackie Leung published the "*Prognostic importance of post-bypass regional wall-motion abnormalities in patients undergoing coronary artery bypass graft surgery. SPI Research Group*" [49]. This small study of 50 patients undergoing elective CABG surgery, used surrogate variables [continuous transesophageal echocardiography (TEE), electrocardiography (ECG, recorded with a Holter monitor), and hemodynamic measurements] during the prebypass, postbypass, and early postoperative intensive care unit (ICU) periods to define outcome. TEE and ECG evidence of ischemia were related to adverse clinical outcomes (postoperative myocardial infarction, ventricular failure, and cardiac death). The association of surrogate markers with hard clinical outcomes was a crucial advance. This pioneering work was a collaborative one between anesthesiology (Leung, O'Kelly, Mangano), medicine (Tubau, Browner), epidemiology (Browner), and cardiology (Hollenberg).

Further analyses of the story of SPI and McSPI, illustrate the opportunities and difficulties inherent in outcomes research. Mangano, the founder of McSPI, has published 147

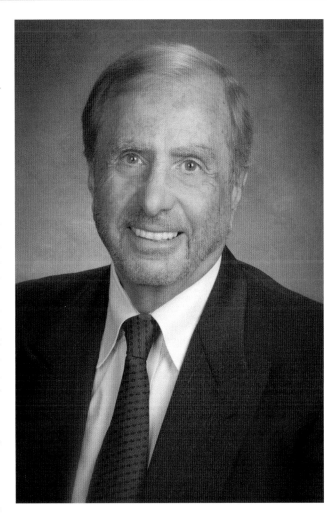

Fig. 43.2 Dennis Mangano. (Courtesy of CBS)

manuscripts as of 2012, the results of which have fundamentally changed the perioperative care of patients with cardiac disease undergoing surgery. After obtaining a doctorate in physics and mathematics, Mangano worked at Bell Laboratories. He then shifted to medicine and anesthesiology. His medical research began with animal studies, small studies of human physiology, and case reports. In 1989, he undertook a larger trial (94 patients) a study of pentastarch that taught him several important lessons [50]. "There were no significant between-group differences, ... indicat(ing) that pentastarch is as safe and effective as 5% albumin for plasma volume expansion after cardiac operations with no apparent adverse effects on coagulation. If commercially available at a lower cost than albumin, it would appear to be a reasonable first choice for colloid therapy in this setting." While this small commercial study did not affect clinical practice, it provided seed money and the concepts needed to begin epidemiologic studies that would fundamentally change anesthetic care of these patients.

SPI, the predecessor to McSPI, started as a collaboration between anesthesiology, cardiology, internal medicine, epidemiology, and surgery, and began with a small prospective study, of the incidence of myocardial ischemia in 50 patients awaiting CABG [51]. The next study evaluated wall motion abnormalities in 50 patients undergoing CABG [49]. These small studies had inadequate power to show a change in either death or myocardial infarction, forcing study design based on either surrogate outcome variables (myocardial ischemia) and/ or composite end points (death and myocardial infarction and congestive heart failure and arrhythmia), rather than a more definitive end point such as death.

1990: Multiple Groups Conduct Outcomes Research

By 1990, multiple groups were conducting outcomes research in anesthesia. Forrest performed a prospective, multi-centered (15 hospitals in the US and Canada) clinical trial in 17,201 patients, randomized to receive enflurane, fentanyl, halothane, or isoflurane anesthesia [52, 53]. This study showed that pooling of data across institutions was possible, and that differences among the four anesthetics could be found for minor clinical outcomes. Nineteen patients died (0.11 %), with the anesthetic possibly contributing in seven of these (0.04 %). The rates of death, myocardial infarction, and stroke in the study population were too small (less than 0.15 %) to allow conclusions regarding the relative rates of these outcomes among the four anesthetic agents. While the rates of 16 of 66 types of adverse outcomes in the study population differed significantly among the four study agents, these outcomes were minor in degree or clinical importance. Ventricular arrhythmias were more common with halothane. Hypertension and bronchospasm were more common with fentanyl, and tachycardia was more common with isoflurane. Recovery from anesthesia during the first 30 min was slowest in patients given halothane. In addition, patients given fentanyl experienced less pain during the first hour in the recovery room.

This study allowed several conclusions. Anesthesiologists could conduct large (17,201 patient), multi-centered, international, randomized clinical trials. Anesthesia had become so safe that there were few major definitive (infarction or death) outcomes (0.11 % mortality) in these mostly healthy patients. The study confirmed what everyone already knew: that halothane was associated with arrhythmias, fentanyl slowed the heart rate and relieved pain, and halothane delayed emergence. To reveal clinically significant differences in major outcome variables would require extremely large sample sizes, or extremely high-risk patients undergoing major surgery, or extremely bad care. Outcome studies in patients undergoing minor surgery, or outpatient surgery, have such low event rates for mortality that enormous sample sizes are required to have adequate statistical power to show a significant result.

1992: A randomized, Prospective Clinical Trial with Desflurane

Early in its history, the SPI group investigated the effects of isoflurane on coronary steal, finding that isoflurane was safe and did not lead to steal [54]. James Helman and the SPI group next examined the new anesthetic desflurane, finding that at high concentrations (10 %) it caused transient pulmonary hypertension, tachycardia, myocardial ischemia, and bronchospasm [55]. The desflurane study again showed that a relatively small (200 patients) outcome study, could demonstrate significant effects if the study used a high risk population (patients with coronary artery disease), undergoing a major operation (CABG), if the anesthetic were given at an excessive dose (inhaled induction), and if surrogate outcome variables (Holter ECG, pulmonary artery pressure, TEE) rather than more definitive outcome measures were used. Indeed, the study compared the incidence of myocardial infarction and death after desflurane, with those in a control group given sufentanil, finding differences in transient myocardial ischemia and pulmonary hypertension, but not in death or myocardial infarction.

1990–1992: Mangano's NIH Non-cardiac Surgery Epidemiologic Study

By linking a surrogate outcome variable (Holter ECG derived myocardial ischemia) to two-year mortality, the study of 474 patients provided the basis for the development of therapies to reduce perioperative risk. This study identified a dynamic risk factor, myocardial ischemia, which could be used in small randomized trials to test possible therapies. Most risk factors, such as age, history of some chronic disease (such as hypertension, diabetes, coronary artery disease, peripheral vascular disease), or some chronic health risk factor (like smoking) are fixed. Fixed risk factors cannot be acutely modified to reduce risk. Myocardial ischemia is different; it can be minimized or abolished immediately via therapies. A clinically validated surrogate outcome variable, allowing design of a small clinical trial to test a therapy, cuts the size and therefore the cost and duration of outcome trials. A validated surrogate outcome variable associated with a definitive outcome such as death, allows the design of smaller, less expensive studies, thus speeding the development of therapies.

The next major development in anesthesia outcomes research from SPI, was the long term follow-up study. The Framingham study had shown the value of longitudinal studies of patients, but this was a new concept in anesthesia outcomes research. Patients in the 474 patient NIH study, the atenolol study, the clonidine study [56], and the EPI-2 study, were followed for at least 5 years and some for as long as 10 years. This long-term follow-up increased the power of these studies to identify differences in more definitive outcomes such as death. If intraoperative death is the only "outcome", short-term studies have to be extremely large, because the event rates are small, even in high-risk cases. Even studies from 1925 to 1945 quoted intra-operative death rates of 0.1 %, an incidence mandating tens to hundreds of thousands of patients in order to detect significant changes. However, if the event rate is 3 to 8 % per year (common in high risk populations), differences in long-term mortality can be seen in 200 high-risk patients studied for 5–10 years—perhaps even less.

The NIH funded the original 474 patient SPI epidemiologic study, and the research produced more than 30 highly cited manuscripts. Two follow-up NIH grants were submitted. One proposed investigating medical therapies for preventing myocardial ischemia in patients undergoing non-cardiac surgery (atenolol and clonidine). This grant scored extremely well but was not funded. Reviewers were concerned that the study population did not include equal numbers of women and men, a problem as the study location (a Veterans Administration Hospital) had only 5 % female patients. This deficiency was corrected by collaborating with the San Francisco Kaiser Hospital, but the revised grant was still not funded after again receiving an excellent score.

The members of SPI met to decide what to do. A schism occurred. Jackie Leung wanted to regroup, downsize the studies, and resubmit. Mangano wanted to pursue commercial funding from drug company studies, using the excess funds generated to do the unfunded clinical studies. Acting on his belief, Mangano took the small organization, the Study of Perioperative Ischemia (SPI) Research Group, and expanded it to the Multi-Centered Study of Perioperative Ischemia (McSPI).

Outcomes research takes many forms. It can be a prospective, randomized, clinical trial to test for specific effects of medications. It can be an epidemiologic study of standard care. A simple and relatively inexpensive way to pursue epidemiological studies is to obtain a database collected for some other purpose, such as the Medicare database, or census data, or computerized medical records. McSPI took a different, vastly more expensive approach. Rather than performing an inexpensive retrospective analysis of available databases, providing records for tens of thousands or millions of patients, McSPI collected detailed, prospective epidemiologic data in a limited number of patients with surrogate outcome variables such as Holter ECG to detect myocardial ischemia. Although cost and work-load were great, and sample sizes were small, the depth of information was extensive. McSPI started small and learned to think big from experiences in a study of 156 patients [57]. The next study included 200 high-risk patients undergoing non-cardiac surgery or coronary artery bypass graft (CABG) surgery [58]. Sample size and risk increased in the subsequent 1990 study, to 474 men with coronary artery disease (243) or at high risk for it (231), all undergoing elective non-cardiac surgery [59]. Sample size would ultimately increase 10-fold. The 474 patient study linked the surrogate outcome variable, myocardial ischemia detected by a Holter ECG monitor, to a composite end point, combining cardiac death, myocardial infarction, unstable angina, congestive heart failure, or ventricular tachycardia. The surrogate outcome variable, Holter ECG, detected myocardial ischemia, which predicted a single long-term outcome, 2-year mortality [60].

1996–2004: Risk Reduction Accomplished with Drugs

McSPI began large, commercially funded studies that applied definitive outcomes. These studies included acadesine in 116 patients [61], 566 patients [62], 2,698 patients [63], and finally a meta-analysis in 4,043 patients [64]. The meta-analysis found that acadesine reduced the risk of perioperative cardiac death, myocardial infarction, and combined adverse cardiovascular outcomes. The 2,698 patient study also showed a decreased long term mortality.

The McSPI system then began trials of atenolol [65, 66], clonidine [56], aspirin, coumadin, epidural versus PCA (patient controlled analgesia), mivazerol [67], dexmedetomidine [68], draflazine, propofol [69], RSR-13, C5B-Inhibitor, and COX-2 inhibitors [70]. Mangano and colleagues also performed multicenter observational studies on thousands of patients undergoing coronary artery surgery, the EPI-1 [71] and EPI-2 [72] studies, investigations that provided data for several researches, including the effects of aprotinin on outcomes (see below). McSPI's studies led to the development of perioperative beta blockade [73, 74] and perioperative clonidine [56] to decrease perioperative cardiac risk. The requirement of definitive end points (myocardial infarction or death) necessitated the need for enormous studies. For example, mivazerol was studied in three phases, a 24 patient, then a 300 patient [73], and finally a 2,854 [67] patient study. The plan to study dexmedetomidine was similar, with a 24 patient, then a 300 patient, and finally a 3000 patient study.

2006: Aprotinin and Outcome

The history of aprotinin shows not only the importance of outcomes research, but highlights the critical importance of meticulous evaluation. Aprotinin is the bovine version of the small protein basic pancreatic trypsin inhibitor, or BPTI, which inhibits trypsin and related proteolytic enzymes. It was originally investigated in the 1960s for the treatment of pancreatitis [75]. Aprotinin's ability to reduce acute fibrinolysis associated with extracorporeal circulatory support, was recognized in 1961 [76]. Clinical observation identified its effects on hemorrhage [77], and it was used to reduce hemorrhage [78]. Fibrinolysis leads to the lysis of clots. Aprotinin inhibits such lysis and thereby should decrease hemorrhage and the need for transfusions. Aprotinin competed with two other antifibrinolytics, the lysine analogues, tranexamic acid and epsilon aminocaproic acid. It became a standard in cardiac anesthesia in Europe, particularly in Germany. FDA approval for US use eventually came in 1993,. By then, more than 30 studies had evaluated aprotinin use in cardiac surgery. Design problems, including non-randomization, lack of a control group, historical controls, and/or small sample size compromised these studies, but the consensus was that aprotinin reduced the severity of hemorrhage and the need for transfusion with cardiac surgery. Aprotinin was thought to be safe although there were instances of anaphylaxis. Study results also suggested that it might increase [79, 80] graft thrombosis, but the small size of many studies hindered the likelihood of identifying this adverse event [80].

The FDA required three US prospective, randomized studies before approval, 2 of which showed efficacy for a reduction in perioperative blood utilization and loss [79, 81, 82]. Bayer began selling aprotinin in the US, and the $1,000 per dose medication was extensively marketed. After approval, Bayer supported an international study addressing the issue of graft patency after cardiac surgery in 796 patients [83]. Aprotinin reduced thoracic drainage volume by 43%, and the requirement for red blood cell administration by 49%, but graft occlusions occurred in 15.4% of aprotinin-treated patients and 10.9% of patients receiving a placebo (P=0.03). The increased risk of graft occlusion was more apparent in European centers. The authors divided the study results by country: "At United States sites, patients had characteristics more favorable for graft patency, and occlusions occurred in 9.4% of the aprotinin group and 9.5% of the placebo group (P=0.72). At Danish and Israeli sites, where patients had more adverse co-morbidities, occlusions occurred in 23.0% of aprotinin- and 12.4% of placebo-treated patients (P=0.01). Aprotinin did not affect the occurrence of myocardial infarction (aprotinin: 2.9%; placebo: 3.8%) or mortality (aprotinin: 1.4%; placebo: 1.6%)." This division of the study by country reduced the statistically significant effects,

decreased the concern regarding risk, and allowed marketing of the drug to continue.

However, if an outcomes study shows an adverse event, dividing the study into sub-studies, reduces the power to show the effect. How were McSPI investigators to deal with this concern? Bayer might be reluctant to fund a study revealing an adverse effect. McSPI investigators collected data in the EPI-2 study that allowed the analysis of the effects of aprotinin versus tranexamic acid, and epsilon-aminocaproic acid, on morbidity and mortality [84]. Elizabeth Ott compared medical care in the US, Canada, UK, and Germany, identifying a surprising result [85]. In-hospital mortality was 1.5% (9/619) in the UK, 2.0% (9/444) in Canada, 2.7% (34/1283) in the US, and 3.8% (32/834) in Germany (P=0.03). Composite outcomes (morbidity and mortality) were 12% in the UK, 16% in Canada, 18% in the US, and 24% in Germany (P<0.001) [85]. Regarding the increased mortality in Germany, Ott found that "the practices associated with adverse outcomes were the intraoperative use of aprotinin, intraoperative transfusion of fresh-frozen plasma or platelets, lack of use of early postoperative aspirin, and use of postoperative heparin." Aprotinin was used in 15% of US cases and 85% of German cases. The effects of aprotinin on renal failure, and morbidity and mortality, were rapidly published [84, 86]. Multinational outcomes research with sufficient power to identify definitive but rare outcomes had found that aprotinin increased the risk of death by a factor of 2.5. The German physicians could not identify the more than doubling of risk with the use of aprotinin because almost every patient having cardiac surgery in Germany (85%) was given aprotinin.

International, or multi-centered studies may be essential to identify practices that increase small risks by 2 to 3 fold. Individual physicians are unlikely to discern such effects. Bayer conducted a 60,000 patient retrospective epidemiologic analysis and found results similar to those of McSPI [81], but publication was delayed [87]. The delay deferred FDA action, and allowed aprotinin to remain on the market for another two years. Ultimately the BART trial (Blood conservation using Antifibrinolytics in a Randomized Trial) [88], a multicenter, blinded trial, randomly assigned 2,331 high-risk cardiac surgical patients to one of three groups: 781 received aprotinin, 770 received tranexamic acid, and 780 received aminocaproic acid. The relative risk of death in the aprotinin group was 1.53 (95% CI, 1.06 to 2.22). The BART trial concluded that "Despite the possibility of a modest reduction in the risk of massive bleeding, the strong and consistent negative mortality trend associated with aprotinin, as compared with the lysine analogues, precludes its use in high-risk cardiac surgery." Aprotinin was removed from the US market. Outcomes research using epidemiologic techniques and a randomized trial had been used to delineate the risks.

But did they? Some researchers began to question the results [89]. The reliability of Mangano's 2006 conclusions were disputed on the basis that the non-randomized, non-blinded observational trial was subject to bias in the choice of aprotinin in some patients [90]. In addition, Mangano's analysis did not include the impact of bypass time, the number of vessels grafted, or whether the procedure was done "off pump.

The more influential BART study has also attracted criticism. Although it was a randomized controlled trial, 137 patients were excluded from analysis for unknown reasons, and the trend in the mortality for these patients was opposite to that for the included patients [91]. A large number of primary outcomes (excessive bleeding) were reclassified from the originally reported data, favoring the lysine analogues [91]. It has also been noted that both the method and control of anticoagulation was inconsistent [92].

Meta-analyses that include the BART data have been published as recently as 2011. However it is now apparent that the weight of the BART study may have inadvertently swayed the conclusions [93–95].

These concerns prompted Health Canada to review the BART study. The conclusion was that the BART study was not a reliable assessment of the safety of aprotinin, and further, that the benefits of the drug in coronary artery bypass surgery outweigh the risks [89, 91]. The Commission on Human Medicines (CHM) has also reviewed the previous studies and arrived at a similar conclusion, leading to the lifting of the suspension of aprotinin in Europe in 2012 [92].

2008: Lessons Learned from POISE

The Peri-Operative Ischemic Evaluation (POISE) [95, 96] study was conducted by PJ Devereaux, who wished to re-evaluate the capacity of perioperative beta blockade to prevent myocardial ischemia. He first conducted a meta-analysis of studies of perioperative beta blockade, which showed that beta-blockade was effective [97]. He then reduced the number of studies included in the meta-analysis until the analysis showed that beta-blockade wasn't effective [97]. The Canadian government and AstraZeneca, the manufacturer of metoprolol XL used in the study, underwrote ($3,000,000) the POISE trial, a 10,000 patient randomized, clinical trial with death, stroke, MI, as well as hypotension, bradycardia, and atrial fibrillation as the primary outcomes [95]. The POISE trial obtained its results from 190 hospitals in 23 countries including Cuba, Iran, China, and India, but not the US. During the study design, investigators reasoned that if the study failed to show an effect, it would be criticized for inadequate drug dose. Accordingly, they chose a dose that

could not be criticized as too low. But every medication has a correct dose and a therapeutic index. Patients in the POISE study received multiple doses of metoprolol XL, apparently 400 mg on the day of surgery, and then 200 mg each day for a month. The 400 mg starting dose exceeded the recommended starting dose for metoprolol XL: 25 mg for hypertension, 100 mg for coronary artery disease, and 12.5 mg for congestive heart failure. A second problem arose. Because of limited funding ($300 per patient), site monitoring was only performed at 6% of centers. This incomplete monitoring revealed that 10% of data were fraudulent, defined as non-existent (no patient actually existed), and the "data" for these "patients" were excluded from analysis.

From the 10,000 planned patients, data from 8,351 patients were included in analyses. Metoprolol decreased the risk of myocardial infarction but increased the risk of hypotension, bradycardia, stroke, and death. Publication of the results from this enormous study initially generated considerable attention, but the limitations noted above curtailed continued interest.

2006–2009: Clean Hands Decreased Infection

The interest among anesthesiologists in surgical site infections, expanded to include research on how anesthesiologists might help prevent all types of Healthcare Associated Infections (HAI). Studies in the 1990s found that central venous catheters, placed by anesthesiologists in the operating room, were more likely to be infected than those placed elsewhere in the hospital, and that careful attention to sterile technique and wide draping substantially reduced the infection rate. Anesthesiologist Peter Pronovost, at Johns Hopkins (named by TIME magazine in 2008 as one of the most influential persons of the year), partnered with a statewide safety initiative in Michigan, to show that implementation of a checklist-based intervention to increase adherence to evidence-based practices, markedly decreased the incidence of catheter-related bloodstream infections [98].

Anesthesiologists Loftus and Koff, and colleagues at Dartmouth, contributed to HAI prevention by evaluating the impact of hand hygiene by anesthesia providers in the operating room [99]. At baseline, anesthesia providers performed hand hygiene (soap and water or alcohol based gel) less than once per hour in the operating room. The anesthesia work area and the patients' intravenous catheters commonly became contaminated with bacteria within a few minutes of the start of a case. Providing a clip-on device that dispensed alcohol gel and provided periodic reminders for hand hygiene, increased the rate of hand hygiene to about 7 times per hour, reduced workspace and intravenous catheter contamination, and reduced HAI.

2006-Present: Does Anesthetic Choice Affect Cancer Recurrence?

In 2006, Exadaktylos et al. reported results from a retrospective study, showing that patients having mastectomy for breast cancer had a greater chance of recurrence if a general as opposed to a regional anesthetic were used [100]. This and other evidence supported the notion that anesthetic management, and particularly choice of drugs and choice of regional vs. general anesthesia, might increase the risk of recurrence in patients with cancer [101], but other studies did not [102]. Some opioids and other anesthetic agents might inhibit host defenses, specifically natural killer cell function. But as of 2012, anesthesiologists Kavanagh and Buggy, found the present evidence for a connection between the effects of anesthetic technique and cancer recurrence to be equivocal [103].A multicenter trial will examine this premise [104].

2010: Arthur Wallace Performs Inexpensive, Retrospective, Epidemiologic Studies Using Analysis of Electronic Medical Records

Outcomes research may be undertaken with retrospective analysis of computerized medical records. Wallace conducted a study in 5,000 patients using McSPI EPI-2 data entitled "*The association of the pattern of use of anti-ischemic agents on morbidity and mortality after coronary artery bypass surgery*" [105]. This study investigated the effects of perioperative beta blockade and other anti-ischemic agents on morbidity and mortality. He repeated the study using VA computerized medical records for 38,779 operations performed between 1996 and 2008 at a cost less than 0.3 % of the cost of the EPI-2 study and found parallel results [106]. The ability to study 7.5 times the number of operations for 0.3 % of the cost, shows the advantages of retrospective epidemiologic analysis of computerized medical records. The EPI-2 study had collected robust data over 5 years, from 70 centers in 17 countries in 5,065 patients, prospectively studied undergoing coronary bypass surgery. The study cost $38,000,000. The advantages of this prospective design included the ability to randomize and collect in depth data, but the cost and human effort disadvantages were enormous. The EPI-2 data set quickly became outdated as the last patient was operated on in June of 2000. The study enrolled patients who had coronary artery bypass surgery using extracorporeal support, excluding the then common "off-pump" CABG, thereby precluding conclusions about relative risks and benefits. Outcomes research based on retrospective analysis of computerized medical records can reduce the cost and difficulty of outcomes studies, and increase the richness of their findings.

Some Reflections

Cardiologists developed large, randomized, prospective, clinical outcomes studies with definitive but rare end points, techniques subsequently adopted by anesthesiologists. The development of pharmacologic techniques to reduce perioperative cardiac risk with beta blockers [74], statins [107], clonidine [56], and aspirin [72], directly flowed from this research. However, such outcome studies were expensive and difficult—and could provide positive results, negative results, and sometimes results with negligible benefit. For example, $11,000,000 and a decade were spent studying the effects of hypothermia on neurologic outcome with cerebral aneurysm surgery, finding that hypothermia did not improve outcome, a negative result that had the salutary effect of sparing future patients from the side effects of hypothermia [108]. The POISE study of more than 8,000 patients consumed $3,000,000, to indicate that although beta sympathetic blockade may decrease myocardial infarction it may increase other untoward effects such as stroke and death. Another interpretation suggested that the POISE study showed only that all drugs have a therapeutic index, and that dose matters, and that the increased incidence of stroke and death resulted from the excessive use of beta blockade. After two decades of work and $45 million, the EPI-1 and EPI-2 studies demonstrated the benefits of aspirin for cardiac surgery, the risks of aprotinin, and clarified the risks of neurologic outcomes with cardiac surgery. Despite the expense and difficulty, outcomes research is essential for the improvement of anesthesia care and the reduction in perioperative risk. Anesthesia outcomes research leads and has led to evidence based medicine that improved anesthetic and medical care.

Acknowledgment We gratefully acknowledge the stories and advice given us by Arthur Wallace, particularly concerning the outcome studies that examined factors affecting the safety of anesthesia in patients at risk of cardiovascular disease. His knowledge of SPI and McSPI was invaluable. Where the telling of these stories adds error, it is error that we have introduced.

References

1. Waters RM. Present status of cyclopropane. Br Med J. 1936;2:1013–7.
2. Rubin A, Metz-Rubin H. The effect of dramamine upon postoperative nausea and vomiting; a controlled study of 250 consecutive surgical patients. Surg Gynecol Obstet. 1951;92:415–8.
3. Hume RH, Wilner WK Jr. The use of dramamine in control of postoperative nausea and vomiting. Anesthesiology. 1952;13:302–5.
4. Dent SJ, Ramachandra V, Stephen CR. Postoperative vomiting: incidence, analysis, and therapeutic measures in 3,000 patients. Anesthesiology. 1955;16:564–72.

5. Bellville JW, Bross ID, Howland WS. Postoperative nausea and vomiting. IV. Factors related to postoperative nausea and vomiting. Anesthesiology. 1960;21:186–93.

6. Bellville JW, Howland WS, Bross ID. Postoperative nausea and vomiting. III. Evaluation of the antiemetic drugs fluphenazine (prolixin) and promethazine (phenergan) and comparison with triflupromazine, (vesprin) and cyclizine (marezine). JAMA. 1960;172:1488–93.

7. Leeser J, Lip H. Prevention of postoperative nausea and vomiting using ondansetron, a new, selective, 5-HT3 receptor antagonist. Anesth Analg. 1991;72:751–5.

8. Doze VA, Westphal LM, White PF. Comparison of propofol with methohexital for outpatient anesthesia. Anesth Analg. 1986;65:1189–95.

9. McKenzie R, Tantisira B, Karambelkar DJ, Riley TJ, Abdelhady H. Comparison of ondansetron with ondansetron plus dexamethasone in the prevention of postoperative nausea and vomiting. Anesth Analg. 1994;79:961–4.

10. Egor EI, II, Kraft ID, Koncling HH A comparicon of atropino, or scopolamine, plus pentobarbital, meperidine. or morphine as pediatric preanesthetic medication. Anesthesiology. 1961;22:962 9.

11. Apfel CC, Korttila K, Abdalla M, Kerger H, Turan A, Vedder I, Zernak C, Danner K, Jokela R, Pocock SJ, Trenkler S, Kredel M, Biedler A, Sessler DI, Roewer N IMPACT, Investigators. A factorial trial of six interventions for the prevention of postoperative nausea and vomiting. N Engl J Med. 2004;350:2441–51.

12. Edwards G. Death on the table, An address to students. Br J Anaesth. 1938;15:87–103.

13. Bishop HF. Operating room deaths. Anesthesiology. 1946;7:651–62.

14. Gregory JE The pathology of sudden and unexpected death under anesthesia. Anesthesiology. 1949;10:105–8.

15. Caplan RA, Posner KL, Ward RJ, Cheney FW. Adverse respiratory events in anesthesia: a closed claims analysis. Anesthesiology. 1990;72:828–33.

16. Caplan RA, Ward RJ, Posner K. Cheney FW Unexpected cardiac arrest during spinal anesthesia: a closed claims analysis of predisposing factors. Anesthesiology. 1988;68:5–11.

17. Cheney FW, Posner K, Caplan RA, Ward RJ. Standard of care and anesthesia liability. JAMA. 1989;261:1599–603.

18. Cheney FW, Posner KL, Caplan RA. Adverse respiratory events infrequently leading to malpractice suits. A closed claims analysis. Anesthesiology. 1991,75.932–9.

19. Beecher HK, Todd DP. A study of the deaths associated with anesthesia and surgery: based on a study of 599, 548 anesthesias in ten institutions 1948–1952, inclusive. Ann Surg. 1954;140:2–35.

20. The Royal College of Physicians and Oxford Brookes University Medical Sciences Video Archive MSVA 145. Professor Cecil Gray CBE KCSG FRCP FRCS FRCA in interview with Dr. Bax Blythe, Oxford, 25th November 1996, Interview Two.

21. Scholler KL. Modification of the effects of chloroform on the rat liver. Brit J Anaesth. 1970;42:603–5.

22. Davies GE. Is halothane hepatotoxicity an allergic reaction to halothane? Proc Royal Soc Med. 1973;66:55–6.

23. Summary of the National Halothane Study. Possible association between halothane anesthesia and postoperative hepatic necrosis. Report by Subcommittee on the National Halothane Study of the Committee on Anesthesia, National Academy of Science. JAMA. 1966;197:775–88.

24. Gall EA. Report of the pathology panel. National halothane study. Anesthesiology. 1968;29:233–48.

25. Martin JL, Plevak DJ, Flannery KD, Charlton M, Poterucha JJ, Humphreys CE, Derfus G, Pohl LR. Hepatotoxicity after desflurane anesthesia. Anesthesiology. 1995;83:1125–9.

26. Katz J, Magee J, Baker B, Eger E I II. Hepatic necrosis associated with herpesvirus after anesthesia with desflurane and nitrous oxide. Anesth Analg. 1994;78:1173–6.

27. Crandell WB, Pappas SG, Macdonald A. Nephrotoxicity associated with methoxyflurane anesthesia. Anesthesiology. 1966;27:591–607.

28. Vandam LD. Report on methoxyflurane. Anesthesiology. 1966;27:534–5.

29. Cousins MJ, Mazze RI. Methoxyflurane nephrotoxicity: A study of dose-response in man. JAMA. 1973;225:1611–6.

30. Goldman L, Caldera DL, Southwick FS, Nussbaum SR, Murray B, O'Malley TA, Goroll AH, Caplan CH, Nolan J, Burke DS, Krogstad D, Carabello B, Slater EE. Cardiac risk factors and complications in non-cardiac surgery. Medicine. 1978;57:357–70.

31. Slogoff S, Keats AS. Does perioperative myocardial ischemia lead to postoperative myocardial infarction? Anesthesiology. 1985;62:107–14.

32. Slogoff S, Keats A. Randomized trial of primary anesthetic agents on outcome of coronary artery bypass operations. Anesthesiology. 1989;70:179–88.

33. Lee LA, Posner KL, Domino KB, Caplan RA, Cheney FW. Injuries associated with regional anesthesia in the 1980s and 1990s: a closed claims analysis. Anesthesiology. 1980s;2004;101;143 52.

34. Gild WM, Posner KL, Caplan RA, Cheney FW. Eye injuries associated with anesthesia. A closed claims analysis. Anesthesiology. 1992;76:204–8.

35. Gild WM. Risk management in cardiac anesthesia: the ASA Closed Claims Project perspective. J Cardiothorac Vasc Anesth. 1994;8:3–6.

36. Cheney FW, Posner KL, Caplan RA, Gild WM. Burns from warming devices in anesthesia. A closed claims analysis. Anesthesiology. 1994;80:806–10.

37. Kent CD, Domino KB. Awareness: practice, standards, and the law. Best practice & research. Clin Anesthesiol. 2007;21:369–83.

38. Peterson GN, Domino KB, Caplan RA, Posner KL, Lee LA, Cheney FW. Management of the difficult airway: a closed claims analysis. Anesthesiology. 2005;103:33–9.

39. Caplan RA, Vistica MF, Posner KL, Cheney FW. Adverse anesthetic outcomes arising from gas delivery equipment: a closed claims analysis. Anesthesiology. 1997;87:741–8.

40. Jimenez N, Posner KL, Cheney FW, Caplan RA, Lee LA, Domino KB. An update on pediatric anesthesia liability: a closed claims analysis. Anesth Analg. 2007;104:147–53.

41. Lee LA, Posner KL, Cheney FW, Caplan RA, Domino KB. Complications associated with eye blocks and peripheral nerve blocks: an american society of anesthesiologists closed claims analysis. Reg Anesth Pain Med. 2008;33:416–22.

42. Cranshaw J, Gupta KJ, Cook TM. Litigation related to drug errors in anaesthesia: an analysis of claims against the NHS in England 1995–2007. Anaesthesia. 2009;64:1317–23.

43. Hindman BJ, Palecek JP, Posner KL, Traynelis VC, Lee LA, Sawin PD, Tredway TL, Todd MM, Domino KB. Cervical spinal cord, root, and bony spine injuries: a closed claims analysis. Anesthesiology. 2011;114:782–95.

44. Rathmell JP, Michna E, Fitzgibbon DR, Stephens LS, Posner KL, Domino KB. Injury and liability associated with cervical procedures for chronic pain. Anesthesiology. 2011;114:918–26.

45. Cooper JB, Newbower RS, Long CD, McPeek B. Preventable anesthesia mishaps: a study of human factors. Anesthesiology. 1978;49:399–406.

46. Cooper JB, Newbower RS, Kitz RJ. An analysis of major errors and equipment failures in anesthesia management: Considerations for prevention and detection. Anesthesiology. 1984;60:34–42.

47. Pegalis SE, Bal BS. Closed medical negligence claims can drive patient safety and reduce litigation. Clin Orthop Relat Res. 2012;470:1398–404.

48. Moody ML, Kremer MJ. Preinduction activities: a closed malpractice claims perspective. AANA. 2001;69:461–5.

49. Leung JM, O'Kelly B, Browner WS, Tubau J, Hollenberg M, Mangano DT. Prognostic importance of postbypass regional wall-

motion abnormalities in patients undergoing coronary artery bypass graft surgery. SPI Research Group. Anesthesiology. 1989;71:16–25.

50. London MJ, Ho JS, Triedman JK, Verrier ED, Levin J, Merrick SH, Hanley FL, Browner WS, Mangano DT. A randomized clinical trial of 10 % pentastarch (low molecular weight hydroxyethyl starch) versus 5 % albumin for plasma volume expansion after cardiac operations. J Thorac Cardiovasc Surg. 1989;97:785–97.

51. Knight AA, Hollenberg M, London MJ, Mangano DT. Myocardial ischemia in patients awaiting coronary artery bypass grafting. Am Heart J. 1989;117:1189–95.

52. Forrest JB, Cahalan MK, Rehder K, Goldsmith CH, Levy WJ, Strunin L, Bota W, Boucek CD, Cucchiara RF, Dhamee S et al. Multicenter study of general anesthesia. II. Results. Anesthesiology. 1990;72:262–8.

53. Forrest JB, Rehder K, Goldsmith CH, Cahalan MK, Levy WJ, Strunin L, Bota W, Boucek CD, Cucchiara RF, Dhamee S et al. Multicenter study of general anesthesia. I. Design and patient demography. Anesthesiology. 1990;72:252–61.

54. Leung JM, Goehner P, O'Kelly BF, Hollenberg M, Pineda N, Cason BA, Mangano DT. Isoflurane anesthesia and myocardial ischemia: comparative risk versus sufentanil anesthesia in patients undergoing coronary artery bypass graft surgery. The SPI (Study of Perioperative Ischemia) Research Group. Anesthesiology. 1991;74:838–47.

55. Helman JD, Leung JM, Bellows W, Roach GW, Reeves JD, III, Howse J, McEnany MT, Pineda N, Mangano D, SPI Research, Group. The risk of myocardial ischemia in patients receiving desflurane versus sufentanil anesthesia for coronary artery bypass graft surgery. Anesthesiology. 1992;77:47–62.

56. Wallace AW, Galindez D, Salahieh A, Layug EL, Lazo EA, Haratonik KA, Boisvert DM, Kardatzke D. Effect of clonidine on cardiovascular morbidity and mortality after noncardiac surgery. Anesthesiology. 2004;101:284–93.

57. London MJ, Tubau JF, Wong MG, Layug E, Hollenberg M, Krupski WC, Rapp JH, Browner WS, Mangano DT. The "natural history" of segmental wall motion abnormalities in patients undergoing noncardiac surgery. S.P.I. Research Group. Anesthesiology. 1990;73:644–55.

58. Mangano DT. Characteristics of electrocardiographic ischemia in high-risk patients undergoing surgery. Study of Perioperative Ischemia (SPI) Research Group. J Electrocardiol. 1990;23 Suppl:20–7.

59. Mangano DT, Browner WS, Hollenberg M, London MJ, Tubau JF, Tateo IM. Association of perioperative myocardial ischemia with cardiac morbidity and mortality in men undergoing noncardiac surgery. The Study of Perioperative Ischemia Research Group. N Engl J Med. 1990;323:1781–8.

60. Mangano DT, Browner WS, Hollenberg M, Li J, Tateo IM. Long-term cardiac prognosis following noncardiac surgery. The Study of Perioperative Ischemia Research Group. JAMA. 1992;268:233–9.

61. Leung JM, Stanley T 3rd, Mathew J, Curling P, Barash P, Salmenpera M, Reves JG, Hollenberg M, Mangano DT. An initial multicenter, randomized controlled trial on the safety and efficacy of acadesine in patients undergoing coronary artery bypass graft surgery. SPI Research Group. Anesth Analg. 1994;78:420–34.

62. Jain U, Laflamme CJ, Aggarwal A, Ramsay JG, Comunale ME, Ghoshal S, Ngo L, Ziola K, Hollenberg M, Mangano DT. Electrocardiographic and hemodynamic changes and their association with myocardial infarction during coronary artery bypass surgery. A multicenter study. Multicenter Study of Perioperative Ischemia (McSPI) Research Group. Anesthesiology. 1997;86:576–91.

63. Mangano DT, Miao Y, Tudor IC, Dietzel C. Post-reperfusion myocardial infarction: long-term survival improvement using adenosine regulation with acadesine. J Am Coll Cardiol. 2006;48:206–14.

64. Mangano DT. Effects of acadesine on myocardial infarction, stroke, and death following surgery. A meta-analysis of the 5 international randomized trials. The Multicenter Study of Perioperative Ischemia (McSPI) Research Group. JAMA. 1997;277:325–32.

65. Wallace A, Layug B, Tateo I, Li J, Hollenberg M, Browner W, Miller D, Mangano D. Prophylactic atenolol reduces postoperative myocardial ischemia. McSPI Research Group. Anesthesiology. 1998;88:7–17.

66. Mangano DT, Layug EL, Wallace A, Tateo I. Effect of atenolol on mortality and cardiovascular morbidity after noncardiac surgery. Multicenter Study of Perioperative Ischemia Research Group. N Engl J Med. 1996;335:1713–20.

67. Oliver MF, Goldman L, Julian DG, Holme I. Effect of mivazerol on perioperative cardiac complications during non-cardiac surgery in patients with coronary heart disease: the European Mivazerol Trial (EMIT). Anesthesiology. 1999;91:951–61.

68. Talke P, Li J, Jain U, Leung J, Drasner K, Hollenberg M, Mangano DT. Effects of perioperative dexmedetomidine infusion in patients undergoing vascular surgery. The Study of Perioperative Ischemia Research Group. Anesthesiology. 1995;82:620–33.

69. Jain U, Body SC, Bellows W, Wolman R, Mangano CM, Mathew J, Youngs E, Wilson R, Zhang A, Mangano DT. Multicenter study of target-controlled infusion of propofol-sufentanil or sufentanil-midazolam for coronary artery bypass graft surgery. Multicenter Study of Perioperative Ischemia (McSPI) Research Group. Anesthesiology. 1996;85:522–35.

70. Nussmeier NA, Whelton AA, Brown MT, Joshi GP, Langford RM, Singla NK, Boye ME, Verburg KM. Safety and efficacy of the cyclooxygenase-2 inhibitors parecoxib and valdecoxib after noncardiac surgery. Anesthesiology. 2006;104:518–26.

71. Mangano CM, Diamondstone LS, Ramsay JG, Aggarwal A, Herskowitz A, Mangano DT. Renal dysfunction after myocardial revascularization: risk factors, adverse outcomes, and hospital resource utilization. The Multicenter Study of Perioperative Ischemia Research Group. Ann Intern Med. 1998;128:194–203.

72. Mangano DT. Aspirin and mortality from coronary bypass surgery. N Engl J Med. 2002;347:1309–17.

73. Perioperative sympatholysis. Beneficial effects of the alpha 2-adrenoceptor agonist mivazerol on hemodynamic stability and myocardial ischemia. McSPI—Europe Research Group. Anesthesiology. 1997;86:346–63.

74. Poldermans D, Boersma E, Bax JJ, Thomson IR, Paelinck B, van de Ven LL, Scheffer MG, Trocino G, Vigna C, Baars HF, van Urk H, Roelandt JR. Bisoprolol reduces cardiac death and myocardial infarction in high-risk patients as long as 2 years after successful major vascular surgery. Eur Heart J. 2001;22:1353–8.

75. Asang E. Changes in the therapy of inflammatory diseases of the pancreas. A report on 1 year of therapy and prophylaxis with the kallikrein- and trypsin inactivator trasylol (Bayer). Langenbecks Arch Klin Chir Ver Dtsch Z Chir. 1960;293:645–70.

76. Derom F, Derom E, Meirsma N-Roobroeck G, Rolly G. Rolly-Penninck J. Extracorporeal circulation followed by acute fibrinolysis successfully treated with Trasylol. Acta Chir Belg. 1961;60:695–701.

77. Kaeser, H. Hemorrhagic Syndrome in Labor. Geburtshilfe Frauenheilkd. 1963;23:1026.

78. Marggraf W. Blood preservation with trasylol, a method for preventing proteolytic enzyme activation. Bibl Haematol. 1963;16:259–64.

79. Cosgrove DM 3rd, Heric B, Lytle BW, Taylor PC, Novoa R, Golding LA, Stewart RW, McCarthy PM, Loop FD. Aprotinin therapy for reoperative myocardial revascularization: a placebo-controlled study. Ann Thorac Surg. 1992;54:1031–6; discussion 1036–8.

80. van der Meer J, Hillege HL, Ascoop CA, Dunselman PH, Mulder BJ, van Ommen GV, Pfisterer M, van Gilst WH, Lie KI. Aprotinin in aortocoronary bypass surgery: increased risk of vein-graft occlusion and myocardial infarction? Supportive evidence from a retrospective study. Thromb Haemost. 1996;75:1–3.

81. Daily PO, Lamphere JA, Dembitsky WP, Adamson RM, Dans NF. Effect of prophylactic epsilon-aminocaproic acid on blood loss and transfusion requirements in patients undergoing first-time coronary

artery bypass grafting. A randomized, prospective, double-blind study. J Thorac Cardiovasc Surg. 1994;108:99–106; discussion 106–8.

82. Murkin JM, Lux J, Shannon NA, Guiraudon GM, Menkis AH, McKenzie FN, Novick RJ. Aprotinin significantly decreases bleeding and transfusion requirements in patients receiving aspirin and undergoing cardiac operations. J Thorac Cardiovasc Surg. 1994;107:554–61.

83. Alderman EL, Levy JH, Rich JB, Nili M, Vidne B, Schaff H, Uretzky G, Pettersson G, Thiis JJ, Hantler CB, Chaitman B, Nadel A. Analyses of coronary graft patency after aprotinin use: results from the International Multicenter Aprotinin Graft Patency Experience (IMAGE) trial. J Thorac Cardiovasc Surg. 1998;116:716–30.

84. Mangano DT, Tudor IC, Dietzel C. The risk associated with aprotinin in cardiac surgery. N Engl J Med. 2006;354:353–65.

85. Ott E, Mazer CD, Tudor IC, Shore-Lesserson L, Snyder-Ramos SA, Finegan BA, Mohnle P, Hantler CB, Bottiger BW, Latimer RD, Browner WS, Levin J, Mangano DT. Coronary artery bypass graft surgery—care globalization:the impact of national care on fatal and nonfatal outcome. J Thorac Cardiovasc Surg. 2007;133:1242–51.

86. Mangano DT, Miao Y, Vuylsteke A, Tudor IC, Juneja R, Filipescu D, Hoeft A, Fontes ML, Hillel Z, Ott E, Titov T, Dietzel C, Levin J. Mortality associated with aprotinin during 5 years following coronary artery bypass graft surgery. JAMA. 2007;297:471–9.

87. Schneeweiss S, Seeger JD, Landon J, Walker AM. Aprotinin during coronary-artery bypass grafting and risk of death. N Engl J Med. 2008;358:771–83.

88. Fergusson DA, Hebert PC, Mazer CD, Fremes S, MacAdams C, Murkin JM, Teoh K, Duke PC, Arellano R, Blajchman MA, Bussieres JS, Cote D, Karski J, Martineau R, Robblee JA, Rodger M, Wells G, Clinch J, Pretorius R. A comparison of aprotinin and lysine analogues in high-risk cardiac surgery. N Engl J Med. 2008;358:2319–31.

89. McMullan V, Alston RP III. Aprotinin and cardiac surgery: a sorry tale of evidence misused. Br J Anaesth. 2013;110:675–8.

90. The Committee of the Association of Cardiothoracic Anaesthetists. Statement on the use of aprotinin in cardiac surgery 2011. Available from http://www.acta.org.uk/store/docs/publications/ACTA_aprotinin_response_160306–762321–31–08-2011.pdf (accessed 8 July 2012).

91. Health Canada. Final report—expert advisory panel on Trasylol (aprotinin) 2011. Available from http://hc-sc.gc.ca/dhp-mps/medeff/advise-consult/eap-gce_trasylol/final_rep-rap-eng.phpn (accessed 8 July 2012).

92. European Medicines Agency. European Medicines Agency recommends lifting suspension of aprotinin 2012. Available from http://www.ema.europa.eu/docs/en_GB/document_library/Press_release/2012/02/WC500122914.pdf (accessed 4 May 2012).

93. Henry DA, Carless PA, Moxey AJ, O'Connell D, Stokes BJ, Fergusson DA, Ker K. Anti-fibrinolytic use for minimising perioperative allogeneic blood transfusion. Cochrane database of systematic reviews 2011: CD001886.

94. Takagi H, Manabe H, Kawai N, Goto SN, Umemoto T. Aprotinin increases mortality as compared with tranexamic acid in cardiac surgery: a meta-analysis of randomized head-to-head trials. Interact Cardiovasc Thorac Surg. 2009;9:98–101.

95. Devereaux PJ, Yang H, Guyatt GH, Leslie K, Villar JC, Monteri VM, Choi P, Giles JW, Yusuf S. Rationale, design, and organization of the PeriOperative ISchemic Evaluation (POISE) trial: a randomized controlled trial of metoprolol versus placebo in patients undergoing noncardiac surgery. Am Heart J. 2006;152:223–30.

96. Devereaux PJ, Yang H, Yusuf S, Guyatt G, Leslie K, Villar JC, Xavier D, Chrolavicius S, Greenspan L, Pogue J, Pais P, Liu L, Xu S, Malaga G, Avezum A, Chan M, Montori VM, Jacka M, Choi P. Effects of extended-release metoprolol succinate in patients undergoing non-cardiac surgery (POISE trial): a randomised controlled trial. Lancet. 2008;371:1839–47.

97. Devereaux PJ, Beattie WS, Choi PT, Badner NH, Guyatt GH, Villar JC, Cina CS, Leslie K, Jacka MJ, Montori VM, Bhandari M, Avezum A, Cavalcanti AB, Giles JW, Schricker T, Yang H, Jakobsen CJ, Yusuf S. How strong is the evidence for the use of perioperative beta blockers in non-cardiac surgery? Systematic review and meta-analysis of randomised controlled trials. BMJ. 2005;331:313–21.

98. Pronovost P, Needham D, Berenholtz S, Sinopoli D, Chu H, Cosgrove S, Sexton B, Hyzy R, Welsh R, Roth G, Bander J, Kepros J, Goeschel C. An intervention to decrease catheter-related bloodstream infections in the ICU. N Engl J Med. 2006;355:2725–32.

99. Koff MD, Loftus RW, Burchman CC, Schwartzman JD, Read ME, Henry ES, Beach ML. Reduction in intraoperative bacterial contamination of peripheral intravenous tubing through the use of a novel device. Anesthesiology. 2009;110:978–85.

100. Exadaktylos AK, Buggy DJ, Moriarty DC, Mascha E, Sessler DI. Can anesthetic technique for primary breast cancer surgery affect recurrence or metastasis? Anesthesiology. 2006;105:660–4.

101. Snyder GL, Greenberg S. Effect of anaesthetic technique and other perioperative factors on cancer recurrence. BJA. 2010;105:106–15.

102. Tsui BC, Rashiq S, Schopflocher D, Murtha A, Broemling S, Pillay J, Finucane BT. Epidural anesthesia and cancer recurrence rates after radical prostatectomy. Can J Anaesth. 2010;57:107–12.

103. Kavanagh T, Buggy DJ. Can anaesthetic technique effect postoperative outcome? Curr Opin Anaesthesiol. 2012;25:185–98.

104. Sessler DI, Ben-Eliyahu S, Mascha EJ, Parat MO, Buggy DJ. Can regional analgesia reduce the risk of recurrence after breast cancer? Methodology of a multicenter randomized trial. Contemp Clin Trials. 2008;29:517–26.

105. Wallace A, Fontes M, Mathew J, Sonntag H, Scholz J, Drenger B, Tonner P, Wang S. The association of the pattern of use of anti-ischemic agents on morbidity and mortality after coronary artery bypass surgery. ASA Abstracts, 2003.

106. Wallace AW, Au S, Cason BA. Perioperative beta-blockade: atenolol is associated with reduced mortality when compared to metoprolol. Anesthesiology. 2011;114:824–36.

107. Kertai MD, Boersma E, Westerhout CM, Klein J, Van Urk H, Bax JJ, Roelandt JR, Poldermans D. A combination of statins and beta-blockers is independently associated with a reduction in the incidence of perioperative mortality and nonfatal myocardial infarction in patients undergoing abdominal aortic aneurysm surgery. Eur J Vasc Endovasc Surg. 2004;28:343–52.

108. Nguyen HP, Zaroff JG, Bayman EO, Gelb AW, Todd MM, Hindman BJ. Perioperative hypothermia (33 degrees C) does not increase the occurrence of cardiovascular events in patients undergoing cerebral aneurysm surgery: findings from the Intraoperative Hypothermia for Aneurysm Surgery Trial. Anesthesiology. 2010;113:327–42.

A History of Pharmacogenomics Related to Anesthesiology

44

John C. Kraft, Jerry Kim, Debra A. Schwinn and Ruth Landau

Summary

Medical genetics began with the twentieth century rediscovery of Gregor Mendel's nineteenth century work on plant genetics [1]. In the early 1900s, British scientist Archibald Garrod made the first major advance in human genetics by identifying inborn errors of metabolism as a recessive trait [2], leading to George Beadle and Edward Tatum's 1941 promulgation of the 'one gene, one enzyme' theory [3]. In a landmark 1949 paper [4], Linus Pauling's group linked sickle cell anemia to a specific protein derangement, the first proof that genetic changes could produce human disease. This set the stage for the birth of pharmacogenetics, described by Arno Motulsky in 1957 [5], named by Friedrich Vogel in 1959 [6], and established by Werner Kalow's monograph in 1962 [7]. The next sections of this history provide exemplars of pharmacogenetic discoveries having major implications in anesthesia.

Introduction

Approximately 50 years ago, pharmacogenetics (defined as how genetic makeup may influence response to a drug) began to be applied to explain drug action in humans, increasingly revealing that genetic variation present in deoxyribonucleic acid (DNA) ultimately determines drug metabolism and effectiveness via encoded proteins, providing hope that individually tailored medical therapy might improve outcome and safety, the essence of personalized medicine. We begin with the birth of pharmacogenetics and continue by describing events surrounding clinical observations on 3 genetic pathologies important in anesthesiology: prolonged apnea with succinylcholine, malignant hyperthermia, and hepatic drug metabolism by a cytochrome P450 (CYP) enzyme CYP2D6 (Fig. 44.1). Next, we highlight some pharmacogenetic studies, particularly genetic variation in adrenergic and opioid receptor genes, followed by reflections on how modern genome science methods may provide insights that underlie aspects of perioperative patient care. We conclude by discussing future directions.

Prolonged Apnea After Succinylcholine

The depolarizing muscle relaxant succinylcholine entered clinical practice in 1951. Paralysis from succinylcholine peaks in approximately 45 seconds and usually lasts for 2 to 6 minutes, convenient for facilitating tracheal intubation. In 1952, anesthesiologists reported rare cases of prolonged paralysis after its use. Biochemical studies revealed why. Plasma butyrylcholinesterase (BChE, also called pseudocholinesterase) hydrolyzes succinylcholine to inactive components. Succinylcholine acts quickly and briefly in individuals with normal BChE activity, but abnormal BChE activity in 1:2500 (0.04%) of Caucasians [8, 9] prolongs succinylcholine activity—and paralysis—by 5 to 10-fold. In 1952, Bourne et al. [10] reported that "those patients who recover slowly from succinylcholine had significantly lower pseudocholinesterase levels than did patients recovering at the normal speed." Lehmann and Evans, and Kalow independently established the mechanism. Lehmann's group detected decreased levels of BChE in patients with prolonged paralysis [11], leading to their suggestion that a genetic cause, rather than chronic disease or chemical

R. Landau (✉)
Obstetric Anesthesia & Clinical Genetics Research, Department of Anesthesiology & Pain Medicine,University of Washington, Box 356540, 1959 NE Pacific Street HSB, BB-1415, Seattle, WA, USA
e-mail: n.franks@imperial.ac.uk

J. C. Kraft
Department of Anesthesiology & Pain Medicine, University of Washington, Box 356540, 1959 NE Pacific Street, BB-1469, Seattle, WA 98195-6540, USA

J. Kim
Department of Anesthesiology & Pain Medicine, Seattle Children's Hospital, University of Washington, Box 356540, 1959 NE Pacific Street, BB-1469, Seattle, WA 98195-6540, USA

D. A. Schwinn
The University of Iowa
212 CMAB, 451 Newton Road
Iowa City, Iowa 52242-1101, USA
e-mail: debra-schwinn@uiowa.edu

E. I Eger II et al. (eds.), *The Wondrous Story of Anesthesia*, DOI 10.1007/978-1-4614-8441-7_44, © Edmond I Eger, MD 2014

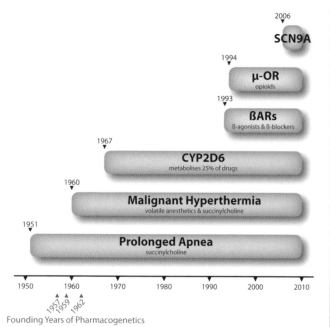

Fig. 44.1 Historical overview of influence of pharmacogenetics on anesthesia. *ßARs* β-adrenergic receptors, *μ-OR* μ-opioid receptor, *SCN9A* sodium channel mutation

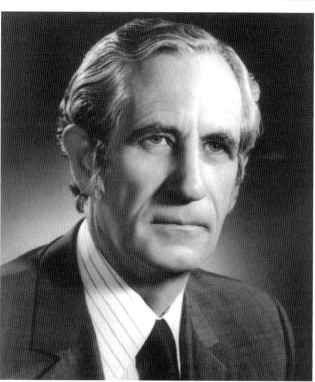

Fig. 44.2 Werner Kalow (1917–2008) joined the University of Toronto, Canada, in 1951, and remained active in academics as a pharmacologist until the year of his death. (From Kalow W: Atypical plasma cholinesterase. A personal discovery story: a tale of three cities. Can J Anaesth 2004; 51: 206–11, with permission.)

poisoning, altered BChE activity. In their 1956 landmark publication, Lehmann and Evans investigated families of 5 unrelated patients having prolonged responses to succinylcholine [12], finding otherwise healthy family members with low BChE activity without any reason for such levels. These findings provided a genetic link to prolonged paralysis after succinylcholine.

In 1951, Werner Kalow (Fig. 44.2) proved that procaineesterase was actually BChE. He provided a more efficient method to measure esterase activity. Serendipitously, he contacted Donald Gunn, a physician using low-dose succinylcholine to dampen muscular contractions during electric shock therapy. Gunn noted that a few patients remained relaxed for almost an hour rather than 2 to 6 minutes. Kalow discovered that BChE enzymes from 2 of these patients behaved differently from normal BChE, and inferred that a genetic change caused a structural difference in the enzyme. In the families of these two patients, Kalow found differential inhibition of BChE by a local anesthetic called dibucaine (also known as cinchocaine or nupercaine). Dibucaine inhibited 79 % of normal BChE activity. In both parents of the two patients, inhibition was only 62 %, and minimal inhibition (16 %) occurred in patients having a prolonged effect of succinylcholine. Such patients had two abnormal genes for BChE (homozygous trait); the parents were heterozygous with one normal and one abnormal gene, and the average person had two normal genes. Succinylcholine was one of the first drugs whose metabolism was shown to be affected by genes displaying simple Mendelian patterns of inheritance [13].

Kalow and his co-workers then demonstrated that individuals having a prolonged response to succinylcholine had abnormally functioning BChE rather than a low quantity of enzyme. They had a genetically determined defect in BChE—a so-called dibucaine resistant enzyme, or atypical enzyme—causing the abnormal reaction to succinylcholine. Kalow's use of dibucaine inhibition percentage remains the standard for classifying heterozygous, homozygous, and wild-type phenotypes of BChE. His findings and his study of other examples of varied responses to drugs, motivated him to write his 1962 book "Pharmacogenetics: Heredity and the Response to Drugs" [7] establishing pharmacogenetics as a new scientific discipline. Subsequently, over 40 polymorphisms associated with BChE deficiency were described, the most common being the A and the K enzyme variants. The A (for "atypical") variant has an altered activity while the K variant (after Kalow) results in a lesser production of enzyme. Although prolonged paralysis following succinylcholine is now a rare but easily managed clinical problem, the finding of prolonged muscle relaxation with succinylcholine in specific individuals provided the first evidence for serious clinical effects from genetic variation, and highlighted anesthesiology as a discipline wherein genetics had immediate clinical implications.

Malignant Hyperthermia

Succinylcholine contributed to another anesthesia-related pharmacogenetic discovery. Malignant hyperthermia (MH) is an uncommon adverse pharmacogenetic syndrome associated with administration of succinylcholine and/or inhaled volatile anesthetics [14]. The mechanism triggering this reaction remains unknown (severe stress alone can trigger MH). When triggered, MH increases cytosolic Ca^{2+} in skeletal muscle cells, and this increase can produce hyperthermia, hypermetabolism, muscle rigidity, breakdown of muscle tissue, and death [15].

Here is the story of the discovery of MH. On 8 April 1960, a car hit a 21 year old student, fracturing his right tibia and fibula [16]. Upon arrival at the casualty department of the Royal Melbourne Hospital, in Victoria, Australia, he and his mother expressed more concern about the anesthesia than his leg. Ten family members (3 cousins and 7 aunts and uncles), out of 38, had died during or shortly after receiving ether anesthesia. This family history caused the student's mother to request a local anesthetic when the boy had an appendectomy at age 12. The consultant anesthesiologist on 8 April was James Villiers. Having heard the story, he and the surgeon learned that the patient's cousin had recently been safely anesthetized with a "modern anesthetic" at the nearby children's hospital. After excluding porphyria, the only condition known at the time to affect anesthesia, Villiers believed that the deaths must have been due to "ether convulsions" and recommended using a new, possibly safer anesthetic, halothane—plus vigilant monitoring. Ten minutes into anesthesia, hypotension, tachycardia, cyanosis, and hyperventilation occurred, and the soda lime canister became very hot. The fractures were quickly set, and anesthesia administration discontinued. The patient remained cyanotic and unresponsive and became hot and sweaty. He was immediately packed in ice from a nearby cardiac theater, and within an hour, he was awake and alert. His subsequent course was uneventful. He was the first recorded patient to have had—and survive—MH [17].

Villiers referred the patient to Richard Lovell, who, in turn asked his research assistant, Michael Denborough (Fig. 44.3), to see the patient. Denborough had an interest in genetics, and the familial history led him to suspect a previously unrecognized inborn error of metabolism. When the student again required anesthesia for an impacted renal calculus in 1961, John Forster of the Royal Melbourne Hospital gave him an uneventful spinal anesthetic [16].

In 1964, deaths were noted to have occurred during anesthesia in a large Wisconsin (USA) family. One child had died in Toronto, Canada, and Beverly Britt, the anesthesiologist, along with Kalow and RA Gordon, a professor of anesthesia, organized inquiries throughout Canada. This led to presentation of 13 cases of MH at a 1966 symposium in Toronto [18].

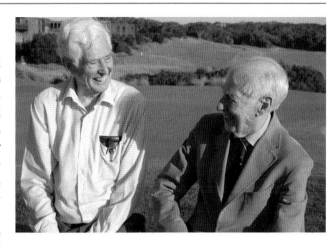

Fig. 44.3 Michael Denborough (*left*) and James Villiers (*right*), photographed in 2012. (Courtesy of Christine Ball)

These patients had evinced two common features: muscle rigidity and high temperature. The first description in the American literature of a patient with MH, with reported blood gas data, was similar to that of Villiers in that the patient survived after being packed in ice [19]. When this case was presented at the annual American Medical Association meeting, several in the audience reported caring for similar patients who had received halothane and succinylcholine.

In November 1969, a patient at the Royal Melbourne Hospital received halothane and succinylcholine and died from MH [20]. This patient's right arm had became rigid, prompting a test of plasma creatine kinase activity, an enzyme involved in energy production in muscle fibers. Creatine kinase activity was increased, indicating muscle breakdown. The original student who had broken his leg in 1960, and some of his relatives also were found to have increased serum creatine kinase activity—evidence of a generalized muscular disease [21]. In 1970, in Johannesburg South Africa, H Isaacs and M Barlow independently observed increased serum creatine kinase levels in relatives of MH patients [22]. Impressed by the muscle rigidity, Kalow and Britt tested their muscle samples for contractile force *in vitro*. Muscle from patients with MH exhibited abnormally strong contractions in the presence of caffeine. Caffeine was used because it induces *in vitro* skeletal muscle contraction. This resulted in the first clinically useful test for detection of a predisposition to MH in 1970 [23]. In 1971, F Ellis and colleagues showed that halothane augments muscle contraction in patients who are susceptible to MH [24].

In the early 2000s, molecular genetic testing for MH susceptibility was introduced in Europe [25] and North America [14]. The genetic assessments were based on DNA sequence variations in the skeletal muscle type ryanodine receptor (*RYR1*) gene, which encodes a protein involved in the excitation-contraction process of muscle cells. In 1990, MacLennan *et al.* had identified the *RYR1* gene as a candidate gene that might mediate MH [26]. More than 180 *RYR1* variants have since been documented, with 29 considered mutations predisposing to MH [27, 28]. In 2001, the European Malignant Hyperthermia Group published criteria for proof of causation, and agreed on guidelines for molecular genetic detection for susceptibility to MH. These guidelines are the first to describe genetic screening for testing in anesthesiology [25, 29, 30].

CYP2D6 Enzyme Variation

The next pharmacogenetic discovery relevant to anesthesia came in the late 1960s, in association with a description of an enzyme, now called CYP2D6. CYP2D6 affects metabolism of 25% of the drugs used in medicine, including anesthesiology [31]. CYP2D6 is part of a family of cytochrome P450 (CYP) drug metabolizing enzymes, enzymes involved in metabolism of morphine derivatives, β-blockers, antiarrhythmics, antipsychotics, and antiemetic drugs [31]. Polymorphisms (specific variations in protein structure and function) in *CYP2D6* can affect drug efficacy, side effects, and toxicity. Beginning in 1967, 3 laboratories independently discovered polymorphic CYP2D6.

Folk Sjöqvists' group in Sweden found that metabolism of two CYP2D6 substrates showed considerable inter-individual variation in metabolite plasma levels. Two phenotypes were identified in 1967 [32]. Studies in 19 identical (monozygotic) and 20 fraternal (dizygotic) sets of twins in 1969, suggested the difference was gene-based [33].

At St. Mary's Medical School in London in 1975, Robert Smith studied debrisoquine, a new agent for treating hypertension. Several healthy volunteers, including Smith, received 40 mg of debrisoquine. Everyone but Smith seemed unfazed by the injection, but Smith became severely hypotensive and collapsed. He recovered fully, but his startling reaction prompted further investigation, revealing that his debrisoquine hydroxylase, the enzyme that metabolizes debrisoquine, eliminated only 10% of the drug. The normal enzyme eliminates 80%. Smith then identified 2 medical students with deficient debrisoquine hydroxylase, traced the family histories, and found that the trait was inherited. His team then tested hundreds of volunteers, discovering that 1 in 10 developed hypotension after debrisoquine. Although 10% of the population were homozygous carriers, 45% were heterozygote carriers of the deficient gene and could transmit it to their children. Smith's observations had uncovered a mechanism explaining numerous adverse drug reactions [34].

Finally, Michel Eichelbaum's group in Bonn, Germany, studied the antiarrhythmic effects of sparteine [35]. Two subjects complained of double vision, blurred vision, dizziness, and headache after receiving the drug. Both had 4–5 times higher sparteine plasma levels than other individuals, demonstrating a defect in the capacity to oxidize some drugs, a defect inherited as an autosomal recessive trait. In 1980, Bertilsson *et al.* in Sweden showed that subjects having an impaired metabolism of debrisoquine, also had an impaired metabolism of sparteine [36]. Also in 1980, Kalow found that students of European *versus* Chinese descent differed in their capacity to metabolize debrisoquine and sparteine [37], the first observation of inter-ethnic differences in drug metabolism. Debrisoquine and sparteine metabolism were suspected to be genetically linked [38]. A search then began for the gene underlying their variable pharmacokinetics.

In 1985, Distlerath *et al.* purified the protein—CYP2D6—responsible for the altered metabolism from human liver microsomes [39]. In 1987, Eichelbaum *et al.* localized the gene encoding CYP2D6 to chromosome 22 [40]. CYP2D6 was the first polymorphic P450 to be characterized at a molecular level, initially identified as a gene responsible for altered metabolism of debrisoquine, sparteine, and other drugs [41]. Further study revealed that CYP2D6 is the only non-inducible enzyme of the P450 family of enzymes. Non-inducible means that it is constantly expressed rather than being turned on or off. As a result, a mutation of the enzyme may cause sustained inter-individual variation in enzyme activity [31]. Genotyping for CYP2D6 activity is drug specific, and the need for typing an individual is limited. If genotyping is needed, patients are assigned to one of four categories based on their ability to metabolize CYP2D6 substrates: ultrarapid metabolizers (UM), extensive metabolizers (EM), intermediate metabolizers (IM), and poor metabolizers (PM) [42]. PMs (two non-functional gene alleles) metabolize CYP2D6 substrates less well than their counterparts (IMs, EMs, UMs). UMs possess multiple functional copies of the same normal CYP2D6 gene, and an increase in the number of functional copies in an individual increases the rate of metabolism of CYP2D6 substrates (Fig. 44.4).

CYP2D6 genetic variations have other clinical implications. In 2006, Koren *et al.* [43] described a neonatal death leading to the suggestion that breastfeeding mothers taking codeine for postpartum pain should be genotyped for CYP2D6 activity. CYP2D6 O-demethylates codeine to morphine. Mothers and neonates that are CYP2D6 UMs or EMs may produce toxic blood levels of morphine or its active metabolite morphine-6-glucuronide (M6G). The infant in this case report was a CYP2D6 EM, and had a blood concentration of 70 ng/ml morphine; neonates breastfed by mothers receiving codeine normally have concentrations of 0–2.2 ng/ml [43]. The mother was a CYP2D6 UM, and her breast milk had 87 ng/ml morphine—the normal range being 1.9–20.5 ng/ml at doses of 60 mg codeine every 6 hours [43]. Thus the infant had 2 reasons for increased morphine levels. These findings and those from case-control studies [44] indi-

Fig. 44.4 CYP2D6 activity predicts ability to metabolize a wide range of drugs (see text for details). Clinical doses of nortriptyline (a tryicyclic antidepressant) to be used in different genotypes are indicated. (From Meyer UA: Pharmacogenetics—five decades of therapeutic lessons from genetic diversity. Nat Rev Genet 2004; 5: 669–76 with permission.)

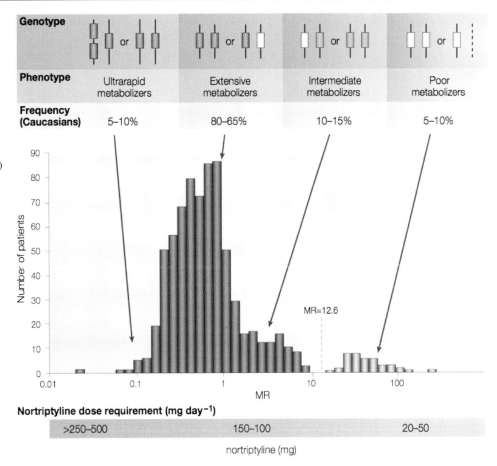

cate that codeine should be avoided in breastfeeding mothers with CYP2D6 EM and UM genotypes.

Genetics and Pharmacodynamic Variation

Pharmacokinetics (what the body does to a drug) and pharmacodynamics (what a drug does to the body) can influence the effectiveness and metabolism of medicines given to produce anesthesia. The previous section concentrated on pharmacokinetics, identifying genetic alterations in drug metabolizing enzymes that change circulating drug levels. The next section explores pharmacodynamic effects, specifically genetic variations in receptor proteins that may alter activation of signaling pathways, despite the presence of constant drug concentration. We present 3 clinically relevant examples.

β-Adrenergic Receptors and Altered Physiologic Responsiveness

β-adrenergic receptors (βARs) influence cardiac contractility, heart rate, and vessel dilation. Anesthesiologists use βAR agonists and antagonists to ensure intraoperative hemodynamic stability and improve perioperative outcome

[45]. β_2AR genetic variants, generally single nucleotide polymorphisms (SNPs), were initially identified in 1993 and 1994, and clinically relevant β_1AR SNPs were identified in 1999 and 2000 [46]. β_1AR and β_2AR antagonist therapy after acute myocardial infarction (MI) decreases *aggregate* patient mortality, a fact known for decades [47]. In 2005 Lanfear *et al.* [48] asked whether specific sub-groups of individuals benefited more than others, from βAR antagonist therapy. Examining four common β_1 and β_2AR SNPs, Lanfear found *increased* mortality with βAR blocker therapy in individuals with genetic variants in the gene encoding the β_2AR (*ADRB2*) (about 25 % of the acute MI population), whereas the remaining patients benefited. Such findings suggest that β_2AR DNA testing might indicate which patients should receive βAR antagonists after MI. If these findings are reproduced, such genetic testing would routinely precede the use of βAR antagonists after MI.

Airway hyper-reactivity associated with asthma is a concern to anesthesiologists. Bronchodilators prescribed to prevent or to treat airway hyper-reactivity interact with β_2ARs. In 1999, Lima *et al.* [49] reported that asthmatic subjects who were homozygous for the Arg16 wild-type (normal) allele in *ADRB2* (i.e., they had 2 copies of the normal gene), initially demonstrated enhanced responsiveness to β_2-agonist bronchodilators, compared to patients homozygous for the

Gly16 variant. However, this acute protective effect of Arg16 differed from results in studies assessing prolonged β-agonist therapy. In 2004, Israel *et al.* [50] showed that mildly asthmatic patients who were homozygous for Gly16, improved with long-term albuterol therapy, a result subsequently confirmed [51]. Our current understanding is that in Arg16 homozygous patients, long-acting β-agonist therapy may increase severe asthma exacerbations. Alternative treatment strategies may better help this subgroup of individuals [52]. This provides another example of how pharmacogenetics may help guide and/or facilitate alternative treatment strategies [53].

μ-Opioid Receptor Variation and Pain Medicine Effectiveness

Opium has been harvested from poppies and smoked to relieve pain and alter mentation for centuries. Morphine, codeine, and non-narcotic alkaloids come from this folk remedy. Opium is also the precursor for recreational drugs such as heroin. Morphine and other clinically relevant opioid analgesics primarily target the μ-opioid receptor (μOR), a receptor whose gene, *OPRM1*, varies extensively. In May of 1998, Wendel and Hoehe described the μOR gene (*OPRM1*) [54]. Three months later, Bond and her colleagues discovered a SNP at position 118 in 10% of their study population, and suggested that this A118G polymorphism (in which guanine substitutes for adenine at position 118 in the receptor protein) alters the extracellular binding site of the μOR, thereby changing the binding affinity of β-endorphins (the natural endogenous biochemical for the opioid receptors) as well as exogenous opioids [55]. Two reports of the functional consequence of the A118G genetic variant came in 2002. Wand *et al.* [56] found that healthy volunteers carrying the G118 variant, had increased cortisol responses when given the opioid-antagonist, naloxone. Days later, Lötsch *et al.* [57, 58] suggested that the A118G polymorphism protects against morphine-6-glucuronide toxicity.

Variants of the μOR gene may explain inter-individual responses to opioid analgesia [59]. An approach to examining the heritable component of pain perception and response to opioids has historically involved twin studies [60]. Other clinical studies relevant to anesthesia have examined the potential pharmacogenetic effect of the common A118G polymorphism, on the response to various opioids after surgery, or when given to women for labor pain during epidural analgesia. Importantly, the dose of intravenous morphine required by post-surgical patients has been shown to vary, based on an individual's μOR genotype [61]. Defining μOR genetic variants is needed to understand complex pain pathways, stratify pain phenotypes into their individual components, and create novel predictive genetic tests for use in pain medicine [62].

Sodium Channel Genetic Variants and Channelopathies

A rare, fascinating, and deadly condition preventing the perception of pain has enhanced our understanding of sodium channels' role in pain perception. It has also entered popular culture (see "The Girl Who Played with Fire" by Stieg Larsson). Survival and protection of the body demands the perception of pain (e.g., to remove one's fingers from a hot object). In 2006, Cox *et al.* [63] described the genetic basis of a congenital inability to experience pain. In unrelated consanguineous Pakistani families, Cox and colleagues identified 3 loss-of-function mutations of *SCN9A*, a gene encoding for the alpha subunit of the voltage-gated $Na_v1.7$ sodium channel, which, along with other voltage-gated sodium channels, subserves the generation and conduction of action potentials that mediate pain. Isolated patients and families subsequently demonstrated similar mutations [64–66]. Presently 15 loss-of-function recessive trait mutations of the channelopathy-associated insensitivity to pain phenotype are known [66].

Genetic and Genomic Methods, Tools, and Their Impact

Variation in response to disease onset and severity, or to drug treatments, may result from augmenting/dampening of cascades of genes. Animal models have facilitated examination of the effect of genetic variability in the context of a whole organism. We now review some of the most common of these non-human models to see how they have advanced the field.

Classic Non-Human Models

The study of genetics began with Mendel's observations of pea plants. Animal models—rats, cats, dogs, and monkeys—have also been used. The most commonly used models today include the nematode Caenorhabditis elegans (C. *elegans*), the fruitfly Drosophila melanogaster (D. *melanogaster*), and genetically engineered mice (knock-out and transgenic mice). These models reflect key discoveries in medicine, as acknowledged by several Nobel Prizes. Below we summarize advances related to the understanding of genetics and anesthetic mechanisms for each of these classic genetic models.

C. *elegans* is a transparent roundworm approximately 1 mm long. It reproduces rapidly allowing generations to be studied quickly. This simple organism was the first multicellular organism with a nervous system to have its genome completely sequenced. Under normal conditions C. *elegans* is almost constantly moving. When exposed to a volatile anesthetic, after an initial phase of increased locomotion, uncoordinated motion progresses to immobility. When *C. elegans* is removed from the anesthetic, motion returns quickly. Phil Morgan and Helmut Cascorbi first described this model as a tool to study the mechanism of action of volatile anesthetics in 1985 [67]. Over the last two decades, Mike Crowder, Phil Morgan, and Marge Sedensky applied this model to study those mechanisms [68]. The two most common endpoints used to measure anesthetic effects in *C. elegans* have been uncoordination (or change in motion caused by anesthetic exposure), and immobility. The mechanisms of the two anesthetic actions are distinct and most likely reflect different aspects of the complex behavioral effects.

Mutations in neuronal proteins (called syntaxin) of *C elegans* significantly alter the sensitivity to volatile anesthetics (a 33-fold range of sensitivity for isoflurane), suggesting that syntaxin is a possible target of volatile anesthetics. Overall, genetic studies suggest that a vast group of molecular targets or pathways determine anesthetic sensitivity. More recent studies have identified additional sites of action of volatile anesthetics, including ion channels and mitochondrial proteins. The implication that mitochondria were involved in anesthetic sensitivity was highlighted by the observation that children anesthetized with sevoflurane to perform muscle biopsies for the diagnosis of suspected mitochondrial defects, had different anesthetic responses as a function of their mitochondrial function. Modification of genes have been used to create anesthesia sensitive and resistant worms, facilitating exploration of mechanisms of anesthetic action [68], such as identifying most recently that complex I of the electron transport chains (ETC) is a possible target of volatile anesthetics [69].

Physical characteristics of *D. melanogaster* such as eye bristles, wing patterns, antenna, and patterns on the head and thorax have been used as phenotypic markers for alterations in specific genes. As with *C. elegans*, the entire genome and several variants of *D. melanogaster* have been sequenced in the last decade. Howard Nash at the NIH, discovered strains of *D. melanogaster* that were either sensitive or resistant to inhaled anesthetics [70]. Genes that regulate states of arousal, gene copy number, and unusual ion channels that serve as a depolarizing leak may underlie resistance and sensitivity. The *D. melanogaster* nervous system stays active during anesthesia and in this, and overall conservation of genes and their function, provides parallels with the human nervous system.

Some of the yet unresolved questions about the mechanism of action of anesthesia are related to the fact that (1) the numerous endpoints associated with the anesthetic state are probably the result of effects at different sites of anesthetic action, (2) 'immobility' as observed in nematodes doesn't reflect the state of 'loss of consciousness and perception of pain' that is the goal of anesthesia, and (3)

genetic studies do not explore all the pathways involved in mechanism of action, such as regulation that occurs downstream.

Mario Capecchi, Martin Evans and Oliver Smithies received the Nobel Prize in Medicine for their 1989 creation of the first knockout mouse, a mouse lacking a specific gene. By inactivating a specific gene, and observing the consequent differences in physiologic expression and phenotype, the function of the gene can be inferred. These models have been used to further our understanding of human biology, including mechanisms of anesthetic action [71]. Such genetic manipulation allows a controlled change heretofore only available as natural variations as described above (e.g., consider the natural variations in the opioid receptor). Knockout mice have been used to assess the relevance of numerous ligand- and voltage-gated channels to mediate the effects of inhaled anesthetics, particularly their capacity to produce immobility in the face of noxious stimulation. However, despite high hopes, a review by Sonner in 2003 [72] and a follow-up review by Eger in 2008 [73] do not suggest that the hopes have been realized. Why? Knockout of a gene affects but one ion channel, and then only one member of what may be a large family. What if anesthesia results from actions on multiple channels? And the body may compensate for the loss of function produced by a knockout, obscuring the consequences of the knockout.

A potential solution to the issue of compensation lies in the use of knockin mice. In contrast to knockout mice, the targeted gene allows the production of an altered channel that responds normally (it is hoped!) to its ligand (e.g., glycine or GABA) but not to, say, an anesthetic. In the early 1990s, several investigators, notably Gregg Homanics, Neil Harrison and Adron Harris produced such mutations and engineered knockin mice from them. In 1997, John Mihic from Harris' laboratory described such a mutation for glycine and GABA [74]. A $GABA_A1$ knockin mouse was made from this mutation. However, a 2007 report on the resulting mouse did not reveal that it was resistant to the immobilizing effect of isoflurane [75]. Results from this mouse suggested that it was resistant to the amnestic effects of isoflurane. One step at a time!

In contrast to the slow progress with inhaled anesthetics, a knockin mouse allowed a dramatic insight into the mechanism underlying one aspect of the actions of etomidate and propofol. In 1999, Uwe Rudolph suggested that the actions of benzodiazepines might lie in specific parts of the $GABA_A$ receptor [76]. Building on this, in a 2003 landmark report, Rachel Jurd from Rudolph's laboratory found that the immobilizing action of etomidate and propofol were virtually eliminated in a knockin mouse in which the response to GABA was "normal", but the capacity of etomidate and propofol to enhance the response of the GABAA receptor was abolished [77].

Human Genetic Studies

Human genetic studies "associate" specific genetic variants and the ensuing altered biologic pathways, with endpoints such as occurrence of disease, altered response to drugs, or death. Three prerequisites must be satisfied to yield meaningful findings: (1) robust clinical phenotyping (e.g., quantifiable physiologic parameters such as blood pressure or heart rate change, pharmacological responses; and/or long term clinical outcomes), (2) expert biostatistical analysis including statistical genetics, and, (3) high quality genetic analysis (i.e. genotyping, sequencing, and genome wide association studies).

Clinical Phenotyping

Specific measures, including vital signs, pain scores, blood chemistries and plasma drug concentrations, can define clinical phenotypes. To be valid, such measures must be reproducible within a given individual. Since many genetic effects are small and additive, "crisp" detailed clinical phenotypes are essential for a valid clinical genetics study. However, "mined" DNA databases combined with vaguely measured phenotypes have had limited power. Well designed genetic association studies that examined cardiovascular outcomes from medication choice usually result in clinically useful findings [48], but reliable and applicable findings have been elusive in studies of genetic influences on pain perception and response to analgesics [78]. Conflicting outcomes in pain studies examining the effect of the A118G polymorphism may relate to the use of subjective visual analog scores rather than measurable outcomes such as blood pressure. In addition to this inter-person variability, there is also complexity underlying the pain phenotype (multifactorial, highly subjective, various pain modalities—experimental pain, labor pain, acute post-operative pain, ischemic pain, inflammatory pain and of course chronic pain).

Integration of Animal and Human Genetic Studies

One method connecting animal models to human disease first identifies relevant genes and proteins in humans, then studies their mechanistic effects in animal models, and finally translates such information back to the clinic to improve outcomes. Jeffrey Mogil, at McGill University proposed such a paradigm for pain research [79]. His work largely focuses on the second step of this paradigm and the human association studies required for translation into the clinic. Mogil *et al.'s* 2003 publication [80] presented a translation of genetic findings from rodent models examining several genetic variants to humans. Women with two variant alleles of the *MC1R* (melanocortin-1 receptor) gene, which deter-

mine fair skin, and red hair [81], and immunomodulation [82], had increased sensitivity to a κ-opioid drug. But drugs acting at the μ-opioid receptor, not the κ-opioid receptor, represent the mainstay of clinical treatment of moderate to severe pain. So Mogil performed an analogous study in 2005 [83] with the μ-opioid receptor morphine metabolite, morphine-6-glucuronide (M6G). Human redheads inheriting two or more inactivating variants of the *MC1R* gene had increased analgesic responsiveness to M6G. In the same year, Liem and colleagues [84] observed that lidocaine was less effective in preventing pain in redheaded women. Also in 2003, Mogil observed that drugs from diverse neurochemical classes (e.g., μ-opioid, κ-opioid, cannabinoid, nicotinic, and α$_2$-adrenergic) had high genetic correlations: mouse strains were either sensitive or resistant to analgesia, regardless of the drug used. This suggests that analgesic pathways may interact to confer sensitivity across drug classes [79].

The next step was high throughput discovery of the involved genes. In 2007, Mogil created the *PainGenes Database* [85], an open-to-all interactive online database cataloging genes whose null mutant has a published pain related phenotype. Each gene and phenotype is derived from knockout mice studies reporting changes in either nociceptive or analgesic sensitivity. It remains to be seen whether the *PainGenes Database* will facilitate translation of pharmacogenetic studies into clinical trials and clinical care.

Exercise to Exhaustion

Are the patterns of the stress response to major surgery in humans unique to surgery or seen with all extremes of human physiology? This is one of multiple questions raised by anesthesiologists and scientists interested in the parallels that can be drawn between the peri-operative period as a model of acute stress, and other 'stressors' that individuals may experience in their life. Studies in the 2000s of exercise to exhaustion, suggest commonalities with perioperative stress. Half-marathon runners have been examined before a race, immediately after the race, and 24 hours later for inflammatory markers. Peripheral blood mononuclear cells (PMBCs) have been examined using a microarray approach, showing upregulation of mitogen-activated protein kinase-activated protein kinase-2 (MAPKAP-K2), L-selectin, IL-1 receptor antagonist (IL-1ra), and thioredoxin (which may play a role in oxidant defense), as well as downregulation of CD81 (which promotes B and T cell activation and T cell maturation) [86]. Others have found increases in cortisol and adrenaline [87, 88], increased cytokines in plasma or urine (levels which decrease by the following day) [89–95], and generation of reactive oxygen/nitrogen species [96]. Acute endurance exercise also affects gene expression of metabolic transcriptional co-activators and transcription factors [97]. Such effects on the immune system and inflammation suggest that exhaustive exercise produces findings similar to those from perioperative stresses.

Sepsis

Similarly, in the 2000s, it was found that severe sepsis provides another challenge to human physiology, paralleling perioperative stresses. The inflammatory response to sepsis was studied by administering bacterial endotoxin IV over 24h to healthy volunteers with measurements of the resulting acute-phase cytokines in serum [98]. And a network-based approach was used to define biologic targets from 200,000 published articles [99]. In general [99], 2–4 hours post endotoxin, secreted proinflammatory cytokines and chemokines increased, consistent with early activation of innate immunity. The 4 to 6h post endotoxin time was critical, with increased expression of transcription factors, both those that initiated and those that limited immune response. In summary, although sepsis provides an initial activation of innate immunity, the resultant whole body response to the stress of infection is remarkably similar to that found in cardiac surgery or exhaustive exercise models. This suggests that, independent of the insult, the human stress response triggers identical changes in genes, proteins, and metabolites.

Gene Expression Studies of Myocardial Preconditioning

In 1986, Murry and co-workers reported that exposure of the heart to a short episode of ischemia/reperfusion affords protection against a subsequent more prolonged period of ischemia. In 1997, Cason's group showed that cardioprotection from "ischemic preconditioning" can also be achieved by administration of isoflurane [100]. In the next few years, other potent inhaled anesthetics were also shown to produce this phenomenon [101]. Indeed, hundreds of reports have appeared showing prolonged protection by diverse inhaled anesthetics. The prolonged nature of protection implies a genetic up or down regulation. Regulation of potassium channels and a recently emerging understanding of the important role of mitochondrial homeostasis, in dampening oxygen free-radical cascades leading to cell apoptosis and death, underlie the protection. Microarrays have been applied to evaluate organ-specific responses to surgical stress, and CPB with cardioplegic arrest [102]. These studies have identified different transcriptional programs activated in ischemic *versus* anesthetic preconditioning, the differential activation resulting in distinct cardioprotective phenotypes [103]. Similarly, characteristic gene expression patterns have been

described in chronic ischemia that differ from those found in experimental induced ischemic preconditioning [104, 105].

Conclusion

Genetics and genomic medicine can be important to anesthesia-related clinical care. Genetic studies have revealed mechanisms underlying malignant hyperthermia, have given us the dibucaine number for testing for the presence of an impairment in succinylcholine degradation, and have aided our understanding of mechanisms of anesthesia action and/or effectiveness of drugs used to induce the anesthetic state. Genetic studies can explain outliers and the "bell-shaped curve" of clinical responses. Our application of genetics to anesthetic delivery will advance in tandem with technical advances such as rapid and relatively inexpensive sequencing of individual genomes. Genetic diagnostics and pharmacogenetic predictions will increasingly define anesthetic practice.

Acknowledgements The authors thank Arno Motulsky for his critical reading of the manuscript and for granting a personal interview where he provided insights into the history and future of pharmacogenetics. We are grateful for his historic contributions to genomic science, and we are honored to have him contribute to this manuscript. The authors also thank Gary Peltz for granting a personal interview and allowing a close examination of his research.

References

1. Weber WW. Pharmacogenetics. New York: Oxford University Press; 1997.
2. Garrod AE. Inborn Errors of Metabolism. London: Oxford University Press; 1909.
3. Beadle GW, Tatum EL. Genetic control of biochemical reactions in neurospora. Proc Natl Acad Sci U S A. 1941;27:499–506.
4. Pauling L, Itano HA, et al. Sickle cell anemia, a molecular disease. Science. 1949;110:543–8.
5. Motulsky AG. Drug reactions enzymes, and biochemical genetics. J Am Med Assoc. 1957;165:835–7.
6. Vogel F. Moderne Problem der Humangenetik. Ergeb Inn Med U Kinderheilk. 1959;12:52–125.
7. Kalow W. Pharmacogenetics; heredity and the response to drugs. Philadelphia: W.B. Saunders Co.; 1962
8. Lockridge O, Masson P. Pesticides and susceptible populations: people with butyrylcholinesterase genetic variants may be at risk. Neurotoxicology. 2000;21:113–26.
9. Ostergaard D, Jensen FS, Jensen E, Skovgaard LT, Viby-Mogensen J. Mivacurium-induced neuromuscular blockade in patients with atypical plasma cholinesterase. Acta Anaesthesiol Scand. 1993;37:314–8.
10. Bourne JG, Collier HO, Somers GF. Succinylcholine (succinoylcholine), muscle-relaxant of short action. Lancet. 1952;1:1225–9.
11. Evans FT, Gray PW, Lehmann H, Silk E. Sensitivity to succinylcholine in relation to serum-cholinesterase. Lancet. 1952;1:1229–30.
12. Lehmann H, Ryan E. The familial incidence of low pseudocholinesterase level. Lancet. 1956;268:124.
13. Kalow W. Atypical plasma cholinesterase. A personal discovery story: a tale of three cities. Can J Anaesth. 2004;51:206–11.

14. Litman RS, Rosenberg H. Malignant hyperthermia: update on susceptibility testing. JAMA. 2005;293:2918–24.
15. Parness J, Bandschapp O, Girard T. The myotonias and susceptibility to malignant hyperthermia. Anesth Analg. 2009;109:1054–64.
16. Denborough MA, Forster JF, Lovell RR, Maplestone PA, Villiers JD. Anaesthetic deaths in a family. Br J Anaesth. 1962;34:395–6.
17. Ball C. Unravelling the mystery of malignant hyperthermia. Anaesth Intensive Care. 2007;35 Suppl 1:26–31.
18. Gordon MA. Malignant hyperpyrexia during general anesthesia. Can Anaesth Soc J. 1996;13:415–6.
19. Saidman LJ, Havard ES, Eger EI 2nd. Hyperthermia during anesthesia. JAMA. 1964;190:1029–32.
20. Denborough MA, Forster JF, Hudson MC, Carter NG, Zapf P. Biochemical changes in malignant hyperpyrexia. Lancet. 1970;1:1137–8.
21. Denborough MA, Ebeling P, King JO, Zapf P. Myopathy and malignant hyperpyrexia. Lancet. 1970;1:1138–40.
22. Isaacs H, Barlow MB. Malignant hyperpyrexia during anaesthesia: possible association with subclinical myopathy. Br Med J. 1970;1:275–7.
23. Kalow W, Britt BA, Terreau ME, Haist C. Metabolic error of muscle metabolism after recovery from malignant hyperthermia. Lancet. 1970;2:895–8.
24. Ellis FR, Harriman DG, Keaney NP, Kyei-Mensah K, Tyrrell JH. Halothane-induced muscle contracture as a cause of hyperpyrexia. Br J Anaesth. 1971;43:721–2.
25. Urwyler A, Deufel T, McCarthy T, West S. Guidelines for molecular genetic detection of susceptibility to malignant hyperthermia. Br J Anaesth. 2001;86:283–7.
26. MacLennan DH, Duff C, Zorzato F, Fujii J, Phillips M, Korneluk RG, Frodis W, Britt BA, Worton RG. Ryanodine receptor gene is a candidate for predisposition to malignant hyperthermia. Nature. 1990;343:559–61.
27. Metra M, Covolo L, Pezzali N, Zaca V, Bugatti S, Lombardi C, Bettari L, Romeo A, Gelatti U, Giubbini R, Donato F, Dei Cas L. Role of beta-adrenergic receptor gene polymorphisms in the long-term effects of beta-blockade with carvedilol in patients with chronic heart failure. Cardiovasc Drugs Ther. 2010;24:49–60.
28. Davis PJ, Brandom BW. The association of malignant hyperthermia and unusual disease: when you're hot you're hot or maybe not. Anesth Analg. 2009;109:1001–3.
29. Mansur AJ, Fontes RS, Canzi RA, Nishimura R, Alencar AP, de Lima AC, Krieger JE, Pereira AC. Beta-2 adrenergic receptor gene polymorphisms Gln27Glu, Arg16Gly in patients with heart failure. BMC Cardiovasc Disord. 2009;9:50.
30. A protocol for the investigation of malignant hyperpyrexia (MH) susceptibility. The European Malignant Hyperpyrexia Group. Br J Anaesth. 1984;56:1267–9.
31. Ingelman-Sundberg M, Sim SC, Gomez A, Rodriguez-Antona C. Influence of cytochrome P450 polymorphisms on drug therapies: pharmacogenetic, pharmacoepigenetic and clinical aspects. Pharmacol Ther. 2007;116:496–526.
32. Hammer W, Sjoqvist F. Plasma levels of monomethylated tricyclic antidepressants during treatment with imipramine-like compounds. Life Sci. 1967;6:1895–903.
33. Alexanderson B, Evans DA, Sjoqvist F. Steady-state plasma levels of nortriptyline in twins: influence of genetic factors and drug therapy. Br Med J. 1969;4:764–8.
34. Mahgoub A, Idle JR, Dring LG, Lancaster R, Smith RL. Polymorphic hydroxylation of Debrisoquine in man. Lancet. 1977;2:584–6.
35. Eichelbaum M, Spannbrucker N, Dengler HJ. A probably genetic defect in the metabolism of sparteine in biological oxidation of nitrogen. In: Gorrow JW, editor. Amsterdam: Elsevier North-Holland Biomedical; 1978. pp. 113–8.
36. Bertilsson L, Dengler HJ, Eichelbaum M, Schulz HU. Pharmacogenetic covariation of defective N-oxidation of sparteine and 4-hydroxylation of debrisoquine. Eur J Clin Pharmacol. 1980;17:153–5.
37. Kalow W, Otton SV, Kadar D, Endrenyi L, Inaba T. Ethnic difference in drug metabolism: debrisoquine 4-hydroxylation in Caucasians and Orientals. Can J Physiol Pharmacol. 1980;58:1142–4.
38. Eichelbaum M, Bertilsson L, Sawe J, Zekorn C. Polymorphic oxidation of sparteine and debrisoquine: related pharmacogenetic entities. Clin Pharmacol Ther. 1982;31:184–6.
39. Distlerath LM, Reilly PE, Martin MV, Davis GG, Wilkinson GR, Guengerich FP. Purification and characterization of the human liver cytochromes P-450 involved in debrisoquine 4-hydroxylation and phenacetin O-deethylation, two prototypes for genetic polymorphism in oxidative drug metabolism. J Biol Chem. 1985;260:9057–67.
40. Eichelbaum M, Baur MP, Dengler HJ, Osikowska-Evers BO, Tieves G, Zekorn C, Rittner C. Chromosomal assignment of human cytochrome P-450 (debrisoquine/sparteine type) to chromosome 22. Br J Clin Pharmacol. 1987;23:455–8.
41. Ingelman-Sundberg M. Genetic polymorphisms of cytochrome P450 2D6 (CYP2D6): clinical consequences, evolutionary aspects and functional diversity. Pharmacogenomics J. 2005;5:6–13.
42. Gardiner SJ, Begg EJ. Pharmacogenetics, drug-metabolizing enzymes, and clinical practice. Pharmacol Rev. 2006;58:521–90.
43. Koren G, Cairns J, Chitayat D, Gaedigk A, Leeder SJ. Pharmacogenetics of morphine poisoning in a breastfed neonate of a codeine-prescribed mother. Lancet. 2006;368:704.
44. Madadi P, Ross CJ, Hayden MR, Carleton BC, Gaedigk A, Leeder JS, Koren G. Pharmacogenetics of neonatal opioid toxicity following maternal use of codeine during breastfeeding: a case-control study. Clin Pharmacol Ther. 2009;85:31–5.
45. Kim JH, Schwinn DA, Landau R. Pharmacogenomics and perioperative medicine–implications for modern clinical practice. Can J Anaesth. 2008;55:799–806.
46. Kirstein SL, Insel PA. Autonomic nervous system pharmacogenomics: a progress report. Pharmacol Rev. 2004;56:31–52.
47. A randomized trial of propranolol in patients with acute myocardial infarction. I. Mortality results. JAMA. 1982;247:1707–14.
48. Lanfear DE, Jones PG, Marsh S, Cresci S, McLeod HL, Spertus JA. Beta2-adrenergic receptor genotype and survival among patients receiving beta-blocker therapy after an acute coronary syndrome. JAMA. 2005;294:1526–33.
49. Lima JJ, Thomason DB, Mohamed MH, Eberle LV, Self TH, Johnson JA. Impact of genetic polymorphisms of the beta2-adrenergic receptor on albuterol bronchodilator pharmacodynamics. Clin Pharmacol Ther. 1999;65:519–25.
50. Israel E, Chinchilli VM, Ford JG, Boushey HA, Cherniack R, Craig TJ, Deykin A, Fagan JK, Fahy JV, Fish J, Kraft M, Kunselman SJ, Lazarus SC, Lemanske RF Jr, Liggett SB, Martin RJ, Mitra N, Peters SP, Silverman E, Sorkness CA, Szefler SJ, Wechsler ME, Weiss ST, Drazen JM. Use of regularly scheduled albuterol treatment in asthma: genotype-stratified, randomised, placebo-controlled cross-over trial. Lancet. 2004;364:1505–12.
51. Wechsler ME, Lehman E, Lazarus SC, Lemanske RF Jr, Boushey HA, Deykin A, Fahy JV, Sorkness CA, Chinchilli VM, Craig TJ, DiMango E, Kraft M, Leone F, Martin RJ, Peters SP, Szefler SJ, Liu W, Israel E. beta-Adrenergic receptor polymorphisms and response to salmeterol. Am J Respir Crit Care Med. 2006;173:519–26.
52. Hawkins GA, Weiss ST, Bleecker ER. Clinical consequences of ADRbeta2 polymorphisms. Pharmacogenomics. 2008;9:349–58.
53. Lima JJ, Blake KV, Tantisira KG, Weiss ST. Pharmacogenetics of asthma. Curr Opin Pulm Med. 2009;15:57–62.
54. Wendel B, Hoehe MR. The human mu opioid receptor gene: 5′ regulatory and intronic sequences. J Mol Med. 1998;76:525–32.
55. Bond C, LaForge KS, Tian M, Melia D, Zhang S, Borg L, Gong J, Schluger J, Strong JA, Leal SM, Tischfield JA, Kreek MJ, Yu L. Single-nucleotide polymorphism in the human mu opioid receptor gene alters beta-endorphin binding and activity: possible implications for opiate addiction. Proc Natl Acad Sci U S A. 1998;95:9608–13.

56. Wand GS, McCaul M, Yang X, Reynolds J, Gotjen D, Lee S, Ali A. The mu-opioid receptor gene polymorphism (A118G) alters HPA axis activation induced by opioid receptor blockade. Neuropsychopharmacology. 2002;26:106–14.

57. Lotsch J, Skarke C, Grosch S, Darimont J, Schmidt H, Geisslinger G. The polymorphism A118G of the human mu-opioid receptor gene decreases the pupil constrictory effect of morphine-6-glucuronide but not that of morphine. Pharmacogenetics. 2002;12:3–9.

58. Lotsch J, Zimmermann M, Darimont J, Marx C, Dudziak R, Skarke C, Geisslinger G. Does the A118G polymorphism at the mu-opioid receptor gene protect against morphine-6-glucuronide toxicity? Anesthesiology. 2002;97:814–9.

59. Landau R, Kraft JC. Pharmacogenetics in obstetric anesthesia. Curr Opin Anaesthesiol. 2010;23:323–9.

60. Angst MS, Phillips NG, Drover DR, Tingle M, Galinkin JL, Christians U, Swan GE, Lazzeroni LC, Clark JD. Opioid pharmacogenomics using a twin study paradigm: methods and procedures for determining familial aggregation and heritability. Twin Res Hum Genet. 2010;13:412–25.

61. Sia AT, Lim Y, Lim EC, Goh RW, Law HY, Landau R, Teo YY, Tan EC. A118G single nucleotide polymorphism of human mu-opioid receptor gene influences pain perception and patient-controlled intravenous morphine consumption after intrathecal morphine for postcesarean analgesia. Anesthesiology. 2008;109:520–6.

62. Holmes MV, Shah T, Vickery C, Smeeth L, Hingorani AD, Casas JP. Fulfilling the promise of personalized medicine? Systematic review and field synopsis of pharmacogenetic studies. PLoS One. 2009;4:e7960.

63. Cox JJ, Reimann F, Nicholas AK, Thornton G, Roberts E, Springell K, Karbani G, Jafri H, Mannan J, Raashid Y, Al-Gazali L, Hamamy H, Valente EM, Gorman S, Williams R, McHale DP, Wood JN, Gribble FM, Woods CG. An SCN9A channelopathy causes congenital inability to experience pain. Nature. 2006;444:894–8.

64. Goldberg YP, MacFarlane J, MacDonald ML, Thompson J, Dube MP, Mattice M, Fraser R, Young C, Hossain S, Pape T, Payne B, Radomski C, Donaldson G, Ives E, Cox J, Younghusband HB, Green R, Duff A, Boltshauser E, Grinspan GA, Dimon JH, Sibley BG, Andria G, Toscano E, Kerdraon J, Bowsher D, Pimstone SN, Samuels ME, Sherrington R, Hayden MR. Loss-of-function mutations in the Nav1.7 gene underlie congenital indifference to pain in multiple human populations. Clin Genet. 2007;71:311–9.

65. Dib-Hajj SD, Cummins TR, Black JA, Waxman SG. From genes to pain: Na v 1.7 and human pain disorders. Trends Neurosci. 2007;30:555–63.

66. Nilsen KB, Nicholas AK, Woods CG, Mellgren SI, Nebuchennykh M, Aasly J. Two novel SCN9A mutations causing insensitivity to pain. Pain. 2009;143:155–8.

67. Morgan PG, Cascorbi HF. Effect of anesthetics and a convulsant on normal and mutant *Caenorhabditis elegans*. Anesthesiology. 1985;62:738–44.

68. Morgan PG, Kayser EB, Sedensky MM. *C. elegans* and volatile anesthetics. WormBook 2007:1–11.

69. Kayser EB, Suthammarak W, Morgan PG, Sedensky MM. Isoflurane selectively inhibits distal mitochondrial complex I in *Caenorhabditis elegans*. Anesth Analg. 2011;112:1321–9.

70. Alone DP, Rodriguez JC, Noland CL, Nash HA. Impact of gene copy number variation on anesthesia in *Drosophila melanogaster*. Anesthesiology. 2009;111:15–24.

71. Campagna JA, Miller KW, Forman SA. Mechanisms of actions of inhaled anesthetics. N Engl J Med. 2003;348:2110–24.

72. Sonner JM, Antognini JF, Dutton RC, Flood P, Gray AT, Harris RA, Homanics GE, Kendig J, Orser B, Raines DE, Rampil IJ, Trudell J, Vissel B, Eger EI 2nd. Inhaled anesthetics and immobility: mechanisms, mysteries, and minimum alveolar anesthetic concentration. Anesth Analg. 2003;97:718–40.

73. Eger EI 2nd, Raines DE, Shafer SL, Hemmings HC Jr, Sonner JM. Is a new paradigm needed to explain how inhaled anesthetics produce immobility? Anesth Analg. 2008;107:832–48.

74. Mihic SJ, Ye Q, Wick MJ, Koltchine VV, Krasowski MD, Finn SE, Mascia MP, Valenzuela CF, Hanson KK, Greenblatt EP, Harris RA, Harrison NL. Sites of alcohol and volatile anaesthetic action on GABA(A) and glycine receptors. Nature. 1997;389:385–9.

75. Sonner JM, Werner DF, Elsen FP, Xing Y, Liao M, Harris RA, Harrison NL, Fanselow MS, Eger EI 2nd, Homanics GE. Effect of isoflurane and other potent inhaled anesthetics on minimum alveolar concentration, learning, and the righting reflex in mice engineered to express alpha1 gamma-aminobutyric acid type A receptors unresponsive to isoflurane. Anesthesiology. 2007;106:107–13.

76. Rudolph U, Crestani F, Benke D, Brunig I, Benson JA, Fritschy JM, Martin JR, Bluethmann H, Mohler H. Benzodiazepine actions mediated by specific gamma-aminobutyric acid(A) receptor subtypes. Nature. 1999;401:796–800.

77. Jurd R, Arras M, Lambert S, Drexler B, Siegwart R, Crestani F, Zaugg M, Vogt KE, Ledermann B, Antkowiak B, Rudolph U. General anesthetic actions in vivo strongly attenuated by a point mutation in the GABA(A) receptor beta3 subunit. FASEB J. 2003;17:250–2.

78. Walter C, Lotsch J. Meta-analysis of the relevance of the OPRM1 118A > G genetic variant for pain treatment. Pain. 2009;146:270–5.

79. Lacroix-Fralish ML, Mogil JS. Progress in genetic studies of pain and analgesia. Annu Rev Pharmacol Toxicol. 2009;49:97–121.

80. Mogil JS, Wilson SG, Chesler EJ, Rankin AL, Nemmani KV, Lariviere WR, Groce MK, Wallace MR, Kaplan L, Staud R, Ness TJ, Glover TL, Stankova M, Mayorov A, Hruby VJ, Grisel JE, Fillingim RB. The melanocortin-1 receptor gene mediates female-specific mechanisms of analgesia in mice and humans. Proc Natl Acad Sci U S A. 2003;100:4867–72.

81. Rees JL, Birch-Machin M, Flanagan N, Healy E, Phillips S, Todd C. Genetic studies of the human melanocortin-1 receptor. Ann N Y Acad Sci. 1999;885:134–42.

82. Tatro JB. Receptor biology of the melanocortins, a family of neuroimmunomodulatory peptides. Neuroimmunomodulation. 1996;3:259–84.

83. Mogil JS, Ritchie J, Smith SB, Strasburg K, Kaplan L, Wallace MR, Romberg RR, Bijl H, Sarton EY, Fillingim RB, Dahan A. Melanocortin-1 receptor gene variants affect pain and mu-opioid analgesia in mice and humans. J Med Genet. 2005;42:583–7.

84. Liem EB, Joiner TV, Tsueda K, Sessler DI. Increased sensitivity to thermal pain and reduced subcutaneous lidocaine efficacy in redheads. Anesthesiology. 2005;102:509–14.

85. Lacroix-Fralish ML, Ledoux JB, Mogil JS. The Pain Genes Database: an interactive web browser of pain-related transgenic knockout studies. Pain. 2007;131:3.e1–4.

86. Zieker D, Elvira F, Dietzsch J, Fliegner J, Waidmann M, Nieselt K, Gebicke-Haerter P, Spanagel R, Simon P, Niess AM, Northoff H. cDNA microarray analysis reveals novel candidate genes expressed in human peripheral blood following exhaustive exercise. Physiol Genomics. 2005;23:287–94.

87. Hoffman-Goetz L, Quadrilatero J. Treadmill exercise in mice increases intestinal lymphocyte loss via apoptosis. Acta Physiol Scand. 2003;179:289–97.

88. Pedersen BK, Hoffman-Goetz L. Exercise and the immune system: regulation, integration, and adaptation. Physiol Rev. 2000;80:1055–81.

89. Hoffman-Goetz L, Pedersen BK. Exercise and the immune system: a medel of the stress response? Immunol Today. 1994;15:382–7.

90. Niess AM, Passek F, Lorenz I, Schneider EM, Dickhuth HH, Northoff H, Fehrenbach E. Expression of the antioxidant stress protein heme oxygenase-1 (HO-1) in human leukocytes. Free Radic Biol Med. 1999;26:184–92.

91. Northoff H, Weinstock C, Berg A. The cytokine response to strenuous exercise. Int J Sports Med. 1994;15:S167–71.

92. Suzuki K, Nakaji S, Yamada M, Totsuka M, Sato K, Sugawara K. Systemic inflammatory response to exhaustive exercise. Cytokine Kinetics Exerc Immunol Rev. 2002;8:6–48.

93. Vikingsson A, Pedderson K, Muller D. Enumeration of IFN-g producing lymphocytes by flow cytometry and correlation with quantitative measurement of IFN-g. J Immunol Methods. 1994;173:219–28.

94. Ronsen O, Lea T, Bahr R, Pedersen BK. Enhanced plasma IL-6 and IL-1ra responses to repeated vs. single bouts of prolonged cycling in elite athletes. J Appl Physiol. 2002;92:2547–53.

95. Steenberg A, Fischer CP, Keller C, Moller K, Pedersen BK. IL-6 enhances plasma IL-1ra, IL-10, and cortisol in humans. Am J Physiol Endocrinol Metab. 2003;285:E433–7.

96. Niess AM, Dickhuth HH, Northoff H, Fehrenbach E. Free radicals and oxidative stress in exercise–immulogic aspects. Exerc Immunol Rev. 1999;5:22–56.

97. Russell AP, Hesselink MKC, Lo SK, Schrauwen P. Regulation of metabolic transcriptional co-activators and transcription factors with acute exercise. FASEB J. 2005;19:986–8.

98. Talwar S, Munson PJ, Barb J, Fiuza C, Cintron AP, Logun C, Tropea M, Khan S, Reda D, Shelhamer JH, Danner RL, Suffredini AF. Gene expression profiles of peripheral blood leukocytes after endotoxin challenge in humans. Physiol Genomics. 2006;25:203–15.

99. Calvano SE, Xiao W, Richards DR, Felciano RM, Baker HV, Cho RJ, Chen RO, Brownstein BH, Cobb JP, Tschoeke SK, Miller-Graziano C, Moldawer LL, Mindrinos MN, Davis RW, Tompkins RG, Lowry SF, Program IHRtILSCR. A network-based analysis of systemic inflammation in humans. Nature. 2005;437:1032–7.

100. Cason BA, Gamperl AK, Slocum RE, Hickey RF. Anesthetic-induced preconditioning: previous administration of isoflurane decreases myocardial infarct size in rabbits. Anesthesiology. 1997;87:1182–90.

101. Zaugg M, Lucchinetti E, Spahn DR, Pasch T, Schaub MC. Volatile anesthetics mimic cardiac preconditioning by priming the activation of mitochondrial K(ATP) channels via multiple signaling pathways. Anesthesiology. 2002;97:4–14.

102. Podgoreanu MV, Schwinn DA. New paradigms in cardiovascular medicine: emerging technologies and practices: perioperative genomics. J Am Coll Cardiol. 2005;46:1965–77.

103. Lucchinetti E, Aguirre J, Feng J, Zhu M, Suter M, Spahn DR, Harter L, Zaugg M. Molecular evidence of late preconditioning after sevoflurane inhalation in healthy volunteers. Anesth Analg. 2007;105:629–40.

104. Shen YT, Depre C, Yan L, Park JY, Tian B, Jain K, Chen L, Zhang Y, Kudej RK, Zhao X, Sadoshima J, Vatner DE, Vatner SF. Repetitive ischemia by coronary stenosis induces a novel window of ischemic preconditioning. Circulation. 2008;118:1961–9.

105. Depre C, Park JY, Shen YT, Zhao X, Qiu H, Yan L, Tian B, Vatner SF, Vatner DE. Molecular mechanisms mediating preconditioning following chronic ischemia differ from those in classical second window. Am J Physiol Heart Circ Physiol. 2010;299:H752–62.

The Unfolding Story of How General Anesthetics Act

Nicholas P. Franks

Summary

Soon after Morton's 1846 demonstration of ether anesthesia, von Bibra and Harless proposed that ether acted by extracting brain lipids. In 1901, Overton noted that this theory did not explain the rapid reversibility of narcosis and proposed that anesthetics acted by dissolving in the lipids, not *vice versa*. In support of this theory, Meyer and Overton showed that anesthetic potency correlated with partitioning between water and lipid. In the next half century, not all agreed with their theory. Harris' 1951 book, for example, suggested that anesthetics might act by impeding diffusion through membranes, or by diminishing metabolism, or by asphyxiation.

In the early 1900s, women in labor might receive morphine and scopolamine to produce "twilight sleep". They might thrash and scream, but not recall pain, an early example of different mechanisms mediating different components of anesthesia.

In 1961, Pauling and Miller proposed that anesthetics acted by forming hydrates of water at membrane surfaces… but many inhaled anesthetics did not produce hydrates. In 1963, Merkel and Eger described "MAC", a measure of inhaled anesthetic equipotency. MAC gave the partial pressure at the site governing a crucial anesthetic endpoint, immobility, in the process also producing amnesia. Further undermining the hydrate theory, Eger et al. found a poor correlation between MAC and the anesthetic partial pressure required to form hydrates.

Investigators in the 1970s embraced the Meyer and Overton hypothesis, offering four "lipid theories". Anesthetics might change bilayer dimensions (volume or thickness), increase bilayer fluidity, induce phase transitions in bilayer lipids, or alter bilayer permeability. Mullins suggested that anesthetics acted by expanding the membrane, a beguiling theory that might explain the remarkable ability of high pressures (e.g., a hundred atmospheres) to antagonize anesthesia. But in the early 1970s, Lieb and I tested how anesthetics altered membrane bilayers, by 1978 finding they didn't. We turned our attention to protein sites of action. By 1982, the evidence against lipid theories was convincing, while evidence for protein theories was thin. But in 1984, we showed that anesthetics inhibited a protein, firefly luciferase, at anesthetizing concentrations—a Meyer-Overton correlation, except that no lipids were involved. Our studies of stereoselectivity in the 1990s were also consistent with a protein site of anesthetic action.

The debate became "which protein?" By the early 1990s, studies showed that propofol and etomidate potentiated GABA$_A$ receptor responses, and that specific receptor amino acids influenced effects of inhaled anesthetics and etomidate. In 1993, both Antognini and Rampil found that the spinal cord mediated immobility caused by inhaled anesthetics. In 2005, Jinks showed that central pattern generators in the ventral horn were the specific targets. By the 2000s, most investigators agreed that specific molecular targets for inhaled anesthetics must exist, but did not agree as to which targets mediated particular endpoints.

The Greatest Challenge

Understanding how general anesthetics reversibly remove consciousness and sensibility to pain has been one of the great challenges in pharmacology and neuroscience. The extraordinary diversity of anesthetics (ranging from noble gases to complex steroids), together with the intangible nature of human consciousness, makes this a particularly difficult problem to solve. Until relatively recently, most research into how general anesthetics act has been directed at the molecular level, [1–6] and this will be a primary focus of this chapter[1].

N. P. Franks (✉)
Biophysics Section, Blackett Laboratory, Imperial College, South Kensington, SW7 2AZ, London, UK
e-mail: n.franks@imperial.ac.uk

[1] Readers looking for scholarly accounts of anesthetic mechanisms should read the reviews I have cited in the text. What they will find here is a personal account of how the field has changed during the past 35 years from my own, inevitably biased, perspective.

E. I Eger II et al. (eds.), *The Wondrous Story of Anesthesia*, DOI 10.1007/978-1-4614-8441-7_45, © Edmond I Eger, MD 2014

Within one year of the public demonstration in Boston of the use of ether as an anesthetic, Ernst von Bibra and Emil Harless proposed the first mechanism of anesthetic action, suggesting that ether extracted fatty components of brain cells, and these fatty components then accumulated in the liver [7]. Moreover, they argued that other compounds with this property would be anesthetic—the first physicochemical theory. This work influenced the thinking of both Hans Horst Meyer and Charles Ernest Overton who independently proposed a new, and highly influential, theory of anesthetic action that was also based on an interaction between anesthetics and lipids [8, 9].

The Meyer-Overton Hypothesis

Overton recognized two major difficulties with the notion that anesthetics extracted brain lipids. First, this could not easily account for the rapid reversibility of narcosis upon removal of the anesthetic. Second, lipids would in fact be insoluble in dilute aqueous solutions of ether. Overton turned the idea on its head and proposed that anesthetics dissolved in the lipids, and not *vice versa*. This changed the physical state of brain cell lipids, thereby producing narcosis. Overton clearly regarded this as the critical causal step in the induction of anesthesia. In support of this idea, both Meyer and Overton showed that the potency of an anesthetic in animals closely correlated with its partitioning between water and lipid (using olive oil, a complex mixture of triglycerides, as a convenient model lipid).

Importantly, the correlation between anesthetic potency and lipid partitioning had a slope of unity, meaning that at the point of anesthesia, the concentration in the lipid would be the same for all anesthetics (Fig. 45.1). Hence was born the influential lipid theory of anesthesia (refined and made more quantitative by Meyer's son, Kurt Meyer). Kurt Meyer summarized the theory [10]: "Narcosis commences when any chemically indifferent substance has attained a certain molar concentration in the lipoids of the cell". However, Kurt Meyer cautiously avoided describing this as a mechanistic theory—"it is not really a theory which explains the mechanism of narcosis but rather the expression of an experimentally observed regularity, a rule of which every theory must take account". The simplest interpretation of this observation is that whatever determines the solubility of anesthetics in olive oil, also determines their solubility at their sites of action in the brain. The most parsimonious idea, of course, as originally stated by Overton, was that these sites in the brain *were* membrane lipids and that something must be happening to these lipids which caused anesthesia. This idea has two fundamental problems. The first is that the data on which it was based were incomplete. The second is that it is wrong. More to that point in a moment.

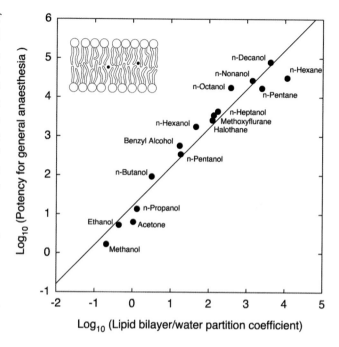

Fig. 45.1 The Meyer-Overton correlation between anesthetic potency in animals and partitioning between water and lipid bilayers

Twilight Sleep

In the early 1900s, women in labor might receive a combination of morphine and scopolamine to produce something called "twilight sleep" (see Chapter 48. A History of Pain Relief during Childbirth). Delivery might occur with thrashing and screaming, but afterwards the mother would recall nothing, believing that she had experienced a pain-free delivery. This supplied an early modern example of the possibility that different mechanisms might mediate the components of anesthesia. In this case, scopolamine blocked remembrance (produced amnesia), but neither scopolamine nor morphine sufficiently blocked the perception of, and motor/movement response to, noxious stimulation.

The Variable Impact of Meyer and Overton (And Hermann)

In the next half century, Meyer and Overton's hypothesis appears to have received a mixed reception. In 1930, Henderson [11] suggested it was important and pointed to the site of anesthetic action, but a 768-page book by TAB Harris entitled The Mode of Action of Anaesthetics [12] published in 1951 suggested otherwise. Eger says that this book was the most exciting text he read in his residency (1956–1958) because it was full of ideas on how things acted. No matter that the ideas usually were, in retrospect, incorrect. Harris noted that an LR Hermann had thought of the Meyer-Overton Hypothesis in 1866.

More importantly, in his single page (p 51) devoted to the Hypothesis, Harris concluded that Meyer and Overton were wrong: "This generalization does not bear criticism, for there are drugs—such as many of the benzol derivatives—which have a high oil/water partition coefficient, but do not produce narcosis", a thought anticipating the cut-off for large alcohols and the non-immobilizers as contradictions to the Hypothesis.

Harris focused on many other things in his text, considering in detail the importance of kinetics to achievement of an anesthetic effect. He noted suggestions that anesthetics might act by impeding diffusion through membranes, a recurring theme in theories of narcosis. He focused on the capacity of anesthetics to diminish metabolism, and argued (p 103) that "it is impossible to escape the suggestion that the state of narcosis must be attributed to the diminution of cell energy which results from the inhibition of the oxidation of glucose, lactate and pyruvate." He gave credence to the notion that some (not all) anesthetics "act…as a simple asphyxiant gas(es)." (p 164)

Two Inventions in the Early 1960s

In 1963, Giles Merkel and Eger published [13] a description of "a method for determining equipotency", a method using dogs that was applied two years later to humans [14]. They called the standard "MAC" (the minimum alveolar concentration that abolished movement in response to noxious stimulation in 50% of subjects).

This invention had several implications for mechanisms of anesthetic action. First, it dealt with kinetics and metabolism as confounding factors in measures of potency. The alveolar concentration (really the partial pressure) was assumed to be in equilibrium with the partial pressure in arterial blood, and given sufficient time for equilibrium, the partial pressure at the site of anesthetic action. That is, with those caveats, MAC gave the partial pressure at the site of anesthetic action, wherever that might be.

Second, the endpoint chosen, absence of movement in response to noxious stimulation, was a crucial clinical endpoint, one required for any operation. It also exceeded the concentration required to abolish memory, thus providing a two-for-one: production of immobility virtually guaranteed production of amnesia.

Third, it forced a consideration of what constituted anesthesia.

Fourth, MAC and the technique that underlay it, spawned similar measures of other clinically meaningful endpoints such as MAC-awake, the alveolar concentration eliminating appropriate response to command in 50% of subjects—a measure of consciousness.

Finally, the data producing MAC imposed another requirement for theories of narcosis. They had to explain the extraordinarily steep dose-response relationship associated with the production of immobility: at a concentration 10% less than MAC, 90% of subjects might move; but at a concentration 10% greater than MAC, 90% would not move. MAC was not a theory of narcosis, but it provided a powerful tool to investigate theories. (For experimental studies with animals, many used and continue to use the loss of righting reflex, an easily measured endpoint of central nervous system depression by anesthetics which correlates well with loss of consciousness in humans [6], but is not of such direct relevance clinically.)

Linus Pauling [15] and, independently, Stanley Miller [16] supplied a second invention in 1961, this one a theory of narcosis, an alternative to the lipid-based theories. They proposed that anesthetics formed microcrystals of water, or "icebergs" as Miller put it, hydrates perhaps stabilized by protein side chains, which disrupted membrane or enzyme function, possibly by effectively thickening membranes. In support of their theory they noted that the partial pressure required to produce anesthesia by several gaseous anesthetics correlated with the partial pressure required to produce the hydrate. Eger remembers a 1961 meeting of the Association of University Anesthetists (later Anesthesiologists) at which Pauling presented his hypothesis. A great showman, he pulled models of his icebergs (he called them clathrates), molecules connected with springs, from a small sports bag he had carried to the podium. "With a snap, each iceberg grew before our eyes. There it was! Visual proof of the theory!"

But the iceberg theory never took hold and remained largely forgotten as one of many ingenious, but unsupported, theories. Well, not just unsupported; there was evidence against it [17, 18]. Many inhaled anesthetics failed to produce the requisite icebergs.

Biophysical Table-Talk

Many investigators were less inclined than TAB Harris to dismiss the correlation found by Meyer and Overton. They sought to give the correlation a mechanistic basis. In 1982, my colleague Bill Lieb and I summarized what we thought were the shortcomings of such lipid theories [2]. An unimpressed reviewer[2] of the submitted manuscript described our analysis as "biophysical table-talk". This marvelous phrase has lived with me ever since and I happily use it here to describe the lipid theories based on the central observations of Meyer and Overton.

[2]This reviewer was not the only person who was unimpressed by our review. We received a letter from Linus Pauling telling us that, in fact, he had solved the problem of how anesthetic acted many years previously (see above).

Lipid theories fell broadly into four different camps. Anesthetics were said to change the dimensions of the bilayer (volume or thickness), increase the fluidity of the hydrocarbon chains, induce phase transitions in the bilayer lipids, or alter bilayer permeability. Lorin Mullins made an early and long-lasting suggestion that anesthesia occurred when anesthetics had expanded the membrane by a critical amount. This Critical Volume Hypothesis, refined and extended by Keith Miller and Brian Smith in the 1970s [19], became one of the best-known concepts. It was particularly beguiling because it might explain the remarkable ability of high pressures (e.g., a hundred atmospheres pressure) to antagonize general anesthesia—the so-called Pressure Reversal of Anesthesia.

Also in the 1970s, the concept of lipid fluidity was all the rage. Theories proposed that altered bilayer fluidity underlay anesthesia. It was suggested that anesthetics induced chain-melting phase-transitions in membrane lipids, similar to those known to occur in pure, artificial lipid bilayers. Jim Trudell proposed the most sophisticated version of this [20], suggesting that anesthetics disrupted the lateral phase separation of lipids. Finally, there were theories arguing that anesthetics compromised permeability of the lipid bilayer portion of nerve membranes [21].

It is impossible to do justice to the hundreds of papers written in support of various lipid theories. The array of possible explanations for anesthesia were bewildering, but when I became interested in the problem while pursuing my PhD with Maurice Wilkins in the early 1970s, I had little doubt that one of these lipid theories must be correct. I had been using and developing the techniques of X-ray and neutron scattering to study lecithin-cholesterol lipid bilayers, and we had the highest resolution structural description available [22, 23].

My first project (and, as it turned out, the direction of my subsequent career) began with an argument with Bill Lieb over coffee. Lieb[3], an expert on membrane permeability working in the lab as a postdoctoral Fellow, explained that anesthetics would thicken lipid bilayers because the anesthetics would tend to accumulate in the center of the bilayer where the packing density was lowest. I argued the opposite—the increased fluidity of the lipids would reduce the effective hydrocarbon chain-length, and the bilayer would get thinner. We decided to do the experiment. We started work in January 1975 (and worked together for 30 years until his death in 2005).

Our results were a shock. I vividly remember looking at the first diffraction pattern, expecting to see an obvious change in the pattern of intensities, but it looked exactly the same as the control. A detailed analysis showed no detectable changes in bilayer structure at clinically relevant concentrations. Neither of us had considered that *both* of our predictions might be wrong. It took a long time and more experiments to convince us that this result was correct. We used both X-ray and neutron diffraction, tried various anesthetics, and explored all artifacts we could think of. Three years later, we sent a paper describing our work to *Nature* [24], which had just published a paper by Denis Haydon, claiming that anesthetics caused membrane thickening [25].

We were not alone in questioning the validity of lipid bilayer theories. In 1976, Boggs et al. [26] showed that fluidity changes caused by anesthetics were extremely small and that they did not correlate with the size of the reduction in fluidity produced by pressures reversing anesthesia in animals. Nonetheless, the tide took a long time to turn.

There were both quantitative and qualitative problems with lipid theories. First, the concentrations of anesthetics causing anesthesia in animals produced either undetectable or extremely small effects in lipid bilayers. So small, in fact, that a slight rise in temperature could usually mimic the effect. Some proponents of lipid theories argued that the effects of temperature and anesthetics can never be exactly equated. True, but for simple biophysical theories claiming that bilayer properties such as volume or fluidity were critical, it was difficult to ignore their predictions regarding the effects of temperature. More importantly, the decrease in anesthetic potency found with increasing temperature [27, 28] was a major qualitative problem because almost all lipid theories predicted the opposite.

Second, the exceptions to the Meyer-Overton correlation were usually ignored. The most notable at the time were the long-chain alcohols, compounds that were highly soluble in olive oil and lipid bilayers, but were not anesthetics. As Miller and Smith wrote in 1973, this was "a feature that defies explanation in terms of the lipid solubility model" [29]. The fact that some fluorinated compounds also lack anesthetic activity, despite their lipid solubility, was exploited in the 1990s by Eger to investigate anesthetic mechanisms [30–32].

Third, lipid theories have difficulty explaining why anesthetic enantiomers (mirror-image isomers) may have different potencies in animals. This was known for barbiturates [33] in the 1970s, but interpretation of the data was not straightforward because of the potentially confounding effect of differential rates of metabolism.

Perhaps the most unsatisfactory aspect of almost all the lipid theories was that they provided no plausible mechanistic explanation of how the postulated changes in bilayer properties affected the functioning of membrane proteins

---

[3] Lieb was a native of Chicago and had a novel, an effective, way of avoiding jet-lag. He simply stayed on Chicago time all his life. He therefore arrived in the lab at around 2 in the afternoon and we would work together until the evening. He would then continue until the early hours when he would write me a letter telling me what he had been up to. This modus operandi persisted for the 30 years that we worked together.

which (almost) everyone believed to be the ultimate target. The explanations were usually along the lines of "… and then a miracle happens". Miller put it more soberly in an editorial [34] in 1977: "… although we can be quite precise about the lipid perturbations, we know comparatively little about the protein's involvement."

Why were lipid theories so popular? Probably because they grew naturally out of the Meyer-Overton correlation which, as Kurt Meyer pointed out [10], has to be accounted for by any successful theory. There was another reason— lipid theories possibly explained the remarkable observation that high pressures (of the order of 100 atm) could antagonize the actions of general anesthetics. During the 1970s and 1980s, anesthetic action and pressure reversal went hand in hand; explain one and you must explain the other. However, the concentration-response curves for general anesthesia are extremely steep, as mentioned above. Consequently, a small change in potency can cause a dramatic "reversal" (i.e., a big change in anesthetic effect), but the shift in the anesthetic dose-response relationship may be small. For mice, for example, the shift for a range of simple gases is only about 30% [2].

Does pressure cause a true pharmacological antagonism, directly reversing the molecular effects of anesthetics, or is the effect physiological, with pressure causing incidental changes in the animal (for example, by increasing the general level of excitability), and thereby decreasing anesthetic potency? The possibility that it is caused by a physiological antagonism is, I now believe, the most plausible explanation. I recall Brian Smith, at a meeting in Calgary in 1984, conceding that an anesthetized mouse restored to "normality" by pressure "didn't look like it would be too good at mental arithmetic". In the absence of anesthetics, pressure causes an increased excitability called the "High Pressure Nervous Syndrome." A generalized increase in excitable tone would explain why pressure can reverse the actions of not just simple gases, but also highly selective intravenous agents [35] which bind to specific receptors with minimal changes in system volume, where a pharmacological antagonism is most difficult to imagine.

Model Proteins

Although by 1982 the evidence against lipid theories was convincing, at least for Bill Lieb and me, evidence favoring the alternative—that anesthetics bound directly to protein targets—was thin. This was not an original notion, but had not taken off, partly because of the pre-eminence of the Meyer-Overton hypothesis, and partly because the diversity of chemicals causing anesthesia seemed inconsistent with the specificity of enzyme and protein action. In our 1982 review [2] we highlighted one class of proteins, the luciferase enzymes,

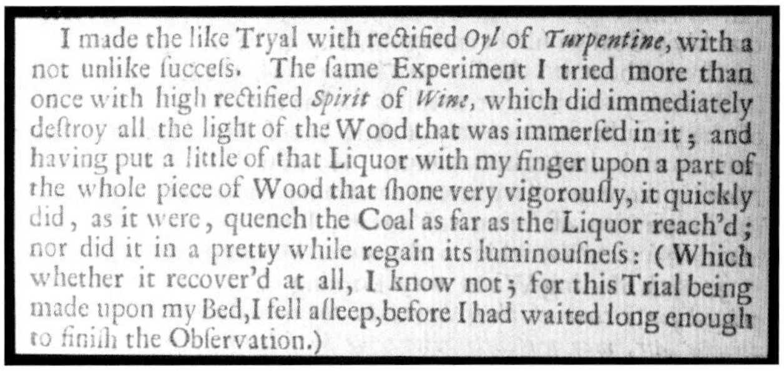

Fig. 45.2 The first anesthetic experiment on a luciferase enzyme as described by Robert Boyle [36]. Boyle was contrasting the light emitted by burning coals and that emitted by wood that had been infected by a bioluminescent fungus ("shining wood") and tried the effects of ethanol ("high rectified spirit of wine"). (From Boyle R: Observations and tryals about the resemblances and differences between burning coal and shining wood. Phil Trans. 1667;2:605–612, with permission.)

that looked to be sensitive to anesthetics, and we decided to work on these. We met with skepticism from local and more distant colleagues. Keith Miller, who represented mainstream thinking, wrote to us in January 1983 "I don't share your optimism about finding a protein site that behaves like a lipid bilayer!…. if you present me with a new example that works, then so be it." Nothing could have stimulated us more.

Work from Princeton by Frank Johnson, Woody Hastings, Henry Eyring, WD McElroy, and their colleagues from the 1940s, furthered our enthusiasm to work on luciferase enzymes. They had studied various luciferase enzymes, in intact organisms and in crude cell-free extracts. Indeed, centuries earlier, Robert Boyle had reported [36] that ethanol inhibited bioluminescence (Fig. 45.2). Eyring, had developed absolute rate theory for enzyme reactions in the 1930s and had also helped develop a curious way of looking at the inhibition of enzymes which centered around the involvement of a thermally-denatured form of the protein that was said to co-exist with the native form [37]. We pointed out that anesthetic binding directly to the native form provided a more plausible explanation for their data [2] and gave more plausible values for binding entropy and enthalpy. This analysis was a turning point in our thinking and pointed the way forward for our research.

We chose to work on the enzyme from the firefly, because Issaku Ueda in Salt Lake City had shown [38] that the bioluminescence from crude extracts of firefly tails was as anesthetic-sensitive as that in bacterial enzymes, and because pure crystalline protein could be prepared using simple affinity chromatography [39]. We purchased lots of firefly tails, purified the luciferase enzyme, and built the apparatus necessary to rapidly mix the enzyme with its substrates and record the resulting flash of light with a photomultiplier. The results were spectacular. Every simple anesthetic compound we picked off the shelf inhibited the enzyme at its anesthetic concentration in animals (Fig. 45.3). We had our

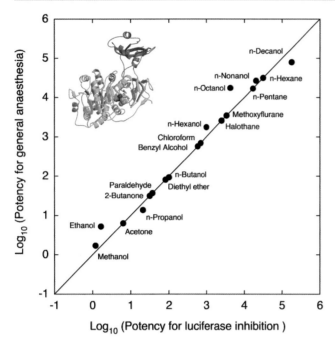

Fig. 45.3 The correlation between anesthetic potency in animals and the inhibition of the soluble enzyme, firefly luciferase

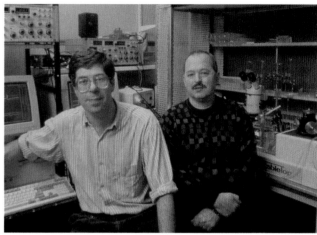

Fig. 45.4 This photograph of Bill Lieb (*right*) and myself was taken at Imperial College in 1992 to accompany an article about our work [48]. The caption to the photograph described us as "Lipid Theory Skeptics". Photograph taken by Nick Jackson. (From Matthews R: A low-fat theory of anesthesia. Science. 1992;255:156–157 with permission.)

own Meyer-Overton correlation, except that this time, no lipids were involved. The fact that inhibition of the enzyme was purely competitive in nature (the anesthetics simply competing for the binding of the endogenous ligand, luciferin) made this result immediately generalizable. If the architecture of a protein pocket on luciferase could account for anesthetic potency, then surely a similar site could exist amongst the thousands of proteins in the central nervous system.

We sent our results to *Nature* including, in our excitement (hubris?), a suggestion for the cover. The paper was immediately rejected without review. On appeal it went out for review and eventual publication [40]. The results were first presented at the Third International Conference on Molecular and Cellular Mechanisms of Anesthesia, held at Calgary in 1984, and a commentary [41] on the meeting described our results as "an interesting departure from the mainstream" and concluded, rather grudgingly we thought, that "it appears, in principle, that protein sites cannot be ruled out".

We went on to study the long-chain alcohols and found that, unlike lipid bilayer solubility [42], firefly luciferase displayed cutoffs in anesthetic potency for both alkanes and alcohols mimicking those seen in animals [43]. Our later work using X-ray crystallography also showed the anesthetic binding sites on the enzyme [44], and that the enzyme had a similar temperature dependence of anesthetic potency to animals [45], although it did not show pressure reversal.

The keystone for a new paradigm was in place, but further building blocks and at least another decade of work were required, before the idea that anesthetics acted by binding directly to proteins became the mainstream view. One argument

involved the stereoselectivity of action of those anesthetics that were "chiral", or in other words existed as two mirror-image forms (enantiomers). If anesthetics bound to sites on proteins, then one might expect that the two mirror-image enantiomers would act differently. As mentioned earlier, it had been appreciated since the 1970s that the enantiomers of various barbiturates differed in their anesthetic potencies, but this could have been explained by differential binding to their target sites, or by different rates of metabolism. To avoid metabolism (or kinetics) as a confounding problem, in 1989 we studied the difference in potencies of the enantiomers of isoflurane. Don Halpern, of Anaquest, part of the BOC Group, based in Murray Hill, New Jersey, synthesized the enantiomers of isoflurane. After the purified enantiomers arrived in London, they remained unopened for several months in a refrigerator while we screwed up courage to test whether they differentially affected ion channels, as a protein binding site would predict. Our first experiment in August 1989 revealed (to our great relief) that the S(+) enantiomer of isoflurane was about twice as potent as the R(−) enantiomer in opening an anesthetic-activated potassium channel and in inhibiting nicotinic acetylcholine receptors. Because the enantiomers affected lipid bilayers equally, this seemed to us good evidence that, even for the less potent inhaled agents, general anesthetics bound directly to protein targets. Work in 1998 reinforced this point using the intravenous anesthetic etomidate [46].

A few months after our 1991 paper [47] was published, an article [48] appeared in the same journal about our work. Bill Lieb and I were pictured (Fig. 45.4) with the caption "Lipid theory skeptics". This editorial gave a fair reflection of the mood at that time. For Keith Miller, it was "still too early to write off the lipid theory". "None of the experiments are absolute proof" said a skeptical Adron Harris. But by now, we had no doubts and turned our attention to characterizing anesthetic binding sites on proteins using X-ray crystallography [49] and, more importantly, tried to develop strategies for identifying which were the relevant protein targets in the central nervous system [3].

Which Proteins in the Central Nervous System Are Relevant Targets?

In the 1990s, the emphasis shifted from the "lipid vs. protein" debate to the question of "which proteins?" For some, this had always been the focus. A decade earlier, Roger Nicoll, Jeff Barker, Bob Macdonald and Richard Olsen had argued that anesthetic-potentiation of the inhibitory $GABA_A$ receptor was a possible mechanism underlying neuronal inhibition [50]. In 1982, Nicoll and Madison suggested that an unidentified anesthetic-activated potassium channel was a plausible target for inhaled anesthetics [51].

Over the past two-to-three decades, numerous studies examined the effects of diverse anesthetics on putative targets. In 1994, Bill Lieb and I wrote another review, but this time focused on which protein targets were or were not relevant to anesthesia [3]. We concluded that "General anaesthetics are much more selective than is usually appreciated and may act by binding to a small number of targets in the central nervous system." We highlighted the importance of a few targets including $GABA_A$ receptors, glycine receptors, NMDA receptors and anesthetic-activated potassium channels. Since then, two themes emerged from studies on putative targets. One came from investigations focused on intravenous anesthetics, concluding that these highly selective drugs may act on only a single target. Another theme emerged from (some) investigations of inhaled anesthetics, one that emphasized non-selectivity. It is convenient to tell these two stories separately.

Targets for Intravenous Anesthetics

Definitive work has been done with propofol and etomidate. Electrophysiological studies in the late 1980s, and early 1990s showed that both drugs potently potentiated responses of the $GABA_A$ receptor to GABA [52, 53]. Concurrently, heterologous expression systems such as the *Xenopus* oocyte and the HEK cell line enabled expression and characterization of neuronal ion channels and the effects of general anesthetics. Adron Harris, Neil Harrison and Jerry Lambert vigorously applied this technique, studying receptors with defined subunit compositions *in vitro*. This lovely approach allowed testing of the effect of site-specific mutations of amino acids on anesthetic sensitivity. Two 1997 papers proved most influential. By using chimeric ion channels

composed of sensitive and insensitive forms, followed by site-directed mutagenesis, Adron Harris and Neil Harrison demonstrated that specific amino acids influenced the effects of inhaled anesthetics acting on $GABA_A$ and glycine receptors [54]. The second study by Paul Whiting, Jerry Lambert and colleagues came to the same conclusion for etomidate [55].

For etomidate, the first step was the demonstration that the β subunit plays a critical role [56] Etomidate has a roughly ten-fold greater effect on $GABA_A$ receptors containing β2 or β3 subunits versus β1 subunits. This 1997 discovery [56] was followed by the discovery [55] that mutation of a single amino acid in the β3 subunit (Asn289) to its β1 equivalent (Ser) markedly decreased the actions of etomidate. While the sensitivity of $GABA_A$ receptors to etomidate greatly depended upon the type of beta subunit, propofol showed little subunit dependence. Nonetheless, the same mutations in β2 or β3 subunits affected both anesthetics [57]. This finding led, in 2003, to the production of "knock-in" mice [58, 59] containing mutations in either β2 or β3 subunits that were expected to render the animals insensitive to etomidate and/or propofol but "normally" sensitive to GABA. The resulting β3(N265M) mice were dramatically resistant to both etomidate and propofol for the anesthetic endpoint of withdrawal from a painful stimulus, but retained their normal sensitivity to alphaxalone. These data reflected the *in vitro* data for sensitivity, and showed that a single target is responsible for this endpoint for etomidate and propofol. But other endpoints (e.g., the duration of loss of righting reflex) were less affected or not affected at all, suggesting that etomidate and propofol had additional targets.

These results demonstrated that β3-containing $GABA_A$ receptors are crucial targets for etomidate and propofol for the loss of response to a painful stimulus and that both β2- and β3-containing $GABA_A$ receptors mediate the loss of righting reflex caused by etomidate. I believe that these fundamental conclusions are sound, although I suspect that the presumed "silence" of the mutations is an oversimplification. Our understanding of how propofol and etomidate act at the molecular level is more advanced than that for any other anesthetic (with the possible exception of dexmedetomidine, which is a highly selective α_2-adrenergic agonist with anesthetic properties [60]), but our understanding of which targets are important for inhaled agents is much less complete.

Targets for Inhaled Anesthetics

In 1993, Joseph Antognini and Ira Rampil independently made one of the great advances in defining the gross anatomic target of inhaled anesthetics, finding that the spinal cord and not the brain mediated immobility produced by inhaled anesthetics [61, 62]. A dozen years later, Steve Jinks showed that central pattern generators within the ventral horn of the spinal core were the specific targets [63].

LJS, one of the editors of this book recalls that similar to the initial rejection by *Nature* of Franks and Lieb's paper [40]. The paper by Rampil was also initially rejected for publication by LJS—the then Editor of *Anesthesiology* who responded to the compelling argument by the authors to solicit an additional review, resulting in its publication.

But identification of the definitive molecular targets for inhaled anesthetics has progressed slowly. Since the late 1990s, most of us have assumed that, as with intravenous agents, specific targets must exist. What is not agreed, however, is what these targets are and which ones significantly contribute to particular anesthetic endpoints. While opinions currently differ about how many targets are relevant for inhaled anesthetics, certain ion channels and receptors appear more likely to play a role than others [1, 3, 5, 6].

The 1997 work of Harris and Harrison [54] mentioned above, laid the foundations for a continuing theme of work. They found that specific mutations in $GABA_A$ and glycine receptors could ablate their potentiation by inhaled anesthetics and alcohols. What emerged from a large body of work was a bewildering complexity serving to emphasize how difficult it is to interpret the effects of "simple" alterations to allosteric proteins. Nonetheless, a plausible case emerged for a specific binding site of the $GABA_A$ and glycine receptor for inhaled anesthetics [64]. This work did not directly bear on whether or not these receptors contributed to anesthesia in whole animals. However, because potentiation of $GABA_A$ receptors containing β2 and β3 subunits was sufficient at least for etomidate and propofol, and because many inhaled anesthetics (e.g. halothane, isoflurane and sevoflurane) potentiated exactly the same receptors (see, e.g. ref. [65]), it seemed reasonable to postulate that this would contribute to the anesthesia caused by these inhaled anesthetics. Because the potentiation caused by volatile anesthetics is usually smaller (typically half) than that observed with etomidate and propofol (at equi-anesthetic concentrations) then $GABA_A$ receptors containing β2 and β3 subunits cannot be the only target.

Perhaps not surprisingly in view of the low potencies of volatile agents, stereoselectivity has provided less guidance as to which targets are most likely. Nonetheless, stereoselectivity has been observed in animals with isoflurane [66–69] (although this might depend upon the endpoint), and a similar degree of stereoselectivity is found in potentiating the $GABA_A$ receptor [70].

Volatile anesthetics show no absolute requirement for particular $GABA_A$ subunits for their potentiating effects, and generally show little subunit dependence. This may explain why the successful knock-in approach with etomidate (see above) has not proven to be so straightforward for inhaled

agents. Nonetheless, the β3(N265M) mice discussed above show a significant increase in MAC for halothane, enflurane and isoflurane, although no changes in their loss of righting reflex [71]. These data support the idea that $GABA_A$ receptors play some role in the actions of volatile agents although others disagree [72].

While during the last fifteen years, $GABA_A$ receptors have taken center stage, other potential targets have also been investigated. For example, glycine receptors, which are often co-localized with $GABA_A$ receptors, and of particular importance in lower brain centers and the spinal cord, are a plausible target for inhaled agents [73–75]. Glycine receptors can exist as αβ heteromers or α homomers. Their plausibility as a target is particularly strong for the loss of response to a painful stimulus which appears to be determined predominantly by actions in the spinal cord [5]. In both expression systems [75] and neurons [73, 74], low concentrations for all of the volatile agents potentiated the action of glycine on glycine receptors, but there was no evidence of stereoselectivity [73]. Definitive data, genetic or otherwise, proving the role of glycine receptors in general anesthesia, have yet to be published.

The so-called two-pore-domain potassium channels regulate membrane excitability and thereby provide another plausible target for inhaled general anesthetics. In 1982, Nicol and Madison suggested that inhaled anesthetics might work by activating potassium channels [51] and in 1988, we provided further supporting evidence in identified neurons of the pond snail Lymnaea stagnalis [76] Among the 15 mammalian subunits so far identified, volatile and gaseous anesthetics activated TREK, TASK and TRESK channels, although the activation was anesthetic specific [77, 78].

Data from a knock-out mouse from Michel Lazdunski's laboratory [79] published in 2004 supported a role for TREK-1. This work culminated from a series of studies by Eric Honoré and Amanda Patel and their colleagues [78, 80] showing that TREK-1 was sensitive to diverse inhaled anesthetics. Knock-out increased MAC by less than 10 % to nearly 50 % and minimally affected the loss of righting reflex. However, the increases in MAC did not correlate with the effect on *in vitro* current in wild-type receptors.

In the past few years, we found that mice lacking TASK channels were significantly less sensitive to anesthetic-induced loss of righting reflex and response to a painful stimulus [81, 82]. Furthermore, selective ablation of TASK channels from cholinergic neurons (including the cholinergic motor neurons of the spinal cord), changed MAC by essentially the same amount as did whole-animal knock-out [81].

As with all knock-out data, one has to be cautious in interpretation because compensatory changes can occur. Data on knock-in animals or on conditional knock-outs where TREK-1 or TASK expression is eliminated only in certain anatomical sites will be required before the data on knock-out animals can be considered to be the final word on the role of this channel in general anesthesia.

How Many Targets Are Relevant for Inhaled Anesthetics?

During the last fifteen years, two views emerged regarding the number of plausible targets for inhaled anesthetics: one believed that only a few targets were important (Eger and I are in this camp [3, 83]) and the other believed that anesthesia resulted from small effects at many targets [84].

The use of inappropriately high concentrations for *in vitro* experiments has long been a problem in this field. Many experimenters have used aqueous concentrations of anesthetics without translating them to gas phase concentrations reflecting activity. This is surprising, given the widespread acceptance of MAC as a precise measure of anesthetic potency for inhaled anesthetics [85]. An added complication has been that many *in vitro* experiments were conducted at room temperature whereas anesthetic potencies were usually established (for mammals) at 37 °C. Because MAC decreases with decreasing temperature [27, 28], this means that these gas-phase concentrations were excessive for room-temperature experiments, leading to the perception that more targets were "sensitive", and therefore relevant, than is probably the case.

Another argument invoked by Eger in particular, has been that one should be able to test the importance of any given target by testing how anesthetic potency changes when that target has been perturbed in some way (modified by a knock-in or inhibited by another drug, for example). This systematic approach over the last several decades has tended to conclude that no single target is particularly important. The results with this approach may be particularly convincing where a receptor has been removed or blocked without affecting MAC (i.e., a negative result). Two examples: In 1978, Marilyn Harper with Eger showed that a wide range of opioid antagonist doses have no effect on MAC, indicating that opioid receptors do not mediate the immobility produced by inhaled anesthetics [86]. Similar studies using blockers in 2002 indicated that acetylcholine receptors were irrelevant to inhaled anesthetic-induced immobility [87]. This last study illustrates the importance of the anesthetic endpoint to the issue of mechanisms. Acetylcholine receptors do not mediate the immobility produced by inhaled anesthetics but may have a great deal to do with the mediation of the amnesia produced by inhaled anesthetics. Inhaled anesthetics potently block transmission at acetylcholine receptors at sub-MAC concentrations [88, 89]. Overall, these results were consistent with the more profound clinical effect of inhaled anesthetics on memory than on immobility.

But what about studies that might not produce a definitively negative result? The problem is that, if more than three or four targets are involved, then perturbing only one of them by, say, knockout may cause too small a change in potency to be measured against a control animal whose baseline excitability has, almost inevitably, been disrupted. Eger might respond by arguing that at least for MAC, differences of 10 % can be defined with relatively few animals, as few as five to ten, arguing further that changes in baseline activity can be dealt with by assuring that the control and knockout animals only differ in the specific receptor knocked out.

The question of the exact number of targets for inhaled anesthetics remains an open one although I retain my prejudice, based in part on Occam's Razor, that a small number of targets is most likely. (Although I hear the warning of Bill Paton—"God does not shave with Occam's Razor".)

And what if…?

Over the past three decades, mainstream thinking has shifted from lipid to protein theories of narcosis, from membrane bilayers to protein receptors and channels. For some injected anesthetics (etomidate and propofol and opioids and dexmedetomidine), the proof that a single protein can explain most of the narcotic effect seems overwhelming. Less clear is whether a few or many proteins mediate particular inhaled anesthetic endpoints. A few voices in the wilderness would have us return to the days of yesteryear, to a lipid theory of narcosis. In 2003, Robert Cantor argued that in addition to binding to and activating their receptors, neurotransmitters modulate their receptors by an action on the adjacent membrane [90]. He postulated that anesthetics might act by mimicking the membrane-based non-specific effect of neurotransmitters. In 2007, Jim Sonner's group provided results consistent with Cantor's notion [91]. The group found that applying GABA to glycine receptors at GABA concentrations that had little or no direct effect on the glycine receptors, nonetheless potentiated the effect of glycine by over 100 %. The reverse also was true: glycine potentiated the effect of GABA on $GABA_A$ receptors. And finally, background acetylcholine concentrations that did not affect NMDA receptor currents decreased the current produced by glutamate (plus glycine) application by up to 50 %. Others have argued [92], however, that the actions of GABA on glycine receptors is simply accounted for by GABA binding directly to the glycine receptor and acting as a weak agonist. No doubt future work will establish exactly how one neurotransmitter can affect the actions of another and hence determine whether or not these observations have any relevance to anesthetic mechanisms.

Combatants and Collaborators

Before making some final remarks, I want to mention some important drivers of the research into anesthetic mechanisms, at least during the time that I have been involved. I believe that the polarization of a field into two opposing camps (such as lipid *vs.* protein) can be highly productive. Notwithstanding its potential dangers, Bill Lieb and I have had great fun sparring with Keith Miller and many others. It was usually good natured and respectful. In contrast to this combative spirit which I have tended to adopt, others have taken a more collaborative approach (and the one does not exclude the other). A notable example has been the series of Anesthetic Mechanisms conferences started by Raymond Fink and which grew into the international conferences that continue to this day. Ray was a remarkable individual who single-handedly organized the first few meetings before they were taken on by others, particularly Sheldon Roth and Keith Miller. I recall Ray telling me towards the end of his long life, with tears in his eyes, how the death of a young patient of his in South Africa during World War II, was the catalyst for him to understand the scientific basis of his practice as well as he could. The "Fink Meetings" as I think of them, are one of his many legacies. Other examples of the collaborative approach were the large Program Project Grants on anesthetic mechanisms funded by the US National Institutes of Health. The Programs of Miller, Evers, Eckenhoff, Lynch and Eger have been collaborative enterprises that have had a major impact on our understanding of how anesthetics act. Collectively these brought together some of the best workers in the field and spawned countless novel approaches and collaborations. I was fortunate to be an occasional visitor to the meetings of Principal Investigators on the Program, organized by Eger, which was aimed at understanding inhalational anesthesia. This group was an eclectic mix of scientists including mainstream neuroscientists as well as chemists and physical chemists, some of whom still held the torch for lipid-based theories. Eger was there as the ringmaster to challenge and cajole.

Final Remarks

In this chapter I have focused on molecular mechanisms of anesthesia, mainly because this aspect of anesthesia has fascinated me most, but also because it has been the main focus of the field during the last 50 years. Many questions remain to be answered at the molecular level: which targets are *really* important for inhaled anesthetics, where are the molecular binding sites on the relevant receptors, and how does binding translate into changed channel function, to name but three. The long-awaited publication [93] of a crystal structure of general anesthetics (sevoflurane and propofol) binding to a transmembrane receptor was, at least for me, a crucial landmark along the road towards understanding anesthetic action at a molecular level. While this work at the molecular level will take its course, attention in the field of anesthetic mechanisms is beginning to shift once again. If anesthetics act at a limited number of protein targets, then it is reasonable to ask whether this specificity extends to the level of neuronal networks. This will, I'm sure, be a main focus of research in the next decade and beyond, with the ultimate goal of identifying the neuronal networks in the brain and spinal cord that mediate anesthetic endpoints ranging from amnesia, to unconsciousness, to immobility.

Acknowledgement Although this chapter only bears my name, I want to acknowledge the many contributions and suggestions made by the Editors (particularly Ted Eger).

References

1. Campagna JA, Miller KW, Forman SA. Mechanisms of actions of inhaled anesthetics. N Engl J Med. 2003;348:2110–24.
2. Franks NP, Lieb WR. Molecular mechanisms of general anaesthesia. Nature. 1982;300:487–93.
3. Franks NP, Lieb WR. Molecular and cellular mechanisms of general anaesthesia. Nature. 1994;367:607–14.
4. Rudolph U, Antkowiak B. Molecular and neuronal substrates for general anaesthetics. Nat Rev Neurosci. 2004;5:709–20.
5. Sonner JM, Antognini JF, Dutton RC, Flood P, Gray AT, Harris RA, Homanics GE, Kendig J, Orser B, Raines DE, Rampil IJ, Trudell J, Vissel B, Eger EI 2nd. Inhaled anesthetics and immobility: mechanisms, mysteries, and minimum alveolar anesthetic concentration. Anesth Analg. 2003;97:718–40.
6. Franks NP. General anaesthesia: from molecular targets to neuronal pathways of sleep and arousal. Nat Rev Neurosci. 2008;9:370–86.
7. Hintzenstern U, Petermann H, Schwarz W. Frühe Erlanger Beiträge zur Theorie und Praxis der Äther- und Chloroformnarkose. Anaesthetist. 2001;50:869–80.
8. Meyer H. Welche Eigenschaft der Anästhetica bedingt ihre narkotische Wirkung? Naunyn-Schmiedebergs Arch. Exp. Pathol. Pharmakol. 1899;42:109–18.
9. Overton E. Studien über die Narkose, zugleich ein Beitrag zur allgemeiner Pharmakologie. Jena: Gustav Fischer; 1901.
10. Meyer K. Contributions to the theory of narcosis. Trans. Faraday Soc. 1937;33:1062–4.
11. Henderson VE. The present status of the theories of narcosis. Physiol Rev. 1930;10:171–220.
12. Harris TAB. The mode of action of anesthetics. Baltimore: Williams and Wilkins, p. 1951
13. Merkel G, Eger EI 2nd. A comparative study of halothane and halopropane anesthesia including method for determining equipotency. Anesthesiology. 1963;24:346–57.
14. Eger EI 2nd, Saidman LJ, Brandstater B. Minimum alveolar anesthetic concentration: a standard of anesthetic potency. Anesthesiology. 1965;26:756–63.
15. Pauling L. A molecular theory of general anesthesia. Science. 1961;134:15–21.
16. Miller SL. A theory of gaseous anesthetics. Proc Natl Acad Sci U S A. 1961;47:1515–24.
17. Eger EI 2nd, Lundgren C, Miller SL, Stevens WC. Anesthetic potencies of sulfur hexafluoride, carbon tetrafluoride, chloroform and Ethrane in dogs: correlation with the hydrate and lipid theories of anesthetic action. Anesthesiology. 1969;30:129–35.
18. Miller KW, Paton WD, Smith EB. Site of action of general anaesthetics. Nature. 1965;206:574–7.
19. Miller KW, Paton WD, Smith RA, Smith EB. The pressure reversal of general anesthesia and the critical volume hypothesis. Mol Pharmacol. 1973;9:131–43.

20. Trudell JR. A unitary theory of anesthesia based on lateral phase separations in nerve membranes. Anesthesiology. 1977;46:5–10.
21. Bangham AD, Mason WT. Anesthetics may act by collapsing pH gradients. Anesthesiology. 1980;53:135–41.
22. Franks NP. Structural analysis of hydrated egg lecithin and cholesterol bilayers. I. X-ray diffraction. J Mol Biol. 1976;100:345–58.
23. Worcester DL, Franks NP. Structural analysis of hydrated egg lecithin and cholesterol bilayers. II. Neutrol diffraction. J Mol Biol. 1976;100:359–78.
24. Franks NP, Lieb WR. Where do general anaesthetics act? Nature. 1978;274:339–42.
25. Haydon DA, Hendry BM, Levinson SR, Requena J. The molecular mechanisms of anaesthesia. Nature. 1977;268:356–8.
26. Boggs JM, Yoong T, Hsia JC. Site and mechanism of anesthetic action. I. Effect of anesthetics and pressure on fluidity of spin-labeled lipid vesicles. Mol Pharmacol. 1976;12:127–35.
27. Eger EI 2nd, Saidman LJ, Brandstater B. Temperature dependence of halothane and cyclopropane anesthesia in dogs: correlation with some theories of anesthetic action. Anesthesiology. 1965;26:764–70.
28. Franks NP, Lieb WR. Temperature dependence of the potency of volatile general anesthetics: implications for *in vitro* experiments. Anesthesiology. 1996;84:716–20.
29. Miller K, Smith E. Intermolecular forces and the pharmacology of simple molecules. In: Featherstone RA, editors. A guide to molecular pharmacology-toxicology. New York: Marcel Dekker, 1973, pp 427–75.
30. Eger EI 2nd, Liu J, Koblin DD, Laster MJ, Taheri S, Halsey MJ, Ionescu P, Chortkoff BS, Hudlicky T. Molecular properties of the "ideal" inhaled anesthetic: studies of fluorinated methanes, ethanes, propanes, and butanes. Anesth Analg. 1994;79:245–51.
31. Koblin DD, Chortkoff BS, Laster MJ, Eger EI 2nd, Halsey MJ, Ionescu P. Polyhalogenated and perfluorinated compounds that disobey the Meyer-Overton hypothesis. Anesth Analg. 1994;79:1043–8.
32. Liu J, Laster MJ, Koblin DD, Eger EI 2nd, Halsey MJ, Taheri S, Chortkoff B. A cutoff in potency exists in the perfluoroalkanes. Anesth Analg. 1994;79:238–44.
33. Freudenthal RI, Martin J. Correlation of brain levels of barbiturate enantiomers with reported differences in duration of sleep. J Pharmacol Exp Ther. 1975;193:664–8.
34. Miller KW. Towards the molecular bases of anesthetic action. Anesthesiology. 1977;46:2–4.
35. Tonner PH, Scholz J, Koch C, Schulte am Esch J. The anesthetic effect of dexmedetomidine does not adhere to the Meyer-Overton rule but is reversed by hydrostatic pressure. Anesth Analg. 1997;84:618–22.
36. Boyle R. Observations and tryals about the resemblances and differences between burning coal and shining wood. Phil Trans. 1667;2:605–12.
37. Johnson F, Eyring H, Polissar M. The kinetic basis of molecular biology. New York: Wiley; 1954.
38. Ueda I, Kamaya H. Kinetic and thermodynamic aspects of the mechanism of general anesthesia in a model system of firefly luminescence in vitro. Anesthesiology. 1973;38:425–36.
39. Branchini BR, Marschner TM, Montemurro AM. A convenient affinity chromatography-based purification of firefly luciferase. Anal Biochem. 1980;104:386–96.
40. Franks NP, Lieb WR. Do general anaesthetics act by competitive binding to specific receptors? Nature. 1984;310:599–601.
41. Brett RS, Firestone LL. Morpheus in Calgary. Trends Pharmacol Sci. 1985;6:146–8.
42. Franks NP, Lieb WR. Partitioning of long-chain alcohols into lipid bilayers: implications for mechanisms of general anesthesia. Proc Natl Acad Sci U S A. 1986;83:5116–20.
43. Franks NP, Lieb WR. Mapping of general anaesthetic target sites provides a molecular basis for cutoff effects. Nature. 1985;316:349–51.
44. Franks NP, Jenkins A, Conti E, Lieb WR, Brick P. Structural basis for the inhibition of firefly luciferase by a general anesthetic. Biophys J. 1998;75:2205–11.
45. Dickinson R, Franks NP, Lieb WR. Thermodynamics of anesthetic/protein interactions. Temperature studies on firefly luciferase. Biophys J. 1993;64:1264–71.
46. Tomlin SL, Jenkins A, Lieb WR, Franks NP. Stereoselective effects of etomidate optical isomers on gamma-aminobutyric acid type A receptors and animals. Anesthesiology. 1998;88:708–17.
47. Franks NP, Lieb WR. Stereospecific effects of inhalational general anesthetic optical isomers on nerve ion channels. Science. 1991;254:427–30.
48. Matthews R. A low-fat theory of anesthesia. Science. 1992;255:156–7.
49. Bhattacharya AA, Curry S, Franks NP. Binding of the general anesthetics propofol and halothane to human serum albumin. High resolution crystal structures. J Biol Chem. 2000;275:38731–8.
50. Franks NP. Molecular targets underlying general anaesthesia. Br J Pharmacol. 2006;147 Suppl 1:72–81.
51. Nicoll RA, Madison DV. General anesthetics hyperpolarize neurons in the vertebrate central nervous system. Science. 1982;217:1055–7.
52. Hales TG, Lambert JJ. The actions of propofol on inhibitory amino acid receptors of bovine adrenomedullary chromaffin cells and rodent central neurones. Br J Pharmacol. 1991;104:619–28.
53. Proctor WR, Mynlieff M, Dunwiddie TV. Facilitatory action of etomidate and pentobarbital on recurrent inhibition in rat hippocampal pyramidal neurons. J Neurosci. 1986;6:3161–8.
54. Mihic SJ, Ye Q, Wick MJ, Koltchine VV, Krasowski MD, Finn SE, Mascia MP, Valenzuela CF, Hanson KK, Greenblatt EP, Harris RA, Harrison NL. Sites of alcohol and volatile anaesthetic action on $GABA_A$ and glycine receptors. Nature. 1997;389:385–9.
55. Belelli D, Lambert JJ, Peters JA, Wafford K. Whiting PJ: The interaction of the general anesthetic etomidate with the $GABA_A$ receptor is influenced by a single amino acid. Proc Natl Acad Sci U S A. 1997;94:11031–6.
56. Hill-Venning C, Belelli D, Peters JA, Lambert JJ. Subunit-dependent interaction of the general anaesthetic etomidate with the $GABA_A$ receptor. Br J Pharmacol. 1997;120:749–56.
57. Siegwart R, Jurd R, Rudolph U. Molecular determinants for the action of general anesthetics at recombinant alpha(2)beta(3) gamma(2)gamma-aminobutyric acid(A) receptors. J Neurochem. 2002;80:140–8.
58. Jurd R, Arras M, Lambert S, Drexler B, Siegwart R, Crestani F, Zaugg M, Vogt KE, Ledermann B, Antkowiak B, Rudolph U. General anesthetic actions in vivo strongly attenuated by a point mutation in the GABA(A) receptor beta3 subunit. FASEB J. 2003;17:250–2.
59. Reynolds DS, Rosahl TW, Cirone J, O'Meara GF, Haythornthwaite A, Newman RJ, Myers J, Sur C, Howell O, Rutter AR, Atack J, Macaulay AJ, Hadingham KL, Hutson PH, Belelli D, Lambert JJ, Dawson GR, McKernan R, Whiting PJ, Wafford KA. Sedation and anesthesia mediated by distinct $GABA_A$ receptor isoforms. J Neurosci. 2003;23:8608–17.
60. Correa-Sales C, Rabin BC, Maze M. A hypnotic response to dexmedetomidine, an alpha 2 agonist, is mediated in the locus coeruleus in rats. Anesthesiology. 1992;76:948–52.
61. Antognini JF, Schwartz K. Exaggerated anesthetic requirements in the preferentially anesthetized brain. Anesthesiology. 1993;79:1244–9.
62. Rampil IJ, Mason P, Singh H. Anesthetic potency (MAC) is independent of forebrain structures in the rat. Anesthesiology. 1993;78:707–12.
63. Jinks SL, Atherley RJ, Dominguez CL, Sigvardt KA, Antognini JF. Isoflurane disrupts central pattern generator activity and coordination in the lamprey isolated spinal cord. Anesthesiology. 2005;103:567–75.
64. Jenkins A, Greenblatt EP, Faulkner HJ, Bertaccini E, Light A, Lin A, Andreasen A, Viner A, Trudell JR, Harrison NL. Evidence for

a common binding cavity for three general anesthetics within the GABA$_A$ receptor. J Neurosci. 2001;21:RC136.

65. Nishikawa K, Jenkins A, Paraskevakis I, Harrison NL. Volatile anesthetic actions on the GABA$_A$ receptors: contrasting effects of alpha 1(S270) and beta 2(N265) point mutations. Neuropharmacology. 2002;42:337–45.

66. Harris B, Moody E, Skolnick P. Isoflurane anesthesia is stereoselective. Eur J Pharmacol. 1992;217:215–6.

67. Eger EI 2nd, Koblin DD, Laster MJ, Schurig V, Juza M, Ionescu P, Gong D. Minimum alveolar anesthetic concentration values for the enantiomers of isoflurane differ minimally. Anesth Analg. 1997;85:188–92.

68. Dickinson R, White I, Lieb WR, Franks NP. Stereoselective loss of righting reflex in rats by isoflurane. Anesthesiology. 2000;93:837–43.

69. Lysko GS, Robinson JL, Casto R, Ferrone RA. The stereospecific effects of isoflurane isomers in vivo. Eur J Pharmacol. 1994;263:25–9.

70. Hall AC, Lieb WR, Franks NP. Stereoselective and non-stereoselective actions of isoflurane on the GABA$_A$ receptor. Br J Pharmacol. 1994;112:906–10.

71. Lambert S, Arras M, Vogt KE, Rudolph U. Isoflurane-induced surgical tolerance mediated only in part by beta3-containing GABA$_A$ receptors. Eur J Pharmacol. 2005;516:23–7.

72. Liao M, Sonner JM, Jurd R, Rudolph U, Borghese CM, Harris RA, Laster MJ, Eger EI 2nd. Beta3-containing gamma-aminobutyric acidA receptors are not major targets for the amnesic and immobilizing actions of isoflurane. Anesth Analg. 2005;101:412–8.

73. Downie DL, Hall AC, Lieb WR, Franks NP. Effects of inhalational general anaesthetics on native glycine receptors in rat medullary neurones and recombinant glycine receptors in Xenopus oocytes. Br J Pharmacol. 1996;118:493–502.

74. Harrison NL, Kugler JL, Jones MV, Greenblatt EP, Pritchett DB. Positive modulation of human GABA$_A$ and glycine receptors by the inhalation anesthetic isoflurane. Mol Pharmacol. 1993;44:628–32.

75. Mascia MP, Machu TK, Harris RA. Enhancement of homomeric glycine receptor function by long-chain alcohols and anaesthetics. Br J Pharmacol. 1996;119:1331–6.

76. Franks NP, Lieb WR. Volatile general anaesthetics activate a novel neuronal K$^+$ current. Nature. 1988;333:662–4.

77. Gruss M, Bushell TJ, Bright DP, Lieb WR, Mathie A, Franks NP. Two-pore-domain K$^+$ channels are a novel target for the anesthetic gases xenon, nitrous oxide, and cyclopropane. Mol Pharmacol. 2004;65:443–52.

78. Patel AJ, Honore E. Anesthetic-sensitive 2P domain K$^+$ channels. Anesthesiology. 2001;95:1013–21.

79. Heurteaux C, Guy N, Laigle C, Blondeau N, Duprat F, Mazzuca M, Lang-Lazdunski L, Widmann C, Zanzouri M, Romey G, Lazdunski M. TREK-1, a K$^+$ channel involved in neuroprotection and general anesthesia. EMBO J. 2004;23:2684–95.

80. Patel AJ, Honore E, Lesage F, Fink M, Romey G, Lazdunski M. Inhalational anesthetics activate two-pore-domain background K$^+$ channels. Nat Neurosci. 1999;2:422–6.

81. Lazarenko RM, Willcox SC, Shu S, Berg AP, Jevtovic-Todorovic V, Talley EM, Chen X, Bayliss DA. Motoneuronal TASK channels contribute to immobilizing effects of inhalational general anesthetics. J Neurosci. 2010;30:7691–704.

82. Pang DS, Robledo CJ, Carr DR, Gent TC, Vyssotski AL, Caley A, Zecharia AY, Wisden W, Brickley SG, Franks NP. An unexpected role for TASK-3 potassium channels in network oscillations with implications for sleep mechanisms and anesthetic action. Proc Natl Acad Sci U S A. 2009;106:17546–51.

83. Eger EI 2nd, Fisher DM, Dilger JP, Sonner JM, Evers A, Franks NP, Harris RA, Kendig JJ, Lieb WR, Yamakura T. Relevant concentrations of inhaled anesthetics for in vitro studies of anesthetic mechanisms. Anesthesiology. 2001;94:915–21.

84. Eckenhoff RG. Promiscuous ligands and attractive cavities: how do the inhaled anesthetics work? Mol Interv. 2001;1:258–68.

85. Quasha AL, Eger EI 2nd, Tinker JH. Determination and applications of MAC. Anesthesiology. 1980;53:315–34.

86. Harper MH, Winter PM, Johnson BH, Eger EI 2nd. Naloxone does not antagonize general anesthesia in the rat. Anesthesiology. 1978;49:3–5.

87. Eger EI 2nd, Gong D, Xing Y, Raines DE, Flood P. Acetylcholine receptors and thresholds for convulsions from flurothyl and 1,2-dichlorohexafluorocyclobutane. Anesth Analg. 2002;95:1611–5.

88. Flood P, Ramirez-Latorre J, Role L. Alpha 4 beta 2 neuronal nicotinic acetylcholine receptors in the central nervous system are inhibited by isoflurane and propofol, but alpha 7-type nicotinic acetylcholine receptors are unaffected. Anesthesiology. 1997;86:859–65.

89. Violet JM, Downie DL, Nakisa RC, Lieb WR, Franks NP. Differential sensitivities of mammalian neuronal and muscle nicotinic acetylcholine receptors to general anesthetics. Anesthesiology. 1997;86:866–74.

90. Cantor RS. Receptor desensitization by neurotransmitters in membranes: are neurotransmitters the endogenous anesthetics? Biochemistry. 2003;42:11891–7.

91. Milutinovic PS, Yang L, Cantor RS, Eger EI 2nd, Sonner JM. Anesthetic-like modulation of a gamma-aminobutyric acid type A, strychnine-sensitive glycine, and N-methyl-d-aspartate receptors by coreleased neurotransmitters. Anesth Analg. 2007;105:386–92.

92. Lu T, Rubio ME, Trussell LO. Glycinergic transmission shaped by the corelease of GABA in a mammalian auditory synapse. Neuron. 2008;57:524–35.

93. Nury H, Van Renterghem C, Weng Y, Tran A, Baaden M, Dufresne V, Changeux JP, Sonner JM, Delarue M, Corringer PJ. X-ray structures of general anaesthetics bound to a pentameric ligand-gated ion channel. Nature. 2010;469:428–31.

A History of Inhaled Anesthetics

46

Ron Jones

Summary

Valerius Cordus synthesized diethyl ether in 1540 and shortly thereafter Theophrastus Bombastus von Hohenheim (Paracelsus) noted that it could diminish pain. Priestley synthesized nitrous oxide in 1774, and in 1800, Davy found that it decreased pain and suggested its use for surgery. In the 1820s, Hickman advanced the notion of anesthesia, but Davy quashed Hickman's idea. Von Liebig synthesized chloroform in 1831.

The recreational use of diethyl ether and nitrous oxide and a desire to eliminate the pain of surgery, initially led to unsuccessful (nitrous oxide) demonstrations or unreported use in patients undergoing surgery. Long's experience with ether in 1842 is as famous as his failure to publicize the discovery. Anesthesia was born on 16 Oct 1846 (Ether Day) with Morton's public demonstration of ether anesthesia. Simpson's 1847 discovery of the anesthetic effects of chloroform followed. Nitrous oxide (restored to favor in the 1860s) and ether combined with oxygen provided anesthesia for a century, with modest competition in the 1930s to 1950s from divinyl ether, cyclopropane and trichloroethylene.

World War II advances in fluorine chemistry enabled development of compounds halogenated with fluorine to eliminate flammability. The major advance was Suckling's synthesis of halothane in the early 1950s. Released for clinical use in the mid-1950s, halothane swept away its pungent, toxic, flammable predecessors, dominating anesthesia for more than a decade. Its use in newly developed vaporizers (Copper Kettle and Fluotec) allowed the precise control of anesthetic concentrations, contributing to its safety and popularity.

World War II also gave birth to methods, particularly the infrared analyzer, to continuously analyze inhaled anesthetics. This facilitated the measurement of the Minimum Alveolar Concentration (MAC) required to eliminate movement in response to noxious stimulation in 50% of subjects, an anesthetic EC50.

Halothane was less than perfect. It caused a rare, immunologically-based and potentially fatal hepatic injury. This spurred the synthesis of progressively less metabolized, less toxic, and less soluble (faster recovery) anesthetics. Enflurane came first, and displaced halothane in the US in the 1970s. However, enflurane could cause convulsions and in the 1980s, isoflurane, a compound less soluble and without convulsant properties, replaced enflurane. The rise of ambulatory, day case surgery in the 1980s increased the demand for more rapid awakening from anesthesia, and the 1990s saw the release of the poorly soluble anesthetics, sevoflurane and desflurane.

Two decades have passed since the clinical release of a new inhaled anesthetic. What we have is very good, but it seems wrong to stop just short of perfect.

The Foundations Are Laid: Why Ether?

Ether Day, 16 Oct 1846, introduced anesthesia to the world. It had to be ether—and nitrous oxide and chloroform—all inhaled anesthetics, because no useful alternative existed. Drugs that might produce anesthesia by intravenous delivery either did not exist or were too dangerous in their actions. Furthermore, the hypodermic syringe had yet to be invented. What about swallowed drugs? Ingestion of opium could de-

crease pain, but ingestion sufficient to minimize the pain of surgery would stop breathing. Alcohol also could produce insensibility, but control over its dosing was too crude. The patient ingesting too little might have an exaggerated response to stimulation (surgery), and the patient ingesting too much might die. And once inebriation set in, one could not add more or subtract from what had been given. No, inhaled anesthetics, especially ether or chloroform were the only possibility. Their application required no complicated device; a handkerchief would do. And their effect could be controlled. The anesthetist could give more to produce a greater effect, or stop administration and the patient would eliminate the anesthetic by breathing. As long as the anesthetic hadn't stopped the patient from breathing, the anesthetic would float away.

R. Jones (✉)
Imperial College of Science, Technology and Medicine,
University of London, London, UK
e-mail: candrj@btinternet.com

E. I Eger II et al. (eds.), *The Wondrous Story of Anesthesia*, DOI 10.1007/978-1-4614-8441-7_46, © Edmond I Eger, MD 2014

The Age of Enlightenment

But why 16 Oct 1846? Part of the answer may lie in the social, theological, and scientific circumstances of the late eighteenth and early nineteenth centuries—the Age of Enlightenment. The Age of Enlightenment was the name given to the eighteenth century philosophical movement that placed greater emphasis on reason and observation than on tradition and theological dogma. This movement profoundly influenced later eighteenth and early nineteenth century science. No idea, no belief was exempt from scrutiny, making Western Civilization the tolerant, science and idea based society it is today.

The humanist philosophers of the Enlightenment such as Jeremy Bentham, David Hume, and Voltaire questioned the moral basis of many accepted practices including religion, slavery, and cruelty. Bentham (1748–1832) helped found London University and University College, London. After his death, his clothed skeleton was fitted with a wax model of his head and kept in a glass fronted cabinet at University College, his natural but shrunken head being placed at his feet. To this day, during meetings of the College Council, the cabinet's door is opened so that his spirit can be present. Bentham stated: "*The greatest happiness of the greatest number is the foundation of morals and legislation.*" And "*Nature has placed mankind under the governance of two sovereign masters, pain and pleasure*" [1].

At the end of the eighteenth century, few accepted the notion that sensation could be abolished without endangering life. From a scientific perspective, pain was viewed as an essential aspect of physiology and necessary to healing. And in Christian theology pain entered the world after Eve's disobedience in the Garden of Eden. Thus, the philosophical advances of the Enlightenment conflicted with scientific and theological paradigms. Enlightenment philosophers abhorred pain and suffering whereas scientific and religious thinking accepted pain as a necessary part of life. The late Emanuel (Manny) Papper, of the University of Miami, summed up this crucial change in social attitudes in this way. "*The discovery of anesthesia required the flowering of the view that the individual was important and deserved to have happiness. If only the group was important, the suffering of individuals was not and anesthesia was not something to be sought*" [2].

Studies of the anatomy and physiology of the nervous system, at the beginning of the nineteenth century, engendered a change in the attitude of science. Charles Bell and Francois Magendie established that specific parts of the brain controlled specific functions, that different nerves conducted sensation versus movement, and that vital functions (e.g., of the heart and lungs) were governed independently. If pain was a process independent from vital functions, then pain might be abolished without affecting vital functions, a belief required to make a search for anesthesia reasonable.

The Birmingham Lunar Society

At this time of changing scientific, moral and social attitudes toward pain and suffering, three individuals laid the foundations needed for the subsequent development of inhaled anesthetics; the scientist Joseph Priestley, the physician Thomas Beddoes and the philosopher and social reformer Jeremy Bentham, noted above. All were members of the Birmingham Lunar Society, so named because meetings were held at the time of the full moon, so that afterwards its members could better navigate their way home. Its diverse membership included James Watt (the steam engine), Josiah Wedgewood (pottery), Samuel Taylor Coleridge (poet) and Erasmus Darwin, grandfather of Charles.

The Birmingham Lunar Society financially supported Joseph Priestley (1733–1804), famed for his 1770s discoveries of oxygen and nitrous oxide. Priestley termed what the French chemist Lavoisier later called oxygen, 'dephlogisticated air'. Lavoisier was guillotined in 1797, after the French Revolution. The politically radical Priestley vigorously supported the Revolution. His attitude later forced him to flee his hometown and eventually, his country. Thus, the French revolution significantly altered the lives of both these pioneers of chemistry, pioneers linked by oxygen.

Joseph Priestley, from the English county of Yorkshire, was a scientist and radical political thinker (his application to join Captain James Cook's 1772 Antarctic expedition was rejected because of his political and religious views). He influenced, and in turn was influenced by Bentham. Priestley produced nitrous oxide—or 'gaseous oxyd of azote'—in 1772, by exposing nitric oxide to a mixture of iron filings, sulfur and water. He noted that nitrous oxide delayed decay of animal tissues (perhaps by excluding oxygen), a potentially useful finding in an age of no refrigeration. He also suggested that "*…considerable use might be made of it in medicine….*" [3]. Later he became a correspondent and friend of Benjamin Franklin. On the second anniversary of the fall of the Bastille, his political sympathies led a Royalist mob to ransack his home, library and scientific apparatus, and he fled to London. Ostracized by his scientific colleagues, he left Britain in 1794 to join his sons in Northumberland, Pennsylvania and took up farming. Hilaire Belloc, the poet and historian, was a great-grandson.

Beddoes, Davy, and the Pneumatic Institution

Like Priestley, Thomas Beddoes (1760–1808) had radical political and social views and supported the French Revolution. He was of short stature, short temper and large girth. In the latter part of the eighteenth century, pneumatic medicine came into vogue. Various gases were given by various routes, including as enemas, in the hope of some therapeutic action.

Beddoes' radical views were not well received in conservative Oxford where he lectured in chemistry, so he moved to Bristol which had a reputation for tolerance. With the financial support of the Lunar Society, he founded the Pneumatic Medical Institution intent on investigating the medicinal effects of gases, including nitrous oxide, particularly on tuberculosis. In 1798, Beddoes recruited as his assistant, a young apothecary's apprentice from Cornwall, *Humphrey Davy*, who at age 20 started to experiment on himself with nitrous oxide.

By 1800, Beddoes and Davy had demonstrated both euphoric and analgesic effects of nitrous oxide. Members of the Lunar Society, including the poet, Samuel Coleridge, and Peter Roget, famous for his Thesaurus, visited the Institute to breathe nitrous oxide. Coleridge, known for his supernatural poems, '*The Rime of the Ancient Mariner*' and '*Kubla Khan*' inhaled nitrous oxide at the Pneumatic Institute and observed: "*I had recollections of such unmingled pleasure than I ever had before experienced*". This observation probably relates to the lack of hangover effects associated with nitrous oxide compared with opium—to which he was addicted.

Davy (1778–1829) found that nitrous oxide could relieve the pain of toothache and stated: "*As nitrous oxide in its extensive operation appears capable of destroying physical pain, it may probably be used with advantage during surgical operations in which no great effusion of blood takes place* [4]." Davy was a hands-on scientist who studied the effects of nitrous oxide on himself. In one experiment he was put into a box-like chamber whilst an assistant added aliquots of nitrous oxide. His lively description of the effects of the gas need to be interpreted in the light of the fact that oxygen was not co-administered [5]. Thus everything was in place in 1800 for the emergence of anesthesia. Yet nearly 50 years passed before Davy's prediction became reality. Why? In 1960, writing about the first 100 years of anesthesia, WS Sykes commented: "*What is surprising is that* (Davy's) *suggestion was ignored by the very people whom it should have interested most: that surgeons should have continued for nearly fifty years longer to operate on screaming, struggling patients in full consciousness. Surely a lasting testimonial to their thickheadedness*" [6].

Davy left the Pneumatic Institute in 1801. He was politically conventional and became a respected part of the British scientific establishment. He subsequently made a negative contribution to the development of inhaled anesthetics, by his unenthusiastic reception of a communication sent to the Royal Society, of whom he was a sometime President, a communication from a Shropshire doctor, Henry Hill Hickman.

The Sorry Story of Henry Hickman

While in Shifnal, Shropshire, Beddoes birthplace, Hickman (1800–1830) became interested in Pneumatic Medicine. He was thus aware of the work of Beddoes and Davy (who later contributed to his undoing). Driven by a desire to relieve pain during surgery, Hickman experimented on the '*torpid state*' or suspended animation caused by inhalation of carbon dioxide. Despite some success in relieving pain during surgery in animals under the 'torpid state', the largely London based scientific and medical establishments of the day did not accept his views. In 1824, he wrote to the Royal Society: "*…something has not been thought of whereby the fears (of the patient) may not be tranquilized and suffering relieved*" [7]. The snub given by Humphrey Davy and others may be explained in parochial terms. Shropshire is a rural county, which many Englishmen would be hard pressed to place. Undeterred, Hickman took his claims of pain free surgery to the French '*Academie Royale de Medicine*', France, having at the time a reputation for medical innovation. But he fared no better with that medical establishment. Rejected and depressed, Hickman committed suicide in 1830, at age 31. Whether his studies were relevant remains unclear (administration of carbon dioxide can cause anesthesia, but the concentrations needed could compromise oxygen delivery). His importance lay in his view of pain-free surgery as an achievable goal.

Everything Comes Together: The 1840s in the United States

Coleridge's dependence on opium was not unusual for his time. In Europe and America, the recreational use of drugs was relatively common. Recall the parties at the Bristol Pneumatic Institution where nitrous oxide was inhaled for its euphoric effects. So popular was nitrous oxide that in some circles it replaced champagne. One visitor at such a party, skeptical of the effects of the gas breathed 'quite a sufficiency' and: "*…he began to dance and devastate the adjoining flower-bed in his ecstasy* [8]." And there is a parallel in diethyl ether ("ether"), synthesized in 1540 by Valerius Cordus. Ether was sold by chemists as 'sweet (oil of) vitriol' and used, like nitrous oxide, as a recreational drug ('ether frolics'). Now to Crawford Long in rural Georgia, in a small town called Jefferson.

Crawford Long and Ether-Sniffing in Jefferson, Georgia, 1842

Crawford Long (1815–1878), a native of Jefferson Georgia, studied medicine at the University of Pennsylvania. He attended ether frolics as a student and in the early 1840s introduced such frolics to the citizens of Jefferson, including his friend and patient, James Venable. Long purchased ether from a pharmacist in Athens, Georgia, Robert Goodman, and anecdotally, Long told Goodman in November 1841, that pain free surgery might be possible after inhaling ether [9].

Venable complained of a large cyst on his neck, wanting it removed but fearful of the pain that removal would cause. Long, appreciating the analgesic effects of ether, reportedly advised: *"Breathe ether then I'll cut off the cyst"* [10]. Familiarity with ether sniffing made Venable receptive to the suggestion. Thus, on 30 March 1842, the date usually taken as that of the first successful general anesthetic in a human, Long removed Venable's cyst without pain. Long remembered:

> *"When giving it to Venable, with one hand I held the towel over his mouth and nose permitting him to breathe a little air as he inhaled the drug; my other hand I kept on his pulse. When he became insensible to the prick of a pin I operated. As an inducement to Venable to allow himself to be the subject of the experiment, my charge for the operation was nominal, $2.00 Ether, 25 cents"* [9].

Although the date, 30 March 1842, is generally acknowledged to be that of the first successful use of ether in surgery, there is a report that in January of that year William Clarke, a medical student from Rochester, New York, and a regular ether sniffer, used ether during a dental extraction, the patient being Miss Hobbie and the dentist, Elijah Pope [11].

Although Long used ether several times in ensuing years he did not publicize his achievements. By the time (1849) he told the world, Boston had seen successful public demonstrations of general anesthesia. Long comes off well in this history. Modestly, he never claimed to be the one who should have been given credit for the discovery of anesthesia. He died a happy man.

Colton, Wells, and the Grand Exhibition at Union Hall, Hartford, 10 Dec 1844

Gardner Colton, a medical student at Columbia University, sought to subsidize his medical career with exhibitions of the inebriating effects of nitrous oxide, one such in Hartford Connecticut in December 1844. A local dentist, Horace Wells (1815–1848), attended the exhibition, as did a Samuel Cooley, who, under the influence of nitrous oxide, ran against a bench and cut his leg. Wells noticed that Cooley did not appear to feel any pain from his collision with the bench, and Cooley confirmed Wells' observation.

Wells wished to enlarge his practice by providing pain-free dentistry. Wells had an abscessed tooth and persuaded Colton to bring a bag of nitrous oxide to Wells' office the next day. Wells breathed the nitrous oxide, and while under its influence, a colleague, John Riggs, painlessly (according to Wells) extracted the abscessed tooth. Wells subsequently experimented with the manufacture and use of nitrous oxide in his dental practice with uneven success. Undaunted, he ar-

ranged to demonstrate the anesthetic effects of nitrous oxide before the faculty and students of Harvard University, including the surgeon in chief of the Massachusetts General Hospital, John Collins Warren. A student agreed to have a tooth extracted, but the demonstration was less than successful. According to Wells, he removed the mask too soon. The student groaned toward the end of the extraction and this was taken as a failure by an audience all too ready to label the experiment unsuccessful. Wells *"heard the word 'Humbug' called out over and over again* [12]." He later wrote that "*…several expressed their opinion that it was a humbug affair (which in fact was all the thanks I got for this gratuitous service)…*." [12]. Wells never recovered from this failure and died, a suicide in January 1848.

Wells' failure demonstrates a fundamental problem of nitrous oxide anesthesia; limited potency. By itself, it is a weak anesthetic or in modern parlance, the minimum alveolar concentration needed for anesthesia is 105%—more than can be obtained at sea level [13]. Thus, used alone it is at the limits of its ability to produce anesthesia, as Wells in front of his skeptical audience, found to his cost. And, when given at 100% of an atmosphere (the greatest partial pressure possible at sea level), part of the effect is not anesthesia but lack of oxygen. Indeed, a pupil of Claude Bernard's in Paris, Paul Bert, understood that 100% nitrous oxide could not be administered without causing hypoxia and undertook animal studies conducted in a hyperbaric chamber, a technique that was then used in patients, but was too cumbersome for routine use [14].

Morton, Jackson, and Anesthesia. Who Made the discovery?

William GT Morton (1819–1868) had been a student and then partner of Wells. In their partnership they used a solder invented by Riggs (the dentist who extracted Wells' tooth on 11 December 1844) in the manufacture of an improved denture. The solder used by Wells, Morton and Riggs was endorsed by a well known Boston physician, Charles Jackson (1805–1880), with whom Morton was destined to disagree over who should be acknowledged as the discoverer of anesthesia.

Morton was present at Wells' failed attempt to demonstrate nitrous oxide anesthesia in 1844, and was convinced that the principle was sound. Greed prompted him to continue pursuit of pain free dental surgery. Advances in dental techniques had introduced far superior artificial teeth but fitting them necessitated the removal of not only the stumps and remnants of the originals but also their roots. Many patients could not bear the pain and fled before completion of the surgery. Morton knew about Wells' work with nitrous oxide and had heard first hand, accounts of its efficacy from his patients. So Morton discussed the matter further with his colleague Charles Jackson. Jackson suggested to Morton that ether could produce some numbing effect if applied around a tooth to be extracted, not realizing that inhalation of the vaporized ether would be the cause of the "numbing". Morton experimented with the use of ether in animals and on himself, and extracted the tooth of Eben Frost in his Boston office on 30 September 1846. Morton subsequently undertook several extractions successfully with ether, and like Wells, sought to demonstrate his finding publicly [15].

Henry Bigelow, a surgeon at the Massachusetts General Hospital, had read about Morton's activities and had witnessed extractions under ether. He arranged with Warren (who had witnessed Wells' failed attempt to demonstrate anesthesia with nitrous oxide) a parallel attempt using ether on 16 October 1846, Ether Day. Warren was one time Dean of Harvard Medical School and founder, with others, of the Massachusetts General Hospital in 1821. He initiated the Boston Medical and Surgical Journal which became the New England Journal of Medicine.

The patient, Gilbert Abbott had an arterio-venous malformation in his neck. But Morton's apparatus for administering ether was not quite ready and Morton was tardy. Warren was losing patience when Morton arrived with his apparatus, a glass flask with two necks and a sponge contained within the flask. The sponge ensured the saturation of the air breathed by Abbott with ether vapor, and prevented the aspiration of liquid ether. Warren testily remarked: "Your patient is ready, sir!" Morton had Abbott breathe the ether for a few minutes, and then returned Warren's comment, word for word. The operation began, initially with no response from Abbott. As with the attempted demonstration of anesthesia with nitrous oxide, toward the end of surgery Abbott moved and vocalized but when asked afterwards, he confirmed that he had felt no pain. Warren then supposedly provided the most famous quotation in anesthesia: "*Gentlemen, this is no humbug*". Abbott stayed in hospital nearly two months after the surgery. A century and a half later he would have left that day.

Superficially, Morton's demonstration was no more successful than that of Wells two years earlier. But Morton was a greater extrovert, he was not as rushed, and he used an agent that was more potent and had a longer lasting effect—being 25 times more soluble in blood than nitrous oxide [16, 17]. He supplied anesthesia for a longer procedure. And in Henry Bigelow, he had the backing of a member of the Boston medical establishment. A second demonstration on the following day, using a slightly modified apparatus, was also successful and the world, or at least the Boston medical world, was convinced of Morton's discovery. From November onwards, ether was used extensively in Boston and environs.

Morton and Jackson disputed who discovered anesthesia. The details are complex and do not appreciably add to this narrative. The underlying motivations appear to have been Morton's longing for a fortune (greed) and Jackson's enormous ego. Clever Charles Jackson graduated with honors from Harvard University in 1829. He became a prominent geologist, hard working and ambitious. Ambition led him to pursue imaginative, perhaps inappropriate, methods to enhance his reputation. An example: Traveling by ship from France to America in 1832, Jackson met Samuel Morse, an American portrait painter who was also interested in the electric telegraph. Morse devised a code to be transmitted by electromagnetic relays. The American Congress gave Morse financial support. In 1843, a line was constructed from Washington DC to Baltimore. The famous message: "*What hath God Wrought*" was sent on 24 May 1844 using his system of dots and dashes. Imagine Morse's surprise to find in a Boston paper: "*…that the electro-magnetic telegraph which SFB Morse of New York claims to have made, was really made by our fellow citizen Charles T Jackson*". It took several years for Morse to correct the situation just as it took several years for Morton to be recognized as the discoverer of *etherization* for pain free surgery. After Morton's death, Jackson became possessed with what he saw as his just and rightful recognition. But the momentum of history, and probably justice, conspired against him. Jackson ended his days in an institution for the mentally insane, perhaps brooding on the injustices heaped upon him by Morse, Morton, and the world in general.

Although Morton is generally credited with the discovery, he never made the fortune he had hoped might be his. He tried to publicize his cause in 1847, by administering ether to American soldiers fighting Mexicans off the port of Vera Cruz, and to soldiers at the battles of Fredericksburg (December 1862) and Wilderness (May 1864), just a few years before his death in 1868. He hoped to receive a $100,000 award from the US Congress, but Congress happily did nothing, finding that several citizens (Wells, Jackson, and Morton) had made conflicting claims. In addition, the US Civil War preoccupied Congress much of the time.

Oliver Wendell Holmes Coins "Anaesthesia"

And what of the word "Anesthesia"? The professor of Anatomy and one time Dean of Harvard Medical School was Oliver Wendell Holmes, better known today as an essayist. From the Greek for sensation, *aesthesia*, he christened this new phenomenon '*anaesthesia*', or lack of sensation. The first Academic Department in our specialty in the UK was at Oxford University. The then University Registrar, Sir Douglas Beale, told the Chair, Robert Macintosh, that the Department would be named 'Anaesthe*tics*' to be consistent with poli*tics* and econom*ics*. The linguistic authority, Peter Cuff, Vice Regent of Pembroke College Oxford, noted that the word 'Anaesthesia' meant loss of feeling. He added…"*I cannot see how it would be right to have a professor of that state, any more than a Professor of Amnesia.*" He went on to review alternatives: "*Anaesthesiology: the subject and practice of Anaesthesia and Anaesthetics. The word first occurs in Steadman's Medical Dictionary 1914*". Cuff continued to state that the term 'Anaesthesiology' was too clumsy and recent for Oxford.

News Travels to Liverpool

News of Morton's discovery traveled fast. A wooden paddle steamer of the Cunard Line, the '*Acadia*', arrived with the news in Liverpool on December 16, providing the basis for an account of Morton's use of ether that was reported in the Liverpool Mercury. The ship's surgeon, William Fraser, went home to Dumfries where his news prompted the use of ether for setting a leg fracture on 19 December. On that day, the American physician Francis Boott, living in London, received a letter from Henry Bigelow, describing Morton's 'discovery', carried aboard the *Acadia*. He convinced a dentist, James Robinson, to give ether to his niece, a Miss Lonsdale, for a molar extraction. After Robinson's successful painless extraction, Boott persuaded the Professor of Surgery at University College Hospital, Robert Liston, to operate using ether. On 21 December, a medical student, William Squire, provided ether anesthesia to Frederick Churchill while Liston uneventfully amputated Churchill's leg. Liston commented that: "*This Yankee Dodge, gentlemen, beats mesmerism hollow*". The operation provoked considerable publicity and ether's role in the UK was assured.

It is noteworthy that Liston immediately compared ether anesthesia with mesmerism. Mesmeric anesthesia was practiced widely in Europe and the US in the nineteenth century, and its followers did not take well to the introduction of etherization. Introduced by Austrian, Franz Anton Mesmer (described as stubborn, secretive, an opportunist and plagiarist) [18], mesmerism was a mystical 'science' in which the practitioner placed himself between energizing heavenly 'fluidism' and human disease. John Elliotson was a proponent of mesmeric anesthesia and editor of '*Zoist*' *A Journal of Cerebral Physiology and Mesmerism and Their Applications to Human Welfare*. *Zoist* was published until 1855. Mesmeric anesthesia had a strong following in the Southern US. That popularity may have contributed to Long's reluctance to advertise his activities.

The use of ether anesthesia spread well beyond the US and the UK. Here is an example concerning the first anesthetic given in Singapore in August 1847.

"On Monday last Kling (Indian) boatman was brought to Mr Little, Surgeon, with a large splinter of wood run in his hand, and suffering much pain. Mr Little tried to extract the splinter by several means during which poor Kling suffered much pain. So Little resolved to try ether as this appeared a good case to test its powers. The man's own hubble-bubble was then brought, into which a few ounces of Ether were poured. Mr Little then closed Kling's nostrils by means of a flat letter clip and asked the patient to inhale the ether from his hubble-bubble. After extensive surgery, during which Mr Kling was quite insensible the paper clip was removed from the patient's nose and water thrown in his face. Kling declared he had felt no pain and was much struck with the sight of his bandaged hand" [19].

Ether had limitations however. Being highly soluble in blood and pungent, it produced a slow onset of anesthesia, often marred by excitement. Therefore, some skill was needed in its successful administration, a skill that many surgeons lacked, and presumably such individuals may have abandoned its use. However, John Snow (1813–1858), the first specialist anesthetist, reported that he did not have a single failure administering ether anesthesia. Snow's safe use of ether doubtless stems from his scientific background in chemistry and physiology as well as being one of the first to recognize the importance of the use of an inhaler for its quantitative delivery, as opposed to the 'rag and bottle' approach which delivered an unknown concentration. Still, the quest for a less pungent agent continued. Here we leave America, with the principal protagonists in bitter dispute about priority, committing suicide or going mad, and travel back across the Atlantic to the sober capital of Scotland, Edinburgh.

Simpson, Snow, and Chloroform

In 1831, von Liebig in Germany described a new compound called 'perchloride of formyl'. Dumas termed it chloroform in 1834. Chloroform ($CHCl_3$) was used, like nitrous oxide and ether, as a recreational drug. Horace Wells' addiction to chloroform played a part in his suicide. However, social uses played no part in its discovery as an anesthetic. James Simpson (1811–1870), nicknamed 'Young' because of his youthful appearance, was Professor of Midwifery in Edinburgh. He used ether on 17 January 1847, at the Edinburgh Infirmary, to relieve the pain of labor. Because of its slow onset of action, ether seemed less than optimum to Simpson—who began a search for a less pungent alternative.

Simpson sequestered a variety of liquid compounds in an oak dresser in his morning room at 52 Queen Street, Edinburgh. Among these was chloroform, which his colleague, James Waldie, had recently synthesized in Liverpool. From June 1847, Simpson and his associates, including James Duncan, would breathe the vapors from the bottles in the oak dresser. On 4 November, Duncan was at the bottles and reported to his sister that he: "…*found himself awakening slowly and pleasantly from an unconscious sleep, which the timepiece showed must have lasted about quarter of an hour*

[20]." That night Simpson, Duncan and another colleague, Thomas Keith, filled their glasses with the pleasant smelling liquid and after a brief period of disinhibition and excitement, narcosis intervened. Simpson awoke to exclaim: "*This is far stronger and better than ether*". The next day Simpson used this stronger and better agent successfully to relieve pain during labor. By 10 November, he had compiled sufficient successful cases to report to the Edinburgh Medical and Chirurgical Society, and on 15 November he published a paper; '*On a new anaesthetic agent, more efficient than sulphuric ether*', which sold 4,000 copies.

The Duchess of Sutherland sent one copy to Queen Victoria, and Snow soon started using chloroform. Snow presciently observed: "*It certainly has greater advantages for patients but greater care is necessary in its use to avoid accidents* [21]." Victoria requested chloroform for the birth of two of her children.

It is a myth that the Church had staunchly opposed chloroform's use during childbirth on theological grounds [*e.g.*, *"In sorrow thou shalt bring forth children"* (Genesis iii, 16)] until Victoria's use in childbirth subdued the opposition. Derek Farr, a student of Colin Russell of the Open University in England, searched for documents indicating that the Church objected to pain free labor. He found little supporting evidence. Explanations for the myth were presented at the 8th Priestley Conference at the Royal Society of Chemistry in London, on 22–24 April 1997 [22]. Opposition to anesthesia for laboring woman came from the medical community, often disguised in religious terms. Reasons for opposition may have varied from honestly held physiological objections—pain is necessary for effective labor—to less charitable interpretations. No objector was a woman.

By Christmas of 1847, chloroform featured in children's pantomimes, and in 1849, the first of several chloroform muggings were reported by 'HN' in the Times (of London) newspaper. With respect to an elderly relative of his: "*Coming round after an agreeable dream, he hazily recollected three men. His purse, keys, spectacles, and gold eye glass were gone and his pockets ransacked*" [23].

Chloroform Kills

We know now that chloroform has potent cardiovascular effects, can cause the heart to beat erratically, and may lethally damage the liver and kidney. In October 1847, 15 year old Hannah Greener had a toenail removed under ether anesthesia. Illegitimate and abused, Hannah led a hard life and had long suffered from painful feet. On 28 January 1848, she had another toenail removed, but this time chloroform was used. Within moments of breathing chloroform, Hannah was dead. The Times reported her death, the first of many associated with chloroform anesthesia [24]. After a post-mortem enquiry, the jury concluded that: "*Hannah Greener died of congestion of the lungs produced by the direct effects of chloroform*." The true cause of death cannot be known, but it is likely that she died from the tendency of chloroform to cause cardiac arrhythmias. Vomiting and aspiration of vomit offer another possibility.

The ease of use by the non-trained, the '*rag and bottle*' method, whereby chloroform was dropped onto a simple face mask or a handkerchief, made chloroform popular. (My father, not a specialist anesthetist, used chloroform frequently by this method aboard the World War II cruiser HMS Belfast, now moored near Tower Bridge on the river Thames. It is worth a visit as the old 'sick bay', complete with operating theatre and anesthetic equipment is well preserved.)

Simpson and Snow disagreed on why patients died during or after chloroform, citing either its respiratory or cardiac effects. And they disagreed on how to give it. Simpson argued that: "*Inhaling instruments frighten patients, whilst the handkerchief does not* [25]." Snow advocated inhalers as safer because of the control offered over delivered chloroform concentrations. Although Snow was correct, their disagreements outlasted both of them.

The greatest protagonist for the safety of chloroform given by simple means was Lieutenant-Colonel Edward Lawrie (1846–1915). As the senior medical officer and driving force for sixteen years, at the medical school in Hyderabad, he followed unfailingly, the teachings of his hero and former chief, Professor James Syme (1799–1870). While most of the profession concerned about the deaths from chloroform argued that the cause was cardiac, Lawrie maintained that the cause was asphyxia or overdose. The findings of the first (1888) and second Hyderabad commissions (1890) reinforced Lawrie's view. However, the commissions were financed by Lawrie's benefactor, the Nizam of Hyderabad, and chaired by Lawrie himself. The science was dubious. Lawrie, who claimed to have safely given 40,000 to 50,000 administrations, engaged in prolific correspondence to the British Medical Journal and the Lancet [26]. An example of his single-mindedness may be seen in his reply to comments in The Lancet in 1889: "I have no wish to say anything to give offence to those who hold the same view as the writer of the annotation, but I hold that those views are wrong, and that there is no such thing as chloroform syncope [27]."

Augustus Waller (1856–1922), lecturer in physiology at St Mary's Medical School in West London, advocated administration of chloroform in concentrations between 1% and 2% [28]. Others advocated safe use of concentrations up to 3%, and a variety of inhalers were developed to achieve its accurate administration. In 1901, Waller joined the Chloroform Commission convened by the British Medical Association (BMA). The commission did not issue its final report until 1910, by which time Edward Embley (1861–1924) had published the results of his extensive research in Melbourne, Australia [29–31]. In the 25 pages devoted to his research, he pointed out defects in Lawrie's case. He proved conclusively that sudden death during chloroform administration was due to the effect of chloroform on the heart, not the respiration. This paved the way for A Goodman Levy (1866–1954), whose research established that ventricular fibrillation was the actual cause [32]. Lawrie remained unconvinced to his death.

Remember that chloroform was the "British" anesthetic and ether the "American" anesthetic. Perhaps it is not surprising that a decade later, the Committee on Anesthesia of the American Medical Association (AMA) concluded that: "*The use of chloroform as an anesthetic could no longer be justified.*" Despite Embley, Levy, the BMA, and the AMA, chloroform continued to be used for another half-century in the US. Eger remembers being asked if he wanted to use it in his residency in 1957. He declined. With the introduction of the safer halothane, chloroform and ether both disappeared as anesthetics in the US.

However, ether remained in use in other parts of the world (often for economic reasons), well into the 1980s. One reason for its continued use, well past its "sell by date" in the UK, was a technique of rapid induction of anesthesia with ether as taught by Harry Churchill-Davidson of St Thomas's Hospital (situated opposite the Houses of Parliament in London). Harry C-D, as he was known, was a larger than life, English gentleman. He had the patient breathe 10 % carbon dioxide in oxygen for 5 min, ensuring profound hyperventilation. The ether dial was then turned to maximum over the next 10 breaths and the energetic breathing ensured a rapid induction with the added benefit that the tracheal tube was sucked into place by the patient. Ether was still used in the UK in the mid 1980s; I'm told that an enthusiast (perhaps John Snow's ghost) gave ether at St. Bartholomew's Hospital in London as late as 1985.

Before we leave the year 1847 one further topic deserves mention. In this year the first theory of the neuro-physiological basis of anesthesia was proposed. Mike Halsey, who had worked with Eger and John Nunn on the molecular basis of anesthetic action, noted that, von Bibra, Harless, and von Herman suggested that the dissolution of fat within neurons caused the state of anesthesia [33]. The theory did not explain how recovery from anesthesia occurred.

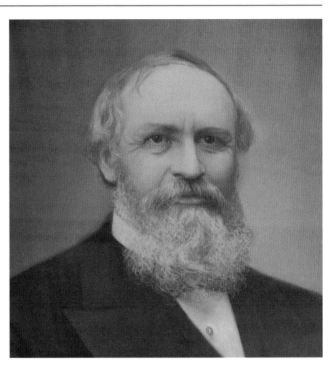

Fig. 46.1 Edmund Andrews. (Photograph of portrait, Feinberg School of Medicine Library, courtesy of the EIE collection)

remained in use ever since. The surgeon, Edmund Andrews (Fig. 46.1), suggested that the concurrent addition of oxygen would enhance the safety and usefulness of nitrous oxide [34]. The effective use of this suggestion required the development of compressed gases, containers that withstood high pressures, and a means for the controlled delivery of the gases, toward the end of the nineteenth century. The non-pungent nitrous oxide was then used to smooth and hasten the induction of anesthesia with the more pungent ether. In most developed countries, ether gained in popularity as skill in its administration increased and its greater safety was recognized. The lesser safety of chloroform probably prompted differences in the skills of US versus Commonwealth anesthetists. Its dangers mandated that medically knowledgeable persons, particularly physicians, give chloroform, but in the US, anyone could and did give ether. In the US, the safest anesthesia was probably given by nurse anesthetists trained in the art (see Chapter 22). And so, for a time, anesthesia advanced more rapidly in the UK than in the land of its discovery.

Inhaled Anesthetic Developments in the Second Half of the Nineteenth Century

Ether and chloroform continued as mainstays of anesthetic delivery for a century after their introduction. Nitrous oxide temporarily fell from favor after Wells' failed demonstration, but Gardner Colton re-introduced it in 1862, and it has

The First Half of the Twentieth Century

The first half of the twentieth century saw the discovery of several new inhaled anesthetics, most being but marginal improvements on ether. Consider ethylene, or ethene, the first member of the alkene series (C_2H_4), the polymer being polyethylene. In 1908, growers noted that carnations failed to flower in greenhouses where there had been a leak of ethylene, used for illumination. The expression 'go to sleep' was used to describe the condition of the ethylene contaminated carnations. This chance finding that ethylene induced 'sleep' in carnations prompted Arno Luckhardt to trial its use as an anesthetic. Ethylene entered clinical practice around 1923 [35]. As it was more potent than nitrous oxide, and thus could be administered with greater oxygen concentrations, it transiently became popular in the US. However, ethylene is highly flammable and by the early 1930s, several explosions had occurred. This, along with the introduction of the more potent cyclopropane, caused its use to wane. However, Eger remembers with awe, a presence of history while giving ethylene at Chicago's Presbyterian Hospital in the early 1950s for emergency surgery. The Presbyterian Hospital was the site of the first use of ethylene in patients.

Cyclopropane's introduction as a general anesthetic was also initiated by a chance finding. Cyclopropane was synthesized in 1882. George Lucas and Velyien Henderson in Toronto thought that a contaminant of a cylinder of propylene might have resulted in toxic reactions. Two kittens put in a jar with the contaminant, cyclopropane, were anesthetized and recovered uneventfully [36]. Henderson was the first human subject anesthetized with the gas. Cyclopropane had several advantages. It was potent, having a MAC of approximately 10% [37]. Because of its potency, poor blood solubility, and lack of irritant properties, it induced anesthesia quickly. It did not depress the heart; in fact it increased blood pressure. However, it could explode, it caused the heart to sometimes beat irregularly, and it depressed breathing. Indeed, as early as 1956, the Ministry of Health in the UK set up a working party to investigate fires and explosions associated with anesthesia and reported a total of 36 explosions and three deaths between 1947 and 1954. These limitations and the advent of the nonflammable halothane eventually led to the abandonment of cyclopropane. However, as late as the 1980s, it continued to be used, especially in children, and in patients who needed support of their blood pressure. Eger remembers in the 1960s, promising volunteers that if they would breathe 10 breaths of 50% cyclopropane they would fall asleep by the tenth breath. He lied. They all fell asleep by the third breath.

Vinethene (Vinesthine, Vinydan), the commercial name for divinyl ether (CH_2CH-O-$CHCH_2$), was the first inhaled anesthetic developed with some notion of a relationship of structure to activity (a precedent sometimes, erroneously in my opinion, accorded halothane). Leake and Chen deliberately combined the advantageous properties of ether (high potency) and ethylene (absent pungency and low solubility), substituting two ethylene moieties for the two ethane moieties in ether to produce divinyl ether [38]. Its primary advantage was that it was one-quarter as soluble in blood as ether [39]. It was used for approximately 40 years, particu-

larly to smooth the induction of anesthesia with ether. Larry Saidman remembers that it was still in use for this purpose in the early 1960s. He recalls that some skill was needed to hold both the divinyl ether bottle and the ether can in the right hand and maintain the airway with the left hand all the time using an open drop ether mask!

In the late 1930s, the degreasing and dry cleaning agent, trichloroethylene (CCl_2CHCl) or Trilene, was introduced as an anesthetic by the London anesthetist Langton Hewer, finding favor mostly in the UK [40]. It had been sniffed illicitly by thrill seekers and had found a place in medicine as a treatment for trigeminal neuralgia. Trilene possessed innate analgesic properties, and was inexpensive and easy to administer. Perhaps most attractive, it was non-explosive, a particular advantage because of the increasing use of electrocautery by surgeons to stop bleeding. But Trilene produced a high incidence of postoperative nausea and vomiting and had the potential to be hepatotoxic. It had to be used in an open (high-flow) system because it reacted with carbon dioxide absorbents to produce the nerve gas phosgene. Nevertheless, Trilene continued to be used by cost conscious anesthesiologists for many years after the introduction of halothane.

Changes in society in the early part of the twentieth century drove the search for improved inhaled anesthetics. Doctors wanted to improve the patient experience during and after surgery, and patients expected more. Anesthetics used before World War II were toxic (especially chloroform and Trilene), associated with postoperative nausea and vomiting (all anesthetics), or explosive (ether, ethylene, cyclopropane, Vinethene), or had a combination of these unwanted effects. Nitrous oxide caused nausea and vomiting, had a subtle toxicity, and lacked sufficient potency to produce surgical anesthesia. Chloroform use provided an example of how prevailing societal attitudes influenced anesthetic use. Although chloroform was easy to use, produced a pleasanter induction than ether, and was non-explosive, death from cardiovascular side effects or liver or renal injury were relatively common. As the twentieth century advanced, 'patient safety' became a concern of doctors and of society in general. Litigation motivated some of the changes. Chloroform continued to be used commonly in the UK and the Southern US, as opposed to the Northern US where litigation was increasingly an issue. Indeed, I'm unaware of any British anesthetist being sued following a chloroform-induced death even though the jury at Hannah Greener's inquest clearly believed that chloroform caused her demise.

Even before World War II, we knew where to search for a better inhaled anesthetic. In a prophetic introduction to their studies on fluorine derivatives of chloroform in 1932, Harold Booth and E May Bixby of Western Reserve University in Cleveland stated: "*A survey of the properties of 166 known gases suggests that the best possibility of finding a new non-combustible anesthetic gas lay in the field of organic fluoride compounds. Fluorine substitution for other halogens lowers the boiling point, increases stability and generally decreases toxicity* [41]." Every time I read this, especially the last sentence, I marvel at Booth and Bixby's perspicacity. We knew what should be done, but the great electronegativity and reactivity of fluorine made it difficult to study, and we lacked sufficient expertise in its control in the 1930s. Then war broke out, and we found the expertise.

Advances in Fluorine Chemistry During World War II

Scheele identified fluorine in 1771, but it was not isolated until 1886 because fluorine is the most electronegative of all elements, and is very reactive. Like all halogens (five non-metallic elements which form simple salts like sodium chloride or table salt—the word 'halogen' derives from the Greek 'salt producing') fluorine is not found in the free state in nature. Chemists in the 1930s could synthesize but few fluorine-containing compounds that might have anesthetic activity.

Two military goals greatly advanced fluorine chemistry, and led to the synthesis of the first fluorinated anesthetic, methoxyflurane. First, the huge increase in demand for high octane aviation fuel necessitated production of a catalyst—hydrogen fluoride. Second, in 1942, the best chemists available in the US were recruited to the Manhattan Project to develop the atomic bomb containing the fissile U[235]isotope of uranium. U[235]had to be separated from its natural, non-fissile isotope, U[238]. To do this required making the uranium volatile—a gas! And that could be done by combining uranium with fluorine to make uranium hexafluoride (UF_6). The rest was simple: just use a jillion centrifuges to separate U[235]$F_6$from U[238]$F_6$and then remove the fluorine. The atomic bomb detonated 300m above Hiroshima on 6 August 1945, contained U[235]. Thus, great advances in fluorine chemistry occurred, advances enabling the synthesis of diverse, potentially anesthetic compounds. The aphorism '*Every evil hath its good, every sweet its sour*' was never more apposite (attributed to Oliver Wendell Holmes Jr. whose father, as previously noted, coined the term 'anaesthesia').

Two developments linked the Manhattan Project and fluorinated anesthetics. The first led to methoxyflurane (CH_3-O-CF_2-$CHCl_2$). As part of the Manhattan Project, William Miller, Edward Fager, and Paul Griswold synthesized several fluorinated methyl ethyl ethers [42]. Methoxyflurane was synthesized in 1944 but went unnoticed. Miller and his colleagues were working for the Manhattan Project at SAM Laboratories, Columbia University, under contract number W-7405-Eng-50 and at SAM Laboratories Carbide and Carbon Chemicals Corporation, New York City under contract number W-7405-Eng-26, Supplement No 4. The details of methoxyflurane's synthesis were published in Volume 1 of Division VII of the Manhattan Project Technical Series. I in-

clude the contract numbers to demonstrate that fluorinated anesthetics directly resulted from nuclear weapons research. I'm unaware that this has previously been noted in the anesthetic literature. Miller submitted the details of his synthesis to the Journal of the American Chemical Society, when I was six days old (submitted to JACS 30 April 1947). Ten years were to pass before its rediscovery as an anesthetic. Miller, later of Cornell University, thereby became the first to synthesize a fluorinated inhaled anesthetic. But he did not realize or pursue its anesthetic possibilities; he was pre-occupied in developing weapons of mass destruction.

Second, in a search for a better anesthetic, Earl McBee (who worked on U[235]) synthesized 46 fluorine-containing ethanes, propanes, butanes, and an ether for the Mallinckrodt Chemical Works. Mallinckrodt gave these compounds to Benjamin Robbins, the first Chairman of Anesthesia at Vanderbilt University and a member of the Pharmacology Department, to test for anesthetic activity. The Pharmacology Department at Vanderbilt had historical close links with the Mallinckrodt Chemical Works which is why Robbins was involved with their assessment. The Mallinckrodt Chemical Works manufactured ether and cyclopropane, and thus had an interest in anesthesia. The founder, Edward Mallinckrodt Jr., went to school with Paul Lamson, who became Chairman of Pharmacology at Vanderbilt. He gave his old school friend a grant of $25,000 a year, to fund research related to anesthesia.

In 1946, Robbins published his preliminary report [43]. Although no compound was a useful anesthetic, three compound structures differed but slightly from halothane. In two, a single chlorine substitution for either hydrogen or bromine would have produced halothane—as would the addition of a single fluorine and alteration of the position of chlorine in the third. The race was still on.

Julius Shukys synthesized the first fluorinated anesthetic to enter practice, an ethyl vinyl ether (CF_3-CH_2-O-$CHCH_2$) named fluroxene (Vinamar, Fluoromar). John Krantz in Maryland studied it in the late 1940s [44], and it entered practice in 1953. However, it was not ideal, producing rapid breathing and heart rate, it was flammable, and it could injure the liver. Indeed, although toxicity in primates was small, it was lethal to many other species [45]! Larry Saidman also remembers its propensity to cause nausea and vomiting, hence its alternative names 'Vomomar' and "Fluorobarf" Had fluroxene been subjected to today's standards, it never would have been tested in humans. The search for a better agent crossed the Atlantic back to Britain.

Chance and Science Come Together: The Story of Halothane

Imperial Chemical Industries (ICI), in Cheshire in the North of England, founded a pharmaceutical division in 1944, having previously synthesized fluorine containing compounds in the 1930s for use as refrigerants. Chance again played a crucial role. In the 1930s, John Ferguson, later to become ICI's Research Director of the General Chemical Division, tested agrochemical agents that might be used to fumigate grain silos to rid them of weevils and beetles. Some of the agents stunned but did not kill the weevils. Remembering this in 1951, he prompted a young fluorine chemist working at ICI, Charles Suckling (with whom I have discussed the subject) to explore fluorinated compounds as anesthetics. Suckling set about searching for an anesthetic, combining the multi-perspectives of patient, surgeon, anesthetist, and manufacturer. Although Suckling synthesized and selected the compounds for testing, recognize that Ferguson's earlier chance observations set Suckling on the road leading to the synthesis of the halogenated alkane (CF_3-CHClBr) called halothane. Suckling succeeded surprisingly quickly, halothane being the ninth of twelve compounds tested for anesthetic activity [46]. Suckling then asked the pharmacologist, James Raventos, to determine the relevant pharmacology. Suckling described Raventos as: *"Wise with an impish sense of humour and an infectious chuckle, cautious until sure of his facts"*. Raventos found in animals that the new hydrocarbon had desirable properties; non-flammability, absent pungency, high potency (close to that of chloroform), no obvious toxicity, and could produce a rapid induction of and recovery from anesthesia [47]. Although halothane had significant cardiovascular effects (it could predispose to irregular beating of the heart and could depress the heart), its dangers were far less than those of the other eleven 'highly cardiotoxic' compounds synthesized by Suckling.

The laboratories of ICI are in Widnes, Cheshire, close to the Manchester Royal Infirmary where an anesthetist, Michael Johnstone, worked. Johnstone had witnessed the limitations of 'rag and bottle' chloroform anesthesia and this experience determined his career choice, believing that as an anesthetist he could improve the lot of the patient. On January 20, 1956, Suckling received a telephone call from Raventos, who was in the operating theater with Johnstone to witness the first use of halothane in a patient. Ethical approval was not sought, and preclinical investigation had not been undertaken as was standard practice for the time. Raventos related that everything had gone satisfactorily, and in turn, Suckling relayed the message to Ferguson. Unknown at that moment, chance had played yet another role in the successful development of halothane. The first patient scheduled for operation, the one that would have received halothane, had awakened unwell, and her surgery was postponed. The second patient received halothane in her stead. The next morning the first scheduled patient developed jaundice! Had the patient received halothane, surely the halothane would have been blamed, ending halothane's use forever. To paraphrase Lefty Gomez, an American baseball player, "it is better to be lucky than good".

Johnstone continued the early trials [48], and by September of 1956, over 500 patients had received halothane. The trials were widened before its release in the UK in 1957, and the US in 1958. In the initial trials, halothane was given by the open drop method, but a calibrated vaporizer, the Fluotec, was soon developed by a small engineering firm, Cyprane, and this vaporizer facilitated the commercial success of halothane. In the US, fortuitously, another vaporizer, the Copper Kettle had already been developed [49]. Both of these vaporizers allowed anesthetists to control the depth of anesthesia, quickly and predictably. Due to the combination of high vapor pressure, lower blood solubility, and high potency, precise control was essential to the safe delivery of this new potent inhaled anesthetic.

The advantages of the new alkane rapidly placed it as the anesthetic of choice world wide. But within four years of its release, cases of unexplained postoperative liver failure emerged. Bunker and Blumenfeld reported that a 16 year old school girl had died in the Sutter Community Hospital in Sacramento, of liver failure, 13 days after being exposed to halothane for a minor surgery [50]. Gerald Brody (pathologist) and Robert Sweet (anesthesiologist) reported four cases of severe hepatic injury after halothane anesthesia [51]. Such observations prompted Bunker to propose that the National Academy of Sciences in Washington organize a study of the safety of halothane, a study that would define the risk imposed on our patients by this extraordinarily useful anesthetic. One thing seemed clear: although halothane might cause severe injury to the liver, the incidence appeared to be less than that seen with chloroform. But how much less? A large epidemiological study would be needed to sort out the incidence and the characteristics, the phenotype, associated with "halothane hepatitis". A large scale retrospective analysis was undertaken and the results published in 1966 [52], with more detailed results published in 1969 [53]. Only 3 patients out of 367,000 given halothane gave clear evidence of a direct cause and effect relationship. The anesthesia community breathed a sigh of relief.

Mounting evidence indicated that halothane-induced liver damage took two forms [54]. One was mild, transient and sub-clinical, measurable only by changes in liver function tests. The rare second form resulted in fulminant injury to the liver and a high mortality. Between 1978 and 1985, the UK Committee on Safety of Medicines (CSM) received 84 reports of liver injury after halothane with adequate histories in 62 patients. Of the 62, 41 had been exposed to halothane more than once. The mortality rate was 29% in patients given but one anesthetic with halothane; 41% after two exposures; and 56% in those given more than two. Not only did mortality increase with repeated exposures, the time to the appearance of injury shortened. These relationships suggested an immune-mediated, allergic-type reaction, with the following sequence mediating injury [55]. The liver metabolizes halothane to a reactive form of trifluoracetyl (CF_3-COO-) which by virtue of its reactivity can combine with liver proteins (liver proteins because they are nearby). The addition of the trifluoracetyl group to the protein changes the immune character of the protein which is no longer recognized as "self" or normal, but as "foreign". The body's immune system produces antibodies that attack the "foreign" proteins and, thereby, injure the liver. A greater immune response is mounted with repeated exposures to halothane, as would occur with repeated vaccinations. The precise sequence of events is complicated. Although the incidence of fatal halothane-induced hepatitis was small, it enormously impacted on the use of halothane. Halothane is now available in the UK only to special order. Use of halothane continues in developing countries where costs trump the rare risk of severe injury of the liver.

ICI did not attempt to produce a better inhaled anesthetic to follow up on their success with halothane. However, in 1983 they introduced an alternative to thiopental, propofol (isopropylphenol) for intravenous induction and maintenance of anesthesia. Thus, the early 1980s saw the end of a nearly 150 year era, in which inhaled agents were the invariable foundations of general anesthesia and total intravenous anesthesia became a viable alternative.

The introduction of halothane also marked a new era in anesthetic pharmacology. Twenty years earlier, Booth and Bixby had predicted part of halothane's beneficial and detrimental effects: fluorine substitution produced an anesthetic that was non-explosive and less toxic than chloroform. The rare association with hepatic failure initiated epidemiological surveys (outcome studies, studies required for our present goal of evidence-based medicine) and extensive studies into the immunological basis of unpredicted side effects.

Methoxyflurane

Although Miller (later at Cornell) and colleagues synthesized methoxyflurane under a Manhattan Project contract in 1944, only in 1960 did Joseph Artusio and Alan Van Poznac, also at Cornell publish their results of studies of methoxyflurane in humans [56]. Methoxyflurane was non-explosive, extremely potent with a MAC of 0.16%, and purportedly a good analgesic. This latter property gave it a place in obstetric analgesia (licensed for use in obstetrics in 1970 in the UK). But problems with methoxyflurane limited its use. It was too soluble in blood to allow a rapid induction and recovery [57]. The liver metabolized more than 50%, perhaps even 75% of the methoxyflurane taken into the body [58], with metabolites excreted in the urine for up to 12 days postoperatively. Prolonged use—3 MAC-hours or longer—could cause high output kidney failure [59]. The French had a nice term for this 'Diabetes Insipidus Fluorique'. Methoxyflu-

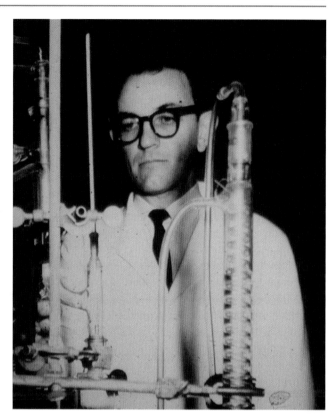

Fig. 46.2 A young Ross Terrell, probably in the 1960s. (Courtesy of Airco files)

rane never gained widespread acceptance in the US, and its use slowly withered away. Licenses for its use have lapsed in the UK and North America. However, in Australia, paramedical personnel, the military, and emergency departments still use it regularly for analgesia. Self-administered by means of a disposable device allowing a maximum dose of 6 ml over 50 to 55 min, it remains registered for use in Australia, New Zealand and the Middle East. The only manufacturing facility is now in Australia [60].

The next fluorinated anesthetic to be introduced came from the efforts of the chemist Ross Terrell (Fig. 46.2), from a sustained project, underwritten by the Ohio Chemical Corporation, dedicated to the development of a better inhaled anesthetic [61]. But first we need to review the topic of depth of anesthesia and how to measure it. The discovery of the measurement was concurrent with and partially driven by the rise of halothane as the predominant anesthetic of the day.

Defining Anesthetic Depth: The Minimum Alveolar Concentration or MAC

In 1847, by dint of painstaking observation, John Snow defined depth as a succession of five degrees, the fourth being the degree commonly used to facilitate the progress of surgery. During World War I, Arthur Guedel refined Snow's concepts, arriving at a scheme of four stages, the third being that used for surgery [62]. The introduction of premedication, the use of opioids and then muscle relaxants provoked a debate concerning what the term 'anesthesia' meant—what did it encompass and could depth be scientifically measured? Cedric Prys-Roberts observed that anesthesia is the state in which, as a result of drug induced unconsciousness, the patient neither perceives nor recalls noxious stimuli [63]. The motor response to noxious stimuli is essentially an all or none one with motor activity resulting from stimulation of the inadequately anesthetized patient. Snow observed that his third degree permitted such movement but the fourth degree did not [64].

Eger, Saidman and Brandstater used this motor reflex as an end point in defining the minimum alveolar concentration (MAC) of anesthetic needed to inhibit movement in 50 % of subjects [65]. This concentration is greater than that required to produce unconsciousness. The concept of MAC, developed by Eger and his colleagues in San Francisco, was an important contribution to the anesthetist's ability to conceptualize and thus modify depth of anesthesia and use different inhaled agents safely. It enabled quantitative comparisons of the effects of inhaled anesthetics and the ability to define factors affecting the depth of anesthesia.

A Search for Metabolically Stable Ethers

Like his predecessors searching for a better anesthetic, Ross Terrell synthesized several series of fluorinated compounds including alkanes, alcohols and various ethers. A potentially useful compound would produce a "smooth" anesthetic state, preferably without also producing convulsions. A useful compound would be stable, would resist degradation by the liver or by carbon dioxide absorbents, and would not be toxic. He quickly discarded alkanes because they predisposed to irregular beating of the heart, and focused (because they did not so predispose) on ethers, particularly methyl ethyl ethers. Terrell worked with dogged persistence—remember halothane was Suckling's 9th compound. In 1963 Terrell synthesized a methyl ethyl ether (CHF_2-O-CF_2-CHFCl) that had the code name Investigational Compound Number 347 or I-347 because it was the 347[th]structure he synthesized. A first report of its anesthetic characteristics appeared in 1966 [66], and it was given the generic name 'enflurane'.

Enflurane

Compared with halothane, enflurane had two immediately apparent, indeed predictable advantages, and other disadvantages that became clearer with time. First, it was a fluo-

rinated methyl ethyl ether, and ethers, unlike alkanes, tend not to cause cardiac arrhythmias. Second, only 2–3 % of the enflurane taken up was metabolized, and thus it was less likely to cause injury from potentially toxic metabolites. That is, the relatively low metabolism meant that defluorination was small, far smaller than with methoxyflurane, and cases of postoperative renal insufficiency did not appear. So enflurane provided a potentially safer alternative to either halothane or methoxyflurane. Not predicted, was the early finding of an association of enflurane anesthesia with tonic and clonic muscular activity [67]. Indeed, EEG epileptiform activity was common, although frank seizure activity was uncommon.

By the mid 1970s, enflurane supplanted halothane in much of the developed world except that halothane continued to be used for anesthesia in children because of halothane's absence of pungency. Methoxyflurane and Trilene had hardly any followers and a few stalwarts refused to give up ether. The non-flammable, minimally toxic, potent characteristics of enflurane increasingly made it the leader.

At this juncture two trends increasingly influenced anesthetic practice, trends ensuring a persistent search for alternatives to halothane and enflurane. First, advances in anesthetic and surgical techniques, coupled with economic considerations, increased the demand for and scope of day case (patients being both admitted and discharged the day of surgery) surgery. By the 1980s, surgery was increasingly being performed on a day case basis, and in the US, by the 1990s, this increased to a majority. Second, obesity rates in prosperous nations steadily increased. In 1980, I left the UK to work at the University of Michigan Medical Center in Ann Arbor. I remember being stunned at the high proportion of obese patients. Eventually, the rest of the world caught up with this epidemic of obesity. The increasing use of day case surgery and increasing girth of the population dictated a need for anesthetics that were eliminated rapidly to speed the rate of recovery. Those were not the only goals of the ideal anesthetic. Additionally, it should be non-flammable, lack toxicity (for both patient and operating room personnel), and have minimal cardiorespiratory effects. Also, it should be inexpensive. Both enflurane and halothane fell short of the ideal.

A Search for Less Soluble Anesthetics

Terrell's team synthesized more than 700 compounds in the 1950s and 60s, in pursuit of a better inhaled anesthetic. They synthesized the 469[th]compound in 1965, two years after having synthesized the structural isomer enflurane. I-469 (CHF_2-O-CHCl-CF_3) was given the generic name, isoflurane (from the term 'isomer').

Table 46.1 Year introduced, solubility, and metabolism

Year	Anesthetic	Blood solubility[a]	Percent metabolized[b]
1844	Nitrous Oxide	0.47	0.00
1846	Diethyl Ether ("Ether")	12	
1847	Chloroform	8.4	
1950s	Halothane	2.4	20–40
1960s	Methoxyflurane	12	75
1970s	Enflurane	1.8	3
1980s	Isoflurane	1.4	0.2
1990s	Sevoflurane	0.65	3
1990s	Desflurane	0.45	0.02

[a] Defined as the blood/gas partition coefficient: the concentration of anesthetic in blood divided by the concentration in the overlying gas when the anesthetic is in equilibrium between the two phases (gas and blood)

[b] The percent metabolized indicates the percent of the anesthetic taken up that is metabolized. With occasional aberrations (e.g., methoxyflurane), the trend has been to develop progressively less soluble and less metabolized inhaled anesthetics

Isoflurane

Isoflurane continued the trend towards a lower solubility and a greater resistance to metabolism (Table 46.1). In animals, it had a good "anesthetic syndrome" without evidence of the convulsive activity seen with enflurane. It was stable to UV light and alkali, including soda lime. It thus looked promising. However, the manufacturing process required purification by distillation, and the isomers of I-469 have boiling points close together. Thus a large number of distillations were initially needed to obtain the pure compound, and the expense of such distillations nearly led to the abandonment of isoflurane.

However, these problems were overcome, and Eger and colleagues in San Francisco reported on the first clinical trials in 1971 [68]. They confirmed the attractive characteristics of isoflurane. There was no innate convulsant activity, and more rapid elimination ensured faster recovery than with enflurane. Being a structural isomer of enflurane, isoflurane was predicted to have a similar MAC, but this was not so. The lesser potency of enflurane compared with isoflurane possibly resulted from enflurane's capacity to stimulate the brain—to cause convulsions. Only an ethereal odor marred isoflurane's clinical profile and gaseous induction of anesthesia remained smoother with halothane, especially in less experienced hands.

Isoflurane was scheduled for release to the anesthesia community in the mid-1970s. And then disaster struck. Eger got a phone call from Thomas Corbett at the University of Michigan. Corbett had studied the potential carcinogenicity of isoflurane, believing he had found evidence for such a terrible possibility [69]. Corbett's study was flawed in several respects. For example, there were insufficient control animals, an absence of blinding of the investigators to experimental versus control animals, failure to use peer animals as controls, inadequate statistical analysis, and absence of a comparator anesthetic. And if isoflurane caused cancer, was this an effect of all anesthetics or was it—as Corbett thought—most dangerous with isoflurane? One could not tell from Corbett's study whether isoflurane presented a problem of carcinoge-

nicity, but in the absence of certainty, the release of isoflurane was cancelled.

Wendell Stevens and Eger, with Corbett's help, set out to repeat Corbett's study, correcting the errors of that study. Using Corbett's general methodology but expanding control comparisons and adding studies of all the then used inhaled anesthetics, they studied the carcinogenicity of anesthetics in thousands of mice. Corbett participated in the analysis, examining each specimen for evidence of the development of cancer. But in this case, Corbett was blinded to the origin of the animal (i.e., whether the animal had been exposed to an anesthetic or not). The experiment took two years to complete, and the findings exonerated all anesthetics except, possibly, methoxyflurane [70].

Exonerated, isoflurane was released for clinical use in 1980/1. Although more expensive than enflurane, its superior properties caused it to displace enflurane. Halothane still had a place, chiefly for inhalation induction of anesthesia in children. But its use in children worried many anesthetists as it was argued, perhaps fancifully, that anyone should only be anesthetized once with halothane, and it was best not to use up this opportunity(!) Inhalation induction apart, the only property of concern with isoflurane was that it decreased arterial pressure by opening up blood vessels—as opposed to halothane which decreased pressure by depressing the heart. This vascular dilation included the coronary vessels, which sounds beneficial, but a report suggested that in patients with pre-existing coronary narrowing, isoflurane could cause 'stealing' of coronary blood away from those areas less able to dilate [71]. A debate about coronary steal commenced which was lively at the time, but subsequent studies did not support the original report. Coronary steal seems not to overly concern contemporary anesthetists.

More than 30 years after its introduction, isoflurane continues to be popular, a testament to the excellence of the compound Terrell synthesized in 1965. But it was not the ideal inhaled anesthetic. Even lesser solubility could be an advantage in longer-duration day case surgery, and in the

Fig. 46.3 Prof. Kazuyuki Ikeda administering the first sevoflurane anesthetic to a patient. (Prof Ikeda to EIE)

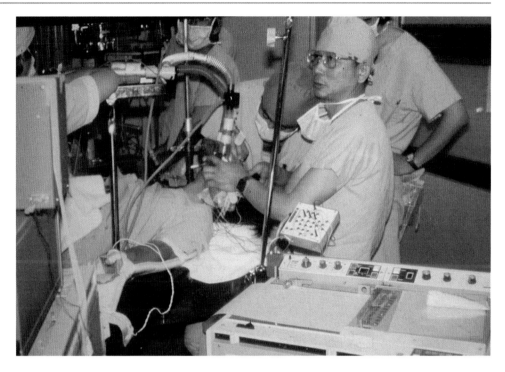

obese patient. Less metabolism would bring with it theoretical, and possibly, clinical advantages as would absence of pungency—important to an inhaled induction of anesthesia, particularly in children. Each of the next two inhaled anesthetics to be used clinically, sevoflurane and desflurane, supplied some of these desirable characteristics.

Sevoflurane

Although synthesized after desflurane, the fluorinated methyl propyl ether sevoflurane [CH_2F-O-$CH(CF_3)_2$] was evaluated earlier and so appears first in our chronological review. At Travenol Laboratories, Richard Wallin and Bernard (Barney) Regan (a skilled synthetic organic chemist with a profound interest in anesthesia and understanding of anesthetic literature) synthesized sevoflurane. Terrell had also synthesized sevoflurane, but had set it aside because it was not stable in soda lime. Wallin and Martha Napoli, pharmacologists with Travenol Laboratories Inc at Morton Grove in Illinois, described its pharmacology in abstract form in 1971, and in 1975, a full report followed [72].

This comprehensive evaluation reported that sevoflurane's cardiorespiratory effects were unremarkable but drew attention to two problems. Sevoflurane is not stable in bases such as soda lime. And the fluorine atom on the methyl group is vulnerable to cleavage. Although less metabolized than methoxyflurane, the cleavage raised the possibility of kidney injury. Indeed, in 1976 Russell Van Dyke of the Mayo Clinic, commented [73] on a paper from Dick Mazze and his colleagues in Palo Alto [74] comparing the renal effects and me-

tabolism of sevoflurane and methoxyflurane in rats: "*Unfortunately, the study of sevoflurane may be rendered academic, since the compound appears to be unstable in base, a characteristic shared by several halogenated hydrocarbons.*"

Nevertheless, sevoflurane continued into volunteer studies which found that induction was rapid and smooth [75]. Several subjects volunteered that a sense of the odor of the anesthetic preceded loss of consciousness, all before the fifth breath. However, subsequent clinical trials in the US were halted. The decision was influenced by experiences with methoxyflurane and to some extent halothane, drugs significantly metabolized and toxic to liver, kidney or both. Beyond metabolism of sevoflurane to fluoride ions, base-containing carbon dioxide absorbents like soda lime degraded sevoflurane to two vinyl ethers, termed Compounds A and B, and these compounds were thought to have toxic potential. And it didn't help that about this time, a study showing that if rats were given phenobarbital and then anesthetized with sevoflurane, they died or had severe injury to their livers and kidneys [76].

So sevoflurane went away (See Chapter 31)—to Japan. Maruishi, a small pharmaceutical company, continued the development of sevoflurane (Fig. 46.3). Drug registration in Japan nearly 30 years ago differed from that in the US or Europe. The opinion of a small number of influential individuals could determine the receipt of a license for clinical use. Soon after application was made, sevoflurane appeared for clinical use in Japan, and by the later 1980s was probably the most widely used inhaled anesthetic in that country. The predicted postoperative renal problems did not materialize. Eventually sevoflurane would re-emerge on the world stage (reviewed later), but meantime developments were taking place in the US.

Desflurane

Two issues prompted US based pharmaceutical companies to continue to search for a new inhaled anesthetic. First, was a perceived need for an agent less soluble than isoflurane and maybe sevoflurane (see Table 46.1). It would also be desirable if the anesthetic were stable in soda lime, insignificantly metabolized, and non-pungent. Second, patent protection of isoflurane was coming to an end, and commercial interests suggested that a better replacement for isoflurane would be of economic as well as clinical value. So in the mid 1980s, Terrell and Eger re-examined Terrell's 700 compounds with these criteria in mind. They focused on a later compound in the series, the 653rd, synthesized in 1966. It was difficult and dangerous to synthesize (synthesis involved the use of elemental fluorine, an explosive atom) and had a vapor pressure close to one atmosphere, precluding its use in the then standard variable-bypass vaporizer. However, this compound was halogenated entirely with fluorine and was predicted to have the desired low solubility and to have great stability.

A digression. I was returning one evening with Ross Terrell to our downtown hotel in San Francisco, in a cab driven by a morbidly obese taxi driver. Hearing our conversation he was keen to tell us about his recent stomach stapling operation, and stopped the cab to talk. For reasons not immediately relevant to this essay, our conversation turned to philosophy, specifically to that of the Austrian philosopher, Ludwig Wittgenstein who in 1941, had worked as a porter in the pharmacy of Guy's Hospital in London (where the first volunteer studies of desflurane were to take place). I was at Guy's in the 1980s and not only had I read Wittgenstein's opaque '*Tractatus Logico Philosophicus*' but so had the taxi driver. We instantly bonded. Both of us having only a layman's knowledge of twentieth century philosophy, the conversation eventually waned, and he wanted to know why we were in town. Ross explained that we were reviewing inhaled anesthetics and had been discussing future developments. Not only did our new friend appreciate twentieth century philosophy, but when, at his request, Ross drew the isoflurane molecule, it was clear that he was also a gifted amateur chemist. He pronounced the molecule 'ugly' in view of the presence of the chlorine atom on the alpha ethyl carbon and suggested that were it to be replaced by a fluorine atom, then it would be better looking, and with fluorine having a lower atomic weight than chlorine, it would have a lower molecular weight, which he appeared to appreciate was an advantage. Ross mentioned that he had already synthesized this molecule and had discussed it with Eger at the University of San Francisco. It is comforting to think, that perhaps for one last time, chance (remember Lefty Gomez: "I'd rather be lucky than good!") in the guise of the coming together of a morbidly obese taxi driver, the spirit of philosopher Lud-

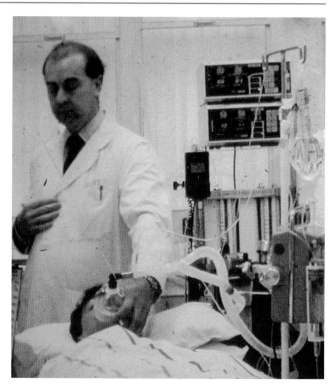

Fig. 46.4 Ron Jones poses as Napoleon while Jeremy Cashman breathes desflurane. Cashman was the first human subject anesthetized with desflurane (late 1980s). (Courtesy of the author)

wig Wittgenstein, an anesthetist from Guy's Hospital, and a skilled fluorine chemist, had a place in the development of CF_3-CHF-O-CHF_2, Investigational Compound Number 653, desflurane.

The first reports on the pharmacology of desflurane appeared in 1987 [77, 78], and the initial volunteer studies were performed at Guy's Hospital in 1988 [79]. The first volunteer, Jeremy Cashman (Fig. 46.4), then Lecturer in Anaesthetics at Guy's Hospital, was studied on 10 October 1988. It became apparent over the next few years that desflurane approached the ideal in many, but not all, characteristics. Its blood:gas partition coefficient of 0.42–0.48 was less than that of sevoflurane, enabling the most rapid recovery achievable with a potent inhaled anesthetic. And the molecule seemed indestructible. Thus there was virtually no metabolism, and in clear distinction from sevoflurane, the molecule was stable in bases such as soda lime. The MAC value was around 6% and so was compatible with high concentrations of oxygen, unlike nitrous oxide.

However, it was not an ideal anesthetic. Concentrations of desflurane exceeding MAC could irritate the respiratory tract making it unsuitable for a rapid inhaled induction. And a rapid increase in concentration beyond MAC could provoke considerable, albeit usually transient, increases in blood pressure and heart rate. In adults, the popularity of desflurane was second only to that of sevoflurane in the

US. It found a particular place in surgery in obese patients because of the fast recovery associated with its use. It also had an advantage in prolonged anesthesia, again because of the low solubility and rapid recovery. One last disadvantage was that desiccated carbon dioxide absorbents, particularly an absorbent called Baralyme®, could degrade desflurane to carbon monoxide. Baralyme® has since been removed from clinical practice, and so, apparently, has the problem.

The Return of Sevoflurane

After nearly a decade of apparently safe use in Japan, sevoflurane was again re-evaluated in the US and the UK. Burnell Brown, at the University of Arizona, led the re-evaluation of sevoflurane. He emphasized two issues that needed examination. After prolonged anesthesia what range of concentrations of inorganic fluoride ions might be anticipated? And was sevoflurane's use in soda lime or any alternative base such as Baralyme contraindicated because of breakdown to the vinyl ethers, Compounds A and B? Essentially, the answer seemed to be that despite all the theoretical issues involved, there did not appear to be a clinically important incidence of postoperative renal complications following even prolonged sevoflurane anesthesia [80]. Indeed the authoritative 2009 British National Formulary has this statement: "*However in spite of extensive use, no cases of sevoflurane-induced permanent renal injury have been reported*". It is an unhappy coincidence that two of the most crucial personalities in the development of sevoflurane, the synthesizing chemist Barney Regan and the lead clinician in its re-evaluation, Burnell Brown, died before their retirement, and before the agent became established as a popular choice the world over.

I fondly remember Burnell Brown. He had a particular love of nineteenth century romantic music and was an accomplished pianist. In Brussels one day, we were looking around an old music shop, and he found an early manuscript of a chamber piece by the Russian composer, Alexander Borodin. Burnell was especially pleased as Borodin was a chemist and founder of a medical school in Moscow.

Other Developments of the Second Half of the Twentieth Century

Aliflurane [CH_3-O-c(CFCClFCF$_2$)] was an ether, like enflurane and isoflurane, halogenated with chlorine as well as fluorine. The compound progressed as far as volunteer assessment by Holaday et al. around 1978 [81]. It had properties not dissimilar from isoflurane, but it was more soluble than isoflurane in blood, and it was flammable in oxygen at 3 to 4 %. Its development did not progress further.

Xenon was shown to have anesthetic properties in mice in 1946 [82], and Stuart Cullen and Erwin Gross anesthetized two patients with it in 1950 [83]. It had a low solubility in blood (blood:gas solubility coefficient 0.11) and a potency that produced anesthesia, without depriving the patient of oxygen [84]. As a noble gas, it was invulnerable to degradation and was unlikely to injure any tissue. High cost and limited availability restricted its application. Nonetheless, it has attracted attention as a potential niche anesthetic for patients at risk of inadequate blood flow to certain vital organs. It may protect the brain against transient lack of oxygen [85], or trauma to the brain [86]. Unlike some anesthetics, it seems to have no untoward effects on the developing brain [87].

However, it appears to have a particular drawback, the capacity to produce considerable postanesthetic nausea and vomiting [88]. The British Oxygen Company asked me and my colleagues to undertake a volunteer trial using xenon alone for induction and maintenance of anesthesia. All our volunteers either felt sick or had prolonged nausea and vomiting after exposure to xenon alone, and after discussion and observation by the ethical committee, we abandoned the trial. Whether xenon will find a clinical place in anesthesia remains unclear.

Inhaled Anesthetics and the Environment

And what of the environmental impact of the inhaled anesthetics that we release into the atmosphere? Two issues need to be considered. First, there is the global warming potential which is calculated for 1kg of agent in the gaseous phase over a time period relative to carbon dioxide. Using this ratio the global warming potential of nitrous oxide is 300, isoflurane 1100, sevoflurane 1600 and desflurane 1900. The relative potency of the different agents adds complexity to the situation. Thus, although nitrous oxide has a low global warming potential, the sheer volume of its use compared with other agents more than compensates for this and in absolute terms it is the most damaging of all. However, the vast majority of nitrous oxide release is from agricultural and industrial processes. Second, we need to consider ozone depletion in the upper atmosphere, which is related to chlorine atoms. Hence, desflurane and sevoflurane have no effect, whereas isoflurane has some ozone depleting potential. Were it still in use, Trilene or chloroform would have the most ozone depleting activity, as the molecules contain three chlorine atoms.

Previous discussions have considered the negative influence of inhaled agents on the environment, but intravenous agents also may have an effect. No one knows how much carbon dioxide is produced in the production of propofol, but it is not negligible. Although the step in its manufacture from phenol is simple, manufacture of the lipid medium used to dissolve propofol must generate appreciable amounts of carbon dioxide. Policies prompting a move to total intravenous anesthesia (with propofol) to decrease carbon production may do the reverse, and thus aggravate rather than alleviate climate change. When assessing the overall effect of the processes of anesthesia, simple calculations and assumptions may result in a green paradox.

Concluding Thoughts

At the beginning of the second decade of the twenty-first millennium, the three inhaled agents having clear roles in contemporary anesthetic practice are: isoflurane, the most cost effective for routine procedures; sevoflurane, particularly useful in pediatric anesthesia and when inhaled anesthetic induction is indicated; and desflurane which has a place in prolonged surgery, or surgery for the obese patient, in low flow anesthetic systems, or when rapid emergence from anesthesia is of paramount importance. These three agents taken together possess the characteristics wanted in an ideal inhaled anesthetic, but none alone possesses all the wished for traits. The anesthetic market is not a large one compared with others such as those for chemotherapeutic agents or antibiotics. The commercial rewards are not there, and thus it is difficult to envisage much time and effort being invested in an attempt to bring together the useful characteristics of these three agents in one ideal agent. What a pity.

References

1. Benthem J. Elogia. Commonplace Books, Complete Works, Volume X. 1781–1785.
2. Papper EM. The influence of romantic literature on the medical understanding of pain and suffering – the stimulus to the discovery of anesthesia. Perspectives Biol Med. 1992;35:401–15.
3. Priestley J. Experiments and observations on different kinds of air. London: J Johnson; 1775.
4. Davy H. Researches, chemical and philosophical; chiefly concerning nitrous oxide or dephlogisticated nitrous air and It's respiration. Bristol: Biggs and Cottle; 1800. pp. 1–580.
5. Smith WDA. Extract of a letter from H Davy published in Nicholson's Journal 3, 93. Br J Anaesth. 1965;37:790–8.
6. Sykes WS. Essays on the First 100 Years of Anaesthesia. Volume 1. Edinburgh, Livingstone, 1960, p 125.
7. Hickman HH. Letter from Henry Hill Hickman to Thomas Andrew Knight, 21 February 1824, held at the Wellcome Trust Library, London.
8. Smith WDA. Under the Influence. London, Macmillan, 1982, p 35.
9. Taylor FL. Long and the discovery of ether anaesthesia. New York: Paul B Hoeber, Inc; 1928.
10. Snow SJ. Blessed Days of Anaesthesia; How Anaesthetics Changed the World. Oxford: Oxford University Press; 2008. p. 23.
11. Atkinson RS, Rushman GB, Davies NJH, editors. Quoted in Lee's Synopsis of Anaesthesia (11th edition). Oxford: Butterworth-Heinemann; 1993. p. 880.
12. Fenster J. Ether day: The strange tale of America's greatest medical discovery and the haunted men who made it. New York: Harper Collins; 2001. p. 64.
13. Hornbein TF, Eger EI II, Winter PM, Smith G, Wetstone D, Smith KH. The minimum alveolar concentration of nitrous oxide in man. Anesth Analg. 1982;61:553–6.
14. Bert P. Sur la possibilite d'obtenir, a l'aide du protoxyde d'azote, une insensibilite de longue duree, et sur l'innocuite de cet anesthesique. Compt Rendu Acad Sci (Paris) 1878;87:728–30.
15. Kitz RJ, Vandam LD. Scope of Modern Anaesthesia. In: Miller RD, editor. Anesthesia, 3rd edition. New York: Churchill Livingstone; 1990. P. 5.
16. Eger EI II, Shargel RO, Merkel G. Solubility of diethyl ether in water, blood and oil. Anesthesiology. 1963;24:676–8.
17. Kety SS, Harmel MH, Broomell HT, Rhode CB. Solubility of nitrous oxide in blood and brain. J Biol Chem. 1948;173:487–96.
18. Thomson GE. Mesmer, Mozart and music an anesthesiology. ASA Newsletter. 1995;59:16.
19. Little R. Singapore Free Press, 5 Aug 1847, in Singapore.
20. Wilkinson D. A strange little book. Anaesthesia. 2003;58:36–41.
21. Snow J. The Lancet 1847;II:575–6.
22. Russell CA. Objections to anaesthesia: The case of James Young Simpson. In: Smith EB, Daniels S, editors. Gases in medicine. London: The Royal Society of Chemistry; 1998. pp. 181–7.
23. HN. The Times. 5 October 1849, p. 3.
24. The Times. 3 February 1848, p. 8.
25. Snow SJ. Operations without pain: The practice and science of anaesthesia in Victorian Britain. London: Palgrave Macmillan; 2006. p. 84.
26. Sykes WS. Essays on the First 100 Years of Anaesthesia. Park Ridge, Illinois: Wood Memorial Library and Museum; 1982.
27. Lawrie E. The Hyderbad Chloroform Commission. Lancet 1889;1:952–3.
28. Waller AD. Remarks on the dosage of chloroform. Br Med J 1898:1057–62.
29. Embley EH. The causation of death during the administration of chloroform. Br Med J. 1902;2:817–21.
30. Embley EH. The causation of death during the administration of chloroform. Br Med J. 1902;1(2154):885–93.
31. Embley EH. The causation of death during the administration of chloroform. Br Med J. 1902;1(2155):951–61.
32. Levy AG. Sudden death under light chloroform anaesthesia. Proc Roy Soc Med. 1914;7:57–84.
33. Halsey MJ. The molecular basis of anaesthesia. In: Nimmo WS, Rowbotham DJ, Smith G, editors. Anaesthesia (volume 1, second edition). pp. 21–32.
34. Lichtenstein ME, Method H. Edmund Andrews, M.D., a biographical sketch with historical notes concerning nitrous oxide anesthesia. Q Bull Northwest Univ Med Sch. 1953;27(4):337–52.
35. Luckhardt AB, Carter JB. The physiological effects of ethylene. JAMA. 1923;80:765–70.
36. Lucas GHW, Henderson VE. New anaesthetic gas: cyclopropane; preliminary report. Can Med Assoc J. 1929;21:173–5.
37. Saidman LJ, Eger EI II, Munson ES, Babad AA, Muallem M. Minimum alveolar concentrations of methoxyflurane, halothane, ether and cyclopropane in man: Correlation with theories of anesthesia. Anesthesiology. 1967;28:994–1002.
38. Mazurekr MJ. Dr. Chauncery Leake and the development of divinyl oxide from bench to bedside. Calif Soc Anes Bull. 2007;55:86–9.
39. Eger EI II, Larson CP Jr. Anaesthetic solubility in blood and tissues: Values and significance. Br J Anaesth. 1964;36:140–9.
40. Atkinson RS, Rushman GB, Davies NJH. Agents and techniques no longer in use. Lee's Synopsis of Anaesthesia (11th edition). Oxford: Butterworth-Heinemann; 1993. pp. 919.

41. Booth HS, Bixby EM. Fluorine derivatives of chloroform. J Ind Eng Chem. 1932;24:637–41.

42. Miller WT Jr, Fager EW, Griswald PH. The addition of methyl alcohol to fluoroethylenes. J Amer Chem Soc. 1948;70:431–2.

43. Robbins BH. Preliminary studies of the anesthetic activity of fluorinated hydrocarbons. J Pharmacol Exp Therap. 1946;86:197–204.

44. Krantz JC Jr, Carr CJ, Lu G, Bell FK. Anesthesia. XL. The anesthetic action of trifluoroethyl vinyl ether. J Pharmacol Exp Ther. 1953;108:488–95.

45. Johnston RR, Cromwell TH, Eger EI II, Cullen D, Stevens WC, Joas T. The toxicity of fluroxene in animals and man. Anesthesiology. 1973;38:313–9.

46. Suckling CW. Some chemical and physical features in the development of Fluothane. Br J Anaesth. 1957;29:466–70.

47. Raventos J. The action of Fluothane – a new volatile anaesthetic. Br J Pharmacol. 1956;11:394–410.

48. Johnstone M. The human cardiovascular response to Fluothane anaesthesia. Br J Anaesth. 1956;28:392–410.

49. Morris LE. A new vaporizer for liquid anesthetic agents. Anesthesiology. 1952;13:587–93.

50. Bunker JP, Blumenfeld CM. Liver necrosis after halothane anesthesia. N Eng J Med. 1963;268:531–4.

51. Brody GL, Sweet RB. Halothane anesthesia as a possible cause of massive hepatic necrosis. Anesthesiology. 1963;24:29–37.

52. Summary of the National Halothane Study. Possible association between halothane anesthesia and postoperative hepatic necrosis. Report by Subcommittee on the National Halothane Study of the Committee on Anesthesia, National Academy of Science. JAMA. 1966;197:775–88.

53. Bunker JP, Forrest WH, Moesteller F, Vandam L. The National Halothane Study. Bethesda, National Institute of Health, 1969.

54. Ray DC, Drummond GB. Halothane hepatitis. Br J Anaesth. 1991;67:84–99.

55. Jones RM. Volatile anaesthetic agents. In: Nimmo WS, Rowbotham DJ, Smith G, editors. Anaesthesia (2nd Edition). Oxford: Blackwell Scientific Publications; 1994. pp. 59–60.

56. Artusio JF Jr, Van Poznak A, Hunt RE, Tiers RM, Alexander M. A clinical evaluation of methoxyflurane in man. Anesthesiology. 1960;21:512–7.

57. Eger EI II, Shargel R. The solubility of methoxyflurane in human blood and tissue homogenates. Anesthesiology. 1963;24:625–7.

58. Carpenter RL, Eger EI II, Johnson BH, Unadkat JD, Sheiner LB. Pharmacokinetics of inhaled anesthetics in humans: Measurements during and after the simultaneous administration of enflurane, halothane, isoflurane, methoxyflurane, and nitrous oxide. Anesth Analg. 1986;65:575–82.

59. Crandall WB, Pappas SG, Macdonald A. Nephrotoxicity associated with methoxyflurane anesthesia. Anesthesiology. 1966;27:591–607.

60. Ball C, Westhorpe RN. Cover note – Methoxyflurane: Then and now. Anaesth Int Care. 2007;35:161.

61. Vitcha JF. A history of Forane®. Anesthesiology. 1971;35:4–7.

62. Guedel AE. Inhalation anesthesia: A fundamental guide. New York: Macmillan Co; 1937. pp. 172.

63. Prys-Roberts C. Anaesthesia: a practical or impractical construct? Br J Anaesth. 1987;59:1341–5.

64. Snow J. On the Inhalation Of The Vapour Of Ether In Surgical Operations: Containing A Description Of The Various Stages Of Etherization, And A Statement Of The Result Of Nearly Eighty Operations In Which Ether Has Been Employed In St. George's And University College Hospitals. London: John Churchill; 1847. pp. 1–88.

65. Eger EI II, Saidman LJ, Brandstater B. Minimum alveolar anesthetic concentration: A standard of anesthetic potency. Anesthesiology. 1965;26:756–63.

66. Virtue RW, Lund LO, McKinley P Jr, Vogel JHK, Beckwitt H, Heron M. Difluoromethyl 1,1,2-trifluoro-2-chloroethyl ether as an anaesthetic agent: Results with dogs, and a preliminary note on observations with man. Can Anaesth Soc J. 1966;13:233–41.

67. Clark DL, Hosick EC, Rosner BS. Neurophysiological effects of different anesthetics in unconscious man. J Appl Physiol. 1971;31:884–91.

68. Cromwell TH, Eger EI II, Stevens WC, Dolan WM. Forane uptake, excretion and blood solubility in man. Anesthesiology. 1971;35:401–8.

69. Corbett TH. Cancer and congenital anomalies associated with anesthetics. Ann NY Acad Sci. 1976;271:58–66.

70. Eger EI II, White AE, Brown CL, Biava CG, Corbett TH, Stevens WC. A test of the carcinogenicity of enflurane, isoflurane, halothane, methoxyflurane, and nitrous oxide in mice. Anesth Analg. 1978;57:678–94.

71. Reiz S, Balfors E, Sorensen MB, Ariola S Jr, Friedman A, Truedsson H. Isoflurane — A powerful coronary vasodilator in patients with coronary artery disease. Anesthesiology. 1983;59:91–7.

72. Wallin RF, Regan BM, Napoli MD, Stern IJ. Sevoflurane: A new inhalational anesthetic agent. Anesth Analg. 1975;54:758–65.

73. VanDyke RA. (Guest discussion). Anesth Analg. 1975;54:835.

74. Cook TL, Beppu WJ, Hitt BA, Kosek JC, Mazze RI. A comparison of renal effects and metabolism of sevoflurane and methoxyflurane in enzyme-induced rats. Anesth Analg. 1975;54:829–35.

75. Holaday DA, Smith FR. Clinical characteristics and biotransformation of sevoflurane in healthy human volunteers. Anesthesiology. 1981;54:100–6.

76. Hitt BA, Mazze RI, Cook TL, Beppu WJ, Kosek JC. Thermoregulatory defect in rats during anesthesia. Anesth Analg. 1977;56:9–14.

77. Eger EI II. Partition coefficients of I-653 in human blood, saline, and olive oil. Anesth Analg. 1987;66:971–3.

78. Eger EI II, Johnson BH, Ferrell LD. Comparison of the toxicity of I-653 and isoflurane in rats: A test of the effect of repeated anesthesia and use of dry soda lime. Anesth Analg. 1987;66:1230–3.

79. Jones RM, Cashman JN, Mant TGK. Clinical impressions and cardiorespiratory effects of a new fluorinated inhalation anaesthetic, desflurane (I-653), in volunteers. Br J Anaesth. 1990;64:11–5.

80. Munday IT, Stoddart PA, Jones RM, Lytle J, Cross MR. Serum fluoride concentration and urine oxmolality after enflurane and sevoflurane anesthesia in male volunteers. Anesth Analg. 1995;81:353–9.

81. Holaday DA, Jardines MC, Greenwood WH. Uptake and biotransformation of aliflurane (1-chloro-2-methoxy-1,2,3,3-tetra-fluorocyclopropane, compound 26-p) in man. Anesthesiology. 1979;51:548–50.

82. Lawrence JH, Loomis WF, Tobias CA, Turpin FH. Preliminary observations on the narcotic effect of xenon with a review of values for solubilities of gases in water and oils. J Physiol. 1946;105:197–204.

83. Cullen SC, Gross EG. The anesthetic properties of xenon in animals and human beings, with additional observations on krypton. Science. 1951;113:580–2.

84. Eger EI II, Brandstater B, Saidman LJ, Regan MJ, Severinghaus JW, Munson ES. Equipotent alveolar concentrations of methoxyflurane, halothane, diethyl ether, fluroxene, cyclopropane, xenon and nitrous oxide in the dog. Anesthesiology. 1965;26:771–7.

85. Homi HM, Yokoo N, Ma D, Warner DS, Franks NP, Maze M, Grocott HP. The neuroprotective effect of xenon administration during transient middle cerebral artery occlusion in mice. Anesthesiology. 2003;99:876–81.

86. Coburn M, Maze M, Franks NP. The neuroprotective effects of xenon and helium in an in vitro model of traumatic brain injury. Crit Care Med. 2008;36:588–95.

87. Ma D, Williamson P, Januszewski A, Nogaro MC, Hossain M, Ong LP, Shu Y, Franks NP, Maze M. Xenon mitigates isoflurane-induced neuronal apoptosis in the developing rodent brain. Anesthesiology. 2007;106:746–53.

88. Petersen-Felix S, Luginbuhl M, Schnider TW, Curatolo M, Arendt-Nielsen L, Zbinden AM. Comparison of the analgesic potency of xenon and nitrous oxide in humans evaluated by experimental pain. Br J Anaesth. 1998;81:742–7.

A History of Intravenous Anesthesia

Paul F. White

Summary

Wren began intravenous (IV) anesthesia in 1656, using a goose quill and a bladder to inject wine and ale into a dog's vein. Invention of the hollow needle in 1843 and the hypodermic syringe in 1853 allowed IV administration of drugs. By the 1900s, diverse drugs, including ether, had been given IV for sedation.

Redonnet made the first IV barbiturate, Somnifen, in 1920. Weese and Scharpff synthesized the short-acting hexobarbital in 1932, but the introduction of thiopental by Lundy and Tovell in 1934 provided the greater advance, dominating induction of anesthesia for the next half century. Price suggested in 1960 that thiopental redistribution from brain to muscle, rather than to fat, explained the rapid awakening from thiopental. This work underlay many subsequent pharmacokinetic and pharmacodynamic concepts. Thiopental decreased cerebral metabolism and cerebral blood flow, leading to its use in the 1970s to protect the brain from hypoxic insult. Methohexital, a shorter-acting barbiturate with central nervous system-stimulating properties, was introduced in 1956 and remains a popular anesthetic for electroconvulsive therapy (ECT).

Etomidate was synthesized in 1964. It had desirable cardiovascular properties, but untoward corticosteroid effects limited its use. Introduced in 1965, ketamine maintained blood pressure in hypovolemic patients, but psychomimetic side effects restricted its use. Benzodiazepines underwent trials in the 1960s and 1970s. In the 1970s, steroid anesthetics enjoyed restricted interest. None of these drugs displaced thiopental.

Glen and colleagues at ICI synthesized propofol in 1973. It took another decade to solubilize it safely. Introduced in 1983 in a phospholipid formulation, propofol displaced thiopental because of its favorable early recovery profile and low incidence of postoperative side effects. Its rapid degradation enabled the use of continuous infusions to maintain sedation or anesthesia without unduly prolonging recovery. Propofol infusions became popular for maintenance of general anesthesia as part of "balanced" and total IV anesthesia (TIVA) techniques. As sedation practices continued to expand, propofol became used for most minor surgical and diagnostic procedures performed outside the operating room, and for ventilator-dependent patients in intensive care units.

In the 1980, Schwilden and others introduced computer-assisted titration of intravenous anesthesia and the first "target controlled infusion" (TCI) system. From the late 1980s, sedation and TIVA techniques increasingly utilized pharmacokinetic-based computer controlled devices for administering IV anesthesia—except in the US.

Current research is focused on propofol-like IV anesthetics that are devoid of pain on injection or cardiovascular depression. Closed-loop TCI systems are also being developed using non-invasive cerebral function monitoring devices.

Introduction

Sedative-hypnotic drugs are the 'foundation' of intravenous (IV) anesthesia. They are used for induction and maintenance of general anesthesia as part of 'balanced' or total IV anesthesia (TIVA) techniques, or for IV sedation during local and regional anesthesia. Sedative-hypnotics are frequently combined with other drugs including volatile agents, opioid and non-opioid analgesics, muscle relaxants, cardiovascular drugs and local anesthetics. This essay focuses on the historical development of sedative-hypnotic drugs in anesthesiology.

Modern hypnotic drugs produce dose-related sedation, progressing to loss of consciousness or hypnosis (i.e., artificially-induced sleep), after the Greek god of sleep, *Hypnos*. As with inhaled anesthetics, some hypnotics can provide immobility and muscle relaxation, and directly or indirectly affect other major organ systems as a result of their cardiovascular and/or metabolic effects. As with inhaled anesthetics, steep dose-response curves characterize most IV anesthetic effects, allowing clinicians to precisely achieve the desired sedative or hypnotic (unconscious) state. Despite

P. F. White (✉)
Department of Anesthesia, Cedars-Sinai Medical Center
in Los Angeles, Los Angeles, USA
e-mail: paul.white@cshs.org

many similarities among IV anesthetics, there are clinically important differences which this chapter will review from a historical perspective.

Before 1900

Intravenous (IV) anesthesia and analgesia began in 1656 with the English architect and founder of the Royal Society, Christopher Wren (1632–1723). Wren used a syringe consisting of a dog's bladder and a needle formed from a goose quill, while Robert Boyle (1627–1691; of gas law fame) from Oxford provided a large dog and assistants to restrain it [1]. Wren wrote "I have injected wine and ale in a living dog into the mass of blood by a veine, in good quantities, till I have made him extremely drunk, but soon after he pisseth it out." The dog survived the experiment! Wren and Robert Major were the first to conceive of injecting centrally-active compounds intravenously [2]. Wren later injected opium intravenously [1, 3]. However, he was not the first to administer opium intravenously to humans, a distinction belonging to Sigismund Elsholtz (1623–1686) from Brandenburg, Germany, in 1665 [3].

Facilitating administration of IV drugs were Irish surgeon Francis Rynd's (1801–61) invention of the hollow needle in 1844, and French surgeon Charles Pravaz's (1791–1853) invention of the syringe in 1853. Concurrently, Scottish physician Alexander Wood (1817–1884) developed the first true hypodermic syringe and used it to inject morphine into painful joints [4]. Notwithstanding Wren's demonstration, IV anesthesia *per se* did not begin until the second half of the 19th century. In 1864, Adolf von Baeyer (1835–1917) synthesized malonylurea by condensing urea (an animal waste product) with diethyl malonate (an ester derivative of the acid of apples). Von Baeyer and his German colleagues celebrated their discovery in a local tavern commemorating the feast of Saint Barbara, prompting their decision to name their new compound 'Barbituric acid' (by amalgamating Barbara + urea). Although barbituric acid itself did not affect the central nervous system (CNS), it led scientists working at the Bayer Company (no relation to von Baeyer) to subsequently develop many different barbiturate compounds with sedative and hypnotic properties.

In 1869, Oskar Liebreich (1839–1908), a German physician and pharmacologist, reported that chloral hydrate (which when combined with alcohol later became known as a 'Mickey Finn') could be used as an IV anesthetic [5]. In 1872, Pierre-Cyprien Oré described IV anesthesia using choral hydrate at the Société Chirurgicale de Paris [6]. Despite Oré's enthusiasm, the high mortality rate associated with IV chloral hydrate limited its popularity for IV anesthesia until the next century.

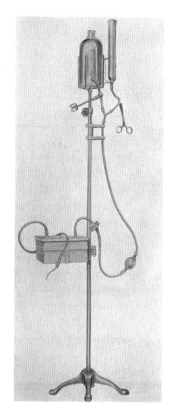

Fig. 47.1 This apparatus was designed by the Kny-Scheerer Co. for use with any type of IV anesthetic drug. As described in a report on Intravenous Anesthesia by two New York surgeons, William Honan and J Wylis Hassler, read at the American Association of Anaesthetists meeting in June, 1913: "the narrow tube by the side of the reservoir was for the introduction of hedonal or isopral preliminary to the employment of a solution of ether."

1900–1940

In an essay read before the American Association of Anaesthetists in June, 1913 (Published in a supplement to the Ann Surg 1913:58, 900–16), New York surgeons William Honan and J. Wyllis Hassler described ether as an "anaesthetic veneer", noting that with "the usual methods of inhalation anaesthesia, a robust patient may go to an operating room for an operation of an hour's duration only to emerge beaten, broken and shattered, and in such condition that months (or even years) may intervene before he recovers his normal status of health." In their lengthy essay, they described in detail the technical approach to administering IV anesthesia, including early IV delivery systems (Fig. 47.1).

Hedonal, Ether, Paraldehyde, Magnesium, and Alcohol

In 1909, Russian pharmacologist Nicholas Krawkow (1865–1924) demonstrated the anesthetic properties of hedonal in St. Petersburg. Hedonal was a urethane derivative used primarily to treat insomnia. It was the first agent given intravenously that produced surgical anesthesia with "a moderate degree of safety" [7]. Unfortunately, hedonal dissolved minimally in water, had a slow onset, and a long duration of hypnotic action. In 1909, Ludwig Burkhardt in Wurzburg, Germany, described IV administration of ether and chloroform for surgical anesthesia [8]. Subsequently, in 1911, Felix Rood in England gave a 5% solution of ether in saline intravenously to 18 patients [9], reporting that it enabled great flexibility of anesthetic depth, and was accompanied by minimal postoperative vomiting or pulmonary irritation. In 1913, HLC Noel and HS Souttar described the anesthetic effects of IV paraldehyde (Paral) [10], and shortly after, CH Peck and SJ Meltzer described the anesthetic effects of magnesium sulfate given by continuous IV infusion [11]. K Naragawa used ethyl alcohol for IV anesthesia in 1921 [12], as did H Cardot and H Laugier in 1922 [13]. However, none of these anesthetics became popular in clinical practice.

The First Effective Barbiturates

In 1903, Nobel laureate Emil Fischer (1852–1919) and Joseph von Mering (1849–1908), two German chemists working at Bayer, synthesized the first derivative of barbituric acid (diethyl-barbituric acid) possessing sedative and hypnotic properties, an oral sedative named "Veronal", named after Mt Verona where Fischer had recently spent a holiday [14]. In 1921, the French anesthesiologist, Daniel Bardet reported the first clinical use of an IV barbiturate, Somnifen, a mixture of diethyl-barbituric acid (Veronal) and diallyl-barbituric acid (Dial), for induction of anesthesia [15]. However, low solubility in water and a long duration of hypnotic action limited the clinical use of Somnifen. In 1929, JH Fjelde reported his use of a smaller dose of Somnifen for 'induction' before ethylene anesthesia [16].

> "The patient is put to sleep right in his room, a distinct advantage which further relieves him of further thoughts of the coming operation. When awakening they are back in their own bed and have no recollection of having been to the operating room at all. A wonderful feature (of the drug)!"

Introduced in 1927, a more water-soluble barbituric acid derivative called Pernoston (originally Pernocton), gained acceptance for induction of general anesthesia—as part of the increasing acceptance of intravenous induction of anesthesia [17]. H Weese and W Scharpff synthesized the first rapid and short-acting barbiturate, hexobarbital (Evipan, Evipal) in 1932 [18]. Despite producing prominent excitatory side effects, hexobarbital was widely used in Europe. LG Zerfas described the intravenous use of soluble sodium amytal (amobarbital) in 1930 [19]. Although Zerfas cautioned users regarding the prominent cardiorespiratory depressant properties of amobarbital, it became the most popular intravenous anesthetic in North America until the introduction of thiopental.

Thiopental and Methohexital

Fischer and von Mering described the sulfur-containing barbiturates in 1903 [17]. They administered a single dose to a dog which promptly died, leading them to conclude that sulfur made the compound toxic. They immediately discontinued this avenue of research. In the early 1930s, Ernest Volwiler and Donalee Tabern, working at Abbott Laboratories, resumed studies on the sulfur-containing barbiturates. After trials in animals, two compounds were presented to the American anesthesiologist John Lundy (1894–1973) to investigate at the Mayo Clinic, namely sodium allyl-sec-butyl-thiobarbiturate (also known as thiosebutal), and sodium ethyl (1-methyl-butyl)-thiobarbiturate, a sulfur derivative of pentobarbital (Nembutal), which was called thionembutal or "Hypnotic 8064". In 1934, Lundy and Ralph Tovell reported their initial clinical experience with thionembutal in 2207 patients [20]. They observed that rapid injection of thionembutal led to respiratory depression which was monitored by taping a fluffy piece of cotton to the patient's upper lip and using the movement of the cotton to measure the respiratory rate. This monitoring technique was subsequently referred to as "Lundy's butterfly". Two years later, Ralph Waters' group in Madison, Wisconsin published results of their study of thionembutal [21], subsequently renamed sodium thiopental or thiopentone [Pentothal]). Thiopental rapidly replaced other barbiturates for intravenous induction of anesthesia, particularly in the Americas.

1940–1960

Thiopental

Anesthesia folklore suggested that after the Japanese attack on Pearl Harbor in 1941, "more USA servicemen died from thiopental than war-related injuries", but no direct evidence supports that assertion. It is true that large doses of thiopental administered to hypovolemic but otherwise healthy traumatized patients could produce profound hypotension. When administered as the sole anesthetic during World War II, the cardiorespiratory depressant effects led to deaths, and FJ Halford, a surgeon, suggested that IV anesthesia with thiopental was "an ideal method for euthanasia" [22]. He also wrote "While intravenous anesthesia would seem ideal for war injuries because of its compactness, ease of preparation, and non-explosive characteristics, it should clearly be recognized that under war conditions, anesthetics cannot always be given by highly skilled anesthesiologists, but have to be given by doctors, nurses and even orderlies, for whom the art is strange…." What a wonderfully perceptive statement! But an analysis by FE Bennetts [23] suggested that the number killed, missing or fatally injured as a result of the attack on Pearl Harbor was 2403 and despite shortages of oxygen and transfusion supplies, thiopental caused few deaths.

The German pharmacologist Helmut Weese (1897–1954), the director of research at the Bayer Co., introduced another thiobarbiturate, known as Baytenal or buthalitone, with a 'brief' recovery time. In Britain, it was marketed as Transithal or Ulbreval. As with hexobarbital, a high incidence of involuntary muscle movement led to its abandonment. In Germany, ethyl-secbutyl-thiobarbiturate, known as Inaktin, produced actions similar to thiopental and was briefly popular in the 1950s. Pharmacologists Zima, von Werder and Hotovy attempted to accelerate the breakdown of the barbiturate molecule by substituting a methyl thioethyl group at position five [24]. The resulting drug, called Nercval in the US and Thiogenal in Germany, was very short-acting but less effective than thiopental as an induction agent.

The rapid onset of hexobarbital's action was considered to be due to the methyl group on the molecule. This stimulated further research into methylated barbiturates, and researchers at Eli Lilly Laboratories developed Lilly 22,451 in 1956. The drug showed greater potency and faster recovery than thiopental, but also possessed convulsive properties. Further modification led to Lilly 25,398, known as methohexital (Brevital). Methohexital continues as a popular IV anesthetic for dental and short procedures, in particular where less suppression of CNS electrical activity is desirable (e.g., surgery for seizure disorders and electroconvulsive therapy). Although methohexital allowed a more rapid recovery of consciousness than thiopental (or its chemical analog, thiamylal, also known as Surital), the occurrence of excitatory side effects made methohexital less attractive for short-lasting surgical procedures following the discovery of propofol. Despite its well-known cardiovascular and respiratory depressant side effects, thiopental dominated IV anesthesia from the mid-1930s until the introduction of propofol in the mid-1980s. In 1982, Dundee and McIlroy wrote "Thiopentone.....will be hard to replace by non-barbiturate agents... methohexitone still holds a place for brief procedures, but this agent may be replaced by a shorter-acting non-barbiturate" [14]. They did not mention propofol.

Steroid Anesthetics

In the early 1940s, Hans Selye (1907–82) discovered that glucocorticoid steroids such as progesterone could produce sleep in rodents [25]. Selye found anesthetic properties required the presence of an oxygen atom at either end of the steroid molecule. While pregnanedione was the most potent of the steroids tested, it was poorly soluble in water

and irritated veins—and never reached clinical practice. Hydroxydione (marketed as Viadril and Presuren), a water-soluble steroid, came into clinical practice in the mid-1950s. However, its slow onset (3–5 min), high incidence of thrombophlebitis, and prolonged recovery times limited acceptance.

1960–1980

IV Inhaled Anesthetics

As Burkhardt, Rood, Honan and Hassler reported in the early 1900s [8–10], inhaled (volatile) anesthetics such as diethyl ether and chloroform could be given intravenously. A half century later, the modern 'Godfather' of inhalation anesthesia, Edmond ("Ted") Eger from UCSF, confirmed these observations [26]. Although this route of administration avoided airway irritation, the anesthetic state it produced was no better than that produced by inhalation of ether, and required fluid volumes occasionally producing pulmonary edema. Although interest in IV infusion of volatile anesthetics recently returned [27], it is unlikely to gain widespread clinical acceptance in the future.

Thiopental

Henry Price (1922–2002) pioneered the effort to connect the pharmacokinetic (PK) effects of IV anesthetics to their pharmacodynamic (PD) effects. In 1960, he suggested that redistribution of thiopental from vessel-rich tissues (e.g., brain) to less well-perfused tissues (especially muscle)—rather than elimination of the drug from the body or uptake by fat—governed the initial rapid awakening from thiopental [28]. Cedric Prys-Roberts and Chris Hull in England, and Don Stanski in the US, used these pharmacokinetic-dynamic concepts to expand our understanding of the clinical properties of newer IV drugs (see Chapter 40).

Thiopental was used to induce a deep coma-like state in patients with traumatic head injuries (or strokes), the rationale being that thiopental possessed 'brain protecting effects' because of its ability to decrease cerebral metabolism and intra-cranial pressure. In 1962, Ellison ("Jeep") Pierce and colleagues at the University of Pennsylvania demonstrated that thiopental proportionally decreased cerebral metabolic rate and cerebral blood flow, and increased cerebral vascular resistance [29]. In 1973, Jack Michenfelder (1931–2004) and Richard Theye (1923–1977) at the Mayo Clinic, showed that thiopental diminished cerebral energy requirements by reducing metabolic activity, thereby affording some degree of protection of the functioning brain (i.e., the brain in which thiopental could decrease metabolic rate) [30]. Unfortunately, in the absence of brain function (i.e., in the case of severe [global] hypoxic brain injury), thiopental provided no improvement in clinical outcome. Nevertheless, thiopental-induced coma remains a common treatment for acutely head-injured and post-cardiac arrest patients.

Etomidate

The cardio-respiratory depressant effects of thiopental prompted a search for a more 'ideal' IV anesthetic, one having thiopental's good characteristics but not its limitations. In 1964, Paul Janssen (1926–2003) and colleagues reported their synthesis of etomidate, a new IV anesthetic, with a chemical structure unrelated to that of any other IV anesthetic. Alfred Doenicke described early clinical studies with etomidate in 1974 [31]. An aqueous solution of etomidate (Amidate) was unstable at physiologic pH, and etomidate was formulated as a 0.2% solution with 35% propylene glycol at a pH of 6.9, a combination producing pain on injection. In 2006, a lipid emulsion formulation (Etomidate-Lipuro) was introduced in Europe which produced less pain on injection [32]. Etomidate advocates pointed to a major advantage compared to thiopental: minimal cardio-respiratory depression even in patients with clinically-significant cardiovascular disease [33]. Many anesthetists considered it to be the induction agent of choice for high-risk patients who would benefit from preservation of a normal blood pressure during induction of anesthesia (i.e., patients with clinically-significant cardiac and cerebrovascular disease), from so called 'stress-free' anesthesia. My research group at Stanford University subsequently demonstrated that etomidate's ability to maintain a 'stress-free' state was not due to its central effect, but rather to a peripheral action, namely inhibition of adrenal steroidogenesis.

Propanidid

A chance observation that eugenol, a centrally-active compound derived from the oil of cloves and cinnamon exhibited anesthetic properties, led Jean Thuillier and Robert Domenjoz to use a congener of eugenol for IV anesthesia [34]. Propanidid [Epontol, Fabontal], a phenoxyacetic acid derivative of eugenol, was introduced into clinical practice in Europe in the 1960s as the first non-barbiturate IV anesthetic. This so-called ultra short-acting anesthetic became popular for brief day-surgery (ambulatory) procedures. Unfortunately, this poorly water-soluble compound was formulated in a Cremophor EL solution causing hypersensitivity reactions that led to the withdrawal of propanidid from clinical practice.

Steroid Anesthetics

In the early 1970s, Glaxo Research examined many pregnanedione derivatives, eventually leading to the development of CT-1341, a mixture of two steroids, alphaxalone and alphadolone in a Cremophor EL solution, and eventually marketed in 1973 as Althesin (also Alfathesin) [35]. Alphaxalone provided the anesthetic activity, and alphadolone enhanced the solubility of alphaxolone. Althesin became a popular anesthetic in Europe and elsewhere for short day-surgery procedures, but was never marketed in the US. Its brief duration of action facilitated control over the hypnotic state when administered as a continuous infusion for maintenance of anesthesia [36]. Unfortunately, as with propanidid, the Cremophor EL solubilizing agent produced rare but dangerous hypersensitivity reactions, resulting in Althesin's withdrawal from the market in 1984.

Minoxalone, a water-soluble, rapid-acting steroid was developed in 1979. However, excitatory reactions and more prolonged recovery times limited its use. Most recently, the steroid anesthetic pregnanolone (eltanolone), a naturally occurring metabolite of progesterone, solubilized in the lipid emulsion used to dissolve propofol, was tested for its anesthetic properties. Although it rapidly induced an hypnotic state [37], eltanolone produced longer recovery times than propofol, and it was never approved for clinical use.

Phencyclidine (PCP) and Ketamine

PCP was synthesized in 1928. Investigations into the clinical use of cyclohexylamines began in 1958, with two compounds produced by the Parke-Davis Company, CI 395 and CI 400. Both drugs produced disorientation, agitation and hallucinations. According to Vincent Collins, CI 400 produced "reverbigeration" (i.e., selecting a phrase that would then be repeated rapidly, sometimes for the entire duration of the procedure) [38]. Although rejected for use in humans because it produced hallucinations, mania, delirium and disorientation, CI 395 (Sernyl, [the name it was given prior to clinical testing is said to be derived from 'serenity']) was approved for use in veterinary medicine in 1962 [39].

Calvin Stevens, working at Parke Davis Laboratories, synthesized the 'sister' drug of Sernyl known as CI 581, later called ketamine (Ketalar or Ketaject). After relocating to the US and entering the practice of anesthesia, Guenter Corssen (1916–1990) became an active investigator and passionate advocate of new IV anesthetic drugs and delivery systems. In 1965, he and Ed Domino (father of Karen Domino (author of chapter 18 in this book) at the University of Michigan first used ketamine clinically [40]. They noted that "CI 581 appears to produce a state resembling cataplexy where patients felt as though they were in outer space, or had no arms and legs." They proposed the term "dissociative anesthesia" to describe an unconscious state with profound analgesia but devoid of the cardio-respiratory depressant effects associated with the commonly used barbiturate compounds [41].

In the early 1970s, as a graduate student in pharmacology at the University of California, San Francisco, I became interested in IV anesthesia, initially investigating the pharmacologic properties of ketamine and its interactions with the volatile anesthetics [42]. Ketamine was a racemic mixture of two optical isomers and in a preliminary clinical trial we performed at UCSF in the late 1970s, it was found that the S(+) isomer possessed more potent hypnotic and analgesic properties than the R(−) isomer [43]. The S(+) enantiomer also produced less prominent psychomimetic properties and allowed a faster recovery of cognitive functioning [44].

Subanesthetic doses of ketamine produced profound analgesia and amnesia without suppressing consciousness and protective reflexes, useful properties in patients having emergency surgery. Analogous to PCP, anesthetic doses of ketamine could produce untoward psychomimetic side effects. A surgical colleague asked a young Eger to anesthetize an elderly VIP with diabetes and significant vascular disease, for debridement of a gangrenous big toe. Eger suggested to the patient that a spinal anesthetic might be just what was needed, but the patient demurred, observing that the surgeon had suggested this new anesthetic, called ketamine. Prompted by youth, arrogance, and an absence of any experience with ketamine, Eger agreed, supplying what generously might be called an "uneven" anesthetic. Nonetheless, he and the patient survived. A month later, his surgical colleague called on Eger to again anesthetize this patient. Eger had barely entered the room for his preoperative visit when the patient pointed his finger at him and said "Don't you give me that stuff again. I wasn't right in my head for two days."

Luis Vasconez (a prominent plastic surgeon at UCSF) and I, developed a ketamine-based sedation-analgesic technique for patients having cosmetic surgery procedures [45]. The technique consisted of an intravenous benzodiazepine followed by sub-hypnotic doses of IV ketamine in combination with local analgesia. With this technique, patients breathed spontaneously and maintained good oxygenation without requiring ventilatory assistance or supplemental oxygen. Many patients reported vivid dreams (e.g., one elderly San Francisco matriarch commented in a beautifully composed 'Thank You' card [that had a flock of multi-colored birds flying through the sky on the cover] that she felt she was flying above the operating table throughout the procedure). Although some patients reported dreams akin to "near death" experiences (e.g., descending down a dark tunnel with a bright light at the end), most patients found the dreams interesting and many reported pleasant experiences.

In 1999, Manzo Suzuki and colleagues described the opioid-sparing effects of low-doses of IV ketamine (50–100 µg/kg) given to supplement opioid analgesics [46]. More recently, several investigative groups have described the use of 100–200 µg/kg to minimize or replace opioids as part of an IV anesthestic technique, thereby decreasing respiratory depression [47]. These small doses of ketamine produce analgesia without the untoward psychological sequelae associated with 'anesthetic' doses.

Benzodiazepines

In 1961, Sternbach and Reeder at Hoffman-La Roche Laboratories synthesized the first IV benzodiazepine—diazepam (Valium). Released for clinical use in 1963, psychiatrists used it to relieve chronic anxiety, neurologists to control seizure disorders, and anesthesiologists to relieve acute situational anxiety prior to surgery. In 1965, Stovner and Endresen in Oslo reported on its use IV as an induction agent [48]. However, diazepam's solubilizing agent, proplylene glycol, produced pain on injection and venous irritation (i.e., thrombophlebitis). These properties and a prolonged recovery after short surgical procedures limited its popularity.

In 1971, lorazepam (Ativan, Temesta) was developed at Wyeth Laboratories and introduced into anesthesia practice for use as a premedication, but this benzodiazepine produced prolonged postoperative amnesia and fell into disfavor when elective surgery shifted from a hospital-based to an ambulatory setting. As with diazepam, lorazepam produced significant pain and venous irritation following IV administration.

In 1976, Rodney Freyer and Armin Walser at Hoffman-LaRoche Laboratories synthesized midazolam (Versed or Dormicum), a water-soluble IV benzodiazepine. Jerry Reves and his associates at the University of Alabama conducted the first trials in 1978, concluding that "Ro 21-3981 is a promising intravenous anesthetic agent. It appears superior to the closely related benzodiazepine, diazepam, in that it is more potent, less irritating, and shorter-acting" [49]. However, induction of anesthesia with midazolam produced a more prolonged recovery than did thiopental (or ketamine) [50], and it never became popular for that purpose. Nevertheless, it quickly became widely used as a sedative-hypnotic agent for premedication and IV sedation.

At a meeting held on Hilton Head Island immediately before the launch of midazolam, Roche's anesthesia advisory board warned the company that the availability of the higher concentration (5 mg/ml) of midazolam used for induction of anesthesia might lead to excessive dosing of the drug when given for IV sedation. The company ignored these warnings, and the FDA almost withdrew approval of this valuable drug following reports of multiple deaths due to ventilatory depression after IV administration (at doses similar to those used with diazepam) for sedation by non-anesthesiologists. These clinicians were unaware of the more rapid onset, greater potency, 'steeper' dose-response curve, and more profound respiratory depressant effects of midazolam compared to diazepam [45].

1980–Present

Propofol

Iain Glen and colleagues at Imperial Chemical Industries (ICI) Laboratories in Macclesfield, England synthesized ICI 35-868, or propofol (2,6-diisopropylphenol) in 1973. The poor solubility in water prompted its initial solution in Cremophor EL and ethyl alcohol (the alcohol was soon removed). Preliminary studies in humans by Brian Kay and George Rolly in 1977 confirmed the excellence of propofol for induction of anesthesia, offering a rapid onset and short duration of action [51]. Pain on injection and possible anaphylactic reactions led these investigators to suggest that "Should further work in man confirm that ICI 35-868 has a desirable anaesthetic profile, it is hoped that an alternative formulation can be developed…." In 1983, propofol was reformulated in an Intralipid solution and subsequently marketed as Diprivan. Kay in the UK and Bob Fragen in the US performed the initial studies of the new formulation for induction of anesthesia [52, 53]. The major limitation seemed to be pain on injection, especially when injected into small veins.

A more serious problem appeared shortly after its introduction into clinical practice in 1986. Severe systemic infections associated with bacterial contamination of the injected propofol solution occurred when anesthetists attempted to 'avoid wasting' this expensive new anesthetic [54]. An anesthesiologist in New Zealand had saved the unused propofol from his cases on a Friday, and administered it to patients on the following Monday. Seven patients developed systemic infections with the same organism. Similar findings were reported in Canada. In the US, the Center for Disease Control reported post-surgical infections from contaminated propofol in Michigan, Maine, Illinois and California. Awareness of the problem led to an immediate solution—discarding all unused propofol at the end of the day. The manufacturers of commercial propofol took additional measures, namely adding excipients to retard bacterial growth (e.g., EDTA or bisulfite).

As a young academician at Stanford University, I met one of the international leaders in IV anesthesia, Professor John Dundee from Belfast, Ireland at an international meeting in Vienna in the early 1980s. We discussed our mutual interests in the barbiturates, ketamine, midazolam and propofol (even though propofol was not available for clinical investigation in the US at that time). Dundee strongly encouraged me to conduct clinical studies with this novel IV anesthetic for

day-surgery cases. When I returned to Stanford University, I contacted the medical director at Stuart Pharmaceuticals (the company which was responsible for developing propofol [Diprivan] for clinical use in the US) to discuss a research proposal to compare propofol with methohexital for induction and maintenance of anesthesia for short ambulatory surgical procedures. After obtaining IRB approval, I initiated the randomized, prospective study at Stanford.

Approximately one week after initiating the study, the US representative for ICI in the UK contacted me and advised against pursuing this study because the company had serious concerns about using the drug for maintenance of anesthesia. They felt that propofol might adhere to the volumetric drip chamber and IV tubing, and a negative outcome from this study might delay its approval by the US Food & Drug Administration for induction of anesthesia. The company's primary interest at that time was to introduce propofol [Diprivan] in the US as an alternative to thiopental for routine induction of anesthesia. Fortunately, I convinced them to allow me to continue my study by arguing that the maintenance period for brief ambulatory procedures was so short that the maintenance infusion could also be considered as a 'slow bolus injection' (over 15–20 min). As it turned out, their fears were groundless and subsequent clinical studies confirmed the safety and efficacy of propofol infusions for maintenance of general anesthesia as part of balanced and total intravenous anesthetic techniques.

In the 1980s, outpatient (ambulatory) surgery became increasingly popular for elective surgical procedures. In this context, propofol offered clinically significant advantages over both inhaled and other IV anesthetics [55, 56]. Propofol produced less residual postoperative sedation and less nausea and vomiting (PONV), side effects that were known to delay discharge after ambulatory surgical procedures. Post-anesthesia care unit (PACU) nurses commented that patients given propofol were more alert and clear-headed (i.e., less drowsy) and not infrequently displayed behavior consistent with a mood elevation ('euphoria'). Rapid awakening and absent PONV were important because efficiency and economy assume greater importance in the ambulatory setting and compensated for the initial greater expense of proprietary propofol (Diprivan).

The early awakening after a single (induction) dose of propofol might equal that after a similar induction dose of thiopental because initial recovery (i.e., awakening or emergence) resulted from re-distribution of drug from brain to muscle and subsequently to fat, as described earlier for thiopental by Price [28]. Although redistribution occurred almost as rapidly with thiopental as with propofol, later recovery events were more dependent on drug metabolism and elimination (i.e., hepatic and renal clearance). Hepatic clearance of propofol was approximately 10 times greater than that of thiopental [56]. This latter factor increasingly influenced recovery from its sedative-hypnotic effects as the duration of administration increased (as with a prolonged propofol infusion for sedation of ventilator-dependent patients in the intensive care unit (ICU).

In 1980, Cedric Prys-Roberts from Bristol, England, introduced the concept of continuous intravenous anesthesia and the need for an index comparable to the minimum alveolar concentration (MAC) for volatile anesthetics [57]. He emphasized the importance of knowing the pharmacokinetics of an intravenous anesthetic in optimizing the continuous infusion technique. In 1985, Jerry Reves and his colleagues at the University of Alabama developed one of the first computer-assisted continuous infusion (CACI) devices [58]. In 1990, Gavin Kenny and his colleagues in the UK introduced the concept of target-controlled infusion (TCI) to facilitate administration of a propofol infusion for maintenance of general anesthesia [59]. In order to develop a computerized delivery system for propofol, information regarding the plasma (blood) propofol concentration, and the theoretical 'target' concentration in the brain or the "effect site" to produce the desired anesthetic state, was needed. One of the early studies describing propofol's pharmacokinetic-dynamic profile was performed by my research group at Stanford University [60].

Although the availability of TCI systems facilitated the use of IV anesthesia throughout the world, no pharmacokinetic-based drug delivery system has been approved for clinical use by the US FDA. One FDA concern was that these systems are based on theoretical models derived from groups rather than actual measured concentrations of the drug in the blood and/or brain of the individual patient. A monitor measuring hypnotic effect (e.g., bispectral index [BIS] monitor) could potentially provide a surrogate endpoint for monitoring propofol's effect on the brain. Using this EEG-based cerebral function monitor to assess propofol's cerebral effects during balanced and TIVA anesthesia, a colleague of mine from Japan created a closed-loop delivery system providing for a prompt emergence from anesthesia even after prolonged administration of a large dose of propofol [61]. Other clinical studies have demonstrated that the use of BIS monitoring may reduce the average infusion rate of propofol during the maintenance period, thereby facilitating a faster emergence from general anesthesia [62].

I obtained an investigator-sponsored IND from the FDA in 1986, to study propofol for IV sedation during local and regional anesthesia, as part of a monitored anesthesia care technique [63]. Propofol provided for a more rapid recovery of cognitive function than midazolam, even when flumazenil was administered after midazolam [64]. Steve Shafer utilized data from our original propofol sedation study [63] to develop the dosing guidelines in the Diprivan package insert. The use of propofol for IV sedation progressively expanded worldwide, and in 2013, over 70% of propofol is administered for IV sedation in the operating room, and for diagnos-

tic and therapeutic procedures in locations remote from the OR (including the ICU).

With prolonged administration of propofol to critically ill neonates and adult patients in the ICU, cases of fatal lactic acidosis and hyperlipidemia were reported. This led to efforts to develop a lower lipid formulation of propofol (e.g., Ampofol [Amphastar Pharmaceuticals]). Unfortunately, this formulation was associated with increased pain on IV injection [65].

Etomidate

Untoward effects (e.g., nausea and vomiting) limited the clinical acceptance of etomidate for induction of anesthesia and IV sedation [66]. More importantly and unexpectedly, in 1984, an increased mortality was reported in critically-ill patients sedated with etomidate infusions in the ICU [67]. This finding was surprising in light of etomidate's favorable hemodynamic profile and its alleged ability to produce a 'stress free' anesthetic state associated with low levels of cortisol and circulating catecholamines. Subsequent research at Stanford University demonstrated that etomidate inhibits 11-β-hydroxylase, an enzyme in the adrenal cortex responsible for the synthesis of cortisol, aldosterone, 17-hydroxyprogesterone, and corticosterone [68]. Etomidate suppressed adrenocortical function, and suppression persisted for 5–8 hr after even a single induction dose of etomidate [69]. Nevertheless, there may be hope for a "new" etomidate derivative. Cotton and colleagues reported that an analog of etomidate, methoxycarbonyl-etomidate, retains etomidate's favorable pharmacologic properties but is so rapidly metabolized that it does not produce prolonged adrenocortical suppression after a single bolus injection [70].

S (+) Ketamine

Doenicke and his German colleagues [71] 're-discovered' S(+)-ketamine more than a decade after our initial clinical study [43]. S(+)-ketamine was approved for clinical use in Europe in the late 1990s and is currently under clinical investigation in the US. However, the racemic mixture remains the most commonly used formulation of ketamine in most parts of the world [72].

Flumazenil

Unique among IV sedative-hypnotic drugs, the benzodiazepines possess a receptor specific antagonist, flumazenil (Romazicon, Anexate). Flumazenil was developed by scientists at Roche Laboratories and was introduced into clinical practice in 1987 for reversal of residual midazolam-induced sedation and benzodiazepine overdosage. Unfortunately, due to its rapid elimination relative to the benzodiazepine agonist, flumazenil therapy is associated with frequent 're-sedation, [73], and it is rarely used clinically except as an antidote for treating massive benzodiazepine overdose in the emergency department and to treat iatrogenic overdoses in diagnostic suites.

Total IV Anesthesia (TIVA)

In Chapter 40 by Fisher and Shafer entitled "Pharmacokinetic and Pharmacodynamic Modeling in Anesthesia", these authors describe the 'key players' responsible for describing the PK-PD concepts that led to the development of modern TIVA. The clinical application of these PK-PD models improved the ability of clinicians to administer IV anesthesia and led to its growing acceptance throughout the world.

During the French–Indo-Chinese war in the late 1940s, two French anesthesiologists, Laborit and Huguenard developed a "lytic cocktail" to prevent circulatory shock in the wounded [74]. The so-called state of "artificial hibernation" (or "neuroplegia") was induced by the simultaneous injection of a barbiturate; an analgesic, meperidine; and the tranquilizer chlorpromazine (L'Argactil), and was described as "a state of stress-free suspended animation". The concept was characterized as "neurolept-analgesia," a term Oliver Wendell Holmes had considered in 1846, before suggesting the term 'anaesthesia' to describe the newly demonstrated phenomenon. George DeCastro and associates in Belgium replaced chlorpromazine with the butyrophenone, haloperidol, and meperidine was replaced by the potent opioid analgesic fentanyl to produce another variant of neurolept analgesia [75]. Paul Janssen (1926–2003) and his colleagues at Janssen Pharmaceutica mixed another butyrophenone, droperidol, with fentanyl to produce the neurolept-anesthetic drug combination marketed as Innovar [76]. Although the FDA subsequently placed a 'Black Box Warning' on droperidol because of its ability to produce dose-related QT prolongation, there has not been a single case report describing 'torsade de pointes' or cardiac arrhythmias in the operating room even when large doses of droperidol were administered as part of a neurolept anesthetic technique [77]. A common observation was that patients given large doses of Innovar would lie quietly, awake and perfectly still, the picture of tranquility. When later asked how they felt, many would reply that it seemed as if they were in a 'chemical straight-jacket'. Eger remembers patients given Innovar who commented that they believed that they were "going to die!" Because of the untoward psychotropic effects associated with droperidol (and other butyrophenones), many anesthesia practitioners abandoned neurolept-anesthesia. However,

small doses of droperidol (0.625–1.25 mg IV) remain in use for the prevention of PONV [77].

A feared complication of TIVA is the occurrence of awareness (recall) during the operation. Historical data suggests that awareness occurs more frequently during IV anesthesia than during general anesthesia with inhaled (volatile) anesthetics, in particular when patients receive neuromuscular blocking drugs [78]. Recent large scale clinical studies have reported that cerebral monitoring with the BIS device can reduce the incidence of intraoperative recall [79, 80]. However, a recent study by Avidan and colleagues found that use of a BIS monitor offered no significant advantage when end-tidal anesthetic gas monitoring was utilized during volatile anesthesia [80].

In addition to general anesthesia with TIVA, the use of lower dosages of IV sedative-analgesic drug infusions (e.g., propofol-remifentanil or propofol-ketamine), in combination with local or regional analgesic techniques, represents an increasingly popular form of IV sedation, commonly referred to as monitored anesthesia care [81]. However, if the infusion rates of these sedative-analgesic drugs are too high or the patient is unusually sensitive to the CNS depressant effects of these compounds, the patient can rapidly progress from a state of 'deep' sedation to unconsciousness and the technique becomes yet another form of TIVA.

To facilitate a better understanding of IV anesthesia techniques, an international group of anesthesiologists, led by Elmer Zsigmond from Chicago, formed the Society for Neurolept Anesthesia (SONLA) in the 1980s. Recognizing the growing importance of other forms of IV anesthesia (e.g., TIVA and monitored anesthesia care), we changed the name of the society to the Society for Intravenous Anesthesia (SIVA), and it later became the International Society for Anesthetic Pharmacology (ISAP) [82]. The latter name change indicated the attempt to bring together experts in both IV and volatile anesthetic drugs in an attempt to improve anesthesia by combining the strengths of both techniques. At a scientific meeting in Cadiz, Spain in 1995, Steve Shafer described the advantages and disadvantages of inhalation versus intravenous anesthesia in a fictitious debate between Professor El Eger II ('Edmundo Eger Segundo') and myself ('Pablo Blanco'), a former graduate/medical student at UCSF who worked with Eger's research group in the 1970s [83]. Neither anesthetic technique nor their proponents survived unscathed.

Reprise

Intravenous anesthesia, specifically TIVA, evolved from a technique used to induce anesthesia, to one providing ongoing unconsciousness and amnesia for surgical procedures performed under local, regional, and general anesthesia [84].

The use of propofol for induction and maintenance of anesthesia has grown remarkably during the last three decades, and in some parts of the world is now the standard for both sedation and general anesthesia [85]. However, the use of combined IV and inhaled (volatile), so-called 'balanced' anesthetic techniques, remains the most popular approach for general anesthesia in the US and other countries where computer-based IV drug delivery systems are not routinely available. Finally, the search continues for a more ideal IV anesthetic than propofol (e.g., a 'painless' propofol-type drug possessing analgesic properties but without cardio-respiratory depression).

References

1. Dagnino J. Wren, Boyle, and the origins of intravenous injections and the Royal Society of London. Anesthesiology. 2009;111:923–4.
2. Major DJ. Chirurgia infusoria placidis CL: vivorium dubiis impugnata, cun modesta ad Eadem, Responsione. Kiloni, 1667.
3. Boulton TB. The development of the syringe. In Essays on the history of anaesthesia. International Congress and Symposium series 213. Royal Society of Medicine. 1996. pp. 79–84.
4. Wood A. A new method of treating neuralgia by the direct application of opiates into painful joints. Edinburgh Med Surg J. 1855;82:265–81.
5. Liebreich O. Observations on the action and uses of croton-chloral hydrate. Br Med J. 1873;20:677–713.
6. Etudes OPC, cliniques sur l'anesthesie chirurgicale par la method des injection de choral dans les veines. Paris: JB Balliere et Fils, 1875.
7. Kissin I, Wright AJ. The introduction of hedonal: a Russian contribution to intravenous anesthesia. Anesthesiology. 1988;69:242–5.
8. Burkhardt L. Uber chloroform and aethernarkose durch intravenose injektion. Arch Exper Path Pharmakol. 1909;61:323.
9. Rood F. Infusion anaesthesia: the use of normal saline as a means of administering ether. Br Med J. 1911;21:974–6.
10. Noel H, Souttar HS. The anesthetic effects of intravenous injection of paraldehyde. Ann Surg. 1913;57:64–7.
11. Peck CH, Meltzer SJ. Anesthesia in human beings by intravenous injection of magnesium sulphate. JAMA. 1916;67:1131–3.
12. Naragawa K. Experimentelle studien uber die intravenose infusions narkose mittels alcohols. J Exp Med. 1921;2:81–126.
13. Cardot H, Laugier H. Anesthesie par injection intrareineuse d'un mélange alcool-chloroform-solution physiologique chez le chien. C R Seances Soc Biol. 1922;87:889–92.
14. Dundee JW, McIlroy PD. The history of the barbiturates. Anaesthesia. 1982;37:726–34.
15. Bardet D. Sur l'utilisation, comme anesthesique general, d'un produit nouveau. le diethyl-diallyl-barbiturate de diethylamine. Bull Gen Ther Med Chir Obstet Pharm. 1921;172:27–33.
16. Fjelde JH. The production of obstetrical and surgical anaesthesia by the use of barbituric acid compounds. Anesth Analg. 1929;8:40–7.
17. Fischer E, Mering J von. Uber eine neue klasse von schlafmitteln. Ther Gengenwart. 1903;44:97–101.
18. Weese H, Scharpff W. Evipan, cin neuartiges Einschlafmittel. Deut Med Wochenschr. 1932;58:1205–7.
19. Zerfas LG. Sodium amytal and other derivatives of barbituric acid. Brit Med J. 1930;2:897–902.
20. Lundy JS, Tovell RM. Some of the newer local and general anesthetic agents: methods of their administration. Northwest Med (Seattle). 1934:33:308–11.
21. Platt TW, Tatum AL, Hathaway HR, Waters RM. Sodium ethyl (alpha-methyl butyl) thiobarbiturate: preliminary experimental and clinical study. Am J Surg. 1936;31:464–6.
22. Halford FJ. A critique of intravenous anesthesia in war surgery. Anesthesiology. 1943;4:67–9.
23. Bennetts FE. Thiopentone anaesthesia at Pearl Harbour. BJA. 1995;75:366–8.
24. Zima O, Von Werder F, Hotovy R. Methylthioethyl-2′-pentyl-thiobarbituric acid sodium (thiogenal), a new short acting anesthetic. Der Anaesthesist. 1954;3:244–5.
25. Selye H. Anesthetic effects of steroid hormones. Proc Soc Exp Biol Med. 1941;46:116–20.
26. Eger EI II, Johnson EA, Larson CP. Severinghaus JW: The uptake and distribution of intravenous ether. Anesthesiology. 1962;23:647–50.
27. Yang XL, Ma HX, Yang ZB, Liu AJ, Luo NF, Zhang WS, Wang L, Jiang XH, Li J, Liu J. Comparison of minimum alveolar concentration between intravenous isoflurane lipid emulsion and inhaled isoflurane in dogs. Anesthesiology. 2006;104:482–7.
28. Price HL. A dynamic concept of the distribution of thiopental in the human body. Anesthesiology. 1960;21:40–5.
29. Pierce EC Jr, Lambertsen CJ, Deutsch S, Chase PE, Linde HW, Dripps RD, Price HL. Cerebral circulation and metabolism during thiopental anesthesia and hyper-ventilation in man. J Clin Invest. 1962;41:1664–71.
30. Michenfelder JD, Theye RA. Cerebral protection by thiopental during hypoxia. Anesthesiology. 1973;39:510–7.
31. Etomidate DA. A new intravenous hypnotic. Acta Anaesthesiol Belg. 1974;25:307–15.
32. Mayer M, Doenicke A, Nebauer AE, Hepting L. Propofol and etomidate-Lipuro for induction of general anesthesia. Hemodynamics, vascular compatibility, subjective findings and postoperative nausea. Anaesthesist. 1996;45:1082–4.
33. Gooding JM, Corssen G. Effect of etomidate on the cardiovascular system. Anesth Analg. 1977;56:717–9.
34. Thuillier MJ, Domenjoz R. Pharmacology of intravenous short anesthesia with 2-methoxy-4-allylphenoxyacetic acid-N, N-diethylamide (G 29505). Anaesthesist. 1957;6:163–7.
35. Davis B, Pearce DR. An introduction to Althesin (CT 1341). Postgrad Med J. 1972;48:13–7.
36. Savege TM, Ramsay MA, Curran JP, Cotter J, Walling PT, Simpson BR. Intravenous anaesthesia by infusion. A technique using alphaxolone/alphadolone (Althesin). Anaesthesia. 1975;30:757–64.
37. Tang J, Qi J, White PF, Wang B, Wender RH. Eltanolone as an alternative to propofol for ambulatory anesthesia. Anesth Analg. 1997;85:801–7.
38. Collins VJ, Gorospe CA, Rovenstine EA. Intravenous non-barbiturate non-narcotic analgesics: Preliminary Studies. 1. Cyclohexylamines. Anesth Analg. 1960;39:302–6.
39. Camilleri JG. The use of phencyclidine (C1-395) in obstetric procedures. A preliminary communication. Anaesthesia. 1962;17:422–6.
40. Domino EF, Chodoff P, Corssen G. Pharmacologic effects of CI-581: a new disscoiative anesthetic in man. Clin Pharmacol Ther. 1965;6:279–91.
41. Corssen G, Miyasaka M, Domino EF. Changing concepts in pain control during surgery: dissociative anesthesia with CI-581. A progress report. Anesth Analg. 1968;47:746–59.
42. White PF, Johnston RR, Pudwill CR. Interaction of ketamine and halothane in rats. Anesthesiology. 1975;42:179–86.
43. White PF, Ham J, Way WL, Trevor AJ. Pharmacology of ketamine isomers in surgical patients. Anesthesiology. 1980;52:231–9.
44. White PF, Schüttler J, Shafer A, Stanski DR, Horai Y, Trevor AJ. Comparative pharmacology of 2 ketamine isomers. Studies in volunteers. Br J Anaesth. 1985;57:197–203.
45. White PF, Vasconez LO, Mathes SA, Way WL, Wender LA. Comparison of midazolam and diazepam for sedation during plastic surgery. Plast Reconstr Surg. 1988;81:703–12.

46. Suzuki M, Tsueda K, Lansing PS, Tolan MM, Fuhrman TM, Ignacio CI, Sheppard RA. Small-dose ketamine enhances morphine-induced analgesia after outpatient surgery. Anesth Analg. 1999;89:98–103.

47. Blakeley KR, Klein KW, White PF, Trott S, Rohrich RJ. A total intravenous anesthetic technique for outpatient facial laser resurfacing. Anesth Analg. 1998;87:827–9.

48. Stovner J, Endresen R. Diazepam in intravenous anaesthesia. Lancet. 1965;2:1298–9.

49. Reves JG, Corssen G, Holcomb C. Comparison of two benzodiazepines for anesthesia induction: midazolam and diazepam. Can Anaesth Soc J. 1978;25:211–4.

50. White PF. Comparative evaluation of intravenous agents for rapid sequence induction—thiopental, ketamine, and midazolam. Anesthesiology. 1982;57:279–84.

51. B K, G R. ICI 35 868, a new intravenous induction agent. Acta Anaes Belg. 1977;28:303–16.

52. Kay B, Stephenson DK. ICI 35868 (Diprivan): a new intravenous anaesthetic. A comparison with Althesin. Anaesthesia. 1980;35:1182–7.

53. Fragen RJ, Grood PM de, Robertson EN, Booij LH, Crul JF. Effects of premedication on diprivan induction. Br J Anaesth. 1982;54:913–6.

54. Henry B, Plante-Jenkins C, Ostrowska K. An outbreak of Serratia marcescens associated with the anesthetic agent propofol. Am J Infect Control. 2001;29:312–5.

55. Doze VA, Westphal LM, White PF. Comparison of propofol with methohexital for outpatient anesthesia. Anesth Analg. 1986;65:1189–95.

56. Doze VA, Shafer A, White PF. Propofol-nitrous oxide versus thiopental-isoflurane-nitrous oxide for general anesthesia. Anesthesiology. 1988;69:63–71.

57. Prys-Roberts C. Practical and pharmacological implications of continuous intravenous anesthesia. Acta Anaesthesiol Belg. 1980;31:225–30.

58. Alvis JM, Reves JG, Govier AV, Menkhaus PG, Henling CE, Spain JA, Bradley E. Computer-assisted continuous infusions of fentanyl during cardiac anesthesia: comparison with a manual method. Anesthesiology. 1985;63:41–9.

59. White M, Kenny G. Intravenous propofol anaesthesia using a computerised infusion system. Anaesthesia. 1990;45:204–9.

60. Shafer A, Doze VA, Shafer SL, White PF. Pharmacokinetics and pharmacodynamics of propofol infusions during general anesthesia. Anesthesiology. 1988;69:348–56.

61. Sakai T, Matsuki A, White PF, Giesecke AH. Use of an EEG-bispectral closed-loop delivery system for administering propofol. Acta Anaesthesiol Scand. 2000;44:1007–10.

62. Gan TJ, Glass PS, Windsor A, Payne F, Rosow C, Sebel P, Manberg P. Bispectral index monitoring allows faster emergence and improved recovery from propofol, alfentanil, and nitrous oxide anesthesia. Anesthesiology. 1997;87:808–15.

63. White PF, Negus JB. Sedative infusions during local and regional anesthesia: a comparison of midazolam and propofol. J Clin Anesth. 1991;3:32–9.

64. Ghouri AF, Ruiz MA, White PF. Effect of flumazenil on recovery after midazolam and propofol sedation. Anesthesiology. 1994;81:333–9.

65. Song D, Hamza MA, White PF, Byerly SI, Jones SB, Macaluso AD. Comparison of a lower-lipid propofol emulsion with the standard emulsion for sedation during monitored anesthesia care. Anesthesiology. 2004;100:1072–5.

66. Urquhart ML, White PF. Comparison of sedative infusions during regional anesthesia–methohexital, etomidate, and midazolam. Anesth Analg. 1989;68:249–54.

67. Watt I, Ledingham IM. Mortality amongst multiple trauma patients admitted to an intensive therapy unit. Anaesthesia. 1984;39:973–81.

68. Wagner RL, White PF, Kan PB, Rosenthal MH, Feldman D. Inhibition of adrenal steroidogenesis by the anesthetic etomidate. N Engl J Med. 1984;310:1415–21.

69. Wagner RL, White PF. Etomidate inhibits adrenocortical function in surgical patients. Anesthesiology. 1984;61:647–51.

70. Cotten JF, Forman SA, Laha JK, Cuny GD, Husain SS, Miller KW, Nguyen HH, Kelly EW, Stewart D, Liu A, Raines DE. Carboetomidate: a pyrrole analog of etomidate designed not to suppress adrenocortical function. Anesthesiology. 2010;112:637–44.

71. Doenicke A, Kugler J, Mayer M, Angster R, Hoffmann P. Ketamine racemate or S-(+)-ketamine and midazolam. The effect on vigilance, efficacy and subjective findings. Anaesthesist. 1992;41:610–8.

72. White PF, Way WL, Trevor AJ. Ketamine—its pharmacology and therapeutic uses. Anesthesiology. 1982;56:119–36.

73. Ghouri AF, Ruiz MA, White PF. Effect of flumazenil on recovery after midazolam and propofol sedation. Anesthesiology. 1994;81:333–9.

74. Laborit H, Huguenard P. Pratique de l'hibernotherapie en chirurgie et medicine. Paris: Masson; 1954. pp. 267–71.

75. DeCastro G, Mundeleer P, Bauduin T. Crtical evaluation of ventilation and acid-base balance during neuroleptanalgesia. Ann Anaesthesiol Fr. 1964;5:425–34.

76. Spoerel WE, Chan WS. Innovar in surgical anaesthesia. Can Anaesth Soc J. 1965;12:622–33.

77. White PF. Droperidol: a cost-effective antiemetic for over thirty years. Anesth Analg. 2002;95:789–90.

78. Ekman A, Lindholm ML, Lennmarken C, Sandin R. Reduction in the incidence of awareness using BIS monitoring. Acta Anaesthesiol Scand. 2004;48:20–6.

79. Myles PS, Leslie K, McNeil J, Forbes A, Chan MT. Bispectral index monitoring to prevent awareness during anaesthesia: the B-Aware randomised controlled trial. Lancet. 2004;363:1757–63.

80. Avidan MS, Zhang L, Burnside BA, Finkel KJ, Searleman AC, Selvidge JA, Saager L, Turner MS, Rao S, Bottros M, Hantler C, Jacobsohn E, Evers AS. Anesthesia awareness and the bispectral index. N Engl J Med. 2008;358:1097–108.

81. Sá Rêgo MM, Watcha MF, White PF. The changing role of monitored anesthesia care in the ambulatory setting. Anesth Analg. 1997;85:1020–36.

82. White PF, Bovill JG. From SIVA to ISAP!—a logical evolution. Anesth Analg. 2001;92:1–2.

83. Shafer SL, Gambús PL. Inhalation versus intravenous anesthesia: a fictitious debate between E.I. Eger II and P.F. White. J Clin Anesth. 1996;8:38S–41S.

84. White PF, Editor. Textbook of intravenous anesthesia. Baltimore: Williams & Wilkins; 1997. pp 1–617.

85. Smith I, White PF, Nathanson M, Gouldson R. Propofol. An update on its clinical use. Anesthesiology. 1994;81:1005–43.

The History of Opioid Use in Anesthetic Delivery

Theodore H. Stanley

Summary

"Opioids" relieved pain for 6,000 years. In 1805, Serturner isolated morphine from opium. In the last half of the nineteenth century, morphine pre-anesthetic medication shortened induction and decreased anesthetic requirement.

Several new opioids were synthesized between World Wars I and II. In 1942, the opioid antagonist nalorphine was synthesized. Using meperidine as a template, Janssen produced fentanyl in 1960 adding sufentanil and carfentanil in 1974 and alfentanil in 1976. In the late 1980s, Glaxo synthesized remifentanil.

In the mid twentieth century, opioids were combined with sedatives, tranquilizers, and other drugs to produce "neuroleptanalgesia", "neuroleptanesthesia", and "artificial hibernation". One form of this theme combined small doses of morphine and then fentanyl with halothane-nitrous oxide anesthesia in the 1950s and 1960s.

High-dose morphine "anesthesia" appeared early in the 1960s, becoming popular in patients having valvular heart surgery despite incomplete amnesia, histamine release with marked venodilation, and postoperative respiratory depression. Substitution of fentanyl for morphine produced less histamine release and less hypotension. Fentanyl doses up to 50 µg/kg minimized perioperative cardiovascular and stress hormonal changes.

The terms "effect site" and "context-sensitive half-time" arose in the early 1990s, displacing concepts such as half-life as guidelines for administering opioids and other anesthetics. The introduction of remifentanil in the mid 1990s decreased the reliance on degradation and redistribution to terminate opioid effect. Rapid metabolic clearance terminated remifentanil's presence, providing a short duration of effect irrespective of the duration of infusion.

The introduction of short onset, short duration, intravenous anesthetics (particularly propofol and remifentanil) led to the development of total intravenous anesthesia (TIVA). Quantification of the pharmacokinetics of these compounds, invention of "anesthetic depth" monitors, and availability of "smart" infusion pumps enabled Schwilden and others to show that kinetic models can predict effect-site concentrations for populations.

Until the 1970s, little research focused on perioperative pain management, particularly during the postoperative period. Postoperative analgesia consisted of fixed modest intramuscular doses of opioid given at set intervals, often resulting in inadequate analgesia. The 1970s discovery of spinal opioid receptors opened a new path to pain management. The 1970s also saw the invention of patient controlled analgesia. In the 1980s, transdermal patches and transmucosal delivery systems expanded the means of opioid delivery and improved pain control.

Early History

"Opioids" constitute the oldest class of compounds still routinely used to relieve pain [1–4]. For 6,000 or more years, patients swallowed or inhaled opium obtained from the poppy plant, Papaver somniferum [1–4]. Ancient Egyptians used it to ease pain and induce sleep [1, 2]. Avicenna (Ibn Sīnā, 980–1037), an 11th century CE Persian physician, philosopher, and scientist, described opium as the most powerful of stupor producing substances [1]. For centuries, the dried

milky juice of the poppy's seed pod, mixed with brandy or wine or the juices of mandragora, hemlock, hemp, or henbane [1–4], might be swallowed to minimize the agony of surgery. Few patients drinking these confections however, had event-free, reliable anesthesia [1–4]. These inadequacies led some countries (France) to condemn (for witchcraft) physicians attempting to create anesthesia with potions, later declaring the practice illegal [1, 2].

To make a "sleeping sponge" in the Middle Ages, a sea sponge was soaked with the juices of opium, mandragora, henbane root and more [1]. Patients were told to breathe through the sponge and swallow any juices leaking from it. Despite some popularity, "sleeping sponges" were minimally successful. If unconsciousness did supervene (perhaps from ingesting opium and alcohol), application of a vinegar-

T. H. Stanley (✉)
Department of Anesthesiology, School of Medicine,
University of Utah, Salt Lake City, UT, USA
e-mail: Theodore.Stanley@hsc.utah.edu

soaked sponge to the face supposedly revived the patient [1–4].

In 1656, Christopher Wren gave solutions of opium (and other compounds) intravenously via a quill inserted into a dog's vein. He caused unconsciousness in some dogs but killed others. Anesthetic and surgical practice did not change as a result [2]. In the 18th century, tincture of raw opium (laudanum or paregoric elixir) was injested to produce analgesia. A Dutch chemist named Le Mort formulated the first of these preparations in 1715 [5].

Opioids in the Nineteenth and Early Twentieth Centuries

Advancing the controlled administration of opioids, Serturner isolated morphine from opium in 1803 [1–4, 6], Francis Rynd introduced the hollow needle in 1844, and Charles Pravaz made the piston syringe in 1853 [1–4, 7]. Using the needle and syringe, Alexander Wood initiated intramuscular delivery of medications, injecting morphine in measured amounts to treat neuralgias [8].

Codeine (o-methyl morphine) is one of 20 pharmacologically active opioids in opium. It is found in concentrations of 0.9–3.0 % in raw opium and was first isolated in 1832 in France by Pierre Robiquet. Morphine, the most common alkaloid, represents 4–23 % of opium [9]. Codeine was originally used for its anti-tussive and anti-diarrheal actions, and is currently one of the most widely used opioids in the world. Its popularity reflects a wide margin of safety; the ability to be used alone or in combination with non-opioid analgesics (acetaminophen, Tylenol, aspirin); and efficacy as a peri-operative analgesic (for mild to moderate pain), cough suppressant and anti-diarrheal agent.

By the mid 1850s, ether and chloroform anesthesia were used world-wide [1] with often slow and sometimes stormy anesthetic inductions. Intramuscular injection of 10–15 mg of morphine made anesthestic induction faster and smoother [1–3, 10–12]. The addition of atropine or scopolamine intramuscularly further smoothed induction by reducing airway secretions. Preanesthetic injection of the combination became routine in the late 1800s. Morphine was the first premedicant used before general anesthesia [10, 11]—unless one considers the occasional fortifying slug of alcohol.

Alder Wright, an English chemist working in St. Mary's Hospital Medical School in London synthesized heroin (diamorphine or diacetyl morphine) in 1874 [13]. It was not introduced clinically until resynthesized 23 years later by Felix Hoffman, working for the German pharmaceutical company today called Bayer. Diacetyl morphine is 1.5–2.0 times as potent as morphine. Bayer marketed the compound as a non-addictive morphine substitute and cough suppressant from 1898 to 1910, under the trademark "Heroin". The Bayer Company also marketed Heroin as a cure for morphine addiction until it was discovered that it is rapidly metabolized into morphine and is essentially a more rapid acting form of morphine. The Heroin story became a historic blunder for Bayer [14]. Because of its popularity as a recreational drug, heroin is now only legally available for use as a peri-operative intravenous analgesic in the UK and a few European countries.

Between 1895 and 1905, some clinicians in Europe and the US noticed that increasing the dose of morphine premedication shortened the time for induction and decreased the amount of inhaled anesthetic needed [11, 12]. Extrapolating from these observations led to a morphine-scopolamine anesthesia or "twilight sleep" [11, 12, 15, 16]. Large doses of morphine (sometimes as much as 1–2 mg/kg) plus scopolamine (0.01–0.04 mg/kg) injected in divided doses provided complete anesthesia for surgical procedures and obstetric deliveries. This approach to anesthesia was initially popular [11, 12, 15, 16], a remarkable outcome given the profound respiratory depression caused by these doses of morphine and the concurrent absence of assisted or controlled ventilation. The technique was abandoned after 1915 because of associated operative morbidity and mortality. From 1915 to 1947, intraoperative opioid use virtually disappeared in the US [2–4, 10–12, 15, 16]. When hydromorphone (Dilaudid) and hydrocodone (Dicodid) were introduced in 1926 and 1943 respectively, they were used almost exclusively before or after surgery [2–4]. Introduction of the short-acting barbiturates and especially thiopental in 1935 [1, 10, 17, 18], and the popularization of "balanced anesthesia" ultimately renewed enthusiasm for the intraoperative use of opioids in the late 1940s [19, 20].

Balanced Anesthesia and the Introduction of Meperidine

The concept of "Balanced Anesthesia" originated with George Crile's 1910 theory of "Anoci-association" [18]. Crile believed that light general anesthesia blocked the psychic stimuli associated with surgery while local anesthetic agents injected around or dripped onto nerves blocked painful stimuli.

John Lundy introduced the term "balanced anesthesia" in 1926 [19] to describe the balance of agents and techniques needed to produce the different components of anesthesia (analgesia, amnesia, muscle relaxation and blockade of autonomic reflexes). Of course in the 1920s and 1930s, neuromuscular blocking agents had yet to be introduced, and surgeons' resistance to the intra-operative

Table 48.1 Opioids synthesized in Germany from 1914 to 1937

Opioid	Year synthesized	Chemist and/or company[a]
Oxymorphone (Numorphone)	1914	
Oxycodone	1916	Freud and Speyer, University of Frankfurt, 1917
Hydrocodone	1920	Mannich and Lowenheim
Hydromorphone (Dilaudid)	1924	Launched by Knoll, 1926[+]
Meperidine (pethidine-Demerol)	1932	Eisleb, launched by IG Farber 1938–1939[+]
Methadone	1937	Launched by IG Farber, 1939[+]

[+]First used clinically, if known
[a]If known

use of morphine (because of the problems of morphine-scopolamine anesthesia) meant that opioids rarely (except as part of premedication) supplied the analgesic component of balanced anesthesia. Nitrous oxide, diethyl ether or a local anesthetic supplied analgesia [4, 10]. This changed with the introduction of meperidine in the US after World War II [20].

Preparing for World War II in the 1930s, the German government sought a synthetic opioid that could replace morphine. Morphine had proven useful in managing pain from battle injuries, but was only available (at that time) from outside Germany. Blockade could impede access to morphine. In 1932, while searching for a synthetic anticholinergic drug, the German chemical industry made a synthetic opioid, meperidine (called pethidine in Europe) [21, 22]. In 1946, meperidine became available in America. In 1947, William Neff in California reported that meperidine provided the analgesia needed in N_2O-O_2 techniques [20]. Two years later, English anesthetists Mushin and Rendell-Baker described the use of meperidine as an analgesic supplement during N_2O-O_2 anesthesia [22].

Initially in the US and UK, opioids were used with N_2O-O_2 after induction with thiopental [4, 10, 20, 23, 24]. Later, in the 1950s and 1960s, small amounts of morphine and then fentanyl were used to supply analgesia during halothane–nitrous oxide anesthesia [4, 10, 20, 25]. Greater amounts of opioids were given with enflurane (1970s) and isoflurane (1980s) to supply analgesia and decrease the amount of inhaled agent required. In addition, their action on the central vagal nucleus in the brain minimized tachycardia [26, 27]. These approaches continued with sevoflurane and desflurane (1990s to present) [10, 28]. Some form of balanced anesthesia that includes administration of an opioid is perhaps the most common anesthesia technique used today in adult patients in the US and elsewhere. Its popularity is based on evidence that combinations of opioids and inhaled anesthetics allow the use of lower doses and/or concentrations of each [10]. Less depression of the cardiovascular and other systems, a more rapid recovery, and possibly less post-operative side effects may result.

Germany and World Events Impact Anesthesia, Science, Thinking and Commercial Development in the US, UK, and Europe

As noted above, the failure of heroin to be "the new and superior morphine of the future" embarrassed Bayer in the 1910–1914 period. The beginning of World War I in June of 1914, and the political events leading to World War II, stimulated German universities and pharmaceutical companies to synthesize new opioid analogues or opioid like compounds with strong analgesic activity. Most chemists of the period chose either morphine, thebane or codeine (all components of opium) for their starting point, hoping to produce semi-synthetic compounds having less addictive properties, fewer side effects, and as much or more analgesic, anti-tussive and anti-diarrheal activities. New semi-synthetic opioids (oxymorphone, oxycodone, hydrocodone, and hydromorphone) and opioid-like compounds (meperidine and methadone) all resulted between 1914 and 1937 (Table 48.1). A few of these made it to the US before the end of World War II (hydromorphone [Dilaudid], late 1920s; oxycodone, 1939; hydrocodone, 1943), and fewer made it to the UK, but most remained unavailable in these two countries until after the war (Personal communication with Dr. Paul Janssen and Dr. Jorge de Castro).

After the war, the Allies confiscated German patents, trademarks and research records. Some research records were slowly released over the next two decades, slowing the post-war introduction of these opioids into the UK, and North and South America. In contrast, the availability, use, and experience of clinicians in Continental Europe with the German opioids before, during and after World War II, allowed physicians in these countries to become familiar with intravenous opioids and opioid-like analgesics as analgesic supplements. This accelerated European acceptance of the Janssen opioids introduced in the late 1950s–1980s. First came dextromoramide (Palfrum), followed by phenoperidine and then fentanyl, alfentanil and sufentanil, some mixed with new intravenous hypnotics, tranquilizers, sedatives, and amnestics as early forms of balanced anesthesia. The successes of German companies with the new opioids, and the popularity of ultra short acting barbiturates stimulated many European pharmaceutical companies to pursue the development of similar compounds from the late 1940s through to the 1960s.

During this period, the situation in the US and the UK differed significantly from that in Europe. The German opioids synthesized between 1914 and 1937 were either not available or had limited impact on anesthesia practice (perhaps partly due to surgeons' resistance to the use of intra-operative opioids as mentioned previously) in these countries. In addition, most companies in the US and UK anesthesia related business (British Oxygen Company, Ohio Medical, von Foregger, Heidbrink, McKesson and others) sold anesthetic machines which delivered anesthetic gases contained in tanks (also sold by the companies) or volatile liquids delivered from vaporizers on their machines. Inhalation anesthesia was a US and UK invention, and to an extent is still a more important part of anesthetic practice in the US and UK than intravenous anesthesia, the reverse being true in Europe (see section on total intravenous anesthesia). Finally, the capital cost of the machines required to deliver an inhaled anesthetic exceeded that required to deliver an intravenous anesthetic, a significant factor for Europe, recovering from an economically disastrous war. Thus in the first two decades after World War II, European but not North American companies vigorously pursued development of new intravenous opioid and non-opioid anesthetic compounds.

Neurolept Analgesia—Anesthesia

In the late 1940s and early 1950s, European investigators re-examined inhalation anesthesia [4, 29–33], believing they might create a better state of general anesthesia with less organ system depression by substituting or adding intravenous compounds. The success of the barbiturates in the 1930s and early 1940s stimulated several European companies to look at other "intravenous anesthetics" as potential alternatives to inhalation agents. These approaches sought a "better anesthetic state," one that provided analgesia (and thus was more effective at blocking the "stresses of surgery"), anxiolysis, sedation and hopefully amnesia without disturbing (or minimally altering) cardiovascular, respiratory, and other vital organ functions [4, 29, 30].

In 1954 in France, Laborit and Huygenard introduced the idea of artificial hibernation [29]. They attempted to inhibit cellular, autonomic, and endocrine mechanisms that are normally activated in response to stress. They developed a "lytic cocktail" containing an analgesic (meperidine), two tranquilizers (chlorpromazine and promethazine), and atropine [29, 30]. The resultant "artificial hibernation" (also called ganglioplegia or neuroplegia) often produced circulatory depression and delayed awakening, and did not achieve widespread popularity [4]. Another approach called "ataralgesia" nominally provided tranquility and freedom from pain by

combining an analgesic (meperidine), a tranquilizer (mepazine), and an analeptic (aminophenazole). A related cocktail called "narco-ataralgesia" used diazepam, phenoperidine, and droperidol. Neither was widely accepted for reasons similar to those described above [4].

Janssen synthesized haloperidol, the first member of a new series of tranquilizer compounds called butyrophenones in the late 1950s. It induced a syndrome called "neurolepsis" [4, 32] consisting of inhibition of psychic, vegetative, and motor functions (patients became cataleptic) and suppression of apomorphine-induced vomiting. In 1959, de Castro and Mundeleer combined haloperidol with the new narcotic analgesic, phenoperidine in the first demonstration of neurolept analgesia (NLA)—a detached, pain-free state without marked circulatory depression [33]. In the 1960s, NLA with haloperidol and phenoperidine achieved significant popularity in Europe as an alternative to anesthesia using potent inhaled agents [4, 31, 34]. Janssen and colleagues then produced even more potent drugs, the butyrophenone droperidol, and the opioid fentanyl [4]. In 1963, de Castro and Mundeleer found the fentanyl–droperidol combination superior to haloperidol and phenoperidine for NLA, with more rapid onset of analgesia, less respiratory depression and fewer extrapyramidal side-effects [4, 31, 34]. Use of NLA with fentanyl and droperidol became widespread throughout Europe in the 1970s and early 1980s. When N_2O was added to the mixture in the early 1960s (to improve analgesia and amnesia), the technique was called neurolept anesthesia (NLAN).

Besides droperidol and haloperidol, a phenothiazine (usually chlorpromazine and promethazine) or sometimes diazepam were used with fentanyl for neurolept analgesia in Europe during the 1960s–1980s. Some historians believe the numerous variations in NLA techniques developed during this interval deterred further popularization of the technique. Reasons cited include confusion about the choice, timing, and dosage of drugs to be administered, and the unclear indications for and contraindications to NLA [4]. It is also possible that NLA and NLAN are inferior approaches to anesthesia. That might explain the numerous variants developed in a search for something better. As a result, many European clinicians lost confidence in the efficacy of NLA and NLAN. In the US, neither NLA nor NLAN became popular because of the aforementioned concerns, the lack of experience, and the unavailability of many of the compounds [4, 10].

Opioid Antagonists and Agonist-Antagonists

Pohl synthesized the first opioid antagonist, N-allylnorcodeine in 1914 while attempting to improve the analgesic properties of codeine [4, 10]. The discovery that this compound mildly antagonized the respiratory depression produced by morphine went unnoticed for 26 years, until

McCawley and co-workers (in 1940) in search of a strong analgesic with "built in" antagonistic action, attempted to prepare N-allylnormorphine (nalorphine) [4, 10]. Weyland and Erickson successfully synthesized nalorphine in 1942, and then found that the drug blocked all actions of morphine [4, 10]. In 1950, Schnider and Hellerback, found that nalorphine possessed strong analgesic properties in humans [4, 10, 35], but the doses needed to provide analgesia also yielded severe psychotomimetic effects, rendering it clinically unsuitable as an analgesic.

In 1960, naloxone was synthesized and found to be a more potent and less toxic opioid antagonist than nalorphine [4, 10, 36]. Naloxone produced no dysphoria at any dose but had a short duration of action [35]. By the 1970s, it had largely replaced nalorphine in the peri-operative period [4, 10]. In the 1980s, a longer lasting pure opioid antagonist called nalmefene was introduced for clinicians needing prolonged opioid antagonistic activity [10].

The discovery of nalorphine stimulated a search for other agonist-antagonist drugs in the 1950s. Most chemists focused on replacing the methyl (CH_3) group attached to the N of the piperidine structure in morphine (Fig. 48.1) or oxymorphone. Pentazocine (also known as Fortral or Talwin) was the first successful agonist-antagonist produced [4, 10, 37]. Synthesized by the Sterling-Winthrop Research Institute of the Sterling Drug Company of Rensselaer, New York in 1958, it was approved by the FDA in 1967 and released in mid-1967 in the US, England, Mexico, and Argentina. The hope was that pentazocine (which acts principally at k rather than at μ receptors) would provide analgesia with less respiratory depression than morphine, and less liability for abuse. Although the potential for abuse is less and a ceiling for respiratory depression does occur at doses of 30–70 mg, the compound is only one-half to one-fourth as potent as morphine, resulting in maximal analgesia at a dose similar to that causing respiratory depression. It can also cause dysphoric side effects similar to those of nalorphine. None of the other agonist-antagonists found clinical or commercial success.

Re-introduction of High-Dose Opioid Anesthesia

Morbidity and mortality, likely from inadequate ventilation, caused the abandonment of twilight sleep by 1915. By the 1960s, assisting and controlling ventilation had become commonplace, enabling the re-introduction of high dose opioid administration. In the early 1960s, the cardiac anesthesia group at the Massachusetts General Hospital (MGH) in Boston, and de Castro in Brussels independently experimented with high-dose "opioid anesthesia" [38–41]. The Boston group used morphine and de Castro used fentanyl. Both used opioids to produce anesthesia without compromising cardiovascular stability. Their patient populations differed

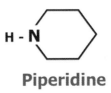

Fig. 48.1 Morphine and meperidine shared characteristics that made them analgesics and provided clues in the search for a better opioid analgesic

however: the sickly Boston patients had surgery for end stage cardiac valvular disease while De Castro's had routine surgical procedures such as cholecystectomy or bowel resection.

The cardiac anesthesia group at MGH contended with end stage rheumatic aortic and/or mitral valvular heart disease, low cardiac indices, and pulmonary dysfunction [38, 39]. The then standard induction of anesthesia, carefully performed with thiopental and succinylcholine, followed by N_2O, halothane and curare, frequently produced hypotension and arrhythmias, and cardiac arrest was not uncommon. Death during or soon after surgery was distressingly frequent. All patients required mechanical ventilation in the Respiratory Care Unit and most received morphine to enable them to tolerate their tracheal tubes. The anesthesiologists caring for these patients made a surprising observation: tens of milligrams of morphine were usually required for tracheal tube tolerance in the post operative period, but these huge doses had minimal circulatory effects, and often resulted in unconsciousness [38, 39].

From this observation, Myron Laver, one of the cardiac team, reasoned that morphine might substitute for barbiturates and inhalation anesthetics for induction of anesthesia, and the team moved from small to large doses of morphine, first with additional inhalation anesthetics and then with only oxygen plus a neuromuscular blocking agent and scopolamine. Few of the patients anesthetized with the new technique reported awareness or pain. The high-dose morphine technique changed induction of anesthesia from an anxiety filled period to a calm controlled one that also set the stage for an orderly transition to postoperative mechanical ventilation.

After using the technique in 1,000 patients, the MGH cardiac anesthesia team formally studied 15 patients (7 with aortic-valve disease and 8 without major heart or lung disease) [39]. Published in December of 1969, the report confirmed the benign nature of a large dose of morphine in severely compromised patients. The 15 patients breathed 100% oxygen while 1 mg/kg of morphine was slowly infused [39]. The anesthetist had to shout at the patient to prompt continued breathing. Hemodynamics, measured frequently, remained stable, and additional morphine, sometimes up to 3.0 mg/kg was given. As the patients became unresponsive, they were paralyzed and the trachea intubated. Results of the study were "startling and pleasing" [38, 39]. The control patients (no heart or lung disease) had no consistent hemodynamic response; those with aortic valve disease experienced increased cardiac output and decreased systemic vascular resistance. The report changed the practice of anesthesia for patients with severe cardiac disease. Within months, clinicians throughout the US experimented with high-dose morphine-oxygen anesthesia in patients having cardiac surgery, and similar patients having major non-cardiac procedures, and reported positive results. Lowenstein's classic article was rejected for presentation at the annual meeting of the American Society of Anesthesiologists.

Meanwhile in Brussels in the early 1960s, de Castro looked for ways to provide anesthesia that minimally altered cardiovascular dynamics and also blocked the "stress hormonal" responses to major surgery [40, 41]. He was not a cardiac anesthesiologist but did provide anesthesia for patients undergoing most kinds of surgery. He used large doses of the newly-introduced fentanyl (up to 50 µg/kg) plus oxygen to produce what he called analgesic anesthesia [40, 41]. He gave analgesic anesthesia to patients having cholecystectomy, gastric resection, bowel surgery, and similar operations, finding minimal cardiovascular and stress hormonal changes during and after surgery. He suggested that analgesic anesthesia had advantages beyond minimal cardiovascular and stress hormonal changes; simplicity (no need for hypnotics);

lack of side effects (no histamine release which can occur after morphine) and a high therapeutic index (safety margin 400 vs. 70 for morphine). His patients did not report awareness but their lungs often required mechanical ventilation for up to 3 hours after surgery, before tracheal extubation could be accomplished. He reported his results at the World Congress of Anesthesiology in Mexico City in 1976 [40]. He was unable to publish his results in a major anesthesia journal but did publish them in a regional European journal [41]. Because his work remained unknown to most anesthesiologists, it had little impact on the world anesthesia community.

Between December 1969 and 1975, numerous reports extolled the virtues of morphine-oxygen anesthesia in severely ill patients [42–47]. Stanley studied the effects of high (1–3 mg/kg) and ultra-high (8–11 mg/kg) doses of morphine in patients undergoing cardiac surgery, finding advantages and disadvantages [43, 44]. The ultra-high doses decreased the need for non-opioid pharmaceutical supplementation and ensured that patients were "unaware", but produced increased veno-vasodilation, requiring markedly greater crystalloid and or/colloid fluid replacement to maintain stable intra and postoperative hemodynamics and adequate urinary output. The greater infusion of fluids increased tissue edema. High dose morphine anesthesia became particularly popular in sick patients having valvular heart surgery [4, 10, 42–49]. However, nothing's perfect! Problems with incomplete amnesia, histamine release, prolonged postoperative respiratory depression, increased blood volume requirements secondary to marked venodilation, and hypotension and hypertension limited the popularity of morphine as a sole anesthetic [4, 10, 42–49].

The problems with high-dose morphine prompted studies of high-dose fentanyl anesthesia in animals [50–53], and then in patients having first valvular and later coronary artery surgery [54–56]. Clinical success in the late 1970s and early 1980s dramatically increased fentanyl usage. Sales in the US increased 10-fold during the first year the drug was off-patent (1981) [34]. Why? Before the reports of high-dose fentanyl anesthesia, fentanyl was infrequently used in a dose exceeding 50 µg for an entire operation. However, after the reports, fentanyl doses used in cardiac operations increased to 50–100 µg/kg [34, 42]. High-dose fentanyl anesthesia rapidly replaced high-dose morphine for both cardiac patients having valvular heart surgery and patients undergoing the new coronary artery bypass operations in the 1980s [10, 42]. Fentanyl's advantages over morphine were its greater potency and ease of use (it could be safely administered rapidly in a minute or less), its shorter onset and duration of action, and an absence of histamine release and venodilation. As a result, induction of anesthesia was faster. There was less hypo and hypertension, blood and crystalloid volume requirements were not increased, and tracheal extubation and post-operative recovery occurred sooner [10, 42].

The marked increase in fentanyl usage throughout the world in the early 1980s spurred the Janssen Company to develop sufentanil and alfentanil [4, 10, 34, 42, 57–61]. Glaxo experimented with new opioids, resulting in remifentanil [62], and Anaquest of the British Oxygen Company developed its own series of opioids that are on the brink of being introduced for wild life immobilization [63]. Alza and Anesta (young drug delivery companies in the mid 1980s) began experiments with fentanyl in transdermal patches and oral mucosal lozenges [64–68].

Paul Janssen and the Fentanyl Family of Analgesics

Janssen ("Dr. Paul" to friends and colleagues) was born (1926), raised, and educated in Belgium. After graduating from medical school, he gained a PhD while working with Nobel Prize winner Corneille Heymans at the University of Ghent [34]. His father, Conrad Janssen, much influenced Dr. Paul. His father started his professional life as a family doctor, later selling pharmaceutical products [34], mostly tonics, stimulants, vitamin preparations and organic extracts. During college, Dr. Paul, perhaps because of exposure to his father's business, saw the importance of chemistry to medicine, what he called "medicinal chemistry." He realized that selling only generic medicines limited the future of the company, and this heightened his interest in new drugs. He also understood that chemical structure determined action. In 1953, after visiting several US and European pharmaceutical companies and pharmacologists, Dr. Paul started Janssen Pharmaceutica. An early interest was the pain produced by muscle spasms. In 1955, he introduced the fifth of his newly synthesized compounds, ambucetamide (Neomeritine), a uterine antispasmodic still marketed for the relief of menstrual pain.

In 1953, morphine (Fig. 48.1) was the standard analgesic. Dr. Paul knew about the synthetic alternative, the less potent meperidine (see above). Both meperidine and morphine contain a piperidine ring (Fig. 48.1), and Dr. Paul conjectured that this was important to the production of analgesia. Working with meperidine as the lead molecule (because it was less complex and easier to manipulate than morphine), they began a search for molecules that were more powerful and specific analgesics, molecules with fewer unwanted side effects [34].

In 1956, the Janssen team thought that meperidine was one-tenth as potent as morphine because it poorly penetrated the blood-brain barrier.[1] To overcome this limitation, they believed a more fat soluble derivative was needed, leading

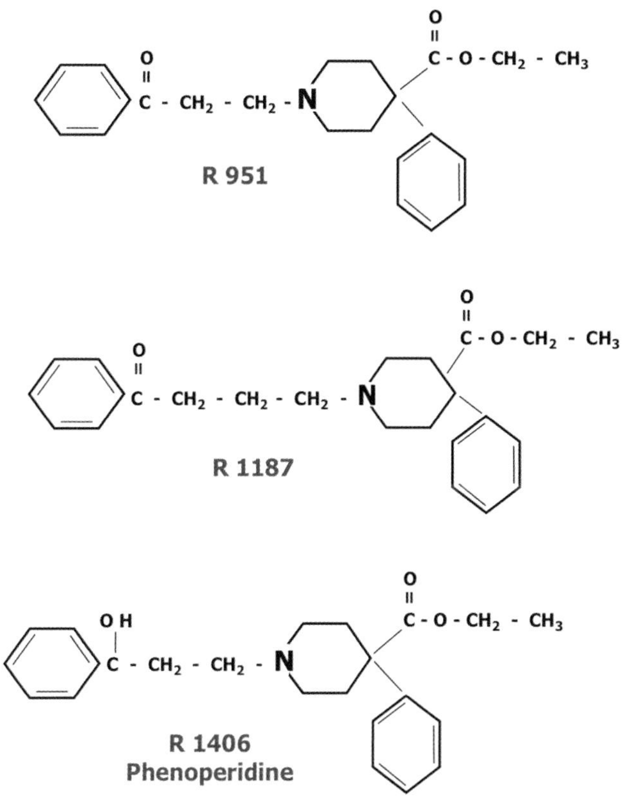

[1] In retrospect, we know that they got it backwards. Morphine penetrates more slowly than meperidine. But the rationale doesn't matter to the end result.

Fig. 48.2 Various experimental steps led to a new opioid, and ultimately to the useful series shown in Fig. 48.3

them to replaced the methyl (CH$_3$) group attached to the N at the extreme left of the meperidine molecule (Fig. 48.1) with a benzene ring. They then added a C=O in combination with two CH$_2$ groups between the left benzene and piperidine rings of the first new compound. The resulting compound R951 (Fig. 48.2), showed a greater analgesic potency. Addition of another CH$_2$ group between the benzene and piperidine rings in R951 produced R1187 (Fig. 48.2), a less analgesic compound than R951. In 1957, Janssen chemists changed the C=O group attached to the left benzene ring in R951 to a C–OH group, producing R1406 (phenoperidine; Fig. 48.2). At that time phenoperidine was the most potent opioid in the world, having 20 times the potency of morphine [34]. It was introduced into Europe in 1964, but not the US, as a potent, fast acting, short lasting analgesic for anesthetic use. It is still used in Europe.

In 1960, the Janssen team modified the phenoperidine molecule to produce fentanyl (Fig. 48.3). Fentanyl was approved for use in Europe 3 years later [34, 57]. Subsequently, the Janssen team created sufentanil (synthesized in 1974, introduced into Europe in 1979 and the US in 1985), alfentanil (synthesized in 1976, introduced into Europe in 1983 and the US in 1987) and carfentanil (synthesized in 1974 introduced into veterinary [wild life immobilization] medicine in 1986; Fig. 48.3; Table 48.2) [57–61].

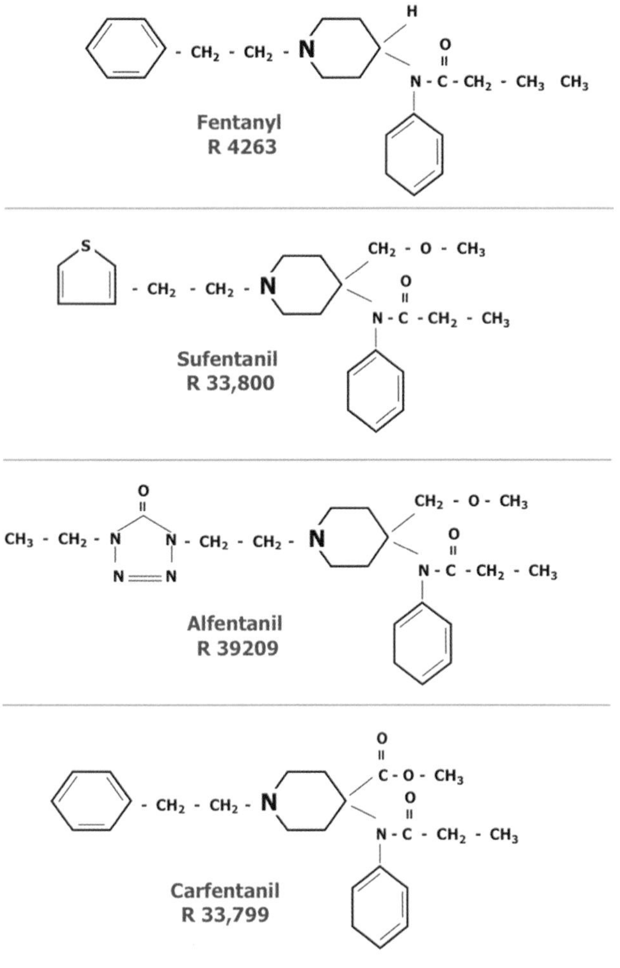

Fig. 48.3 Clinically useful opioids that resulted from the steps suggested in the previous figure. The first three were used in humans, the last, carfentanil, was used to produce immobilization in animals

Fentanyl's Approval in the US

The international healthcare conglomerate, Johnson & Johnson (J&J), purchased Janssen Pharmaceutica in July 1961 [34], providing Janssen with financial security and access to individuals within the J&J family, including Robert McNeill, the founder of the Philadelphia Company, McNeill Laboratories, purchased by J&J in 1959. In the mid 1960s, Janssen successfully launched fentanyl and droperidol as independent drugs in Europe [32–34, 57]. Janssen could not however, get Food and Drug Administration (FDA) approval for fentanyl in the US [34]. Robert Dripps, Professor of Anesthesiology at the University of Pennsylvania, felt that fentanyl was too potent, and caused muscle rigidity. These effects, he thought, increased the need for tracheal intubation and would lead to abuse problems. McNeill knew Dripps and introduced Dripps to Janssen, beginning a dialogue that led to a compromise. Fentanyl would be submitted for approval in combination with droperidol. When approved by the FDA in 1968, fentanyl became available combined with droperidol

in a ratio of 50:1 droperidol to fentanyl. The combination was called Innovar in the US and Thalamonal in other countries.

Why with droperidol, and why a 50:1 ratio? Janssen had consulted with Belgian anesthesiologist, George de Castro [34]. De Castro had tested Janssen's intravenous (IV) analgesics, hypnotics, and sedatives in patients—after animal testing in the Janssen laboratories. He used fentanyl in combination with droperidol in a neurolept-anesthesia technique popular in some Western European countries in the early to mid 1960s. Reviewing his clinical practice, he found that he used fentanyl and droperidol in approximately a 50:1 ratio, the ratio then suggested by Janssen to Dripps. Both knew that the recreational use of droperidol produced a "bad high" and believed that mixing droperidol and fentanyl would minimize any abuse potential. The FDA agreed and Innovar was approved for use in the US in early 1968 (personal communication, P. Janssen and T. Stanley). Four years later, fentanyl became available alone but for the next six years only as a 1 ml vial containing 50 μg [34].

Opioids as Supplements to Induction of General Anesthesia

Todays anesthetists often use opioids to enhance the induction of general anesthesia [10, 42, 62, 69, 70]. They use doses of opioids during induction that exceed those used for entire surgical cases in the 1950s, 1960s and 1970s, thereby providing analgesia and decreasing tachycardia and hypertension during induction (including rapid sequence induction) and maintenance of anesthesia. Such administration also reduces the requirements for hypnotics during anesthetic induction and maintenance as well. Such benefits explain the present popularity of opioid use [10, 42].

The transition from infrequent small doses of opioids during the 1960s and 1970s to the more frequent and larger doses used today took place largely during the 1980s [10, 42]. In November of 1979, Ted Stanley, having introduced high-dose fentanyl and oxygen anesthesia in the US [54–56], was invited to join Simon de Lange at the University of Leiden to evaluate the then new opioids, sufentanil and alfentanil. They first visited de Castro in Belgium since he had great experience with these and most other opioids. They discussed the properties and advantages of alfentanil and sufentanil with de Castro and watched him administer both agents during various surgical procedures in order to gain insight into his experience with them.

De Castro was most impressed with alfentanil because of its rapid onset of action (60–90 s) and short duration (3–5 min) after a bolus injection. In December 1979, he suggested that alfentanil should be effective as a sole anesthetic induction agent, as an analgesic component of nitrous oxide–opioid "balanced" anesthesia, and possibly as a sole opioid

Table 48.2 Potency and safety comparisons of morphine, meperidine and some Janssen analgesic compounds. (From Janssen Pharmaceutica and de Castro et al. [60], with permission)	Compound	Tail withdrawal reflex ED50 (mg/kg)	Potency ratio[a]	LD50 (mg/kg)	Therapeutic index
	Meperidine	6.15	1.00	29.0	4.72
	Morphine	3.15	1.95	223	71.0
	Phenoperidine	0.12	51.3	4.69	39.1
	Alfentanil	0.044	140	47.5	1,080
	Fentanyl	0.011	559	3.05	277
	Sufentanil	0.00067	9,180	17.9	26,700
	Carfentanil	0.00037	16,200	3.13	8,460

[a] Relative to meperidine

anesthetic for cardiac surgery. He was also impressed with the potency and ability of relatively high doses of sufentanil to block hemodynamic and hormonal responses to "surgical stress." He thought it would be useful as a sole or principal opioid anesthetic for cardiac and major vascular surgery. De Lange, Stanley, Stanski and others began a series of studies with alfentanil and sufentanil in January 1980 that spread to other centers in the US and Europe, changing the way clinicians viewed and used opioids [71–80]. It became clear that both alfentanil and sufentanil could be administered (like fentanyl) in doses that resulted in unconsciousness in less than five minutes (<2 min with alfentanil) without appreciable change in heart rate and arterial blood pressure.

Publication of hundreds of papers in the 1970s studying large doses of morphine as an "anesthetic", and then similar studies with fentanyl in the late 1970s and early 1980s, began a new anesthetic paradigm. This continued with studies evaluating alfentanil and sufentanil as induction agents, as sole opioid anesthetics for cardiac surgical and other procedures in the 1980s. With regulatory approval and introduction of alfentanil and sufentanil into clinical practice in the mid-1980s, clinicians (especially those in the UK and US) became more comfortable with larger doses of the potent opioids. While no opioid became popular as a "sole induction agent" (other than in high-dose opioid–oxygen anesthesia for cardiac or major vascular surgery), a large dose use of these compounds to provide analgesia before and during induction/intubation and during the maintenance of anesthesia, did catch on.

Sufentanil

The remarkable increase of sales in fentanyl as it went "off patent" stimulated sales of generic versions of the drug in the early 1980s. Concurrently, the Janssen research and development team had another newer opioid, sufentanil (Fig. 48.3), that they felt was superior to fentanyl and had a patent life that extended until the mid 1990s [34]. They believed sufentanil would be a better opioid for cardiac and major vascular surgery than fentanyl because early studies indicated that sufentanil provided more cardiovascular stability and greater

suppression of hormonal stress responses than fentanyl [10, 42, 71]. In addition, sufentanil was significantly more potent (which at the time was considered the explanation for its hemodynamic and stress hormonal superiority), had a markedly higher therapeutic index (which they reasoned would make it a safer drug for clinicians), had a similar or possibly faster onset time and shorter duration of action than fentanyl, and did not increase plasma histamine or cause venodilation [34, 42, 71, 72].

While subsequent studies generally confirmed the advantages of sufentanil over fentanyl [81, 82], its approval by American and European regulatory authorities (in 1982 in Europe and 1985 in the US) and introduction into clinical practice, did not have a major impact on clinicians. Sufentanil was usually priced significantly higher than fentanyl, impeding its acceptance. In addition, the introduction of the beta blocking drugs at about the same time neutralized sufentanil's hemodynamic and stress hormonal advantages over fentanyl. While sufentanil did and still does find a place in many cardiac anesthesiologists' practices, it was never a major commercial success. Sufentanil and alfentanil's poor commercial performances in the late 1980s and early 1990s convinced the Janssen company that further research in opioids for anesthesiology was not worthwhile. The similarly poor commercial performances of etomidate and droperidol caused the company to leave the anesthesiology field entirely in the mid 1990s.

Alfentanil

Janssen synthesized alfentanil in 1976 and introduced it in Europe in 1983, and in the US in 1987 (Fig. 48.3). Alfentanil offered a rapid onset (60–90 s), short duration (5–10 min when used as a bolus) and a high therapeutic index (1080), (Table 48.2) [34, 42, 73–79]. These features caused the Janssen Company to envision alfentanil as the perfect opioid for short surgical and outpatient procedures and the increasingly popular total intravenous delivery of anesthesia [34, 42]. When alfentanil was introduced in the US in 1987, the possibility of a "blockbuster" was considered likely. It didn't work out that way.

Although a large bolus dose of alfentanil produced unconsciousness in a minute or so, it also produced muscle rigidity in 70–80% of patients [74]. As a result, alfentanil did not become popular as an induction agent. Alfentanil's quick onset and short duration has been valuable in single or few bolus doses as a sole analgesic agent or in combination with inhaled or intravenous hypnotics for balanced anesthesia. However, when used for 45–60 min or longer, either as a continuous infusion or as many boluses, alfentanil accumulates in tissues and its duration becomes prolonged [79, 80, 83]. This made alfentanil less desirable for TIVA (see below) especially relative to remifentanil which was introduced into clinical practice in 1996 [84–86]. Alfentanil has a niche today as a rapid onset/offset analgesic IV bolus prior to short painful procedures [10], but even in that application, remifentanil often supplants alfentanil.

Total Intravenous Anesthesia (TIVA) and Opioids

By definition, TIVA is used for both anesthetic induction and maintainance with intravenous drugs alone [87]. Therefore TIVA excludes the use of nitrous oxide or volatile anesthetics. While the first intravenous anesthetic, chloral hydrate, introduced by Pierre-Cyprien Oré in Paris in 1872, could produce complete anesthesia, mortality associated with its use dampened enthusiasm for its application and for the development of other intravenous anesthetics until the twentieth century [87]. The first intravenous non-opioids developed for anesthesia in the early 1900s (hedonal, a urethane derivative introduced in 1909) and the early barbituates (in the beginning of the 1920s) were slow in onset, had a long duration of action (or both) and were not successful in clinical practice [87]. The 1930s introduction of the ultra-short acting barbituates changed anesthetic induction in adults.

The re-introduction of opioids into operating rooms, especially in the US and the UK, the increasing popularity of "balanced anesthesia" worldwide, and the introduction of neurolept analgesia (anesthesia) in Europe in the 1950s, set the stage for TIVA. The first TIVA advocates (they did not call it TIVA) introduced "artificial hibernation," "ataralgesia," "narco-ataralgesia" and neurolept analgesia. These approaches used an opioid (usually meperidine, phenoperidine, or fentanyl) plus non-opioid intravenous hypnotics (tranquilizers, benzodiazepines and other similar compounds). The theory was to independently regulate each anesthetic component (unconsciousness, amnesia, the sympathetic nervous system, and muscle relaxation) with intravenous agents that targeted the specific component. But the cumulative effects of the intravenous agents of the times and inadequate methods of administration (intermittent-bolus administration) resulted in delayed awakening and often circulatory

depression. Accordingly, interest in TIVA waned until the 1980s when the introduction of computerized pharmacokinetic-driven infusion devices combined with better drugs stimulated new research [87].

In 1981, Helmut Schwilden showed that a computer-controlled infusion pump guided by the published pharmacokinetics of the drug could produce target plasma anesthetic (and analgesic) concentrations in specific populations [88]. This began the application of target-controlled infusion (TCI) which is also sometimes called computer-assisted continuous infusion (CACI). Jacobs, Reves and Glass coined the latter terminology in 1991 [89]. With this technique, the anesthesiologist chooses a plasma concentration of both a hypnotic and an analgesic, usually an opioid. The technique accounts for the patient's characteristics and the degree of anticipated surgical stimulation. The computer-driven infusion pump then adjusts the drug infusion rate to obtain the targeted plasma concentration as predicted by pharmacokinetic information known for a similar population of patients.

In 1992, Shafer and Stanski showed that computer simulation programs of continuous infusions of intravenous anesthetics (including opioids) increased the understanding of these drugs' clinical pharmacokinetics [90]. It became clear that the terminal half-life of an intravenous anesthetic does not predict the rate of decrease of its plasma concentration after discontinuation of administration. In 1991, Shafer and Varvel found that the duration of drug infusion influenced the immediate rate of decline of fentanyl, alfentanil and sufentanil effect-site concentrations during recovery [91]. In 1992, Hughes and colleagues introduced the concept of "context-sensitive half-times" (the time it takes for the plasma concentration of an opioid to decrease by 50% after its infusion is discontinued). The concept was also confirmed with intravenous hypnotics [92]. In 1994, Young and Shafer proposed the desirable pharmacokinetic properties that an intravenous opioid should posses for rapid onset and recovery [93].

Some advocates of TIVA believe that ultimate acceptance of the technique depends on closed-loop administration [87]. The development of a feedback control system for maintaining neuromuscular blockade using neuromuscular blocking agents (pancuronium) was first described in 1980 and was considered a breakthrough [94]. The absence of an adequate feedback signal for the development of closed-loop systems for the control of other components of the anesthetic state, hypnotic depth, and especially a measure of analgesia, have impeded the development of closed-loop TIVA systems [87, 95]. TIVA has become increasingly popular in Europe in the last decade despite less than ideal closed-loop systems. This has resulted from the introduction of short onset, short duration intravenous agents (particularly propofol and remifentanil), and the quantification of their pharmacokinetics, the invention of "brain monitoring devices", and the development of "smart" infusion pumps.

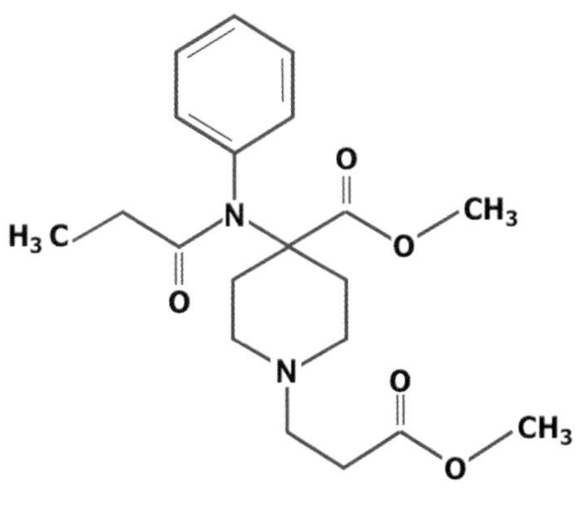

Remifentanil

Fig. 48.4 Remifentanil shares several molecular characteristics with its sister opioids fentanyl, sufentanil, and alfentanil (see Fig. 48.3)

Modern infusion systems permit a controlled delivery of intravenous drugs that is superior to intermittent manual injections [4, 10, 96, 97]. However, some clinicians argue that the benefits may not justify the increased cost of the drugs and devices, and the complexity of the systems utilized. Another argument against TIVA is predictability. As Schwilden (and others) have shown, kinetic models can be used to fairly accurately predict effect-site concentrations, but these are for populations, and individuals may deviate considerably from population predictions. At present, TIVA is more popular in Western Europe than the US and the rest of the Americas. An important reason for this is that the US FDA has not yet approved a TIVA device or infusion system whereas several systems have been approved in Europe.

Remifentanil

Commercial disappointment was Janssen's principal reason for terminating research into opioids for anesthesiology in the early 1990s. In contrast, the commercial popularity of propofol as a component of TIVA induced Glaxo to seek an intravenous opioid that was superior to alfentanil and more like propofol [10, 83]. In the late 1980s, chemists at Glaxo (and concurrently at a US Army laboratory) synthesized phenylpiperidine compounds with significant analgesic activity that underwent ester hydrolysis by both plasma and tissue esterases [10, 83–86]. The best of the Glaxo series of compounds was remifentanil (Fig. 48.4), a lipid-soluble weak base (octanol/water portion co-efficient of 19.9 at pH 7.4). It's pKa of 7.1 means that a significant amount of remifentanil exists in the un-ionized form at physiological pH, which explains its rapid onset of action. Remifentanil is a typical μ receptor specific agonist. It is slightly less potent than fentanyl and has respiratory and cardiovascular actions like other fentanyl cogeners. Remifentanil has the highest

therapeutic index (33,000) of any opioid and possibly any intravenous agent ever evaluated in rats. This is probably related to its extremely short duration of action [10, 83–86].

Remifentanil is the first true "ultra-short acting" opioid and was approved for use by the US FDA and many Western European countries in 1996–1997. Remifentanil's introduction in Europe in the late 1990s succeeded principally because of the popularity of TIVA in many European countries and the usefulness that a rapid onset, short duration, "very titratable" opioid brings to clinicians experienced and skilled in TIVA [10]. In contrast, remifentanil's introduction in the US was considered by Glaxo to be a failure. Sales of the drug were far less than Glaxo had hoped they would be and within a few years Abbott Laboratories bought the US rights to the drug. Remifentanil is still not extensively employed in the US, being largely confined to a handful of centers where TIVA and TIVA-like techniques are common. It has also gained popularity for neurosurgical cases requiring both intense analgesia during surgery as well as rapid dissipation of the opioid effect and rapid awakening following anesthesia.

For clinicians not experienced with TIVA, the rapid recovery after either a bolus or infusion of remifentanil is often a liability rather than an advantage since patients may have little or no postoperative analgesia unless the infusion is continued or another opioid is administered toward the end of the surgical procedure [98]. One subtle untoward effect accrues from the use of high infusion rates of remifentanil, an effect appreciated in the past decade. The high blood levels of remifentanil present during administration increase the tolerance to opioids in the postoperative period [99]. The resulting increased need for opioids to control postoperative pain can increase unwanted side effects such as postoperative nausea and vomiting.

Opioids and Perioperative Pain Control

Perioperative opioid use began in the mid-nineteenth century when (as described previously) morphine was administered intramuscularly in the preanesthetic period to speed induction and decrease ether or chloroform requirements [10–12, 15, 16]. In the first 70–80 years of the twentieth century, morphine and other opioids (hydrocodone and hydromorphine in the 1920s and meperidine in the 1950s) were used for postoperative analgesia. In contrast to this clinical use, little research focused on perioperative, particularly postoperative, pain management. This changed radically in the last 50 years [100].

The concept of perioperative pain management by anesthesiologists is now well established [100–102]. In the 1960s, post operative analgesia usually consisted of a fixed modest intramuscular dose of morphine or meperidine given at set intervals prescribed by the surgeon in the "post operative pain orders." In 1973, Marks and Sachar [103] showed that more than 50% of patients were under-treated with this approach. In 1968, Roe demonstrated that small IV doses of opioids provided more effective pain relief than did conventional IM injections [104]. Nonetheless, in the 1970s, many surgeons considered IM opioid injections safe, useful and adequate and resisted changes to this form of delivery [100–102].

Studies in 1980 by Austin, Stapleton, and Mather [105, 106] showed that a fixed IM dose of meperidine produced 5-fold differences in peak blood concentrations, 7-fold differences in times to reach peak concentrations and 4-fold differences in serum meperidine concentrations required to produce analgesia in different patients. Other studies confirmed these findings with other opioids [100–102, 107]. As long ago as 1971, Bellville and colleagues showed that there was no correlation between gender and analgesic requirement and no justification for calculating analgesic doses based on body weight or surface area [108]. More recent work confirmed these findings [107]. Still, surgeons resisted change. In 1985, Catley et al. [109] and in 1989 Brose and co-workers [110] showed that apnea and abnormal respiratory patterns occurred frequently, and hemoglobin oxygen desaturation could be severe following IM opioid administration. Resistance to change then began to diminish.

Forrest et al. [111] in 1970 and Catling and co-workers [112] in 1980, showed that small intermittent intravenous bolus doses of opioids could abolish wide swings in blood concentrations of these drugs, minimize respiratory depression, and permit the titration of the drug to the needs of individual patients. This method of delivering opioids set the stage for the introduction of patient-controlled analgesia (PCA) [111, 112].

Patient Controlled Analgesia (PCA)

Recognition of the variability in postoperative opioid requirements due to differences in individual patient opioid pharmacokinetics and, pharmacodynamics, as well as anthropometric and personality factors (first noted in the late 1960s and early 1970s by Sechzer [113, 114] and Forrest [111] and later by others [112, 115]) led to a new approach to managing postoperative pain. This approach was initially called "demand anesthesia" and later "patient controlled anesthesia" (PCA). It employed negative feedback. When patients experienced pain they gave themselves pain medication, and when pain decreased they did not [112, 114].

Sechzer pioneered on-demand or PCA in 1968 by evaluating the quality of the analgesic response to small intravenous doses of opioids given by a nurse, on patient demand [113]. In 1971, the study was repeated except that a machine gave the opioids [114]. Sechzer noted that his "demand

anesthesia" system provided pain relief with smaller total drug dosages than that with conventional IM therapy. He also observed that post-operative analgesic requirements of patients were often cyclical and varied greatly among individuals [113, 114]. Clearly the frequent administration of IV doses of opioids by nurses to large numbers of patients was impractical and costly. As a result the late 1960s witnessed the development of new PCA technologies [107].

Three investigators developed the first PCA prototypes: Forrest et al in 1970 [111] (The Demand Drop master that automatically administered IV analgesic drugs when activated by pressing a button in a handgrip); Sechzer in 1971 [114]; and Kerri-Szanto in 1971 [115] (The Demanalg). These early devices consisted of electronically controlled infusion pumps connected to timing devices triggered by patients [107, 111, 114–117]. When triggered, each device delivered a preset amount of opioid medication [111–121]. These devices decreased the incidence of moderate/severe post-operative pain from 20–40% to less than 5% when compared to conventional IM therapy [111–122]. The first commercially available PCA pump, the "Cardiff Palliator" was developed at the Welsh National School of Medicine in 1976 [107, 117, 123]. Digital electronics controlled the dose and imposed a lockout interval (to minimize the possibility of an overdose), and recorded the time of dosing.

In the mid 1970s, pharmaceutical companies recognized the market possibilities for these devices [117], and the associated potential for sales of their opioid analgesics. Thus, Janssen's Scientific Instruments division introduced the On-Demand Analgesic Computer (ODAC), and Pharmacia AB of Sweden developed the Prominject. The ODAC had the most sophisticated microprocessor of the time controlling its PCA device. The ODAC also had a pneumograph suspending drug administration if the patients' respiratory rate decreased to less than a critical value. The ODAC could administer opioids at a low (background) fixed rate and/or at a rate that varied automatically with patient demand. These forays of Janssen and Pharmacia into PCA devices stimulated entry of other companies in the late 1970s and 1980s with increasingly sophisticated microprocessor-based devices [117]. These companies included Abbott with its LifeCare PCA, Bard with its Harvard PCA, and Leicester with its Mircopalliator and its Programmable On-Demand Analgesia Computer called PROPAC. With the acceptance of PCA as a superior method of providing postoperative pain relief, the PCA concept spread to the treatment of cancer pain, obstetric pain, and as an investigative tool in drug trials and comparisons of analgesic techniques [107, 117].

In the last 5 years, simplified non-electric, disposable PCA systems have been evaluated and some introduced into clinical practice [117, 124]. These cost-effective devices are appearing in outpatient settings and patients' homes as well as hospitals. While On Demand or PCA therapy was initially only administered via the intravenous route, because of advantages to patients and caregivers it is now used with alternative methods that include oral, inhaled, nasal, buccal, transmucosal, transcutaneous, subcutaneous, and epidural approaches [107, 117, 118, 125].

Alternative Methods of Opioid Delivery

In the last 20 years the cost of inventing and developing new drugs including opioids and other analgesic compounds has dramatically increased, with total costs exceeding a billion dollars [10, 67, 126]. The result is that most large pharmaceutical companies will only invest in drugs with potential annual sales of more than a billion dollars. For smaller pharmaceutical companies, developing older drugs in patentable newer drug delivery systems (especially if these systems provide advantages to patients and/or caregivers) is an attractive alternative to developing new drugs [10, 126], because today's cost of developing an older drug in a new delivery system ranges from only 15–35 million dollars [10, 67, 126].

Opioid Transdermal Drug Delivery

Although dermal ointments and creams for local (transdermal) application have been used for hundreds of years, the first transdermal patents were only issued in 1971. The FDA approved a scopolamine transdermal patch in 1979, for management of nausea [67]. Its advantages compared to oral administration included decreased GI degradation and first-pass hepatic metabolism, more stable plasma concentrations, and an impressive improvement in patient compliance through greater ease of administration. Its modest success convinced the Alza Corporation in the mid-1980s that an opioid pain patch might provide similar advantages [67, 126]. The Alza researchers recognized that a good transdermal opioid would have a high potency, low molecular weight, be highly soluble in both water and lipid (because of the lipid content of the skin), and produce little or no skin irritation [67, 126, 127]. Fentanyl had these characteristics [127–131]. A fentanyl patch was first studied in patients with acute post-operative pain but produced too much respiratory depression [129]. The first fentanyl patch (Duragesic) approved by the FDA and European regulatory authorities was used in opioid-tolerant patients having cancer induced chronic pain in the early 1990s [10, 126].

At the time of the fentanyl patch development in the mid 1980s, Alza was a small California company without a sales force. Alza approached Janssen Pharmaceutica to help sell its new drug. Janssen's US marketing and sales people conducted an in depth market analysis that predicted peak sales of approximately 80 million dollars/year (a large amount at that time), but they had a hard time convincing Dr. Paul that this new way of giving fentanyl would be successful. Finally, he allowed the partnership to proceed. The resulting Duragesic eventually became the most successful analgesic/anesthetic pharmaceutical product ever introduced, with sales in 2004 (its last year of patent life) exceeding 2.4 billion dollars. The success of the patch caused generic companies to copy the Duragesic once it went "off patent", adding alternative opioids including sufentanil.

The fentanyl patch succeeded in chronic pain management because one patch lasted for 2–3 days. It was less useful for acute pain because it took 14–18 hours to produce steady state concentrations. This prompted some investigators (Ashburn, Streisand, Zhang and others) [132, 133] and companies (Alza, J&J, and Cadence) to study methods that would speed opioid passage across the skin. These efforts started in the late 1980s and continue to the present (Ted Schroeder, President and CEO Cadence Pharmacuticals Inc. personal communication) [10, 132, 133]. Iontophoresis augments drug passage through the skin with a small electric current applied to salts such as morphine HCL and fentanyl citrate [132]. Using this technique, analgesic doses were effectively delivered to patients with post-operative pain and opioid plasma levels were shown to be directly proportional to the electric current utilized [132, 133]. Reliability of these devices has however been erratic and no iontophoretic device for opioid delivery has been approved for use in the US or Europe.

Oral Opioid Transmucosal Drug Delivery

Sufentanil's 1985 approval in the US and many European countries allowed research into delivery by nasal, buccal, or ocular mucosa as a premedicant or to produce rapid onset analgesia for acute pain [10, 34, 66–68, 126, 134–136]. These studies in adults and children proved that sufentanil could be useful for such indications. Since the compound had many years of patent life remaining, cooperation of the Janssen Company was required for development of an approved product. The Janssen company preferred to focus on sufentanil's approved intravenous uses rather than on novel methods of delivery and this halted further efforts in the mid to late 1980s.

Similarly, in 1984, Stanley thought to put fentanyl in a "child friendly" red lollipop-like form, a sweetened lozenge on a stick which was later called an "Oralet", but the Janssen company declined involvment [65–67, 126, 137–140]. Undeterred, Stanley persisted, forming a small new company, Anesta, to develop oral transmucosal fentanyl citrate (OTFC). Stanley believed that this simple non-invasive, easy to titrate approach could be quickly and easily removed by the patient or clinician when the desired effect was evident. It would offer a rapid onset (5–15) minutes and relatively short duration (1–2 hours).

The Oralet (Fig. 48.5) gained regulatory approval in 1993 for use as a premedicant before surgery and for painful procedures in children and adults [65–68, 137–142]. It was introduced later in 1993, but achieved only modest commercial success. OTFC was also studied and approved by the FDA in 1998 for breakthrough cancer pain [137, 140–142] in a different form called Actiq (Fig. 48.5). Actiq was a commercial success in the 2000s, and stimulated other pharmaceutical companies to develop competitive products (e.g., Cephalon's Fentora and Prostraken's Abstral) in the late 1990s. In 2012 there were six oral transmucosal products available for providing rapid onset analgesia. They included:

- Abstral®: a sublingual tablet
- Actiq: the original lozenge
- Fentora: a buccal tablet
- Onsolis: a buccal soluble film
- Subsys: a sublingual spray

Nasal Transmucosal Delivery

The nasal mucosa offers a larger area for drug absorption (400–600 cm^2) than the buccal cavity and thus a potential for faster onset of drug action. The venous system atop the nasal cavity drains through the cribiform plate, directly into the forebrain. Accordingly, some investigators and small drug companies (in the late 1990s and 2000s) considered evaluating opioid nasal transmucosal products for premedication and analgesia and postoperative PCA [10, 126, 143–147]. However, weather (humidity changes) and infection can alter the nasal mucosal surface, and thus absorption can be changed (decreased) sometimes dramatically [66, 68, 125]. Several potent opioids administered by nasal sprays have been studied as analgesic premedicants before operation and for pain relief after surgery. Only butorphanol and fentanyl nasal sprays have achieved regulatory approval in the US. Fentanyl also as a nasal spray has been recently approved for PCA in some Western European countries. The difficulties of getting new opioid products through the regulatory bodies of the US and European countries (because of current fears of illicit use and abuse liability) has discouraged investment by pharmaceutical companies.

Opioid Delivery Through Other Tissue Surfaces

Over the last 10–15 years occasional researchers and companies (Inhaled Therapeutics, Alexa Pharmaceuticals) have considered the potential advantages (speed of onset, ease of use, low cost, improved safety) of delivering opioids to the trachea and the alveoli of the lung using hand held devices that provide inhaled powders, mists, vapors, crystals, or liposomes [66, 126, 148–152]. The devices produce particles sized so as to deposit in bronchioles or alveoli. Successful inhalation and absorption requires proper coordination with inspiration and some devices include strategies facilitating this goal. The same factors that govern control of other forms

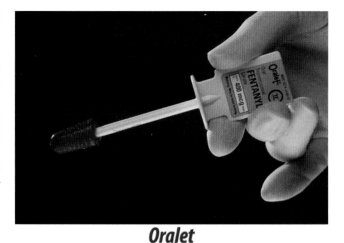

Oralet

Actiq

Fig. 48.5 The Oralet mucosal delivery system had as its intended use opioid (fentanyl) premedication for anesthesia. The Actiq was to be used in the management of pain in patients suffering from chronic pain such as that resulting from cancer

of PCA apply. Presently, no pulmonary inhalant device providing an opioid for pain or premedication has successfully navigated the European or US regulatory process.

The rectal mucosa offers another surface for opioid delivery [153–155]. Rectal sedatives and hypnotics (methohexital, tribromethanol) were used in the past to premedicate children [154]. Rectal suppositories containing morphine, hydro-morphine, oxymorphine, and oxycodone have also been studied and are currently available. Although the hydrogel formulation of rectal morphine has been used for premedication and analgesia in children [154], the rapid turnover of most outpatient and hospital pediatric surgical services make use of rectal administration of opioids impractical.

Oral Controlled-Release Medications

In the 1990s, Purdue Fredrick, a large privately held International Pharmaceutical Company developed a sustained release morphine that achieved great popularity because one or two pills per day produced analgesia for patients with chronic pain. Oxycodone was also studied and approved in an oral time-release tablet for chronic pain in the late 1990s. Several other companies developed similar morphine and other opioid sustained release products for chronic pain [156–162]. Some of these products have also been evaluated for premedication and post-operative analgesia, but have shown little advantage, although some data suggest that side effects may be less frequent after oral controlled release use of some opioids. Some time-release opioid products (oxycontin) have been abused, stimulating the development of abuse resistant controlled-release oxycodone pain capsules [162]. One was approved by the FDA in 2009 and another in 2011.

Delivery of Opioids to the Spinal Cord

In the 1980s, opioids, initially morphine, were delivered to the spinal cord via either intrathecal or epidural routes to produce long-term analgesia. A discussion of the history of this administration is found in Chapter 60 on pain management.

Some Final Thoughts on the History of Opioids

Opioids were given for pain relief in surgery for millenia before the demonstration of anesthesia by Morton in 1846. Morton's discovery transiently diminished the use of opioids for anesthetic purposes, but even in Snow's time the advantages accruing to the addition of morphine to ether or chloroform became obvious (see Chapter 49)—a greater ease of anesthetic induction and a decrease in the need for those vapors. The addition of scopolamine to morphine made for a lovely premedication, and some clinicians in the early 1900s used the combination to the exclusion of the inhaled anesthetics to produce "twilight sleep". But the price was too great, increasing morbidity and mortality, probably from respiratory depression.

The use of opioids to complement or replace general anesthetics was also limited by morphine's slowness of entry into and departure from the brain, leading to a slowness of onset and offset of effect. The synthesis of new opioids, meperidine in the 1930s–1940s, fentanyl in the 1960s, and later its "sisters and brothers", overcame these problems. Opening the door to an increasing intraoperative use of opioids, this culminated in the use of enormous ("industrial sized") doses for anesthetic or near-anesthetic effects. Further facilitating the use of opioids was the discovery of opioid antagonists that could reverse unwanted effects such as respiratory depression. It also helped that drugs were developed to manage side effects such as nausea and vomiting.

Drugs complimenting the "anesthetic" effects of opioids were discovered. Propofol produced sleep and amnesia. The capacity to produce sleep and amnesia was far weaker in opioids, but opioids could produce analgesia where propofol could not. Both propofol and some of the newer opioids had kinetic properties allowing moment to moment control of their effect. In the 1980s, this led to the combined infusion of propofol and opioids to give total intravenous anesthesia (TIVA).

Finally, in the past few decades, new approaches in opioid delivery have broadened and enhanced their use. Think of patient controlled analgesia where pain is treated as it arises by the patient rather than by a person who can only ask about the extent of the pain suffered. Think of opioids introduced through mucous membranes for a rapid effect without the psychological trauma associated with the stick of a needle. Think of patches placed on the skin that deliver opioids to provide long term relief of postoperative pain, or more importantly, chronic pain from disease. And think of attacking pain by placing an opioid where receptors for the transmission of pain live, receptors in the spinal cord. It is almost magical.

References

1. Keys TE. The history of surgical anesthesia. Wood Library—Museum of Anesthesiology, Park Ridge, Illinois, original publication 1945, reprinted 1996.
2. Foldes FF, Swerdlow M, Siker ES, editors. Narcotics and narcotic antagonists. Springfield, IL: Charles C. Thomas; 1964.
3. Macht DI. The history of opium and some of its preparations and alkaloids. J Am Med Assoc. 1915;64:477–81.
4. Corssen G, Reves JG, Stanley TH. Intravenous anesthesia and analgesia. Philadelphia, PA: Lea & Febiger; 1988.
5. Lerner AM. The abuse of paregoric in Detroit, Michigan (1956–1965). UNDOC Bull Narc. 1966;3:13–9.
6. Serturner FWA. Ueber das Morphin, eine neue salzfahige Grundlage, und die Mekonsaure, als Haupbestandteile des Opiums. Annalen der Physik. 1817;56–89.
7. Pravaz C. Sur un Nouveau d'operer la Coagulation du Sangue dans Aerteres, Applicable a la Guerison des Aneurismes. Compt Rend Acad Sci Paris. 1853;36:88–91.
8. Wood A. On a new method of treating neuralgia. Edinb Med Surg. 1855;5:265–81.
9. Srimvason V, Wielbo D, Tebbett IR. Analgesic Effects of Codeine–IG-glucuronide after intravenous administration. Europ J Pain. 1997;1:185–90.
10. Bailey PL, Egan TD, Stanley TH. Intravenous opioid anesthetics. In: Miller RD, editor. Anesthesia. 5th Ed. Philadelphia, PA: Churchill Livingston; 2000 (Chapter 23).
11. Van Hoosen BA. Scopolamine–morphine anesthesia. Chicago, IL: The House of Manz; 1915.
12. Smith RR. Scopolamine–morphine anesthesia with report of two hundred and twenty-nine cases. Surg Gyne Obstet. 1908;7:414 (abstract).
13. Wright CRA. On the action of organic acids and their anhydrides on the natural alkaloids. J Chem Soc. 1874;27:1031–43.
14. Sawynok J. The therapeutic use of heroin: a review of the pharmacological literature. Can J Physical Pharmacol. 1986;64:1–6.
15. Sexton JC. Death following scopolamine–morphine injection. Lancet Clin. 1905;55:582–5.

16. Gauss CJ. Die Anwendung des Skopolamin – Morphium Dammer-schlafes in der Geburtshilfe. Med Klin. 1906;2:136–8.
17. Lundy JS. Intravenous anesthesia: preliminary report of the use of two new thiobarbiturates. Proc Staff Meeting Mayo Clinic. 1935;10:536–43.
18. Crile GW. Phylogenetic association in relation to certain medical problems. Boston Med Surg J. 1910;163:893–4.
19. Lundy JS. Balanced anesthesia. Minn Med. 1926;9:299.
20. Neff W, Mayer EC, de la Luz Pecales M. Nitrous oxide and oxygen anesthesia with curare relaxation. Calif Med J. 1947;66:67–9.
21. Eisleb O, Schaumann O. Dolantin, lin neuartiges spasmolytikum und analgeticum. Dtsch Med Wochenschr. 1939;65:967.
22. Mushin WW, Rendell-Baker L. Pethidine as a supplement to nitrous oxide anesthesia. Brit Med J. 1949;2:472.
23. Brotman M, Cullen SC. Supplementation with Demerol during nitrous oxide anesthesia. Anesthesiology. 1949;10:696–705.
24. Siker ES, Foldes FF, Pahk NM, Swerdlow M. Nisentil (1,3,dimethyl-4-phenyl-4-propionoxypiperidine): a new supplement for nitrous oxide oxygen thiopentone (Pentothal sodium) anesthesia. Brit J Anaesth. 1954;26:405–10.
25. Dundee JW, Brown SS, Hamilton RC, McDowell SA. Analgesic supplementation of light general anesthesia: a study of its advantages using sequential analysis. Anaesthesia. 1969;24:52–61.
26. Hall RI, Szlan F, Hug CC Jr. The enflurane-sparing effect of alfentanil in dogs. Anesth Analg. 1987;66:1287–91.
27. McEwan AI, Smith C, Dyar O, Ancas FC, Goodman D, Smith LR, Glass PS. Isoflurane minimum alveolar concentration reduction by fentanyl. Anesthesiology. 1993;78:864–9.
28. Glass PSA, Gan TJ, Howell S, Ginsberg B. Drug interactions: volatile anesthetics and opioids. J Clin Anesth. 1997;9:18S.
29. Laborit H, Huygenard P. Pratique de l'hibernotherape en Chirurgie et en Medicine. Paris: Massom; 1954.
30. Laborit H. Stress and cellular function. Philadelphia: Lippincot; 1959.
31. Edmonds-Seal J, Prys-Roberts C. Pharmacology of drugs used in neurolept analgesia. Br J Anaesth. 1970;42:207–16.
32. Nilsson E, Janssen PAF. Neurolept-analgesia an alternative to general anesthesia. Acta Anaesth Scand. 1961;5:73–84.
33. De Castro J, Mundeleer R. Anesthesia san barbiturates: la neurolept analgesie. Anesth Analg (Paris). 1959;16:1022–56.
34. Stanley TH, Egan TD, Van Aken H. A tribute to Paul A. J. Janssen: entrepreneur extraordinaire, innovative scientist, and significant contributor to anesthesiology. Anesth Analg. 2008;106:451–62.
35. Paul D, Pick CG, Tive LA, Pasternok GW. Pharmacological characterization of Nalorphine: a kappa 3 analgesic. J Pharmocol Exp Ther. 1991;257:1–7.
36. Ngai SH, Berkowitz BA, Yang JC. Pharmacokinetics of Naloxone in rats and man. Anesthesiology. 1976;44:398–401.
37. Jasinski DR, Martin WR, Hoeldtke RD. Effects of short and long term administration of Pentazorine in man. Clin Pharmocol Ther. 1970;11:385–406.
38. Lowenstein E. The birth of opioid anesthesia. Anesthesiology. 2004;100:1013–5.
39. Lowenstein E, Hallowell P, Levine FH, Daggett WM, Austen WG, Lover MB. Cardiovascular response to large doses of intravenous morphine in man. N Engl J Med. 1969;281:1389–93.
40. de Castro and Parmentier. Pure analgesic anaesthesia and its limitations, VI World Congress of Anaesthesiology; 1976, Mexico. V, p. 214 (abstract).
41. Castro J de. Analgesic anesthesia. Anesth Analg Reanim. 1969;26:145–50.
42. Bovil JG, Sebel PS, Stanley TH. Opioid analgesics in anesthesia: with special reference to their use in cardiovascular anesthesia. Anesthesiology. 1984;61:731–55.
43. Stanley TH, Gray NH, Stanford W, Armstrong R. The effects of high dose morphine on fluid and blood requirements in open-heart operations. Anesthesiology. 1973;38:536–41.
44. Stanley TH, Gray NH, Isern-Amaral JH, Patton C. Comparison of blood requirements during morphine and halothane anesthesia for open-heart surgery. Anesthesiology. 1974;41:34–8.
45. Hasbrouck JD. Morphine anesthesia for open-heart surgery. Ann Thorac Surg. 1970;10:364–9.
46. Wong KC, Martin WE, Hornbein TF, Freund FG, Everett J. The cardiovascular effects of morphine sulfate with oxygen and with nitrous oxide in man. Anesthesiology. 1973;38:542–9.
47. McDermott RW, Stanley TH. The cardiovascular effects of low concentrations of nitrous oxide during morphine anesthesia. Anesthesiology. 1974;41:89–91.
48. Stanley TH. Anesthesia with high doses of analgesics. In Spierdijk J, Bennebroek-Gravenhorst J, Feldman SA, Mathe H, editors. Analgesia in anesthesia and obstetrics. Leiden: Dicenda Medics Astra; 1980. pp. 62–3.
49. Stanley TH, editor. An International Symposium on Intravenous Anesthesia. Chicago: Grune-Stratton; 1980. pp. 367–84.
50. Liu W, Bidwai AV, Stanley TH, Isern-Amaral J. Cardiovascular dynamics after large doses of fentanyl and fentanyl plus N_2O in the dog. Anesth Analg. 1976;55:168–72.
51. Bidwai AV, Liu W, Stanley TH, Bidwai V, Loeser EA, Shaw CL. The effects of large doses of fentanyl and fentanyl with nitrous oxide on renal function in the dog. Can Anaesth Soc J. 1976;23:296–302.
52. Freye E. The effect of fentanyl on the resistance and capacitance vessels of the dog's hindlimb. Arzneimittelforschung. 1977;27:1037–9.
53. Liu W, Bidwai AV, Lunn JK, Stanley TH. Urine catecholamine excretion after large doses of fentanyl, fentanyl and diazepam and fentanyl, diazepam and pancuronium. Can Anaesth Soc J. 1977;24:371–9.
54. Stanley TH, Webster LR. Anesthetic requirements and cardiovascular effects of fentanyl–oxygen and fentanyl–diazepam–oxygen anesthesia in man. Anesth Analg. 1978;57:411–6.
55. Stanley TH, Philbin DM, Coggins CH. Fentanyl–oxygen anesthesia for coronary artery surgery: cardiovascular and anti-diuretic hormone responses. Can Anaesth Soc J. 1979;26:168–72.
56. Lunn JK, Stanley TH, Eisele J, Webster LWoodwardA. High dose fentanyl anesthesia for coronary artery surgery: plasma fentanyl concentrations and influence of nitrous oxide on cardiovascular responses. Anesth Analg. 1979;58:390–5.
57. Janssen PAJ, Niemegeers CJE, Dong JGH. The inhibitory effect of fentanyl and other morphine-like analgesics on the warm water induced tail withdrawal reflex in rats. Arzneimittel-Forschung. 1963;13:502–7.
58. Niemegeers CJE, Schellekens JHL, Bever WFM van, Janssen PAF. Sufentanil, a very potent and extremely safe intravenous morphine-like compound in mice, rats and dogs. Arzneimittel-Forschung. 1976;26:1551–6.
59. Van Bever WFM, Niemegeers CJE, Schellekens KHL, Janssen PAF. N-(4-substituted-1-(2-arylethyl)-4-piperidinyl)-N-phenyl-propan-amides, a novel series of extremely potent analgesics with unusually high safety margin. Arzneimittel-Forschung. 1976;26:1548–51.
60. De Castro J, Water A van de, Wouters A, Xhonnrux R, Reneman R, Kay B. Comparative study of cardiovascular, neurological, and metabolic side effects of eight narcotics in dogs. Acta Anaesthesiolog Belg. 1979;30:5–99.
61. Niemegeers CJE, Janssen PAF. Alfentanil (R39209) a particularly short-acting intravenous narcotic analgesic in rats. Drug Dev Res. 1981;1:83–8.
62. Egan T. The clinical pharmacology of remifentanil: a brief review. J Anesthesia. 1998;12:195–204.
63. Burns W. Personal communication. 1988.
64. Stanley TH. Anesthesiology in the 21st century: analgesic sedative and anesthetic focusing. J Clin Monit Comput. 1986;3:21–5.
65. Nelson PS, Streisand JB, Mulder SN, Pace NL, Stanley TH. Comparison of oral transmucosal fentanyl citrate and an oral solution of meperidine, diazepam and atropine for premedication in children. Anesthesiology. 1989;70:616–21.

66. Stanley TH. Novel drug delivery systems: oral transmucosal and intranasal transmucosal. J Pain Symptom Manaage. 1992;7:163–71.
67. Tarver SD, Stanley TH. Alternative routes of drug administration and new drug delivery systems. Adv Anesth. 1989;7:337–68.
68. Streisand JB, Stanley TH. Opioids: new techniques in routes of administration. Curr Opin Anaesthesiol. 1989;2:456–62.
69. Clark NJ, Meuleman T, Liu W, Zwanikken P, Pace NL, Stanley TH. Comparison of sufentanil-N2O and fentanyl-N2O in patients without cardiac disease undergoing general surgery. Anesthesiology. 1987;66:130–5.
70. White PF, Coe V, Shafer A, Sung ML. Comparison of alfentanil with fentanyl for outpatient anesthesia. Anesthesiology. 1986;64:99–107.
71. Lange S de, Boscoe MJ, Stanley TH. Comparison of sufentanil–O2 and fentanyl–O2 for coronary artery surgery. Anesthesiology. 1982;56:112–8.
72. Lange S de, Boscoe JM, Stanley TH, de Bruijn N, Philbin DM, Coggins CH. Anti-diuretic and growth hormone responses during coronary artery surgery with sufentanil–oxygen and alfentanil–oxygen anesthesia in man. Anesth Analg. 1982;61:434–8.
73. Lange S de, Stanley TH, Boscoe JM. Alfentanil–oxygen anaesthesia for coronary artery surgery. Br J Anaesth. 1981;53:1167–72.
74. Nauta J, Lange S de, Koopman D, Spierdijk J, Kleff J van, Stanley TH. Anesthetic induction with alfentanil: a new short-acting narcotic analgesic. Anesth Analg. 1982;61:267–72.
75. Kay B, Pleurry B. Human volunteer studies of alfentanil (R39209), a new short-acting narcotic analgesic. Anaesthesia. 1980;35:952–6.
76. Van Leeuwen L, Deen L. Alfentanil, a new potent and very short-acting morphinomimetic for minor operative procedures: a pilot study. Anaesthetist. 1981;30:115–7.
77. Bruijn N de, Christian C, Frograeus L, Freedman B, Davis GF, Hamm DP, Everson CT, Pellom GL, Wechsler AS. The effects of alfentanil on global ventricular mechanics. Anesthesiology. 1983;A59 (abstract).
78. Bovill JG, Sebel PS, Blackburn CL, Heykantz J. The pharmacokinetics of alfentanil (R39209): a new opioid analgesic. Anesthesiology. 1982;57:439–43.
79. Stanley TH, Pace NL, Liu WS, Gillmor ST, Willard KF. Alfentanil–N2O vs fentanyl–N2O balanced anesthesia: comparison of plasma hormonal changes, early postoperative respiratory function and speed of postoperative recovery. Anesth Analg. 1983;62:285 (abstract).
80. Stanski DR, Hug CC Jr. Alfentanil—a kinetically predictable narcotic analgesic (editorial). Anesthesiology. 1982;57:435–8.
81. Anand KJS, Philbin D, Hickey PR. Halothane-morphine compared with high-dose sufentanil for anesthesia and postoperative analgesia in neonatal cardiac surgery. N Eng J Med. 1992;326:1–9.
82. Mangano DT, Siliciano D, Hollenberg M, Leung JM, Browner WS, Goehner P, Merrick S, Verrier E. Postoperative myocardial ischemia: therapeutic trials using intensive analgesia following surgery. Anesthesiology. 1992;76:342–53.
83. Egan TD, Minto CF, Hermann DJ, Ban J, Muir KT, Shafer S, Barr J. Remifentanil versus alfentanil: comparative pharmacokinetics and pharmacodynamics in healthy adult male volunteers. Anesthesiology. 1996;84:821–33.
84. Rosow C. Remifentanil: a unique opioid analgesic (editorial). Anesthesiology. 1993;79:875–6.
85. Egan TD. Remifentanil pharmacokinetics and pharmacodynamics: a preliminary appraisal. Clin Pharmacokinet. 1995;29:80–94.
86. Egan T, Lemmens HJM, Fiset P, Hermann DJ, Muir KT, Stanski DR, Shafer SL. The pharmacokinetics of the new short-acting opioid remifentanil (G187084B) in healthy adult male volunteers. Anesthesiology. 1993;79:881–92.
87. White PF. Intravenous anesthesia. Baltimore: MD Williams and Williams; 1997.
88. Schwilden H. A general method for calculating the dosage scheme in linear pharmacokinetics. Eur J Clin Pharmacol. 1981;20:379–86.
89. Jacobs JR, Reves JG, Gloss PSA. Continuous infusions for maintaining for maintaining anesthesia. Int Anesth Clin. 1991;29.
90. Shafer SL, Stanski DR. Improving the clinical utility of anesthetic drug pharmacokinetics. Anesthesiology. 1992;76:327–30.
91. Shafer SL, Varvel JR. Pharmacokinetics, pharmacodynamics, and rational opioid selection. Anesthesiology. 1991;74:53–63.
92. Hughes MA, Glass PSA, Jacobs JR. Context sensitive half-times in multi-compartment pharmacokinetic models for intravenous anesthetic drugs. Anesthesiology. 1992;76:334–41.
93. Young E, Shafer SL. Pharamacokinetic parameters relevant to recovery from opioids. Anesthesiology. 1994;81:833–42.
94. Brown BH, Perks R, Anthony M, Asbury J, Linkers DA. Closed-loop control of muscle relaxation during surgery. Clin Phyo Physical Meas. 1980;1:203–10.
95. Stanski DR. Monitoring depth in anesthesia. In: Miller RD, editor. Anesthesia. 4th ed. New York: Churchill Livingstone; 1994. pp. 1127–59.
96. Ausems ME, Vuyk J, Hug CC Jr, Stanski DR. Comparison of a computer-assisted infusion versus intermittent bolus administration of alfentanil as a supplement to nitrous oxide for lower abdominal surgery. Anesthesiology. 1988;68:851–61.
97. Alvis JM, Reves JG, Govier AV, Menkhaus PG, Henling C, Spain JA, Bradley E. Computer-assisted continuous infusions of fentanyl during cardiac anesthesia: comparison with a manual method. Anesthesiology. 1985;63:41–9..
98. Yarmush J, D'Angelo R, Kirkhart B, O'Leary C, Pitts MC II, Grafe G, Sebel P, Watkins WD, Miguel R, Streisand J, Maysick LK, Vujis D. A comparison of remifentanil and morphine sulfate for acute postoperative analgesia after total intravenous anesthesia with remifentanil and propofol. Anesthesiology. 1997;87:235–43.
99. Crawford MW, Hickey C, Zaarour C, Howard A, Naser B. Development of acute opioid tolerance during infusion of remifentanil for pediatric scoliosis surgery. Anesth Analg. 2006;102:1662–7.
100. Ready LB. Acute perioperative pain. In: Miller RD, editor. Anesthesia. 5th ed. Philadelphia, PA: Churchill Livingston; 2000 (Chapter 69).
101. Ready LB, Oden R, Chadwick HS, Benedetti C, Rooke GA, Caplan R, Wild LM. Development of an anesthesiology-based postoperative pain management service. Anesthesiology. 1988;68:100–6.
102. Cartwright PD, Helfinger RC, Howell JJ, Scepmann KK. Introducing an acute pain service: Department of Anaesthesia, Princess Royal Hospital, Telford. Anaesthesia. 1991;46:188–91..
103. Marks RM, Sachar ES. Under treatment of medical inpatients with narcotic analgesics. Ann Intern Med. 1973;78:173–81..
104. Roe BB. Are postoperative narcotics necessary? Arch Surg. 1963;88:912–5.
105. Austin KL, Stapleton JV, Mather LE. Multiple intramuscular injections: a major source of variability in analgesia response to meperidine. Pain. 1980;47:8.
106. Austin KL, Stapleton JV, Mather LE. Relationship between blood meperidine concentrations and analgesic response. Anesthesiology. 1980;53:460–6.
107. Grass JA. Patient-controlled analgesia. Anesth Analg. 2005;101:544–61.
108. Bellville JW, Forrest WH, Miller E, Brown BW Jr. Influence of age on pain relief from analgesics. JAMA. 1971;217:1835–41.
109. Catley DM, Thorton C, Jordan C, Lehane JR, Royston D, Jones JG. Pronounced episodic oxygen desaturation in the postoperative period: Its association with ventilatory pattern and analgesic regimen. Anesthesiology. 1985;63:20–8.
110. Brose WG, Cohn SE. Oxyhemoglobin saturation following Cesarean section in patients receiving epidural morphine, PCA or IM meperidine analgesia. Anesthesiology. 1989;70:948–53.

111. Forest WH, Smethurst PWR, Kienitz ME. Self-administration of intravenous analgesics. Anesthesiology. 1970;33:363–5.
112. Catling JA, Pinto DM, Jordan C, Jones JG. Respiratory effects of analgesia after cholescystectomy: comparison of continuous and intermittent papaveretum. Br Med J. 1980;281:478–80.
113. Sechzer PH. Objective measurement of pain. Anesthesiology. 1968;29:209–10.
114. Sechzer PH. Studies in pain with the analgesic-demand system. Anesth Analg. 1971;50:1–10.
115. Kerri-Szanto M. Apparatus for demand analgesia. Can Anaesth Soc J. 1971;18:581–2.
116. White PF. Use of patient-controlled analgesia for management of acute pain. JAMA. 1988;259:243–7.
117. White PF. Patient-controlled analgesia (Part I): historical perspective. In: Astrburri MA, Fine PG, Stanley TH, editors. Pain management and anesthesiology. Dordrecht: Kluwer Academic Piblishers; 1998.
118. White WD, Pearce DJ, Norman J. Postoperative analgesia: a comparison of intravenous on-demand fentanyl with epidural bupivacaine. Br Med J. 1979;2:166–7.
119. Tamsen A, Hartvig P, Fagerlund C, Dahllstrom B, Bondesson U. Patient controlled analgesia therapy: clinical experience. Acta Anaesthesiol Scand Suppl. 1982;26:157–60.
120. Ellis R, Haines D, Shah R, Cotton BR, Smith G. Pain relief after abdominal surgery: comparison of IM morphine, sublingual buprenorphene and self-administered IV pethidine. Br J Anaesth. 1982;54:421–8.
121. Welchew EA. On-demand analgesia: a double-blind comparison of on-demand intravenous fentanyl with regular intramuscular morphine. Anaesthesia. 1983;38:19–25.
122. White PF, Parker RK. Is the risk of using "basal" infusion with patient-controlled analgesia therapy justified (letter)? Anesthesiology. 1992;76:489.
123. Evans JM, Rosen M, MacCarthey J, Hogg MI. Apparatus for patient-controlled administration of intravenous narcotics during labour. Lancet. 1976;1:17–8.
124. Blumenthal S, Dullen A, Rensch K, Borgeat A. Continuous infusion of ropivacaine for pain relief after iliac crest bone grafting for shoulder surgery. Anesthesiology. 2005;102:392–7..
125. Striebel HW, Koenigs D, Kromen J. Postoperative pain management by intranasal demand–adopted fentanyl titration. Anesthesiology. 1992;77:281–5..
126. Stanley TH. Personal communication with Paul Janssen.
127. Duthie DJR, Rowbotham DJ, Wyld R, Henderson PD, Nimmo WS. Plasma fentanyl contentrations during transdermal delivery of fentanyl to surgical patients. Br J Anaesth. 1988;60:614–8.
128. Rowtotham DJ, Wyld R, Peacock JE, Duthie JR, Nimmo WS. Transdermal fentanyl for the relief of pain after upper abdominal surgery. Br J Anaesth. 1989;63:56–9.
129. Sandler AN, Baxter AD, Katz J, Samson B, Freidlander M, Norman P, Koren G, Roger S, Hull K, Klein J. A double-blind placebo-controlled trial of transdermal fentanyl after abdominal hysterectomy. Anesthesiology. 1994;81:1169–80.
130. Varvel JR, Shafer SL, Hwang SS, Coen PA, Stanski DR. Absorption characteristics of transdermally administered fentanyl. Anesthesiology. 1989;70:928–34.
131. Rolf D. Chemical and physical methods of enhancing transdermal drug delivery. Pharm Tech. 1988;12:131–40.
132. Ashburn MA, Stephen RL, Petelenz TJ. Controlled iontophoretic delivery of morphine HCl for postoperative pain relief. Anesthesiology. 1988;69:A348.
133. Ashburn MA, Streisand J, Zhang J, Love G, Rowin M, Niu S, Kievit JK, Kroep JR, Mertens MJ. The ion + ophoresis of fentanyl citrate in humans. Anesthesiology. 1995;82:1146–53.
134. Ralley FE. Intranasal opiates: old route for new drugs (editorial). Can J Anaesth. 1989;36:491–2.

135. Henderson JM, Brodsky DA, Fisher DM, Brett CM, Hertzka RE. Pre-induction of anesthesia in pediatric patients with nasally administered sufentanil. Anesthesiology. 1988;68:671–5.
136. Karl HW, Keifer AT, Rosenberger JL, Laroch MG, Ruffle JM. Comparison of the safety and efficacy of intranasal midazolam or sufentanil for pre-induction of anesthesia in pediatric patients. Anesthesiology. 1992;76:209–15.
137. Stanley TH, Hague B, Mock DL, Streisand JB, Bubbers S, Dzelzkalns RR, Bailey PL, Pace NL, East KA, Ashburn MA. Oral transmucosal fentanyl citrate (lollipop) premedication in human volunteers. Anesth Analg. 1989;69:21–7.
138. Streisand JB, Stanley TH, Hague B, Vreeswijk H van, Ho GH, Pace NL. Oral transmucosal fentanyl citrate premedication in children. Anesth Analg. 1989;69:28–34..
139. Stanley TH, Leiman BC, Rawal N, Marcus MA, Nieuwenhuyzen M van den, Walford A, Cronau LH, Pace NL. The effects of oral transmucosal fentanyl citrate premedication on preoperative behavioral responses and gastric volume and acidity in children. Anesth Analg. 1989;69:328–35.
140. Streisand JB, Varvel JR, Stanski DR, LeMarie L, Ashburn MA, Hague BI, Tarver SD, Stanley TH. Absorption and bioavailability of oral transmucosal fentanyl citrate. Anesthesiology. 1991;75:223–9.
141. Ashburn MA, Fine PG, Stanley TH. Oral transmucosal fentanyl citrate for the treatment of breakthrough cancer pain: a case report. Anesthesiology. 1989;71:615–7.
142. Egan TD, Sharma A, Ashburn MA, Kievit J, Pace NL, Streisand JB. Multiple dose pharmacokinetics of oral transmucosal fentanyl citrate in healthy volunteers. Anesthesiology. 2000;92:665–73..
143. Abboud TK, Zhu J, Gangolly J, Longhitano M, Swart F, Makar A, Chu G, Cool M, Mantilla M, Kurtz N. Transnasal butorphanol: a new method of pain relief in post-Cesarean section pain. Acta Anaesthesiol Scan. 1991;35:14.
144. Zacny JP, Lichtor JL, Klafta JM, Alessi R, Apfelbaum JL. The effects of transnasal butorphanol on mood and psychomotor functioning in healthy volunteers. Anesth Analg. 1996;82:931–5.
145. Striebel HW, Bonillo B, Schwagmeier R, Dopjans D, Spies C. Self-administered intranasal meperidine for postoperative pain management. Can J Anaesth. 1995;42:287–91.
146. Striebel HW, Oelmann T, Spies C, Rieger R, Schwagmeier R. Patient-controlled intranasal analgesia: a method for noninvasive postoperative pain management. Anesth Analg. 1996;83:548–51.
147. Takala A, Kaasalainen V, Seppala T, Kalso E, Olkkola KT. Pharmacokinetic comparison of intravenous and intranasal administration of oxycodone. Acta Anaesthesiol Scand. 1997;41:309–12.
148. Worsley MH, Macleod AD, Brodie MJ, Ashbury AJ, Clark C. Inhaled fentanyl as a method of analgesia. Anaesthesia. 1990;45:449–51.
149. Hung OR, Whynot SC, Varvel JR, Shafer SL, Mezei M. Pharmacokinetics of inhaled liposome-encapsulated fentanyl. Anesthesiology. 1995;83:277–84.
150. Higgins MJ, Ashbury MB, Brodie MJ. Inhaled nebulized fentanyl for postoperative analgesia. Anaesthesia. 1991;46:973.
151. Thipphawong JB, Babul N, Moushige RJ, Findlay HK, Raber KR, Millwood GJ, Otulana B. Analgesic efficacy of inhaled morphine in patients after bunionectomy surgery. Anesthesiology. 2003;99:693–700.
152. Selami AO, Erol K, Gonca CT, Ismali D, Alpay HC, Levent A. Preliminary findings for pre-emptive analgesia with inhaled morphine: efficacy in septoplasty and septorhimoplasty cases. Otolatungol Head Neck Surg. 2006;135:85–9.
153. Lindahl S, Olsson AK, Thomson D. Rectal premedication in children. Use of diazepam, morphine and hyoscine. Anaesthesia. 1981;36:376–9.
154. Hanning CD, Vickers AP, Smith G, Graham NM, McNeil ME. The morphine hydrogel suppository. Br J Anaesth. 1988;61:221–7.

155. Lundeberg S, Beck O, Olsson GL, Boreus LO. Rectal administration of morphine in children: pharmacokinetic evaluation after a single dose. Acta Anaesthesiol Scand. 1996;40:445–51.
156. Simpson KH, Dearden MJ, Ellis FR, Jack TM. Premedication with slow release morphine (MST) and adjuvants. Br J Anaesth. 1988;60:825–30.
157. Banning AM, Schmidt JF, Chroemmen-Jorgensen B, Risbo A. Comparison of oral-release morphine and epidural morphine in the management of postoperative pain. Anesth Analg. 1986;65:385–8.
158. Derbyshire DR, Bell A, Parry PA, Smith G. Morphine sulfate slow release: a comparison with IM morphine for postoperative analgesia. Br J Anaesth. 1985;57:858–65.
159. Khojasteh A, Evans W, Reynolds RD, Thomas G, Savarese JJ. Controlled-release oral morphine sulfate in the treatment of cancer pain with pharmacokinetic correlation. J Clin Oncol. 1987;5:956–61.
160. Hoskin PJ, Poulain P, Hanks GW. Controlled-release morphine in cancer pain. Anaesthesia. 1989;44:897–901.
161. Riley J, Eisenberg E, Miller-Schwefe G, Drewes AM, Arendt-Nielsen L. Oxycodone: a review of its use in the management of pain. Curr Med Res Opin. 2008;24:175–92.
162. Friedman N, Klutzaritz V, Webster L. Long term safety of Remoxy (extend release Oxycodone) in patients with moderate to severe chronic osteo arthritis or low back pain. Pain Med. 2011;12:755–60.

The Evolution of Premedication

49

Robert K. Stoelting

Summary

Morton's demonstration of the anesthetic effects of diethyl ether (ether) made painless surgery possible, but ether irritated the airways, often initiating laryngospasm and stimulating production of secretions. Premedication—the administration of drugs before induction of anesthesia—alleviated such problems.

Over the latter half of the nineteenth century, clinicians increasingly injected morphine and scopolamine or atropine before ether anesthesia. The capacity of morphine to depress breathing was of limited concern because ether did not appear to depress breathing. The rationale for using premedication before chloroform, was less compelling. Chloroform depressed breathing and did not irritate the airway or promote secretions. However, morphine plus scopolamine could decrease preoperative apprehension before anesthesia with either ether or chloroform.

Introduced in 1934, pentobarbital might be given as premedication in place of or in addition to morphine. It offered two advantages over morphine: greater sedation and much less postoperative nausea and vomiting.

The 1950s introduction of the non-pungent anesthetic halothane changed how and when premedication was used. The elimination of airway irritation on induction removed the need to diminish airway responses, leaving the issues of apprehension and the smooth transition from wakefulness to anesthesia.

The subsequent use of premedication reflected the advantages offered by new drugs, the increased use of same-day surgery, and the extended limits of patient age and suitability for surgical procedures. Perhaps most importantly, the focus of premedication shifted in timing. In the 1970s and 1980s, intramuscular injection of the longer-acting, slower-onset morphine or pentobarbital an hour before the induction of anesthesia gave way to intravenous injection of the shorter-acting, more rapid onset fentanyl (synthesized in 1960), moments before induction to diminish the sympathetic response to tracheal intubation. Similarly, in the 1980s, the new benzodiazepine, midazolam, was given intravenously shortly before induction of anesthesia to relieve apprehension, decrease nausea, and produce amnesia. Midazolam replaced older drugs because of shorter duration and less venous irritation. In children, midazolam was given orally to produce somnolence allowing easier separation from parents. The "pre" of premedication has become an integral part of the anesthesia process.

Introduction

Diverse reasons and changing purposes explain the history of preanesthetic medication—commonly described as "premedication"—the administration of drugs before anesthesia. The goals of premedication and the drugs used to achieve these goals evolved in parallel with (1) the changing pharmacologic profile of drugs used to produce anesthesia, (2) the availability of new drugs for premedication, (3) changing surgical practice (e.g., outpatient surgery/anesthesia), and (4) changing aims (e.g., a greater focus on reduction of patient anxiety) [1].

Misconceptions have been and remain prevalent concerning premedication. Indeed, even today the use of certain drugs for premedication (principally belladonna drugs) continues although these drugs are no longer routinely indicated. Furthermore, evidence supporting the perceived value and effects of premedication at times is absent. Premedication may be ordered empirically, perhaps reflecting more the tradition and the habits of the practitioner (instilled from others during training) than evidence supporting these practices. In a 1955 editorial discussing premedication, Henry Beecher (Fig. 49.1) observed, *"Empirical procedures firmly entrenched in the habits of good doctors seem to have a vigor and life, not to say immortality of their own"* [2].

The author preserved the use of the word *narcotic* in this chapter as used by the authors of the articles referenced, recognizing that the current accepted designation is *opioid*.

R. K. Stoelting (✉)
Department of Anesthesia, Indiana University School of Medicine, Indianapolis, IN, USA
e-mail: Stoelting@apsf.org

Anesthesia Patient Safety Foundation, 8007 South Meridian Street, Building One, Suite Two, Indianapolis, IN 46217, USA

E. I Eger II et al. (eds.), *The Wondrous Story of Anesthesia,* DOI 10.1007/978-1-4614-8441-7_49, © Edmond I Eger, MD 2014

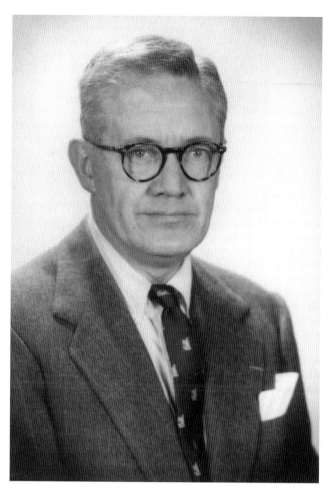

Fig. 49.1 Henry K. Beecher (1904–1976). (Courtesy of the Wood Library-Museum of Anesthesiology, Park Ridge, IL.)

Premedication is part of the history of anesthesia and thus deserves inclusion in our story. But it is more than part, more than a recitation of the drugs used at various times. Premedication responded to the anesthetics used, the evolution of anesthetic practice (e.g., the elimination of the preanesthetic visit; the shift to outpatient anesthesia), a greater focus on patient demands, and an increasing knowledge of drug pharmacokinetics and dynamics. As such the history of premedication also reflects the history of anesthesia.

Ancient Times

Prior to the discovery of anesthesia, alcohol and opium might be given before surgery,. These could not substitute for anesthesia, but provided some comfort. Wedel suggested that "Opium in a moderate draft (might be given) to the patient on the night preceding the operation (amputation), for thus he bears the burning and cutting of the limb with a readier spirit, and various symptoms will be averted" [3]. But this

could hardly be called premedication in anticipation of anesthesia. The controlled administration of drugs before the induction of anesthesia—demanded the invention of a precision means of delivery, the hollow needle, invented by Francis Rynd in 1844, and the hypodermic syringe, introduced by Charles Pravaz in 1853 [4].

Premedication: The Ether and Chloroform Era

Induction of ether anesthesia is slow. Its pungency can cause coughing, breath holding and laryngospasm (closure of the larynx). It stimulates salivary secretions which, in turn, add to the potential for coughing, breath holding and laryngospasm. An inhalation induction of anesthesia with ether has one other drawback—it can be frightening, invoking a sense of claustrophobia and suffocation, a feeling of swirling down into a black hole. One of the editors (LJS) has never forgotten two terrifying childhood experiences—in each being restrained while desperately trying to breathe in the face of ether's pungency. He heard a buzzing sound that increased to a crescendo in association with visual hallucinations—until unconsciousness blessedly intervened. Administration of a drug producing anxiolysis might have had a salutary effect on such fears. Anesthetists often ignored some of these untoward effects for a century, effects that should have mandated the use of drugs to speed induction, decrease the perception of pungency, decrease anxiety, and prevent secretions.

Over the last half of the nineteenth century clinicians increasingly injected morphine and scopolamine or atropine before ether anesthesia, scopolamine and atropine minimizing the production of secretions [5, 6]. We know from modern studies that premedication with morphine (and the siblings of morphine—opioids such as fentanyl) can minimize some of the problems noted in the preceding paragraph. Premedication with a standard dose of morphine decreases anesthetic (i.e., ether) requirement by approximately 10% [7]. That is, premedication with morphine provides a head start in the induction process. It also decreases the perception of pungency. Premedication with morphine or fentanyl decreases the incidence of coughing on induction of anesthesia with desflurane, an inhaled anesthetic that, like ether, is pungent (Fig. 49.2) [8].

Chloroform presents different problems. It is more potent and less pungent than ether, but it can induce premature ventricular contractions, especially in the anxious patient. Even with chloroform, the need to facilitate the induction of anesthesia remained. As with ether, morphine and atropine evolved as the premedication drugs most commonly selected for patients about to receive chloroform.

Premedication might be used for particularly difficult patients. Carl Uterhart (1835–1895)

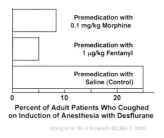

Fig. 49.2 Premedication with either morphine or fentanyl decreases the incidence of coughing on induction of anesthesia with the pungent anesthetic desflurane by 65 to 80 %. (From Kong CF, Chew STH, Ip-Yam PC: Intravenous opioids reduce airway irritation during induction of anaesthesia with desflurane in adults. Br J Anaesth 2000; 85: 364–7, with permission.)

> "…observed that the onset of the chloroform narcosis, which in alcoholics is known to be preceded by a severe and dangerous state of excitement, was extremely easy…after a small dose (of morphine). The state of excitement failed to appear; a quiet sleep with complete relaxation of all muscles occurred immediately after use of a few drams of chloroform" [9].

And we admire the advice of Joseph Clover, who in 1874 said

> "I like to give a teaspoonful of brandy, without water, a few minutes beforehand, but not so much as a tablespoonful. If wine be given or if the patient must have some water in the brandy, then they should be given half an hour before inhaling, to allow time for absorption" [10].

In 1881, Henry Lyman gave similar advice for care preceding anesthesia with ether [11]:

> "…there are many nervous individuals who cannot contemplate the approaching danger of operation without the greatest degree of agitation. Every possible effort should be made to calm such apprehensions. The tact of the surgeon will guide him to the methods best calculated to effect his purpose in this particular. The administration of a few doses of an alcoholic stimulant before inhalation is highly recommended as a means of tranquilizing a timid patient."

In 1850, Lorenzo Bruno of Turin (Fig. 49.3) reported injection of morphine 1 hour before induction of chloroform anesthesia to "lessen psychic trauma" [12]. Claude Bernard (Fig. 49.4), Professor of Physiology at the Sorbonne had worked in Bruno's clinic. In 1869, Bernard gave a series of lectures at the College de France describing the injection of morphine into animals to decrease the amount of chloroform needed for deep anesthesia [1, 13]. This led Labbé and Guyon to use morphine before chloroform anesthesia in humans, and in 1872 they described their experiences in four patients to the Académie des Sciences [14]. In the same year, Demarquay presented to the Académie des Sciences, his experience giving morphine before chloroform anesthesia [15]. He concluded that this practice added to the dangers of anesthesia and should not be done, but did not indicate the basis for his

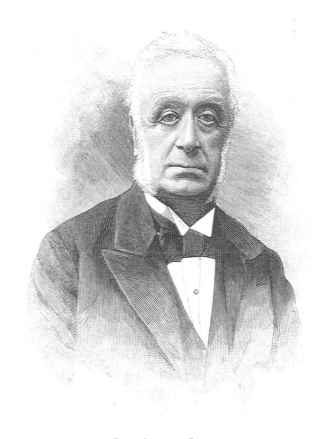

Prof. Lorenzo Bruno.
(Fotografia Alessandro Pasta, di Torino).

Fig. 49.3 Lorenzo Bruno (1821–1900). (Courtesy of http://www.comune.murazzano.cn.it/Contatti/tabid/1146/Default.aspx, *"L'illustrazione italiana"*, Milano, Fratelli Treves, Bibl. Sen. 308/37 p. 356.)

conclusion. Perhaps he considered that morphine's ability to depress breathing and thereby induce hypercapnia and hypoxia might lead to cardiac dysrhythmias in the presence of chloroform. Despite these explorations with premedication, its use was apparently not widespread before 1900.

In her review of developments in the last half of the nineteenth century, Duncum noted some peculiar beliefs regarding the combination of morphine and a belladonna drug, views that continued to the time (1956) when one of the editors (EIE) was a resident [16]. The view was that each drug counteracted the untoward effect of the other drug. For example, giving atropine or scopolamine would prevent the vomiting often associated with morphine. But some data suggested otherwise [17].

The 1880s to the 1950s

Like morphine, using atropine as part of the premedication has a long history. Professor Dastre, a French Physiologist

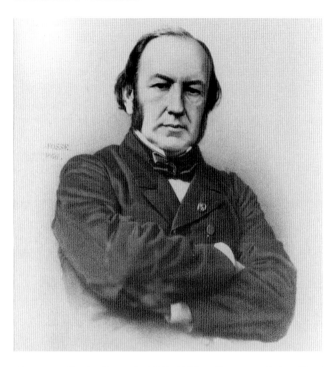

Fig. 49.4 Claude Bernard (1813–1878). (Courtesy of the Wood Library-Museum of Anesthesiology, Park Ridge, IL.)

who had worked with Claude Bernard, recognized that atropine prevented chloroform-induced vagal slowing of the heart [1]. In 1878 he described the use of atropine in his animal experiments, conducted under morphine narcosis and a small dose of chloroform [18]. Dastre could not interest Paris surgeons in his method but Aubert, a surgeon from Lyons, embraced Dastre's suggestions and described giving atropine 0.5 mg with morphine 10 mg to his patients 20 to 30 minutes before chloroform anesthesia [19]. He viewed its advantages as safety, rapid induction, quietness of the patient and reduced postoperative sickness.

In 1880, E.A Schäfer wrote that

> "It is well known that atropin paralyses the cardiac inhibitory apparatus, and since it is probable that death in these (chloroform anesthesia) cases results from a stimulation of this apparatus…there undoubtedly seems good reason for the employment of atropin. But clearly, it should be given immediately before the administration of the chloroform, as a preventive…" [20].

Despite such advocacy, European surgeons were slow to embrace the use of premedication. There was also little enthusiasm in Britain. G Cockburn Smith investigated the action of hyoscine in France. In a letter to the Lancet in 1891, he wrote "…the extreme kindness of the (French) surgeons has enabled me to satisfy myself that the dangers of ether and chloroform can be greatly, if not entirely, removed by the injection of one centigramme of hydrochlorate of morphia and one milligramme of sulphate of atropia some twenty five minutes previously to their administration in adults" [21]. Smith's advice fell on deaf ears.

In 1900, Schneiderlin, of Emmendingen, Germany, introduced the combined injection of morphine and hyoscine prior to anesthesia. He had previously used the combination as a sedative to treat mental patients. He recommended small doses repeated several times, beginning sometimes on the day before operation. However it was the recommendations of Carl Hartog, who in 1903, advised routine administration half to three quarters of an hour before ether, that encouraged the increasing use of premedication in Europe.

In England, Dudley Buxton was the first to promote the use of morphine and hyoscine. In 1909, he wrote

> "…a terrified patient after a sleepless night is in the worst condition for an anaesthetic and an operation. In such patients, I am convinced that the use of scopolamine and morphine injections before a general anaesthetic is valuable" [22].

The first enthusiasm for morphine and scopolamine premedication in the US arose in 1910. Clifford Collins of Peoria, Illinois reported on more than 1000 cases:

> "Tablets are obtained containing a combination of scopolamin, 1/100 grain (0.065 mg), and morphin 1/6 grain (11 mg), and the solution is made just before it is administered hypodermically, which is done one and a half hours before the operation is begun…all necessary manipulations and handling of the patient in the preparation are completed before the hypodermic is administered. The room is darkened and everything is kept quiet, and he falls into a tranquil slumber. About twenty minutes before the operation, a layer of damp cotton is placed over the eyes and the patient is taken to the operating room and placed on the operating table…" [23].

A Sea Change Should Have Resulted from the Use of Intravenous Barbiturates and Less Soluble, Less Pungent Inhaled Anesthetics

In the mid-1930s, Waters' group [24] and Lundy and Tovel [25] reported that thiopental (Pentothal®), a short-acting intravenous anesthetic circumvented the claustrophobia and irritant effects associated with induction of anesthesia with ether. Anesthesia now could be induced quickly ("Count backwards from 100, please") and pleasantly. And in the 1920s and 30s, non-pungent inhaled anesthetics such as ethylene [26] and cyclopropane [27] were introduced into clinical practice. They were wonderful except that they exploded when touched by a spark. Still, just two or three breaths of cyclopropane could induce anesthesia.

Thus, the need for morphine and atropine before anesthesia was much diminished, perhaps gone. However, these discoveries of intravenous and non-pungent inhaled anesthetics did little to alter patterns of use that persisted in spite of diminished pharmacological need. Inertia is indeed a powerful force.

Halogenated Anesthetics and the Need for Routine Morphine Premedication

Fluorinated volatile anesthetics initially appeared in the early 1950s, presenting new pharmacologic characteristics (more potent, more rapid awakening, less airway irritation and fewer associated secretions). This altered the potential need for morphine and atropine. In 1951, RT Stormont, Secretary of the American Medical Association observed [28]:

> "Narcotic drugs are often employed more or less routinely for preanesthetic medication without a full appreciation of their relative value for this purpose. The Council (Council on Pharmacy and Chemistry of the American Medical Association) has authorized publication of the following report with the view of encouraging additional well-controlled and critical studies in this and related fields."

The report referred to by Stormont was: "Narcotics in Preanesthetic Medication" and the authors were Ellis N. Cohen and Henry K. Beecher (Fig. 49.1) [28]. These authors began by observing that the:

> "Use of narcotics to support patients about to undergo anesthesia has a very long history; nevertheless there are adequate reasons for examining this practice objectively. Such an examination begins logically with questions as to the purposes of the practice, its undesirable effects, and whether or not there are better ways to attain the desired results."

Cohen and Beecher observed that in the 1930s, some practitioners found that morphine decreased the quantity of anesthetic needed to achieve a desired level of cyclopropane and ether anesthesia [29, 30], while others reported that morphine contributed little, or not at all, to a reduction of the amount of ether required for a given plane of anesthesia [31, 32]. Given the ubiquitous use of morphine premedication (in 1951), Cohen and Beecher asked whether the basis for such use was valid. Accordingly, they studied 558 hospitalized patients undergoing surgery [28]. Three premedication solutions were given intramuscularly (one injection per patient): 15 mg morphine and 0.6 mg atropine, 90 mg pentobarbital and 0.6 mg atropine, or 0.6 mg atropine. The contents of the solutions were unknown to the floor nurse, patient and anesthesiologist. A preoperative interview was carried out in the operating room and the anesthesiologist recorded his/her view of whether morphine had been used in the premedication.

From the anesthesiologist's perspective the characteristics of induction were similar in all three groups and there was equal satisfaction with all the premedication solutions including atropine alone [28]. Furthermore, 47% of the time the anesthesiologist could not determine if morphine had been administered and there was an equal tendency to confuse the presence of pentobarbital with that of morphine. Moreover, the anesthesiologist mistakenly thought 34% of the atropine group had received morphine. The premedication did not affect venous blood concentrations of ether or cyclopropane during surgical anesthesia (i.e., did not appear to decrease anesthetic requirements).

Cohen and Beecher concluded that pentobarbital premedication was an effective and satisfactory substitute for morphine and was viewed as having fewer hazards. They further observed that their results should not imply that morphine was to be discarded entirely, but rather its use should be restricted to the few patients coming to surgery who were in pain.

This author (RKS) wonders if Cohen and Beecher would have reached the same conclusions if scopolamine rather than atropine had been administered with morphine in their study patients? When a calm and sedated patient is desirable, as before major and sometimes life-threatening surgery, the combination of scopolamine with morphine is highly effective and predictable.

Beecher further expanded his views on premedication in a 1955 editorial, emphasizing the need to reappraise the use of morphine [2]. He challenged traditional medical teaching that morphine produces euphoria in normal patients, citing "unpublished data" that morphine produced euphoria in only 10% of patients and dysphoria in 80%. Beecher argued that pentobarbital was better at producing euphoria. Furthermore, opioids like morphine produce nausea and vomiting while pentobarbital does the opposite [17]. In the editorial, the use of atropine for premedication was endorsed as promoting safety, by reducing airway secretions and blocking troublesome vagal reflexes.

In summary, Beecher concluded that narcotics were useful premedicants for the few patients in pain immediately preceding anesthesia [2]. For the typical patient, the oral use of a hypnotic on the evening before surgery (to promote a good night's sleep), and again early on the morning of surgery, was desirable. According to Beecher, the best premedication consisted of a barbiturate (instead of a narcotic) given intramuscularly along with atropine.

An Alternate View of Premedication in the 1950s

Not everyone agreed with Cohen and Beecher. A 1959 report by John Adriani (Fig. 49.5) and O. Horace Yarberry [33] argued that misconceptions concerning premedication were prevalent, and that it was often ordered empirically and without a rational basis. Their perception of premedication often differed from those of Cohen and Beecher [28], although both groups had the same premedicants in mind. Adriani and Yarberry argued for the use of depressants (narcotics and hypnotics) to provide psychic sedation (anxiolysis) and belladonna alkaloids to suppress secretions:

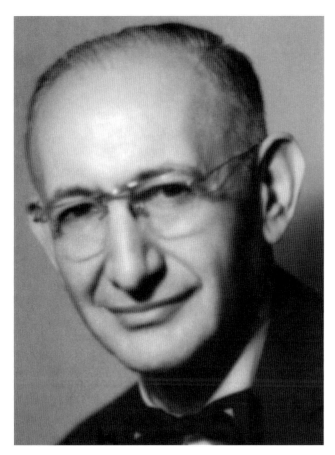

Fig. 49.5 John Adriani (1908–1988). (Courtesy of the Wood Library-Museum of Anesthesiology, Park Ridge, IL.)

"Despite prejudice against narcotics they remain the most effective agents available [2, 28]. Premedication should relieve anxiety. Narcotics produce euphoria and an air of indifference unmatched by other depressant drugs. (and) Barbiturates are largely hypnotic. They do not alter the patient's attitude toward his environment as well as the narcotics." All these views disagreed with those of Cohen and Beecher.

Adriani and Yarberry believed that premedication supplied four important elements: psychic sedation, decreased secretions, decreased requirement for general anesthetics (especially important with less potent anesthetics such as nitrous oxide and ethylene which otherwise might limit oxygen availability), and suppressed vagal and other autonomic reflex activity. They argued for individualizing premedication for a particular patient and anesthetic technique. One of the editors of the present book (EIE) remembers the preanesthetic "rounds" guided by an individual faculty, and the vigorous discussion of what and how much premedication should be given to the patients having anesthesia the next day. "It probably was overkill, but we had great fun!"

Adriani and Yarberry argued both for and against present practices. They agreed with the importance of psychic sedation, choosing narcotics and hypnotics for this purpose and

giving belladonna alkaloids to all patients. On the other hand, they believed that "Obviously, newborns, small infants, the aged, and patients who are anoxic, in shock, or otherwise acutely ill are intolerant to and should not have narcotics or other depressant drugs." Today's anesthetist might have a more sanguine view. Adriani and Yarberry believed that "Scopolamine enhances the effects of narcotics and hypnotics and produces amnesia. (It clearly does produce amnesia, but enhancement of narcotics is questionable.) Also, it has superior drying effects and causes less increase in pulse rate. Atropine accelerates the pulse." [This author (RKS), again notes that Cohen and Beecher did not consider this perceived advantage of scopolamine, in evaluating only atropine] [28].

Scopolamine use can come with a price. EIE remembers that in his residency (1956–8)

"Someone from the Department of Pharmacology at the University of Iowa called the anesthesia attending in the operating room and said they'd made a mistake. They'd intended to give medical students 0.1 mg scopolamine to illustrate its drying effect but they slipped a decimal point and gave 1.0 mg, and now they had a lot of loony students and could the Department of Anesthesia help, please? I think the students stayed in the recovery room for several hours. They all returned to sanity, and I believe all got A's in their pharmacology course."

Adriani and Yarberry concluded that premedication was part of the anesthetic [33]. The desired goal of premedication was tranquility and amnesia without loss of consciousness. They argued that narcotics combined with belladonna alkaloids constituted the most reliable agents for premedication. They contradicted the conclusions of Cohen and Beecher [28].

In Great Britain and many other non-US countries, the common premedication narcotic at mid-century was papaveretum, marketed as Omnopon or Pantopon. Papaveretum is a mixture of alkaloids, but is primarily morphine with small amounts of papaverine and codeine. It was usually given in combination with scopolamine in a mixture commonly known as "Om and Scop".

A Personal Anecdote from the 1950s

Premedication comes in many flavors. One unusual flavor may be the technique described to RKS by an anesthesiologist and close friend (VK Stoelting) for managing patients considered to be at risk of thyroid storm (a dangerous condition that produces hyperactivity) on induction of anesthesia. It was thought that patient apprehension engendered the storm. Such patients would be admitted to the hospital several days before the scheduled surgery. Every morning a nurse would administer a saline enema, and the patient ultimately accepted this as routine. On the morning of the scheduled surgery (schedule not known to the patient), the nurse administered an anesthetic (Avertin®) rather than saline in the enema and the patient "was delivered to the operating room" deeply sedated and at a lowered risk of thyroid storm. This was known as "stealing the patient to the operating room."

Rectal Premedication

In 1913, James Gwathmey proposed premedication with rectal chloretone or paraldehyde in olive oil, followed 30 minutes later by an injection of morphine and atropine. Chloretone is a combination of chloroform and acetone.

Avertin was developed in the late 1920s and was used as a rectal premedication or anesthetic as indicated by the above anecdote, particularly in Europe. The rapid-acting barbiturates introduced in the 1930s could also be given rectally to produce sedation, and partially displaced this use of Avertin. However, Avertin continued to be used, especially in Germany, as a background narcotic, amnesic and antiemetic. The introduction of midazolam for anesthetic purposes late in the 1970s, extended to premedication via the rectal route, an approach popular in children in many countries, especially in Scandinavia and the US.

Pre-anesthetic Visits Recognized as Premedication in the 1960s and 1970s

Up to the 1960s and 1970s, anesthesiologists prepared their patients emotionally for anesthesia and surgery with various combinations of narcotics and hypnotics. Egbert et al. evaluated the psychological effects of the preoperative visit by the anesthesiologist versus pentobarbital for premedication [34]. Patients receiving pentobarbital 1 hour before an operation became drowsy, but it could not be shown that they became calm. Patients having a preoperative visit by an anesthesiologist who informed them about the events that were to take place and the type of anesthetic to be administered, were not drowsy but were more likely to be calm preoperatively. Eckenhoff and Helrich observed that "the anesthetist should never underestimate the value of the pre-anesthetic visit" [35].

Leigh et al. further supported the value of the preoperative visit. They measured anxiety levels in patients who received preoperative reassurance from a member of the hospital staff versus a control group given no such support [36]. The group given preoperative reassurance had lower anxiety levels than those not receiving reassurance either from a member of staff or from an information booklet.

The increasing frequency of outpatient surgery and admission to hospital on the day of elective surgery, has limited the opportunity for anesthesia professionals to visit with the patient preoperatively. It is no longer possible to predictably make use of the calming value of the preoperative visit.

Today's anesthesia professional may first meet the patient a few minutes before the scheduled surgery, and premedication, if any, is pharmacologic rather than psychological.

Fluorinated Anesthetics and Barbiturates Decrease the Need for Routine Atropine and Other Premedication

As halothane in the 1960s (later supplanted by enflurane in the 1970s, and isoflurane in the 1980s) complemented by thiopental for induction of anesthesia replaced chloroform, ether and cyclopropane, the routine use of premedication with atropine waned. Several investigations challenged its use, suggesting that undesirable effects outweighed potential benefits [37–39]. In a double-blind investigation in 250 adult males 0.6 mg atropine did not alter the incidence of traction reflexes (slow heart rate and low blood pressure), bradycardia (slow heart rate), or cardiac dysrhythmias compared with patients not receiving atropine [38]. Although secretions were decreased, eliminating ether from practice removed the need for atropine, at least for a time. The development of the pungent anesthetic desflurane might suggest otherwise. Still, premedication with atropine is rare today.

In 1977, Forrest et al. [40] characterized preoperative medication as a combination of two or more drugs from different pharmacologic groups (sedative, tranquilizer, analgesic, vagolytic) with a variety of combinations prescribed for patients facing essentially the same type of operation. The variety suggested an absence of agreement about indications for premedication. Another reason for the variety was that clinical investigations of drug efficacies lacked both definition and persuasiveness, despite the use of objective measures or because of the use of subjective responses [40]. To overcome these limitations, Forrest et al. [40] designed a controlled, double-blind study of six commonly used premedicants, evaluating their effects on sleepiness, apprehension, restlessness and confusion, and determined the incidence of side effects. The medications were barbiturates (pentobarbital, secobarbital), diazepam, hydroxyzine, and opioids (morphine and meperidine) administered at different doses and compared to a placebo.

The results were surprising. All the drugs except diazepam increased patients' subjective ratings of sleepiness. None significantly affected patient reports of apprehension compared with placebo. These results conflicted with clinical impressions and with other reports that these drugs decreased preoperative anxiety (e.g., see Eger and Keasling) [41]. Anesthesiologists rated all treatments, including placebo, as satisfactory for ease of induction of anesthesia. This probably reflected the use of potent intravenous induction drugs which obviated the need for the assistance of premedication in the induction process. The only frequently observed side

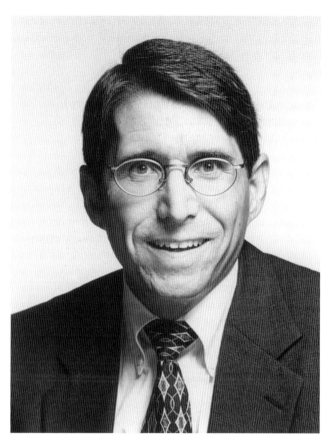

Fig. 49.6 Paul White. (Courtesy of the Wood Library-Museum of Anesthesiology, Park Ridge, IL.)

effects found with all six drugs *and the placebo group* were dry mouth and slurred speech [40, 42].

Pharmacologic and Clinical Goals of Premedication in the Present Era

In 1986, Paul White (Fig. 49.6) reviewed the pharmacologic and clinical goals of premedication [42]. He observed that the rationale for preoperative medication arose during the days of ether and cyclopropane anesthesia. To minimize side effects of induction of anesthesia by inhalation of these anesthetics (i.e., without induction of anesthesia with barbiturates), anesthesiologists brought patients heavily sedated and with a dry mouth to the operating room. Inertia and conservatism perpetuated the choice of drugs to the 1980s, often continuing the use of a sedative-hypnotics, opioids, tranquilizer, and/or belladonna drugs. As noted above, there was no general agreement about the indications for premedication although it was generally agreed that patient apprehension was a major factor that should be controlled in the preoperative period.

White argued that the rational use of drugs for premedication allowed the patient to enter the operating room with minimal apprehension, sedated but easily aroused and co-

operative without uncomfortable side effects. From the patient's point of view, lack of recall and relief of anxiety were the primary objectives of premedication. White saw additional new goals: to decrease gastric fluid pH and volume (histamine H_2-receptor antagonists, antacids, gastrokinetics), and to prevent postoperative emesis. Further, he saw that premedication for outpatients might differ from premedication for patients having operations in the traditional hospital setting. White's views might contrast with those of others who prefer to limit sedation in order to accomplish a more rapid and complete early recovery from anesthesia. There are no unmixed blessings!

White's review antedated the use of propofol, the intravenous drug now used for induction, and sometimes maintenance, of anesthesia in most adult patients. Propofol is an antiemetic, considerably decreasing patients' tendency to nausea and vomiting. Propofol has an added benefit—its effects are more short-lived than those of any other intravenous induction agent.

The now prevalent use of the anxiolytic drug midazolam also provides antiemesis as an additional benefit. Currently, it is sometimes the sole premedication used. It belongs to a class of drugs called benzodiazepines, a class that also includes diazepam (Valium®). But again, nothing is for free; benzodiazepine premedication may increase the incidence of postoperative agitation (Fig. 49.7) [43].

Although not traditional premedication, other drugs are often administered at the time of premedication. For example, oral medications that the patient may be taking for control of medical diseases (antihypertensives, antidysrhythmics, antidepressants, statins, steroids etc.) may be administered with up to 150 ml of water in the hour preceding induction of anesthesia [44]. For insulin-dependent diabetics, it is common to administer insulin in the perioperative period. For patients with known or suspected coronary artery disease, preoperative beta-blockers may be added to the premedication. Protection is probably the result of a drug class effect or hemodynamic effect rather than use of a specific beta blocker. Like beta-blockers, statins have been recommended preoperatively in patients with cardiovascular disease [45]. Prophylactic antibiotics are often administered immediately before induction of anesthesia. And anticoagulents may be given prior to anesthesia to reduce the likelihood of postoperative deep venous thrombosis. Administration of such drugs broadens our notion of what constitutes premedication [43].

Reprise

Preanesthetic medication, the giving of drugs before anesthesia, evolved from trial and error in the days of ether and chloroform to a somewhat amorphous present state that invokes both "art and science" [46]. Newer anesthetics, inhaled

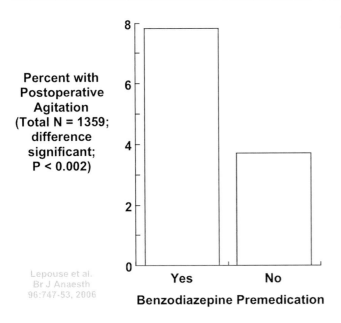

Fig. 49.7 Premedication with benzodiazepines may increase postoperative agitation.
(From Lepouse C, Lautner CA, Liu L, Gomis P, Leon A: Emergence delirium in adults in the post-anaesthesia care unit. Br J Anaesth 2006; 96: 747–53, with permission.)

and intravenous, influenced the choice of premedication. A further modifying choice was the mid-twentieth century recognition of the importance of the pre-anesthesia visit by the anesthetist. Prompting still further change, was the evolution of outpatient anesthesia and the discovery of newer premedicants such as midazolam.

Initially, premedication didn't exist other than as the occasional oral administration of a dollop of alcohol or a bit of opium/morphine. With time, the properties of ether and chloroform prompted administration of various premedications. Atropine or scopolamine were used to decrease the secretions induced by ether. Morphine was used to decrease the perception of pungency and accelerate induction. Morphine also hastened recovery, because less ether and chloroform were required. Things might have—but didn't—change with the 1920s-1930s introduction of non-pungent anesthetics and especially intravenous inductions of anesthesia with barbiturates. Inertia supported the continued use of a belladonna-morphine-hypnotic triumvirate. This support eroded with the addition of modern (fluorinated) inhaled anesthetics, most notably halothane, to the smooth induction provided by thiopental. The need for atropine disappeared. Outpatient anesthesia arose in the 1970s and 1980s, imposing realities of economic and time constraints limiting the ability of the anesthesia professional to provide psychological preparation or administer of drugs more than a few minutes before the scheduled surgery. We've come nearly full circle from the initial days of anesthesia with no premedication, through a period of considerable premedication to a present time of perhaps a single drug to allay apprehension.

References

1. Shearer WM. The evolution of premedication. Br J Anaesth. 1960;32:554.
2. Beecher HK. Preanesthetic medication; guest editorial. J Am Med Assoc. 1955;157:242–3.
3. Wedel GW. Opiologia ad mentem academiae naturae curiosorum. Jena 1682.
4. Pravaz C. Sur un Nouveau d'operer la Coagulation du Sangue dans Aerteres, Applicable a la Guerison des Aneurismes. Compt Rend Acad Sci. Paris. 1853;36:88–91.
5. Macht DI. The history of opium and some of its preparations and alkaloids. JAMA. 1915;64:477–81.
6. Smith RR. Scopolamine—morphine anesthesia with report of two hundred and twenty-nine cases. Surg Gyn Obs. 1908;7:414 (abstract)
7. Saidman LJ, Eger EI II. Effect of nitrous oxide and of narcotic premedication on the alveolar concentration of halothane required for anesthesia. Anesthesiology. 1964;25:302–6.
8. Kong CF, Chew STH. Ip-Yam PC: intravenous opioids reduce airway irritation during induction of anaesthesia with desflurane in adults. Br J Anaesth. 2000;85:364–7.
9. Uterhart CES. Mittheilungen aus der chirurgischen Klinik des Rostocker Krakenhauses (Communication from the Surgical Clinic of the Rostock Hospital). Berliner Klinische Wochenschrift. 1868;32:329–30.
10. Clover JT. Br Med J 1874;1:202.
11. Lyman HM. Artificial anaesthesia and anaesthetics. New York: William Wood & Company; 1881. p. 20.
12. Bruno L. In: Dogliotti AM, editor. Anesthesia: narcosis, local, regional, spinal (translated by CS Scuderi). Chicago: S.B. Debour Co; 1939. p. 20.
13. Bernard C. Des effects physiologiques de la morphine et de leur combinaison avec ceux du chloroforme. Bull Gen de Therap. 1869;77:241.
14. Labbe I, Guyon E. Medical Times (London). 1872;1:350.
15. Demarquay. Medical Times (London). 1872;1:334
16. Duncum BM. 'Mixed Anaesthesia' and premedication. Chapter XIII. In: The development of inhalation anaesthesia with special reference to the years 1846–1900. London: Oxford University Press; 1947. pp. 375–404
17. Eger EI II, Kraft ID, Keasling HH. A comparison of atropine, or scopolamine, plus pentobarbital, meperidine, or morphine as pediatric preanesthetic medication. Anesthesiology. 1961;22:962–9.
18. Dastre. Comptes Rendus Acad Sci. Paris. 1878;86:1303.
19. Aubert. Comptes Rendus Soc Biol. Paris. 1883;5:242.
20. Schäfer EA. Letter to the Editor. Br Med J. 1880;II:620.
21. Smith GC. Letter to the editor. Lancet. 1891;II:843.
22. Buxton D. Proc Roy Soc Med. 1908–9;2(i)(Sect Anaesth):60.
23. Collins C. JAMA. 1910;54:1051.
24. Pratt T, Tatum A, Hathaway H, Waters R. Sodium ethyl (1-methyl butyl) thiobarbiturate. Am J Surg. 1936;31:464–6.
25. Lundy J, Tovell R. Some of the newer local and general anesthetic agents. Methods of their administration. Northwest Med (Seattle). 1934;33:308–11.
26. Luckhardt AB, Carter JB. Ethylene as a gas anesthetic: preliminary communication. Clinical experience in 106 surgical operations. JAMA. 1923;80:1440–3.
27. Stiles J, Neff W, Rovenstine E, Waters R. Cyclopropane as an anesthetic agent: a preliminary report. Anesth Analg. 1934;13:56–60.
28. Cohen EN, Beecher HK. Narcotics in preanesthetic medication; a controlled study. J Am Med Assoc. 1951;147:1664–8.
29. Robbins BH, Baxter JH, Fitzhugh GG. The effects of morphine, barbital and amytal upon the concentration of cyclopropane in the blood required for anesthesia and respiratory arrest. J Pharmacol Exp Ther. 1939;65:136.

30. Seevers MH, Meek WJ, Rovenstine E, Stiles JA. A study of cyclo-propane anesthesia with especial reference to gas concentrations, respiratory and electrocardiographic changes. J Pharmacol Exp Ther. 1934;51:1.

31. Calderone FA. Studies on ether dosage after preanesthetic medication with narcotics (barbiturates, magnesium sulfate and morphine). J Pharmacol Exp Ther. 1935;55:24.

32. Potter R, Livingstone H, Andrews E, Light G. Blood ether levels in surgical anesthesia. Surgery. 1941;10:757.

33. Adriani J, Yarberry OH Jr. Preanesthetic medication; old and new concepts. Arch Surg. 1959;79:976–80.

34. Egbert LD, Battit G, Turndorf H, Beecher HK. The value of the pre-operative visit by an anesthetist. A study of doctor-patient rapport. JAMA. 1963;185:553–5.

35. Eckenhoff JE, Helrich M. Study of narcotics and sedatives for use in preanesthetic medication. J Am Med Assoc. 1958;167:415–22.

36. Leigh JM, Walker J, Janaganathan P. Effect of preoperative anaes-thetic visit on anxiety. Br Med J. 1977;2:987–9.

37. Holt AT. Premedication with atropine should not be routine. Lancet. 1962;2:984–5.

38. Middleton MJ, Zitzer JM, Urbach KF. Is atropine always necessary before general anesthesia? Anesth Analg. 1967;46:51–5.

39. Falick YS, Smiler BG. Is anticholinergic premedication necessary? Anesthesiology. 1975;43:472–3.

40. Forrest WH Jr, Brown CR. Brown BW. Subjective responses to six common preoperative medications. Anesthesiology. 1977;47:241–7.

41. Eger EI II, Keasling HH. Comparison of meprobamate, pentobar-bital, and placebo as preanesthetic medication for regional proce-dures. Anesthesiology. 1959;20:1–9.

42. White PF. Pharmacologic and clinical aspects of preoperative medi-cation. Anesth Analg. 1986;65:963–74.

43. Lepouse C, Lautner CA, Liu L, Gomis P, Leon A. emergence delirium in adults in the post-anaesthesia care unit. Br J Anaesth. 2006;96:747–53.

44. Soreide E, Holst-Larsen H, Reite K, Mikkelsen H, Soreide JA, Steen PA. Effects of giving water 20–450 ml with oral diazepam premedi-cation 1–2 h before operation. Br J Anaesth. 1993;71:503–6.

45. Huffmyer JL, Mauermann WJ, Thiele RH, Ma JZ, Nemergut EC. Preoperative statin administration is associated with lower mortal-ity and decreased need for postoperative hemodialysis in patients undergoing coronary artery bypass graft surgery. J Cardiothorac Vasc Anesth. 2009;23:468–73.

46. Dotson R, Wiener-Kronish JP, Ajayi T. Preoperative evaluation and medication. In: Stoelting RK, Miller RD, editors. Basics of anesthe-sia. Philadelphia: Churchill Livingstone/Elsevier. 2007. p. 157.

A History of Neuromuscular Block and Its Antagonism

50

James E. Caldwell

Summary

Fifteenth century South American explorers knew of the arrowhead poison "ourari" or curare. The eighteenth century physician Bancroft brought samples of crude curare from South America, and in 1808 Brodie showed that it was safe if ventilation continued artificially. In 1846, Bernard demonstrated that curare acted where the nerve impulse reached the muscle, the neuromuscular junction.

In 1912, surgeon Lawen used curare for tracheal intubation and surgical procedures. The idea did not catch on! In the 1930s, Gill brought curare from South America to the US. With Squibb chemists, pharmacologist McIntyre purified the crude extract as Intocostrin, which Holaday assayed for potency with the rabbit head drop test. By standardizing the concentration, this allowed "Intocostrin's" study. In 1939, psychiatrist Bennet reported that Intocostrin prevented compression fractures from convulsive therapy. Cullen then tried Intocostrin in dogs, but because it seemed to cause bronchspasm said it had "*no place in anesthesia.*"

In 1942, anesthesiologists Griffith and Johnson safely gave Intocostrin to 25 patients anesthetized with cyclopropane. In 1946, several investigators given curare noted that it did not decrease consciousness. In 1954, Beecher and Todd reported "curare" deaths, and it was soon appreciated that curare's safe use required control of ventilation and neostigmine to antagonize residual effects.

Succinylcholine was introduced in 1951, after Bovet observed its paralyzing action. Bowman developed the long-acting and cardiovascularly active aminosteroid relaxant pancuronium in the 1960s. Savage designed a relaxant to supplant pancuronium, leading to the 1980s release of vecuronium. Payne and Hughes then described atracurium, whose chemical breakdown via Hofmann elimination could terminate its action. In 1988, Savarese described the short acting mivacurium, but slow onset ensured a limited commercial life. Rocuronium, a nondepolarizing drug with a faster onset and lack of adverse effects, was released in the 1990s. Cisatracurium was released in the 1990s. It had fewer side-effects than atracurium. In 1999, the fast onset rapacuronium was released but was soon withdrawn because it caused bronchospasm in children.

The need for clinical monitoring of neuromuscular blockade led Ali, Utting, and Gray to develop the train-of-four ratio test in the 1970s. In the late 1970s and the 1980s, Miller, Benet, and Sheiner invented concepts explaining the interaction of relaxant pharmacokinetics and pharmacodynamics.

In 2001, Bom described sugammadex, a drug with a ring structure that inactivated rocuronium by capturing every rocuronium molecule, thereby quickly and completely reversing blockade. In 2004, Savarese and his group described relaxants rapidly inactivated by endogenous or exogenous cysteine.

The First Few Centuries: 1495–1900

It took 450 years from European observations of curare poisoning to the introduction in 1942 of a purified extract of curare into anesthesia practice. In subsequent years, more than 30 different muscle relaxants (we will use "muscle relaxants" or just "relaxants" in place of the more correct "neuromuscular blocking drugs") were tried in clinical practice (Table 50.1)

[1]. Most failed to achieve widespread use, and successful relaxants often fell into disuse, superseded by superior drugs. This essay traces the path that took these compounds from "poisons" to mainstays of modern anesthesia practice.

In the Beginning

"*The natives poisoned their arrows with the juice of a death-dealing herb. In a twinkling the forty-seven Spaniards were pierced with arrow-wounds, before they could protect themselves with their shields. There was but one man who survived, all the rest perishing from the effects of the poison.*"

J. E. Caldwell (✉)
Department of Anesthesia and Perioperative Medicine,
University of California, 521 Parnassus Avenue, San Francisco,
CA 94143-0648, USA
e-mail: jimnche@gmail.com

E. I Eger II et al. (eds.), *The Wondrous Story of Anesthesia*, DOI 10.1007/978-1-4614-8441-7_50, © Edmond I Eger, MD 2014

Table 50.1 Relaxant and reversal drugs used clinically at some time

Relaxants			Reversal Drugs
Alcuronium	Diadonium	*PANCURONIUM*	*NEOSTIGMINE*
Amidonium	Dipyrandium	Pipecuronium	Edrophonium
Anatruxonium	Duador	Quilidium	Pyridostigmine
ATRACURIUM	Fazadinium	Rapacuronium	Galanthamine
Benzoquinonium	Laudexium	*ROCURONIUM*	4-aminopyridine
C-Toxiferin	Maluetin	Stercuronium	3:4-diaminopyridine
CISATRACURIUM	Metocurine	*SUCCINYLCHOLINE*	*SUGAMMADEX*
Cycobutonium	*MIVACURIUM*	Tercuronium	
Dacuronium	Myanesin	Toxiferine	
Decadonium	Mytolon	Tubocurarine	
Decamethonium	N-methyl Tubocurarine	*VECURONIUM*	
Doxacurium	Nubitanium		

Drugs in capitalized italics are in current use

Thus was the existence of a paralyzing drug revealed to Europeans by Pieter Martyr D'Anghere in his fifteenth century treatise De Orbe Novo. Rather than traveling with the conquistadores like embedded modern day correspondents, D'Anghere simply interviewed those returning from the "New World." A century later, in 1594, Sir Walter Raleigh returned from an incursion into now Venezuela and described a tribe he encountered, the Aroras, as *"people who used strong poison in their arrows."* Lawrence Keynes, one of Raleigh's lieutenants, named this strong poison "ourari", literally the "bird-killer." One can imagine the transliteration of ourari into curare.

Two plant groups, Chondodendron Tomentosum and Strychnos Toxifera supplied the poison. The ritual preparation of the poison took several days. An apocryphal story has it that some tribes sequestered old women with the necessary knowledge and skills throughout the process of manufacture. The resulting condition of the women defined the potency of the tarry substance produced. If they still stood and appeared relatively healthy, the batch was deemed insufficiently potent and discarded. In contrast, if the women were weak, unable to stand, the poison was deemed acceptable. Given these working conditions, it is surprising that any of these women lived to become old and experienced. Having passed this first potency test, a frog was pricked with the poison, and the number of leaps the frog then made, before expiring, quantified the potency. The laborious process, and the limited availability of old women, made the toxin valuable. Its use was commonly restricted to hunting and not warfare.

Although von Humboldt in one place in his book partially confirms the above apocryphal story in which old women made and were the test subjects for establishment of potency of the curare preparation, in another place he denies that such testing could be possible [2]. Charles Waterton adds to the latter view, stating that women and young girls were excluded from the preparation of the curare concentrate [2].

Given the highly ionized nature of curare and other muscle relaxants, it is difficult to imagine how curare could be vaporized. If this is correct, then inhalation of curare in the vapors made in the process of purification seems unlikely.

Over the next four centuries, more reports and crucial observations were made. The poison was not toxic if ingested, inhaled, or applied directly to or injected into a nerve [3]. Also, after poisoning with curare, the heart continued to beat, and artificial respiration saved the animal from death [4, 5].

Eighteenth and Nineteenth Centuries: Early Scientific Investigations

Explorers Discover and Bring Back Curare

Explorer-scientists, including Charles-Marie De La Condamine, Edwin Bancroft, and Charles Waterton, travelled extensively in different areas of South America. They provided the raw material to European pharmacologists and physiologists who undertook the initial studies of curare. These hardy explorers often put themselves at personal risk; the Amazonian forest was an inhospitable place, and working with the raw material was dangerous. The French scientist FD Herissant describes how he and his assistant became weak and almost unconscious while boiling the crude curare extract in order to create a concentrated mixture. *"A pint of good wine and sugar"* cured both investigators.

The eighteenth century physician, Edwin Bancroft, brought back samples of crude curare from South America for study. He was the first to thoroughly report the diverse tribal methods of preparation and storage of the curare. The natives used a variety of vessels for storage of the curare preparation: a clay pot (pot curare), a calabash gourd (calabash curare), or a hollow piece of bamboo (tube curare, hence "tubocurare"). His son, Edward Bancroft provided samples to the English surgeon, Benjamin Brodie, who made the crucial observation that animals poisoned with curare could be kept alive by inflating their lungs [5]. Brodie also suggested treatment of tetanus with curare [6].

1814

No early explorer was more colorful than Charles Waterton, an English nobleman who managed his family's estates in South America. His exploits included scaling the dome of St. Peter's Cathedral in Rome, much to the displeasure of the Pope. While in Guiana, he showed that curare was effective in many species, including large animals. He witnessed Brodie and William Sewell's famous 1814 public demonstration of the effect of curare on a donkey.

> "*A she ass received the wourali poison in the shoulder and died in apparently 10 minutes. An incision was made in its windpipe, and through it the lungs were regularly inflated for two hours with a pair of bellows. Suspended animation returned. The ass held up her head and looked around.*"

The ass "now named Wouralia" was put out to graze at Walton Hall, on the estate of Earl Percy, who stated, "*No burden shall be placed on her and she shall end her days in peace.*" Wouralia lived on in this happy state for almost 25 more years [7].

1838

Twenty years after the "Wouralia" demonstration, Sewell, a veterinary surgeon, used curare to treat two horses with tetanus. Both animals died. Despite this failure, curare was later used in humans to treat disorders involving spasticity. None proved successful.

1846

In 1846, the French polymath Claude Bernard (1813–1878) discovered the site of action of curare (Fig. 50.1) [8]. In curarized (paralyzed) frogs, he noted that electrical impulses still passed down the motor nerves [8], and that electrical impulses applied directly to the muscle caused contraction. He concluded that curare acted where the nerve impulse reached the muscle, the neuromuscular junction. It was not until the 1930s that Henry Dale and others showed that acetylcholine released from the motor nerve terminal effected neuromuscular transmission, and curare acted by blocking acetylcholine receptors.

1858

The surgeon Lewis Sayre, and his house officer FA Burrell, at Bellevue Hospital New York, took up Brodie's suggestion that curare might be used to treat tetanus. In a patient with tetanus, the standard treatments of brandy, beef tea, (by both

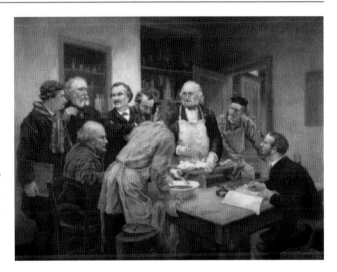

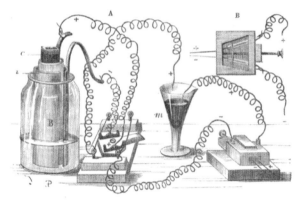

Fig. 50.1 Claude Bernard in his laboratory. The drawing shows the equipment he used to demonstrate the site of action of curare at the neuromuscular junction. (Courtesy of Wellcome Images UK.)

mouth and per rectum) had failed. Four applications of a dilute solution of the "*woorari*" poison were applied directly onto the hand wound through which the original infection occurred. The patient died during a severe spasm shortly thereafter [9]. Despite such setbacks, the search for a therapeutic use of curare in spastic conditions such as chorea, rabies, epilepsy and strychnine poisoning continued. But curare extract sufficient to decrease spasticity inevitably produced fatal respiratory failure.

1860s

The Edinburgh scientists Thomas Fraser and Alexander Brown made the next breakthrough demonstrating that conversion of alkaloids with tertiary (three atom) nitrogen groups (e.g., atropine or morphine) to a quaternary (four atom) form produced compounds with curare-like activity [10]. This first demonstration of a structure-activity relationship in medicine was fundamental to drug development a century later.

Fig. 50.2 Two scientists at either end of the Hofmann elimination story. August Hofmann (*left*) described the reaction that bears his name, in 1907 (photograph from fineartamerica.com). John Stenlake (*right*) used the reaction described by Hofmann in the development of atracurium more than 70 years later (1981). (Image of August Hoffman is courtesy of Wellcome Images UK.)

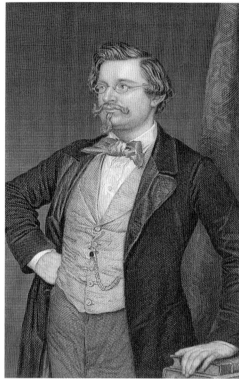 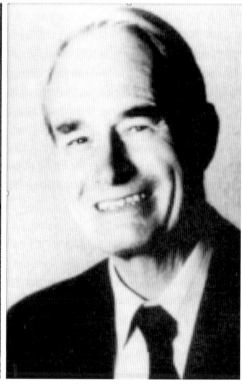

1900–1940: Some False Starts

First Medical Trials with Curare

Despite poor therapeutic experiences, many considered using the curare "poison" for medical purposes, but its inherent dangers made it unsuitable as a drug for *trial and error* experimentation. Nonetheless, we were getting nearer to the discovery of the beneficial uses of curare.

1906

In 1906, the chemist August von Hofmann synthesized quaternary amines (Fig. 50.2). Muscle relaxants have this structure [11]. He also described the capacity of increased pH and temperature to break down a quaternary amine to a tertiary amine, the eponymous Hofmann reaction. More than seventy years later, John Stenlake (Fig. 50.2) at the University of Strathclyde in Glasgow made use of this reaction in the design of the then revolutionary drug, atracurium [12].

Also in 1906, the pharmacologists R Hunt and R Taveau synthesized succinylcholine and studied it in animals [13]. However, their anesthetized animals had already been paralyzed with curare, and thus they did not observe succinylcholine's neuromuscular effects. They did observe that it slowed the heart but otherwise thought it an uninteresting drug. In 1941, D Glick noted that cholinesterase metabolized succinylcholine, but again missed succinylcholine's neuromuscular blocking properties [14].

1912

Arthur Lawen (a colleague of the more famous Trendelenberg), a surgeon in Leipzig, used curare to "soften" the abdominal muscles to facilitate wound closure. He even practiced tracheal intubation and controlled ventilation. However, supplies of curare were unreliable and its potency variable so he abandoned the practice [15]. Some anesthesiologists might find it hard to accept that the first physician to use curare in the operating room was a surgeon.

1928

Francis de Caux, an anesthetist at the North Middlesex Hospital in London, gave curare to patients [16]. Supplies and purity were variable, and he treated only 7 patients:

> "When I used Curare in 1928 I used a watery extract of crude curare made by the North Middlesex Hospital Dispensary. It was because there was no method of standardization that we dropped the method because of the inconsistent results obtained—I wrote to two firms Hoffman la Roche and Zimmermans, I believe, who were not very helpful."

He did not publish his results, and 14 years passed before Griffith and Johnson repeated his experiment in Montreal.

1930s

The use of curare was refined by trial and error until it could be applied safely, but not successfully, in patients with tetanus and other spastic disorders. Interestingly, a group of pathologists (no doubt familiar with the consequences of the failed treatments of tetanus) led by Howard Florey suggested the

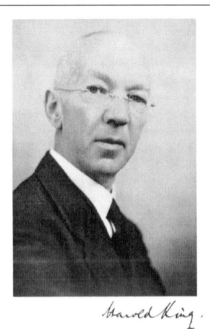

Fig. 50.3 Harold King was the first to isolate and describe the structure of curare. He actually made a minor error and described the group circled as quaternary when in fact it is a protonated tertiary group. This misled scientists for the next three decades to incorrectly think that drugs that had a tertiary group at this site would not be relaxants

Nitrogen group originally described as quaternary by King in 1935. In fact, *in vivo*, it is a protonated tertiary group.

humane treatment of patients with tetanus by a combination of general anesthesia, paralysis with curare, and artificial ventilation with an iron lung. Although they never tried it, they had predicted what would become standard ICU practice [17].

1935

In 1935, Harold King (1887–1956) extracted tubocurarine from a crude preparation of unknown origin. From the information he gathered, he published an erroneous chemical structure of tubocurarine (Fig. 50.3) [18]. King proposed that curare had quaternary nitrogen groups at each end of the molecule (i.e. it was *bis*quaternary). This notion underlay the subsequent development of new muscle relaxants [18]. Discovery of this error in 1970 facilitated development of a new generation of monoquaternary relaxants, the prototype being vecuronium. Although in 1935, large-scale production of tubocurarine was not possible, there followed a string of fortunate circumstances, leading to the first public demonstration of curare in humans.

1938

Richard Gill solved the problem of inadequate supplies of crude curare. In the course of South American travels, Gill learned how to make crude curare, becoming an honorary witch doctor in the process. When he developed multiple sclerosis he saw the potential for a cure in curare. He brought substantial supplies of curare extract back from Ecuador but the firm Merck that had agreed to process his samples changed their mind and instead pursued investigations into a different plant alkaloid, "erythroidine".

Gill then offered his supplies to various investigators, including AR McIntyre, Chair of Pharmacology at the University of Nebraska. McIntyre had a research grant from the

pharmaceutical company Squibb, and they collaborated to purify the crude extract. A Squibb chemist, Horace Holaday, devised the rabbit head drop test (the name describes the test) to assay the potency of the purified drug [19]. Aliquots of the Intocostrin were administered to the rabbit until the neck muscles no longer kept the head up. Purifying the curare and defining its potency opened the door to therapeutic success.

Success at Last

The psychiatrist Abram Bennet was a colleague of Michael Burman, an orthopedic surgeon who had reported his use of curare in childhood spasticity. Bennet saw a potential for the use of curare to minimize the traumatic consequences of convulsive shock therapy [2, 20]. Metrazol-induced convulsions produced a 40–50% incidence of compressive spinal fractures. As reported by Bennet, curare prevented these fractures [20], Such results showed the effectiveness of curare, and probably preserved the practice of convulsive therapy.

The 1940s: It All Comes Together

Because de Caux had not pubished his results, the work had gone unnoticed, and curare was not used in anesthetic practice. Serendipity triggered a change. In 1940, Bennett showed a film of his use of curare to the 91st annual session of the New Jersey Academy of Science. Present was Lewis Wright, Medical Advisor to the pharmaceutical company Squibb. Wright thought curare might be useful in anesthesia. He obtained a preparation of curare, Intocostrin, and donated some to EA Rovenstine at New York University.

Rovenstine instructed his resident EM Papper to try Intocostrin in two patients. Both patients became apneic, and Papper had to manually ventilate their lungs overnight. Stuart Cullen at the University of Iowa, also received Intocostrin, used it in dogs, and pronounced "*Intocostrin has no place in anesthesia*" because the dogs developed bronchospasm. Things did not look good for curare, but this then changed dramatically.

1942   Griffith and Johnson: The Report That Changed Everything

In 1942, a modest paper, brief and to the point, altered forever the practice of anesthesia [21]. With little fanfare, no IRB approval, no oversight, and no previous experience, Harold Griffith and Enid Johnson at the Homeopathic Hospital of Montreal administered Intocostrin to 25 patients anesthetized with cyclopropane. All patients breathed spontaneously throughout surgery, none had their tracheas intubated, and some were challenging (e.g., a 112 kg patient for hemorrhoidectomy and an "*...extremely obese woman...*" for dilatation and curettage.) Griffith opined: "*we have been so much impressed by the dramatic effect produced in every one of our patients that we believe this investigation should be continued.*" It is tempting to speculate on what might have followed had any of these patients died from what Beecher might have labeled a "curare death" (see below).

In 1943, two chemists at Squibb purified d-tubocurarine from the bark of Chondodendron Tomentosum. King had extracted the same compound in 1935 but had not known the source of his preparation. The purified d-tubocurarine had 6 times the potency of Intocostrin, and soon replaced it.

1946
In Great Britain, TC Gray and J Halton published an enthusiastic report of the use of both Intocostrin and the purified d-tubocurarine [22]. In 1946 and for sometime thereafter, most patients given curare breathed spontaneously, often without tracheal intubation. It required great skill and vigilance to administer the drug safely, a point made forcibly by Gray and Halton. By 1952, it was appreciated that safe use required control of ventilation [23]. Safety also mandated the postoperative use of doses of up to 5 mg neostigmine to antagonize the residual effect, a use advocated in 1946 [24].

What Does Paralysis Feel Like?

To better understand the patient's potential perception of curare's effects, some doughty clinicians submitted to paralysis while awake. In 1943, Helen Barnes underwent laryngoscopy after her colleagues gave her 4 ml of Intocostrin IV while she was awake. Her colleagues passed a laryngoscope and viewed her vocal cords with ease. She then used Intocostrin to facilitate tracheal intubation in 5 patients [25], recognizing that these doses of curare necessitated pharmacologic reversal with neostigmine. In 1946, Frederick Prescott, a pharmacologist at the Westminster hospital in London, submitted to awake paralysis with Intocostrin, a reportedly unpleasant experience during which he remained aware [24].

Despite the reports of Barnes and Prescott, some clinicians believed that curare depressed the central nervous system and could produce anesthesia, and many patients suffered awareness under anesthesia in those early years. "I...*was awakened by the most excruciating pain in my tummy. It felt as if my whole insides were being pulled out...*" [26].

Scott Smith, a pediatric anesthesiologist in Salt Lake City thought that curare anesthetized babies because they remained immobile during surgery. To test his belief he had colleagues completely paralyze him with curare with support of his respiration by bag and mask [27]. In contrast to what he expected, he perceived touch and pain throughout his paralysis and required tracheal intubation.

Many anesthetists initially thought that the use of muscle relaxants was inherently unsafe, a correct perception for partially paralyzed patients allowed to breathe spontaneously and whose tracheas were not intubated. Some suggested that curare had inherent cardiotoxicity [28]. However in the ten years following its introduction, it became clear that inappropriate use rather than curare caused the problems.

1947
The enthusiastic adoption of curare soon strained supplies, and the need for a synthetic drug became apparent. In response, the Swiss chemist, Daniel Bovet (1907–1992), and his group created gallamine [29]. Gallamine had some clinical success, but Bovet's work in the next decade with the older drug, succinylcholine, had a much greater impact.

The 1950s: Things Nearly Come Undone

Succinylcholine Appears in 1951

The decade opened propitiously, with the 1951 clinical introduction of succinylcholine. Although succinylcholine was first synthesized in 1906, it fell to Bovet in 1949 to observe its paralyzing action [30]. This observation, and his earlier discovery of gallamine, resulted in his 1957 Nobel Prize for Medicine.

In contrast to Intocostrin, succinylcholine received a warm welcome. Frances Foldes stated "*Its use is not accompanied by unwanted side-effects and the incidence of post-operative complications after its use is low*"[31]. But first impressions can be deceptive. Subsequently, numerous adverse effects of succinylcholine were identified [6]. One, prolonged block in patients with plasma cholinesterase deficiency, was an early example of the influence of pharmacogenetics, a term coined in 1957 (see Chapter 44 on A History of Pharmacogenomics Related to Anesthesiology). The familial nature of prolonged block was soon identified [32], and its relation to atypical cholinesterase demonstrated [33].

Curare and Mortality

In 1954, the "honeymoon" ended. Beecher and Todd reported a six-fold increase in "anesthesia-related" deaths in patients receiving "curare" [28]. To Beecher and Todd, "curare" encompassed d-tubocurarine, Intocostrin, dimethyl-tubocurarine (metubine), gallamine, succinylcholine, and decamethonium: the overall risk of death from anesthesia at that time was 1 in 2100 (far greater than today), but in a patient given curare the risk increased to 1 in 370. No cause was determined, and the increased mortality was not related to the patient's medical status, experience of the provider, or any other factor that could be identified. Reversal with an anticholinesterase was not reported in the study and presumably was not accomplished. The failure to administer neostigmine almost certainly underlay the lethality of the administration of curare, but in the opinion of the authors, most of the anesthesia-related deaths were from cardiovascular collapse, not respiratory insufficiency. This finding could have ended the clinical use of muscle relaxants, but Beecher and Todd wisely avoided simplistic conclusions. Although the use of relaxants increased anesthesia-related mortality, it did not appear to increase, indeed possibly decreased, overall operative mortality, a point argued forcefully by Abajian and colleagues in a rebuttal paper [34]. Beecher and Todd presciently reasoned that if curare caused an anesthesia-specific problem then the professionalism of anesthesiologists would compel them to investigate, understand, and resolve it.

Mechanisms and Murder in 1956

The depolarizing action of succinylcholine was not immediately appreciated. William Paton delineated relaxants into depolarizing and non-depolarizing drugs in 1956 [35]. Non-depolarizing drugs had a bulky structure (were pachycurares); depolarizing drugs had a long narrow structure (were leptocurares). We are still not sure how relaxants work. Do they enter and plug up ion channels? Do they compete with acetylcholine for receptors on the motor nerve terminal? Do they block the release of acetylcholine? Probably all of the above, and more [36].

In the body, succinylcholine quickly degraded to the naturally occurring compounds choline and succinate. Their natural nature made them nearly undetectable and possibly made succinylcholine the "ideal murder weapon." Lurid cases of suspected murder by succinylcholine have occurred. In 2007 a Nevada jury convicted critical care nurse, Chaz Higgs, of first degree murder in the death of his wife, Kathy Augustine, a prominent Nevada political figure. The murder weapon was a syringe of succinylcholine [37].

1958

One limitation of curare had been its capacity to cause histamine release and ganglionic blockade—with subsequent low blood pressure and bronchospasm (asthma). One plant species providing raw curare was Strychnos Toxifera. Another alkaloid, *alcuronium*, extracted from this plant was introduced in 1958. Alcuronium had properties similar to tubocurare but significantly less propensity to produce histamine release and ganglion blockade [38].

The 1960s: Pancuronium, Drug Design, and David Savage

Structure-Function and Steroidal Molecules

This decade saw structure-function analysis applied to drug design. The discovery of a steroidal alkaloid malouetine prompted development of steroid molecules with curare-like effects. In 1935, King had described the structure he thought was required in a neuromuscular blocking drug: two quaternary nitrogen groups separated by a distance (interonium) of 1.4 to 1.5 nm. The interonium distance proved to be more flexible than King predicted, for pancuronium being 1.05 nm and for fazadinium 0.7 nm [39, 40]. The general structure had two acetylcholine-like groups separated by an appropriate distance, and had to be bulky (pachycurare) to confer non-depolarizing characteristics. William "Bill" Bowman was a gifted pharmacologist at the University of Strathclyde in Glasgow, Scotland, who had worked with Paton on curare-like drugs. Bowman considered that the rigid steroidal androstane molecule was the perfect skeleton on which to place the quaternary nitrogen groups to create a muscle relaxant drug.

It was these structural "rules" and Bowman's idea to use the androstane nucleus that led to the development of the aminosteroid relaxant pancuronium by Hewett and Savage [41]. Pancuronium obeyed the rules except for its short interonium distance. This shortness conferred high potency and was long enough to avoid producing ganglionic blockade. Soon after the report of its clinical use in 1967 [42], pancuronium supplanted curare and gallamine for use in patients. Although devoid of ganglionic blocking effects, it had both vagolytic and sympathomimetic activity, but did not

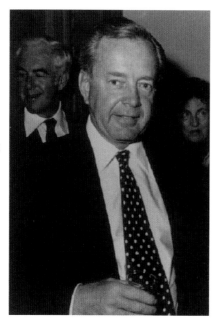

Fig. 50.4 David Savage and his creations, pancuronium and vecuronium. Vecuronium was originally rejected because it was monoquaternary (one *red* group) as opposed to the *bis*quaternary pancuronium (two *red* groups). Sadly, the laboratory where he worked, and where these drugs plus rocuronium and sugammadex were developed has recently closed due to mergers within the pharmaceutical industry

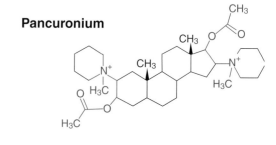

produce the hypotension associated with d-tubocurarine, or as much tachycardia as seen with gallamine.

David Savage

The success of pancuronium heralded the emergence of West Scotland as the epicenter for muscle relaxant development for the next 25 years. Leading this effort was David Savage, the principal chemist-scientist working on these compounds at Organon's research laboratories (Fig. 50.4). He had notable and inventive enthusiasm. He claimed, a bit (but just a bit) tongue in cheek, that using an androstane (steroid) backbone he could create a drug that would work at any receptor. He said that for fun he had made and tested a steroidal appetite suppressant in rats. It was all too good; the rats starved to death! He was also a *bon viveur*. For one particular experiment he needed a small pressure vessel to contain the reaction. The ideal vessel turned out to be a champagne bottle, and of course the contents had to be drunk first.

Savage had the then novel insight that scientists and clinicians should work together to develop drugs clinicians needed. So he worked closely with anesthesiologists: Leslie Baird at Glasgow Royal Infirmary, and Ronald Miller in San Francisco. There is a story that one of the brain storming sessions occurred at a local bar. Purely by chance, David Savage and a local anesthesiologist struck up a conversation, and started discussing curare and the neuromuscular junction. In the course of the conversation many novel drug structures, probably including a pancuronium prototype, were written down on paper napkins. So engrossed were the two men that they had to be asked to leave several hours later, as the bartender wanted to close up. Many clinician colleagues of David Savage describe similar "design" sessions, where they would

articulate their needs for a drug, and David would draw putative structures. To further scientist/clinician interaction, Savage organized the 1st International Neuromuscular Meeting, bringing clinicians and scientists together in London in 1975.

Like its peers, pancuronium had too long a duration of action because its elimination was primarily via the kidney. Continued research at the Scottish facility solved this problem, leading to the development of two successful drugs, vecuronium and rocuronium, and one ill-fated drug, rapacuronium [43].

Up to the 1970s, clinicians had no practical way of monitoring relaxant effect, except for subjective clinical signs such as abdominal muscle relaxation or adequacy of spontaneous respiration. The need to develop a method of monitoring the residual effects of such powerful drugs was addressed in the next decade.

The 1970s: Monitoring; Ideal Drug; Pharmacokinetics and Pharmacodynamics

Monitoring

In the 1950s and 1960s, clinical acumen and judicious dosing guided the administration of muscle relaxants. The first monitors of neuromuscular function were simple nerve stimulators [44]. They required subcutaneous needles for nerve stimulation, The need to define a control response before relaxant administration made them impractical for normal clinical use. In the 1970s, this led Hassan Ali to develop the train-of-four ratio (TOF; Fig. 50.5) [45]. Ali used the known effect of repeated stimulation (repeated stimulation produces a decreasing contraction in a partly paralyzed muscle) in a clinically useful way [46]. Patients received four stimuli at 2 Hz (0.5 s intervals) and the ratio of the fourth response (T4)

Fig. 50.5 Significant figures in the modern history of neuromuscular function. Hassan Ali in Boston developed the concept of the train-of-four ratio to quantify block. Jørgen Viby-Mogensen in Copenhagen took this work further and developed the techniques of post-tetanic count to quantify profound block, and double burst stimulation to facilitate clinical detection of low levels of residual block. John Savarese, originally in Boston and later in New York developed mivacurium and has had a career-long pursuit of a type A fast-onset short acting non-depolarizer muscle relaxant. Finally, Anton "Ton" Bom, a native of Holland, working in Scotland, changed the whole concept of relaxant reversal with the discovery and development of sugammadex

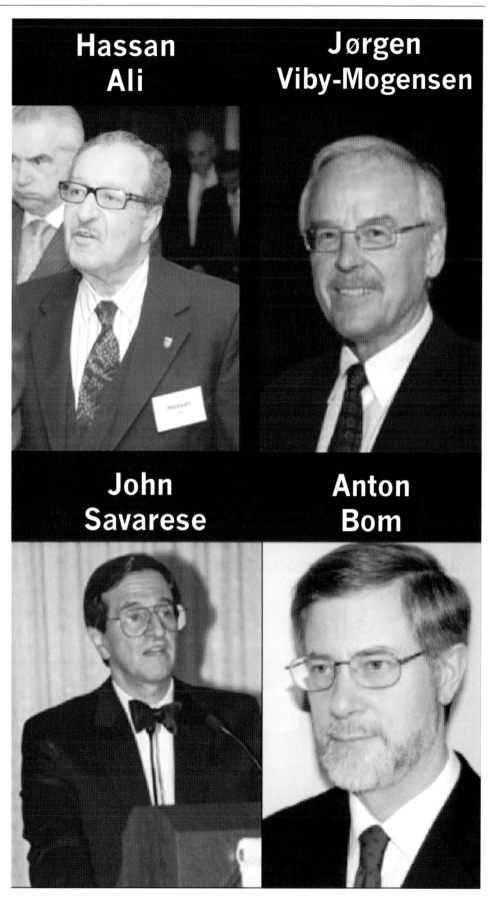

Fig. 50.6 The three most common stimulation modalities in neuromuscular monitoring are single twitch height, train-of-four and tetanus at 50 Hz. They have a fairly reproducible relationship to one another and to the fraction of acetylcholine receptors that need to be blocked (occupied) by the muscle relaxant for a given effect. (From an online lecture Thompson C: Monitoring the Neuromuscular Junction, University of Sydney, 2010, with permission.)

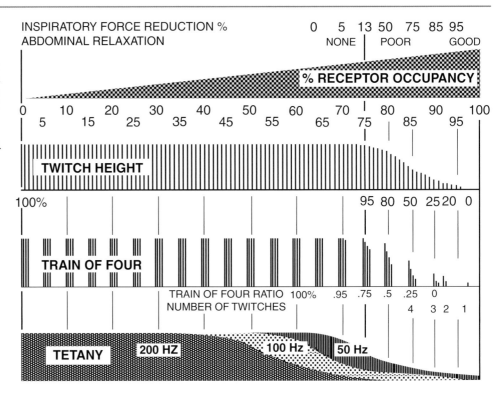

to the first (T1) was measured. A material decrease, especially below 0.7, indicated residual paralysis.

This useful ratio (Fig. 50.6) correlated with other indices of muscle function, including the absolute decrease in strength of the muscle contraction, the decrease in response to tetanic stimulation, and deteriorating pulmonary function [47, 48]. Because it provided its own internal control, it did not require a baseline measurement. The response could be either mechanical force, or electromyography. It also discriminated between succinylcholine-induced block (minimal fade) and depolarizing (marked fade) block. TOF assessment persists as the mainstay of clinical monitoring.

The Ideal Drug

In the 1970s, clinicians could choose a short-acting drug (succinylcholine) or longer acting (nondepolarizing) drugs. All had side effects. This unsatisfactory situation led to the concept of the ideal drug by Karis and Gissen in 1971 [49]. Their criteria have stood the test of time and are still quoted today (Table 50.2), with the notable exception that a demand for fast onset was absent.

Savarese and Kitz elaborated on these concepts in 1975 [50], adding their belief that one drug could not be ideal for all clinical situations. They defined three categories of ideal drug, A, B and C. Type A was a non-depolarizing succinylcholine (rapid onset, rapid offset). Type B had a duration of action approximately half that of curare or pancuronium, and soon became a reality with the introduction

Table 50.2 Definition of the "Ideal Drug" Karis and Gissen

Criterion	Comment
1. Competitive non-depolarizing	Avoided complications of depolarizing action
2. Recovery not organ-dependent	Fulfilled by atracurium and mivacurium
3. Breakdown products inactive	Fulfilled by rocuronium and cisatracurium
4. Relatively short duration	Fulfilled by intermediate acting drugs
5. Highly specific	Delayed development of drugs with fast onset
6. Reversible by anticholinesterase	Did not foresee alternatives

of vecuronium and atracurium. Type C was long acting and without adverse cardiovascular effects, anticipating pipecuronium and doxacurium which arrived approximately 15 years later. John Savarese has crusaded for a Type A drug, and, as we shall see, his efforts may be close to fruition.

Defining the direction for new drugs pressured the pharmaceutical industry to synthesize products that would meet the challenges implied by the definitions. As noted earlier, Savage facilitated the dialogue between clinicians and industry by organizing the 1st Neuromuscular Meeting in London in 1975, just when the concept of the "ideal relaxant" was described. Few at the meeting appreciated the impending "revolution" in neuromuscular pharmacology—the era of the intermediate-acting relaxant was about to dawn.

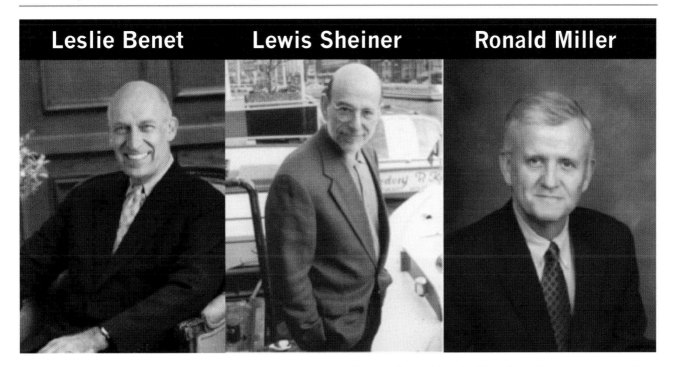

Fig. 50.7 The University of California San Francisco threesome that significantly advanced the scientific understanding of the pharmacokinetics and pharmacodynamics of muscle relaxants in the 1970s. Leslie Benet created the pharmacokinetic concept of "*Clearance.*" Concurrently, Lewis Sheiner pursued the science of drug concentration-effect relationships, developing sophisticated modeling tools. Finally, a young clinician/scientist Ronald Miller, freshly back from Vietnam, had many questions relating to the clinical behavior of muscle relaxants and their antagonists. Good fortune brought together a clinician with important questions and scientists with the talents to develop the tools to address those questions

Pharmacokinetics and Pharmacodynamics

Until the 1970s, there was but a rudimentary understanding of drug actions, and of the interaction of biodisposition (pharmacokinetics) and effect (pharmacodynamics). Developments at the University of California San Francisco (UCSF) changed this (Fig. 50.7). Leslie Benet developed and refined the science of pharmacokinetics and pharmacodynamics, creating the concept of drug "Clearance." Concurrently, Lewis Sheiner pursued the science of drug concentration-effect relationships. And a young clinician/scientist Ronald Miller, freshly back from Vietnam, had a mind full of questions relating to the clinical behavior of muscle relaxants and their antagonists. These circumstances fortuitously combined a clinician with important questions and scientists with the talents to develop the tools to address those questions. The breakthrough was to measure both the effect of a drug and the concentrations associated with the effect, and to make inferences as to how underlying conditions (e.g., renal or hepatic failure) influenced these. The first paper applying these techniques focused on the impact of renal failure on the pharmacokinetics of tubocurare [51].

A problem remained: the concurrent measurement of the concentration of a drug at its site of action (e.g., the neuromuscular junction) and the effect of that concentration. The researcher couldn't sample the neuromuscular junction. Sur-

rogate measures (e.g., the concentration in blood) had to serve instead. That was fine (sort of) if there were equilibrium between the blood and the neuromuscular junction, but how could one be sure? Sheiner and Stanski published an important paper in 1979 that provided the "missing link" between concentration and effect [52]. The authors in this paper recognized that initially the concentration at the neuromuscular junction (and the effect) lagged behind what the anesthetist gave and was in the blood. During recovery, the opposite was true. The paper demonstrated how one could calculate the concentration and effect at the neuromuscular junction by knowing the effect during input and output. This model has broad applicability to any situation where the drug concentration is measured in one place and its effect takes place at another.

The 1980s: Advances, Complacency, and Monitoring Techniques

1980: Vecuronium

Jan Crul and Leo Booij published the first clinical report of vecuronium's actions in 1980 [53]. Vecuronium provided the first major advance in non-depolarizing muscle relaxants since 1942. Clinicians now had a relaxant with an intermediate duration of action. Two critical observations enabled the development of vecuronium. First, Everett et al. corrected the error in tubocurare's structure that King had made [39], leading to renewed interest in monoquaternary drugs such as vecuronium. Second, it was realized that the vagolytic and neuromuscular blocking effects of pancuronium could be separated by specifically designing a molecule with greater affinity for the acetylcholine receptors at the neuromuscular junction than at other sites [54, 55]. These insights led to vecuronium, a drug with the same neuromuscular blocking potency as pancuronium, but with only 1/20th the vagolytic effect. To this day vecuronium remains the model for a "clean" (relatively few side effects) relaxant.

Vecuronium had another important property, a duration of action less than half that of pancuronium. Its monoquaternary structure permitted elimination by both the liver and the kidneys (pancuronium elimination is predominantly renal), leading to a shorter and more certain duration of action [56].

1981: Atracurium

As vecuronium emerged from Organon's laboratories, a similar major advance, the synthesis of atracurium, was under development at the University of Strathclyde in Glasgow. Like vecuronium, it had an intermediate duration of action, but one based on a unique method of elimination [12]. August Hofmann synthesized the first quaternary amines, the general group to which all muscle relaxants belong [11], in 1851. He described a novel reaction in the degradation of such amines ("Hofmann Elimination"), in which two parts of the molecule fall off, leaving behind a double bond. But the reaction only took place at high temperatures (e.g., 100 °C), and in an extreme alkaline environment (pH 12–14), thus seemingly having no immediate application in biology. A hundred years later, John Stenlake searched for a neuromuscular blocking drug that would break down *in vivo* by Hofmann elimination (Fig. 50.2) [12].

The observation that the plant alkaloid petaline could degrade by Hofmann elimination at physiologic pH and temperature prompted the search, culminating in the creation of atracurium. Atracurium was the first muscle relaxant whose elimination depended on neither enzyme nor organ function; a remarkable breakthrough [57]. Previously, muscle relaxants could only be eliminated when in the circulation, exposed to either enzyme degradation (succinylcholine) or elimination by kidney and/or liver (all the non-depolarizing drugs). Because atracurium broke down at body pH and temperature, its elimination occurred everywhere in the body [57].

In 1981, James Payne and Robert Hughes reported the first application of atracurium in patients [58]. Clinical neuromuscular block had entered a "golden age": vecuronium had no cardiac effects, and atracurium elimination did not depend on organ function. Savarese and Kitz's Type B ideal relaxant had been realized. However, whether vecuronium and atracurium were free of biologically active by-products (criterion # 3 of Karis and Gissen; Table 50.2) remained a question.

Vecuronium undergoes deacetylation to an active metabolite with 50 % of vecuronium's potency [59]. This might be a clinical problem for prolonged relaxation as in the ICU, and we will hear more of that later. Atracurium's metabolism by Hofmann elimination produced a compound called laudanosine, an analeptic. Could it antagonize anesthesia or cause seizures [60]? This argument, debated over several years, was finally settled with the conclusion that there was nothing to worry about in the operating room. There remained in some people's minds, a concern about long-term use in the ICU, but that use was about to end anyway.

Mivacurium

As vecuronium and atracurium were pursued in Scotland, John Savarese and his group in Boston synthesized bulky bisquaternary esters looking for drugs with a short duration of action [61], an enduring interest of Savarese (Fig. 50.5) [62]. Not surprisingly he defined Type A as a necessary element of an ideal relaxant. This so-called "non-depolarizing succinylcholine" proved difficult to develop. Savarese's collaboration with Burroughs-Wellcome would lead to the introduction of mivacurium, which like succinylcholine is metabolized by plasma cholinesterase.

While mivacurium had the sought-after short duration of action [63], it did not have a fast onset, and this limited interest in its use. Mivacurium took about twice as long as succinylcholine to act, its duration of action was twice as long, and if the patient had a cholinesterase deficiency, block would last twice as long. With shorter duration, onset time took up a greater proportion of the total duration. To get a faster onset and better intubating conditions, clinicians increased the dose but then ran into problems with histamine release. Mivacurium's manufacture in the US ended in 2006 because of insufficient demand. It continues to be available in other countries.

Failure of Doxacurium and Pipecuronium

The 1980s also saw the introduction of two ultimately unsuccessful drugs, pipecuronium and doxacurium. Vecuronium's popularity, lack of cardiovascular effect, and modest duration of action suggested the possibility that there might be a clinical need for a "clean" long-acting relaxant (*i.e.* pancuronium without side effects), the Type C drug described by Savarese and Kitz in 1975. The steroidal drug pipecuronium from Hungary, and the benzylisoquinolinium drug doxacurium from the US resulted [64, 65]. But both drugs arrived ten years too late because clearly vecuronium and atracurium met any clinical need that doxacurium or pipecuronium might serve. They were doomed to obscurity.

New Monitoring Modalities

The Danish anesthesiologist Jørgen Viby-Mogensen (Fig. 50.5) and his creative and productive research group had a particular interest in monitoring neuromuscular block. In the 1980s and 1990s, they built on the work of Ali to develop new monitoring modalities. Perhaps the intermediate duration of action of vecuronium and atracurium led to a fascination with deep levels of block. Monitoring post-tetanic responses enabled measurement of block in the absence of Ali's train-of-four (TOF) responses [66]. By monitoring post-tetanic responses, clinicians could control administration of enormous doses of relaxant, doses paralyzing even the diaphragm [67]. Neuroanesthesiologists used this technique to eliminate all possibility of movement during neurosurgery. Inevitably, this technique delayed reversal of the block [68].

Double-burst stimulation added another modality: two short tetanic bursts were felt as two responses [69]. Double-burst stimulation proved more sensitive than TOF at identifying residual block [69]. While these monitoring techniques are used quite commonly in academic centers in Europe they have had little penetration in other types of practice, or in other parts of the world.

Children Get Attention

In the 1980s, neuromuscular studies in pediatric patients started in earnest [70–74]. Up to this time there were few studies in children, perhaps in part because of the emotional stress surrounding informed consent from parents, and assent from older children. In addition, the smaller blood volume of children and infants limited studies requiring blood sampling. Notwithstanding these difficulties, the UCSF mathematician-pediatric anesthesiologist, Dennis Fisher and his colleagues characterized the pharmacodynamic/kinetic effects of both relaxants and antagonists in children, and studied placental transfer of vecuronium and pancuronium.

Various studies in the 1980s showed that children are not simply small adults. Younger children are more likely to have greater sensitivity to relaxants, and to have altered biodisposition and rate of elimination [72, 75, 76]. Onset of paralysis is shorter and duration longer in infants than in children and adults [71]. Fisher et al. also showed that, contrary to popular belief, children do not need disproportionately large doses of neostigmine, but in fact responded in much the same way as adults [73]. During Caesarean section under general anesthesia, there is measurable placental transmission of muscle

relaxant to the fetus, but there do not appear to be adverse clinical effects on the newborn [70].

In the 1990s, the effects of relaxants in children would be studied in the OR, the ICU and the Emergency Department [77–79], and the unique response of children to monitoring would be evaluated [80]. For the first time, children were included in early Phase 3 clinical trials, specifically during the assessment of rapacuronium [81]. Subsequent events would show the irony of this development.

Antagonists

The need to give drugs that reversed the paralyzing effects of muscle relaxants—to "unparalyze" patients at the end of surgery—has been appreciated since the early days of relaxant administration. Reversal drugs have been the neglected half of the muscle relaxant/reversal combination. They fall into three categories, anticholinesterase drugs (that block the destruction of acetylcholine), the aminopyridines (that increase acetylcholine release), and sugammadex (which captures and thereby inactivates the relaxant.) Aminopyridines have found little clinical application for this use and will not be discussed further.

The pharmacokinetics and dynamics of anticholinesterase drugs were largely defined in the 1980s using the tools developed at UCSF (Fig. 50.7). Several conclusions resulted. First, the anticholinesterase effect of these drugs underlies their action [82]. Second, neostigmine more effectively antagonizes profound block than does edrophonium [83]. Third, their actions usually outlast those of the muscle relaxant [82]. Finally, there is a ceiling to their capacity to produce reversal, resulting in inadequate reversal of profound block [83, 84]. One might think of inadequate reversal as consequent to three factors. First, there is a maximum rate at which acetylcholine that can be released from the motor nerve terminal. Second, even in the absence of cholinesterase, the acetylcholine will rapidly diffuse out of the neuromuscular junction and the equilibrium between rate of release and rate of diffusion away sets an upper limit to the concentration that can be achieved at the neuromuscular junction. Finally, because the interaction between muscle relaxant and acetylcholine is competitive, if the maximum acetylcholine concentration is insufficient to antagonize the concentration of relaxant, then inadequate reversal will be the consequence.

Inadequate reversal in some patients has been a long-known clinical fact of life, a fact potentially leading to disasters, including death. The introduction of vecuronium and atracurium led to complacency. Their short duration of action might be thought to guarantee recovery, but Bevan and others showed that this was not the case [84]. Indeed, not even the short-acting mivacurium was immune from inadequate recovery if reversal was omitted [85]. Adequate reversal was

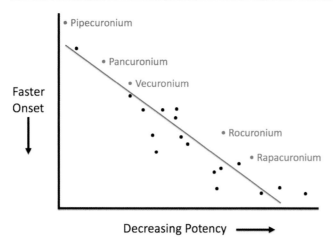

Fig. 50.8 The striking relationship between the potency of a neuromuscular blocking drug and its onset time [84] for the aminosteroid group of relaxant compounds. The fast onset drugs rocuronium and rapacuronium were not in the original study, and are included for reference. A similar relationship is found for the benzylisoquinoline compounds. (Created with data from Bowman et al. 1988 [84].)

an area in need of pharmacological innovation. This came in the 2000s with the development of sugammadex.

Potency Versus Onset Time

By the end of the 1980s, clinicians had type B and type C, but not type A drugs. Indeed, fast onset continued to elude the chemists. In part this was due to condition #5, high selectivity, set by Karis and Gissen [49]. This had always been assumed to correlate with high potency. High potency and greater selectivity for one receptor over others would be accompanied by fewer adverse effects. William (Bill) Bowman, a physiologist at the University of Strathclyde then made an observation that reversed this view.

The Organon R&D laboratories had synthesized many relaxant compounds in the steroidal series. Bowman observed that their potencies correlated inversely with onset time (Fig. 50.8) [86]: the more potent a relaxant, the slower its onset. This observation undermined the search for drugs with greater potency. As a result, ORG 9426 was identified and released in the 1990s as rocuronium, a nondepolarizing drug with a faster onset.

The 1990s: Fast Onset At Last; Problems in the Intensive Care Unit (ICU)

Rocuronium

Rocuronium showed that low potency, fast onset, and lack of adverse effects could be combined. Because it had an onset

time approaching that of succinylcholine, a nondepolarizing drug could be used for rapid-sequence intubation [87]. Doses of 1.0–1.2 mg/kg produced good conditions for rapid-sequence tracheal intubation, a first for a non-depolarizing drug [88].

Another new drug further illustrated the link between onset and potency. Cisatracurium was a single isomer isolated from atracurium, itself a mixture of 10 isomers [89]. Having a 5-fold greater potency than atracurium, it had a lesser tendency to release histamine [90]. However, the greater potency slowed onset, requiring larger doses to give acceptably brief onset times [91]. It has succeeded clinically because it is a "cleaner" atracurium and because, like atracurium, its elimination is largely organ independent.

Which to choose between the new guys on the block, rocuronium or cisatracurium? For some clinicians the onset time of rocuronium was most important; for others the more predictable recovery of cisatracurium was of overriding concern [92]. Most clinicians are happy to have both available.

ICU Problems

The otherwise "safe" use of muscle relaxant in the operating room motivated expansion of their use into ICUs. Rather than give patients depressant sedative drugs, paralysis could be used to facilitate ventilation. Relaxants, usually pancuronium and vecuronium, were used in virtually every ICU in the 1980s and 1990s [93]. Although Barnes, Prescott and Smith in the 1940s had shown that muscle relaxants did not provide sedative or analgesic effects, remarkable misconceptions existed among ICU caregivers regarding the properties of muscle relaxants. A 1980 study revealed that 5% of ICU physicians thought that pancuronium had analgesic properties, and 50% thought it was an anxiolytic [94]. A different effect provided another problem.

In 1985 Op de Coul identified significantly prolonged paralysis in patients receiving large doses of muscle relaxants in the ICU [95]. Weakness persisted for weeks after cessation of relaxant administration. Others confirmed the existence of this problem, finding that it occurred with all relaxants. Drugs that were safe and efficacious when used short-term in the operating room assumed a different safety profile with long-term use [96].

Patients recovered from the problem that brought them to the ICU, but were left with a paralysis that could last for weeks or months. Particularly bad was the combination of muscle relaxants plus steroids for treatment of severe asthma, a treatment requiring tracheal intubation and artificial ventilation [96]. After Segredo et al. published their work in the *New England Journal of Medicine* in 1992, the problem received greater notice [97]. The weakness had more than one form, including prolonged neuromuscular block, or motor neuropathy (something wrong with the nerve going to the muscle), or myopathy (something wrong with the muscle). As might be imagined, risk increased with larger relaxant doses, longer durations of administration, concomitant use of steroids, and renal failure. The use of muscle relaxants in ICUs decreased dramatically. When relaxants were indicated, the doses were kept small, and drug "holidays" were allowed, to permit the neuromuscular junction to have intermittent periods of normal function. The problem then largely disappeared.

Tracheal Intubation Without Relaxant

The 1990s proved yet again that tracheal intubation doesn't require relaxants [98]. In the era before relaxants, tracheal intubation was accomplished under deep, usually ether, anesthesia. The existence of propofol, potent short-acting opioids and sevoflurane enabled a return to those days of yesteryear.

In adults, propofol and remifentanil could provide excellent intubation conditions. The price was cardiovascular depression, since intubation depended on "deep" anesthesia [98]. In children, intubation solely with sevoflurane was successful, and remains a mainstream clinical technique [99]. In adults, intubation without relaxant fell out of favor since, compared to techniques using a muscle relaxant, it was associated with a greater risk of laryngeal injury [100, 101].

1999 and Rapacuronium

The decade went out with a bang. It appeared that the Type A drug had been found. The inverse relationship between potency and onset was pushed even further with the development of the drug rapacuronium. Its low potency enabled a fast onset, and it had a duration of action that made it a type A drug [102].

By the end of the 1990s we were feeling pretty good. We had drugs for virtually every clinical situation and good monitoring techniques. We thought we had solved all the problems, and that there was perhaps not much more going to happen in the world of muscle relaxants. We were in for unpleasant surprises.

The New Millenium: Uncertainty and a Revolution (Sugammadex)

Rapacuronium Withdrawn

A stunner opened the 2000s. The manufacturer of rapacuronium, the first true Type A drug, abruptly withdrew the drug on 27 March 2001 because of reports of severe bronchospasm, particularly in children [103]. Because the incidence was small, the number of subjects in the clinical trials preceding rapacuronium's release was insufficient to reveal the problem. However, when approved and used in hundreds of thousands of patients, this rare but serious problem became apparent.

Histamine release did not underlie the bronchospasm, also conspiring to conceal the cause. Measurements of histamine revealed nothing. It was reported in 2005 that rapacuronium activated cholinergic M3 receptors in the smooth muscle of the lung [104]. Karis and Gissen (condition #5; Table 50.2) had recognized that less potent drugs might be less specific for their primary target and risk being active at similar receptors in other systems. Such was the case with rapacuronium.

Allergic Responses?

The withdrawal of rapacuronium was first in a series of setbacks for muscle relaxant drugs. Reports came from France [105] and then Norway [106] concerning severe allergic responses to rocuronium. Reports from other European countries were few. In the largest market, the US, rocuronium seemed free of reports of allergic responses. What was going on? The fascinating story combined a real effect with some over-zealous diagnosis.

The diagnoses of rocuronium sensitivity were made using a skin test with a high sensitivity and low specificity, translating into a lot of false positive results [107]. After refining the skin tests the incidence of false positives decreased significantly [107, 108]. A clinically reliable test would be to repeat administration of a small dose of rocuronium (provocation test), in those who had putatively suffered an allergic response, to observe any recurrence of a reaction. This test was not performed because it was believed that the risk was not justified.

A current explanation for the geographic mal-distribution of individuals having the allergic responses is that some non-relaxant drugs provide a sensitizing exposure that makes a patient vulnerable to the subsequent administration of a muscle relaxant. Such a drug is pholcodine, which was in common use in Norway and France as a cough suppressant. It was not available in Denmark, which had no substantiated reports of allergy to rocuronium.

The false perception remains that muscle relaxants are the commonest cause of severe allergic responses in the operating room. However, some results from Denmark challenge this belief, and results from two studies are particularly important [109, 110]. First, data gathered by the central allergy response unit in Denmark suggest that muscle relaxants cause fewer allergic responses than first thought, muscle relaxants being third after chlorhexidine and fentanyl. The second paper examined whether the drug reported to cause the allergic response was in fact the cause. The drug originally reported as the cause was incorrect in more than half the cases [110].

Why Can't We Reverse Relaxant Block?

Since publication of the TOF ratio method in the 1970s, a TOF ratio of 0.7 had been accepted as indicating adequate recovery of neuromuscular function [111]. Lars Eriksson and then Aaron Kopman challenged that belief at the end of the 1990s [112, 113]. Complete recovery of neuromuscular function had not occurred at a TOF of 0.7, and in fact required a TOF ratio of greater than 0.9. In addition, even careful intraoperative monitoring of neuromuscular function could not eliminate the occurrence of residual block [114].

Entering the 2000s, many anesthetists considered that neuromuscular function in a patient given a muscle relaxant (with the exception of succinylcholine) could not be rapidly restored to the pre-relaxant state. They considered that pharmacological reversal with neostigmine, was not as reliable as previously thought [115]. A full reversal dose of neostigmine, given even after 4 TOF responses were present, did not guarantee rapid recovery to a TOF ratio of 0.7, and particularly not to the newly recommended ratio of 0.9. The age of uncertainty about relaxant reversal was upon us [116].

The method of antagonism of block had significant limitations, most prominently incomplete efficacy against profound levels of block. Users of intermediate-duration relaxants had incorrectly believed that residual paralysis would not be a problem. This belief sometimes led to failure to antagonize residual block, with a consequent persistent incidence of some degree of paralysis with all neuromuscular blocking drugs [117]. As patients became increasingly obese, with less pulmonary reserve (and especially after abdominal or thoracic surgery), the problem of inadequate reversal became more apparent, and of greater clinical import [118].

In particular circumstances, neostigmine might itself produce paradoxical weakness. In 1980, Payne and others showed that neostigmine alone, without previous administration of a relaxant, could produce mild weakness [119]. Caldwell later found that administration of neostigmine to a patient with a TOF ratio equal to or greater than 0.9 could decrease the TOF ratio [120]. In studies of airway muscle [121, 122], Eikermann elegantly showed that excessive neostigmine could decrease pharyngeal muscle tone, and diminish the ability to maintain an open airway.

Nonetheless, clinicians continued using the same drug, neostigmine, that they had used in the 1940s, a drug that could not be guaranteed to produce adequate recovery, even with careful attention to monitoring relaxant effect. In contrast, over the same period, muscle relaxants had gone through quite dramatic development and improvement. The time was ripe for new pharmacology applied to relaxant reversal.

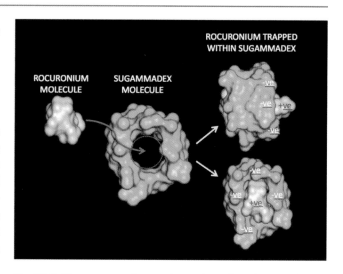

Fig. 50.9 How sugammadex terminates the action of rocuronium. In brief, the sugammadex molecule was designed specifically to accommodate (encapsulate) one molecule of rocuronium. Once the bulk of the rocuronium molecule enters the sugammadex molecule, negatively charged groups (−ve) on the sugammadex molecule are attracted to the positively charged terminal group (+ve) of the rocuronium, and lock it in place. If sufficient sugammadex is given to encapsulate all rocuronium molecules, reversal of block is almost immediate and complete. This was the first major pharmacological breakthrough in reversal since the introduction of muscle relaxants to anesthesia in 1942

2001

There was little indication of the excitement to come when the 7th International; Neuromuscular Meeting opened in Belfast in 2001. At that meeting, the Dutch pharmaceutical chemist Anton "Ton" Bom (Fig. 50.5) made a fascinating presentation. He had been conducting experiments with rocuronium, at the Organon research laboratories in Scotland, and things were not going well. He was having difficulty dissolving rocuronium in the medium he was using. From a brief literature review, he discovered a group of compounds, the cyclodextrins that had been used as solubilizing agents. The cyclodextrins are doughnut shaped molecules that solubilize drugs by incorporating the drugs' lipophilic part inside the hole in the doughnut, leaving only the hydrophilic end exposed. However, he found that after mixing with cyclodextrin his rocuronium solution had lost potency. Bom then had a "Eureka" moment. He realized that if he could design a cyclodextrin that would similarly attract and then trap rocuronium then he had a perfect mechanism for reversal of neuromuscular block (Fig. 50.9). His insight produced the first significant pharmacologic development in relaxant reversal in 60 years.

He and his collaborators experimented with different cyclodextrins, finally arriving at the drug sugammadex. Sugammadex is a gamma cyclodextrin, a ring structure composed of eight sugar molecules. Since each sugammadex molecule captures one rocuronium molecule, any concentration of rocuronium could be inactivated by an appropriate dose of sugammadex. If that reasoning was correct, it would be possible to quickly restore the patient's neuromuscular junction to the state before muscle relaxant had been given *i.e.* there should be complete reversal of neuromuscular block. Several experiments supported that view [123]. We now had two drugs; rocuronium and sugammadex, which when used in combination provided the "ideal drug". This new pharmacologic approach may be the most innovative discovery since the introduction of muscle relaxants to clinical practice.

2008

Sugammadex was approved for clinical use in 2008 and is now available in over 50 countries—but not the US. The failure of the Food and Drug Administration to approve sugammadex was a great surprise to all who had been involved in the drug's development. The official reason was concern over the possibility of hypersensitivity reactions in some of the experimental subjects. To the best knowledge of the author, there had been no serious adverse events with the drug during the clinical trials. Of note, there have been few reports of adverse clinical events with sugammadex from the more than 50 countries where it is now approved.

Gantacurium and Cysteine Adduction

Concurrent with the development of sugammadex, as part of their 30-year quest for a Type A drug, Savarese and his group continued their development of benzylisoquinolinium compounds [124]. The chlorofumarate compounds gantacurium and CV002 resulted from these efforts [125]. These compounds bear a resemblance to mivacurium and undergo a unique, rapid inactivation *in vivo* by adduction to endogenous cysteine. In addition, administration of exogenous cysteine accelerates their inactivation. As with sugammadex, the combination of gantacurium, and exogenous cysteine administration has the potential to rapidly return neuromuscular function to a normal state. This drug combination is currently in clinical trials.

The Future

It took five centuries from the first reports of "death-dealing" arrow poison to the clinical use of curare. The next 70 years saw the evolution of newer, safer, better relaxants and an increased understanding of their actions. The discovery of sugammadex and chlorofumarate drugs reveals continuing innovation in neuromuscular pharmacology.

Where will the next generations of drugs that provide skeletal muscle relaxation act? Perhaps these drugs will work on the spinal cord or in the brain. Might we have drugs working preferentially at one or more groups of muscles, for example the laryngeal adductors, to facilitate tracheal intubation—but not the diaphragm—so breathing would remain normal. Even further out, might we develop inactive pro-drugs, which would be activated only when needed, and turned off when no longer required?

Reflections and Conclusions

Curare had a long gestation period from the fifteenth century until its birth into anesthesia practice in 1942. In the last century we have witnessed the evolution of one of anesthesia's greatest stories—unraveling the mysteries of neuromuscular blocking drugs and their use in everyday clinical practice. Some characteristic patterns have marked the development of these drugs.

Little Is New Under the Sun (At Least Not Very Often)

Each generation thinks it is first with a particular idea. Most ideas have been conceived before, but with poor timing. In 1912, a surgeon Arthur Lawen used curare, tracheal intubation, and assisted ventilation for surgical procedures i.e. long before this became standard practice in anesthesia. The idea did not catch on at first.

Every Change Carries the Risk of Unintended Consequences

A good, even revolutionary, drug may produce effects that outweigh its benefits. Doubtless many patients died from the effects of curare in the 1940s and 1950s. Later during the decades of the 1960s–80s, patients in intensive care units were certainly harmed by drugs that, at the time, had a good record of safety in the operating room. Finally, in the past decade rapacuronium, despite its unique properties, was withdrawn because of rare but serious adverse affects.

Many Major Breakthroughs Are Accidental

The first formal use of curare in anesthesia in 1942 resulted from a series of coincidences rather than a directed program of research and development. Fast onset was developed after a simple insight by Bowman in the 1990s, an insight contrary to accepted wisdom. At the beginning of this decade, sugammadex resulted from Bom's openness to the chance discovery of an interaction that no one had been pursuing. The next major discovery may be just as revolutionary—and fortuitous—for someone open to the discovery.

Persistence Pays Dividends

In the 1930s, it was the persistence of Richard Gill in pursuit of a cure for his multiple sclerosis that led him to bring from South America, sufficient curare extract to enable its development for clinical use. It was Stenlake's tenacity in the 1970s that resulted in the development of atracurium. He was able to create a drug that degraded via Hofmann elimination, a process that previously functioned only in temperature and pH ranges far outside the physiologic domain. Finally, John Savarese and his group may be on the verge of developing a fast onset, short-acting nondepolarizing drug, more than 30 years after he first described the clinical need for such a compound.

Acknowledgment This work was supported by the University of California Department of Anesthesia and Perioperative Care.

References

1. Bevan DR. Fifty years of muscle relaxants. Acta Anaesthesiol Scand Suppl. 1995;106:2–6.
2. Alexander von Humboldt. Personal Narrative of Travels to the Equinoctial Regions of America, During the Years 1799–1804–Volume 2, reproduced courtesy of Google's Project Gutenberg. And Charles Waterton, Wanderings in South America, the Noth-West of the United States, and the Antilles, in the years 1812, 1816, 1820 and 1824. Published in1825 by J Mawman, London. pp. 239.
3. Betcher AM. The civilizing of curare: a history of its development and introduction into anesthesiology. Anesth Analg. 1977;56:305–19.
4. Brocklesby RA. Concerning the Indian poison sent over from M. de la Condamine. Edited by Society PotR. London, Philos Trans Royal Soc Lond, 1747, pp. 407–12.
5. Brodie BC. Further experiments and observations on the actions of poisons on the animal systems. Philos Trans. 1812;102:205–27.
6. Dorkins HR. Suxamethonium-the development of a modern drug from 1906 to the present day. Med Hist. 1982;26:145–68.
7. Sykes K, Bunker J. Curare: the Indian arrow poison. In: Sykes K, Bunker J, editors. Anaesthesia and the practoce of medicine: Historical perspectives. London: Royal Society of Medicine Press Ltd.; 2007. pp. 105–20.
8. Bernard C. Analyse physiologiquedes propriétiés des systèmes musculaire et nerveux au moyen de curare. CR Acad Sci (Paris). 1856;43:825–9.
9. Sayres LA. Two cases of traumatic tetanus. NY J Med. 1858;4:250–3.
10. Raghavendra T. Neuromuscular blocking drugs: discovery and development. J R Soc Med. 2002;95:363–7.
11. Alston TA. The contributions of A. W. Hofmann. Anesth Analg. 2003;96:622–5.
12. Stenlake JB. Atracurium: design and function, medicinal chemistry. London: Academic Press Inc.; 1985. pp. 143–65.
13. Hunt R, Taveau R. On the physiological action of certain choline derivaties and new methods for detecting cholin. Br Med J. 1906;2:1788–91.
14. Glick D. Some additional observations on the specificity of cholinesterase. J Biol Chem. 1941;137:357–62.
15. Lawen A. Ueber die verbindung der lokalanesthesie mit der narkose, uber hohe extraduralanasthesie und epidurale injektionen anasthesia render losungen bei tabischen magenkrisen. Beitr Klin Chir. 1912;80:168–89.
16. Wilkinson DJ. Dr F.P. de Caux—the first user of curare for anesthesia in England. Anaesthesia. 1991;46:49–51.
17. Sykes K. Treating severe tetanus with muscle paralysis and intermittent positive pressure ventilation. Eur J Anaesthesiol. 1998;15:380.
18. King H. Curare alkaloids. Part 1—tubocurarine. J Chem Soc. 1935;5:1381–9.
19. Varney RF, Linegar CR, Holaday HA. The assay of curare by the rabbit head-drop method. J Pharmacol Exp Ther. 1949;97:72–83.
20. Hansa WR, Bennett AE. Traumatic complications of convulsive therapy. A method of preventing fractures of the spine and lower extremities. JAMA. 1939;114:2244–6.
21. Griffith HR, Johnson GE. The use of curare in general anesthesia. Anesthesiology. 1942;3:418–20.
22. Gray TC, Halton J. A milestone in anaesthesia?: (d-tubocurarine chloride). Proc R Soc Med. 1946;39:400–10.
23. Gray TC, Rees GJ. The role of apnoea in anaesthesia for major surgery. Br Med J. 1952;2:891–2.
24. Prescott F, Organe G, Rowbotham S. Tubocurarine as an adjunct to anaesthesia. Lancet. 1946;2:80–4.
25. Barnes H. Use of curare for direct oral intubation. Lancet. 1943;241:478.
26. Whitacre RJ, Fisher AJ. Clinical observations on the use of curare in anesthesia. Anesthesiology. 1945;6:124–30.
27. Smith SM, Brown HO, Toman JEP, Goodman LS. The lack of cerebral effects of d-tubocurarine. Anesthesiology. 1947;8:1–14.
28. Beecher HK, Todd DP. A study of the deaths associated with anesthesia and surgery: based on a study of 599, 548 anesthesias in ten institutions 1948–1952, inclusive. Ann Surg. 1954;140:2–35.
29. Ball C, Westhorpe R. The first synthetic nondepolarizing muscle relaxant—gallamine. Anaesth Intensive Care. 2005;33:557.
30. Bovet D, Bovet-Nitti F, HGuarino S, Longo VG. Proprietà farmacodinamiche di alcuni derivati della succinilcoline dotati di azione curarica. RC 1st Sup Sanita Roma. 1949;12:106–37.
31. Foldes FF, McNall PG, Borrego-Hinojosa JM. Succinylcholine: a new approach to muscular relaxation in anesthesiology. N Engl J Med. 1952;247:596–600.
32. Lehmann H, Ryan E. The familial incidence of low pseudocholinesterase level. Lancet. 1956;271:124.
33. Kalow W, Staron N. On distribution and inheritance of atypical forms of human serum cholinesterase, as indicated by dibucaine numbers. Can J Biochem Physiol. 1957;35:1305–20.
34. Abajian J, Arrowood JG, Barrett RH, Dwyer CS, Eversole UH, Fine JH, Hand LV, Howrie WC, Marcus PS, Martin SJ, Nicholson MJ, Saklad E, Saklad M, Sellman P, Smith RM, Woodbridge PD. Critique of "A Study of the Deaths Associated with Anesthesia and Surgery". Ann Surg. 1955;142:138–41.
35. Paton WD. Mode of action of neuromuscular blocking agents. Br J Anaesth. 1956;28:470–80.
36. Bowman WC. Neuromuscular block. Br J Pharmacol. 2006;147 Suppl 1:S277–86.
37. Rother C. Poisoned love. NY: Pinnacle, Kensington Publishing Corp.; 2005.
38. Bernauer K. Über die Konstitition der Calebassen-Alkaloide C-Dihydrotoxiferin und C-Toxiferin I und des Alkaloids Curarin V aus Strychnos Toxifera. Helv Chim Acta. 1958;41:2293.
39. Everett AJ, Lowe LA, Wilkinson S. Revision of the structures of (+)-tubocurarine and (+)-chondrocurine. J Chem Soc Chem Commun. 1970:1020–1.
40. Pauling P, Petcher TJ. Neuromuscular blocking agents: structure and activity. Chem Biol Interact. 1973;6:351–65.
41. Hewett CL, Savage DS, Lewis JJ, Sugrue MF. Anticonvulsant and interneuronal blocking activity in some synthetic amino-steroids. J Pharm Pharmacol. 1964;16:765–7.

42. Baird WL, Reid AM. The neuromuscular blocking properties of a new steroid compound, pancuronium bromide. A pilot study in man. Br J Anaesth. 1967;39:775–80.

43. Tuba Z, Maho S, Vizi ES. Synthesis and structure-activity relationships of neuromuscular blocking agents. Curr Med Chem. 2002;9:1507–36.

44. Churchill-Davidson HC, Christie TH. The diagnosis of neuromuscular block in man. Br J Anaesth. 1959;31:290–301.

45. Ali HH, Utting JE, Gray C. Stimulus frequency in the detection of neuromuscular block in humans. Br J Anaesth. 1970;42:967–78.

46. Ali HH, Utting JE, Nightingale DA, Gray C. Quantitative assessment of residual curarization in humans. Br J Anaesth. 1970;42:802–3.

47. Ali HH, Savarese JJ, Lebowitz PW, Ramsey FM. Twitch, tetanus and train-of-four as indices of recovery from nondepolarizing neuromuscular blockade. Anesthesiology. 1981;54:294–7.

48. Ali HH, Wilson RS, Savarese JJ, Kitz RJ. The effect of tubocurarine on indirectly elicited train-of-four muscle response and respiratory measurements in humans. Br J Anaesth. 1975;47:570–4.

49. Karis JH, Gissen AJ. Evaluation of new neuromuscular blocking agents. Anesthesiology. 1971;35:149–57.

50. Savarese JJ, Kitz RJ. Does clinical anesthesia need new neuromuscular blocking agents? Anesthesiology. 1975;42:236–9.

51. Miller RD, Matteo RS, Benet LZ, Sohn YJ. The pharmacokinetics of d-tubocurarine in man with and without renal failure. J Pharmacol Exp Ther. 1977;202:1–7.

52. Sheiner LB, Stanski DR, Vozeh S, Miller RD, Ham J. Simultaneous modeling of pharmacokinetics and pharmacodynamics: application to d-tubocurarine. Clin Pharmacol Ther. 1979;25:358–71.

53. Crul JF, Booij LH. First clinical experiences with ORG NC 45. Br J Anaesth. 1980;52 Suppl 1:49S–52S.

54. Durant NN, Marshall IG, Savage DS, Nelson DJ, Sleigh T, Carlyle IC. The neuromuscular and autonomic blocking activities of pancuronium, Org NC 45, and other pancuronium analogues, in the cat. J Pharm Pharmacol. 1979;31:831–6.

55. Savage DS, Sleigh T, Carlyle I. The emergence of ORG NC 45, 1-[2 beta,3 alpha,5 alpha,16 beta,17 beta]-3, 17-bis(acetyloxy)-2-(1-piperidinyl)-androstan-16-yl]-1-methylpiperidinium bromide, from the pancuronium series. Br J Anaesth. 1980;52 Suppl 1:3S-9S.

56. Shanks CA. Pharmacokinetics of the nondepolarizing neuromuscular relaxants applied to calculation of bolus and infusion dosage regimens. Anesthesiology. 1986;64:72–86.

57. Fisher DM, Canfell PC, Fahey MR, Rosen JI, Rupp SM, Sheiner LB, Miller RD. Elimination of atracurium in humans: contribution of Hofmann elimination and ester hydrolysis versus organ-based elimination. Anesthesiology. 1986;65:6–12.

58. Payne JP, Hughes R. Evaluation of atracurium in anaesthetized man. Br J Anaesth. 1981;53:45–54.

59. Caldwell JE, Szenohradszky J, Segredo V, Wright PM, McLoughlin C, Sharma ML, Gruenke LD, Fisher DM, Miller RD. The pharmacodynamics and pharmacokinetics of the metabolite 3-desacetylvecuronium (ORG 7268) and its parent compound, vecuronium, in human volunteers. J Pharmacol Exp Ther. 1994;270:1216–22.

60. Chapple DJ, Miller AA, Ward JB, Wheatley PL. Cardiovascular and neurological effects of laudanosine. Studies in mice and rats, and in conscious and anaesthetized dogs. Br J Anaesth. 1987;59:218–25.

61. Savarese JJ, Ali HH, Basta SJ, Sunder N, Moss J, Gionfriddo MA, Lineberry CG, Wastila WB, El-Sayad HA, Montague D, Braswell L. The clinical pharmacology of BW A444U. A nondepolarizing ester relaxant of intermediate duration. Anesthesiology. 1983;58:333–41.

62. Savarese JJ, Kitz RJ. The quest for a short-acting nondepolarizing neuromuscular blocking agent. Acta Anaesthesiol Scand Suppl. 1973;53:43–58.

63. Savarese JJ, Ali HH, Basta SJ, Embree PB, Scott RP, Sunder N, Weakly JN, Wastila WB, el-Sayad HA. The clinical neuromuscular pharmacology of mivacurium chloride (BW B1090U). A short-acting nondepolarizing ester neuromuscular blocking drug. Anesthesiology. 1988;68:723–32.

64. Alant O, Darvas K, Pulay I, Weltner J, Bihari I. First clinical experience with a new neuromuscular blocker pipecurium bromide. Arzneimittelforschung. 1980;30:374–9.

65. Basta SJ, Savarese JJ, Ali HH, Embree PB, Schwartz AF, Rudd GD, Wastila WB. Clinical pharmacology of doxacurium chloride. A new long-acting nondepolarizing muscle relaxant. Anesthesiology. 1988;69:478–86.

66. Viby-Mogensen J, Howardy-Hansen P, Chraemmer-Jorgensen B, Ording H, Engbaek J, Nielsen A. Posttetanic count (PTC): a new method of evaluating an intense nondepolarizing neuromuscular blockade. Anesthesiology. 1981;55:458–61.

67. Werba A, Klezl M, Schramm W, Langenecker S, Muller C, Gosch M, Spiss CK. The level of neuromuscular block needed to suppress diaphragmatic movement during tracheal suction in patients with raised intracranial pressure: a study with vecuronium and atracurium. Anaesthesia. 1993;48:301–3.

68. Engbaek J, Ostergaard D, Skovgaard LT, Viby-Mogensen J. Reversal of intense neuromuscular blockade following infusion of atracurium. Anesthesiology. 1990;72:803–6.

69. Drenck NE, Ueda N, Olsen NV, Engbaek J, Jensen E, Skovgaard LT, Viby-Mogensen J. Manual evaluation of residual curarization using double burst stimulation: a comparison with train-of-four. Anesthesiology. 1989;70:578–81.

70. Dailey PA, Fisher DM, Shnider SM, Baysinger CL, Shinohara Y, Miller RD, Abboud TK, Kim KC. Pharmacokinetics, placental transfer, and neonatal effects of vecuronium and pancuronium administered during cesarean section. Anesthesiology. 1984;60:569–74.

71. Fisher DM, Miller RD. Neuromuscular effects of vecuronium (ORG NC45) in infants and children during N_2O, halothane anesthesia. Anesthesiology. 1983;58:519–23.

72. Fisher DM, O'Keeffe C, Stanski DR, Cronnelly R, Miller RD, Gregory GA. Pharmacokinetics and pharmacodynamics of d-tubocurarine in infants, children, and adults. Anesthesiology. 1982;57:203–8.

73. Fisher DM, Cronnelly R, Miller RD, Sharma M. The neuromuscular pharmacology of neostigmine in infants and children. Anesthesiology. 1983;59:220–5.

74. Fisher DM, Cronnelly R, Sharma M, Miller RD. Clinical pharmacology of edrophonium in infants and children. Anesthesiology. 1984;61:428–33.

75. Fisher DM, Canfell PC, Spellman MJ, Miller RD. Pharmacokinetics and pharmacodynamics of atracurium in infants and children. Anesthesiology. 1990;73:33–7.

76. Fisher DM, Castagnoli K, Miller RD. Vecuronium kinetics and dynamics in anesthetized infants and children. Clin Pharmacol Ther. 1985;37:402–6.

77. Gerardi MJ, Sacchetti AD, Cantor RM, Santamaria JP, Gausche M, Lucid W, Foltin GL. Rapid-sequence intubation of the pediatric patient. Pediatric Emergency Medicine Committee of the American College of Emergency Physicians. Ann Emerg Med. 1996;28:55–74.

78. Gronert BJ, Brandom BW. Neuromuscular blocking drugs in infants and children. Pediatr Clin North Am. 1994;41:73–91.

79. Movius AJ, Martin LD. Sedation, analgesia, and neuromuscular blockade during pediatric mechanical ventilation. Respir Care Clin N Am. 1996;2:509–43.

80. Goudsouzian NG. Comparison of train-of-four and posttetanic response as guides for endotracheal intubation in children. J Clin Anesth. 1991;3:438–41.

81. Kaplan RF, Fletcher JE, Hannallah RS, Bui DT, Slaven JS, Darrow EJ, Tsai KT. The potency (ED50) and cardiovascular effects of rapacuronium (Org 9487) during narcotic-nitrous oxide-propofol anesthesia in neonates, infants, and children. Anesth Analg. 1999;89:1172–6.

82. Bowman WC. Mechanisms of action of reversal agents. In: Fukushima K, Ochiai R, editors. Muscle relaxants: physiologic and pharmacologic aspects. Tokyo: Springer; 1995. pp. 19–30.

83. Donati F, Lahoud J, McCready D, Bevan DR. Neostigmine, pyridostigmine and edrophonium as antagonists of deep pancuronium blockade. Can J Anaesth. 1987;34:589–93.

84. Bevan DR, Smith CE, Donati F. Postoperative neuromuscular blockade: a comparison between atracurium, vecuronium, and pancuronium. Anesthesiology. 1988;69:272–6.

85. Bevan DR, Kahwaji R, Ansermino JM, Reimer E, Smith MF, O'Connor GA, Bevan JC. Residual block after mivacurium with or without edrophonium reversal in adults and children. Anesthesiology. 1996;84:362–7.

86. Bowman WC, Rodger IW, Houston J, Marshall RJ, McIndewar I. Structure: action relationships among some desacetoxy analogues of pancuronium and vecuronium in the anesthetized cat. Anesthesiology. 1988;69:57–62.

87. Andrews JI, Kumar N, van den Brom RH, Olkkola KT, Roest GJ, Wright PM. A large simple randomized trial of rocuronium versus succinylcholine in rapid-sequence induction of anaesthesia along with propofol. Acta Anaesthesiol Scand. 1999;43:4–8.

88. Perry J, Lee J, Wells G. Rocuronium versus succinylcholine for rapid sequence induction intubation. Cochrane Database Syst Rev. 2003:CD002788.

89. Lien CA, Schmith VD, Belmont MR, Abalos A, Kisor DF, Savarese JJ. Pharmacokinetics of cisatracurium in patients receiving nitrous oxide/opioid/barbiturate anesthesia. Anesthesiology. 1996;84:300–8.

90. Bryson HM, Faulds D. Cisatracurium besilate. A review of its pharmacology and clinical potential in anaesthetic practice. Drugs. 1997;53:848–66.

91. Mellinghoff H, Radbruch L, Diefenbach C, Buzello W. A comparison of cisatracurium and atracurium: onset of neuromuscular block after bolus injection and recovery after subsequent infusion. Anesth Analg. 1996;83:1072–5.

92. Lighthall GK, Jamieson MA, Katolik J, Brock-Utne JG. A comparison of the onset and clinical duration of high doses of cisatracurium and rocuronium. J Clin Anesth. 1999;11:220–5.

93. Hansen-Flaschen JH, Brazinsky S, Basile C, Lanken PN. Use of sedating drugs and neuromuscular blocking agents in patients requiring mechanical ventilation for respiratory failure. A national survey. JAMA. 1991;266:2870–5.

94. Loper KA, Butler S, Nessly M, Wild L. Paralyzed with pain: the need for education. Pain. 1989;37:315–6.

95. Op de Coul AA, Lambregts PC, Koeman J, van Puyenbroek MJ, Ter Laak HJ, Gabreels-Festen AA. Neuromuscular complications in patients given Pavulon (pancuronium bromide) during artificial ventilation. Clin Neurol Neurosurg. 1985;87:17–22.

96. Tousignant CP, Bevan DR, Eisen AA, Fenwick JC, Tweedale MG. Acute quadriparesis in an asthmatic treated with atracurium. Can J Anaesth. 1995;42:224–7.

97. Segredo V, Caldwell JE, Matthay MA, Sharma ML, Gruenke LD, Miller RD. Persistent paralysis in critically ill patients after long-term administration of vecuronium. N Engl J Med. 1992;327:524–8.

98. Erhan E, Ugur G, Alper I, Gunusen I, Ozyar B. Tracheal intubation without muscle relaxants: remifentanil or alfentanil in combination with propofol. Eur J Anaesthesiol. 2003;20:37–43.

99. Inomata S, Watanabe S, Taguchi M, Okada M. End-tidal sevoflurane concentration for tracheal intubation and minimum alveolar concentration in pediatric patients. Anesthesiology. 1994;80:93–6.

100. Mencke T, Echternach M, Plinkert PK, Johann U, Afan N, Rensing H, Noeldge-Schomburg G, Knoll H, Larsen R. Does the timing of tracheal intubation based on neuromuscular monitoring decrease laryngeal injury? A randomized, prospective, controlled trial. Anesth Analg. 2006;102:306–12.

101. Mencke T, Echternach M, Kleinschmidt S, Lux P, Barth V, Plinkert PK, Fuchs-Buder T. Laryngeal morbidity and quality of tracheal intubation: a randomized controlled trial. Anesthesiology. 2003;98:1049–56.

102. Fleming NW, Chung F, Glass PS, Kitts JB, Kirkegaard-Nielsen H, Gronert GA, Chan V, Gan TJ, Cicutti N, Caldwell JE. Comparison of the intubation conditions provided by rapacuronium (ORG 9487) or succinylcholine in humans during anesthesia with fentanyl and propofol. Anesthesiology. 1999;91:1311–7.

103. Rajchert DM, Pasquariello CA, Watcha MF, Schreiner MS. Rapacuronium and the risk of bronchospasm in pediatric patients. Anesth Analg. 2002;94:488–93.

104. Jooste EH, Sharma A, Zhang Y, Emala CW. Rapacuronium augments acetylcholine-induced bronchoconstriction via positive allosteric interactions at the M3 muscarinic receptor. Anesthesiology. 2005;103:1195–203.

105. Laxenaire MC, Mertes PM. Anaphylaxis during anaesthesia. Results of a two-year survey in France. Br J Anaesth. 2001; 87:549–58.

106. Heier T, Guttormsen AB. Anaphylactic reactions during induction of anaesthesia using rocuronium for muscle relaxation: a report including 3 cases. Acta Anaesthesiol Scand. 2000;44:775–81.

107. Berg CM, Heier T, Wilhelmsen V, Florvaag E. Rocuronium and cisatracurium-positive skin tests in non-allergic volunteers: determination of drug concentration thresholds using a dilution titration technique. Acta Anaesthesiol Scand. 2003;47:576–82.

108. Levy JH, Gottge M, Szlam F, Zaffer R, McCall C. Weal and flare responses to intradermal rocuronium and cisatracurium in humans. Br J Anaesth. 2000;85:844–9.

109. Garvey LH, Roed-Petersen J, Menne T, Husum B. Danish Anaesthesia Allergy Centre—preliminary results. Acta Anaesthesiol Scand. 2001;45:1204–9.

110. Kroigaard M, Garvey LH, Menne T, Husum B. Allergic reactions in anaesthesia: are suspected causes confirmed on subsequent testing? Br J Anaesth. 2005;95:468–71.

111. Brand JB, Cullen DJ, Wilson NE, Ali HH. Spontaneous recovery from nondepolarizing neuromuscular blockade: correlation between clinical and evoked responses. Anesth Analg. 1977;56:55–8.

112. Eriksson LI, Sundman E, Olsson R, Nilsson L, Witt H, Ekberg O, Kuylenstierna R. Functional assessment of the pharynx at rest and during swallowing in partially paralyzed humans: simultaneous videomanometry and mechanomyography of awake human volunteers. Anesthesiology. 1997;87:1035–43.

113. Kopman AF, Yee PS, Neuman GG. Relationship of the train-of-four fade ratio to clinical signs and symptoms of residual paralysis in awake volunteers. Anesthesiology. 1997;86:765–71.

114. Fruergaard K, Viby-Mogensen J, Berg H, el-Mahdy AM. Tactile evaluation of the response to double burst stimulation decreases, but does not eliminate, the problem of postoperative residual paralysis. Acta Anaesthesiol Scand. 1998;42:1168–74.

115. Kirkegaard H, Heier T, Caldwell JE. Efficacy of tactile-guided reversal from cisatracurium-induced neuromuscular block. Anesthesiology. 2002;96:45–50.

116. Naguib M, Kopman AF, Lien CA, Hunter JM, Lopez A, Brull SJ. A survey of current management of neuromuscular block in the United States and Europe. Anesth Analg. 20010;111:110–9.

117. Debaene B, Plaud B, Dilly MP, Donati F. Residual paralysis in the PACU after a single intubating dose of nondepolarizing muscle relaxant with an intermediate duration of action. Anesthesiology. 2003;98:1042–8.

118. Arbous MS, Meursing AE, van Kleef JW, de Lange JJ, Spoormans HH, Touw P, Werner FM, Grobbee DE. Impact of anesthesia management characteristics on severe morbidity and mortality. Anesthesiology. 2005;102:257–68; quiz 491–2.

119. Payne JP, Hughes R, Al Azawi S. Neuromuscular blockade by neostigmine in anaesthetized man. Br J Anaesth. 1980;52:69–76.

120. Caldwell JE. Reversal of residual neuromuscular block with neostigmine at one to four hours after a single intubating dose of vecuronium. Anesth Analg. 1995;80:1168–74.

121. Eikermann M, Fassbender P, Malhotra A, Takahashi M, Kubo S, Jordan AS, Gautam S, White DP, Chamberlin NL. Unwarranted administration of acetylcholinesterase inhibitors can impair genioglossus and diaphragm muscle function. Anesthesiology. 2007;107:621–9.

122. Eikermann M, Zaremba S, Malhotra A, Jordan AS, Rosow C, Chamberlin NL. Neostigmine but not sugammadex impairs upper airway dilator muscle activity and breathing. Br J Anaesth. 2008;101:344–9.

123. Jones RK, Caldwell JE, Brull SJ, Soto RG. Reversal of profound rocuronium-induced blockade with sugammadex: a randomized comparison with neostigmine. Anesthesiology. 2008;109:816–24.

124. Belmont MR, Lien CA, Tjan J, Bradley E, Stein B, Patel SS, Savarese JJ. Clinical pharmacology of GW280430A in humans. Anesthesiology. 2004;100:768–73.

125. Lien CA, Savard P, Belmont M, Sunaga H, Savarese JJ. Fumarates: unique nondepolarizing neuromuscular blocking agents that are antagonized by cysteine. J Crit Care. 2009;24:50–7.

The Development of Local Anesthetics

Kenneth Drasner

Summary

In 1862, von Schroff found that cocaine numbed the tongue. In 1880, von Anrep recommended testing cocaine as a local anesthetic. No one listened. Koller's 1884 report that cocaine induced corneal insensibility enabled ophthalmological procedures and marked the discovery of local anesthesia. In 1884, Halsted and Hall produced peripheral nerve blocks with cocaine. Corning in 1885 and Bier in 1898 used it for spinal anesthesia. Increasing reports of central nervous system and cardiac toxicity accompanied cocaine's expanded use. Toxicity and addiction stimulated the search for alternative local anesthetics.

Einhorn patented the first new useful local anesthetic, the ester procaine, in 1904. Procaine's short duration of action limited clinical utility, a limitation Eisleb's 1928 synthesis of tetracaine overcame. However, tetracaine proved toxic if used in high-volume peripheral blocks. Lidocaine, introduced in 1948, had an amide rather than an ester linkage, imparting greater stability and eliminating concern of allergic reactions from p-aminobenzoic acid, a breakdown product of the ester compounds. Ironically, chloroprocaine (released in 1952) reverted to the ester linkage, but its rapid degradation by plasma esterases decreased the risk of systemic toxicity. Regrettably, neural injury occurred when a large dose of chloroprocaine intended for the epidural space was administered intrathecally.

Bupivacaine, a longer-acting amide anesthetic was released in 1963. Associated untoward cardiac effects were reported in the 1970s. Modifications in practice decreased the risk of these effects. Stereochemical strategies further decreased risk, resulting in levobupivacaine which had less affinity for cardiac sodium channels. The 1996 release of ropivacaine, an S (–) enantiomer followed these observations. In 1998, Weinberg suggested that intravenous infusion of lipid could decrease the availability of local anesthetics and thereby treat toxicity.

Toxic reactions with spinal lidocaine resulted in its near abandonment as a spinal anesthetic. Toxicity took two forms: a rare serious neurologic injury reported in 1991; and a frequent postoperative pain/dysesthesia reported in 1993. Ironically, chloroprocaine, once the "poster child" for local anesthetic toxicity, appears from studies reported in 2004, to be a serious contender to replace lidocaine. The dose required for spinal anesthesia is 10-fold less than that associated with injury following inadvertant intrathecal injection during epidural anesthesia.

As apparent from this story, toxicity, rather than efficacy, directed the evolution of these compounds. Importantly, present data suggest that neurotoxicity does not result from blockade of voltage-gated sodium channels, thus opening the way to the development of local anesthetics with therapeutic advantages.

The Origins of Local Anesthesia

Just as Morton's historic use of ether four decades previously marked the birth of general anesthesia, Joseph Brettauer's (1835–1905) demonstration of cocaine-induced numbing of the cornea on September 15, 1884, marked the birth of local anesthesia [1]. The event took place before the Ophthalmological Congress in Heidelberg, on a patient from the Heidelberg Eye Clinic. Carl Koller (1857–1944; Fig. 51.1),

Brettauer's Viennese colleague, had performed the work enabling this demonstration, but lacked the funds to attend the meeting. This demonstration prompted an immediate wave of experimentation, development, and clinical application. Henry Noyes (1832–1900), a renowned American ophthalmologist, attended the meeting and sent an account in a letter published less than a month later in the New York Medical Record. He commented, "The future which this discovery opens up in ophthalmological surgery and medication is obvious. The momentous value of the discovery seems likely to be in eye practice of more significance than has been the discovery of anesthesia by chloroform or ether in general surgery and medicine". More than 60 publications concerning the use of cocaine as a local anesthetic appeared in 1885 [2].

K. Drasner (✉)
Department of Anesthesia and Perioperative Care, San Francisco General Hospital, University of California, Room 3C-38, San Francisco, California, USA
e-mail: kdrasner@anesthesia.ucsf.edu

E. I Eger II et al. (eds.), *The Wondrous Story of Anesthesia*, DOI 10.1007/978-1-4614-8441-7_51, © Edmond I Eger, MD 2014

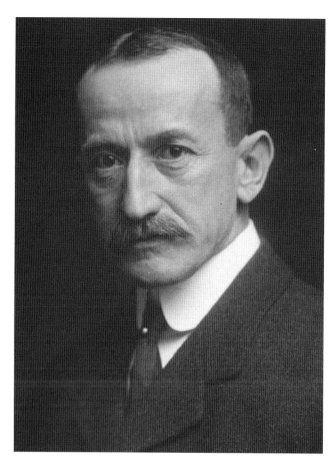

Fig. 51.1 Carl Koller (1857–1944) is recognized as the discoverer of the usefulness of cocaine for local anesthesia. (Courtesy of the National Library of Medicine, Bethesda, MD)

While Koller is recognized as the "discoverer of local anesthesia", this title may be no more valid than recognizing Christopher Columbus as the discoverer of America. Other investigators had noted the local anesthetic properties of cocaine and its potential uses before Koller's experiments and clinical application. Nonetheless, Koller was responsible for delivering cocaine as a local anesthetic into clinical practice. Perhaps a more appropriate title might be "discoverer of clinical local anesthesia". As with the ether story, a surprisingly long time extended from the recognition of cocaine's potential as an anesthetic, to the translational event bringing it into clinical use.

Although the first verified use of the coca plant (*Erythroxylum coca*) around 500 CE was established by its presence in an ancient Peruvian gravesite [3], its stimulant properties were recognized more that two millennia earlier. The Incas considered the plant to be divine, referring to the plant as khoka, or "the plant", translating to the term coca by Europeans [4]. It was used in religious ceremonies, and described as "that heavenly plant which satisfies the hungry, strengthens the weak, and makes men forget their misfortunes" [5]. Some early European explorers shared such sen-

timents. For example, Paolo Mantegazza (1831–1910), was an Italian pathologist, anthropologist, writer, and member of Parliament who worked in Argentina from 1854 to 1858. He had extensive experience with coca, and published a monograph on his return to Italy "On the hygienic and medicinal virtues of coca". His descriptions are astounding:

> "….some of the images I tried to describe in the first part of my delerium were full of poetry. I sneered at mere mortals condemned to live in this valley of tears while I, carried on the wind of two leaves of coca, went flying through the spaces of 77,438 worlds, each more splendid than the one before. An hour later, I was sufficiently calm to write these words in a steady hand 'God is unjust because he made man incapable of sustaining the effect of coca all life long. I would rather have a life span of ten years with coca than one of 1000000….(and here I have inserted a line of zeros) centuries without coca'."

The German chemist Friedrich Gardeke (1828–1890) was first to extract the active ingredient of the coca plant, doing so in 1855. He named it erythroxyline [1]. Shortly thereafter, Carl von Scherzer (1821–1903), returning from an expedition on the frigate Novarra, delivered an abundant supply of the plant to the chemist, Friedrich Woehler (1800–1882), who asked his assistant, Albert Niemann (1880–1921) to extract the alkaloid [6]. Niemann or perhaps Woehler named the product cocaine, a name with greater appeal than erythroxyline. Niemann also chewed some of the isolated compound and reported, "It numbs the tongue, and takes away both feeling and taste" [7]. In 1862, Karl von Schroff (1802–1887) reported to the Viennese Medical Society, describing the numbness cocaine produced when applied to the tongue. However, no Viennese then applied cocaine for the relief of surgical pain.

In 1868, T Moreno y Maiz [8], later the Physician-in-Chief of the Peruvian Army, reported the first systematic investigations of the anesthetic properties of cocaine. In frogs he noted that,

> "Notwithstanding that the spinal cord remains intact, we nevertheless observe disappearance of sensibility in the injected limb. It is therefore on peripheral sensibility that cocaine acetate appears to act. Furthermore the local action of the substance is very evident. Could it be used as a local anesthetic? One cannot reply on the basis of so few experiments; it is the future that will decide." [8]

These animal experiments also described cocaine's capacity to produce generalized irritability and convulsions, and self-experimentation confirmed the induction of a feeling of well-being, but Moreno y Maiz did not apply cocaine for the relief of surgical pain. Missed the gold ring, he did.

In 1880, an Estonian, B. von Anrep [9] (1852–1927) described the potential of cocaine to produce anesthesia, but failed to recognize the importance of this observation:

> "After studying the physiological actions of cocaine in animals I had intended to investigate it also in man. Various other activities have so far prevented me from doing so. Although

the experiments on animals have not had any practical consequences, I would recommend that cocaine be tested as a local anesthetic." [9]

Von Anrep did not take his own advice, with respect to surgical anesthesia although he did use it for the treatment of pain.

Koller's interest in cocaine came by way of Sigmund Freud (1856–1939), a senior colleague and friend. Freud was interested in cocaine taken orally as a possible therapeutic for various conditions including fatigue, dyspepsia, hysteria, and headaches. He also advocated its use for management of morphine addiction, prescribing it for his colleague, the notable pathologist Ernst Fleischl von Marxow (1846–1891). Von Marxow had become addicted to morphine used to treat neuropathic pain after a thumb amputation [2]. Although cocaine addiction substituted for morphine addiction, it also resulted in Von Marxow's untimely death.

While primarily interested in cocaine's systemic effects, Freud alluded to its anesthetic properties in his 1884 publication *Uber Cocain*, commenting "Indeed, the anesthetizing properties of cocaine should make it suitable for a good many further applications". He encouraged two colleagues, Leopold Konigstein and Koller, to investigate cocaine's use in ophthalmological surgery, but the former's interests focused on the treatment of pathological conditions. Freud's role in prompting Koller's investigations of cocaine are not entirely clear, but what is clear is Freud's comment, that the discovery of topical surgical anesthesia belongs to Koller [10].

A colleague of Koller's remarked on cocaine's numbing effect on the tongue [1]. Koller confirmed the resulting lack of sensitivity with self-experimentation, commenting, "At that moment it flashed upon me that I was carrying in my pocket the local anesthetic for which I had searched some years earlier. I went straight to the laboratory… and instilled this into the eye of the animal." He performed the first surgical procedure under cocaine anesthesia on a patient with glaucoma on 11 September 1884, four days before the historic Heidelberg demonstration.

It is difficult to understand the inordinate time passing between the recognition of cocaine's anesthetic properties and its clinical application. Perhaps Winston Churchill summarized it: "Men occasionally stumble over the truth, but most will pick themselves up, and hurry along as if nothing happened".

Although Koller won fame for his introduction of one of the most important contributions to medicine, he never obtained a much-desired assistantship in the University of Vienna Eye Clinic. In addition to being Jewish (hardly an asset during that period in Austria), his daughter described him as "a tempestuous young man, and one who could never be compelled to speak diplomatically even for his own good " [1]. Any hope for an appointment evaporated with an incident that put his career in jeopardy. A disagreement over

patient management caused another physician to call him either a "Jewish swine" or an "Impudent Jew." Koller hit the offender in the face. The two were reserve officers in the Austrian army and settled the matter with a sabre duel—ending after three thrusts, with Koller inflicting wounds on his opponent's head and upper arm. Koller was not wounded, at least physically, but was charged with criminal offences, which were later withdrawn [1]. Koller emigrated to New York, where he maintained a successful practice and died in 1944. He was awarded the American Ophthalmological Society's first Gold medal in 1921.

Cocaine's ability to induce insensibility was soon used for other clinical applications, including topical anesthesia in diverse areas (e.g., mucosal surfaces of the nose, throat, and urethra). Techniques for spinal anesthesia and peripheral nerve blocks were also developed, the former championed by J. Leonard Corning (1855–1923) and August Bier (1861–1949), and the latter by William Halsted (1852–1922) and Richard Hall (1856–1897).

The Emergence of Toxicity

At its introduction into clinical medicine, cocaine was thought to be remarkably safe, indeed, beneficial to health. It enjoyed widespread popularity outside mainstream medicine, notably in Vin Mariani (Fig. 51.2), a popular French tonic composed of Bordeaux wine infused with coca leaves. Such notables as Thomas Edison, Jules Verne, Rodin, HG Wells, and Pope Leo XIII (Fig. 51.3) consumed and endorsed the drink. Robert Louis Stevenson is supposed to have written "Dr Jekyll and Mr Hyde" under the influence of cocaine. It inspired John Pemberton's Coca Wine in Atlanta, Georgia. And after the introduction of prohibition in Atlanta and Fullerton County in 1886, a non-alcoholic version of the drink premiered as Coca Cola. Coca Cola continued to contain cocaine until 1903.

Many physicians also initially believed cocaine was relatively innocuous. As late as 1886, one practitioner reported to the New York Neurological Society that "I do not believe that any dose could be taken that would be dangerous" [11]. However, increasing reports of central nervous system and cardiac toxicity accompanied its expanding use. In 1887, speaking before the Kings County Medical Society, Jansen Mattison (1845-?) related 50 cases of toxicity, including 4 fatal cases. By 1891, this number had increased to 126 [11]. The significance of these complications can be appreciated by Mattison's comment that "the risk of untoward results have robbed this peerless drug of much favor in the minds of many surgeons, and so deprived them of a most valued ally." Mattison dismissed the often-held belief that toxicity was due to impurities: "It has a killing power, per se, and the purer the product, the more decided this may be."

Fig. 51.2 Vin Mariani "fortified and refreshed body & brain" with its wine and cocaine content. (A lithograph created by Jules Cheret, printed in 1894)

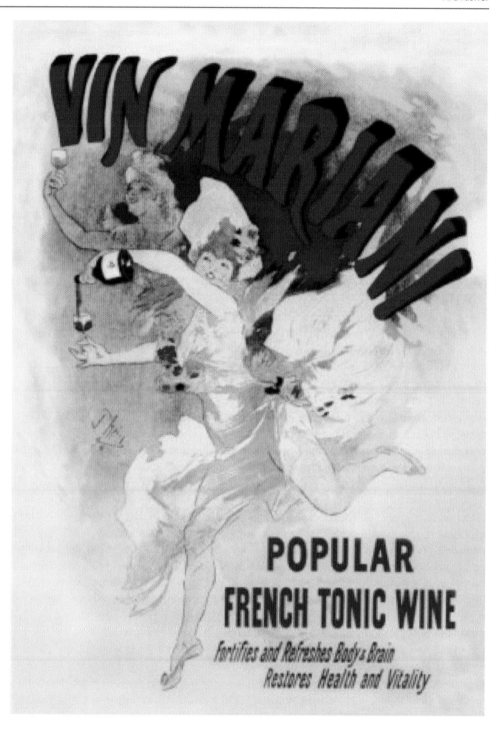

The Search for Less Toxic Local Anesthetics Begins

Toxicity and emerging issues of addiction stimulated the search for alternative topical-local anesthetics. Early investigations of natural products identified tropocaine, an alkaloid isolated from a different variety of coca, but this compound had no therapeutic advantage over cocaine [4]. Synthetic chemistry proved more fruitful. Mimicking the chemical structure of cocaine, synthetic strategies focused on benzoic acid esters. In 1890, Eduard Ritsert created benzocaine. However, its poor water solubility made it suitable only for topical anesthesia, an application sunburn sufferers still find useful. Similar synthetic efforts by Alfred Einhorn (1856–1917) and colleagues (in the employ of the Bayer Company, originally a dye works founded by Friedrich Bayer and Johann Weskott in 1863[1]) resulted in procaine, one of 18 related compounds patented in 1904 [7].

---

[1] It has no connection to Adolf von Baeyer.

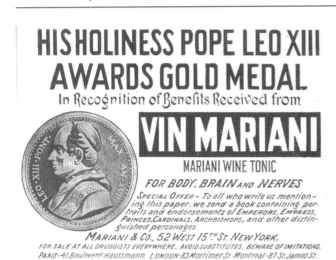

HIS HOLINESS POPE LEO XIII
AWARDS GOLD MEDAL
In Recognition of Benefits Received from
VIN MARIANI
MARIANI WINE TONIC
FOR BODY, BRAIN AND NERVES

SPECIAL OFFER – To all who write us mentioning this paper, we send a book containing por-
traits and endorsements of EMPERORS, EMPRESS,
PRINCES, CARDINALS, ARCHBISHOPS, and other distinguished personages.

MARIANI & CO., 52 WEST 15TH St. NEW YORK.
FOR SALE AT ALL DRUGGISTS EVERYWHERE. AVOID SUBSTITUTES. BEWARE OF IMITATIONS.
PARIS-41 Boulevard Haussmann, LONDON-83 Mortimer St. Montreal-87 St. James St.

Fig. 51.3 Pope Leo XIII recognized the benefits received from Vin Mariani. (From an advertisement that was printed in 1899)

Shortly after its introduction, Heinrich Braun documented the effectiveness and reduced toxicity of procaine relative to cocaine [12]. Procaine however, lacked cocaine's vasoconstrictive properties (which slow its removal into the bloodstream), and Braun made prescient comments concerning toxicity and the potential utility of epinephrine:

> "The new drug by itself cannot substitute for cocaine. To obtain results similar to those with cocaine one would have to increase the concentration and dose so much that the lower toxicity would be rendered illusionary. Fortunately, this drawback can be readily overcome with the addition of epinephrine." [12]

Although procaine had a greater therapeutic index than cocaine, this advantage did not eliminate concerns for toxicity. In response, the American Medical Association established the Committee for the Study of Toxic Effects of Local Anesthetics, under the leadership of Emil Mayer. The first publication of the committee described 43 deaths associated with the use of local anesthetics. The anesthetic was judged to have caused all but 3 deaths, including 2 that clinicians had attributed to "status lymphaticus" [13].

Although seizures (convulsions) or respiratory failure were usually the first or sole manifestation of toxicity, in some cases cardiac arrest occurred before apnea, and without convulsions. Medical errors (administration of the wrong drug or of an overdose) caused several deaths. Frequently, incorrect drug administration followed misinterpretation of verbal orders. Excessive doses of anesthetic were also administered due to lack of labeling of anesthetic solutions. The resulting recommendations for preventing such incidents (e.g., solutions should be uniquely identifiable with respect to drug and concentration, verbal orders should be minimized) paralleled modern National Patient Safety Goals. (The more things change the more they remain the same.) The committee's

review appeared to confirm cocaine's greater toxicity: although it was used less often than procaine, cocaine was associated with the majority of cases. The committee did not recommend abandoning the use of cocaine, but its recommendations effectively eliminated widespread use of cocaine as an injectable anesthetic.

The report by Mayer's committee did much to change practice and reduce the toxic manifestations of local anesthetics. However, procaine's short duration of action limited its clinical utility. This set the stage for the introduction of tetracaine, a compound synthesized in 1928 by Eisleb, and introduced into clinical practice four years later [14]. While tetracaine represented a step forward (it had a longer duration of effect than procaine), it was toxic if used in a high volume for peripheral blocks. As with procaine, its ester linkage rendered it somewhat unstable and thus not amenable to repeated sterilization by autoclaving. These characteristics ultimately led to more limited use, primarily as a spinal anesthetic, for which it still finds some application. A similar fate befell dibucaine, a compound synthesized by Meischer and introduced into clinical practice by Uhlmann.

The Woolley and Roe Case: A Major Setback for Local Anesthesia

Spinal anesthesia served as the spearhead for local anesthetic development. Sporadic reports of neurological sequelae may have tempered enthusiasm but did little to impact the use of this invaluable technique. However, the tragic occurrence of paraplegia in two patients (Albert Woolley and Cecil Roe) on a single day in 1947 at Chesterfield Royal Hospital culminated in a landmark legal case, which would profoundly impact spinal anesthesia, not just in the UK, but also throughout the world. The court ruled in the physician's favor, believing the weight of evidence overwhelming supported contamination of the anesthetic as the etiology of injury [15]. This was thought to occur from phenol used for sterilization penetrating through invisible cracks in the anesthetic ampoules. Although others have challenged this theory, alternative explanations have largely focused on contamination of the equipment used to deliver the local anesthetic rather than the anesthetic solution, again exonerating the local anesthetic [15]. Most critically, more modern techniques of ensuring sterility eliminated such risk, enabling spinal anesthesia to be conducted with impressive safely in modern practice.

Introduction of Amide Anesthetics

The commercial release of lidocaine in 1948 heralded the modern local anesthetics. Unlike procaine and tetracaine which had ester linkages, lidocaine had an amide linkage, and consequently a greater stability and longer shelf life. And unlike procaine, it did not break down to p-aminobenzoic acid, a compound believed responsible for allergic reactions. Lidocaine was not the first amide anesthetic; Niraquine, a compound abandoned because of its local irritant properties was introduced in 1898 [4].

The development of lidocaine emerged from studies of mutant barley [16, 17]. Synthesis of analogs of alkaloid isolated from these plants yielded LL30, named for the two chemists responsible for the synthesis and discovery of local anesthetic properties, Nils Löfgren (1913–1967) and Bengt Lundqvist. Lundqvist was a young chemistry student, who came to Löfgren's laboratory after the latter had synthesized LL30. Lundqvist sought something that he could experiment with, and Löfgren gave him some of the LL30. With little research money available, and no laboratory animals, Lundqvist borrowed some texts on local anesthesia from a medical student friend, and took the LL30 home. There he supposedly performed digital and spinal blocks on himself! How he would perform a spinal block on himself is unclear—it is said that he used a mirror; perhaps he had help! He then told Löfgren that LL30 was the best local anesthetic substance that existed. Also interesting is the opportunity that Pharmacia passed up by not buying the patent when it was offered to them! LL30 was named Xylocaine, or lignocaine or lidocaine.

Lofgren was a dedicated researcher, brilliant lecturer, and gifted musician. He became wealthy as a result of his discovery of lidocaine, but was increasingly frustrated with academic bureaucracy. During an episode of depression, he took his life in 1967. Lundqvist was a champion fencer, and keen sailor. At the age of 30, he suffered a head injury from which he died. His family used the royalties from his discovery to establish a fund to pay for the studies of many young and promising chemistry students [18].

In 1943, Astra Pharmaceuticals acquired the rights to lidocaine. Torsten Gordh Sr. (1907–2010) commented (personal communication): "Before lidocaine, Astra was a small local drug firm. Lidocaine was the start of ASTRA as a world wide company." The initial animal experiments performed by Leonard Goldberg, and the clinical studies undertaken by Gordh in 1945, showed that lidocaine had a greater therapeutic index than procaine [17]. Gordh (personal communication) described his studies as follows:

> "Several hundred intracutaneous and subcutaneous tests were carried out in volunteers, using different concentrations of lidocaine versus procaine, all in a double blind fashion. Then 400 clinical infiltration anesthetics were given with lidocaine without adrenaline, and another 405 with addition of adrenaline. Effects were also assessed in brachial plexus blocks, sacral blocks, and spinal anesthetics."

For the next half century, lidocaine stood as the "gold standard" for safety, enjoying enormous popularity, and provid-

ing a template for future local anesthetic synthesis. The full "Lidocaine story" is in "Xylocaine—a discovery, a drama, an industry" by Lundkvist and Sundling—1993, published at the 50-year anniversary of the original synthesis of lidocaine.

A Late-Arriving Ester

Although chloroprocaine was a reversion to the ester linkage, it became popular because of, rather than despite, its inherent instability. Francis Foldes and co-workers demonstrated that plasma esterases degraded chloroprocaine four times faster than procaine, translating to a lethal dose twice that of procaine despite chloroprocaine's greater potency [19]. Confirming this reduced potential for systemic toxicity, Ansbro et al. found that the incidence of toxic reactions with epidural administration of chloroprocaine was roughly 1/20th that of lidocaine [20]. Chloroprocaine gained widespread use in obstetrics, where its rapid degradation virtually eliminated concerns for fetal exposure.

The Long Acting, Lipid-Soluble Amides and Cardiotoxicity

The next major milestone in local anesthetic history was the development of bupivacaine, a longer-acting, lipid-soluble anesthetic released into clinical practice in Scandinavia in 1963. A similar agent, etidocaine was released shortly thereafter, but failed because it inhibited motor function more than sensory function (i.e., a patient might feel but not be able to move!) In laboratory studies, bupivacaine's systemic toxicity appeared to be equivalent to that of tetracaine and four times greater than that of mepivacaine (paralleling their relative potency) [21].

Unfortunately, clinical experiences revealed a particular potential for cardiotoxicity with bupivacaine. The first serious adverse events were reports of bradycardia and fetal demise after paracervical blocks. However, this complication was not unique to bupivacaine, nor was this complication initially described with bupivacaine [22]. In fact, it remains unsettled as to whether bupivacaine poses a greater risk than other anesthetics used for this procedure. Other early reports of adverse events associated with these lipid soluble anesthetics seemed to reflect the expected incidence of central nervous system toxicity, cardiovascular effects consistent with the physiological effects of anesthetic block, or more serious complications ascribed to patient morbidity. None of these explanations accounted for the cardiac arrest of a healthy 31-year-old man following caudal anesthesia reported by Prentiss in 1979 [23]. Despite a negative test dose, convulsions progressed almost immediately to ventricular fibrillation after administration of 25 ml of 1% etidocaine. The patient's complete recovery following a 75-minute re-suscitation is a tribute to remarkable care. Prentiss dismissed hypoxia as a potential cause, and his insightful conclusions regarding the direct effect of this lipid- soluble, highly-bound anesthetic were eclipsed by the seminal editorial published by George Albright [24] later that year.

Albright's editorial reviewed the cardiac arrest reported by Prentiss and five other similar cases, four of which had not been previously reported. Albright proposed that these local anesthetics were uniquely cardiotoxic, in that they could induce simultaneous seizures and arrest, in the ab-sence of hypoxia. Although the editorial was harshly criti-cized, experimental studies and clinical experience proved Albright correct. For example, de Jong found that doses of bupivacaine and etidocaine as low as 2/3 of those produc-ing convulsions could induce arrhythmias, while the margin between central nervous system and cardiac toxicity for lido-caine was 2.5 times wider [25].

Within 4 years, the Food and Drug Administration learned of 12 cases of cardiac arrest (10 fatal) associated with obstetrical use of 0.75% bupivacaine (the highest concentration available) [26]. Albright reported an ad-ditional 8 cases (6 fatal). The FDA then banned the use of 0.75% bupivacaine for obstetrical anesthesia, and ad-vised against the use of any concentration for paracervical blocks or intravenous regional anesthesia [27]. The reports surrounding these cases also led to widespread use of the test dose and incremental injections as standards for anes-thetic practice. These modifications proved effective, but not foolproof.

Chloroprocaine Neurotoxicity

Add a new crisis to the toxicity story. Ravindran [28] and Reisner [29] described neurologic deficits following inad-vertent intrathecal injection of solutions of Nesacaine-CE (a chloroprocaine solution containing 0.2% sodium bisulfite) intended for epidural administration. Although some of the cases lacked definitive evidence for intrathecal injection, and hypotension or total spinal anesthesia complicated other cases, it seemed clear that injury resulted from the toxicity of the anesthetic solution. Subsequent experimental studies produced conflicting results: some implicated the anesthetic, others suggested the bisulfite preservative was responsible [30]. This controversy regarding the potential neurotoxicity of Nesacaine-CE resembled earlier concerns generated by problems associated with the use of hyperbaric Durocaine for spinal anesthesia reported by Ferguson and Watkins in 1937 [31]. Here, too, the issue of whether toxicity resided in the anesthetic (10% procaine) or the vehicle components (15% ethanol, glycerine, and gum acacia) was never fully

resolved, although some experiments in cats demonstrated that 10% procaine induced similar neurologic impairment, while the vehicle did not [32].

These reports of injury associated with the use of epidural chloroprocaine led to more restricted use—but stay tuned, chloroprocaine did not disappear.

Synthetic Strategies to Reduce the Risk of Systemic Toxicity

Pharmaceutical company-supported research turned to de-creasing the cardiotoxic potential of the long-acting amides while maintaining their desirable qualities. One method re-lied on stereochemistry. Isomeric compounds have the same molecular formula. Isomers having atoms connected by the same sequence of bonds but with different spatial orienta-tions are called stereoisomers. Enantiomers are a subset of stereoisomers existing as mirror images. Enantiomers have identical physical properties except for the direction of the rotation of the plane of polarized light. This property is used to classify the enantiomer as dextrorotatory (+) if the ro-tation is to the right or clockwise, and as levorotatory (−) if it is to the left or counterclockwise. A racemic mixture contains equal parts of enantiomers and is optically inactive because the rotation caused by the molecules of one isomer cancels the opposite rotation of its enantiomer. Such chiral compounds can also be classified by their absolute configu-ration: R (Latin: rectus, or right) or S (Latin: sinistra, or left). The term chiral is derived from the Greek word for "hand," because, like right and left hands, these forms are non-super-imposable mirror images.

Bupivacaine is a racemic mixture, and investigations re-vealed that the S (−) enantiomer was less cardiotoxic than its R (+) mirror image, with subsequent marketing as (generic and trade names) levobupivacaine and Chirocaine®, respec-tively. Marketing of ropivacaine, an S (−) enantiomer, with slightly lesser potency than bupivacaine shortly followed. The substantial literature regarding the relative cardiotoxic-ity of these compounds indicates that the S (−) enantiomer is modestly less toxic [33]. In addition to this more favorable affinity for neuronal vs. cardiac sodium channels, ropiva-caine has a greater propensity to produce vasoconstriction, which might reduce cardiotoxicity. Some electrophysiologic evidence suggests the possibility that ropivacaine preferen-tially blocks C fibers, implying a greater differential block (sensory > motor). However, when reduced potency is fac-tored in, clinical studies suggest that any benefit over bu-pivacaine with respect to differential block is marginal, at best. As might be anticipated, these enantiomeric anesthetics have found their greatest use in epidural anesthesia and high-volume peripheral blocks.

Lidocaine's Fall from Grace for Spinal Anesthesia

A 1991 report described four cases of cauda equina syndrome (a clinical manifestation of injury of the nerves emerging from the end of the spinal cord) after continuous spinal anesthesia. This expanded concerns for anesthetic neurotoxicity beyond the use of chloroprocaine. Surprisingly, three of these cases, and several subsequently reported, implicated lidocaine, the "gold standard" of safety for nearly half a century [34]. In these cases, relatively large doses of lidocaine were administered through newly marketed small-bore (28-gauge) catheters designed specifically for continuous spinal anesthesia. Ken Drasner in collaboration with Kendall Healthcare's R&D team headed by Jim Cianci developed the catheters. The manuscript describing the use of the new catheter was never published. It was replaced with a manuscript describing the cases of injury collected by Drasner from three institutions, and first-authored by his research fellow, Mark Rigler [34]. This report suggested that repetitive injections, in combination with maldistribution of anesthetic, led to localized toxic concentrations in the subarachnoid space. Within a year, 8 additional cases were reported, leading to withdrawal of the catheter from the market [35].

The new catheter was not the only culprit. A case of injury to the lumbosacral roots (cauda equina syndrome) resulted when lidocaine was injected intrathecally as a (larger) dose intended for epidural administration [36]. A subsequent prospective study of regional anesthesia in France by Auroy et al. generated concern that lidocaine, itself, might induce permanent neurologic deficits, even at doses recommended for single-injection spinal anesthesia [37]. These findings led to recommendations for a reduction in the maximum acceptable dose [38].

In addition to the rare permanent spinal nerve injury associated with large doses of intrathecal lidocaine, it soon became evident that minor complications commonly follow modest doses of spinal lidocaine. In 1993, Markus Schneider and colleagues reported cases in which pain and/or dysesthesia in the buttocks and lower extremities appeared after a single intrathecal injection of lidocaine [39]. They suggested that these symptoms represented a transient neurotoxic effect of lidocaine and proposed the term "transient radicular irritation", later changed to the less specific "transient neurologic symptoms" (TNS). Karl Hampl et al., found a remarkable 37% incidence of TNS with lidocaine, while only 1 of 150 patients receiving bupivacaine was symptomatic [40, 41]. Julia Pollock and colleagues confirmed these findings [41], suggesting that the position of the patient's legs during knee arthroscopy was a risk factor for symptoms, similar to that associated with lithotomy identified by the Basel group. A large epidemiological study of 1863 patients organized by Drasner and John Freedman identified two additional risk factors, outpatient status and obesity [42]. The reason for

the enhanced risk in outpatients has yet to be established. Perhaps it results from greater invasive surgery performed on inpatients, where more intense postoperative pain could serve to distract or require more aggressive pain management, thus masking these symptoms.

Chloroprocaine Spinal Anesthesia: Back to the Future

The rare major injury with spinal lidocaine coupled with the common occurrence of TNS, created dissatisfaction with lidocaine as a spinal anesthetic. Although little evidence linked bupivacaine to toxicity, the long recovery time after its intrathecal injection made it less than ideal for short duration or outpatient procedures, procedures increasingly more common. The need for a suitable short-acting spinal anesthetic rekindled interest in chloroprocaine. How ironic that attention focused on an anesthetic, long considered the "poster child" of anesthetic neurotoxicity, to replace the "gold standard" of safety, lidocaine! Dan Kopacz, whose group at Virginia Mason conducted rigorous systematic investigations of chloroprocaine, championed its use in 2004 [43]. Published in two series of several manuscripts, their results give a picture of a spinal anesthetic well suited for outpatient procedures: a duration of action shorter than lidocaine with minimal, if any, risk of TNS.

The rationale for using chloroprocaine despite prior reports of neurologic deficits was based on the assumption that the previous injuries resulted from the bisulfite preservative and not chloroprocaine. As discussed earlier, previous work did not necessarily support this assumption. However, the most widely referenced work, experiments reported in 1984 by Gissen from an in vitro model, appeared to exonerate the anesthetic [44]. A 2004 report using a more representative in vivo model not only failed to support this conclusion, but demonstrated bisulfite to be neuroprotective [45], which may not be surprising given that it is an antioxidant. What might the reader carry away concerning the current use of chloroprocaine? On a mg for mg basis, chloroprocaine is most likely as toxic as lidocaine [29], and if modest doses are used (≤60 mg), the risk of neurotoxicity is likely to be low. This concept is currently being tested in clinical practice by off label use. As the role of bisulfite remains a little uncertain, and the entire supportive off label clinical experience has been with a preservative-free formulation, current recommendations suggest the use of a solution devoid of preservatives.

Lipid Resuscitation

Is there a remedy to local anesthetic induced cardiotoxicity? Apparent cardiotoxicity followed administration of an extremely low dose of bupivacaine (22 mg) in a patient with carnitine deficiency. Weinberg postulated that this metabolic derangement enhanced toxicity because of myocardial accumulation of fatty acids [46]. He hypothesized that giving lipid would *potentiate* cardiotoxicity. But his experiments to test this hypothesis gave an opposite answer—administering lipid afforded protection [47]. His follow-up studies confirmed this observation [48], and clinical confirmation came eight years later in a sentinel case reported by Rosenblatt [49]. The mechanisms by which lipid is effective is incompletely understood, though the predominant effect likely derives from lipid in the blood combining with local anesthetic, thereby removing it from where it causes harm (i.e., the lipid acts as a "sink"). Thus, it not only may be effective against local anesthetic central nervous system toxicity [50], but against untoward effects of non-anesthetic as well as anesthetic lipophilic drugs [51].

Systemic Local Anesthetics: Not Always a Bad Thing

Although this chapter has focused on the use of the local anesthetics to induce neural blockade resulting in anesthesia in a restricted region, these compounds also have potential beneficial effects that can be achieved through systemic administration. In addition to the well exploited effects of lidocaine on cardiac conduction, relatively low concentrations can decrease anesthetic requirement [52], reduce postoperative pain [53], and decrease chronic pain [54, 55]. The last of these derives from the fact that local anesthetics can suppress abnormal ectopic discharge by blocking sodium channels at concentrations much lower than those needed to block propagation of action potentials in normal nerves. Therefore, these drugs can be given systemically to produce salutary effects without inducing failure of normal nerve conduction. With respect to systemic effects, the following rank ordering of anesthetic effects on pain has been suggested: (1) small doses may suppress ectopic impulse generation in chronically injured peripheral nerves; (2) moderate doses may suppress central sensitization and central neuronal hyperexcitability; (3) large doses have general analgesic effects; (d) very large doses are associated with seizure activity, cardiac arrhythmias, and cardiovascular collapse [56].

The Future

Two pharmacophores, compounds with amide versus ester linkages, have supplied most of the local anesthetics of the last century. Much of their history has been driven by the discovery of individual members of each family and by exploration of issues of safety, rather than efficacy. Despite their seeming safety, these compounds have a relatively narrow therapeutic index. A fundamental question is whether a common mechanism mediates toxicity and effect. If so, they are inextricably linked, and a narrow therapeutic index is inevitable. However, Shinichi Sakura in Drasner's lab demonstrated that neurotoxicity does not result from blockade of the voltage-gated sodium channel [57], the basis for local anesthesia. Development of anesthetics with greater therapeutic advantage is thus a realistic goal.

References

1. Becker HK. Carl Koller and cocaine. Psychoanal Q. 1963;32:309–73.
2. Grzybowski A. Cocaine and the eye: a historical overview. Ophthalmologica. 2008;222:296–301.
3. Goldberg R. Drugs across the spectrum. 5th ed. Belmont: Thomson; 2006.
4. Ruetsch YA, Boni T, Borgeat A. From cocaine to ropivacaine: the history of local anesthetic drugs. Curr Top Med Chem. 2001;1:175–82.
5. Russell SA. The new anaesthetic—chloride of cocaine. Albany Med Ann. 1884;5:333–8.
6. Woehler F. Ueber eine organische Base in der Coca. Justus Liebig's Annalen der Chemie. 1860;114:213–17.
7. Ring ME. The history of local anesthesia. J Calif Dent Assoc. 2007;35(4):275–82.
8. Morenoy MT. Recherches chimiques et physiologigues sure l'erythroxylon coca du Perou et la cocaine. Paris 1868:77.
9. Anrep Bv. Ueber die physiologische Wirkung des Cocain. Pflueger's Archiv fuer die gesamte Physiologie. 1879;21:38–77.
10. Galbis-Reig D. Sigmund Freud and Carl Koller: the controversy surrounding the discovery of local anesthesia. International Congress Series. 2002;1242:571–5.
11. Mattison JB. Cocaine poisoning. Med Surg Rep. 1891;115:645–50.
12. Braun H. Ueber einige neue ortliche Anaesthetica (Stovain, Alypin, Novocain). Deutsche klinische Wochenschrift. 1905;31:1667–1.
13. Mayer E. The toxic effects following the use of local anesthetics. JAMA. 1924;82:876–85.
14. Brown DL, Fink BR. The history of neural blockad and pain management. In: Cousins MJ, Bridenbaugh LD, Editors. Neural blockade in clinical anesthesia and management of pain. 3rd ed. Philadelphia: Lippincott-Raven; 1998. pp. 3–27.
15. Hutter CD. The Woolley and Roe case: a reassessment. Anaesthesia. 1990;45:859–64.
16. Gordh T. Xylocain GT. A new local analgesic. Anaesthesia. 1949;4:4–9.
17. Holmdahl MH. Xylocain (lidocaine, lignocaine), its discovery and Gordh's contribution to its clinical use. Acta Anaesthesiol Scand Suppl. 1998;113:8–12.
18. Lunqvist K, Sundling S. Xylocaine—a discovery—a Drama—an industry. Astra 1993.
19. Foldes FF, Mc NP. 2-Chloroprocaine: a new local anesthetic agent. Anesthesiology. 1952;13(3):287–96.
20. Ansbro FP, Blundell AE, Furlong RE, Pillion JW, Bodell B. Chloroprocaine (nesacaine); its relative nontoxicity as demonstrated by epidural anesthesia. AMA Arch Surg. 1959;78:75–8.
21. Henn F, Brattsand R. Some pharmacological and toxicological properties of a new long-acting local analgesic, LAC-43 (marcaine), in comparison with mepivacaine and tetracaine. Acta Anaesthesiol Scand Suppl. 1966;21:9–30.
22. Nyirjesy I, Hawks BL, Hebert JE, Hopwood HG Jr, Falls HC. Hazards of the Use of Paracervical Block Anesthesia in Obstetrics. Am J Obstet Gynecol. 1963;87:231–5.

23. Prentiss JE. Cardiac arrest following caudal anesthesia. Anesthesiology. 1979;50:51–3.

24. Albright GA. Cardiac arrest following regional anesthesia with etidocaine or bupivacaine. Anesthesiology. 1979;51:285–7.

25. Jong RH de, Ronfeld RA, DeRosa RA. Cardiovascular effects of convulsant and supraconvulsant doses of amide local anesthetics. Anesth Analg. 1982;61(1):3–9.

26. Adverse Reactions with Bupivacaine. FDA Drug Bull 1984;13:23.

27. Administration FaD. Adverse reactions with bupivacaine. FDA Drug Bull. 1983;12:23.

28. Ravindran RS, Turner MS, Muller J. Neurologic effects of subarachnoid administration of 2-chloroprocaine- CE, bupivacaine, and low pH normal saline in dogs. Anesth Analg. 1982;61:279–83.

29. Reisner LS, Hochman BN, Plumer MH. Persistent neurologic deficit and adhesive arachnoiditis following intrathecal 2-chloroprocaine injection. Anesth Analg. 1980;59:452–4.

30. Drasner K. Chloroprocaine spinal anesthesia: back to the future? Anesth Analg. 2005;100:549–52.

31. Ferguson F, Watkins K. Paralysis of the bladder and associated neurologic sequelae of spinal anaesthesia (cauda equina syndrome). Br J Surg. 1937;25:735–52.

32. Macdonald A, Watkins K. An experimental investigation into the cause of paralysis following spinal anesthesia. Br J Surg. 1937;25:879.

33. Heavner JE. Cardiac toxicity of local anesthetics in the intact isolated heart model: a review. Reg Anesth Pain Med. 2002;27:545–55.

34. Rigler ML, Drasner K, Krejcie TC, Yelich SJ, Scholnick FT, DeFontes J, et al. Cauda equina syndrome after continuous spinal anesthesia. Anesth Analg. 1991;72:275–81.

35. Safety Alert FDA. Cauda equina syndrome associated with the use of small-bore catheters in continuous spinal anesthesia; May 29, 1992.

36. Drasner K, Rigler ML, Sessler DI, Stoller ML. Cauda equina syndrome following intended epidural anesthesia. Anesthesiology. 1992;77:582–5.

37. Auroy Y, Narchi P, Messiah A, Litt L, Rouvier B, Samii K. Serious complications related to regional anesthesia: results of a prospective survey in France. Anesthesiology. 1997;87:479–86.

38. Drasner K. Lidocaine spinal anesthesia: a vanishing therapeutic index? Anesthesiology. 1997;87:469–72.

39. Schneider M, Ettlin T, Kaufmann M, Schumacher P, Urwyler A, Hampl K, et al. Transient neurologic toxicity after hyperbaric subarachnoid anesthesia with 5 % lidocaine. Anesth Analg. 1993;76:1154–7.

40. Hampl KF, Schneider MC, Ummenhofer W, Drewe J. Transient neurologic symptoms after spinal anesthesia. Anesth Analg. 1995;81:1148–53.

41. Pollock JE, Neal JM, Stephenson CA, Wiley CE. Prospective study of the incidence of transient radicular irritation in patients undergoing spinal anesthesia. Anesthesiology. 1996;84:1361–7.

42. Freedman JM, Li DK, Drasner K, Jaskela MC, Larsen B, Wi S. Transient neurologic symptoms after spinal anesthesia: an epidemiologic study of 1,863 patients. Anesthesiology. 1998;89:633–41.

43. Kouri ME, Kopacz DJ. Spinal 2-chloroprocaine: a comparison with lidocaine in volunteers. Anesth Analg. 2004;98:75–80.

44. Gissen A, Datta S, Lambert D. The chloroprocaine controversy. II. Is chloroprocaine neurotoxic? Reg Anesth. 1984;9:135–44.

45. Taniguchi M, Bollen AW, Drasner K. Sodium bisulfite: scapegoat for chloroprocaine neurotoxicity? Anesthesiology. 2004;100:85–91.

46. Weinberg GL, Laurito CE, Geldner P, Pygon BH, Burton BK. Malignant ventricular dysrhythmias in a patient with isovaleric acidemia receiving general and local anesthesia for suction lipectomy. J Clin Anesth. 1997;9:668–70.

47. Weinberg GL, VadeBoncouer T, Ramaraju GA, Garcia-Amaro MF, Cwik MJ. Pretreatment or resuscitation with a lipid infusion shifts the dose-response to bupivacaine-induced asystole in rats. Anesthesiology. 1998;88:1071–5.

48. Weinberg G, Ripper R, Feinstein DL, Hoffman W. Lipid emulsion infusion rescues dogs from bupivacaine-induced cardiac toxicity. Reg Anesth Pain Med. 2003;28:198–202.

49. Rosenblatt MA, Abel M, Fischer GW, Itzkovich CJ, Eisenkraft JB. Successful use of a 20 % lipid emulsion to resuscitate a patient after a presumed bupivacaine-related cardiac arrest. Anesthesiology. 2006;105:217–8.

50. Spence AG. Lipid reversal of central nervous system symptoms of bupivacaine toxicity. Anesthesiology. 2007;107:516–7.

51. Cave G, Harvey M. Intravenous lipid emulsion as antidote beyond local anesthetic toxicity: a systematic review. Acad Emerg Med. 2009;16:815–24.

52. Himes RS Jr, DiFazio CA, Burney RG. Effects of lidocaine on the anesthetic requirements for nitrous oxide and halothane. Anesthesiology. 1977;47:437–40.

53. Cassuto J, Wallin G, Hogstrom S, Faxen A, Rimback G. Inhibition of postoperative pain by continuous low-dose intravenous infusion of lidocaine. Anesth Analg. 1985;64:971–4.

54. Abram SE, Yaksh TL. Systemic lidocaine blocks nerve injuryinduced hyperalgesia and nociceptor-driven spinal sensitization in the rat. Anesthesiology. 1994;80:383–91. (Discussion 25A).

55. Tremont-Lukats IW, Challapalli V, McNicol ED, Lau J, Carr DB. Systemic administration of local anesthetics to relieve neuropathic pain: a systematic review and meta-analysis. Anesth Analg. 2005;101:1738–49.

56. Dirks J, Fabricius P, Petersen KL, Rowbotham MC, Dahl JB. The effect of systemic lidocaine on pain and secondary hyperalgesia associated with the heat/capsaicin sensitization model in healthy volunteers. Anesth Analg. 2000;91:967–72.

57. Sakura S, Bollen AW, Ciriales R, Drasner K. Local anesthetic neurotoxicity does not result from blockade of voltage-gated sodium channels. Anesth Analg. 1995;81:338–46.

Anesthesia Machines and Breathing Systems: An Evolutionary Success Story

52

Jerry A. Dorsch and Susan E. Dorsch

Summary

The first anesthetists delivered ether and chloroform from handkerchiefs, towels or inhalers, and nitrous oxide from large reservoirs such as bladders. In 1847, Snow devised a temperature-compensated vaporizer that delivered fully saturated ether in air. Clover improved matters in 1877 by adding liquid chloroform to a large measured gas volume to produce a known concentration. Except for the French Ombrédanne ether inhaler, the United Kingdom provided most advances in vaporizer equipment. Delivered concentrations of anesthetic were usually inexact until 1951 when Morris introduced the Copper Kettle vaporizer to deliver a concentration that could be precisely calculated. In the mid-1950s, Cyprane produced the Fluotec, a "variable bypass vaporizer" that allowed the user to set any desired concentration, eliminating the calculations required with the Copper Kettle.

Early nitrous oxide anesthesia produced insensibility partly from hypoxia. In 1868, Andrews suggested adding oxygen, but no convenient method to do so was available until the 1880s when steel cylinders to contain liquid nitrous oxide and compressed oxygen enabled the delivery of roughly controlled nitrous oxide concentrations. Flowmeters were needed. Cotton and Boothby devised a sight-feed device for visualizing gas flow. In 1913, Gwathmey adapted this as a bubble flowmeter, and Heidbrink improved this device. In 1908, Kuppers introduced what became the primary method of measuring gas flow for most of the twentieth century, the rotameter. In the twenty-first century, electronic flow control replaced the rotameter.

Anesthesia breathing systems replaced simple inhalers. Anesthesia providers increasingly used carbon dioxide absorption systems to minimize delivery of expensive or explosive anesthetics. Water's to-and-fro system competed with the circle system suggested by Jackson in 1916. In 1926, Dragerwerk of Germany developed the first circle breathing system for use on their anesthesia machine. In 1954, Mapleson classified and clarified the function of breathing systems without absorbents. Perhaps the most important development shaping today's anesthesia machines was the 1979 adoption of an anesthesia machine standard written jointly by clinicians and industry engineers. This standard eliminated potential dangers with previous machines.

For many years, anesthesia machines and monitors were sold separately. Displays, controls and alarms of different devices varied, predisposing to confusion and difficulty in management. In the 1990s the distinction between anesthesia machine, ventilator and monitors started to blur. All were integrated into an "anesthesia workstation" so that all modalities were controlled and displayed consistently and in one place, with alarms coordinated and prioritized. Anesthesia delivery systems continue to evolve in ways that improve safety.

Introduction: Early Inhalers

On 16 October 1846, William Morton conducted the first successful public demonstration of surgical anesthesia [1]. That demonstration had two crucial elements. The first was ether's miraculous anesthetic effect. The second was a device that delivered ether in concentrations sufficient to produce anesthesia without killing the patient. The original device (Fig. 52.1) was a glass globe with two necks. The patient breathed in from a brass tube attached to one neck and air entered through the other. The globe usually contained a sponge soaked with ether [2]. The sponge restrained the liquid within the globe—otherwise if tipped the wrong way, the patient might inhale liquid ether. Completing the device were two leather valves in the brass tube, directing the flow of the ether-containing air to the patient, and diverting the expired breath into the room.

Morton's carefully made device (he was late for the first demonstration because his instrument maker was adding last-minute improvements) provided no way of accurately

S. E. Dorsch (✉)
Orange Park, FL, USA
e-mail: jdors556@bellsouth.net

J. A. Dorsch
Mayo Clinic Jacksonville, Jacksonville, FL, USA

E. I Eger II et al. (eds.), *The Wondrous Story of Anesthesia*, DOI 10.1007/978-1-4614-8441-7_52, © Edmond I Eger, MD 2014

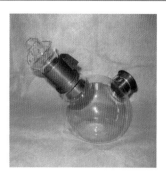

Fig. 52.1 This replica of Morton's Inhaler shows the reservoir (globe) that contained the ether. The mouthpiece is to the left. A sponge was often placed in the globe, increasing the surface available for vaporization, but more importantly holding the ether so that liquid anesthetic would not be inhaled. (Courtesy of Wood Library-Museum of Anesthesiology, Park Ridge, IL.)

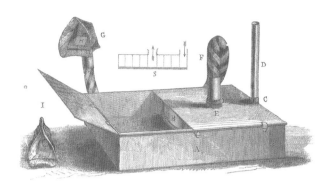

controlling the ether concentration inhaled by the patient. It was made of glass, a poor conductor of heat. Cooling of the ether caused by its vaporization decreased the delivered concentration. Morton had little or no understanding of the physics involved. This limitation did not apply to the next character in our story.

News of the discovery of anesthesia quickly reached Britain. Physician John Snow appreciated the great significance of the discovery and set out to apply it in his practice. Unlike Morton, Snow understood the physical principles needed to deliver a controlled concentration of ether (or chloroform) and in 1847 constructed an elegant ether inhaler (Fig. 52.2). Air entered the vaporizer and passed through a metal spiral to maximize contact between the air and the ether, thus ensuring a saturated output (i.e., a constant output if the temperature was held constant). Snow immersed the vaporizing chamber in a water bath, to stabilize the temperature. He added a crude means (see below) to dilute the concentration delivered to the patient and connected the vaporizer to the patient with tubing of sufficient width to minimize resistance to breathing. This tubing was connected to a mask edged with leather that molded to fit the patient's face. Some of these features in Snow's vaporizer applied principles used in modern vaporizers.

Snow's vaporizer allowed administration of a constant maximum concentration of anesthetic, useful for induction of anesthesia with ether, the agent for which it was originally devised. The high solubility of ether in blood limited the rate at which induction could be accomplished, and although high concentrations could irritate the airway, they hastened the process. Induction was the principal focus because early in the history of anesthesia, most operations were brief. The introduction of chloroform changed things. Airway irritation was minimal. Unlike ether, chloroform profoundly depressed the heart, making it important to not deliver a maximum concentration for too long. Snow solved this problem by adding a valve on his facemask that could be opened to dilute the delivered anesthetic with room air. Still, control over the delivered concentration was crude.

Joseph Clover solved some of these problems but added others. In 1877, he invented an "inhaler" for chloroform. By

Fig. 52.2 Snow's Inhaler. The air inlet was on the peripheral side (at the right). The drum contained a metal spiral with five turns. This allowed the air to become saturated with anesthetic vapor. Note the wide bore tube which extended from the center to the patient mask. (From Snow J: On the Inhalation of the Vapour of Ether in Surgical Operations: Containing a Description of the Various Stages of Etherization, and a Statement of the Result of Nearly Eighty Operations in Which Ether Has Been Employed In St. George's and University College Hospitals. London: John Churchill; 1847. pp 1–88.)

putting a measured amount of liquid chloroform into a large reservoir bag of known volume, he could produce a large amount of chloroform vapor in air at a known concentration. The bag was connected to a face mask, including a leaflet valve that allowed exhalation into the operating room. Air could be admitted from the room (thereby diluting the chloroform concentration) by turning the leaflet to the side. Interestingly, the mask and bag connectors had 22 mm diameters, the dimension used today and one that did not impose significant resistance to breathing. Unfortunately Clover's device was cumbersome and had limited popularity. Clover died in 1882 and was buried 200 yards from Snow's grave. One wonders what conversations they have when all is quiet.

Nitrous Oxide

Horace Wells had failed in his January 1845 attempt to demonstrate the anesthetic properties of nitrous oxide. The audience ridiculed Wells, calling the demonstration a humbug, and for nearly two decades nitrous oxide lapsed into obscurity. Gardner Colton resurrected nitrous oxide in the early 1860s. He gave it to more than 100,000 patients for dental procedures without, it is said, a fatality–a remarkable record.

Several problems surrounded the early use of nitrous oxide. First, in normal patients, the anesthetizing partial pressure exceeds atmospheric pressure. To achieve anesthesia, the earliest users administered 100% nitrous oxide, a lethal concentration if given for more than a minute or two because of the associated lack of oxygen. Nonetheless, nitrous oxide in air or occasionally 100% nitrous oxide for induction was used until the 1940s, with anesthesia resulting from a combination of nitrous oxide and hypoxia.

Second, because nitrous oxide was a gas, it could not be conveniently stored. It could be manufactured on the spot by heating (with great care, as the process could result in an explosion) ammonium nitrate in a retort [3]. The resulting nitrous oxide was purified by washing it in various reagents and stored in a reservoir—at first a bag made from oiled silk or animal bladders, and later in a gasometer (a small version of the enormous cylinders we see that are used to store natural gas). In 1865, the SS White Dental Manufacturing Co of Philadelphia made a storage bag. A valve was attached to the bag to control the release of the gas to the patient through a wooden mouthpiece. The patient held the mouthpiece with one hand while the nostrils were held closed with the other hand or a nose clip, in order to prevent air dilution. The clumsiness of this system limited its popularity.

The development of low pressure compressed gas cylinders in 1868 decreased the clumsiness; away with the cumbersome bladder/bag. In 1870, nitrous oxide was liquefied. Liquid nitrous oxide was supplied in cylinders by both Coxeter and Son, and Barth in Great Britain. By 1873, Johnson Brothers of New York were supplying similar cylinders to the American market. An attachment to the cylinder led to a large reservoir bag attached to a mask [4]. There was a supplemental bag, a valve to admit nitrous oxide directly into the mask, and an evacuation valve.

Why were these considerable efforts made, to overcome the difficulties and limitations imposed by the large volumes of nitrous oxide needed to provide anesthesia? Nitrous oxide offered two advantages over the then-popular ether: it acted quickly and didn't irritate the airway. These properties complemented those of ether, reducing the slowness and untoward respiratory effects of ether, which were particularly problematic during induction. Around 1876, Clover designed a portable apparatus to deliver nitrous oxide and ether. A nitrous oxide cylinder supplied gas to an ether vessel (vaporizer) with a 6 liter bag connecting the vaporizer to a mask. Air or the nitrous oxide-ether combination could be admitted to the bag. Inadequate oxygen (hypoxia) evidenced by cyanosis caused the patient to breathe more, accelerating the uptake of anesthetic. When marked cyanosis occurred, fresh air was admitted by lifting the face mask.

A few perceptive people recognized the problems imposed by the lack of oxygen. It is not known when oxygen was first used with chloroform, but Snow used it in an unsuccessful resuscitation of a patient given chloroform. In 1868, Edmund Andrews, a Northwestern University surgeon, suggested adding oxygen to nitrous oxide. So did Paul Bert and Clover. In 1879, Bert combined 15 % oxygen with 85 % nitrous oxide to produce anesthesia in a pressure (hyperbaric) chamber. But such an approach was a logistical nightmare. A more practical solution was to go back to a combination of nitrous oxide, oxygen, and ether (called gas, oxygen and ether or GOE). Such a solution was not practical before 1885 when oxygen became available in cylinders. But GOE was not immediately adopted because the importance of using oxygen with nitrous oxide was not widely appreciated until after the turn of the twentieth century. Anesthesia providers continued to use nitrous oxide and air, not recognizing the potential negative effect on patient intelligence.

The availability of both nitrous oxide and oxygen in cylinders meant that large volumes of each could be stored efficiently, and this allowed development of apparatus delivering both. In 1886, Viennese dentist HT Hillischer produced the first machine dispensing both nitrous oxide and oxygen and coined the term "Schlafgas" (sleeping gas) to describe nitrous oxide. He found it best in most cases to commence with 10 percent oxygen/90 percent nitrous oxide, and to gradually increase this to 15 or even 20 percent oxygen. In dealing with alcoholic subjects and others resistant to the influence of nitrous oxide with 10 percent oxygen, he reduced the oxygen to 5 percent or even lower. If breathing became labored, or cyanosis appeared, he increased the percentage of oxygen. Hillischer used a proportioning valve to achieve the target percentages of oxygen. But his proportioning valve was a crude device. Something better was needed.

In 1885, SS White patented what today's clinicians might recognize as an anesthesia machine. Gases were supplied from cylinders to separate inflatable bags then directed to a mixing chamber between the oxygen and nitrous oxide controls and delivered to the patient through wide bore tubing. The tap on the nitrous oxide bag needed to be fully opened, and a similar tap for oxygen allowed a variable flow according to uncalibrated gradations on a semi-circular gauge plate. By 1910 the SS White anesthesia machine had yokes for 4 cylinders, and reducing valves (pressure regulators) that decreased the high but variable pressure of gas from cylinders to a lower more constant level [5].

Gas Flow Measurement

Early anesthetic apparatus lacked a means to deliver precisely known flows (and therefore concentrations) of oxygen and nitrous oxide in the gases presented to the patient [6]. In 1902, dentist Charles Teter developed a gas machine that delivered a variable mixture of oxygen and nitrous oxide, each controlled by separate but coarse valves. There was no indicator of percentage or flow [7]. In 1916, after observing the principles of a mercury sphygmomanometer, Teter added mercury columns to his machine, calibrated to indicate gas flows.

Another dentist, Jay Heidbrink, purchased one of Teter's machines in 1906, and set about improving it. He reasoned that better accuracy could be achieved by equalizing the pressure in the two bags supplying gas from the cylinders to the adjustable valves, and that the valves could be engineered to give finer control. An additional problem was moisture in the nitrous oxide, which often led to freezing of the nitrous oxide valve. Heidbrink solved this by placing an electric light bulb in the mixing chamber. Still, the machine had no indicator of gas flow. He achieved an acceptable calibration of flow control by adopting commercially available pressure-reducing valves and further refining the control valves. His first commercial machine was the Model A, introduced in 1912. He sold them for $1 per pound weight, $32 each.

In 1911, Frederick Cotton and Walter Boothby developed the first anesthesia machine that provided a visible indication of the rate of flow of nitrous oxide and oxygen. Each gas was fed separately into a water-filled glass mixing chamber. The rate of bubbling in the "bubble bottle" allowed an estimation of the flow and proportion of the gases. After exiting the first mixing chamber, a portion of the gas mixture could be directed through another chamber containing ether before rejoining the main gas stream.

In the following year, James Gwathmey improved on Cotton and Boothby's idea by placing "bubble tubes" for each gas within the water sight feed bottle. Each tube had five holes, allowing from one to five streams of bubbles to be seen, thus indicating the gas flow. This was the forerunner of the 1917 Boyle apparatus, developed by Henry Boyle after meeting Gwathmey and purchasing one of his machines in 1912. James Gwathmey was one of the first physicians to practice anesthesia full time. He was president of the New York Society of Anesthesiologists, the forerunner of the American Society of Anesthesiologists.

Richard von Foregger (1872–1960), was born in Vienna, studied chemistry and emigrated to the US in 1898 [8]. In 1905, he began development of an oxygen generator using "oxone" or fused sodium peroxide. In 1907, he met Gwathmey, by which time the oxygen generator was a commercial success. In 1909, they produced an ether-oxygen device using an oxygen generator. On several occasions, Foregger and Gwathmey took the generator to Madison Square and administered oxygen to runners in 10-mile relay races and 6-day bicycle races. In 1914, Foregger established the Foregger Company and began manufacturing Gwathmey's anesthesia machines.

Foregger later developed the water depression flowmeter A competing CIG flowmeter is shown in Fig. 52.3. Gas flowing past a restriction in the top of the flowmeter depressed the water level in a tube submerged in a water-filled container, in proportion to the gas flow. This worked

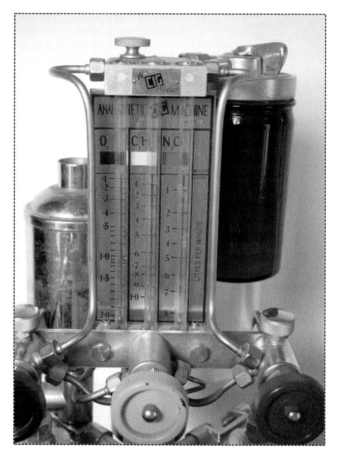

Fig. 52.3 In these CIG water depression flowmeters, the water meniscus was at the black line just above the mark indicating a 1 liter per minute flow rate when there was no gas flow. Flow depressed the meniscus non-linearly, with the greatest change occurring at the higher flows (the opposite of what might be desired)

well as long as the flow did not exceed that which produced the maximum intended depression of the water level in the tube. Flows exceeding that limit forced gas into the water-filled container with a violence that depended on the flow. In some training programs no resident entered the "anesthetic brotherhood" until he had fully opened the oxygen valve to the flowmeter, blowing water all over the operating room.

Dry Flowmeters

Karl Kuppers in Germany, introduced the rotating bobbin flowmeter, the "Rotamesser", in 1909 for industrial purposes, and gynecologist Maximillian Neu used it in an anesthesia apparatus in 1910 [9]. It went into commercial production, but did not become widely known. Rotameters were not used again until 1937, when once more they were adapted to anesthesia machines, this time in Britain.

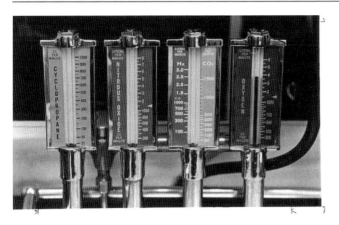

Fig. 52.4 As shown on the oxygen flowmeter on the right, gas flow through these Heidbrink flowmeters caused the indicator to rise in the tube. Note that one flowmeter (flowmeter number 3 in the illustration) could be used for either helium or carbon dioxide

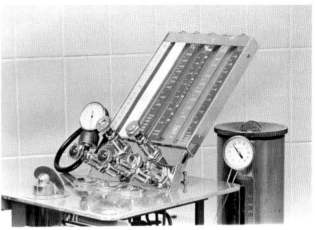

Fig. 52.5 In Foregger and Connell flowmeters one or two balls rose with increasing flow, and the flow was read at the juncture of the two balls. At the right is a Copper Kettle vaporizer. At the front of the machine is the on-off valve that controlled flow to the vaporizer. The flowmeter for the Copper Kettle is at the left. Note the thermometer at the top of the Copper Kettle

American anesthesia providers working in British hospitals during World War II gained experience with rotameters and recognized their advantages. They were first used in American machines in 1950 by Foregger, and quickly became the gold standard for measuring gas flows.

In 1933, Heidbrink invented a tapered tube flowmeter (Fig. 52.4; really a variant of the rotameter), where a disc was attached to a stem, the disc rising in the tapered tube with increasing gas flows, the tip of the stem indicating the flow on a calibrated scale. It presented a graded visual display of flows for oxygen and nitrous oxide, the gases merging as they exited from the flowmeters. An improved version appeared on his Heidbrink machine in 1938.

The Coxeter dry bobbin flowmeter (1933) consisted of a glass tube of uniform diameter with 24 small holes in the wall. An H-shaped bobbin in the tube rose with increasing gas flow, the flow exiting the tube through the holes. As flow increased, the bobbin rose and more gas left the tube through the holes. This flowmeter was relatively inaccurate because friction or dirt between the bobbin and the wall impeded the rise or fall of the bobbin. Since the bobbin moved in steps from hole to hole, it could not measure intermediate flows, and was inaccurate at low flows. These flowmeters were used in the 1933 Boyle machine that was the forerunner of the modern anesthesia machine. It is said that Boyle placed the oxygen flowmeter on the left because he was left handed. Machines manufactured in the US placed it on the right.

The Connell flowmeter was patented in 1934. The six-inch flow tube contained two ball bearings that rose with increasing flow inside a tilted glass tube with a tapered bore. Two ball bearings were needed to ensure steady movement and prevent each ball from oscillating in the tube. Gas flow was noted by the point where the two balls touched. Foregger also marketed a flowmeter that was inclined at an angle

and used a ball indicator (Fig. 52.5). It also had shape-coded flow control knobs.

Ultimately, the rotameter became the most popular means of measuring gas flow in anesthesia, appearing on virtually all anesthesia machines up to the end of the twentieth century, when electronic measurement devices and displays replaced tapered tubes.

Intermittent Flow Machines: A Digression

The machines described above delivered a constant flow of gas, much of which was wasted [10, 11]. Intermittent flow machines were devised to decrease this waste, and supply only what the patient needed. They delivered a controlled mixture of gases in a volume "demanded" by the spontaneously breathing patient. They featured a mixing device for oxygen and nitrous oxide. The McKesson Nargraf machine (see Fig. 6.3) was the most popular. It could be set to deliver an oxygen percentage from 0% to 100%. The negative pressure generated by the patient during inhalation initiated gas flow from the machine. The flow ended when the patient stopped inhaling. A one-way valve at the patient end of the breathing system opened, so that exhalation to the room could occur.

One of McKesson's techniques, referred to as secondary saturation, used 100% nitrous oxide until severe cyanosis and muscular rigidity or spasm appeared. Oxygen was then added to the inhaled mixture. It was an exciting approach to anesthesia, but most anesthesia providers preferred not to bring their patients so close to death. Also, it was difficult to deliver a potent anesthetic [12]. Of note, with this apparatus and technique, anesthesia with halothane could be induced in 11 seconds. There is much more to the McKesson history, including the fact that the McKesson Nargraf machine in 1930 incorporated automated anesthesia record keeping.

The Evolving Anesthesia Machine

Anesthesia machines began to take the form initiated by the Boyle machine. In early machines, the Boyle bottle and direct-reading vaporizers like the Fluotec could be placed in the tubing between the machine outlet and the breathing system. If the gas flow in the fresh delivery tubing from the machine was attached (incorrectly) to the outflow connection to the vaporizer, a higher-than-expected output could result. In addition, these vaporizers handled the high flow from the oxygen flush poorly. Coxeters, the manufacturers of the Boyle machine, continuously modified and improved it. By 1927, the rubber hoses had been replaced by a large bore rigid tube between the flowmeters and the vaporizers. Later, the whole apparatus was incorporated into a table on wheels. The Boyle configuration persisted until the 1990s when major changes in anesthesia machines began to appear.

In 1978, Jeff Cooper and his colleagues at the Massachusetts General Hospital exhibited a completely computer-controlled anesthesia machine (the Boston Anesthesia System or MGH machine) [13]. It was never used for humans but was the first to suggest that a computerized machine was possible. In the 1990s anesthesia machines began to incorporate microprocessor-based technology. Computerized ventilators allowing the choice of various ventilatory modes appeared on many machines, and computer-controlled flowmeters working from flow sensors began to replace the rotameter.

Vaporizers

As noted earlier, Snow devised a vaporizer/inhaler for ether that incorporated many features present in modern vaporizers. They included a spiral gas passage to ensure saturation of gases flowing through the vaporizer, and a water bath surrounding the vaporizer to provide better temperature stabilization. Snow differed with another anesthetic great, Sir James Simpson, who said that simpler was better, that a few drops of chloroform on a handkerchief sufficed, and all that complicated apparatus was unnecessary. Simpson's simplistic view often prevailed in the early days of anesthesia. Anesthesia was frequently delivered by a handkerchief or a more sanitary variant that used a gauze placed over a wire frame, such as the Schimmelbusch mask (Fig. 52.6), into the 1950s.

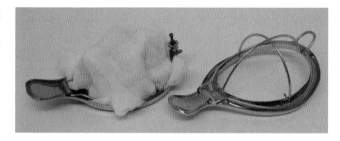

Fig. 52.6 This Schimmelbusch Mask was used to administer ether or chloroform. A gauze or handkerchief was placed over the wire frame and liquid anesthetic dripped onto it. One problem was that as fluid was poured onto the gauze or handkerchief it flowed down to the sides, leaving a dry patch through which the patient breathed. The rim served as a trough to catch surplus fluid

For a time, Snow's ideas were largely forgotten. Apparatus for vaporizing liquid anesthetic agents was crude and inexact. Of necessity, the anesthesia provider's observations of the patient's anesthetic depth (e.g., Snow's degrees and Guedel's signs and stages of anesthesia) were used to determine the amount of anesthetic to deliver.

In 1902, Dragerwerk developed a drip feed injector to administer ether or chloroform. The drops could be counted and thus the volume of agent added to the gases breathed by the patient could be calculated. But who had time to count the drops and then calculate (taking into account the flow of diluent gases) the actual concentration of anesthetic inhaled by the patient? Observations of the patient's clinical signs still governed the amount of anesthetic delivered.

A Parisian surgeon, Louis Ombrédanne, introduced a new ether inhaler in 1908 [14]. He criticized previous inhalers *"....as these are not provided with means of admission of fresh air, they rapidly produce cyanosis if one does not constantly raise the mask from the face."* Ombrédanne's inhaler/vaporizer avoided delivery of hypoxic gas mixtures by admitting air. It became the most commonly used apparatus for ether delivery in France and Latin America, and aided in the conversion from chloroform to ether. It continued to be used for a half century.

The Boyle Bottle (Fig. 52.7) appeared in 1917, and consisted of a glass bottle (the vaporizing chamber) that held the liquid anesthetic (any could be used). A controllable fraction of the gas to be delivered was diverted through the bottle, which was fitted with a plunger and cowl that could direct the gas flow close to the surface of the liquid—or under the liquid surface, resulting in a greater amount of agent being vaporized. Heat loss occurred during vaporization, and the decreased temperature decreased vaporization of the liquid anesthetic, and thus the concentration added to the diverted gases. The anesthesia provider often placed a pan of hot water around the outside of the bottle (there was a formal arrangement that permitted this to be done easily) to warm it, but the

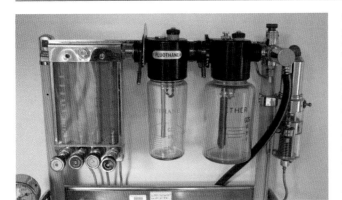

Fig. 52.7 Rotameters were used on this Boyle machine. Gas issued to the right of the flowmeter bank through valve-levers that could direct none to all of the flow through each of the two glass Boyle bottles (one here for halothane and the other for ether) in series to its right. In this photograph, the levers are down (off). Vaporization could also be increased by lowering a plunger that forced the gas directed through the vaporizing chamber to bubble through the liquid anesthetic

Fig. 52.8 Ohio #8 bottles were placed in the breathing circuit, usually on the inspiratory side. The gases flowing past the vaporizer could be diverted through the glass bottle by rotating the lever atop the vaporizer. The amount of gas diverted was proportional to the degree to which the lever was turned. Note the wick used to increase vaporization. As with the Boyle bottle, one could increase or decrease the amount of anesthetic administered (by increasing or decreasing diversion), but the resulting concentration delivered to the patient was unknown

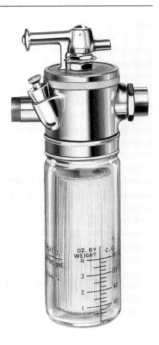

bottle was composed of glass, a poor heat conductor. Snow also incorporated a pan of water around his vaporizer, but he made his vaporizer of copper, a good conductor of heat. The anesthesia provider using the Boyle Bottle could not know the concentration of anesthetic delivered. The patient's clinical signs guided how much should be administered.

The Boyle bottle could be placed inside a rebreathing absorption system ("in-circuit"), but was normally outside the system or used with a non-absorption system (no carbon dioxide absorption by soda lime). Simpler versions of the Boyle bottle with small liquid capacities (Rowbotham, Goldman) were used in British circle breathing systems.

The Ohio #8 bottle (Fig. 52.8) was one of the most popular in-circuit vaporizers in the 1940s and 1950s in North America. Its sister, the Goldman, was used throughout the rest of the world. Both were glass bottles containing a wick to maximize the surface available for vaporization of the liquid anesthetic, usually ether. There was no way to provide temperature compensation. A control dial atop the vaporizer allowed the anesthesia provider to divert any proportion from none to all of the inspired gases through the vaporizing chamber. Since this was an in-circuit vaporizer, some anesthetic vapor returned to it during the next inspiration, adding to the imprecision of vapor delivery. This could be dangerous because vaporizer output was directly tied to minute ventilation, and lethal concentrations of anesthetic could be delivered, especially with controlled ventilation. This device was especially dangerous when used with a potent volatile anesthetic having relatively low blood solubility and a relatively high vapor pressure such as halothane. Again, the patient's clinical signs were used to guide the amount of anesthetic delivered. Exhaled gases contain water vapor,

and when passing through the vaporizer the water would dissolve in the liquid anesthetic. Large amounts of water can dissolve in ether. The ether would be diluted and its vapor pressure lowered, limiting the level of anesthetic that might be achieved at a particular setting of the indicator dial.

In the 1950s, a major advance occurred with the development of the Copper Kettle vaporizer by Lucien Morris [15]. This change was so important that Chapter 53 in this book is devoted to this invention. The Copper Kettle vaporizer was the first to deliver a known output of anesthetic at any flow rate or vaporizer temperature. As with the Boyle bottle, any liquid anesthetic could be used. There were two gas flows. One was independent of the vaporizer (the diluent or bypass flow), and the other was the flow through the kettle. The kettle containing liquid anesthetic was made of copper attached to a copper tabletop (hence the name). Copper was chosen because of its high thermal conductivity, allowing the temperature (and therefore the vapor pressure) of the liquid anesthetic within the kettle to remain relatively constant (as in Snow's inhaler—at last someone listened). The anesthesia provider knew the flow to the kettle and its temperature from a thermometer in the vaporizer wall. Assuming that the gas exiting the kettle was fully saturated with anesthetic, calculation of the added volume of anesthetic was possible. For example, if 100 ml of gas were directed to a kettle containing halothane, then the exiting gas would contain 33 % of an atmosphere of halothane (its vapor pressure) and the volume of halothane vapor would be 50 ml (i.e., 50/(100+50)=0.33 or 33 %). Add this to a diluent flow of 5,000 ml and the delivered concentration approximated 1 %. Vapor output remained constant with the Copper Kettle.

Most clinicians were accustomed to the concentration decreasing as the liquid cooled, and sometimes were surprised to achieve a greater-than-expected anesthetic depth when using the Copper Kettle.

Ohio Medical Products Corporation soon marketed a vaporizer called the Vernitrol that was similar to the Copper Kettle. Two Vernitrol's (for two anesthetics, perhaps halothane and ether) could be placed on an anesthesia machine, each with its own flowmeter. Copper Kettle and Vernitrol vaporizers continued in common use until the 1980s. The Ohio DM 5000 anesthesia machine, introduced in the late 1960s, featured the last of the kettle-type vaporizers. The vaporizer was heated to maintain a constant temperature and provide an accurate agent concentration. On this machine, the vaporizer flowmeter indicated ml of vapor emanating from the vaporizer rather than ml of oxygen going into the vaporizer, as was the case with the Copper Kettle. If the same calculations as those for the Copper Kettle were used with the DM 5000, the patient would receive a much higher anesthetic concentration. Having a mix of machines within an OR suite sometimes resulted in anesthesia providers moving from one operating room to another without realizing that the output of the vaporizer was double or one half of that in the room from whence they came. This resulted in several deaths and a number of cases of patient awareness. Some anesthesia providers called the DM 5000 "the widow maker".

In the 1950s, Cyprane in England produced the Fluotec vaporizer (Fig. 52.9), a so-called "variable bypass vaporizer" that allowed the user to directly set the desired percentage of agent—thus eliminating the calculations associated with the Copper Kettle and Vernitrol. Incremental improvements further increased the output stability, so that it remained relatively constant despite variations in fresh gas flow and temperature. It was the first vaporizer designed and calibrated for use with only one anesthetic agent. Other companies also developed direct-reading vaporizers, such as the Foregger Fluomatic and the Dragerwerk Vapor. A potential problem with the Fluotec (and other "Tec" type vaporizers) was that any volatile anesthetic could be poured into the vaporizing chamber. Of course this would result in an anesthetic concentration different than that on the dial—greater if the vapor pressure of the agent was greater than that of the agent for which the vaporizer was calibrated, and vice versa. This problem was partially solved using a keyed system on both the bottle and the vaporizer (see also Chapter 66 on the contributions of industry to the history of anesthesia.).

Desflurane was introduced in the late 1980s. Since it had a boiling point near room temperature, it could not be used in the usual variable bypass vaporizer. This problem could be solved by either cooling the agent to a point well below room temperature, or by heating it to well above room temperature so that the vaporizing chamber delivered 100 % agent as a gas. Heating was chosen. An amount of pure vapor,

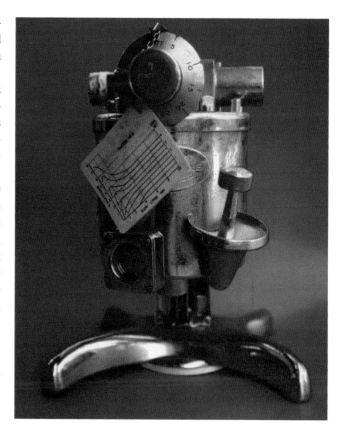

Fig. 52.9 Fluotec Mark II Vaporizer. Note the card chained to the vaporizer with a graph showing how fresh gas flow affected the vaporizer output. A predictable (flat line) output was accomplished at inflow rates of 1–2 l/min or more for this early model. Later versions produced constant known outputs at flows as low as a few 100 ml/min

determined by the concentration dial, was added to the fresh gas passing through the vaporizer.

Until the middle 1990s, vaporizers were mechanically controlled by altering the relative flows through the bypass and the vaporizing chamber. The Physioflex anesthesia machine was the first to use computer control of vapor concentration in a totally closed rebreathing absorption circuit with constantly circulating gas. Using feedback from agent monitors, a computer directed the vaporizer to inject liquid anesthetic directly into the gas stream in an amount sufficient to produce the agent concentration dialed on the anesthesia machine.

A new variable bypass vaporizer, the ADU, became popular in the 2000s [16]. It differed from the "Tec-type" devices in that the output was governed by computer control of the flow issuing from the vaporizer sump and the flow that bypassed the sump, doing so in a manner that produced the output concentration of anesthetic prescribed by the dial setting. This meant that any volatile anesthetic, including desflurane, could be used. The ADU vaporizer was separate from the anesthetic sump. A given sump was specific for a given anesthetic, and when the sump was attached to the vaporizer, the vaporizer recognized the anesthetic by the identity of the sump (oh, those computers!)

Breathing Systems

Systems Without Carbon Dioxide Absorption

The preceding discussions focused on the anesthetic machine, the large and expensive device concocting a mixture of known concentrations at a controlled flow rate. In order to produce anesthesia, this mixture must be transported to the patient. The delivery vehicle is the breathing system with the interface being a mask, a supraglottic airway device (such as the laryngeal mask airway) or a tracheal tube.

Morton, Snow and Simpson used non-rebreathing systems where the anesthetic mixture was inhaled and then exhaled to ambient air. There were exceptions. Patients breathing from bags containing nitrous oxide might rebreathe some of the gas they exhaled. And some of the systems delivering potent vapors did not have valves to prevent rebreathing.

Over the years various other systems developed. In 1954, WW Mapleson analyzed and classified the various systems that did not have carbon dioxide absorption, and suggested the fresh gas flows needed to minimize rebreathing of exhaled carbon dioxide [17]. These seemingly uncomplicated devices had many advantages, being lightweight and relatively simple. Today, however, they have largely disappeared because they required high flows, potentially increasing the cost of anesthetic delivery to $100 per hour or more! High flows also increased contamination of the atmosphere with anesthetic gases and vapors, a matter of rising environmental concern. Some of these systems linger today in the form of the Mapleson D and E systems used for pediatric anesthesia, or to supply oxygen during patient transport or emergency situations when the primary source of anesthesia malfunctions.

Systems with Carbon Dioxide Absorption

In 1903 Dragerwerk developed a device to absorb carbon dioxide from rebreathed gases using soda lime (mostly calcium hydroxide spiked with a bit of sodium and potassium hydroxide). Miners carrying oxygen cylinders used this device underground. Oxygen was added to the breathed gas to make up for the oxygen taken up by the miner. This invention was not immediately applied to anesthesia breathing systems because anesthetics were relatively inexpensive (Crawford Long charged $0.25 for the ether he used to anesthetize James Venable). In addition, chloroform, which was commonly used at that time, reacted with soda lime to produce the nerve gas phosgene.

In 1916, Dennis Jackson demonstrated an apparatus equipped with a device for absorbing carbon dioxide, but he used a solution of alkali, an approach difficult to apply in

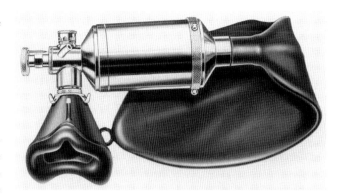

Fig. 52.10 In the to-and-fro system developed by Ralph Waters, the carbon dioxide absorbent was placed in the large canister. The patient breathed back and forth (to and from the reservoir bag attached to the distal end of the canister) through this valveless system. There were two problems with this elegantly simple system: 1) The absorbent at the proximal (patient) end of the canister exhausted first, increasing the dead space. 2) The absorbent tended to settle, resulting in a low resistance pathway at the top of the absorber

practice. In 1923, Ralph Waters introduced a breathing apparatus with an absorber between the reservoir bag and the fresh gas inlet (Fig. 52.10) [18]. The absorber contained soda lime, and although this "to-and-fro" system worked, it was cumbersome and became progressively less efficient (absorbed less carbon dioxide) with continued use. Although it remained of academic interest and was buoyed by Waters' great imprimatur, it gradually fell out of favor. It was used as recently as the 1970s for patients with pulmonary infections since it could be cleaned easily.

In 1926, Dragerwerk of Germany developed the first circle breathing system for use with their Model A anesthesia machine. There were separate hoses for inhalation and exhalation; low resistance, thin mica unidirectional valves that forced the gases to move in a circle; a canister for the soda lime; a reservoir bag, and a pressure-limiting valve—all components found in circle systems today. It also included an absorber bypass to allow deliberate rebreathing of carbon dioxide. The bypass was included in many systems, but caused problems because it was often inadvertently left in the bypass position. As a result, it was removed from circle systems in the US. It was reintroduced in the twenty-first century, to allow the absorbent to be changed during an anesthetic. The risk associated with its being inadvertently left in the bypass position was lessened by the routine use of carbon dioxide monitoring.

For a time, large absorbent canisters were in vogue. Wrongfully, it was thought that soda lime would regenerate since the color indicator (indicating exhaustion of the absorbent) returned to white after a period of non-use. James Elam and Elwyn Brown designed and advocated the use of large absorbers, particularly two large canisters in series [19].

These allowed nearly complete absorbent exhaustion before the upstream canister needed to be changed. The presence of the second canister ensured that no carbon dioxide would be rebreathed.

A controversy arose in the 1990s regarding the reaction of sevoflurane with an absorbent—either Baralyme® or soda lime - to produce a nephrotoxin called compound A [20], and the reaction of several anesthetics (particularly desflurane) with desiccated Baralyme® or soda lime to produce carbon monoxide [21]. These problems led to the development of new absorbents (e.g., Amsorb® in 1999) that, even when desiccated, did not react with the anesthetic [22]. In the early 2000s, several fires and explosions occurred during the use of sevoflurane [23]. The problem was traced to a triple combination of sevoflurane, desiccated but otherwise fresh Baralyme®, and low fresh gas flows. Baralyme® was removed from the market and the problem disappeared.

Scavenging Systems

Before the late 1960s there was little concern about the effects of occupational exposure to trace concentrations of anesthetic gases. Then a report on health problems in Russian workers exposed to anesthetic gases and vapors was published [24]. Investigators from other countries confirmed that there might be adverse effects in anesthesia providers. As a result, devices for scavenging and removing gases from the operating room quickly came into use.

Corrugated Tubing and the Reservoir Bag

Winston Churchill said "Out of intense complexities, intense simplicities emerge." The anesthetic circuit has evolved by trial and error into a system of considerable efficiency and utility. Some of the principles of the anesthetic circuit have been known since the time of Snow who maintained that significant resistance to breathing should not be imposed by the anesthesia system. Thus the tubing used to conduct gases to and from the patient must be of large diameter. Pictures of early devices do not show a crucial characteristic of modern tubing: corrugation. A corrugated tube resists kinking, and for the better part of the last century, corrugated tubing has been used.

The circle system became more popular after ethylene and cyclopropane were introduced into anesthesia practice, in 1923 and 1934. Exposing these gases to a spark could produce an explosion that could kill or injure patients and clinicians, a disaster that led to the cessation of the use of cyclopropane in Latin America in the late 1930s. To minimize the chance of a spark from a static electric charge, the anesthetic machine and everything connected to it were made conductive. Thus the corrugated tubing and bags were composed of black (carbon) conductive rubber. Anesthesia personnel wore conductive shoes that grounded the clinician to the floor, and wet sheets were draped around the anesthesia machine and operating room table, as well as on the floor, for personnel to stand on to prevent static sparks from being generated. Special non-sparking electrical power switches, using mercury in a sealed glass tube, were used in operating rooms. As the 1960s came to an end, so did use of ether, ethylene, and cyclopropane—and the need for conductive rubber and other measures. Halothane swept all the explosive anesthetics aside and lightweight disposable tubes and bags came into vogue.

And what of the mundane reservoir bag? To best serve the anesthesia provider and patient, it needs to be of sufficient size to hold enough gas to allow deep respiration. In the 1950s, 10 L reservoir bags were available. These were cumbersome, difficult for the anesthesia provider to grasp, and made it difficult to see how deeply the patient was breathing. As Goldilocks would say, the reservoir bag should be not too small, not too large, but just right. And so, today, it is usually three liters for adults, and smaller for children.

Standardization, Information Technology, and Modern Anesthetic Machines

Perhaps the most important development shaping today's anesthesia machines was the 1979 adoption of the first anesthesia machine standard. Clinicians and industry engineers examined problems with previous machines that could have or did lead to patient mortality and morbidity. The standard aimed to eliminate or warn of serious problems. Some of the requirements in the standard included flowmeters in series instead of in parallel, fluted oxygen flow control knobs for tactile feedback, a means to prevent administration of a hypoxic mixture, and color-coded flowmeters. Machines manufactured after publication of this standard needed to meet all the requirements of the standard.

For many years, anesthesia machines and monitors were sold separately. Buying the "best of breed" equipment for each use allowed healthcare facilities to distribute spending over time. But monitors stacked on anesthesia machines or separate carts were difficult to manage. Cables from different monitors caused what came to be known as the "spaghetti syndrome", and the whole array was referred to as a "Christmas tree" [25]. The combined collection of devices could turn into a discotheque of buzzers, bells and flashing alarm lights, with important information scattered over the separate units. Displays, controls and alarms of different devices varied, leading to confusion and management problems. In the 1990s, the distinction between anesthesia machine, ventilator and monitors started to blur. All were integrated into an "anesthesia

Table 52.1 Timeline

1846 William Morton publically demonstrates ether anesthesia.

1847 John Snow constructs an inhaler for constant vaporization of ether.

1865 SS White manufactures a storage bag for nitrous oxide.

1868 The Coxeter and Barth companies provide compressed gas in a cylinder.

1868 Edmond Andrews suggests adding O_2 to N_2O.

1870 Cylinders of liquefied N_2O become available.

1877 Joseph Clover invents a chloroform inhaler giving a known concentration.

1879 Paul Bert gives 15% O_2 with N_2O to produce anesthesia in a pressure chamber.

1885 Coxeter of London makes O_2 available in cylinders.

1885 SS White develops the first machine where O_2 and N_2O are mixed in a chamber and then administered to the patient.

1886 Hillischer develops a machine to deliver both O_2 and N_2O.

1886 Gwathmey develops a nitrous oxide-oxygen apparatus with control valves for the gases and a bubble flowmeter.

1893 Hewitt develops a N_2O-oxygen stopcock which becomes available in 1897.

1893 Hewitt's anesthesia apparatus uses cylinders for nitrous oxide and O_2.

1902 Drager develops a drip-feed vaporizer.

1903 Dragerwerk describes the first breathing system with CO_2 absorbent.

1906 Heidbrink develops an O_2-N_2O anesthesia machine.

1909 Kuppers develops the rotameter.

1910 Neu uses the rotameter in anesthesia

1910 SS White anesthesia machine has yokes for 4 cylinders but does not estimate gas concentration or flow.

1912 Boothby develops the bubble bottle flowmeter.

1913 Heidbrink develops the disc flowmeter.

1914 The Foregger Company builds the Gwathmey apparatus.

1916 Dennis Jackson describes a breathing system that absorbs CO_2 using an alkali solution.

1923 Ralph Waters introduces to-and-fro rebreathing systems with CO_2 absorption.

1926 Heidbrink offers the first mass-produced anesthesia machine, the Model A.

1926 Dragerwerk develops the circle rebreathing system.

Late 1920s Foregger develops the water depression flowmeter.

1930 Coxeter dry bobbin flowmeter is developed.

1934 Connell double ball flowmeter is developed.

1950 Rotameters are introduced into US anesthesia machines.

1952 Lucien Morris invents the Copper Kettle vaporizer.

1954 Mapleson categorizes non-rebreathing anesthesia circuits.

1957 Fluotec vaporizer is released.

1978 The Boston Anesthesia System is described.

workstation". These workstations were designed to solve some problems by integration so that all modalities were controlled and displayed consistently and in one place, with alarms coordinated and prioritized. The whole setup could be purchased from and serviced by a single manufacturer.

And what of the future? It seems likely that the anesthesia workstation will someday be part of an information network for the entire healthcare facility. Other tasks, including anesthesia recordkeeping, will increasingly become automated.

Reprise

In the beginning, anesthetists delivered ether and chloroform from various devices ranging from handkerchiefs to inhalers, while nitrous oxide was inhaled from a bladder (see Table 52.1). The inhalers underwent improvements in their control over the delivered anesthetic concentration. Today's vaporizers accurately deliver the anesthetic concentration dialed by the anesthesia provider at any fresh gas flow rate and at any temperature, an achievement attained by the mid-twentieth century. The use of nitrous oxide to complement the action of the potent inhaled anesthetics was delayed for several decades after the discovery of anesthesia in 1846, until a means to efficiently store it and combine it with oxygen (also requiring an effective means of storage) were developed. The needed technology was applied in the latter part of the nineteenth century, and was combined with gas flow measurement to give birth to the anesthetic machine. Gas flow measurement was first accomplished using a water sight flowmeter where bubbles indicated the gas flow. Water depression and dry bobbin flowmeters were replaced by the rotameter. Electronic flow controls replaced rotameters in the twenty-first century.

The machines supplied the anesthetic mixture, but a breathing system was needed for the interface between the machine and the patient. Many early breathing systems were non-rebreathing devices (e.g., open drop delivery of ether or chloroform). Most mask inhalers relied on rebreathing, some to a potentially dangerous level. All these devices released the exhaled gases into the operating room. With the need to minimize delivery of expensive or explosive anesthetics, in the first half of the twentieth century, anesthesia providers turned to rebreathing systems with carbon dioxide absorption—except for anesthetics such as trichloroethylene where the potential for production of phosgene from the reaction of absorbent with trichloroethylene discouraged the use of such absorption. To-and-fro systems competed with circle systems in the first half of the twentieth century, with circle systems winning out. Carbon dioxide absorbents developed in ways that decreased the likelihood of degradation of potent inhaled anesthetics. Other components of the circle system (the corrugated tubing, valves, and reservoir bag) evolved in ways that minimized resistance to gas flow, and unwieldiness. In the latter portion of the twentieth century, concerns regarding the health implications to operating room personnel of breathing exhaled anesthetics led to the scavenging of excess gases.

References

1. Fenster J. Ether day: the strange tale of America's greatest medical discovery and the haunted men who made it. New York: Harper Collins; 2001.
2. Petty C. History of the development of the anesthesia machine. The Anesthesia machine. New York: Churchill Livingstone; 1987. pp. 1–19.
3. Mushin WW, Jones PL. Some practical aspects of anaesthetic apparatus and vaporizers. Physics for the anaesthetist. Oxford: Blackwell; 1987. pp 340–63.
4. Thomas KB The 2 oxide series. The development of anaesthetic apparatus. Oxford: Blackwell; 1975. pp 103–74.
5. Epstein HG, Hunter AR. Anaesthetic apparatus. A pictorial review of the development of the modern anaesthetic machine. Br J Anaesth. 1968;40:636–47.
6. Mushin WW, Jones PL. Pressure regulators. Physics for the Anaesthetist. Oxford: Blackwell; 1987. pp 185–221.
7. Stebbins HM, Teter CK. J Am Dent Soc Anesthesiol. 1958;5:15–6.
8. Foregger R. Richard von Foregger, Ph.D., 1872–1960. Manufacturer of anesthesia equipment. Anesthesiology. 1996;84:190–200.
9. Ball CM, Westhorpe R. Historical notes on anaesthesia and intensive care. Sydney: Australian Society of Anaesthetists; 2012. pp 212–3.
10. Ward CS. Intermittent flow apparatus—demand flow. Anaesthetic equipment. Physical principles and maintenance. Baltimore: Williams & Wilkins; 1975. pp 146–70.
11. Dorsch J, Dorsch S. The intermittent flow machine. Understanding anesthesia equipment. Baltimore: Williams & Wilkins; 1975. pp 72–83.
12. Young TM. Vaporizers for dental anaesthesia modified by the addition of a wick: an evaluation of performance. Br J Anaesth. 1969;41:120–9.
13. Cooper JB, Newbower RS, Moore JW, Trautman ED. A new anesthesia delivery system. Anesthesiology. 1978;49:310–8.
14. Ombrédanne L. Un Appareil pour l'anesthésie par l'éther. Gaz des Hopitaux. 1908;81:S1095.
15. Morris LE. A new vaporizer for liquid anesthetic agents. Anesthesiology. 1952;13:587–93.
16. Hendrickx JFA, De Cooman S, Deloof R, Vandeput D, Coddens J, De Wolf AM. The ADU vaporizing unit: a new vaporizer. Anesth Analg. 2001;93:391–5.
17. Mapleson WW. Fifty years after–reflections on 'The elimination of rebreathing in various semi-closed anaesthetic systems'. Br J Anaesth. 2004;93:319–21.
18. Waters RM. Clinical scope and utility of carbon dioxide filtration in inhalation anesthesia. Anesth Analg. 1924;3:20–2.
19. Elam JO, Brown ES, Ten Pas RH. Carbon dioxide homeostasis during anesthesia. I. Instrumentation. Anesthesiology. 1955;16:876–85.
20. Morio M, Fujii K, Satoh N, Imai M, Kawakami U, Mizuno T, Kawai Y, Ogasawara Y, Tamura T, Negishi A, Kumagai Y, Kawai T. Reaction of sevoflurane and its degradation products with soda lime. Toxicity of the byproducts. Anesthesiology. 1992;77:1155–64.
21. Stabernack CR, Brown R, Laster MJ, Dudziak R, Eger EI II. Absorbents differ enormously in their capacity to produce compound A and carbon monoxide. Anesth Analg. 2000;90:1428–35.
22. Murray JM, Renfrew CW, Bedi A, McCrystal CB, Jones DS, Fee JPH. Amsorb. A new carbon dioxide absorbent for use in anesthetic breathing systems. Anesthesiology. 1999;91:1342–8.
23. Wu J, Previte JP, Adler E, Myers T, Ball J, Gunter JB. Spontaneous ignition, explosion, and fire with sevoflurane and barium hydroxide lime. Anesthesiology. 2004;101:534–7.
24. Vaisman AI. [Working conditions in the operating room and their effect on the health of anesthetists]. Eksp Khir Anesteziol. 1967;12:44–9.
25. Westhorpe RN. The anesthetic machine in the 1990s. Anesthesiol Rev. 1992;19:46–55.

The Development of the Copper Kettle with Comments on Vaporizers that Preceded and Followed

53

Lucien E. Morris and Donald C. Morris

Summary

Chance and personal interest led me (LEM) sequentially to chemistry, medicine (graduating in 1943), anesthesia, and Ralph Waters who offered me a residency. World War II intervened, and being drafted into the US Army delayed the residency. I managed to practice anesthesia despite a limited knowledge of the art, in 1944 becoming chief of the anesthesia and operating room section at the US Army 103rd General Hospital in England.

In 1946, I began residency, working regularly with Waters in the operating room. In my second year, I participated in the ongoing 1947 departmental study of chloroform as though it were a brand new anesthetic agent. The poor control over chloroform vapor concentration frustrated me, and I foolishly publically lamented that "anyone ought to be able to make a better vaporizer than this". Waters persuaded me to try.

I applied principles John Snow used 100 years earlier: adequate anesthetic vaporization and control over vapor pressure. I added the goals of delivery of a known concentration of anesthetic at a measured inflow rate. To achieve these ends I controlled the liquid anesthetic temperature by housing it in a copper sump (reservoir) and delivered two precisely known flows – one to the sump and the other bypassing the sump. Flow through the sump passed through a sintered bubbler, ensuring complete vapor equilibration with the flow. Knowing the liquid anesthetic temperatures and the two flows allowed a precise calculation of the anesthetic concentration delivered.

The Foregger Company manufactured the prototype of the Copper Kettle, delivering the first version late in the summer of 1948. The first satisfactory commercial model of the vaporizer appeared in late 1951. It was described in *Anesthesiology* in 1952 and now resides in the Guedel Memorial Anesthesia Center in San Francisco.

The Copper Kettle could be used with any volatile anesthetic, and so it was used for ether and then halothane and enflurane anesthesia. Imitations of the Copper Kettle were made in the US, Japan, South America, and the United Kingdom, and motivated development of variable by-pass, Tec-type vaporizers in the mid-1950s. The principles of operation were the same as those for the Copper Kettle. All had two flows through the vaporizer, the by-pass flow and the flow through the sump containing the liquid anesthetic. Over the next decade or two, these vaporizers replaced the Copper Kettle because they were simpler to use, and required no calculations. They flattered the Copper Kettle with their imitation.

The Story

My increasing dissatisfaction with existing equipment, an interest in chemistry and physics, and a personal challenge led to the creation of what became the Copper Kettle vaporizer. How did it begin? I long had an affection for chemistry and physics, an affection that may have attracted me to anesthesia and certainly influenced my invention of the Copper Kettle. I fondly remember spending time as a child in the laboratory with my father, who was the professor and head of the Department of Biochemistry at Western Reserve University. After graduating in 1936 from Oberlin College with a bachelor's degree in chemistry, I enrolled as a graduate student at Western Reserve University in biochemistry,

Lucien Morris lived from November 30, 1914 to November 15, 2011. By the time he died, he had created and completed this essay with the help of his son and co-author, Donald Morris. Lucien was effectively blind from macular degeneration in his last years, and much of the story was told from memory. It is a lovely story, a personal story of an invention that helped advance anesthesia from art to science. It also paints a picture of part of anesthesia in the US at mid-century.

D. C. Morris (✉)
The Washington Group, Inc., Seattle WA, USA
e-mail: dcm@dcmseattle.com

L. E. Morris
Anesthesiology, Medical College of Ohio, Toledo OH, USA

intending to teach biochemistry to medical students. Because I thought I might better understand what medical students needed to know if I saw biochemistry through their eyes, I enrolled into the medical college, continuing as a laboratory assistant in the Biochemistry Department until the beginning of my senior year. I graduated as an MD in February 1943.

My internship at Grasslands Hospital, Westchester County, New York provided my first exposure to anesthesia, a one-on-one tutoring that in hindsight led to an appreciation of how my basic science training would support my future interests in anesthesia. Not yet realizing that I was destined to become an anesthesiologist, I applied for a residency in women's diseases, an area of study that I felt had been neglected during my internship. My letters of inquiry evoked a single response from a small private hospital in Madison, Wisconsin. En route to Madison, I learned that all the house officers for that hospital had been called into active military duty and the post of being the only resident was offered to me. I accepted it because I felt that as the sole resident, I might choose my opportunities based on what interested me.

After reporting for duty in Madison, and while exploring the hospital, I met a surgeon who asked if I had any experience with anesthesia. When I said I had some experience as an intern, he explained that all nurse anesthetists were busy and requested that I provide "just a touch of Pentothal for a short case". Wanting to be helpful, I unwisely acquiesced. Because the three CRNA's were using all available machines, I hurried to find an intravenous drip, suction equipment, an oropharyngeal airway, an oxygen tank fitted with a flow meter and a bag and mask. Finding these essentials in unfamiliar surroundings took about fifteen minutes. The displeased surgeon berated me for the delay. The "short case" lasted nearly four hours, compounding my and his unease. I managed to keep the patient quiescent with a total of three and a half grams of thiopental. Later that evening, after listening to my grumbling about the case, an extern, a medical student from the University of Wisconsin, suggested, "If you're that interested in anesthesia why don't you go and see Dr. Waters" (1883–1979)? Perceiving my ignorance about Dr. Waters, he told me about the excellent residency program in anesthesia at Wisconsin, and why students held Prof. Waters in high regard.

Shortly thereafter, I received notice to report for active military duty. I called Dr. Waters and requested an urgent interview. He responded quickly, graciously inviting me to his home that evening. After an hour and a half interview we agreed that if I survived the war, I would return as his resident for advanced training in clinical anesthesia.

A week later I was in the Army. Following a few weeks of indoctrination, those of us who had received a war-truncated nine month internship were ordered to an army general hospital in upper New York State where we were to spend two

weeks each on surgery and medicine, and a third two weeks on an elective option. I asked to have an anesthetic elective for the first two week stint, and then asked the chief of surgery to have the second two weeks on anesthesia instead of surgery. After obtaining his agreement, I presented the chief of medicine with a similar request, which was also granted. I suspect that these men complied because they then had one less naïve transient to keep out of trouble. Although the anesthesiologist in charge taught poorly and lacked enthusiasm, I was delighted to have six weeks experience in anesthesia, and grateful to learn how to use a Heidbrink machine to give a satisfactory GOE [gas (nitrous oxide)-oxygen-ether] anesthesia. My next assignment was to O'Halloran General Hospital on Staten Island where I learned a variety of anesthetic blocks. After two and a half weeks, I joined the 103rd General Hospital, in preparation for deployment to England.

On arrival in England, all doctors were interviewed by Lt. Col. Morton. Because another Morton first publically demonstrated ether anesthesia, I took it as a favorable sign, saluting and saying "Lt. Morris reporting, Sir". He looked up, seemingly startled and said, "Lucien Morris is it?" I said, "Yes sir". I felt certain he had started to say, "We've been looking for you", but the rest of the interview was unremarkable. The next day I was interviewed by a full colonel, William S. Middleton, who probed my background and experience, ending with a discussion of mutual friends and acquaintances in medicine. I later learned he was the Dean of the Medical School at the University of Wisconsin – on military leave of absence. The next day my name was posted, indicating my assignment as chief of the anesthesia and operating room section at the 103rd General Hospital.

From the beginning, the 103rd General Hospital received soldiers injured in the European Theatre. In eight and a half months in 1944–45, we provided nearly 5,000 anesthetics. I personally administered more than 700 anesthetics and, in addition, supervised and assisted a staff of nurse anesthetists and other physicians who dealt with the remainder. Although relatively few cases required tracheal intubation, we did enough that the team and I began to feel reasonably confident in the use of the Guedel laryngoscope. No deaths could be either directly or remotely related to the administration of anesthesia. This reflected the health and youth of our patient population with war wounds of the extremities. Patients with life threatening injuries of head, thorax, or abdomen were sent elsewhere.

With the end of the European conflict and then VJ Day (14 August 1945), I was redeployed onto home territory. The final months of my more than two and one-half years of active military service were spread among assignments to several small army hospitals in the eastern and southeastern US.

Returning to Madison in late August 1946 to begin the residency program, I worked with Dr. Waters in the operating room on a daily basis, quickly learning about the

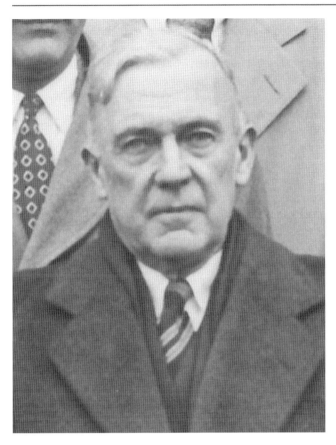

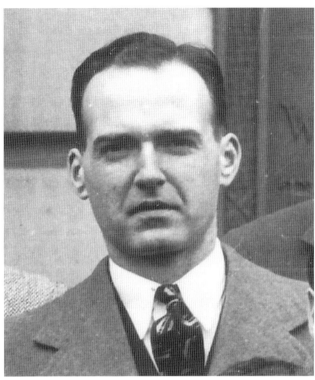

Fig. 53.2 A young Lucien Morris from a group photograph of his residency mates and the faculty at the University of Wisconsin. (From the personal collection of the author)

Fig. 53.1 Dr. Ralph Waters at age 65 in 1948 from the same group picture that included Lucien Morris (Fig. 53.2). (From the personal collection of the author)

pharmacological and psychological preparation of the patient. Dr. Waters routinely gave an amnesic drug as part of his pre-medication routine, because he believed it facilitated the use of less anesthesia and diminished patient recollection of problems with the anesthetic induction. Dr. Waters would have a friendly conversation with the patient as the patient moved to the operating table. The conversation always indicated Dr. Waters' concern for the patient's well being and often included a suggestion that the patient make a conscious effort to relax. He used the positioning of the blood pressure cuff as the signal that this was a part of the routine. A pillow under the patient's head had another purpose: it helped to support the to-and-fro carbon dioxide absorption canister (see Figs. 52.10 and 57.1) [9]. Part of Dr. Waters' conversation was intended to distract the patient, and part assure them that he was their advocate and would look after their well being during anesthesia. During the surgical procedure, Dr. Waters' attention to patient well-being included tracking pulse, blood pressure and urinary output. Throughout his esteemed career, Dr. Waters advocated teaching by example, continuing this daily pattern until he retired in 1948 on the day he turned 65 (Fig. 53.1).

In my second year at Madison (Fig. 53.2), I participated in the ongoing departmental study of chloroform, which was subjected to scrutiny as though it were a brand new anesthetic agent [1]. I worked closely with Dr. Waters on the chloroform cases, becoming increasingly frustrated by the poor control over chloroform vapor concentration, and lamenting in the operating room that "anyone ought to be able to make a better vaporizer than this". Several weeks later, while in Florida, Dr. Waters sent a postcard to the staff and residents with a single question: "Has Morris made a new vaporizer yet?" With that encouragement, I set out to solve the problem.

Though not known by me at the start of this quest, John Snow (1813–1858) had noted the importance of several principles that I eventually applied. He observed that there had to be an anesthetic surface area sufficient to ensure equilibrium of anesthetic with the air passing through it. He knew that temperature affected vaporization and to stabilize temperature he made his vaporizer of copper and surrounded it with a water jacket (water because it has a great capacity to hold heat) (see Fig. 52.2). But his and the contemporaneous vaporizer developed by Joseph Thomas Clover (1825–1882) were "non-rebreathing" systems that lacked the economy needed in modern vaporizers [2, 3]. Other vaporizers developed in the last half of the nineteenth century had one

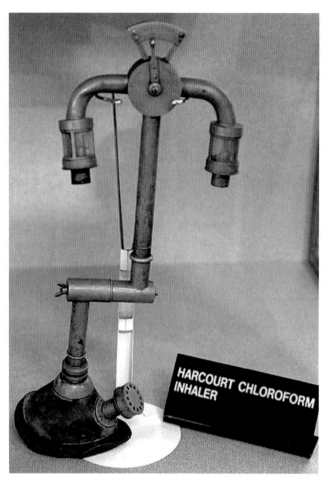

Fig. 53.3 The Harcourt vaporizer was designed to produce a known delivered concentration of chloroform. Two glass bulbs, probably long since broken, were attached to the two arms. The vaporizer compensated for the effect of the temperature of the chloroform on the concentration produced. (Courtesy of the Wood Library-Museum of Anesthesiology, Park Ridge, IL)

or more deficiencies. Vernon Harcourt (1834–1919) for example, built an accurate chloroform vaporizer that was easily broken and its glass components did not lend themselves to temperature stability (Fig. 53.3).

In the first half of the twentieth century, volatile anesthetic concentrations were often provided to patients from gauze masks onto which the liquid anesthetic was dropped. There was no way to estimate the anesthetic concentration breathed by the patient. Alternatively, anesthetic concentrations were produced by anesthetic machines with metered gas flows to which anesthetic vapor was added. In these machines, vapor was added by diverting a coarsely variable portion of the total flow of gases breathed and rebreathed by the patient over or through liquid anesthetic contained in an "in-circuit" vaporizer. These diverted gases were returned to the mixture of fresh and rebreathed gas, ultimately delivered to the patient. Vapor concentration and anesthetic effect could not be predicted, and could produce excessive or inadequate

concentrations. The Boyle's vaporizer (bottle), invented by Henry Boyle (1875–1941), is an example of such a vaporizer. The glass with which it was made insulated the liquid anesthetic which thus would cool (although a water jacket surrounded the glass and limited the cooling). It provided a limited anesthetic surface area, and the control for the diversion of gases through the vaporizer was qualitative at best, indicating administration of more or less anesthetic, but not how much more or how much less. Other vaporizers, including one built by Victor Goldman (1903–1994), had some modern characteristics, but like many previous devices, they were usually designed for nonrebreathing use and did not provide for the quantitative delivery of anesthetic. Generations of anesthetists learned to cope with these deficiencies. I wanted something better.

In retrospect the desirability of producing precisely known concentrations of vapor for addition to the respired gas mixture is clear. My laboratory notebook contained several designs to achieve that end, but they all contained one notion – a separate measured flow of carrier gas, all of which bubbled through the vaporizer. In disguise, this principle continues to be applied in vaporizers used today (see below), long after the demise of the Copper Kettle. Oxygen was chosen as the carrier gas so that if the oxygen supply failed the addition of anesthetic vapor would cease (Fig. 53.4).

The new vaporizer had two important additional components. First, to provide the heat necessary for vaporization, and thereby prevent undue chilling of the anesthetic, I replaced the nearly ubiquitous glass bottle of previous decades with a copper container (Figs. 53.4 and 53.5). Copper was used because of its considerable capacity to conduct heat. I further increased temperature stability by attaching the copper container to a copper tabletop. Secondly, the metered gas was directed through a sintered bronze bubbler (see POREX in Fig. 53.4) at the bottom of the copper container with a resulting dispersion into a multitude of fine bubbles. This provided an enormous combined surface area, a large gas-liquid interface, one providing rapid saturation of the bubbling gas with anesthetic.

The output of this vaporizer, the Copper Kettle, was added to an independent, precisely metered flow of other gases such as oxygen with or without nitrous oxide. Thus the entire system delivered three gases to the anesthetic circuit from which the patient breathed. First, there was the measured flow of fresh gas (A) directed to the Copper Kettle. Second, there was the vaporized anesthetic gas (B) added to A. Third, there was the independent precisely metered flow of other fresh gases (C) that had bypassed the vaporizer. A and B were added to C. The fractional concentration of anesthetic could then be calculated as $B/(A+B+C)$. If one wanted percent, one multiplied the fractional concentration by 100.

But how to calculate B, the volume of entrained vapor per unit of carrier gas? B depended upon the saturated

Fig. 53.4 The photograph of an early Copper Kettle on the left is from the ASA Newsletter 62:1998. The schematic on the right shows a precisely known flow of oxygen that enters through a diffuser leading to a porex filter that caused the gas to break into small bubbles, assuring that a maximum concentration of anesthetic was achieved in the gas, which then passed through an outflow tube, ultimately to be mixed with a second precisely known gas flow. Note the less safe filling funnel at the top of the vaporizer, a position that would permit the careless anesthetist to overfill the vaporizer and allow liquid anesthetic to enter the carrier gas stream, thereby potentially producing a lethal anesthetic concentration. Contrast this with the vaporizer shown in Fig. 53.7. (From the personal collection of the author)

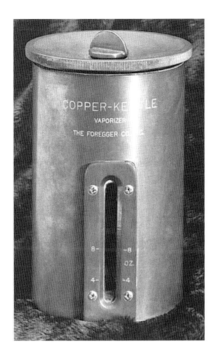 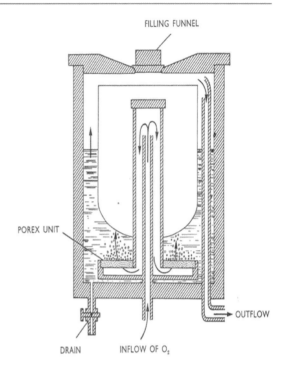

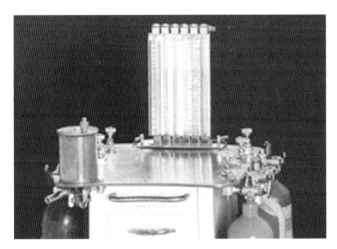

Fig. 53.5 This photograph shows the first commercial Copper Kettle that was made by the Foregger Company. The Copper Kettle placement at the front left of the tabletop (itself to be made of copper to increase the heat sink for and thus temperature stability of the anesthetic) was changed in later models to the rear of the tabletop. The panel at the rear of the tabletop consisted of the two flowmeters (plus other flowmeters) needed in the design of the Copper Kettle. (From the ASA Newsletter. 62:1998)

vapor pressure of anesthetic at the observed temperature (temperature in the Copper Kettle was measured separately). Each anesthetic has its own characteristic vapor pressure-temperature curve, and this had to be applied to accurately calculate the delivered concentration. For example, suppose isoflurane had a saturated pressure of 250 mm Hg and the total ambient pressure was 750 mm Hg, then the effluent concentration would be 250/750 or 1/3rd of an atmo-

sphere. That is, every third molecule issuing from the vaporizer would be isoflurane. For 100 ml of metered carrier gas flowing into the vaporizer, 50 ml of isoflurane plus the 100 ml of metered gas would emerge (i.e., the output would equal 50/(100 + 50)). This highly concentrated output of 33% is roughly thirty times an appropriate anesthetic concentration. Such a concentrated output must be properly diluted by the other metered gases (the "C" gases, above) in the total flow offered to the patient.

The Foregger Company, New York, made the first apparatus that included many of the design principles of this new vaporizing system. They delivered it to us in the late summer of 1948 (Fig. 53.5). We chose Foregger because they made their staff and facilities available for prototype manufacturing. This prototype now resides in the Wood Library-Museum in Park Ridge, Illinois. Although it had the separate metered vaporizing circuit and the copper container for anesthetic liquid, it did not meet all our criteria, specifically omitting certain safety features such as prevention of vaporizer overfilling or pressurization. However, it allowed us to gain clinical experience and pursue further laboratory studies. Persuading the manufacturer to incorporate all the design features of this new apparatus was not easy. Many letters of explanation and several vigorous face-to-face discussions with the owner, Richard von Foregger, Ph.D. (Fig. 53.6), produced a grudging agreement to include all of the features of my design. I received the first satisfactory commercial model of the Copper Kettle vaporizer (Fig. 53.5) in late 1951. The apparatus was described in *Anesthesiology* in 1952 [4], and now resides in the Guedel Memorial Anesthesia Center in San Francisco.

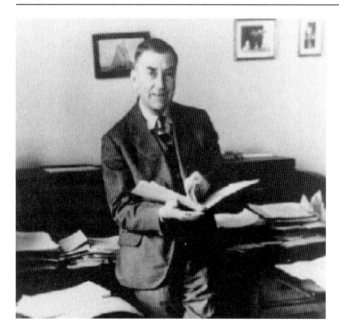

Fig. 53.6 Richard von Foregger in his office. (From an internet tribute for Richard von Foregger, Ph.D., 1872–1960)

Further clinical trials and laboratory studies resulted in additional modifications motivated by safety considerations, most notably a side arm funnel (Fig. 53.7) for filling the liquid container (to prevent over filling), and a double cam valve for the positive exclusion of both the outflow and inflow of the vaporizing chamber. This valve precluded entrainment of vapor or build up of pressure in the vaporizer – which otherwise might cause a surge in vapor output after an oxygen flush.

A need for better control over *chloroform* vapor delivery motivated the design of this innovative vaporizer. But why stop there? This versatile precision equipment could deliver any volatile anesthetic that was liquid at room temperature. It was soon applied to administration of diethyl ether. The ability to smoothly and gradually increase ether vapor concentrations sped inductions and decreased patient discomfort that sometimes accompanied induction of anesthesia with ether. It also became evident that it was easy to overdose a patient with ether: "Good old safe ether" was less safe when ether was improperly administered from the Copper Kettle. Concern regarding the ease of over-dosage with misuse caused us to advise the use of the Copper Kettle primarily in high flow and semi-closed systems. It also seemed best to limit its use to spontaneously breathing patients (that is, without the help of a ventilator or manual ventilation) and to carefully adjust the dosage in accordance with patient response and surgical needs.

Halothane, introduced in the late 1950s, rapidly replaced ether as the anesthetic of choice. Again the Copper Kettle was widely used for its administration – and for administration of other liquid anesthetic agents as well.

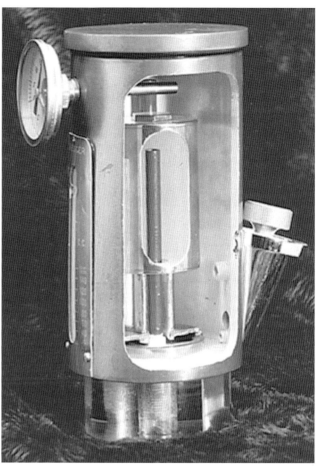

Fig. 53.7 In this picture of the revised Copper Kettle, the opening used to fill the vaporizer with anesthetic is placed low on the side (*right side* in this picture) of the vaporizer, precluding overfilling of the vaporizer. (Picture from the ASA Newsletter 62:1998)

Several reports [5–7] following the original publication [4], enlarged our understanding of the concepts and underlying principles embodied in the design of this versatile vaporizer as a precision tool for the administration of anesthetic vapors. The Copper Kettle rapidly became popular and remained the preferred vaporizer in many US teaching hospitals for many years. The Foregger Company developed several models incorporating the principles of the Copper Kettle, but after the death of Richard von Foregger in 1960 [8], the company made some inappropriate modifications, such as a multiple selection anesthetic turntable, likely intended to simplify agent selection, without regard for potential human error of unknowingly mixing anesthetic agents. Such decisions may have been indicative of problems in management. The company was sold in 1968 and went out of business in 1984 [8].

Imitations of the Copper Kettle were made in the US (especially the Vernitrol® vaporizer), Japan, South America, and the United Kingdom. Most of these ignored one or more of the underlying principles that were part of the original design. In England for instance, a so-called copy utilized the separate carrier gas flow, but used a glass bottle rather than a copper container. As a result, some users never gained a full appreciation of the benefits of the Copper Kettle.

Introduction of the Copper Kettle motivated commercial competition, mostly agent-specific, temperature- and flow-compensated direct reading percentage vaporizers (i.e., variable by-pass, Tec-type vaporizers). The earliest variable by-pass vaporizers were often faulty and imprecise, and were originally intended for use with high flow systems, precluding the application of economical low flow and closed absorption techniques. Compounding the lesser economy, these vaporizers were intended for use with a specific anesthetic rather than the general use possible with the Copper Kettle. However, they had one (perceived) advantage over the Copper Kettle. The anesthetist did not need to calculate and recalculate the concentration of anesthetic obtained at the initiation of anesthesia, or after changes in inflow rate or dialed concentration. Life was simpler, and this fact contributed to their now universal adoption. In the process, we have lost more than the flexibility and economy of the Copper Kettle. The need to calculate the concentration of anesthetic educated a generation of anesthetists concerning the physics underlying anesthetic delivery—a great loss.

We should not leave this history without noting that variable by-pass vaporizers are, in fact, imitations of the Copper Kettle. Like the Copper Kettle, variable by-pass vaporizers have two flows through the vaporizer, although seemingly there is but one: The by-pass flow and the flow through the sump (reservoir) containing the liquid anesthetic, each, as with the Copper Kettle, metered precisely. As with the Copper Kettle, the variable-by-pass vaporizer ensures complete equilibrium of the gas passing through the sump. Finally, as with the Copper Kettle, the variable by-pass vaporizer accounts for the temperature of the anesthetic and the total flow delivered. These marvelous devices have now been perfected to eliminate the inadequacies of earlier models. They flatter the Copper Kettle with their imitation.

And what about the revival of chloroform, a revival that motivated the invention of the Copper Kettle? The Copper Kettle allowed control over the delivery of chloroform that was not possible with previous approaches. But that control did not alter the inherent toxicity of chloroform. Still, we have chloroform to thank for the invention, without which the anesthetic community would be the poorer.

The Copper Kettle proved to be a versatile tool for administration of all anesthetic vapors, and was in general use in the US for about twenty-five years. It went out of favor, in part, because of the development of variable bypass vaporizers that supplied an easy alternative to the requirement that the anesthetist calculate the delivered concentration. It also may have gone out of favor, in part because of ill-advised modifications made by the manufacturer, and in part because of misuse and lack of appreciation of the dangers of over-dosage. *Just as with a jet airplane or car, the best safety device of any potentially harmful equipment is the knowledge and full attention of the operator!* In contrast to variable by-pass (direct reading percentage) vaporizers which may encourage "cookbook" administration of anesthesia, the Copper Kettle encouraged users to think in terms of patient response, partial pressures and volume of vapor in the vaporizer output, which (when used in a closed absorption system) leads to a clearer understanding of uptake of anesthetics in the patient; important points for anesthetists and patient care even today.

Acknowledgment The authors wish to thank Mark E. Schroeder, MD, for his helpful editorial consultation, and advice.

References

1. Waters R. Chloroform; a study after 100 years. Madison: University of Wisconsin Press; 1951.
2. Snow J. On chloroform and other anaesthetics: their action and administration. London: John Churchill, New Burlington Street; 1858. pp. 1–443.
3. Snow J. On the inhalation of the vapour of ether in surgical operations: containing a description of the various stages of etherization, and a statement of the result of nearly eighty operations in which ether has been Employed In St. George's And University College Hospitals. London: John Churchill; 1847. pp 1–88.
4. Morris LE. A new vaporizer for liquid anesthetic agents. Anesthesiology. 1952;13:587–93.
5. Feldman SA. Morris LE: Vaporization of halothane and ether in the copper kettle. Anesthesiology. 1958;19:650–5.
6. Morris LE. Feldman SA: Considerations in the design and function of anesthetic vaporizers. Anesthesiology. 1958;19:642–9.
7. Morris LE. Feldman SA: Evaluation of a new anaesthetic vaporizer. Anaesthesia. 1962;17:21–8.
8. Foregger R. Death of a company. Posted on the internet by Richard Foregger; 1997.

The Development of Techniques for Airway Management

54

Carin A. Hagberg, Amna A. Ghouse and Dawn G. Iannucci

Summary

For a century, gauze masks served as the vehicle for vaporizing ether and chloroform. The anesthetist controlled anesthesia by regulating the drops of anesthetic applied to the gauze. Solid masks (leather, metal, rubber, and modern disposable plastic masks) fitted to the face allowed a more controlled delivery of anesthetic from vaporizers and gas flowmeters.

Ventilation and anesthetic delivery require an unobstructed airway. In 1873, Heiberg suggested jaw thrust, and in 1880, Howard added head tilt and extension. Artificial airways, tubes introduced through the nose (Faure 1859) or mouth (Hewitt 1908) replaced tongue forceps that might draw the tongue forward but also often damaged the tongue. Guedel and Waters produced the modern oropharyncal airway in the 1930s, and Shipway introduced a cuffed oropharyngeal airway in 1935, predating Brain's 1983 laryngeal mask airway.

Tracheal intubation provided a more secure airway. In 1796, Herholdt and Rafn used blind digitally-guided tracheal intubation to resuscitate drowning victims. Babbington viewed the glottis in 1829 by indirect laryngoscopy. Macewen pioneered blind tracheal intubation for anesthetic delivery in 1878, and in 1882, O'Dwyer used a tube to relieve obstruction from diphtheria. Kirstein reported laryngoscopy in 1895 with the "autoscope", used by Killian in 1897 to extract a foreign body from a bronchus. Jackson invented a direct laryngoscope in 1910. Miller and Macintosh described their blades for viewing the larynx by direct and indirect elevation of the epiglottis in the 1940s. Indirect laryngoscopy returned as an aid to intubation in 1980, with Bullard's rigid fiberoptic laryngoscope. Subsequently, advances in fiberoptic and video technology applied to laryngoscopes and bronchoscopy improved portability and ease of use.

Tracheal intubation began with rigid, then flexible, metal tubes. In 1898, van Stockum fitted his tube with an inflatable cuff, Reports of cuffed tracheal tubes appeared over the next three decades. In 1919, Magill and Rowbotham inserted a narrow rubber tube into the trachea for insufflation, later adding an exit tube. Flagg (1927) and Magill (1938) concluded that one wide-bore tube should work equally well. Magill made his tube from mineralized red rubber tubing. Polyvinyl chloride tubes were introduced in 1964.

Early thoracic surgeons operated on moving lungs. In 1931, Waters and Gale solved this problem by ventilating only the non-operated lung. Magill suggested the bronchial blocker in 1936. Carlens' invented the double-lumen tube in 1949 for bronchospirometry. It was later used in anesthetized patients.

In 1984, the Cormack-Lehane Laryngoscopy Grading System provided the first systematic approach to prediction of difficult intubation. Mallampati suggested an alternative the following year.

Introduction

Egyptian tablets from 3600 BCE (before the common era—equivalent to BC) describe tracheostomy, a surgical procedure which subsequently fell into and out of popularity [1–3]. Avicenna (also known as Ibn Sīnā), an Arabian physician, described tracheal intubation or an oropharyngeal airway in his book *Liber Canonis*: "when necessary, a cannula of gold, silver or suitable material is advanced down the throat to support inspiration." [3–5] Airway management attracted increasing interest after the 1846 discovery of anesthesia. A diverse assortment of physicians, priests, engineers, ministers and even musicians, made subsequent inventions and discoveries in airway management [1]. The use of the neuromuscular blocking drug, curare, to produce relaxation changed anesthetic delivery and launched further developments in airway management [6].

C. A. Hagberg (✉) · A. A. Ghouse · D. G. Iannucci
Department of Anesthesiology, The University of Texas
Medical School at Houston, Houston, TX, USA
e-mail: carin.a.hagberg@uth.tmc.edu

D. G. Iannucci
School of Public Health, The University of Texas
Health Science Center at Houston, Houston, TX, USA

Tracheostomy

Currently accepted as the last line of airway defense, a surgically obtained airway—tracheostomy or cricothyrotomy—is the oldest form of airway management. It remains the final pathway in "cannot intubate-cannot ventilate" circumstances [7–9].

Following the above-noted 3600 BCE Egyptian tablets, 2000 BCE Hindu scriptures mention tracheostomy, and around 100 BCE, Asclepiades is said to have performed a non-emergency tracheostomy [10–12]. Near to 100 CE, the Greek surgeon, Antyllus suggested bypassing upper airway obstruction by transverse tracheostomy. In 160 CE, the great Greek philosopher, Galen, described a technique similar to today's vertical tracheotomies [2, 3, 10], finding that "if you take a dead animal and blow air through its larynx (through a reed) you will fill its bronchi and watch its lungs attain the greatest dimensions." [3, 11]

In 1543, 28-year-old Andreas Vesalius published *de humani corporis Fabrica*, a 7-volume book, providing anatomic descriptions of the human body, including a detailed depiction of how to perform a tracheostomy in an animal. Because performing autopsies was considered scandalous, his dissections were performed in secrecy. Ironically, his demonstration of ventilation on the fresh cadaver of a Spanish nobleman led to Vesalius' death. Allegedly, while performing the tracheostomy and artificial ventilation, the nobleman's heart began to beat, outraging the general and medical community. Vesalius was exiled and while escaping, his boat capsized and he drowned [4, 5, 11, 13].

In 1546, Antonio Brasavola, an Italian physician, described the first successful use of a tracheostomy to bypass tonsillar obstruction in a human [5, 10]. In the early 1600s, Italian anatomist, Fabricius of Aquapedent, stated that few surgical procedures could so quickly revive a person as a tracheostomy [5, 10]. No evidence of regular use, however, appeared, and a 2001 review found published descriptions of only 50 tracheostomies before 1800 [3].

An early 1800s epidemic of diphtheria prompted the performance of tracheostomies, led by French internist, Armand Trousseau [5, 11, 13]. Desperate to save lives, Trousseau personally conducted more than 200 tracheostomies in afflicted children by 1833 [2, 5, 11]. Unfortunately, his method often produced tracheal stenosis which had a 50 % mortality rate. High perhaps, but better than the nearly 100 % mortality from diphtheria-induced suffocation [13, 14].

The use of a tracheostomy to facilitate anesthetic delivery began soon after the discovery of anesthesia. In 1853, John Snow administered chloroform to rabbits through a tracheostomy tube [4, 5]. In 1871, Friedrich Trendelenburg used this technique on humans, solving the problem of aspiration with his cuffed tracheostomy tube and funnel apparatus (Fig. 54.1) [4, 5, 11].

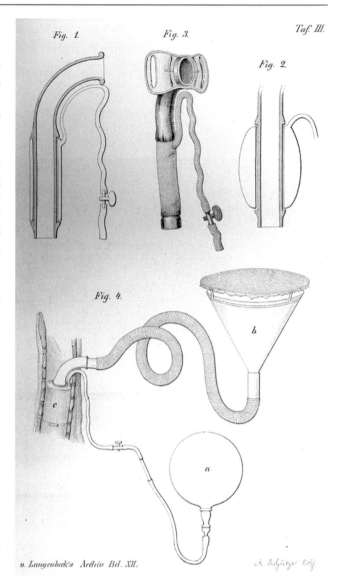

Fig. 54.1 Trendelenburg apparatus. (Courtesy of American Society of Anesthesiologists, ASA Newsletter Vol 72, Sep 2008, p. 9)

In 1909, Chevalier Jackson advanced the performance of tracheostomy by describing what are now modern techniques and principles (optimizing airway control before surgery; employing local anesthesia; using a well-designed tube; and applying meticulous surgical technique and postoperative care). These principles decreased mortality to 3 % and increased the acceptance of the procedure [10, 14, 15].

Cricothyrotomy

In 1805, French surgeon and anatomist Vicq d'Azyr described cricothyrotomy [16]. Initially ignored, these "high tracheostomies" increased in popularity in parallel with tracheostomies. However, concerned about the associated risk of subglottic stenosis, Chevalier Jackson decried cricothyrotomy. His objections hindered the performance of cricothyrotomy for over half a century [13, 14, 17].

In 1976, Colorado cardiothoracic surgeons Charles Brantigan and John Grow, Sr. published results of cricothyrotomies in 655 patients, with no incidence of chronic subglottic stenosis. Published complication rates of traditional tracheostomy exceeded the overall complication rate of 6.1%. Brantigan and Grow concluded that cricothyrotomy was faster, easier, and less likely to bleed [16]. Today, although the use of either tracheostomy or cricothyrotomy has decreased, they remain the preferred techniques when all other approaches have failed [7–9].

Anesthesia Facemasks and Upper Airway Obstruction

For more than a century, the facemask provided the primary interface to the anesthetic system for spontaneously breathing patients, and for most of those receiving positive pressure ventilation. After the 1950s, tracheal tubes increasingly displaced the facemask. Ventilation via a facemask remains an essential component of all difficult airway algorithms [7–9]. Modern transparent, high-volume, low pressure disposable plastic facemasks minimize dead space, maximize seal, and allow prompt recognition of regurgitation—as the ideal facemask should [18–20].

The facemasks created soon after the discovery of anesthesia took two forms. One provided a gauze surface (sometimes simply a handkerchief) onto which ether or chloroform was dripped or poured, and through which the patient might breathe, acquiring anesthetic in the process. The gauze might be supported by a wire frame, such as that devised by Thomas Skinner, a Scottish obstetrician [21]. These devices evolved into many variations, the most popular being the Yankauer and Schimmelbusch masks. Facemasks made of gauze had the advantages of simplicity and minimal cost, but the operating room became contaminated with anesthetic vapor (wasting anesthetic in the process) and positive pressure ventilation was not possible.

Skinner's reason for designing the wire frame mask was truly advanced for his time. Although the antisepsis debate developed eight years later, Skinner felt that facepieces preceding his design were "disgusting". Typically, a mask would be used and reused, without cleaning, without considering whether it had been applied to a patient with a possibly contagious infection before applying it to the next patient. Skinner's mask came with multiple flannel cloth coverings that could easily be replaced allowing each patient to have a clean mask [22, 23].

The second form of facemask, like that devised by Snow, might be recognized as the forerunner of the modern mask. It was made with harder material—leather or leather edged

metal. In the latter part of the nineteenth century, most masks (often in the form of "inhalers") were made of metal, sometimes with a rubber rim. Masks in the first half of the twentieth century were made of rubber, softer than leather or metal, but far harder than today's masks.

In the late 1950s, pediatric facemasks were miniature versions of adult masks. Because an infant's face differs from an adult's, these masks provided a poor seal and imposed a deadspace that might equal an infant's tidal exchange. Anesthesiologist Leslie Rendell-Baker and dental student Donald Soucek, (both from Western Reserve University) designed a better facemask from plaster moulds of infants' faces. They eliminated the cuffed rim and added a partitioned adapter that further minimized deadspace. Their 1961 result produced the still popular RBS facemask for children ≤5 years old [24, 25].

Adequate ventilation via facemask requires both a good seal and an unobstructed airway [18, 19]. In the late 1800s, Joseph Clover, Jacob Heiberg and Johannes Von Esmarch each recommended jaw thrust to relieve obstruction [20, 26, 27]. In 1894, surgeon Theodor Kocher advocated jaw thrust and chin lift for all anesthetized patients [28]. Jaw thrust became known as Esmarch's maneuver although it was first described by Heiberg [26, 27]. In 1880, Benjamin Howard found that head tilt and neck extension opened the airway by lifting the epiglottis and tongue [27]. In the 1950s and 1960s, radiologic studies documented that chin lift, head tilt, and jaw thrust opened the airway [18, 20].

Position change was used to resolve some forms of upper airway obstruction. Snow argued that the recumbent position permitted surgical debris to pool in the back of the throat where it might pass down the esophagus—never mind that it might also enter the glottis. If the anesthesiologist heard gurgling sounds, the patient's head should be tilted forward or sideways to empty accumulated debris [4, 29, 30]. British anesthetist Alexander Wilson tied his patients to a rocking chair for surgeries of the tongue, thereby allowing an array of positions: reclined for induction; seated for surgery; and, body/head tilted forward to clear the pharynx of debris [29, 30]. James Murphy described an 1894 Parisian patient position—supine with his head hanging over the end of the operating table, using gravity to protect the airway against aspiration. In 1904, operating tables were fitted with special headrests to simulate Murphy's position [30]. Trendelenburg's downward tilt was similarly used to drain debris from the airway [31].

Devices Used to Manage Upper Airway Obstruction

Tongue Forceps

In an 1856 letter describing "never before pointed out impediments of respiration," Marshall Hall observed that

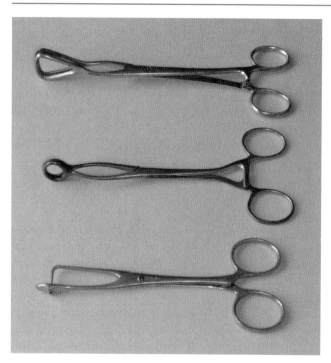

Fig. 54.2 Various tongue forceps were devised to allow the user to pull the subject's tongue forward, sometimes damaging tongue and teeth in the process. (Courtesy of Rod N. Westhorpe and the Geoffrey Kaye Museum of Anaesthetic History)

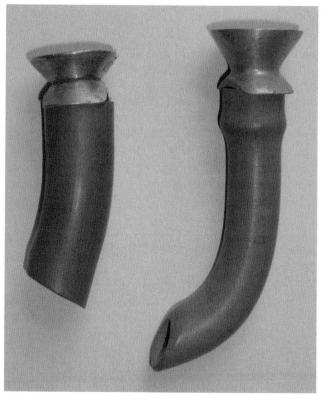

Fig. 54.3 Hewitt oropharyngeal airway, original straight version on left. (Courtesy of Rod N. Westhorpe and the Geoffrey Kaye Museum of Anaesthetic History)

glottic obstruction sometimes occurred in supine patients. He believed that relaxation of the tongue caused the epiglottis to block the glottis [26]. In seeming support of Hall's suggestion in 1880, Benjamin Howard found that traction on the tongue to displace it from the posterior pharyngeal wall could relieve obstruction (actually implying that the tongue and not the epiglottis was the problem) [27].

Accordingly, tongue forceps were invented (Fig. 54.2). But in 1874, Jacob Heiberg gave a frightful image of forceps-based management of airway obstruction. Their use broke teeth and injured the tongue. Injury could impair speaking and/or swallowing and cause prolonged pain [26]. Despite the English Suspended Animation Committee's 1879 objection to these devices—recommending instead Esmarch's maneuver—tongue forceps continued in use into the 1930s [26, 32].

Oropharyngeal and Nasopharyngeal Airways

An oropharyngeal or nasopharyngeal airway may be used to assist in opening the upper airway [18, 19]. In 1859, Faure of Paris inserted a long rubber tube through the nares, a primitive nasopharyngeal airway, to create a passage for chloroform delivery [33]. Similarly, Joseph Clover in 1881 connected his chloroform/nitrous oxide bag to an India-rubber nasal tube to deliver anesthesia during jaw surgery [32–34]. In 1913, Karl Connell, a Columbia University surgeon,

described anesthetic delivery through either a single or double nasopharyngeal airway [32, 35].

Frederic Hewitt's classic 1890 summary noted the frequency and danger of upper airway obstruction. In 1908, dissatisfied with the use of tongue forceps and acknowledging that Esmarch's maneuver sometimes failed, he described the first oropharyngeal airway, the Hewitt Airway (Fig. 54.3). The tube was less than 8 cm long, ideally connecting the oral opening to the hypopharynx [27, 30, 36]. Within a year, a longer curved version replaced the first, straight model. The Hewitt Airway anticipated many subsequent oropharyngeal airway designs [4, 27, 32].

Improvements and increased use of the oropharyngeal airway followed World War I [32]. In 1930, Ralph Waters, the first Chairman of an Anesthesiology department in the US (University of Wisconsin), designed an airway made of metal, further differing from Hewitt's design by being oval in shape and later including a side tube for insufflation [34, 37, 38].

Although Arthur Guedel and Waters never worked at the same institution, they corresponded and collaborated on research projects [39, 40]. Guedel, at the University of Southern California, believed that steel oropharyngeal airways caused oral trauma [38–40], and that it could be better contoured to fit the shape of the pharynx [32, 40]. Thus he made his airway of rubber, sufficiently soft to be flexible and perhaps less traumatic, yet rigid enough to maintain a patent airway. It included a metal piece at the level of the incisors as a bite block [39, 40]. A wide rubber flange at the oral opening prevented over insertion and allowed easy retrieval [40]. Guedel wrote to Waters "As I use the rubber airway more and more, I am growing to like its action better and even as well as or better than the metal (Waters) airway. I am proud of the idea…" [40]

Resident Robert Berman had an incident with a Guedel Oral Airway which resulted in a new oropharyngeal airway [41]. He had placed a Guedel Airway in a shirt pocket that also contained safety pins (safety pins were often used to puncture the lead tops of containers of ether; they formed a wick that facilitated the controlled delivery of ether). After using the oropharyngeal airway during induction, he performed laryngoscopy and noticed a safety pin in the posterior pharynx. The opacity of the black rubber had hidden the presence of the safety pin, which had been dislodged by the force of ventilation [41]. Berman discussed the problem with his neighbor, Meyer Moch, a plastic fabricator. Excited by the problem and seeing a solution, Moch and Berman retired to Moch's basement where they softened butyrate tubing, formed it into the shape of an airway, and sanded it smooth. Since Moch lacked pharyngeal reflexes, they immediately tested its fitting and function on him [41]. In 1951, Berman and Moch officially introduced the airway. The final version differed from Guedel's in having no closed tube that might trap foreign bodies. Instead, it had a central longitudinal strut with upper and lower flanges [41, 42]. See Fig. 54.4 for a view of the different types of oropharyngeal airways.

While these oropharyngeal airways could overcome upper airway obstruction, their use did not preclude aspiration. Without tracheal intubation, packing with gauze, sponges, or repositioning of the patient was used to manage this complication. Such management was imperfect and gauze and sponges could be swallowed or inhaled. An alternative solution was required [43]. Just before retiring in 1935, Francis Shipway, anesthetist to King George V, designed the Shipway Oropharyngeal Airway (Fig. 54.5). The Shipway Airway added an inflatable cuff to the Hewitt Airway. It was specifically designed to prevent aspiration of blood during intranasal surgery [30, 43, 44]. A special fitting permitted the connection of the Shipway Airway directly to an anesthetic circuit [30, 43, 44].

In 1937, Canadian Beverly Leech invented the Leech Pharyngeal Bulb Gasway. A solid rubber bulbous plug with a hollow core surrounded the distal end of this metal oropharyngeal airway, the assembly fitting closely to the pharyngeal tissues to provide an airtight seal [32, 44–46]. While not an inflatable cuff, the plug served a similar function and is often called a "cuffed device". Its design was based on studies of pharyngeal anatomy [30, 32, 45]. Used to deliver

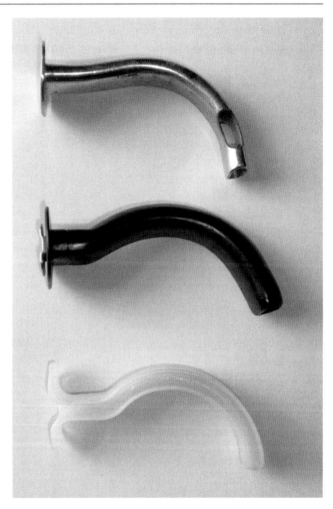

Fig. 54.4 Oropharyngeal airways. From top to bottom, Connell, Guedel, and Berman oral airways. (Courtesy of Rod N. Westhorpe, and the Geoffrey Kaye Museum of Anaesthetic History)

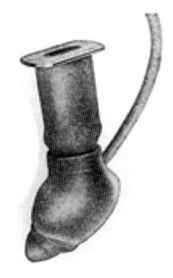

Fig. 54.5 Shipway cuffed oropharyngeal airway. (From [44])

closed circuit cyclopropane anesthesia, it remained popular until tracheal intubation rendered it obsolete in the mid-1950s [45].

In 1991, Robert Greenberg, at John Hopkins developed the Cuffed Oropharyngeal Airway, a Guedel oral airway which included an inflatable cuff and a 15 mm connector for attaching to an anesthesia circuit. The cuffed oropharyngeal airway was prone to dislodgement when the cuff was inflated [45]. Removal with its cuff inflated helped prevent aspiration of blood or secretions.

Cuffed oropharyngeal airways were an important part of airway management history, serving as an inspiration for future supra-laryngeal airways [18, 43, 44], but interest in these airways was not sustained. They gave way to tracheal intubation and supralaryngeal airways.

Supralaryngeal Airway Devices

Before the 1980s, ventilation via a facemask supplied the primary alternative for tracheal intubation. However, ventilation via a facemask did not preclude aspiration of gastric contents. Securing an airtight seal could also be difficult [4, 47, 48]. After 1981, progress in supralaryngeal airway devices increasingly overcame these shortcomings.

Determined to develop an airway minimizing the limitations of facemask-assisted ventilation, British anesthetist Archie Brain invented a device connecting the natural airway to an artificial airway that did not require insertion equipment, and did not demand the use of muscle relaxants [4, 34, 47, 48]. Brain noticed that the shapes of plaster casts of a cadaver's pharynx resembled the Goldman nasal masks used in dental anesthesia. Brain created his first laryngeal mask airway (LMA) by attaching a Goldman nasal mask to a diagonally cut end of a 10 mm Portex tracheal tube, joining them with acrylic adhesive [47–49]. In the summer of 1981, Brain blindly inserted the LMA prototype in a patient undergoing a routine hernia repair under halothane anesthesia, achieving a clear airway that allowed positive pressure ventilation [48, 49]. Success! A pilot study in 23 patients undergoing various operations, including gynecological laparoscopic procedures requiring positive pressure ventilation, showed that the device could supply a patent protected airway without requiring muscle relaxants to facilitate placement. Published in the British Journal of Anaesthesia in 1983, the results received surprisingly little attention from the medical or manufacturing community [47–50]. Undeterred, Brain soon filed a dozen patents [4, 47].

Despite the lack of commercial interest, Brain continued to modify his invention, experimenting with diverse materials before settling on silicone for the LMA-Classic (cLMA) [47, 48]. So strange were some designs that several early prototypes were mistaken for exotic rubber condoms by members of the cleaning staff at Brain's laboratory in Newham General Hospital [47]. Over the next seven years, Brain produced hundreds of prototypes testing them in approximately 7,000 patients [47–49].

The large number of prototypes and long development process reflected Brain's quest to balance ease of use, efficacy and safety [48, 49]. While one modification improved one aspect of the LMA, it might sacrifice another [48, 49]. For example, increasing surface mucosal contact with the cuff provided greater seal pressure but caused ischemia of the tongue. Also, the use of an insertion device eased placement, but increased the risk of trauma. With clinically acceptable seal pressures of 20 cm H_2O, the cLMA became commercially available in 1988 [49, 51, 52]. Following a demonstration of the new device, Colin Alexander, a British anesthetist and chair at the Royal East Sussex Hospital, acquired the cLMA for his hospital and published his experiences in a letter to *Anaesthesia* [47, 49]. Within 2 years, the LMA was available in every hospital in the UK [34, 48]. It was marketed in Australia and New Zealand in 1989. Ronald Katz at UCLA received a prototype LMA in 1985. He quickly wrote of his experiences, sparking interest in the US [49]. The cLMA had been used in more than 2 million cases when approved by the FDA in 1991 [48, 49]. Commercial release of the LMA in the US occurred in 1992.

British anesthetist, John Nunn, assisted Brain in marketing the cLMA in the UK [47, 48]. US anesthesiologists Jonathan Benumof, Paul White and Andranik Ovasspian paved the way for North American recognition. White and his team demonstrated that the cLMA was a useful airway device for routine anesthetic cases. Ovassapian and Benumof tested its use for "cannot intubate, cannot ventilate" patients. They argued that the cLMA provided a "second-last-ditch" effort for cases of failed intubation when a surgical airway was the only other remaining option [48]. With their influence, the LMA was added to the ASA Difficult Airway Algorithm in 1993, with an expanded role in the 1996 and 2003 algorithms [7–9, 51, 53]. It is currently listed in difficult airway algorithms throughout the world [9]. The American Heart Association's 2000 Guidelines for CPR and Emergency Medicine Cardiovascular Care incorporated the disposable LMA-Unique (uLMA) as an essential airway rescue device [52]. Development of the LMA has been touted as one of the greatest advancements in anesthesia since the advent of the tracheal tube. It has changed airway management in emergency, critical care, and ambulatory medicine, as well as anesthesia. For his efforts, Brain received numerous awards and accolades [4, 47, 48].

Brain revolutionized the use of the supralaryngeal airway, but he was not the first to conceive of the idea [4, 48, 49]. Oropharyngeal airways (1908) and the Fell-O'Dwyer apparatus (1882) took advantage of placing the tip of an artificial airway into the pharynx rather than the trachea. Some argue that the Leech Gasway (1937) was father to all supralaryngeal airway devices, including the LMA [2, 4, 34]. Brain's device differed in a crucial attribute—its approach to sealing the airway. While the LMA used a soft inflatable "mask over the larynx" whose tip is positioned in the esophagus, at least one previous device surrounded the tube at the glottic opening with a solid plug [2, 4, 34].

While some supralaryngeal airway devices were similar to Brain's LMA design, others resembled a tracheal tube that enabled pulmonary ventilation without passing through the vocal cords. In 1968, Don Michael developed the first of such devices, the Esophageal Obturator Airway. It had a distal balloon blocking the esophagus and sixteen holes for ventilation between this and a proximal balloon. Difficulties arose in using the Esophageal Obturator Airway and comparative studies with tracheal tubes revealed no advantages, thus the device disappeared [34, 54, 55].

Austrian internist, Michael Frass, with Reainhard Frenzer and Jonas Zahler envisioned a need for an airway device that could ventilate the lungs regardless of whether the device entered the glottis or esophagus. In 1987, they invented the Esophageal Tracheal Combitube (Fig. 54.6), a device with two lumens separated at the proximal end, allowing attachment of the airway circuit to either [52, 54–56]. The esophageal lumen is closed at the tip and has eight perforations between a proximal and a distal cuff. The alternative lumen, the tracheal lumen, is open at the end and when placed in the glottis, functions essentially as a tracheal tube. Thus, regardless of where the device is positioned, the Esophageal Tracheal Combitube provides a patent airway. No time is lost to repositioning, making it particularly useful in prehospital and emergency care settings, where time may be crucial [52, 54–56].

Developed in 2003, the EasyTube was functionally the same as the Esophageal Tracheal Combitube but had a smaller tip and the pharyngeal cuff had a lower volume. The redesigned pharyngeal aperture allowed for easier passage of a flexible fiberoptic bronchoscope, gum elastic bougie or tracheal suction catheter and uses polyvinyl chloride in the large oropharyngeal cuff [34, 52, 56] Both devices are included in guidelines for difficult airway management and emergency resuscitation throughout the world [9].

Similar in appearance to the Esophageal Tracheal Combitube, the King Laryngeal Tube (King LT) is a supralaryngeal airway device introduced in Europe in 1999 by VBM Medizintechnik. Redesigned by King Systems, it received FDA approval in 2003 [56]. It differs slightly from other supralaryngeal airways in that it consists of a reusable, dual-cuffed single-lumen tube with a blind distal tip. Two anterior ventilation outlets between the low-pressure distal (esophageal) and proximal (oropharyngeal) cuffs allow the device to function as a supralaryngeal airway. Unlike the Esophageal Tracheal Combitube or EasyTube, both cuffs are inflated through a single valve [52, 55, 56]. The King LT can be used during both positive pressure ventilation and spontaneous ventilation. The King LTS (reusable) and King LTS-D (disposable)

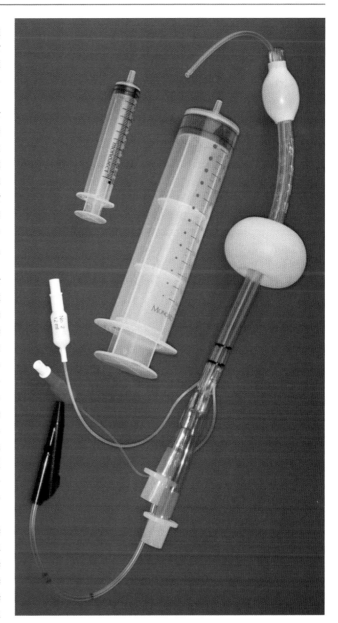

Fig. 54.6 Esophageal-Tracheal Combitube (Frass M et al. [54]) esophageal/endotracheal double-lumen airway: the combitube and the easytube. (From Hagberg C (ed.) *Benumof's and Hagberg's Airway Management: Principles and Practice 3rd edition*. Mosby, Inc., St. Louis, 2012)

devices released in 2003 added an opening in their distal tip for esophageal access. Like the pLMA, the King LTS and LTS-D allow for passage of a gastric tube. The King LT family of devices has gained popularity in emergency medicine and prehospital care settings [52, 55, 56].

Laryngoscopy, Laryngoscopes, and Tracheal Tubes

Initial visualization of the larynx occurred outside the operating room, and was prompted by curiosity concerning voice production. In 1829, Benjamin Babington, a British physician, used sunlight reflected off a hand mirror and a small mirror attached to the end of a spatula to view the vocal cords in action. A colleague called Babington's device a "laryngoscope" while Babington called it a glottiscope. He reported his findings to a disbelieving Hunterian Society, his peers certain that the vocal cords could not be seen in a living person [57, 58].

A quarter century later, Manuel Garcia, a famous singing teacher at the Royal Academy of Music in London, wanted to see his own vocal cords. Benefiting from naturally obtunded gag reflexes, Garcia performed laryngoscopy of his active vocal cords using a dental mirror positioned in his oropharynx and a hand mirror to simultaneously reflect light and visualize the image in the dental mirror. He meticulously documented observations of his vocalization and that of others, and in 1855, presented his results to the Royal Society. This time, indirect laryngoscopy was met with interest [33, 58–60].

After witnessing Garcia's demonstration, Austrian neurologist, Ludwig Turck, began using laryngeal mirrors in his hospital practice. Attaining indirect laryngoscopy was cumbersome, often requiring cooperative patients to assist with a self-applied tongue depressor and/or forceps, while Turck positioned the mirrors. Turck claimed to see the mucosal surface of the posterior tracheal wall, the bifurcation of the trachea and even the first six circular cartilages of the bronchi in optimal cases. His colleagues considered these assertions exaggerated [33, 58–60]. Hungarian physiologist and physician, Johann Czermak, expanded the studies of indirect laryngoscopy, popularizing the technique. His work introduced laryngoscopy as a new branch of surgery [58–60].

Tracheal Intubation

Indirect laryngoscopy allowed a view of the glottis but did not immediately lead to tracheal intubation. After Avicenna, tracheal intubation was mostly performed to aid in the resuscitation of drowning victims and to treat patients with diphtheria. In 1796, Herholdt and Rafn described blind digitally assisted tracheal intubation to resuscitate drowning victims, their work receiving little notice until the mid-1980s [61]. In 1788, the British physician, Charles Kite, described a metal orotracheal tube bent like a male urethral catheter, passed blindly through the glottis, and then connected to a bellows [4, 62, 63]. Encouragement by European and British medical societies in the late 18th century prompted development of new airway devices for artificial ventilation. These were widely distributed, primarily for use in victims of drowning. However, experiments performed by Jean Leroy d'Etoilles in the late 1820s, revealed the danger of developing a tension pneumothorax from forced inflation of the lungs caused by the use of the bellows in the resuscitation of drowned victims.

Although Leroy modified the bellows to be safer, the Royal Humane Society retracted their support of artificial ventilation, temporarily delaying the advancement of airway management and the use of positive pressure ventilation [11, 64].

Scottish surgeon William Macewen pioneered elective tracheal intubation for anesthetic delivery [60, 65–67]. In 1878, he practiced blind digitally assisted orotracheal and nasotracheal intubation on cadavers. He abandoned nasotracheal intubation as impractical, probably because of the size and stiffness of his metal tubes [33, 60, 66]. He hoped to deliver anesthetic without contaminating the surgical field and to protect the lungs from aspiration without performing a tracheostomy. Orotracheal intubation would also resolve the conflict between surgeon and anesthesiologist for access to the mouth and airway [1, 33, 61, 66]. He used his index finger to depress the epiglottis and guide a rigid, curved brass tracheal tube of his design [1, 61, 68] over his finger and into the larynx [33]. In July 1878, he performed his first tracheal intubation in a patient undergoing removal of an epithelioma of the tongue, right anterior pillar of fauces and posterior pharyngeal wall [33, 60, 68]. Topical anesthesia awaited discovery, and Macewen practiced several awake tracheal intubations in the unanesthetized patient before the day of surgery [33, 61, 66, 68]. Other than bouts of coughing both during and immediately after placement of the tracheal tube, the patient tolerated the intubation, and Macewen proceeded with anesthesia [33, 60]. With sponges packed into the pharynx to prevent aspiration, the extensive surgical procedure, including sawing through the lower jaw, concluded successfully [1, 33, 60, 66]. The patient maintained spontaneous ventilation and showed no signs of pain [60]. As did others, Macewen advocated viewing the glottis via indirect laryngoscopy to determine oropharyngeal pathology before performing intubation.

Between 1878 and 1880, Macewen described two additional successful tracheal intubations for glottic obstruction [60, 66, 68]. His fourth patient, the second scheduled for anesthesia and surgery following tracheal intubation, resulted in a fatality [33, 60, 68]. Like the first case, the patient had an epithelioma of the tongue—but also had bronchitis [60]. Although Macewen successfully practiced awake intubations in the patient before the day of surgery, on the day of surgery the patient pulled out the tube and pleaded for its placement after induction with chloroform [60, 66, 68]. The patient struggled with induction, and once achieved, Macewen inserted the tube [60, 66]. Within minutes, the radial pulse and spontaneous ventilation ceased [36, 60, 66]. An autopsy revealed cerebral hemorrhage, probably stress-related [36, 66]. This was the last tracheal intubation reported by Macewen [33, 60, 66, 68].

Joseph O'Dwyer, a physician at the Foundling Hospital in New York, found the mortality from diphtheria to be unacceptable. He studied autopsies to define alternatives to tracheostomy [2, 60, 69], and from these investigations developed the O'Dwyer endolaryngeal tubes. He first used these clinically in 1882 and by 1885 had perfected his skills and tubes. The metal tubes came as a set in a range of sizes and featured a collar, designed to rest within the pharynx against the false vocal cords, to prevent the tube from advancing down the trachea [1, 68]. O'Dwyer is credited with publicizing tracheal (actually endolaryngeal) intubation, albeit not for anesthetic purposes [4, 60].

In 1885, a young woman with known laryngeal stenosis, approached O'Dwyer requesting an alternative to tracheostomy. O'Dwyer accommodated her request, by inserting one of his tubes. Similar cases followed [33]. In 1887, the New York physician George Fell modified his breathing apparatus supplying positive pressure ventilation using a bellows and mask, by attaching it to a tracheotomy tube. Fell's apparatus was specifically used to treat narcotic overdose. Learning of Fell's modifications, O'Dwyer altered his tube to permit controlled ventilation with Fell's device, hence the Fell-O'Dwyer Apparatus [1, 4, 68]. (Fig. 54.7) Theodore Tuffier, a French surgeon, and Rudolph Matas, a Texas and Louisiana surgeon, made further modifications for positive pressure ventilation during intrathoracic surgery [1, 33, 68].

In 1893, Karl Maydl, Professor of Surgery at the University of Prague, suggested that intubation of the larynx, and packing gauze around the glottic opening would prevent aspiration of blood [33, 66]. Although Macewen had advocated this technique, little was known of Macewen's work [33]. Maydl knew however, of O'Dwyer's work and adopted O'Dwyer's intubation techniques for otorhinolaryngological surgical procedures [1, 33, 66].

In 1896, German surgeon Franz Kuhn found that rigidity of existing tracheal tubes was limiting [68, 70]. Using coiled metal similar to that found in spouts of old gasoline cans, he made a tracheal tube that was flexible, yet resisted compression [36, 68, 70]. Like Macewen, Kuhn performed blind, digitally-assisted awake tracheal intubation with the aid of a rigid curved introducer [60, 68, 70]. His method was easier than Macewen's because topical anesthesia with cocaine had been discovered. Topical anesthesia allowed great advances in nasotracheal intubation after World War I [1, 66, 70].

Kuhn surrounded his tracheal tube with a supralaryngeal flange to prevent over-insertion [60, 66, 68]. Kuhn acknowledged the existence of tracheal tube cuffs but preferred to pack the larynx with oil-soaked gauze [30, 36, 60, 68] which also helped secure the tube in place [60]. Kuhn pioneered suctioning of tracheal blood and secretions [68, 71]. Most tubes at this time were narrow and were used for insufflation (blowing air plus ether or chloroform vapor into the trachea). He preferred larger tubes because they allowed bidirectional respiration. During World War II, English prisoners of war found Kuhn's technique and tracheal tubes beneficial. One

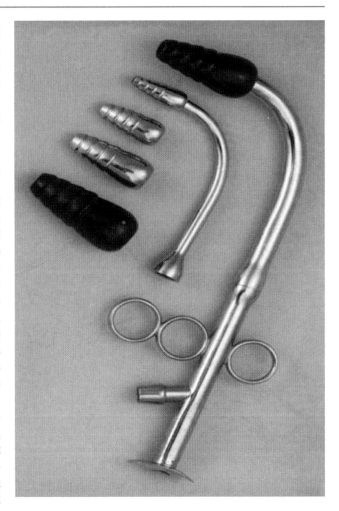

Fig. 54.7 Modified O'Dwyer's tubes intended for insertion into the larynx. Combined with Fell's foot bellows and air hose, they comprised the Fell-O'Dwyer apparatus. (Courtesy of Science Museum London/Science and Society Picture Library, London, England)

advantage touted for this technique was that batteries which were in short supply were not required [30, 60].

In 1902, Kuhn pioneered nasotracheal intubation in living patients [66, 69, 72]. He argued that the anatomy of the nasal route provided a more direct approach to the glottic opening [66], prevented the tracheal tube from being bitten, and left the mouth unoccupied [66, 68]. However, he ultimately viewed orotracheal intubation as better suited to his patients' needs, probably because the metallic composition of his tubes might traumatize the nasal mucosa despite its flexibility [66].

Before 1900, placement of a tracheal tube usually required a blind digitally assisted orotracheal intubation, a difficult maneuver requiring extensive practice and involving significant risk to the intubator whose finger might be bitten and become infected [2, 36]. Widespread use of blind nasotracheal intubation awaited development of soft flexible tracheal tubes. The introduction of direct laryngoscopy during the 1910s overcame these limitations.

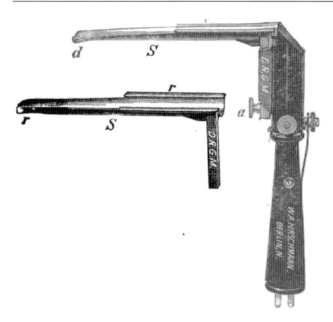

Fig. 54.8 Alfred Kirstein's "Autoscope". (From [73])

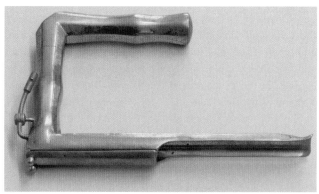

Fig. 54.9 Chevalier Jackson's U-shaped laryngoscope. (Courtesy of Sheffield Teaching Hospitals NHS Trust Dept of Anaesthesia, Sheffield, UK)

Laryngoscopy

Direct laryngoscopy originated with Alfred Kirstein's 1895 article describing his "autoscope" (Fig. 54.8) [58, 73, 74]. A colleague's accidental placement of an esophagoscope into the trachea sparked Kirstein's interest. Initially, he directly visualized the larynx by shortening an esophagoscope and attaching an electric lamp to the handle, deflecting light down the lumen by a prism taken from Caspar's electroscope. The enclosed "O" shape of this original autoscope limited the view of the glottis, leading to a redesigned blade with an open crescent shape and an improved distal width and thickness for direct or indirect positioning of the epiglottis [33, 59, 68]. Notwithstanding this work, Kirstein never performed tracheal intubation or bronchoscopy. But in 1897, his student, Gustav Killian, used the autoscope to extract a foreign body from a patient's bronchus. This case and his subsequent work made Killian the "father of bronchoscopy." [59]

By 1910, Chevalier Jackson had invented a U-Shaped direct laryngoscope (Fig. 54.9) for examining the esophagus and airway. He became renowned for his ability to remove foreign bodies from the airway, and patients came from all over the world to obtain his services—often performed at little to no cost to the patient. In 1912, Charles Elsberg used the Jackson laryngoscope for tracheal intubation and insufflation. This prompted Jackson to publish a paper advocating examining vocal cords for pathology before intubation and ascertaining the proper size of tube to be used. His work furthered the popularity that laryngoscopy gained over the succeeding decades [15, 75, 76].

Appreciating the benefits of illumination, Jackson added a light bulb to the distal end of the blade. Cords from a large dry cell battery powered the light, which, however, added the risk of an explosion if a short circuit caused a spark in the presence of ether. Nonetheless, this Jackson laryngoscope gained great popularity over the next three decades [1, 59, 60, 68]. New York anesthesiologist, Henry Janeway, solved the sparking problem in 1913 with a laryngoscope powered by batteries located in the handle, but his laryngoscope never achieved the popularity of Jackson's [60, 68].

Laryngoscope blades remained largely unchanged until Robert Miller and Robert Macintosh described their inventions for direct and indirect elevation of the epiglottis in the 1940s. Blades did evolve (Fig. 54.10). Straight blades are traditionally called Miller-type blades, but the straight blades devised by Magill, Flagg and Guedel all predate Miller's [59]. Miller introduced his modification in 1941. In 1943, Macintosh developed a curved blade which when placed into the angle made by the epiglottis and the base of the tongue indirectly lifted the epiglottis, potentially reducing the risk of trauma. Macintosh contended that the blade could be used at a lighter level of anesthesia (perhaps because it caused less stimulation of the epiglottis.).

It became apparent that patient position affected the ease of tracheal intubation. Initially, patients assumed the sitting position, useful in awake patients but problematic in anesthetized patients. In 1913, Jackson advocated the "classical position" placing the patient supine on a flat surface with the head and neck fully extended. In 1933, he amended this to have patients "sniffing the air" (aka, "sniffing position"): head extended with the neck flexed, accomplished by placing a 10 cm thick pillow underneath the head [59].

In 1944, British anesthetist Freda Bannister and British otolaryngologist Ronald MacBeth proposed a theory of best position for visualisation of the larynx, defined by three longitudinal axes: the oral, pharyngeal and laryngeal axes. From

Fig. 54.10 Evolution of laryngoscopy. (From Anesthesia & Analgesia, April 2010 journal cover, with permission)

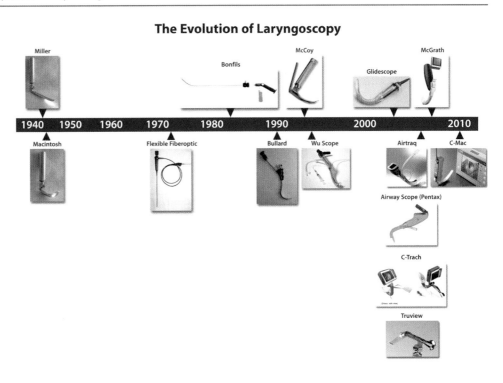

The Evolution of Laryngoscopy

radiographic studies they confirmed Jacksons conclusion that the sniffing position created the ideal position by aligning these axes [59]. In 1964, Frederic Adnet and colleagues reviewed the original radiographs, and obtained new images, concluding that the classical position produces optimal positioning [59]. This debate continues.

While the art of direct laryngoscopy blossomed, major advancements were also made in the techniques and tubes used for nasotracheal intubation. In 1919, British anesthetist Ivan Magill, and his colleague Edgar Rowbotham, an anesthetist in the Royal Army Medical Corps, were stationed at the Queen's Hospital for Facial and Jaw Injuries. They managed patients undergoing prolonged surgeries requiring a secure airway that did not obstruct surgical access [1, 36, 72, 77]. Anesthesia for these patients had been ether in oil administered rectally. Beyond the drawbacks of prolonged induction and emergence plus minimal control over the depth of anesthesia, this approach left the airway unprotected [1, 68, 78].

Insufflation offered a better solution. A narrow tube was inserted via the mouth or nose through the glottic opening. Anesthetic vapor delivered via this tube was inspired, and, escaped around the tube [4, 68, 77]. The surgeons appreciated the more secure airway and greater control over anesthesia, but were not enthralled with vapor-laden air blown into their faces or blood occasionally sprayed from the surgical site [68, 77, 78]. However this technique required that the insufflated air freely escape to avoid a fatal pneumothorax. The means to assure such an escape while also diverting the

excess became apparent in 1922. A facial deformity prevented air from properly escaping, leading Magill and Rowbotham to pass a second tube through the nose into the trachea parallel to the first one. The benefit of this "exhaust" tube was immediately obvious [77].

Magill and Rowbotham adopted this two-tube intubation system for routine cases using either another insufflation catheter or Silk's wide-bore rubber pharyngeal tube [67, 71, 77]. This second, exit tube allowed the surgeons to pack the pharynx with gauze to protect against aspiration [1, 4, 66]. Magill and Rowbotham learned that placing the semi-rigid insufflation catheters in hot water softened them, decreasing nasal trauma during insertion [66, 68, 72]. Nasotracheal intubation became standard practice.

In New York, Paluel Flagg learned of Magill's and Rowbotham's two-tube system and concluded that one wide-bore tube should work equally well. The result was Flagg's tracheal tube: a single, wide-bore tube useful for either orotracheal or nasotracheal intubation [78]. Unaware of Flagg's work, Magill reached a similar conclusion in 1928. Magill sought a tube allowing for bidirectional airflow and rigid enough to hold the curve necessary for nasotracheal intubation without traumatizing nasal tissues [68, 72, 77]. The solution came to him in a local hardware store selling rubber gas tubing [72]. The natural curve in the tubing formed by their storage in coils was ideal for passage through the nose [67, 71, 72]. He customized the length of each tube to each patient—twice the distance from the tip of the earlobe to the tip of the nose. He beveled the tip, lubricated its surface with paraffin wax and smoothed it with emery sandpaper [67, 72, 77]. It took him several years to secure a company to manufacture stiffer mineralized rubber tubes to his specifications [77]. Between 1928 and 1932, his method of tracheal anesthesia, coinciding with his introduction of the "Magill circuit" (later known as the Mapleson A breathing system), gradually replaced insufflation [66, 71, 77].

Magill and Rowbotham perfected their technique for blind nasotracheal intubation. They rediscovered the advantages of airway cocainization, which allowed tracheal intubation with the patient awake or lightly sedated [68, 72, 77]. As they practiced their skills, they noticed that as it left the nasopharynx, the tracheal tube naturally entered the trachea [68, 72, 77, 78]. To deal with circumstances when this failed, Magill designed curved forceps (aka Magill forceps) used to guide the tracheal tube tip into the glottis, facilitated if necessary by laryngoscopy [60, 66, 77]. Because blind awake nasotracheal intubation required frequent use and practice to perform well, the technique initially met resistance. Acceptance gradually increased in the 1930s [36, 60, 77]. Until the 1980s, blind nasotracheal intubation was an essential skill needed to circumvent difficult or contraindicated laryngoscopy, but the advent of fiberoptic endoscopy eliminated this need.

In the 1940s, Francis Murphy, Chief Anesthesiologist at the University of California San Francisco, designed tubes with a rounded tip to prevent the tip from catching on the vocal cords, as bevel-tipped tubes often did. In addition, the rounded tip had one or two small side holes, referred to as Murphy eyes, which allowed continued ventilation if the distal opening abutted the tracheal or bronchial wall. The famous Murphy eye exists in the design of many later tracheal tubes [36, 79].

Cuffed Tracheal Tubes

Maydl protected against aspiration of surgical debris and/or gastric contents by surrounding the orotracheal tube with oil-soaked gauze as it passed through the oropharynx. In 1893, Austrian physician Victor Eisenmenger added an inflatable cuff, like the one used with Trendelenburg's tracheostomy tubes, to his curved tracheal tube made of hard rubber [1, 4, 33, 66]. In 1898, Dutch physician WJ van Stockum, aware of both Maydl's and Eisenmenger's work, constructed a wide-bore tracheal tube fitted with an inflatable cuff. He combined both techniques, packing the airway with a collar of sponges above an inflated cuff [33, 66]. Over the next three decades, reports of cuffed tracheal tubes would appear and disappear, but had little practical impact, perhaps because of the lack of a significant market.

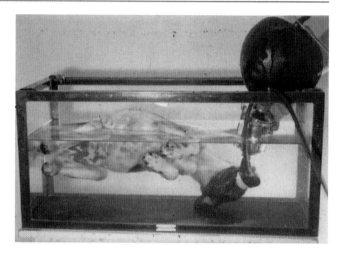

Fig. 54.11 "Airway" the subject of the Dunked Dog Experiment. (Courtesy of Guedel Memorial Center, San Franscisco, CA)

In the early 1900s, approximately 100 physicians regularly practiced anesthesia in the US [68]. Only otolaryngologists performed intubations, usually for emergency purposes [68]. Not until the 1930s, when the work of Guedel and Waters became known, did the use of cuffed tracheal tubes become common as pathways for anesthetic delivery. Anesthesia needed to emerge as a specialty chosen by increasing numbers of physicians.

Guedel made his first cuffs by gluing the fingers of surgical gloves, and later condoms, to the outer wall of a tracheal tube [39, 68]. He experimented with position: the cuff above, below and at the level of the vocal cords, concluding that just below the cords provided the best seal of the airway and allowed access to fluid that might accumulate above the cuff [39, 68]. The design for the cuff, however, eluded him until Waters recommended a detachable cuff made of two layers of soft rubber cemented together at the edge, allowing it to easily slip over the end of the tracheal tube. And a detachable cuff could be replaced if it malfunctioned [67, 68].

By 1928, Guedel and Waters became satisfied with their cuff and began exhibiting its use. Initially, Guedel demonstrated its effectiveness and safety by filling an anesthetized patient's oropharyngeal cavity with water following intubation and cuff inflation. He would remove the water with suction before extubation. Unfortunately, during the second demonstration, his assistant neglected to apply suction, and the patient experienced bronchospasm from inhaling the water [39, 40, 68].

Guedel subsequently performed experiments on his dog, "Airway". He anesthetized and intubated Airway's trachea, connected the tracheal tube to a Waters carbon dioxide absorption canister and rebreathing bag, and placed Airway under water in an aquarium. He performed the first public "dunked dog" experiment (Fig. 54.11) in 1928, at the Indiana University School of Medicine. Airway was submerged for an hour. He was then removed from the tank and allowed to awaken. He showed that he was unharmed by shaking-off on the audience. He then pranced out of the room for an afternoon nap. This "dunked dog" experiment became a popular display that introduced carbon dioxide absorption and cuffed tracheal tubes into clinical practice [36, 39, 40, 60, 68]. After retiring from show business, Airway happily lived out his life at the Waters' family home [39].

While tracheal intubation protected patients' lungs from aspiration once the cuffed tracheal tube was placed, they were at risk prior to intubation. To reduce this, in 1961, British anesthetist Brian Sellick, suggested applying pressure to the cricoid cartilage during induction [63, 80]. This "Sellick maneuver" (or simply cricoid pressure) was not original to Sellick. In the eighteenth century, Charles Kite and James Curry suggested the application of cricoid pressure to prevent air from entering the stomach of drowning victims during their resuscitation. In contrast, Sellick hoped to prevent the gastric contents from entering the lungs [63].

By the time Sellick had developed this maneuver, it had already been recognized that aspiration of acidic gastric contents had disastrous consequences, particularly in obstetric patients and non-fasting patients requiring emergency surgery [63]. Correctly applied, Sellick's maneuver obliterated the esophageal lumen and prevented ejection of stomach contents [63, 80]. Sellick warned against performing his maneuver in an actively vomiting patient because the resulting high pressures in the esophagus might rupture the esophagus [80]. With this caveat, "Sellick's maneuver" was quickly adopted internationally [63]. Although the effectiveness of cricoid pressure is currently debated, it has continued as standard practice for over 50 years in the performance of rapid sequence or modified rapid sequence induction of general anesthesia.

The limited supply of rubber during World War II prompted the evolution from reusable rubber tracheal tubes to disposable plastic tubes. In 1940, Sydney Leader, a London dental surgeon, started the company, Portland Plastics, later Portex. He sought to replace the ceramic and glass used in medical and dental equipment with plastic. He began producing plastics, such as polyvinyl chloride, polyethylene and acrylic as substitutes for the natural rubber and shellacs used in dentures, artificial eyes and flexible dental tubing [67, 71].

Working with Major HL Thornton of the Royal Army Medical Corps, Leader substituted disposable polyvinyl chloride for rubber tracheal tubes, publishing reports on the first clinical trials in 1944 [71]. Initially, Leader supplied lengths of polyvinyl chloride tubing which anesthesiologists customized for each patient. Eventually, Portex marketed tubes with predetermined specifications [71]. Polyvinyl chloride tubes quickly replaced rubber tubes because polyvinyl chloride tubes were less apt to kink (occlude) when bent to acute angles; and polyvinyl chloride softened as it

warmed to body temperature, molding to the shape of the airway, thereby reducing pressure on laryngeal and tracheal tissues [67, 71].

An American, David Sheridan, contributed to the evolution of disposable tracheal tubes because of his concern that cross-contamination increased the risk of infection. Sheridan had to learn how to extrude plastic, which he originally did in his home. He pioneered the addition of centimeter markings on the tube to assist in determining the insertion depth. This decreased the risks of both accidental bronchial intubation and inadvertent extubation [68].

Advancements in disposable tracheal tubes continued with the introduction of the polyvinyl chloride cuff in 1964. The original version copied the less than ideal thickness and spherical shape found with older rubber cuffs [67, 71, 81]. Around the same time, polyvinyl chloride was shown to allow prolonged intubation with minimal injury to airway tissues. Tissue injury still occurred due to high intracuff pressures leading to the introduction of high-volume, low-pressure cuffs by Niels Lomholt in 1967 [71]. In 1969, Benny Geffin and Henning Pontopiddan found that pre-stretching the standard polyvinyl chloride cuff in boiling water produced a thinner cuff that better adapted to airway contours and decreased injury to tracheal tissue. By 1973, the cuff became more oblong, larger in diameter and decreased in thickness [67, 71].

Although these modifications decreased the incidence of tissue damage, injury still occurred during prolonged intubation. In 1975, British anesthetists Brian Crawley and David Cross, sought techniques that further reduced tracheal tissue damage yet maintained protection against aspiration. They introduced the concept of minimal intracuff pressure [67, 71]. The 1977 research of U Nordin found that intracuff pressures exceeding 40 cm H_2O caused tissue damage. By 1984, this value was reduced to 30 cm H_2O [71].

In the 1950s and 1960s, the ventilation paradigm for delivery of general anesthesia switched from spontaneous ventilation via a mask, to positive pressure ventilation via a tracheal tube [20, 65]. This was an essential development for the advancement of thoracic surgery and the associated need for one-lung ventilation [65].

When intrathoracic surgery began, no provision existed to prevent potentially lethal lung collapse. Although drowned victims had long benefited from artificial respiration with bellows, thoracic surgery was performed with the patient spontaneously breathing. Surgical speed and dexterity favored survival, but if the surgery could not be completed before the lung(s) collapsed, the patient died [64]. Much of the apprehension in using artificial respiration throughout the medical community, including use in thoracic surgery, came from the adverse reports of Leroy d'Etoilles regarding the risk of pneumothorax [64]. Consequently, surgeons accepted costly and/or inconvenient solutions [82].

To preclude lung collapse, in 1896, Ernst Sauerbruch, a German thoracic surgeon, developed the Sauerbruch Box, a negative-pressure chamber housing the body of the patient, as well as the surgical team. The head of the patient and the anesthesiologist remained outside the box at normal atmospheric pressure. This was considered a great feat for intrathoracic surgery. Surgeons using the Sauerbruch Box could take more time to carefully perform surgery, dramatically decreasing the overall mortality rate [36, 64, 82].

Sauerbruch's colleague, Ludolf Brauer, developed a positive pressure chamber to maintain lung expansion. Brauer placed just the patient's head into a box and pumped in pressurized oxygen and chloroform from a Roth-Drager apparatus. Of course, with the chest open the patient could not breathe, so the delivery of anesthetic was irrelevant. Clinically, the results were the same as with Sauerbruch's box, but using positive pressure added advantages of smallness and greater portability [64].

The inconvenience of these devices ultimately caused surgeons and anesthesiologists to return to tracheal intubation. This cheaper, convenient solution initially was used to insufflate gases and later used to produce positive pressure controlled ventilation. Franz Kuhn of Germany, Rudolph Matas and FW Parham of the US, and Theodore Tuffier of France pioneered this evolution. Kuhn, Tuffier and Matas modified the Fell-O'Dwyer apparatus to provide tracheal anesthesia for patients undergoing thoracic surgery. The pharynx was packed to form an air-tight seal, and the tracheal (actually endolaryngeal) tube was connected to a bellows providing positive pressure ventilation [4, 33, 66, 82].

In 1899, Matas experimented with the modified Fell-O'Dwyer apparatus in animals paralyzed with curare [1, 83]. In fact, Matas believed O'Dwyer's intubation system was so ingenious, he wrote "O'Dwyer's resurrection of…intubation and his magical transformation of the bloody and tragic picture of tracheotomy in diphtheria into a simple, painless, and bloodless bit of technical jugglery by his perfected method of intubation has practically closed for all time one of the most conspicuous chapters in the history of surgery." [64] Matas believed "The procedure that promises the most benefit in preventing pulmonary collapse in operations of the chest is the artificial inflation of the lung and the rhythmical maintenance of artificial respiration by a tube in the glottis directly connected with a bellow." [64] Matas' colleague, Frederick Parham, applied Matas' work to humans and reported on a comparison of two patients for the removal of intrathoracic tumors, one anesthetized via open drop ether versus a second where anesthesia was delivered via the Fell-O'Dwyer apparatus. In the first case, the lungs collapsed and the patient nearly died. In the second case, the open drop technique was initially used, but Parham then intubated the trachea using a modified Fell-O'Dwyer apparatus. Surgery

proceeded with greater ease than in the first case [1, 83]. Despite this, it would take almost 30 years for Matas' work to enter clinical practice [64].

Providing controlled positive pressure ventilation required the thoracic surgeon to operate on moving (ventilated) lungs. In 1931, Waters and Joseph Gale accidentally placed a standard tracheal tube into the right main bronchus. They immediately recognized that such placement offered the benefit of one-lung ventilation [4, 68, 82]. Learning of his friend's "misadventure", Guedel proposed the construction of a double-cuffed, elongated tracheal tube to isolate the ventilation of the right and left lungs. Emory Rovenstine later put the idea into practice [4, 68, 82].

Magill moved from facial to thoracic anesthesia, in 1936 describing insertion of a cuffed catheter into the bronchus of the operated side. Inflation of the cuff would close off the main bronchus, allowing tracheal anesthesia to and suctioning of the other lung. Thus was born the bronchial blocker. He preferred this method of one-lung ventilation because it could be extended to cordon off just the lower lobe for lobectomies [36, 77, 78, 82].

Now consider the invention of the double-lumen tracheal tube, two long D-shaped tracheal tubes fused together. One of the D-shaped tracheal tubes extends into a main bronchus and has a cuff that fits in the bronchus, allowing ventilation of the lung served by that bronchus. The opening of the second D-shaped tracheal tube ends (if the tube is placed properly) in the trachea, just above the carina. A cuff just proximal to this opening surrounds both D-shaped tracheal tubes just as would a cuff on an ordinary tracheal tube. This array allows ventilation to be limited to one lung or both [81]. In 1949, Eric Carlens, a Swedish physiologist, designed the first double-lumen tube for use in bronchospirometry [36, 82]. By 1950, he and Bjork had modified the tube specifically for use in anesthetized patients undergoing intrathoracic surgery [68, 82, 84]. His tube included a hook designed to sit on the carina to ensure proper placement, stabilize the tube, and prevent dislodgement during patient movement [81, 82, 84]. In 1962, Frank Robertshaw designed the double-lumen tracheal tube commonly used today, differing from Carlens' tube by removal of the carinal hook [36, 69, 82]. Special versions of both tubes have been developed for positioning in the right main bronchus to prevent occlusion of the right upper lobe bronchus [81].

In 1982, Hiroshi Inoue invented the Univent Tube, a tracheal tube providing a separate catheter passing via the main lumen into the bronchus to be blocked. The separate catheter had a cuff for bronchial blockade and a channel that permitted suction or high-frequency jet ventilation [81, 82].

Like thoracic surgery, otorhinolaryngeal surgery, surgery involving the mouth or nose, can pose special challenges. The standard tracheal tube may impair the surgeon's view. To solve this problem, British anesthetist, Alsop developed the right angled "Oxford" tube in 1955. Sylvia Duck-worth published the experience with 18,000 cases in 1962 [83]. Improving on these rigid rubber tubes, Utah pediatric anesthesiologists, Wallace Ring, John Adair and Richard Elwin invented RAE tubes, pre-shaped tracheal tubes bent to hug the chin or nose. They performed 10,000 intubations with their prototype before publishing their results in 1975 [81, 85]. Since the introduction of plastic in the early 1960s, more diverse airways and tracheal tubes have been invented and produced than can be discussed here [81].

As tracheal intubation became the standard of care for most surgeries, a problem arose; not all patient's tracheas could be successfully intubated using direct laryngoscopy. For such patients, a tracheostomy was often their only option. In 1960, New York surgeons Frank Butler and Anchise Cirilo, suggested an alternative technique, retrograde intubation [86–88]. In 1963, D Waters, a British anesthetist at the University of Ibadan in Nigeria, performed retrograde intubation in a patient with "cancrum oris" (gangrenous condition of the oral cavity). Through a Tuohy epidural needle passed through the cricothyroid membrane, he threaded an epidural catheter back into the nasopharynx. Waters retrieved the catheter from the nasopharynx and used it as a guide for delivering the tracheal tube through the nose into the trachea [87, 88].

The invasiveness and potential complications from puncturing the cricothyroid membrane limited the popularity of retrograde tracheal intubation [87, 88]. By the mid-1990s, studies showed that retrograde intubation was an easy and reliable technique; however, only approximately 500 cases had been reported, over half in cadavers [87]. Despite its infrequent use, retrograde intubation was incorporated into the ASA Difficult Airway Algorithm in 1993 [8, 34, 88]. In 1990, with the assistance of Antonio Sanchez, a California anesthesiologist, Cook Critical Care developed a preassembled kit for retrograde intubation [88, 89]. It has been successfully used in human patients, and was adapted for use in a llama when Sanchez consulted at the San Diego Zoo [90].

Intubating Stylets

As mentioned previously, the intubating stylet, or gum elastic bougie, provided another tool for guiding the tracheal tube into the glottic opening. The Portex Venn Tracheal Tube Introducer, previously known as the Eschmann Endotracheal Tube Introducer, is commonly referred to as a gum elastic bougie—a misnomer, as it is neither made of gum elastic nor used as a bougie (a dilator). In 1973, Paul Venn, a British anesthetist and advisor to the original Eschmann company, developed the tracheal tube introducer. Venn was inspired by Robert Macintosh's 1949 report of tracheal intubation using a real gum elastic bougie, a urinary catheter made of

gum elastic and originally intended for dilating urethral strictures [91–93]. Several other intubating guides/stylets act like the Portex Venn Tracheal Tube Introducer, but are made of different materials and have different features. Most of these guides and stylets are disposable, including the present Portex Venn Tracheal Tube Introducer.

Macintosh did not invent the intubating stylet. O'Dwyer, Kuhn and Maydl used curved metal stylets around a hundred years ago [33, 68, 69]. During World War I, Rowbotham designed a "guiding rod" to facilitate nasotracheal intubation [36, 68, 69]. In 1941, Murphy used a metal stylet to keep tracheal tubes rigid while intubating under direct laryngoscopy [79]. The malleable stylet continues to be a part of routine tracheal intubation and is an essential adjunct to many alternative intubating devices.

In 1957, Macintosh and his colleague, Harry Richards, described the lighted tracheal tube introducer, a device they used to assist tracheal tube placement during direct laryngoscopy [93]. However, they did not describe the technique of trans-illumination. This fell to Hideo Yamamura and colleagues, who in 1959 described trans-illumination (the transmission of a bright light from the tip of a catheter, visible through the skin of the neck, thus indicating the location of the catheter tip) during nasotracheal intubation.[93] Since then, lighted stylets or "lightwands" have been used to assist blind intubation during difficult and routine airway management [89, 93].

Lighted stylets for trans-illumination increased in popularity after 1977, when British anesthetist CA Foster had a special trans-illuminating fiberoptic bundle designed to facilitate tracheal intubation in a young child with trismus [93, 94]. (In 1978, M Ducrow used a flexible surgical light, the Flexi-lum, to achieve the same result. After achieving trans-illumination with the lighted stylet, Ducrow passed a guide (two plastic suction catheters connected end to end) into the trachea followed by passage of the tracheal tube over the guide. It was not until a year later that it was noted that the Flexi-lum could be placed inside the tracheal tube, thus acting as a guide for the tube. The Flexi-lum became the first commercial lightwand [93–95]. In 1986, the Flexi-lum evolved into the Tube-stat which included a sleeve surrounding the bulb designed to prevent bulb loss/detachment. Although originally limited to use in children, a longer, more flexible version was developed for adult nasotracheal intubation [93–95].

Despite growing interest in these devices, limitations, such as diminished light intensity, short length, and absence of a connector to secure the tube, became apparent [93]. Released in 1995 for blind intubation, the Trachlight was designed to overcome limitations of the previous devices. It consisted of two pieces, a reusable handle with an internal light source and a disposable, retractable stylet providing rigidity during insertion but flexibility during withdrawal [93–95]. Several other lighted stylets have since been introduced and removed from clinical practice [94]. However, limited transmission of light especially in obese patients with thick necks remains as a limitation of the technique.

In 1969, Peter Murphy, a British anesthetist, introduced the optical stylet, a flexible fiberoptic choledochoscope that he used to aid in nasotracheal intubation of a patient with Still's disease [59, 96]. Optical stylets further evolved in 1979 when George Berci and Ronald Katz, published the use of a straight endoscope as a tracheal tube stylet that featured a proximal viewing element and a sliding tracheal tube adapter with a Luer-lock inlet through which oxygen or air could be insufflated [59, 96]. This publication coined the term "optical stylet" [96].

Fiberoptic Devices

Flexible fiberoptic intubation continued the evolution of advances in airway management, particularly for viewing the airway and introducing tubes into the airway. Bronchoscopy dates to 1887, when Gustav Killian devised a rigid bronchoscope to extract a foreign object from the respiratory tract of a farmer. In 1904, his student, Chevalier Jackson, added a distal tungsten light bulb and suction channel [97]. John Baird, a Scottish electrical engineer and pioneer of fiberoptics, television and radar technology, conceived of fiberoptic bronchoscopy in the late 1920s. His patented idea used hollow, thin, flexible, glass rods bundled together in a honeycomb-type collection that transmitted images by internal reflection down their entire length. Not requiring a lens or mirror, fiberoptic devices could be much smaller than their predecessors [98]. In 1954, fiberoptic technology made its way into the medical field, when Basil Hirschowitz, a Michigan gastroenterologist, developed the first fiberoptic endoscope [4, 98].

Shigo Ikeda, a Japanese thoracic surgeon and "father" of fiberoptic bronchoscopy proposed the concept of using fiberoptic technology for flexible bronchoscopy, to the Machida Endoscope Company in 1964, and then the Olympus Company in 1965 [99, 100]. Based on Ikeda's recommendations, Machida Endoscope developed the first prototype of the flexible fiberoptic bronchoscope in 1966. It was initially used in conjunction with a rigid bronchoscope [5, 100]. One month later, Olympus developed its own flexible fiberoptic bronchoscope, a stand-alone device that included a maneuverable working channel allowing the use of cytology brushes. Ikeda described his work at the International Congress on Diseases of the Chest in 1966, and reported on his new flexible fiberoptic bronchoscope in 1971 [100, 101].

In 1972, a flexible fiberoptic bronchoscope was used for nasotracheal intubation in a patient in whom rheumatoid arthritis had precluded orotracheal intubation [102]. In 1972, California anesthesiologist Claire Stiles and colleagues published a report of the first 100 cases using flexible fiberoptic bronchoscopy for tracheal intubation, demonstrating that intubation could be performed in less than 60 seconds, making it a viable option for difficult intubations [103]. The use of flexible fiberoptic bronchoscopy expanded to include the confirmation of tracheal tube positioning, [104] placement of left-sided and right-sided double-lumen bronchial tubes, [105, 106] and evaluation of the upper and lower airway. Andranik Ovassapian was a pioneer in teaching the proper use of flexible fiberoptic bronchoscopy, especially for awake tracheal intubation, creating workshops for training and simulation that were critical in accomplishing its universal acceptance [51, 107].

Specialized oropharyngeal airways were developed to offer all the benefits and simplicity of the traditional oropharyngeal airway during flexible fiberoptic intubation [108, 109]. They protected the flexible fiberoptic bronchoscope from physical damage from teeth, offered a clear passageway for the flexible fiberoptic bronchoscope, and aligned the tracheal tube with the glottic opening [34, 108, 109].

Transtracheal Ventilation

In the rare patient, after induction of anesthesia, adequate airway and ventilation cannot be established. Time is needed to allow the patient to awaken and recover their airway control. If supraglottic airway devices, such as the LMA, are inappropriate or unsuccessful, the anesthesiologist has two options—surgical/percutaneous airway or the less invasive transtracheal jet ventilation [34].

Robert Hooke in 1667 and Meltzer and Auer in 1909 demonstrated transtracheal ventilation of paralyzed dogs [66, 110]. Ohio anesthesiologist Jay Jacoby and colleagues revisited the idea in 1951, examining the safety and efficacy of oxygen insufflation through a 13 gauge transtracheal needle in dogs [110]. In 1956, Jacoby and colleagues performed transtracheal resuscitation in an anesthetized patient with complete respiratory obstruction [111]. Oxygen insufflated via a cricothyrotomy catheter provided adequate oxygenation but caused carbon dioxide retention. In 1971, Spoerel and coworkers introduced the concept of intermittent jet ventilation via a percutaneous transtracheal catheter in adults undergoing general anesthesia [112]. Jonathan Benumof, became a strong advocate of transtracheal jet ventilation as a life-saving technique. His 1989 review encouraged all US hospitals to stock the jet ventilation equipment needed for the unexpected "cannot intubate, cannot ventilate" scenario, including how to accomplish emergency jet ventilation when appropriate kits were unavailable [113]. He ensured inclusion of transtracheal jet ventilation in the ASA Difficult Airway Algorithm [7–9].

Airway Exchange Catheters

Placement of a tracheal tube, especially a cuffed tracheal tube, secures the airway. What should be done if the tracheal tube requires exchange in the patient whose trachea was difficult to intubate? This issue led to invention of airway exchange catheters.

In 1978, Brendan Finucan and Hilton Kupshik at Emory University in Georgia performed a blind awake nasal intubation in a patient with an unstable cervical fracture. After beginning anesthesia, they discovered a significant cuff leak requiring tracheal reintubation. Having just placed a Sorenson central venous pressure catheter, they had the outer protective sheath in which the catheter was packaged. It was long and narrow and fitted inside the faulty tracheal tube. They inserted the sheath deeply within the tracheal tube; withdrew the tracheal tube; and slid a new tracheal tube over the sheath, down the nose, and into the trachea, the sheath guiding the way. Voila! The first airway exchange catheter [114].

In 1980, Sukunar Desai and Vladimir Fencl, at the Peter Bent Brigham Hospital in Massachusetts, used a flexible fiberoptic bronchoscope to guide the exchange of faulty tracheal tubes. Because of the limited length of the flexible fiberoptic bronchoscope, such an exchange required cutting the replacement and original tracheal tubes to the shortest length possible, [115] a less than ideal solution.

In 1987, Irving Mizus invented a catheter specifically for the purpose of exchanging tracheal tubes, the Mizus Endotracheal Tube Replacement Obturator (METTRO). The METTRO was a long, polyethylene, solid core, bougie that had distance markings and a flexible tip. The use of the METTRO did not necessitate the use of a cut tracheal tube and the anesthesiologist knew exactly how deeply it had been inserted. Other uses for the METTRO (which applied to all airway exchange catheters) included the removal of a tracheal tube during a tracheostomy procedure, and tentative extubation of patients who might need reintubation [116].

But the METTRO was not hollow, precluding the use of insufflation or jet ventilation. Development of the hollow Cook Airway Exchange Catheter in 1990 by Cook Critical Care solved this problem. An adapter allowed the catheter to be attached to an Ambu bag or airway circuit [90].

Advances in technology prompted new requirements for exchanging airways. While the Cook airway exchange catheter was hollow, its long and narrow lumen precluded passage of a flexible fiberoptic bronchoscope. The desire to use flexible fiberoptic bronchoscopy in exchanging a supralaryngeal airway for a tracheal tube, prompted the development of a new airway exchange catheter device by Peter Charters, a British anesthetist at Aintree Hospital. Introduced into clinical practice in 1997, the Aintree Intubation Catheter allowed enough exposure of the distal fiberoptic bronchoscope for

the operator to steer the tip into the glottis and trachea. Beyond acting as an airway exchange catheter, it could be used as a tracheal tube introducer, or applied to facilitate extubation [90, 117, 118].

Indirect Laryngoscopes

Indirect rigid laryngoscopy using mirrors and prisms figured in the initial efforts to view the larynx but gave way to less cumbersome approaches that used direct laryngoscopy. New technology restored indirect laryngoscopy as an aid to intubation. Modern indirect rigid laryngoscopes enable a view of the laryngeal inlet through fiberoptic bundles or other optical aids such as mirrors and prisms packaged into a single unit and easily operated by one person. Their advantage is the reduction of anatomic stress needed for direct laryngoscopy; they enable vision "around the corner" of the tongue.

In 1980, Georgia anesthesiologist Roger Bullard designed the first indirect rigid fiberoptic laryngoscope introduced into anesthetic practice. A rigid L-shaped blade incorporating fiberoptic bundles transmitted an image to an eye piece. The most recent version, the Bullard Elite Laryngoscope, can be used with a conventional laryngoscope handle, and the eye piece can accept a video camera attachment [19, 34, 59, 89].

Two historically important, now extinct, indirect fiberoptic rigid laryngoscopes were the 1994 Wu Scope and the 1996 Upsher Scope [34, 59]. Although neither the Wu-Scope or the Upsher scope gained widespread use, they represented devices used during the transition between the Bullard rigid laryngoscope and the soon to arrive videolaryngoscopes in the early 2000s. In 2006, King Systems Corporation developed the Airtraq, an indirect rigid laryngoscope that provided a view of the glottis without requiring alignment of the 3 axes. Unlike indirect rigid fiberoptic laryngoscopes, images were transmitted to a proximal viewfinder by lenses and prisms. Versions of the Airtraq also provided for nasotracheal intubation and double lumen tube placement. A snap-on video system allowed viewing on an external screen [34, 89, 119].

Videolaryngoscopy

Video imaging during bronchoscopy began immediately before World War II when British surgeon John McGibbon obtained photographs and a video of the epiglottis, carina, and trachea using a rigid bronchoscope fitted with a camera lens [120]. Flexible fiberoptic bronchoscopy added external cameras to record the view or to allow visualization on external monitors. In the late 1980s, the charge coupled device (CCD) video microchip became available, placing video technology inside the scope. This costly device required bulky cables [34, 51]. In 1987, Ikeda worked with the Asahi Corporation to develop the prototype of the flexible video endoscope, thereby revolutionizing the bronchoscope [100]. Pentax, then Olympus and Machida-Toshiba made the first commercial video endoscopes. Otolaryngologists and pulmonologists quickly adopted these devices, but their use by anesthesiologists for tracheal intubation lagged, eventually becoming popular at the end of the 1990s.

Around 2006, mobile phone technology required a smaller and less expensive CMOS camera chip. Video endoscopes and laryngoscopes soon incorporated this new technology, which offered better image resolution [34, 121]. Placing the chip within the device also decreased weight and reduced the number of cables extending from the device, or permitted the incorporation of the monitor into the device itself.

In 2009, Olympus introduced this built-in video monitor into the portable Olympus MAF Flexible Endoscope with a built-in, long-life, white LED light source and a 2.5 inch color LCD display monitor incorporated into the proximal end of the scope, replacing the eyepiece. A rechargeable lithium battery could power the MAF endoscope for 60 minutes [122].

Flexible fiberoptic bronchoscopes and video endoscopes require time-consuming and potentially costly disinfection [123]. To solve this problem, Vision Science developed the BRS-5000 Video Bronchoscope with EndoSheath Technology, a single-use, disposable, sterile sheath that isolates the scope from the patient. With replacement of the sheath, the BRS-5000 is immediately ready for re-use [123].

A disposable, flexible, video endoscope provided another solution to the problem of endoscope disinfection. In 2007, the Ambu engineering team sought the world-wide assistance of airway experts to develop the aScope, a disposable video endoscope with a flexible, steerable tip plus the expected refinements for high resolution viewing and recording. The aScope became available in 2009 [121, 123].

Video Laryngoscopes

Application of advances in video technology to laryngoscopes provided improved views of the glottis and an enlarged image of the tracheal tube as it passed through the glottic opening. The video laryngoscope consists of a traditional laryngoscope design with a miniature video camera or fiberoptic bundle embedded within the blade to capture an image of the laryngeal inlet. The image is transmitted to a monitor mounted either on the handle or separately [59, 119, 124, 125].

Around 1999, George Berci, a California surgeon and a pioneer in endoscopic surgery; John Pacey, a Canadian surgeon; Markus Weiss, a Swiss anesthesiologist; and Jon Berall, a US military Internist, independently produced distinctive video laryngoscopy systems. Weiss invented the Angulated Video Intubating Laryngoscope, primarily for use in children. Although Weiss wrote the first paper on video la-

ryngoscopy in 2001, his device never became commercially available in the US [126].

Pacey invented the first commercially available video laryngoscope, introduced into clinical practice in 2001. After observing a tediously difficult intubation by two highly skilled anesthesiologists, Pacey realized that the video technology that had revolutionized minimally invasive surgery might be applied to facilitate intubation [127]. His idea spawned the GlideScope, a single-piece handle and blade made from medical-grade plastic. A video camera with an LED and antifogging mechanism was mounted at the distal end of the blade. The captured image was transmitted to a color LCD monitor [34, 59, 128]. Many versions of the GlideScope appeared subsequently, as did a special stylet, the GlideRite® Auto Stylet, with a pre-curved shape that matched the angle of the Glidescope blades [59, 128]. Studies comparing the GlideScope systems with traditional direct laryngoscopy, confirmed the usefulness of the GlideScope, especially in patients with a potentially difficult airway [59, 128, 129].

Berci, with anesthesiologist Marshal Kaplan, invented the most diverse of the initial video laryngoscopy systems, the Berci-Kaplan DCI Video Laryngoscope (DCI; direct coupler interface). In 1999, Berci and Kaplan made the first direct coupler interface prototype. It allowed a limited tubular view similar to that seen during direct laryngoscopy. In 2000, a second prototype incorporated a panoramic view that improved visualization. The final version appeared in clinical practice in 2003, as a hybrid device using fiberoptic bundles in a channel of the laryngoscope blade, to deliver an image to a camera located in the handle.

The advantage of the initial direct coupler interface over other video laryngoscopes, was that it used traditionally shaped blades and allowed direct or indirect viewing of the larynx. Several makers of video laryngoscopes, such as the GlideScope Direct recognized these advantages and incorporated them into their own devices [119, 125].

A 2009 version of this system, the CMAC video laryngoscope, had an integrated video camera in the blade, and like its predecessor, provided a wide viewing arc. Data are delivered by cable to an accompanying battery-powered, portable, 7 inch monitor with the usual options for recording images [59, 119, 125]. Studies indicated the ease of use and versatility of the direct coupler interface and CMAC systems, especially as aids for teaching tracheal intubation [130, 131].

Berall invented the last of the original video laryngoscopes, the Coopdech C-Scope Video Laryngoscope, available in Europe and Japan since 2005. The handle of the laryngoscope contained the 3.5 inch LCD video monitor, included a high-intensity white LED light source, and was powered by a rechargeable lithium ion battery. The C-Scope could be fitted with disposable plastic blade covers to minimize cross-contamination [132].

Airway Assessment Techniques

In the 1960s and 1970s, Ronald Cormack and John Lehane found that anesthetic deaths due to aspiration were often associated with a failure to perform tracheal intubation. They offered two key conclusions: 1) although specific diseases might predispose to difficult intubation, difficulty was also seen in apparently normal/healthy individuals; and 2) if difficulty was not always predictable, then anesthesiologists must learn how to master the art of difficult intubation. This research produced the 1984 Cormack-Lehane Laryngoscopy Grading System. The system divided the view during laryngoscopy into four grades defined by how much of the vocal cords and surrounding tissue were visible, 1-to-4 indicating minimal to maximal view of the larynx [83, 133]. The concept received immediate international acceptance.

Seshagiri Mallampati, at Harvard Medical School, suggested an alternative Grading System. In 1983, he published a letter describing an unexpectedly difficult intubation in a female whose mouth could be opened widely but whose tongue obstructed the view of her faucial pillars and uvula, leaving only her soft palate visible. Subsequently, he asked his patients to open their mouths and stick out their tongues. He found that the resulting view correlated with the difficulty of intubation. In 1985, he published the results of his study of 210 patients. The original Mallampati scoring system had three classes that ascended with decreasing visualization of the faucial pillars, soft palate, and uvula and correlated inversely with the ease of intubation [134]. Samsoon and Young added a fourth class (more difficult intubation) where the soft palate was not visible [134, 135]. A fifth (but easier intubation) class was suggested for patients whose epiglottis could be seen [136].

Conclusion

While anesthesia began in the mid-1800s, the history of airway management is as old as medicine itself. Surgical airway management dates back to 3600 BCE. Major contributions to the many techniques and devices for airway management came from dentists, priests, engineers, musicians—and physicians.

Discoveries evolved concurrently in multiple parts of the world, but early limitations in communication invited controversy in claims of priority. Ideas might be invented and reinvented. While tracheostomies date to 3600 BCE, they were repeatedly rediscovered, finally becoming popular in the 1900s. Although tracheal intubation was first described in the 1 century, it was rarely, if ever performed in humans until the 1700s, and not for airway management during surgery until the late 1800s. It did not become popular until the early 1900s. With the invention of the LMA in the 1980s, the most recent addition to airway management, the supralaryngeal airway was born, but the idea was formed long before with the concept of the oropharyngeal airway and the Fell-O'Dwyer apparatus, both of which are positioned either at, or above, the vocal cords.

Modern anesthesia owes a great deal to these past inventors, for their contributions to the many airway devices and techniques mentioned throughout this chapter. Their inquisitive nature and skills of observations revolutionized how and what surgeries could be performed. Future inventors will only further their progress.

References

1. Keys T. The history of surgical anesthesia. New York: Schuman's; 1945.
2. Doyle DJ. A brief history of clinical airway management. Anesthesiology News. 2008;34:9–14.
3. Sittig SE, Pringnitz JE. Tracheostomy: evolution of an airway. AARC Times. 2001;25:48–51.
4. Shephard D. From craft to specialty: a medical social history of anesthesia and its changing role in health care. Ontario: York Point Publishing; 2009.
5. Szmuk P, Ezri T, Evron S, Roth Y, Katz J. A brief history of tracheostomy and tracheal intubation, from the Bronze Age to the Space Age. Intensive Care Med. 2008;34:222–8.
6. Griffith H, Johnson G. The use of curare in general anesthesia. Anesthesiology. 1942;3:418–20.
7. American Society of Anesthesiologists Task Force on Management of the Difficult Airway. Practice guidelines for management of the difficult airway: an updated report by the American Society of Anesthesiologists Task Force on Management of the Difficult Airway. Anesthesiology. 2003;98:1269–77.
8. American Society of Anesthesiologists Task Force on Management of the Difficult Airway. Practice guidelines for management of the difficult airway. A report by the American Society of Anesthesiologists Task Force on Management of the Difficult Airway. Anesthesiology. 1993;78:597–602.
9. Frova G, Sorbello M. Algorithms for difficult airway management: a review. Minerva Anestesiol. 2009;75:201–9.
10. Stock CR. What is past is prologue: a short history of the development of tracheostomy. Ear Nose Throat J. 1987;66:166–9.
11. Stoller JK. The history of intubation, tracheotomy, and airway appliances. Respir Care. 1999;44:595–601.
12. Yapijakis C. Hippocrates of Kos, the father of clinical medicine, and Asclepiades of Bithynia, the father 2 molecular medicine. In Vivo. 2009;23:507–14.
13. Melker RJ, Kost K. Percutaneous dilational cricothyrotomy and tracheostomy. In: Hagberg CA, editor. Benumof's airway management: principles and practice. Philadelphia: Elsevier; 2007. pp. 240–77.
14. Gibbs M, Walls RM. Surgical airway. In: Hagberg CA, editor. Benumof's airway management: principles and practice. Philadelphia: Elsevier; 2007. pp. 678–96.
15. Jackson C. The life of Chevalier Jackson: an autobiograph. New York: Macmillian; 1938.
16. Brantigan CO, Grow JB. Cricothyrotomy. Elective use in respiratory problems requiring tracheotomy. J Thorac Cardiovasc Surg. 1976;71:72–81.
17. Jackson C. High tracheotomy and other errors: the chief cause of chronic laryngeal stenosis. Surg Gynecol Obstet. 1923;32:292.

18. McGee JP, Vender JS. Nonintubation management of the airway: mask ventilation. In: Hagberg CA, editor. Benumof's airway management: principles and practices. 2nd ed. Philadelphia: Elsevier; 2007. pp. 345–70.
19. Henderson J. Airway management in the adult. In: Miller RD, Fleisher LA, Wiener-Kronish JP, Young WL, Eriksson LI, editors. Miller's Anesthesia. 7th ed. Philadelphia: Elsevier; 2009. pp. 1573–610.
20. Matioc AA. The adult ergonomic face mask concept: historical and theoretical perspectives. J Clin Anesth. 2009;21:300–4.
21. Frost P. Thomas Skinner. In: Barr AM, Boulton TB, Wilkinson DJ, editors. Essays on the hisotry of anaesthesia. London: Royal Society of Medicine; 1996. pp. 146–8.
22. Gray TC. History of anaesthesia in Liverpool. Med His. 1972;16:375–82.
23. Westhorpe R. Skinner's chloroform mask. Anaesth Intensive Care. 1995;23:3.
24. Rendell-Baker L, Soucek DH. New paediatric face masks and anaesthetic equipment. Br Med J. 1962;1:1690.
25. Rendell-Baker L. Rendell-Baker-Soucek mask: Leslie Rendell-Baker (1917). In: Maltby JR, editor. Notable names in anaesthesia. London: Royal Society of Medicine; 2002. pp. 173–5.
26. Ball C, Westhorpe R. Clearing the airway—tongue forceps. Anaesth Intensive Care. 1997;25:105.
27. McGoldrick KE. Sir Fedreric William Hewitt: the man and his airway. ASA Newsl. 2008;72:10–3.
28. Kocher TH. Operative surgery. New York: Williams Wood; 1894.
29. Westhorpe R. Clearing the airway—probangs. Anaesth Intensive Care. 1997;25:3.
30. Sykes WS. Essays on the first hundred years of anaesthesia. Park Ridge: American Society of Anesthesiologists; 1982.
31. Maltby JR. Trendelenburg position: Friedrich Trendelenburg (1844–1924). In: Maltby JR, editor. Notable names in anaesthesia. London: Royal Society of Medicine; 2002. pp. 213–5.
32. McIntyre JW. Oropharyngeal and nasopharyngeal airways: I (1880–1995). Can J Anaesth. 1996;43:629–35.
33. Duncum BM. The development of inhalation anaesthesia: with special reference to the years 1846–1900. London:Oxford University Press; 1947.
34. Rosenblatt WH. Airway management. In: Barash PG, Cullen BF, Stoelting RK, Cahalan MK, Stock MC, editors. Clinical anesthesia. Philadelphia: Lippincott Williams & Wilkins; 2009. pp. 751–89.
35. Thomas KB. The development of anaesthetic apparatus: a history based on the Charles King collection of the association of anaesthetists of Great Britain and Ireland. Oxford: Blackwell Scientific; 1975.
36. Larson MS. History of anesthetic practice. In: Miller RD, Fleisher LA, Wiener-Kronish JP, Young WL, Eriksson LI, editors. Miller's Anesthesia. 7th ed. Philadelphia: Elsevier; 2009. pp. 3–43.
37. Morris L. Waters circuit: Ralph Milton Waters (1883–1979). In: Maltby JR, editor. Notable names in anaesthesia. London: Royal Society of Medicine; 2002. pp. 219–21.
38. Ball C, Westhorpe R. Clearing the airway—the development of the pharyngeal airway. Anaesth Intensive Care. 1997;25:451.
39. Maltby JR. Guedel oral airway, guedel signs of ether anaesthesia: Arthur E. Guedel (1883–1956). In: Maltby JR, editor. Notable names in anaesthesia. London: Royal Society of Medicine; 2002. pp. 84–6.
40. Dr CSH. Arthur Guedel's contributions. ASA Newsl. 2008;72:14–6.
41. Berman JC. Berman airway: Rovert Alvin Berman (1914–1999). In: Maltby JR, editor. Notable names in anaesthesia. London: Royal Society of Medicine; 2002. pp. 16–8.
42. Berman JC. Robert Alvin Berman, M.D.: airway inventor. ASA Newsl. 1999;63.
43. Ball C, Westhorpe R. Clearing the airway—the cuffed pharyngeal airway. Anaesth Intensive Care. 1997;25:603.
44. Rendell-Baker L. From something old something new. Anesthesiology. 2000;92:913–8.
45. Maltby JR, Rubins J. Leech pharyngeal bulb gasway. Bull Anesth His. 2002;20:2, 11.
46. Shephard DA. Beverly Charles Leech (1898–1960). Can J Anaesth. 1990;37:689.
47. Brain AI. Laryngeal mask airway: Archie Brain (1942–). In: Maltby JR, editor. Notable names in anaesthesia. London: Royal Society of Medicine; 2002. pp. 28–30.
48. Brimacombe JR, Brain AIJ, Berry AM. The laryngeal mask airway: a review and practical guide. London: W. B. Saunders; 1997.
49. Ferson DZ, Brain AI. Laryngeal mask airway. In: Hagberg CA, editor. Benumof's airway management: principles and practice. 2nd ed. Philadelphia: Elsevier; 2007. pp. 476–502.
50. Brain AI. The laryngeal mask—a new concept in airway management. Br J Anaesth. 1983;55:801–5.
51. Ferson D, Chi TL. Developments in general airway management. Thorac Surg Clin. 2005;15:39–53.
52. Cook TM. Facemask and supraglottic airway devices. In: Calder I, Pearce AC, editors. Core topics in airway management. 2nd ed. Cambridge: Cambridge University; 2011. pp. 73–90.
53. Benumof JL. Laryngeal mask airway and the ASA difficult airway algorithm. Anesthesiology. 1996;84:686–99.
54. Frass M, Urtubia RM, Hagberg CA. The combitube esophageal-tracheal double-lumen airway. In: Hagberg CA, editor. Benumof's airway management: principles and practice. 2nd ed. Philadelphia: Elsevier; 2007. pp. 594–615.
55. Sinha PK, Misra S. Supraglottic airway devices other than laryngeal mask airway and its prototypes. Indian J Anaesth. 2005;49:281–2.
56. Agro FE, Cataldo R, Mattei A. New devices and techniques for airway management. Minerva Anestesiol. 2009;75:141–9.
57. Conlay LA, Sim PP. Anesthetics in history, from ingestion to inhalation: recent significant acquisitions of the Wood Library-Museum. ASA Newsl. 2008;42:24–7, 33.
58. Jahn A, Blitzer A. A short history of laryngoscopy. Logoped Phoniatr Vocol. 1996;21:181–5.
59. Law JA, Hagberg CA. The evolution of upper airway retraction: new and old laryngoscope blades. In: Hagberg CA, editor. Benumof's airway management: principles and practice. 2nd ed. Philadelphia: Elsevier; 2007. pp. 532–75.
60. Sykes WS. Essays on the first hundred years of anaesthesia. Endinburgh: E & S Livingston; 1961.
61. Christodoulou CC, Murphy MF, Hung OR. Blind digital intubation. In: Hagberg CA, editor. Benumof's airway management: principles and practice. 2nd ed. Philadelphia: Elsevier; 2007. pp. 393–8.
62. Brandt L. The first reported oral intubation of the human trachea. Anesth Analg. 1987;66:1198–9.
63. Wilkinson DJ. Brian A. Sellick, M.D.: father of cricoids pressure maneuver (1918–1996). ASA Newsl. 1999;63.
64. Mayer JA. Unterdruck and Überdruck, 1904. Ann Thorac Surg. 1989;47:933–8.
65. Kemp EN. Elementary anesthesia. Baltimore: Williams & Wilkins; 1848.
66. Gillespie NA. Endotracheal anaenesthesia. 2nd ed. Madison: The University of Wisconsin; 1948.
67. Watson WF. Development of the PVC endotracheal tube. BioMaterials. 1980;1:41–6.
68. Calverley RK. Intubation in anaesthesia. In: Atkinson RS, Boulton TB, editors. The history of anaesthesia. London: Royal Society of Medicine; 1989. pp. 333–41.
69. Ezri T, Warters RD. Indications for tracheal intubation. In: Hagberg CA, editor. Benumof's airway management: principles and practice. 2nd ed. Philadelphia: Elsevier; 2007. pp. 371–8.
70. Thierbach A. Franz Kuhn, his contribution to anaesthesia and emergency medicine. Resuscitation. 2001;48:193–7.
71. Russell CA. Developments in thermoplastic tracheal tubes. In: Barr AM, Boulton TB, Wilkinson DJ, editors. Essays on the history of anaesthesia. London: Royal Society of Medicine; 1996, pp. 94–7.

72. Jacob AK, Kopp SL, Bacon DR, Smith HM. The history of anesthesia. In: Barash PG, Cullen BF, Stoelting RK, Cahalan MK, Stock MC, editors. Clinical anesthesia. 6th ed. Philadelphia: Lippincott Williams & Wilkins; 2009. pp. 4–26.

73. Kirstein A, Thorner M. Autoscopy of the larynx and the trachea. Philadelphia: The F. A. Davis Co.; 1897.

74. Hirsch NP, Smith GB, Hirsch PO. Alfred Kirstein. Pioneer of direct laryngoscopy. Anaesthesia. 1986;41:42–5.

75. Bouse GS. WLM's Nicholas Samponaro, M.D. collection. Indirect gifts from airway pioneer Chevalier Jackson. ASA Newsl. 2008;72:18–9.

76. Tandy CC. Personal reflections: a boy meets an airway pioneer…the 'hard' way. ASA Newsl. 2008;72:20–1.

77. McLachlan G. Sir Ivan Magill KCVO, DSc MB, BCh BAO, FRCS. FFARCS (Hon), FFARCSI (Hon), DA, (1888–1986). Ulster Med J. 2008;77:146–52.

78. Maltby JR. Magill forceps: Sir Ivan Whiteside Magill (1888–1986). In: Maltby JR, editor. Notable names in anaesthesia. London: Royal Society of Medicine; 2002. pp. 123–5.

79. Maltby JR. Murphy eye: Francis John Murphy (1889–1974). In: Maltby JR, editor. Notable names in anaesthesia. London: Royal Society of Medicine; 2002. pp. 151–3.

80. Maltby JR. Sellick Manoevre: Brian Arthur Sellick (1918–1996). In: Maltby JR, editor. Notable names in anaesthesia. London: Royal Society of Medicine; 2002. pp. 196–8.

81. Jaeger JM, Durbin CG. Special purpose endotracheal tubes. Respir Care. 1999;44:661–83.

82. Brodsky JB. The evolution of thoracic anesthesia. Thorac Surg Clin. 2005;15:1–10.

83. Duckworth SI. The Oxford non-kinking endotracheal tube. Anaesthesia. 1962;17:208–14.

84. Maltby JR, Settergren G. Carlens catheter: Eric Carlens (1908–1990). In: Maltby JR, editor. Notable names in anaesthesia. London: Royal Society of Medicine; 2002. pp. 35–8.

85. Ring WH. RAE (Ring, Adair, Elwyn) endotracheal tubes: Wallace Harold Ring (1932–). In: Maltby JR, editor. Notable names in anaesthesia. London: Royal Society of Medicine; 2002. pp. 167–9.

86. Butler FS, Cirillo AA. Retrograde tracheal intubation. Anesth Analg. 1960;39:333–8.

87. Pearce AC. Retrograde intubation. In: Calder I, Pearce AC, editors. Core topics in airway management. Cambridge: Cambridge University Press; 2005. pp. 105–8.

88. Sanchez A. Retrograde intubation technique. In: Hagberg CA, editor. Benumof's airway management: principles and practice. 2nd ed. Philadelphia: Elsevier; 2007. pp. 439–62.

89. Hagberg CA. Current concepts in the management of the difficult airway. Anesthesiology News. 2010;Special Edition:49–72.

90. Hagberg CA MD, editors. Re: development of the METTRO, CAEC, Aintree, Frova, Retrograde Intubation Kit edition. Clinical Representative, Cook Critical Care. 2011.

91. El-Orbany M, Salem MR. The eschmann tracheal tube introducer is not an airway exchange device. Anesth Analg. 2004;99:1269–70. author reply 1270.

92. Henderson JJ. Development of the 'gum-elastic bougie'. Anaesthesia. 2003;58:103–4.

93. Hung OR. Intubating stylets. In: Hagberg CA, editor. Benumof's airway management: principles and practice. 2nd ed. Philadelphia: Elsevier; 2007. pp. 463–75.

94. Davis L, Cook-Sather SD, Schreiner MS. Lighted stylet tracheal intubation: a review. Anesth Analg. 2000;90:745–56.

95. Murphy MF, Hung OR. Lighted stylet intubation. In: Walls RM, Murphy MF, editors. Manual of emergency airway management. 3rd ed. Philadelphia: Lippincott Williams & Wilkins; 2008. pp. 140–8.

96. Liem EB, Bjoraker DG, Gravenstein D. New options for airway management: intubating fibreoptic stylets. Br J Anaesth. 2003;91:408–18.

97. Burkle CM, Walsh MT, Harrison BA, Curry TB, Rose SH. Airway management after failure to intubate by direct laryngoscopy: outcomes in a large teaching hospital. Can J Anaesth. 2005;52:634–40.

98. Calder I, Ovassapian A. Calder N. John Logie Baird–fibreoptic pioneer. J R Soc Med. 2000;93:438–9.

99. Ikeda S, Yanai N, Ishikawa S. Flexible bronchofiberscope. Keio J Med. 1968;17:1–16.

100. Miyazawa T. History of the flexible bronchoscope. In: Bolliger CT, Mathur PN, editors. Progress in respiratory research: interventional bronchoscopy. Basel: Krager; 2000. pp. 16–21.

101. Ikeda S, Tsuboi E, Ono R, Ishikawa S. Flexible bronchofiberscope. Jpn J Clin Oncol. 2010;40:e55–64.

102. Conyers AB, Wallace DH, Mulder DS. Use of the fiber optic bronchoscope for nasotracheal intubation: case report. Can Anaesth Soc J. 1972;19:654–6.

103. Stiles CM, Stiles QR, Denson JS. A flexible fiber optic laryngoscope. JAMA. 1972;221:1246–7.

104. Davis NJ. A new fiberoptic laryngoscope for nasal intubation. Anesth Analg. 1973;52:807–8.

105. Ovassapian A, Schrader SC. Fiberoptic aided tracheal intubation. Semin Anesth. 1987;6:133.

106. Raj PP, Forestner J, Watson TD, Morris RE, Jenkins MT. Technics for fiberoptic laryngoscopy in anesthesia. Anesth Analg. 1974;53:708–14.

107. Ovassapian A, Yelich SJ, Dykes MH, Goldman ME. Learning fiberoptic intubation: use of simulators vs. traditional teaching. Br J Anaesth. 1988;15:237–9.

108. Atlas GM. A comparison of fiberoptic-compatible oral airways. J Clin Anesth. 2004;16:66–73.

109. Greenland KB, Irwin MG. The Williams airway intubator, the Ovassapian airway and the Berman airway as upper airway conduits for fiberoptic bronchoscopy in patients with difficult airways. Curr Opin Anaesthesiol. 2004;17:505–10.

110. Reed JP, Kemph JP, Hamelberg W, Hitchcock FA, Jacoby J. Studies with transtracheal artificial respiration. Anesthesiology. 1954;15:28–41.

111. Jacoby JJ, Hamelberg W, Ziegler CH, Flory FA, Jones JR. Transtracheal resuscitation. JAMA. 1956;162:625–8.

112. Spoerel WE, Narayanan PS, Singh NP. Transtracheal ventilation. Br J Anaesth. 1971;43:932–9.

113. Benumof JL, Scheller MS. The importance of transtracheal jet ventilation in the management of the difficult airway. Anesthesiology. 1989;71:769–78.

114. Finucane BT, Kupshik HL. A flexible stilette for replacing damaged tracheal tubes. Can Anaesth Soc J. 1978;25:153–4.

115. Desai SP, Fencl V. A safe technique for changing endotracheal tubes. Anesthesiology. 1980;53:267.

116. Audenaert SM, Montgomery CL, Slayton D, Berger R. Application of the Mizus endotracheal obturator in tracheostomy and tentative extubation. J Clin Anesth. 1991;3:418–21.

117. Cook TM, Seller C, Gupta K, Thornton M, O'Sullivan E. Nonconventional uses of the Aintree Intubating Catheter in management of the difficult airway. Anaesthesia. 2007;62:169–74.

118. Cattano D, Hagberg CA. A comparison of two laryngeal masks as a conduit for fiberoptic tube exchange. Anaesthesia Product News. 2009;17:28–9.

119. Law JA, Hagberg CA. Video laryngoscopy and the difficult airway-Image is everything. Anesthesiology News. 2008;34:91–8.

120. McGibbon JEB. Cinebronchography. Lancet. 1940;235:1083.

121. Hagberg CA MD, editor. Clinical representative, Ambu A/S. 2011.

122. Hagberg CA MD, editor. Clinical representative, Olympus. 2011.

123. Piepho T, Werner C, Noppens RR. Evaluation of the novel, single-use, flexible aScope for tracheal intubation in the simulated difficult airway and first clinical experiences. Anaesthesia. 2010;65:820–5.

124. Agres T. Video laryngoscopes: the airway management tool for the masses? Anesthesiology News. 2007;33.

125. Cattano D, Hagberg CA. Video laryngoscopy in obese patients. Anesthesiology News. 2010;36.

126. Weiss M, Hartmann K, Fischer J, Gerber AC. Video-intuboscopic assistance is a useful aid to tracheal intubation in pediatric patients. Can J Anaesth. 2001;48:691–6.

127. Diagnostic Ultrasound, Maker of BladderScan Bladder Volume Instruments. Acquires GlideScope Manufacturer, Staurn Biomedical Systems. [Press Release]; 2006.

128. Jones PM, Armstrong KP, Armstrong PM, Cherry RA, Harle CC, Hoogstra J, Turkstra TP. A comparison of glidescope videolaryngoscopy to direct laryngoscopy for nasotracheal intubation. Anesth Analg. 2008;107:144–8.

129. Roberts JL, Reed WR, Mathew OP, Menon AA, Thach BT. Assessment of pharyngeal airway stability in normal and micrognathic infants. J Appl Physiol. 1985;58:290–9.

130. Kaplan MB, Hagberg CA, Ward DS, Brambrink A, Chhibber AK, Heidegger T, Lozada L, Ovassapian A, Parsons D, Ramsay J, Wilhelm W, Zwissler B, Gerig HJ, Hofstetter C, Karan S, Kreisler N, Pousman RM, Thierbach A, Wrobel M, Berci G. Comparison of direct and video-assisted views of the larynx during routine intubation. J Clin Anesth. 2006;18:357–62.

131. Kaplan MB, Ward DS, Berci G. A new video laryngoscope-an aid to intubation and teaching. J Clin Anesth. 2002;14:620–6.

132. Jon Berall MD. Re: development of the C-Scope Video Laryngoscope edition. Edited by Carin A. Hagberg MD; 2010.

133. Cormack RS, Lehane J. Cormack-Lehane laryngoscopy grades: Ronald Sidney Cormack (1930–) & John Robert Lehane (1945–). In: Maltby JR, editor. Notable names in anaesthesia. London: Royal Society of Medicine; 2002. pp. 43–5.

134. Mallampati R, Maltby JR. Mallampati score: Seshagiri Rao Mallampati (1941–). In: Maltby JR, editor. Notable names in anaesthesia. London: Royal Society of Medicine; 2002. pp. 126–8.

135. Samsoon GL, Young JR. Difficult tracheal intubation: a retrospective study. Anaesthesia. 1987;42:487–90.

136. Ezri T, Warters RD, Szmuk P, Saad-Eddin H, Geva D, Katz J, Hagberg C. The incidence of class "zero" airway and the impact of Mallampati score, age, sex, and body mass index on prediction of laryngoscopy grade. Anesth Analg. 2001;93:1073–5.

John W. Severinghaus

Summary

Before 1950, anesthetists assessed adequacy of ventilation by watching or rarely measuring gas volume exchange or chest movements. About 1950, infrared (IR) light absorption by CO_2 was used to continuously measure expired CO_2, a first real monitor of respiration. It was dubbed capnometry, and remains the basis of all respiratory gas monitors. Gaseous oxygen was first monitored in anesthetic circuits using a polarographic oxygen electrode, made available about 1960. Mass spectrometers that could continuously measure O_2, CO_2, N_2O and anesthetic gases were rarely used until 1975 when methods were introduced to use one mass spectrometer to sequentially measure gases sampled through long catheters from many patients. In the late 1980s, infra red detectors of CO_2 and anesthetic vapors were combined with polarographic O_2 electrodes to make the modern operating room gas monitoring devices.

Blood gas analysis never became a continuous monitoring procedure except in cardio-pulmonary by-pass oxygenators. Invention in 1954 of a blood CO_2 electrode and in 1956 of a blood O_2 electrode led to rapid, if not continuous, blood PO_2, PCO_2 and pH analysis, introduced in 1958 and soon made available in most operating, recovery and other critical care areas.

Transcutaneous estimation of blood PO_2 and PCO_2 was developed in the early 1970s to protect premature infants from either too much or too little oxygen. It played little role in anesthesia monitoring.

Oximetry was occasionally used in anesthesia after World War II, but only became widely used following the development of pulse oximetry about 1985, 10 years after its serendipitous invention in Japan.

Anesthesia Monitoring Before Polio and Transistors

During the first century of anesthesia, the only variables that anesthetists monitored routinely were chest movements, skin color and pulse. S Riva Rocci (1863–1937) invented blood pressure measurement using an inflatable cuff in 1896. In 1905 N Korotkoff (1874–1920) reported that the arterial sounds heard through a stethoscope placed over the brachial artery during occlusion and release of pressure in a cuff surrounding the arm could be used to measure diastolic as well as arterial pressure. Harvey Cushing applied these in his newly invented anesthetic record in the early 1900s.

Monitoring was still minimal in 1927, when academic anesthesia training began in Madison, Wisconsin under Ralph Waters (1883–1979), the world's first academic anesthesia department chair. In 1950, Stuart Cullen (1909–1979), Professor of Anesthesia at the University of Iowa, taught inhalational anesthesia methods at the WHO training course for 3rd world physicians in Copenhagen (Fig. 55.1). Watched by Waters and 4 young Danish anesthetists (each a future department chair), the only monitors to be seen were Cullen's finger on the pulse and his view of the motion of the rebreathing bag. Pupil sifze was used to gauge the depth of ether anesthesia, the legacy of Arthur Guedel (1883–1956). At the time, mortality primarily due to anesthesia in the US was 3.7–11.7 per 10,000 anesthetics [1, 2].

In the 1950s, ether and cyclopropane flammability precluded the use of most electrical apparatus near the patient. Operating rooms in the US and elsewhere had conductive floors, and anesthesia machines had chains or wires touching the floor to discharge static charges. To avoid explosions, ECG monitoring required construction of a pressurized cathode ray tube electrocardiograph in a bullet-like cylinder, supplied with a bicycle tire pump to sustain its internal pressure. Low voltage thermistors in flexible catheters were used to monitor rectal or esophageal temperature in the early days of hypothermic anesthesia for cardiac and neurosurgery. Non-electrical ventilatory volume monitors became incorporated in some new anesthesia machines, particularly if artificial ventilators were used.

Introduction of the transistor in 1954 removed the danger of sparks and permitted low voltage amplifying devices to

J. W. Severinghaus (✉)
Anesthesia and Cardiovascular Research Institute,
University of California, San Francisco, CA, USA
e-mail: jwseps@comcast.net

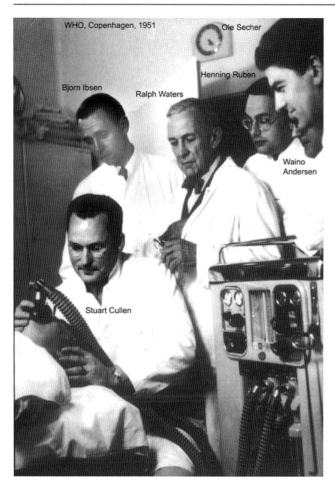

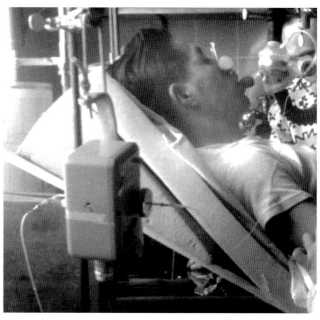

Fig. 55.2 Luft CO_2 detector principle was used in Beckman infrared CO_2 analyzers for research and operating room use, 1950. (Courtesy of the author's collection.)

Fig. 55.1 Stuart Cullen demonstrated inhalation anesthesia in Copenhagen to Ralph Waters and several of the Danish anesthesia faculty of the World Health Organization Anesthesia training course for 3rd world doctors in 1951. Absence of monitoring equipment is notable. (Courtesy of the author's collection.)

be used, thus initiating the modern use of monitoring. The introduction of curare and other muscle relaxants, the poliomyelitis epidemics of the 1950s, positive pressure ventilators, cardio-pulmonary bypass, and of course, the fatality rate, stimulated development of monitoring devices.

Airway Monitoring of Respiratory and Anesthetic Gases

Capnometry

John Tyndall (1820–1893) Professor of Natural Philosophy at the Royal Institution, was the first to discover and report that CO_2 gas absorbs infra red light [3]. He built a device to measure this absorption. August Pfund (1879–1949) developed an analyser in 1939, to measure concentrations of carbon dioxide and carbon monoxide [4]. Radiation from a heated nickel chrome wire was directed through a sample cell into a detector cell containing a 3 % carbon dioxide

mixture, where the temperature was measured. The presence of carbon dioxide in the sample cell caused less radiation to reach the detector cell resulting in a smaller rise in temperature.

Karl Luft (1909–1999) deserves the credit for developing the modern infrared capnograph. Working with the German BASF company in 1937, he invented a clever principle to detect the infra-red (IR) light passing through an unknown gas sample [5]. His "Luft cell" incorporated two IR light sources, one beam directed through a reference cell, the other through a sample cell filled with a stream of the unknown gas (Fig. 55.2). The IR light beams then entered a two-chambered detector cell, each containing 3 % CO_2. The relative heating induced by the incoming IR light beams moved a membrane separating the two chambers. An electrical capacitance sensor detected the membrane motion. The IR beams were "chopped" by a rotating shutter, providing an AC signal proportional to the decrease in IR light entering the detector on the sample side.

Shortage of components before and during World War II limited the manufacture of Luft cells to several hundred. Some were used for environmental monitoring in submarines. Others, stored in salt mines, were confiscated and removed to the US and England after the war. The Germans also telescopically tracked their buzz-bombs by the CO_2 absorption of IR light from the exhaust of the bomb.

In the 1950s, an infra-red respiratory CO_2 analyzer was designed by Max Liston (1924–2004) using German patents confiscated at the end of WWII. He was guided and encouraged by James Elam (1918–1995) and associates to apply it to operating room monitoring [6]. The Beckman Co.

marketed the capnograph. Like the ECG bullet, its cast aluminum "head" near the airway was pressurized. The unpressurized capnograph amplifier control was supposed to be mounted at least 6 ft above the OR floor, a rule that assumed leaking explosive agents were heavier than air thus settling at a lower level.

The device was widely used for research but little used for patient safety monitoring. In the 1960s, the Beckman LB-1 capnometer was modified to analyze N_2O, ether, halothane or other anesthetics, for research (only one gas per instrument) [7].

Multi-Patient Anesthetic Mass Spectrometry

Francis Aston (1877–1945), a student of Joseph (JJ) Thomson (1856–1940) at the Cavendish Laboratory at Cambridge, devised the first mass spectrometer to separate isotopes of elements in 1919. Aston was awarded the Nobel Prize in Chemistry in 1922 for his discovery. A mass spectrometer ionized substances (in a vacuum) and accelerated a beam of charged particles (elements or compounds). The beam passed through a magnetic field to bend and separate heavier from lighter particles, each weight being collected in separate metal cups from which the ion current was measured. For respiratory gas studies, an extremely small leak continuously admitted a stream of sample gas into the ionizer, providing continuous concentration information.

In the late 1950s, in order to continuously monitor many artificially ventilated ICU patients (particularly polio victims suffering from long term paralysis), several institutions used a single centrally located respiratory mass spectrometer connected through long sampling catheters to the airways to provide sequential and frequent analysis of inspired and end tidal PCO_2 [8]. The data were typically displayed on the central nursing desk. N Davies and D Denison [9] investigated the performance of long sampling catheters, and concluded that they introduced no important errors.

Mass spectrometers could also analyze inhalational anesthetics, but were too expensive and too difficult to maintain for continuous use in each operating room. However, the monitoring cost per patient could be reduced significantly by using one mass spectrometer for many patients, as in the ICU systems. In the mid 1970s at UCSF, Gerald Ozanne (1941-), Bill Young (1954-) and I installed a single mass spectrometer to sequentially sample airway gases from each patient in the 10 room OR suite of Moffitt Hospital [10]. Long nylon catheters were installed thru the OR ceilings. Young, a recent Oberlin college graduate with talents in both physical chemistry and computer programming, enthusiastically took on the design and programming tasks. We found that patient airway gases could be continuously and slowly sampled from each patient through 30 m long catheters, accurately storing in the catheters about 20 sec of data. When a catheter

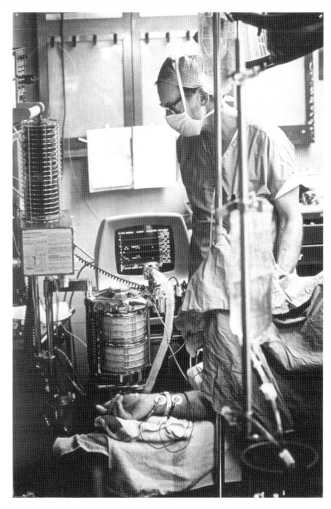

Fig. 55.3 Mass spectrometer anesthetic and respiratory gas analysis operating room display screen in Moffitt Hospital with author, 1978. (Courtesy of the author's collection.)

was switched to the mass spectrometer inlet, gas stored in the catheter was drawn into the mass spectrometer within 6 sec by a lower pressure. The inspired and end tidal concentrations of respiratory gases and the anesthetic vapor were reported on a display in each OR about once per minute (Fig. 55.3). In each OR, by default, the display was a time plot of 30 min of end tidal PCO_2 and halothane %, and a table of current values of all sampled end-tidal gases. The mass spectrometer terminal in each operating room became a communication system before the Web. It permitted Bill Young to monitor each operating room after he moved to New York. He called me one day, worried about operating room 5. I called the attending anesthesiologist and said, "New York wants to know why your patient in room 5 has a PCO_2 of 80."

Anesthetists at UCSF became dependent on (addicted to) this device. So did researchers. A couple of things flowed from this dependence. One was a demand for such analysis by other institutions. At one point, several hundred of these multiplexed multi-OR systems were in use at institutions, mostly in the U.S. The second was that the device needed competent technician care and was susceptible to occasional breakdown, affecting all the operating rooms. Not good for anesthetists addicted to minute by minute analyses of anesthetic concentrations. This stimulated various manufacturers to develop cheaper stand-alone respiratory gas monitors, using the infrared principle already described.

Infrared Analyzers

The absorption spectrum of each anesthetic vapor is unique, especially in the far IR band from 8–9 μm wavelength. The technology for inhaled anesthetic analysis was slowly improved, primarily by the Datex Co, until mixtures of several halogenated vapor anesthetics, CO_2 and N_2O could be successfully analyzed with a single Luft type IR detector cell, including correcting for overlap of the IR absorption peaks [11]. With the addition of an internal polarographic O_2 electrode, end-tidal gas monitoring in every operating room became widely employed. These monitors were less expensive to maintain than the mass spectrometer systems, a failing unit could rapidly be replaced, and only affected one OR. By 1995, multiplexed mass spectrometers had been replaced by stand-alone infra-red gas analyzers [12].

Blood Gas Analysis

Gas Bubble Analysis

In 1801, John Dalton (1766–1844), the Quaker English chemist, meteorologist and physicist, observed that the total pressure exerted by a mixture of gases is the sum of the "partial pressures" of each component gas. In 1803, he described the role of partial pressure in absorption of gases by water and other liquids. The concept of partial pressures gradually stimulated interest in measuring the partial pressures of oxygen (PO_2) and carbon dioxide (PCO_2) in blood in the late nineteenth century. In 1872, Eduard Pflüger (1829–1910) in Bonn equilibrated a small gas bubble with a large volume of blood at body temperature, and then analyzed the O_2 and CO_2 in the bubble using volume loss by chemical absorption [13]. Bubble analysis was developed into a clinical and laboratory method in 1945 by Richard Riley (1911–2001) [14]. He used a specially adapted syringe with a capillary attached, that had been invented by FJW (Jack) Roughton (1899–1972) and Per Scholander (1905–1980) during World War II [15]. Riley's method worked reasonably well for PCO_2 but poorly for PO_2, especially for blood nearly saturated with oxygen.

Acid Base Balance and Carbon Dioxide

Even before Robert Boyle's time in the 1660s, fermentation and respiration were recognized as producing "fixed

air" or "gas", early names for CO_2. The alchemists had used acids and bases in the middle ages, and in Paris, Hilaire-Martin Rouelle (1718–1779) discovered the alkalinity of blood, using titration and color indicators. In 1831, William O'Shaughnessy (1809–1889), an Irish physician working in India, showed that the major pathologic effect of cholera was loss of blood "free alkali" [16]. In 1877, Friedrich Walter (1850-?) established the relationship between the carbon dioxide content of blood and its alkalinity in his 1877 thesis, while studying in Strasbourg under fellow Latvian, Oswald Schmiedeberg (1838–1921) [17]. Walter's finding made it possible to measure a patient's abnormality of alkalinity (now called metabolic acid-base balance) by analyzing blood carbon dioxide content.

Methods Underlying Blood Gas and Acid Base Analysis

The electrodes now used for rapid analysis of oxygen, CO_2 and pH, and all the derived acid-base balance data, come from the science of physical (electro) chemistry, born in the 1880s by two discoveries; ionization and osmotic pressure theory.

Ionic Theory and the Hydrogen Ion

Jacobus van't Hoff (1852–1911) initiated the development of electrochemical theory in 1889, by discovering that the long known gas laws applied to osmotic pressure [18]. The concept of ionization of salts into cations and anions, although first suggested by Michael Faraday (1791–1867) in 1830, was thought to be imaginary until 1887, when Svante Arrhenius (1859–1927) in Uppsala published a thesis proving, by measuring solution conductivity, that some salts dissociated as their concentration was reduced [19]. His discovery was the first to link acid strength to the hydrogen ion concentration. It stimulated Wilhelm Ostwald (1853–1932) to make the first electrometric measurement of H^+ ions by the potential on a platinum electrode in solutions saturated with hydrogen gas [20]. By combining the van't Hoff osmotic theory with the new ionic theory, Ostwald's student, Walter Nernst (1864–1941), discovered the energetic equivalence of Faraday's constant, F, to the gas laws, thereby mathematically linking electrometric ion activity to the behavior of gases [21]. For these discoveries, Nobel prizes in chemistry were awarded to van't Hoff (1901), Arrhenius (1903), Ostwald (1909), and Nernst (1920).

Introduction of pH for Hydrogen Ion Activity

Søren Sørensen [22] (1868–1939) proposed the term pH, the negative logarithm of H^+ concentration, as a simplification. The pH terminology quickly came to be used more than nanomoles of hydrogen ion concentration because the behavior of a substance in a chemical system is proportional to its energy (chemical potential), a logarithmic function of the activity (or concentration) of the substance. A pH electrode responds to the chemical potential of H^+, and thus the instrument provides a precise and readily obtained measurement of the chemical behavior of H^+.

Development of the Glass pH Electrode

In 1906, Max Cremer (1865–1935) discovered an electrical potential across thin glass membranes, proportional to the acid concentration difference on each side, implying that the glass is actually permeable to H^+ ions[23]. By 1909, glass H^+ ion (pH) electrodes had been constructed [24]. In London in 1925, Phyllis Kerridge built the first blood pH electrode designed to prevent CO2 escape from the sample [25]. Corning Glass marketed the first precise pH glass capillary electrode in 1932, and it was still the best when I started a blood gas laboratory at NIH in 1953 [26].

Buffers: The Relationships of Bicarbonate, Hydrogen Ion and Carbonic Acid

In 1907, the remarkable ability of blood to neutralize large amounts of acid, led Lawrence Henderson (1878–1942), then an instructor in biochemistry at Harvard University, to investigate the relationship of bicarbonate to dissolved carbon dioxide gas, and how they acted as buffers of fixed acids [27]. It was his insight that helped chemists and physiologists realize that when acids are added to blood, the hydrogen ions react with blood bicarbonate, generating CO_2 gas that is then excreted by the lungs, almost eliminating the increased acidity. The computer equations in all modern blood gas analyzers derive from Henderson [28] who rewrote the laws of mass action for weak acids and their salts, in the case of carbonic acid as: $k = [H^+][HCO_3^-]/[H_2CO_3]$. In 1917, Karl Hasselbalch (1874–1962) converted Henderson's equation to log form, the Henderson-Hasselbalch equation, $pH = pK' + \log[HCO3^-/(S \cdot PCO_2)]$ [29].

Until the mid 1950s, PCO_2 was computed from this equation by measuring the blood pH and plasma CO_2 content using the manometric apparatus developed by Donald van Slyke (1883–1971), head of the laboratory at the Rockefeller Institute in New York [30].

The World Wide 1952 Polio Epidemic Leads to Blood Gas Analysis

Severinghaus' Memories of Ibsen, Astrup and the Polio Epidemic

I was invited by Bjørn Ibsen (1915–2007; Fig. 55.4) to dine in his apartment with his wife, shortly after arrival for my first sabbatical in Copenhagen, in 1964–5. I was there to

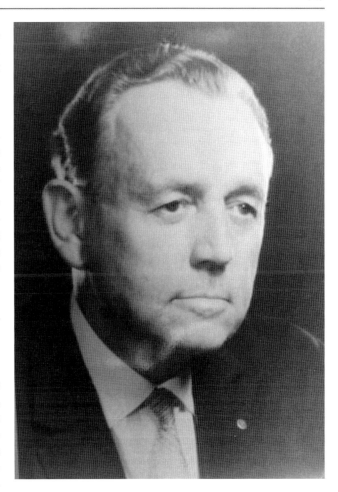

Fig. 55.4 Bjørn Ibsen, creator and director of world's first intensive care unit during the 1950's polio epidemic in Copenhagen. (Courtesy of the author's collection.)

study the possible active transport of something, presumably HCO_3^-, across the blood brain barrier to account for the rapid reduction in CSF HCO_3^- and relatively constant, slightly increased pH found during altitude acclimatization. I had met Poul Astrup (1915–2000; Fig. 55.5) in London in December, 1958, at the Ciba Symposium on blood gas analysis organized by John Nunn (1923-). I collaborated with Astrup and Ole Siggaard Andersen (1932-) on acid base problems, and taught 3rd world WHO anesthesia students in an ongoing program, mostly taught by well trained Danish anesthesiologists (Fig. 55.6).

A vicious polio epidemic struck Copenhagen in 1952–3. Hundreds of people, especially the young, were sent for isolation to the communicable disease Blegdams hospital just across Tagensvej from Rigshospitalet. The director, Professor HCA Lassen, was overwhelmed. He and his associate Mogens Bjørneboe had not understood the cause of many deaths. High CO_2 concentrations in blood samples led him to assume that the patients were somehow developing a metabolic alkalosis.

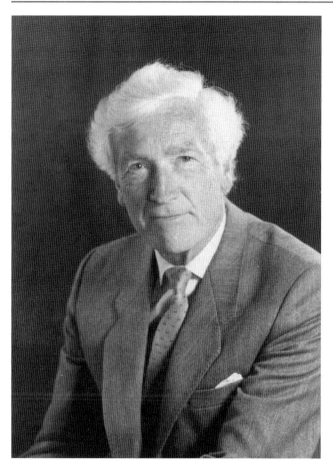

Fig. 55.5 Poul Astrup, who invented a new method to analyze blood PCO_2 in response to the need to control artificial ventilation during the polio epidemic. (Courtesy of the author's collection.)

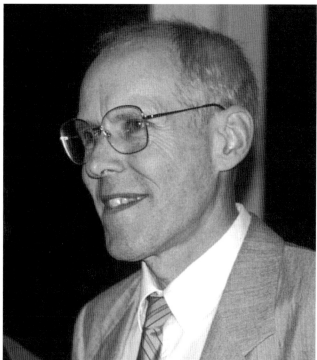

Fig. 55.6 Ole Siggaard Andersen, student of Astrup, developer of acid-base apparatus, theory and Base Excess and Standard Base Excess definitions and terms. (Courtesy of the author's collection.)

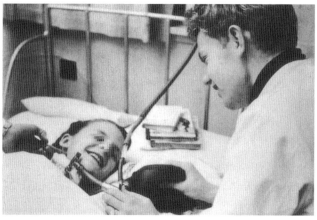

Fig. 55.7 A smiling 12 year-old polio patient ventilated via a tracheostomy by a medical student. (Courtesy of the author's collection.)

After a suggestion from Bjørneboe, Lassen asked Ibsen, a young anesthesiologist (who had trained at the Massachusetts General Hospital) at Rigshospitalet to help. Ibsen, looking at the blood studies, that did not include pH, realized that the diagnosis was not metabolic alkalosis but hypoventilation, with CO_2 retention and resulting severe hypoxia [31]. Blegdam hospital had only one iron lung and some almost useless cuirass ventilators. Ibsen initiated ventilation in a 12-year-old girl (Fig. 55.7), at first by an anesthesia bag and mask, then later ventilation powered by hand via a tracheotomy. She survived.

Ibsen was not sure how much ventilation the patients needed. He asked Poul Astrup for help by determining what the arterial PCO_2 was in some of the patients in order to guide adjustments needed to maintain PCO_2 at the normal level of 5 % (or 40 mm Hg). Astrup was a young clinical chemist in charge of the laboratory at Rigshospitalet. He had no routine way of measuring PCO_2 but knew the method: Measure arterial pH, and measure plasma or serum CO_2 content using a Van Slyke manometric analyser. Compute PCO_2 by the Henderson-Hasselbalch equation, formalized in Copenhagen 35 years earlier by Hasselbalch.

Astrup knew that the pH of blood must be measured at body temperature. No temperature controlled pH meters were available so Astrup took his lab pH meter into his 37 °C culture room, and waited while the meter and the blood sample warmed. He soon became involved in speeding up the analysis of large numbers of samples, doing arterial punctures, transporting the warm blood, in a syringe wrapped in a blanket, to his culture room, computing PCO_2 and sending the result to help the student adjust the ventilation toward a more normal level.

Astrup sought a better method of measuring PCO_2. His solution became known as the "equilibration method". He modified one of Hasselbalch's ideas: Measuring "reduced pH" after equilibration of a blood sample to 40 mm Hg PCO_2. Astrup modified Van Slyke's graph showing the linear relationship of log PCO_2 to pH after equilibration of blood with differing PCO_2 gases [32]. Displacement of this straight line by added acid or base permitted Astrup, and his student and associate Ole Siggaard Andersen (1932-), to estimate not only PCO_2 but also the acid-base abnormality of the blood, later named base excess.

Astrup and Svend Schroeder of the Radiometer Co. designed and built an apparatus to measure pH at 37 °C before and after equilibration with gases of known CO_2 content. Over the next decade, it was modified by Siggaard Andersen [33], improved, marketed by Radiometer, and widely used as the "Astrup Apparatus" (Fig. 55.8). The Stow-Severinghaus PCO_2 electrode gradually made it obsolete.

Acid-Base Nomenclature

The term base excess (BE) was originally introduced to define blood metabolic (non-respiratory) acid base balance [34]. Some clinicians rejected BE because it changed with altered PCO_2 as plasma bicarbonate equilibrated readily with all the body's extracellular fluid (ECF), about 3 times the blood volume. To obtain an index independent of acute changes in PCO_2, in 1966, Siggaard Andersen introduced a modified index termed Standard Base Excess (SBE) and published a modified Van Slyke equation to compute SBE now used in most blood gas analyzers [35]. SBE is nearly independent of acute changes in PCO_2, and applies to the ECF of the entire body by assuming a total ECF hemoglobin concentration of 5 g/dl.

The CO_2 Electrode

A CO_2 electrode was first described by physiologists Robert Gesell (1886–1954) and Daniel McGinty at the University of Michigan in 1926, for use in expired air, but not in blood [36]. It used the effect of CO_2 on the pH of a film of peritoneal membrane, wet with a salt solution, and wrapped over an antimony pH electrode.

In Columbus, Ohio, a physical chemist, Richard Stow (1916-), in the department of Physical Medicine, Ohio State University, (Fig. 55.9), needed to measure blood PCO_2 to guide the setting of mechanical ventilators in the care of polio patients in 1951–3. In the library, he found several Macy reports about ion-specific electrodes. They triggered an idea. He knew that carbon dioxide permeated rubber freely and

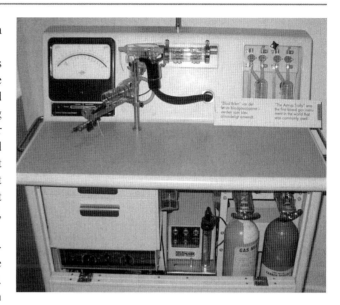

Fig. 55.8 Blood gas analyzer using the Astrup equilibration method for PCO_2, with micro-capillary pH electrode and equilibrators designed by Siggaard Andersen, and the Clark electrode for PO_2 analysis. "S": sampling tip on hand-held pH electrode, also used to connect pH sample to KCl reference electrode. *(Radiometer Co, Copenhagen, ~1960).* (Courtesy of the author's collection.)

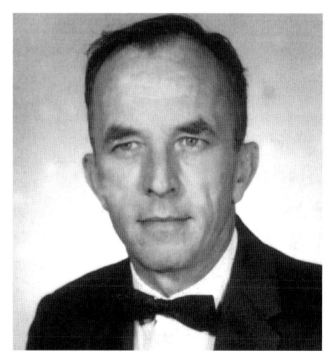

Fig. 55.9 Richard Stow, the inventor of a blood PCO_2 electrode. (Courtesy of the author's collection.)

that it acidified water. He conceived of an electrode for measuring PCO_2 using a latex film to separate a blood sample from a glass pH electrode wet with distilled water. Being an expert glass blower, he constructed his own combined

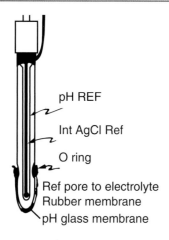

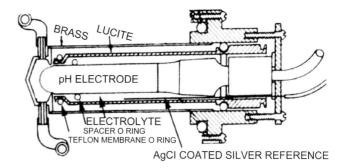

Fig. 55.11 First working PCO_2 electrode, stabilized and made practical by author, 1954. (Courtesy of the author's collection.)

Fig. 55.10 Stow's combined glass pH and reference electrode. (Courtesy of the author's collection.)

glass pH and reference electrode (Fig. 55.10). He immediately confirmed that the pH electrode potential increased in response to increasing PCO_2 in either gas or liquid. As he expected, pH was a logarithmic function of PCO_2.

In August 1954, Stow reported his design at the fall meeting of the American Physiologic Society in Madison, Wisconsin [37]. He had been unable to prevent significant drift, and therefore concluded that his electrode probably could not be useful. During the question period after his talk, I asked Stow whether he had considered adding bicarbonate to the distilled water electrolyte. He said he had assumed that bicarbonate was a buffer that would prevent any change of pH when PCO_2 varied. I realized that, despite his doctorate in physical chemistry, Stow clearly did not grasp the differences between fixed and volatile buffering systems. We agreed that I would construct and investigate a CO_2 electrode with a bicarbonate electrolyte [38].

A few days later, using a Stow type pH and reference electrode, I found that a 25 mM sodium bicarbonate electrolyte solution stabilized the pH signal and doubled the PCO_2 sensitivity such that a 10 fold change in PCO_2 altered pH by almost 1 pH unit. A spacer of cellophane was needed to hold a wet film between the non-conductive rubber membrane, and the pH glass surface (Fig. 55.11). In 1959, Forrest Bird (1921-), inventor of a popular ventilator, arranged for his firm, the National Welding Co, to make my CO_2 electrodes commercially available. The unpatented design concept was soon copied and marketed by Beckman, Radiometer, Instrumentation Labs and several other firms in the US, Europe and Japan.

The Polarographic Oxygen Electrode

The method now called polarography originated in Nernst's laboratory in Göttingen, Germany. Nernst suggested to his assistant Heinrich Danneel (1867–1942), that he investigate the properties of single noble metal electrodes (gold,

platinum) in solutions, by using large and non-polarizable reference electrodes to maintain a constant and known solution potential. Danneel soon noted that oxygen in the solution interfered with measurements whenever the test metal was cathodic (negative). In studying this, he showed that the reaction of oxygen with a negatively charged metal (cathode) was approximately a linear function of the oxygen pressure in the solution [39]. Danneel's work was soon forgotten because the noble metal surface was easily contaminated or 'poisoned' by organic substances but his work had identified the basis of the polarographic oxygen electrode.

Jaroslav Heyrovsky (1890–1967), in Prague, avoided 'poisoning' by using polarized mercury in a continuously refreshed droplet surface exiting a tiny capillary. Heyrovsky coined the name "polarography" to describe his automatic recording apparatus for plotting the relationship between applied voltage and resulting current, the polarogram [40]. After removing all the O_2, Heyrovsky found that this device could be used for measuring the concentrations of very small quantities of the most diverse substances. Heyrovsky was awarded the Nobel Prize in chemistry in 1959 for his discovery of the then widely used polarographic analysis.

J Percy Baumberger (1892–1973) at Stanford, first applied the dropping mercury polarographic method for blood oxygen measurements in 1938 [41], in order to study the oxygen dissociation curve of the blood of insects, his scientific interest. Henry K. Beecher (1904–1976), as a young researcher in anesthesia at Harvard, devised a dropping mercury apparatus to measure PO_2 in plasma separated from blood [42].

The Membrane Covered Polarographic Oxygen Electrode

The solution to the problem of measurement of PO_2 in blood and other liquids is attributed to Leland Clark (1918–2005), a biochemist, physiologist and inventor (Fig. 55.12), working at the Fels Research Institute of Antioch College, Ohio. While investigating enzyme and steroid chemistry in perfused

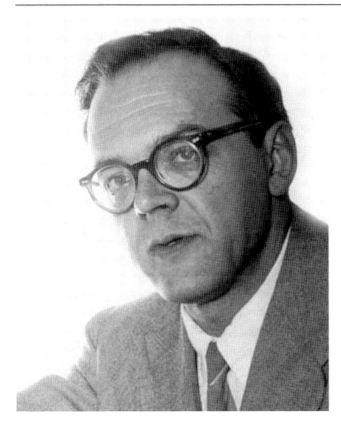

Fig. 55.12 Leland Clark, inventor of the membrane covered polarographic oxygen electrode. (Courtesy of the author's collection.)

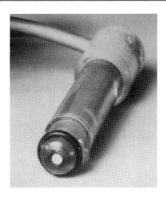

Fig. 55.13 Clark's oxygen electrode, 1956. (Courtesy of the author's collection.)

liver, he used Heyrovsky's dropping mercury polarography, becoming aware that oxygen had to be removed because it reacted first with a negatively charged cathode. In order to perfuse a liver with oxygenated blood for testosterone studies, he built a bubble oxygenator. He discovered that silicone covered glass wool was effective in breaking the foam created by bubbles. The oxygenator was so successful that Clark and Frank Gollan (1909–1988) built a whole animal cardiac bypass apparatus [43] and demonstrated its use in animals. In collaboration with surgeons in 1950, they developed one of the first successful clinical oxygenators. Their paper, submitted to Science, was initially rejected because they had not measured the blood oxygen levels before and after oxygenation. In response, Clark covered a polarographic platinum oxygen electrode with cellophane to avoid cathode poisoning by blood protein. He obtained sufficient data to satisfy the Science editors but found that the electrode was incapable of accurate oxygen analysis because the permeable cellophane resulted in very high cathode oxygen consumption [44].

Clark's Aha Moment

In October, 1954, Clark suddenly realized that he could combine a platinum cathode with a silver reference wire coated with silver chloride in a self contained electrode,

avoiding having the reference electrode in the blood sample. This made possible the use of an electrically non-conducting and much less permeable polyethylene membrane over the tip. He promptly wrote a patent application and sold it to the Beckman Co. The Yellow Springs Instrument Co. made these electrodes, using Clark's design of a 2 mm diameter platinum disk cathode sealed in the tip of glass. He submitted an abstract describing his new electrode to the Society for Artificial Organs that he had just founded. Its first meeting was held at the Federation meetings in Atlantic City on April 18, 1956 [45]. By chance, I had invited Clark and some 30 other respiratory physiologists who had been trying to measure blood PO_2 to an ad-hoc meeting at FASEB on the same day. Before our meeting began, Clark pulled his electrode out of his pocket for us to inspect (Fig. 55.13). Our meeting adjourned, each of us realizing that Clark had solved the problem of measuring blood PO_2. Clark's electrode was immediately in demand, and impacted the subsequent scientific careers of dozens of physiologists.

Clark's invention was the historic turning point in blood gas analysis and all of respiratory physiology. It has been applied in anesthesia, aviation, transcutaneous blood gas analysis, blood oxygen content determination, cell metabolism, and in food, sewage, wine, and various other industrial applications.

Applying Clark's Electrode to Blood Gas Analysis

The Clark electrode had to be calibrated with blood equilibrated at 37 °C with a known gas PO_2, and read in a cuvette with a stirring paddle. In 1957, I built a thermostat water bath for the CO_2 electrode and the Clark O_2 electrode [46]. This first blood gas analyzer was exhibited at the 1957 ASA annual meeting, and at the Atlantic City FASEB spring meeting in 1958 (Fig. 55.14). The need for stirring blood was eliminated by reducing the diameter of the platinum cathode from 2 mm to 10 microns in commercial versions of Clark's

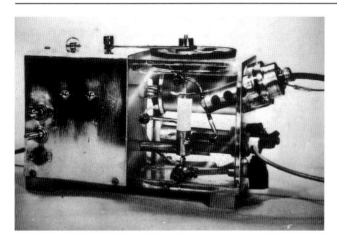

Fig. 55.14 First 2-function blood gas apparatus for PCO_2 and PO_2 analysis by author, 1957. (Courtesy of the author's collection.)

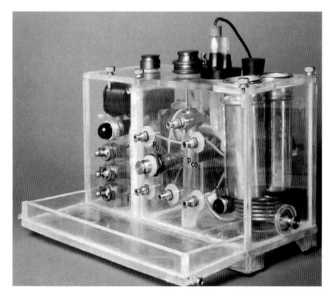

Fig. 55.15 First 3-function blood gas apparatus, with added pH electrode, by author, 1958. (Courtesy of the author's collection.)

electrode. This reduced the O_2 consumption from samples to about 2 % difference between stirred and unstirred blood. In 1958, I added a pH electrode, the first three-function blood gas apparatus (Fig. 55.15) [47].

Transcutaneous (tc) Blood Gas Analysis

Transcutaneous PO_2
In the early 1960s, when airway positive pressure ventilation with oxygen was introduced to save very premature infants, many of the saved infants became blind. This blindness was originally termed RLF (retrolental fibroplasia) but now ROP (retinopathy of prematurity). It created an urgent need for continuous non-invasive monitoring of premature infant

blood oxygen [48]. Physiologists studying skin respiration had shown that human skin breathes, taking up oxygen and giving off CO_2 to the air. If skin is covered (as by a flat unheated PO_2 electrode) the surface PO_2 decreases to zero in a few minutes. However, in 1951, Baumberger and Goodfriend showed that if skin blood flow is greatly increased by the highest tolerable heat, the surface PO_2 increases to approximate PaO_2 (arterial blood) [48].

Within a year after Clark announced his invention of the membrane covered platinum polarographic electrode, studies with polarographic electrodes confirmed the Baumberger report [49]. In Marburg, Germany, Dietrich Lübbers (1917–2005) and students vaso-dilated the skin under an oxygen electrode by heating the electrode to 43–45 °C [50]. The resulting "transcutaneous" $PtcO_2$ was remarkably similar to arterial blood PO_2 in infants [51, 52]. Transcutaneous oxygen monitoring was soon made commercially available by many firms and used in other clinical and critical care situations. It was also useful although less accurate in older children and adults, especially at high PO_2 [53].

Transcutaneous PCO_2
The success of transcutaneous measurement of oxygen led to the design and testing of electrodes to measure $PtcCO_2$ by Beran et al. [54, 55], Huch et al. [56], and me [57]. Interestingly, we found that PO_2 and PCO_2 electrodes could be combined, sharing the same electrolyte and reference electrode because the very small O_2 current had no effect on the pH at the CO_2 electrode surface [58, 59].

Combined Earlobe SpO_2 and $PtcCO_2$
In 2002, Eberhard et al. developed a surprisingly small and light-weight earlobe probe containing both a pulse oximeter and a heated transcutaneous $PtcCO_2$ electrode, cleverly dubbed TOSCA (Transcutaneous Oxygen Saturation and CO_2 Analyzer) [60]. The heating of the skin, needed for $PtcCO_2$, improved the pulse signal strength and speed of response of the pulse oximeter.

Oximetry

Before 1950, physicians estimated adequacy of oxygenation by looking for cyanosis. In good light and with adequate hemoglobin concentration, a keen observer could detect cyanosis at desaturations exceeding 15 % of the hemoglobin [61]. More accurate measures were clearly needed.

Optical Physics Underlying Oximetry
In 1860, Robert Bunsen (1811–1899), professor of chemistry at Heidelberg, and his colleague Gustav Kirchhoff (1824–1887), professor of physics, invented the spectroscope [62]. They showed that each element, when in a flame, gives off

its own specific, identifying wavelengths of light that they called the emission spectrum.

The observation that light influenced electricity is attributed to Alexandre Becquerel (1820–1891), who showed in 1839 that the potential between two electrodes in a solution was altered when one electrode was illuminated. This was the forerunner of the photocell.

In 1760, Johann Lambert (1728–1777) described the relationship of the absorption of light to the amount of absorbent. August Beer (1825–1863) further investigated the relationship in colored flowing solutions in 1852, and from these studies came the Lambert-Beer law: The transmission of light is a logarithmic function of the density or concentration of the absorbent, since each absorbing molecule absorbs an equal fraction of a particular wavelength of the incident light [63, 64].

George Stokes (1819–1903) discovered that the colored substance in blood was the carrier of oxygen [65]. Felix Hoppe-Seyler (1825–1895), professor of applied chemistry in Tübingen and the founder of physiological chemistry in Germany, crystallized the blood pigment and coined the term hemoglobin in 1864. He proved that hemoglobin caused the absorption of green and blue light from the solar spectrum, the "Soret band," and that this absorption changed when he shook the solution with air. He then showed that oxygen and hemoglobin formed a loose, dissociable compound that he called oxyhemoglobin [66].

Hemoglobin's strongest absorption bands are in the blue-green region, so opaque that blood must be diluted to measure optical density, and this changes the oxygen saturation. Optical density is less in the red band from 600 to 750 nm where reduction increases density. In the infrared region, at 805 nm, no change in light absorption occurs with oxygenation, and is called the isobestic point. At greater wavelengths, oxyhemoglobin absorbs more infrared light than that absorbed by reduced hemoglobin.

Origins of In Vivo Oximetry

In 1876, using Bunsen and Kirchhoff's spectrometer, Karl von Vierordt (1818–1884) studied the spectrum of light transmitted through hemoglobin and oxyhemoglobin in solutions and in tissues (his hand) [67]. He found that after stopping circulation in the hand using a tourniquet, the two bands of oxyhemoglobin disappeared and the band of deoxygenated hemoglobin appeared. He measured the hand's oxygen consumption by timing this change in transmitted light. His methods were not used again for 55 years.

In 1931, Ludwig Nicolai (1904-?) initiated the quantitative spectrophotometric investigation of light transmitted through human skin in an effort to understand the dynamics of tissue oxygen consumption [68]. By occluding the circulation, he measured the rate of decay of oxyhemoglobin, and the increase in reduced hemoglobin.

In 1934, Nicolai's associate, K Kramer reported the first precise measurements of oxygen saturation in cuvettes through which blood flowed [69]. He confirmed that the Lambert-Beer law was precisely correct in hemoglobin solutions, and approximately correct in whole blood in cuvettes. In 1935, Kramer continuously recorded the oxygen saturation of blood flowing through unopened vessels in animals [70]. These oxygen saturation measurements had an accuracy of $\pm 1\%$ compared with Van Slyke analyses.

In 1935 in Leipzig, Karl Matthes (1905–1962), constructed the first device to continuously measure the saturation of human blood in vivo by transillumination of the ear or other tissue, based on Nicolai's prior studies [71]. He and Franz Gross were the first to use two spectral regions, one not affected by oxygen, to compensate for changes in tissue thickness, blood content, light intensity, and other variables [72, 73]. They first used blue-green light, following Nicolai's lead, but later switched to infrared. In 1939, they described the first red and infrared ear oxygen saturation meter [74].

In 1940, J Squire at University College Hospital in London, built an oxygen saturation meter for use on the web of the hand [75]. Squire measured the light transmission while compressing the tissue to squeeze out the blood, and again after restoring blood flow. This was a first step toward the absolute reading oximeter. Squire was the first to suggest that the changes of light transmission caused by return of blood should permit an absolute calibration.

Development of oximetry in the US and Britain was stimulated by the needs of World War II fighter aircraft, most of which lacked pressurized cabins but carried O_2 and masks. In 1941, Glen Millikan developed a lightweight ear oxygen meter for which he coined the term oximeter (Fig. 55.16) [76]. However, because measurement was with a motion sensitive galvanometer, his oximeter could not be used in aviation. The earliest studies on the effect of the depth of anesthesia on the electroencephalogram used Millikan's oximeter in a positive pressure chamber, in subjects receiving nitrous oxide anesthesia [77].

Calibration Problems

For calibration, the Millikan oximeter was initially set to read 100%, while the subject breathed oxygen, but it was not calibrated at low saturation. Earl Wood (1912–2009) (Fig. 55.17) at the Mayo Clinic needed oxygen saturation measurements during human centrifuge studies. He knew that in vitro studies had shown that the ratio of the red and IR optical densities of hemoglobin solutions was a unique function of saturation, and he knew of Squire's use of pneumatic tissue compression. He and J Geraci modified Millikan's earpiece, improving the infrared filter and adding an inflatable balloon with which the ear could be made bloodless [78]. Wood recorded the changes of the ear optical density at

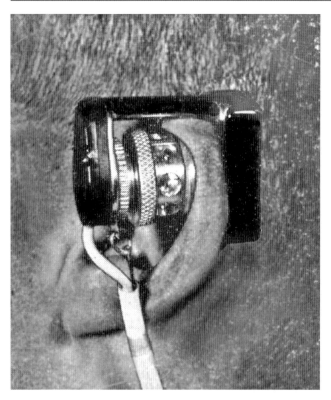

Fig. 55.16 Milliken's ear oximeter, 1941. (Courtesy of the author's collection.)

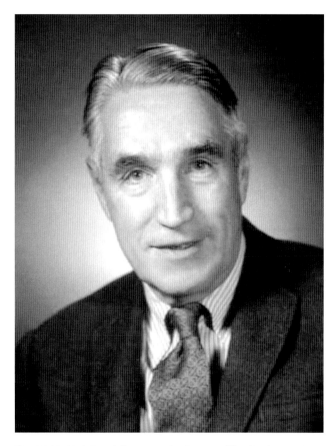

Fig. 55.17 Earl Wood, inventor of oximeter calibration by ear tissue pneumatic compression, a key to the later discovery of pulse oximetry. (Courtesy of the author's collection.)

the two wavelengths when blood was readmitted to the ear, using the resulting 4 values to compute oxygen saturation.

By 1950, Wood's group had reported use of the new oximeter in newborns, in thoracic surgical operations, in cardiac diagnostic procedures, in exercise testing of congenital heart defects, in the human centrifuge and in catheterization (with the cuvette oximeter) [79, 80]. Wood's calibration method failed because the barrier layer photocells were non-uniform in spectral sensitivity, and variable with time, the light was too unsteady and the galvanometer resistance caused photocell output voltage to change with signal. But Wood's insight was crucial to the later discovery by Aoyagi of the pulse oximeter.

Ear Oximetry

R Shaw, a surgeon, engineer and inventor in San Francisco, in 1963–4, invented an ear oximeter using eight-wavelengths to avoid the need for calibration. It successfully tracked SaO_2 to within 1 % over the range from 100 % down at least to 50 %. Because of its large earpiece and great expense (Hewlett Packard, > $ 12,000), it was seldom used for clinical monitoring but was used in physiological research and in cardiac catheterization and pulmonary function laboratories.

Pulse Oximetry

The concept of pulse oximetry may be considered a development of the technique of Squire and Wood. Each had compressed the tissue pneumatically at the beginning of measurement to set the bloodless density for both wavelengths. When blood was readmitted, one could assume that all the light absorption was produced by blood, thereby eliminating tissue pigments and thickness as factors. Wood used the ratio of ratios of the changes in light at the two wavelengths, to compute saturation of the readmitted arterial blood.

Discovery of Pulse Oximetry

The realization that the arterial pulsatile light variation could be used to measure arterial oxygen saturation first occurred to Japanese physiological bioengineer Takuo Aoyagi (Fig. 55.18) [81]. Aoyagi was born on 14 February 1936, in Niigata Prefecture, Japan, and graduated in 1958 from the Faculty of Engineering at Niigata University with a degree in electrical engineering. While working on dye dilution technology at the Shimadzu Corp, he was stimulated by a summer course, "Classical Physiology with Modern Instrumentation," taught at Baylor University, Waco, Texas, by H Hoff and L Geddes. This led him, in February 1971, to join the Research Division of Nihon Kohden Corporation. He tried to use an earpiece densitometer for the measurement of cardiac output by dye dilution to avoid arterial blood sampling. The light signal transmitted through the ear contained pulsatile variations that prevented accurate extrapolation during washout. The effort to eliminate these artifacts led Aoyagi to the possibility of using them to measure oxygen saturation,

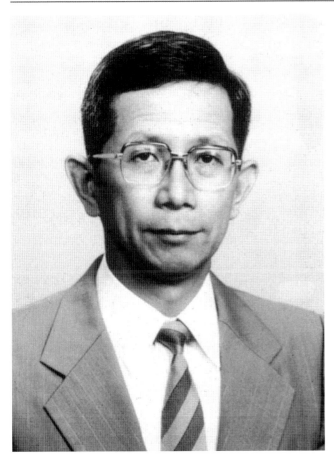

Fig. 55.18 Takuo Aoyagi, inventor of pulse oximetry, 1971. (Courtesy of the author's collection.)

a classic example of the adage that "one man's noise is another man's signal". In 1971, Aoyagi suddenly realized that the pulse-induced variation in detected red and infrared light was equivalent to Wood's use of the pneumatic cuff to induce the change of ear blood volume, and thereby obtain the 4 data points used to directly compute oxygen saturation by the ratio of ratios. Aoyagi's insight made pulse oximetry possible.

Aoyagi tested various wavelengths and methods of implementing the device. He selected the 630-nm wavelength, at which red light transmission was most sensitive to saturation, and he balanced this against a 900-nm infrared wavelength, which is not absorbed by dye. The maximum density of the dye occurs at 805 nm, the isobestic point of hemoglobin and oxyhemoglobin absorption (i.e., the point of equal absorptions). Wood and other workers had chosen 805 nm as the optimal oxygen-insensitive wavelength to balance the 650-nm oxygen-sensing red light for oximetry, and 805 nm would have been useful as the third wavelength in an earpiece designed for recording both dye dilution curves and oxygen saturation. However, Aoyagi had seen oxygen sensitivity without using the usual oximeter red wavelengths around 650 nm. He had compared light at 805 and 900 nm. Thus the 900-nm light was found to be sensitive to oxygen.

Its response proved to be opposite in direction to the effect of oxygen in the red wavelengths; that is, desaturation increased the infrared light transmission of blood but decreased the red light transmission. Thus the now universal choice of infrared light in pulse oximetry arose fortuitously from Aoyagi's work with dye dilution.

On April 26, 1974, Aoyagi presented "Improvement of the Earpiece Oximeter," to the Japanese Society of Medical Electronics and Biological Engineering, representing the development team of Aoyagi, M Kishi, K Yamaguchi, and S Watanabe.

In early 1973, S Nakajima, a surgeon working at the Sapporo Minami National Sanatorium, heard about Aoyagi's idea from Aoyagi's supervisor, Y Sugiyama. Nakajima ordered the as-yet-undeveloped apparatus from Nihon Kohden. In September 1973, Nakajima tested Aoyagi's prototype pulse oximeter in Sapporo. Nakajima and his associates used a revised instrument in February 1974, and their initial publication included the developers as authors [82]. Aoyagi and his associates delivered the first commercial instrument, the OLV-5100, to Nakajima on 13 March 1974. It used an earpiece with incandescent light, filters, and photocells like those of Millikan's 1940 oximeter.

However, Nihon Kohden did not continue to develop or market this instrument and made no effort to patent it abroad. Aoyagi was transferred to a post as assistant manager in the patient monitoring division of Nihon Kohden in September 1975, and the research and development of the pulse oximeter was assigned to another worker. Finally, in September 1985 Aoyagi was permitted to resume research and development of his pulse spectrophotometer, a dye dilution method to measure cardiac output, plasma volume and liver blood flow.

In the late 1970s, the Minolta Co in Japan marketed the Oximet MET-1471, a version of Aoyagi's pulse oximeter, and it was tested in the US where several groups began developmental work using Aoyagi's idea. However, few foresaw its value during anesthesia, intensive care, and other emerging venues, probably because conventional oximetry had never been convenient or inexpensive enough for these uses.

Michael Hickey, Scott Wilber, and Bill Moe founded Biox Technology in 1979. Chief engineer-scientist Wilbur introduced and patented the use of red and infrared light emitting diodes (LED's) and "normalization circuitry". Biox marketed the first pulse oximeters in the US in 1980, mainly for respiratory therapy, but soon noted that anesthesiologists were using them in the operating room. Ohmeda Corporation soon purchased Biox and marketed the Ohmeda-Biox 3700. Stanford University anesthesiologist William New was among the first to recognize the tremendous need for pulse oximetry. In 1981 with Jack Lloyd and Jim Corenham, he founded Nellcor. Their first pulse oximeter was marketed in 1983 [83]. Fortunately, light-emitting diodes provided the wavelengths permitting the construction of small finger or ear probes. Furthermore these diodes could turn on and off at high frequencies, enabling the device to use a single photocell sensitive to both wavelengths by turning on one light at a time. A further advantage was that ambient light, being continuous, was not sensed and amplified by the gated AC amplifiers detecting current pulses from the photocell. Technological developments occurred at critical times for pulse oximetry and account for some of its growth.

Role of Pulse Oximetry in Patient Safety

Pulse oximetry is arguably the most important technological advance ever made in monitoring the well-being and safety of patients during anesthesia, recovery, and critical care. Its simplicity, portability, low cost and permanent calibration made its use nearly universal in patients having potentially impaired gas exchange. Physicians now monitor and control oxygen saturation (SpO_2), rather than PO_2.

The more than 10 fold reduction in deaths attributed to anesthesia in the US since 1980 coincided with the widespread use of pulse oximetry. In an effort to link these events, a Danish Anesthesia group initiated multi-institutional double blind studies of anesthesia in which the anesthesiologist was unaware of the pulse oximeter readings in half the patients [84]. Four groups have repeated this for a total of 23,000 study patients. None of these studies revealed a beneficial role of pulse oximetry!

No conclusive explanation has been offered for this anomaly. Perhaps even a brief experience with a pulse oximeter and the resulting better understanding of the importance of cardio-respiratory physiology provoked anesthesiologists to pay more careful attention to their patients. And in all these double blind studies the anesthesiologists were aware that they were involved in a study.

References

1. Beecher HK, Todd DP. A study of the deaths associated with anesthesia and surgery: based on a study of 599, 548 anesthesias in ten institutions 1948–1952, inclusive. Ann Surg. 1954;140:2–35.
2. Dripps RD, Lamont A, Eckenhoff JE. The role of anesthesia in surgical mortality. JAMA. 1961;178:261–6.
3. Tyndall J. On the transmission of heat of different qualities through gases of different kinds. Proc R Inst G B. 1859;3:155–8.
4. Pfund AH, Gemmill CL. An infrared absorption method for the quantitative analysis of respiratory and other gases. Bull Johns Hopkins Hosp. 1940;67:61–5.
5. Luft K. Über eine neue Methode der registrierenden Gasanalyse mit Hilfe der Absorption ultraroter Strahlen ohne spektrale Zerlegung. Ztschrf Techn Phys. 1943;24:97–104.
6. Elam JO, Brown ES, Ten Pas RH. Carbon dioxide homeostasis during anesthesia. I. Instrumentation. Anesthesiology. 1955;16:876–85.
7. Eger EI II, Saidman LJ, Brandstater B. Minimum alveolar anesthetic concentration: a standard of anesthetic potency. Anesthesiology. 1965;26:756–63.
8. Fowler KT. The respiratory mass spectrometer. Phys Med Biol. 1969;14:185–99.
9. Davies NJ, Denison DM. The uses of long sampling probes in respiratory mass spectrometry. Respir Physiol. 1979;37:335–46.
10. Ozanne GM, Young WG, Mazzei WJ, Severinghaus JW. Multipatient anesthetic mass spectrometry: rapid analysis of data stored in long catheters. Anesthesiology. 1981;55:62–70.
11. Hendrickx JFA, Hendrikus JM, Lemmens RC, DeWolf AM, Saidman LJ. Can modern infrared analyzers replace gas chromatography to measure anesthetic vapor concentrations? BMC Anesthesiology. 2008;8:2.
12. Ilsley AH, Runciman WB. An evaluation of fourteen oxygen analysers for use in patient breathing circuits. Anaesth Intensive Care. 1986;14:431–6.
13. Pflüger EFW. Über die Diffusion des Sauerstoffs, den Ort und die Gesetze der Oxydationsprozesse im tierischen Organismus. Arch gesamte Physiol. 1872;6:43–64.
14. Riley RL, Campbell EJ, Shepard RH. A bubble method for estimation of PCO_2 and PO_2 in whole blood. J Appl Physiol. 1957;11:245–9.
15. Vogt Lorentzen F, Brinch Johnsen T. Quantitative gas determination in the Scholander-Roughton syringe. Scand J Clin Lab Invest. 1951;3:241–3.
16. O'Shaughnessy WB. Experiments on the blood in cholera. Lancet. 1831;17:490.
17. Walter F. Untersuchungen über die Wirkung der Saüren auf den thierisch on Organimus. Archiv f exper Pathol u Phar. 1877;5:148–55.
18. van't Hoff JH. The function of osmotic pressure in the analogy between solutions and gases (translated by W. Ramsay). Philos Mag. 1888;26:81–105.
19. Arrhenius SA. Über die Dissociation der in Wasser gelösten Stoffe. Z Physik Chemie. 1887;1:631–58.
20. Ostwald WF. Die Dissocation des Wassers. Z Physik Chemie. 1893;11:521.
21. Nernst WH. Die elektromotorische Wirksamkeit de Jonen. Z Physik Chemie. 1889;4:129–81.
22. Sørensen SPL. Enzymstudien II. Mitteilung über die Messung und die Bedeutung der Wasserstoffionen-konzentration bein enzymatischen Prozessen. Biochem Z. 1909;21:131–4.
23. Cremer M. Über die Ursache der elektromotorischen Eigenschaften der Gewebe. zugleich ein Beitrag zur Lehre von den polyphasischen Elektrolytketten. Z Biol. 1909;47:562–608.
24. Haber F, Klemensiewicz Z. Über elektrische Phasengrenzkrafte. Z Phys Chem. 1909;77:385–97.
25. Kerridge PM. The use of the glass electrode in biochemistry. Biochem J. 1925;19:611–7.
26. McInnes DA, Belcher D. A durable glass electrode. Ind Eng Chem Anal Ed. 1933;5:199–200.
27. Henderson LJ. Das Gleichgewicht zwischen Basen und Sauren im tierischen Organismus. Ergebn Physiol. 1909;8:254–325.
28. Henderson LJ. Blood as a physicochemical system. J Biol Chem. 1921;26:411–9.
29. Hasselbalch KA. Die Berechnung der Wasserstoffzahle des Blutes aus der freien und gebundenen Kohlensaure desselben und die Sauerstoffbindung des Blutes als Funktion des Wasserstoffzahl. Biochem Z. 1917;78:112–44.
30. Van Slyke DD, Neill JM. The determination of gases in blood and other solutions by vacuum extraction and manometric measurement. J Biol Chem. 1924;61:523–73.
31. Ibsen B. The anaesthetist's viewpoint on the treatment of respiratory complications in poliomyelitis during the epidemic in Copenhagen, 1952. Proc R Soc Med. 1954;47:72–4.
32. Astrup P. A simple electrometric technique for the determination of carbon dioxide tension in blood and plasma, total content of carbon dioxide in plasma and bicarbonate content in separated plasma at a fixed carbon dioxide tension. Scand J Clin Lab Invest. 1956;8:33–44.
33. Siggaard Andersen O, Engel K, Jorgensen K, Astrup P. A micro method for determination of pH, carbon dioxide tension, base excess and standard bicarbonate in capillary blood. Scand J Clin Lab Invest. 1960;12:172–6.
34. Siggaard Andersen O. The acid-base status of the blood. Scand J Clin Lab Invest. 1963;15(Suppl 70):92–6.

35. Siggaard Andersen O. The van Slyke equation. Scand J Clin Lab Invest Suppl. 1977;146:15–20.
36. Gesell R, McGinty DA. Regulation of respiration: VI. Continuous electrometric methods of recording changes in expired carbon dioxide and oxygen. Am J Physiol. 1926;79:72–90.
37. Stow RW, Randall BF. Electrical measurement of the PCO_2 of blood. Am J Physiol. 1954;179:678. (abstract).
38. Severinghaus JW, Astrup PB. History of blood gas analysis. Int Anesthesiol Clin. 1987;25:1–224.
39. Danneel HL. Über den durch diffundierende Gase hervorgerufenen Reststrom. Z Elektrochem. 1897;98:227–42.
40. Heyrovsky J. Electrolysis with the dropping mercury electrode. Chemicke Listy. 1922;16:256–304.
41. Baumberger JP, Goodfriend RB. Determination of arterial oxygen tension in man by equilibration through intact skin. Fed Proc. 1951;10:10. (abstract).
42. Beecher HK, Follansbee R, Murphy AJ, Craig FN. Determination of the oxygen content of small quantities of body fluids by polarographic analysis. J Biol Chem. 1942;146:197–206.
43. Clark LC, Gollan F, Gupta VB. The oxygenation of blood by gas dispersion. Science. 1950;111:85–7.
44. Clark LC Jr, Wolf R, Granger D, Taylor Z. Continuous recording of blood oxygen tensions by polarography. J Appl Physiol. 1953;6:189–93.
45. Clark LC. Monitor and control of blood and tissue O_2 tensions. Trans Am Soc Artif Intern Organs. 1956;2:41–8.
46. Severinghaus JW, Bradley AF. Electrodes for blood PO_2 and PCO_2 determination. J Appl Physiol. 1958;13:515–20.
47. Severinghaus JW. Electrodes for blood and gas PCO_2, PO_2, and blood pH. Acta Anesth Scand Suppl. 1962;11:207–20.
48. Avery ME. Presidential address. What is good for children is good for mankind: the role of imagination in discovery. Science. 2004;306:2212–3.
49. Rooth G, Sjostedt S, Caligara F. Bloodless determination of arterial oxygen tension by polarography. Sci Tools LKW Instrument J. 1957;4:37–9.
50. Huch R, Huch A, Lübbers DW. Transcutaneous measurement of blood Po2 (tcPo2) -- xMethod and application in perinatal medicine. J Perinat Med. 1973;1:183–91.
51. Huch R, Lübbers DW, Huch A. Quantitative continuous measurement of partial oxygen pressure on the skin of adults and new-born babies. Pflügers Arch. 1972;337:185–98.
52. Eberhard P, Mindt W. Continuous PO_2 monitoring of newborns by skin electrodes. Med Biol Eng. 1975;13;436–42.
53. Palmisano BW, Severinghaus JW. Transcutaneous PCO_2 and PO_2: a multicenter study of accuracy. J Clin Monit. 1990;6:189–95.
54. Beran AV, Huxtable RF, Sperling DR. Electrochemical sensor for continuous transcutaneous PCO_2 measurement. J Appl Physiol. 1976;41:442–7.
55. Beran AV, Shigezawa GY, Yeung HN, Huxtable RF. An improved sensor and a method for transcutaneous CO_2 monitoring. Acta Anaesthesiol Scand Suppl. 1978;68:111–7.
56. Huch A, Seiler D, Meinzer K, Huch R, Galster H, Lubbers DW. Transcutaneous PCO_2 measurement with a miniaturised electrode. Lancet. 1977;1:982–3.
57. Severinghaus JW, Stafford M, Bradley AF. tcPCO2 electrode design, calibration and temperature gradient problems. Acta Anaesthesiol Scand Suppl. 1978;68:118–22.
58. Parker D, Delpy DT, Reynolds EO. Single electrochemical sensor for transcutaneous measurement of PO_2 and PCO_2. Birth Defects Orig Artic Ser. 1979;15:109–16.
59. Severinghaus JW. A combined transcutaneous PO_2-PCO_2 electrode with electrochemical HCO_3^- stabilization. J Appl Physiol. 1981;51:1027–32.
60. Eberhard P, Gisiger PA, Gardaz JP, Spahn DR. Combining transcutaneous blood gas measurement and pulse oximetry. Anesth Analg. 2002;94:S76–80.
61. Comroe JH, Botelho S. The unreliability of cyanosis in the recognition of arterial anoxemia. Am J Med Sci. 1947;124:1–6.
62. Kirchhoff GR, Bunsen RWE. Chemische Analyse durch Spectralbeobachtungen. Leipzig, Engelmann; 1860, p. 98.
63. Lambert JH. Photometria, siva de mensura et gradibus luminis, colorum et umbrae (1760), Klassiker der exakten Wissenschafter. Edited by O W. Leipzig, W. Engelmann; 1892, pp. 31–3.
64. Beer A. Bestimmung der Absorption des rothen Lichts in farbigen Flüssigkeiten. Ann Phys Chem. 1852:86;78–88.
65. Stokes GG. On the reduction and oxygenation of the colouring matter of the blood. Proc Roy Soc. 1864;13:355–64.
66. Hoppe-Seyler F. Über das Verhalten des Blutfarbstoffes im Spektrum des Sonnenlichtes. Virchow's Arch. 1862;23:446–9.
67. Vierordt K. Die quantitative Spektralanalyse in ihrer Anwendung auf Physiologie, Chemie und Technologie. (Ger). Tubingen, H. Laupp'sche Buchhandlung; 1876.
68. Nicolai L. Über Sichbarmachung, Verlauf und chemische Kinetik der Oxyhemoglobinreduktion im lebenden Gewebe. besonders in der menschlichen Haut. Arch Ges Physiol. 1932;229:372–89.
69. Kramer K. Bestimmung des Sauerstoffgehaltes und der Hämoglobin Konzentration in Hämoglobinloslungen und hämolysierten Blut auf lichtelektrischen Wege (Ger). Z Biol. 1934;95:126–34.
70. Kramer K. Ein Verfahren zur fortlaufenden Messung des Sauerstoffgehaltes im stromenden Blute an uneroffneten Gefassen. Z Biol. 1935;96:61–75.
71. Matthes K. Untersuchungen uber die Sauerstoffsattingungen des menschlichen Arterienblutes. Arch Exp Pathol Pharmacol. 1935;179:698–711.
72. Matthes K, Gross F. Untersuchunger über die Absorption von rotem und ultraotem Licht durch kohlenoxydesattigtes und reduziertes Blut. Arch Exp Pathol Pharmacol. 1939;191:369–90.
73. Matthes K, Gross F. Fortlaufende Registrierung der Lichtabsorption des Blutes in zwei verschiedenen. Arch Exp Pathol Pharmacol. 1939;191:381–90.
74. Matthes K, Gross F. Zur methode der fortlaufenden Registrierung der Farbe des menschlichen Blutes. Arch Exp Pathol Pharmacol. 1939;191:523–8.
75. Squire JR. Instrument for measuring quantity of blood and its degree of oxygenation in web of the hand. Clin Sci. 1940;4:331–9.
76. Millikan GA. The oximeter: an instrument for measuring continuously oxygen saturation of arterial blood in man. Rev Sci Instr. 1942;13:434–44.
77. Faulconer A, Pender JW, Bickford RG. The influence of partial pressure of nitrous oxide on the depth of anesthesia and the electroencephalogram in man. Anesthesiology. 1949;10:601–9.
78. Wood EH, Geraci JE. Photoelectric determination of arterial oxygen saturation in man. J Lab Clin Med. 1949;34:387–401.
79. Wood EH. Oximetry, medical physics, Vol 2. Edited by O Glasser. Chicago, Year Book; 1950. pp. 664–80.
80. Burchell HB. Symposium on in vivo photometry of blood in human beings. Proc Mayo Clin. 1950;25:377–412.
81. Aoyagi T. Pulse oximetry: its invention, theory, and future. J Anesth. 2003;17:259–66.
82. Nakajima S, Harai Y, Takase H. Performances of new pulse wave earpiece oximeter. Respir Circ. 1975;23:41–5.
83. Yelderman M, New W Jr. Evaluation of pulse oximetry. Anesthesiology. 1983;59:349–52.
84. Moller JT, Pedersen T, Rasmussen LS, Jensen PF, Pedersen BD, Ravlo O, Rasmussen NH, Espersen K, Johannessen NW, Cooper JB et al. Randomized evaluation of pulse oximetry in 20,802 patients: I. Design, demography, pulse oximetry failure rate, and overall complication rate. Anesthesiology. 1993;78:436–44.

The Story of Artificial Ventilation

Keith Sykes

Summary

In 1543, Vesalius found that lung collapse resulting from opening the chest soon caused the heart to stop, but Hooke showed in 1667, that blowing air down the windpipe and out through punctures in the lungs sustained life. In 1744, Tossach reported saving a suffocated miner with expired air (mouth-to-mouth) resuscitation (EAR).

Between the 1850s and the 1940s there were over 70 descriptions of diverse, rarely successful manual methods of artificial ventilation. A few methods were effective, including the Swedish Holger Nielson technique (external chest compression and expansion) that came to be recommended. In 1954, Elam showed that individuals taught to maintain an open airway in a patient without a tracheal tube could maintain normal levels of oxygen and carbon dioxide with EAR. In 1958–9, Safar showed that lay personnel could open the airway by thrusting the jaw forwards and tilting the head backwards. Rescue organizations slowly adopted the new techniques.

In 1876, Woillez described a chamber that enclosed the body below the neck and enabled the lungs to be inflated by intermittent manual reduction of the pressure surrounding the chest. In 1929, Drinker and McKann produced a mechanical version. Over the next 30 years, these "iron lungs" saved many lives, but cost limited their availability and they restricted access to the patient.

In the severe polio epidemic in the UK in 1938 there were too few iron lungs to treat patients with respiratory paralysis. On the advice of Macintosh (Professor of Anaesthetics at Oxford), Lord Nuffield, owner of the Morris car factory, offered to provide a tank ventilator for every Commonwealth hospital. Australian, Ted Both, designer of a simple wooden version of the Drinker "iron lung", volunteered his design. The Morris factory built 1,750 Both ventilators by 1947.

Disadvantages of the iron lung led to its replacement by intermittent positive pressure ventilation (IPPV). In 1887, Fell used IPPV from a bellows via a tracheostomy to inflate the lungs. Later he substituted a facemask for the tracheostomy. In 1904, German surgeon Sauerbruch maintained lung inflation (but not ventilation) by enclosing the patient's body and the operating team within a giant chamber having a negative pressure of 5 cm of water, the patient's head protruding from the chamber. In 1907, Dräger produced the Pulmotor, a compressed gas powered ventilator designed for rescuing miners. Between 1906 and 1910, Green and Janeway demonstrated the advantages of controlled (as opposed to assisted) ventilation but prematurely discontinued their groundbreaking work. For the next 20 years, surgeons used the technique of insufflation introduced by Meltzer and Auer in 1909.

In 1916, Giertz reported in Swedish the advantages of IPPV. In 1934, Anderson, Frenckner and Crafoord, described the Spiropulsator ventilator, making Giertz' work known outside Sweden. Blease, in England, produced a prototype mechanical ventilator in 1947, and a commercial model in 1950. Other events promoted the use of ventilators, including the 1942 introduction of neuromuscular blocking drugs, the expansion of thoracic surgery, and the use of cardiopulmonary bypass machines in the 1950s.

Introduction

In this and the next chapter, we trace the development of methods of artificially ventilating the lungs. This chapter examines how various methods for resuscitating the apparently dead eventually led to the 1960s introduction of the ABCs of resuscitation—Airway, Breathing and Cardiac compression. We then deal with the development of tank ventilators or "iron lungs", large machines that create sub-atmospheric pressures around the chest to inflate the lungs in patients with poliomyelitis. The final section describes the development of controlled ventilation and the use of intermittent positive pressure ventilation for thoracic and other types of surgery.

In the next chapter the remarkable story of how the 1952 epidemic of poliomyelitis in Copenhagen initially overwhelmed the medical facilities is told along with how the

K. Sykes (✉)
Emeritus Professor, University of Oxford, Oxford, UK
e-mail: k@mksykes.co.uk

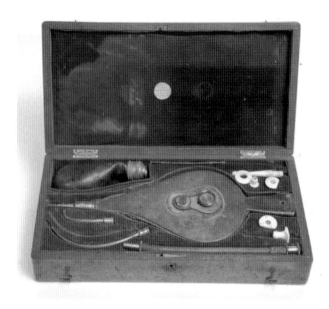

Fig. 56.1 Royal Humane Society box containing bellows and oral and nasal tubes—late 18th century. (Courtesy of Nuffield Department of Anaesthetics, Oxford, UK)

anaesthetist, Bjørn Ibsen, saved the day by applying methods of airway care and artificial ventilation used during anaesthesia. The realization that these techniques could save lives led to the development of critical care as we know it today.

Artificial Ventilation

Two methods may be used to artificially expand the lungs. One applies positive pressure to the airway (intermittent positive pressure ventilation, or IPPV), and the second creates a sub-atmospheric or "negative" pressure around the chest (intermittent negative pressure ventilation or INPV). Both techniques rely on the natural elasticity of the lungs to produce expiration.

Intermittent Positive Pressure Ventilation

Mouth-to-mouth respiration (now called expired air resuscitation or EAR) provides a simple and effective way to restore ventilation in apnoeic subjects. The technique may have been practised in biblical times (11 Kings 4, v.34–5) and was later used by midwives to resuscitate newborn babies [1]. The carbon dioxide and decreased oxygen in the rescuer's breath do not compromise the effectiveness of the technique. It requires no apparatus and can be applied immediately, preventing the brain damage occurring with oxygen deprivation exceeding 2–3 min. But it is sometimes difficult to maintain a clear airway and rescuers may not like either kissing a potential corpse, or a live but possibly infected person!

A negative intrapleural pressure of 5 to 10 cm of water normally holds the lung against the inside of the chest wall, but if the chest is opened, air rushes in and the lungs collapse, ultimately looking like liver. In 1543, Andreas Vesalius, the great Italian anatomist, opened the chest of a live animal, observing that when the lungs collapsed, the heart would beat irregularly and eventually stop. In his famous work *De humanis corporis fabrica* (*On the fabric of the body*) [2] he wrote:

> *"That life may in a manner of speaking be restored to the animal, an opening must be attempted in the trunk of the trachea, into which a tube of reed or cane should be put; you will then blow into this, so that the lung may rise again and the animal take in air. Indeed with a slight breath in the case of the living animal, the lung will swell to the full extent of the thoracic cavity, and the heart will become strong and exhibit a wondrous variety of motions".*

Robert Hooke, (a polymath who designed and performed experiments for meetings of the Royal Society in London, and who helped Christopher Wren redesign London after the Great Fire of 1666), repeated the experiments of Vesalius in 1664. In 1667, he performed an extraordinary sequel: he opened a dog's chest and held the lungs inflated by blowing air down the windpipe and out through holes drilled in the lungs. The animal stayed alive, even though the lungs were still. However, when Hooke stopped the airflow, the lungs collapsed and the heart faltered, only to recover when the flow of air was restored. Anaesthesia had not been invented, and these horrific experiments were performed in a conscious animal. The suffering of the animal so upset Hooke that he vowed never to repeat the experiment. The result however, was of great importance, unquestionably demonstrating that the gases entering and leaving the lungs, and not the movement of the lungs (as had previously been thought) sustained life.

Because 18th century life expectancy was low, deaths from cardiovascular disease were uncommon. Infections, accidents, drowning and smoke inhalation caused most deaths. In 1744, a Scottish physician, William Tossach, described his 1732 resuscitation of a suffocated miner with mouth-to-mouth ventilation [1]. Although mouth-to-mouth ventilation persisted in midwifery, the public did not adopt it.

The many canals in Amsterdam made drowning a particular problem, and in 1767, some citizens formed a Society for the Resuscitation of the Apparently Drowned. Similar societies were formed in Venice and Milan in 1768, Paris in 1771 and London in 1774. Some bizarre treatments were suggested (e.g. insufflation of tobacco smoke into the rectum). The Amsterdam Society recommended using a fireside bellows to provide artificial respiration, and the English surgeon John Hunter investigated the use of a double bellows to produce inspiration and expiration [3]. Although many rescuers attempted to use a bellows (Fig. 56.1), it proved difficult to provide an airtight connection with the lungs. Diverse tubes were designed to join the bellows to the nose or windpipe, but only the highly skilled could use them effectively. Successful resuscitations were reported, but there was considerable doubt about the efficacy of the technique. In 1827 and 1828, J Leroy in Paris, showed that over-inflation with a bellows could damage the lungs, and the use of a bellows soon ceased [4].

Manual Methods of Artificial Ventilation

From the 1850s to the 1940s, more than 70 different manual methods of artificial ventilation were described. These expanded the lungs by lifting the upper limbs, thus stretching the muscles attached to the chest wall. Compressing the thorax or abdomen then caused deflation. Although rarely successful, these techniques became sacrosanct. Attempts to introduce EAR to police and rescue organisations in the early 1960s met enormous opposition, despite demonstrating superior results. Surprisingly, some opposition came from distinguished scientists.

Between 1930–1950, several investigators compared the effectiveness of various manual techniques in apnoeic subjects, including those with drug overdose and anaesthesia, and even in warm corpses without rigor mortis [5]. These studies demonstrated that some manual methods were effective and The Council on Physical Medicine and Rehabilitation then recommended adoption of the Swedish Holger Nielson technique [6]. This seemed to be the last word, but nothing in science stays still.

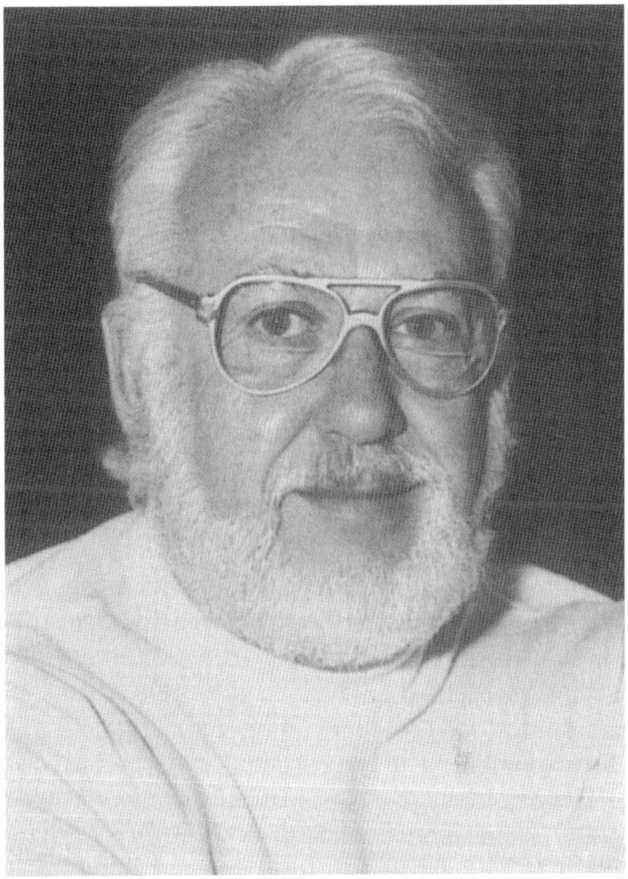

Fig. 56.2 James O Elam (1918–1995), the innovative but controversial anaesthesiologist from Buffalo who had a contract with the US Army to study methods of resuscitating victims of nerve gas poisoning, and who subsequently led the campaign to re-instate expired air resuscitation. (From [7])

Expired Air Resuscitation (EAR) Returns

In all these studies, a tracheal tube maintained the airway, permitting direct measurement of the volume of air moved. But, as James Elam (Fig. 56.2) an anaesthesiologist from Buffalo observed, tracheal intubation invalidated the results [7]. Why? Because with loss of consciousness, the tongue falls back obstructing the airway while the tube prevents the obstruction! Elam then showed that EAR performed by individuals taught to maintain a clear airway without a tracheal tube, could provide normal levels of oxygen and carbon dioxide in an apnoeic victim for prolonged periods [8, 9].

In 1954, Elam met Baltimore anaesthesiologist Peter Safar at a mid-west meeting. Safar gave Elam a lift back to Baltimore. During the journey, Elam persuaded Safar to join the crusade to convince the establishment that EAR provided optimum rescue ventilation for apnoeic subjects. The key to success was Safar's demonstration that the tongue obstructed the airway in the unconscious patient, and that thrusting the jaw forwards and tilting the head backwards,

a technique that anaesthesiologists use routinely, opened the airway [10]. Safar next conducted several daring studies on anaesthetized-paralysed human volunteers who were not intubated, demonstrating that after a brief period of training, firemen, boy scouts, and almost anyone could establish a clear airway and provide effective ventilation (Fig. 56.3) [11]. Another anaesthesiologist, Archer Gordon of the University of Illinois, who had conducted many studies on techniques of artificial ventilation and who had been a strong advocate of manual methods, also became convinced that expired air resuscitation was the technique of choice, and produced incontrovertible evidence that the method worked in both children and adults [12]. Two years later, Kouvenhoven, Jude and Knickerbocker dramatically demonstrated that compressing the chest could produce effective artificial circulation after a cardiac arrest—completing the triad of Airway, Breathing and Cardiac compression (A, B, C) that was the basis for the emergency treatment of cardiac arrest for the next half-century [13, 14]. Although cardiac

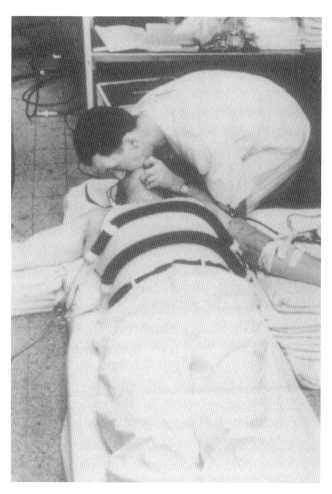

Fig. 56.3 Peter Safar (1924–2003) performing expired air resuscitation during one of his studies on anaesthetized, paralysed volunteers in 1957. Tidal volume was derived from the change in pressure within the two corrugated tubes surrounding the chest. (Photo donated to the author by Safar in 1976)

compression produces some ventilation, the American Heart Association still recommends that there should be 2 breaths to 30 heart compressions. However, it is now recognised that the reluctance of bystanders to perform EAR reduces survival, and that survival rates with some types of cardiac arrest are probably increased if cardiac compression is used as the primary treatment [15].

Intermittent Negative Pressure Ventilation

In the nineteenth century several attempts were made to inflate the lungs by reducing the pressure surrounding the chest. A Woillez in France was among the first to describe an effective negative pressure ventilator in 1876 [16, 17]. His "spirophore", consisted of a metal chamber surrounding the patient's body, the head protruding through a rubber collar that provided an airtight seal at the neck (Fig. 56.4).

Moving a lever connected to a flexible diaphragm that sealed the foot end of the box expanded the patient's lungs. Opposite movement of the lever allowed deflation. His device had problems: an ineffective neck seal; inadequate decreases in chamber pressure; and reliance on manual power. Drinker and McKhann in Boston Massachusetts, solved these problems in 1929, with a machine powered by vacuum pumps (Fig. 65.9) [18]. However, Drinker's machines cost about $3,000, a lot of money in those days. In 1931, John ("Jack") Emerson, an engineer working in Boston, manufactured a similar, but more efficient, machine from standard plumbing, electrical and automotive parts; that cost about $1,000 [19]. Drinker sued Emerson, charging patent infringement, but Emerson fought back, showing that the principle had been described previously. After Harvard University intervened, Emerson was allowed to continue production. He made incremental improvements for the next 25 years and travelled country-wide for months at a time, with demonstration models in a motor home trailer.

Over the next thirty years these "iron lung" ventilators saved many lives during the poliomyelitis epidemics that repeatedly scourged the world (Fig. 56.5). Some patients (like Emerson himself) had only a transient paralysis, but in others a permanent paralysis meant a lifetime in the iron lung [20]. Cost limited availability of these machines. Only the huge popular support for the "March of Dimes Fund" enabled purchase of enough machines to cope with the epidemics of polio that recurred in the US until the Salk and Sabine vaccines were introduced in the late 1950s.

The Iron Lung in England: Morris and Macintosh

In 1930, a Drinker iron lung was imported into England. Similar machines were constructed under license. Attempts were also made to support breathing with a cuirass respirator This generated intermittent negative pressures beneath a shell applied over the chest and upper abdomen, but achievement of an airtight seal was difficult and it was less effective than the tank ventilator.

In 1938 there was another severe epidemic of poliomyelitis in England. William Morris (later Lord Nuffield), a bicycle maker who developed the Morris Motor Company and who had made many philanthropic gifts to medicine, was concerned about the shortage of equipment and turned to his friend Robert Macintosh for advice. Macintosh, a New Zealander who had served in the British air force in World War I, been shot down and taken prisoner, and made remarkable escapes from various prisoner-of-war camps in Germany [21]. After training in medicine at Guy's Hospital, London, Macintosh began training in surgery. To pay for his studies, he gave nitrous oxide ("laughing gas") anaesthetics for teeth extractions in dental surgeries. His skill resulted

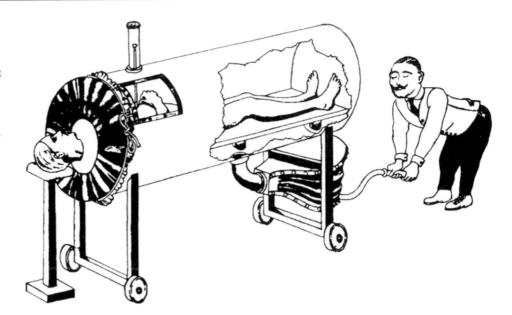

Fig. 56.4 The Woillez spirophore (1876). This drawing was made by one of Emerson's assistants in the 1930s to illustrate that the principle of the iron lung had been described long before Drinker had patented his device. (From The evolution of iron lungs. JH Emerson Company, 1957. Wood Library-Museum of Anesthesiology, Park Ridge, IL)

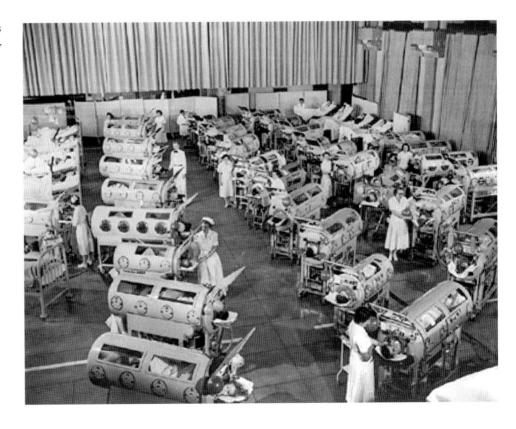

Fig. 56.5 Patients in Iron lungs at Rancho Los Alamos Hospital, Downey, California during a polio epidemic in 1953

in a lucrative Harley Street private practice. Shortly after the new intravenous agent Evipan (hexobarbital) had been introduced, Macintosh administered it to Nuffield. The experience was markedly different to the dreaming and struggling that characterised the "laughing gas" anaesthetics that Nuffield had suffered for removal of teeth in his youth. Thus began a friendship that influenced the course of anaesthesia in England and the world.

Macintosh and other doctors from Guy's Hospital played golf at Nuffield's club near Oxford. Nuffield sought their advice when considering his many medical benefactions. In 1936, he said he would finance the creation of a Postgraduate Medical School at Oxford, and that he had earmarked funds to provide chairs in Medicine, Surgery and Obstetrics and Gynaecology. Macintosh jested: "I see that anaesthetics has been left out again". Saying nothing, Nuffield then added a

Fig. 56.6 Professor Robert Macintosh (left) and Lord Nuffield putting a "patient" (Richard Salt, Chief technician) into a Both ventilator made in the Morris works at Cowley, Oxford in 1938. Salt was Macintosh's assistant in London and later became a Chief Technician in the Nuffield Department of Anaesthetics, Oxford. He made many of the prototypes of apparatus developed in the department from 1937 to the 1970s. (Courtesy of Nuffield Department of Anaesthetics, Oxford, UK)

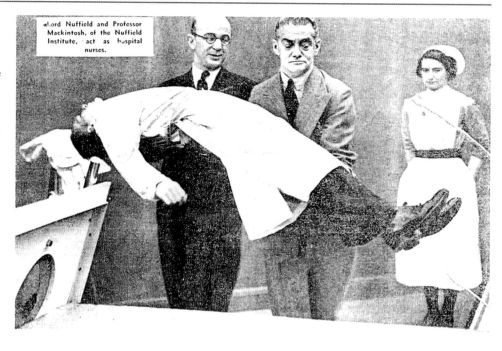

Chair in Anaesthetics to his benefaction. The University resisted this addition because anaesthetics was not considered to be an academic subject. Nuffield responded: no anaesthetics, no benefaction. In 1937, Macintosh was appointed to the Nuffield Chair of Anaesthetics at Oxford, the first such Chair in the Commonwealth, and the second in the World.[1]

There were only 6 iron lungs in the country when the 1938 polio epidemic started. Seeing a need for machines to support breathing, Nuffield turned to Macintosh for advice. C Pratt, a physiologist in the Nuffield department, produced a film to show Nuffield the available devices, and Nuffield responded by offering to provide a tank ventilator for every British Commonwealth hospital requesting one. Fortuitously, an ingenious Australian engineer, Ted Both, was in England to try and interest the Ministry of Health in his new direct-writing ECG. He had recently designed and built a simple wooden version of the Drinker "iron lung" in Australia, and agreed to allow Nuffield to use his design (Fig. 56.6). By 1947 the Morris car factory had built 1,750 Both ventilators (450 for British hospitals). This was a remarkable achievement, considering the wartime limitation on the supply of materials and labour, and the fact that the factory was concurrently producing Oxford vaporizers for anaesthesia, and mine-sinkers and other armaments for war purposes.

The Nuffield Department of Anaesthetics assumed responsibility for training medical and nursing staff in the use of the Both ventilator, and within five years of its introduction, the ventilator had supported respiration in patients with snakebite poisoning, diphtheritic diaphragmatic pa-

ralysis, and barbiturate poisoning, as well as poliomyelitis. In 1940, Macintosh attempted to tackle postoperative pain with large doses of morphine, treating the resultant respiratory depression with a Both ventilator. As he later wryly commented, "The idea did not catch on, since neither the patient nor the surgeon liked the idea of a patient waking up in a coffin."

Disadvantages of Intermittent Negative Pressure Ventilation

The iron lung had major disadvantages: patients had to synchronise swallowing and phonation with the machine's rhythm; the machine was bulky and expensive; the rigid walls of the device limited access to the patient and thereby hindered nursing care; and achievement of a satisfactory neck seal could cause discomfort and ulceration of the skin. Furthermore, paralysis of laryngeal or pharyngeal muscles often resulted in the aspiration of mouth secretions, lung collapse, pneumonia, and death. Inserting a tracheostomy tube could prevent aspiration, but the rubber neck seal on the iron lung impeded care of the tracheostomy. These disadvantages ultimately resulted in the demise of INPV.

Intermittent Positive Pressure Ventilators

Toward the end of the nineteenth century, surgeons started to operate within the chest but opening the chest caused the lungs to collapse. In 1887, George Fell of Buffalo advocated the use a bellows and tracheostomy to inflate the lungs. Later

---

[1] The first Chair was created for Ralph Waters, in Madison, Wisconsin in 1933.

he substituted a face mask for the tracheostomy. The next year Joseph O'Dwyer of New York (who had developed laryngeal tubes to maintain the airway in diphtheria) modified the technique by using a foot bellows that was connected to a laryngeal tube, and in 1899, Rudolph Matas, the innovative New Orleans vascular surgeon, reported that he had successfully used an anaesthetic modification of this apparatus to provide anaesthesia and ventilation during an operation to remove a chest wall tumour. He remarked at that time, that it was curious that surgeons had failed to use a technique that had been in use in the physiology laboratory since the time of Magendie [22].

News of these advances had probably not reached Germany, for in 1903, the great German surgeon Ferdinand Sauerbruch (1875–1951) adopted a grotesque, inadequate solution. To maintain lung inflation he enclosed the patient's body and the operating team within a giant chamber having a negative pressure of about 5 cm of water, the patient's head protruding from the chamber. This technique maintained lung inflation but since there was no mechanical link between the lungs and chest wall, ventilation was grossly inadequate. With the stubbornness characterising European professors of the time, Sauerbruch continued to use this method to support the performance of intrathoracic operations for many years.

In 1907, the innovative German engineer Bernard Dräger, produced the Pulmotor, a compressed gas powered intermittent positive pressure ventilator designed to breathe for subjects rescued in mines. Although several thousand Pulmotors were produced, and although fire and rescue squads were trained in its use, most of the medical establishment ignored it. In 1910, Läwen and Sievers, assistants to the surgeon Friedrich Trendelenburg (1844–1924) in Leipzig, Germany, developed an electrically driven piston type ventilator to provide intermittent positive pressure during pulmonary embolectomy [23]. World War I however, precluded further progress in Germany.

Between 1906 and 1910 in New York, Nathan Green and Henry Janeway built machines to deliver intermittent positive pressure to the lungs through a box enclosing the head, or through a tracheal tube. This technique provided satisfactory operating conditions for oesophageal surgery in animals, and Green and Janeway made the important observation that apnoea resulted if they increased the rate or depth of breathing. Their technique, which they named *controlled ventilation*, greatly facilitated surgery because they could control the rate and volume of each breath, and because they could also control lung distension with positive airway pressures imposed during expiration [24]. Unfortunately, Green and Janeway did not continue their groundbreaking work, and for the next twenty years surgeons utilised the technique of insufflation introduced by Meltzer and Auer in 1909 [25]. The high flow of anaesthetic gas mixture blown down a narrow tube in the trachea, washed CO_2 out of the trachea,

reduced tidal volumes and produced a positive pressure in the airways. Although lung expansion was maintained, CO_2 removal became inadequate when the chest was opened, even if the lungs were intermittently deflated.

In 1927, the pharmacologist, Dennis Jackson of Cincinnati, Ohio (who had described CO_2 absorption during anaesthesia in 1915), reported on the combined use of an anaesthetic machine and mechanical ventilator [26]. Jackson repeatedly demonstrated the technique in animals, but no one was interested in using it in humans. The normally patient Jackson wrote:

> "378 years ago Vesalius had demonstrated what artificial respiration may often accomplish…It would appear, however, that the interval of time required for artificial respiration in the dog to evolute into artificial respiration in man may be almost as great as that required for an animal comparable to a dog to evolute into man" [27].

Anaesthesiologists Arthur Guedel and David Treweek in Madison, Wisconsin rediscovered controlled ventilation in 1934 [28]. The technique quickly achieved acceptance for lung ventilation during thoracic surgery. Parallel progress had been made in Sweden. In 1916, the surgeon K Giertz described the advantages of IPPV over the Sauerbruch method, but his publication was in Swedish [29]. Not until 1934, when the engineer S Anderson, and the surgeons Paul Frenckner and Clarence Crafoord described the Spiropulsator ventilator [30], did Giertz' work became known outside Sweden. The ventilator initially utilised the flasher mechanisms from nautical buoys to provide rhythmical inflation of the lungs. For many years it was used successfully for thoracic surgery by Crafoord in Stockholm [31]. Although Crafoord demonstrated his methods in Los Angeles in 1940, and F Mautz developed a ventilator and anaesthetic machine in the US [32], most thoracic anaesthetists continued to ventilate the lungs by squeezing the reservoir bag.

The innovative Copenhagen anaesthetist, Trier Mørch (Fig. 56.7), knew of Crafoord's work, and during the World War II German occupation, built a piston ventilator out of an iron water pipe. Emigrating to the US after the war, he built a new piston ventilator and became one of the first anaesthetists to promulgate the use of IPPV for anaesthesia and prolonged mechanical ventilation [33, 34].

Lung secretions provided a major problem for pioneer thoracic anaesthetists and in 1944, a Manchester anaesthetist, K Pinson, (inventor of the "ether bomb" vaporizer) described a combined anaesthetic machine, suction apparatus and mechanical ventilator for use during thoracic surgery (Fig. 56.8). Mørch spent some time in England shortly after the war, and went to see it demonstrated. The machine was too large to pass through the door of the operating room and had to be taken apart and re-assembled before the demonstration could proceed. In nearby Liverpool, a city also being

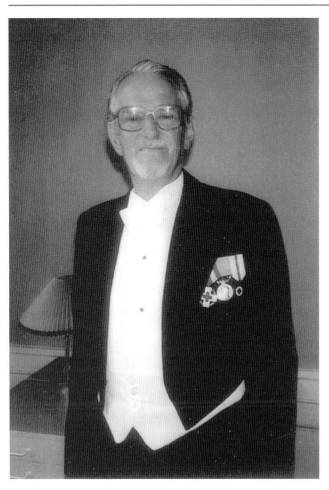

Fig. 56.7 Ernst Trier Mørch 1908–1996. He was one of the first anaesthesiologists to build a ventilator in Denmark during the German occupation in World War 2 and subsequently emigrated to the USA where he pioneered the use of intermittent positive pressure ventilation. His remarkable life is described elsewhere. (From [34], with permission)

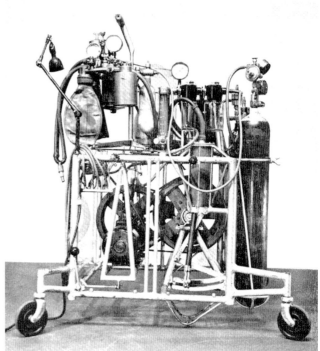

Fig. 56.8 The Pinson anaesthesia machine and ventilator designed for thoracic anaesthesia. Since excessive secretions were a major problem in patients in the industrial north of England, the machine incorporated a suction apparatus for tracheal aspiration. (From [36] with permission)

pounded by German bombs, a motor engineer, JH Blease (Fig. 56.9), who had manufactured apparatus for an anaesthetist friend, helped the hard-pressed medical staff by giving anaesthetics! Bored with bag-squeezing, he built a mechanical ventilator to do the job. He demonstrated the prototype at Wallasey Cottage Hospital in 1947, and produced a commercial model in 1950 (Fig. 56.10). This became the first successful anaesthetic ventilator in the UK. Blease continued to produce new ventilators for the next 30 years [35].

When thoracic surgeons began to operate routinely on the lungs and heart in the 1930s, anaesthetists assisted spontaneous breathing by gently squeezing the reservoir bag in time with the patient's inspiration (*assisted ventilation*). However, they soon learnt, as had Green and Janeway, that *controlled ventilation* provided better operating conditions, and by the 1940s, most UK and Scandinavian thoracic anaesthetists used manually controlled ventilation. Because no real-time methods allowed measurement of oxygen and carbon dioxide levels in blood or expired air, anaesthetists

used patient responses to gauge the adequacy of ventilation, increasing ventilation until spontaneous respiration ceased. When the surgeon had closed the chest, the anaesthetist reduced ventilation until spontaneous breathing returned. They then turned off the anaesthetic, and removed the tracheal tube as the patient recovered consciousness.

In the 1950s, in the US, manually assisted ventilation was still the norm in thoracic anaesthesia, but cardiac surgeons Gibbon, Dennis and Allbritten realised the need for mechanical ventilation during surgery with the open chest. They remembered Crafoord's demonstration of the Spiropulsator in Los Angeles in 1940, tried the latest version of this machine and that of Mautz, and then developed their own ventilator [38]. The original device (Fig. 56.11) was driven by a windscreen wiper motor, but the ventilator developed from this prototype, the well-known Jefferson ventilator produced in 1955, used a mechanism powered by compressed gas.

One other factor stimulated the development of mechanical ventilation. In the mid-19th century, physiologists administered the muscle relaxant curare to immobilize animals during experiments. This barbarous practice led to the 1876 Cruelty to Animals Act in the UK, limiting the use of muscle relaxants and ensuring the effective provision of anaesthesia for experimental procedures. Since curare impaired respiration, various devices were developed to maintain adequate gas exchange. In 1926, the physiologist EH Starling

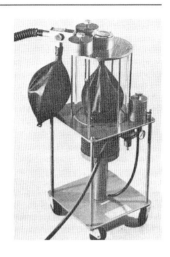

Fig. 56.11 Prototype of Jefferson ventilator. This was powered by a car windscreen motor. (From [37], p. 208, with permission)

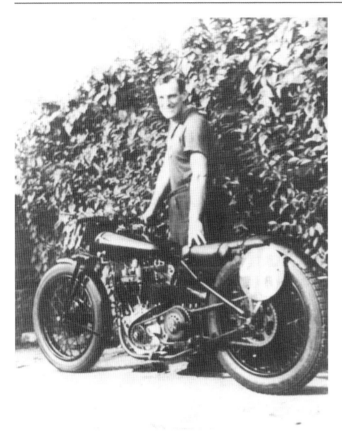

Fig. 56.9 The motor engineer John Blease (1906–1985) with the 1000 cc motorcycle that he built in the 1930s and raced very successfully on sand beaches. (From [34], with permission)

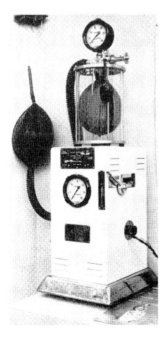

Fig. 56.10 The prototype Blease ventilator. The 1950 model became the first commercially available ventilator in the UK. JH Blease continued to develop new ventilators and respiratory equipment for the next 30 years. (From [37], p. 204, with permission)

described a simple, reliable piston ventilator, one used by many researchers for experiments in animals. In the absence of other suitable ventilators, this was used on 50 infants and children in 1960–1 [39].

The introduction of curare into anaesthesia in 1942 (see Chapter 50) increased the incentive to control ventilation. Initially, curare was given in small doses, to enhance the relaxation produced by ether or cyclopropane, while the anaesthetist augmented each spontaneous inspiration by squeezing the reservoir bag. In 1946, Cecil Gray and John Halton in Liverpool successfully applied this technique in 1000 cases [40]. However, increasing familiarity with curare prompted the use of larger, paralyzing doses mandating controlled ventilation. Anaesthesia with thiopental, nitrous oxide, oxygen, curare and hyperventilation, reduced arterial PCO_2 and respiratory drive, and it was claimed that this produced superior operating conditions, reducing the quantity of anaesthetic drug required to maintain unconsciousness [41]. Within a few years, controlled ventilation became an integral component of the thiopental-nitrous oxide-oxygen-intravenous analgesic-muscle relaxant sequence, still used today. Although the use of such light levels of anaesthesia increases the risk of awareness, a problem that is still engaging the profession, the use of controlled ventilation is a key component of modern anaesthesia. It was this technique that Bjørn Ibsen introduced into Blegdams infectious diseases hospital during the Copenhagen poliomyelitis epidemic of 1952. It was an event that completely changed the treatment of respiratory failure.

References

1. Trubuhovich RV. History of mouth-to-mouth rescue breathing. Part 1: Crit Care Resusc. 2005;7:250–257. Part 2: the 18th century. Crit Care Resusc. 2006;8:157–171. Part 3: the 19th to mid-20th centuries and rediscovery. Crit Care Resusc. 2007;9:1–17.

2. Vesalius A. *De humanis corporis fabrica. Basle 1543.*
3. Hunter J. Proposals for the recovery of people apparently drowned. Philosophical Transactions. 1776;66:412.
4. Leroy J. Rechérches sur l'asphyxie. Journal de Physiologie. 1827;7:45–65, and 1828;8:97–135.
5. *See papers in* J Appl Physiol 1951;4:403–95.
6. Council on Physical Medicine and Rehabilitation. JAMA 1951;147:1454–5.
7. Safar P. The resuscitation greats. James O. Elam MD, 1918–1995. Resuscitation. 2001;50:249–56.
8. Elam JO, Brown ES, Elder JD. Artificial respiration by mouth-to-mask method. A study of the respiratory gas exchange of paralyzed patients ventilated by operator's expired air. N Engl J Med. 1954;250:749–54.
9. Elam JO, Greene DG, Brown ES, Clements JA. Oxygen and carbon dioxide exchange and energy cost of expired air resuscitation. JAMA. 1958;167:328–34.
10. Safar P, Escarraga LA, Chang F. Upper airway obstruction in the unconscious patient. J Appl Physiol. 1959;14:760–4.
11. Safar P, Escarraga LA, Elam JO. A comparison of the mouth-to-mouth and mouth-to-airway methods of artificial respiration with the chest pressure arm-lift methods. N Engl J Med. 1958;258:671–7.
12. Gordon AS, Frye CW, Gittelson L, Sadove MS, Beattie EJ. Mouth-to-mouth versus manual artificial respiration in children and adults. JAMA. 1958;167:320–8.
13. Kouwenhoven WB, Jude JR, Knickerbocker GG. Closed chest cardiac massage. JAMA. 1960;173:1064–7.
14. Jude JR, Kouwenhoven WB, Knickerbocker GG. Cardiac arrest: report of application of external cardiac massage in 118 patients. JAMA. 1961;178:1063–71.
15. Eisenberg MS, Psaty BM. Cardiopulmonary resuscitation: celebration and challenges. JAMA. 2010;304(1):87–8.
16. Woollam CHM. The development of apparatus for intermittent negative pressure ventilation. (1) 1832–1918. Anaesthesia. 1976;31:537–47.
17. Woollam CHM. The development of apparatus for intermittent negative pressure ventilation. (2) 1919–1976, with special reference to the development and uses of cuirass respirators. Anaesthesia. 1976;31:666–85.
18. Drinker PA, McKhann CF 3rd. The iron lung. First practical means of respiratory support. JAMA. 1986;255:1476–80.
19. Branson RD. Jack Emerson: Notes on his life and contributions to respiratory care. Resp Care. 1998;43:567–8.
20. Gould T. A summer plague. Polio and its survivors. New Haven and London: Yale University Press; 1995.
21. Hervey HE. Cagebirds. London:Penguin; 1940.
22. Mushin W, Rendell-Baker L The principles of thoracic anaesthesia. Past and present. Oxford: Blackwell Scientific Publications; 1953, p. 45.
23. Läwen und Sievers. Zur praktischen Anwendung der instrumentellen künstlichen Respiration am Menschen. Muench Med Wochenschr. 1910;59(43):2221–5.
24. Janeway HH, Green NW. Experimental intrathoracic esophageal surgery. JAMA. 1909;53:1975–8.
25. Meltzer SJ, Auer J. Continuous respiration without respiratory movements. J Exp Med. 1909;11:622–5.
26. Jackson DE. A universal artificial respiration and closed anesthesia machine. J Lab Clin Med. 1927;12:998–1002.
27. Jackson DE The use of artificial 2 in man. Report of a case. J Med. 1930; December 3–7, Cincinnati, Ohio.
28. Guedel AE, Treweek DN. Ether apnoeas. Anesth Analg. 1934;13:263–4.
29. Giertz KH. Studier Ofver Tryckdifferensandning (rytmisk luftenblassning) via intrathoracala operationer. Uppsala Lakaref Forh. 1916–1917;22:Suppl 1–176. Ommexperientella lungsextirpationer. Uppsala Lakaref Forh. 1916–1917;22:1–109.
30. Frenckner P. Bronchial and tracheal catheterization and its clinical applicability. Acta Otololaryngol (Stockh). 1934;suppl 20:1–134.
31. Crafoord C. Pulmonary ventilation and anesthesia in major chest surgery. J Thoracic Surg. 1940;9:237–53.
32. Mautz FR. Mechanical respirator as adjunct to closed system anesthesia. Proc Soc Exp Biol (NY). 1939;42:190–2.
33. Mörch ET. History of mechanical ventilation. In: Kirby RR, Banner MJ, Downs JB, editors. Clinical applications of ventilatory support. Edinburgh: Churchill Livingstone; 1990. S. 1–62.
34. Rosenberg H, Axelrod JK. Ernst Trier Mørch: Inventor, medical pioneer, heroic freedom fighter. Anesth Analg. 2000;90:218–21.
35. McKenzie AG. The inventions of John Blease. BJA. 2000;85:928–35.
36. Allbritten FF, Haupt GJ, Amadeo JH. The change in pulmonary alveolar ventilation achieved by aiding the deflation phase of respiration during anaesthesia for surgical operations. Ann Surg. 1954;140:569–82.
37. Mushin WW et al. Automatic ventilation of the lungs. 2nd ed. Oxford: Wiley-Blackwell; 1969. p. 205.
38. Mushin WW et al. Automatic ventilation of the lungs. 3rd ed. Oxford: Wiley-Blackwell; 1980.
39. Monro JA, Scurr CF. The Starling pump as a ventilator for infants and children. Anaesthesia. 1961;16:151–9.
40. Gray TC, Halton J. A milestone in anaesthesia? (*d*-tubocurarine chloride). Proc Roy Soc Med. 1946;39:400–8.
41. Gray TC, Rees GJ. The role of apnoea in anaesthesia for major surgery. BMJ. 1951;2:891–2.

From Copenhagen to Critical Care

57

Keith Sykes

Summary

In 1952, a poliomyelitis epidemic struck Copenhagen, causing 2,722 hospital admissions. In those with spinal and bulbar paralysis, anaesthetist Bjørn Aage Ibsen implemented tracheostomy and manual intermittent positive pressure ventilation (IPPV) to manage respiratory failure, thereby markedly decreasing mortality. His experience led him to develop the world's first intensive care unit (ICU) in 1953. Further, it led to the creation of intensive care medicine. Intensive respiratory support was soon applied to patients with diverse diseases. In 1954, Lassen et al and Honey et al reported survival of patients with severe tetanus treated with curare and mechanical ventilation. In 1955, Björk and Engström used IPPV to provide adequate ventilation after thoracic surgery. In 1956, Mørch applied IPPV to manage a crush injury of the chest.

Following the Copenhagen epidemic, several physicians helped design their own ventilators. Many were primitive yet enjoyed widespread and long use (e.g., the Radcliffe ventilator introduced in 1953). Engström invented one of the world's most successful mechanical ventilators, tested in the 1952 Copenhagen and 1953 Swedish polio epidemics. The British parallel to the Engström was the Smith-Clarke, the 1962 Cape-Waine version of which was used in anaesthesia. Diverse and often less expensive ventilators followed (e.g., the Howells, Manley, and Barnet.) In the 1950s, US engineers Bird and Bennett developed ventilators powered by compressed gas where the patient could trigger inspiration. In 1965, Emerson, with anaesthesiologists Benson and Pontoppidan, produced the first dedicated postoperative/ICU ventilator in the US.

In 1967, Nash *et al.* described lung damage with prolonged ventilation at high airway pressures and high concentrations of oxygen. In the 1970s, techniques were designed to minimise the harmful pulmonary and circulatory effects of PEEP, including continuous positive airway pressure (CPAP) during spontaneous ventilation and the addition of "mandatory breaths". In the 1970s and 1980s, microprocessors allowed synchronized ventilation. Swedish physicians introduced high frequency positive pressure ventilation in 1971. Repeated opening and closing of small air sacs could damage lungs, leading to Hickling's 1984 use of end-expiratory pressure sufficient to prevent alveolar collapse with a decrease in peak inspiratory pressures. Although this caused hypercapnia (*permissive hypercapnia*), it shortened the duration of mechanical ventilation and decreased mortality.

For the past 70 years, US anaesthesiologists used rebreathing CO_2 absorption systems, whereas many European anaesthesiologists used non-rebreathing systems. Rebreathing systems provided mechanical ventilation by replacing the reservoir bag with a bag- or bellows-in-bottle system, the bag being compressed by the ventilator. Some manufacturers now make piston type ventilators that deliver precise tidal volumes despite changes in airway resistance or compliance.

Ventilators became increasingly complex. Physicians, particularly in the US, increasingly delegated ventilator settings to specialist technicians who developed new techniques and significantly contributed to the literature.

It Started with Polio

Egyptian images suggest that poliomyelitis is an ancient disease. The twentieth century saw many epidemics throughout the world, but in 1952, there was an epidemic in Copenhagen, Denmark, exceeding all others in severity. The scale is

K. Sykes (✉)
Emeritus Professor University of Oxford, Oxford, UK
e-mail: k@mksykes.co.uk

difficult to imagine. Of the 1.2 million citizens of Copenhagen, 2,899 developed polio, an attack rate far exceeding that in previous severe epidemics in New York in 1916, 1931 and 1944. Of the 2,722 patients admitted to Blegdam Infectious Diseases Hospital, an unusually high percentage had paralyzed pharyngeal and laryngeal muscles (bulbar paralysis) combined with paralysis of respiratory and limb muscles (spinal paralysis). Oral secretions entered the tracheobroncheal tree, causing collapse of areas of lung and pneumonia.

E. I Eger II et al. (eds.), *The Wondrous Story of Anesthesia*, DOI 10.1007/978-1-4614-8441-7_57, © Edmond I Eger, MD 2014

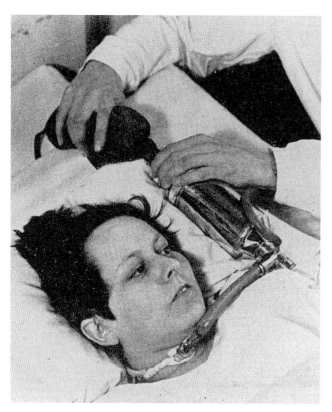

Fig. 57.1 Patient with respiratory paralysis in the 1952 polio epidemic being manually ventilated with a Waters CO_2 absorption system

Mortality exceeded 80% in patients with spinal and bulbar paralysis. Death, it was thought, was due to an overwhelming viral infection of the base of the brain [1, 2].

Six cuirass ventilators and one (Emerson) iron lung were available; woefully inadequate resources. By the end of the third week of the epidemic, Henry Cai Alexander Lassen, the Chief Physician at the Blegdam Hospital, realised that this epidemic differed from previous ones and that desperate measures were needed. Although it was not usual for Chief physicians to ask others for advice, his assistant, Mogens Bjørneboe, eventually persuaded him to call in the anaesthetist, Bjørn Ibsen, who had recently returned from a year in the anaesthesia department at the Massachusetts General Hospital, Boston (see Fig. 55.4). After examining some patients and the records and autopsy reports of those who had died, Ibsen concluded that the polio patients were dying from respiratory failure and not from an overwhelming viral infection. He suggested that IPPV would provide an effective treatment. Ibsen proposed to insert a cuffed tracheostomy tube in all patients with respiratory failure, thus providing an airway and preventing secretions entering the trachea. He also proposed that the lungs should be ventilated manually using the standard Waters breathing system and carbon dioxide absorber (Fig. 57.1). Two days after the

initial consultation, Ibsen demonstrated the technique on a 12 year-old girl and used a Brinkman carbovisor and a Millikan ear oximeter to show that the patient had severe CO_2 retention and that blood gas values could be returned to normal when adequate ventilation was provided. Lassen realised that Ibsen's plan might just work, and together they implemented it.

Logistics now became the problem. First, supplies of cuffed tracheostomy tubes, suction apparatus, anaesthetic breathing systems, and gas cylinders had to be obtained. Second, patients whose lungs required ventilating had to be concentrated in the hospital area containing the requisite resources. Third, trained teams of internists, surgeons, and anaesthetists had to provide skilled care continuously. Fortunately, the World Health Organisation had started an anaesthesia training centre in Copenhagen in 1950, and a number of these trainee anaesthetists were drafted to help supervise patient care. More help was needed: people to aspirate tracheal secretions, and manually compress the anaesthetic reservoir bags 24 hours a day for two to three months. Copenhagen medical students volunteered and soon organized their 6-hour shifts. Such care was a heavy responsibility for such untrained personnel: they not only had to maintain artificial ventilation, but also had to monitor the patient's condition and alert doctors to problems.

At the peak of the epidemic, the lungs of 70 patients were simultaneously receiving manual ventilation. From 28 August to 3 September, 335 patients were admitted to Blegdam with polio—48 per day. By November, the number of medical students became insufficient, so Lassen drafted dental students too. In total, 1,500 students put in 165,000 hours ventilating patients' lungs. Mortality in the severely affected patients decreased from about 80% to approximately 25%, a remarkable achievement.

A Defining Moment

The Copenhagen epidemic was a defining moment in the history of controlled ventilation. First, it demonstrated that airway control, secretion removal, and intermittent positive pressure ventilation could save the lives of patients in respiratory failure. Second, it stimulated development of mechanical ventilators. Third, it demonstrated the value of concentrating trained staff and essential facilities in one area, leading Ibsen to set up the world's first ICU in his hospital in 1953 [3]. Fourth, it convinced Poul Astrup, who had performed blood tests during the epidemic, that new techniques of determining acid-base balance were needed [4]. Fifth, it demonstrated a need for new methods of safely transporting seriously ill patients. And sixth, it led to the creation of the speciality of intensive care medicine.

The Immediate Aftermath of the Epidemic

European doctors responsible for the care of polio patients visited Copenhagen to learn and apply the new techniques. On returning home, many of these physicians enrolled engineers to build mechanical ventilators. They began to treat patients with other causes of respiratory failure, including a 16 year-old girl admitted to the Radcliffe Infirmary in Oxford in August 1953. Initially diagnosed as having polio, she was treated in a tank ventilator but developed swallowing difficulties and chest complications. W Ritchie Russell and John Spalding, two Oxford neurologists who had visited Copenhagen, ordered a tracheostomy and mechanical ventilation using the prototype Radcliffe ventilator. Within a few days she was only able to communicate by small movements of her eyes. Several physicians questioned the ethics of keeping her alive. Not Russell and Spalding.

Fortunately, the paralysis was due to acute toxic polyneuritis (Guillain-Barré syndrome) and not to poliomyelitis. The patient recovered and was discharged from hospital 6 weeks later. She became a nurse, worked in the respiration unit, married a farmer and had four children. Kudos came to the doctors looking after her, and society benefited because her story advanced the adoption of this form of treatment [5].

Another disease in which IPPV proved to be life-saving was tetanus (lockjaw). Tetanus may cause severe, sometimes fatal, muscle spasms. In 1952, Woolmer and Cates in the UK, abolished the spasms in an afflicted patient, using succinylcholine to relax the muscles and manually ventilating the patient's lungs for five days until the spasms wore off [6]. In 1954, Lassen *et al* in Copenhagen and Honey *et al* in Oxford, reported survival of patients with severe tetanus who received curare and whose lungs were ventilated mechanically [7, 8]. This technique also saved newborn babies with severe tetanus in Capetown, South Africa [9] and a randomized controlled trial in Durban showed that neonatal mortality could be reduced from more than 80%, to 40% [10, 11].

In 1955, Viking Björk and Carl-Gunnar Engström reported the use of the Engström ventilator to support patients breathing inadequately after thoracic surgery [12]. Three years later one of the pioneers of Swedish anaesthesia, Olof Norlander, and colleagues working in other hospitals, described the use of ventilator support to treat patients with other causes of respiratory failure [13].

In 1956, a 51-year-old Chicago railway worker was crushed and rolled in an 8 inch (20 cm) space: "Like piedough under a rolling pin his body diameter was reduced to the size of this space". The patient was in shock with multiple rib and other fractures, air in both pleural cavities, crush injuries to the liver and genitourinary tract, and gastrointestinal paralysis. Attempts were made to stabilise the chest by applying traction to the ribs, but only when Trier Mørch (recently

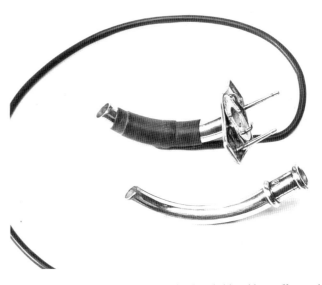

Fig. 57.2 Metal tracheostomy tube with detachable rubber cuff around outer tube and inner tube with extension to connect to ventilation system. Trier Mørch later used a similar tube but without a cuff. This enabled the patient to speak during inflation of the lungs

emigrated to Chicago from Copenhagen) connected his piston ventilator to the cuffed tracheostomy tube, did the patient's condition improve. Intermittent positive pressure kept the lungs inflated, providing an internal splint while the rib fractures healed. IPPV was continued for 30 days. The patient left hospital 51 days later, without apparent respiratory impairment. This incredible story revolutionised the treatment of crushed chest injuries [14]. The successful outcomes described above encouraged the development of ICUs with dedicated facilities and specially trained staff [15–17]. These early studies demonstrated successful treatments in patients with diverse types of respiratory failure, and resulted in the creation of numerous general and specialised ICUs over the next two decades.

Technical Developments After Copenhagen

The Airway

The standard metal tracheostomy tube used in Copenhagen was modified with an extension allowing connection to the breathing system, and an inflatable rubber cuff was applied over the lower end of the tube to provide an airtight seal with the trachea (Fig. 57.2). However, the tracheostomy tube and its modifications brought new problems. Bypass of the warming and moistening normally supplied by the nose, caused drying of secretions that became difficult to aspirate. The cuff tended to slip off the tube and traction from the breathing system pulled the tube from the trachea. These problems led to development of right-angled rubber, and later plastic, tubes with integral cuffs.

Humidification

Blockage of the tracheostomy tube from the drying of secretions prompted development of systems to warm and humidify the inspired gas. Marshall and Spalding in Oxford [18] examined possible methods and developed a simple hot water humidifier based on a biscuit tin with a thermostat and electric kettle element: this proved to be extremely effective but, since the inspired gas temperature varied with flow rate, it was necessary to monitor the inspired temperature close to the patient Y-piece. In 1971, a washing machine manufacturer in Auckland, New Zealand, produced the sophisticated Fisher and Paykel hot water humidifier that solved the problem [19]. Subsequently, heat and moisture exchangers were developed that could be connected to the tracheostomy tube and so function as an artificial nose.

Sterilization

In the 1960s, bacteria were found in the ventilator, humidifier and breathing systems. To overcome this problem, formaldehyde or ethylene oxide gas was recirculated around the ventilator circuit for 12 to 24 hours before use in a patient. The ventilator then had to be left running for another 24 hours to eliminate residual sterilizing agent. These problems initially forced manufacturers to design ventilators with autoclavable patient circuits (e.g. the Engström 300, and the Penlon Oxford ventilator). However, in the mid-1970s, improved low-volume bacterial filters that could be placed at the patient Y-piece became available, reducing the need for sterilization.

The AMBU Bag

In the hospital setting, manual ventilation with oxygen can normally be provided by a Waters circuit and expiratory valve with or without a CO_2 absorber, but in 1956 there was a strike of gasoline truck drivers in Denmark that threatened hospital oxygen supplies. What was needed was a means of providing artificial ventilation with air. The anaesthetist, Henning Ruben, took up the challenge. Ruben had qualified as a dentist before the war, and utilised his talents as a ballroom dancer, champion fencer, magician and thought-reader to pay his way through college. In 1943, he had to escape from Copenhagen in a fishing boat, when the Nazi occupiers started to round up the Jews. The escapees lay under a false bottom in the fish hold and children were sedated with barbiturate suppositories to keep them quiet during the voyage to Sweden. It is said that Trier Mørch and a pharmacist friend developed a mixture of rabbit blood and cocaine that was sprinkled on the deck to abolish the sense of smell in the

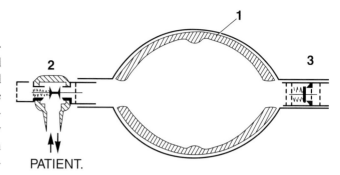

Fig. 57.3 The AMBU bag developed by Henning Ruben in 1956–1957. *1* Foam lining. *2* Ruben non-rebreathing valve. *3* Inlet valve. Oxygen could be added to a reservoir attached to *3*. (Reproduced from Mushin WW et al. Automatic ventilation of the lungs, 3rd edition, 1980, p. 762, with permission from Wiley-Blackwell)

tracker dogs that searched the boats before departure to the fishing grounds. After the war, Ruben returned to Copenhagen, qualified in medicine and trained as an anaesthetist. He spent 6 months with Lucien Morris at the University of Iowa, and met James Elam. The two developed a lasting friendship and Ruben went on to demonstrate that neck extension, as practised in anaesthesia, provided a simple way of maintaining an airway in the unconscious patient.

Ruben developed numerous medical devices among which were a non-rebreathing valve and a portable suction apparatus. The latter was manufactured by the Danish company AMBU-TESTA, and it was this company that produced his next invention—a self-inflating bag. His first prototype consisted of a double-ended bag that was kept open by three bent bicycle wheel spokes, and was fitted with his non-rebreathing valve at one end and an air inlet valve at the other. Later, he filled the bag with lumps of foam rubber, the final version having a foam rubber lining to the bag (Fig. 57.3). Oxygen could be added to a reservoir attached to the air inlet. Many variants of this design have since been produced, and it has proved invaluable, not only in emergencies, but as a routine method of transporting patients with respiratory insufficiency [20].

The Development of Mechanical Ventilators After the Epidemic

Space limitations preclude a comprehensive description of ventilator development after the Copenhagen epidemic. This section is restricted to significant developments in Scandinavia, the UK and the US, although similar developments took place in many European countries, and the British Commonwealth. Readers desiring more information should refer to standard works [21–24]. Here I summarize the evolution of ventilators from the simple mechanical pumps of the 1950s, to the sophisticated computer-controlled machines of today, and I describe how increasing knowledge of the physiology of mechanical ventilation and the pathophysiology of respiratory failure, influenced design considerations.

Many early ventilators were used in both the operating room and ICU. Those that utilised a non-rebreathing circuit, required a fresh gas flow equal to the patient's minute volume [25]. Others were connected to a CO_2 absorber circuit and so required a smaller flow of fresh gases. From the 1970s onwards, the introduction of microprocessor-controlled ventilators facilitated the development of new techniques of respiratory support in the ICU, but since these techniques were not needed in the operating room, anaesthesia ventilators remained relatively simple. Most anaesthesia ventilators now compress a bag or bellows in a rigid chamber connected to a standard CO_2 absorption circuit, so that low fresh gas flows can be used. This minimises environmental pollution with anaesthetic vapours and gases, and cuts the cost of expensive agents. There has however, been a recent trend to use sophisticated piston type ventilators to cope with the ventilatory problems introduced by the insufflation of CO_2 into the abdominal cavity and the extreme changes of body position required for laparoscopic surgery.

Ventilator Specifications

By 1950, it was known that that inflation of the lungs, whether by application of positive pressure to the airway or subatmospheric pressure to the chest wall, impeded venous return and so could impair cardiac output. It was also known that high inflation pressures could damage the lung. These findings suggested that: peak airway pressures should not exceed 25–30 cm H_2O; the duration of inspiration should be less than the duration of expiration; and airway pressure should be zero during expiration. Machines were designed to produce a normal range of tidal volumes and breathing frequencies with an inspiratory:expiratory time ratio of 1:2, and most ventilators incorporated a pressure relief valve set to 30 cm H_2O. These early machines ventilated normal lungs satisfactorily, but could fail to produce adequate ventilation when lung compliance decreased or airway resistance increased.

Because of the concern that the application of IPPV might decrease cardiac output, many early ventilators could also generate a subatmospheric pressure during expiration. However, it was soon found that a negative phase had little effect on the circulation and often impaired gas exchange, so cardiac output was optimized by infusing vasoconstrictor drugs or by increasing blood volume. Heart filling pressures were initially monitored by a central venous catheter

but from the 1970s onwards, the Swan-Ganz (pulmonary artery) catheter was increasingly used in critically ill patients. Although this catheter enabled left heart filling pressures to be monitored, its use was associated with a number of complications and there is no firm evidence to indicate that it reduces mortality in severely ill patients [26]. Indeed, some authors suggest that the use of the catheter increases morbidity and mortality [27].

Until the late 1950s, PCO_2 could only be measured by the tedious Van Slyke analysis and the use of rather crude pH electrodes. Thus, ventilators were usually set to provide a minute volume that was 20–30 % more than the norms calculated from the Radford or Herzog ventilation nomograms[28, 29]. These nomograms were designed for patients with normal lungs and it would be expected that patients with diseased lungs would require more ventilation. But how much more? Because of this uncertainty, patients with respiratory failure were hyperventilated until apnea occurred, apnea being the sign that ventilation was sufficient. Apnea also ensured that the patient did not fight the ventilator. If ventilatory drive still prevented synchronisation with the ventilator, apnea was produced by the administration of opioids or muscle relaxants. The introduction of the rebreathing technique for measurement of PCO_2, the Astrup interpolation technique, and the development of O_2 and CO_2 electrodes in the late 1950s, revolutionised treatment and encouraged the attempt to produce normal blood gas values. In patients with severe lung disease, this often resulted in the use of high inflation pressures. Peak airway pressures increased further in the early 1970s, when it became known that the application of a positive end-expiratory pressure could improve gas exchange in the lung by preventing alveolar collapse during expiration. It soon became apparent however, that these high pressures (up to 70 cm H_2O) produced lung damage, leading to the development of techniques designed to minimise such harmful effects. These will be discussed later.

Post-1952 European Ventilators

Several of the physicians visiting Copenhagen during and after the 1952 epidemic, recruited local engineers to build their own mechanical ventilators, to provide long term respiratory support. Many were primitive. For example, the Radcliffe ventilator, introduced in 1953, was based on the Oxford Inflating bellows developed in the Nuffield Department of Anaesthetics. Oxygen was added to air in a T-piece reservoir and the mixture sucked into a weighted bellows by a mechanism driven by an electric motor. The weights then forced the gas into the lungs through a pressure-operated non-rebreathing valve. The motors were powered by mains

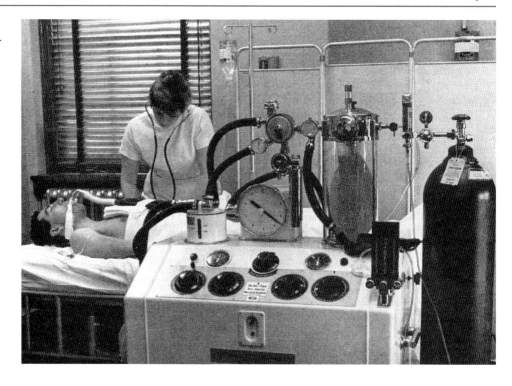

Fig. 57.4 Engström 150 ventilator in a Swedish Hospital. The warmed water humidifier is on the left and the gas meter recorded expired volume breath-by-breath. (From Safar P, Respiratory Therapy. by kind permission of the Publishers, F A Davis Company)

electricity or a 12-volt car battery, and 8 ventilation rates could be selected with a bicycle gear change and a hand-operated clutch. The latter allowed the ventilator to be powered by turning a gramophone handle in case of power failure. The non-rebreathing valve situated close to the patient sometimes failed when wet, and was later replaced by cam-operated valves in the machine. Since the Radcliffe ventilator was cheap, simple, robust and could be maintained by any bicycle mechanic, it was widely used in the UK and developing countries for over 30 years [30]. In 1962, the ventilator was modified so that it could be used both in the operating room and ICU. This flexibility resulted in its widespread use throughout the UK and Commonwealth [31]. The Radcliffe was classified as a *pressure generator* since the weights on the bellows produced a constant pressure during inspiration; the tidal volume depended on the compliance (stiffness of the lungs), the airway resistance and the duration of inspiration. Since the lung characteristics could change rapidly it was essential to monitor the expired volume at regular intervals.

Other ventilators, often powered by compressed gases or an electrically driven piston or bellows, produced a fixed pattern of flow (*flow generators*). In these machines (*e.g.* Engström, Blease, Smith-Clarke), changes in lung compliance or airway resistance resulted in changes in airway pressure, though tidal volume was maintained. Since a knowledge of ventilator characteristics is essential for effective therapy, the Cardiff anaesthesia department physicist, WW Mapleson, utilised these and other major differences in functional characteristics (such as methods of initiating or controlling the duration of inspiration and expiration) to produce a classification of ventilator mechanisms that remains valid to this day [32]. In the course of his investigations, Mapleson found that many ventilators did not perform as predicted and over the next 20 years British and International Standards Organisations developed test lungs and procedures that revealed deficiencies in design and improved safety standards [33].

One man who did understand ventilator mechanics was Carl-Gunnar Engström, a doctor working in a Swedish infectious diseases hospital during the 1949 and 1950 polio epidemics [34]. He invented one of the world's most successful mechanical ventilators (Fig. 57.4). With remarkable percipience, he recognised that patients died because of inadequate ventilation and designed an intermittent positive pressure ventilator that delivered breaths of controllable volume and frequency. This ventilator was used successfully in Copenhagen towards the end of the 1952 epidemic, and the Swedish government then ordered several machines, no doubt anticipating the Swedish polio epidemic in 1953, where they demonstrated their effectiveness. The machine proved lifesaving in other conditions including respiratory insufficiency due to skull trauma, brain tumour, and barbiturate intoxication. It was also adapted to provide controlled ventilation during anaesthesia with either a non-rebreathing or partially closed circuit. Though the precision Swedish engineering made this machine and its successors expensive, they were and are widely used throughout Europe and other parts of the world.

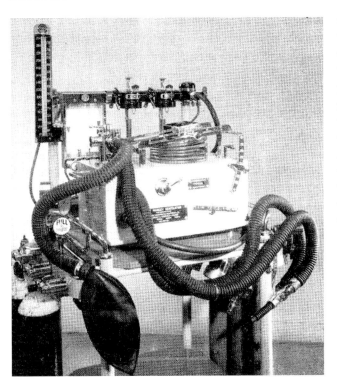

Fig. 57.5 The Manley ventilator that normally sat on the bottom shelf of the Boyle's anaesthetic machine. (Courtesy of the author.)

The British answer to this machine was the Smith-Clarke, designed by the ex-chief engineer of the Alvis motor company. Like the Rolls Royce car, the ventilator came with a mahogany box containing an oilcan, but the operator had to supply his own engine driver's cap to fully enjoy oiling the cams. The Cape ventilator was the popular successor to this machine and incorporated an efficient, low-volume, hot-water humidifier. The Cape-Waine version of this ventilator was designed for use in anaesthesia with CO_2 absorption [35].

In the UK, two other ventilator systems were commonly used during anaesthesia. In one, the ventilator was part of a non-rebreathing system, the fresh gas being led into a weight- or spring-loaded bellows and intermittently discharged into the patient. In the Howells and Manley ventilators the inspiratory and expiratory valves were pneumatically controlled whereas in the Barnet they were controlled by solenoids. These ventilators sat comfortably on the lower shelf of the ubiquitous Boyle's anaesthetic machine, were relatively cheap, safe and simple to operate (Fig. 57.5). Some models could also be used in intensive care [36, 37].

The second type of ventilator system used during anaesthesia in the UK was based on the Bain (Mapleson D) breathing system. The anaesthetic gas mixture was delivered to the patient via a narrow bore tube situated concentrically within a light-weight 22 mm corrugated tube and the ventilator was attached to a fitting that replaced the Bain expira-

tory valve by means of a 1.5 m length of corrugated tube. This prevented dilution with the gases delivered by the ventilator. Interestingly, when tidal volume was set to 10 ml/kg body weight, CO_2 levels could be controlled by adjusting the fresh gas flow, an inflow of 70 ml/kg body weight providing normocapnia [38, 39]. An advantage of this system was that the delivery tubes could be lengthened so that the ventilator could be situated some distance from the patient (for example during magnetic resonance imaging), and it could be used with almost any ventilator. It was commonly used with the Pneupac, a simple, compact, fluid logic ventilator that was originally designed for resuscitation. There were four models, the one designed for anaesthesia having controls for flow rate and inspiratory and expiratory times [40]. This compact system was eventually displaced by the new generation of anaesthetic machines, fitted with integral ventilators and rapid response gas monitors that enabled low gas flows to be used safely, thus conserving expensive volatile agents and reducing pollution of the environment with anaesthetic gases and vapours.

Early US Intensive Care Ventilators

Two engineers (Bird and Bennett) devoted to the problems of flying at high altitude during World War II, developed popular ventilators in the US. Compressed oxygen drove the ventilators and the patient triggered inspiration. Although neither machine was developed for use in the ICU, both were widely used in ICUs when these opened in the US in the late 1950s [16].

Forrest Bird, an American aviator and inventor, was awarded the Presidential Citizens Medal by President George W Bush in 2008 and, the National Medal of Technology and Innovation by President Barack Obama in 2009. He developed his ventilator in Palm Springs, California for patients undergoing bronchodilator therapy for chronic respiratory diseases, the prototype being built from three tin cans and a doorknob (Fig. 57.6). Although Bird and Bennett ventilators dominated the US market until the late 1960s, the early versions of the Bird were not very suitable for long-term use. The control of oxygen concentration was poor, the nebulizer provided inadequate humidification, and mechanical delay and relative insensitivity of the triggering mechanism sometimes caused distress to patients. Bird discovered that he could administer drugs other than bronchodilators via the nebulizer, and once told the author that with a demanding patient he was sometimes tempted to replace the bronchodilator with cascara sagrada—but he never did.

The Bennett PR2 ventilator was developed from one of some forty devices that Ray Bennett and his colleagues produced to help treat polio patients (Fig. 57.7). These significantly decreased mortality [41]. The unique feature of

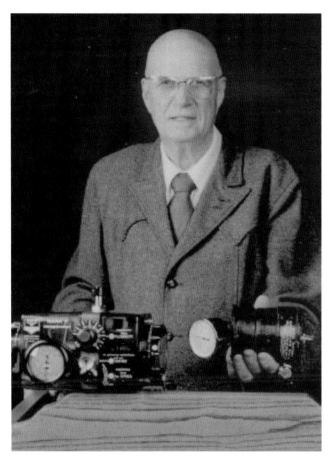

Fig. 57.6 Dr Forrest M. Bird with the prototype (in his left hand) and Mk 7 versions of his ventilator. (Courtesy of Dr Bird.)

Bennett's ventilator was a flow-sensitive valve that initiated inspiratory flow from the ventilator when the patient inhaled, and terminated flow when it had decreased to a predetermined level. The device was originally intended to augment ventilation of patients in tank ventilators when the patient developed lung complications and the tank could not provide sufficient ventilation, but it was subsequently used to provide IPPV to patients in the ICU independent of the tank. Although the Bird and Bennett machines could nebulize a bronchodilator drug, they could not supply adequate humidification. Bennett subsequently designed many other respiratory assist devices including the Puritan-Bennett MA-1 ventilator, one of the first electronically controlled devices, that was widely used in the 1970–80s.

Credit for the first dedicated ICU ventilator in the US goes to Jack Emerson of Boston, who cooperated with anaesthesiologists Donald Benson in Baltimore, and Henning Pontoppidan in Boston, to produce the Emerson postoperative ventilator in 1965. An electrically driven piston with a variable stroke drove gas into the lungs. Varying the motor speed throughout the cycle controlled the inspiratory

and expiratory times. Later, Emerson designed a ventilator allowing the patient to trigger each breath. Emerson's ventilator included a hot water humidification system that ensured that lung secretions could be aspirated easily. Another of Emerson's machines featured a sigh mechanism that intermittently increased tidal volume for a few breaths. This feature was introduced because the group at the Massachusetts General Hospital believed that such a sigh could re-expand collapsed alveoli in patients requiring long-term ventilation.

US Anaesthesia Ventilators

American anaesthesiologists have used anaesthesia machines with circle CO_2 absorption systems and relatively low fresh gas flows (thought of as 2 to 4 l/min in Europe and 2 l/min or less in the US), whereas in many European countries the non-rebreathing system has been more popular. The use of low fresh gas flows conserves anaesthetic agents, but the composition of gases entering the lung may differ from that in the fresh gas delivered from the machine. With a CO_2 absorption system, the obvious way to provide mechanical ventilation was to replace the reservoir bag with a bag-in-bottle system, the bag being compressed by the ventilator mechanism. The Jefferson ventilator was an early example of this system The Bennett B_2A assistor introduced in 1957 utilised a hanging bellows instead of a bag and, despite its name, was one of the first US ventilators that could be adjusted to provide controlled ventilation with a predetermined tidal volume (Fig. 57.8).

The hanging bellows had the advantage that there was no impedance to expiration but, in the 1970s, it was realised that a leak in the circuit could dilute the anaesthetic mixture. As a result, manufacturers introduced bellows that expanded upwards in expiration. Failure to expand demonstrated the presence of a leak, but the bellows had to be made of light material to minimise the resistance to expiration. With the increasing sophistication of measurement techniques and the use of very low fresh gas flows to conserve expensive volatile agents and reduce pollution, manufacturers began to realise that bag- or bellows- in-bottle systems contained a large volume of gas that was compressed during each inflation. This not only reduced the tidal volume delivered to the patient, but also distorted the inspiratory flow pattern.

To counter these criticisms, manufacturers such as the Draeger company now use directly driven piston type ventilators that have minimal internal compliance and can be accurately calibrated to deliver precise tidal volumes, despite changes in airway resistance or compliance, With such devices and the sophisticated monitoring incorporated in modern machines, low fresh gas flows can now be used safely.

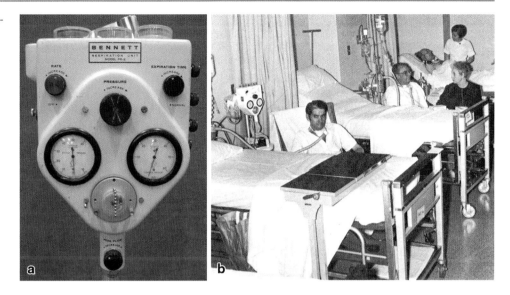

Fig. 57.7 a Bennett PR2 ventilator. **b** Bennett PR2 ventilators being used in an early Intensive Therapy Unit

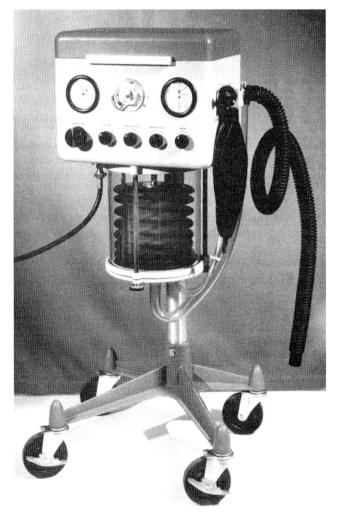

Fig. 57.8 Bennett assistor. This was one of the first effective US anaesthesia ventilators and could provide controlled as well as assisted ventilation. (From Mushin WW et al. Automatic ventilation of the lungs, 2nd edition, 1969, p. 328, with permission from Wiley-Blackwell)

Neonatal Ventilators

In 1953, Ian Donald, a Scottish obstetrician at the Hammersmith Hospital and Postgraduate Medical School in West London, recognised that many infants died of respiratory inadequacy at birth and that a mechanical device was needed to replace the midwives' use of mouth-to-mouth ventilation. There were many problems in developing apparatus for such a difficult clinical situation and the electronically controlled pneumotron ventilator that he designed met with only limited success [42]. The British Oxygen Company subsequently manufactured a patient-cycled intermittent positive pressure machine (the Pneumotron) that never achieved popularity. In the US, Goddard *et al.* also attempted to ventilate neonates, but again results were poor [43]. In 1958, Swedish workers used adult machines adapted to produce small tidal volumes, and reported the survival of three babies treated with IPPV [44]. In 1959, when the author attempted to treat neonatal tetanus using curare-induced paralysis and IPPV with the Smith-Clarke ventilator (minimum tidal volume 250 ml), he had to decrease the volume delivered to approximately 16 ml by adding a parallel compliance—a 500 ml reservoir bag sandwiched between two pieces of hardboard held together by elastic bands [45]. With the gradual development of appropriate apparatus and new techniques, neonatal resuscitation became a successful enterprise and the author recently had the great pleasure of seeing his 32 weeks-gestation grandson, who was ventilated for 8 days, depart for university. A Wellcome Trust Witness Seminar has nicely chronicled the development of neonatal intensive care in the UK [46].

Ventilator, Airway, and Vascular Pressures

During the 1960s, new ventilators were introduced, and research demonstrated how IPPV affected circulation and gas exchange. In 1967, Ashbaugh and colleagues [47]. described the adult respiratory distress syndrome (later called the acute respiratory distress syndrome or ARDS) in patients who had multiple injuries, shock or severe sepsis. ARDS reflected widespread damage to the lung, and severe impairment of oxygen transfer. It was often fatal. Increasing lung volume by applying positive pressure to the airway during expiration (positive end-expiratory pressure or PEEP) improved oxygenation by preventing collapse of the damaged air sacs. This was soon applied to improve oxygenation in ARDS, but it increased end-inspiratory and mean pressures throughout the respiratory cycle. The increased pressures in the airways and thus the inside of the chest, decreased the return of blood to the heart, decreased the output of the heart, and decreased blood pressure. Using monitoring of arterial and venous pressures, physicians learnt to restore heart output by increasing venous pressure, by transfusing fluid or using drugs to constrict the veins. The introduction of the Swan-Ganz catheter in 1970 enabled pulmonary artery and left atrial pressures to be measured at the bedside, but a 2006 Cochrane review concluded that the knowledge gained therefrom did not appear to improve patient outcome [48].

New Techniques of Respiratory Support

High airway pressures imposed other serious effects. In 1967, Nash *et al.* [49] described lung damage in adults whose lungs were ventilated for long periods with high airway pressures and high concentrations of oxygen. Northway *et al.* [50] also described lung damage in neonates mechanically ventilated to treat respiratory problems at birth. So, the 1970s saw the development of techniques of ventilation designed to minimise the harmful pulmonary and circulatory effects of high airway pressures, and minimize lung damage [51].

Since many patients with acute lung disease have alveolar collapse, reduced functional residual capacity and increased shunt, the first move was to increase lung volume by applying continuous positive airway pressure (CPAP) during spontaneous ventilation. This often increased oxygenation but in many patients the $PaCO_2$ increased, necessitating additional respiratory support [52]. The next development added "mandatory breaths" of predetermined volume delivered by the ventilator without any attempt to synchronise them with the patient's spontaneous ventilation (intermittent mandatory ventilation or IMV). The BabyBird ventilator described in 1971 was first to use this technique [53, 54]. When patient-triggering technology improved in the 1970s, it became possible to synchronise these breaths with one of the spontane-

ous breaths (synchronized intermittent mandatory ventilation or SIMV). The volume of the mandatory breath was initially preset, but with the later introduction of *pressure support* the patient's spontaneous breath could be augmented by a predetermined level of pressure developed by the ventilator. This technique is frequently used in current practice. Two other techniques that have been widely used in some centres are: airway pressure release ventilation (APRV), where the patient respires spontaneously at a high level of CPAP and elimination of carbon dioxide is assisted by allowing the lung to deflate to a lower CPAP level at regular intervals; and biphasic positive pressure ventilation (BIPAP) where the patient breaths spontaneously at two different levels of CPAP, the lower CPAP levels helping carbon dioxide elimination and the higher levels preventing lung collapse.

Microprocessor Controlled Ventilators

The introduction of the microprocessor-controlled ventilator made these techniques possible. The first such ventilator in Europe was the Siemens Servo 900 series, introduced in 1971. In the US, the earliest machines were the Puritan Bennett 7220 (1984), the Bear 5 (1985) and the Hamilton Veolar (1986). Unique to these new ventilators were their high sensitivity and the rapid response of the sensors and valve mechanisms. These eliminated the mechanical delay that vitiated patient-triggering in earlier ventilators.

Respiratory Therapists

Alas, these new machines were complex, offering many controls, and adjustment of one control often affected the impact of another. Those unfamiliar with the intricacies of a machine could worsen the patient's condition by wrong adjustment of the settings. In Europe, doctors working in ICUs usually retained control of ventilator settings, but in the US, respiratory therapists assumed this aspect of treatment.

The development of respiratory therapy as a sub-specialty has two origins. First, in the pre-ICU era many American hospitals employed oxygen therapy technicians to set up oxygen tents and maintain supplies of oxygen. This service provided income for departments accepting responsibility for its organisation. The increasing tendency to concentrate seriously ill patients in a special unit, created a parallel need for technicians to service and sterilize mechanical ventilators and other respiratory equipment. The increased responsibilities of these tasks attracted more sophisticated technicians, and as ventilators became more complex, doctors increasingly left their settings to the technician. In the 1970s, the speciality of critical care developed, embracing emergency care, resuscitation and intensive care. This attracted physicians from other disciplines and anaesthetists gradually returned from intensive care to the more lucrative practice of anaesthesia. Since intensive care physicians had less interest in technical devices than anaesthesiologists, respiratory therapists gained more control over ventilator therapy. These increasingly sophisticated workers have helped with the development of new techniques and the design of new ventilators, and indeed have made significant contributions to the literature.

High Frequency Ventilation

Another way to decrease airway pressures was to use high frequency ventilation, providing the same ventilation with smaller tidal volumes. Since the dead space didn't change significantly with frequencies of up to 100 breaths per minute, large minute volumes were required to maintain the same alveolar ventilation and CO_2 removal. Swedish doctors introduced the first technique (high frequency positive pressure ventilation or HFPPV) in 1971 to decrease the cyclical effects of IPPV during experiments on the brain circulation. A second technique, high frequency jet ventilation (HFJV) used a high gas pressure and a solenoid-controlled valve to produce jet pulses of 60 to 300 breaths per minute. Directed into a tube inserted into the trachea, the jet created the positive pressure that inflated the lungs. The resulting uncertain tidal volume depended on the design of the jet, the driving pressure, the entrainment of surrounding gas, and pulmonary compliance and airway resistance. Minute volumes were large and humidification difficult. The technique has proven useful in selected applications such as surgery on the larynx or in the trachea, where the absence of a tracheal tube facilitated surgery. Lunkenheimer, a Berlin physiologist, introduced a third technique, high frequency sinusoidal oscillations at 300–1800 (!) breaths per minute [55]. How the resulting small tidal volumes achieved gas exchange is unclear, but the technique has proven useful to sustain ventilation in infants who have suffered severe lung damage at birth [56]. Once again, Emerson had beaten the field, since he had noted the panting of a dog and applied for a patent of a device to emulate this pattern of breathing in 1954–5 [57].

Extracorporeal Membrane Oxygenator (ECMO) Support

Not surprisingly, some centres used a heart lung machine to maintain patients with extremely severe acute lung disease, hoping to buy the time needed to allow a natural recovery. Even ignoring the immense technical difficulties, trials have not shown a significant advantage over conventional treatments [58]. The technique may be of value in babies with neonatal respiratory distress, but treatment with nitric oxide

inhalation, surfactant replacement therapy and high frequency oscillation has decreased the use of ECMO in such patients.

In 1978, Kolobow and colleagues suggested separating oxygenation and carbon dioxide removal by passing only 20 % of the cardiac output through a membrane artificial lung optimized for carbon dioxide removal. Oxygenation was accomplished by the patient's lungs plus the membrane lung [59]. Although Gattinoni and colleagues in Italy, and several other European centres achieved some success with the method, complexity and cost prevented its widespread application [60].

Permissive Hypercapnia and Low Volume Ventilation

Many patients with respiratory failure tolerate moderately increased levels of carbon dioxide without undue distress, but treatment with mechanical ventilation usually aims to accomplish normal levels. During the 1980s and 1990s, several studies confirmed that high inspiratory pressures could further damage lungs of patients with lung disease. It also appeared that repeated opening and closing of small air sacs at each breath could damage lungs, leading to the suggestion that end-expiratory pressure should be sufficient to prevent alveolar collapse, and that peak inspiratory pressure should be decreased by reducing tidal volume. In 1984, Hickling *et al* applied this pattern of ventilation, perforce moderately increasing carbon dioxide levels. They called this technique *permissive hypercapnia,* and showed that it shortened the duration of ventilator use and decreased mortality. Positive end expiratory pressure plus limited tidal volume producing permissive hypercapnia is now standard treatment for severe lung disease [61].

Non-Invasive Ventilation

Effective IPPV in severe lung disease requires tracheal intubation or tracheostomy. But intubation and tracheostomy may produce complications, thereby increasing interest in non-invasive methods of respiratory support using nasal or full-face masks. There are two main applications: IPPV to augment spontaneous breathing during acute attacks of respiratory infection in patients with chronic obstructive lung disease; and nasal CPAP to treat snoring and obstructive sleep apnoea. The problem with these approaches is air-leak at the mask-patient interface. A large capacity pressure-generating ventilator can increase flow to maintain the pressure profile despite a large leak. Modern lightweight plastic masks have decreased leakage, but success still depends on good nursing care and encouragement. The use of nasal

CPAP for treatment of obstructive sleep apnoea is usually successful, and greatly reduces daytime somnolence because of improved sleep.

Afterthoughts

The development of Intensive Care was recently reviewed by doctors and nurses who pioneered the speciality in the UK [62]. Doctors increasingly adopted mechanical IPPV after the Copenhagen polio epidemic. Over the next two decades much was learnt about the physiological effects of IPPV. It was shown to decrease mortality in many types of respiratory failure. Studies in the late 1960s demonstrated that high airway pressures could impair circulatory stability and damage the lungs. Techniques of respiratory support that limited mean and peak pressures reduced these complications. The advent of microprocessor-controlled ventilators facilitated the increased use of a spontaneous breathing component, further decreasing the circulatory effects of IPPV and possibly improving the distribution of ventilation. The use of CAT scans by Luciano Gattinoni and his colleagues in Milan from the 1980s, revolutionised our understanding of the pathophysiological changes accompanying the acute respiratory distress syndrome and other lung diseases [63, 64]. Other studies identified the mechanism of lung damage with IPPV and suggested methods by which such damage could be minimised. Although there is still much to be learnt about mechanisms of lung damage and the effectiveness of the various therapeutic options, there is no doubt that the use of mechanical ventilation can greatly decrease mortality in the seriously ill patient.

References

1. Lassen HCA. A preliminary report on the 1952 epidemic of poliomyelitis in Copenhagen with special reference to the treatment of acute respiratory insufficiency. Lancet. 1953;1:37–41.
2. Wackers GL. Modern anaesthesiological principles for bulbar polio: manual IPPR in the 1952 polio-epidemic in Copenhagen. Acta Anaesthesiol Scand. 1994;38:420–31.
3. Berthelsen PG, Cronquist M. The first intensive care unit in the world. Copenhagen 1953. Acta Anaesthesiol Scand. 2003;47(10):1190–5.
4. Astrup P, Severinghaus JW. The history of blood gases, acids and bases. Copenhagen: Munksgaard; 1986.
5. Beinart J. The Nuffield Department of Anaesthetics 1937–87. Oxford: University Press; 1987. p. 112–8.
6. Woolmer R, Cates JE. Succinylcholine in the treatment of tetanus. Lancet. 1952;2:808–9.
7. Lassen HCA, Bjørnboe M, Ibsen B, Neukirch F. Treatment of tetanus with curarisation, general anaesthesia, and intra-tracheal positive pressure ventilation. Lancet. 1954;267:1040–4.
8. Honey GE, Dwyer BE, Smith AC, Spalding JMK. Tetanus treated with tubocurarine and intermittent positive-pressure respiration. BMJ 1954;2:442–3.
9. Smythe PM, Bull A. Treatment of tetanus neonatorum with intermittent positive pressure respiration. BMJ 1959;2:107–13.

10. Wright R, Sykes MK, Jackson BG, Mann NM, Adams EB. Intermittent positive pressure respiration in tetanus neonatorum. Lancet. 1961;2:678–80.
11. Adams EB, Holloway R, Thambiran AK, Desai SD. Usefulness of intermittent positive-pressure respiration in the treatment of tetanus. Lancet. 1966;2:1176–80.
12. Björk VO, Engström CG. The treatment of ventilatory insufficiency after pulmonary resection with tracheostomy and prolonged artificial respiration. J Thorac Surg. 1955;30:356–67.
13. Norlander OP, Björk VO, Crafoord C, Friberg O, Hohlmdahl M, Swensson A, Widman B. Controlled ventilation in medical practice. Anaesthesia. 1961;16:285–307.
14. Avery EE, Mörch ET, Benson DW. Critically crushed chests: a new method of treatment with continuous mechanical hyperventilation to produce alkalotic apnea and internal pneumatic stabilization. J Thorac Surg. 1956;32:291–311.
15. Pearce DJ. Experiences in a small respiratory unit of a general hospital. With special reference to the treatment of tetanus. Anaesthesia. 1961;16:308–16.
16. Safar P, DeKornfeld TJ, Pearson JW, Redding JS. The intensive care unit. A three year experience in Baltimore city hospitals. Anaesthesia. 1961;16:275–84.
17. Fairley HB. The Toronto General Hospital Respiratory Unit. Anaesthesia. 1961;16:267–74.
18. Marshall J, Spalding JMK. Humidification in positive-pressure respiration for bulbospinal paralysis. Lancet. 1953;265:1022–4.
19. Spence M, Melville AW. A new humidifier. Anesthesiology. 1972;36:89–93.
20. Baskett P, Zorab J, Henning R. The Ruben valve and the AMBU Bag. In: Baskett PJF, Baskett T, editors. Resuscitation greats. Bristol: Clinical Press; 2007. p. 257–61.
21. Mushin WW, Rendell-Baker L, Thompson PW, Mapleson WW. Automatic ventilation of the lungs. 2nd ed. Oxford: Blackwell; 1969 (3rd ed., 1980).
22. Rendell-Baker L, Pettis JL. The development of positive pressure ventilators. In: Atkinson RS, Boulton TB, editors. The History of anaesthesia. Royal Society of Medicine International Congress and Symposium Series. No. 134. 1989. p. 402–25.
23. Mörch ET. History of mechanical ventilation. In: Kirby RR, Banner MJ, Downs JB. Clinical applications of respiratory support. London: Churchill Livingstone; 1990.
24. Tobin MJ. Principles and practice of mechanical ventilation. 2nd ed. New York: McGraw-Hill; 2006.
25. Adams AP. Ventilators for use in anaesthesia. Br J Hosp Med. 1968 Nov; Equipment supplement:23–31.
26. Mathews L, Kalyan Singh RK. Swan-Ganz catheter in hemodynamic monitoring. J Anaesth Clin Pharmacol. 2006;22:335–45.
27. Bashein G, Ivey TD. Con: A pulmonary artery catheter is not indicated for all coronary artery surgery. J Cardiothorac Anesth 1987;1:362–5.
28. Radford EP. Ventilation standards for use in artificial respiration. J Appl Physiol. 1955;7:451–60.
29. Engström C-G, Herzog P. Ventilation nomogram for practical use with the Engström respirator. Acta Chir Scand. 1959; Suppl 245:37.
30. Russell WR, Schuster E, Smith AC, Spalding JMK. Radcliffe respiration pumps. Lancet. 1956;270:539–4.
31. Sykes MK. The East-Radcliffe ventilator adapted for anaesthesia. Br J Anaesth. 1962;34:203–6.
32. Mapleson WW. The effect of changes of lung characteristics on the functioning of automatic ventilators. Anaesthesia. 1962;17:300–14.
33. Loh L, Sykes MK, Chakrabarti MK. The assessment of ventilator performance. Br J Anaesth. 1978;50:63–71.
34. Engström C-G. Treatment of severe cases of respiratory paralysis by the Engström Universal Respirator. BMJ. 1954;2:666–9.
35. Waine TE, Fox DER. A new and versatile closed circuit anaesthetic machine with automatic and manual ventilation. Br J Anaesth. 1962;34:410–6.

36. Manley RW. A new mechanical ventilator. Anaesthesia. 1981;16:317–23.
37. English ICW, Manley REW. The Brompton system of artificial ventilation. Anaesthesia. 1970;25:541–7.
38. Bain JA, Spoerel WE. A streamlined anaesthetic system. Can Anaesth Soc J. 1972;19:426–35.
39. Henville JD, Adams AP. The Bain anaesthetic system: an assessment during controlled ventilation. Anaesthesia. 1976;31:247–56.
40. Adams AP, Henville J. A new generation of anaesthetic ventilators. The Pneupac and Penlon A-P. Anaesthesia. 1977;32:34–40.
41. Trubuhovitch RV. On the very first large-scale, long-term use of IPPV. Crit Care Resusc. 2007;9:91–100.
42. Donald I, Lord J. Augmented respiration studies in atelectasis neonatorum. Lancet. 1953;1:9–16.
43. Goddard RF, Clark JPE, Bennett VR. Newer concepts of infant resuscitation and positive pressure therapy in pediatrics. Am J Dis Child. 1953;89:70–97.
44. Benson F, Celander O, Haglund G, Nilsson L, Paulsen L, Renk L. Positive-pressure respirator treatment of severe pulmonary insufficiency in the newborn infant. Acta Anaesthiol Scand. 1958;2:37–43.
45. Sykes MK. Intermittent positive pressure respiration in tetanus neonatorum. Anaesthesia. 1960;15:401–10.
46. Christie DA, Tansey EM, editors. Origins of neonatal intensive care. (Wellcome Trust Witness Seminar. No 9). London: The Wellcome Trust Centre for the History of Medicine at UCL; 2001.
47. Ashbaugh DG, Bigelow DB, Petty TL, Levine BE. Acute respiratory distress in adults. Lancet. 1967;2:319–23.
48. Harvey S, Young D, Brampton W, et al. Pulmonary artery catheters for adult patients in intensive care. Cochrane Database Syst Rev. 2006 Jul 19;3:CD003408.
49. Nash G, Blennerhassett JB, Pontoppidan H. Pulmonary lesions associated with oxygen therapy and artificial ventilation. N Engl J Med. 1967;276:368–74.
50. Northway WH, Rosan RC, Porter DY. Pulmonary disease following respiratory therapy of hyaline membrane disease. N Engl J Med. 1967;276:357–68.
51. Sykes K, Young JD. Respiratory support in intensive care. 2nd ed. London: BMJ Publications; 1999.
52. Kumar A, Falke KJ, Geffin B, Aldredge CF, Laver MB, Lowenstein E, et al. Continuous positive–pressure ventilation in acute respiratory failure. Effects on hemodymics and lung function. N Engl J Med. 1970;283:1430–6.
53. Kirby RR, Robison E, Shulz J, de Lemos RA. A new pediatric volume ventilator. Anesth Analg. 1971;50:533–7.
54. Kirby RR, Robison E, Shulz J, de Lemos RA. Continuous flow ventilation as an alternative to assisted or controlled ventilation in infants. Anesth Analg. 1972;51:871–5.
55. Lunkenheimer PP, Whimster WF, Sykes MK, editors. High frequency ventilation 20 years of endeavour reviewed: final stress or departure to achievement. Acta Anaesthesiol Scand. 1989;33 Suppl 90.
56. Courtney SE, Durand DJ, Asselin JM, Hudak ML, Aschner JL, Shoemaker CT. High-frequency oscillatory ventilation versus conventional mechanical ventilation for very-low-birth-weight infants. N Engl J Med. 2002;347:643–52.
57. Branson RD. Jack Emerson: notes on his life and contributions to respiratory care. Resp Care. 1998;43:567–8.
58. Lewandowski K. Extracorporeal membrane oxygenation for severe acute respiratory failure. Crit Care. 2000;4:156–68.
59. Kolobow T, Gattinoni L, Tomlinson T, Pierce JE. An alternative to breathing. J Thorac Cardiovasc Surg. 1978;75:261–6.
60. Peek JG, Mugford M, Tiruvoipati R, et al. Efficacy and economic assessment of conventional ventilatory support versus extracorporeal membrane oxygenation for severe adult respiratory failure (CESAR): a multicentre randomised controlled trial. Lancet. 2009;374:1351–63.
61. Girard TD, Bernard GR. Mechanical ventilation in ARDS: a state-of-the-art review. Chest. 2007;131:921–9.
62. Reynolds LA, Tansey EM, editors. History of British intensive care, c. 1950–c. 2000. (Wellcome Witnesses to Twentieth Century Medicine, Vol. 42). London: School of History, Queen Mary, University of London; 2011 (ISBN: 978 0902238756).
63. Gattinoni L, Chiumello D, Cressoni M, Valenza F. Pulmonary computed tomography and adult respiratory distress syndrome. Swiss Med Wkly. 2005;135:169–74.
64. Gattinoni L, Caironi P, Pelosi P, Goodman LR. What has computed tomography taught us about the acute respiratory distress syndrome? Am J Resp Crit Care Med. 2001;164:1701–11.

A History of Intensive Care Medicine

58

Jukka Takala

Summary

Most historians believe that Bjørn Ibsen's response to the 1952 polio epidemic in Copenhagen led to intensive care medicine (ICM) and intensive care units (ICUs). The epidemic involved thousands of patients, many dying from respiratory failure. Ibsen convinced his skeptical colleagues to concentrate all patients with respiratory failure in one area and institute tracheostomy and manual positive pressure ventilation in these patients. Attempts to understand the pathophysiology of respiratory failure and monitor its treatment accelerated the development of blood gas analysis by Poul Astrup.

Modern ICUs arose from the application of the concepts of managing respiratory failure from polio; intermittent positive pressure ventilation with mechanical ventilators; and locating all human resources and patients requiring high level care into a single location. Mechanical ventilation was an important theme, but the French, particularly Rapin in the 1960s, also focused on infections, with the world following suit decades later.

Many advances accompanied the development of ICUs. Cournand's work in the late 1940s suggested that positive end-expiratory pressure (PEEP) decreased cardiac output. However, in 1967, Ashbaugh and Petty reported that PEEP corrected severe hypoxemia during mechanical ventilation in patients with hypoxemia refractory to mechanical ventilation without PEEP, probably by expanding otherwise collapsed bronchi or alveoli.

The evolution of ICM in the 1970s and 1980s led to recognition of multiple organ failure. Patients now survived the acute phase of single organ failure but subsequently died from a poorly defined but clinically recognizable syndrome of failure of several organs, with sepsis as a postulated underlying cause. Knaus suggested that chronic diseases, combined with the severity of physiologic abnormalities during the first 24 hrs of intensive care, could predict outcome. Thus was born the APACHE scoring system in 1981, and then APACHE II, in 1984. Other scoring systems followed.

Until the early 1980s, research in intensive care medicine developed slowly. Large randomized controlled trials towards the end of the 1980s presaged the 1990s application of evidence-based medicine. Notwithstanding the high hopes placed on large randomized controlled trials, their results in intensive care medicine have largely been disappointing; new therapeutic interventions have not improved outcome. Some have even been harmful, and some positive results have not been reproducible. Perhaps these difficulties should have been expected, considering the complexity of underlying clinical problems in ICU patients. Several factors complicated ICM: poorly definable syndromes rather than clear-cut diseases, the heterogeneity of disease severity and treatment, and poorly understood but highly relevant interactions between treatments and underlying pathophysiology. There is still much work to do.

In the Beginnings

As a medical specialty or special area of competence, Intensive Care Medicine (ICM) is young—even compared with anesthesiology, one of its essential parents and partner specialties. Surgery, internal medicine, and pulmonology have also volunteered for parenthood. The present place of ICM in the spectrum of medical specialties varies in different countries. In some, it is an independent specialty. In others, it is a superspecialty open to multiple base specialties, a subspecialty anchored to a specific basic specialty, or integrated within a specialty (e.g., anesthesiology). Some presently regard it as a special competence, based on a common skill-mix acquired by a competence-based training program open to physicians from multiple specialties. How did we get there?

It is tempting to outline the history of ICM based on "firsts". However, in trying to do this, I found myself confronted by difficulties with definitions, conflicting dates, controversial and perhaps competing claims, and geographical and cultural bias. In contrast to the "firsts" of say, ether anesthesia, open heart surgery, or the discovery of penicillin, intensive care is defined by care processes and organization—issues of continuing importance to ICM. ICM can be defined as prevention, reduction, and

J. Takala (✉)
Department of Intensive Care Medicine, University Hospital Bern (Inselspital) and University of Bern, 3010 Bern, Switzerland
e-mail: jukka.takala@insel.ch

E. I Eger II et al. (eds.), *The Wondrous Story of Anesthesia*, DOI 10.1007/978-1-4614-8441-7_58, © Edmond I Eger, MD 2014

Fig. 58.1 British nurse Florence Nightingale during the Crimean War in the 1850s, is credited by many with having established the first intensive care unit. (Florence Nightingale (1820–1910) in the Military Hospital at Scutari during the Crimean War, 1856 (color litho) by Joseph-Austin Benwell (fl.1865–86). National Army Museum, London/ The Bridgeman Art Library. Nationality/copyright status: English/out of copyright.)

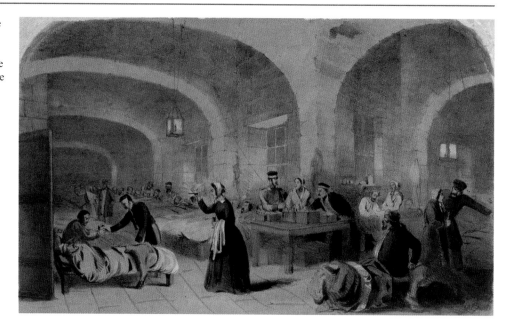

removal of the temporary risk of death. A concentrated investment of human, material, and technological resources for monitoring and treatment are employed to defeat death and morbidity. This view of ICM facilitates tracing its evolution.

Although the evolution of ICM took place just recently— the last half century, selecting the individuals associated with major contributions is difficult, partly because of the problem of fairly ranking of colleagues still actively contributing and practicing, and partly because of the evolutionary rather than revolutionary development of ICM. I have therefore approached the evolution in terms of ideas, themes and concepts, naming only some of the individuals involved. Due to this essayist's admitted bias, some of those who undoubtedly should have been included (either based on their own view or that of others) have been omitted, whereas other less famous individuals have been included to illustrate specific aspects of the story.

Cohorting and the Basic Concepts of High-Dependency Care

The need to treat war casualties or victims of major deadly epidemics, probably prompted the idea of concentrating cohorts of sick patients to enhance their monitoring and care. Many regard Florence Nightingale, the famous British nurse, as the first to establish an ICU (Fig. 58.1) [1]. During the Crimean war in the 1850s, she collected the most severely injured casualties in one area to observe them more effectively, and intervene when needed.

Some authors refer to an earlier postoperative ward in the Newcastle Infirmary, England, around 1801, with "two five-bed rooms adjacent to the operating theatre", reserved for the sickest patients and those recovering from surgery [2]. If the latter is correct, then the first efforts in high-dependency care preceded both Nightingale's efforts and the introduction of general anesthesia by several decades. Recovery rooms for patients undergoing ether anesthesia were introduced in the 1870s, in the Massachusetts General Hospital in the US. These facilities probably provided immediate care after anesthesia, and thus cannot be regarded as predecessors of ICUs. Postoperative high-dependency care units appeared on both sides of the Atlantic in the 1920s in parallel with the development of more complex surgical procedures.

Early Steps in Technological (R)evolution

In addition to the concentration of human resources, the application of technology and use of invasive therapeutic interventions have been associated with ICM. General anesthesia, airway management, mechanical ventilation and vascular access in the nineteenth and early twentieth centuries developed in parallel, and independently rather than evolving in association with high-dependency care concepts. Nevertheless, these parallel developments laid the foundation for ICM as we know it today. Ake Grenvik, one of the pioneers of critical care medicine in the US, and Michael Pinsky recently reviewed the evolution of the ICU as a clinical center, and ICM as a discipline, using the development of technology as the main reference [3]. According to Grenvik, "intensive care medicine owes its roots to the support of failing ventilation."

If so, perhaps it began with Vesalius, who described the use of positive pressure ventilation in the sixteenth century (a partial translation of the original reference "*De Humani Corporis Fabrica*" by Vesalius is available on the Internet at http://www.ncbi.nlm.nih.gov/pmc/articles/PMC1965933/pdf/bullnyacadmed00859-0008.pdf):

> "*That life may in a manner of speaking be restored to the animal, an opening must be attempted in the trunk of the trachea, into which a tube of reed or cane should be put; you will then blow into this, so that the lung may rise again and the animal take in air. Indeed with a slight breath in the case of the living animal, the lung will swell to the full extent of the thoracic cavity, and the heart will become strong and exhibit a wondrous variety of motions.*"

It was then forgotten for centuries.

New trends and techniques in thoracic surgery in the early twentieth century triggered the next major steps in technology related to sustained artificial ventilation. Ferdinand Sauerbruch (1875–1951)—probably as notorious as he was famous for his surgical skills—influenced the evolution of future intensive care technologies [4] (Fig. 58.2). In 1904 he used a subatmospheric surgical chamber to inflate the lungs of patients undergoing thoracic surgery, but he forbade the addition of positive pressure ventilation. The patient's head was outside the chamber, with the neck tightly sealed, and the patient's body and the surgical team were inside the chamber. This created conditions equivalent to continuous positive airway pressure (CPAP), maintaining lung volume and supporting oxygenation by preventing atelectasis and thereby shunting, while the chest was open. Although the lungs might be inflated, diaphragmatic movement produced minimal ventilation when the chest was opened, and supplementary oxygen was necessary to prevent cyanosis—indicating progressive hypoventilation and increased alveolar pCO_2. Sauerbruch thus advanced the development of future intensive care technology by demonstrating some of the beneficial effects of CPAP. At the same time, he may also have delayed other developments, most notably the use of tracheal intubation, positive pressure ventilation, and, as we will see later, vascular access. The sub-atmospheric surgical chamber shows Sauerbruch as the brilliant surgeon and innovator; the hindering of tracheal intubation and vascular access exemplify Sauerbruch's negative influence.

Franz Kuhn (1866–1929), a German surgeon, described orotracheal intubation in 1902–1911 [5]. Others proposing tracheal intubation at the end of the nineteenth century included Karl Maydl (1853–1903), a Prague surgeon, and the Viennese physician Viktor Eisenmenger (1864–1932), but their ideas did not receive the attention that they deserved. Sauerbruch vigorously opposed the use of orotracheal intubation, and effectively delayed its introduction to clinical practice. Orotracheal intubation came into wide-spread use in the 1940s after the introduction of curare into anesthesia.

In the late 1920s, the first device suitable for prolonged artificial ventilation, the iron lung, was invented. Unlike

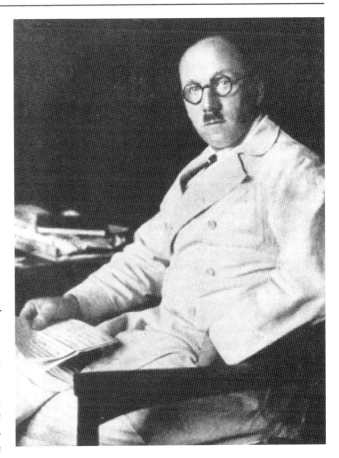

Fig. 58.2 In the early 1900s, German surgeon Ferdinand Sauerbruch invented a subatmospheric surgical chamber to prevent lung collapse in patients undergoing thoracic surgery, thereby demonstrating the benefits of continuous positive airway pressure. [Photo originally published as Plate 5 in *The Dismissal: the Last Days of Ferdinand Sauerbruch, Surgeon*, by Jurgen Thorwald. Thames & Hudson: London, 1961. Original copy owned by the National Library of Australia. Instructions also say to include persistent identifier or call number, possibly 610.92 SAU (2555658)]

the inventors of the surgical negative pressure chamber, the inventors of the iron lung—Philip Drinker and Louis Shaw—were interested in more than a short-term solution: their 1929 paper was appropriately titled "An apparatus for the prolonged administration of artificial respiration" [6]. John Emerson, the founder of the JH Emerson Co further developed their invention for larger-scale commercial production [7]. The iron lung (or tank respirator) enclosed the patient within a metal cylinder up to the head and neck, with an airtight collar surrounding the neck. Cyclic intermittent negative pressure around the body within the cylinder effected ventilation. Major problems in long-term use related to reliability, respiratory tract care, accessing the abdomen and thorax and comfort. Cuirass negative pressure ventilators were a modification of the iron lung, restricted to enclosing only the thorax. Although the cuirass allowed better access and was far less expensive, it was less effective as a ventilator, and nursing care and comfort remained problematic.

Neither device solved the crucial problem of the patient who could not maintain their own airway.

Major developments in vascular access paralleled the early steps of ventilatory support. The young German surgeon-in-training Werner Forssmann (1904–1979) summarized the problems related to the lack of central vascular access in the introduction of his 1929 paper "*Die Sondierung des rechten Herzens*" [8] (*Right heart catheterization*; freely translated from German by me): "In acute dangerous situations, where the patient is at risk of cardiac arrest, i.e. by acute collapse, in cardiac failure, or through complications of anesthesia or poisoning, rapid treatment with drugs locally is necessary. In such cases, attempting an intracardiac injection is often the only possibility to save the patient." Forssmann then described the complications of cardiac puncture and proposed right heart catheterization as the solution [9]. He tested the feasibility of such a procedure during autopsies. Then, with the help of a "friendly colleague", Forssmann advanced a well-lubricated ureteral catheter via his right brachial vein to a depth of 35 cm and verified the intrathoracic position of the catheter using X-ray. At this stage he broke off the experiment at the urging of the colleague, who considered the procedure too risky. One week later, Forssmann advanced a 65-cm-long ureteric catheter through his own left brachial vein to its full length, verifying the catheter tip in the right atrium by chest X-ray—he was disappointed that he did not choose a longer catheter. He then described the first clinical use in a patient in severe septic shock who initially responded favorably to fluids and drugs but died after a few hours. Sauerbruch rewarded Forssmann by firing him. Undeterred, Forssmann continued to develop right heart catheterization and pulmonary angiography as a diagnostic tool.

According to Forssmann [9], O Klein made the first measurements of cardiac output using a right heart catheter and the Fick principle in 1930 [10]. Next, Andre Cournand advanced his special catheters into the pulmonary circulation in the late 1930s and early 1940s, and shared the Nobel Prize in physiology/medicine with Forssmann in 1956 [11]. It took more than 40 years after Forssmann's initial experiments to convert these tools to practical monitoring devices.

Polio Epidemics Jump Start Modern ICM

An outbreak of polio in California in the late 1940s resulted in many patients needing tank and cuirass ventilators and intermittent positive pressure ventilation. There is inconsistency in the reported numbers of patients that were treated with the different methods. Albert Bower and Ray Bennett reported their experiences with ventilator support in nearly 300 cases in 1948 [12].

The Californian epidemic was vastly overshadowed by the catastrophic polio epidemics in the early 1950s prompting

the next important technological and clinical developments in prolonged mechanical ventilation. The response to the epidemics, particularly the 1952 epidemic in Copenhagen, led to the development of ICM.

Numerous authors have debated details surrounding the Copenhagen polio epidemics and the roles of the various players [13–15]. The doctors, nurses, and other personnel confronted with the initial high mortality, and the large number of new patients arriving daily, had priorities that precluded precise record keeping. It is also meaningless to debate the "firsts". The heroic efforts of individuals worldwide, especially Bjørn Ibsen, the pioneering intensivist [13–16], have been described in detail, and are also surrounded by folklore. I will summarize the framework, give an approximate temporal sequence of events, and then try to explain why the Copenhagen polio epidemic was so special and why it had such a large impact on the evolution of ICM.

As detailed elsewhere in this book, the late 1940s was an era of rapid development in anesthesiology. Departments of Anesthesia had been established in major hospitals, and the first positive pressure ventilators had been introduced for perioperative use during thoracic surgery. The role of anesthetists in Europe was undergoing a major change. European anesthetists visited the US, going especially to the Massachusetts General Hospital for training. Concurrently, various anesthesia-related activities commenced in Europe—particularly in Sweden. A commission for future organization of anesthetic services in Copenhagen recommended the establishment of independent departments of anesthesia for each hospital. The World Health Organization founded the Anaesthesiology Centre Copenhagen, in May 1950, drawing leading anesthetists from the UK, Sweden and the USA to teach in a one-year anesthesia training course. The "*primus motor*" ("prime mover") of this course was Erik Husfeld, a thoracic surgeon, who served as the course director from the first course until 1973. Thus, perhaps fortuitously, there was already a considerable focus in Copenhagen, on this "specialty in the making [14]."

The scale of the epidemic, and the ultimate success in saving lives in Copenhagen, received much publicity. The struggle with polio elsewhere is less well known. During the polio epidemic in many other countries, medical communities endured frustrating experiences treating the severely paralyzed patients. In postwar Europe, resources were scarce, and innovative solutions were badly needed. In Germany, Alfred Dönhart, a pulmonologist from Hamburg, together with the Dräger company, converted old submarine torpedo-tubes into iron lungs (Fig. 58.3). Dräger became a major producer of ventilators, anesthesia machines, and other medical equipment.

In California, clinician Bower and engineer Ray Bennett described a comprehensive approach to the patient with respiratory failure, in their 1950 [9] paper reporting the results of their treatment of more than 70 polio patients with

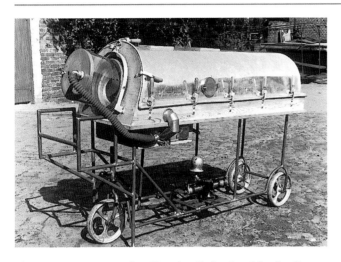

Fig. 58.3 A prototype of an "iron lung", developed by the German firm Dräger in 1947. (Courtesy of Drägerwerk AG & Co. KgaA.)

their combined approach, reporting improved outcomes with positive pressure ventilation in comparison with the use of the tank ventilator alone. They developed different types of positive pressure devices, primarily for use in combination with the tank ventilator, but also capable of supporting ventilation via mask during nursing care. Why they insisted on the combined use of the tank ventilator and the positive pressure device is unclear. They also developed tracheostomy tubes specifically for prolonged assisted ventilation. Blood gas analyses were used to assess the adequacy of ventilation. Humidifiers, monitoring devices and alarm systems were added. Special mechanical mattresses were developed to prevent pressure sores.

Until recently, these accomplishments received surprisingly little attention, although Ibsen, the pioneer in the subsequent Copenhagen epidemics, gave Bower and Bennett the credit they deserved. Bennett established a company manufacturing positive pressure ventilators, and the successor of his original company (Puritan-Bennett), became a market leader in intensive care ventilators worldwide.

The Danish polio epidemic began in August 1952, and by the end in in April 1953, almost 5700 polio cases had been registered throughout the country. In Copenhagen, Blegdam Hospital received many of the more seriously ill victims, including 345 patients with either breathing or swallowing difficulties or both. During the second half of August 1952, the number of cases, especially those with paralysis, increased at an alarming rate. Eighty-seven percent of patients with bulbar polio (27 of 31) died. Most physicians incorrectly thought that these patients died from irreversible cerebral lesions of polio. Tank or cuirass negative pressure ventilators were used to support ventilation in patients with respiratory paralysis, but only one tank and 6 cuirass respirators were available.

The high mortality rate and rapid increase in new cases persuaded the chief of the hospital and professor of epidemiology, HC Lassen, to consult with Bjørn Ibsen—an anesthetist. Aware of the reports of Brower and Bennett from the California polio outbreak, Ibsen became convinced that the patients suffered from progressive severe hypercapnia, not irreversible brain injury. He believed that the high blood CO_2 content resulted from hypoventilation and not metabolic alkalosis, as was thought at the time. Ibsen convinced his skeptical colleagues to undertake a trial in a test patient, with tracheostomy and manual positive pressure ventilation. After initial difficulties (it was initially impossible to inflate the patient's lungs due to secretions and bronchospasm, followed by hypovolemic shock), the patient's condition was stabilized. Temporarily transferring the patient back to the cuirass resulted in cyanosis, which disappeared on returning to positive pressure ventilation. This convinced Lassen and his colleagues that Ibsen was correct. The new strategy was then applied to all polio patients with respiratory failure. This was no simple task, since at the peak of the epidemic, 30 to 50 new patients per day were admitted to Blegdams, 6 to 12 with breathing or swallowing problems or both. 1500 students were enlisted over the course of the epidemic to manually ventilate the patient's lungs around the clock. [17] The new strategy decreased mortality from 90 to 25 % in those severe cases. The personal memoir of one of the student "ventilators" gives special insight into the circumstances in Copenhagen [17].

I believe that the success of Ibsen, Lassen, and co-workers illustrates the approaches needed to solve problems in critically ill patients. First, Ibsen used clinical observations based on sound physiologic concepts. Second, he introduced a novel application of existing methodology. Third, he developed a treatment strategy. Fourth, he convinced the decision makers to supply substantial resources. Fifth, a multidisciplinary team was used. Sixth, the logistics necessary for the prolonged treatment of large numbers of patients were established. Seventh, the outcomes of the new strategy were carefully assessed.

The use of positive pressure ventilator support for polio patients with respiratory failure spread rapidly in Scandinavia, continental Europe, and the United Kingdom. It stimulated the development of positive pressure ventilators. The prototype of the Engström ventilator had already been tested in Copenhagen, and was further developed by Carl-Gunnar Engström before the 1953 Swedish polio epidemic. [15] Engström's company became a major ventilator manufacturer, and was subsequently acquired by Datex—the Finnish manufacturer of anesthesia and intensive care technology and later by General Electric.

The need to understand the pathophysiology of respiratory failure, and monitor its treatment, accelerated the development of blood gas analysis technology. Analysis of blood gases in the early 1950s was applied during the Copenhagen polio epidemic, but required a glass electrode to measure blood pH, a Van Slyke apparatus to measure CO_2 content, and application of the Henderson-Hasselbalch equation to calculate pCO_2. To circumvent this cumbersome and labor-intensive analysis, Poul Astrup introduced a new approach based on the linear relationship between blood pH and the logarithm of the pCO_2 [18]. This was subsequently used by the Radiometer company—a leading producer of blood gas analyzers today. A more detailed description of this development appears in Chapter 41.

ICUs Arise in the Post-polio Era

Modern ICUs arose in the wake of the polio epidemic. It was not a "big bang" but rather an evolution in which the concepts of managing respiratory failure from polio were applied to a wider patient population: providing intermittent positive pressure ventilation with mechanical ventilators, concentrating human resources, and congregating patients requiring intensive care, thus enabling continuous treatment and monitoring. Among many "firsts", it appears that the first ICU started at Kommunehospitalet, the Municipal Hospital of Copenhagen, in December 1953, under Ibsen's leadership.

In the next decade, ICUs developed in Europe, the US, and Australasia. The new possibilities for prolonged mechanical support of breathing made mechanical ventilation and management of respiratory problems a hallmark of ICUs. In parallel, it became apparent that concentrating human and technological resources covering a range of special skills enhanced care for severely ill patients.

This evolution is evident in the National Academy of Sciences—National Research Council Committee on Anesthesia's "Workshop on Intensive Care Units", held 14 October 1963 [19]. The pioneers attending the meeting pointed out problems related to intensive care that remain challenging today: the role of different specialties in the treatment of patients with multidisciplinary problems; the need for special training of nurses and doctors; and the need for attending specialists to be directly responsible for patient care.

John Kinney, a future pioneer in metabolic research in the critically ill [20] at Columbia Presbyterian Medical Center, New York, pointed out that no single physician can attend to a critically ill patient 24 hours a day for 5–6 days. Yet, this was an average length of stay in many units then, and now, necessitating shared responsibility—a fact still denied in many hospitals today. Henning Pontoppidan from the Massachusetts General Hospital, also best known for his contributions to management of acute respiratory failure [21], presented one of the first patient classification systems relevant for ICM. He defined "critical care" as care of patients actually or potentially needing life-saving devices or activities,

and needing highly skilled nursing care and close and frequent, if not constant, nursing observation. Peter Safar, who developed ICM in Baltimore and Pittsburgh, summarized the prerequisites for smooth functioning of intensive care: interdepartmental cooperation, well-defined responsibilities and authority, efficient design of ICU facilities, and standardization of certain procedures—principles that are all applicable today.

The topics discussed at the 1963 "Workshop on Intensive Care Units" reflected important international developments in intensive care. An influx of European anesthesiologists facilitated the adoption of the innovations of Ibsen and his colleagues in the US, after an initial delay, European anesthetists had already established connections in the US in the late 1940s, through training in anesthesiology, particularly at the Massachusetts General Hospital (MGH). Henrik Bendixen came to Boston to start his anesthesia residency in 1954, having graduated in Copenhagen in 1951. Henning Pontoppidan graduated one year later and also came to the MGH. Myron Laver and John Hedley-White shared Bendixen's and Pontopiddan's interests in respiratory and cardiovascular pathophysiology. This group of innovators produced physiologic and clinical research that established the basic tenets underlying mechanical ventilation in the operating room and in ICM [22–23]. They helped found the first respiratory ICU at the MGH in 1966.

Until the mid-1960s, mechanical ventilation with continuous positive pressure was avoided, largely because Cournand's early work in the late 1940s indicated that continuous positive pressure decreased cardiac output. But then David Ashbaugh and Thomas Petty published "*Acute Respiratory Distress in Adults*" (ARDS) in the *Lancet* in 1967 [24], reportedly after rejection by three major American journals. They described the use of positive end-expiratory pressure (PEEP) to correct severe hypoxemia during mechanical ventilation, in 12 patients with hypoxemia refractory to mechanical ventilation without PEEP. This led several groups of researchers, including the Boston group, to study the underlying mechanisms. By the early 1970s Pontopiddan, Laver, and co-workers established that the functional residual capacity of the lungs in ARDS was dramatically reduced, and that it could, at least in part, be restored by applying continuous positive pressure [25]. More Europeans came to Boston, among them Konrad Falke from Germany, who after participating in some of the important studies on PEEP [26], became a leader in using extracorporeal lung support in Europe, and a long-term Editor-in-Chief of *Intensive Care Medicine*.

ICM Evolution in Europe

Europeans who went to the US defined much of the evolution of ICM in North America, and ICM in Europe profited from knowledge contributed by intensivists returning from the US. Still, the 1950s to the 1970s produced less interaction between English-speaking and non-English-speaking medical communities than today—partly due to language and cultural barriers.

In Germany, the first ICUs appeared in the late 1950s [27], well after 1953 reports of a large case series of patients requiring prolonged ventilation using the iron lung. Mechanical ventilation was an important theme in France as well—however, the French focused early on infections, with the rest of the world following suit decades later. Creative individuals in France had a decisive impact. One such person was Maurice Rapin in Paris who along with his colleagues applied mechanical ventilation to a broad spectrum of patients. His first publications on the use of prolonged mechanical ventilation stem from 1955, in patients with tetanus [28]. They were followed by applications in post-pneumonectomy respiratory failure [29], various paralytic conditions including polio, and postoperative respiratory failure of various etiologies. In 1958, he published two papers outlining the problems of respiratory failure in patients with chronic obstructive pulmonary disease (COPD) [30, 31]. Published in French, neither paper received the attention it deserved. Rapin then published several papers on barbiturate intoxication, and in 1960, his first paper on septic shock. In 1963, he described the risks of nosocomial infections ("Infectious complications in respiratory resuscitation. Etiological, symptomatic and therapeutic data") [32].

Rapin placed an increasing emphasis on infections, with intoxications and tetanus as his "hobbies". In 1967, he played a central role in organizing and publishing a Round Table report on "Indications and limits in medical resuscitation"—a first step in the continuing strong French tradition in ethics issues—published in French. At the time he had authored and co-authored nearly 200 papers on various aspects of ICM—all in French—a loss for the non-French-speaking medical community! Rapin and the institution he developed, subsequently produced several internationally prominent French intensivist-scientists, who made major contributions to the scientific basis of modern ICM: Francois Lemaire (respiratory failure, ethics), Christian Brun-Buisson (infectious diseases issues in intensive care), and Laurent Brochard (artificial ventilation). Both Lemaire and Brochard held the Editor-in-Chief position for *Intensive Care Medicine*.

Shifting from Lungs Alone to the Circulation: The 1970s

A conceptual turning point in the approach to caring for patients with acute respiratory failure and ARDS was the concept of "best" PEEP, published in 1975 by Peter Suter, H.

Barrie Fairley and Michael Isenberg [33]. Fairley pioneered respiratory intensive care at the Toronto General Hospital Respiratory Unit, a multidisciplinary respiratory ICU established in 1958 [34]. In the mid 1960s, Fairley moved to San Francisco, and in the early 1970s, Suter, a Swiss combat pilot and physician, joined Fairley's group as a research fellow. According to Fairley, and described in his "how it really happened" report in 2001, [35] they showed that "the level of PEEP applied during mechanical ventilation could be adjusted in each patient to optimize the balance between recruitment of atelectatic lung and overdistension, and that this…coincided with optimal pulmonary gas exchange". Their study should be seen as a fundamental change in thinking in intensive care, shifting from a focus on single organ failure (lung), to an emphasis on the body as a whole: for the first time, pulmonary gas exchange was considered relative to whole body oxygen delivery.

Cournand used right heart catheterization to study the physiology and pathophysiology of the circulation. Catheterization of the right and left heart was used routinely in the 1950s and 1960s. In 1967, Jeremy Swan, a California cardiologist, conceived of a catheter that would "sail through the heart", while standing on a beach in Santa Monica watching sailboats. He and his cardiology colleague, William Ganz, described their eponymous catheter (Swan-Ganz pulmonary artery catheter) in 1970 [36]. Edwards Laboratories introduced the catheter commercially, and it was rapidly adopted for clinical monitoring in intensive care, and later during surgery. This invention facilitated bedside assessment and monitoring of cardiovascular and respiratory function, and oxygen transport.

The paper of Suter et al. [33], one of the first studies in intensive care using the Swan-Ganz catheter to measure oxygen transport, produced a new concept—that lung mechanics, gas exchange, and cardiovascular function interacted. Their finding that individuals differed in their responses to specific PEEP levels, indicated the need for individual titration based on physiologic response instead of a "one-size-fits-all" approach.

If studies in the 1950s and 1960s focused on mechanical ventilation, those in the 1970s and 1980s focused on circulation and cardiovascular function. Guyton, Cournand, Starling, and other twentieth Century physiologists established the central physiologic concepts of cardiovascular function and pathophysiology in the preceding decades. Subsequent pioneers in ICM began clinical research in cardiovascular pathophysiology in the 1950s and 1960s. Max Weil, a Californian cardiologist-internist (Fig. 58.4), and William Shoemaker, a Chicago surgeon (Fig. 58.5), investigated various types of shock in the mid 1950s. They recognized the importance of continuous monitoring to understand the pathophysiology of cardiovascular problems in unstable, critically ill patients. Both applied methods normally

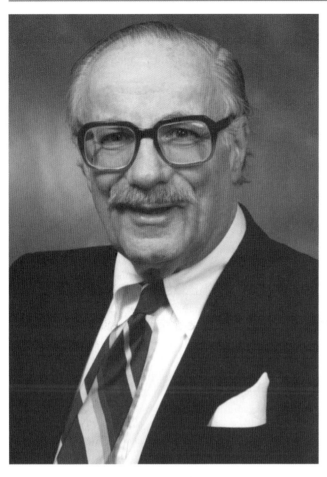

Fig. 58.4 California cardiologist-internist Max Harry Weil, a founder and first President of the Society of Critical Care Medicine (SCCM). (Courtesy of the Weil Institute of Critical Care Medicine.)

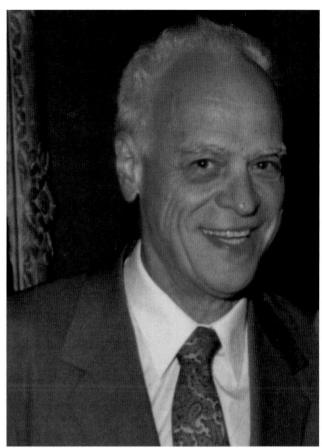

Fig. 58.5 Chicago surgeon William Shoemaker, an SCCM founder and the first Editor-in-Chief of SCCM's journal, *Critical Care Medicine.* (Reproduced with permission of the publisher. Courtesy of the Society of Critical Care Medicine.)

available in the physiology laboratory, such as cardiac output measurement using dye dilution at the bedside—even before the new Swan-Ganz pulmonary artery catheter was available [37, 38]. Once the Swan-Ganz catheter was marketed, both applied it enthusiastically in patient care.

Weil's contribution to the evolution of ICM extended beyond shock [39], cardiovascular management, and cardiopulmonary resuscitation. In 1970, he and 28 other like-minded physicians founded the Society of Critical Care Medicine (SCCM), becoming the first President. Many of his trainees became leaders in ICM. Shoemaker was also an SCCM founder and President, and the Editor-in-Chief of SCCM's journal, *Critical Care Medicine*—a post he held for 18 years, from the first issue in 1973. Shoemaker left Chicago and moved via New York to California, where he studied oxygen transport variables as therapeutic targets for high-risk surgical patients [40–43]. In large-scale observational studies [40–42], he found that survivors had greater oxygen delivery and oxygen consumption values than non-survivors. He assumed that the lower values in non-survivors caused an oxygen debt. Using survivors' oxygen delivery

values as targets led to improved outcomes in high-risk surgical patients [43]. Although his studies may lack the methodological rigor expected today, he established the concept that avoiding tissue hypoperfusion improved outcome in at-risk patients. This concept led to several studies using "the Shoemaker goals", with controversial results. Studies using a pre-emptive approach in high-risk patients mostly supported the original concept. But studies using "supranormal" oxygen transport targets in patients with cardiovascular or other organ function instability usually failed to improve, or even worsened outcome. Shoemaker left us the notion that it is best to prevent clinical instability, rather than intervene after instability has ensued.

The enthusiasm for invasively assessing the circulation had its down-side. Invasive hemodynamic monitoring was used to excess—partly from revenue-driven motivation. The pendulum swung to the other extreme: after the enthusiasm of the 1970s and 1980s, intensivists in the 1990s called for a moratorium on invasive hemodynamic monitoring. Since then, a new balance has started to develop, and despite new, less invasive monitoring technologies,

Fig. 58.6 Max Harry Weil (center, with stethoscope in pocket) and his many protégés, including Jean-Louis Vincent (second from the left in the second row). (Courtesy of Jean-Louis Vincent.)

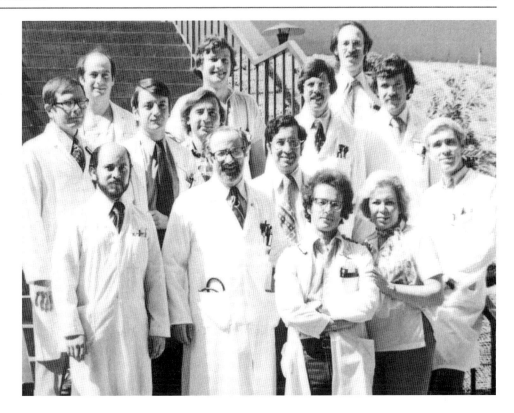

invasive hemodynamic monitoring will return to the armamentarium of the intensivist. Ironically, Weil and Shoemaker actively advocated less invasive monitoring technologies in the 1980s—not to replace, but to complement invasive methods.

A New Generation in the 1980s

The concepts of organization of intensive care advocated by the pioneers became established in many institutions in the 1970s and 1980s. Safar moved to Pittsburgh to become the founding chairman of the department of anesthesiology and first director of the ICU at the Presbyterian University Hospital. Grenvik joined Safar in Pittsburgh in 1968– one more European to become a leader in ICM in the US and internationally [44]. Grenvik became Safar's successor in the ICU, and established a major academic interdisciplinary training program in ICM in Pittsburgh. This led to the formation of the first independent academic Department of Critical Care Medicine in the US. When he retired after 40 years of service, Grenvik had educated more than 400 trainees, many of whom became major figures in ICM.

Meanwhile, in Europe, a new generation of intensivists evolved—some with clinical and research training in the US, others home grown. In 1982, a group of enthusiastic young intensivists founded the European Society of Intensive Care Medicine (ESICM), among them Peter Suter, who became the first President. In a long career in clinical and academic

ICM, he held several leadership positions, including the Presidency of the Swiss Academy of Medical Sciences. He has helped shape ICM in Europe and currently contributes to health care reform in Switzerland. Another founding member was Jean-Louis Vincent, who trained with Max Weil (Fig. 58.6). An entrepreneur with endless energy and wit, he founded numerous journals and imported Weil's successful model of an annual scientific meeting to Brussels. With 30 years of continuing success, his meeting has become an institution and is one of the largest intensive care meetings in the world [45].

Luciano Gattinoni was also a founder of ESICM. Gattinoni applied extracorporeal lung support in the late 1970s; pioneered the use of computed tomography for studies of lung pathophysiology in ARDS [46]; and established a large network for multicenter trials in Italy. If he ever tired of ICM, he could switch at any time to professional piano playing!

Scoring Systems to Assess Prognosis

The 1980s and 1990s saw fundamental changes in ICM, particularly the development of severity of illness scoring systems, the concept of multiorgan failure or dysfunction as a syndrome with high mortality, and the concept of sepsis as an entity with high mortality, including a new approach to grading sepsis. Towards the end of the 1980s, large randomized controlled trials arrived, followed by the appearance of evidence-based medicine in the 1990s.

ICM is one of the pioneer specialties in medicine in assessing prognosis, outcome, and resource utilization—probably due to the cost of resources and survival from immediately life-threatening conditions as its most important outcome. William Knaus from Washington, DC, is the undisputed pioneer in severity-of-illness assessment and outcome prediction. In 1974, anesthesiologist David Cullen at the MGH, and surgeon Joseph Civetta at the University of Miami, introduced their Therapeutic Intervention Scoring System (TISS) for assessment of resource utilization, with the idea that the TISS could also reflect the severity of illness [47]. Knaus went further, suggesting that the underlying chronic diseases plus the severity of physiologic abnormalities during the first 24 hrs of intensive care could be used to predict outcome. Thus was born the first APACHE scoring system, introduced in 1981 [48] and its revision, APACHE II, in 1984. Others followed: the European SAPS system, developed by Jean-Roger LeGall from France, and the MPM system of Stanley Lemeshow from Boston. The various systems now extend to third to fourth generations. All use the same principle: assess severity of illness based on statistical models created and validated in large patient populations. These systems have helped us understand the case mix of ICU patients, facilitated comparisons of performance between ICUs, and provided a basis for classification of patients for clinical trials.

The evolution of ICM led to a new problem: multiple organ failure (MOF), multiple systems organ failure (MSOF), multiorgan dysfunction syndrome (MODS) ... various names (and acronyms!) for the same problem. Patients who previously died from single organ failure survived the acute phase and progressed to a poorly defined but clinically recognizable syndrome of simultaneous or sequential failure of several organs—a syndrome with high mortality. Shoemaker noted this in a 1973 editorial [49]. By the 1980s, the syndrome was well recognized, thanks to the work of surgeon-intensivists like Arthur Baue and Donald Fry. MOF was described as "a syndrome of the 1980s".

Surgeon-intensivists observed MOF in surgical patients concurrently displaying infectious complications, and suspected that MOF reflected uncontrolled infection—although a causal relationship could not be proven. In parallel, intensivists with non-surgical specialty backgrounds had also connected severe infections to the pathogenesis of organ failures and mortality. In the 1980s, the first large sepsis trials, using new agents such as endotoxin- and other antibodies were completed. Definitions of sepsis were perceived as being too vague and too variable between trials. Roger Bone, a Chicago-based medical intensivist and researcher, with a special interest in ARDS and sepsis, proposed new definitions for sepsis in a series of opinion papers [50, 51]. Additional motivation to search for better definitions was the increasing number of new drugs needing assessment in clinical trials. The American College of Chest Physicians and the Society of Critical Care Medicine held a consensus conference, launching new definitions of sepsis, severe sepsis, septic shock, multiple organ dysfunction syndrome, and systemic inflammatory response syndrome (SIRS) [52]. Although these new definitions helped to better conceptualize sepsis, they were not universally accepted, and consensus conferences often featured disagreements as much as consensus. As Bone et al. pointed out in an accompanying editorial, one of the items on the agenda was "to provide maximum flexibility in classifying patients for identification and treatment in both the clinical and research settings [53]."

Confrontation with Evidence-based Medicine

Until the early 1980s, research in ICM focused largely on evaluation of physiologic and pathophysiologic responses in small patient series, or on reporting selected case series on specific clinical conditions. Using the search terms "intensive care OR critical care" and the limits "clinical trial" and "randomized controlled trial" (RCT) in PubMed yields 84 papers between 1970 and 1980 increasing to 10,493 for 2000 to 2010 (Fig. 58.7). This rough quantification shows the enormous increase in intensive care research during the past decades.

Several reasons underlie the rapid proliferation of large-scale clinical RCTs in ICM. RCTs have been widely accepted as the "ultimate proof" in most fields of medicine, and ICM has accepted this trend. The new pharmacologic agents developed by industry and introduced for the treatment of sepsis, required support by larger RCTs often undertaken by investigator-initiated clinical trial networks. The most successful in performing and publishing larger RCT's in intensive care patients include the Australian and New Zealand Intensive Care Society Clinical Trials Group, the Canadian Critical Care Trial Group, and the National Heart, Lung and Blood Institute's ARDS Clinical Network in the US. Notwithstanding the high hopes placed on these large RCTs, the results from most have been disappointing: new therapeutic interventions have not improved outcome, or have even been harmful, or the results have not been reproducible [54]. Controversies have developed over the validity and safety of study designs, and interpretations of some benchmark studies have been questioned [55]. Perhaps these difficulties should have been expected considering the complexity of the underlying clinical problems, the presence of poorly definable syndromes rather than clear-cut diseases, the heterogeneity of disease severity and treatment, and the poorly understood but highly relevant interactions between treatments and underlying pathophysiology.

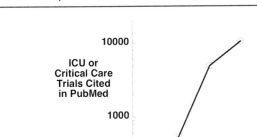

Fig. 58.7 The number of ICU or critical care trials has grown exponentially over the past 4 decades, only recently showing a flattening of this trend

Evidence-based medicine was enthusiastically introduced to ICM in the mid-1990s [56]. However, the argument for evidence-based medicine did not convince everybody. The characterization of evidence-based medicine by its founders, as "de-emphasizing reasoning based on pathophysiologic rationale [57]" sounded odd. Martin Tobin, the former Editor-in-Chief of the *American Journal of Respiratory and Critical Care Medicine*, summarized these doubts: "...we are talking about a practice of medicine divorced from the scientific principles that are its foundation [58]." If the pendulum swung to one extreme in the early days of evidence-based medicine, it seems to have reached a more neutral position in the first decade of this century.

Focus on Organization and Care Processes

The introduction of scoring systems for the severity of injury in the 1980s and their subsequent large-scale use in quality and benchmarking initiatives in the next decades, revealed diverse results of severity-adjusted outcomes, (standardized mortality rates) and severity-adjusted resource utilization (standardized resource utilization) [59]. Hospital survival rates between individual ICUs for patients with similar severity of illness varied 2–3 fold. The resources needed for producing similar survival rates for patients with a specific severity of illness varied up to 6-fold. Variations in case mix, available resources, and structural factors could not explain such differences, suggesting that other factors, perhaps related to organization and care processes, may have a large impact. The differences in performance exceeded what might realistically be expected from any single therapeutic intervention.

Some clinicians applied treatment protocols based on individual components of patient care, such as sedation [60] or weaning from mechanical ventilation [61]. Others evaluated the impact of organizational issues, such as staffing patterns, on outcomes [62]. All these efforts blurred the distinction between classical hypothesis-driven research, and quality improvement and process control. Nevertheless, the use of these approaches has improved patient care. A prime example is the dramatic reduction in catheter-related infections when simple measures of cleanliness and check-lists are applied, as demonstrated by Peter Pronovost [63]. Concerns over both safety and efficiency have been major drivers behind the various efforts of quality and process improvement. Treatment guidelines based on consensus opinions of experts is a present trend [64]. But consensus opinions often lack the backing of solid evidence. Clearly, this trend has not yet reached its peak. Conclusions based on expert opinions ignore the probability that experts tend to share opinions and that experts as a group can be dead wrong. They ignore the basic rule taught in Logic 101: never appeal to authority to support/prove an argument.

The Forgotten Brain

The lungs, the cardiovascular system, and the immune system (in the context of sepsis) had received the lion's share of attention in the decades preceding the new millennium. New imaging technologies facilitated monitoring and diagnosis of brain dysfunction, thereby adding a new group of patients to ICUs. They have helped us understand the pathophysiology of traumatic brain injury, and guide its treatment. Finally, the work of Peter Safar in the 1960s led to a breakthrough 40 years later—namely, cerebral protection after cardiopulmonary resuscitation that hypothermia offers. In 2002, mild therapeutic hypothermia after cardiac arrest was shown to improve outcome in a multicenter randomized controlled trial [65]. Despite this long delay from bench to bedside, Peter Safar could comment on this development in an accompanying editorial before he died in 2003 [66]. Subsequently, therapeutic hypothermia became an integral part of current treatment guidelines for cardiac arrest [67].

Training in ICM

Despite the early recognition of the need for a multidisciplinary approach to ICM, and the necessary broad skill-mix, training programs in ICM have remained highly variable, often fragmented, and unable to provide a uniform skill-mix and competencies. Australia was a pioneer in establishing formal qualifications for intensivists, and the Australian

Faculty of Anaesthesists organized the first examination for intensivists in 1979. In many European countries and in the US, several surgical and medical specialties as well as anesthesiology developed their own training programs, resulting in subspecialties of intensive care within a main specialty. In the Nordic countries and Italy, ICM developed as a natural extension of anesthesiology, although formal training programs in ICM were established relatively late, for example, in the late 1990s in Scandinavia. ICM has been established as a primary specialty in Spain and Switzerland, in the latter with multidisciplinary access, and the United Kingdom has been a leader in Europe in developing competence-based training in ICM, with access from multiple basic specialties. This approach emphasizes skills and competencies rather than knowledge alone. Competence-based training has been supported by the European Union, and the European Society of Intensive Care Medicine has played a leading role in its further development (http://www.cobatrice.org/en/index.asp). Consequently, the European Diploma of Intensive Care has been accepted by several countries as the official examination for intensive care.

Epilogue

Has ICM reached maturity? Ideas and principles presented by the pioneers in the 1950s and 1960s concerning organization, structure, responsibility, and training have been institutionalized. ICM has achieved recognition as an independent specialty. Competence-based training programs are growing, and open access to training in ICM. Ownership debates may have been relegated to the past.

In looking back, the description of intensive care, in Shoemaker's editorial for the third issue of the journal *Critical Care Medicine* in 1973, still seems apt today [49]:

> "Traditionally, complicated cases are handled by calling for consultations. When the complications are few and they appear in staggered fashion, this approach may function reasonably well. But management of the critically ill patient with multiple vital organ failures often requires maximum coordination of a wide range of professional activities and close monitoring of the patient's course. This can best be attained in a multidisciplinary ICU where the maximum input of specialties may be coordinated with continuous surveillance and laboratory support. The patient with multiple injuries and the acutely ill patient with multiple vital organ failure have many common physiologic problems. As the same therapeutic modalities are used, the multidisciplinary team approach is optimally suited to coordinate therapy for multiple organ failure."

Acknowledgments Thanks to Jeannie Wurz, Medical Writer/Editor, Dept. of Intensive Care Medicine, for research support and careful editing of the manuscript.

References

1. Gill CJ, Gill GC. Nightingale in Scutari: her legacy reexamined. Clin Infect Dis. 2005;40:1799–805.
2. Barone CP, Pablo CS, Barone GW. A history of the PACU. J Peri-Anesth Nurs. 2003;18:237–41.
3. Grenvik A, Pinsky MR. Evolution of the intensive care unit as a clinical center and critical care medicine as a discipline. Crit Care Clin. 2009;25:239–50.
4. Cherian SM, Nicks R, Lord RSA. Ernst ferdinand sauerbruch: rise and fall of the pioneer of thoracic surgery. World J Surg. 2001;25:1012–20.
5. Thierbach A. The resuscitation greats: Franz Kuhn, his contribution to anaesthesia and emergency medicine. Resuscitation. 2001;48:193–7.
6. Drinker P, Shaw LA. An apparatus for the prolonged administration of artificial respiration. J Clin Invest. 1929;7:229–47.
7. Banner MJ, Kirby RR, Block AJ. Mr. Jack Emerson—a matter of life and breath. Chest. 1997;112:307–8.
8. Forssmann W. Die sondierung des rechten herzens. Klin Wochenschr. 1929;8(45):2085–7.
9. Forssmann W. Historical development and methodology of heart catheterization; its application, with special reference to lung diseases. (In german) Geschichtliche entwicklung- und methodik der herzkatheterung; ihr anwendungsgebiet unter besonderer berücksichtigung der lungenerkrankungen. Langenbecks Arch Klin Chir Ver Dtsch Z Chir. 1954;279:450–73.
10. Klein O Zur bestimmung des zirkulatorischen minutenvolumens beim menschen nach dem fickschen prinzip. Gewinnung des gemischten venösen blutes mittels herzsondierung. Münchner Med Wochenschr. 1930;77(31):1311–12.
11. Raju TN. The nobel chronicles.1956: Werner Forssmann (1904–79); André Frédéric Cournand (1895–1988); and Dickinson Woodruff Richards, Jr (1895–1973). Lancet. 1999;353:1891.
12. Bower AG, Bennett VR, Dillon JB, Axelrod B. Part I.: investigation on the care and treatment of poliomyelitis patients. Ann West Med Surg. 1950;4(10):561–82.
13. Lassen HCA. The epidemic of poliomyelitis in Copenhagen, 1952. Proceedings of the royal society of medicine. 1953;47:67–71.
14. Berthelsen PG, Cronqvist M. The first intensive care unit in the world: Copenhagen 1953. Acta Anaesthesiol Scand. 2003;47:1190–5.
15. Trubuhovich RV. In the beginning. The 1952–1953 Danish epidemic of poliomyelitis and Bjørn Ibsen. Crit Care Resusc. 2003;5:227–30.
16. Zorab J. The Resuscitation Greats: Bjørn Ibsen. Resuscitation. 2003;57:3–9.
17. West JB. The physiological challenges of the 1952 Copenhagen poliomyelitis epidemic and a renaissance in clinical respiratory physiology. J Appl Physiol. 2005;99:424–32.
18. Severinghaus J, Astrup P, Murray JF. Blood gas analysis and critical care medicine. Am J Respir Crit Care Med. 1998;157:114–22.
19. National Academy of Sciences. National research council committee on anesthesia: workshop on intensive care units. Anesthesiology. 1964;25:192–222.
20. Kinney JM. Nutrition in the intensive care patient. Crit Care Clin. 1987;3:1–10. (Review).
21. Pontoppidan H, Wilson RS, Rie MA, Schneider RC. Respiratory intensive care. Anesthesiology. 1977;47:96–116.
22. Bendixen HH, Laver MB, Flacke WE. Influence of respiratory acidosis on circulatory effect of epinephrine in dogs. Circ Res. 1963;13:64–70.
23. Pontoppidan H. From continuous positive-pressure breathing to ventilator-induced lung injury. Anesthesiology. 2004;101:1015–7.
24. Ashbaugh DG, Bigelow DB, Petty TL, Levine BE. Acute respiratory distress in adults. The Lancet. 1967;2:319–23.

25. Falke KJ, Pontoppidan H, Kumar A, Leith DE, Geffin B, Laver MB. Ventilation with end-expiratory pressure in acute lung disease. J Clin Invest. 1972;51:2315–23.

26. Falke KJ. The introduction of positive endexpiratory pressure into mechanical ventilation: a retrospective. Intensive Care Med. 2003;29:1233–6.

27. Schuster HP. Zur Entwicklung der Intensivmedizin in Deutschland—von den anfängen bis heute. Wien Klin Wochenschr. 2007;119:6–12.

28. Mollaret P, Bastin R, Damoiseau B, Goulon M, Pocidalo JJ, Rapin M. Heroic treatment of severe tetanus: maximum curarization without anesthesia but with tracheostomy and artificial respiration by internal volumeric control of the changes of pressure; (first four cases). Presse Med. 1955;63:1413–6.

29. Bastin R, Goulon M, Le Brigand H, Liot F, Pocidalo JJ, Ranson-Bitker B, Rapin M. Severe respiratory insufficiency following pneumonectomy; treatment by tracheotomy and artificial respiration. J Fr Med Chir Thorac. 1956;10:562–71. (French).

30. Mollaret P, Bastin R, Rapin M, Pocidalo JJ, Goulon M, Lissac J, Liot F. Artificial respiration in acute respiratory insufficiency during bronchopneumopathies with chronic cor pulmonale. I. Clinical and biological data. Presse Med. 1958 65:1271–3. (French).

31. Mollaret P, Bastin R, Rapin M, Pocidalo JJ, Goulon M, Lissac J, Liot F. Artificial respiration in acute respiratory insufficiency during bronchopneumopathies with chronic cor pulmonale. II. Therapeutic conclusions. Presse Med. 1958;66:1326–8. (French).

32. Rapin M, Lissac J, Lamelin JP. Infectious complications in respiratory resuscitation. Etiological, symptomatic and therapeutic data. Presse Med. 1963;71:2139–42.

33. Suter PM, Fairley HB, Isenberg MD. Optimum end-expiratory airway pressure in patients with acute pulmonary failure. N Engl J Med. 1975;292:284–9.

34. Fairley HB, Safar P, Norlander P, et al. Reports to the second congress of the world federation of societies of anesthesiologists, Toronto 1960. Anaesthesia. 1961;16:267–316.

35. Fairley HB. Ventilating the acutely injured lung. Am J Respir Crit Care Med. 2001;163:1049–50.

36. Swan HJ, Ganz W, Forrester J, Marcus H, Diamond G, Chonette D. Catheterization of the heart in man with use of a flow directed balloon tipped catheter. N Engl J Med. 1970;283:447–51.

37. Brown RS, Carey JS, Mohr PA, Monson DO, Shoemaker WC. Comparative evaluation of sympathomimetic amines in clinical shock. Circ Shock. 1966;20:281–90.

38. Weil MH, Bradley EC. Circulatory effects of vasoactive drugs in current use for treatment of shock: a reclassification based on experimental and clinical study of their selective arterial and venous effects. Bull NY Acad Med. 1966;42:1023–36.

39. Chernow B, Carlson RW, Rackow EC. Giants of critical care: a tribute to Max Harry Weil, MD, PhD. Crit Care Med. 1992;20:915–6.

40. Shoemaker WC, Carey JS, Mohr PA, Brown RS, Monson DO, Yao ST, Kho LK, Stevenson A. Hemodynamic measurements in various types of clinical shock. Analysis of cardiac output and derived calculations in 100 surgical patients. Arch Surg. 1966;93:189–95.

41. Shoemaker WC, Printen KJ, Amato JJ, Monson DO, Carey JS, O'Connor K. Hemodynamic patterns after acute anesthetized and unanesthetized trauma. Evaluation of the sequence of changes in cardiac output and derived calculations. Arch Surg. 1967;95:492–9.

42. Shoemaker WC, Montgomery ES, Kaplan E, Elwyn DH. Physiologic patterns in surviving and nonsurviving shock patients. Use of sequential cardiorespiratory variables in defining criteria for therapeutic goals and early warning of death. Arch Surg. 1973;106:630–6.

43. Shoemaker WC, Appel PL, Kram HB, Waxman K, Lee TS. Prospective trial of supranormal values of survivors as therapeutic goals in high-risk surgical patients. Chest. 1988;94:1176–86.

44. Snyder JV. Giants of critical care: a tribute to Ake N. A. Grenvik, MD, PhD, FCCM, DSP. Crit Care Med. 1996;24:1602.

45. Vincent JL, Singer M, Marini JJ, Moreno R, Levy M, Matthay MA, Pinsky M, Rhodes A, Ferguson ND, Evans T, Annane D, Hall JB. Thirty years of critical care medicine. Crit Care. 2010;14:311.

46. Gattinoni L, Caironi P, Pelosi P, Goodman LR. What has computed tomography taught us about the acute respiratory distress syndrome? Am J Respir Crit Care Med. 2001;164:1701–11.

47. Cullen DJ, Civetta JM, Briggs BA, Ferrara LC. Therapeutic Intervention Scoring System: a method for quantitative comparison of patient care. Crit Care Med. 1974;2:57–60.

48. Knaus WA, Zimmerman JE, Wagner DP, Draper EA, Lawrence DE. APACHE-acute physiology and chronic health evaluation: a physiologically based classification system. Crit Care Med. 1981;9:591–7.

49. Shoemaker WC. Multiple injuries and multiple organ failure. Crit Care Med. 1973;1:157.

50. Bone RC. Let's agree on terminology: definitions of sepsis. Crit Care Med. 1991;19:973–6.

51. Bone RC. Sepsis, the sepsis syndrome, multi-organ failure: a plea for comparable definitions. Ann Intern Med. 1991;114:332–3.

52. Bone RC, Balk RA, Cerra FB, Dellinger RP, Fein AM, Knaus WA, Schein RM, Sibbald WJ. Definitions for sepsis and organ failure and guidelines for the use of innovative therapies in sepsis. The ACCP/SCCM consensus conference committee. American college of chest physicians/pociety of critical care medicine. Chest. 1992;101:1644–55.

53. Bone RC, Sibbald WJ, Sprung CL. The ACCP-SCCM consensus conference on sepsis and organ failure. Chest. 1992;10:1481–3.

54. Takala J. Better conduct of clinical trials: the control group in critical care trials. Crit Care Med 2009;37:S80–90.

55. Deans KJ, Minneci PC, Suffredini AF, Danner RL, Hoffman WD, Ciu X, Klein HG, Schechter AN, Banks SM, Eichacker PQ, Natanson C. Randomization in clinical trials of titrated therapies: unintended consequences of using fixed treatment protocols. Crit Care Med. 2007;35:1509–16.

55. Cook DJ, Sibbald WJ, Vincent JL, Cerra FB. Evidence based medicine in critical care group: evidence based critical care medicine; what is it and what can it do for us? Crit Care Med. 1996;24:334–7.

57. Evidence-Based Medicine Working Group. Evidence-based medicine: a new approach to teaching the practice of medicine. JAMA. 1992;268:2420–25.

58. Tobin MJ. The role of a journal in a scientific controversy. Am J Respir Crit Care Med. 2003;168:511–14.

59. Rothen HU, Stricker K, Einfalt J, Bauer P, Metnitz PG, Moreno RP, Takala J. Variability in outcome and resource use in intensive care units. Intensive Care Med. 2007;33:1329–36. (Epub 2007 Jun 1).

60. Kress JP, Pohlman AS, O'Connor MF, Hall JB. Daily interruption of sedative infusions in critically ill patients undergoing mechanical ventilation. N Engl J Med. 2000;342:1471–7.

61. Kollef MH, Shapiro SD, Silver P, St John RE, Prentice D, Sauer S, Ahrens TS, Shannon W, Baker-Clinkscale D. A randomized, controlled trial of protocol-directed versus physician-directed weaning from mechanical ventilation. Crit Care Med. 1997;25:567–74.

62. Pronovost PJ, Angus DC, Dorman T, Robinson KA, Dremsizov TT, and Young TL. Physician staffing patterns and clinical outcomes in critically ill patients: a systematic review. JAMA. 2002;288:2151–62.

63. Pronovost P, Needham D, Berenholtz S, Sinopoli D, Chu H, Cosgrove S, Sexton B, Hyzy R, Welsh R, Roth G, Bander J, Kepros J, Goeschel C. An intervention to decrease catheter-related bloodstream infections in the ICU. N Engl J Med 2006;355:2725–32. Erratum in: N Engl J Med. 2007;356:2660.

64. Dellinger RP, Levy MM, Carlet JM, Bion J, Parker MM, Jaeschke R, Reinhart K, Angus DC, Brun-Buisson C, Beale R, Calandra T,

Dhainaut JF, Gerlach H, Harvey M, Marini JJ, Marshall J, Ranieri M, Ramsay G, Sevransky J, Thompson BT, Townsend S, Vender JS, Zimmerman JL, Vincent JL. Surviving sepsis campaign: international guidelines for management of severe sepsis and septic shock: 2008. intensive care med 2008; 34: 17–60. Epub 2007 Dec 4. Erratum in: Intensive Care Med. 2008 Apr;34:783–5.

65. Hypothermia after Cardiac Arrest Study Group. Mild therapeutic hypothermia to improve the neurologic outcome after cardiac arrest. N Engl J Med. 2002;346:549–56. Erratum in: N Engl J Med 2002;346:1756.

66. Safar PJ, Kochanek PM. Therapeutic hypothermia after cardiac arrest. N Engl J Med. 2002;346:612–3.

67. Nolan JP, Hazinski MF, Billi JE, Boettiger BW, Bossaert L, de Caen AR, et al. Part 1: executive summary: 2010 International consensus on cardiopulmonary resuscitation and emergency cardiovascular care science with treatment recommendations. Resuscitation. 2010;81(suppl 1):e1–e25.

The Development of Ambulatory and Office-Based Anesthesia

59

Kathryn E. McGoldrick

Summary

Long, Wells, and Morton provided outpatient anesthesia in the 1840s. Nicoll in Scotland and Waters in the US gave outpatient anesthesia in the early twentieth century. Modern outpatient anesthesia began in 1959, with Canadian anesthetists Webb and Graves' report of their 6-month experience with 494 surgical patients, cared for as outpatients. In 1962 at UCLA, Cohen and Dillon opened the first ambulatory surgery program, in 1966 describing the safety and economic advantage of their approach. Free-standing outpatient surgical facilities followed in 1968 in Rhode Island, and in 1969 in Arizona.

Ambulatory surgery grew rapidly, by the 1990s overshadowing in-hospital surgery. Important advances included new drugs providing rapid onset and offset of effect, management of postoperative pain without the nausea associated with opioids, antiemetics developed in the 1980s, the 1987 release of the laryngeal mask airway, and increasing use of regional anesthesia.

Studies during the 1980s estimated that ambulatory surgery centers (ASCs) decreased the cost per case by 25–75 % relative to comparable inpatient care. In 2004, Ansell and Montgomery reported that ASA III patients had no obvious increase in morbidity or mortality relative to ASA I or II patients. Today, approximately 80 % of elective surgical and diagnostic procedures in the US are performed on an outpatient basis.

Established in the US in 1984, the Society for Ambulatory Anesthesia (SAMBA) furthered the development of ambulatory anesthesiology as a subspecialty. Wetchler's *Anesthesia for Ambulatory Surgery* was published in 1985. The journal *Ambulatory Surgery* was introduced in 1993.

Until the late 1980s, local laws and third-party payers limited reimbursement for office-based procedures. Once that obstacle was removed, office-based surgery in the US grew rapidly, increasing from less than 2 % in 1984 to an estimated 25 % of all outpatient procedures in 2010. Financial, regulatory and safety factors limited acceptance of office-based anesthesia outside the US. In Australia and the UK comprehensive standards on facility, equipment, and practice requirements apply wherever anesthesia is conducted. In 2003, Vila and colleagues reported a 10-fold greater incidence of morbidity and death in patients anesthetized in offices versus ASCs in the US. An anesthesiologist was present in only 15 % of cases resulting in death. The burgeoning growth of office-based surgery in the face of demonstrated risks may reflect the motivational strength of cost containment.

Historical Influences

The history of ambulatory anesthesia is as old as the history of anesthesia. Crawford Long, Horace Wells, and William Morton all administered anesthesia in office settings in the 1840s. Outpatient surgery and attempts at anesthesia go back to mankind's ancient attempts to treat illness invasively [1]. Drawings from 3500 BCE depict amputations and skull trephination performed in primitive surroundings long before hospitals existed.

K. E. McGoldrick (✉)
Society for Ambulatory Anesthesia, New York Medical College,
40 Sunshine Cottage Rd, Valhalla, NY 10595, USA
e-mail: Kathryn_McGoldrick@nymc.edu

Centuries before the discovery of anesthesia, hospitals were established to care for the sick, particularly to treat military conscripts and the indigent. Anesthesia enabled a gradual increase in the numbers of operations performed but, as before the discovery of anesthesia, surgery predominantly corrected problems on body surfaces and extremities—cataract removal, manipulations of fractures and dislocations, and lightning-fast amputations. A byproduct of the slow advances in surgery was a dependence upon hospitals to provide care.

Hospitals were a mixed blessing. A major deterrent to hospital-based care was infection, or "hospitalism" as it was termed in the pre-antibiotic era. (In recent years, however, the term "hospitalism" has expanded to include iatrogenic maladies acquired by hospitalized patients, maladies that are often more threatening than the primary condition) [2].

E. I Eger II et al. (eds.), *The Wondrous Story of Anesthesia*, DOI 10.1007/978-1-4614-8441-7_59, © Edmond I Eger, MD 2014

Consequently, the affluent arranged treatment, if possible, in their homes. Koller's 1884 introduction of cocaine, and subsequent local anesthetics facilitated use of the physician's office for minor surgery. With the application of Lister's 1867 demonstration of antisepsis and then Bergmann's 1886 application of asepsis, objections to hospitalization receded [1], and the hospital became the dominant site for advanced medical and surgical care

'Modern' ambulatory surgical and anesthetic practices largely evolved from the early work of itinerant dental surgeons, traveling their circuits by horseback and later on trains. They frequently operated from hotel rooms and then moved on. Only the fortunate (usually urban-located) dentist worked from an office, which was typically in the dentist's home. Those using anesthesia from 1846 to 1862, gave ether or chloroform via the drop-bottle method. In 1862, Gardner Colton resurrected the use of dentist-generated (baking of ammonium nitrate) nitrous oxide for near-asphyxial 100% nitrous oxide anesthetics (personal communication, George Bause). The cumulative effect of catastrophes from ether fires and chloroform-related mortalities increased interest in using local anesthesia with cocaine in dental offices after 1884. Gradually, local anesthetics other than cocaine became available, but it was not until 1904 that the first genuine alternative, stovaine, appeared.

Ambulatory Surgery Truly Began in 1899

In 1909, James Nicoll (Fig. 59.1), a pediatric surgeon in Scotland, wrote of his experiences with ambulatory anesthesia and surgery on nearly 9,000 children as outpatients, during a 10-year interval at Glasgow Royal Hospital for Sick Children [3]. Operations included cleft lip and palate repair, correction of pyloric stenosis, mastoidectomy, repair of inguinal and umbilical hernias, and even management of spina bifida and depressed skull fractures. Nicoll offered no details concerning surgical morbidity or mortality, or the results of the operations *per se*. Nearly one-half of the children were less than three years of age, and many were less than one year of age. Nicoll emphasized the disadvantages of hospitalization and the benefits of home care for convalescence, especially for frail children and nursing mothers.

Nicoll pleaded with his fellow surgeons to perform more pediatric operations on an outpatient basis. He thought that "…a large number of the cases at present treated in-door constitutes a waste of the resources of a children's hospital…. The results obtained in the out-patient department at a tithe (small part) of the cost are equally good [3]." He also stated that certain cases were unsuitable as outpatients. He believed that "as a rule" unsuitable cases tended to involve children as opposed to infants. "Cleft palate operations in suckling infants do well as out-patients, but the child of 3 or 4 must go into the wards, where care can be taken to prevent his putting

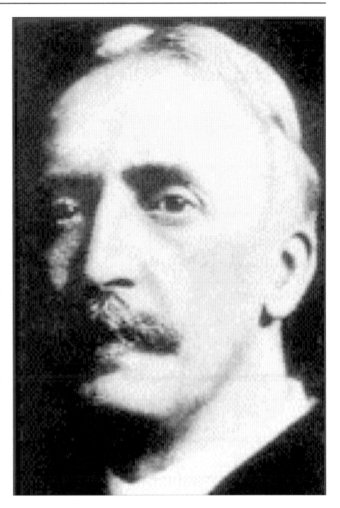

Fig. 59.1 A picture of James H. Nicoll. Nicoll was arguably the father of modern ambulatory anesthesia. (From Young DG, Carachi R. James H. Nicoll, MB, CM Glasg, FRFPS Glasg. Legion of Honour France. Father of Day Surgery. SMJ [Scottish Medical Journal] 2006:51; 48–50, with permission.)

hard edibles into his mouth." He commented that "Infants and young children in a ward are noisy, and not infrequently malodorous." Nicoll doubted that these babies benefited from "trained" nursing, arguing that they rested more quietly and comfortably at home, nursing in the arms of their mothers. The prescient Nicoll further commented that his experience with pediatric ambulatory herniotomy and other operations, suggested that similar cases in adults are kept too long in bed and that the average recumbent period should be "something under a week." In light of the scope of the operations performed and the primitive state of anesthesia, Nicoll's report is impressive.

Waters Came Second

The next pioneering communication came from Ralph Waters (Fig. 59.2), who in 1919, described the care of patients for ambulatory surgery, commenting that patient evaluation

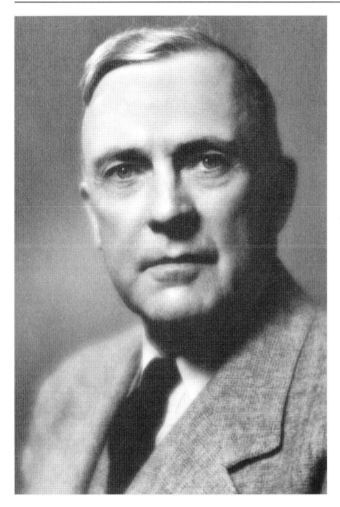

Fig. 59.2 Ralph Waters, an icon of American anesthesiology, was a pioneer in the field of ambulatory anesthesia. Among his many accomplishments was his establishment at the University of Wisconsin of the first academic program for training anesthesiologists, but before that he developed an office-based practice of anesthesia. (Courtesy of the Wood Library-Museum of Anesthesiology, Park Ridge, IL.)

Sioux City, Iowa, and apparently did not insist that patients be accompanied by a responsible adult when discharged. He advertised the economic benefits of his approach for all concerned parties.

Waters had an astute business sense, and he offered no apologies for his focus on the bottom line. He sought "to give satisfaction to operator and patient and charge a fee that will pay expenses and a good profit." He had no fixed fee schedule and charged according to the cost of materials and the time involved with the procedure. He appeared proud of the fact that "Many patients and some doctors object to the fees but they come back and their friends come back. Satisfactory anesthesia and too large fees work better than bargain sale fees and unsatisfactory anesthesia." Waters was keenly aware of the importance of pleasing his referral base, claiming "As for *business getting* activity, it is all with the dentists and physicians. The place is for their use and their convenience, and consideration for them comes first." Waters' Clinic, which offered anesthesia care for dental and minor surgical procedures, is the prototype for the modern free-standing ambulatory surgery facility.

Dentists and surgeons contributed substantially to the early progress in ambulatory anesthesia. Most important *clinical* advances in anesthesia emanated from surgeons (e.g., August Bier and William Halsted) and dentists (think of Wells and Morton) or obstetricians (e.g., John Cleland and James Simpson). A meager few of those practicing anesthesia made technical improvements involving innovations in technique or equipment. Most functioned largely as technicians making minimal contributions to advancing our understanding of the principles of physiology, pharmacology, physics, and chemistry that are the foundation of anesthesia practice.

required "…careful physical examination on all suspicious risks [4]." Medical conditions had to be well controlled before surgery, and certain unspecified medical conditions precluded outpatient care. "Initially a modest office was equipped with a waiting room and a small operating room with an adjoining room containing a cot on which a patient could lie down after his anesthetic….In due time the place became popular and we moved……" [4] Waters used nitrous oxide liberally, and occasionally administered morphine and scopolamine sublingually. He allowed consumption of clear liquids until immediately before surgery and permitted patients having late morning or early afternoon surgery to ingest a light breakfast. With regard to his rather liberal fasting guidelines, Waters bluntly stated, "As to the preoperative preparation of the patient we worry little about it." Waters meticulously documented perioperative variables, including patient satisfaction. He did not use regional anesthesia in his Downtown Anesthesia Clinic in

Hospital-Based Outpatient Surgery

In 1959, two Canadian anesthetists, Eric Webb and Horace Graves, were concerned about a shortage of hospital beds in Vancouver, British Columbia, and proposed outpatient surgery as an alternative to inpatient care. They reported their experience with 494 patients cared for successfully during a 6-month period [5]. In fact, their experience with outpatient surgery began in 1949, but the expansion initially proceeded slowly. An estimated 12,000 patients, or 5 % of all surgical patients, underwent outpatient procedures from 1949 to 1959.

Building on the experience of Webb and Graves, ambulatory surgical care developed momentum in the 1960s. In 1962, the first so-described ambulatory surgery program, under the direction of David Cohen and John Dillon, opened at the University of California Los Angeles [6]. In 1967, Mary Louise Levy and Charles Coakley [7], at George Washington University, reported a similar experience, again in a hospital-based ambulatory surgery program that had opened in 1966. Cohen and Dillon [6] perceived a shortage of hospital beds and a rapidly growing population in the Los Angles area, and postulated that outpatient surgery would redress this imbalance. They noted, moreover, that regulatory obstacles impeded efficient use of hospital beds and hindered creation of a favorable (more pleasant) environment for ambulatory surgery. For example, patients were admitted to the hospital for minor surgery because insurance only covered inpatients, or because they needed "major" anesthesia and the hospital's rules mandated postoperative admission (insurance companies were not the only entities swayed by the profit motive). Further, insurance carriers required admission to the hospital for at least 18 hours, paradoxically increasing cost.

In 1966, Cohen and Dillon described the first two years of their experience [6]. The surgeon selected outpatients, based on the prediction that the patient should require only brief postoperative observation, owing to minimal likelihood of postoperative bleeding. Neither general nor regional anesthesia excluded prospective candidates. Only complications necessitated hospitalization. Types of surgical procedures were limited and most patients were healthy. However, some patients who were not in good health were accepted, if they were stable and "under good control [6]." Their personal physician completed a history and physical examination one week before surgery, and the anesthesiologist undertook a preoperative evaluation on the morning of surgery. In contrast to the criteria Waters described 40 years earlier, patients were enjoined to fast preoperatively, recruit a responsible accompanying adult, and not drive in the immediate postoperative period. Of their 804 patients, 31 (3.9%) were admitted overnight for administrative or surgical issues. There were no serious anesthetic complications, and only two patients (0.25%) were admitted for anesthetic reasons (prolonged emergence from general anesthesia). The use of ambulatory surgery produced savings that varied from case to case, but typically ranged from 30 to 46% [6].

The editorial board of the *Journal of the American Medical Association (JAMA)* initially rejected the Cohen-Dillon manuscript that described their experiences, because they considered that outpatient surgery was not "good practice of medicine." Dillon responded that it was permissible to criticize his grammar or spelling, but that it was not acceptable to criticize something that was the future of medicine. He insisted that outpatient surgery was too important to ignore and *JAMA* finally acceded [8].

North America was not the only venue where freestanding units within hospitals were established. An existing hut at Hammersmith Hospital in London was converted in 1969 to a small outpatient surgery facility that provided care to about 750 patients annually. Despite the restricted space, this renovation enabled the waiting list for plastic surgery to be reduced by 1970 to nearly half of the 1968

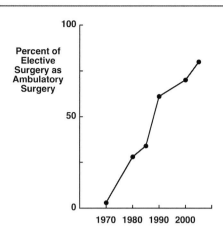

Fig. 59.3 Growth of ambulatory surgery as a percent of elective surgery in the US grew linearly from 1970 to 2000, driven by economic forces and abetted by the development of drugs and devices that facilitated and made safe such practice

figure [9]. In March 1970, a former maternity ward at Gulson Hospital in Coventry opened as a surgical day unit [10]. The unit managed cases involving general, otorhinolaryngologic, orthopedic, dental, and plastic surgery. Vitually immediately, this facility greatly decompressed the long waiting lists for most minor and "intermediate" operations. Specifically, the waiting list for varicose vein operations, which was nearly 600 in 1970, was under 50 patients by 1972. Economic benefits were considerable, with initial annual savings of £40,000, and considerable sparing of nursing staff.

Starting in the 1980s, the number of patients undergoing ambulatory anesthesia and surgery in the US grew rapidly, and by the 1990s overshadowed in-hospital anesthesia and surgery (Fig. 59.3). A confluence of economic, technologic and pharmacologic factors contributed to this rapid growth. Pharmacologic advances included development of drugs facilitating rapid onset and offset, with fewer unpleasant side effects (Table 59.1). Improved analgesic agents enhanced the management of postoperative pain. Concern about escalating health care costs prompted the Medicare program to pay for care in freestanding ambulatory surgery centers. The development of a prospective payment system, based on diagnostic-related groups, created financial incentives for hospitals to shift less complicated surgery to outpatient facilities. Other insurers followed Medicare's lead. Studies during the 1980s estimated that ambulatory surgery decreased the cost per case by 25 to 75%, relative to comparable inpatient care [11, 12]. And in a government-based health care system, ambulatory surgery decreased the waiting time for elective operations [13].

Such changes and motivations were not limited to the US. For example, in Australia, the motivation to expand outpatient surgery was primarily economic, and financial realities were a powerful impetus to the development of ambulatory surgery in other countries as well.

Table 59.1 Examples of pharmacologic advances enhancing the growth and safety of ambulatory anesthesia and surgery

Traditional agent (s)	Improved profile agent (s)
Diazepam	Midazolam
Thiopental	Propofol
Curare, pancuronium	Atracurium, cisatracurium, rocuronium
Halothane, Isoflurane	Desflurane, Sevoflurane
Morphine, meperidine	Fentanyl, sufentanil, remifentanil
Labetalol	Esmolol
Droperidol	Ondansetron, aprepitant
Acetaminophen	Ketorolac, celecoxib
Bupivacaine	Ropivacaine, levobupivacaine

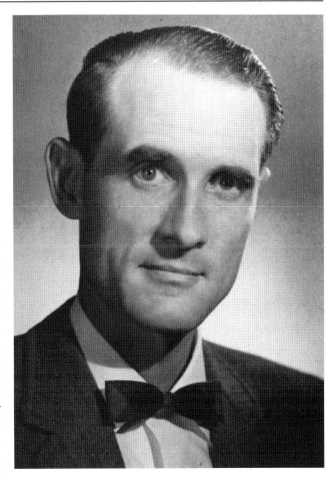

Fig. 59.4 Wallace Reed (pictured) and John Ford, co-founded the first modern free-standing outpatient surgery clinic, the Surgicenter,® which opened in Phoenix in 1970. (Courtesy of the Wood Library-Museum of Anesthesiology, Park Ridge, IL.)

However, some economists worried that the ability to treat more patients in a given interval might increase total expenditures, the so-called "efficiency trap [14]." Analyzing direct and indirect costs of substituting ambulatory for inpatient care, Aviva Berk and Thomas Chalmers [15] concluded that putative savings largely depended on the closure of hospital wings or entire hospitals. If vacated beds were used to meet previously unmet demand for more hospitalization, then more care would be provided at a higher total cost [15]. In 1981, Detmer [16] observed that "Whether money is ultimately saved at the level of the health care system is difficult to determine....Since we do not know what will happen to system-wide costs, a national policy with incentives favoring free-standing units over hospital-based units seems inappropriate." Detmer further cautioned that the unlimited growth of independent free-standing surgical units might undermine the economic viability of traditional community and teaching hospitals. Even today, hospital administrators resent "cherry picking" by ambulatory surgery facilities, facilities not required to provide complex services 24/7, nor care for critically ill or indigent patients.

But by the mid-1980s, it seemed clear that ambulatory surgery offered relief from skyrocketing health care expenditures, and a 1985 survey of Fortune 500 companies ranked outpatient surgery as the most critical of 15 possible options for health care expenditure containment [17]. Insurance carriers and the federal government recognized the economic advantages of outpatient surgical care as reflected by their denial of reimbursement for some procedures, such as cataract surgery or inguinal herniorrhaphy, when performed on an inpatient basis.

Free-Standing Outpatient Surgical Facilities

Charles Hill, familiar with the efforts of Ralph Waters, reintroduced the concept of a free-standing ambulatory facility in 1968 [18]. In a medical office suite in Providence, Rhode Island, he opened a fully-equipped operating suite with a recovery room. However, the facility failed financially owing to lack of support from the State of Rhode Island Health Department, which maintained that the suite was a physician's office. Blue Cross and other third party insurance carriers also denied support.

In 1969, in Phoenix, Arizona, John Ford and Wallace Reed [19] (Fig. 59.4) established the first modern, free-standing outpatient surgical clinic, (Surgicenter®), in the mode of Ralph Waters' "Downtown Anesthesia Clinic." They argued that almost any patient whose operation does not involve major trespass into the cranial vault, thorax, or abdomen is a candidate for outpatient surgery. They appeared to place more emphasis on the type of surgical procedure, than on the patient's physical status, when determining suitability for care at Surgicenter.® However, in a 1976 publication, they wrote that their "...patients are good risk [20]."

Ford and Reed successfully anticipated obstacles before, and after, their Surgicenter® opened in 1970. These visionaries obtained clearance from the local health planning council, the Maricopa County Medical Society, and state planning authorities, complied with local building requirements and zoning codes, and obtained approval from third-party insurers, including Medicare and Medicaid. By mandating that their surgeons were credentialed to perform a given surgical procedure at an inpatient institution, and by implementing procedures for quality assurance, the facility demonstrated that it functioned like a hospital, enabling payers to fund the surgical care rendered.

They created economies that seem obvious. They did not require a preoperative visit to Surgicenter.® Having been carefully screened by their surgeons as appropriate candidates for outpatient surgery, patients were instructed to arrive no more than one hour before surgery to undergo preoperative evaluation by the anesthesiologist. Ford and Reed did not require that ingrown toenails or infant foreskins be sent to a pathologist. They created staggered shifts for personnel to enable an employee/patient ratio of 1:1, as opposed to the 2.5 to 3:1 ratio associated with hospitals. They eliminated unnecessary preoperative laboratory testing and counterproductive premedication with long-lasting drugs. Safety was comparable to that in hospitals, but costs were considerably less. In their 1976 publication, Ford and Reed pointed out that they had cared for more than 33,000 patients since the opening of their facility, without a single death or malpractice suit [20]. Reed wisely arranged with a nearby hospital to admit patients who developed complications. He also relied on an increasingly sophisticated public to assume a greater share of its own care at home. This successful Surgicenter® became the model for similar facilities, both in the US and internationally.

In 1972, Reed and Ford received the Gerard B. Lambert Award from the Lambert Foundation for their contribution to medical care in the US. Gerard Lambert, whose father discovered Listerine and founded Lambert Pharmacal Company of St. Louis, was interested in honoring innovative ideas in health care delivery, especially if they originated from or pertained to hospitals. After he devised the compound that would eventually be known as Listerine, the senior Lambert, a chemist by training, scraped together sufficient funds to travel to London and there invested his last dollar in a beautiful carriage with a liveried coachman. Fortified by this elegant equipage, he coaxed from Lord Lister, the developer of antiseptic surgery, the right to christen the new formula with the great man's name.

Competition in the health care arena came to be viewed favorably, the *Federal Register* in 1982 stating:

> "These proposed regulations would permit a new class of facilities, ambulatory surgical centers to compete with hospitals in providing ambulatory surgical services to Medicare beneficiaries….We believe….that the extension of coverage of reimbursement to ambulatory surgical centers will give beneficiaries and their physicians important additional options in their selection of sites for surgery. These options in turn will enhance the competition between ambulatory surgical centers and hospitals [21]."

The increase in outpatient surgery was not without opposition. The Wood Library-Museum of Anesthesiology offers a historical DVD wherein Reed and Ford chronicle some of the unsavory conflicts developing between them and local hospital administrators [22]. Once the negative financial impact of a free-standing competitor was appreciated, hospital administrators in the Phoenix area complained that Surgicenter® would be "skimming the cream," leaving their institutions with all the "…high overhead items of cost and poor reimbursement." (Steve Morris, former Administrator of Good Samaritan Hospital). A rate battle ensued, even before the first case was performed at Surgicenter.® Reed commented, "…in applying for similar approval to do outpatients in hospital-affiliated units, the hospitals somehow acquired copies of our schedules, used the same schedules with the same spelling errors, and reduced the price by five or ten dollars just to show that they were going to be less expensive than the outpatient facility." The hospital administrators also resorted to negative reinforcement, suggesting to surgeons that if they transferred their loyalty to Surgicenter,® they would no longer receive preferential treatment at this or that hospital (Daniel Cloud, Pediatric Surgeon and former President of the AMA) [22]. The situation became tense, despite Reed's assertion that he did not wish to endanger the hospitals' financial viability, because it was in the best interest of the entire community that a tertiary care facility be maintained. A few years after Surgicenter® opened, Reed wrote to Ralph Waters (then 90 years old), proudly informing him of its success. Waters responded in a handwritten note. "Just why the idea of 'outpatient service' did not progress I can't say. I always thought the idea was sound."

The invention of the laryngeal mask airway (LMA) and the cuffed oropharyngeal airway (COPA) enlarged the options for airway management, decreasing the need to administer muscle relaxants and their attendant reversal agents solely to secure the patient's airway. Also, surgeons increasingly embraced minimally invasive surgery. In 1988, the first meeting of the Society for Minimally Invasive Therapy, a multidisciplinary international group composed of surgeons, anesthetists, and radiologists, convened in London. The impressive development of endoscopic surgical techniques and the growth of this organization were inextricably linked, and added to the explosive growth of outpatient surgery.

Free-standing ambulatory surgery centers (ASCs) continue to proliferate to this day, when currently approximately 80% of all elective surgical and diagnostic procedures in the US are performed on an outpatient basis. Notably, the rate of visits to freestanding ASCs tripled from 1996 to 2006, while the number of visits to hospital-based ambulatory surgery centers remained unchanged. In the US in 2006, an estimated 19.9 million (57.2%) of the ambulatory surgery visits occurred in hospitals and 14.9 million (42.8%) occurred in freestanding ASCs [23].

Influence of Professional Organizations

The prescient Waters knew the importance of formal organizations defining and overseeing standards of education and practice. Establishment of the Society for Ambulatory Anesthesia (SAMBA) in the US in 1984, led to the development of ambulatory anesthesiology as a subspecialty. Early leaders of SAMBA included Bernard Wetchler (Fig. 59.5), Burton Epstein, Paul White, and Wallace Reed. Wetchler became President of the American Society of Anesthesiologists (ASA) from 1994 to 1995 and received the ASA's 2002 Distinguished Service Award. Epstein was the recipient of the ASA's 1999 Distinguished Service Award.

Textbooks on ambulatory anesthesia followed its recognition as a distinct subspecialty. Wetchler led the way in 1985 with *Anesthesia for Ambulatory Surgery* [24] and White's *Outpatient Anesthesia* [25] appeared in 1990. In 1995, Kathryn McGoldrick produced *Ambulatory Anesthesiology: A Problem-Oriented Approach* [26]. A handbook by Rebecca Twersky titled *The Ambulatory Anesthesia Handbook* [27] appeared in 1995. The journal *Ambulatory Surgery* was introduced in 1993, with Paul White and British surgeon Paul Jarrett as coeditors.

SAMBA first met in 1985 and now draws approximately 500 registrants to its Annual Meeting. SAMBA gained recognition as a leader in ambulatory anesthesia education. In addition to its annual spring meeting, SAMBA holds a one-day session before the ASA Annual Meeting, and a one and a half day meeting at the same venue as the World Congress of Anaesthesiologists. Shortly after 2000, the ASA Annual Meeting introduced an "ambulatory track." SAMBA also holds a seat on the Council of the International Association for Ambulatory Surgery.

An industry sprouted to address perceived needs associated with outpatient perioperative care [28]. Vendors, accrediting organizations, publishers, for-profit companies, consultants, and professional societies for physicians (SAMBA), nurses, and administrators all claimed a share of the action. In 1994, for example, certification for nurses caring for ambulatory surgical patients was created (Certified Ambulatory Perianesthesia Nurses [CAPAs]).

Clinical research in the subspecialty began to flourish. A multimodal preemptive approach to postoperative complications such as nausea and vomiting, and pain management, evolved [29–32]. Patients considered at high risk for postoperative nausea and vomiting now routinely receive prophylactic therapy with three antiemetics that have different mechanisms of action, such as low-dose droperidol, ondansetron, and dexamethasone. This approach has resulted in postoperative emesis rates of less than 10% [29]. Similarly, anesthesiologists and surgeons increasingly use multimodal analgesic regimens that incorporate non-opioid analgesics (e.g., local anesthetics, nonsteroidal anti-inflammatory

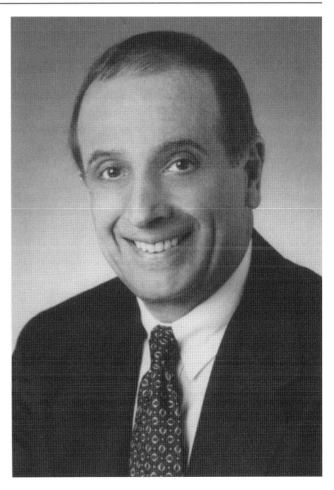

Fig. 59.5 Bernard Wetchler was one of the early founders of the Society for Ambulatory Anesthesia. He also served as President of the American Society of Anesthesiologists from 1994 to 1995. (Courtesy of the Wood Library-Museum of Anesthesiology, Park Ridge, IL.)

drugs, acetaminophen, ketamine, and alpha$_2$ agonists) to supplement or replace opioid analgesics [30].

Criteria for acceptance of patients for ambulatory surgery expanded from the initial restriction to ASA physical status I and II patients. A review of ASA PS III patients compared with ASA PS I or II patients having outpatient surgery identified no subsequent increase in unplanned admissions and postoperative complications [33]. Increasingly invasive and lengthy procedures were performed successfully in the outpatient milieu, and creative arrangements for 23-hour postoperative stays developed. Other innovations enabling further expansion of outpatient surgery included freestanding recovery care units and hospital hotels. Home health care nurses assisted families postoperatively, administering intravenous antibiotics and analgesics. A 1993 study of more than 38,000 consecutive patients undergoing ambulatory anesthesia provided one-month followup data [34]. Four patients died (1:11,273), two in automobile accidents, and two of myocardial infarction.

Ambulatory surgery also grew in most economically developed countries. Credit much of this development to outreach efforts of the International Association for Ambulatory Surgery (IAAS), an "organization of organizations" that held its first meeting in Brussels, Belgium in 1995. The IAAS exists to provide international practitioners with state-of-the-art information about types of patients and procedures that are appropriate for outpatient surgery, recognizing that socio-political and economic factors guide local decisions. For example, although Germany is a highly developed country, ambulatory surgery has not advanced as rapidly as one might expect, owing to financial and organizational issues. The German health care system favors inpatient treatment, which provides remuneration 3–10 times greater than that for ambulatory treatment [35]. Thus, only 3% of all the ambulatory surgery in Germany is performed in hospitals because hospitals would rather focus on more lucrative inpatient care, and 97% is conducted in freestanding ASCs. Since 1 January 2004, however, a new law opened part of the social health insurance (SHI) to the free market, partially limiting the "wall" between hospitals and day clinics by allowing contracts that individual sickness funds can sign with panel doctors for single or multiple procedures. These contracts are based predominantly upon the diagnostic related group (DRG) system, and the ambulatory payments typically amount to 50–90% of the DRGs for inpatient treatment [35].

In Australia, as of 2006, approximately 50% of all procedures were conducted as day surgery, either in hospitals or in freestanding ASCs. There were 248 freestanding ASCs. Nonetheless, ambulatory surgery has not reached its full potential, in part perhaps owing to the absence of extended (overnight) recovery in day surgery centers/units, and the absence of post-discharge convalescent limited-care accommodation facilities (medimotels) [36].

Evolution of Processes

Patient selection criteria, preoperative evaluation and preparation, intraoperative anesthetic techniques, and postoperative care have evolved. Dillon [37] stated in 1967 that diabetes, vascular insufficiency, or anemia precluded outpatient surgery. Not today. It is now common to care for optimally stabilized ASA physical status III and IV patients on an outpatient basis. Patient selection tends to be location-specific based on the facility's resources and capability. As the complexity of patients' medical conditions and surgical procedures have increased, so too has the importance of a thoughtful preoperative evaluation geared toward realistic risk stratification and minimization.

Until recently, most outpatients received a general anesthetic. Increasingly however, regional anesthesia and monitored anesthesia care are used, partially an outgrowth

of the increasing availability of minimally invasive surgery and advancement of endoscopic diagnostic/therapeutic procedures. The history of regional anesthesia has moved from the placement of local anesthetic based on anatomical landmarks to placement guided by paresthesia, to placement by nerve stimulation and, most recently, to placement by ultrasound guidance. Outpatient anesthesia has evolved with these changes and with the realization that regional anesthesia offers particular advantages to the patient having outpatient surgery. For example, effective analgesia lasting several days postoperatively is now provided in the home using mechanical or programmable pumps delivering local anesthetics through peripheral catheters [38]. Research on encapsulated formulations of local anesthetics that provide long-lasting postoperative analgesia may allow elimination of the pumps [39, 40]. These developments may further expand the types of procedures that can be successfully performed in the outpatient venue.

Office-Based Anesthesia

Interest in office-based surgery represents a return to the origins of ambulatory surgery, following in the footsteps of Long, Wells, Morton, and Waters. *Plus ça change, plus c'est la même chose.* Lewis Ferguson's 1947 text, directed to surgeons and internists caring for minor surgical conditions in the office [41], discussed anesthetic techniques and agents, and issues germane to patient selection and recovery. Thiopental, he said, was unsuitable for ambulatory surgery owing to slow emergence, and he advocated using divinyl ether, as opposed to diethyl ether, because the former afforded a more rapid induction and emergence. He cautioned against administration of cyclopropane by anyone other than an experienced anesthesiologist. He also presented techniques and agents for local and regional anesthesia. Ferguson no doubt hoped that his observations and recommendations would be useful to surgeons and internists because there was not a great deal of interest on the part of anesthesiologists to participate in office anesthesia during the 1940s and 1950s. Despite sporadic publications in the surgical literature, anesthesiologists made minimal efforts to pursue office-based opportunities until the 1980s when financial concerns prompted a re-evaluation.

Dillon stated in 1967, that outpatient surgery could be conducted in any facility that carefully selected appropriate patients [37]. The same forces propelling the expansion of outpatient surgery have driven the growth of office-based anesthesia [42]. Costs are less than in a free-standing surgery center, being the lowest overhead costs of all types of surgical locations. Nonetheless, until the late 1980s and early 1990s, local laws and third-party payers limited reimbursement for office-based procedures. Once that obstacle was removed, office-based surgery grew and is currently the most rapidly expanding subset of anesthesia practice. In the US between 1984 and 1990, the number of office-based procedures increased from less than 2 % to almost 5 %, and by 1994, 8.5 % of all procedures were performed in offices [43]. By the year 2000, approximately 15–20 % of all outpatient procedures were performed in offices [44], and the 2010 estimate is that approximately 25 % of all ambulatory procedures (which account for approximately 80 % of all surgical procedures) are conducted in offices [45].

And in Australia, New Zealand and Other Parts of the World?

The current situation in Australia underscores the importance of financial considerations. Office-based surgery is not yet fully established, largely owing to the failure of health insurers to provide a facility rebate. Australian surgeon Lindsay Roberts states, "A large number of more minor operations/procedures, possibly 20–25 %, could be carried out in such units and the Australian Day Surgery Council (ADSC) has published comprehensive *Guidelines for the Accreditation of Office-Based Surgical Facilities* to ensure that standards of quality and safety are not compromised [36]." Although the absence of this rebate is an important disincentive causing many healthy patients having relatively simple procedures to be cared for currently in day surgery centers at much greater expense, the situation is more complex.

It is not quite as simple as Roberts says. The Australian and New Zealand College of Anaesthetists (ANZCA) publishes comprehensive standards on facility, equipment, and practice requirements that apply no matter where anesthesia is carried out. (The standards are obtainable on the ANZCA website).

The most recent guidelines issued by the ADSC describe office surgery as surgery performed under local anesthesia, with or without sedation. The guidelines also state that if general anesthesia is to be provided, then the standards issued by ANZCA should be adhered to. In addition, it should be noted that the ANZCA standards are recognized by the Australian Council on Health Care Standards, the national accrediting body for health facilities. The ADSC guidelines are not seen in the same light. Hence, it is not surprising that insurers have not embraced "office" surgery, since few offices meet the required standards. Compounding this is a continuing trickle of disasters typically involving "cosmetic surgeons" operating in unaccredited facilities, usually without an anesthetist present.

Australia and New Zealand are not the only countries where more stringent guidelines apply to facilities and staffing for outpatient anesthesia. A similar situation applies in the UK, where regulations and published standards also exist.

Is Office-Based Anesthesia Safe?

Both patients and surgeons value the convenience of surgery performed in the office. Nonetheless, this can be a "double-edged sword". Because most offices function without regulatory oversight, physicians have extraordinary autonomy, performing any surgical procedure without a need for credentialing. This freedom can, and has, resulted in tragedies [46, 47]. Three decades ago, anesthesia-related mortality was generally cited as approximately 1 per 10,000 healthy anesthetized patients. Now the commonly quoted figure is approximately 1 per 200,000–400,000, although these estimates may be optimistic [48]. However, the death rate for office-based surgery in Florida a decade ago was estimated at 1 in 8,500, and a 1999 report found that the mortality rate for patients undergoing liposuction may be as great as 1 in 5,000 [46]. Despite subsequent implementation by the Florida Board of Medicine of corrective actions, Vila and colleagues [49] recently reported a 10-fold greater rate of adverse incidents (66 in 100,000 versus 5.3 in 100,000) and deaths (9.2 in 100,000 versus 0.78 in 100,000) when comparing offices and ASCs, respectively, during the period from 1 April 2000 to 1 April 2002. An anesthesiologist was present in only 15 % of cases that resulted in death. Unfortunately, we have no data indicating the percent of cases not resulting in death where an anesthesiologist was present. These lacunae underscore the need to create a mandatory national computerized database assembling this vital information.

However, Hoefflin et al [50] reported no office deaths in more than 23,000 cases in their accredited office staffed with board-certified anesthesiologists and surgeons, a level of care superior to most of the other comparison reports. The fact that anesthesiologists are present in nearly all ASCs and were present in the favorable 2003 report by Hoefflin et al. [50] emphasizes the importance of their presence for patient safety. In April 2002, the Florida Board of Medicine mandated the presence of an anesthesiologist for all office cases involving general anesthesia, regional anesthesia, and deep sedation. After implementation of this directive, injuries declined by 65 % and deaths by 58 % during the period from April 2002 through March 2003 [51].

Data from the ASA Closed Claims Project database are similarly instructive. Although most ambulatory malpractice claims involve relatively minor injuries, 60 % of office-based anesthesia claims are for death. Moreover, more than 90 % of office-based claims resulted in payment and ASA Closed Claims experts deemed most injuries preventable [52]. Despite formidable risks, about two-thirds of anesthesia practices provide some variety of office services [53]. Medicare has approved more than 2,500 procedures for the office setting. Most of the 9 million cosmetic surgical procedures performed annually in the US are done in physician's offices. Approximately 25 % of all elective outpatient procedures in the US may be conducted in offices [45]. The burgeoning growth of office-based surgery in the face of demonstrated risks reflects the motivational strength of cost containment and convenience in contemporary society.

As office-based anesthesia gained acceptance during the last two decades, ASA and SAMBA jointly advocated for patient safety, and in 1999 developed the ASA Guidelines for Office-Based Anesthesia. Additionally, many states (with dates of enactment) including New Jersey (1998), Pennsylvania (1999), Texas (2000), California (2001), Florida (2002), Alabama, Connecticut and Virginia (2003), Ohio (2004), Tennessee (2005), and New York (2007) enacted legislation regulating office surgical practice. Many other states have safety guidelines that are not, however, legally binding. Accrediting bodies now include the Joint Commission, the Accreditation Association for Ambulatory Health Care (AAAHC), and the American Association for Accreditation of Ambulatory Surgical Facilities (AAAASF).

Accredited offices must maintain safety standards similar to those in a hospital or free-standing surgicenter [54, 55]. Office-based surgery is safe in carefully selected patients having appropriate procedures performed by highly qualified practitioners [54, 55]. More than 1.1 million operative procedures in *AAAASF-accredited* office-based facilities were studied from 2001 to 2006. Deaths were infrequent, occurring in 2.02 of 100,000 procedures or 0.002%, which is comparable to the overall risks of such procedures performed in hospital surgery facilities [56, 57]. Most deaths were due to pulmonary embolism rather than anesthesia-related complications. Only one death was attributable to an anesthetic event, an event which occurred in the absence of an anesthesiologist.

Conclusions

Although the history of ambulatory anesthesia is as old as the history of anesthesia, ambulatory anesthesia in the US grew little until the 1960s, increasing thereafter to the point where it represented 34% of all surgical cases in the mid-1980s, and 75–80% of all procedures today. Medical and economic forces combined to translocate patients from hospitals to freestanding ambulatory centers and offices. The medical advances enabling this translocation included improvements in anesthesia allowing patients to regain consciousness more quickly, with fewer complications, and the development of better analgesics and techniques for relief of postoperative pain. In addition, minimally invasive and noninvasive procedures, such as laparoscopy, laser surgery, and endoscopy, were developed and are being used with increasing regularity, thereby facilitating the movement from inpatient to ambulatory venues.

Contemporaneously, concern regarding increased health care expenditures led to changes in the Medicare program that encouraged the expansion of ambulatory surgery. In the early 1980s, Medicare began to reimburse for care in ambulatory surgery centers, and adopted a prospective payment system based on diagnostic-related groups for hospital inpatient care. These changes generated financial incentives for hospitals to shift less complex surgery to outpatient settings. This trend will probably continue until hospitals care for only the most complex patients having highly invasive, complicated surgery. As the US enters an era of health care reform, more comprehensive epidemiologic data on the utilization of medical resources and the outcomes of medical interventions will be carefully analyzed to make health care policy decisions. The effect of this analysis on the future growth of ambulatory surgery remains to be seen.

Acknowledgments The author thanks the late Patrick Sim, the Paul M. Wood Distinguished Librarian of the Wood Library-Museum of Anesthesiology (WLM), Karen Bieterman, Managing Librarian at the WLM, and Shawn Manning, Librarian at New York Medical College for their invaluable assistance in obtaining historical literature relevant to ambulatory and office-based anesthesia. She also thanks Felicia Reilly, Archivist of the WLM, and Margie Jenkins of the WLM for their gracious help in providing photographs of some of the pioneers in the field.

References

1. Vandam LD. A history of ambulatory anesthesia. Anesthesiol Clin North America. 1987;5:1–13.
2. Goldman L. Hospitalists as cure for hospitalism. Trans Am Clin Climatol Assoc. 2003;114:37–48.
3. Nicoll JH. The surgery of infancy. Br Med J. 1909;18:753–4.
4. Waters RM. The down-town anesthesia clinic. Am J Surg. 1919;39 Suppl:71–3.
5. Webb E, Graves H. Anesthesia for the ambulatory patient. Anesth Analg. 1959;38:359–63.
6. Cohen D, Dillion JB. Anesthesia for outpatient surgery. JAMA. 1966;196:98–100.
7. Levy ML, Coakley CS. Survey of in and out surgery—first year. South Med J. 1967;61:995–8.
8. Calmes, SH. Dr, John Dillon and the founding of the UCLA Department of Anesthesiology. CSA Bulletin. 2000;49:52–4.
9. Calnan J, Martin P. Development and practice of an autonomous minor surgery unit in a general hospital. Br Med J. 1971;4:92–6.
10. Berrill TH. A year in the life of a surgical day unit. Br Med J. 1972;4:348–9.
11. Kaye KW, Gonzalez R, Fraley EE. Microsurgical vasovasostomy—an outpatient procedure under local anesthesia. J Urol. 1983;129:992.
12. Kitz DS, Slusarz-Ladden C, Lecky JH. Hospital resources used for inpatients and ambulatory surgery. Anesthesiology. 1988;69:383–6.
13. White PF, editor. Ambulatory anesthesia and surgery: past, present, and future. London: Saunders; 1997. p. 3–34.
14. Haworth EA, Balarajan R. Day surgery—does it add to or replace inpatient surgery? Br Med J. 1987;294:133–5.
15. Berk AA, Chalmers TC. Cost and efficacy of the substitution of ambulatory for inpatient care. N Engl J Med. 1981;304:393–7.

16. Detmer DE. Ambulatory surgery. N Engl J Med. 1985;305:1406–9.
17. Rhodes RS. Ambulatory surgery and the societal cost of surgery. Surgery. 1994;116(5):938–40.
18. Hill CL. Surgery in an office suite (letter). Med Econ. 1968 Oct;28:61–2.
19. Ford JL, Reed WA. The surgicenter—an innovation in the delivery and cost of medical care. Ariz Med. 1969;26:801–4.
20. Reed WA, Ford JL. Development of an independent outpatient surgical center. Int Anesthesiol Clin. 1976;14(2):113–30.
21. Federal Register. 23 March 1982. 12,583, section VIII.
22. History of the first surgicenter. DVD available from the Wood Library-Museum of Anesthesiology Living History of Anesthesiology series. Revised version for PHX Channel 11; 1 March 1994.
23. Cullen KA, Hall MJ, Golosinskiy A. Ambulatory surgery in the United States, 2006. National health statistics reports; no 11. Revised. Hyattsville, MD, National Center for Health Statistics; 2009.
24. Wetchler BV, editor. Anesthesia for ambulatory surgery. Philadelphia: Lippincott; 1985.
25. White PF. editor. Outpatient anesthesia. New York: Churchill Livingstone; 1990.
26. McGoldrick KE. editor. Ambulatory anesthesia: a problem-oriented approach. Baltimore: Williams & Wilkins; 1995.
27. Twersky RS. editor. The ambulatory anesthesia handbook. St. Louis: Mosby; 1995.
28. Burden N. Outpatient surgery: a view through history. J Perianesth Nurs. 2005;20(6):435–7.
29. Skledar SJ, Williams BA, Vallejo MC, et al. Eliminating postoperative nausea and vomiting in outpatient surgery with multimodal strategies including low doses of nonsedating, off-patent antiemetics: Is "zero tolerance" achievable? Sci World J. 2007;7:959–77.
30. White PF. The changing role of non-opioid analgesic techniques in the management of postoperative pain. Anesth Analg. 2005;101 Suppl:S5–22.
31. Power I. Recent advances in postoperative pain therapy. Br J Anaesth. 2005;95:43–51.
32. Hurley RW, Cohen SP, Williams KA, Rowlingson AJ, Wu CL. The analgesic effects of perioperative gabapentin on postoperative pain: a meta-analysis. Reg Anesth Pain Med. 2006;31:237–47.
33. Ansell GL, Montgomery JE. Outcome of ASA III patients undergoing day case surgery. Br J Anaesth. 2004;92:71–4.
34. Warner MA, Shields SE, Chute CG. Major morbidity and mortality within 1 month of ambulatory surgery and anesthesia. JAMA. 1993;270:1437–41.
35. Brökelmann J. Ambulatory surgery in Germany. and historical aspects. J Ambul Surg. 2006;12:173–6.
36. Roberts L. Day surgery—national and international: from the past to the future. J Ambul Surg. 2006;12:143–5.
37. Dillon JB. Anesthetic management of the outpatient. Anesth Rounds. 1967;2:1–15.
38. Chelly JE, Gebhard R, Coupe K, et al. Local anesthetic delivered via a femoral catheter by patient-controlled analgesia pump for pain relief after an anterior cruciate ligament outpatient procedure. Am J Anesthesiol. 2001;28:192–4.
39. Grant G, Bansinath M. Liposomal delivery systems for local anesthetics. Reg Anesth Pain Med. 2001;26:61–3.
40. Franz-Montan M, Silva ALR, Cogo K, et al. Liposome-encapsulated ropivacaine for topical anesthesia of the human oral mucosa. Anesth Analg. 2007;104:1528–31.
41. Ferguson LK. Anesthesia: surgery of the ambulatory patient. Philadelphia: Lippincott; 1947. p. 18–59.
42. Pregler JL, Kapur PA. The development of ambulatory anesthesia and future challenges. Anesthesiol Clin North America. 2003;21:207–28.
43. Lazarov SJ. Office-based surgery and anesthesia: where are we now? World J Urol. 1998;16:384–5.
44. Pandit SK. Ambulatory anesthesia and surgery in America: a historical background and recent innovations. J Perianesth Nurs. 1999;14:270–4.
45. Hausman LM, Rosenblatt MA. Office-based anesthesia. In: Barash PG, Cullen BF, Stoelting RK, Cahalan MK, Stock MC, editors. Clinical anesthesia. 6th ed. Philadelphia: Lippincott; 2009. p. 847–60.
46. Rao RB, Ely SF, Hoffman RS. Deaths related to liposuction. N Engl J Med. 1999;340:1471–5.
47. McGoldrick KE. Is "risk" just another four-letter word? (editorial). SAMBA Newsl. 2005;20:1, 5.
48. Lagasse RS. Anesthesia safety: model or myth? A review of the published literature and analysis of current and original data. Anesthesiology. 2002;97:1609–17.
49. Vila H, Soto R, Cantor AB, Mackey D. Comparative outcomes analysis of procedures performed in physician offices and ambulatory surgery centers. Arch Surg. 2003;138:991–5.
50. Hoefflin SM, Bornstein JB, Gordon M. General anesthesia in an office-based plastic surgery facility: a report on more than 23,000 consecutive office-based procedures under general anesthesia with no significant anesthetic complications. Plast Reconstr Surg. 2001;107:243–57.
51. Vila H, Soto RG, Miguel RV, et al. 2003 update: outcomes analysis of procedures performed in Florida physician offices and ambulatory surgery centers. Anesthesiology. 2003;99:A1364.
52. Domino KB. Office-based anesthesia: lessons learned from the closed claims project. ASA Newsl. 2001;65(6):9–11, 15.
53. Koch ME, Giannuzzi R, Goldstein RC. Office anesthesiology: an overview. Anesthesiol Clin North America. 1999;17:395–405.
54. American Society of Anesthesiologists: Directory of Members. Park Ridge: ASA; 2000. p. 480.
55. Stoelting RK. Office-based anesthesia growth provokes safety fears. APSF Newsl. 2000;15:1–2.
56. Keyes GR, Singer R, Iverson RE, et al. Mortality in outpatient surgery. Plast Reconstr Surg. 2008;122:245–50.
57. Hancock JG, Venkat AP, Coldiron B, et al. The safety of office-based surgery. Arch Dermatol. 2004;140:1379–82.

The Anesthesiologist and Pain: A Historical Memoir

60

Daniel B. Carr and Michael J Cousins

Summary

Pain has forever troubled humankind. Elucidation of nociceptive mechanisms and pathways, and appreciation of their diversity and adaptability, have been essential to understanding pain. Anesthesiologists have furthered such understanding and treatment, and advanced the appreciation of pain as a public health issue.

During the twentieth century, the concepts of post-injury sensitization and hyperalgesia were developed, and the role of humoral mediators recognized. The 1950s saw the emergence of anesthesia departments, facilitating research into acute and chronic pain by specialists whose daily task originated with the elimination of pain during operations.

Henry Beecher observed injured soldiers during World War II, noting that post-injury pain intensity and the dose of opioids needed to control their pain were both less than with comparable civilian injuries. He argued that the meaning of the injury, not the injury *per se,* dictates the intensity of pain. In the 1960s, Melzack and Wall described the gate control theory, providing a neurological basis to Beecher's concept. They proposed that rostral descending pathways modulate nociceptive afferent traffic at the spinal segmental level.

John Bonica pioneered pain advocacy, research and practice. His comprehensive 1953 monograph summarized available knowledge on pain. In 1973, he convened an international meeting that led to the formation of the International Association for the Study of Pain (IASP) and founding of the journal *Pain.* Anesthesiologists were influential in widening the focus of IASP from chronic pain to acute and cancer pain. Recognition that physical, psychological and environmental factors play a key role in all pain and its treatment remains Bonica's lasting legacy.

From 1950 to 1990, control of acute and postoperative pain received inadequate attention despite knowledge of effective treatments. Ready's watershed description of an organized acute pain service in 1988 accelerated the initiation of multidisciplinary pain teams in developed countries. Increasing understanding of the pharmacokinetic and pharmacodynamic properties of opioids and other analgesic drugs, together with an appreciation of the neural mechanisms governing pain perception, led to the use of multiple classes of analgesic and adjuvant drugs. This "multimodal approach" aims to optimize acute pain management and prevent the transition from acute to chronic pain. The IASP published *Management of Acute Pain: a Practical Guide* in 1992.

Anesthesiologists have advanced new concepts in pain management during the past 40 years, reported their findings in thousands of studies, and applied them to improve outcomes. In 2010, the IASP, through the Declaration of Montreal, affirmed that access to pain management is a fundamental human right.

Introduction

Since prehistory, pain has driven sufferers to pursue relief by any available means. Anesthesiologists have played a central role in advancing the understanding and treatment of pain, a primal experience shaped by meaning, and social and religious contexts [1–10]. This chapter describes pioneers in anesthesiology who extended pain management outside the operating room, to improve pain sufferers' quality of life by applying lessons learned from anatomy, physiology, pharmacology, neuroscience, and the study of human behavior [11]. We also describe how anesthesiologists recently framed pain as a public health problem and played an advocacy role in achieving access to pain management as a fundamental

D. B. Carr (✉)
Program on Pain Research, Education and
Policy, Tufts University School of Medicine,
136 Harrison Avenue, 02111 Boston, MA USA
e-mail: daniel.carr@tufts.edu

M. J Cousins
Department of Anaesthesia and Pain Management,
Royal North Shore Hospital, University of Sydney
Sydney, Australia
e-mail: mcousins@nsccahs.health.nsw.gov.au

human right [12]. Anesthesiologists have led governmental and nongovernmental initiatives, championed pain education for health professionals and the public, [13, 14] and elevated the standard of pain research and its subsequent translation into clinical practice [15].

In 1954, John Bonica described two roles for the anesthesiologist managing pain: first, as a technician skilled in performing specific diagnostic or therapeutic procedures "whose contribution will, of necessity, be an exercise rather than a discipline"; second, "as the individual who is responsible for the over-all management of the patient" [16]. The development of methods and techniques for regional anesthesia and neural blockade *per se* are described elsewhere in this volume. In the spirit of Bonica's distinction, the present chapter focuses on the anesthesiologist's roles in advancing the science of pain and translating new knowledge to benefit patients.

Numerous publications describe the history of pain from scientific, philosophical and literary perspectives. Bibliometric analyses provide objective measures of the number of published articles on pain, the evolution of popular topics, and the impact of these publications (defined as the number of citations according to article, subject or author) [17–21]. We intend to present a personal perspective, emphasizing people, places and events that we have known first-hand. In defense of this approach, we note that Thucydides himself conceded possible bias in writing at greater length about military campaigns in which he had fought, or political debates in which he had participated, but he claimed that the benefit of an eyewitness narrative outweighed the risk of myopic emphasis.

Antecedents

Anesthesiologists and anesthesia have woven much of the fabric of modern pain management. Long before the specialty was recognized as such, inhalational and local anesthetics transformed medical practice. In his graduate thesis in English and Comparative Literature, written in retirement after a distinguished academic career in anesthesiology, Emanuel Papper recounted Davy's and others' observations of the analgesic effects of nitrous oxide, a half-century before its clinical application [22]. Papper argued that attitudes of the emerging Romantic era, particularly its focus on the happiness of the individual independent of the group, prompted Western society to overcome prior disinterest in relieving individual suffering. By 1884, when Koller first described local anesthesia, the desirability of relieving intraoperative pain was no longer questioned. Early techniques for neural blockade applied cocaine to surgically exposed peripheral nerves or plexuses [23, 24]. The advent of percutaneous approaches to peripheral and neuraxial blockade expanded surgeons' interest in and techniques of blockade during the late 19th century and early 20th century.

By the outbreak of World War II, differentiated anesthesia units had formed in some academic centers [23–26]. A few of these focused upon neural blockade (e.g., Mayo Clinic [27] or Bellevue Hospital [23–24]. In Europe, Leriche linked division of sympathetic ganglia and plexuses with improved blood flow to ischemic limbs and reduction of some forms of chronic pain. These included causalgias or phantom limb pain that had been observed for millennia, but were first described systematically during the US Civil War. By the mid-20th century, the anatomy of nociception was understood well enough to provide a rationale for neurosurgical division of spinal (cordotomy) or central (cingulotomy) pathways, among other neurosurgical techniques for pain relief [28, 29].

The German pain researcher Goldscheider questioned Von Frey's and Muller's 19th century hypothesis of specific receptors for pain. Goldscheider proposed that a single set of nerve receptors mediated both the sensation of non-painful touch and its central summation to become pain [30]. In the early 20th century, Henry Head, a British neurologist, distinguished between rapid, well-localized touch sensations ("epicritic"), and the slower onset of dull, poorly localized, highly aversive sensations ("protopathic"), characteristic of regenerating injured nerves. Sherrington, a contemporary of Head, introduced the term "nociceptor" and the concept of descending inhibition. Working in St Louis, Missouri in the 1930s, Erlanger and Gasser identified distinct neuronal populations with differing conduction velocities, within peripheral nerves. Their classification of neurons, using Roman letters A to D to describe groups according to axonal conduction velocity, and Greek letters alpha to gamma to delineate subgroups, remains in use today. During these studies, Zotterman and Adrian employed the oscilloscope to record an action potential from a single nociceptive neuron.

In the first half of the 20th century, researchers investigated phenomena we now term post-injury sensitization and hyperalgesia [30–31]. Anticipating the current practice of multimodal analgesia, the UK internist, Lewis, postulated in the 1930s and 1940s that humoral mediators (including histamine, bradykinin and substance P) of injury, in the vicinity of a primary lesion, enhanced sensitivity to stimuli. Others during these pre-war decades, including Livingstone in Oregon, and Hardy and Wolff at Yale University, focused upon activation of a neuronal pool of variable excitability within the spinal cord, as the basis for post-injury hyperalgesia (excessive sensitivity to pain). Research on hyperalgesia and sensitization echoed prescient clinical observations at the beginning of the 20th century by George Crile, surgeon and founder of the Cleveland Clinic [32]. Crile proposed that using local anesthesia to block transmission of nociceptive impulses from the periphery to the central nervous system, could avert the debilitating effects of surgery or trauma. Crile's hypothesis ("anoci-association") anticipated not only the concept of central sensitization, but also the benefit of regional anesthesia in inhibiting what were later identified as catabolic and immunosuppressive postoperative stress responses. He argued that untreated pain facilitated the development of central sensitization and the stress responses (see below). Not surprisingly, recognition of the importance of regional anesthesia and pain control by its leadership, led the Cleveland Clinic to continuing prominence in these fields.

Thus, by World War II, a substantial foundation supported the growth of pain research and treatment. Observations of combatants and veterans during World War II were pivotal to the careers of pioneers such as Henry Beecher and John Bonica. Progress in this field accelerated in postwar developed nations witnessing the return of veterans (many of them with chronic pain from wounds), and a baby boom demanding better obstetric pain relief. By the 1950s, many departments of anesthesiology had differentiated from their surgical antecedents. Circumstances were ripe for clinicians, clinical researchers, and research scientists in or affiliated with these departments to address major gaps in scientific knowledge and clinical practice. Bacon documented the relatively low, constant number of citations to both pain and conduction anesthesia from the early part of the 20th century until about 1950, [23] when a steady upsurge of citations began, roughly doubling in each subsequent decade [11]. We describe how this progress unfolded in the past 60 years using selected highlights of pain research and practice in which anesthesiologists and their basic science collaborators have changed medical practice.

Boston: Beecher, Analgesic Trials, and the Placebo Effect

Beecher was a Midwesterner born with the improbable surname of Unangst [33]. A month before entering Harvard Medical School, he legally changed his surname to Beecher (the maiden name of his maternal great-grandmother) perhaps to be more acceptable to Boston's Brahmin society, and possibly to distance himself from his irresponsible father with whom he had a strained relationship. Beecher was a high-energy iconoclast. His research was influenced by early positions teaching chemistry and physiology, award-winning laboratory studies in respiratory physiology as a medical student, and a year (1935) studying in Copenhagen with the 1920 Nobel laureate in medicine August Krogh. In 1936, and without training in clinical anesthesia, Beecher became the first Anesthetist-in-Chief at the Massachusetts General Hospital (MGH), and chairman of this new department within the Department of Surgery. In 1938, he published a 388-page monograph on the physiology of anesthesia.

During World War II, Beecher was mobilized to Europe where he made an insightful observation concerning pain at the 1944 Anzio beachhead. Beecher noticed that battlefield casualties had less intense pain and required less morphine than civilian counterparts suffering equally severe injuries. He surmised that the soldiers thought, "I have survived and will go home and not return to the front line!" Despite major nociception, the soldiers' pain was minimal—implying that the meaning of the injury and not the injury *per se* dictates the intensity of pain. Two decades later, when working at MIT, on the other side of the Charles River from Boston, Melzack and Wall supplied a neurological basis for Beecher's insight in their now classic 1965 paper describing the gate-control theory [34]. They proposed that rostral descending pathways modulate nociceptive afferent traffic at the spinal segmental level.

Pain research fascinated Melzack, and he generously encouraged others involved in such research. He became President of the International Association for the Study of Pain (IASP). Wall could be intimidating on first meeting, and in his role as the first Editor-in-Chief of the journal *Pain*. He could be devastatingly critical of sloppy work or adherence to outdated concepts. Both he and Melzack became warm friends of the current authors (MJC & DBC), and inspired many pain researchers who remain active to this day.

Beecher's personal library was placed "up for grabs" before it was to be discarded by his successor Richard Kitz, on Kitz's retirement [25]. A young staff anesthesiologist, DBC, grabbed as many books as he could. These volumes covered neurochemistry, central nervous system metabolism, regional blood flow, oxygen consumption, pharmacology and physiology, mental health issues including opioid addiction, mathematical biophysics modeling synaptic conduction, and the biological basis of fatigue and stress. Just as Beecher's group found that a single pencil stroke made by a patient on a visual analog pain scale could offer insight into that person's perceptions, Beecher's underlining and marginal scrawls in these rescued volumes document a deep, career-long interest in neuroscience. One of the earliest of the volumes is a 1929 printing of Haldane's and Huxley's *Animal Biology* [35]. Unlike later volumes that all bear the stamp "Property of the Department of Anesthesia of the Massachusetts General Hospital" along with the purchase date and Beecher's signature, this has none, suggesting that it was acquired before the department was organized. The handwritten notes are identical in appearance (including sole use of pencil, never pen) to those in later volumes bearing the MGH stamp. The notes are concentrated in sections on neuronal physiology. A copy of Page's 1937 monograph *The Chemistry of the Brain*, purchased in 1940, shows Beecher's questions about the validity of the methods then used to assess cerebral metabolism, particularly their inability to observe regional vasoconstriction [36]. Bartley's and Chute's 1947 monograph on *Fatigue and Impairment in Man* [37] is heavily underlined in sections on sleep deprivation as a means to induce psychosis. A 1953 research monograph on metabolic and toxic diseases of the nervous system, [38] is densely highlighted—but only in the chapter on psychoses produced by administration of drugs, with stars drawn alongside specific descriptions of the effects of LSD and mescaline. "Get" is scrawled next to several chapter references on delirium and clinical studies of hallucinogens. Of the latter, one of these has "8/17/57" written alongside—just four days after the volume's receipt date. The near-immediate attention Beecher gave to this chapter coincides with his active, secret research funded by the Central Intelligence Agency (see below).

Beecher assembled a remarkable team to initiate modern analgesic trials. Many methods they introduced or refined remain in use today. Louis Lasagna, the first author of this group's influential 1954 study quantifying the magnitude of the placebo response in postoperative analgesic trials, [39] became "the father of modern clinical pharmacology", an FDA advisor (one of three consultants who developed the current regulatory framework of phase 1–3 trials to demonstrate safety and efficacy of medications prior to FDA approval), and a pain researcher in his own right (e.g., inventor of the vertical "pain thermometer" scale) [40]. Lasagna advocated rigorously controlled clinical trials, yet privately described such trials as "hothouse medicine" whose results were often over generalized to real-world patients. In print, he pleaded for "the naturalistic study of medicines", anticipating the current emphasis on comparative effectiveness research. Lasagna later became a graduate dean at Tufts, where he founded its Center for the Study of Drug Development, and was instrumental in inaugurating its Master of Science program in pain research, education and policy. In the mid 1990s DBC heard a lecture by Lasagna, during which he uncomfortably revealed that in the Cold War era of the 1950s, Beecher and his group conducted secret studies of the effects of LSD in healthy subjects, research supported by the Central Intelligence Agency. Each week's results would be placed in a sealed envelope and handed to a government courier in civilian garb who had traveled from Washington to Boston solely to receive them. Perhaps it was a sense of guilt at participation in this classified program—identified 50 years later in newly declassified documents as the CIA's notorious MKULTRA project, exploring drugs for mind control—that led Beecher in the 1960s to advocate for the ethical conduct of clinical trials [41]. Beecher not only underlined those sections in his books focusing on hallucinogens, sleep deprivation and other means to induce psychosis, but devoted a lengthy chapter to psychotomimetic drugs in his classic 1959 text *The Measurement of Subjective Responses in Man* [42]. In retrospect, the almost disproportionate comprehensiveness of that chapter is another clue to his intense yet clandestine Cold War research.

Statistical Studies and the Emergence of International Collaboration

Donald Todd, a Beecher protégé and co-author of the 1954 study of deaths associated with nearly 600,000 anesthetics in 10 institutions, [43] devoted his later career to clinical care of patients with pain. DBC once asked Todd why death was selected as the sole outcome analyzed in the 1954 study. He chuckled and replied "because it was the only outcome whose definition everyone could agree upon". His use of regional anesthesia to diagnose and treat painful conditions dated from a 1940s collaboration with William Sweet, a neurosurgeon and pioneer in pain studies. This collaboration led him to provide anesthesia care for trigeminal thermal or glycerol ablations, cingulotomies, and to test the effect of local anesthetic sympathetic blocks prior to planned surgical sympathectomy. Todd formed a "diagnostic and therapeutic nerve block unit" that DBC joined in 1986, at Kitz's suggestion. The suggestion acknowledged DBC's prior research fellowship in endocrinology and peptide chemistry, measuring β-endorphin. That work resulted in reports on neuro-immune interactions and the effects of physical exercise upon β-endorphin secretion (the 1981 "runner's endorphin" publication) [44]. The nerve block unit expanded to a multidisciplinary pain clinic following the Seattle model (see below), to which a clinical fellowship was subsequently added. The blueprint for the evolution of this nerve block unit into a multidisciplinary center was provided in the mid-1980s, through a comprehensive consultation arranged by Kitz with his friend MJC. At that time, in his capacity as President of the IASP, Cousins was codifying desirable features for various types of pain treatment facilities worldwide. The authors' personal interactions and multiple collaborations date from this time.

Frederick Mosteller developed the statistical methods for Beecher's (and hence the field's) early analgesic trials. Later, with his colleague Tom Chalmers, Mosteller originated the technique of meta-analysis. In 1990, DBC co-chaired the first US federal clinical practice guideline panel; its topic was acute pain [45]. Mosteller and Chalmers provided support with systematic reviews and meta-analyses, for example, of patient-controlled analgesia [46] and the respiratory benefits of postoperative epidural analgesia [47]. Bucknam McPeek, another Beecher protégé, personal medical advisor to Mosteller, and senior member of the MGH acute pain team, facilitated an expanded international co-operation. McPeek's European connections included Edmond Neugebauer and Stefan Schug from Germany, whose productivity in translational pain research, particularly in relation to acute pain and often based upon international collaborations, led them to organize IASP's Acute Pain Special Interest Group (APSIG) in the months leading up to its 2005 World Congress in Sydney. The APSIG's inaugural meeting took place at that World Congress. DBC, currently Chair of the APSIG, enjoyed additional collaborations with French and Greek clinical scientists. Chalmers and Mosteller continued to support evidence-based analyses for a subsequent guideline on cancer pain, after which their protégé Joseph Lau at Tufts picked up the task, becoming Director of Tufts' Evidence-based Practice Center, funded by the Agency for Healthcare Research and Quality [48]. Anesthesiologists were not only involved in the first evidence-based US federal guidelines, but to this day have participated in numerous international evidence syntheses [15] and related policy efforts such as providing expert guidance and testimony to the US FDA.

The pioneering advances of Beecher and his collaborators continue to guide how medical science worldwide quantifies subjective responses, conducts regulatory affairs such as drug approval, and monitors pain in everyday practice [49]. Today's routine uses of placebo or sham comparators in analgesic trials, and current neuroscience research on placebo, also reflect Beecher's influence. One indication of this impact is the selection of publications from Beecher, Lasagna and Mosteller (on placebo) and Lau (on cumulative meta-analysis) by the Editor of *The Lancet* for his personal 27-item "core canon of medical literature" [50]. Others so selected included Hippocrates, Galen and Koch.

In the 1960s, Todd's colleagues cautiously began using small doses of morphine as an antitussive for patients requiring prolonged controlled ventilation following cardiac surgery [51]. The patients did so well that larger and larger doses of morphine (and later, fentanyl) were given earlier in their course, culminating in what for the time were unprecedented large doses of opioids being given routinely during cardiac anesthesia, as reported by Edward Lowenstein in 1969 [52]. That practice was adopted worldwide.

Boston is replete with academic medical activity, facilitating cross-fertilization. Benjamin Covino—in the 1970s a senior executive at Astra, a global pharmaceutical firm self-termed "the house of regional anesthesia"—decided to pursue clinical training in anesthesiology after years as a clinical researcher and pharmaceutical executive. He completed his anesthesiology residency at the MGH, occasionally swapping on-call dates to catch a flight overseas to a corporate board meeting. Upon completing his residency in 1977, he became the first and still only MGH anesthesia trainee whose initial post-residency position was as an academic chairman (at the University of Massachusetts). In 1979, he succeeded Leroy Vandam as Chairman of Anesthesiology at the Brigham and Women's Hospital. That hospital's patients included many with arthritis undergoing joint replacements under regional anesthesia, and many parturients whose labor pain was managed with epidurals. Covino's department included stellar clinicians along with clinical and preclinical scientists, including Gary Strichartz, the 1987 ASA Excellence in Research Awardee, honored for his work on mechanisms of action of local anesthetics [53] and other pain-related topics. Many Brigham graduates advanced pain research and practice, including two Past Presidents of ASRA-PM, Michael Ferrante and Mark Lema. Lema, an MD with a PhD in pharmacology, is also a Past President of the ASA. As the long-term Chair of Roswell Park Cancer Institute's Department of Anesthesiology, Critical Care & Pain Medicine, he has focused upon cancer pain control. He has mentored prominent clinician-researchers including Oscar de Leon-Casasola. Carol Warfield, the Edward Lowenstein Professor (see above) of Anesthesiology at the Beth Israel Deaconess Medical Center, is another Boston-based leader in pain medicine known for numerous educational and organizational activities and a multi-edition textbook on pain.

Other major metropolitan centers had their own pioneers in pain treatment and research. In New York's Bellevue Hospital, Emery Rovenstine established one of the nation's first outpatient pain clinics in 1936, focusing on nerve blockade. About a mile away, Raymond Houde's group at Cornell and Memorial Sloan Kettering Cancer Center advanced analgesic trial design and produced leaders in opioid research. The growth of pain research and care in recent generations led many centers to assemble critical masses of pain clinicians and researchers not only in the Americas but also in the United Kingdom, the European continent, and Asia including Australia (in Adelaide, Brisbane and Sydney).

Bonica, Chronic Pain as Disease, Multidisciplinary Pain Clinics, and IASP

John Bonica, working in Tacoma and Seattle, was the second pioneer of the current worldwide era of clinical pain research and treatment. Like Beecher, he rose from humble beginnings to join the first generation of academic anesthesiologists. Although Giovanni Giuseppe Bonica's parents Americanized their 12-year-old's name to John Joseph Bonica when they fled Mussolini's Italy and emigrated to the US, unlike Beecher, Bonica never discarded his ethnicity [54]. MJC recalls that Bonica's forceful personality sometimes evoked suspicions of a subterranean connection with a powerful Italian organization, a link for which no justification existed, but that Bonica chose not to refute.

Remarkable physical strength and endurance complemented Bonica's dominating personality. Apart from Resh Lakish in imperial Rome, and Bonica in democratic America, history offers few examples of professional wrestlers who went on to careers as distinguished scholars [55]. Bonica began wrestling in secondary school, became New York City's high school middleweight champion, and two years later the regional intercollegiate champion. His biography in the Professional Wrestling Hall of Fame describes his competing as Johnny "Bull" Walker, and once defeating all 36 members of a college wrestling team in a single day. He wrestled professionally for 14 years (1936–1950), including as "The Masked Marvel" during military service. In 1939, he won the light heavyweight championship of Canada and in 1941 was world champion at that weight. He fought in 1485 professional bouts, and 2000 additional matches in carnivals and circuses where he earned money for medical school tuition by taking on all comers. Chaperoned by her mother Angela, his wife Emma often sold tickets at these carnivals. His wrestling career and numerous consequent operations, including hip replacements, left him with lifelong pain that underlay his interest in pain management.

As with Beecher, clinical observations in World War II proved fundamental to Bonica's career. In 1944, Bonica entered the Army directly from residency, and was assigned to the then largest military hospital in the world, the 7700-bed Madigan Army Medical Center in Fort Lewis, Washington. His orders stated "You will be in charge of pain control". He read classic works, corresponded extensively, yet was baffled by the many pain problems in wounded soldiers under his care [56]. He began a regular lunch meeting to which he invited an orthopedist, a neurosurgeon and a psychiatrist to discuss such cases. Years later, he stated "These early experiences convinced me that complex pain problems could be more effectively treated by a multidisciplinary/ interdisciplinary team, each member of which would contribute his/ her specialized knowledge and skills to the common goal of making a correct diagnosis in developing the most effective therapeutic strategy" [56]. From this came the multidisciplinary pain clinic. He continued such a clinic as Chairman of Anesthesiology at Tacoma General Hospital after Army service, and later in 1960, as founding Chairman of the Department of Anesthesiology at the University of Washington in Seattle. Influenced in part by early visionaries such as Leriche, Bonica considered chronic pain to be a disease entity *per se* (see below) in which psychosocial features were substantial. The "father" of operant conditioning, the psychologist William Fordyce, oversaw Bonica's pain rehabilitation program [57].

The concept that chronic pain has important psychological and systemic comorbidities is an ancient one. The Roman general and emperor Marcus Aurelius wrote in his *Meditations* that "many other things which we find uncomfortable are of the same nature as pain: feelings of lethargy, or a feverish temperature, or loss of appetite" [58]. Robert Burton, in his voluminous 17th-century *Anatomy of Melancholy* voiced similar observations, [59] as did the US Civil War physician Weir Mitchell. These insights appear to have been nearly forgotten by early 20th century medical research. The slender 1948 monograph on pain by Wolff and Wolf, for ex-

ample, describes pain solely in nociceptive terms without mention of psychological factors [60]. Its single index entries for both "brain" and "cortex" refer simply to the insensibility of each to direct stimulation. It was the "charismatic entrepreneur" [2] Bonica who laid the foundation for today's view of chronic pain as a disease entity best treated in a multidisciplinary fashion.

Building upon Bonica's early work, MJC and Philip Siddall were the first to assemble and integrate a wide range of basic and clinical (including psychological) evidence that chronic pain is a disease entity *per se* [61]. They observed that "continuing nociceptive inputs result in a multitude of consequences that impact on the individual, ranging from changes in receptor function to mood dysfunction, inappropriate cognitions, and social disruption" [61]. They maintained that the changes brought about in multiple bodily systems "as a consequence of continuing nociceptive inputs argue for the consideration of persistent pain as a disease entity in its own right." Anticipating the current interest in pain and its control from the perspective of public health (see below), Siddall and Cousins pointed out that "the best outcomes will be obtained when those involved in the treatment of persistent pain recognize and also tackle the variety of environmental factors that may be contributing to the presence of persistent pain."

Bonica's desire to optimize acute postoperative pain control (see below) led to the formation of one of the earliest organized acute pain services based in anesthesiology, described in 1988 by Brian Ready and colleagues [62]. His work on chronic pain led to the founding and expansion of the IASP (see below), now the single largest global interdisciplinary organization focused upon pain. In 1953, Bonica authored a 1500-page monograph summarizing the world's preclinical and clinical knowledge of pain and emphasizing the distinctive nature of chronic pain [63]. He accomplished this while working full-time in Tacoma! A major theme of this watershed text was that "whereas in acute pain, the pain is a symptom of the disease or injury, in chronic pain the pain itself is the disease" [64]. He lectured extensively about his ideas and served as President of the ASA and the World Federation of Societies of Anaesthesiologists (WFSA). As Baszanger [2] and others [65] pointed out, a less obvious but ongoing powerful factor was the worldwide assignment of increasing importance to the wishes of patients and their families for enhanced quality of life and hence improved pain control.

In 1972, Bonica invited an international group of researchers to a meeting, with the goal of founding a global organization to establish pain as a differentiated field of study. To organize the meeting, he recruited his department's editor, Louisa Jones. The May 1973 meeting attracted 102 international speakers and 237 other delegates to Issaquah, Washington, where the IASP charter (modeled after the charter of WFSA) was promulgated [66]. A Council was established, and planning began for a new journal, *Pain*. Jones asked Bonica what to do next. His simple response was "You handle it" [66]. Although Jones said Bonica had a reputation as a difficult supervisor, the two worked well together. Jones attributed their collegiality to a similar outlook, resulting from having grown up within a half mile of each other in Brooklyn, New York. DBC and MJC interacted with Jones for decades, in awe of her administrative and editorial capacities and her work ethic, noting her unofficial maternal counseling of members of IASP including its officers.

MJC's close relationship with Bonica extended from the 1970s into the 1990s. He recalls that:

"I first met Bonica in 1970 when I visited Seattle to discuss my acute pain research carried out under the supervision of Bromage in Montreal. I knew that Bonica had a reputation for being 'imposing' and engendered a feeling that one did not want to be 'on the wrong side of him'. He had a handshake like a steel clamp and had shoulders almost equal in breadth to his height. He listened with some apparent irritation to my research findings and then fired off a series of staccato questions which dashed my hopes of his approval (even though the editors of *Surgery, Gynecology and Obstetrics* had already agreed to publish my manuscript). In the end he said 'Not bad. Keep up the good work. Follow me and I will show you what we do here'. Before I left he gave me some advice for the future 'Remember always to get your facts straight…and never, never give up'. Subsequently Bonica appointed me as a Regional Vice President and then IASP Councilor. I learned as a junior Councilor 'Never say no to Bonica'. He involved people from diverse specialties and balanced basic with clinical input. His tireless work in fostering the development of the careers of many IASP members besides myself spanned many others too numerous to name.

"Some interpreted Bonica's apparent 'grumpiness' as being 'difficult'. More likely the underlying cause was injuries from his wrestling career resulting in his having close to 50 operations and severe chronic pain. His ability to pursue 'active approaches to pain control' by keeping busy was an object lesson to any pain patient—he just kept going even after 70 years of age. However, when his beloved wife Emma died he did not persevere much longer. He took the unusual step of calling me, and his other close friends, to say goodbye about 24 hours prior to his death—as always he was in control of the situation."

We can only speculate to what degree Bonica's drive to establish the field of Pain Medicine resulted from his own chronic severe pain, poor postoperative pain control after his dozens of operations, or Emma's near-fatal response to a general anesthetic, poorly administered during delivery [54]. Perhaps part was a reaction to his earning a livelihood for decades by defeating opponents in hand-to-hand combat.

He did not comment upon his personal motivations when he wrote "the anaesthetist in his daily practice sees and cares for patients who fear pain and consequently he naturally develops a sympathetic understanding, a considerate feeling for those who suffer. This is, without doubt, the most important and greatest single qualifying attribute" [67].

As more people entered the fields of pain research and treatment, they built on the contributions of individual postwar pioneers such as Beecher and Bonica, resulting in group efforts on a national or international scale. This pattern of pioneers succeeded by numerous followers is typical of the diffusion of all types of knowledge [17–21, 68].

Early Years of the IASP

Anesthesiologists played an integral role in IASP from its beginning. Bonica sought to link basic researchers to clinicians and thus asked Denise Albe-Fessard, PhD (head of a basic pain neurophysiology research group at INSERM, in Paris) to be the First President of IASP. Bonica became President-elect, ensuring long service in three consecutive presidential positions: President-elect, 2nd President and Past-President. He also would continue to serve on IASP's Executive for that organization's first nine formative years [69]. Another anesthesiologist from Bonica's department in Seattle, B Raymond ("Ray") Fink, served as the first IASP Secretary. Still other anesthesiologists on the first Council were Fausto Molina (Argentina), Joseph Sodipo (Nigeria), Jean Lassner (France) and Hideo Yamamura (Japan). Bonica achieved his vision of IASP fostering interaction among basic scientists and clinicians. IASP presently has more than 8000 members in 126 countries and chapters in 85 countries. Of 12 IASP Presidents to date, besides Bonica only two (MJC and Eija Kalso) were anesthesiologists. On the other hand, given IASP's tradition of nominating preclinical scientists alternating with clinicians for President, that figure corresponds to half of the clinicians elected.

During Melzack's and MJC's Presidencies (1984–1990), IASP's brief increased from a focus largely on chronic pain, to include acute pain and cancer pain. An official NGO relationship was developed with the World Health Organization, with the Norwegian anesthesiologist and researcher, Harald Breivik, in the long-term liaison role. Several task forces were formed by MJC including Acute Pain Management (1984); Pain in the Workforce (1987); Core Curriculum for Professional Education in Pain (1987); and Undergraduate Curriculum in Pain (1987). Membership in IASP was extended to those from developing countries and countries with currency difficulties—increasing international interactions. Anesthesiologists comprised the majority of the considerable increase in IASP membership during this time.

Acute Pain: Services, Multimodal Control, Pre-emption, and Prevention

Anesthesiologists drew attention to inadequacies of traditional acute pain management. Ferrante and Covino (see below) assembled a historical "core literature" of 18 reports, in 1990 documenting the inadequacy of conventional intramuscular injections of opioids for postoperative pain [70]. The earliest of these reports, published in 1952, was a collaboration between anesthesiologists Papper and Rovenstine and the clinical pharmacologist Brodie [71]. This paper reported that a third of conventionally managed patients experienced inadequate postoperative analgesia. Arthur Keats reported a similar incidence (range 26–53%) in 1956 [72]. In 1961, Roy Simpson's group in London (University College) pioneered the use of postoperative thoracic epidural analgesia, [73] as did Bruce Scott's group later in Edinburgh [74]. Two internists, Marks and Sachar, in 1973 found that fewer than half of adult medical inpatients with acute pain received adequate pain relief [75]. An Australian 1983 study by Mather and Mackie (the first in children) similarly reported that 50% of children did not receive adequate pain relief [76]– a disturbing statistic given the universal instinct to comfort the young. In 1986, MJC and Phillips reported on acute pain management in critical care patients, a neglected area with few research publications appearing subsequently [77]. The consistent theme from this literature, is the documentation of poorly controlled acute pain in numerous research studies and editorials, from the 1950s until the first report of a formal acute pain service by Ready in 1988 [62]. Knowledge, drugs and techniques existed to successfully treat 90% of postoperative and other acute pain, [77, 78] but only a third to a half of patients were adequately treated [70]. In developing countries, undertreatment of acute pain remains the rule [12].

Correlative opioid pharmacokinetic-pharmacodynamic (PK-PD) studies on patient-controlled opioid analgesia by Mather at Flinders Medical Centre in Adelaide [79, 80] (and see below), focused attention on management of postoperative and other forms of acute pain. Thus, an increasingly sophisticated "acute pain service" began to evolve in 1975. Relying entirely on clinician researchers and research staff of the Flinders Academic Department of Anaesthesia & Intensive Care, the improvement in acute pain management, and encouragement of the surgeons who witnessed the benefit, increasingly drew clinicians into involvement in the acute pain service. Some surgeons initially believed that their residents could handle opioid infusions, resulting in numerous cases of under-dosing and a few overdoses and acute admissions to the ICU.

On commencing his Presidency of IASP in 1987, MJC appointed a Task Force on Management of Acute Pain. Concurrently, the National Health & Medical Research Council (NHMRC) of Australia established a Working Party (including MJC) on management of all forms of pain. The NHMRC recommended a team approach to acute pain management. MJC appointed anesthesiologist Brian Ready from Seattle to Chair the IASP Task Force, resulting in the IASP Document on Acute Pain. Ready's team, including a nurse, anesthesiologist, and anesthesiology fellow, had published their experience in postoperative pain in 1988 [62] followed by Macintyre's 1990 publication from Australia, [81] Sinatra's from New Haven (US) in 1998, [82] Schug's from New Zealand in 1995, [83] and Rawal's from Sweden in 2005 [78]. In retrospect, the delay in establishing such anesthesiology-based services is surprising, since the scientific basis of acute pain management had long been known. Patient-controlled analgesia devices, for example, were first described in the late 1960s and early 1970s [84–86]. Publication of correlative PK-PD studies occurred with nearly a 10-year time lag until their application. One might speculate that routine use of PCA devices was awaiting development of clinically useful pulse oximetry, permitting continuous monitoring of the patient's ventilatory status. The issue of postoperative monitoring to detect opioid-induced hypoventilation remains an ongoing one.

The IASP document "Management of Acute Pain: a Practical Guide" was published in 1992. The Royal College of Surgeons of England and the College of Anaesthetists concurrently published a collaborative "white paper" on pain control after surgery [87]. Also in 1992, a US Government effort to link evidence to recommendations resulted in the first federal clinical practice guideline on any topic. Its focus was acute pain management after operative or medical procedures and trauma. DBC co-chaired the panel preparing this report, with contributions from many anesthesiologists [45]. In 1995, Australia's NHMRC appointed a Working Party (chaired by MJC) which reported in 1998 on the current management, scientific evidence and recommendations for improved treatment of all forms of acute pain. The Australian & New Zealand College of Anaesthetists published a second edition in 2005, with a third edition in 2010 [88]. No other English language evidence-based exhaustive document on all types of acute pain currently exists—resulting in multidisciplinary and multinational endorsement of the document. Similarly comprehensive documents have been prepared following parallel French and German efforts. The ASA prepared an evidence-based clinical practice guideline on acute postoperative pain in 1995, updated in 2004 and 2012 [89]. The ASA produced and updated companion guidelines for cancer pain and chronic non-cancer pain, with an authorship consistent with the many contributions that anesthesiologists have made to these latter two classes of pain.

Acute Pain Services became common during the late 1980s, facilitated by the then-new, patient-controlled analgesia that with specialized supervision could, for the most part, be safely used in general wards. Patient-controlled epidural analgesia could be implemented on general surgical wards using low dose local anesthetic and opioid combinations. However, safe deployment of such neuraxial modalities required development of clinical protocols, education of staff, and appropriate monitoring. The trend towards multimodal perioperative therapy required knowledge of the properties of opioids, NSAIDs, COX-2 inhibitors, anticonvulsants, antidepressants and more. Thus the anesthesiologist on the Acute Pain Service became the clinical pharmacologist, and the acute care internist who managed concurrent acute medical problems in surgical patients. Increasing numbers of anesthesiology departments renamed themselves to include "Anesthesiology, Pain Medicine, and Perioperative Care". To the detriment of Acute Pain Services, recent fiscal pressures have obliged some anesthesiologists to minimize time spent outside of the Operating Room.

Multiple factors determine the risk that acute pain from surgery might evolve to chronic pain. Hence, "multimodal analgesia"—the use of multiple (including non-drug) strategies acting concurrently through multiple pathways and mechanisms—is logical. As Egbert, Battit and colleagues described in 1964, [90] a multimodal strategy may include allaying pre-operative anxiety by a clear explanation of the operation, expected adverse effects, and plans for pain relief. A pharmacological multimodal approach uses different drug classes aimed at different analgesic targets. Appreciation of the different neural mechanisms involved in pain perception, has led to the use of two or more classes of analgesic and "adjuvant" drugs, drugs with different mechanisms and/or sites of action. This approach aims to maximize pain relief, particularly for pain associated with movement, while minimizing side effects. Acute pain management occurs in the context of factors such as wound care, drain placement, temperature maintenance, hydration, provision of nutrition (particularly protein), glycemic control, and early mobilization—which together with pain management embodies a multidisciplinary strategy of "acute rehabilitation". Anesthesiologists have developed and applied these concepts over the past 30 years to improve outcomes, [91] including the quality of recovery [92].The results have shortened postoperative stays sufficiently to perform many previously inpatient operations on an outpatient basis [93].

Studies of the benefit of multimodal systemic analgesia were shown in 1960, for the addition of an NSAID to an opioid [94]. The 1992 review of evidence by DBC and colleagues confirmed the safety and efficacy of the combined use of opioids and NSAIDs in postoperative pain [45]. The then-recent availability of an injectable NSAID (ketorolac) further encouraged the use of this combination. In 2005, a meta-analyses by Marret, Bonnet, and other French colleagues added support for perioperative opioid-sparing, and the decrease of some opioid side effects by use of diverse injectable NSAIDs, including acetaminophen (paracetamol) [95].

By the late 1980s, the WHO had developed a simplified, step-wise "Analgesic Ladder" for the management of cancer pain: acetaminophen+/- NSAIDS+/- opioids, supplemented with adjuvant drugs at any step of the ladder. Space limitations do not permit discussion of the important ways in which anesthesiologists brought specialized skills to bear on the relief of cancer pain, e.g., through neurolytic blockade or intrathecal drug delivery. Most anesthesiologists dealt with acute pain differently from cancer pain, and thus the WHO publication on cancer pain relief had limited impact on the management of acute pain. Since the release of the AHCPR and NHMRC documents, there have been numerous studies of multimodal treatment. In addition to NSAIDs, evidence supports the use of intravenous lidocaine, low-dose ketamine, and anticonvulsants such as gabapentin and pregabalin to provide postoperative opioid sparing, and thereby a reduction in opioid side effects. The 1996 development by Brennan of an animal model that replicated essential features of postoperative incisional pain, has furthered progress in understanding the preclinical pathophysiology of acute postoperative pain [96].This model imposes a plantar incision into a rat hind paw followed by closure of the incision with sutures [96]. It is now employed worldwide to elucidate the cascade of cellular responses evoked by incisional pain [97].

The increasing use of patient-controlled and epidural opioids to provide postoperative pain relief (see below) saw a parallel increase in the incidence of catastrophic respiratory depression [98]. This led to recent initiatives spearheaded by the Anesthesia Patient Safety Foundation (APSF) in the US [100] and elsewhere (e.g., by Pamela Macintyre and David Scott of the Australian and New Zealand College of Anaesthetists). These initiatives call for close monitoring of patients receiving postoperative opioids, including frequent checking of their level of sedation, or the use of oximetry and capnography to trigger alarms when blood oxygen and carbon dioxide levels move outside safe ranges [99].

Pediatric Pain Control

The Boston Children's Hospital established the position of Chief of Anesthesia immediately after World War II, a role filled by Robert Smith from 1946 until his retirement in 1980. Smith was a founding father of pediatric anesthesiology in the US, training more than 800 residents and fellows, many remaining in the Boston area to advance pediatric anesthesiology and develop early pain treatment services. The second generation of such clinicians involved in pediatric pain included Charles Cote and John Ryan. Well into the 1980s, it was commonly taught worldwide that newborn infants had immature nervous systems and required muscle relaxation but not analgesia to undergo surgery. Attracted by the opportunity to extend his earlier studies on pediatric pain at Oxford in the 1980s, Kanwal ("Sunny") Anand accepted a research fellowship at Boston Children's Hospital. During that fellowship his studies of pediatric stress responses to surgery and their inhibition by analgesia, demonstrated infants' sensitivity to noxious stimuli and the benefit of analgesics to blunt their catabolic perioperative stress responses. Charles Berde, a contemporary of Anand, developed Boston Children's multidisciplinary program to treat chronic pain in children, and conducted laboratory studies leading to novel extended-release delivery systems for injected local anesthetics.

Clifford Woolf, a student of Patrick Wall in London, immigrated to Boston in 1997 as the first Richard Kitz Professor of Pain Research at the MGH, moving in 2010 to work at Children's Hospital with Berde. His initial research established the importance of central (e.g., spinal) sensitization in the amplification and persistence of pain resulting from noxious stimuli in the periphery (see below). More recently his laboratory has identified specific genes and gene products, such as intracellular enzymes whose presence and/or activation make their bearers more likely to experience a transition from acute to chronic pain. His distinguished research career was honored by the ASA's 2004 Excellence in Research Award.

Concern regarding pain in burned children led to the establishment of "Project Pain" in 1980, at the MGH and the adjoining Shriners Burns Institute, directed by Stan Szyfelbein. Clinical studies involving a pharmacologist, Patricia Osgood, and a pain nurse, Nancy Atchison, commenced along with a laboratory research program [100–101]. Resulting innovations included the use of low concentrations of epinephrine and lidocaine injected under skin graft donor sites to reduce pain and blood loss, daily multidisciplinary pain rounds by a physician, nurse and pharmacologist to assess pain using a large "thermometer" scale easily read by children within bacterial isolation units, and formulation of the concept of burn pain as a neuropathic entity arising from the newly coined term "phantom skin". Most importantly, through careful correlations of burn depth and extent with pain intensity, they overthrew the prevailing view that third degree burns don't hurt—they do! In retrospect it is hard to believe that conventional wisdom could have been blind to the obvious agony of severely burned children.

Sensitization and Pre-emptive Pain Management

It is a small step to extend the concept of treating pain as soon as possible after it occurs, to applying preoperative interventions such as neural blockade to avert surgical pain. As noted above, in the 1900s, the surgeon George Crile introduced a concept he termed "anoci-association" [32, 102]. He used peripheral neural blockade to prevent afferent noxious signals from reaching the spinal cord and brain lest they trigger harmful neurohumoral responses and compromise recovery from injury or surgery. Crile, and later, O'Shaugnessy and Slome, [103] produced evidence supporting this concept, including experiments with spinal anesthesia in traumatized patients. The Montreal anesthesiologist Philip Bromage picked up this concept, reporting in 1971 that epidural blockade blunted neurohumoral responses to surgery [104].

In 1976, Danish gastrointestinal surgeon Henrik Kehlet began to explore stress responses to surgery [105]. His studies of hormonal changes associated with surgery and postoperative pain, found that epidural local anesthesia begun before surgery and continued postoperatively, could attenuate the catabolic (i.e., protein-wasting) effects of surgery. At issue was whether trauma or surgery would trigger "central sensitization" unless afferent nociceptive traffic were blocked completely. In general, the response was "yes"; avoiding central sensitization requires a sufficiently dense neural afferent blockade for a sufficient time, over a sufficient spatial extent. Clifford Woolf, a clinician-turned-researcher, like his mentor Patrick Wall, reported in 1983 that post-injury sensitization could be averted if spinal analgesia was in place pre-injury [106]. Wall supported these concepts in multiple editorials and lectures. Subsequent clinical studies designed to compare analgesia given before or immediately after surgery (often continued only briefly after surgery) frequently failed to show a favorable effect because they did not provide a sufficiently dense neural blockade, extended over a duration outlasting the tissue injury response. Thus, Moiniche's 2002 evaluation of published studies purporting to test the efficacy of pre-emptive analgesia was negative [107]. Later studies with a more effective pre-emptive intervention, using a more powerful analgesic regimen (e.g., epidural neural blockade, systemic ketamine) over a longer time course, did report reduction of pain and decreased use of supplemental analgesia. For example, Lavan d'homme reported that perioperative epidural analgesia combined with intravenous ketamine decreased hyperalgesia and long term pain for up to one year after colon surgery, compared with intravenous analgesia alone [108]. The importance and frequency of chronic postsurgical pain had not previously been appreciated, nor had the consequent significant disability.

"Protective analgesia" applies techniques that reduce sequelae of central sensitization, such as secondary hyperalgesia. "Preventive analgesia" is the modern terminology for what Crile and Wall espoused, namely, applying measures sufficient to avoid central sensitization in the first place. To be effective, preventive treatment must be continued for as long as the injury response is active. This appears to be for at least 3 days following major surgery. Such an approach holds the best hope for reducing the development of persistent post-surgical pain. As James Eisenach noted in 2010, anesthesiologists and other pain researchers have joined with the US NIH, and pharmaceutical companies to answer the question "can effective acute pain management prevent transition to chronic pain?" [109].

Contrary to prior views that acute pain is separate from chronic pain, it now appears that acute pain triggers cascades of neuronal processes initiating the transition to chronic pain. Some of these processes occur in nearly all people while others are specific to an individual's genes. Physical, psychological and environmental factors also influence the transition from acute to chronic postoperative pain. Indeed, in the 1990s, Kehlet and Rathmell [110] and anesthesiologist William Macrae [111] identified risk factors for this transition, including severity of pain, repeat surgery, preoperative anxiety, female gender, genetic predisposition, surgical technique, radiation therapy to the surgical area, neurotoxic chemotherapy, depression, psychological vulnerability (e.g., a tendency to perceive even minor setbacks as heralding catastrophe), and postoperative anxiety. Coordinated management by a team consisting of surgeons, anesthesiologists, nurses, clinical psychologists and other healthcare professionals can minimize the impact of these risk factors on the transition from acute to chronic pain.

Intriguingly, as suggested in another chapter, preclinical studies and retrospective surveys suggest the possibility of another major long-term benefit of optimal perioperative analgesia, achieved using regional anesthesia to decrease stress responses and lower morphine requirements during cancer resection. Not yet confirmed clinically, the possible benefit is a lower likelihood of cancer recurrence, attributed to better immune function in patients whose pain and stress responses are minimized, and opioid requirement decreased, by regional anesthesia [112].

Spinal Analgesia and the Gate Control Theory

The development of caudal and lumbar epidural as well as spinal subarachnoid blocks intertwines with the history of obstetric analgesia and conduction anesthesia [23, 24, 113]—topics that are dealt with in other chapters of this volume, and that will not be duplicated here. For the sake of the present narrative focusing upon pain, we note that texts by Bromage [114] and Nicholas Greene [115] in the 1950s, presented the scientific and practical bases of central neuraxial analgesia. In 1967, Bromage described the use of a thoracic extradural catheter for analgesia following chest trauma, thereby implying that extradural analgesia at an appropriate spinal level could successfully treat acute pain. In 1969, working with surgeon Wright and Bromage at McGill, MJC found that perioperative epidural analgesia improved graft blood flow in patients undergoing lower limb vascular surgery [116].

Increasing attention to spinal and other central modulation of afferent nociceptive stimuli during the late 1960s, culminated in the most influential pain research paper ever published: Melzack's and Wall's 1965 description of the Gate Control Theory of Pain [34]. Initially this new theory drew little attention. However, a 1967 report by Wall and MGH neurosurgeon William Sweet, described abolition of pain by vibration devices in human volunteers, aimed at activating Aβ fibers that in turn would "close the gate" [117]. This demonstration of the applicability of the Gate Control Theory prompted a resurgence of interest in transcutaneous electrical nerve stimulation (TENS), and led to the development of spinal cord stimulation (SCS) for pain control. In the present era of close attention to early patenting and commercial development of scientific advances by academic investigators, it is noteworthy that Melzack revealed to MJC that neither he nor Wall sought or received any royalties for the development of TENS, SCS or other applications of the "Gate Theory".

In 1974, Brazilian Octavio Calvillo (also a prior "Fellow" at McGill) studied cats, finding arguably the first evidence of a spinal action of morphine [118]. Also in 1974, anesthesiologist Luke Kitahata described a spinal action of morphine but inferred that the specific site of action was lamina V rather than the substantia gelatinosa [119]. In 1976, neuroscientists Arthur Duggan and Tony Yaksh provided unequivocal evidence of the spinal site of action of morphine. Duggan described morphine/enkephalin effects on the substantia gelatinosa [120] and Yaksh reported the "direct spinal action of narcotics" [121].

By the late 1970s, informed by advances in applying patient-controlled analgesia and spinal opioid analgesia, Mather and colleagues observed that "the plethora of new parenteral agents which the pharmaceutical companies have introduced over the past 25 years is *not* a reminder that we have not found the right drug but a reminder that we have not found the optimal mode of administration of perfectly adequate analgesic drugs" [122]. With this perspective in mind, when MJC moved to Adelaide in 1975, he recruited basic scientist/pharmacokineticist Mather, who in 1976–79 studied the PK/ PD of oral, intramuscular and intravenous administration, including PCA. Wang and colleagues [123] conducted a small case series of intrathecal morphine in 1979, prompting MJC et al. to begin concurrent PK-PD studies of intrathecal and epidural opioids—research that has continued to the present and has included "combination" intrathecal analgesia using concurrently administered opioid and non-opioid drugs [124].

In the meantime, Wall, while visiting Israel, stimulated Florella Magora and her colleagues to administer morphine epidurally to decrease various types of pain. Their results were published in a letter to *The Lancet* on 10 March 1979 [125]. Seeing that publication prompted MJC's group to issue a preliminary report of the PK-PD study of intrathecal morphine and pethidine (meperidine in the US), and epidural pethidine. Since the blood and CSF PK-PD data, and neurological assessment strongly suggested a spinal site, with sparing of normal non-noxious sensation, motor power and sympathetic function, MJC titled the Letter "Selective Spinal Analgesia" [126]. The letter was accepted 24 hours after receipt and published on 26 May 1979. In the same volume, a letter [127] from Samii and colleagues in Paris reported hyperbaric intrathecal injections of 20 mg morphine (6–20 times the doses in MJC's study). All patients had complete pain relief. Others soon began to report delayed respiratory depression after intrathecal morphine, and lower intrathecal doses of 0.25–0.5 mg morphine subsequently emerged as a safer standard for opioid naïve patients [128]. MJC's group published the full data from the 1979 Lancet letter, in 1981 [129].

Anesthesiologists undertook most of the research on efficacy and side effects of spinal opioids from the 1980s onward. Continuing to extend the scientific foundation to guide clinical dosing of increasing numbers of opioids administered by various routes, Torda *et al* from Sydney demonstrated in 1980 that epidural administration of opioids provided longer-lasting and more efficacious analgesia than intramuscular administration [130]. In 1983, Swedes Nordberg *et al*, described cerebrospinal fluid (CSF) concentrations of morphine after spinal injection, [131] confirming the results of the Adelaide group that analgesia correlated with CSF concentrations of opioid, not blood concentrations. In 1984, Rawal and colleagues [132] observed patients undergoing gastroplasty for obesity. They found that, compared to those receiving intramuscular morphine, those given epidural morphine postoperatively were better able to sit, stand, or walk unassisted within 6,12, and 24 hr, respectively, and that they better tolerated vigorous physiotherapy, resulting in fewer pulmonary complications. Earlier postoperative recovery of peak expiratory flow and bowel function in the epidural group contributed to a shorter hospital stay. This second major contribution from Sweden did much to support the ongoing clinical use of spinal opioids. The status of spinal opioids as a clinical entity can be gauged by the numerous citations of articles on this topic in citation analyses of the literature on anesthesiology and pain [17]. The 1984 review [133] of intrathecal and epidural administration of opioids, by Cousins & Mather, was by far the most frequently cited paper.

Pain as a Public Health Issue: Education, Evidence, Global Health Policy and Human Rights

Although Bonica's statement of future needs and goals in his monograph did not employ the phrase "public health", the points he made concerning the prevalence and societal burden of pain do so *de facto*. In particular, he wrote that "the challenge to the biomedical scientific community, health professionals and society as a whole is to organize, mount and support a multipronged program" [65]. Included in this program, was the need "to markedly increase our efforts in the education and training of students, house officers, and physicians and other health professionals in order to improve the care of patients suffering from pain." Responding to Bonica's call, in the 1990s both DBC and MJC established inter-professional educational programs at their institutions to supplement anesthesiology-based physician fellowships [13, 14].

Prophetically, in 1999, pain physician Rollin Gallagher wrote "Chronic pain is a public health problem crying out for a reorganization of the manner in which the health care system manages pain" [134]. Pain is a public health problem because it affects many people. In addition, pain is linked with other aspects of health through complex networks. Pain is amenable to preventive efforts such as education, exacts a higher burden on the lower socioeconomic population, and access to pain relief has a social justice dimension. Pain is now on the agenda of mainstream healthcare, governmental and nongovernmental organizations. In the US, the Joint Commission has advocated for pain management as a standard of care, and provides resources for health care systems to support this standard [135]. Both the World Health Organization (WHO) and the US Institute of Medicine (IOM), describe pain as a public health problem [136]. Anesthesiologists have actively participated in high-profile initiatives (including development of educational materials) by all of these organizations. Through the efforts of the anesthesiologist Michael Ashburn (then a health policy fellow in the office of a senior US senator) in late 2000, Congress declared the ten-year period that began 1 January 2001 to be the Decade of Pain Control and Research. This successful legislation continues to influence governmental activities such as funding for pain research and the recent establishment of an NIH pain consortium.

Repositories of clinical trial data and their analysis in systematic reviews provide a basis for evidence-guided care [137]. The Oxford group at Churchill Hospital, led by anesthesiologists Henry McQuay and Andrew Moore, [15] and their former research fellows including anesthesiologists Eija Kalso and Martin Tramer, have made major contributions to aggregating relevant clinical evidence through the Cochrane Collaboration. Registration of a specific new Cochrane review group on pain, palliative and supportive care, followed a 1997 visit by the Oxford pharmacist Phil Wiffen with DBC in which the two began drafting their application. Registration was approved the following year. Ewan McNicol, a pharmacist in Tufts' Department of Anesthesiology and 2001 graduate of Tufts' pain education program, succeeded DBC as an editor for this group, whose reviews include many prepared by anesthesiologists.

A pivotal chapter in the relationship between IASP and WHO occurred when DBC heard a lecture by Christopher Murray of Harvard Medical School, describing a long-term WHO project to assess the worldwide disease burden of major conditions. WHO had previously been unresponsive to IASP's request for collaboration, arguing that it had no resources to devote to pain while it confronted a world full of killer diseases. Hearing Murray's lecture, DBC realized that the WHO's own data would, if analyzed in greater detail, establish pain as integral to the worldwide disease burdens of conditions such as cancer, diabetes, war trauma, and HIV. DBC contacted the IASP's liaison to WHO, the anesthesiologist Harald Breivik of Oslo, who then visited DBC in Boston. Together they outlined a strategy to present to the WHO, based upon WHO's own data [138]. As a result, the WHO supported IASP's inaugural Global Day Against Pain, held in Geneva in 2004.

In 2010, at the urging of MJC, and chaired by him, the IASP convened the first International Pain Summit during its World Congress on Pain in Montreal. This summit resulted in the Declaration of Montreal, affirming that access to pain management is a fundamental human right [139]. Further initiatives including those seeking to improve pain control internationally on the basis of a quality improvement strategy, [140] and to reduce disparities in access to pain assessment and treatment, [141] are now occurring. MJC's efforts to enlist the Australian public as an ally to improve pain control led him to prepare the first national-level detailed pain strategy and to establish Painaustralia, a nonprofit organization, in 2011 to implement it [142]. One early success of Painaustralia was the commitment of 26 million Australian dollars by the New South Wales Ministry of Health and Medical Research to advance pain care services, research and education. In the US, California and Massachusetts now mandate several hours of continuing professional education in pain and related topics, such as opioid prescribing, for every physician (and many non-physicians) to maintain an active license. These examples from the authors' personal experience illustrate the many national and international initiatives to advance pain-related research, education and policy now taking place worldwide.

In 2011, in its report *Relieving Pain in America*, the IOM summarized findings of a multidisciplinary blue ribbon panel that included anesthesiologists such as Stanford's Sean Mackey and other professionals with primary appointments in departments of anesthesiology nationwide [136]. Describing pain as "a public health challenge" the IOM called for a "population-level prevention and management strategy". This strategy aims to

"heighten awareness about pain and its health consequences; emphasize the prevention of pain; improve pain assessment and management in the delivery of health care and financing programs of the federal government; use public health communication strategies to inform patients on how

to manage their own pain; and address disparities in the experience of pain among subgroups of Americans."

Back to the Future?

In 1956, Eckenhoff published a prophetic essay on the anesthesiologist and the management of pain, in the *Journal of Chronic Diseases* (even the choice of journal was far-sighted) [143]. In words current today, he pointed out that

"anesthesiologists have made highly significant advances to our understanding of pain and its treatment. This has been particularly true within the last decade. New local anesthetics have been introduced and tested; simplification and popularization of regional nerve blocks has been widespread among the specialty; inquiries into the action, effectiveness, and limitations of analgesics and sedatives have been made; investigations concerning the effect of drugs upon the intangibles of mood and mind have been published; diagnostic tests employing spinal anesthesia have been reported; researches into the sites of action of intravenously injected local anesthetics have been made; and a major reference work on pain has been published. As a comparatively new specialty, anesthesiology can be proud of its already significant contributions to ourknowledge and treatment of pain."

Eckenhoff's essay suggested how far we had come by mid-century, but the 1950s marked just the beginning of the modern era of pain research and management. With World War II succeeded by the less destructive Cold War, the world entered an era of relative peace and progress. Watson and Crick published their model of DNA. The first computers were marketed, the integrated circuit was invented, and the first widely adopted high-level programming language (FORTRAN) enabled persons with limited training to harness computers for personal purposes. The Beat Generation energized music and literature. Capturing the spirit of the times, Kerouac wrote, "We had finally found the magic land at the end of the road and we never dreamed the extent of the magic" [146].

Eckenhoff clearly felt in the 1950s that anesthesiology had traveled far towards understanding and treating pain. Yet we doubt that he, Beecher or Bonica dreamed the extent of what anesthesiologists and basic scientists working in collaboration would achieve. These pioneers might well have viewed as magical the precision with which molecular pain research has elucidated mechanisms of normal and disordered nociception, e.g., genotyping to identify patients at risk for persistent pain after operations or lumbar disc herniation, or those likely to need sub- or supranormal doses of opioid analgesics. The design and interpretation of analgesic trials have advanced to a high degree of sophistication. Modern computers that allow clinicians, scientists and patients to explore massive databases have transformed every corner of science. Biomedical informatics allows discernment of relationships from the level of DNA through large clinical populations, and consolidation of results from worldwide clinical experience to guide bedside clinical decisions. Real-time computational power supports functional MRI studies of awake and conversant human subjects. Mobile phones' data capture and transfer capacities now surpass those of mainframe computers 20 years ago, and allow real-time monitoring of individual patient outcomes including physical activity.

Key advances since the 1950s include the current trend towards shared decision-making between clinicians and patients. Patients increasingly have access to knowledge and guidance (albeit not all equally credible, and some frankly erroneous) over the Internet, and participate in online chat rooms and blogs to reduce social isolation. Patient-centered outcomes including satisfaction with care are now an integral part of clinical analgesic trials and routine hospital-based quality assurance — the latter influencing quality-based payment. Patients' personal illness narratives are now being elicited, heard and read.

Anesthesiologists and their preclinical collaborators have led and will lead in the ongoing advances described in this chapter. A recent glimpse into the future of medicine by senior editors of the *New England Journal of Medicine* merits reading by all who practice pain medicine. Echoing Bonica's insight that "a considerate feeling for those who suffer…is, without doubt, the most important…attribute" of the pain physician, [67] their comments also bring to mind new challenges such as the need to balance freer prescribing of opioids for pain, versus undesired consequences such as rising drug diversion and abuse. "The high-technology, information-rich medicine of the future will provide powerful and useful tools…(but) will not, of course, solve all problems, and it cannot prevent violent or self-destructive human behaviors. Patients will continue to rely on physicians and the medical community for the guidance, support, and help that only a skilled and caring health professional can offer" [147].

Acknowledgment The authors thank Helen Johnston for administrative assistance during the preparation of this manuscript.

References

1. Fülöp-Miller R. Triumph over pain. New York: the literary guild of America Inc.; 1938. pp 1–438.
2. Baszanger I. Translated by Isabelle Baszanger. Inventing pain medicine. From the laboratory to the clinic. New Brunswick:Rutgers University Press; 1998. pp 1–348.
3. Carr DB, Loeser JD, Morris DB, editors. Narrative, pain, and suffering. Progress in pain research and management, vol. 34. Seattle:IASP Press; 2005. pp 1–362.
4. Morris DB. The culture of pain. Berkeley:University of California Press;1991. pp 1–342.
5. Fishman S, Berger L. The war on pain. New York: HarperCollins; 2000. pp 1–301.
6. Resnik DB, Rehm M, Minard RB. The undertreatment of pain: scientific, clinical, cultural, and philosophical factors. Med Health Care Philos. 2001;4:277–88.
7. Rey R. Translated by Louise Elliott Wallace, JA Cadden, SW Cadden. The history of pain. Cambridge:Harvard University Press; 1995. pp 1–394.
8. Scarry E. The body in pain: the making and unmaking of the world. New York: Oxford University Press; 1985. pp 1–385.
9. Sontag S. Regarding the pain of others. New York:Farrar, Straus and Giroux; 2003. pp 1–131.
10. Thernstrom M. The pain chronicles. New York, Farrar, Straus and Giroux; 2010. pp 1–364.
11. Gallagher RM, Fishman SM. Pain medicine: history, emergence as a medical specialty, and evolution of the multidisciplinary approach. In: Cousins MJ, Bridenbaugh PO, Carr DB, Horlocker TT editors. Cousins & Bridenbaugh's neural blockade in clinical anesthesia and management of pain, 4th edn. Philadelphia:Lippincott Williams & Wilkins; 2009. pp 631–43.
12. Brennan F, Carr DB, Cousins MJ. Pain management: a fundamental human right. Anesth Analg. 2007;105:205–21.
13. Lasch KE, Greenhill A, Wilkes G, Carr D, Lee M, Blanchard R. Why study pain? A qualitative analysis of medical and nursing faculty and students' knowledge of and attitudes to cancer pain management. J Palliat Med. 2002;5:57–7114.
14. Devonshire E, Siddall P. Joining forces: collaborating internationally to deliver high-quality, online postgraduate education in pain management. Pain Res Manage. 2011;16:411–15.
15. McQuay HJ, Moore RA. An evidence-based resource for pain relief. Oxford: Oxford University Press; 1998. pp 1–264.
16. Bonica JJ. The role of the anaesthetist in the management of intractable pain. Proc Roy Soc Med. 1954;47:1029–32.
17. Strassels SC, Carr DB, Meldrum M, Cousins MJ. Toward a canon of the pain and analgesia literature: A citation analysis. Anesth Analg. 1999;89:1528–33.
18. Baños JE, Ruiz G, Guardiola E. An analysis of articles on neonatal pain published from. to 1965 1999. Pain Res Manage. 2001;6:45–50.
19. Keefe FJ, Lumley MA, Buffington ALH, Carson JW, Studts JL, Edwards CL, Macklem DJ, Aspnes AK, Fox L, Steffey D. Changing face of pain: evolution of pain research in psychosomatic medicine. Psychosom Med. 2002;64:921–38.
20. Mogil JS, Simmonds K, Simmonds MJ. Pain research from 1975–2007: a categorial and bibliometric meta-trend analysis of every research paper published in the journal Pain. Pain. 2009;142:48–58.
21. Robert C, Wilson CS, Donnadieu S, Gaudy J-F, Arreto C-D. Bibliometric analysis of the scientific literature on pain research: a 2006 study. Pain. 2008;138:250–4.
22. Papper EM. Romance, poetry, and surgical sleep. Literature influences medicine. Westport: Greenwood Press; 1995 (Contributions in Medical Studies, No. 42). pp 1–162.
23. Bacon DL. Regional anesthesia and chronic pain therapy: a history. In: Brown DL, editor. Regional anesthesia and analgesia. Philadelphia: Saunders, 1996. pp 10–22.
24. Brown DL, Fink BR. The history of regional anesthesia. In: Cousins MJ, Bridenbaugh PO, Carr DB, Horlocker TT, editors. Cousins & Bridenbaugh's Neural Blockade in Clinical Anesthesia and Management of Pain, 4th edn. Philadelphia:Lippincott Williams & Wilkins; 2009. pp 1–23.
25. McPeek B: Henry K. Beecher and the early years of the Anesthesia Service. In: Kitz RJ, editor. "This is No Humbug!" reminiscences from the department of anesthesia at the Massachusetts General Hospital—a history. Atlasbooks Distribution Serv; 2003. pp 107–12.
26. Cope DK. Intellectual milestones in our understanding and treatment of pain. In: Fishman SM, Ballantyne JC, Rathmell JR, editors. Bonica's Management of Pain. Philadelphia: Wolters Kluwer/ Lippincott Williams & Wilkins; 2010. pp 1–12.

27. Weingarten TN, Martin DP, Bacon DR. The origins of the modern pain clinic at the Mayo Clinic. Bulletin Anesth History. 2011;29:34–9.

28. White JC, Sweet WH. Pain and the neurosurgeon: a forty-year experience. Springfield (IL): Charles C. Thomas; 1969. pp 1–1000.

29. Burchiel K. Surgical management of pain. New York: Thieme; 2002. pp 1–992.

30. Zimmermann M. The history of pain concepts and treatment before IASP. In: Merskey H, Loeser JD, Dubner R, editors. The paths of pain 1975–2005. Seattle: IASP Press; 2005. pp 1–22.

31. Murphy PM, Cousins MJ. Neural blockade and neuromodulation in persistent pain. In: Merskey H, Loeser JD, Dubner R, editors. The paths of pain 1975–2005. Seattle: IASP Press, pp 447–68.

32. Crile GW. Phylogenetic association in relation to certain medical problems. Boston Med Surg J. 1910;163:893–904.

33. Lowenstein E, McPeek B, editors. Enduring contributions of Henry K. Beecher to medicine, science, and society. Parts I and II. International anesthesiology clinics: vol. 45, Number 4, fall 2007, and vol. 46, Number 1, winter 2008. Philadelphia: Lippincott Williams & Wilkins.

34. Melzack R, Wall PD. Pain mechanisms: a new theory. Science. 1965;150:971–9.

35. Haldane JBS, Huxley J. Animal biology. Oxford: Oxford University Press; 1929. pp 28–38.

36. Page IH. Chemistry of the Brain. Springfield: Chalres C Thomas; 1937. pp 336–8.

37. Bartley SH, Chute E. Fatigue and Impairment in Man. New York: McGraw-Ill; 1947. pp 240–79.

38. Hoch PH, Pennes HH, Cattell JP. Psychoses produced by the administration of drugs. In: Merritt HH, Hare CC, editors. Metabolic and toxic diseases of the nervous system. Res Publ Assoc Nerv Ment Dis, vol. 32. Baltimore: Wiliams & Wilkins; 1953. pp 287–96.

39. Lasagna L, Mosteller F, Felsinger JM von, Beecher HK. A study of the placebo response. Am J Med. 1954;16:770–9.

40. Erill S, editor. Clinical pharmacology through the pen of Louis Lasagna. Barcelona: Prous Science; 1997 (Pharmacology Revisited: An Esteve Foundation Series, No. 1). pp 1–223.

41. Mashour GA. From LSD to the IRB: Henry Beecher's psychedelic research and the foundation of clinical ethics. In: Lowenstein E, McPeek B, editors. Enduring contributions of Henry K. Beecher to medicine, science, and society. Parts I and II. International Anesthesiology Clinics, vol. 45, Number 4, fall 2007, and vol. 46, Number 1, winter 2008. Philadelphia: Lippincott Williams & Wilkins, pp 105–11.

42. Beecher HK. Psychotomimetic drugs. In: Beecher HK, editor. Measurement of subjective responses: quantitative effects of drugs. New York: Oxford University Press; 1959. pp 286–320.

43. Beecher HK, Todd DP. A study of the deaths associated with anesthesia and surgery. Ann Surg. 1954;140:2–33.

44. Carr DB, Bullen BA, Skrinar GS, Arnold MA, Rosenblatt M, Beitins IZ, Martin JB, McArthur JW. Physical conditioning facilitates the exercise-induced secretion of beta-endorphin and beta-lipotropin in women. N Engl J Med. 1981;305:560–3.

45. Carr DB, Jacox AK, Chapman CR, Ferrell BR, Fields HL, Heidrich G III, Hester NK, Hill CS Jr, Lipman AG, McGarvey CL, Miaskowski CA, Mulder DS, Payne R, Schechter N, Shapiro BS, Smith RS, Tsou CV, Vecchiarelli L. Acute pain management: operative or medical procedures and trauma. Clinical practice guideline number 1. Rockville: Agency for Health Care Policy and Research, U.S. Department of Health & Human Services;1992.

46. Ballantyne JC, Carr DB, Chalmers TC, Dear KB, Angelillo IF, Mosteller F. Postoperative patient-controlled analgesia: meta-analyses of initial randomized control trials. J Clin Anesth. 1993;5:182–93.

47. Ballantyne JC, Carr DB, deFerranti S, Suarez T, Lau J, Chalmers TC, Angelillo IF, Mosteller F. The comparative effects of postoperative analgesic therapies on pulmonary outcome: cumulative meta-analyses of randomized, controlled trials. Anesth Analg. 1998;86:598–612.

48. Kirby T. Joseph Lau: mastering the meta-analysis. Lancet. 2012;379:403.

49. Lasagna L. Clinical analgesic research: a historical perspective. In: Max MB, Portenoy RK, Laska EM, editors. The design of analgesic clinical trials. Advance in pain resaerch and therapy, vol. 18, New York: Raven Press; 1991. pp 1–7.

50. Horton R. A manifesto for reading medicine. Lancet. 1997;349:872–4.

51. Lowenstein E: Narcotics in anesthesia: past, present, and future. In: Estafanous FG, editor. Opioids in anesthesia. Boston: Butterworth; 1984, pp 3–6.

52. Lowenstein E, Hallowell P, Levine FH, Daggett WM, Austen WG, Laver MB. Cardiovascular response to large doses of intravenous morphine in man. N Engl J Med. 1969;281:1389–93.

53. Strichartz G, Pastijn E, Sugimoto K. Neural physiology and local anesthetic action. In: Cousins MJ, Bridenbaugh PO, Carr DB, Horlocker TT, editors. Cousins & Bridenbaugh's neural blockade in clinical anesthesia and management of pain, 4th edn. Philadelphia: Lippincott Williams & Wilkins; 2009, pp 26–47.

54. Liebeskind J, Meldrum ML. John J. Bonica, world champion of pain. In: Jensen TS, Turner JA, Wiesenfeld-Hallin Z, editors. Proceedings of the 8th world congress on pain. Progress in pain research and management, vol. 8. Seattle: IASP Press; 1997, pp 19–32.

55. Steinsaltz A. Resh Lakish: chapter 11 in Steinsaltz A. Talmadic Images. New Milford: Maggid Books; 2010, pp 79–84.

56. Bonica JJ. Evolution of pain concepts and pain clinics. In: Brena SF, Chapman SL, editors. Chronic pain management: principles. Clinics in Anaesthesiology vol. 3. Philadelphia:Saunders; 1985. pp 1–16.

57. Loeser JD. Multidisciplinary pain management. In: Merskey H, Loeser JD, Dubner R, editors. The paths of pain 1975–2005. Seattle: IASP Press, pp 503–11.

58. Aurelius M. Meditations. Staniforth M, translator. London: Penguin Books; 1964. p 116

59. Burton R. The anatomy of melancholy. New York: New York Review Books; 2001. p 1–547.

60. Wolff HG, Wolf S. Pain. Springfield: Charles C Thomas; 1948 (American lecture series, publication number 5. A monograph in American lectures in physiology). pp 1–86.

61. Siddall PJ. Cousins MJ: Persistent pain as a disease entity: implications for clinical management. Anesth Analg. 2004;99:510–20.

62. Ready LB, Oden R, Chadwick HS, Benedetti C, Rooke GA, Caplan R, Wild L. Development of an anesthesiology-based postoperative pain management service. Anesthesiology. 1988;68:100–6.

63. Bonica JJ. The management of pain, with special emphasis on the use of analgesic block in diagnosis, prognosis and therapy. Philadelphia: Lea & Febiger; 1953. pp 1–1533.

64. Bonica JJ, editor. The management of pain, 2nd edn. Philadelphia: Lea & Febiger; 1990. pp 11–7.

65. Carr DB. The development of national guidelines for pain control: synopsis and commentary. Eur J Pain. 2001;5(Suppl. A):91–8.

66. Jones LE. First steps: the early years of IASP 1973–1984. Seattle: IASP Press; 2010. pp 4–6

67. Bonica JJ. The role of the anaesthetist in the management of intractable pain. Proc Roy Soc Med. 1954;47:1029–32.

68. Rogers EM. Diffusion of innovations, 5th edn. New York: Free Press; 2003. p 273.

69. Loeser J. How a founder's vision became IASP. IASP Insight. 2012;1:6–10.

70. Ferrante FM, Covino BG. Patient-controlled analgesia: a historical perspective. In: Ferrante FM, Ostheimer GW, Covino BG, editors. Patient-controlled analgesia. Boston:Blackwell; 1990. pp 3–9.

71. Papper EM, Brodie BB, Rovenstine EA. Postoperative pain: its use in comparative evaluation of analgesics. Surgery. 1952;32:107–9.

72. Keats AS. Postoperative pain: research and treatment. J Chronic Dis. 1956;4:72–83.

73. Simpson BR, Parkhouse J, Marshall R, Lambrechts W. Extradural analgesia and the prevention of postoperative respiratory complications. Br J Anaesth. 1961;33:628–41.

74. Scott DB, Schweitzer S, Thorn J. Epidural block in postoperative pain relief. Regional Anesth. 1982;7:135–9.

75. Marks RM, Sachar EJ. Undertreatment of medical inpatients with narcotic analgesics. Ann Intern Med. 1973;78:173–81.

76. Mather L, Mackie J. The incidence of post-operative pain in children. Pain. 1983;15:271–82.

77. Bryan-Brown C. Development of pain management in critical care. In: Cousins MJ, Phillips GD, editors. Acute pain management. Clinics in critical care medicine. New York:Churchill Livingstone; 1986. pp 1–20.

78. Rawal N. Organization, function and implementation of acute pain service. Anesthesiol Clin North America. 2005;23:211–25.

79. Austin KL, Stapleton JV, Mather LE. Multiple intramuscular injections: a major source of variability in analgesic response to meperidine. Pain. 1980;8:47–62.

80. Austin KL, Stapleton JV, Mather LE. Relationship between blood meperidine concentrations and analgesic response: a preliminary report. Anesthesiology. 1980;53:460–6.

81. Macintyre PE, Runciman WB, Webb RK. An acute pain service in an Australian teaching hospital: the first year. Med J Aust. 1990;153:417–21.

82. Sinatra RS. Acute pain management and acute pain services. In: Cousins MJ, Bridenbaugh PO, editors. Neural blockade in clinical anesthesia and pain management, 3rd edn. Philadelphia: Lippincott;1998. pp 793–835.

83. Schug SA, Torrie JJ. Safety assessment of postoperative pain management by an acute pain service. Pain. 1995;55:387–91.

84. Forrest WH Jr, Smethurst PWR, Kienitz ME. Self-administration of intravenous analgesics. Anesthesiology. 1970;33:363–5.

85. Keeri-Szanto M. Apparatus for demand analgesia. Can Anaesth Soc J. 1971;18:581–2.

86. Sechzer PH. Studies in pain with the analgesic-demand system. Anesth Analg. 1971;50:1–10.

87. Royal College of Surgeons and College of Anaesthetists. Pain after surgery. London: Royal College of Surgeons of England; 1990.

88. Macintyre PE, Schug SA, Scott DA, Visser EJ, Walker SM; APM:SE working group of the Australian and New Zealand college of anaesthetists and faculty of pain medicine. Acute pain management: scientific evidence. 3rd edn. Melbourne: ANZCA & FPM; 2010.

89. American society of anesthesiologists task force on acute pain management. Practice guidelines for acute pain management in the perioperative setting: an updated report by the American society of anesthesiologists task force on acute pain management. Anesthesiology. 2012;116:248–73.

90. Egbert LD, Battit GE, Welch CE, Bartlett MK. Reduction of postoperative pain by encouragement and instruction of patients: a study of doctor-patient rapport. N Engl J Med. 1964;270:825–7.

91. Liu SS, Wu CL. Effect of postoperative analgesia on major postoperative complications: a systematic update of the evidence. Anesth Analg. 2007;104:689–702.

92. Myles PS, Weitkamp B, Jones K, Melick J, Hensen S. Validity and reliability of a postoperative quality of recovery score: the QoR-40. Br J Anaesth. 2000;84:11–5.

93. White PF, Kehlet H, Neal JM, Schricker T, Carr DB, Carli F, the Fast-track surgery study group. The role of the anesthesiologist in fast-track surgery: from multimodal analgesia to perioperative medical care. Anesth Analg. 2007;104:1380–96.

94. Houde RW, Wallenstein SL, Rogers A. Clinical pharmacology of analgesics: I. a method of assaying analgesic effect. Clin Pharmacol Ther. 1960;1:163–74.

95. Marret E, Kurdi O, Zufferey P, Bonnet F. Effects of nonsteroidal anti-inflammatory drugs on patient-controlled analgesia morphine side effects: meta-analysis of randomized controlled trials. Anesthesiology. 2005;102:1249–60.

96. Brennan TJ, Vandermeulen EP, Gebhart GF. Characterization of a rat model of incisional pain. Pain. 1996;64:493–501.

97. Spofford CM, Brennan TJ. Gene expression in skin, muscle and dorsal root ganglion after plantar incision in the rat. Anesthesiology. 2012;117:161–72.

98. Glynn CJ, Mather LE, Cousins MJ, Wilson PR, Graham JR. Spinal narcotics and respiratory depression. Lancet. 1979;2:356–7.

99. Weinger MB, Lee LA. "No patient shall be harmed by opioid-induced respiratory depression". APSF Newsletter, Fall 2011. http://www.apsf.org/newsletters/html/2011/fall/01_opioid.htm. Accessed Oct. 2012.

100. Atchison NE, Osgood PF, Carr DB, Szyfelbein SK. Pain during burn dressing change in children: relationship to burn area, depth and analgesic regimens. Pain. 1991;47:41–5.

101. Carr DB, Osgood PF, Szyfelbein SK. Treatment of pain in acutely burned children. In: Schechter NL, Berde CB, Yaster M, editors. Pain in Infants, children, and adolescents. Baltimore: Williams & Wilkins; 1993. pp 495–504.

102. Crile GW, Lower WE. Anoci-Association. Philadelphia: Saunders; 1914. pp 223–5.

103. O'Shaughnessy L, Slome D. Etiology of traumatic shock. Br J Surg. 1934;22:589–618.

104. Bromage PR, Shibata HR, Willoughby HW. Influence of prolonged epidural blockade on blood sugar and cortisol responses to operations upon the upper part of the abdomen and thorax. Surg Gynecol Obstet. 1971;132:1051–6.

105. Kehlet H. Clinical course and hypothalamic-pituitary-adrenocortical function in glucocorticoid-treated patients. Copenhagen, FADL's Forlag, 1976.

106. Woolf CJ. Evidence for a central component of post-injury pain hypersensitivity. Nature. 1983;306:686–8.

107. Moiniche S, Kehlet H, Dahl JB. A qualitative and quantitative systematic review of pre-emptive analgesia for postoperative pain relief: the role of timing of analgesia. Anesthesiology. 2002;96:725–41.

108. Lavand'homme P, De Kock M, Waterloos H. Intraoperative epidural analgesia combined with ketamine provides effective preventive analgesia in patients undergoing major digestive surgery. Anesthesiology. 2005;103:813–20.

109. Eisenach JC. Action on the prevention of chronic pain after surgery: public-private partnerships. Anesthesiology. 2010;112:509–18.

110. Kehlet H, Rathmell JP. Persistent post surgical pain: the path forward through better design of clinical studies. Anesthesiology. 2010;112:514–5.

111. Macrae WA. Chronic post-surgical pain. 10 years on. Br J Anaesth. 2008;101:77–86.

112. Jacob AK, Kopp SL. The impact of regional anesthesia on cancer recurrence: is it real? ASA Newsletter. 2012;76:14–7.

113. Cousins MJ. History of the development of pain management with spinal opioid and non-opioid drugs. In: Meldrum M, editor. Opioids and pain relief: a historical perspective. Progress in pain research and management, vol. 25. Seattle: IASP Press; 2003. pp 141–55.

114. Bromage PR. Spinal epidural analgesia. Edinburgh: Livingstone; 1954. pp 1–123.

115. Greene NR. Physiology of spinal anesthesia. Baltimore: Williams & Wilkins; 1958. pp 1–195.

116. Cousins MJ, Wright CJ. Graft, muscle and skin blood flow after epidural blocks in vascular surgical procedures. Surg Gynecol Obstet. 1971;133:59–64.

117. Wall PD, Sweet WH. Temporary abolition of pain in man. Science. 1967;155:108–9.

118. Calvillo O, Jenry JL, Neuman RS. Effects of morphine and naloxone on dorsal horn neurones in the cat. Can J Physiol Pharm. 1974;61:82–8.

119. Kitahata LM, Kosaka Y, Taub A, Bonikos K, Hoffert M. Lamina specific suppression of dorsal horn unit activity by morphine sulphate. Anesthesiology. 1974;41:39–48.

120. Duggan AW, Hall JG, Headley PM. Morphine, enkephalin and the substantia gelatinosa. Nature. 1976;264:456–8.

121. Yaksh TL, Rudy TA. Analgesia mediated by a direct spinal action of narcotics. Science. 1976;192:135–7.
122. Stapleton JV, Austin KL, Mather LE. Postoperative pain [letter]. Br Med J. 1978;2:1499.
123. Wang JW, Nauss LA, Thomas JE. Pain relief by intrathecally applied morphine in man. Anesthesiology. 1979;50:149–51.
124. Walker SM, Goudas LC, Cousins MJ, Carr DB. Combination spinal analgesic chemotherapy: a systematic review. Anesth Analg. 2002;95:674–715.
125. Behar M, Magora F, Olswang D, Davidson JT. Epidural morphine in the treatment of pain. Lancet. 1979;1:527–9.
126. Cousins MJ, Mather LE, Glynn CJ, Wilson PR, Graham JR. Selective spinal analgesia. Lancet. 1979;1:1141.
127. Samii K, Feret J, Harari A, Viars P. Selective spinal analgesia. Lancet. 1979;1:1142.
128. Carr DB, Cousins MJ. Spinal route of analgesia: opioids and future options for spinal analgesic chemotherapy. In: Cousins MJ, Bridenbaugh PO, Carr DB, Horlocker TT, editors. Cousins & Bridenbaugh's Neural Blockade In: Clinical Anesthesia and Management of Pain, 4th ed. Philadelphia: Lippincott Williams & Wilkins; 2009. pp 886–947.
129. Glynn CJ, Mather LE, Cousins MJ, Graham JR, Wilson PR. Peridural meperidine in humans: analgetic response, pharmacokinetics, and transmission into CSF. Anesthesiology. 1981;55:520–6.
130. Torda TA, Pybus DA, Liberman H, Clark M, Crawford M. Experimental comparison of extradural and IM morphine. Br J. Anaesth. 1980;52:939–43.
131. Nordberg G, Hedner T, Mellstrandt T, Dahlström B. Pharmacokinetic aspects of epidural morphine analgesia. Anesthesiology. 1983;58:545–51.
132. Rawal N, Sjostrand U, Christofferson E, Dahlstrom B, Arvill A, Rydman H. Comparison of intramuscular and epidural morphine for postoperative analgesia in the grossly obese: influence on postoperative ambulation and pulmonary function. Anesth Analg. 1984;63:583–92.
133. Cousins MJ, Mather LE. Intrathecal and epidural administration of opioids. Anesthesiology. 1984;61:276–310.
134. Gallagher RM. Primary care and pain medicine: a community solution to the public health problem of chronic pain. In: Gallagher RM, editor. Chronic Pain. Philadelphia: W. B. Saunders. Med Clin N Amer. 1999;83:555–83.
135. Foreward CDB. In: Porche R, editor. Approaches to pain management: an essential guide for clinical leaders, 2nd edn. Oakbrook Terrace: Joint Commission Resources; 2010. pp v–vi.
136. IOM (Institute of Medicine). Relieving pain in America: a blueprint for transforming prevention, care, education, and research. Washington: The National Academies Press;pp 1–364. Viewable at http://books.nap.edu/openbook.php?record_id = 13172. Accessed Sep. 10. 2012.
137. Uppington J. Guidelines, recommendations, protocols, and practice. In: Shorten G, Carr DB, Harmon D, Puig MM, Browne J, editors. Postoperative pain management: an evidence-based guide to practice. Philadelphia: Saunders Elsevier; 2006. pp 12–26.
138. Breivik H, Bond M. Why pain control matters in a world full of killer diseases. In: Wittink HM, Carr DB, editors. Pain management: evidence, outcomes and quality of life. St. Louis:Elsevier; 2008. pp 407–11.
139. Cousins M, Lynch M. The declaration of montreal: access to pain management is a fundamental human right. Pain. 2011;152:2673–4.
140. Painout. Improvement in postoperative pain outcome. http://pain-out.med.uni-jena.de/index.php/component/content/frontpage. Accessed Sep. 10. 2012.
141. Green CR, Anderson KO, Baker TA, Campbell LC, Decker S, Fillingim RB, Kaloukalani DA, Lasch KE, Myers C, Tait RC, Todd KH, Vallerand AH. The unequal burden of pain: confronting racial and ethnic disparities in pain. Pain Med. 2003;4:277–94.
142. Painaustralia. Working to prevent and manage pain. http://www.painaustralia.org.au. Accessed Sep. 10. 2012.
143. Eckenhoff JE. The anesthesiologist and the management of pain. J Chron Dis. 1956;4:96–101.
144. Chapin H, Bagarinao E, Mackey S. Real-time fMRI applied to pain management. Neurosci Lett. 2012;520(2):174–81.
145. Brown EN, Lydic R, Schiff ND. General anesthesia, sleep, and coma. N Engl J Med. 2010;363:2638–50.
146. Kerouac J. On the road: 50th anniversary edition. New York:Viking/ Penguin; 2007. p 276.
147. Kohane IS, Drazen JM, Campion EW. A glimpse of the next 100 years of medicine. N Engl J Med. 2012;367:2538–9.

A History of Cardiac Anesthesiology

Edward Lowenstein and J. G. Reves

Summary

In 1953, Gibbon used a heart-lung machine to allow closure of an atrial septal defect under direct vision. In 1967, Barnard performed the first heart transplant. In 1973, surgeons stopped the heart beating (cardioplegia), thereby protecting it, by infusing cold hyperkalemic solutions into the coronary arteries.

Advances in cardiac surgery spurred the development of cardiac anesthesiology. We changed from open drop ether to modern anesthetics and ventilation via tracheal tubes. In 1951, Keown described anesthetic management with hypothermia for the conduct of mitral commissurotomy. In 1964, Wynands used postoperative tracheal intubation and mechanical ventilation to increase survival.

In 1972, Civetta and Gabel described the use of the pulmonary artery (Swan-Ganz) catheter intra and postoperatively. The results were inconsistent, sometimes suggesting increased risk. Matsumoto introduced M-mode (one dimensional) transesophageal echocardiography (TEE) in 1980, followed in 1982 by Cahalan's description of 2-dimensional TEE, and deBruijn and colleagues' report of color-flow Doppler TEE in 1987. TEE made cardiac anesthesiologists into intraoperative cardiac diagnosticians who guided the surgeon.

Before 1969, cyclopropane, ether, or halothane dominated cardiac anesthesia. Lowenstein reported the use of high dose morphine for cardiac anesthesia in 1969, and Stanley reported use of high dose fentanyl in 1973, suggesting benefit in patients with valvular and congenital disease. Two randomized trials in 1973 found no advantage with morphine compared with halothane or ketamine. Studies in the 1970s and 1980s did not reveal an ideal "cardiac anesthetic". While anesthetic choice might matter little, in 1989 Slogoff and Keats reported that the choice of anesthesiologist did matter. Finally, research at Duke in the 1980s suggested that protecting central nervous system function from the deleterious effect of cardiac surgery required multiple strategies.

In the 1980s, Slogoff and Keats showed that increased heart rate endangered the myocardium of patients with coronary artery disease (CAD). Cardiac anesthesiologists then showed that beta blockers decreased long term mortality after non-cardiac surgery. In 2006, Mangano's group demonstrated that although aprotinin decreased transfusion requirements in patients undergoing open heart surgery, it increased the incidence of kidney failure and death. Anesthesiologists and surgeons added and removed "fads" such as early extubation (in the 1970s) and "off-pump" coronary artery bypass (in the 1990s).

Maturity of cardiac anesthesia required new technologies and knowledge promulgated in books and journals (e.g., *The Journal of Cardiothoracic Anesthesia,* first published in 1987). It required the development of leaders, training programs, and a sufficient cohort of practitioners. The Society of Cardiovascular Anesthesia, founded in 1978, now has 7,000 members.

Introduction

"A surgeon who would attempt such an operation [cardiac suture] should lose the respect of his colleagues." Billroth [1]

"No discovery can overcome the natural difficulties that attend to a wound of the heart." Padget [2]

"In the late fifties, the cardiologist…surrendered the patient to the surgeon after administration of the last rites." Teasdale-Scott [3]

"The production of relief of pain for the patient and provision of good operating conditions for the surgeon are relatively minor problems for the anesthesiologist compared with his problem of keeping the patient alive and safe." Pender [4]

"Since before recorded history, people died from narrowing (stenosis) of the heart valves, obstructing blood flow. Stenosis of the mitral valve predisposes to flooding of the lungs and people with stenosis might struggle for each breath. In 1956, an apparently healthy young woman with mitral stenosis suddenly had difficulty breathing while climbing the Pyramid of the Sun God in Mexico. She was flown to Boston for an emergency operation on her heart."

J. G. Reves (✉)
Medical University of South Carolina, 167 Ashley Avenue Suite 301, Charleston, SC 29425, USA
e-mail: revesj@musc.edu

E. Lowenstein
Dept. of Anesthesia, Critical Care and Pain Medicine, Massachusetts General Hospital, 55 Fruit Street, Boston, MA 02114, USA
e-mail: elowenstein1@partners.org

E. I Eger II et al. (eds.), *The Wondrous Story of Anesthesia,* DOI 10.1007/978-1-4614-8441-7_61, © Edmond I Eger, MD 2014

"Such patients often died during induction of anesthesia because their apprehension of surgery caused their heart to beat faster and flood the lungs. Mindful of this danger, the anesthesiologist Burton Briggs went to their hospital rooms to deliver small increments of intravenous thiopental; small enough to avoid cardiovascular collapse but large enough to sedate the patient and prevent the increased heart rate. There followed a race to the operating room, where the actual anesthetic was meticulously delivered so the surgeon could split the fused, narrowed valve, enabling natural blood flow through the valve. The patient lived a subsequently normal life." (Personal Communication EL)

This anecdote from the early years of heart surgery indicates the challenges faced by anesthesiologists—the need to preserve life while enabling an operation on the heart. The first operations were not performed on adults, but on infants and children with congenital malformations of the heart and great vessels, malformations that if uncorrected, caused early death. Surgeons and their anesthesiology peers next addressed the correction/replacement of damaged heart valves, and then the treatment of coronary artery disease. We then accomplished heart transplantation and used artificial pump devices to sustain life. The measures that preserved life in these patients were next applied to patients with similar heart diseases but undergoing non-cardiac surgical operations previously considered too dangerous to apply.

Hessel's review [5] supplies an authoritative rendering of the history of cardiac anesthesiology, and Mushin [6] and Benunof [7] similarly describe the related field of thoracic anesthesiology. A portion of our essay derives from such sources. We shall convey aspects of this history from a participatory perspective, spanning nearly half a century, the life of contemporary cardiac anesthesiology. The story includes anecdotes not easily found elsewhere.

Maintaining Life in the Presence of an Open Chest

Wounds allowing air into the chest—the "pneumothorax problem"—can fatally compromise breathing [6, 7]. Before we learned to breathe for such patients, surgeons only operated on the chest wall. Nineteenth century physiologists performed intrathoracic surgery in animals by inserting a tube into the trachea and rhythmically inflating the lungs through the tube with a bellows. Tuffier and Hallion reported to the Societé de Biologie in 1896 on "Intrathoracic operations with artificial respiration by insufflation," using a rhythmic inflation method. Surgeons applied these principles to humans many decades later [6].

The "pneumothorax problem" compromises oxygen delivery to the lungs, a delivery needed for survival. Surgeons initially expanded the lungs by a negative pressure chamber around the body (leaving the head exposed) or applied positive pressure around the head. These cumbersome techniques might expand but did not ventilate (intermittently

bring oxygen into and remove carbon dioxide from) the lungs. Chest surgery was thus rare and hazardous in the last decade of the nineteenth century.

We learned to insufflate, blow gas—including oxygen—continuously into the trachea, and this led naturally to tubes into the trachea and then to effective ventilation. William Macewen in Scotland described tracheal intubation in 1878; and in 1899, American physician scientist, Rudolph Matas pioneered intermittent positive pressure ventilation (the rhythmic application of pressure to the gases delivered to the lungs).

In 1906, Franz Kuhn (1866–1929) developed an intermittent positive pressure apparatus which he used with tracheal intubation. Tiegel, in 1908, used a face-mask, with an ingenious system to collect vomit (overcoming one of the major problems with early positive pressure ventilation). His system used a rebreathing bag allowing the addition of ether or chloroform. However it took Guedel and Waters in the United States and Nosworthy in Great Britain, in the 1930s, to allow successful surgery inside the chest by applying Macewen and Matas' principles, using tracheal tubes and rebreathing bags [6].

The safe use of the respiratory depressant anesthetic gas, cyclopropane, in the 1930s, and the introduction of pharmacologically induced paralysis in the 1940s, necessitated the increasing application of positive pressure ventilation. It demanded control of ventilation—and facilitated the subsequent development of surgery on intrathoracic great vessels that began modern cardiac surgery and anesthesiology *(vide infra).*

Major Historical Events in Cardiac Surgery

In 1896, the year that Padget predicted the impossibility of cardiac surgery [2], Rehn in Frankfurt sutured a wound to the heart [6]. Luther Hill repeated the feat in Montgomery, Alabama in 1902 [5]. Fig. 61.1 demonstrates the symbiotic relationship of cardiac surgery and anesthesia, showing the parallel landmark advances in each specialty.

Modern cardiac surgery began with operations on intrathoracic blood vessels—rather than on the heart itself. In 1938, at the Children's Hospital of Boston, surgical resident Robert Gross (1905–1988) successfully ligated a patent ductus arteriosus, a daring unsupervised feat. William Ladd, "the surgeon," was away on holiday! In 1944, Clarence Crafoord (1899–1983) repaired a coarctation (narrowing) of the aorta in Stockholm [5].

In Baltimore, in 1944 Alfred Blalock (1899–1964) performed the first palliative surgical procedure for cyanotic congenital heart disease (blue baby). The Blalock-Taussig operation involved creating an artificial connection (shunt) between one of the major systemic arteries and the

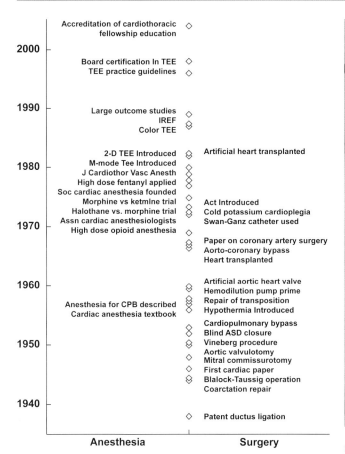

Fig. 61.1 timeline (Anesthesia / Surgery):

Year	Anesthesia	Surgery
2000	Accreditation of cardiothoracic fellowship education ◇	
	Board certification In TEE ◇	
	TEE practice guidelines ◇	
1990	Large outcome studies ◇	
	IREF ◈	
	Color TEE	
1980	2-D TEE Introduced ◈	Artificial heart transplanted
	M-mode Tee Introduced ◈	
	J Cardiothor Vasc Anesth ◈	
	High dose fentanyl applied ◈	
	Soc cardiac anesthesia founded ◇	
	Morphine vs ketmine trial ◇	Act Introduced
	Halothane vs. morphine trial ◈	Cold potassium cardioplegia
1970	Assn cardiac anesthesiologists	Swan-Ganz catheter used
	High dose opioid anesthesia ◇	
		Paper on coronary artery surgery
	◈	Aorto-coronary bypass
		Heart transplanted
1960		Artificial aortic heart valve
	◈	Hemodilution pump prime
	Anesthesia for CPB described ◈	Repair of transposition
	Cardiac anesthesia textbook ◇	Hypothermia Introduced
		Cardiopulmonary bypass
	◈	Blind ASD closure
1950	◈	Vineberg procedure
	◇	Aortic valvulotomy
	◇	Mitral commissurotomy
		First cardiac paper
	◈	Blalock-Taussig operation
		Coarctation repair
1940		
	◇	Patent ductus ligation

Anesthesia   Surgery

Fig. 61.1 A timeline of advances in cardiac anesthesia and surgery. Anesthesia by Morton enabled modern surgery, allowed the development of myriad new surgical procedures. Conversely, as Fig. 61.1 shows, the development of new surgical procedures, in this case those on the heart, came before and animated the development of people, techniques, and pharmacological approaches to support the work of the surgeon, developments led especially by anesthesiologists. Note that the figure does not include three events of import in the nineteenth century: tracheal intubation, first heart surgery, and positive pressure ventilation, all accomplished by surgeons

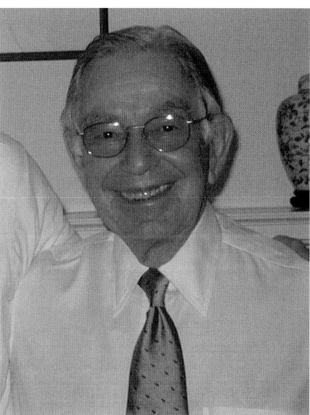

Fig. 61.2 Merel Harmel was the first to administer anesthesia for the successful paliation of Tetrology of Fallot. (Photograph from the private collection of J. Reves)

pulmonary artery, enabling greater mixing of the oxygenated and deoxygenated blood in the circulation. In 1946, Merel Harmel (1917-; Fig. 61.2) and Austin Lamont (1905–1969) described the anesthesia for the first 100 Blalock-Taussig Operations, the first cardiac anesthesiology paper [8]. Here follows an abridged contemporary memoire from Harmel (personal communication):

"About two weeks before the operation, Lamont mentioned that we might be faced with operations upon the heart and/or great vessels. Imagine my surprise, apprehension and excitement, when shortly before the operation was scheduled, he informed me that Dr. Blalock proposed to operate upon a 15 month old cyanotic infant with a tetralogy of Fallot, weighing 4 Kg. Earlier, Lamont had refused to anesthetize the infant for some minor operation because he felt she would not survive. So the prospect of a major experimental procedure involving a thoracotomy would surely hasten the baby's death. Blalock however was determined to operate. He had discussed the seriousness of the operation with the family, telling them the operation had never

been attempted before and the chances were good that the child might die on the operating table. (This is a sterling example of providing informed consent years before the requirement was widely recognized! EL and JGR)

"The day the operation was posted, Lamont offered me the 'opportunity' to anesthetize the baby! He would of course be with me in the operating room. He thought that the experience of anesthetizing this infant would be educational (I was just completing my 11th month of training). In 1944, at Hopkins there was no appropriate equipment for conducting endotracheal anesthesia in 4 Kg. infants. We thought to fashion an endotracheal tube from a large bore urethral catheter should intubation be necessary.

"On the 29th of November, Eileen Saxon was brought to the operating room. She was anesthetized with open drop ether, and oxygen was delivered by catheter under the mask. The only monitor was a finger on the carotid pulse. Blalock had Vivian Thomas (an African American laboratory assistant who had devised the procedure in Blalock's dog lab and who is credited with much of the success of the operation) at his side during the procedure. William Longmire (later the Chairman of Surgery at UCLA) and Denton Cooley (subsequetly a pioneering cardiac surgeon in Houston) assisted Blalock, performing a subclavian to pulmonary artery anastomosis in 1 hour and 45 minutes. Helen Taussig who had proposed the concept of the operation to Blalock was also in the room. When the subclavian and pulmonary arteries were clamped, the pulse became slow and almost imperceptible. Breathing became shallower and cyanosis deepened. The outlook appeared dismal, but she rallied and the operation continued. Toward the end of the operation we thought she might be obstructed and attempted unsuccessfully to intubate her trachea with our makeshift catheter. Positive pressure was applied with our smallest mask in an effort to re-expand her lung. At the end of the procedure her color dramatically improved. The atmosphere was jubilant. Against seemingly insuperable odds, she had miraculously survived and dramatically improved. Eileen recovered and was discharged almost two months later.

"A palpable excitement accompanied the operation, a feeling that something historic was happening. The initial presentation by Blalock and Taussig to the Hopkins Medical and Surgical Association meeting was accompanied by a standing ovation. The "blue baby" turning pink caught the hearts and imagination of parents, surgeons and the general populace. Surgeons from around the world came to see Blalock operate, and patients were referred from home and abroad. By 1946, when our article was published, we had completed over 200 operations, most with an anesthetic technique suggested by Elisabeth Lank (Fig. 61.3), the nurse anesthetist at the Boston Children's Hospital who had demonstrated the advantages of managing infants with intubation and anesthesia with cyclopropane."

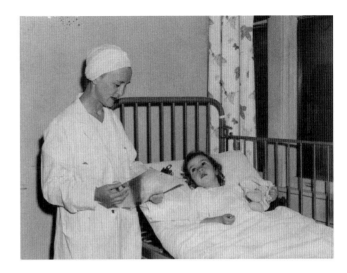

Fig. 61.3 Elizabeth (Bessie) Lank was a nurse anesthetist of enormous clinical skill. She taught many anesthesiologists who later became leaders in cardiac and pediatric anesthesia. As indicated in the text, she gave the anesthesia for many "firsts" in cardiac surgery. (Courtesy of Mark Rockoff and the archives of Boston Children's Hospital)

Before 1948, except for repairs of wounds to the heart during World War II, cardiovascular surgeons did not invade the heart or touch its valves. The temptation however, to relieve mitral stenosis (a narrowing of the valve joining the two chambers of the left side of the heart) by dilating the narrowed valve, was great. On January 29, 1948, Horace Smithy of Charleston (Medical University of South Carolina) successfully performed the first mitral commissurotomy using a device he designed [9]. The commissurotomy was performed "closed," blindly reaching the deformed valve through a small hole made in the heart's left atrium. Smithy's affliction with mitral stenosis, from which he died at age 34, surely animated this heroic effort. Smithy had tried to convince Blalock to perform the operation on him, but Blalock refused.

In 1950, Charles Bailey (1910–1993) attacked aortic valve stenosis, performing a closed aortic valvotomy in Philadelphia [10]. With both major left sided heart valves surgically accessible, cardiac surgery had reached major milestones of palliating and/or correcting congenital and valvular heart disease.

Two fears daunted these early cardiac surgeons. One was fear of damage to the heart, either physical damage or damage consequent to impaired blood flow to the heart, injuring the heart muscle so it could not pump effectively. A second parallel fear was concern that they might impair blood flow to the brain and injure that vital organ.

The cardiac surgeon and anesthesiologist extended the time to safely abolish blood flow to the heart and brain by cooling the patient. Cold protects the bloodless brain or heart by decreasing tissue metabolism and oxygen consumption. In the "early days", i.e., the 1950s,—the anesthetized patient was lowered into a tub of ice water with ice cubes floating in the tub—a tricky business because if the patient became too cold, the heart might stop and not start again. This limited

the lowest temperature to about 28 °C. Furthermore, with insufficient anesthesia, the patient shivered, opposing cooling. Cooling for cardiac surgery was debated and even transiently abandoned over the past 50 years. Conventional practice now uses moderate cooling (to 32–34 °C).

A few procedures required cessation of blood flow to heart and/or brain, and for these a much lower temperature was achieved, sometimes in just the heart by application of cardioplegia (see below) [11]. Sometimes so called deep hypothermic cardiac arrest (DHCA) was required for brain protection [12]. In DHCA the entire body was cooled to <20 °C and the circulation halted, while complex congenital anomalies in infants, and (rarely) the aorta in adults, were repaired.

Coronary artery disease, the limitation of arterial blood flow to the heart causing oxygen deprivation, and inadequate function or death of the heart muscle, became recognized as the greatest killer in industrialized countries. It was a topic of surgical attention as early as the 1930s [13]. How could the cardiac surgeon fix this problem?

Two early operations were developed by Vineberg. The first interrupted the two internal mammary arteries, coursing down the back of the sternum or breast bone, on the premise that bilateral ligation (BIMAL) of these vessels "downstream" of the heart would increase "upstream" flow to the coronary arteries. This operation achieved increasing popularity in the mid to late 1950s because it was simple, safe and *some* patients experienced decreased severity and/or frequency of angina pectoris. However, animal studies failed to confirm the premise, and many doubted the improvement. Two groups then performed randomized, "double blind" placebo controlled studies in a total of 35 patients [14, 15]. The control patients had a sham operation consisting of only a skin incision. These studies each revealed random and equivalent improvements of angina among patients who had undergone the placebo operation and internal mammary ligation, proving the ineffectiveness of the operation and putting an end to its performance. These results prompted anesthesiologist Henry Beecher's landmark article, arguing that it was unethical to perform new surgical operations *without* first establishing effectiveness [16]. Unfortunately, this call has been largely unheeded.

Contemporary cardiac surgery lacks placebo-controlled, sham operated studies of effectiveness, a reluctance based largely on claims that performing hazardous sham operations is unethical. Whether this is a wise decision, or whether more lives would be preserved and fewer people subjected to hazardous and ineffective operations by conducting sham studies in fully informed cardiac surgical candidates, remains an ethical conundrum that probably will not be confronted.

The second Vineberg operation for relief of angina pectoris actually improved (albeit not immediately) blood flow to the heart in both experimental animals and patients. Devised in the 1940s, and performed in patients in the 1950s and 1960s, the Vineberg operation implanted an internal mammary into the heart muscle [17], and over a period of weeks thereby brought new collateral vessels to the heart. These patients posed a challenge to the anesthetist because the heart lacked adequate blood flow, the muscle was injured by the operation itself and no immediate improvement in flow accompanied the additional stress of surgical trauma. Managing these patients inspired Earl Wynands (Fig. 61.4) to develop principles for anesthetic management of patients with severe coronary artery disease that are valid to this day [18]. Most importantly, Wynands sought to maintain coronary artery perfusion pressure by infusing phenylephrine as needed. He was the first to recognize that patients with unstable angina sustained a higher mortality rate than those with stable angina. Another major contribution was his observation that a resting electrocardiogram was of no use in predicting which patients would experience perioperative problems. Finally, he promoted the life-saving notion of maintaining tracheal intubation and ventilatory support postoperatively.

The inability of the Vineberg procedure to immediately improve coronary blood flow led, in 1967, to a third operation, one constructing a vascular (initially a vein but later a segment of artery) conduit between the ascending aorta and the diseased coronary artery segment, the coronary artery bypass graft operation or CABG [19]. It achieved almost immediate acceptance, and has been performed (without placebo controlled proof of effectiveness) upon millions of people worldwide.

Now we retreat to the 1950s to describe developments enabling modern cardiac surgery on the valves and vessels of the heart. In 1952, Gross (now having graduated from residency) performed the first true "open heart surgery",

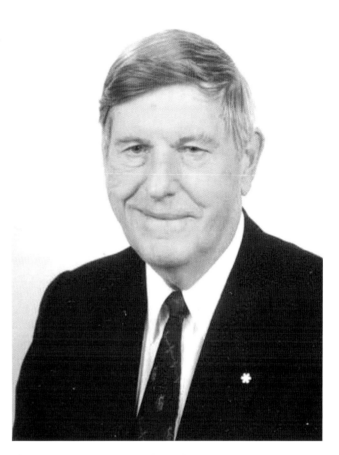

Fig. 61.4 Earl Wynands who advanced cardiac anesthesiology despite being more or less blind from macular degeneration

repairing an atrial septal defect (a hole between the right and left sides of the heart). Widely opening the right atrium and attaching a "well" to avoid the lethal entrainment of air into the circulation, he closed the hole in the septum, blindly suturing below the air-blood interface in the well [5].

However, applying the axiom that "necessity demands invention", widespread conduct of open heart surgery required invention of the heart-lung machine (cardiopulmonary bypass). This device collected venous blood, oxygenated it, removed carbon dioxide, and pumped the nourishing arterialized blood back into the aorta (i.e., back to the body). Thus, while the heart was not pumping and the lungs were not functioning circulation of oxygenated blood to the body was continued., Such a device permitted operations on the heart using direct vision. While a premedical student in 1952, one of the authors, EL, heard with great excitement that this seemingly impossible feat of stopping the heart and repairing it without killing the patient would soon become feasible. Indeed, it became a reality within the year.

On May 6, 1953, John Gibbon Jr (1903–1973) at Jefferson Medical College in Philadelphia, first successfully used a heart-lung machine in a patient in whom he closed an atrial septal defect in an empty heart under direct vision [20]. He and his wife Mary had taken two decades to develop the machine beginning the age of true invasive open heart surgery. He found minimal support for his initial work in the Department of Surgery at the Massachusetts General Hospital (MGH)—his chief, Edward Churchill, suggested that it had little promise. This prompted Gibbon to relocate to Jefferson Medical College in Philadelphia. During the ensuing 20 years, he addressed problems concerning filtration and coagulation of blood, and reestablishing normal coagulation after completion of the surgery. He had to enable oxygen and carbon dioxide gas exchange (as in the alveoli), and devise a pump that could reliably and controllably perfuse the systemic circulation.

Gibbon's invention, refined and adopted by many, revolutionized cardiac surgery by giving the surgeon a bloodless field and a time limited by how long a hypothermic heart could tolerate no coronary blood flow (about 30 minutes). The reintroduction in 1973, of myocardial protection techniques with a cold hyperkalemic (high potassium concentration) solution (cardioplegia) facilitated the expansion of cardiac surgery [11], giving surgeons well over an hour to perform their work. Because the heart resists longer periods of ischemia than does the brain, Arthur Keats (1923–2007) commented: "The heart is a very tough organ, and when it malfunctions, we simply cannot look to a brief period of ischemia for its failure" [21]. However, the heart is not invincible, and prolonged ischemia during intra-cardiac surgery required a protective strategy. Cardioplegia during intentional interruption of coronary blood flow to the heart was second only to the invention of the heart-lung machine as a factor in the development of cardiac surgery.

Perhaps the last major surgical accomplishment was heart transplantation. Christian Barnard (1922–2001) performed the first cardiac transplant in Capetown, SA in 1967 [5]. The anesthesiologist, J Ozinsky reported: "From the anesthetist's point of view, it was not anticipated that we would be faced with anything we had not been faced with before, and the anesthesia was conducted with optimism" [22]. Ozinsky and Barnard did not fear their daring venture into the unknown. Perhaps, however, they ventured too soon. Barnard's patient lived but a short time. Norman Shumway (1923–2006) of Stanford University thought the effort was premature. He believed that success required the development of a multidisciplinary team, one particularly focused on issues of tissue rejection. Indeed, the discovery of the immunosuppressive drug cyclosporine, provided the key to success [21].

Cardiac Anesthesiology

"Anesthesia for patients undergoing cardiac surgery" differs, in our minds, from "cardiac anesthesiology." Skillful physicians and nurses provide the former; individuals developing the science and art so that others may practice it more safely comprise the latter. Using this definition, we can point to a number of cardiac anesthesiologists. Kenneth Keown's 1951 description of the anesthetic management and hypothermia for patients undergoing mitral commissurotomy [23] recognized the importance of light anesthesia with minimal cardiac depression, and the benefit of letting the temperature drift down, i.e. of producing mild hypothermia. Artusio's use in the early 1950s of "ether analgesia" during mitral commisurotomy may be the ultimate in light anesthesia. Patients managed in this fashion responded appropriately to questions and commands during the procedure but experienced no pain or recall [24]. Patrick et al.'s 1957 [25] description of anesthesia for patients undergoing cardiopulmonary bypass, merits special attention, because they used animal experimentation to test hypotheses regarding control of physiologic variables such as pump flow, temperature, and blood gas management during cardiopulmonary bypass. They surmised that these factors were of greater interest than the anesthetic management per se': "The management of anesthesia for patients undergoing intracardiac surgery by means of a Gibbon type pump-oxygenator differs in no important respect from the anesthesia management of patients for ordinary intrathoracic procedures." Their work established the principle, that attaining physiologic ends was paramount rather than the means to achieve them.

Monitoring

The first patients undergoing cardiac surgery were anesthetized with minimal monitoring, such as a finger on a temporal or carotid artery! However, as the surgery became more complex, and particularly after cardiopulmonary bypass was employed, monitoring of hemodynamic variables became an important component of cardiac anesthesiology. In 1972, Civetta and Gabel described the use of the pulmonary artery (Swan-Ganz) catheter intra and postoperatively [26], and in 1973 Lappas et al. demonstrated that pulmonary capillary wedge pressure accurately reflected left atrial pressure intraoperatively, which in turn reflected left heart filling and function [27]. Indeed, invasive monitoring and expertise sometimes seemed to define cardiac anesthesiologists, who demonstrated their expertise by their ability to "slip in" invasive lines quickly and deftly, equating this skill, perhaps erroneously, with superior knowledge. The need for arterial pressure measurement and access to arterial blood samples provided sufficient reason for inserting an indwelling arterial catheter. Measurement of central venous pressure seemed similarly beneficial in helping estimate adequacy of blood volume and heart function, although echocardiography is now considered a better reflection. At the MGH, Laver (personal communication) explained the philosophy of hemodynamic measurement versus the clinician's intuition: "If the measurements contradict your clinical impression, change your clinical impression!"

The introduction of the pulmonary artery catheter in the early 1970s provoked vigorous controversy. Some outstanding cardiac anesthesiologists considered this technology essential for optimal intra- and postoperative management. Others eschewed the routine use of such costly catheters, fearing the complications they could bring (e.g., death), or unconvinced that the additional data facilitated a positive outcome. Reports in 1987 indicated that information supplied from a pulmonary artery catheter added little to the successful management of many cardiac surgical patients [28, 29]. Like all tools and drugs, the risks and benefits needed to be balanced. In selected patients, particularly those with impaired pumping function of the heart at any perioperative stage, the use of a pulmonary artery catheter facilitated successful management, but in many others it imposed unnecessary risks and expense [28, 29].

Until recently, monitoring in cardiac anesthesia practice lacked visualization of the anatomy of the heart. Anatomy is crucially important because many operations propose to repair or palliate anatomic defects such as incompetent mitral valves or ventricular septal defects, and because visualization of malfunctioning areas of the heart can provide clues to explain impaired circulation. Cardiac anesthesiologists and surgeons had no view of the internal anatomy of the heart as complexity of surgery progressed. Transesophageal echocardiography (TEE) changed that.

The 1980 introduction of M-mode (one dimensional) TEE by Matsumoto [30] was followed in 1982 by Cahalan's description of 2-dimensional TEE [31], and deBruijn and colleagues' report of color-flow Doppler TEE in 1987 [32]. Each of these gave different information. M-mode alone was least useful, almost uninterpretable in real time. Two dimensional TEE allowed a rapid meaningful interpretation of structure. Color Doppler TEE enabled visualization of flow allowing anatomic and physiologic interpretations (e.g. seeing turbulent backward flow through an aortic valve means significant aortic valve regurgitation.) Most recently, TEE allows a 3-dimensional view of structures and even better visualization [33]. TEE has permitted cardiac anesthesiologists to literally look into the heart and become intraoperative cardiac diagnosticians, the intraoperative counterpart of the cardiologists providing the preoperative diagnosis guiding the surgeon to the appropriate procedure. Cardiac anesthesiologists can now inform surgeons in real time, of new intraoperative findings, make new diagnoses, confirm proper repair of the cardiac lesion, and specify needs for further immediate surgical management [21].

TEE has transformed the intraoperative experience for patients, anesthesiologists and surgeons alike, particularly in congenital [22] and valvular surgery. Clinical anecdotes demonstrate its value: A surgeon believes a ventricular septal defect in a 6-year-old child has been successfully closed. However, when preparing to terminate cardiopulmonary bypass, high pulmonary artery pressures and blood gas analysis indicate a continuing left to right shunt, and examination by TEE reveals the precise location of a second major but previously unappreciated hole in the ventricular septum. Before the advent of TEE, the second hole would have awaited an emergency postoperative cardiac catheterization, and would have required a second operation to obtain a satisfactory result. Likewise in adults with mitral valve rupture, the anesthesiologist determines which valve leaflet is flailing and whether it is repairable or requires a prosthesis. Once the repair is done, the anesthesiologist assesses valvular integrity. This diagnostic information has reduced re-operations and prevented further heart damage. No other monitoring technology has provided comparable benefit to intra-operative decision making.

Anesthetic Drug Regimen (or Anesthetic Pharmacology)

Before 1969, cyclopropane, ether or halothane dominated anesthesia for cardiac surgical patients. The flammability of the first two led to dominance of the non-explosive halothane. Death during induction of anesthesia, and inability to differentiate cardiac from pulmonary failure after cardiopulmonary bypass and postoperatively, were common. A search for better approaches to anesthesia led to the introduction, at MGH, of high dose morphine. This was the era before coronary revascularization; cardiac surgical patients had primarily valvular or congenital disease. Reminiscing about this introduction, Lowenstein (Fig. 61.5) wrote: "At least three things were necessary to set the stage for a new concept of anesthesia for our most ill patients: an environment that tolerated and even encouraged radically creative solutions; a clinical problem that caused an unacceptably high death rate; and a cast of characters with imagination, vision, courage, and clinical credibility" [34]. It was noted that large doses of intravenous (IV) morphine given postoperatively could relieve pain and, by depressing ventilation, could enable patients to tolerate tracheal intubation and mechanical ventilation. Morphine had recently been demonstrated to not depress heart contraction [35]. Why not deliver large doses of morphine *preoperatively* to produce insensibility yet not impose cardiovascular collapse during induction? Continuing this regimen postoperatively would produce the already appreciated salutary benefits.

The paper, published in 1969 in the *New England Journal of Medicine*, documented the hemodynamic effects of enormous doses of morphine in patients with valvular heart disease and patients without heart disease, and changed the

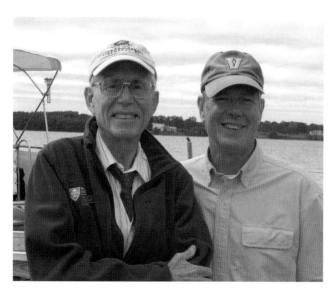

Fig. 61.5 A photograph of Edward Lowenstein (*left*) and Jerry Reves, happily at the water's edge

conduct of cardiac anesthesia [36]. It increased interest in the physiological consequences of drugs used to conduct cardiac anesthesia, for example, documenting a different hemodynamic response to the same drug in patients with and without valvular heart disease. Valvular heart disease leads to heart failure and large blood volumes that predispose to pulmonary edema. Morphine improved the circulation of these patients by causing vasodilation, decreasing systemic vascular resistance and reducing the work required of the heart. On the other hand, patients with uncomplicated coronary artery disease had neither increased blood volume nor cardiac failure, nor had they adapted to the continual release of endogenous catecholamines as had patients with valvular heart disease. Thus, in patients with uncomplicated ischemic heart disease, surgical stimulation during morphine anesthesia was accompanied by increased blood pressures and heart rates, dangerous changes that increased myocardial oxygen demand and consumption.

The increasing number of patients with coronary artery disease prompted a search for better cardiac anesthesia techniques. In retrospect, this was ironic since Wynands' 1967 article had defined many of the optimal principles, if not specific drugs, for managing such patients [18]. "Recipes" followed, each describing different "ideal" anesthetic regimens. However, two randomized trials in the early 1970s failed to demonstrate an outcome difference with different anesthetic drug regimens [37, 38]. A 1978 trial advocated "industrial-sized" doses of fentanyl, a synthetic opioid devoid of the histamine liberating effect of morphine, to provide "stress-free" anesthesia [39].

The originators of high-dose "opioid anesthesia" documented limitations of the technique including patient awareness [40, 41]. Patient awareness may occur more commonly in cardiac surgery than in other settings, because less anesthetic may be given to avoid cardiac depression, and because high opioid doses provide unreliable amnesia. As early as 1951—before opioid use as anesthetics—awareness was recognized as a possible outcome: "At the time of the pre-anesthetic examination, and again before anesthesia is induced, an attempt is made to explain the stages of the procedure of which the patient may be aware during operation" [23]. It continues to be a problem. In 2007, Pollard described the incidence of awareness in 87,361 surgical patients [42]. Of the six who remembered events, 4 had undergone cardiac surgery.

The obligatory period of postoperative ventilation was an initial stimulus for using high-dose opioids. While advantageous in many patients, it proved to be unnecessary in others, and may be accompanied by awareness. Subsequent small and then large studies revealed, not surprisingly, that there is no single ideal "cardiac anesthetic" [37, 38, 43, 44]. Harmel and Lamont recognized this in 1946: "…one cannot be dogmatic in regard to choice of anesthetic agent and technique" [4]. Optimal care for any given patient requires matching patient pathophysiology with the pharmacology of anesthetic and other drugs by knowledgeable and skilled clinicians [45].

The Cardiac Anesthesiologist

While choice of anesthetic regimen may matter little, Slogoff and Keats at the Texas Heart Institute found that the choice of anesthesiologist did [46]. In their study of postoperative myocardial infarction as a function of anesthetic choice, in patients operated upon for coronary artery disease, they incidentally found that outcomes of patients anesthetized by one of the nine attending anesthesiologist's stood out. The frequency of myocardial infarction associated with "Anesthesiologist Number Seven," significantly exceeded that for the other eight [34]. Patients anesthetized by number seven had more variability of blood pressure and heart rate, the two factors most affecting myocardial supply and demand. Whether this was due to inattention, pharmacologic ignorance, poor choice of drugs or drug doses, or chance, is not known.

Present day cardiac anesthesiologists deliver a mixture of drugs. Moderate doses of an opioid (usually fentanyl or sufentanil) are used to minimize adrenergic responses to noxious stimulation. Muscle relaxants keep patients from moving. Potent inhaled anesthetics augment relaxant effect, protect the heart [47], modify hemodynamic perturbations, and together with benzodiazepines, curtail memory of intraoperative events.

Vexations in the Present Care of the Cardiac Surgical Patient

The level of blood pressure during cardiopulmonary bypass has periodically been a matter of much controversy—the primary concern being whether inadequate brain perfusion during non-pulsatile CPB produced postoperative brain damage. After several decades addressing this issue, Newman et al demonstrated in 1994, that cerebral blood flow is well preserved during cardiopulmonary bypass as long as CO_2 levels are normal and perfusion pressure is maintained within the autoregulatory range of 50 to 90 mmHg [48]. The controversy disappeared.

How long should postoperative tracheal intubation continue? In his 1967 study of anesthesia for patients undergoing Vineberg operations, Wynands discovered that postoperative tracheal intubation and elective mechanical ventilation increased survival [18]. In 1968, John Viljoen at the Cleveland Clinic confirmed this result in a larger surgical population, decreasing mortality from 10 to 2% [49]. Such findings strengthened the case for high-dose opioid anesthesia. Immediate removal of tracheal tubes and resumption of spontaneous breathing after cardiac surgery became rare.

But nothing comes for free. Prolonged controlled ventilation through a tracheal tube also carried risks of injury to the trachea, trauma to the lung, and pulmonary infection. Newer shorter-acting opioids and anesthetics decreased the need for prolonged ventilation that the large doses of morphine had imposed. In the 1970s, when aortocoronary bypass graft operations in patients with normal heart function became common, earlier tracheal extubation was advocated to minimize complications. This also decreased intensive care unit (ICU) and hospital stay and costs. But policy then went too far. Many "fit" patients having coronary artery grafts had tracheal extubation in the operating room, as though they had just undergone a simple herniorraphy. If it was possible, it was done…and frequently…for a while. However, urgent postoperative reintubation sometimes followed tracheal extubation in the operating room. Reintubation was required because of respiratory insufficiency, cardiac arrhythmias or dysfunction, or bleeding. Rather than waiting a few hours after establishing satisfactory postoperative conditions, tracheal extubation in the operating room did not improve patient outcomes, nor did it reduce ICU or hospital stay, or cost. The fad passed.

"Off-pump" coronary artery bypass to treat coronary artery disease became a popular deviation from optimum care in the late 1990s. As cardiologists expanded catheter-based methods to treat coronary artery disease, surgeons responded with their own approaches. Coronary artery bypass graft (CABG) surgery was performed without cardiopulmonary bypass ("off-pump CABG"), prompted by the notion that avoiding cardiopulmonary bypass (CPB) would prevent the adverse consequences of CPB on the brain. The lack of CPB required that the heart continue pumping while in unnatural positions and while grafts were placed in difficult-to-reach locations. These positions often compromised venous return and cardiac output, requiring vasopressors to maintain blood pressure and avoid myocardial ischemia. Surgeon Denton Cooley quipped: "We have successfully made cardiac surgery more painful for the surgeon (and anesthesiologist) than

the patient." Studies subsequently established that the revascularization achieved was less effective, and that the brain did not benefit [50]. This fad has also faded.

Influential Individuals and Groups

The authors of this chapter are not professional historians, and have wrestled with the problem of how to recognize contributions made by individuals, versus those made by groups united by their motivation to improve the care and outcome of patients. By its very nature, cardiac anesthesiology must be practiced collaboratively, if only because surgeons, nurses, perfusionists, cardiologists and laboratories are requisites. Nevertheless, we have done our best to differentiate individuals versus groups making particularly important contributions. The historian also tends to provide a chronologic tale. We found this challenging due to the brief period we describe, the fact that many individuals and groups emphasized different activities during this period, and affiliations changed as people worked in different institutions and with different people.

Thus, arbitrarily, we have divided this section into Individuals and Groups who, in our opinion, most altered the development of cardiac anesthesiology (Table 61.1 and Fig. 61.6). The former tend to be those either working alone or with a small group, or who made contributions despite moving to different environments, whereas the latter tended to be gatherings of investigators whose collaborations appeared to synergize each other to make the effort stronger.

Individuals

As documented above, Harmel together with Austin Lamont successfully managed blue babies with cyclopropane, tracheal intubation, and intermittent positive pressure ventilation. They used IV morphine to suppress spontaneous gasping respiration that they attributed to cerebral hypoxia, secondary to hypotension during the repair [8]. They achieved a mortality rate of 23%, considered astoundingly low since no previous treatment had been available for these afflicted babies. They attributed this to the "immediate benefit" of the operation.

In 1951, and two years out of residency, Kenneth Keown et al. published a report describing anesthesia for patients undergoing mitral commisurotomy. Anesthesia began with atropine premedication, followed by establishing IV access by surgical cutdown of the anterior tibial vein. They used a continuous procaine infusion for both sedation and arrythmia suppression, thiopental, decamethonium for neuromuscular blockade, tracheal intubation, and a nitrous oxide oxygen mixture with "augmented respiratory function whenever indicated" [23]. This anesthetic regimen used non-explosive

Table 61.1 Groups and Individuals Influencing the Development of Cardiac Anesthesiology

Initial year & duration of activity	Faculty[a]	School, city
1938–1959	Lank, Smith	Boston Children's Hosp, Boston
1951–1967	Keown	Hahnemann, Philadelphia
1952–1977	Buckley, VanBergen	University of Minnesota, Minneapolis
1957–1978	Theye, Patrick, Tarhan, Tinker, Moffitt	Mayo Clinic, Rochester
1958–1980	Sykes[b]	Hammersmith
1960–1967	Wynands	McGill University, Montreal
1966–1998	Viljoen, Estafanous	Cleveland Clinic, Cleveland
1966–2000	Laver, Lowenstein, Bland, Hallowell, Dalton	MGH, Boston
1966–2004	Prys-Roberts, Foëx, Sykes	Oxford University
1968–1988	Ream, Garman	Stanford University, Stanford
1968–1993	Branthwaite	University College, London
1972–2002	Lell, Reves, Samuelson, Allarde, Oget	University of Alabama, Birmingham
1976–present	Barash, Hines	Yale University, New Haven
1977–1996	Keats, Slogoff	Texas Heart Institute, Houston
1978–2010	Sonntag, Kettler	Göttingen, Germany
1978–present	Coriat	Hospital Pitié-Salpêtrière, Paris
1979–present	Cahalan, Mangano, Wallace, Cason	UCSF
1979–present	Kaplan, Waller, Zaidan, Hug, Levy	Emory University, Atlanta
1984–present	Reves, deBruijn, Clements, Newman, Mathew	Duke University, Durham

[a] The listing of multiple faculty does not indicate that faculty attended the associated institution for the inclusive dates, only that one or more faculty were present during those dates
[b] Hammersmith to 1980; Oxford thereafter

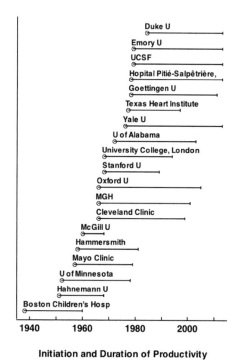

Initiation and Duration of Productivity

Fig. 61.6 Dozens of institutions and greater numbers of individuals contributed to the advancement of cardiovascular anesthesia and the management of patients with cardiovascular disease. This figure indicates many of those institutions and *roughly* illustrates when the individuals in those institutions began their contributions, and the period over which they had their greatest impact

agents, years before halothane was available. The trachea was extubated at the end of the surgical procedure, and the IV catheter was removed to avoid the "temptation to administer excessive IV fluids." Keown published the first cardiac anesthesia textbook in 1956 [51]. Keown, first in Philadelphia and after 1957 at the University of Missouri, may be considered the father of *academic* cardiac anesthesia.

In contrast to the Keown regimen, Pender, reporting on the Mayo Clinic experience in patients undergoing mitral commisurotomy, avoided atropine for fear of tachycardia and avoided procaine because of its capacity to cause myocardial depression [4]. He noted, "our past opinion about what constitutes a safe minimal blood pressure during anesthesia has been too high," "the depth of anesthesia seems much more important than the agent employed" and "little anesthetic agent is necessary." These two contrasting descriptions make the point that empiricism, and trial and error, enabled markedly different but equally successful regimens. Keats praised these pioneers: "These (early cardiac anesthetists) were heroes, because of their courage to face new challenges without guidance or precedence, without sophisticated monitors or equipment, and with only their intelligence and clinical acumen to contribute to the surgical outcome" [21].

At the Mayo Clinic in the 1950s, Richard Theye profoundly influenced the advancement of cardiac surgery with cardiopulmonary bypass [52, 53]. Anesthesiologist Emerson Moffit supported cardiologist HJC Swan and physiologist Earl Wood in studying 45 patients undergoing open heart surgery with cardiopulmonary bypass [53, 54]. This interdisciplinary team worked in a collegial environment that surgeon John Kirklin created at Mayo, and later reproduced at the University of Alabama in Birmingham.

Robert Smith, a pioneering pediatric anesthesiologist, worked at Boston Children's Hospital after World War II with Robert Gross. In 1951, he published an exhaustive article on the circulatory factors affecting anesthesia in congenital heart disease. His 1959 textbook on pediatric anesthesia included further experience with anesthetic techniques for palliative and corrective repairs of congenital defects in infants and children [55]. Smith followed a remarkable nurse anesthetist. Elizabeth (Bessie) Lank came to Boston Children's Hospital in 1935, after 3 months of training in anesthesia. For decades, she anesthetized most of Gross' cardiac surgical patients, including the first child for ligation of a patent ductus arteriosus in 1938, when Gross was a resident acting without supervision [56]. She also taught Harmel and Lamont to use cyclopropane and perform tracheal intubation. (For more on the extraordinary Ms. Lank, see Harmel's memoire above, and George Gregory's Chapter 51 in this book). Smith's and Keown's books, were the standard reference texts for—and thus profoundly influenced the development of—the fledgling field.

As noted above, Earl Wynands in Montreal published his notable 1967 paper describing the anesthetic care of patients undergoing Vineberg's novel operation for myocardial revascularization [18]. These patients presented extraordinary challenges: they had severe ischemic heart disease, marginal cardiac reserve, and postoperative heart function worsened by the surgery.

Wynands accomplishments are remarkable given his development of bilateral macular degeneration (Doynes' maculopathy) during medical school. He had only peripheral vision! The following reflections speak to his pioneering spirit and courage (Personal communication from Wynands):

"I wasn't sure how long my career would last but decided to give it a shot. At this point I could barely read with a magnifying glass and did not know how much further my vision would deteriorate.

"Mr. Pierre Morin challenged me to do a blind cannulation of the artery. In spite of my efforts to hide my visual problems he was obviously aware that I inserted needles and plastic cannulas into veins by feel. He told me outright that I should be able to insert one into an artery by feeling the pulse and I took up his challenge. I was successful on the first attempt and that put an end to the surgeons doing a cut down on the radial artery and limiting blood flow to the hand."

Wynands was awarded the Order of Canada and remains vibrant and active to this day.

Arthur Keats, who trained at the MGH and started his career with a primary academic interest in pain and narcotics. He arrived at Baylor University in Houston as Professor and Chief of Anesthesia in the early 1950s. There were two competing surgeons (DeBakey and Cooley) and surgical programs (Methodist and St Lukes Hospitals) within that system that he bridged for twenty-five years before continuing with just one (Cooley). He became an integral and crucial member of the success of that program, pioneering advances in vascular surgery and adult and pediatric cardiac surgery. Keats possessed a towering intellect and was a protean contributor. He mentored several junior associates who went on to productive careers, but achieved his most striking scholarly advances together with his trainee, Steven Slogoff. Between 1977 and 1991, they reported on randomized, controlled trials defining the effect of different anesthetics and beta blocker management, steal prone anatomy, prebypass ischemia, cardiopulmonary bypass flow and pressure, and prebypass hemodynamic variables, postoperative myocardial infarction, and renal and cerebral outcomes [46]. These series of reports included as many as 1000 patients, extremely large for that time.

Slogoff and Keats observed that tachycardia was the most deleterious, and in their hands, the *only* hemodynamic parameter associated with adverse outcomes [46]. They debunked several ill-founded but widely believed clinical dogmas, such as the hazard of continuing beta adrenergic blockers until the time of surgery [57], and the hazard of isoflurane in patients with coronary-steal prone anatomy [58, 59]. Their work can be considered as an important positive incremental step between studies using surrogate markers rather than true outcomes, and between small series that lacked power to draw conclusions and larger series from which generalizations could be made. They presaged the large series (though primarily observational) of Mangano, and the even larger but randomized, controlled studies of Devereaux (see below).

Keats questioned conventional wisdom. In his 1983 Rovenstine Lecture, he examined the collaboration of surgeon and anesthesiologist in the development of the field, noting that surgeons led the way. He advocated that only important questions be addressed, and identified and discussed unimportant ones on which much time and effort had been wasted. He challenged our emerging field to stop talking to itself in its publications, and to populate non-anesthesiology journals with the new knowledge that we had generated [21]. He served as Editor-in-Chief of *Anesthesiology* and President of the American Board of Anesthesiology. His achievements and his firm leadership make him, in our opinion, the single-most important figure in the history of cardiac anesthesiology.

Dennis Mangano, a native of New York, earned a BS in electrical engineering and PhD in physics from New York Polytechnic Institute. After working at Bell Laboratories, where he developed a mathematical theory of physical acoustic phenomena using a multivariate statistical model, he earned an MD in 1974 from the University of Miami in their innovative program for PhDs, and joined the faculty at UCSF after completing the anesthesiology residency.

Starting with basic cardiac physiologic research in cardiac surgical patients, Mangano soon recognized the importance of myocardial ischemia as a determinant of survival and well being, and began studies in both non-cardiac and cardiac surgical patients. He has determined predictors of myocardial infarction in non-cardiac surgical patients, revealing in 1990, that postoperative ECG changes are the best predictor of adverse cardiac outcomes in high risk patients undergoing non-cardiac surgery [60]. This led him to search for methods of preventing postoperative ischemia. His two hundred patient, randomized, double-blind study of perioperative beta adrenergic blockade claimed a two year survival advantage for blockade. For many years, it was a major impetus for widespread acceptance of this class of drugs as a standard treatment despite criticism due to exclusion from the analysis of in-hospital deaths [61]. It fundamentally changed management of patients at risk of developing perioperative myocardial ischemia, and formed the basis for the American College of Cardiology-American Heart Association Guidelines for Perioperative Cardiovascular Evaluation and Care for Noncardiac Surgery [62].

In the late 1980s, Mangano organized two non-profit independent, international research organizations, Ischemia Research and Education Foundation (IREF) and Multicenter Study of Perioperative Ischemia (McSPI). Over two decades, they performed observational studies of more than 7,000 patients, producing two comprehensive data bases, developing the careers of many investigators, and affecting the conduct of anesthesia and of cardiology and cardiac surgery.

The resulting publications changed our understanding and management of patients with myocardial ischemia and decreased morbidity and mortality. Important examples include the demonstration that aspirin after CABG surgery decreased mortality, heart attack, stroke, and gastrointestinal bleeding without increasing hemorrhage, gastritis or delaying wound healing [63]. This elicited an editorial in the *NEJM* entitled "Aspirin with Bypass Surgery-From Taboo to New Standard of Care" [64]. Another study demonstrated a reduced mortality after CABG in patients receiving preoperative statin therapy. Remarkably, Mangano demonstrated that impeccably conducted observational studies can be used in place of randomized Phase IV studies—studies often mandated by the FDA but almost never conducted. An editorial in the *New England Journal of Medicine* commenting on the aprotinin study described below stated "Mangano and colleagues provide an example of the type of study that may be a model for the future" [65]. The paper to which the editorial referred had found that aprotinin, a controversial substance intended to decrease bleeding and transfusion, was associated with an increased incidence of kidney failure and death [66]. Aprotinin had been vigorously marketed and had gained widespread acceptance. Shortly

following an FDA meeting at which the manufacturer contested the findings, the manufacturer admitted withholding data supporting these complications. Aprotonin was withdrawn worldwide about two years later. Mangano commented that

> "Good medicine demands you protect the patient. That's the issue, not the drug and not the profit margin…Approximately 22,000 lives could have been saved if the drug had been withdrawn in 2006 (when the data were published)…."[1]

Even larger randomized, placebo controlled trials have been conducted after the turn of the twentieth Century, by cardiologist-epidemiologists PJ Devereaux, Salim Yusuf, and colleagues at MacMaster University. Yusuf was one of three Oxford University investigators revolutionizing cardiology research in the 1980s with ISIS-1, the International Study of Infarct Salvage [67]. Stimulated by cancer epidemiologist Richard Peto (of Doll and Peto/lung cancer fame) they conducted a 16,000 patient randomized, placebo controlled study of beta adrenergic blockade, in patients with acute myocardial infarction. This demonstrated a remarkable 20% decrease in mortality. In addition, it led to the practice of using acronyms to name studies!

Yusuf and his student Devereaux turned their attention to perioperative administration of beta blockers, after performing a meta-analysis establishing equipoise, despite the widespread perioperative acceptance of beta blockers. The 8,000 patient Perioperative Ischemia Evaluation Study (POISE) documented a decreased incidence of myocardial infarction, but higher stroke and death rates in patients receiving metoprolol [68]. Thus, beta blockade was effective in decreasing the primary outcome of the study but had unanticipated safety issues. Controversy exists regarding whether this is an intrinsic issue with beta blockade, or is a result of using uniform and possibly excessive metoprolol dosage rather than titration to effect. The adverse effects appeared to be related to prolonged postoperative hypotension. This led the authors to search for a method of controlling postoperative heart rate to prevent heart attacks, not associated with hypotension in the ongoing POISE 2 trial. Thus, Keats' call for large studies using true outcomes, rather than surrogate markers, has come progressively closer to fruition, and yielded enhanced insights and patient safety.

Cardiac Anesthesia Groups

The MGH Group

The seeds for the first and perhaps the most influential academic cardiac anesthesia program, were sown at the MGH in the 1950s and 1960s. Two groups of physician-scientists laid

---

[1] Interview 17 Feb 2008 on "60 Minutes"

the foundations. Keats later noted that "Most of the important conceptual advances in cardiovascular surgery occurred in (this golden era in) the 1950s" [21].

First, in 1951, three faculty members were charged with initiating a program to provide anesthesia for patients undergoing closed mitral valvulotomy. One of those, William Brewster, demonstrated that ether depressed the myocardium of dogs that had sympathetic blockade from total spinal anesthesia, but not that of dogs with intact sympathetic systems [69]. This revealed why patients with low cardiac reserve but intact adrenergic systems tolerated ether well. Initially, the equipment used for this research performed in dogs was wiped clean and taken to the operating room to monitor the patients' cardiovascular responses to anesthesia and surgery! This established the practice of intra-operative research grade monitoring of cardiac surgical patients at MGH, and facilitated clinical research.

Second, four individuals at MGH established the RICU, or Respiratory Intensive Care Unit in 1961. Henrik Bendixen (later chair at UCSD and then Chair and Dean at Columbia) and Henning Pontoppidan (perennial Director of the RICU and later Jenney Professor at Harvard), had participated in the ventilation by hand (the anesthetist's hand squeezing the reservoir bag) of polio patients in the 1952 Copenhagen polio epidemic (see also chapters 43 and 44). Added to this pair, were Myron Laver (later professor at Harvard and University of Basel) and John Hedley-Whyte (A British anaesthetist who had taken a second anesthesia residency at MGH and who was later Sheridan Professor and Chief at Beth Israel Hospital in Boston). These physicians focused primarily on the nascent field of intensive care, and saw cardiac surgery/anesthesia as one aspect of that area.

When Richard Kitz became MGH Anesthetist-in-Chief, in early 1969, he assured Ed Lowenstein, (who had replaced Hedley-Whyte when Hedley-Whyte left to found the department at Beth Israel Hospital), that he could continue to concentrate on cardiovascular anesthesia if he stayed at MGH, rather than accept a position he had been offered elsewhere. The first formal cardiac anesthesia group (CAG) meeting was held before Kitz arrived on 31 July 1969, almost two decades after the initial steps. Tasks were assumed, challenges of the field discussed, and plans developed to address the challenges. Lowenstein was elected to head the group. He wrote: "Without realizing the implications, we had formed the first (1969) academic organization devoted exclusively to the anesthetic management for patients undergoing cardiac surgery" [70]. The first articles from the Group were published in 1971 in *Anesthesiology* [40] and the *New England Journal of Medicine* [71].

Emblematic of the CAG was its sense of mission and control of its destiny. There was pleasure working in a multidisciplinary environment with colleagues from cardiology, cardiac surgery, radiology and pathology who valued each others' opinions and contributions. This culture recurred in many CAGs formed subsequently at other institutions.

In these early days of cardiac anesthesia and surgery (truly frontiers at that time), the participants relished the excitement and challenge. Their common aspiration was to be "cardiac doctors" who understood the heart and circulatory system, and who collegially interacted within the entire spectrum constituting the cardiac surgical environment. Clinical and research excellence were equally respected. Laver, the intellectual leader at MGH, was a charismatic and fearless clinician who worked hardest and longest. He was recognized for his brilliance, but did not monopolize the glory. He jokingly said (personal communication), "I don't care who does the work as long as I get the credit." Indeed, each member believed that good work would be rewarded appropriately and resources seemed generous if not unlimited. There was a spirit of give and take among the surgeons and anesthesiologists, who often made observations about something in the other's realm that improved care, observations that were accepted with gratitude. Lowenstein characterized education of cardiac anesthesia fellows as the greatest contribution of the MGH to cardiac anesthesiology [70]. Through these fellows, MGH influenced cardiac anesthesiology development worldwide. Between 1972 and 1983, 50 fellows completed the program: 15 became professors, 12 led cardiac anesthesia groups (which they usually started), 12 became department chairs, and 3 became vice chairs.

The Emory Group

A second leading Division of Cardiothoracic Anesthesia was started at Emory University and initially directed in 1974 by Joel Kaplan, who had served his residency at the University of Pennsylvania, and served in the armed forces at Wilford Hall Air Force Hospital. Kaplan was an energetic leader who with his colleagues Carl Hug, John Waller, Jim Zaidan and later Jerrold Levy (the latter three, MGH trainees) developed a fellowship rivaling and larger than that at MGH. Approximately half of their trainees stayed in academic practice.

Kaplan organized and edited the "standard" textbook of cardiac anesthesia (now in its sixth edition). The first, 1979 edition, was entirely written by the Emory faculty, while subsequent editions have included national and international authors [72]. Kaplan and his colleagues published and popularized clinical measurements and interventions such as the use of the modified V lead for ischemia monitoring [73], and described the use of IV nitroglycerine for moment to moment control of myocardial ischemia [74]. While nitroglycerine had previously been administered intramuscularly by Viljoen at Cleveland Clinic, and sublingually by Lappas at MGH, IV administration added a degree of controllability that made it far more effective. This experience facilitated approval by the FDA. Kaplan became an active leader in cardiac anesthesia organizations, and in 1987, he founded the first journal devoted to cardiac anesthesiology, *The Journal of Cardiothoracic Anesthesia*.

Following Kaplan's move in 1984 to Mt. Sinai Hospital in New York, the Emory Division of Cardiothoracic anesthesia remained active in education, clinical work and scholarship. It was subsequently directed by Carl Hug, a Michigan trained pharmacist, pharmacologist, and anesthesiologist with particular expertise in opioids, and who has spent his entire career at Emory. He used minimal doses of morphine, avoided neuromuscular blockers in cardiac surgical patients, and would elicit patient responses intraoperatively including during cardiopulmonary bypass, much as Artusio had done using ether analgesia in patients undergoing mitral commisurotomy. He did much to elucidate the "ceiling effect" of opioids; no matter how large a dose is administered, break through responses to stimulation occur despite analgesia, differentiating it from true anesthesia [75]. Hug delighted in describing Boston (personal communication) as "the city where both ether and morphine were rediscovered," referring to the fact that ether anesthesia had been used by Crawford Long in Georgia years before it was publicly demonstrated at MGH.

The Duke University Group

The third cardiac anesthesia group we cite is at Duke, a group initiated by Jerry Reves (Fig. 61.5) and succeeded by his former trainee, Mark Newman. Reves spent two years at the US Naval Hospital in Bethesda, MD, where he and Bill Lell, the first MGH clinical fellow in cardiac anesthesia worked together "doing hearts." They performed but belatedly published an early randomized study comparing outcomes between two anesthetic regimens [38].

Pioneering cardiac surgeon, John Kirklin, had left Mayo Clinic and started an outstanding cardiac surgical program in the 1970s at the University of Alabama. After discharge from the Navy, Lell joined Kirklin as Chief of Cardiac Anesthesia. Reves followed, and in 1975 joined him and performed translational pharmacologic research, including introduction of the ultra short acting beta blocker esmolol, for control of heart rate during extreme surgical stimulation [76].

Most importantly however, Reves and the UAB group began investigations of the impact of cardiac surgery on cerebral blood flow and neurological function, with the object of making cardiopulmonary bypass and cardiac surgery safer for the brain [77]. Early cardiac surgeons and anesthesiologists had observed brain damage and attributed it to air emboli streaming to the brain because the inside of the heart had been exposed to the air. But with CABG, the inside of the heart was not exposed, and brain damage disappeared from the consciousness of cardiac surgeons and cardiac anesthesiologists (though not from the patients!). The UAB program resurrected this focus by beginning systematic examinations of the association between alterations in cerebral blood flow during surgery and changes in subsequent neurological function—work that Reves continued at Duke University, after moving there in 1984 to head cardiac anesthesia.

Research at Duke led by Reves and then by Mark Newman in the following decade, revealed several strategies that decreased the deleterious cerebral effects of cardiac surgery [78]. These included maintaining cerebral perfusion, minimizing cerebral embolization, temperature management, acid-base management, metabolic control (e.g. tight control of glucose), and advanced neurologic monitoring (e.g. near infared spectroscopy, EEG) [78].

However, despite these understandings, cognitive decline after CABG remains common as the age of surgical patients increases. Cognitive dysfunction is present in 40% of patients five years after surgery, according to careful prospective investigations by Newman and Reves [48]. Early postoperative neurocognitive decline is a strong predictor of late neurocognitve deteriorioation. This occurs at a greater rate than that following noncardiac surgery. Their work has been at the forefront of making the entire physician community aware of this devastating effect, and rekindling interest in avoiding it.

Subsequent investigations from the Duke group have continued to define hazards to cerebral function. A randomized study demonstrated that older patients were more susceptible to cognitive decline with profound hemodilution [79]. Current investigations are defining the role of genetic variants in post cardiac surgical cognitive decline. The tragedy of cognitive impairment in the face of improved heart function, gives particular importance to these investigations.

The Duke group adopted and investigated echocardiography in the early 1980s. Reves introduced a mandatory year of research in addition to a clinical year for all cardiac anesthesia fellows, a first in the US. This program produced a number of outstanding contributors, including Debbie Schwinn, now Dean at the University of Iowa School of Medicine. Mark Newman, who headed the cardiac anesthesia division after Reves, and succeeded him as Chairman of Anesthesiology, is an outstanding example of the success of this two year fellowship. The Cardiac Anesthesia Division at Duke appears to be the most productive in the US today, as defined by numbers of fellows educated each year, research publications, presentations at scientific meetings and external research funding.

Thus, in the 1970s and early 1980s, the field "took off" in America and around the world. Although many groups and individuals influenced the development of cardiac anesthesia during this period [5], we consider those in Table 61.1 most noteworthy.

Important Organizations and Institutional (Organizational) Developments

Validation of a specialty in medicine requires "academic homes" responsible for disseminating knowledge created by that specialty. Do scientific organizations, meetings, textbooks, journals, accredited educational programs, and certifications distinguish the specialty? For cardiac anesthesiology, the answer is indeed, yes.

The Association of Cardiac Anesthesiologists, the first professional organization of the subspecialty, formed in 1972 after a 1970 survey by Brian Dalton of the MGH, revealed that twelve centers in the United States performed more than 200 cardiac surgical cases per year and that a small number of anesthesiologists focused on that area [80]. First envisioned as a discussion group to promote interchanges and to encourage education and research, the membership was restricted to 50 members, with the intention of forming additional chapters when membership exceeded fifty. However, multiple chapters never developed, and the association continues as a small active group of self-selected authorities in cardiac anesthesia, with emeritus members such as your essayists.

The smallness of "the Association" indicated a need for a larger organization open to all who were interested in cardiac anesthesiology. In 1978, Robert Marino, George Burgess and Martin Peuler of the Oschner Clinic, founded the Society of Cardiovascular Anesthesia (SCA) in New Orleans. The organization grew rapidly, (Fig. 61.7) and membership now exceeds 7,000, reflecting national and international interest in the field [81]. The progressively richer annual scientific meetings and workshops have been fully subscribed from inception. They have covered cardiopulmonary bypass, coagulation issues, transesophageal echocardiography and more

The SCA initially sought joint publication with the *Journal of Thoracic and Cardiovascular Surgery* (JTCVS). However, after promising discussions, the editor in chief of JTCVS, John Kirklin, who had led the planning with the SCA, unexpectedly vetoed the plan. Determined not to create a new subspecialty journal, in 1994, the SCA agreed with the International Anesthesia Research Society to publish a cardiac anesthesiology "journal" within *Anesthesia and Analgesia*, one of the oldest English language anesthesia journals. In the inaugural issue of this joint publication, Editor-in-Chief, Ron Miller and Ed Lowenstein, Chair of the SCA Publications Committee wrote, "Principles elucidated by anesthesiologists concentrating their efforts in the care of patients with cardiovascular disease should be within the scientific province of all anesthesiologists" [82].

Prompted by SCA leaders, the National Board of Medical Examiners® approved Board certification in transesophageal echocardiography in 1998. An effort led by Alan Schwartz and Daniel Thys, to secure fellowship status for cardiothoracic anesthesia, saw success July 1, 2008, when the Accreditation Council for Graduate Medical Education approved accreditation. We hesitate to prophesize about accreditation of the subspeciality by the American Board of Anesthesiology, but others believe it should happen.

North American Emphasis of This Chapter

In this chapter, we have stressed the advancements originating in North America, almost to the exclusion of the rest of

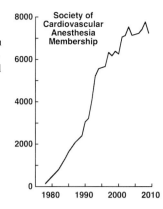

Fig. 61.7 Membership in the Society of Cardiovascular Anesthesia grew rapidly from its inception in 1976, recently stabilizing at approximately 7,000. (Data obtained from the Society by JGR.)

the world. As opposed to earlier advances in thoracic surgery and anesthesia, both cardiac surgery and cardiac anesthesia largely started in North America before spreading to other countries as distinct entities. In this respect, they represent a microcosm of scientific medicine including cardiac surgery and anesthesiology after World War II. The US emerged from the war as a singularly wealthy, powerful and ambitious nation, with leaders determined to grow the medical-scientific enterprise required to develop cardiac surgery. As British cardiac surgeon W P Cleland wrote in 1983 [83], "There seems little doubt that in the realm of cardiac surgery the United Kingdom has been a follower rather than a leader and it has been the United States that that has made most of the running. Undoubtedly, this is largely due to the greater efforts and money into research and development."

This is not to imply that there has been an absence of scientific effort regarding cardiovascular anesthesia in locations other than North America. For instance, Melrose in Great Britain had developed a pump oxygenator that was used in 1953 some months after Gibbon's initial use [84]. He also used potassium citrate to provide cardioplegia in 1955 [85]. Hans Sonntag of the University of Göttingen, was documenting the coronary blood flow response to anesthetics in human beings with and without coronary artery disease in the late 1970s [86]. Margaret Branthwaite in London, was studying filling pressures and differential function of the two sides of the heart after open heart surgery, as well as cerebral blood flow during, and neurologic complications after, open heart surgery [87, 88]. Beta adrenergic blockers were developed by Imperial Chemical Co in the UK, where Cedric Prys-Roberts and Pierre Foëx performed in the 1970s, the first studies documenting their effects upon the heart and myocardial ischemia during anesthetic induction [89].

In the 1980s, the number of anesthesiology articles from continental Europe and Asia to American anesthesiology journals increased progressively. Since then, anesthesiology, including cardiac anesthesiology has become truly international. In particular, a myriad of investigators from every continent have been active and productive in the influential multicenter observational studies of cardiac anesthesia performed by McSPI.

Why Did Cardiac Anesthesia Develop?

Three factors explain the development of this subspecialty. First, severe heart disease imposes special, perhaps unique, demands on the anesthesiologist, dictating a need for greater in-depth knowledge of these conditions than most generalist anesthesiologists possess. Cardiac anesthesiologists are cardiac doctors who are also anesthesiologists and manage patients with heart disease throughout the perioperative period. Quoting Myron Laver, in 1984 Keats wrote: "Anesthesiology is at its best when the observations it makes on the sample of patients we care for apply equally to all patients and contribute benefits to medicine at large" [21].

Second, the cardiac surgical environment presents unusual technological demands, including management of anticoagulation, knowledge of cardiac assist devices and pacemakers, and interpretation of measurements obtained from pulmonary artery catheters and of echocardiography images. The expertise demanded of the cardiac anesthesiologist exceeds that possessed by the generalist, requiring the constant use, reinforcement, experience and education obtained in the cardiac surgical environment. Does the technology focus of cardiac anesthesiology cause scholarly research in the field to suffer? As JGR asked: "Do we run trade schools or professional ones where all are imbued with, or at least honor, the thirst for new knowledge through true scholarship?" [90].

Third, successful cardiac surgery demands a collegial relationship among surgeons, cardiologists, perfusionists, nurses, intensivists, and of course anesthesiologists. O'Donnell and McDermott commented on the need for this team approach in 1955: "These are cases in which the affected specialties working as a harmonious team can contribute a great deal to the patient's welfare" [91], indeed to life or death. The cardiac anesthesiologist contributes crucially to this team, as noted in 1979 by Charles Hatcher, Jr., former chief of cardiac surgery at Emory: "A major factor, if not *the* major factor, in the current remarkably low operative mortality for open heart surgery has been the emergence of the cardiac anesthesiologist" [92]. Surgeon John Kirklin made a similar case nearly a decade later: "For the anesthesiologist to reach his or her potential and for the patient to receive the best care, the anesthesiologist should be a specialist in cardiovascular anesthesia and supportive treatment" [93].

Conclusion

This essay is primarily about the past. We recognize that "the future is important because we have to live and work in it, and it will be what we make of it" [94]. Nevertheless, there are individuals, who if not remembered now, will fade from memory even though their contributions have been responsible for the present and the future.

References

1. Litwak RS. The growth of cardiac surgery: historical notes. Cardiovasc Clin. 1971;3:5–50.
2. Paget S. Surgery of the chest. (pl 2.1). Bristol: John Wright & Co.; 1896.
3. Wynands JE. The contribution of Canadian anaesthetists to the evolution of cardiac surgery. Can J Anaesth. 1996;43:518–34.
4. Pender JW. Anesthesia for mitral commissurotomy. Anesthesiology. 1953;14:77–84.
5. Hessell EA. History of cardiac surgery and anesthesia. In: Barash PG, Estafanous FG, Reves JG, editors. Cardiac anesthesia principles and clinical practice. 2nd ed. Philadelphia: JB Lippincott Co; 2001. pp 1–35.
6. Mushin WW. Thoracic Anaesthesia. Philadelphia: FA Davis Co.; 1963.
7. Benumof JL. History of anesthesia for thoracic anesthesia. In: Anesthesia for thoracic surgery. Philadelphia: Saunders; 1987. pp 1–14.
8. Harmel MH, Lamont A. Anesthesia in the surgical treatment of congenital pulmonic stenosis. Anesthesiology. 1946;7:477–98.
9. Smithy HG, Boone JA, Stallworth JM. Surgical treatment of constrictive valvular disease of the heart. Surg Gynecol Obstet. 1950;90:175–92.
10. Bailey CP, Redondo Ramirez HP, Larzelere HB. Surgical treatment of aortic stenosis. J Am Med Assoc. 1952;150:1647–52.
11. Gay WA Jr, Ebert PA. Aorta-to-right pulmonary artery anastomosis causing obstruction of the right pulmonary artery. Management during correction of tetralogy of Fallot. Ann Thorac Surg. 1973;16:402–10.
12. Drew CE, Anderson IM. Profound hypothermia in cardiac surgery: report of three cases. Lancet. 1959;1:748–50.
13. Beck CS. New developments in surgery of the heart. Postgrad Med. 1947;1:421–3.
14. Glover RP, Davila JC, Kyle RH, Beard JC Jr, Trout RG, Kitchell JR. Ligation of the internal mammary arteries as a means of increasing blood supply to the myocardium. J Thorac Surg. 1957;34:661–78.
15. Dimond EG, Kittle CF, Crockett JE. Comparison of internal mammary artery ligation and sham operation for angina pectoris. Am J Cardiol. 1960;5:483–6.
16. Beecher HK. Surgery as placebo. A quantitative study of bias. JAMA. 1961;176:1102–7.
17. Vineberg A. Formation of a third coronary artery by internal mammary artery implant. Geriatrics. 1953;8:579–95.
18. Wynands JE, Sheridan CA, Kelkar K. Coronary artery disease and anaesthesia (experience in 120 patients for revascularization of the heart). Can J Anaesth. 1967;14:382–98.
19. Favaloro RG. Saphenous vein autograft replacement of severe segmental coronary artery occlusion: operative technique. J Thorac Surg. 1968;5:334–9.
20. Gibbon JH Jr. Application of a mechanical heart and lung apparatus to cardiac surgery. Minn Med. 1954;37:171–85.
21. Keats AS. The Rovenstine Lecture, 1983: cardiovascular anesthesia: perceptions and perspectives. Anesthesiology. 1984;60:467–74.
22. Ozinsky J. Cardiac transplantation–the anaesthetist's view: a case report. S Afr Med J. 1967;41:1268–70.
23. Keown KK, Grove D, Ruth HS. Anesthesia for commissurotomy for mitral setnosis; preliminary report. JAMA. 1951;146:446–50.
24. Artusio JF Jr. Ether analgesia during major surgery. J Am Med Assoc. 1955;157:33–6.
25. Patrick RT, Theye RA, Moffitt EA. Studies in extracorporeal circulation. V. Anesthesia and supportive care during intracardiac surgery with the Gibbon-type pump-oxygenator. Anesthesiology. 1957;18:673–85.
26. Civetta JM, Gabel JC. Flow directed-pulmonary artery catheterization in surgical patients: indications and modifications of technic. Ann Surg. 1972;176:753–6.

27. Lappas D, Lell WA, Gabel JC, Civetta JM. Lowenstein E. Indirect measurement of left-atrial pressure in surgical patients–pulmonary-capillary wedge and pulmonary-artery diastolic pressures compared with left-atrial pressure. Anesthesiology. 1973;38:394–7.

28. Bashein G, Ivey TD. Con: a pulmonary artery catheter is not indicated for all coronary artery surgery. J Cardiothorac Anesth. 1987;1:362–5.

29. Weintraub AC, Barash PG. Pro: a pulmonary artery catheter is indicated in all patients for coronary artery surgery. J Cardiothorac Anesth. 1987;1:358–61.

30. Matsumoto M, Oka Y, Strom J, Frishman W, Kadish A, Becker RM, Frater RW, Sonnenblick EH. Application of transesophageal echocardiography to continuous intraoperative monitoring of left ventricular performance. Am J Cardiol. 1980;46:95–105.

31. Cahalan MK, Kremer P, Schiller NB, et al. Intraoperative monitoring with two dimendional transesophageal echocardiography. Anesthesiology. 1982;57:A152.

32. de Bruijn NP, Clements FM, Kisslo JA. Intraoperative transesophageal color flow mapping: initial experience. Anesth Analg. 1987;66:386–90.

33. Kwak J, Andrawes M, Garvin S, D'Ambra MN. 3D transesophageal echocardiography: a review of recent literature 2007–2009. Curr Opi Anaesthesiol. 2010;23:80–8.

34. Raja SN, Lowenstein E. The birth of opioid anesthesia. Anesthesiology. 2004;100:1013–5.

35. Vasko JS, Henney RP, Brawley RK, Oldham HN, Morrow AG. Effects of morphine on ventricular function and myocardial contractile force. Am J Physiol. 1966;210:329–34.

36. Lowenstein E, Hallowell P, Levine FH, Daggett WM, Austen WG, Laver MB. Cardiovascular response to large doses of intravenous morphine in man. N Engl J Med. 1969;281:1389–93.

37. Conahan TJ 3rd, Ominsky AJ, Wollman H, Stroh RA. A prospective random comparison of halothane and morphine for open-heart anesthesia: one year's experience. Anesthesiology. 1973;38:528–35.

38. Reves JG, Lell WA, McCracken LE Jr, Kravetz RA, Prough DS. Comparison of morphine and ketamine anesthetic technics for coronary surgery: a randomized study. South Med J. 1978;71:33–6.

39. Stanley TH, Webster LR. Anesthetic requirements and cardiovascular effects of fentanyl-oxygen and fentanyl-diazepam-oxygen anesthesia in man. Anesth Analg. 1978;57:411–6.

40. Lowenstein E. Morphine "anesthesia"–a perspective. Anesthesiology. 1971;35:563–5.

41. Philbin DM, Rosow CE, Schneider RC, Koski G, D'Ambra MN. Fentanyl and sufentanil anesthesia revisited: how much is enough? Anesthesiology. 1990;73:5–11.

42. Pollard RJ, Coyle JP, Gilbert RL, Beck JE. Intraoperative awareness in a regional medical system: a review of 3 years' data. Anesthesiology. 2007;106:269–74.

43. Tuman K, McCarthy R, Spiess B, DaValle M, Dabir R, Ivankovich A. Does choice of anesthetic agent significantly affect outcome after coronary artery surgery? Anesthesiology. 1989;70:189–98.

44. Slogoff S, Keats AS. Does perioperative myocardial ischemia lead to postoperative myocardial infarction? Anesthesiology. 1985;62:107–14.

45. Reves JG, Sladen RN, Newman MF. Cardiac anesthetic: is it unique? Anesth Analg. 1995;81:895–6.

46. Slogoff S, Keats A. Randomized trial of primary anesthetic agents on outcome of coronary artery bypass operations. Anesthesiology. 1989;70:179–88.

47. Warltier DC, al-Wathiqui MH, Kampine JP, Schmeling WT. Recovery of contractile function of stunned myocardium in chronically instrumented dogs is enhanced by halothane or isoflurane. Anesthesiology. 1988;69:552–65.

48. Newman MF, Croughwell ND, Blumenthal JA, White WD, Lewis JB, Smith LR, Frasco P, Towner EA, Schell RM, Hurwitz BJ, et al. Effect of aging on cerebral autoregulation during cardiopulmonary bypass. Association with postoperative cognitive dysfunction. Circulation. 1994;90:II243–9.

49. Viljoen JF. Anaesthesia for internal mammary implant surgery. Anaesthesia. 1968;23:515–20.

50. Sellke FW, DiMaio JM, Caplan LR, Ferguson TB, Gardner TJ, Hiratzka LF, Isselbacher EM, Lytle BW, Mack MJ, Murkin JM, Robbins RC. Comparing on-pump and off-pump coronary artery bypass grafting: numerous studies but few conclusions: a scientific statement from the American Heart Association council on cardiovascular surgery and anesthesia in collaboration with the interdisciplinary working group on quality of care and outcomes research. Circulation. 2005;111:2858–64.

51. Keown KK. Anesthesia for surgery of the heart. Springfield: Thomas; 1956.

52. Theye RA, Patrick RT, Kirklin JW. The electro-encephalogram in patients undergoing open intracardiac operations with the aid of extracorporeal circulation. J Thorac Surg. 1957;34:709–17.

53. Theye RA, Moffitt EA, Kirklin JW. Anesthetic management during open intracardiac surgery. Anesthesiology. 1962;23:823–7.

54. Moffitt EA, Theye RA. Management of anaesthesia, perfusion and supportive care during open intracardiac operations and extracorporeal circulation. Br J Anaesth. 1959;31:411–6.

55. Smith RR. Anesthesia for infants and children. St. Louis: Mosby; 1959.

56. Galvin S, Dewan J, Rockoff MA. Betty Lank: a kind and gentle anesthetist devoted to children. AANA journal. 2009;77:176–80.

57. Slogoff S, Keats AS, Ott E. Preoperative propranolol therapy and aortocoronary bypass operation. JAMA. 1978;240:1487–90.

58. Slogoff S, Keats AS, Dear WE, Abadia A, Lawyer JT, Moulds JP, Williams TM. Steal-prone coronary anatomy and myocardial ischemia associated with four primary anesthetic agents in humans. Anesth Analg. 1991;72:22–7.

59. Becker L. Is isoflurane dangerous for the patient with coronary artery disease. Anesthesiology. 1987;66:259–61.

60. Mangano DT, Browner WS, Hollenberg M, London MJ, Tubau JF, Tateo IM. Association of perioperative myocardial ischemia with cardiac morbidity and mortality in men undergoing noncardiac surgery. The Study of Perioperative Ischemia Research Group. N Engl J Med. 1990;323:1781–8.

61. Mangano DT, Layug EL, Wallace A, Tateo I. Effect of atenolol on mortality and cardiovascular morbidity after noncardiac surgery. Multicenter Study of Perioperative Ischemia Research Group. N Engl J Med. 1996;335:1713–20.

62. Fleisher LA, Beckman JA, Brown KA, Calkins H, Chaikof EL, Fleischmann KE, Freeman WK, Froehlich JB, Kasper EK, Kersten JR, Riegel B, Robb JF, Smith SC Jr, Jacobs AK, Adams CD, Anderson JL, Antman EM, Buller CE, Creager MA, Ettinger SM, Faxon DP, Fuster V, Halperin JL, Hiratzka LF, Hunt SA, Lytle BW, Nishimura R, Ornato JP, Page RL, Tarkington LG, Yancy CW. ACC/AHA 2007 guidelines on perioperative cardiovascular evaluation and care for noncardiac surgery: a report of the American College of Cardiology/American Heart Association Task Force on Practice Guidelines (Writing Committee to Revise the 2002 Guidelines on Perioperative Cardiovascular Evaluation for Noncardiac Surgery) developed in collaboration with the American Society of Echocardiography, American Society of Nuclear Cardiology, Heart Rhythm Society, Society of Cardiovascular Anesthesiologists, Society for Cardiovascular Angiography and Interventions, Society for Vascular Medicine and Biology, and Society for Vascular Surgery. J Am Coll Cardiol. 2007;50:e159–241.

63. Mangano DT. Aspirin and mortality from coronary bypass surgery. N Engl J Med. 2002;347:1309–17.

64. Topol EJ. Aspirin with bypass surgery–from taboo to new standard of care. N Engl J Med. 2002;347:1359–60.

65. Vlahakes GJ. The value of phase 4 clinical testing. N Engl J Med. 2006;354:413–5.

66. Mangano DT, Tudor IC, Dietzel C. The risk associated with aprotinin in cardiac surgery. N Engl J Med. 2006;354:353–65.

67. Randomised trial of intravenous atenolol among 16 027 cases of suspected acute myocardial infarction: ISIS-1. First International Study of Infarct Survival Collaborative Group. Lancet. 1986;2:57–66.

68. Devereaux PJ, Yang H, Yusuf S, Guyatt G, Leslie K, Villar JC, Xavier D, Chrolavicius S, Greenspan L, Pogue J, Pais P, Liu L, Xu S, Malaga G, Avezum A, Chan M, Montori VM, Jacka M, Choi P. Effects of extended-release metoprolol succinate in patients undergoing non-cardiac surgery (POISE trial): a randomised controlled trial. Lancet. 2008;371:1839–47.

69. Brewster WR Jr, Isaacs JP, Waino-Andersen T. Depressant effect of ether on myocardium of the dog and its modification by reflex release of epinephrine and nor-epinephrine. Am J Physiol. 1953;175:399–414.

70. Lowenstein E. A journey of the heart: cardiac anesthesia. In: Kitz Richard J, editor. "This is no humbug!" Reminiscences of the Department of Anesthesia at the Massachusetts General Hospital. A History. Boston: Massachusetts General Hospital; 2003. pp. 269–330.

71. Lowenstein E, Little JW 3rd, Lo HH. Prevention of cerebral embolization from flushing radial-artery cannulas. N Engl J Med. 1971;285:1414–5.

72. Kaplan JA. Cardiac anesthesia. Philadelphia: Saunders; 1979.

73. Kaplan JA, King SB 3rd. The precordial electrocardiographic lead (V5) in patients who have coronary-artery disease. Anesthesiology. 1976;45:570–4.

74. Kaplan JA, Dunbar RW, Jones EL. Nitroglycerin infusion during coronary-artery surgery. Anesthesiology. 1976;45:14–21.

75. Murphy MR, Hug CC Jr. The anesthetic potency of fentanyl in terms of its reduction of enflurane MAC. Anesthesiology. 1982;57:485–8.

76. Menkhaus PG, Reves JG, Kissin I, Alvis JM, Govier AV, Samuelson PN, Lell WA, Henling CE, Bradley E. Cardiovascular effects of esmolol in anesthetized humans. Anesth Analg. 1985;64:327–34.

77. Govier AV, Reves JG, McKay RD, Karp RB, Zorn GL, Morawetz RB, Smith LR, Adams M, Freeman AM. Factors and their influence on regional cerebral blood flow during nonpulsatile cardiopulmonary bypass. Ann Thorac Surg. 1984;38:592–600.

78. Arrowsmith JE, Grocott HP, Reves JG, Newman MF. Central nervous system complications of cardiac surgery. Br J Anaesth. 2000;84:378–93.

79. Mathew JP, Mackensen GB, Phillips-Bute B, Stafford-Smith M, Podgoreanu MV, Grocott HP, Hill SE, Smith PK, Blumenthal JA, Reves JG, Newman MF. Effects of extreme hemodilution during cardiac surgery on cognitive function in the elderly. Anesthesiology. 2007;107:577–84.

80. Dalton B. Anesthesia for cardiac surgery. Anesthesiology. 1972;36:521–2.

81. Thys DM. Cardiac anesthesia: thirty years later–the second annual Arthur E. Weyman lecture. Anesth Analg. 2009;109:1782–90.

82. Lowenstein E, Miller RD. The International Anesthesia Research Society and the Society of Cardiovascular Anesthesiologists: a new partnership. Anesth Analg. 1994;78:1–2.

83. Cleland WP. The evolution of cardiac surgery in the United Kingdom. Thorax. 1983;38:887–96.

84. Melrose DG. A mechanical heart-lung for use in man. Br Med J. 1953;2:57–62.

85. Melrose DG, Dreyer B, Bentall HH, Baker JB. Elective cardiac arrest. Lancet. 1955;269:21–2.

86. Sonntag H. Actions of anesthetics on the coronary circulation in normal subjects and patients with ischemic heart disease. Int Anesthesiol Clin. 1980;18:111–35.

87. Jenkins BS. Branthwaite MA. Bradley RD Cardiac function after open heart surgery. Relation between the performance of the two sides of the heart. Cardiovasc Res. 1973;7:297–305.

88. Branthwaite MA. Detection of neurological damage during open-heart surgery. Thorax. 1973;8:464–72.

89. Prys-Roberts C. Foex P. Biro GP. Roberts JG. Studies of anaesthesia in relation to hypertension. V. Adrenergic beta-receptor blockade. Br J Anaesth. 1973;45:671–81.

90. Reves JG. We are what we make: transforming research in anesthesiology: the 45th Rovenstine Lecture. Anesthesiology. 2007;106:826–35.

91. O'Donnell JA, McDermott TF. Anesthetic problems of surgical correction of aortic insufficiency. Anesthesiology. 1955;16:343–54.

92. Hatcher CR. A cardiac surgeon's view of cardiac anesthesia. In: Kaplan JA. Cardiac anesthesia. Philadelphia: Saunders; 1979. pp xi–xii.

93. Kirklin JW, Barratt-Boyes BG. The Operating Room Team. In: Kirklin JW, Barratt-Boyes BG, editors. Cardiac surgery. New York: Wiley, 1986. p. 61.

94. Reves JG. The future of cardiac anesthesiology: personal observations and prognostications. innovations in cardiovascular care (DVD). In: Cook DJ, editor. Society of cardiovascular anesthesiologist monograph. Philadelphia: Lippincott Williams & Wilkins; 2006. p. 13.

A History of Pain Relief During Childbirth

62

William Camann

Summary

Women's quest to relieve the pain of childbirth is timeless. A few religious leaders opposed the relief of childbirth pain, but most clergy did not, nor did lay people. In 1847, Fanny Longfellow, the poet's wife, received ether to aid in delivery. In 1853, Queen Victoria chose chloroform to relieve labor pain during the birth of Prince Leopold, ending any moral opposition to pain relief during childbirth. In 1956, Pope Pius XII approved pain relief during childbirth.

US and British movements advanced obstetric anesthesia from the early 1900s to the present. Women lobbied to assure pain relief during labor and sought greater control over delivery. The medical establishment haltingly increased anesthetic availability. In 1914, some US women organized the National Twilight Sleep Association, bringing this popular European technique to the US. But when one of its prominent advocates died during childbirth in 1915 while using twilight sleep, the Association came to an end. Some use of twilight sleep persisted in the US until the 1960s. In the 1920s, one in two hundred British women died during childbirth. In 1928, British women formed the National Birthday Trust Fund to decrease mortality, and make modern pain relief during childbirth available.

In the 1940s, Hershenson established the first "Division of Obstetric Anesthesia" in the US at the Boston Lying-In Hospital. In 1953, Apgar invented her simple "score", "the Apgar", which defines the condition of all of today's new babies, and correlates with their immediate outcome. In 1968, 6 physicians formed the Society for Obstetric Anesthesia and Perinatology (SOAP), the primary advocate for the world-wide interests of obstetric anesthesia. It now boasts more than 1000 members world-wide.

In the first half of the twentieth century, some mothers and physicians (e.g., Dick-Read, the father of the modern natural childbirth movement) sought a natural birth experience. In the late 1940s, Bradley included the husband as an active *participant* in the birth process. In the 1980s and 1990s, women increasingly demanded a pain-free childbirth, replacing the generation seeking natural childbirth. The percentage of mothers given spinal or epidural analgesia during childbirth tripled to 66% or greater. Infusions of low concentrations of local anesthetics, use of the local-anesthetic sparing properties of epidural opioids, and the advent of patient-controlled techniques, collectively increased safety and efficacy, and hence popularity, of epidural analgesia.

In the 2000s, approaches to obstetric anesthesia increasingly combined regional anesthesia with "alternative" medicine. Women requesting epidural analgesia tried hypnosis, water immersion, aromatherapy, birth balls (big plastic balls similar to those used in exercise training), upright posture during labor and birth, acupuncture, and doulas (trained birthing coaches). The attitude that epidural analgesia is at least compatible with, perhaps synergistic with, various non-medical techniques contributed to the popularity of a blended approach.

Introduction

"Medical men may oppose for a time the use of anaesthesia during childbirth, but they will oppose it in vain; for certainly our patients themselves will force use of it upon the professions. The whole question is, even now, one merely of time."—James Young Simpson, who in 1847 became the first physician to use anesthesia during childbirth [1].

W. Camann (✉)
Department of Anesthesiology, Brigham and Women's Hospital,
75 Francis Street, Boston, MA 02115, USA
e-mail: wcamann@partners.org

Childbirth literature sometimes suggests, incorrectly, that women's quest for labor pain relief is a modern phenomenon. *"Women have been giving birth for centuries without the benefit of modern pain relief"* has been argued. What isn't stated as often, is that women in almost every culture and at every time have sought effective *relief for* pain during childbirth.

But why should a natural event, childbirth, be painful? Does pain confer a survival benefit; is it protective—and therefore should it be welcomed? Have the anatomic characteristics of evolution conferred pain during labor upon humans (creatures with big heads) in ways not seen in other animals? Or is pain an unnatural development of the human intellect, a fearful response to the birthing process? These issues remain unsettled. Regardless of the origin of pain during labor, regardless of any advantage it may confer, women's quest to relieve the pain of childbirth is timeless. Some methods used for centuries were innovative, some were quaint, some hazardous, and some were odd. This chapter will discuss the attitudes towards pain relief during childbirth at different points throughout history.

Pain Relief *Before* Anesthesia's Discovery: Including the Odd and Unusual

Anesthesia began 16 October 1846, with the public demonstration of ether given to a patient undergoing surgery, at Massachusetts General Hospital, in Boston. How did women lessen the pain of childbirth before this discovery? The ancient civilizations of Babylon, Egypt, China and Palestine tried to relieve labor pain [2]. They applied positive thinking, using magical rings, necklaces, and charms. These may have diminished the *anticipation* of pain, rather than help with the *actual* pain during delivery; and they may have supplied a placebo effect. In ancient cultures, laboring women inhaled concoctions made of poppy extract and hemp (perhaps not so unusual, as opioids remain the most commonly used labor analgesic medication), drank herbal tea mixtures or a beverage sprinkled with powdered sow's dung, sometimes mixed with honey wine [3]. Such primitive methods, methods that distracted women's attention from labor pain, paralleled some modern methods, such as hypnosis, warm compresses, massage and herbal teas.

Donald Caton (1937), an academic historian on obstetric anesthesiology, described an early version of the warm compress and massage during labor.

> "One of the earliest references to the management of childbirth pain appeared in a gynecologic text written in the first century CE, by a Greek physician. He suggested that physicians should 'soothe the pains by touching with warm hands and afterwards drench pieces of cloth with warm, sweet olive oil and put them over the abdomen as well as the labia and keep them saturated with the warm oil for some time, and one must also place bladders (containers) filled with warm oil along side.'"

Caton described the pain relief potions recommended by a Puritan Minister well-versed in medicine, Cotton Mather (1663–1728), who advised women to use potions such as the 'livers and galls of eels, dried slowly in an oven,' or 'date, stone, amber and cumin seeds' [4].

Mesmeric Pain Relief (Hypnosis)

In 1836, a decade before the introduction of anesthesia, a French physician and hypnotist, Grubert, suggested

that "magnetic sleep" (a euphemism for hypnosis), might provide labor pain relief [5]. Hypnosis had been tried for surgery, with mixed results, and it did not gain immediate popularity for use during childbirth. A decade later, however, two successful cases of pain relief through the use of hypnosis were recorded. William Fahnestock (ca. 1880) of Lancaster, Pennsylvania, reported the American case, but his report did not stimulate widespread application, possibly because of the therapy's ineffectiveness. Today, such techniques have some popularity, and are often taught in modern childbirth classes, under monikers such as "hypnobabies" or "hypnobirthing".

Blood Letting (Leeches)

In the early nineteenth century, American physician Benjamin Rush (1745–1813), a statesman who signed the Declaration of Independence, recommended the use of leeches to remove three or more pints of blood a day to minimize labor pain. He reasoned that the pain of childbirth could stimulate the woman's central nervous system, and thereby cause harm. Bloodletting, he proposed, would depress the mother's nervous system and avoid the danger. Although absurd in light of today's knowledge, this technique followed the then popular use of bloodletting for treatment of a variety of medical conditions.

Attitudes Toward the Introduction of Pain Relief During Childbirth

Long before the introduction of anesthesia during labor, and for some time after, religion affected the experience of childbirth. A few religious leaders, men who strongly influenced society's laws and social mores, opposed the relief of childbirth pain. They argued that pain was God's punishment to Eve and her descendants (all women) for having disobeyed Him in the Garden of Eden; Genesis 3:16, "*I will greatly multiply thy sorrow and thy conception; in sorrow thou shalt bring forth children.*" To avoid the pain of childbirth was to disobey the will of God. In Germany, in 1521, a physician dressed in women's clothes (men were not allowed to participate in childbirth care at that time) entered the labor room of a woman to provide pain relief. He was discovered and burned at the stake for his offense [6]. It is oft-cited in medical historical literature that the religious objections to pain relief in labor were widely implicated. Simpson did indeed publish a pamphlet answering religious objections to the use of pain relief during childbirth, but there is little evidence that this was a serious concern among clergy or the populace at large [7, 8].

Physicians used opium for centuries for pain relief, and morphine was discovered in the early 1800s, but neither was given to women during childbirth, in part probably because physicians correctly surmised that such drugs might pose risks to both the mother and infant. In addition to questionable historical religious attitudes against the use of pain relief in childbirth, some physicians believed that the pain of childbirth was a natural phenomenon, not requiring intervention. The interpretation of labor pain as God's punishment has been challenged in modern times, and most modern religious leaders do not see pain relief during childbirth as contradicting God's will. In a major address in 1956, Pope Pius XII (1876–1958) gave approval for pain relief during childbirth. John Bonica (1917–1994), the father of modern pain management, assisted in the preparation of this address, (more to follow on Bonica). Modern interpretation by biblical scholars of the Genesis passage 3:16 translates the words concerning childbirth to mean women will bring forth children "in toil or labor," signifying hard work, rather than pain [9].

Anesthesia, a Blessing for Humankind, Emerges: A Brief Timeline

The 1846 demonstration of anesthesia enabled the painless performance of surgical procedures. Today we take anesthesia for granted, but for thousands of years, surgery and other painful medical interventions caused agony in fully aware, conscious patients—although it is possible that many were less than conscious because they had been given alcohol or other mind-altering potions. The discovery of anesthesia profoundly benefited surgical patients and laboring women.

In 1847, four months after the first successful demonstration of anesthesia for surgery, James Simpson, (1811–1870; Fig. 62.1) a Scottish obstetrician, used ether to successfully relieve the pain of childbirth for a woman with a deformed pelvis. Subsequently, he devoted his career to the advancement of anesthesia used during childbirth, increasing the number of pain relief substances by his discovery of the anesthetic properties of chloroform, improving techniques of the day, and enhancing the birth experience of women throughout Europe and the US. Simpson was created a Baronet in 1866, by Queen Victoria [4].

The First Women to Benefit from Anesthesia: The Royal and the Wealthy

In 1853, Queen Victoria's use of chloroform to relieve her labor pain during the birth of her eighth child, Prince Leopold, ended any lingering moral opposition to the relief of pain during childbirth. She also received chloroform in 1857 for the birth of her ninth child, Princess Beatrice. It is reported by the Queen's biographer, Elisabeth Longford, that she wrote in her diary after the delivery of Prince Leopold: "Dr. Snow gave the blessed chloroform and the effect was soothing, quieting and delightful beyond measure."

Those fortunate enough to find a physician willing to provide chloroform or ether soon followed the Queen's example. Women with political and economic power began to challenge the medical establishment, demanding pain relief during childbirth in particular, and better maternal and infant care for all women.

In England there was a literary connection [10]:

> "Mrs. Charles Dickens was expecting her eighth child in 1849. Her husband first 'made himself thoroughly acquainted in Edinburgh with the facts of chloroform', and then (as described in a letter to a friend) he insisted on the attendance of a gentleman from Bart's Hospital who administers it in the operations there and has given it four or five thousand times. It saved her all pain (she had no sensation, but of a great display of sky-rockets) and saved the child from all mutilation. It enabled the doctors to do in ten minutes what might otherwise have taken them one and a half hours; the shock to her nervous system was reduced to nothing, and she was to all intents and purposes well, next day. Administered by someone who has nothing else to do, who knows its symptoms thoroughly, who keeps his hand upon the pulse and his eyes upon the face, and uses nothing but a handkerchief, and that lightly, I am convinced that it is as safe in its administration as it is miraculous in its effects."

Obviously, the anesthetist from Bart's (St. Bartholomew's) was John Snow.

> *"I feel proud to be the pioneer to less suffering. This is certainly the greatest blessing of this age and I am glad to have lived at the time of its coming…" Fanny Appleton Longfellow.* 1847, Cambridge Massachusetts [11]

The first American woman to use analgesia during childbirth was Fanny Appleton Longfellow (1817–1861), wife of the famous poet and scholar, Henry Wadsworth Longfellow [12]. For aid in her third delivery, Fanny Longfellow sought out a prominent physician, Nathan Keep (1800–1875), who had experience in the use of ether, and became the Dean of Dentistry at Harvard [11]. In 1847, while under the influence of ether, Fanny Longfellow gave birth to a little girl (also named Fanny) in Cambridge, Massachusetts, and enthusiastically endorsed the use of this new pain relieving substance (see box). Boston, Massachusetts continued to pioneer American obstetric anesthesia; a colleague of Keep's, Walter Channing (1786–1876), gained great popularity with his use of ether to relieve childbirth pains (Fig. 62.2). Channing was from an aristocratic New England family [13]. His

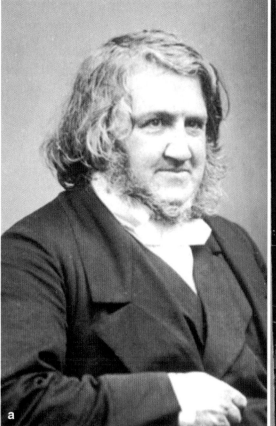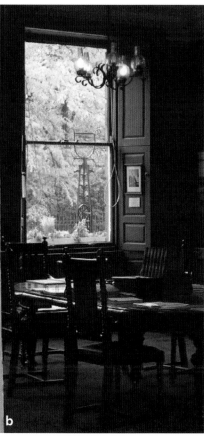

Fig. 62.1 a Scottish obstetrician James Young Simpson was the first to use inhalation anesthesia (ether) for labor pain relief. Shortly thereafter he discovered the anesthetizing capacity of chloroform and applied it, too, for labor pain relief. (Courtesy of http://commons.wikimedia.org/wiki/File:Princes_St_Gardens_James_Young_Simpson.jpg) **b** Dining room of the home of James Young Simpson, in Edinburgh, Scotland, where the initial experiments with anesthetic and euphoric properties of chloroform were noted by Simpson and his friends. (Courtesy of the author)

brother, William Ellery Channing (1780–1842), founded the Unitarian Church, and his grandfather, William Ellery (1727–1820), was a Supreme Court Judge of Rhode Island and a signatory of the Declaration of Independence. Not all these fellows were upright citizens. Harvard College expelled Walter for his participation in a notorious food fight, known as the "Rotten Cabbage Rebellion of 1807", a student-led protest concerning the poor quality of the food served in the dormitories. Harvard College has a long tradition of student-led revolts, and a tree, planted in the late 1700s, at the East end of Hollis Hall, is known as the "Rebellion Elm" (protests often centered around this tree).

After finishing his medical education at the University of Pennsylvania in 1812, Walter Channing returned to Harvard Medical School to become Professor of Obstetrics and Medical Jurisprudence, and then the first Dean of the Medical School, (1816–1847). In 1832, he assisted with the founding of the Boston Lying-In Hospital, a forerunner of today's Brigham & Women's Hospital. Channing detailed his extensive experience with ether during childbirth, in his 1848 book entitled "*A Treatise on Etherization in Childbirth*" [11]. Note that Channing and Keep, the first Deans of both Harvard Medical School and Harvard Dental School respectively (although the term was not used until years later) were anesthesiologists, largely remembered for their work in obstetric pain relief. They reflect the strong tradition of prominent physician practice of pharmacological means of pain relief.

Obstetric Anesthesia From the Start of the Twentieth Century to the Present

Two interconnected threads led to the advancement of obstetric anesthesia from the beginning of the twentieth century to the present. First was the movement to assure pain relief during labor, a movement that took several forms. Some approaches had pain prevention as the immediate goal; others acted as a distraction. Pain prevention included administration of opioids; administration of inhaled anesthetics, particularly ether, chloroform and nitrous oxide, but also ethylene, trichloroethylene, methoxyflurane, and cyclopropane; and finally (and dominant today), administration of epidural analgesia. The application of epidural analgesia required development of methods of anesthetic delivery that provided analgesia with minimal interference in the progress of birth. Second was the movement to give women greater control over their participation in the delivery experience. It increased participation of the father in the birth process.

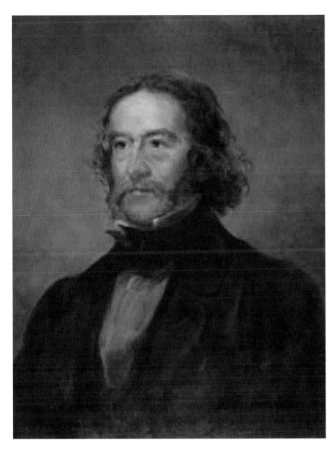

Fig. 62.2 Walter Channing, American professor of midwifery and sometime Dean at Harvard was an early advocate of ether inhalation for labor pain relief. He assisted in the founding of the Boston Lying-In Hospital. (Courtesy of Brigham and Women's Hospital, Boston)

Women's Struggle for Pain Relief During Childbirth in the Early 1900s

In the US and Britain, shortly after the discovery of anesthesia, the quest for pain relief during childbirth became aligned with women's advocacy for the advancement of their own political and economic power. This included demands for better health care for themselves and their children, improved maternal and child health, and a less painful birth experience. Because of the absence of medical birth control, women had many children and spent much of their adulthood pregnant.

Well into the early 1900s, childbirth remained dangerous for women throughout the world, even in medically advanced countries. Physicians contributed to the high mortality rate of women and infants by not washing their hands after examining and treating patients, particularly after conducting autopsies on patients dying from infection. They thereby facilitated the spread of the infectious disease also known as "puerperal", or "childbed" fever. Ignaz Semmelweis (1818–1865), a Hungarian physician, noted in 1847 that far fewer women died from puerperal fever in midwife-led

wards (where no autopsies where performed), than in physician-led wards. His observation preceded the germ theory of infectious disease, and was thus without explanation. Semmelweis' simple admonition to wash the hands offended contemporary physicians (doctors were considered clean, not "dirty"), who ridiculed him. However, even before the advancement of the germ theory, physicians eventually recognized that they might spread infections from one patient to another, and increasingly washed their hands. The number of women dying from infection markedly decreased. Years later, when Pasteur's and Lister's studies explained these results, Semmelweis was given full credit for his insightful observations. As an aside, the Semmelweis Reflex is a rejection of a new idea that confronts what may be thought of as "conventional wisdom" in this case that doctors were considered clean and thus not possibly a source of disease.

Women's rights leaders in the US and Britain fought for a more humane birth experience for all women, not just the wealthy few. During the mid to late 1800s, and well into the early 1900s, only wealthy and well-connected women could benefit from the new "miracle" of a pain-free birth. Several organizations (see below) sought to remedy this social injustice.

> *"One of the most cruel class divisions yet remaining in this country is that rich mothers need not suffer in childbirth as though we were still in the Stone Age, while poorer ones far too often do."* A letter from a British writer, which appeared in the publication, *"The Lady,"* in 1942 [14].

The slowness of the medical establishment to make anesthesia widely available during childbirth frustrated early feminists who championed improved healthcare for all women and children. Some physicians believed that the risks to the mother and infant outweighed the benefits of pain relief, fearing, with good cause, that anesthesia could produce unintended side effects on both mother and newborn. Moreover, some physicians believed that pain was a natural part of the birth process. For example, a noted Russian surgeon who performed the first thyroid surgery under ether anesthesia, Nicolai Pirigoff, (1810–1881) claimed: "Haven't midwives and parturients and indeed all others always viewed the agonies of delivery as an indicator of safety and a well-nigh holy accompaniment of childbirth?" [4] Charles Meigs (1792–1869), one of the most prominent American physicians of the nineteenth century, an outspoken opponent of pain relief in childbirth, and noted for making inflammatory social and cultural comments, pointed out that the "pain of labor had never been great enough to prevent women from having more children" [4]. Several political organizations consequently arose to overcome physician resistance toward the use of anesthesia during childbirth.

> In the early 1900s, American journalists, Marguerite Tracy and Constance Leupp, wrote that the success of the campaign undertaken by women urging physicians to rid women of labor pain would, *"relieve one-half of humanity from its antique burden of suffering which the other half of humanity has never understood."*[4]

The National Twilight Sleep Association

In 1914, several wealthy and politically influential US women formed an organization that sought to bring to all women in the US, a new pain relief technique, reportedly used with success in Europe in the first decade of the twentieth century. The Twilight Sleep method of pain relief combined morphine and scopolamine. Morphine dulled the pain and scopolamine produced memory loss, but had the unintended side effect of lowering women's inhibitions. Laboring women given "twilight sleep" might exhibit bizarre and uncontrolled behavior. The small amount of morphine used was often ineffective against the pain, and women might thrash and scream wildly. ("As an intern, I well recall ordering an intramuscular injection of 10 mg morphine and 0.6 mg scopolamine for a laboring woman who later bit me as I tried to restrain her from climbing over the side rails and who later described the entire experience as absolutely without any discomfort—for her but not me!" *Personal communication, Lawrence J. Saidman*). Unaware of the pain they endured due to the amnesia produced by scopolamine, women often reported a pain free birth experience.

The women who formed the National Twilight Sleep Association successfully campaigned for the use of this technique during childbirth [4]. They held rallies and inspired women to demand that the medical establishment provide twilight sleep—or some form of pain relief—for all laboring women. Their well-organized, well-funded efforts had one critical flaw: twilight sleep did *not consistently* provide adequate pain relief although the scopolamine usually (not always) erased the memory of labor pain. Physicians often put cotton and oil in patient's ears, and blindfolded them to reduce perception of stimuli, but of course the bigger stimulus was that of labor. Often women were restrained to prevent harm to themselves or others. Of note, the husbands were sequestered in waiting rooms, unaware of all this activity. When one of its most prominent and outspoken advocates (Mrs. Francis X Carmody) died during childbirth in 1915, after receiving this method of pain relief, the National Twilight Sleep Association came to an end. Although

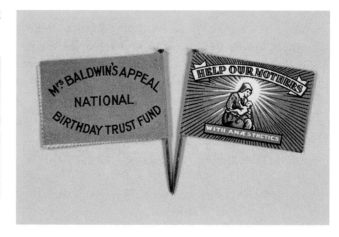

Fig. 62.3 The National Birthday Trust Fund in the UK used promotional materials such as those portrayed here. (Courtesy of the Wellcome Library, London)

twilight sleep probably did not contribute to her death, (which may have been caused by hemorrhage), this tragic event fueled a rising public concern about its safety. Nonetheless, some US hospitals continued to use twilight sleep until the 1960s.

Britain's National Birthday Trust Fund

In 1928, slightly more than a decade after the demise of the Twilight Sleep Association in America, wealthy and politically influential British women formed an organization to improve all aspects of healthcare for women and children [15]. At that time in Britain, nearly one in two hundred women died during childbirth, largely from hemorrhage, sepsis and complications of poor nutrition. The organizers of the National Birthday Trust Fund aimed to reduce this death rate by improving maternity care through programs that would train professional midwives and maternity nurses. The fund also had the goal of making modern pain relief during childbirth available for all women, regardless of their social status or income (Fig. 62.3). The NBTF still exists and continues to support improvement in various women's health issues.

The 1940s to the 1970s: Returning to the Past: from Anesthesia Back to Natural Childbirth

By the 1950s, birth was an institutionalized event for women in the US and parts of Europe. Women had minimal control over the birth process once the hospital and physician assumed responsibility for their care. A new generation of mothers and physicians opposed this institutionalized experience. They sought a more natural birth experience, one free from interventions such as the use of pain relief medications.

A British obstetrician, Grantly Dick-Read (1890–1959) profoundly influenced this shift from advocacy for medical pain relief, to advocacy for a natural birth [16]. He opposed the use of pain relief medications during childbirth, and inspired women to believe that "Healthy childbirth was never intended by the natural law to be painful" and that mothers should be fully conscious and aware, to enjoy childbirth. Fear, he argued, activates a flight-or-fight response, which releases body chemicals, preventing normal functioning of the uterine muscles, causing tension, and resulting in pain. He recognized the importance of keeping baby and mother together after birth and encouraged inclusion of fathers in the birth experience.

Then and today, some physicians challenged Dick-Read's conclusion that only fear causes the pain of contractions, and some denied his claim that information and knowledge about childbirth can eliminate such pain. Nonetheless, he enjoyed popular support among women disheartened by the regimented and institutionalized birth experiences on maternity wards. His book *Childbirth Without Fear*, published in 1933, is still read today, and his theory on the fear-tension-pain syndrome during birth inspired the development of other natural childbirth techniques. Although the physiological explanations for his theories may be questioned, Dick-Read is widely acknowledged as the father of the modern natural childbirth movement.

The US obstetrician, Robert Bradley (1917–1998), developed a natural drug-free childbirth philosophy in the late 1940s. He advocated a birth approach called "Husband-Coached Childbirth." Inclusion of the husband, not just as a witness to the act of birth, but also as an active *participant* in the birth process, was a radically new idea. He taught the use of a particular breathing technique to manage the pain of childbirth, believing that with proper education, preparation and the support of a coach, women could give birth naturally and with minimal pain. By the mid 1960s, the Bradley Method became a popular natural childbirth technique, a technique still used today by women wanting an entirely natural childbirth experience, in the US and around the world.

Parisian obstetrician, Fernand Lamaze (1891–1957), developed a parallel approach to that proposed by Bradley. In the 1940s, Lamaze traveled to Russia, where he observed women using a method called "psychoprophylaxis", simple breathing and relaxation techniques for pain management during childbirth. Lamaze next advanced the idea that controlled rapid breathing during labor would divert attention from the painful contractions, and allow women to give birth without medication. The Lamaze Organization began in the US in the 1960s, and its breathing and relaxation techniques became the most popular approach to the control of pain during birth throughout the country. However, the rapid shallow, "dog-breathing" techniques originally advocated by Lamaze are now recognized as relatively ineffective, and may even cause dangerous degrees of hyperventilation. Today's Lamaze instructors emphasize additional techniques such as movement and position change during labor, labor support personnel such as doulas, massage, dance, water immersion, and other modalities to relieve or diminish pain during labor.

Notable and Quotable Obstetric Anesthetists

Some notable pioneers played crucial roles in the development of obstetric anesthesia as a specialty. In the 1940s, Bert Hershenson was one of a few, perhaps the only, physician to provide obstetric anesthesia full-time (Fig. 62.4). He practiced at the Boston Lying-In Hospital, (the forerunner of the now Brigham and Women's Hospital) where he established the first "Division of Obstetric Anesthesia" in the nation, and served as its director from 1942 until his death in 1956. He wrote the first textbook devoted solely to obstetric anesthesia. Although the anatomical and mechanical tenets of epidural and caudal anesthesia had been developed in the early 1900s for surgical applications, it was not until the 1950s that interest developed in the use of this technique for childbirth pain relief. Jess Weiss, (for whom the "Weiss" epidural needle is named) a successor of Hershenson in Boston, and a future president of the American Society of Anesthesiologists, advocated the use of epidural analgesia, and further promoted obstetric anesthesia as a specialty.

Virginia Apgar's (1909–1974) fame extends beyond anesthesiology, to all of medicine. Her "score", "the Apgar", is used to define the condition of essentially all babies born in the world today (Table 62.1) [17]. "Ginny", began her career at Columbia University in 1938, became the first woman full professor at that institution and directed the division of obstetric anesthesia until 1959. She tirelessly advocated for safe delivery, and safe provision of pain relief in labor. In her later years, she also advocated for women's rights in the medical field, an outcome of her own experiences as a female physician in a male-dominated field, and she worked to prevent crippling birth defects, taking a leadership role in the March of Dimes Foundation. The US Postal Service honored her achievements with a stamp providing her likeness, a rare recognition indeed for an anesthesiologist (Fig. 62.5). She was named the American Society of Anesthesiologists Distinguished Service Awardee in 1961.

The importance of the Apgar Score to the practice of obstetrics, anesthesiology, and pediatrics is enormous. Over the years, some questioned the value of this simple 10-point scale, but the score has stood the test of time, correlating with amazing reliability to the immediate outcome of the newborn. Apgar's contribution, for the first time, allowed physicians and nurses to quickly quantify the condition of a newborn infant. While more probing and complex methods of infant evaluation were developed (e.g., the Brazelton

Obstetrical Anesthesia

ITS PRINCIPLES and PRACTICE

By

BERT B. HERSHENSON, M.D.

Director of Anesthesia
Boston Lying-in Hospital
Clinical Associate in Anesthesia
Harvard Medical School

With a Foreword by

FREDERICK C. IRVING, M.D.

William Lambert Richardson Professor of Obstetrics, Emeritus
Harvard University

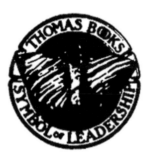

C H A R L E S C T H O M A S · P U B L I S H E R
Springfield · Illinois · U.S.A.

Fig. 62.4 Bert Hershenson wrote the first textbook of obstetrical anesthesia. (Title page given here)

Table 62.1 The Apgar Scoring for Newborns is typically given for each sign at one minute and five minutes after birth[a]

	Sign	0 Points	1 Point	2 Points
A	Appearance (skin color)	Blue-gray, pale all over	Only extremities blue-gray	All body normal color
P	Pulse	Absent	Below 100 bpm	Above 100 bpm
G	Grimace (reflex irritability)	No response	Grimace	Sneezes, coughs, pulls away
A	Activity (muscle tone)	Absent	Arms and legs flexed	Active movement
R	Respiration	Absent	Slow, irregular	Regular breathing, crying

[a]A score of 7–10 is considered normal, while 4–7 possibly indicates a need for some resuscitative measures, and a baby with a score of 3 and below requires immediate resuscitation

Fig. 62.5 Virginia Apgar's image was honored on a US Postal Service stamp

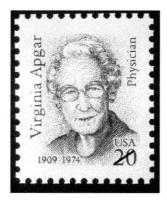

neurobehavioral test), these required specialized training and were rarely applied outside research investigations. Although imperfect as a test for evaluating the effect of drugs or anesthetics on the neonate, or even for determining the extent of resuscitation needed by a neonate, the simplicity of the Apgar score and its excellent correlation with outcomes (in populations, although perhaps less so in individual cases) remain its great strengths. Use of the "Apgar" prompts those involved in childbirth to pay systematic attention to the baby. It is noteworthy that the first description was published (in 1953) in an anesthesia (rather than an obstetric or pediatric) journal *Current Researches in Anesthesia and Analgesia*, the forerunner of *Anesthesia & Analgesia* (Fig. 62.6) [18]. More details of her life, including pictures, can be found at a website maintained by her family: www.apgar.net

John Bonica (1917–1994) practiced in Seattle, first at Tacoma General Hospital and later at the University of Washington, in the 1940s–1970, where he pioneered regional anesthesia techniques, including epidural analgesia, for pain relief in labor. He authored arguably the most comprehensive textbook on regional anesthesia ever published. He devoted the later part of his career to the relief of chronic pain, a deeply personal endeavor. Bonica suffered from injuries incurred as a young man using professional wrestling to supplement his income while also training to become a physician. He had several monikers, including "The Masked Marvel" and "Johnny The Bull Walker" (Fig. 62.7). He had badly injured hips, multiple rib fractures, and chronic back pain. His dear wife Emma nearly died in childbirth in 1943, further prompting his personal interest in obstetric anesthesia. ("I remember his heartbreaking 'Ciao, Emma', at her burial. He died shortly thereafter." *Personal reflection, E. Eger*)

The quintessential development in the specialty of obstetric anesthesia occurred in 1968, with the formation of the Society for Obstetric Anesthesia and Perinatology (SOAP). Six physicians—James Elam, Robert Bauer, Brad Smith, Robert Hustead, Richard Clark, and James Evans met at the Chicago O'Hare airport, and officially held the first organizational meeting of SOAP, which is the primary advocate for the interests of obstetric anesthesia as a specialty in the world today. The Society first met in 1969, in Kansas City, and the first president was Robert Hustead. Today, SOAP boasts over 1000 members world-wide, and has an active annual meeting. More information about the society, including historical information about its founding fathers, can be found at www.soap.org.

One of the more colorful personalities in the specialty of obstetric anesthesia was Gertie Marx (1912–2004). Born and medically trained in Germany, she moved to the US in 1937, initially to the New York Beth Israel Hospital, and in 1955 to New York's Albert Einstein Medical Center, where she remained for the next 40 years. I remember being a visiting professor at Einstein in the early 1990s. Her office was on the 11th floor of the building, and although she was well into her 80s, she made me WALK up the stairs to her office! Tough as nails, she was.

Gertie was a tireless researcher, publishing several hundred articles related to obstetric anesthesia. She was a constant and outspoken fixture at the annual SOAP meetings, and could almost always be counted upon to be at the microphone, her diminutive frame asking some pointed question to a (usually) petrified presenter. Gertie received many awards and accolades during her illustrious career, including the Distinguished Service Award in 1988 from the American Society of Anesthesiologists and the prestigious College Medal of the Royal College of Anaesthetists in London. According to Gerry Bassell, a good friend, (and a former SOAP president) the award reception was attended by Queen Elizabeth II, who asked Gertie what she did. Gertie replied, "*Your Majesty, I take care of mothers and babies*".

Another colorful character was Sol Shnider (1929–1994). Sol, originally from Yorktown, Saskatchewan, Canada, trained in anesthesiology at Columbia University in New York City, where he worked with Virginia Apgar. In 1962, Sol moved to San Francisco, to establish the division of obstetric

Current Researches in Anesthesia and Analgesia—July-August, 1953

A Proposal for a New Method of Evaluation of the
Newborn Infant.*

Virginia Apgar, M.D., New York, N. Y.

*Department of Anesthesiology, Columbia University, College of Physicians and
Surgeons and the Anesthesia Service, The Presbyterian Hospital*

Fig. 62.6 This illustration is from the title page of the original paper describing the Apgar Score, published in 1953 in *Current Researches in Anesthesia and Analgesia*

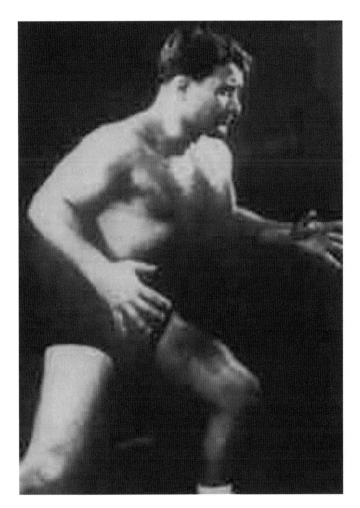

THE MANAGEMENT
OF PAIN

With Special Emphasis on the Use of
Analgesic Block in Diagnosis,
Prognosis, and Therapy

BY

John J. Bonica, M.D.

*Director, Department of Anesthesia, Tacoma General and Pierce County Hospitals;
Clinical Associate, Department of Anatomy, University of Washington Medical
School, Seattle, Washington; Senior Consultant in Anesthesiology, Madigan
Army Hospital, American Lake Veterans Administration Hospital,
Western State Hospital, Northern Pacific Hospital, Doctors
Hospital, U. S. Penitentiary, Tacoma, Washington*

785 Illustrations on 444 Figures

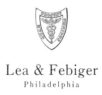

Lea & Febiger
Philadelphia

Fig. 62.7 John Bonica (here in his professional wrestling pose) wrote the classic textbook on pain management

anesthesia at the University of California, San Francisco. He was president of SOAP in 1973. He performed much of the early work on regulation of uterine blood flow and the effects of anesthetic drugs on the uterus and fetus. Shnider also was co-editor (with Gershon Levinson) of one of the major modern obstetric anesthesia textbooks; a work still widely read. In his honor, a popular annual meeting is held in San Francisco, the "Sol Shnider Obstetric Anesthesia Review and Update course". Sol was known for his flamboyant clothes, his love of music, wine, food, and especially opera, and for his mantra "the mother, the baby". As with Gertie Marx, his boundless enthusiasm for obstetric anesthesia motivated

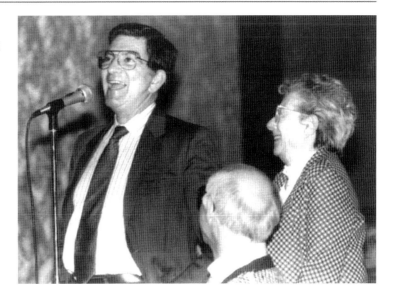

Fig. 62.8 Sol Shnider and Gertie Marx, in a typical scene at the microphone during a discussion session—or was it an entertainment?—at a SOAP meeting. (Author's personal collection)

many fellows and junior faculty, A regular fixture at the microphone at SOAP meetings (usually just behind Gertie) Sol was always ready to ask a pointed question (Fig. 62.8).

The 1980s and 1990s: The Epidural Becomes Popular; Natural Childbirth Declines

In the 1980s and 1990s, the use of epidural analgesia (regional anesthesia) grew dramatically. The offspring of mothers who had given birth without medication, now chose to give birth using medical pain relief, particularly epidural analgesia. A generation of women demanding pain-free childbirth replaced the generation of women who fought for natural childbirth. The "medicalization" of in-hospital childbirth also prompted a rise in popularity of out-of-hospital births, such as at birthing centers and home births. The number of women receiving spinal or epidural analgesia during childbirth increased dramatically from 1981–1997 [19]. In large hospitals nationally, the use of epidurals tripled to 66%, and is higher today. Advances in epidural techniques probably explain the increase. Infusions of low concentrations of local anesthetics, local-anesthetic sparing application of epidural narcotics, and the advent of patient-controlled techniques, collectively increased safety and efficacy, and hence popularity, of epidural analgesia. The epidural allowed women to remain awake, alert, and actively participate in the birth process, without amnesia or drug-induced sedation. This represented a major advantage over previously used forms of labor pain relief, and undoubtedly contributed to the increasing popularity of regional anesthetic techniques for labor pain relief. Concerns that epidural analgesia might adversely affect the progress and outcome of labor have been largely disproven. Secular attitudes may have contributed to the increase in medical labor pain relief; a more technologically sophisticated society easily accepted medical pain relief.

Pain Relief in the 2000s: Medical Pain Relief Advances and Natural Methods Return to Labor and Delivery Rooms

Traditional medical practice has increasingly embraced "alternative" medicine. Increasingly, patients and their physicians accept the idea that non-medical interventions and techniques may promote good health. This trend also affected the childbirth experience. More women, even those requesting epidural analgesia, willingly try techniques that even a few years ago were considered outside of the mainstream. Techniques and devices previously not found on labor and delivery units are now becoming more widely available [20]. These include hypnosis, water immersion, aromatherapy, birth balls (big plastic balls similar to those used in exercise training), advocacy for upright posture during labor and birth, acupuncture, and doulas (trained birthing coaches). The attitude that epidural analgesia is compatible and perhaps synergistic with various non-medical techniques contributes to the popularity of a blended approach. Many leaders in the natural childbirth community accept the role of epidural analgesia. Years ago, many doulas would consider their role finished (even failed) and leave a patient in labor if the patient requested and received epidural analgesia. Today, most doulas remain with their patients throughout labor, regardless of the methods of pain relief chosen, including epidurals; something I refer to as an "epi-doula". Recognition and acceptance by both obstetric anesthesiologists and doulas of the complementary roles of trained labor support personnel and epidural analgesia surely benefits the experience of women in childbirth.

Attitudes toward the use of pain relief, and the actual application of pain relief during childbirth have changed. At present, over eighty percent of women in the US receive some form of medical pain relief during childbirth, but the form taken continues to be debated among caregivers and women themselves. It has been more than 160 years since anesthesia was discovered. What form will the debate over pain-free childbirth take in the next several decades?

References

1. Rae SM, Wildsmith JA. So just who was James "Young" Simpson? Br J Anaesth. 1997;79:271–3.
2. Shchaer HM. History of pain relief in obstetrics. In: Marx GF, Bassell GM, editor. Obstetric analgesia and anesthesia. Amsterdam: Elsevier/North Holland Biomedical Press; 1980. pp. 1–19.
3. French V. Midwives and maternity care in the Roman world. Helios (New Series). 1986;13:69–84.
4. Caton D. What a blessing she had chloroform: the medical and social response to the pain of childbirth from 1800 to the present. New Haven: Yale University Press; 1999. pp. 1–304.
5. Sim PP. To give birth without pain! The first cases of mesmeric pain relief for obstetrics. Amer Soc Anesthesiol Newslett. 1997;61:14–6.
6. Lurie S. Euphemia Maclean, Agnes Sampson and pain relief during labour in 16th century Edinburgh. Anaesthesia. 2004;59:834–5.
7. Farr AD. Religious opposition to obstetric anaesthesia: a myth? Ann Sci. 1983;40:159–77.
8. Adams CN, Maltby JR. Religious objections! Blaming the church, labouring under a micsonception. Proc Hist Anaesth Soc. 2001;39:42–9.
9. Cohen J. Doctor James Young Simpson, Rabbi Abraham De Sola, and Genesis Chapter 3, verse 16. Obstet Gynecol. 1996;88:895–8.
10. Picard L. Victorian London: the life of a city, 1840–1870. London: Weidenfeld & Nicolson; 2006. p. 187.
11. Kannan S. Walter Channing and Nathan Cooley Keep: the first obstetric anesthetics in America. Bull Anesth Hist Assoc. 1998; 1:6–20.
12. Clark R. Fanny Longfellow and Nathan Keep. Amer Soc Anesthesiol Newslett. 1997;61:9.
13. Kass AM. Midwifery and medicine in Boston: Walter Channing, MD, 1786–1876. Boston: Northeastern University Press; 2002. pp. 1–386.
14. Mothers want the princess' drugs. National Birthday Trust Fund. 77 H5/2, Evening Standard. London; 1948.
15. Williams AS. Women and childbirth in the twentieth century: a history of the national birthday trust fund. 1928–93. Stroud: Sutton Publishing; 1997. pp. 1–331.
16. Caton D. Who said childbirth is natural? The medical mission of Grantly Dick Read. Anesthesiology. 1996;84:955–64.
17. Morishima HO. Virginia Apgar (1909–1974). J Pediatr. 1996; 129:768–70.
18. Apgar V. A proposal for a new method of evaluation of the newborn infant. Curr Res Anesth Analg. 1953;32:260–7.
19. Bucklin BA, Hawkins JL, Anderson JR, Ullrich FA. Obstetric anesthesia workforce survey: twenty-year update. Anesthesiology. 2005;103:645–53.
20. Simkin PP, O'Hara M. Nonpharmacologic relief of pain during labor: systematic reviews of five methods. Am J Obstet Gynecol. 2002;186:131–59.

A History of Regional Anesthesia

Michael Mulroy

Summary

South American Indians perhaps applied cocaine as a local anesthetic, long before its importation to Europe in the 1800s. Freud prompted Koller's discovery of topical anesthesia with cocaine, who reported eye surgery under topical anesthesia in 1884. Soon, surgeons applied cocaine anesthesia for eye surgery, local anesthesia, peripheral nerve blockade, and spinal anesthesia. In 1904, Einhorn synthesized procaine, but its effect was brief, and there were allergic responses to its metabolite, para-aminobenzoic acid. Dibucaine (1925) and tetracaine (1928) were useful, but had narrow therapeutic ratios.

In the late 1800s and early 1900s, surgeons popularized regional anesthesia, describing virtually all modern techniques. In 1901, Crile used regional anesthesia to block "surgical shock", presaging "pre-emptive analgesia". Spanish surgeon Pagés-Miravé described lumbar epidural injection in 1921. In 1920, Labat popularized regional anesthesia. His enthusiasm led to organization of the American Society of Regional Anesthesia in 1923. This original ASRA dissolved in 1939. In 1940, Lemmon's malleable needle facilitated development of continuous spinal anesthesia. Hingson and Edwards adapted this technology in 1942 for caudal anesthesia. In 1949, Curbelo placed a ureteral catheter in the epidural space to allow the production of continuous epidural anesthesia.

The use of regional technique reached a nadir in the mid-twentieth century, partly reflecting perceived limitations of regional (especially spinal) anesthesia. But in 1954, Dripps and Vandam found no severe neurologic problem in 10,098 patients given spinal anesthetics, thereby helping revive regional techniques. Moore and Bonica added to the resurrection. The introduction of aminoamide local anesthetics, first lidocaine (1947) and then mepivacaine (1957), prilocaine (1960), and bupivacaine (1963) further increased the use of regional techniques.

In the 1980s, peripheral nerve stimulators facilitated safer and simpler peripheral nerve blockade, and intrathecal and epidural opioids were shown to provide segmental analgesia without anesthetic or systemic effects, other than rare instances of respiratory depression. In the 1990s, University of Vienna investigators identified peripheral nerves using ultrasound, decreasing the volume of anesthetic required, and decreasing patient discomfort from paresthesia-seeking techniques or the motor responses caused by nerve stimulators. Finally, improved techniques (incremental injections), safer new anesthetics (ropivacaine), and "rescue" injection of lipid emulsions overcame concerns in the 1980s regarding the safety of local anesthetics injected intrathecally or intravenously.

In 1973, Winnie revived ASRA whose journal (*Regional Anesthesia*) first appeared in 1976. The European Society of Regional Anesthesia was founded in 1985. the Asian-Oceanic Society of Regional Anesthesia and Pain Medicine in 1991 and the Latin American Society of Regional Anesthesiology in 1995.

Introduction

Regional anesthesia evolved from the cross-currents of fascinating individuals, new drugs, and innovative technologies (Table 63.1). This evolution dictated an inherently overlapping and sometimes redundant narrative. The resulting pathways separated into three arbitrary (and non-distinct) phases—early developments, the "dark ages", and the modern era.

M. Mulroy (✉)
Faculty Anesthesiologist, Department of Anesthesiology,
Virginia Mason Medical Center, Seattle, WA, USA
e-mail: Michael.Mulroy@vmmc.org

The Age of Experimentation

Before anesthesia developed, pressure or ice might be applied to skin overlying peripheral nerves to produce numbness in extremities. True "regional anesthesia" followed the introduction of the first local anesthetic, cocaine. South American Indians knew of the numbing properties of this plant alkaloid long before its importation to Europe in the 1800s. The German chemist Fredrick Gaedcke (1828–1890) isolated cocaine in 1855, and Albert Nieman (1834–1861) achieved further purification in 1860. However, its capacity to produce local numbness and systemic excitation were initially viewed as curiosities, delaying its clinical application.

E. I Eger II et al. (eds.), *The Wondrous Story of Anesthesia,* DOI 10.1007/978-1-4614-8441-7_63, © Edmond I Eger, MD 2014

Table 63.1 Timeline of Historical Developments in Regional Anesthesia

Date	Development
1840s	Importation of coca leaves
1855	Isolation of cocaine
1860	Purification of cocaine
1884	Koller describes the surgical use of cocaine
1884	Halsted, uses cocaine for peripheral nerve block
1885	Corning produces the first epidural anesthetic with cocaine
1889	Bier produces the first subarachnoid block, using cocaine
1901	Sicard treats pain with sacral injections of local anesthetic
1903	Amylocaine (stovaine) synthesized
1904	Procaine synthesized
1921	Pagés-Miravé uses epidural injection
1923	Organization of first American Society of Regional Anesthesia (ASRA)
1925	Dibucaine synthesized
1931	Dogliotti publishes on epidural injections
1932	Tetracaine used clinically
1940	Lemmon introduces the continuous (malleable) spinal needle
1942	Hingson describes continuous caudal anesthesia
1944	Touhy provides continuous spinal anesthesia through a catheter
1947	Curbelo describes continuous epidural anesthesia
1947	Gordh describes the clinical use of lidocaine
1952	2-chloroprocaine used clinically
1957	Mepivacaine used clinically
1960	Prilocaine used clinically
1963	Bupivicaine used clinically
1972	Chapman uses a nerve stimulator to guide local anesthetic injection
1972	Etidocaine used clinically
1975	Organization of second American Society of Regional Anesthesia (ASRA)
1976	Yaksh and Rady describe the use of spinal opioids for analgesia
1977	Selander provides continuous axillary nerve blockade
1979	Cousins et al popularize epidural analgesia
1979	Bupivicaine cardiotoxicity discovered
1980	2-chloroprocaine neurotoxicity described
1985	European Society of Regional Anesthesia founded
1994	Kapral introduces ultrasound detection of nerves
1994	The New York School of Regional Anesthesia website appears
1997	Ropivicaine used clinically
1998	Weinberg describes lipid rescue for local anesthetic cardiotoxicity

Early Pioneers

In 1880, Basil von Anrep reported that injecting cocaine into his arm produced numbing of his skin, but this did not lead to clinical application [1]. Sigmund Freud (1856–1939) prompted the first clinical research into the drug. He had heard of the stimulating effects of cocaine, and began to research those aspects, hoping to find a drug to help a friend overcome his morphine addiction. His initial investigations produced a treatise on cocaine [2]. He subsequently enlisted the help of Carl Koller (1857–1944), a Vienna hospital intern whom he had befriended, Freud gave an envelope containing the powder to Koller, who immediately noticed that his tongue became numb when he licked some spilled powder. Koller, a physician in the ophthalmology clinic in Vienna, recognized the potential use of the numbing effect on the cornea, demonstrating this in animals. Then (true to his nineteenth century medicine tradition), he experimented on himself and a colleague, instilling cocaine into their eyes before touching each others' corneas with the head of a pin. This successful self-experimentation led to an operation under topical cocaine anesthesia, in September of 1884 [3]. Koller reported this triumph a few weeks later to the German Ophthalmological Society Congress in Heidelberg. The paper was read by a colleague because Koller could not afford to attend the Congress. The news spread rapidly, and in that year, ophthalmologists in New York employed cocaine anesthesia for eye surgery. Prominent American surgeons (William Halsted [1852–1922] and Richard Hall [1856–1897]) at the Roosevelt Hospital in New York infiltrated cocaine to numb surgical fields.

In the next year, 60 reports from individual surgeons described successful local anesthesia of the skin. Halsted and Hall were first to describe the use of cocaine to block peripheral nerves, including a report of brachial plexus anesthesia by injection under direct vision. Again, in the tradition of self-experimentation, some of the original investigators, including Freud and Halsted, became addicted to cocaine. Halsted used morphine to end his dependence on cocaine—trading one devil for another. Although he never overcame his addiction, he managed to continue functioning at a high level. He moved to the Johns Hopkins Medical Center in Baltimore, and had a distinguished career as the father of modern surgical training in the US. Halsted's early papers attest to his enthusiasm for the use of conduction anesthesia with the new local anesthetic [4]. After becoming addicted he ceased publishing work related to local anesthesia, and it is unclear whether he continued to use local or regional infiltration techniques in his practice.

Development of Spinal Anesthesia

The application of cocaine dramatically increased after the discovery of its beneficial properties as a spinal anesthetic. An initial report by James Corning (1855–1923) in 1885, of cocaine injected into the spinal column [5] appears, from his description, to have been the first epidural, rather than the first spinal, anesthetic. Corning's injection into a single human subject followed a successful animal injection. No widespread use followed his report.

"Spinal" anesthesia followed from the improved descriptions of spinal anatomy by the German surgeon Heinrich Quincke (1842–1922) who used the spinal canal as an avenue for the treatment of tuberculous meningitis. His descriptions of the anatomy of the dural sac and the spinal cord led to the relatively "safe" insertion of hypodermic needles in the lower lumbar area. His surgical colleague, August Bier (1861–1949), performed the first intentional subarachnoid block [6]. Bier and his assistant, August Hildebrandt, performed subarachnoid injections of 5mg cocaine on each other in 1899. Hildebrandt's initial attempt to inject the drug into Bier failed because the syringe outlet did not fit the hub of the needle. Bier suffered from a spinal headache for nine days. Injection into his assistant resulted in anesthesia of the lower extremities, as evidenced by lack of sensation in response to blows to the shin. Fortunately, the initial subarachnoid injection followed the introduction of aseptic technique, including the routine use of surgical gloves, and infection did not mar the early history of neuraxial block. In 1908, Bier described the first "intravenous regional anesthesia", a technique that did not achieve popularity until the 1960s. Perhaps it was the perceived necessity to expose the veins surgically, or the short duration of procaine that limited enthusiasm, but the report by CM Holmes in 1963 described the percutaneous approach, using the "new" lidocaine, that became an accepted technique.

Bier and Hildebrandt's success with subarachnoid injection addressed concerns regarding the toxicity and short duration of action of cocaine injections; a small dose of drug could profoundly block sensation to half the body. The news of their success spread rapidly to the US, and in 1899, Fredrick Tate and Guido Caglieri in San Francisco, performed surgical procedures under spinal anesthesia [7]. Spinal anesthesia soon became the most popular form of regional anesthesia because of its simplicity and low toxicity. In many countries it was popular because the surgeon could act, sequentially, as anesthetist and surgeon. Surgeons dealt with concerns regarding hypotension by controlling the level of spinal blockade through the use of hyperbaric and hypobaric solutions, and adjustment of patient position.

Some colorful and cavalier European surgeons, such as Thomas Jonnesco (1860–1926) of Bucharest, combined thoracic or cervical level injections of hypobaric stovaine with strychnine, to produce anesthesia for thoracic and even head and neck surgery [8].

> "NEW AID IN SURGERY…Special Cable to The New York Times. LONDON, Nov 20 (1909). The safe use of stovaine as an anaesthetic was proved to-day by a remarkable operation performed by Prof. Thomas Jonnesco, Dean of the University of Bucharest, at the Seamen's Hospital in Greenwich…To-day's operation was the removal of a mass of tubercular glands in the neck…Prof. Jonnesco inserted a small hypodermic needle into the spinal canal, passing it between two of the vertebrae at the base of the neck. Attaching a small syringe to the needle three centigrammes of stovaine and five centigrammes of sulphate of strychnine were injected into the spinal canal. The patient was told to lie down on the operating table. His head and shoulders were lowered, so that the action of gravity would cause the numbing fluid to spread upward. Two minutes later the operation was carried out in an ordinary manner, the patient being perfectly conscious and talking to the surgeon during the whole proceeding. 'Do you feel any pain?' asked one surgeon. 'No, Sir,' replied the patient. 'I am quite comfortable.'…Five minutes after the operation was finished the patient got off the operating table, walked into the next room, and was taken back to bed."

The reader may wonder, "Why strychnine?" The above article explained that "…by coupling with (stovaine) an exhilarating drug like strychnine the bad effect on the heart is neutralized without interfering with the desired numbing influence of the anaesthetic." Most surgeons were content with lumbar level injections, and the judicious use of the new vasoconstrictor, ephedrine, to manage hypotension.

Development of New Local Anesthetics

The inherent drawbacks of cocaine tempered enthusiasm for neural blockade. Cocaine's potential for addiction was well documented. More limiting was its short duration of action (approximately 45 minutes) and relatively small margin of safety. Thus, investigators searched for local anesthetics with minimal issues of toxicity and addiction, and a longer duration.

Niemann's work with cocaine revealed its benzoic acid structural component. The first derivative of this moiety was amylocaine (stovaine), released in 1903. It was used for spinal anesthesia until identified as a nerve irritant. In Germany, Alfred Einhorn (1856–1917) synthesized the amino-ester, procaine, in 1904 [9]. Heinrich Braun (1862–1934) documented procaine's favorable properties compared to those of stovaine. It was not a nerve irritant, and did not have the excitatory and addictive properties of cocaine, and therefore replaced stovaine for clinical use [10]. However, procaine also had a short duration of action, and introduced a new problem, allergic reactions to its metabolite, para-aminobenzoic acid. Other amino esters were synthesized to overcome these issues. Dibucaine (1925) and tetracaine (1928) were clinically useful, but displayed a narrower therapeutic ratio (tetracaine, for example, is 8 times more potent than procaine, but 12 times more toxic, partially related to its slower hydrolysis by plasma esterases). Systemic toxic reactions were more common with tetracaine when used in higher doses for topical anesthesia (bronchoscopy) or peripheral blockade, and thus its use was often limited to spinal anesthesia, where smaller doses of drugs were effective. Further development of regional techniques awaited the synthesis of aminoamide compounds in the 1940s.

Early Leaders

Evangelical-like proponents (e.g., Jonnesco), virtually all surgeons, fathered the development of regional techniques. Braun in Germany published the first textbook describing these techniques in 1905 [11] along with enthusiastic reports of regional anesthesia. Another enthusiastic surgeon, Victor Pauchet (1869–1936) in France, likewise published a textbook of regional anesthesia based on the practice at his surgical theater in Paris. This period of energetic experimentation developed virtually all currently used regional anesthetic techniques, at least in a preliminary form. Subsequent expansion resulted from emergence of new local anesthetics, and new technical equipment for performance of blocks [12].

Gaston Labat (1876–1934) is credited with the wider introduction of regional anesthesia to the US. After graduating from medical school in 1916, he moved to Paris and practiced at the University of Paris under Pauchet. He was the third author of the third edition of Pauchet's textbook on regional anesthesia. Labat was administering anesthesia when Charles Mayo happened to visit Pauchet's surgical clinic, including Labat's operating room in 1920. Impressed with Labat and his regional anesthetic techniques, Mayo invited him to join the faculty at the Mayo Clinic—to teach regional anesthe-

sia and write a textbook in English. Labat moved to Rochester, Minnesota, in October 1920. He expanded interest in regional techniques, and, despite the brevity of his tenure at the Mayo clinic, wrote the textbook. Unfortunately, Labat and the Mayo administration appeared to have disagreed on the publication and royalties of his textbook (although Mayo wrote a positive introduction in the book). Perhaps because of this and perhaps because of marital discord, he left the Mayo Clinic before completing his one-year appointment, and moved to Bellevue Hospital in New York. Labat was a surgeon and there is no record of his assuming the title of "chief" of anesthesia at Bellevue. Emery Rovenstine (1895–1960), who succeeded Labat, established a residency and a department of anesthesia—which he headed. Published in 1922, [13] many of the illustrations and much of the text in Labat's book resembled those in Pauchet's French text. Labat's text was the first comprehensive practical manual of regional techniques in English, and sold 7000 copies in three printings. Labat acknowledged his debt to Pauchet in the preface to the second edition in 1928, which sold an additional 3500 copies [14].

Labat developed a following in New York, including colleagues who met regularly to foster their skills. His enthusiasm led to the establishment of the American Society of Regional Anesthesia (ASRA) in New York in 1923. The organization met quarterly to discuss research in regional anesthesia. Several research papers were subsequently published in the new journal, *Current Researches in Anesthesia and Analgesia,* edited by Francis McMechan. The Society remained small (58 active members in 1937), but changed from a group dominated by surgeons to one including many of the prominent figures in the developing specialty of anesthesiology. The original ASRA then dwindled, voting to dissolve in 1939. Several factors were responsible for the decline in interest, including the development of new general anesthetic drugs (cyclopropane in 1930, thiopental in 1934,) at a time when there was ongoing concern about hypotension with spinal anesthesia and toxicity of the local anesthetics. Another factor was political, involving the positioning of the various societies of anesthesiologists to become the national representative of the specialty [15]. Rovenstine, Labat's successor as president, chose to join the American Society of Anesthetists in endorsing the new American Board of Anesthesiology, and the prominent members of ASRA transferred their interest to those organizations.

Other American Pioneers

Rovenstine, a founder of the ASA, succeeded Labat as chief of anesthesia at Bellevue Hospital in 1935. With the help of a Labat disciple, surgeon Hippolyte Wertheim, Rovenstine continued an emphasis on regional anesthesia at Bellevue [16]. Rovenstine largely abandoned the operating room, to apply regional techniques to patients having problems with pain, presaging a movement that gained momentum in the second half of the century.

George Crile (1864–1943), founder of the Cleveland Clinic and the American College of Surgeons, explored the effects of anesthesia on the phenomenon of "surgical shock" [17] in 1901. Using animals, he found that inhalational anesthetics did not block this physiologic response, while regional techniques prevented nociceptive impulses from reaching the brain, thereby abolishing the response. His concept of "anoci-association" foreshadowed concepts of "pre-emptive analgesia" presently described in conjunction with regional and multimodal analgesic techniques.

The surgeon, George Pitkin (1885–1943), an early American experimenter with spinal anesthetic techniques, shared Crile's interest in reducing surgical stress. In 1927, he invented and popularized a mixture of procaine, strychnine (nominally to act as a vasoconstrictor), and alcohol (the formula was 0.195 gm procaine, 0.0022 gm strychnine, 0.324 gm alcohol, and normal saline to a volume of 2.2 ml) to produce a hypobaric solution which he named "Spinocain" [18, 19]. Spinocain appears to have been widely used, with no suggestion of toxicity. Pitkin described the effect of position and gravity on the spread of spinal anesthesia, and developed a tilt indicator to assist in positioning the patient. He also developed a hyperbaric solution for obstetrical anesthesia. His life-long dedication to regional techniques culminated in his massive tome on *Conduction Anesthesia*, [20] the second major American text on regional anesthesia.

Pitkin's contemporary, William Babock (1872–1963), of Temple University in Philadelphia, also advocated the use of hypobaric spinal anesthesia. He preferred amylocaine (stovaine) mixed with alcohol, strychnine, distilled water and lactic acid, a combination he developed in 1909. Like the Mayo brothers, a visit to France in 1904 had impressed him with the benefits of regional anesthesia. Concern about the hypotension associated with spinal block caused him to advocate measuring the blood pressure and treating hypotension with adrenalin. He preferred spinal anesthesia because of the perceived lower mortality when compared with that of general anesthesia at the time [21].

In 1923, Lincoln Sise (1874–1942), a soft-spoken anesthesiologist, joined the Lahey Clinic in Boston to partner with the renowned surgeon, Frank Lahey. Sise started in general practice but gave anesthesia to supplement his income. He rapidly became a master in anesthesia for patients undergoing abdominal procedures. At the time, regional anesthesia centered on spinal anesthesia because of its short duration and the systemic toxicity associated with peripheral blocks. The introduction of procaine decreased toxicity, but hypotension and post-spinal headaches remained as concerns. Although surgeons appreciated the muscle relaxation provided by "high spinals", a sufficiently high block often precipi-

tated severe hemodynamic changes. Sise pioneered the use of hyperbaric solutions, administered to patients positioned laterally and in a slight Trendelenburg's position, with the head and shoulders elevated. He tilted the table to adjust the block height to an optimum level. Sise deserves the credit for using fluid administration to minimize hypotension. He was also an early proponent of the use of ephedrine to combat hypotension.

Notable was his development of an introducer needle to penetrate the skin and interspinous ligaments, enabling use of a smaller gauge needle for the final dural puncture, thereby decreasing the frequency and severity of headaches. Allowing the spinal needle to bypass the skin may also have reduced the risk of infection, a key consideration in an age preceding antibiotics. And what was the right size needle? Fine gauge needles equaled fewer spinal headaches, but use of finer gauge or malleable needles could lead to broken needles, a phenomenon so common that Sise's partner, Lahey, described how to extract broken needles in 1929 [22]. Other innovators designed new needles, including Green's rounded bevel needle in 1923, subsequently shown to reduce the incidence of headaches. It was not commercially produced until almost sixty years later.

Labat had impressed the surgical staff at the Mayo Clinic. With his departure, they looked for a successor to establish a true department of anesthesia. William Mayo, Charles' brother, accidentally met John Lundy (1874–1973) at a dinner meeting during a visit to Seattle in 1924. Lundy had not performed research or published since graduating from Rush Medical College in 1919, but the young man's enthusiasm and curiosity about anesthetic topics impressed Mayo, and he recruited Lundy to assume the directorship of the anesthesia section at the Clinic. Mayo's decision was based on little evidence, but in hindsight was justified. Lundy went on to introduce thiopental, establish a blood bank, and open the first recovery room. He also established an anatomy laboratory and a strong teaching program. Lundy had never performed a regional anesthetic before he assumed the role of Director of Regional Anesthesia. Nevertheless he joined ASRA, where he met Labat. Lundy continued the tradition of reliance on regional techniques at the Mayo Clinic, often combining regional with general anesthesia. He developed a concept of "balanced anesthesia" wherein a hypnotic agent produced anesthesia, neuromuscular blocking drugs facilitated relaxation, and a regional technique provided postoperative pain relief [23].

Technical Advances: Continuous Analgesia Techniques

The pioneers of spinal anesthesia sought to increase the duration of spinal anesthesia by inserting a needle that could remain in place, and through which repeated doses of local anesthetic could be administered. In 1940, William Lemmon inserted the tip of a flexible (malleable) needle into the subarachnoid space, (SAS) and then had the patient lie on a mattress specially designed to accommodate the protruding needle. This allowed subsequent injections to be made through the needle into the SAS of the supine patient. Such intermittent injections presaged the development of "continuous" spinal anesthesia. Robert Hingson and Waldo Edwards adapted this technology in 1942 for injections into the caudal canal to produce prolonged lower extremity and pelvic analgesia, [24] and extended analgesia for labor and delivery. Hingson taught the technique to Gertie Marx in New York during her training. Edward Tuohy (1908–1959), of the Mayo Clinic, took the next step. Using the needle with a curved tip designed by Huber, Tuohy introduced a small-gauge ureteral catheter into the subarachnoid space to allow continuous spinal anesthesia [25].

Continuous Peridural Techniques

In 1901, Jean Sicard (1872–1929) injected cocaine into the caudal peridural space to treat sciatica, and Ferdinand Cathelin used the technique for surgical anesthesia. The Spanish surgeon, Fidel Pagés-Miravé (1886–1923), was the first to describe lumbar epidural injection, in 1921. The Italian, Achille Dogliotti, (1897–1966) popularized the technique 10 years later [26]. Finally, in 1949, Manuel Curbelo of Cuba used the Tuohy needle to introduce a ureteral catheter into the epidural space enabling the first continuous epidural anesthetic [27].

Beginnings of Obstetrical Anesthesia

John Snow popularized general anesthesia for childbirth, recognizing however, the potential for maternal aspiration of gastric contents. A regional anesthetic technique would minimize the occurrence of this complication. O Kreis in Switzerland and S Marx in the US applied single injection spinal anesthesia in 1900. The approach did not become popular, perhaps because of the short and unpredictable duration of cocaine anesthesia after a single injection. In 1909, the gynecologist, W Stoeckel, used procaine by Cathelin's caudal peridural approach, to produce sacral analgesia for obstetrics, [28] but again the short duration of the single injection limited acceptance. Regional obstetrical analgesia became popular when the continuous techniques mentioned above came into vogue. Hingson's group, and a publication by Manalan in the 1940s, [29] popularized continuous caudal techniques. Gertie Marx (1913–2004) [30] in New York, and John Bonica [31] in Seattle, both employed caudal techniques to provide obstetric analgesia in the 1940s

The Renaissance of Regional Anesthesia

The middle of the twentieth century marked a nadir of regional techniques. Partly this reflected the introduction of improved drugs and techniques for general anesthesia. Thiopental and cyclopropane, agents allowing a more rapid onset and emergence than that associated with diethyl ether, became available by the 1940s. Curare became available in the 1940s to facilitate muscle relaxation. Tracheal tubes were used with increasing frequency. Nonflammable halogenated agents, particularly halothane, arrived in the 1950s, and displaced all previous flammable and more toxic agents.

Regional anesthesia seemed less safe. Peripheral nerve block was of limited duration unless tetracaine was used, and tetracaine could cause systemic toxic reactions because large doses were needed. Overall, anesthetic mortality associated with spinal anesthesia was no greater than with general anesthesia (10–12 deaths per 10,000 anesthetics), but reports of deaths elicited editorial concern, [32] prompting a rebuttal, [33] "A Defense of Spinal Anesthesia" published in 1952. Foster Kennedy, a British-trained American neurologist, published a paper describing what appeared to be another blow to acceptance of spinal anesthesia. In an editorial in the 1950 journal *Surgery, Gynecology and Obstetrics* entitled "The Grave Spinal Cord Paralysis Caused by Spinal Anesthesia," he reported 12 cases of permanent paralysis caused by spinal anesthesia, observing that this "paralysis below the waist is too large a price for a patient to pay in order that the surgeon should have a fine relaxed field of operation." [34] In 1947, the permanent paralysis produced in two British patients had already caused reservations about the use of this technique in Great Britain. Although the cause of their paralysis was never clearly determined, it appeared there may have been contamination of the local anesthetic or the injection equipment. Nevertheless, this internationally publicized disaster precipitated a rapid retreat from regional techniques [35].

Fortunately, some proponents of spinal analgesia scientifically examined these concerns. The Department of Anesthesia at the University of Pennsylvania, led by Robert Dripps and Leroy Vandam, prospectively studied 10,098 spinal anesthetics. No case revealed severe neurologic problems, [36] suggesting the safety of subarachnoid block when performed with tetracaine. Coupled with the introduction of the new aminoamide family of local anesthetics, the Dripps and Vandam findings supported a resurgence of interest in regional techniques in the US.

New Champions, New Drugs

The emergence of new "champions" of regional techniques in Seattle, Washington, Daniel Moore and John Bonica, aided in the resurrection of local anesthetic techniques. So did the development of new local anesthetics.

Daniel Moore (1918-present)

Moore obtained his medical training during World War II in Chicago, at Northwestern University, where he developed an interest in regional anesthetic techniques under the tutelage of anesthesiologist Mary Karp. Senior surgeons at the Virginia Mason Clinic in Seattle, seeking high quality anesthesia for increasingly complex surgical procedures, hired Moore. Moore established a Department of Anesthesia at the Clinic and obtained approval for a residency program in 1948. Within five years, 50 % of patients undergoing surgery at the Clinic received a regional technique. His skill and enthusiasm made him a prominent local and national advocate. In a series of 2,500 patients, he demonstrated the safety of tetracaine for peripheral nerve blocks [37]. He followed this paper with more than 100 publications, primarily on the clinical use of regional techniques for obstetrics, pain management, and surgery. NIH funding supported his studies of local anesthetic blood levels and systemic toxicity. Local anesthetics developed in the 1960s were tested at the Clinic. Moore published his textbook on regional anesthesia in 1952, a richly illustrated practical guide [38]. His election as President of the American Society of Anesthesiologists in 1959, and his colorful presentations in word and in print gave further prominence to the usefulness of regional anesthesia.

John Bonica (1917–1994)

Simultaneous with Moore's arrival at Virginia Mason after World War II, Bonica established a private practice in Tacoma, Washington. Anesthetic complications during his wife's childbirth experience prompted a focus on regional anesthesia with a particular interest in obstetrics and the management of patients with chronic pain. He published the first major American textbooks on both subjects. In 1947, at Tacoma General Hospital, he established the first anesthesia residency in Washington, a residency emphasizing regional anesthesia. In 1960, he assumed the Chairmanship of the Department of Anesthesiology at the University of Washington in Seattle, where he fostered a multidisciplinary pain clinic and formalized the role of the anesthesiologist for the management of complex pain syndromes, including the use of diagnostic and neurolytic nerve blocks. Bonica became a founding member of the International Society of Pain and was a Director of the second American Society of Regional Anesthesia (see below). Though "competitors", Moore and Bonica were lifelong friends, and deserve much of the credit for advancing regional anesthesia immediately after World War II.

New Local Anesthetics

Key to increasing the use of regional techniques was the introduction of the aminoamide local anesthetics. Lidocaine was the first of these. Lofgren and Lundvquist synthesized lidocaine in 1943 and sold the patent to the Astra Pharmaceutical Company in Sweden. Torsten Gordh (1907–2010) at the Karolinska University in Sweden performed volunteer and patient studies leading to the clinical release of lidocaine in 1947. Gordh found that lidocaine acted more rapidly and its anesthetic effects lasted longer than with procaine. Absence of the benzoic moiety in the molecule eliminated the allergic reactions associated with procaine. Subsequent research resulted in the introduction of longer-acting aminoamides, including mepivacaine (1957), prilocaine (1960), and bupivacaine (1963). Bupivacaine offered a larger therapeutic ratio than tetracaine. It provided a longer duration of surgical anesthesia, even extending analgesia into the postoperative period. Extensive clinical studies suggested their safety and efficacy. The aminoamides, with their longer stability in solution than the esters, became the mainstays of regional anesthesia techniques.

The Renaissance—The Modern Age

The early champions of regional anesthesia, combined with new local anesthetics propelled regional anesthesia into new prominence. New champions and technological and organizational developments supported an increasing focus on regional anesthesia.

New Champions

Benjamin Covino (1931–1991) started his career as a physiologist-physician. After obtaining his medical degree in 1962, he joined the small Swedish company, Astra Pharmaceutical Products. As the medical director from 1962–1966, and then as vice-president for scientific affairs until 1974, he oversaw the basic science and clinical research on the new long-acting amino-amide local anesthetics. He completed an anesthesia residency at the Massachusetts General Hospital in 1977, and after a short term at the University of Massachusetts in Worcester (near his old Astra headquarters), he assumed Chairmanship of the Department of Anesthesiology at the Brigham and Womens' Hospital in the Harvard Medical School, from 1979 to his sudden untimely death in 1991. He brought an emphasis on scientific research to the clinical delivery of regional anesthesia, supporting the laboratory work of prominent local anesthetic researchers such as Gary Strichartz, Sanjay Datta and Aaron Gissen. He was a warm and supportive clinical educator who knew all his residents by their first name, and his graduates included many prominent leaders in regional anesthesia such as J Anthony Wildsmith, Mark Lema, Michael Ferrante and William Urmey. As the second Editor-in-Chief of *Regional Anesthesia*, he increased the scientific standards of the published reports. He published 150 papers and five textbooks on regional anesthesia topics, and served as a leader for what he described as the "third phase" of the development of regional anesthesia, the "Scientific Era" [39].

Gerard Ostheimer (1940–1995) a Covino protégé, served as Covino's Vice-Chairman. Ostheimer loved obstetrical anesthesia, which he directed at the Brigham and Women's Hospital, and taught enthusiastically to several generations of residents. He led one of the first studies of the efficacy of epidural blood patches, [40] and was active in the cooperative movement in the 1970s between the ASA and the American Society of Obstetricians and Gynecologists (ACOG) to ensure that anesthesia services were considered as an essential and appropriate part of a delivery service [41]. He was a popular speaker and prolific author, and succeeded Covino as the Editor of *Regional Anesthesia*. He served as a president of the reestablished ASRA, and joined the newly formed (1969) Society for Obstetric Anesthesia and Perinatology (SOAP) (an outgrowth of the interactions between ASA and ACOG), editing their Newsletter. SOAP marked the culmination of efforts to provide a forum for obstetrical issues and recognition, and remains today as a thriving subspecialty organization.

Champions also emerged in Europe. Donald (Bruce) Scott (1925–1998) at the Royal Infirmary in Edinburgh "both practiced and promoted regional anesthesia in the UK at a time when it lay under the cloud of the notorious Woolley and Roe case." [42] He was noted for his research on the management of hypotension in the supine parturient, for his collaboration with Astra Pharmaceuticals (and his friend Ben Covino) in the development of new local anesthetics, and as the founding president of the European Society of Regional Anesthesia (ESRA) in 1979. On the continent, Egor Lanz in Mainz, Germany, performed some of the early work on epidural morphine analgesia, and scientific documentation of the distribution of anesthesia with the various approaches to brachial plexus blockade. In Belgium, Albert van Steenberge (1925–2010) promoted techniques such as low-dose epidural analgesia for obstetrics, and the combined spinal-epidural technique, but his major contribution was as the founding force in ESRA.

Philip Bromage's (1920-present) clinical and research activities straddled two continents. Born in London, he discovered the advantages of regional anesthesia as a wartime ship's medical officer, and eventually trained under J Alfred Lee at Southend Hospital in England. He investigated epidural anesthesia in England, continuing such studies after his move to

Montreal, Canada, in 1956. He published over 80 articles on the anatomy and physiology of epidural blockade (including epidural opioid analgesia), [43] leading to his text on epidural analgesia after his move to Duke University in 1981.

Alon Winnie (1932- present) completed the restoration of regional anesthesia. He was the most productive champion of regional anesthesia in the 1970s. Although crippled by polio during his residency, and confined for life to a wheelchair, he became an articulate advocate and pioneer of regional techniques, notably simplified single-injection techniques for brachial plexus [44] and lumbar plexus anesthesia. Although others later challenged his concept that a "single sheath" enclosed each plexus, his straight-forward illustrations and enthusiastic descriptions led many to undertake regional blocks. His textbook of plexus anesthesia was a popular handbook, [45] and guided many to a first-time attempt of plexus blocks. He became a central figure in the new ASRA, which is perhaps his greatest legacy.

ASRA is Reborn

Renewed interest in regional anesthesia, and emergence of mid-century experts/champions, led to a rebirth of the American Society of Regional Anesthesia. Winnie was frustrated by the lack of an educational forum for regional techniques, feeling that neither the ASA nor the IARS offered sufficient teaching programs for regional blocks. In 1973, he initiated the idea of resurrecting the original ASRA with P Prithvi Raj, and co-opted L Donald Bridenbaugh, Harold Carron, and Jordan Katz, [46] to join together as "founding fathers." The newly reconstituted society, a society dedicated to the promotion, investigation and teaching of regional anesthesia, had its first scientific meeting in March 1976. The society's journal *Regional Anesthesia, (Pain Medicine* was added to the title in 1998) was first distributed in October 1976. Membership grew from 300 original members to 6,500 by 2005, an anesthesia membership second only to that in the ASA. Winnie served as the first president, from 1975–1980. The organization attracted extensive support and expansion of regional anesthesia, and created a Carl Koller Fellowship to encourage junior members to engage in research in regional anesthesia. With the continued expansion of interest in chronic pain management, the Society expanded its educational programs to 2 annual scientific meetings. It has survived twice as long as the original ASRA.

The new ASRA encouraged formation of societies for regional anesthesia in other areas of the world. The European Society of Regional Anesthesia (ESRA) was chartered in 1979, and had its first scientific congress in 1981. The Latin American Society of Regional Anesthesiology, founded in 1993, had its first scientific congress in 1994, and the Asian-Oceanic Society of Regional Anesthesia emerged in 1989, hosting its 11th Congress in 2011. Starting in 1992, these societies have sponsored international symposia in conjunction with each subsequent World Congress of Anesthesiologists. Most recently, the African Society of Regional Anesthesia was established in 2010.

Bumps in the Road

In 1979 and 1980, two challenges described in case reports transiently damaged the standing of regional anesthesia, but eventually improved the drugs available and techniques used. In 1979, [47] cardiotoxicity followed unintentional intravascular injections of bupivacaine. In 1980, an unintended subarachnoid injection of a large dose of preservative-containing 2-chloroprocaine produced neurotoxicity [48]. Animal research demonstrated neurotoxicity from 2-chloroprocaine injected at an acid pH with sodium bisulphite as a preservative. This discovery led to reformulating chloroprocaine in a preservative-free preparation, a safer preparation for either epidural or peripheral nerve injection.

The bupivacaine story is more complex. Results from animal models suggested that the R-enantiomer could produce intractable cardiac arrest, by inducing a prolonged blockade of sodium channels in myocardial tissue, at blood levels slightly greater than those associated with seizures [49]. Three advances, each adding safety, followed identification of this phenomenon and its probable cause. First, safer injection techniques were developed, including careful aspiration, incremental injections, and the use of "test doses" to identify intravascular injection. These techniques alone appear to decrease the incidence of systemic toxic reactions to one percent of the previously reported frequencies [50]. Second, less toxic (than bupivicaine) long-acting aminoamide medications were developed, primarily the levo-enantiomers, ropivacaine and levobupivacaine. Third, was the finding that boluses or an infusion of a lipid emulsion could remove the highly lipid soluble long-acting aminoamides from their channel blocking sites [51]. Intralipid is now stored as a "lipid rescue" drug in locations where high doses of long-acting aminoamides are used.

What about the "safest" of the aminoamides, the original lidocaine, the 'poster' child for safety? Cases of nerve toxicity followed its use with newly developed microcatheters for subarachnoid injection, demonstrating the toxicity of concentrated solutions injected in a localized area. This resulted in removal of microcatheters from the market. These findings increased awareness of the potential toxicity of all local anesthetics in high concentrations. Other investigations revealed a syndrome of Transient Neurologic Symptoms (TNS), consisting of back pain radiating to the legs and persisting for 2–4 days after spinal anesthesia. This transient pain was 4 times more likely when lidocaine was used, particularly for outpatient procedures [52].

Further Technical Developments

New technical developments in the last quarter of the twentieth Century increased the world-wide use of regional anesthesia. Peripheral nerve stimulators now aided nerve localization. A 2 Hz current of 2 mA or less could provoke a motor response in a mixed peripheral nerve without producing sensory stimulation or patient discomfort, a significant advance over the use of paresthesias to identify nerves. Nerve stimulators now allowed delivery of a variable current: a higher "seeking" current could be reduced as the needle approached the nerve. Movement in response to a current of less than 0.5 mA indicated proximity to the nerve sufficient to provide a good anesthetic block. The development of insulated needles, which concentrated the electrical current at the tip of the needle, further improved efficacy of nerve localization. In sum, these incremental advances in the 1980s–1990s, greatly enhanced the performance of peripheral nerve blockade and the anesthetist's confidence.

Simultaneously, the technology of needle and catheter design improved. Better production techniques made disposable equipment a reality. New fine-gauge needles with rounded bevels produced a lower incidence of post-dural puncture headache, reviving this regional technique. Evidence in animals from a study reported in 1993 suggested that new peripheral nerve block needles with a blunter tip than the original Quincke point decreased the incidence of nerve injury [53]. The use of nerve stimulation and ultrasound (below) to localize needle placement further reduced the incidence of nerve injury.

Early catheters for epidural use were adapted from ureteral catheters. Development of smaller gauge Tuohy-type needles in the 1970s–1980s, demanded a parallel development of smaller epidural catheters that passed through an 18 or 19-gauge needle, and were flexible yet rigid enough to maintain patency indefinitely. First adopted for obstetrical anesthesia, these catheters became the mainstay for postoperative analgesia both for continuous peridural blockade, and in the 1990s, for continuous blockade of peripheral nerves for both inpatients and outpatients. They expanded the ability to provide prolonged analgesia.

Pumps

The small catheters prompted the development of portable mechanical and electrical pumps to deliver local anesthetic solutions for 2–3 days. These infusions improved analgesia after major joint replacements and shoulder and knee procedures, expediting a return to movement. Several large series documented the safety and efficacy of these techniques, and by the 2000s they became popular for pain relief following peripheral orthopedic surgery [54].

Epidural Opioid Analgesia

In the 1980s, opioids placed in the spinal and epidural space were shown to provide segmental analgesia without anesthesia or systemic opioid effects. Tony Yaksh demonstrated the analgesic effects of epidural and subarachnoid morphine in rats [55]. Application of these results to humans showed that postoperative epidural opioid infusions provided efficacious pain relief after major abdominal and thoracic surgery [56, 57]. Subsequent clinical studies in the departments of Bonica and Moore demonstrated that these drugs could be given safely on hospital wards [58] with patient-controlled devices [59].

Addition of small concentrations of local anesthetic, such as 0.05–0.0625 % bupivacaine, enhanced analgesia, and hastened the return of bowel function [60] and the ability to ambulate. By 2000, it was accepted that epidural opioid-local anesthetic solutions provided superior analgesia for upper abdominal and thoracic surgery [61]. There was improved patient outcome with reduced pulmonary [62] and cardiac [63] complications, and a reduction in the potential to develop chronic pain syndromes after surgery [64].

Nothing is perfect, however. This approach to pain management can produce rare instances of respiratory depression, with an incidence that may be no greater than following parenteral opioids. It is not yet clear whether lipid soluble opioids (e.g., fentanyl and sufentanil), injected intrathecally, act on spinal cord activity or are effective because of systemic absorption and a subsequent action on the brain—or both.

Ultrasound Nerve Localization

Investigators from the University of Vienna in the 1990s first described ultrasound technology for identification of peripheral nerves [65, 66]. Ultrasound guidance enhanced the ability to identify nerves, enabling reduced volumes of anesthetic to be used, with potentially fewer complications. It was soon widely applied, including for peripheral nerves previously avoided because of their deeper location, e.g., the mid-femoral sciatic nerve. The ultrasound approach decreased patient discomfort, compared with the paresthesia technique or with the muscle contractions associated with the nerve stimulator. More importantly, the approach allowed identification of normal variations in anatomy that had previously presented difficulties in locating nerves using standard surface land-marks. Because this approach allowed observation of the tip of the needle during the entire performance of the block, ultrasound could also increase safety, by facilitating avoidance of intravascular and intraneural injections. Further research is needed to substantiate these advantages, but ultrasound localization is rapidly becoming the technique of choice for identification of peripheral nerves [67]. It is presently limited by the cost of equipment.

The Internet

Internet technology has expanded the teaching of regional techniques. Vincent Chan at the University of Toronto (usra. ca), and Brian Sites at Dartmouth College (dhmc.org) have contributed to this form of information about regional anesthesia. The "New York School of Regional Anesthesia" (NYSORA.com) established by Admir Hadzic in 1994 with Jerry Vloka has a detailed website. This group, based at St. Luke's Roosevelt Hospital (the home of Halsted's original experimentation with cocaine in the 1880s), has established an extensive educational support for regional anesthesia, including workshops, educational programs, and the most recent textbook on the subject.

Reflections

The history of regional anesthesia has been colorful and tumultuous, filled in its early days with self-experimentation, daring and charismatic personalities, and evangelical supporters. The initial enthusiasm retreated before the advance in new general anesthetic drugs and anesthetic adjuvants in the 1930s to 1950s. It took the introduction of long-acting local anesthetics and development of techniques for their safe use in the last quarter of the century that resurrected the fortunes of regional anesthesia. The development of new delivery techniques, particularly ultrasound guidance and continuous epidural and peripheral nerve catheters has supported the renaissance of regional blockade. The detailed and rigorous science of the last 30 years has confirmed a critical role for regional anesthesia and analgesia as a superior perioperative technique, one that the early pioneers may have only partially envisioned, but one they would certainly be pleased with.

References

1. von Anrep B. Über die physiologische Wirkung des Cocain. Pflugers Arch. 1880;21:38.
2. Freud S. Über Coca. Centralbl Gesamte Ther. 1884;289–314.
3. Koller C. On the use of cocaine for producing anaesthesia on the eye. Lancet. 1884;2:990.

4. Halsted W. Practical comments on the use and abuse of cocaine, suggested by its invariably successful employment in more than a thousand minor surgical operations. N Y Med J. 1885;42:327.

5. Corning J. Spinal anaesthesia and local medication of the cord with cocaine. N Y Med J. 1885;42:483.

6. Bier A. Versuche über Cocainisirung des Ruckenmarkes. Dtsch Z chir. 1899;5151:361.

7. Tait D, Caglieri G. Experimental and clinical notes on the subarachnoid space. Transactions Medical Society of California, JAMA. 1900;35:6.

8. Jonnesco T. Remarks on general spinal anesthesia. Brit Med J. 1909;2:1396–401.

9. Link W. Alfred Einhorn. Sc.D., :inventor of novacaine. Dent Radiograph Photogr. 1959;32:1–20.

10. Braun H. Über einige neue ortliche anaesthetica. Dtsch Med Wochenschr. 1905;31:1667–71.

11. Braun H. Local anesthesia: its scientific basis and practical use. 3rd edn. Philadelphia:Lea & Febiger; 1914.

12. Covino B. One hundred years plus two of regional anesthesia. Reg Anesth. 1986;11:105–17.

13. Labat G. Regional anesthesia: its technic and practical application. New York: W. B. Saunders Co.; 1922.

14. Brown DL, Winnie AP. Biography of Louis Gaston Labat, M.D. Regional Anesth. 1992;17:249–62.

15. Mandabach MG, Wright AJ. The American Society of Regional Anesthesia: a concise history of the original group-it's birth, growth, and eventual dissolution. Reg Anesth Pain Med. 2006;31:53–65.

16. Bacon DR, Darwish H. Emery A. Rovenstine and regional anesthesia. Reg Anesth. 1997;22:273–9.

17. Tetzlaff JE, Lautsenheiser F, Estafanous FG. Dr. George Crile—early contributions to the theoretic basis for twenty-first century pain medicine. Reg Anesth Pain Med. 2004;29:600–5.

18. Pitkin GP. Spinocain: the controllable spinal anesthetic. BMJ. 1929;2:183–9.

19. Rosenberg H, Axelrod JK. Two surgeons who popularized spinal anesthesia. Reg Anesth Pain Med. 2001;26:278–82.

20. Pitkin GP. Conduction anesthesia. Philadelphia: Lippincott; 1946.

21. Eckenhoff JE. A wide angle view of anesthesiology. Emery a. Rovenstine Memorial Lecture. Anesthesiology. 1978;48:272.

22. Lahey F. The removal of broken spinal anesthesia needles. JAMA. 1929;93:518–9.

23. Lundy JS. The present states of balanced anesthesia and balanced supportive therapy. Proc Staff Meet Mayo Clin. 1951;26:191–4.

24. Edwards W, Hingson R. Continuous caudal anesthesia in obstetrics. Am J Surg. 1942;57:459–64.

25. Tuohy E. Continuous spinal anesthesia: its usefulness and technique involved. Anesthesiology. 1944;5:142.

26. Dogliotti A. Eine neue Methode der regionaren Anasthesie. Zentralbl Chir. 1931;58:3141–5.

27. Curbelo M. Continuous peridural segmental anesthesia by means of a ureteral catheter. Anesth Analg. 1949;28:13–23.

28. Stoeckel W. Über sakrale anasethesie. Zentralbi Gynaekol. 1909;33:1.

29. Manalan SA. Caudal block anesthesia in obstetrics. J Indiana State Med Assoc. 1942;35:564.

30. Marx GF. Personal reflections on 50 years of obstetric anesthesia. Reg Anesth. 1990;15:232–6.

31. Chadwick H. Obstetric anesthesia—then and now. Minerva Anesthesiol. 2005;71:517–20.

32. The method was good but the patient died, editor (Henry Ruth) Anesthesiology. 1950;11:254–5.

33. Cole F. A defense of spinal anesthesia. Anesthesiology. 1952;13:407–15.

34. Kennedy F, Effron AS, Perry G. The grave spinal cord paralysis caused by spinal anesthesia. SGO. 1950;91:385–98.

35. Cope RW. The Woolley and Roe case. Anaesthesia. 1954;9:249–69.

36. Dripps RD, Vandam LD. Long-term follow-up of patients who received 10,098 spinal anesthetics: failure to discover major neurological sequelae. J Am Med Assoc. 1954;156:1486–91.

37. Moore DC. Pontocaine solutions for regional analgesia other than spinal and epidural block: an analysis of 2,500 cases. JAMA. 1951;146:803–8.

38. Moore DC. Regional block. Springfield: Charles Thomas; 1953.

39. Covino B. One hundred years plus two of regional anesthesia. Reg Anesth. 1986;11:105–17.

40. Ostheimer GW, Palahniuk RJ, Shnider SM. Epidural blood patch for post-lumbar-puncture headache. Anesthesiology. 1974;41:307–8.

41. Marx GE. Obstetric anesthesia organizations in the United States. Anesthesiology. 1974;41:308–10.

42. Wildsmith JAW. Donald Bruce Scott, M.D., F.R.C.A., F.R.C.P.Ed. Reg Anesth Pain Med. 1999;24:195–6.

43. Bromage PR. Epidural analgesia. Philadelphia: W. B. Saunders Co.; 1978.

44. Winnie AP. Interscalene brachial plexus block. Anesth Analg. 1970;49:455–66.

45. Winnie A, Buckhèoj P, Höakansson L. Plexus anesthesia: perivascular techniques of brachial plexus block. Elsevier Health Sciences; 1984.

46. Winnie AP. Diary of a dream: the American Society of Regional Anesthesia (for Surgery, Obstetrics, and Pain Control). Reg Anesth Pain Med. 2006;31:569–74.

47. Albright GA. Cardiac arrest following regional anesthesia with etidocaine or bupivacaine. Anesthesiology. 1979;51:285–7.

48. Reisner LS, Hochman BN, Plumer MH. Persistent neurologic deficit and adhesive arachnoiditis following intrathecal 2-chloroprocaine injection. Anesth Analg. 1980;59:452–4.

49. Clarkson CW, Hondeghem LM. Mechanism for bupivacaine depression of cardiac conduction: fast block of sodium channels during the action potential with slow recovery from block during diastole. Anesthesiology. 1985;62:396–405.

50. Mulroy MF, Norris MC, Liu SS. Safety steps for epidural injection of local anesthetics: review of the literature and recommendations. Anesth Analg. 1997;85:1346–56.

51. Weinberg GL, VadeBoncouer T, Ramaraju GA, Garcia-Amaro MF, Cwik MJ. Pretreatment or resuscitation with a lipid infusion shifts the dose-response to bupivacaine-induced asystole in rats. Anesthesiology. 1998;88:1071–5.

52. Zaric D, Christiansen C, Pace NL, Punjasawadwong Y. Transient neurologic symptoms (TNS) following spinal anaesthesia with lidocaine versus other local anaesthetics. Cochrane Database Syst Rev. 2003;2:CD003006.

53. Selander D. Peripheral nerve injury caused by injection needles. Br J Anaesth. 1993;71:323–5.

54. Richman JM, Liu SS, Courpas G, Wong R, Rowlingson AJ, McGready J, Cohen SR, Wu CL. Does continuous peripheral nerve block provide superior pain control to opioids? A meta-analysis. Anesth Analg. 2006;102:248–57.

55. Yaksh TL, Rudy TA. Analgesia mediated by a direct spinal action of narcotics. Science. 1976 25;192:1357–8.

56. Wang JK, Nauss LA, Thomas JE. Pain relief by intrathecally applied morphine in man. Anesthesiology. 1979;50:149–51.

57. Behar M, Magora F, Olshwang D, Davidson JT. Epidural morphine in treatment of pain. Lancet. 1979 Mar 10;1(8115):527–9.

58. Ready LB, Loper KA, Nessly M, Wild L. Postoperative epidural morphine is safe on surgical wards. Anesthesiology. 1991;75:452–6.

59. Liu SS, Allen HW, Olsson GL. Patient-controlled epidural analgesia with bupivacaine and fentanyl on hospital wards: prospective experience with 1,030 surgical patients. Anesthesiology. 1998;88:688–95.

60. Steinbrook RA. Epidural anesthesia and gastrointestinal motility. Anesth Analg. 1998;86:837–44.

61. Liu SS, Wu CL. The effect of analgesic technique on postoperative patient-reported outcomes including analgesia: a systematic review. Anesth Analg. 2007;105:789–808.

62. Ballantyne JC, Carr DC, deFerranti S et al. The comparative effects of postoperative analgesic therapies on pulmonary outcome: cumulative meta-analyses of randomized, controlled trials. Anesth Analg. 1998;86:598–612.

63. Beattie WS, Badner NH, Choi PT. Meta-analysis demonstrates statistically significant reduction in postoperative myocardial infarction with the use of thoracic epidural analgesia. Anesth Analg. 2003;97:919–2.

64. De Kock M. Expanding our horizons: transition of acute postoperative pain to persistent pain and establishment of chronic postsurgical pain services. Anesthesiology. 2009;111:461–3.

65. Kapral S, Krafft P, Eibenberger K, Fitzgerald R, Gosch M, Weinstabl C. Ultrasound-guided supraclavicular approach for regional anesthesia of the brachial plexus. Anesth Analg. 1994;78:507–13.

66. Marhofer P, Schrögendorfer K, Koinig H, Kapral S, Weinstabl C, Mayer N. Ultrasonographic guidance improves sensory block and onset time of three-in-one blocks. Anesth Analg. 1997;85:854–7.

67. Neal JM, Brull R, Chan VW, Grant SA, Horn JL, Liu SS, McCartney CJ, Narouze SN, Perlas A, Salinas FV, Sites BD, Tsui BC. The ASRA evidence-based medicine assessment of ultrasound-guided regional anesthesia and pain medicine: executive summary. Reg Anesth Pain Med. 2010;35(Suppl 2):S1–9.

A History of Neuroanesthesia

64

Elizabeth A. M. Frost

Summary

Many countries practiced trephination from 10,000 BCE. Cocaine spat in the wound may have minimized pain in Peru. Alcohol, laudanum, henbane, opium or lettuces may have been used in other countries. The 1,700 BCE Edwin Smith Papyrus described the effects of central nervous system trauma.

Surgeons pioneered neurosurgical anesthesia. Horsley in the UK preferred chloroform, and with physical chemist Harcourt, he constructed a vaporizer for chloroform delivery. The Scot Macewen developed metal tubes for tracheal intubation in 1878, and he trained his residents in anesthesia. Cannon monitored intracranial pressure (ICP) in 1901. In the early 1900s, Krause fathered German neurosurgery and introduced operations to treat epilepsy. He used chloroform to produce hypotension and decrease bleeding. Butzengeiger and Eichholtz used tribromethanol in 1923 for neurosurgery as did Dandy in 1931 to decrease ICP. Anesthetists Magill and Rowbotham introduced tracheal intubation to manage neurosurgery in the early 1930s. By 1930, Cushing had decreased neurosurgical mortality from 50–60 % to about 10 %. With Codman, he developed the prototype of today's anesthetic record. White in Boston showed that anesthetics, increased carbon dioxide, and oxygen lack all increased ICP.

Research in neuroanesthesia accelerated in the late 1950s. In 1952, Faulconer developed electroencephalographic monitoring, and Stockard and Bickford's 1972 compressed spectral arrays made EEG patterns comprehensible to most anesthesiologists. In the 1960s, anesthesiologist Wollman and colleagues, defined the cerebrovascular effects of hypotension, hyperventilation and anesthetics. Physiologist Rehder with anesthesiologist Theye, and surgeons Kirklin and MacCarty, applied profound hypothermia during aneurysm clipping. Anesthesiologist Michenfelder fostered neuroanesthesia as a specialty in the US, particularly with his 1969 review. He studied cerebral protection from hypothermia and anesthetics, incidentally devising measures of cerebral blood flow and metabolism. In the 1970s, Shapiro studied ventilation-induced ICP changes, and began neuroanesthetic intensive care. In 1947, Dawson described evoked potential monitoring, and in 1982, Grundy made it popular.

In the UK, Hunter published the first modern book on neuroanesthesia in 1964, and Canadian Gilbert published the second in 1966. 36 anesthesiologists and 4 neurosurgeons formed the Neurosurgical Anesthesia Society in 1973. In 1976, the American Society of Anesthesiologists recognized neuroanesthesia as a subspecialty society. In 1989, the Journal of Neurosurgical Anesthesiology arose from the Newsletter of the Society of Neurosurgical Anesthesia and Critical Care.

Neuroanesthesia resulted from collaboration with other specialists and will be needed to answer questions regarding monitoring of intracranial dynamics, brain survival after head injury, spinal cord regeneration, and long-term cerebral effects of anesthetic agents.

Introduction

Neuroanesthesia would not exist without neurosurgery. Nor would neurosurgery have developed so successfully without advances in anesthesia and other areas. For example, the ubiquitous use of cautery required nonexplosive agents; intracranial maneuvering required meticulous respiratory and hemodynamic control; adaptations had to be made for off site locations; and the patient had to remain immobile for hours but awaken promptly without systemic sequelae. What follows is a chronology of these stories. While surgery on the central nervous system has been practiced for many millennia, the advances made over the past 150 years, many due to developments made by pharmacologists, physiologists, and anesthesiologists, far outweigh any previous progress.

E. A. M. Frost (✉)
Department of Anesthesiology, Icahn Medical
Center at Mount Sinai, New York, NY, USA
e-mail: elzfrost@aol.com

E. I Eger II et al. (eds.), *The Wondrous Story of Anesthesia,* DOI 10.1007/978-1-4614-8441-7_64, © Edmond I Eger, MD 2014

Ancient Times

The oldest known medical papyrus, the Edwin Smith Papyrus, was written in black and red hieratic, the Egyptian cursive form of hieroglyphs. It dates from the seventeenth century BCE and is named for American Egyptologist, Edwin Smith (1822–1906) who purchased the manuscript in two parts from Mustapha Agha in Luxor in 1862 [1]. Some attributed authorship of the manuscript to the writer of a much earlier treatise, the priest and physician of the Old Kingdom, Imhotep (3,000–2,500 BCE). Sixty-nine explanatory notes (glosses) appear to have been added several hundred years after 1,600 BCE [2, 3]. With the medical advice of Arno Luckhardt (of ethylene fame) in 1930, James Breasted provided the first translation of the papyrus [3]. Breasted's translation demonstrated that Egyptian medical care was not limited to the magical modes of healing postulated in other Egyptian medical sources, such as the Ebers Papyrus. Rational, scientific practices followed from observation and examination [4]. The rare book section of the New York Academy of Medicine houses the Smith papyrus (at present on long term loan to the Metropolitan Museum of Art in New York). Allen, the curator at the Metropolitan Museum, undertook subsequent interpretations of the text.

The discourse describes 48 typical (rather than individual) surgical cases, most involving trauma to the head, neck, face and spinal cord. Each case is divided into case or diagnosis, examination, and a treatment decision. Rational surgical treatments are differentiated from the much less employed medico-magical measures. Treatment options are classified as: "An ailment which I will treat"; "An ailment with which I will contend"; or "An ailment not to be treated".

The papyrus also describes the cranial sutures and fontanelles, the meninges, the external surface of the brain, the cerebrospinal fluid, and intracranial pulsations [3, 5]. The symptoms and signs of brain injury are given. Feeble pulse and fever predict hopeless injuries. Deafness and aphasia follow fractures of the temporal region [6]. Immobilization is advised for head and spinal cord injuries, as well as lower body fractures. Surgical stitching of wounds of the lip, throat, and shoulder are described [6]. So are dressings, including the application of fresh meat (to stop bleeding) [6] and honey (honey is still used, especially in war zones, as a type of occlusive and antiseptic dressing). Case 8 describes hemiplegic contractures. Injuries of the cervical spine are noted to change body functions. In Case 31, for example, quadriplegia, urinary incontinence, priapism, and seminal emission followed cervical vertebral dislocation.

Although the patient in Case 4 obviously has pain, the author does not attempt to advise analgesia despite knowledge of drugs such as the poppy [4]. For example:

> "If thou examinest a man having a wound in his temple, penetrating to the bone, (and) perforating his temporal bone, while his two eyes are blood shot, he discharges blood from both his

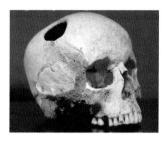

Fig. 64.1 A trephined skull from 3,500 BC demonstrates a rounded edge of the hole, indicating that healing had taken place and that the patient had survived the procedure. (From Wikipedia, accessed 3 June 12)

> nostrils, and a little drops; if thou puttest thy fingers on the mouth of that wound (and) he shudder exceedingly; if thou ask of him concerning his malady and he speak not to thee; Thou shouldst say concerning him: 'One having a wound in his temple, penetrating to the bone, (and) perforating his temporal bone; while he discharges blood from both his nostrils, he suffers with stiffness in his neck, (and) he is speechless. An ailment not to be treated.'"

Trephination: The Cure All

Nowhere does the Edwin Smith treatise mention trephination (trepanation), although it was probably performed in the Mesolithic period (10,000 BCE–5,000 BCE) and continued to modern times. Skulls excavated from graves in all countries of the world except China, Japan, the Malay Peninsula and Australia reveal rounded, often multiple defects, suggestive of trephination. Many show evidence of healing without infection (Fig. 64.1) [7]. A seizure state may have prompted trephination. So might have headache, a passage into manhood, or spiritual or religious reasons such as removal of amulets or postmortem embalming. It may have been used to clean wounds after trauma in battle [8]. Trephination was a form of primitive emergency surgery after head wounds [9] to remove shattered fragments of bone from a fractured skull, and clean out the blood that often pools under the skull after a blow to the head. Such injuries were typical for primitive weaponry such as slingshot projectiles and war clubs. Hippocrates, who also decribed the systemic effects of head injury, recommended trephination for simple skull fractures and for contusions of the brain without fractures, in this latter case to prevent bad consequences [9, 10].

Surgeons believed that boring a hole in a patient's head would increase the brain's metabolism (that is, replace depression with happiness), heighten cranial blood flow (release tension as caused by a hematoma within the cranium), or release evil spirits that resided within the skull. Many "patients" survived, as shown by signs of healing in their skulls [8]. (Fig. 64.1) Individuals undergoing trephination for spiritual reasons reported a new and glorious understanding of themselves and the world around them. In addition, this "third eye" was said to bestow psychic abilities and an understanding of mysticism upon the patient. Some reported that trephination heightened the body's senses.

During the Middle Ages, did the familiar haircut of monks and friars (a ring of hair around the circumference of the head) evolve from holy men who had tops of their heads shaved in preparation for trephination? The phrase, "I need that (some unwanted object) like I need a hole in the head," may be a throwback to trephination.

Trephination, or trepanning as preferred by some authors and cultures, persisted in primitive civilizations until the early twentieth century [11]. Although widely considered to be pseudoscience, the practice of trephination continues in some societies. Proponents point to "recent research" on the increase in cranial compliance following trephination, with increase in blood flow, as justifying the practice. They believe that once the skull is opened, it introduces oxygen, which provides knowledge, significant of a divinity. Some individuals have practiced non-emergency trephination for psychic purposes [12]. A prominent proponent of this view is Peter Halvorson, who, in 1962 drilled a hole in the front of his own skull to increase "brain blood volume" [13]. In 1998, he established the International Trepanation Advocacy Group, which mantains a website and purports to support research into this practice. Theoretical support for the benefits of self-trephination, was offered by Bart Huges (or Hughes, 1934–2004) who claimed that trepanantion increased "brain blood volume" and thereby enhanced cerebral metabolism in a manner similar to cerebral vasodilators such as ginko biloba. No published results support these claims. Huges, a Dutch librarian published "The Mechanism of Brainblood-volume ('BBV')" (also known as "Homo Sapiens Correc-tus") in 1964. Based on an ancient belief, he proposed that when mankind began to walk upright, brains drained of blood while trephination allowed blood to flow in and out of the brain better, causing permanent euphoria.

How was pain minimized for trephination? Coca leaves were widely used in Peru. Perhaps an early anesthetist chewed the leaves and spat in the wound, a technique described for centuries in South America—but possibly ineffective because of the small amount of free cocaine in coca. Or perhaps as in the painting ascribed to Heironymus Bosch (1450–1516), "Extraction of the stone of madness", the figure standing to the side held a jug of wine at the ready (Fig. 64.2). While Bosch was known for his fantastic imagery illustrating moral and religious concepts and narratives, in recent decades, scholars have also viewed his art as reflecting then orthodox religious beliefs.

Peter Treveris is credited with an engraving in the "Handywarke of Surgeri" by Heironymus von Braunschweig, showing the method of trephination in 1525. Treveris also published "The Grete Herball" in two editions in 1526 and 1529. This compendium of herbal and plant remedies was translated from the French "Le Grant Herbier". The author describes laudanum, henbane, opium and lettuces as narcotics for pain relief. These preparations and alcohol may have been used during these procedures.

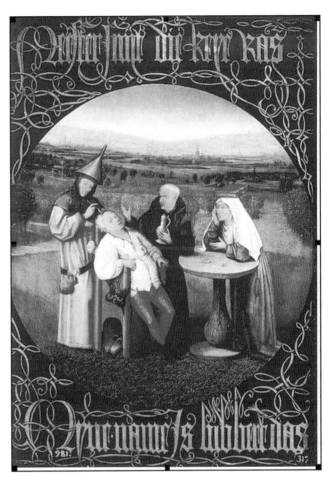

Fig. 64.2 A surgeon makes a hole in the skull while an assistant stands by with a pitcher of wine. (Attributed to Heironymous Bosch, 1450–1516, from "The Extraction of the Stone", 1490, oil painting, Museo del Prado. From Wikipedia, accessed 3 June 12.)

The use of trephination declined in the nineteenth century. In 1829, Astley Cooper, a consulting surgeon to Guy's hospital in London wrote "Trephining in concussion is now so completely abandoned that in the last 4 years I do not know that I have performed it once, while 35 years ago I would have performed it 5 or 6 times a year". More advanced medicine replaced the practice: bleeding, purges and application of leeches [14].

Nineteenth Century and the Discovery of Anesthesia

After the momentous demonstration by William Morton on 16 October 1846, knowledge and application of the benefits of ether, and then chloroform, (James Simpson, 4 November 1847) spread quickly around the world. However, anesthesia for neurosurgical procedures was slow to be accepted, perhaps because it was recognized that the brain does not possess pain endings, and thus unconsciousness might not be necessary. Also the dangers of working within the brain might mandate a responsive patient.

A notable case illustrating the dangers of anesthesia achieved local fame. In Lumberton, New Jersey, on 7 February 1887, Mary Anderson was shot in the head by her thwarted lover [15]. Two weeks later, 4 prominent physicians, Girdner, Spitzka, Pancoast, and Spiller assembled in a tiny cottage, and with a telephonic probe[1] tried to locate and remove the bullet. Under ether anesthesia and breathing spontaneously, her condition rapidly deteriorated as her brain swelled and the procedure was abandoned. She died without regaining consciousness a further 2 weeks later. Her assassin was accused, tried, convicted and executed.

During the nineteenth century, several prominent surgeons, especially neurosurgeons, made important advances in anesthetic techniques for neurosurgery.

Victor Horsley (1857–1916)

In the latter part of the nineteenth century, a few general surgeons performed neurosurgery. Chipault in France and von Bergman and Krause in Germany, Macewen in Scotland, and Keen in the US all performed cranial and spinal procedures as well as general surgery. Victor Horsley studied neurophysiology extensively in his early career. He was also a leader in the temperance movement in the UK, having observed many inebriated head injured patients admitted to hosptial. Horsley was the first neurosurgeon appointed to the hospital in Queen Square, London, now called the National Hospital for Neurology and Neurosurgery—the Victor Horsley Department of Neurosurgery is named in his honor. The Walton Centre for Neurology & Neurosurgery NHS Trust in Liverpool, England, another leading Neurosurgical Hospital dedicated their Intensive Care Unit to Sir Victor Horsley and is called the Horsley ward [16].

Horsley investigated the intracranial effects of chloroform, ether and morphine after experimenting on himself (Fig. 64.3). He concluded that because ether caused hypertension, excessive bleeding, postoperative vomiting and general excitement, it was not to be used in neurosurgery [17]. He considered morphine valuable because of the apparent increase in cerebral blood flow and more readily controlled hemmorhage in the surgical field. The respiratory

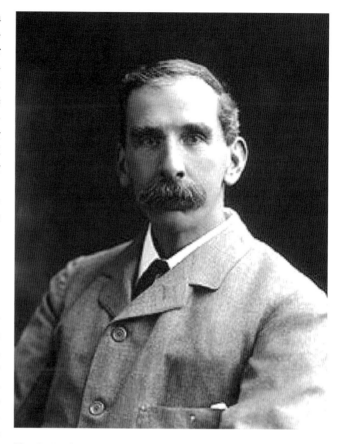

Fig. 64.3 Victor Horsely photograph accessed from Wikimedia Commons, 3 Aug 13.

depression caused by the opioid (an effect that he had noted from self experimentation) could also cause problems. He preferred chloroform, advising the "judicious use of chloroform to control hemmorhage [18]. However, death during chloroform anesthesia was all too common. In 1890, the Hyderabad Commission concluded that death was due to respiratory failure. The need for control of the dose remained unclear, although it was realized that slightly less than 2 % chloroform induced anesthesia and much less allowed maintenance. It was argued that this amount might just as easily be achieved, by sprinkling the liquid onto a cloth. Horsley disagreed and together with a physical chemist, Vernon Harcourt, developed an inhaler that could control the percentage of chloroform administered.

In 1901, the British Medical Association appointed a "Special Chloroform Committee" including Waller, Sherrington, Harcourt, Buxton and Horsley to introduce science to the art of anesthetic administration. The committee concluded that a chloroform dose exceeding 2 % was unsafe because the resulting inhibition of the vagus nerve could cause cardiac arrest. They determined that several inhalers were suitable for administering accurate measures of chloroform including those of Snow, Junker, Clover, Paul Bert, Harcourt, Roth-Drager, Waller and Collingwood [19].

---

[1] On 2 July 1881, President James Garfield was shot in the back while ambling through the Washington railway station. He was 49 years of age and in excellent health. Known for experiments he conducted with metal detectors in England, Alexander Graham Bell was called to the President's bedside. The metal probe which he and a team of assistants had worked to perfect, could not locate the bullet lodged in the President's back, and Garfield died from infection weeks later. Distraught over the President's untimely death, Bell worked tirelessly to create an efficient surgical probe, producing a successful model in October 1881. He named his invention the telephonic probe.

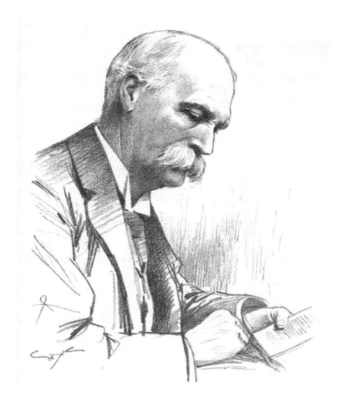

Fig. 64.4 William Macewen. (From Wikimedia commons, accessed 3 June 12.)

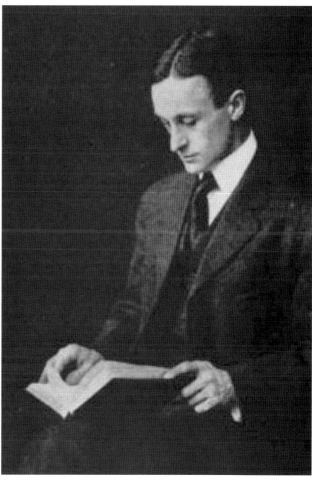

Fig. 64.5 A photograph of Harvey Cushing taken around 1900. (From Wikimedia commons, accessed 3 June 12.)

Harcourt's inhaler delivered no more than 2% chloroform. Horsley believed that administration should be reduced to <0.5% after bone removal during craniotomy, because of potentially adverse effects on intracranial dynamics [18].

William Macewen (1848–1924)

Macewen, medical superintendent of the Glasgow Fever Hospital, dealt with many deaths from respiratory obstruction due to diphtheria. (Fig. 64.4) He developed metal tubes that he inserted into the tracheas of cadavers, and then patients, following the observations of Desault some 100 years previously. He reported the case of a Glaswegian who popped a hot potato into his mouth. A few hours later and after some libation, the man had difficulty breathing and went to the emergency room of the Royal Infirmary. Macewen passed a metal tube into the Glaswegian's trachea and relieved the obstruction. On 5 July 1878, he passed a tube into the larynx of a patient before inducing chloroform anesthesia for removal of an epithelioma from the base of the tongue [20]. He later developed red rubber tubes that were better tolerated by patients, especially those with diphtheria, when the intubation was maintained for 36 hours or longer [19].

After an anesthetic death and much national publicity, a resolution was adopted on 7 March 1883, in Glasgow, requiring training in anesthetics for all medical students and

clerks [21]. Formal anesthetic training was not adopted in the rest of Britain until 1911. In the US, although the American Board of Anesthesiology was established in 1938, formal training for all medical students has only slowly been accepted, and is still not universal, similar to that in many 3rd world countries.

Macewen became a leader in neurosurgery in the UK. He demanded that his patients be anesthetized only by residents that had been appropriately trained and certified under his supervision.

Harvey Cushing (1869–1939)

An American pioneer of neurosurgery and anesthesia, Cushing studied at Yale and Harvard Universities, and trained at Johns Hopkins Hospital with William Halsted (Fig. 64.5). During his residency with Halsted, he became interested in neurosurgery and determined to develop better diagnostic methods, becoming one of the first in American surgery to employ X-rays.

As a medical student he was asked to stand in for the anesthetist Frank Lyman. As recounted in other chapters in this book, Cushing's anesthetic ended in disaster. As the surgery began, the patient vomited, aspirated the vomit, and died.

> "To my perfect amazement I was told it was nothing at all, that I had nothing to do with the man's death, that he had a strangulated hernia and had been vomiting all night anyway, and that sort of thing happened frequently and I had better forget about it and go on with the medical school. I went on with the medical school but I have never forgotten about it [22]."

True to his word, Cushing never forgot this terrible event, and to the benefit of anesthesia, he did something about it [23]. With Codman, Cushing developed the anesthetic record on which anesthetists noted the patient's heart rate and blood pressure (itself, a new measurement in medicine) at five minute intervals, an approach little different from that used in today's anesthetic record. His suggestions were not immediately accepted. In 1903, a Harvard Medical School committee considered "the importance of blood pressure observation in surgical diagnosis and treatment". The committee concluded that the skilled finger was of much greater value clinically for determination of the state of circulation than any pneumatic instrument. They suggested that Cushing's work (and also George Crile's work in Cleveland) should be put aside.

Cushing appeared to agree:

> "I am not so sure that the general use of a blood pressure apparatus in clinical work has done more than harm. Just as Floyer's pulse watch led to two previously unknown diseases, tachycardia and bradycardia, so the sphygmomanometer has led to the uncovering of the diseases of hypertension and hypotension which have vastly added to the number of neuroasthenics in the world" [24].

Cushing became professor of surgery at Harvard Medical School (and chief of surgery at the Peter Bent Brigham Hospital in Boston) in 1912. A perfectionist, he brought to neurosurgery crucial refinements in pre-operative preparation and operative technique. His skill reduced the mortality rate of brain operations from 50–60%, to about 10% by 1930 [25].

In 1898, inspired by Halsted's work with local anesthesia and by observations of deaths under ether anesthesia, Cushing applied local infiltration of cocaine to his surgeries, especially brain cases, but also to hernia and thyroid operations [25]. He kept detailed records of his work, insisting that records similar to current anesthetic records (see above) be maintained on his patients.

Fedor Krause (1857–1937)

The father of German neurosurgery, Krause introduced operations to treat epilepsy into Germany, performing over 400 operations on epileptic patients during his career (Fig. 64.6). He is also remembered for his work in plastic surgery, and

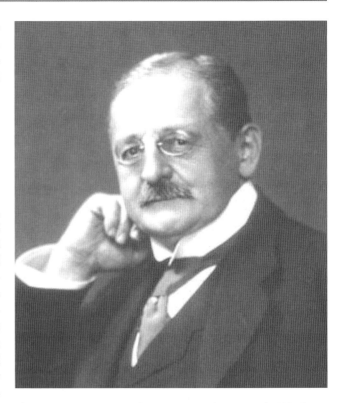

Fig. 64.6 A photograph of Fedor Krause from around 1930. (From Medscape; Source Neurosurg Focus Copyright American Association of Neurological Surgeons.)

was an early practitioner of intraoperative electrostimulation of the cerebral cortex. He developed operative techniques for tumors of the brain and spinal cord.

Krause was also concerned about the neurosurgical implications of anesthetic actions. As an assistant to Richard Volkman, Krause noted the effects of morphine-chloroform anesthesia, and was unconvinced that it offered advantages for neurosurgical procedures. He preferred chloroform alone, [26] but recognized the usefulness of small doses of morphine for postoperative pain relief. He felt that increased venous bleeding offset the safety of ether, and reserved its use for patients with cardiac failure. He advocated increasing the concentration of chloroform to produce controlled hypotension and decrease bleeding during tumor extirpation. He also noted that sudden death might occur if respiration ceased during tumor surgery (respiration was mainly spontaneous or controlled by an assistant under the drapes holding a mask to the patient's face), and he preferred the Roth Drager apparatus that allowed administration of 100% oxygen. Like others, he emphasized that the brain was insensitive to pain, indicating the need for only light planes of narcotization [26]. Nevertheless he did not advocate local anesthesia, believing that pain was not the only problem. Optimum patient preparation for surgery demanded a positive attitude and calmness. Severe anxiety could contribute to death. He concluded that a good outcome required a rapid, aseptic technique, minimal blood loss, normothermia and general

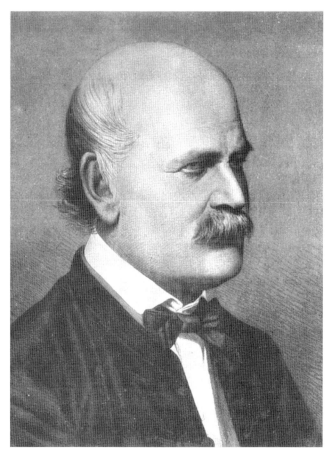

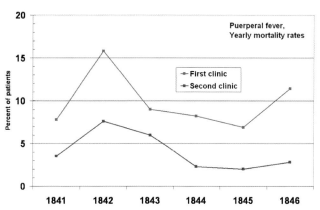

Fig. 64.8 Puerperal fever mortality rates for the first and second clinic at the Vienna General Hospital 1841–6 differed. The first clinic, run by doctors, had a higher mortality rate than did the second, run by mid-wives. (From Wikimedia commons, accessed 3 June 12.)

Fig. 64.7 Ignaz Semmelweis was aged 42 when this pen sketch by Jeno Dopy was made in 1860. (From Wikimedia commons, accessed 3 June 12.)

anesthesia, noting that spinal procedures were amenable to local infiltration [27].

Semmelweis and Clean Hands

The frequency of wound infection, which Horsley found to be as high as 40%, hindered the advancement of surgery and thus also of anesthesia. Ignaz Semmelweis (1818–1865) was a Hungarian physician and early pioneer in the use of antiseptic procedures (Fig. 64.7). Described as the "savior of mothers" [6] Semmelweis discovered that hand disinfection in post partum obstetric clinics drastically decreased the incidence of puerperal fever [28]. In mid-nineteenth-century hospitals, puerperal fever was common and often fatal, with mortality rates of 10%–35%. Semmelweis worked in Vienna General Hospital's First Obstetric Clinic where patients on doctors' wards had three times the mortality of those on the Second Obstetric Clinic, the midwives' wards (Fig. 64.8). He noted that the doctors performed autopsies on patients dying of peurperal fever, but the midwives did not. Semmelweiss postulated that washing of hands and arms with chlorinated lime solutions, especially after cadaveric dissection, would reduce infection rates.

Semmelweis' astounding results showed that hand-washing reduced infection to less than 1%, but such data conflicted with contemporary scientific and medical opinions, and the medical community rejected his ideas. The suggestion that they should wash their hands offended doctors, and Semmelweis could not offer a scientific explanation for his findings. His ideas finally earned widespread acceptance years after his death, when Louis Pasteur (1822–1895) confirmed the germ theory by proving that microorganism (yeast) growth causes fermentation, and that bacteria emerge in nutrient broths from biogenesis and not from spontaneous generation [29]. In 1865, Semmelweis was committed to an asylum, where he died at age 47. It is not clear whether he died of a beating or, ironically, of septicemia.

Lister, von Bergman, Antisepsis and Asepsis

A stream of discoveries provided the knowledge and means to minimize, abolish, and treat infection. In 1867, Joseph Lister (1827–1912), Professor of Surgery at the Royal Infirmary in Glasgow, killed bacteria in the air and on the skin with a carbolic acid spray, thereby giving the world antisepsis. Other antiseptic rituals such as the use of masks, operating gowns, hats, and sterile gloves evolved thereafter. In 1886, Ernst von Bergmann (1836–1907) added asepsis, with his steam sterilization that ensured the sterility of instruments. Alexander Fleming grew penicillin from the mould Penicillium notatum in 1928, thereby beginning the antibiotic revolution. Together with Florey and Chain, who further refined penicillin, Fleming received the Nobel Prize in Medicine in 1945.

Anesthetic improvements had made neurosurgeons bolder, but infection had held them back. Now, advances could leap forward and with them, further anesthetic developments would appear.

Few discoveries, apart from anesthesia, spread as fast as that of X-rays. Röntgen's original paper, "*On A New Kind Of Rays*" (*Über eine neue Art von Strahlen*), appeared on 28 December 1895 [28]. X-rays had an enormous impact on surgery. Soft organs could be visualized by introducing a "contrast material". For the brain, that included the use of air to allow pneumoencepalography, a technique introduced in 1919 by the US neurosurgeon Walter Dandy. Actions of anesthesiologists have enabled the increasing use of interventional neuroradiology in ever more disease states amenable to less invasive therapy. These include interventions such as aneurysm coiling, vertebroplasty, kyphoplasty and carotid stenting. Such offsite venues can be challenging because they may lack OR-oriented personnel or a PACU, and may be equipped with unfamiliar equipment.

Early Twentieth Century

Towards the end of the nineteenth century, many substances were touted as anesthetic agents. In his 1881 textbook, *Artificial Anaesthesia and Anaesthetics*, Henry Lyman listed 47, including benzene, acetone, and kerosene. He also included an intriguing drug, puff ball (also known as Indian bread and tuckahoe), described as a curious fungus found on the roots of fir trees in the southern US [31]. Other means of inducing insensibility included hyperventilation (instructing the patient to breathe 100 times/minute) and electricity. In this last method, an insulated forceps was applied to a tooth, forming the negative electrode, while a positive electrode was held by the patient. A current was applied and the patient became insensitive, and teeth could be extracted. The surgeon directed administration of the anesthetic. Regarding the responsibilities of the anesthetist, Lyman wrote:

> "Death sometimes occurs during the use of an anaesthetic. If inhaled by the decedent in private and of his own motion, was it a case of suicide, or was it an accidental death? If administered by the hand of another…was it given by a person skilled in the theory and practice of etherization or by an individual destitute of these qualifications? [31]" This question remains for legal debate today.

Anesthetic management became an integral part of neurosurgery. In the early 1900s, open drop ether was still the technique of choice. A tourniquet was placed around the skull just above the eyes in an attempt to decrease cutaneous bleeding. Clearly there was no effect on intracranial bleeding. The development of electrocoagulation by William Bovie at Harvard made the use of open circuit explosive agents problematic [32]. Cushing introduced the use of the Bovie, a standard method of halting bleeding today, on 1 October 1926, at the Peter Bent Brigham Hospital, to facilitate removal of a vascular myeloma involving the scalp [33]. He also introduced silver clips to occlude cerebral blood vessels and staunch bleeding.

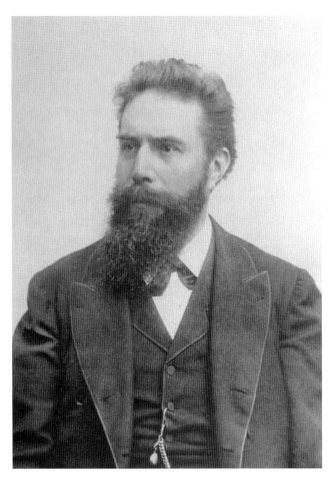

Fig. 64.9 This photograph of Wilhelm Roentgen was taken around 1900, shortly after the discovery of X-rays. (From Wikimedia commons, accessed 3 June 12.)

X-rays

Yet another breakthrough played a major role in the expansion of neuroanesthesia. During 1895, William Röntgen (1845–1923), a German physicist, discovered a new form of electromagnetic radiation while investigating the effect of passing electrical discharges through various vacuum tubes [30]. (Fig. 64.9) He named the new rays, X-rays, a designation for something unknown. Nearly two weeks after his discovery, he took the first picture using x-rays, of the hand of his wife, Anna Bertha. He later reported that at this point he determined to continue his experiments in secrecy, because he feared for his professional reputation if his observations were incorrect. X-rays (Röntgen rays) earned him the first Nobel Prize in Physics in 1901. The resulting development of imaging underlies modern devices such as fluoroscopy, computerized tomography (CT) scans, and magnetic resonance imaging. Röntgen's discovery profoundly altered surgery in more subtle ways than anesthesia and antisepsis. Before X-rays, doctors relied on their five senses. X-Rays provided a sixth sense that facilitated more precise diagnoses.

In 1919, Irish born Ivan Magill (1888–1986), accepted a post as anesthetist at the Queen's Hospital, Sidcup, a hospital established to treat facial injuries sustained by soldiers in World War I. Working with plastic surgeon Harold Gillies, and his colleague in anesthesia, Stanley Rowbotham (1890–1989), Magill developed numerous items of anesthetic equipment but most particularly the single-tube tracheal anesthesia technique, driven by the immense difficulties of using a mask to administer chloroform and ether to men with severe facial injuries. In 1920, Rowbotham described blind nasal intubation, particularly useful for surgery on the oral cavity. Magill and Rowbotham were instrumental in reintroducing tracheal intubation in 1921. Gradually adopted over the next 2 decades (it was in general use in neurosurgery by the early 1930s), it used rubber tubing rather than the flexible metal tube as developed by Macewen [34]. These developments were essential to the furtherance of neuroanesthesia.

Greater understanding of intracranial dynamics developed. The Monro-Kellie doctrine, a synthesis of the works of eighteenth century Scottish anatomist (Alexander Monro) and nineteenth century American physiologist (George Kellie), stated that the cranial cavity is a closed rigid box, and that the quantity of intracranial blood must change through the displacement or replacement of cerebrospinal fluid [35, 36].

Walter Cannon, an American physiologist (who coined the phrase "fight or flight") described intracranial pressure (ICP) monitoring in 1901, as an expansion of the work of Claude Bernard on homeostasis [37]. White et al in Boston, showed in animals, that various anesthetics perturbed ICP and that carbon dioxide accumulation and oxygen lack produced dramatic increases [38]. To minimize these concerns, Andrew Hunter advocated the use of an 8 l/min inflow of 25 % oxygen and nitrous oxide into a semi-closed anesthesia circuit [38]. His preferred opioid was heroin, in 1 mg increments for supretentorial procedures, when reduction in brain bulk was important [39]. Also, some years earlier, CB Courville published a book on adverse effects of nitrous oxide, suggesting that cortical and lenticular damage could be attributed to administration of the gas even if hypoxia had not occurred [40]. In the 1950s–1970s, the Swedish neurosurgeon, Nils Lundberg contributed to our understanding of ICP waves [41, 42]. Lundberg worked with Leksell who developed stereotactic equipment, another important advance that called for flexibility and adjustments by the neuroanesthesiologist.

Various anesthetic techniques were advocated for neurosurgery. Willstaetter and Duisburg synthesized the rectal anesthetic tribromethanol (Avertin) in 1923, and Butzengeiger and Eichholtz used it as the sole anesthetic agent for neurosurgical procedures in the same year. Dandy used it in 1931 to reduce intracranial pressure [43]. Leo Davidoff, professor of neurosurgery at the Albert Einstein College of Medicine in New York, and a former resident with Harvey Cushing, considered that the effects of tribromethanol wore off too

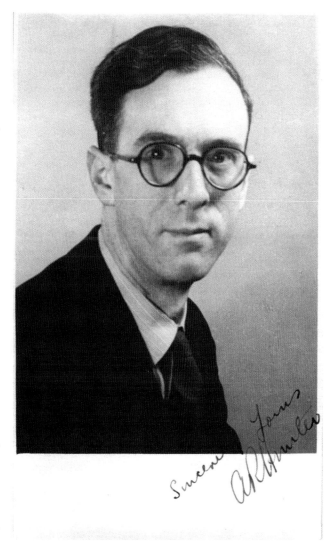

Fig. 64.10 The date of this photograph of Andrew Hunter is unknown. (Photograph courtesy of the Wood Library-Museum and the kind assistance of K. Bieterman)

quickly and advised additional infiltration with local anesthetic [44]. Trichlorethylene with nitrous oxide was popular in the British Commonwealth but not the US or other parts of the world. After DE Jackson described the anesthetic effects of cyclopropane in 1934, BB Hershenson used it for neurosurgery in low concentrations in a closed circuit, publishing his experiences in 1942 [45, 46]. The explosive potential of cyclopropane mandated draping the machine and the patient's head with wet towels. Thiopental, synthesized by Volwiler and Tabern in 1930, was introduced into clinical practice by Waters and Lundy in 1934, and advocated for neurosurgery by Shannon and Gardner in 1946 [47]. The popularity of thiopental as a *sole* agent disappeared with the discovery of fluorinated anesthetics.

Hunter (Fig. 64.10) defined anesthesia for neurosurgery in an address to the diploma candidates in anaesthesia (then a 3 year course) at McGill University in 1947 [38]:

"The anaesthetist whose duties bring him into contact with neurosurgery will find that in this specialty the problems which confront him differ markedly from those which he will meet in other fields of his work. No longer is it necessary to provide profound anaesthesia with extreme relaxation. The primary aim is to find some agent which can be given over periods up to 8 hours or longer with complete safety yet have no tendency to increase intracranial pressure. Further, this drug must be without adverse effects on exsanguinated patients and as electrocoagulation will normally be used to arrest haemorrhage, it should for preference be non-explosive."

A few years later, Hunter, then a visiting anaesthetist at the neurosurgical unit, Royal Infirmary, Manchester, England, noted [48]:

"There is a belief in some quarters that anaesthesia for neurosurgical operations involves merely patience and the use of non-toxic agents…. (But) neurosurgical operations are begun which cannot be completed for reasons directly traceable to the activities of the anaesthetist and…the numbers of such cases varies inversely with his skill…(T)here appear warning signs which only the anaesthetist can detect. If he fails to make the necessary observations…it may well be that the operation which from the surgeon's point of view was technically perfect, results in the death of the patient."

Later Twentieth Century

A major advance for neurosurgery, and anesthesia in general, occurred at the start of the second half of the twentieth century. The main anesthetic gases used at the time were chloroform, cyclopropane and diethyl ether, all of which had drawbacks. When given in oxygen, cyclopropane and ether were explosive, an increasing danger as electrical equipment such as diathermy became more common. Chloroform was toxic to the liver. A British chemist, Charles Suckling, worked on fluorinated compounds during World War II, where they were used in the production of high-octane aviation fuel and the purification of uranium-235. In 1951, while working at Imperial Chemical Industries' (ICI) Central Laboratory in England, Suckling synthesized 12 compounds in a search for a better volatile inhaled anesthetic. Number 9 was halothane [49]. Suckling investigated halothane's anesthetic action in mealworms and houseflies, then sent it to Jaume Raventos, a Catalan pharmacologist, for evaluation in other animals [50, 51]. After Raventos established its pharmacological properties, Michael Johnstone, an anesthetist in Manchester, England, undertook the first clinical trial in 1956. This systematic study of chemical compounds evaluated with a set of pre-defined characteristics, provides one of the first examples of modern drug design. Halothane was quickly incorporated into neurosurgical procedures. However, a few years later, an anonymous report suggested that halothane caused unacceptable increases in ICP (see below).

Controlled ventilation was not used in neurosurgery until the 1960s. Although it was realized that spontaneous ventilation increased intracranial pressure, anesthetists usually tried to preclude adverse situations by maintaining a good airway and improving venous drainage. One benefit of ether was that carbon dioxide remained normal even at deeper levels of anesthesia [38]. However, the introduction of electrocautery required that the machine, breathing system, the patient's face and even part of the anesthesiologist, be covered with wet towels. Halothane was nonflammable but caused respiratory depression. Ventilators gradually came into use for long neurosurgical cases. Hyperventilation was shown to cause cerebral vasoconstriction and was soon introduced in the treatment of head injured victims, as a means to quickly lower intracranial pressure [41]. It took more than 40 years to recognize that cerebral hypoxia accompanied the decrease in intracranial pressure and should not be routinely used for these patients [52].

Neuroanesthesia Emerges as a Specialty

Neuroanesthesia as a specialty emerged slowly, although it was becoming increasingly clear that neurosurgery had special requirements, not met by anesthesia as used in the general surgical arena. Until then, anesthesia had remained a field based largely on clinical skills. Now it was to gradually become founded on scientific enquiry. In the late 1950s, at the University of Pittsburgh, Peter Safar focused on cerebro-cardiac resuscitation, and established national standards that are required knowledge for all health care workers today [53].

Just as in other fields such as obstetrical, pediatric, and cardiac anesthesia, the need for further study and specialization became desirable. AR Hunter published the first modern day textbook on the subject, in England in 1964, and RGB Gilbert in Montreal published the second in 1966 [39, 54]. In 1960, a Commission of Neuroanesthesia, with anesthetists from 9 countries, was formed in Belgium to further research into intracranial dynamics. In 1961, the World Federation of Neurology sponsored a North American working group on neuroanesthesia, composed of Howard Terry (Mayo Clinic), JD Michenfelder (Mayo Clinic), M Albin (Case-Western Reserve), and chaired by Gilbert (McGill). In 1965, Brown of Edinburgh and Hunter in Manchester established the Neuroanaesthetists' Travelling Club of Great Britain. In the US, a review article by Michenfelder (Fig. 64.11) and others appeared in Anesthesiology in 1969. It established the specialty of neuroanesthesia in North America, coining the term "neuroanesthesiologist" (which of couse, remained "neuroanaesthetist" in other countries) [55]. The first US text, now in its fifth edition, was written by Cottrell and Turndorf in 1980, to be followed by *Clinical Anesthesia in*

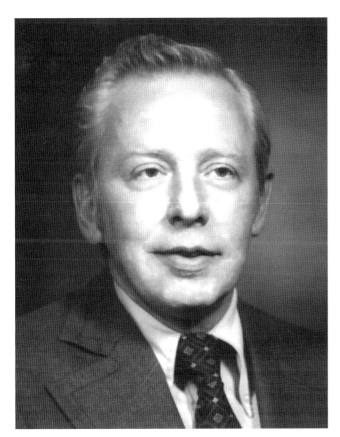

Fig. 64.11 John (Jack) Michenfelder was 58 when this photograph was taken in 1989. (Photograph courtesy of the Wood Library-Museum and the kind assistance of K. Bieterman)

Neurosurgery in 1984 by Frost, and *Clinical Neuroanesthesia* by Cucchiara and Michenfelder in 1990 [56–58].

In the 1960s and 1970s, centers of research arose on both sides of the Atlantic. In Scotland, neuroanaesthetist Gordon McDowell, collaborated with physiologist Murray Harper at the University of Glasgow to study the effects of anesthetics on intracranial dynamics. Two clinical neuroanesthetists, John Barker and William Fitch, took McDowell and Harper's findings into the operating room, showing that anesthetic agents increased cerebral blood flow and decreased metabolism, effects of particular concern in patients with intracranial mass lesions [59–63]. Bryan Jennett, a neurosurgeon famous for the description of the Glasgow Coma Scale, a prognostic indicator of outcome after head injury, joined the team later. He and Graham Teasdale, both professors of neurosurgery at the University of Glasgow's Institute of Neurological Sciences at the city's Southern General Hospital published the scale in 1974 [64].

An unfortunate outcome of this interdisciplinary collaboration may have been an editorial, published anonymously in the British Journal of Anaesthesia, that condemned the use of halothane in neurosurgery, claiming that it increased intracranial pressure despite hyperventilation [65]. The "evidence" was probably obtained from pressures measured in non ventilated supine cats, but nevertheless the "report" inhibited the use of halogenated agents in neurosurgery for years. Intravenous drugs and nitrous oxide combined with muscle relaxants (and often hyperventilation) again became the agents of choice for neurosurgery.

In the US, two centers established neuroanesthesia as a specialty in the 1960s. At the University of Pennsylvania in Philadelphia, Wollman, Pierce, Alexander, Smith, Dripps, and Cohen, studied the cerebrovascular effects of thiopental, cyclopropane, nitrous oxide, neuroleptic agents, and later, halothane and enflurane [66–68]. They also investigated the effects of hypotension and hyperventilation. At the Mayo clinic, in Rochester, Minnesota, Kai Rehder, a research assistant in physiology collaborated with anesthesiologist Richard Theye and surgeons Kirklin and MacCarty, to study the effects of profound hypothermia during aneurysm clipping [69]. Perhaps more than anyone else, neuroanesthesiologist John Michenfelder fostered neuroanesthesia as a specialty in the US. Working clinically in collaboration with neurosurgeons such as Professor Sundt, and in the laboratory, he assessed cerebral protection produced by hypothermia, anesthetic agents, and other pharmacologic agents such as nimodipine. With other physicians (e.g., Lee Milde and William Lanier) from the Mayo Clinic, he investigated means to measure cerebral blood flow and metabolism [69–73].

Michenfelder believed that decreased metabolism, caused by either hypothermia or agents such as barbiturates, could protect the brain. He experimented extensively on several animal models of ischemia. Working with Steen, he showed in a pig model, that barbiturates did not provide protection in complete cerebral ischemia [74]. However, in animals with normoglycemic levels, outcome was improved. The importance of controlling blood glucose levels has recently been re-emphasized in neurosurgical patients [75]. His findings regarding hypothermia were inconclusive, but studies in this area continued. A recently concluded study, the Intraoperative Hypothermia Aneurysm Study Trial (IHAST) indicated that mild hypothermia did not improve outcome in patients [76]. But, given the fact that cerebral metabolism is reduced, and thus should result in a better outcome, studies with hypothermia to different degrees continue, as shown by the multiple on-going studies referenced in a recently published text on stroke research [77]. Michenfelder was later awarded the ASA Award for Excellence in Research.

In the 1970s, Harvey Shapiro in Philadelphia studied intracranial pressure manipulation associated with ventilatory changes. With Kenneth Shulman (a neurosurgeon), Anthony Marmarou (a physiologist), Kenneth Shapiro (another neurosurgeon) and Frost (an anesthesiologist), Shapiro emphasized the importance of respiratory control in brain injured patients, specifically showing that hyperventilation per se, did not improve outcome and that improvement in oxygenation by application of positive end expiratory pressure would reduce raised intracranial pressure [78, 79]. Compartmental analysis of the intracranial space allowed conversion of the compliance curve to a more readily understood straight line [80, 81]. Pre and post pressure measurements after injection or substraction of small amounts of fluid from the intracranial space could, depending on the amount of increase or decrease, determine if the patient was in a potentially dangerous part of the curve. Harvey Shapiro also expanded neuroanesthetic management to intensive care [82, 83]. An intracranial pressure society was established with neurosurgeons from the UK (Douglas Miller) and the US (Kenneth Shulman), but the untimely deaths of the two priniciple investigators led to the demise of this small organization.

By the 1960s, neuroanesthesiology had developed as a specialty in the US. Standard techniques for measurement of cerebral blood flow, cerebral metabolic rate, intracranial pressure and neurochemical moieties were introduced. The physiologic basis of cerebrovascular dynamics was established and instrumentation design leapt ahead. Multidisciplinary research groups in Europe and North America shared findings. In Japan, Takeshita studied the effects of anesthetics on cerebral blood flow and metabolism [84–86]. His life long interest in brain death and resuscitation aided organ transplantation by better defining donors.

While visiting Pittsburgh in 1972, Thomas Langfitt (Professor of Neurosurgery at the University of Pennsylvania) met with anesthesiologist Maurice Albin, to discuss the formation of an organization for neuroanesthesiologists and neursurgeons. Working with James Harp (Chair of Anesthesia at the University of Pennsylvania), they compiled a list of possibly interested parties. An organizational assembly of 36 anesthesiologists and 4 neurosurgeons met in June 1973, in Philadelphia, to form the Neurosurgical Anesthesia Society (NAS) [87]. The Society officially met on 7 October 1973, during the annual meeting of the American Society of Anesthesiologists in San Francisco (annual dues were established at $ 15.00). Michenfelder was elected first president of the fledgling Society of Neurosurgical Anesthesia and Neurological Supportive Care, an immediate name change to acknowledge incorporation of more diverse disciplines. Langfitt included the society in the programs of the Harvey Cushing Society (subsequently named the American Association of Neurologic Surgeons), cementing the collaborative spirit.

Central nervous system trauma was also soon seen as the bailiwick of the neurosurgical team. Head injury kills more young people than any other cause. During the 1970s and early 1980s the National Institute of Health funded four centers (in the Bronx, Houston, San Diego, and Minneapolis/St Paul) to study traumatic brain injury. This multi-institutional study supplied much information, and indeed several subsequent advances have been made. The conclusions included the need to rapidly transfer the injured patient to a tertiary care center (the principle of swoop and scoop took precendence over stay and play), and to avoid hypoxia, hypotension and hyperventilation. Increasing age, male gender, cardiothoracic injury and drug abuse increased risk. The concept of the "Golden Hour" is credited to R Adams Crowley but may have been derived from French military data acquired in World War I. Crowley taught that "There is a golden hour between life and death. If you are critically injured you have less than 60 minutes to survive. You might not die right then; it may be three days or two weeks later—but something has happened in your body that is irreparable [88]." Philip Gildenberg expanded the concept to include brain injury. Gildenberg, a neuorsurgeon with a special interest in anesthesia (perhaps because of his association with the anesthesiologist Burnell Brown in Tucson) showed that immediate tracheal intubation improved survival. Securing the airway within 1 hour of severe brain injury could reduce mortality from around 38 to 22 %, a finding repeatedly confirmed [89, 90].

During the latter part of the twentieth century, technical advances furthered developments in instrumentation. Air embolism, which Gildenberg had earlier quantified, could be detected by a Doppler monitor, transesophageal echocardiography and end tidal CO_2 measurement [91]. In the late 1960s, a system to monitor spinal cord function was prompted by the risks of using Harrington rods during curvature correction for patients with scoliosis. A neurosurgeon, Brodkey, summed the cortical expression of distal peripheral nerve stimulation, a process reported by Dawson in 1947 [92–94]. Combining this knowledge with that of a biomedical engineer, RH Brown, working in the laboratories of Frankel and Burstein at Case Western Reserve, showed that pressure on the cord, time and blood pressure were all critical variables. A stand alone, portable spinal cord monitoring system was produced, at first a 4 channel sysytem that soon expanded to 8 channels with all data stored on a tape for later analysis.

Electroencephalographic monitoring had been advocated as early as 1937, but it was not until Stockard and Bickford described compressed spectral array in 1972, that the patterns became comprehensible to most anesthesiologists [95]. Betty Grundy, an anesthesiologist who was one of the pioneers in spinal cord monitoring, popularized evoked potential monitoring as a standard for anesthesiologists, using the technique Dawson described in 1947 [96].

From the 1950s (and earlier) to the 1980s, posterior fossa procedures and decompressive craniotomies for trigminal neuralgia (the Jannetta procedure) might be performed with the patient in the sitting position (Fig. 64.12) [97, 98]. It became clear that when veins were opened above the level of the heart, air could be entrained. Clinical and laboratory studies identified the pathophysiology, treatment and preventative measures [99, 100]. Because of the potentially catastrophic effects of entrained air,

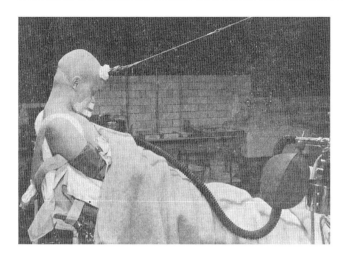

Fig. 64.12 A semi-sitting position produced by adjustment of the operating table, the use of pillows and tape, and the pull of a wire connected to the Crutchfield caliper attached to the patient's head allows access to the posterior fossa [93]. It also facilitates the potentially lethal intrusion of air into veins opened by the act of surgery. (Photograph from the Neurosurgical Department, St Bartholomew's Hospital, probably in the 1950s)

neurosurgeons placed their patients in the lateral position. The sitting position fell out of favor. Recently however, the sitting position has again been used for awake placement of deep brain stimulators. Although the patient does not breathe spontaneously, air can easily be sucked into opened veins. As Professor Albin remarked "We should listen to the drumbeat of history [101]."

In 1972, only 6 anesthesiology training programs in the US and Canada had dedicated neuroanesthesia divisions or sections. Today, the Residency Review Committee requires that all programs provide training in neuroanesthesia. All academic centers have divisions of neuroanesthesia. In 1976, the American Society of Anesthesiologists recognized neuroanesthesia as a subspecialty society. In 1989, the *Journal of Neurosurgical Anesthesiology*, under the editorship of James Cottrell, grew out of the Newsletter of the Society of Neurosurgical Anesthesia and Critical Care. The journal was listed in the Index Medicus and Current Contents by 1993. It is the official journal of 10 societies of neuroanesthesia around the world (including the US) with an Impact Factor greater than 2.

Women in Neuroanesthesia

Female neuroanesthetists have a major presence in the specialty [102]. Hugh Cairns, who had trained with Harvey Cushing, realized the importance of a specialist neuroanesthetist. In 1933, he recruited Olive Jones, a 1928 graduate of the London School of Medicine for Women, as his anesthetist at the London Hospital. She was not only the first neuroanesthetist but also the first full time salaried anesthetist in

the UK. She remained as the sole neuroanesthetist in Oxford until 1967. At the initial meeting of the Neuroanesthetists Travelling Club in 1965, 4 of the 33 neuroanesthetists were women (Olive Jones, Aileen Adams, Betty Everett and Jean Horton). By 1993, 38 of the club's 140 members were women.

Credit must go to two Italian physicians from Milan, Marie Marrubini and Marina Rossande, for the development of neurologic intensive care and the management of severe head injures. In Australia, anesthesiologists Nancy Edwards and Tess Brophy who worked with the neurosurgeon, Ken Jamieson, pioneered management of head injuries in the 1970s–1980s. Female contributors to advances in neuroanesthesia in the US include Jane Matjasko (a founding member of the Society of Neurosurgical Anesthesia and Neurological Supportive Care and the 10th president), Phillipa Newfield (14th president, 1987–8, of the Society of Neurosurgical Anesthesia and Neurological Supportive Care and author of her *Handbook of Neuroanesthesia*, now in the 4th edition), Betty Grundy, Judith Donegan, Elisabeth Abramowicz, Audree Bendo, Rosemary Hickey, Patricia Petrozza, Karen Domino, and Verna Baughman. As Aileen Adams noted, "one of the advantages of being a woman in a man's world is that you are noticeable [102]". I heartily agree.

A Reflection

Neuroanesthesia is less than 130 years old but the practice evolved over thousands of years. Advances resulted from collaboration with other specialists from different fields including surgery, physiology, pharmacology and radiology. Questions regarding precise monitoring of intracranial dynamics, brain survival after head injury, spinal cord regeneration, identification of serum markers of cerebral damage, and long term cerebral effects of anesthetic agents remain to be answered. If progress continues as it has in the past century, these quandaries may soon be solved.

References

1. Nunn F. "Ancient Egyptian Medicine". OK: University of Oklahoma Press; 1996. pp. 26–8.
2. Joost J, Sanchez GM, Burridge AL. The Edwin Smith Papyrus: a clinical reappraisal of the oldest known document on spinal injuries. Eur Spine J. 2010;19:1815–23.
3. Breasted JH. "The Edwin Smith Surgical Papyrus: published in facsimile and hieroglyphic transliteration with translation and commentary in two volumes". (University of Chicago Oriental Institute publications, v. 3–4). Chicago: University of Chicago Press; 1991. pp. xvi, 6, 480–485, 487–489, 446–448, 451–454, 466; 2: pi. XVII, XVIIA.
4. Ghalioungui P. "Magic and Medical Science in Ancient Egypt". New York: Barnes and Noble, Inc; 1965. p 58.
5. Sullivan R. The identity and work of the Ancient Egyptian surgeon. J Roy Soc Med. 1996;89:467–73.

6. Allen JP. "The Art of Medicine in Ancient Egypt". New York: The Metropolitan Museum of Art; 2005. pp. 70–4.

7. Brothwell DR. Digging up Bones; the excavation, treatment and study of human skeletal remains. London: British Museum (Natural History); 1963. p 126. (OCLC 14615536).

8. Weber J, Czarnetzki A. "Trepanationen im frühen Mittelalter im Südwesten von Deutschland – Indikationen, Komplikationen und Outcome" (in German). Zentralblatt für Neurochirurgie. 2001;62:10.

9. Rutkow IM. The origins of modern surgery, surgery-basic science and clinical evidence. New York: Springer Verlag, Inc.; 2001. pp. 2–19.

10. Adams F. The genuine works of Hippocrates translated from the Greek London, the Sydenham Society; 1849. pp. 430,431, 433, 455.

11. Bandelier AF. Aboriginal trephining in Bolivia. Am Anthropol. 1904;6:440–6.

12. http://en.wikipedia.org/wiki/Trepanation. Accessed November 29th 2011.

13. Restak R. "Fixing the Brain". Mysteries of the Mind. Washington, D.C.: National Geographic Society; 2000. (ISBN 0-7922-7941-7. OCLC 43662032)

14. Cooper A. Lectures on the principles and practice of surgery. London: FC Westley; 1829. pp. 123–4.

15. Henderson AR. Prominent medicine convenes at Lumberton, 1887. J Med Soc NJ. 1976;73:18–22.

16. Wikipedia, accessed may 25th 2012.

17. Paget S. Sir Victor Horsley. A study of his life and work. London: Constable; 1919. p. 184.

18. Horsley V. On the technique of operations on the central nervous system. Address in Surgery Toronto Lancet. 1906;2:484–6.

19. ("Final Report Of Special Chloroform Committee". The British Medical Journal 2 (2584). 47–72. 1910–07-09). JSTOR 25291374.)

20. Macewen W. The introduction of tubes into the larynx through the mouth instead of tracheotomy and laryngotomy. Glasgow Med J. 1879;9:72 and 12:218.

21. Frost E. The contributions of Sir William Macewen, a pioneer neurosurgeon, to an early quality assurance survey in anesthesia. J Neuro Anesth. 1991;3:28–33.

22. Shepard DAE. Harvey Cushing and anesthesia. Can Anaes Soc J. 1965;12:431–42.

23. Cushing HW. Anesthesia charts of 1895. Letter to FA Washburn Treedwell Library. Massachusetts Central Hospital, Boston MA.

24. Fulton JF. Harvey Cushing; A Biography. Blackwell: Oxford; 1946. pp. 212–6.

25. Cushing HW. Cocaine anesthesia in the treatment of certain cases of hernia and operations for thyroid tumors. Johns Hopkins Bulletin. 1989;9:192–3.

26. Krause F. Surgery of the brain and spinal cord based on personal experiences. Vol. 1. trans Haubold H, Thorek M. New York: Rebman and Co; 1912. p. 137.

27. Krause F. Surgery of the brain and spinal cord based on personal experiences. Vol. 3. trans Haubold H, Thorek M. New York: Rebman and Co; 1912. p. 957.

28. Hanninen O, Farago M, Monos E. Ignaz Phillipp Semmelweis, the prophet of bacteriology. Infection Control. 1983;4:367–70.

29. Walsh JJ, Pasteur L. Catholic Encyclopedia. New York: Robert Appleton Company; 1913.

30. Glasser, O. Wilhelm Conrad Röntgen and the Early History of the Roentgen Rays. London: John Bale, Sons and Danielsson, Ltd; 1933. p. 305.

31. Lyman HM. Artificial anaesthesia and anaesthetics. New York: William Wood and Co; 1881. pp. 98–330; p. 80.

32. Pollack SV, Carruthers A, Grekin RC. The history of electrosurgery. Dermatologic Surg. 2000;26:904–8.

33. Bovie WT, Cushing H. Electrosurgery as an aid to the removal of intracranial tumors with a preliminary note on a new surgical-current generator. Surg Gynecol Obstet. 1928;47:751–84.

34. Rowbotham ES, Magill I. Anaesthetics in the plastic surgery of the face and jaws. Proc RSM. 1921;14:17–27.

35. Monro A. Observations on the structure and function of the nervous system. Edinburgh: Creech & Johnson; 1783. p. 5.

36. Kelly G. Appearances observed in the dissection of two individuals; death from cold and congestion of the brain. Trans Med Chir Sci Edinb. 1824;1:84–169.

37. Cannon WB, Fraser J, Covell E. The preventive treatment of wound shock. JAMA. 1918;70:618–21.

38. Hunter AR. Anaesthesia for intracranial operations. Canad Med Assoc J. 1948;58:48–53.

39. Hunter AR. Neurosurgical anaesthesia. Phila FA Davis. 1964:86.

40. Courville CB. The untoward effects of nitrous oxide. Pacific Press CA; 1939. pp. 80–7, 122–5.

41. Lundberg N, Kjallquist A, Bien C. Reduction of increased intracranial pressure by hyerventilation. Acta Psychiatr Scand suppl. 1959;34(139):1–64.

42. Lundberg N. Monitoring of intracranial pressure. Proc Roy Soc Med. 1972;65:19–22.

43. Dandy WE. Avertin anesthesia in neurologic surgery. JAMA. 1931;96:1860–4.

44. Davidoff LM. Avertin as a base anesthetic for craniotomy. Bull Neurol Inst. 1934;3:544–50.

45. Jackson DE. A study of analgesia and anesthesia with special reference to such substances as trichlorethylene and vinesthane together with apparatus for their administration. Anesth Analg. 1934;13:198–203.

46. Hershenson BB. Some observations on anesthesia for neurosurgery. NY State J Med. 1942;42:2111–8.

47. Shannon EW, Gardner WJ. Pentothal sodium anesthesia in neurological surgery. N Engl J Med. 1946;234:15–6.

48. Hunter AR. The present position of anaesthesia for neurosurgery. Proc Royal Soc Med. 1952;45:427–34.

49. Suckling CW. Some chemical and physical factors in the development of fluothane. Br J Anaesth. 1957;29:466–72.

50. Raventós J. The action of fluothane—a new volatile anaesthetic. Br J Pharmacol Chemotherapy. 1956;11:394–410.

51. Hervas C. Approach to the scientific work of Jaume Raventos (1905–1982). Rev Esp Anestesiol Reanim. 1992;39:362–70.

52. Soukup J, Bramsiepe I, Brucke M, et al. Evaluation of a bedside monitor of regional CBF as a measure of CO_2 reactivity in neurosurgical intensive care patients. JNA. 2008;20(4):249–55.

53. Safar P, Escarraga L, Elam J. A comparison of the mouth to mouth and mouth to airway methods of artificial respiration with chest pressure arm lift methods. New Eng J Med. 1958;258:6710–7.

54. Gilbert RGB, Brindle GF, Galindo A. Anesthesia for neurosurgery. London: J and A Churchill Co; 1966.

55. Michenfelder JD, Gronert GA, Rehder K. Neuroanesthesia. Anesthesiology. 1969;30:65–100.

56. Cottrell JE, Turndorf H. Anesthesia for neurosurgery. St Louis: Mosby-Yearbook Inc; 1980.

57. Frost EAM. Clinical anesthesia in neurosurgery. Butterworth Stoneham; 1984.

58. Cucchiara RF, Michenfelder JD. Clinical neuroanesthesia. Churchill Livingston. New York. 1990.

59. Fitch W, Barker J, Jennett WB. McDowall DG. The influence of neurolept analgesic drugs on cerebrospinal fluid pressure. Br J Anaesth. 1969;41:800–6.

60. Moss E, McDowell DG. ICP increases with 50 % nitrous oxide in oxygen in severe head injuries during controlled ventilation. Br J Anaesth. 1979;51:757–61.

61. Okuda Y, McDowall DG, Ali MM, Lane MM. Changes in CO_2 responsiveness and in autoregulation of the cerebral circulation during and after halothane induced hypotension. J Neurol Neurosurg Psychiatry. 1976;39:221–30.

62. Harper AM, Bell RA. The effect of metabolic acidosis and alkalosis on the blood flow through the cerebral cortex. J Neurol Neurosurg Psychiatry. 1963;26:341–4.

63. Fitch W, MacKenzie ET, Jones JV, Graham DI, Harper AM. Effect of halothane on teh autoregulation of cerebral blood flow in chronicaly hypertensive baboons. Acta Neurol Scand Suppl. 1977;64:66–7.

64. Teasdale G, Jennett B. Assessment of coma and impaired consciousness. A practical scale Lancet 2. 1974;(7872):81–4.

65. Anonymous: Halothane and neurosurgery (Editorial). Br J Anaesth. 1969;41:277–8.

66. Wollman H, Alexander SC, Cohen PJ. Cerebral circulation and metabolism in anesthetized man. Clin Anesth. 1967;3:1–15.

67. Wollman H, Alexander C, Cohen PJ, Smith TC, Chase PE, Vandermolen R. Cerebral circulation during genral anesthesia and hyperventilation in man: thiopental induction to nitrous oxide and d-tubocurarine. Anesthesiol. 1965;26:329–34.

68. Alexander SC, Wollman H, Cohen PJ, Chase PE, Behar M. Cerebrovascular response to PaCO2 during halothane anesthesia in man. J appl Physiol. 1964;19:561–5.

69. Rehder K, Kirklin JW, MacCarty CS, Theye RA. Physiologic studies following profound hypothermia and circulatory arrest for treatment of intracranial aneurysm. Ann Surg. 1962;156:882–9.

70. Michenfelder JD. Simultaneous cerebral blood flow measured by direct and indirect methods. J Surg Res. 1968;8:475–81.

71. Michenfelder JD, Theye RA. The effects of profound hypocapnia and dilutional anemia on canine cerebral metabolism and blood flow. Anesthesiology. 1969;31:449–57.

72. Theye RA, Michenfelder JD. Effect of nitrous oxide on canine cerebral metabolism. Anesthesiology. 1968;29:1119–24.

73. Theye RA, Michenfelder JD. Effect of halothane on canine cerebral metabolism. Anesthesiology. 1968;29:1113–8.

74. Steen PA, Milde JH, Michenfelder JD. No barbiturate protection in a dog model of complete cerebral ischemia. Ann Neurol. 1979;5:343–9.

75. Pasternak JJ, McGregor DG, Schroeder DR, Lanier WL, Shi Q, Hindman BJ, Clarke WR, Torner JC, Weeks JB, Todd MM, IHAST Investigators. Hyperglycemia in patients undergoing cerebral aneurysm surgery: its association with long-term gross neurologic and neuropsychological function. J Neurosurg. 2012 Mar 9. [Epub ahead of print]

76. Todd MM, Hindman BJ, Clarke WR, Torner JC. Intraoperative hypothermia for aneurysm surgery trial (IHAST) investigators. Mild intraoperative hypothermia during surgery for intracranial aneurysm. N Engl J Med. 2005;352:135–45.

77. Lapchak PA, Zhang JH. Translational stroke research. New York:Springer; 2012.

78. Frost E. The physiopathology of the lung in neurosurgical patients. J Neurosurg. 1979;50:699–714.

79. Frost E, Arancibia CU, Shulman K. Pulmonary shunt as a prognostic indicator in head injury. J Neurosurg. 1979;50:768–72.

80. Marmarou A, Shulman K, LaMorgese J. Compartmental analysis of outflow resistance of the cerebrospinal fluid system. J Neurosurg. 1975;43:523–34.

81. Frost E. Effects of positive end-expiratory pressure on intra-cranial pressure and compliance in brain-injured patients. J Neurosurg. 1977;47:195–200.

82. Shapiro HM. Intracranial hypertension: therapeutic and anesthetic considerarions. Anesthesiology. 1975;43:445–71.

83. Shapiro HM, Aidinis SJ. Neurosurgical anesthesia. Surgical Clinics of North Am. 1975:55:913–28.

84. Takeshita H, Okuda Y, Sari K, Mochizuki K. Recent trends in research on cerebral circulation and metabolism in relation to anesthesia 1. Masui. 1971;20:469–76.

85. Takeshita H, Okuda Y, Sari A, Mochizuki K. Recent trends in research on cerebral circulation and metabolism in relation to anesthesia 2. Masui. 1971;20:579–88.

86. Takeshita H, Okuda Y, Miyazaki H, Fujita S. Problems of "brain death". Masui. 1969;18:277–84.

87. Albin MS. Celebrating silver: the genesis of a neuroanesthesiology society. J Neurosurg Anesthesiol. 1997;9:296–307.

88. Lerner EB, Moscati RM. "The Golden Hour: Scientific Fact or Medical "Urban Legend?"" Academic Emergency Medicine. 2001;8:758–60.

89. Kaufman HH, Makela ME, Lee KF, Haid RW Jr, Gildenberg PL. Gunshot wounds to the head: a perspective. Neurosurgery. 1986;18:689–95.

90. Miraflor E, Chuang K, Miranda MA, et al. Timing is everthing: delayed intubation is associatd with increased mortality in initially stable trauma patients. J Surg Res. 2011;170:286–90.

91. Gildenberg PL, O'Brien RP, Britt WJ, Frost EA. The efficacy of Doppler monitoring for the detection of venous air embolism. J Neurosurg. 1981;54:75–8.

92. Croft TJ, Brodkey JS, Nulsen FE. Reversible spinal cord trauma: a model for electrical monitoring of spinal cord function. J Neurosurg. 1972;36(4):402–6.

93. Brodkey JS, Richards DE, Blasingame JP, Nulsen FE. Reversible spinal cord trauma in cats. Additive effects of direct pressure and ischemia. J Neurosurg. 1972;37(5):591–3.

94. Dawson GD. Cerebral responses to electrical stimulation of peripheral nerve in man. J Neurol Neurosurg Psychiatry. 1947;10:134–40.

95. Bickford RG, Stockard JJ. The compressed spectral array (CSA) a pictorial EEG. Proceedings of the San Diego Biomedical Symposium San Diego, CA; 1972;2:(Abstr)365.

96. Grundy BL. Intraoperative monitoring of sensory-evoked potentials. Anesthesiology. 1983;58:72–87.

97. Jannetta PJ. Arterial compression of the trigeminal nerve at the pons in patients with trigeminal neuralgia. J Neurosurg. 1967;26:159–62.

98. Hewer CL. Recent advances in anaesthesia and analgesia (Including Oxygen Therapy). 7th edn. London: J & A Churchill Ltd; 1953. p. 287.

99. Maroon JC, Albin M. Air embolism diagnosed by Doppler ultrasound. Anesth Analg. 1974;53:399–402.

100. Adornato DC, Gildenberg PL, Ferrario CM, Smart J, Frost E. Pathophysiology of intravenous air embolism in dogs. Anesthesiology. 1978;49:120–7.

101. Albin M. Venous air embolism: a warning not to be complacent-we should listen to the drumbeat of history. Aneshesiology. 2011;115:626–9.

102. Clarke RSJ, Adams AK, Gibbs E, Horton JM, MacDonald R, Robson J, Rollin AM, Willats S. A celebration of women in anaesthesia 1894–1994. J Roy Soc Med. 1995;88:519–21.

Pediatric Anesthesia

65

George Gregory

Summary

Before anesthesia's discovery, children were forcibly restrained during surgery. The introduction of ether in 1846 and chloroform in 1847 quickly led to their use in children. Most nineteenth century pediatric surgery treated minor ailments. The first "giants" initiating development of pediatric anesthesia, emerged in Canada, the US and the UK after World War I. Robson, the father of pediatric anesthesia, became Anaesthetist-in-Chief at Toronto's Hospital for Sick Children. He defined the major problems extant in pediatric anesthesia—and their solutions. Betty Lank, chief Nurse Anesthetist at Boston Children's Hospital, gave anesthesia for several surgical firsts. Robert Smith became head of pediatric anesthesia at Boston Children's Hospital in 1945, noting that Lank "made me a pediatric anesthesiologist." In 1937, Ayre in the UK described his simple "T-piece" and in 1966, Jackson–Rees in the UK added an open-ended bag to Ayre's T-piece. The T-piece required high gas inflows, and thus, gradually gave way in the last half of the twentieth century to rebreathing anesthesia circuits with CO_2 absorption. The US adopted rebreathing circuits early.

In 1952, Deming showed that young children required more anesthesia than older patients, but as late as 1975, some surgeons might operate on infants (e.g., for PDA ligation) receiving little or no anesthesia, believing they felt no pain. In 1987, Redbook magazine put the lie to this belief and changed the practice.

Increasingly, surgery required better airway control. In 1882, New York surgeon O'Dwyer put a metal tube into the glottis to relieve airway obstruction in children with diphtheria. Budin of Paris developed the first neonatal intensive care unit (NICU) in the 1890s. In 1939, Gillespie invented a pediatric laryngoscope. Miller improved this design in 1946, and "Miller" laryngoscopes became fixtures. In 1963, Allen at the Children's Hospital in Adelaide, Australia, introduced nasotracheal intubation for croup, enabling prolonged airway management. To minimize deadspace, Soucek and Rendell–Baker made masks in 1962 that closely fit the faces of children of different ages. Later came the laryngeal mask airway designed by Brain in 1987. In the past 15 years fiberoptic devices facilitated tracheal intubation of infants and children.

The first Pediatric Anesthesia textbook "*Anesthesia in Children*" was published in the UK in 1923. "*Précis Clinique et Opératoire de Chirurgie Infantile*" followed in France in 1925. In 1948, Leigh and Belton wrote the first US book. In 1950, Smith wrote his comprehensive textbook, "*Anesthesia for Infants and Children*". Gregory's 1983 "*Pediatric Anesthesia*" was the first physiology-based textbook.

Societies formed to advance pediatric anesthesia. The Association of Paediatric Anaesthetists was established in the UK in 1973. The Anesthesia and Critical Care section of the American Academy of Pediatrics was established in 1966, and the Society for Pediatric Anesthesia in 1985 in North America.

Introduction

Several reports describe the early chronologies of pediatric anesthesia [1–3]. The present report attends briefly to these, but focuses more on advances that facilitated the modern surgical care of sick infants and children, advances that led to modern pediatric anesthesia.

Surgery Before and soon After the Discovery of Anesthesia

Before the discovery of anesthesia, most surgeries were quick, and brutal [4]; an amputation took a minute or two. Lucky children sucked whisky or poppy juice for pain relief. Unlucky children underwent trephination, extirpation of bladder stones, probing of an imperforate anus, inguinal hernia repair, and circumcision while forcibly restrained. Miraculously, longer procedures were done without anesthesia: cleft lips had been repaired as early as 390 CE. "Anesthetic" remedies for both adults and children were ineffective in the west. The use of scopolamine-like herbal preparations may

G. Gregory (✉)
Department of Anesthesia, University of California, San Francisco, CA 94143–0648, USA
e-mail: gregoryg@anesthesia.ucsf.edu

E. I Eger II et al. (eds.), *The Wondrous Story of Anesthesia,* DOI 10.1007/978-1-4614-8441-7_65, © Edmond I Eger, MD 2014

Table 65.1 Surgeries for which John Snow anesthetized infants and children

	General	Dental	Ophthalmologic	Orthopedic	Plastic	Urologic
Number (Percent)	35 (8.9%)	43 (10.9%)	24 (6.1%)	118 (30.0%)	133 (33.8%)	40 (10.2%)

Table 65.2 Deaths described in Snows casebook. (From [6] with permission)

Patient age	Reason for anesthesia	Comment
3 yrs	Pertussis	Anesthetized for treatment of pertussis—died 1 day post anesthesia
2 yrs	Status epilepticus	Weak, rapid pulse during anesthesia. Died 1 hr after awakening from anesthesia, still in status
1 yr	Meningitis	Seizures and increased intracranial pressure pre-anesthesia. Died with fixed and dilated pupils
16 yrs	Above knee leg amputation	Hemorrhage during and after surgery. Died 4 days after surgery
17 yrs	Typhoid fever	Died post anesthesia—possibly from dehydration

have enabled Japanese surgeons to perform surgery, relying on sedation and amnesia.

Crawford Long (1815–1878) provided the first pediatric general anesthetic, giving ether in 1842 to an eight-year-old child for amputation of a toe. He also anesthetized several adults but waited seven years to report his discovery [5], thereby giving priority in the discovery of anesthesia to William Morton, a dentist who *publicly* demonstrated the anesthetic effectiveness of ether at the Massachusetts General Hospital 16 Oct 1846. The next year in Boston, approximately 80% of children undergoing surgery received ether [3].

James Simpson (1811–1870) discovered the anesthetic effects of chloroform in 1847, and John Snow (1813–1858) used both ether and chloroform (mostly chloroform). Between 1846 and 1858, Snow anesthetized 393 English children (Table 65.1), 186 of whom were less than 1 year of age [6]. Not surprisingly, none had thoracic or abdominal operations. Such procedures were rare at any age.

Amazingly, 98% of Snow's patients survived. Of the five who died, only one underwent surgery, and that death resulted from uncorrected hemorrhage and occurred several days after the surgery (Table 65.2). The other patients had anesthesia for reasons that we would smile upon today.

As Table 65.2 indicates, anesthetic failures joined successes. Shortly after the introduction of chloroform, 15-year-old Hannah Greener died during removal of a toenail under chloroform, the first reported anesthetic death in a child [7]. She had survived a previous anesthetic with ether.

John Snow's remarkable safety record overshadowed that of his peers, both because of his genius and because, in contrast to the occasional anesthetist, he practiced anesthesia nearly full time. Today, 6.5 children die per 100,000 anesthetics (excluding cardiac surgery) [8]. Under Snow's care, 20 per 100,000 died—in a less than friendly environment—mostly homes or surgeon's offices, and without monitoring, intravenous fluids, antibiotics, or postoperative pain relief [6]!

Like adults, children benefited from the introduction of anesthesia. Surgeons were not rushed by patient screams, and previously impossible surgical procedures were now possible: repair of congenital anomalies, gastrostomies, excision of tumors, and increasingly intricate orthopedic procedures. However, for a half-century, surgeons rarely entered the thoracic or abdominal cavities (e.g., see Table 65.1) because of unacceptable post-operative infection rates and pulmonary failure.

For more than a century after the discovery of anesthesia, ether or chloroform given by "rag and bottle" were the primary anesthetics administered to children. Ethyl chloride was a minor addition. It was introduced into Europe as a general anesthetic in 1894, and spread to Britain, the British Commonwealth, and the US in the beginning of the twentieth Century. It was commonly used for dental anesthesia, especially in children (Fig. 65.1). Although Snow recognized the great advantage of control over the concentration of anesthetic delivered, the general use of reliable versions of anesthetic delivery was delayed for a century. Precision vaporizers (e.g., the Copper Kettle) appeared in the 1950s, and radically increased the control over and safety of anesthetic delivery.

Ether stimulated ventilation, an advantage that Snow recognized [9] and Gregory et al. quantified 113 years later [10]. The adult ether masks commonly applied to children, imposed dead space and thus increased rebreathing and carbon dioxide (hypercarbia), and decreased oxygen (hypoxemia). Better to use ether than chloroform since the latter depressed breathing leaving the child more vulnerable to oxygen lack and rebreathing of carbon dioxide. In the 1890s, the concurrent administration of oxygen with ether allowed anesthetists to minimize hypercarbia and hypoxia. Frederick Hewitt (1857–1916) thought this especially helpful for children.

By the early nineteenth century, physicians recognized that children differed from adults in more than size. This recognition led to the development of Children's hospitals

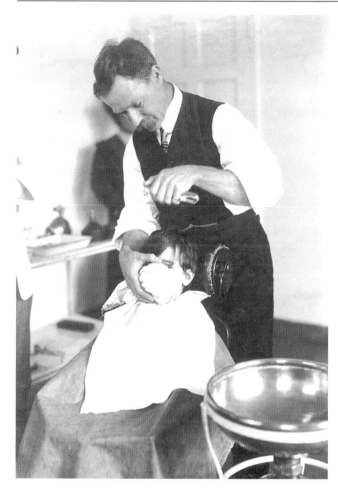

Fig. 65.1 Rupert Hornabrook (Australia's firt full-time anesthesiologist) produces anesthesia with a spray of ethyl chloride to a cloth held to a child's face. (Courtesy of Rod N. Westhorpe and the Geoffrey Kaye Museum of Anaesthetic History)

(Table 65.3) and associated specialties. Just as it took time for anesthesia to be recognized as a medical specialty in its own right, pediatric anesthesia did not develop as a subspecialty until the first half of the twentieth century. Until 1900, it was likely that the hospital physician, the surgeon's assistant, the family doctor or a nurse would administer the anesthetic given to a child.

Most pediatric surgery in the nineteenth century was for minor ailments. Intrathoracic and intra-abdominal surgery awaited the invention of antisepsis and asepsis, developments of the late 1800s. Asepsis and antibiotics were as important to the surgical care of children as they were to adults. Without control and treatment of infections, pediatric surgery (and hence anesthesia) could not advance, especially since the immune system of neonates and infants is less developed than that of older patients [11]. Before asepsis, infection-induced mortality of children following surgery sometimes exceeded 90 %.

With the development of the subspecialty of pediatric anesthesia, it became clear that patients cared for by pediatric

anesthetists had fewer complications and fewer anesthesia-related deaths than patients cared for by adult anesthetists [12, 13]. Those caring for many patients with similar problems provided better results than those caring only occasionally for such patients. Today, children's hospitals in the United States, and elsewhere, are the backbone of pediatric care and research.

Adventurous Surgery

Two congenital anomalies awaiting anesthesia and asepsis for their successful repair were omphalocele (a large midline abdominal hernia) and gastroschisis (an intrauterine vascular accident that produces a large lateral abdominal hernia). For both anomalies the abdominal contents protrude through the abdominal wall at birth. These lesions are easily repaired and today more than 95 % of such infants survive. In the early 1800s, William Hey (1749–1819) and James Hamilton (1749–1835) accomplished the first successful repair, doing so without anesthesia or antibiotics.

In 1889, Joseph O'Dwyer of New York City failed in his attempt to repair an infant's congenital diaphragmatic hernia (CDH). In 1905, Lothar Heidenhain (1860–1940) in Germany successfully repaired the CDH of a 9-year-old. Repair of CDH then and now exacted an invariant heavy price. Mortality exceeded 50 % in 1925 and hasn't changed much since, despite Intensive Care Nurseries (ICNs), mechanical ventilation, and extracorporeal membrane oxygenation (ECMO) [14].

In 1939, William Ladd (1880–1967), in Boston, was the first to repair a tracheo-esophageal fistula (TEF; a connection between the trachea and esophagus), another usually lethal congenital lesion [15]. Ladd favored a two-stage approach (he first closed the fistula and fed the child through a gastrostomy until the child had grown. He later repaired the esophageal atresia). In 1941, Cameron Haight (1901–1970) of the University of Michigan ligated the fistula and did a primary repair of the esophagus as a single procedure [16], inventing the treatment used today. Ether or chloroform given via mask to spontaneously breathing patients supplied the anesthesia for early TEF repairs. Mortality exceeded 70 %. Today nearly all these patients survive if they have no other congenital anomalies.

In 1946, Alfred Blalock (1899–1964), a surgeon, and Helen Taussig (1898–1986), a pediatrician at John Hopkins Medical Center, devised an operation to treat infants with Tetrology of Fallot. Tetrology of Fallot is a congenital defect that diverts blood flow from the lungs, limiting oxygenation of the arterial blood and resulting in a "blue baby" [17]. Merel Harmel (1917–) and Austin Lamont (1905–1969) anesthetized the first 100 of these patients [18], doing so with minimal monitoring (they felt the pulse, counted respiration

Table 65.3 Founders and founding years for early pediatric hospitals

Founded	Hospital	Founder(s)
1778	Hôpital Necker—Enfants Malades (Paris)	Madame Necker
1802	Hospital des Enfant Maladies (Paris)	Conseil général des Hospices
1821	National Children's Hospital (Dublin)	Henry Marsh, Philip Crampton Charles Johnson
1852	Hospital for Sick Children, Great Ormond St (London)	Charles West
1855	Children's Hospital of Philadelphia (Philadelphia)	Francis W Lewis, T Henson Bache, Charles Bingham Penrose
1869	The Boston Children's Hospital (Boston)	Francis Brown and associates
1870	National Hospital, National Medical Center (Washington, DC)	Board of Lady Visitors, DC Busey, F.A. Ashford, William B. Drinkard, & William W. Johnston

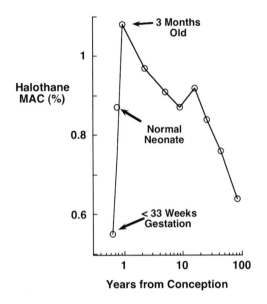

Fig. 65.2 Anesthetic requirement (MAC) for halothane changes with ageing. MAC is the minimum alveolar concentration of anesthetic needed to suppress movement in response to surgery in 50 % of patients

and occasionally measured blood pressure in most cases). Some patients breathed spontaneously via a facemask, even when the chest was open! Patients recovered in the operating room and were cared for on the ward after surgery. Mortality was remarkably only 25 %, a testimony to the skills of the anesthetists and surgeons—and the resilience of young children!

For decades, surgeons sought to repair congenital abnormalities in utero [19], thinking it would improve outcomes. Target lesions included diaphragmatic hernias, teratomas, anomalies of the lung (e.g., cysts), and possibly cleft lips. In utero repair of cleft lips might have the great advantage of leaving no scars. But can we anesthetize the mother without excessive depression of the fetus? Biehl et al. showed that the maternal MAC was considerably greater than the fetal MAC (e.g., see Fig. 65.2) [20]. And fetal surgery may precipitate premature labor—a disaster at 20 weeks gestation because birth at this age is not compatible with extra-uterine life. Fetal surgery remains a tantalizing possibility

for several lesions, and a success for others (e.g., twin-twin transfusion).

Giants Appear

With the end of World War I, came the appearance of the first giants in pediatric anesthesia, anesthetists who prompted the development of the discipline. These included Charles Robson (1884–1969), Betty Lank (1904–2002), Robert Smith (1913–2009), M Digby Leigh (1904–1975), M Kathleen Belton (1916–1980), C Ronald Stephen (1916–2006), Philip Ayre (1902–1980), and Gordon Jackson–Rees (1918–2001; Fig. 65.3). Beyond a focus on children, all of these clinically skilled anesthetists shared a love of teaching, and several advanced the science of pediatric anesthesia.

Robson, considered the father of pediatric anesthesia, returned from World War I to become Anaesthetist-in-Chief at the Hospital for Sick Children in Toronto. He defined the major problems extant in pediatric anesthesia—and their solutions [21]: children differed from adults in their physiology and their response to drugs (e.g., children "take more anesthetic … than do adults" a fact later quantified) [22–24]. Children, he said, require anesthesia equipment designed for their needs (what a concept!), and in conflict with beliefs of some surgeons, he argued that operating on a child without adequate anesthesia was "vivisection".

Robson advocated simple vital aspects of pediatric care, including recognition that induction of anesthesia with an inhaled anesthetic required maintenance of a patent airway. He claimed that "starvation" prior to surgery led to acidosis, and he fed children "strained gruel" up to four hours beforehand, withholding food after that to minimize vomiting, aspiration, and possible lung injury or death. He warned that "accident cases" and patients in pain took longer to empty their stomachs and were at greater risk of vomiting and aspiration. He suggested the insertion of a gastric catheter to relieve the gastric distention of patients who had pyloric stenosis (a constriction at the exit from the stomach). He administered ether as his anesthetic of choice, by open drop or by insufflation via an "ether hook." (i.e., he "blew" ether into the mouth).

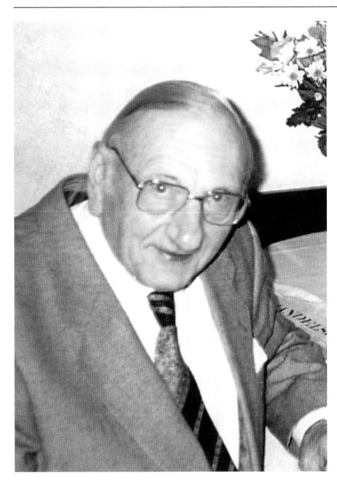

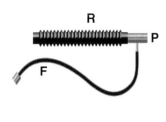

Fig. 65.4 Ayre's "T"-piece consisted of a T connected to the tracheal tube at P and to a reservoir tube, R. Gas containing anesthetic entered the system through F. Intermittently occluding the otherwise open end of R caused ventilation of the patient's lungs. (www.frca.co.uk/ images/ ayre1.gi. Accessed 31/03/2010)

Fig. 65.3 Gordon Jackson-Rees (Courtesy of Rod N. Westhorpe)

He did not hesitate however, to use tracheal intubation, especially when using cyclopropane, a respiratory depressant, for complicated cases.

A little south of Robson, William Ladd (1880–1967) was busy in Boston Children's Hospital developing Pediatric Surgery (he was its "father"). Betty Lank, the Chief Nurse Anesthetist at Children's from 1936 to 1957, enabled Ladd's success [25]. She adapted Riva Roca's measurement of arterial blood pressure to children, initially making the blood pressure cuffs herself. She designed and had built, size-appropriate facemasks and breathing bags for children—later produced by Foregger [26]. She had anesthetic firsts to brag about: Ladd's first patient for tracheo-esophageal fistula repair in 1939; Gross' (1905–1988) first patient for ligation of a patent ducts arteriosus in 1938 [27], and his first patient for repair of a coarctation (narrowing) of the aorta in 1945 [28]. She was the first to administer cyclopropane to children in the United States. She usually gave ether or cyclopropane via mask, even to prone patients (something that would terrify today's anesthetist).

Smith learned anesthesia in a three-month US Army course during World-War II. In 1945, he arrived at the

Boston Children's Hospital "knowing very little" about pediatric anesthesia (Personal communication), his previous patients having been soldiers. Smith said Lank "made me a pediatric anesthesiologist". His first rate training program in Pediatric Anesthesia influenced the development of pediatric anesthesia worldwide.

Leigh, another early force in pediatric anesthesia, asked difficult, intriguing questions. He contributed a one-way valve that reduced the amount of carbon dioxide re-inspired by children during surgery. His textbook "*Pediatric Anesthesiology*," written with Belton in 1948 [29] preceded Smith's book (above) and contained much of what we "know" today, albeit based on an enormous amount of informed speculation.

A fourth early North American (another Canadian) pioneer of pediatric anesthesia—also a product of World War II—was Stephen. An outstanding teacher, he published a small textbook "*Essentials of Pediatric Anesthesia*" in 1954 [30]. He was among the first to (appropriately) raise concerns regarding the effects of operating room temperatures on patient well being. Like Leigh, he developed a valve to prevent carbon dioxide rebreathing.

The first textbook of Pediatric Anesthesia "*Anesthesia in Children*" was published in Great Britain in 1923 [31]. The next such book, "*Précis Clinique et Opératoire de Chirurgie Infantile*" was published in France 1925 [32]. Following the publication of Leigh and Belton's book, in 1950, Smith wrote the first comprehensive textbook on "*Anesthesia for Infants and Children*" and therein, concisely described how to provide anesthesia for infants and children undergoing various surgical procedures [33]. Gregory's textbook "*Pediatric Anesthesia*" was the first physiology-based pediatric anesthesia textbook [34].

The increasing interest in pediatric anesthesia was not confined to North America. The Englishman, Philip Ayre, invented a simple system for delivery of anesthesia to children undergoing craniofacial surgery [35], His "T"-piece (Fig. 65.4) avoided the imposition of increased resistance to breathing, particularly important for infants having cleft lip and palate surgery, and allowed him to get his hands out of the surgical field.

Ayre was a master pediatric anesthetist. Like many of his patients, he had a cleft lip and palate, badly repaired, and he spoke with a "honking" sound that adults found difficult to understand. But his voice apparently mesmerized children, especially during induction of anesthesia, distracting them from the vapors they breathed.

Electronic versions of Ayre's simple device underlie many modern pediatric ventilators. Gordon Jackson–Rees (1918–2001) added an open-ended bag to Ayre's "T"-piece; the bag could be used to control or assist ventilation [36]. We used this modification to provide Continuous Positive Airway Pressure (CPAP) and improve the outcome of premature infants who had hyaline membrane disease (HMD) (See below) [37].

Control of Breathing

Anesthetists recognized early on, that airway obstruction commonly occurred with induction of anesthesia, particularly due to the tongue falling to the back of the oropharynx, and collapse of the upper airway. In 1847, Francis Sibson (1814–1876) applied a jaw thrust (lifting the jaw at its angles) to treat this problem [38], and Snow also suggested maintaining light anesthesia and jaw thrust. In 1908, Frederick Hewitt made an oropharyngeal airway roughly similar to those used today to treat this problem [39].

The increasing demands of surgery, particularly surgery of the chest, abdomen, and cranium, required better control of the airway and a need to protect the airway from contamination with blood, pus, and gastric contents. It required that the anesthetist ensure adequate ventilation and oxygenation. The solution lay in passage of a tube into the trachea, and in this, both surgeons and anesthetists led the charge. In 1882, Joseph O'Dwyer (1841–1898), a New York surgeon, used one of the first "tracheal tubes" (really a tube into the larynx) when he inserted a metal tube into the glottis of children to bypass the pseudo membranes of diphtheria that caused glottic obstruction and death [40]. He adapted the positive pressure artificial respiration apparatus developed by his colleague George Fell, by replacing Fell's mask with O'Dwyer's glottic tube. He was thus able, when necessary, to ventilate the patient's lungs with air supplied by a foot-operated bellows (Fig. 65.5).

After initial failure with a spring-loaded device intended to insert his tube into the glottis of children, O'Dwyer placed the tube blindly by lifting the epiglottis with a finger, sliding the tube along that finger and into the glottis, a technique still occasionally used today (Fig. 65.6).

The Scottish surgeon William Macewen (1848–1924) was the first to use tracheal intubation to deliver anesthesia. He inserted a tube into the trachea of a patient with tongue cancer in 1878, to facilitate excision of the mass [41]. In the early twentieth century, surgeons Charles Elsberg (1872–1948) of New York and Rudolph Matas (1850–1967) of New Orleans,

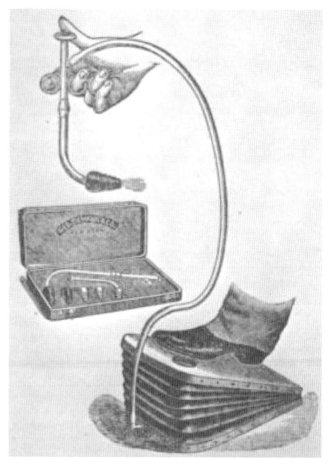

Fig. 65.5 The Fell-O'Dwyer apparatus. The O'Dwyer tube was held in the operator's hand and passed into the glottis. To ventilate the patient's lungs, a bellows was compressed with the foot and the opening on top of the tube occluded with the thumb. During exhalation, the thumb was removed and gas exited the lungs through the opening in the top of the tube. (Courtesy of AATS: Founders)

used blind tracheal intubation and manual ventilation of the lungs to facilitate thoracic surgery. At approximately 1920, Ivan Magill (1888–1996) and Stanley Rowbotham (1878–1979) developed laryngoscopes that allowed anesthetists to visualize the glottis of children [42]. Despite the availability of laryngoscopes and tracheal tubes, neonates and infants seldom underwent tracheal intubation until the advent of pediatric thoracic and cardiac surgery, and even then many were anesthetized with open drop ether! Early tracheal tubes were stiff, often made of hard rubber or latex covered spiraled wire, thick-walled devices that increased resistance to gas flow and caused airway damage.

Cole seemingly solved the resistance problem by making tracheal tubes with a short, narrow distal end that inserted into the trachea. This short end connected to a wide bore, low resistance tube [43] (Fig. 65.7). The shoulder at the junction of the larger and smaller tubes sat on the vocal cords and reduced the incidence of bronchial intubation. However, in

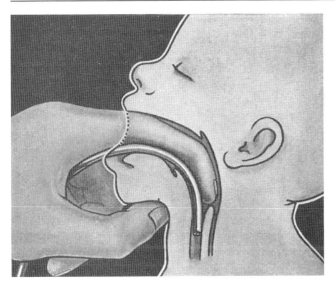

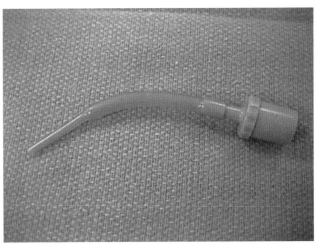

Fig. 65.6 In the "digital" method of tracheal intubation, the index finger was passed into the mouth and the epiglottis was lifted (note identity to the approach used with the MacIntosh blade). A tracheal catheter was passed along the finger and into the trachea. The author was taught this method of tracheal intubation as a medical student before a full time anesthetist (Sol Shnider—1929–1994) directed anesthesia in the delivery room at UCSF and taught us to use a laryngoscope to visualize the glottis for tracheal intubation. (http://www.hmc.org.qa/mejem/mar2002/comm/comm1.htm. Accessed 31/03/2010)

Fig. 65.7 The Cole tube had a wide (low resistance) upper part and a short narrower (higher resistance) lower portion; the short portion was placed into the trachea. The beveled portion rested on (and could distend) the vocal cords. (old.cvm.msu.edu/services/aneth/docs/cat-intu/. Accessed 31/03/2010)

1969, Bernard Brandstater (1929–) reported that downward pressure could force the upper wide portion of the tube between the vocal cords and damage the larynx [44].

Brandstater was one of the pioneers of prolonged intubation in infants. While working at the American University in Beirut in the late 1950s, he achieved encouraging results in 40 infants with tetanus, intubating the trachea with soft polyvinyl chloride tubes, and ventilating their lungs with room air. He used a Harvard sine wave pump from the research laboratory, carefully covering the plaque, which read "For use in laboratory animals only". In 1963, Tom Allen (1923–2011) at the Children's Hospital in Adelaide, Australia, introduced prolonged nasal intubation as an alternative to tracheotomy for croup, and his paper with Ian Steven (1926–2006), published in 1965, paved the way for prolonged airway management in children [45, 46].

Thin-walled plastic tracheal tubes replaced Cole tubes in the 1970s. These low resistance tubes tempted practitioners to leave tubes in the trachea for protracted periods to facilitate mechanical ventilation and avoid tracheotomy. Early on, however, practitioners discovered yet another problem: plasticizers in the tubes damaged the trachea and caused subglottic stenosis (narrowing of the trachea) [47]. Removing the plasticizers allowed safer prolonged tracheal intubation.

In 1939, Noel Gillespie (1904–1955) developed a pediatric laryngoscope. Robert Miller (1906–1976) improved on this design in 1946 [48], and "Miller" laryngoscopes became fixtures

in delivery rooms, neonatal intensive care units, and operating rooms throughout the world. Other designs specifically tailored to pediatric practice were subsequently introduced. In the past 15 years, newly developed fiber optic intubation equipment has proven useful for guiding tracheal intubation of infants and children with upper airway anomalies.

The T-Piece

Before 1937 it was difficult to ventilate the lungs of neonates undergoing head and mouth surgery because the anesthetist competed with the surgeon for airway space. As noted earlier, Ayre solved this problem with his T-piece (Fig. 65.8). He achieved induction of anesthesia via a mask and then intubated the trachea and attached his device to the tracheal tube, thereby removing his hands from the surgical field and out of the "cranky surgeon's" way [49]. Ayre believed this approach decreased pallor, tachypnea (rapid breathing), and respiratory distress during and immediately after surgery. His elegantly simple device imposed little resistance to spontaneous breathing. The T-piece had another virtue—it could be used to ventilate the lungs of patients by intermittently obstructing the gas outflow from the T-piece. In 1963, Keuskamp (1915–1992) of Amsterdam, devised the first pediatric ventilator, the LOOSCO, using a solenoid to intermittently "thumb" the gas outlet from what effectively was an Ayre's T-piece [50]. People called this machine the "electronic thumb". Some modern infant ventilators use this T-piece principle.

Jackson–Rees (1918–2001) modified Ayre's T-piece by adding a bag to the expiratory tube so that he could ventilate

Fig. 65.8 The upper picture is a drawing of the Jackson–Rees modification of the Ayre's "T"-piece. We added an under water "pop off valve" which set an upper limit to the pressure that could be applied and thus minimized the incidence of pneumothorax. The lower picture shows this device applying CPAP to a preterm baby

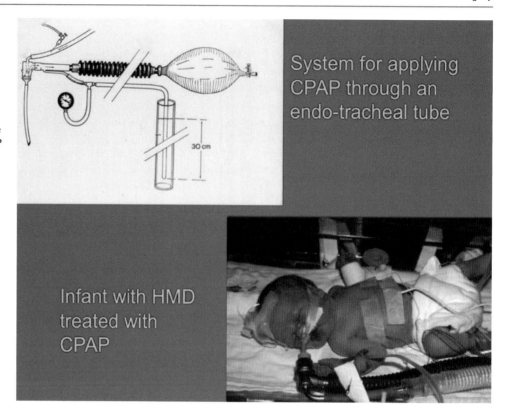

the children's lungs by squeezing the bag. This modification of the Ayre's T-piece facilitated hyperventilation, which was part of Jackson-Rees' "Liverpool Technique" (see below). We used Jackson-Rees' modification of the Ayre's T-piece to create positive end-expiratory pressure while applying CPAP to the lungs of premature infants (Fig. 65.8) [37].

Like all of the Mapleson rebreathing non-absorption circuits (A to E), versions of the Ayre's T-piece (Mapleson E, and the Jackson-Rees modification, often referred to as Mapleson F) are generally used with high gas inflows, often at least twice the patient's minute ventilation, in order to prevent accumulation of CO_2. This wastes potent inhaled anesthetic and carrier gases (air, oxygen, N_2O). And, unless the gases are scavenged, they contaminate the operating room with anesthetic. The relatively recent application of end-tidal gas monitoring allows anesthetists to administer the minimum fresh gas flow needed to maintain the desired end-tidal CO_2, thereby reducing some of the gas wastage.

Today, in most major pediatric centers in developed countries, anesthesia circuits used in children, even in tiny premature babies, are of the "circle" or rebreathing type. The circuits are incorporated into complex modern anesthesia machines with accurate monitoring, largely eliminating wasted gas. The Jackson–Rees modification of the T-piece and the "Liverpool Technique" are still commonly used, however, in developing countries that cannot afford anesthesia machines. They also cannot afford end-tidal CO_2 monitors. Consequently they use

high gas flows, and waste large volumes of fresh gas and anesthetic, which they also cannot afford.

Children's Masks

The use of traditional adult masks for delivery of anesthetic to children, even when reduced in size, resulted in a large volume of "dead space" within the mask. When the child was anesthetized and breathed spontaneously, this could lead to inadequate oxygenation and accumulation of carbon dioxide. In 1960, two pediatric anesthetists were requested by a newly appointed pediatric surgeon to anesthetize his neonatal patients for inguinal hernia surgery, without intubation. The inadequacy of the available masks led Donald Soucek (1935–) and Leslie Rendell Baker (1917–2008) to make alginate casts of the faces of children of different ages, while intubated and anesthetized, and develop the pediatric anesthesia mask that became used universally [51]. The advantage of these masks was that they had very little dead space and reduced rebreathing and hypercarbia.

Anesthetists sought ways to avoid intubation of the larynx and trachea, because of the "delicacy" of these structures. Archie Brain (1942–) accomplished this in 1987 when he introduced the laryngeal mask airway (LMA) as an alternative to tracheal intubation. The mask fits over the glottis (the opening to the larynx), and connects to a wide tube [52].

These devices minimize stimulation of the trachea but in the lightly anesthetized patient still can cause laryngospasm. One day I wondered what the dead-space (volume of inhaled gas that does not take part in alveolar ventilation) was for LMAs of different sizes so I took LMAs and determined the amount of water the mask and connecting tube could contain. The volume of the mask and tube in infants and young children was large. Thus, these devices impose significant amounts of dead-space, making their use less desirable in patients with increased intracranial pressure or respiratory failure. Another problem with the smallest size masks is that they are merely a small version of the adult mask and do not take into account the anatomical difference in the larynx of neonates and young children. This makes seating the masks properly over the larynx uncertain.

Monitoring

In the 1850s, John Snow taught anesthetists to feel the pulse of patients and to observe their skin color, and breathing patterns and rates to detect anesthesia-induced depression of the cardiovascular and respiratory systems [9]. He appreciated that a smaller margin of safety existed for infants, and that it was easier to over anesthetize them and produce apnea, especially when using chloroform. It was this recognition and his exceptional care that allowed him to have excellent outcomes. For the next century, monitoring consisted of palpating the pulse and counting respirations. By the 1960s, anesthetists consistently measured arterial blood pressure (although Cushing advocated such measurement a half century earlier). Betty Lank and Robert Smith were early advocates of doing so during pediatric surgery. Smith and Stuart Cullen (1909–1979) also suggested taping a stethoscope to the chest of patients to monitor heart rate, heart tones, and breathing [53]. Introduction of esophageal stethoscopes by John Inkster (1924–2011) in the 1970s, made it easier to monitor heart tones, breathing, and temperature, but the widespread use of electronic monitors and the increased noise in modern operating rooms have made esophageal stethoscopes obsolete, except in developing countries lacking other forms of monitoring.

Early textbooks made no mention of monitoring, but in the second edition of his book (1959), Smith recommended monitoring the "usual case" with a stethoscope, a sphygmomanometer, and a thermometer [33]. For cardiac surgery, he recommended intra-arterial pressure and ECG measurement. Increases in cardiac and thoracic surgery cases in the 1940s–1960s and the development of intensive care units in the 1960s increased the need for invasive monitoring. Oxygen saturation and end-tidal gas monitors became available in the late twentieth century, and their use decreased anesthesia-related injuries and deaths [54]. The advent of ICUs (see below) increased the need for monitoring and these devices were routinely used in the operating room by the early 1970s.

Infants don't feel Pain, do they?

As late as 1975, some surgeons might operate on infants who were receiving but a small dose of morphine, paralyzed with drugs, and whose lungs were mechanically ventilated. Fearing circulatory depression, anesthetists excused this barbarism, in the belief that infants barely felt pain [55–57]. "And even if they felt pain, no matter, they would not remember it." These notions have now been disproven [58, 59]. I (and countless other parents) knew they were untrue. Once, after I changed my 3-month-old son's diapers, he became inconsolable. I had accidentally stuck a safety pin through his scrotum. Calm returned with removal of the safety pin. Clearly babies feel pain. In 1987, an article in Redbook magazine described surgery in an infant lacking sufficient anesthesia [60]. The resultant publicity caused this practice to change. Infants in developed countries are now appropriately anesthetized, and provided with post-operative pain relief. However, in some developing countries in which I have worked, infants still receive little or no anesthesia, or medication for postoperative pain relief by the local anesthesiologists or anesthetists.

The "Liverpool Technique" commonly used to anesthetize infants and children provided a subtle variant on the "no anesthesia" problem. Originally the technique consisted of "heavy sedation", intravenous induction of anesthesia, muscle paralysis and hyperventilation with oxygen and nitrous oxide [36]. However, many practitioners reduced the technique to hyperventilation with 70% nitrous oxide and muscle paralysis—and no sedation. Anand and Aynsley–Green [58, 61] showed that term and preterm infants anesthetized by this technique had greater hormonal and metabolic stress responses than infants receiving the same "anesthesia" plus fentanyl (a narcotic) [62]. Infants anesthetized with nitrous oxide, muscle paralysis, and hyperventilation alone had approximately nine times more complications after surgery than infants anesthetized by the same technique plus sufentanil. Similarly, administering anesthesia during cardiopulmonary bypass decreased mortality [58].

Despite contrary antique beliefs, young children require more anesthesia than older patients. In 1952, Margery Deming (1914–1998) showed that infants and children had greater concentrations of cyclopropane in their blood than adults, when anesthetized [22], and Snow [9] and Robson [21] intuitively knew that children require more anesthesia. In 1969, Gregory et al [24] and Nicodemas et al [23] showed that minimum anesthetic concentrations (MAC values) for halothane in infants and young children exceed those of adults (Fig. 65.2).

Intravenous Fluids, Blood, and Blood Products

Hemorrhage caused Snow's single surgical death in a child. Both adults and children benefited from advances in intravenous fluid delivery. Anesthetists maintain the internal milieu of the patient during surgery by such administration, and delivery of sterile fluids to maintain intra and extra vascular volumes enabled surgeons to undertake more ambitious surgery. Children may have benefited more because of their smaller fluid volumes, and the fact that smaller fluid losses lead to hypovolemia; children may require seemingly astronomical volumes of fluid to survive some types of surgery.

The invention of plastic intravenous catheters minimized the number of insertions for intravenous infusions, a particular blessing to children and infants who detest needle-sticks, and in whom it is often difficult to find a vein. We are grateful to David Massa (1923–1990), who while an anesthesia resident at the Mayo Clinic, invented the insertable plastic catheter in 1950 [63].

James Gamble (1883–1956) described the fluid compartments of the body and their changes from dehydration, showing that these are not simply proportionate to size in children versus adults [64]. Application of this information improved a child's chance of surviving. Adding to this, Malcolm Holliday (1924–) and William Sager (1898–1951) defined the fluid and glucose requirements of different aged children [65]. It isn't always a perfect world of advances, however. In the 1960s, Tom Shires (1925–2007) described the shifts in extracellular fluid volume occurring during surgery in adults [66]. Misapplication of these findings to infants and children often resulted in fluid overload and congestive heart failure, especially in septic children. Today, fluid is more accurately and safely administered to the smallest infant using infusion pumps. Measurement of electrolytes and serum osmolarity *during* surgery on small volumes of blood (micro liters) guides today's administration of appropriate amounts of fluid.

The ability to transfuse blood, platelets, fresh frozen plasma, and individual clotting factors, makes major pediatric surgery possible. In a premature infant, who may have a blood volume of 80 ml, a loss of 8 ml of blood may be dangerous, and 16 ml disastrous. Transfusion may be needed to sustain life. Without clotting factors and platelets (e.g., as in clotting-factor deficient patients), bleeding from surgical wounds and needle sticks would be excessive. Like John Snow's patient, many would die. The development of safe transfusion was indispensable to the advancement of pediatric anesthesia, and the management of infants and children in pediatric and neonatal intensive care units.

Postanesthesia Care Units

As with transfusions, the development of post anesthesia care units (PACUs) has been essential to the advancement of pediatric anesthesia. PACUs improved outcome for both adult and pediatric patients. The invention of PACUs came earlier than most people realize. In 1801, in an attempt to reduce postoperative complications, English surgeons developed the first PACUs and located them near the operating room [67]. Soon after Morton's demonstration, it was recognized at the Massachusetts General Hospital, that residual anesthetic effects plus longer, complicated and traumatic surgery increased the need for careful postoperative observation, and the first PACU in the United States was built there. Johns Hopkins Hospital had a PACU by the 1920s [68].

But PACUs were not the norm. Well into the early 1940s patients might have surgical procedures, e.g., tonsillectomy, at home, and their parents provided the postoperative care. Into the 1960s, most hospitalized patients, including pediatric patients, received postoperative care on the ward. Beecher (1904–1976) and Todd's (1918–1998) report in 1953, documented fewer deaths in hospitals that had PACUs [69]. Initially infants and children were cared for in adult PACUs in most hospitals. By the 1960s and 1970s, it was realized that it would be better to care for these patients in pediatric PACUs because the problems of children were different from those of adults, and pediatric PACUs became common

Pediatric Intensive Care Units (PICUs)

PICUs enabled the pursuit of complex and traumatic surgery and thus underlay progress in pediatric anesthesia. Anesthetists built and ran the first ICUs in Copenhagen, Denmark, and in Uppsala and Stockholm, Sweden in the 1950s, to care for adults and children suffering from polio (Fig. 65.9).

Drinker tank-type ventilators, which were commonly used for these patients, had considerable limitations. Moreover, during the 1952 polio outbreak in Copenhagen, too few machines existed to meet the needs of the hundreds of patients who required artificial ventilation. Physicians, medical students, and nurses were recruited to manually ventilate these patient's lungs, a heroic but sometimes flawed solution, given human frailties. Positive pressure ventilators were developed to provide a better, more constant and controllable solution. But these early crude devices could cause complications, especially when used to ventilate small children's lungs. Because they were designed to inflate the lungs of adults, they sometimes delivered excessive volumes that ruptured the lungs (pneumothorax), or perversely might inadequately ventilate the lungs of babies who had "stiff" lungs. In the early 1960s, about 30% of babies with stiff lungs receiving mechanical ventilation developed a pneumothorax.

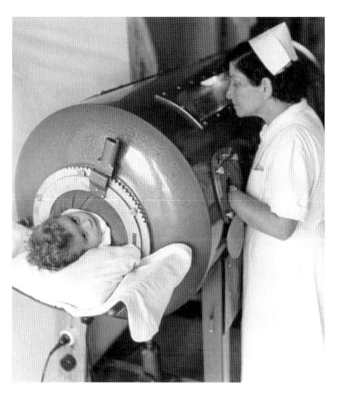

Fig. 65.9 This picture of a child in a Drinker "Iron Lung" exemplifies the devices used to provide ventilation for thousands of patients who could not breathe adequately due to polio. Such artificial ventilation might continue for years. (http://pathmicro.med.sc.edu/lecture/vaccines.htm. Accessed 31/03/2010)

Better ventilators and better understanding of lung diseases decreased this life-threatening event to less than five percent, even in premature infants.

Two factors led anesthetists to develop early PICUs (Table 65.4). First, training in the operating room provided the required knowledge of respiratory and cardiovascular physiology. Second, anesthetists closely observed patients for protracted periods, learning to quickly interpret and act on what they observed. The invention of safer endotracheal tubes, mechanical ventilators, and monitors, and the education of dedicated nurses who understood technology and the physiology of small patients, made possible the PICU care we now take for granted.

New gadgets progressively advanced care [70]. In the 1960s, results from Severinghaus' blood gas and pH electrodes guided changes in mechanical ventilation. Plastic catheters inserted into arteries facilitated the drawing of blood and measurement of arterial blood pressure. Pressures obtained from central venous catheters guided fluid administration. Sometimes a step backwards accompanied a step forward. In 1972, the Swan–Ganz catheter, introduced for adults, was used in pediatric cardiac patients to measure pulmonary artery pressures and cardiac output [71]. Although the derived information improved understanding of the cardiovascular function of ill children, the catheter could cause infections, thrombosis, and lung infarction. Pediatric heart rate and blood pressure monitors became available in the mid 1970s, making possible the ongoing diagnosis and treatment of cardiovascular abnormalities at the bedside. The introduction of echocardiography into PICUs in the 1990s, advanced the diagnosis of congenital heart disease at the bedside, and allowed immediate determination of the effectiveness of treatment. It also decreased the need for cardiac catheterization and provided previously unavailable information about the heart's function and pulmonary vascular resistance.

Neonatal Intensive Care Units (NICUs)

Pierre Budin of Paris (1846–1907) developed the first NICU in the 1890s [72]. Working with a chicken equipment manufacturer, he constructed incubators for premature babies that maintained a relatively constant environmental temperature. Budin appreciated the need of premature babies for warmth, frequent feedings (often only 3 ml at a time), and protection from infection (three hallmarks of modern NICU care). He also recognized the need for specialized nursing care. One of his pupils, Martin Couney (1870–1950), a German physician, exhibited 'incubator babies" at fairs, first in France and then in England and the United States, doing so until 1940 and World War II. Babies of similar size and gestation to those cared for by Couney died in most nurseries around the world, but about 85 % of Cooney's babies survived. Most pediatricians ignored Cooney's work, and between 1940 and 1960 the outcomes of most sick premature babies remained dismal.

Advances Underlying Modern Neonatal Anesthesia and Intensive Care

The period from 1940–1960 laid foundations for great advancement. Geoffrey Dawes' (1918–1996) book "Fetal and Neonatal Physiology" summarized landmark studies carried out at Oxford and in the Caribbean in the 1960s, that defined the circulatory changes that allowed the fetus to move from intra-uterine to extra-uterine life, thereby facilitating the rational resuscitation of troubled neonates [73]. Adamsons et al found that administering glucose and buffers (to correct acidosis) improved resuscitation of acidotic, asphyxiated fetuses [74]. Kenneth Cross (1916–1990) and co-workers showed that the neonate might fail to respond to hypoxia (after all, such an environment was what the neonate faced for 9 months) indicating why asphyxiated neonates require help with their breathing [75].

John Clements (1923–) demonstrated that the low surface tension in the lining of normal alveoli prevented

Table 65.4 Early pediatric intensive care units

Date	Location	Founder
1953	Copenhagen Sweden	Bjørn Ibsen
1955	Gotheburg, Sweden	Goren Hagland
1958	Liverpool, England	Jackson–Rees
1960	Newcastle, England	John Inkster
1961	Stockholm, Sweden	Hans Feychting
1963	Melbourne	John Stocks
1964	Bicêtre, France	G. Huault
1964	Philadelphia, PA	J Downes, L Bachman
1965	Washington, DC	Cheston Berlin

atelectasis [76]. Mary Ellen Avery (1927–2011), a pediatric resident at Harvard, suggested that inadequate quantities of surfactant in the lungs might cause the impaired breathing in preterm infants who had hyaline membrane disease (HMD). Surfactant, a special kind of natural soap, was what induced the low surface tension. Using a Wilhelmy Balance (a device to measure surface tension), she and Jerry Mead (1921–2009) demonstrated that the lungs of infants with HMD lacked surfactant (i.e., lacked the ability to lower surface tension) and indicated that this lack caused the atelectesis and impaired breathing [77]. In an epic 1964 study in Singapore (Singapore because a hospital there had 24,000 births per year), Clements et al insufflated nebulized surfactant into the trachea of these infants in an attempt to improve their outcomes. He also created devices to measure pulmonary blood flow and ventilation while in Singapore (personal communication). Clements and associates documented the predicted decrease in lung volumes (atelectasis), but to their surprise found abnormally low pulmonary blood flows [78]. The infusion of acetylcholine increased pulmonary blood flow. This information added another important piece to the HMD puzzle—in addition to inadequate ventilation, HMD was also associated with reduced pulmonary blood flow.

In 1967, pediatricians William Tooley (1925–1992), Roderic Phibbs (1930–), and Joseph Kitterman (1936–) invited me, an anesthesia resident, to join them in their newly developed NICU at UCSF. They hoped my experience in mechanically ventilating the lungs of adults could be applied to improve the respiratory care of neonates. William Hamilton (1922–), the new Chair of anesthesia allowed me to work in the NICU full time for a year, an adventure that has lasted more than 35 years. Here was the picture in our NICU in 1967. Pediatric ventilators were inadequate, and we were without most neonatal monitors (e.g., heart rate, blood pressure, hemoglobin oxygen saturation monitors) available today. John Severinghaus (1922–) and Freeman Bradley (1932–) (inventors of the CO_2 electrode) [79] made a set of oxygen, CO_2, and pH electrodes for our NICU (Fig. 65.10). Each set of measurements required more than 1 ml of blood,

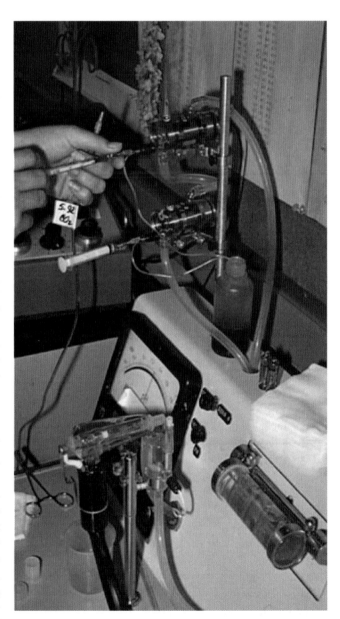

Fig. 65.10 The blood gas and pH electrodes built by Severinghaus and Bradley for use in the ICN at UCSF. (Courtesy of Joseph Kitterman, MD)

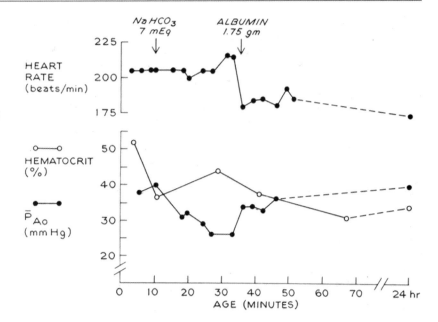

Fig. 65.11 Mean arterial pressure, heart rate, and hematocrit changed in a 1.75 Kg infant during resuscitation. Administration of bicarbonate decreased mean arterial pressure (PA0) and hematocrit, demonstrating that the baby had a low blood volume. Administering albumin and fluid returned the pressure to normal. The hematocrit data indicated a startling 30 % volume deficit. (Courtesy of Joseph Kitterman, MD)

a blood loss necessitating blood transfusion for many infants! Today these analyses plus electrolyte determinations require < 100 micro liters of blood. Residents and faculty made the measurements and repaired the electrodes when they failed. Calibrating standards weren't available, so if the blood gas and pH values conflicted with the patient's clinical picture, I drew blood from my radial artery, and if my measured values differed significantly from what I knew they should be, we changed the electrode membranes (so much for complicated electronics). Since there were no neonatal monitors, we employed the eight-channel Grass Recorder™ used by Clements, et al in Singapore, and measured and recorded arterial and central venous pressures from umbilical artery and venous catheters, doing so at least every five minutes.

We quickly learned what "normal" blood pressures of sick infants were [80], and what constituted hypotension; we used this information to determine whether measures used to correct hypotension were effective or not [81]. While such measurements are routine today, it was new and exciting at the time, because normative data were not available. It was part of the era of phenomenological research. We used arterial pressure determinations to judge the amounts of fluid needed to correct hypovolemia (Fig. 65.11).

We learned that hyperventilation often caused hypotension, and that the combination of hypotension and hyperventilation could be detrimental to the brains of neonates. Such measurements, and others, promoted the care of infants based on physiology, not guesses, and this improved outcomes (Fig. 65.12).

Earlier, I noted some of the problems (e.g., pneumothorax) for sick babies, particularly premature babies, associated with the first commercially available mechanical ventilators. In addition, weaning from the ventilator required

discontinuation of ventilation for progressively longer periods of time to allow spontaneous ventilation. This could precipitate collapse of the lungs (atelectesis) and hypoxemia. In 1968, a report by Harrison et al. led me to devise a way to manage these problems [37]. Harrison et al described the effects of tracheal intubation in infants who had HMD. Before tracheal intubation, these infants grunted during expiration. It was clear to me that they grunted to keep their lungs from collapsing during expiration, and to improve oxygenation. Tracheal intubation prevented grunting, and, instead of making the babies better, made them worse; their oxygenation (PaO2) decreased, the level of carbon dioxide (PaCO2) in their blood increased, and their acidity increased. Removing the tracheal tube made them better.

I combined these thoughts with ones expressed by Hamilton about the "tight bag", a technique for imposing an increased pressure in the airway, and I had an "aha" moment. Why not maintain positive pressure during expiration when the babies were breathing through the tracheal tube (apply "continuous positive airway pressure" or CPAP) and allow the babies to breathe spontaneously? This might improve oxygenation and survival. That night, we tested this proposition in a new patient with a frighteningly low PaO2 of 30 mm Hg (normal is 60–80 mm Hg). After tracheal intubation, we applied an end-expiratory pressure of 8 mm Hg and the PaO2 immediately increased to 88 mmHg. Over the next hour it rose to 230 mm Hg, a remarkable increase, and this very sick infant survived in contrast to those treated previously by us and by others [82]. Of the next 20 patients treated with CPAP, 16 survived! Prior to this therapy, half of such premature babies weighing 1,800 grams at birth had died. Many of the initial babies we cared for were smaller than this, making their odds of survival even smaller. After introducing CPAP,

Fig. 65.12 The percent mortality of preterm infants greatly decreased during a recent 35-year period, probably because of therapies introduced into the ICN. The Y-axis indicates percent mortality and the X-axis, the approximate years for the indicated value. (Courtesy of Joseph Kitterman, MD)

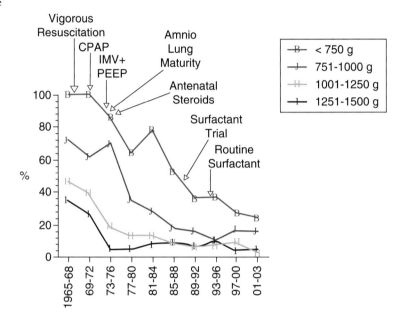

more than 98% of our 1800 g babies survived, without lung injury. Amazingly, none of the original babies treated *only* with CPAP developed chronic lung disease, a finding later confirmed by others [83]. During the same period, Daily [84] reported that those babies surviving mechanical ventilation often developed bronchopulmonary dysplasia (BPD), a newly defined and severe and often fatal form of neonatal lung injury [85].

In the spring of 1970, we presented the effects of CPAP on the outcome in premature infants, at the Society of Pediatric Research. The results prompted Robert Kirby (1938–), an anesthetist at Wilford Hall Hospital at Lackland Air Force Base in San Antonio, Texas, to develop the Baby-Bird Ventilator™. This machine allowed babies to breathe spontaneously between ventilator breaths, and to maintain positive end-expiratory pressure (PEEP). In effect, this machine was both a mechanical ventilator and a means of delivering CPAP. It made separation from the ventilator easier and advanced neonatal mechanical ventilation. However, BPD continued to occur in mechanically ventilated premature babies, and remains a major problem today [86]. Consequently most premature infants are now treated with nasal CPAP when possible. If the patients develop pulmonary hypertension (high blood pressure in the arteries of the lungs) they are now treated with nitric oxide to dilate the pulmonary arteries.

The methods devised in ICNs for the care of preterm infants were subsequently used to care for infants during and after surgery, an example of translational research. Anesthetists improved the outcomes of preterm infants and then applied the information gained in operating rooms. The

Liverpool technique of ventilation had unwittingly provided positive end-expiratory pressure (PEEP), and the good outcome of the patients reported by Nesbit (1926–) and Wilson (1927–1981) in 1958 probably resulted from inadvertent PEEP. Of note, they thought that inadvertent PEEP was detrimental and recommended using zero pressure during expiration [87].

Outreach

During the past 40 years, increasing numbers of anesthetists and surgeons traveled to developing countries to correct lesions, usually congenital anomalies. Among the first to do this was the plastic surgeon Donald Laub (1935–) who, other surgeons, anesthesiologists, and nurses from Stanford University, made weekend trips to Mexico to repair cleft lips and cleft palates. Laub had been moved by Antonio, a 13 year-old boy from Mexicali, who went to Stanford University for cleft surgery. Before surgery Antonio rarely attended school and did poorly when he did attend. After surgery he regularly attended school and did well. Believing that many children like Antonio could benefit from surgery, in 1969 Laub established Interplast (now ReSurge International), an organization dedicated to providing free reconstructive plastic surgery for children in developing countries. Within a few years Interplast had expanded into Vietnam, China, India, Laos, and other countries. Similarly focused organizations, including Operation Smile (1982), Smile Train (1999), and many others have been established. In parallel developments, hundreds of organizations in Europe and the United States now provide free cleft surgery, orthopedic surgery, cardiac surgery, ear nose and throat surgery, eye surgery, and dentistry. These organizations are both large (e.g., Doctors without Borders) and small (sometimes consisting of only two or three people).

The well-known aphorism "if you give a man a fish, he eats for a day while if you teach him to fish, he eats for a lifetime" arose as an issue. At the International Plastic and Reconstructive Surgery Organization meeting in 1990, Ortiz–Minesterio of Mexico, and other surgeons from developing countries requested education that would permit them to perform the surgery themselves. This makes sense because they can do a much better job of preoperative evaluation and follow-up care than groups present for only a week or two. Some organizations responded to this request with outreach programs by the parent group that pay indigenous surgeons, nurses, and anesthesiologists to perform the surgery—once it was clear that the local team can effectively and safely do the repairs. In one-year, Nepalese outreach groups performed nearly 2000 cleft repairs, whereas a traveling surgical group could have performed 75 at most, during their two-week stay. One group, Smile Train, has as its primary goal, the funding of groups to establish outreach programs. This is a daunting task in places lacking consistent electricity and running water and that frequently have no anesthesia machines, monitors, blood pressure cuffs, tracheal tubes, or even stethoscopes.

Societies

Several societies formed to advance knowledge and science in pediatric anesthesia. The Association of Paediatric Anaesthetists was established in Great Britain in 1973. The Anesthesia and Critical Care section of the American Academy of Pediatrics was established in 1966, and the Society for Pediatric Anesthesia in 1985, both in North America. Beyond their educational mandate, these groups address government and other public concerns affecting pediatric patients requiring anesthesia, surgery, and intensive care. Board examination/certification for pediatric anesthesia will begin in 2013 in the US. This will advance the status of pediatric anesthesia and improve patient care, as has specialization and certification advanced critical care.

Conclusions

Pediatric surgery developed in parallel with advances in pediatrics, surgery, and anesthesia. Each group learned from the other and prospered. The ability to safely anesthetize nearly any child allowed the imagination and daring of surgeons to soar. They attempted surgical procedures that they had only dreamt of in the past. The discovery of anesthesia allowed the invention of new operations in adults and children alike. It took half a century and more, for surgery to demand significantly more of anesthesia. Pediatric anesthetists evolved through several steps, first developing safe approaches to anesthetic delivery, modifying advances in techniques and drugs to infants and children. With these approaches codified, pediatric anesthetists expanded development of ideas focused specifically on problems in infants and children. Superimposed on this information, are present research programs investigating basic mechanisms underlying pediatric pathophysiology specific to anesthetic concerns.

In parallel with these developments, the desire to solve new and more complicated problems made it crucial to construct child-centered environments (hospitals) in which surgeons, anesthetists, nurses, and others could work together to improve the care of children. It also allowed those working there to interact and to learn from one another. This interaction advanced knowledge of the differences between children and adults. Anesthesia care benefited greatly from the development of blood banking, antibiotics, electronic monitors and intensive care units. Anesthesiologists gained from, contributed to and continue to contribute to these advances.

Acknowledgment I thank Felicia Reilley of the Wood Library-Museum for her unflagging help in finding references and birth and death dates. Her help, kindness, and expertise are much appreciated.

References

1. Berry FA. Anesthetic management of difficult and routine pediatric patients. New York:Churchill Livingstone; 1986.
2. Downes JJ. Historic origins and role of pediatric anesthesiology in child health care. Pediatr Clin North Am. 1994;41:1–14.
3. Costarino AT, Downes JJ. Pediatric anesthesia historical perspective. Anesthesiol Clin North America. 2005;23:573–95, vii.
4. Stanley P. For fear of pain: British surgery, 1790–1850. New York: Editions Rodopi B; 2003.
5. Long CW. An account of the first use of sulfuric ether by inhalation as an anaesthetic in surgical operations. South Med Surg J. 1849;5:705–13.
6. Ellis RH. The case books of Dr. John Snow. London: Professional and Scientific Publications; 1994.
7. Kalliardou E, Tsiotou AG, Velegrakis D et al. Historical aspects of inhalation anesthesia in children: Ether and chloroform. Paediatr Anaesth. 2006;16:3–10.
8. Braz LG, Braz DG, Cruz DS da et al. Mortality in anesthesia: A systematic review. Clinics (Sao Paulo). 2009;64:999–1006.
9. Snow J. On chloroform and other anaesthetics. London: John Churchill; 1858.
10. Gregory GA, Eger EI, Smith NT, Cullen BF, Cullen DJ. The cardiovascular effects of diethyl ether in man. Anesthesiology. 1971;34:19–24.
11. Avery ME, Taeusch WH. Schafer's diseases of the newborn. 5th ed. Philadelphia: W. B. Saunders Company; 1984.

12. Morray JP, Geiduschek JM, Ramamoorthy C et al Anesthesia-related cardiac arrest in children: Initial findings of the Pediatric Perioperative Cardiac Arrest (POCA) Registry. Anesthesiology. 2000;93:6–14.

13. Morray JP, Posner K. Pediatric perioperative cardiac arrest: In search of definition(s). Anesthesiology. 2007;106:207–8.

14. Hedblom CA. The selective surgical treatment of diaphragmatic hernia. Ann Surg. 1931;94:776–85.

15. Ladd WE. Surgical treatment of esophageal atresia and traceo-esophageal fistulas. N Eng J Med. 1944;230:625–37.

16. Haight C. Congenital atresia of the esophagus with tracheoesophageal fistula: Reconstruction of esophageal continuity by primary anastamosis. Ann Surg. 1944;120:623–52.

17. Blalock A, Taussig HB. The surgical treatment of malformations of the heart in which there is pulmonary stenosis or pulmonary atresia. JAMA. 1945;128:189–202.

18. Harmel MH, Lamont A. Anesthesia in the treatment of congenital pulmonic stenosis. Anesthesiology. 1946;7:477–98.

19. Jancelewicz T, Harrison M. A history of fetal surgery. J Perinatol. 2009;36:1–6.

20. Biehl DR, Côté J, Wade JG, Gregory GA, Sitar D. Uptake of halothane by the foetal lamb in utero. Can Anaesth Soc J. 1983;30:24–7.

21. Robson CH. Anesthesia in Children. Am J Surg. 1936;34:469–73.

22. Deming MVN. Agents and techniques for induction of anesthesia in infants and young children. Curr Res Anesth Analg. 1952;31:113–9.

23. Nicodemus HF, Nassiri–Rahimi C, Bachman L, Smith TC. Median effective doses (ED50) of halothane in adults and children. Anesthesiology. 1969;31:344–8.

24. Gregory GA, Eger EI, Munson ES. The relationship between age and halothane requirement in man. Anesthesiology. 1969;30:488–91.

25. Galvin S, Dewan J, Rockoff MA. Betty Lank: A kind and gentle anesthetist devoted to children. AANA J. 2009;77:176–80.

26. Smith RM. The pediatric anesthetist, 1950–1975. Anesthesiology. 1975;43:144–55.

27. Gross RE. The surgical management of the patent ductus arteriosus: With summary of four surgically treated cases. Ann Surg. 1939;110:321–56.

28. Gross RE. Surgical correction for coarctation of the aorta. Surgery. 1945;18:673–8.

29. Leigh MD, Belton MK. Pediatric anesthesiology. New York: MacMillan; 1948.

30. Stephen CR. Elements of pediatric anesthesia. Springfield: Charles C Thomas; 1954.

31. Hewer L. Anaesthesia in children. London: H.K. Lewis; 1923.

32. Ombredanne L. Precis Clinique et Operatoire de Chirurgie Infantile. 1st ed. Paris: Masson; 1925.

33. Smith RM. Anesthesia for infants and children. Saint Louis: C. V. Mosby; 1950.

34. Gregory GA. Pediatric anesthesia. New York:Churchill Livingstone; 1983.

35. Ayre P. Anaesthesia for hare–lip and cleft palate operations on babies. Br J Surg. 1937;25:131–2.

36. Rees GJ, Owen–Thomas JB. A technique of pulmonary ventilation with a nasotracheal tube. Br J Anaesth. 1966;38:901–6.

37. Gregory GA, Kitterman JA, Phibbs RH, Tooley WH, Hamilton WK. Treatment of the idiopathic respiratory–distress syndrome with continuous positive airway pressure. N Engl J Med. 1971;284:1333–40.

38. Sibson F. On the treatment of facial neuralgia by inhalation of ether, and on a new inhaler. London Med Gaz. 1847;39:358–64.

39. Hewitt F. An artificil "air–way" for use during anaesthesia. Lancet. 1908;1:490–1.

40. O'Dwyer J. Intubation of larynx. New York Med J. 1885;42:145–7.

41. Macewen W. Clinical observations on the introduction of tracheal tubes by the mouth instead of performing tracheostomy or laryngotomy. BMJ. 1880;2:122–4.

42. Magill IW. Technique in endotracheal anaesthesia. BMJ. 1930;2:817–20.

43. Cole F. A new endotracheal tube for infants. Anesthesiology. 1945;6:87–8.

44. Brandstater B. Dilation of the larynx with Cole tubes. Anesthesiology. 1969;31:378–9.

45. Allen T, Steven IM. Prolonged endotracheal intubation in infants and children. Br J Anaesth. 1965;37:566–73.

46. Allen T, Steven IM. Prolonged tracheal intubation in infants and children. Br J Anaesth. 1998;81:474–81.

47. Guess WL, Stetson JB. Tissue reactions to organotin-stabilized polyvinyl chloride (PVC) catheters. JAMA. 1968;204:580–4.

48. Miller R. A new laryngoscope for the intubation of infants. Anesthesiology. 1946;7:205–6.

49. Ayre P. Endotracheal anesthsia for babies, with special references to harelip and cleft palate operations. Anesth Analg. 1937;16:330.

50. Hofland J, Leendertse-Verloop K, Rupreht J. Keuskamp and the Amsterdam infant ventilator. Anaesthesia. 2006;61:705–12.

51. Rendell-Baker L, Soucek D. New paediatric face ask and anestheisia equipment. Br J Anaesth. 1962;1:1690.

52. Brain AI. The laryngeal mask—a new concept in airway management. Br J Anaesth. 1983;55:801–5.

53. Cullen SC. Anesthesia. Chicago: Year Book Medical Publishers Inc.; 1946.

54. Bhananker SM, Ramamoorthy C, Geiduschek JM et al Anesthesia–related cardiac arrest in children: Update from the Pediatric Perioperative Cardiac Arrest Registry. Anesth Analg. 2007;105:344–50.

55. McGraw M. Neural maturation as exemplified in the changing reactions of the infant to pin prick. Child Dev. 1941;12:31–42.

56. Bigelow H. Transactions of the American Medical Association. 1885.

57. Pierson AL. Early operation for harelip. Am J Med Sci. 1852;24:576.

58. Anand K. Metabolic and endocrine effects of surgical ligation of patent ductus arteriosus in the preterm neonate. Mod Problems Pediatr. 1985;23:143–57.

59. Taddio A, Katz J, Ilersich AL, Koren G. Effect of neonatal circumcision on pain response during subsequent routine vaccination. Lancet. 1997;349(9052):599–603.

60. Fischer A. Babies in pain. Redbook. 1987 October;124–25, 184–6.

61. Anand KJ, Brown MJ, Bloom SR, Aynsley–Green A. Studies on the hormonal regulation of fuel metabolism in the human newborn infant undergoing anaesthesia and surgery. Horm Res. 1985;22:115–28.

62. Anand KJ, Hickey PR. Halothane–morphine compared with high–dose sufentanil for anesthesia and postoperative analgesia in neonatal cardiac surgery. N Engl J Med. 1992;326:1–9.

63. Massa DJ, Lundy J, Faulconer AJ, Ridley R. A plastic needle. Mayo Clin Proc. 1950;25:413–5.

64. Gamble JL, Robertson JS, Hannigan CA, Foster CG, Farr LE. Chloride, bromide, sodium, and sucrose spaces in man. J Clin Invest. 1953;32:483–9.

65. Holliday MA, Segar WE. The maintenance need for water in parenteral fluid therapy. Pediatrics. 1957;19:823–32.

66. Shires T. Acute changes in extracellular fluids associated with major surgical procedures. Ann Surg. 1961;154:803–10.

67. Zuck D. Anaesthetic and postoperative recovery rooms. Anaesthesia. 1995;50:435–8.

68. Barone C, Pablo C, Barone G. A history of the PACU. J Perianesthesia Nurs. 2003;18:237–41.

69. Beecher HK, Todd DP. A study of deaths associated with anesthesia and surgery. Ann Surg. 1954;140:2–34.

70. Severinghaus JW. Gadgeteering for health care: The John W. Severinghaus lecture on translational science. Anesthesiology. 2009;110:721–8.

71. Stanger P, Heymann MA, Hoffman JI, Rudolph AM. Use of the Swan–Ganz catheter in cardiac catheterization of infants and children. Am Heart J. 1972;83:749–54.

72. Dunn P. Professor Pierre Budin (1846–1907) of Paris, and modern perinatal care. Arch Dis Childhood (Fetal and Neonatal ed). 1995;73:F193–5.

73. Dawes GS. Foetal and neonatal physiology. 1st ed. Chicago: Year Book Medical Publishers Inc.; 1968.

74. Adamsons K, Dawes GS, Dawkins M, James LS, Ross B. The treatment of acidosis with alkali and glucose during asphyxia in foetal rhesus monkeys. J Physiol. 1963;169:679–89.

75. Cross KW, Oppe TE. The effect of inhalation of high and low concentrations of oxygen on the respiration of the premature infant. J Physiol (London). 1952;117:38–55.

76. Clements JA. Surface tension of lung extract. Proc Soc Exp Biol Med. 1957;95:170–2.

77. Avery ME, Mead J. Surface properties in relation to atelectasis and hyaline membrane disease. J Dis Child. 1959;97:517–23.

78. Chu J, Clements JA, Klaus MH, Sweet A, Tooley WH. Neonatal pulmonary ischemia. Pediatrics. 1967;40:709–82.

79. Severinghaus JW, Bradley AF. Electrodes for blood pO2 and pCO2 determination. J Appl Physiol. 1958;13:515–20.

80. Kitterman JA, Phibbs RH, Tooley WH. Aortic blood pressure in normal newborn infants during the first 12 hours of life. Pediatrics. 1969;44:959–68.

81. Kitterman JA, Phibbs RH. Treated hypotension in extremely low birth weight infants. Pediatrics. 2007;119:220–1.

82. Stahlman MT, Battersby EJ, Shepard FM, Blankenship WJ. Prognosis in hyaline–membrane disease. Use of a linear–discriminant. N Engl J Med. 1967;276:303–9.

83. Stocks J, Godfrey S. The role of artificial ventilation, oxygen, and CPAP in the pathogenesis of lung damage in neonates: assessment by serial measurements of lung function. Pediatrics. 1976;57:352–62.

84. Daily WJ, Sunshine P, Smith PC. Mechanical ventilation of newborn infants. V. Five years' experience. Anesthesiology. 1971;34:132–8.

85. Northway WH, Rosan RC, Porter DY. Pulmonary disease following respirator therapy of hyaline–membrane disease. Bronchopulmonary dysplasia. N Engl J Med. 1967;276:357–68.

86. Sankar MJ, Agarwal R, Deorari AK, Paul VK. Chronic lung disease in newborns. Indian J Pediatr. 2008;75:369–76.

87. Nisbet H, Wilson F. The treatment of respiratory infection in infants. Br J Anaesth. 1958;30:419–34.

Some Examples of Industry Contributions to the History of Anesthesia

66

Richard Leazer, David Needham, John (Iain) Glen and Paul Thomas

Summary

Anesthesia evolved through joint contributions by clinicians, investigators, and industry. For example, physician Squibb formed Squibb Pharmaceutical in 1858, to make a purer form of ether. High pressure cylinders made in the late 1800s enabled the economical use of N_2O and O_2. Dentist-manufacturers developed reducing valves and metering devices, tubing, fittings, and masks—and thus the anesthesia machine.

Shukys at Ohio Chemical/Airco synthesized the first commercial fluorinated inhaled anesthetic, fluroxene, in 1953. In parallel, Suckling, at Imperial Chemical Industries (ICI), synthesized halothane, the anesthetic of the 1960s. Safety required precise control of its concentration. Foregger's support of Morris' 1953 development of the Copper Kettle made this possible. In the 1950s, Edmonson and Jones organized Cyprane Ltd to make the Fluotec, the first variable bypass vaporizer directly indicating the concentration of anesthetic. Ayerst donated the Fluotec to US hospitals to capture the market for both halothane and the Fluotec.

In the mid 1960s, Eger became the de facto "Medical Director" for Airco, illustrating the effective relationship between industry and academia in that era. By 1970, enflurane displaced halothane in the US, but it could produce seizures and (rarely) injure the liver. Isoflurane seemed to have neither problem and became the anesthetic of the 1980s. By 1975, Cyprane produced an estimated 85% of the world's calibrated vaporizers. The 1991 introduction of desflurane challenged vaporizer design. Enter the Tec 6, a vaporizer structured unlike any previous vaporizer. In 1998, the Datex-Ohmeda Anesthesia Delivery Unit (ADU) machine was released, a new form of the variable bypass vaporizer, one that accommodated desflurane.

In 1965, ICI began a search for a replacement for thiopental. In 1973, Glen and James detected hypnotic activity in propofol (2,6-diisopropylphenol), but the vehicle Cremophor EL caused anaphylactoid reactions. In 1981, use of a lipid emulsion formulation, and clinical evaluations allowed launch in May 1986.

In 1981, Schwilden introduced the concept of target-controlled infusion (TCI). UK approval for TCI of propofol by the 'Diprifusor' was given in 1995. Approval has been obtained in most countries of the world, but not in the US.

In the early 1980s, Ohmeda supported a "Safety in Anesthesia" symposium directed by Nick Gravenstein. From this meeting came the Anesthesia Patient Safety Foundation (APSF). Led by Pierce in 1985, the American Society of Anesthesiologists and industry provided financial support. The National Academy of Sciences/NIH cited the APSF for improving quality of care. Industry members also partnered with ASA in the 1986 design and funding of the Foundation for Anesthesia Education and Research (FAER). Dollars given to FAER recipients generated several-fold more dollars in NIH awards.

R. Leazer (✉)
8456 Messerschmidt Drive, Verona, WI 53593, USA
e-mail: dickleazer@gmail.com

D. Needham
Villa Sainte Marie, 525 Ave Henri Matisse, 06140 Vence, France
e-mail: needhamadsl@clara.co.uk

J. (Iain) Glen
Oaklands, 35A Bexton Road, Knutsford, Cheshire WA16 0DZ, UK
e-mail: iglen2@compuserve.com

P. Thomas
7 McKay Drive, Bridgewater, NJ 08807, USA
e-mail: PaulThomas1955@gmail.com

Introduction

Although private sector scientists, engineers and companies have discovered or developed products that advanced anesthetic care, these contributions of industry to the history of anesthesia are rarely considered or recorded. To construct this chapter, I (RL; Fig. 66.1) and special and findable colleagues reviewed selected industry-sourced contributions and added our own recollections. This essay follows an "exemplar" format providing noteworthy examples of successful interactions between industry and our specialty. Through

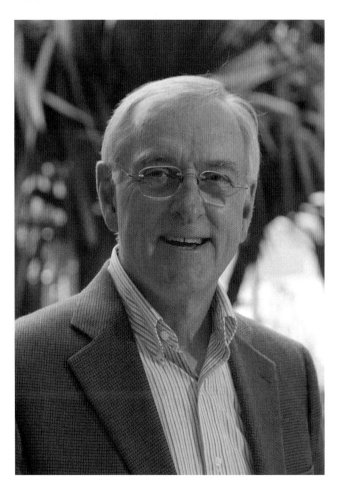

Fig. 66.1 Richard Leazer. (From RL)

this abbreviated—and fragmented (only a small fraction of many tales can be told)—statement of industry contributions, we hope to add information and texture not otherwise available—and perhaps stimulate further chronicles.

The history of industry's contributions to anesthesia, particularly the early history, differs somewhat from that of many other industries because physicians often both invented and used the products. This provided a closed loop guidance system for early manufacturing, arguably accelerating improvements in anesthesia care more than in typical industry models.

Many products, including vaporizers, breathing circuits, anesthesia machines, muscle relaxants, gas analyzers, and inhalation anesthetics, provide examples of joint discovery or invention by physicians and dentists, often stimulated by patient need. More recently, several factors, most notably the increasing demands of regulatory approval, have changed this physician-industry relationship. In addition, as science and technology have become more complex, discoveries and advancements have originated from sources outside the operating room.

In the Beginning…Ether and Nitrous Oxide

An early illustration of the physician-industry interaction arose in the second half of the nineteenth century. Ether had been discovered by Lully in 1275 CE and Morton in 1846 demonstrated its anesthetizing effect. At the time, Jackson cautioned Morton to use a pure ether [1]. Physician Edward Squibb noted this need for ether and other medicines, leading to the 1858 formation of Squibb Pharmaceutical (see uab.edu/Reynolds/cwfigs/squibb). Squibb's contribution (so they said) was to make ether more pure "using an improved production method".

Another early example of a contribution by industry followed progress in the iron and steel industry and the invention of the high pressure gas cylinder in the late nineteenth century. Today, we take for granted the availability of compressed gases for anesthesia, but this was not the case for several decades following the discovery of ether anesthesia. US industrial gas companies were started in the early 1900s, stimulated by the French discovery of new methods of producing various gases at lower cost. Some of these gas companies subsequently developed and manufactured anesthesia equipment and accessories (e.g., Air Products, Puritan Bennett, Airco-Ohio Chemical and Surgical Equipment, and National Cylinder Gas.) In Great Britain, Coxeter and Sons were the first to supply compressed nitrous oxide in steel cylinders. Later, they developed high pressure cylinders for oxygen and until about 1950, were a significant manufacturer of anesthesia equipment of all types.

High-pressure gas cylinders (tanks) solved the problem of storing large amounts of gas in a conveniently small space, but imposed a new problem: how to deal with the huge pressures within the tanks. A full tank of oxygen might have a pressure of 2,200 pounds per square inch, the pressure produced at nearly a mile's depth in the ocean. The development of the tanks also prompted the development of reducing valves and metering devices. To these, manufacturers added tubing, fittings, and masks, all eventually leading to the anesthesia machine.

Along, the way, manufacturers realized the necessity of standards and regulation to make devices safe, consistent, and interchangeable. Standards associations, and groups such as the National Fire Protection Association (formed in 1896), Food and Drug Administration (1906), US Compressed Gas Association (1913), and American Standards Institute (1918) "fit it all together". The chaos of World War II galvanized the effort to improve safety via standards. Anesthesia equipment sent to war zones agonizingly illustrated the dangerous incompatibility of equipment provided by different manufacturers. To preclude operating room fires and explosions, the National Fire Protection Association specified guidelines that would prevent sparks and ignition of flammable inhaled anesthetics in 1941. These developments illustrate the inability of industry and the anesthesia profession to separately deal with joint problems, and the need for such associations and regulatory organizations.

On the other hand, the Pin Index Safety System and Diameter Index Safety System, developed in the 1950s, exemplify successful industry-sourced safety efforts. These systems prevented misconnection of gases to equipment. Prior to their introduction, patients had been killed or injured by mistakes such as connection of a tank of nitrous oxide to a fitting intended for oxygen. Wayne Hay and Harold May invented these safety systems while employed at Ohio Medical and Surgical Equipment Company. The patents were donated to the Compressed Gas Association, thereby facilitating universal use by all manufacturers.

The history of nitrous oxide illustrates the early role of industry in the world of anesthesia. We take the availability of this useful anesthetic for granted, but it wasn't until near the end of the nineteenth century, that industry supplied the wherewithal needed for the practical delivery of nitrous oxide. Large-scale production of nitrous oxide was a daunting task, especially so in the decades prior to sophisticated process control systems. The widely used and economical method involves heating ammonium nitrate to 200 °C, a potentially dangerous process because the process is exothermic (generates heat), and at a somewhat greater temperature, the ammonium nitrate explodes. In 1947, the French registered vessel, SS Grandcamp, with approximately 2,300 tons of ammonium nitrate aboard, caught fire in the port of Texas City. The resulting explosion and onshore fires destroyed Texas City, killing nearly 600 people [2].

Similarly, explosions have occurred at nitrous oxide manufacturing facilities, in some cases causing loss of life. In the 1950s, an explosion occurred at an Ohio Chemical and Surgical Equipment-Airco plant in Montreal, fortunately at night—thus sparing loss of life and injury. However, in the 1980s, an explosion occurred at an Air Products nitrous oxide production facility, resulting in a few fatalities. Ohio Chemical had located a nitrous oxide manufacturing facility at the corner of 10th and Mason in San Francisco, but the San Francisco city fathers remembered the great Texas City explosion. No nitrous plants in the city! An abbreviated daily production system was employed, until the facility relocated to an industrial site in the intrepid town of Berkeley.

The commercialization of nitrous oxide manufacturing required industry to manage the cost and deployment of heavy steel cylinders. Fortunately, nitrous oxide compresses to a liquid at moderate pressures. A cousin of Edgar Allen Poe converted this knowledge into a commercial process in the late nineteenth or early twentieth century in Trenton, New Jersey, but a half-century passed before the implementation of bulk delivery/storage of nitrous oxide at large hospitals. Some hospitals used nitrous oxide in such large quantities that it was economical to take it from the production plant in a bulk tank truck, in liquid form, and transfer it to a bulk liquid storage tank at the hospital, much like the liquid oxygen systems used today.

The memoirs of the dentist, Jay Heidbrink, read at the American Dental Society of Anesthesiology in 1957, testify to the challenges of administering nitrous oxide anesthesia to dental patients in the early 1900s. Heidbrink describes patients who fought with him, one for three bouts, before being subdued or anesthetized! Stimulated by such events he tinkered with an anesthesia machine purchased from Charles Teter in Cleveland, in 1903. The machine apparently provided an inaccurate mixture of oxygen and nitrous oxide, and Heidbrink made improvements to correct the problem. Local Minneapolis physicians and dentists asked him to make machines for their practices. A local machine shop quoted a price of $600 per unit for Heidbrink's device. A second shop asked for $1.00 per pound or $32.00 total. This machine was called the "Model A," and the Heidbrink company was "off and running." His company later became part of "Ohio Chemical and Surgical equipment," with numerous company names to follow.

Of note was the contribution of Elmer McKesson, an anesthesiologist who in the 1910s developed the "McKesson" anesthetic machines, machines particularly devoted to administration of high concentrations of nitrous oxide [3]. McKesson advocated induction of anesthesia with 100 % nitrous oxide. When cyanosis became profound, McKesson machines allowed use of a flush valve that would add enough oxygen to prevent death. The combination of nitrous oxide and transient hypoxia was sufficient to anesthetize patients for brief procedures (e.g., dental extractions). The flush valve was McKesson's lasting contribution to anesthesia. McKesson is an example of the physician-industrialist of a different era. McKesson ran courses for visiting anesthetists, to teach them how to use his machines and learn basic engineering skills, so that they could repair the machines.

Halothane: The First Successful Modern Inhaled Anesthetic

In 1951, Charles Suckling, a chemist at Imperial Chemical Industries (ICI) in Cheshire, England, began work leading to the synthesis of halothane and the world of modern inhaled anesthetics [4]. Pharmacologist James Raventos (1905–1982; Fig. 66.2) tested halothane in animals, finding that it had the desirable properties needed for an inhaled anesthetic—absence of flammability, absence of pungency, high

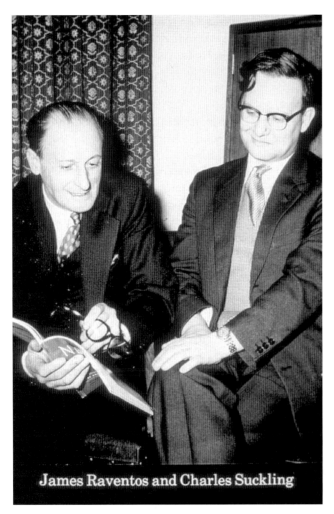

James Raventos and Charles Suckling

Fig. 66.2 James Raventos (on *left*) and Charles Suckling were the key players in the discovery of halothane. (Courtesy of AstraZeneca, Wilmington, DE, USA)

potency, and no obvious toxicity (unlike chloroform, its nonflammable competitor) [5]. Halothane became a smash hit, making millions for ICI, and changing the face of anesthesia from the late 1950s. It wasn't perfect however, as suggested by increasing numbers of reports of hepatotoxicity, starting in the 1960s [6]. The story goes back now to Ohio Chemical.

And Then Enflurane and Isoflurane

In 1906, Justin Scholes founded Ohio Chemical Corp in Cleveland, Ohio. The company developed or manufactured ether and other anesthetic compounds for several decades, with cyclopropane and nitrous oxide being the mainstays for much of its early history. Research at Ohio Medical led to the discovery of several widely used inhaled anesthetics. Around the time of World War II, Airco bought both the Heidbrink Company and Ohio Chemical. The combined entity, Ohio Chemical and Surgical Equipment, continued the develop-

ment of anesthesia apparatus and inhalation products. Today, GE Medical owns much of the equipment portion of Ohio Medical.

Julius Shukys, at Ohio Chemical, synthesized fluroxene, an ethyl vinyl ether in the late 1940s. It was released commercially in 1953, before the introduction of halothane [7]. Another early fluorinated ether discovered by Ohio Chemical, was Indoklon, a convulsant hexafluorodiethyl ether, marketed in the late 1950s as a substitute for electro-shock therapy. However, a convulsant anesthetic is hardly saleable to most anesthetists, and fluroxene couldn't compete with halothane. Other fluorinated ethers had more promising characteristics. These were developed in the 1960s by fluorine chemist Ross Terrell and his small group of colleagues working in Airco's Central Research Laboratories in Murray Hill, New Jersey, rather than at the Ohio Chemical facilities in Cleveland. Terrell et al. would synthesize more than 700 compounds in their search for the perfect inhaled anesthetic. They never found that, but they came close enough, producing the dominant inhaled anesthetics from 1970 to the present [8–10].

A key element in Terrell's program was the establishment of a means to measure the quality of the anesthetic effects produced by his compounds. Accordingly, Ohio Chemical developed a relationship with John Krantz, the chair of Pharmacology at the University of Maryland. One of his graduate students, Freida Rudo (1924–1996) became expert in "screening" the experimental compounds discovered by Terrell and his team. Terrell's program was small in staff and budget, so having an economical means of preliminary animal testing was critical to success. Great expertise at bargain basement price was needed. Each mouse tested was a noted budget expense, and did double duty by serving as a meal for the University of Maryland's snake collection.

Rudo was a favorite with her University and Industry colleagues. She had reportedly won first place in a Miss Puerto Rico beauty contest. Add her personal presence, her statesmanship and her pipe smoking, and she was a memorable personality. She evaluated each new putative anesthetic by placing a few drops of the compound in a one quart Mason jar containing one scrambling mouse. She then observed respiratory and cardiovascular responses (Did the mouse stop breathing? Did it die?), the ease and rate of induction, rigidity and convulsions. She recorded her data on 3 × 5 note cards, an effective if now antiquated data and lab notes management system.

Terrell became an industry legend for his record of successes in inhalation anesthetic discoveries. He synthesized, and Rudo tested, enflurane, isoflurane, sevoflurane and desflurane, in addition to several hundred undeserving compounds. A success rate this great is rare in the pharmaceutical world.

Ohio Medical's clinical and regulatory expertise was modest, especially at the time of the development of their first anesthetic, enflurane. At the outset, Ohio looked for guidance from members of the anesthetic community. In the 1960s, James Vitcha (see below) sought out a surprised Edmond Eger, asking him if he wanted to be involved in Ohio's studies of new anesthetics. Eger remembers that he (Eger) quickly wrote a stellar grant for several hundred thousand dollars and was rewarded with a dinner at Toots Shor's, where Vitcha diplomatically told him that his application was rejected. Eger got it anyway; it just took much longer than he had expected. Eger became involved in the clinical trials for all of the anesthetics that Ohio brought to the market. He was especially effective in arguing for the development of desflurane, noting the need for faster acting anesthetics in a world increasingly focused on ambulatory anesthesia/surgery. The anesthesia community, and especially Eger, played the role of "Medical Director." This was possible in the regulatory world of the last half of the twentieth century, again illustrating the effective relationship between industry and physicians and academia in that era.

James Vitcha had long worked for Ohio Medical, in various capacities in the anesthetics programs, and took on the role of coordinating the clinical studies and preparing in large part, the New Drug Applications for enflurane and isoflurane. He organized clinical anesthesia researchers effectively, created a strong information base for the products upon market introduction, and provided the FDA with information needed for approval reviews.

Vitcha's real role at Ohio Medical/Ohio Chemical/Anaquest, was that of the grain of sand in the oyster leading to the formation of a pearl. Ohio Chemical was poorly equipped in both technical and business experience, to deal with the pharmaceutical world. Jim often threw caution and career future to the wind in arguing for the inhaled anesthetic program, persuading many doubters within the Ohio Medical management team. He followed that with a clinical studies program and FDA submissions effort that was impossible by later standards. Were it not for his unique persistence internally, important inventions might never have seen the market place, or would at least have been delayed for several years.

Although the road from laboratory to marketplace for new compounds was shorter in the 1970s than in the twenty-first century, some unanticipated obstacles impeded progress. The obstacle with halothane was its rare capacity to injure the liver [6]. Enflurane, the 347th compound made by Terrell, had minimal hepatotoxic effects [11], and that advantage gave it a competitive edge over halothane. By 1970, enflurane had largely replaced halothane in the US. However, enflurane had its own problem, the capacity to produce seizures [12]. The incidence of seizure activity with enflurane was low and the number of patients exhibiting seizures was small. Moreover, there were no reports of residual damage from the seizures. The FDA chose a middle of the road solution to this situation. They approved enflurane for sale, on the condition that the package literature fully describe the

risk, and that a " phase 4" study comprising a complaint form be included in the package literature, to be used by anesthesiologists for reporting seizure incidence.

It was clear that the FDA was anxious to have an alternative to halothane, and apparent that they had confidence in the physician's ability to observe and report the condition, to the extent that it was a limitation. This study did not provide alarming findings, and enflurane continued to be widely used.

As indicated above, enflurane largely replaced halothane in the US and some other developed countries (except for anesthesia in children) because enflurane had fewer effects than halothane on the liver. But enflurane was also attacked for its capacity to injure the liver, albeit with a much lower incidence than occurring with halothane [11]. Isoflurane was also tarred with this brush [13]. Anaquest asked Eger to examine each of the rare reported cases of hepatic injury, finding in some patients, that the injury resulted from an infection by a herpes virus [14, 15]. Overall, we were impressed with the small degree of metabolism of isoflurane, and therefore decided to fully investigate and resolve reports of 'toxicity' in patients as they arose, thinking that other causes would most likely be ruled in and isoflurane toxicity ruled out. At worst, no specific cause would be proven or found, and as such, the overall results would keep the product in good stead in the eyes of clinicians. I suppose we were thinking that one patient did not a side effect make.

Sebastian Reiz's 1983 suggestion that isoflurane caused "coronary steal" was a larger concern [16]. This issue had been studied by prominent investigators and was added to the package label. We asked Eger and Cahalan to visit Reiz in Umea, Sweden. Eger remembers it being one of the coldest places he'd ever been, and that Reiz offered him some wild mushrooms to eat (Eger declined). My recollection is that "steal," while not completely irrelevant, did not significantly influence isoflurane usage. The millions of patients, seemingly safely given isoflurane, continued to pile up and significant side effects from any one cause became statistically more remote.

But we've gotten ahead of our story in telling of isoflurane's development. Enflurane was good, but far from perfect, and Terrell and his group searched for something better. In initial trials with compound 469 (isoflurane), made by preparatory chromatograph (personal communication, John Wynne), Rudo found that isoflurane seemed superior in its overall properties. However, a problem in its manufacture nearly killed it. Several hundred pounds were required for additional animal testing, toxicology, and eventually human trials. Wynne was assigned to the process and scale-up work, but was unable to purify the crude final isoflurane to more than 97 % by normal distillation. The problem was the boiling point of a contaminant compound, 1-chloro-2,2,2,-trifluoroethyl monochloro difluoromethyl ether, which at 53 °C was too close to that of isoflurane at 48.5 °C, to enable separation by simple distillation. Louise Speers saved the day, finding that isoflurane forms a high boiling azeotrope with acetone and has a lower volatility, while 1-chloro-2,2,2,-trifluoroethyl monochloro difluoromethyl ether forms a low boiling azeotrope with acetone which can be distilled from isoflurane. As an aside, note that two women, Rudo and Speers, led the way forward in this history of inhaled anesthetics, doing so during an era when female scientists were much less prominent.

Spears took pleasure telling of her interviews for jobs after completion of her PhD in chemistry at Columbia University. During that era, young single women needed a proper escort for their interview travels. Spears' mother filled that role as best she could (I don't think she attended the interviews, themselves). Fortunately for the anesthesia world, her trip from Columbia University to Murray Hill, New Jersey to be interviewed by Terrell was less than 50 miles, causing her to choose a career in anesthetic synthesis and azeotrope distillations!

The submission of the New Drug Application, for approval of isoflurane for clinical use, was a family business. Eger remembers Vitcha proudly talking about several feet of documents on his dining room table, he and his wife sorting and stacking. Isoflurane was his baby.

Towards the mid 1970s, it looked like clear sailing to an approval of isoflurane by the FDA, which had provided a preliminary "approvable" status letter. The celebrations inside Ohio Medical began. Human clinical testing had been well orchestrated by Vitcha and Eger (the shadow Medical Director-Consultant). Vitcha was a friend to numerous investigators in the anesthesia world, investigators providing input to the inhalation anesthetics program. His vigor outside the company was also used inside the company, to argue fiercely for additional funding for the anesthetics program. He usually got what he asked for (although complaining that it never was enough).

And then, isoflurane had an enormous setback. Tom Corbett, at the University of Michigan, had studied the potential of various compounds, particularly alpha chloro ethers to cause cancer [17]. Prompted by this, by considerable intelligence, and by a crusader's zeal, Corbett had conducted a small test on mice which suggested that isoflurane (an alpha chloro ether) had carcinogenic properties [18]. Vitcha, Terrell, and Eger visited Corbett at his laboratory. Convinced that although Corbett's study was fatally flawed (insufficient controls, absence of blinding, inadequate statistical analysis, and failure to use a comparator anesthetic), Airco had no alternative but to stop the release of isoflurane. Corbett had acted with the best of intentions, and with his findings in print there was naught to do but repeat what he had done, eliminating the flaws. Nonetheless, for a time Airco dithered on whether to challenge Corbett, eventually realizing that they would fight a losing battle. In the meantime (and unknown

to us), Eger and Wendell Stevens—with Corbett's help—set about duplicating Corbett's study but correcting the flaws in that study. After several months of indecision, and discussions with the FDA, Airco finally asked Eger and Stevens to conduct the study that they had already set in motion.

So on went the experiment, while Airco and the FDA mused a bit more. And then Eger wryly remembered trouble. Vitcha called and said that the FDA and Anaquest would like to make a minor modification to the protocol—to extend the survival period after anesthetic exposure from 15 to 18 months. However, modification was not possible. The mice were in formaldehyde. There was no way they could grow for an additional three months. It was mea culpa time. So Eger and Stevens met with us and confessed their sins, adding that the data seemed to indicate that no inhaled anesthetic caused cancer. Eger remembers being embarrassed at having deceived me but tickled that he had gotten away with it until we asked for the modification. The final answer came after two years of study; isoflurane was exonerated [19].

A few interesting things resulted from this saga. The FDA enacted and then rescinded a rule specific to isoflurane—to withhold approval based on a flawed study. It was probably a stretch of their authority at that time to enact such rules, and it was discriminatory to isoflurane, relative to rules applied to inhaled anesthetics that followed. Faced with this rule stretching, and its effect to delay the release of isoflurane, we acted to extend isoflurane's patent life. We engaged in lobbying, and I (RL) testified at a congressional hearing conducted by Congressman Kastenmeyer's sub-committee on intellectual property. The life of only 2 patents had previously been extended. One was Ronson lighters; a bribed judge had ruled against their patent. Imagine this, he was in New Jersey! That happened in the first half of the twentieth century. The other patent extension applied to a sweetener that, like isoflurane, had been accused of causing cancer. Legislation extending the isoflurane patent life eventually was bundled into the legislation by Waxman and Hatch, restoring patent life of pharmaceuticals for the amount of time they spent in regulatory review. There was a quid pro quo for that legislation, making it legal for generic manufacturers to use patented processes in preparation for the generic production of products ahead of patent expiration. Prior to that, it was not legal for generic manufacturers to use a patented process ahead of its expiration. Waxman was anxious to have generic competition as early as possible, and manufacturers were anxious to have patent extension for testing period delays.

And Then Desflurane

In 1981, the Ohio Medical Division of BOC placed its anesthetics business in a new division called Anaquest. Anaquest/Ohio Medical had one considerable success, enflurane, and another about-to-be success, isoflurane. These scientific, clinical, and financial achievements prompted and supported the 1983 commitment of BOC, to enormously expand the Research and Development arm of the general anesthetic business, then headed by Ross Terrell, a pioneer in the development of volatile anesthetics. The vision was to become the resource for all the major drugs used to provide the anesthetic state, specifically to invent premier opioids, local anesthetics, neuromuscular blockers and reversal agents. These would compliment Anaquest's inhaled anesthetic offerings, meet the increasing demands of ambulatory surgery, and improve the care of anesthetized patients. It was an extraordinarily ambitious goal.

This goal radically changed Anaquest's drug development program. The small, extremely productive activities of Terrell's team of Speers, Halpern and a few others would be expanded several fold. Experts in pharmacology and toxicology would occupy a wing of rooms at BOC's Murray Hill site in New Jersey. By 1984, it housed fifty scientists plus an accredited animal facility to evaluate new chemical entities (NCEs), including new volatile anesthetics. Ted Spaulding, from Hoechst-Roussel Pharmaceuticals joined with Terrell to head this endeavor, particularly to perform in house validation of the efficacy and safety of intravenous therapeutics. It was thought important to bring biology in close proximity to the expanded synthetic chemistry program. Even with this expansion, Richard Wynn, Frieda Rudo, and Paul Thut continued to test some NCEs in the Pharmacology Department of the School of Dentistry at the University of Maryland. Their experience with inhalation anesthetic and muscle relaxant pharmacology, their enthusiasm for the expanded program, and their role as "biology" teammates were crucial to the advancement of the program.

A parallel move was afoot. In 1984, Eger was asked to review the 700+ compounds that Terrell had made in the 1960s, to see if any might have desirable anesthetic qualities that had been overlooked. Consulting with Terrell (who had no memory of their discussions), Eger searched among a subgroup of ether molecules that were halogenated solely with fluorine atoms, believing that these would have the requisite properties of stability, low solubility, and good anesthetic profile as suggested by the tests performed by Rudo. He found 4 molecules worthy of further testing, but only one passed the test of stability–desflurane. Desflurane had been set aside because it had been dangerous to make, had a relatively low potency, and had a saturated vapor pressure near one atmosphere, making its delivery difficult. Fortunately, Anaquest had thought so little of desflurane that they had not published on its properties, or attempted to patent it. That meant that a new patent and exclusivity for 17 years were possible. Terrell gave Eger all the desflurane that Anaquest had kept on the shelf for 2 decades, approximately 10 ml. Because of the limited availability of compound, Eger recap-

tured the desflurane at the end of each experiment by condensing the gas phase with liquid nitrogen. With careful use, Eger and colleagues conducted several experiments in 1985 and 1986. Anaquest became aware of the possibility that desflurane might supply a desirable alternative to isoflurane.

By late 1986, the synthetic efforts within Ken Spencer's chemistry group had resulted in numerous patents, and first-time-in-human testing of intravenous analgesics and a neuromuscular blocking agent. Because of the development time associated with these new chemical entities (NCEs), efforts to in-license[1] both products and newer technologies in drug delivery systems for its small molecule program were also undertaken. It was hoped that these initiatives would rapidly lead to a portfolio of products supplementing the company's major product isoflurane, whose patent expiry in 1993 was imminent. Times' winged chariot hurried near.

In 1987, Anaquest had taken a year's option with Baxter Laboratories for the right to license sevoflurane. At the same time, as noted above, Eger had explored the properties of desflurane. For several months, Anaquest management debated which agent to pursue. Either choice meant a major financial commitment. The decision to develop the next generation of inhaled anesthetics was a difficult and nuanced choice between desflurane and sevoflurane. In retrospect, Paul Thomas (then product manager, later President of Anaquest) summed up the considerations as follows:

"The context of these deliberations included a need to have an anesthetic with a faster recovery than that from isoflurane, ideally with a lower incidence of postoperative nausea and vomiting, and particularly with minimal or no capacity to irritate the airway (especially relevant in children and with the growing popularity of laryngeal mask airways). It was also important to have an anesthetic that could be safely used with lower flow rates (1–2 l/min) because of potential clinical benefits and cost savings. These thoughts informed our analysis of the relative advantages of desflurane and sevoflurane."

"Desflurane had the lowest—better—blood/gas partition coefficient [20, 21], and this plus tests in rats pointed to a recovery that might be faster than with sevoflurane [22]. Desflurane had the edge in safety, its metabolism producing little fluoride ion, and it didn't break down in soda lime [23] or produce Compound A. Thus desflurane passed muster, but the data for sevoflurane were alarming. And the market's experiences with halothane and methoxflurane made the Anaquest team gun shy of instability and decomposition issues. We feared that the worst-case sevoflurane decomposition scenario would weigh heavily on clinicians, if not the FDA. The patent life advantage went to desflurane (16 yrs) since sevoflurane had only Waxman Hatch protection (5–7 years). And Anaquest owned desflurane, but not sevoflurane. Initial studies in animals did not reveal evidence of airway irritation, but transfer of such evidence to humans is unreliable. Still, this plus the lower blood/gas partition coefficient gave us hope that induction in humans would be more rapid."

---

[1]A business practice of granting a patent license to an invention made by one company for the purpose of further development and commercialization by the company taking the license. One party out-licenses and the other in-licenses.

"But sevoflurane offered counterbalancing advantages. Its lesser MAC [24] meant that sevoflurane would require roughly a third the consumption of desflurane, producing a cost advantage. Sevoflurane could be delivered from a conventional flow vaporizer versus the much more costly vaporizer needed for desflurane. Anaquest would provide vaporizers to anesthetists using either anesthetic, imposing an additional cost with desflurane of tens of millions of dollars. Capital costs—for a plant to manufacture desflurane—were approximately 80 million dollars more than for sevoflurane. And lack of airway irritation in humans was a known fact favoring sevoflurane [25]."

Thus, when it came time to choose between desflurane and sevoflurane, patent life, pharmacology, production costs, licensing fees and more were on the table. There were human data for sevoflurane [25] (a seemingly good clinical anesthetic) but not even preliminary human data for desflurane. Before deciding, should Anaquest commit millions of dollars to get into human trials? Expensive decisions had to be made on limited data. At the decision meeting, probably in 1986, all the information and arguments were presented to an Anaquest management team. Sifting and winnowing swayed to and fro for a couple of hours. Finally I (RL) suggested that the non-sevoflurane favoring group was biased because sevoflurane was "invented there" whereas desflurane "was invented here." In his usual low-key manner, Terrell said "No, sevoflurane had been 'invented *here*' and discarded years ago for the same reason that was of concern now, instability in the presence of soda lime." Those prosaic words seemed to provide a good point for polling of the seven present; not a vote, but a poll because I wanted to reserve the right to act contrary to the majority, to weigh product performance more heavily than financial and business considerations. The result was not unanimous but favored desflurane. I announced we had reached a good consensus and asked that we proceed with desflurane. Thus, the path forward leading to an FDA application for human clinical trials began.

In August 1987, Terrell moved from his executive role to the position of Senior Scientist and Advisor, and Hollis Schoepke joined Anaquest as Vice President of Research. With the emphasis now on product development and regulatory approval leading to market, Schoepke brought to Anaquest the experience of managing pharmaceutical R&D in three major pharmaceutical companies.

Paul Thomas commented regarding the launch of desflurane in October of 1992:

"The market introduction of desflurane and loss of patent protection for isoflurane occurred concurrently, and led to intense generic competition from Abbott Laboratories. The profit impact was profound with the selling price for isoflurane declining in a year from approximately \$100 to about \$60 per bottle, greatly decreasing profitability on isoflurane.

"In the late 1980s and early 1990s, several factors forced a dramatic decrease in research and development. These included the in licensing of nitric oxide, and the acquisition of recombinant albumin and the associated development costs for both products. The anticipated steep profit decline for isoflurane, and

the increased expenses associated with the development and launch of desflurane added further to the pressure on the NCE program, and resulted in elimination of the clinical trials. We sharply decreased our basic research efforts seeking improved anesthetic agents. These efforts had found it difficult to improve upon agents such as rocuronium and fentanyl. The recombinant albumin project became more difficult and expensive to pursue than anticipated. Accordingly, we sold our interest in this enterprise. As part of the project shuffling, we protected our development of inhaled nitric oxide for Persistent Pulmonary Hypertension of the Newborn, which turned out to be the correct decision given the subsequent significant clinical and commercial success of the drug. Unfortunately, inhaled nitric oxide's success was several years later than needed and desired!"

The desflurane project imposed major demands on people and finances at Anaquest. Several nitty-gritty problems had to be faced. Animal and human studies required development of a vaporizer, no small challenge given the saturated vapor pressure of desflurane. Clinicians would also expect to have a monitor that would tell them how much desflurane was being given. It was one thing to produce quantities of desflurane for experimental purposes, but quite another to scale these up for commercial production. A vendor qualified under Good Laboratory Practice guidelines to evaluate safety in animals had to be found. A small group of toxicologists and pharmacokineticists were charged with conducting safety studies, including by this time, studies of mutagenicity. In sum, these studies would be more expensive and comprehensive than those Anaquest had previously undertaken with anesthetics such as enflurane and isoflurane.

Eger presented the safety and efficacy results of desflurane to the NDA Advisory Committee in late 1991. Like presenters at today's Advisory Committee meetings he had hundreds of slides at his disposal, but these were in numerous carousels. He magically knew the location of the one slide needed to answer each committee member's questions. The NDA was approved in 1992.

This delay in new products available for marketing, the increased costs associated with the in-licensed products, coupled with generic isoflurane availabilty resulted in BOC's exit from the business. The BOC Group was primarily an industrial gas company, much more in tune with global strategies for capital intense industries rather than the intense research and regulatory nature of the pharmaceutical industry. BOC decided to divest itself from the health care business. The anesthesia equipment and monitoring businesses (Ohmeda) were sold to Datex Instrumentarium (subsequently GE). The inhalation anesthetics business was sold to Baxter Laboratories. Anesthetic musical chairs!

The BOC decision was similar to those made by Air Products and NCG. Decades earlier it had been cost effective for gas suppliers to make and sell the equipment that delivered gases to patients. As each of the business areas became more complex, specialization became more competitive and cost effective. A single management team found it increasingly difficult to be expert at several major tasks (e.g., equipment manufacture, cryogenics, and development of pharmaceuticals). The economic advantages of specialization overtook the economic advantages of consolidation. For a time, Vitcha's enthusiasm convinced us that we could and should do both equipment manufacturing and pharmaceutical development at the Divisional level, and much more at the corporate level, but ultimately, the forces of specialization won out.

Two decades later, in 2011, Paul Thomas commented on Anaquest's experiences with the introduction of desflurane, saying that:

> "the introduction was modeled after Hernando Cortez's strategy upon arrival in the New World. He burned all of his ships to convince his crew that there was no turning back (i.e., to isoflurane). The New World needed to be conquered (i.e., we needed to convince anesthetists of the value of desflurane). We devoted substantial resources to the desflurane launch (vaporizer placements, clinical support, marketing efforts, sales force commissions) and priced it aggressively to support conversion of the market from isoflurane to desflurane. We were partially successful in our efforts but never fully replaced the profitability lost due to generic isoflurane competition. And then there was the competition that came from the launch of sevoflurane."

> "Our assumptions concerning the safety of sevoflurane and our hopes regarding a lack of laryngospasm with desflurane were in hindsight misplaced. Both anesthetics found a place in anesthesia practice. I don't know if BOC would have supported the simultaneous development of both drugs but clearly we should have pushed for this option!"

And Sevoflurane

Just as had Terrell, Bernard Regan at Baxter independently synthesized sevoflurane, and Richard Wallin (also Baxter) performed several studies of its anesthetic and physical properties [26]. Baxter offered to license sevoflurane to ICI. One of us (JG) was asked to evaluate it.

> "I liked its anaesthetic properties as seen in animals, but noted its marked degradation to a toxic product on contact with soda lime. We were able to show in an experiment in a dog that the degradation product was adsorbed onto soda lime, and changed the colour of the indicator dye, but did not appear to accumulate in the circuit. However, I was concerned that all CO_2 absorbents might not behave in the same way and felt that the degree of chemical instability observed would not be acceptable in a modern anaesthetic. I recommended rejection of the licensing offer in 1977."

So no one wanted this orphan, sevoflurane, until a small fearless Japanese company, Maruishi reopened the issue in the 1980s and successfully brought sevoflurane to market in Japan. In the early 1990s, Maruishi offered to license sevoflurane to Abbott Laboratories who accepted and were enormously successful in sevoflurane's development and sale.

Industry Contributions to Safety

A more recent example of the relationship between industry and the anesthesia specialty is the formation of two US-based anesthesia foundations in the 1980s. The early 1980s were challenging years for anesthesia equipment manufacturers, malpractice insurance companies, and anesthesiologists buying malpractice insurance. Owing to the joint and several liability laws, manufacturers could be held responsible for 99 % of a malpractice award even if their equipment was only 1 % responsible. New machines had safety features that old machines lacked, and manufacturers were sometimes held accountable for human errors resulting from absent safety features in the older machines. For example, in the early 1980s, the TV program 60 Minutes aired an exposé of morbidity and mortality due to adverse anesthesia incidents. This highlighted manufacturers, hospitals and clinicians who failed to develop, obtain and use systems with oxygen monitors. The manufacturer with the oldest equipment in the field (i.e., the one at greatest risk because its equipment might lack specific safety features), Puritan Bennett-Foregger, left the anesthesia business.

In the early 1980s, Ohmeda (formerly Ohio Medical Products) organized a preliminary "Safety in Anesthesia" symposium led by Nick Gravenstein. From this meeting, a commitment was made to create the Anesthesia Patient Safety Foundation (APSF). In 1985, led by Ellison (Jeep) Pierce (1928–2011), the American Society of Anesthesiologists (ASA) and industry members provided financial support for the APSF. This first multi-disciplinary organization, created to improve patient safety in the context of anesthesia, has succeeded in its purpose, as confirmed a decade later by the National Academy of Sciences/National Institutes of Health, who recognized the APSF as a model for improving quality of care within a medical specialty [27].

In 1986, the ASA formed the Foundation for Anesthesia Education and Research (FAER), to expand opportunities for education and research in anesthesia, especially at the post residency level. Funding for basic research from agencies such as the NIH and the National Science Foundation had increased dramatically post World War II, but funding for research in anesthesia had not undergone a commensurate increase. It was intended that FAER would help narrow that gap and thereby ensure the growth of anesthesia as a worthy academic endeavor.

The ASA asked Bill Hamilton to obtain industry support for FAER. He invited me (RL), and Clifford Parrish from Burroughs Wellcome, to a joint discussion in Portland, Oregon. We quickly agreed that education and research were laudable labels and the FAER title was born. Fund raising progressed at a good pace but received a major shot in the arm when the ASA president, Howard Zauder, learned of funding needs and, on the spot, announced a doubling of refresher course fees, from \$5 to \$10 with the increased proceeds devoted primarily to FAER.

FAER has succeeded, as reflected in the return on investment. Every dollar spent by FAER on recipients has generated several-fold greater amounts from the NIH and other granting agencies. Once again, industry members were full partners in the design, funding and implementation of FAER.

Development of Calibrated Anesthetic Vaporizers

Halothane was a game-changing anesthetic. The positives were that it was nearly without pungency, didn't stimulate the circulation, and had a solubility far less than that of diethyl ether, the main potent volatile anesthetic competitor. The negatives were that it was nearly without pungency, didn't stimulate the circulation, and had a solubility far less than that of diethyl ether, the main potent volatile anesthetic competitor. That is, it could induce anesthesia in a thrice and kill patients in two thrices. Its safe use would depend upon precise control of the delivered concentration. Thus, the introduction of halothane by ICI in 1956 prompted development of a calibrated, temperature compensated, and flow-controlled vaporizer. With the exception of the Copper Kettle, invented by Lucien Morris in 1953 (see chapter 39), competing vaporizers offered limited to poor control over the delivered anesthetic concentration. An additional important safety factor of the new vaporizers was that they were positioned outside the anesthetic circle (breathing system) making their output independent of ventilation.

Two entrepreneurs, Bill Edmonson and Wilfred Jones had been employed by Coxeter, a UK manufacturer of anesthetic equipment acquired by British Oxygen Corporation (BOC). Dissatisfied with their new situation, they left BOC in 1949 to found a small company in the north of England. Initially, the entrepreneurs toyed with a new dispensing system for cyclopropane, accordingly coining the name Cyprane Limited for their company. Cyprane never made a cyclopropane dispenser, starting instead with a hand-held inhaler for trichlorethylene, the Cyprane Inhaler, used for analgesia during childbirth (it is still used for that purpose). Concurrently, ICI, based in the northwest of England was developing the new anesthetic, halothane. Only the Pennine hills between Yorkshire and Lancashire separated Cyprane Limited and ICI.

Working closely with ICI, Edmonson and Jones modified a vaporizer that they originally had designed for trichloroethylene (the Tritec). The vaporizer accepted the total flow of delivered gases and produced in these gases the concentration of anesthetic precisely indicated on a control dial, a concentration that nominally was not altered by changes in the flow rate or agent temperature. As halothane had been branded Fluothane by ICI, the vaporizer calibrated for halothane was called the Fluotec, and was used in the clinical evaluation of Fluothane. The Tritec and Fluotec were the world's first fully calibrated vaporizers, devices producing a known anesthetic concentration that was mostly independent of inflow rate and fully compensated for temperature variation. They were the first variable bypass vaporizers.

A minor incident reflects the seriousness and professionalism of the industry. Early in the life of the Fluotec, a clinical report suggested that the control knob had loosened, resulting in delivery of an incorrect, potentially hazardous, concentration. Wilf Jones was devastated by the thought that such a failure was possible. He was convinced that the vaporizer had been dismantled and incorrectly reassembled, but Cyprane recalled all Fluotec vaporizers. Following modification, the vaporizer was re-issued as the Fluotec Mark II.

In the US and Canada, ICI partnered with Ayerst Laboratories and released halothane as Fluothane. In parallel, Cyprane appointed as its agent, Fraser Sweatman Inc, a small supplier of medical equipment which bore the name of its larger-than-life founder. It had a head office in Toronto and a subsidiary in Buffalo, New York. A talented marketing entrepreneur with an infectious enthusiasm for business, Sweatman built a close working relationship with the Cyprane founders. He persuaded Ayerst to offer the Fluotec free to hospitals ordering a minimum annual quantity of halothane. The result successfully promoted both halothane and the Fluotec. Fraser wanted the Fluotec to become the gold standard in the US and promoted its sale to competing producers of anesthesia machines in order to maximize penetration of the Fluotec into the US market. The approach in the US served as a model for the later release of enflurane, isoflurane and desflurane and their corresponding vaporizers in the US.

The Fluotec II was good enough, especially with the marketing plan assembled by Fraser-Sweatman, to capture most of the market. Its primary competitor—and that only in the US—for a flow and temperature compensated vaporizer was the copper kettle. But the copper kettle required calculations to define the concentrations that it produced, and this made it less popular with mathematically challenged anesthetists. Still, the Fluotec II vaporizer was less than precisely accurate, and it failed to compensate for the effect of back-pressure from the breathing circuit. In 1966, Draegerwerk, a German manufacturer of medical equipment, seized on these limitations in its introduction of a vaporizer (named "Vapor") for halothane. For the first time, Cyprane had a serious competitor.

By now relatively wealthy, the Cyprane founders decided in 1967 to sell the business, giving Fraser Sweatman time to produce a financing proposal before seeking other buyers. Sweatman assembled a buy-out financed by a £500,000 equity investment from Industrial and Commercial Finance Corporation (ICFC), a consortium of High Street banks set up by the UK government to promote new start-up business-es. ICFC later became 3i, a noteworthy venture capital firm.

In 1967, Cyprane, with Wilfred Jones, developed the Fluotec III, but the output concentration was not consistent over the design flow range, and the vaporizer was difficult to calibrate, a problem that Sweatman attributed to a lack of consistent internal laminar flow. Jones was not convinced. A determined Sweatman tracked down the designer of the Vapor, Peter Schreiber, and recruited him to join Sweatman's US team.

But Schreiber and Sweatman combined could still not convince the Cyprane design team that there was a problem with the Fluotec III (particularly with laminar flow), and interest turned to another important area, the design of a Safety system to prevent filling of vaporizers with the wrong drug. Meanwhile, reluctant to put at risk his reputation and market position, Sweatman delayed launch of the Fluotec III in the US.

At this point in 1967, in London, Sweatman fortuitously met socially with David Needham (Fig. 66.3), an Imperial College post-doctoral research fellow in laminar flow, albeit at hypersonic speeds. Sweatman persuaded Needham to test his theory. Needham proved Sweatman correct and, better yet, Needham came up with a solution. Needham continued to consult for Cyprane and in 1969 joined the board as technical director, becoming the managing director in 1971. Schreiber then left Fraser Sweatman to form Draeger North America in partnership with his previous employer, thus becoming a direct competitor of Cyprane. Fraser Sweatman replaced Schreiber with Al Bickford, the designer of the Foregger Fluomatic.

Musical Chairs or Incest?

Meanwhile, Abbott Laboratories had developed methoxyflurane (Penthrane), an inhaled anesthetic with strong analgesic properties. Cyprane produced a calibrated vaporizer for Abbott, the Pentec, just in time for clinical trials and an anticipated international launch.

Also in the 1960s, Airco Inc's subsidiary, Ohio Medical Products, turned to Cyprane to produce the Enfluratec for the US launch. Meanwhile, problems of renal toxicity derailed methoxyflurane, and to fill the gap, Abbott licensed the distribution rights for enflurane outside the US from Ohio, and Cyprane supplied the Enfluratec vaporizers.

The possible launch of two new anesthetic agents and an associated possible demand for anesthesia machines capable of dispensing enflurane, halothane or methoxyflurane raised the potential of a disastrous filling of a vaporizer with the wrong anesthetic. This threat prompted development, in approximately 1966, of the safety filling system in which the filler port on the vaporizer and the bottle neck were each uniquely coded for a specific agent.

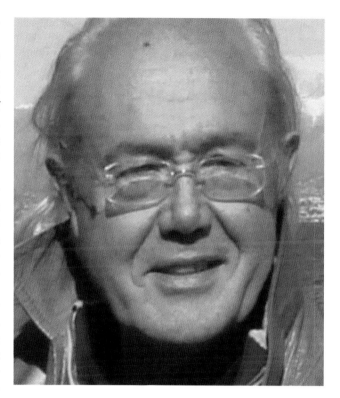

Fig. 66.3 David Needham. (From DN)

The prospect of a worldwide market for vaporizers made Cyprane an acquisition target, and in 1972 the company was sold to the BOC Group, from whom its founders had escaped some 25 years earlier.

Eger's and Stevens' successful experiments "resurrected" isoflurane (now branded Forane), and FDA approval arrived earlier than expected. Ohio's hopes of launching Forane with an in-house vaporizer were dashed when the decision was taken to go to market in the early 1980s. Once again, Cyprane reacted quickly to produce a vaporizer calibrated for isoflurane, named the Fortec, doing so in barely sufficient quantities to support the US launch. (Eger remembers many complaints of delays in receipt of sufficient supplies of vaporizers). DN remembers the struggle at Cyprane to divert common components from the Fluotec line to produce more Fortecs, and the resulting speculative ordering which generated a two-year backlog. All this was against a backdrop of grim economic conditions in the UK with the confrontation between Margaret Thatcher and the striking miners unions, and a government-enforced three-day week to conserve energy stocks. It was, as they say, character building.

Despite these stresses, the company maintained production that met demands, and in the 1970s and 1980s, controlled an estimated 85% of the world market for calibrated vaporizers. The BOC Group now brought together all of its worldwide subsidiaries in medical equipment and consumables, including Cyprane, under the umbrella of a new company, the Medishield Corporation. In 1976, BOC made a successful acquisition bid for Airco Inc., which was immediately blocked by the Federal Trade Commission (FTC) on anti-trust grounds, citing in particular, the combined (Fraser Sweatman-Cyprane) dominance of the anesthesia vaporizer business in the US. Four years later, the FTC objection was removed on the condition that Medishield divest itself of its Fraser Sweatman business in the US, helping to establish Fraser Sweatman as a viable competitor to Cyprane.

1981 and later saw the birth of two new important names in the world of anesthesia, and the end of two others. BOC commenced the task of integrating the Medishield and Ohio Medical businesses under the global name BOC Health Care, thereby creating a $650 million enterprise. The medical equipment companies were brought together under the name Ohmeda, and the Cyprane vaporizer was upgraded to produce the Ohmeda Tec 4 range in 1985. These vaporizers continued to use the basic design of the Fluotec III. The pharmaceutical side of the business emerged as Anaquest and continued the pursuit of new anesthetic agents, particularly desflurane. In the late 1990s, the group was split up and sold to new owners.

Vaporizers continued to be calibrated for each newly introduced anesthetic. Engstrom marketed an anesthetic machine in the mid 1980s, where the bottles of anesthetic agent (halothane, enflurane and isoflurane) were screwed on to indexed ports in a compartment on the rear of the machine. Having selected a concentration to be delivered, the selected agent was electronically and accurately injected into the gas stream. With this exception, the basic vaporizer mechanism remained largely unchanged. Desflurane was a challenge because its saturated vapor pressure of nearly an atmosphere at room temperature precluded the use of the Tec 4 variable bypass technology. An entirely new approach seemed to be required. Enter the Tec 6, a truly new vaporizer, with a structure unlike that of any previous vaporizer. The concept was simple: convert desflurane into a gas (by heating the desflurane) and then meter the gas into a diluent flow of oxygen with or without other gases (e.g., nitrous oxide or air). The concept was simple, but implementing it so that the functional result was the same as with the familiar variable-bypass vaporizer was a challenge. The device had to give an indicated concentration at any diluent inflow rate and at any ambient temperature (within reason). The challenge was met.

The story ends with a return to the future. Through the 1990s, the variable bypass vaporizer had been marginally improved following its release in the 1960s. Accuracy had increased over a wide range of flow rates and temperatures, and a key lock prevented filling with the wrong anesthetic. But it was expensive and could not accommodate desflurane because of the proximity of desflurane's vapor pressure to one atmosphere. In 1998, the Datex-Ohmeda Anesthesia Delivery Unit (ADU) machine was released. It separated the sump holding anesthetic from a control unit. There were different sumps for different anesthetics. Each sump was coded to inform the control unit of the identity of the sump contents. The control unit was programmed to adjust the flows through and past the sump, to produce the concentration indicated on the control knob of the vaporizer. It worked at more than one atmosphere and thus could accommodate desflurane as well as anesthetics with lesser vapor pressures. It was more efficient because the control unit could deal with several cassettes (sumps). General Electric bought the rights to the vaporizer which is now widely used.

The Discovery and Development of Propofol

Around 1965, the search for a novel, short-acting intravenous anesthetic began in the Pharmaceuticals Division of ICI. Thiopental was the standard agent used for induction of anesthesia. ICI sought a new agent reproducing the quality of anesthesia provided by thiopental, but more rapidly metabolized, such that rapid recovery could be obtained if anesthesia were maintained by repeated bolus injections or an infusion. New compounds were screened in mice, and those showing hypnotic activity and an acceptable safety margin were taken forward in other species.

A tension exists for two properties of an intravenous anesthetic: water solubility is needed to facilitate intravenous injection, but access to the brain requires lipophilicity. One solution to this problem is to use compounds that are salts of a weak acid or base. Such salts are soluble in water (blood), but able to dissociate back to the free acid or base needed to enter and act in the brain. Sodium thiopental made into a salt by adding sodium hydroxide is an example. By the end of 1971, the ICI team had studied over 2000 of these compounds but no candidate drug emerged.

A second solution to the solubility problem is to dissolve the putative anesthetic in some lipid-like substance that can be injected safely into blood. In 1972, I (JG; Fig. 66.4) joined the Biology Department at ICI, becoming responsible for the pharmacological evaluation of new compounds. Back in the 1960s in Europe, Bayer Laboratories had introduced the eugenol derivative, propanidid (Epontol), as a short-acting intravenous anesthetic. Propanidid was hydrophobic and was dissolved with the aid of a surfactant, polyoxyethylated castor oil (Cremophor EL), which Bayer also manufactured. This solubilizing agent allowed poorly water-soluble compounds to be injected. Roger James, one of the ICI chemists selected a number of poorly soluble compounds synthesized before 1965 and held in the ICI compound collection, as these could now be tested using this approach. I (JG) did the testing.

In early 1973, hypnotic activity was detected in ICI 43117 (2,6-diethylphenol). No further work was done with

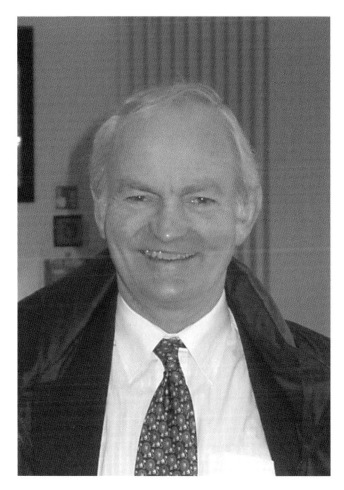

Fig. 66.4 J (Iain) B Glen. (From JB Glen)

this compound because induction of anesthesia in rabbits was slow, but it provided a lead for James to follow. He submitted about 150 related alkylphenols for testing and later that year, I demonstrated the anesthetic activity of propofol (ICI 35,868; 2,6-diisopropylphenol, with the trade name of Diprivan). Many of these compounds had hypnotic activity [28], but propofol had the optimum balance of properties in secondary tests designed to predict rate of onset, duration of effect, rate of recovery, freedom from excitatory effects, absence of accumulation after repeated injection, and clinically acceptable effects on respiration and circulation. Thirteen years elapsed before ICI first marketed propofol, the delay principally reflecting the difficulty in obtaining an acceptable formulation of this highly lipophilic oil.

Around 1972, Glaxo Research Laboratories introduced the combination of two steroids (alphaxalone/alphadolone acetate), named Althesin, again formulated with Cremophor EL, as a new short-acting IV anesthetic. The clinical acceptance of this new agent and Epontol prompted the trial of propofol in Cremophor EL. However, by 1975–76, several severe anaphylactoid reactions had been reported with both Althesin and Epontol. The contribution of Cremophor EL

to these reactions was uncertain; no animal model revealed a deleterious effect of Cremophor. Nevertheless, clinicians began to regard Cremophor with suspicion. It was agreed to proceed to clinical trial of propofol with the Cremophor preparation on the understanding that an alternative non-Cremophor formulation would be developed before marketing the product. No Cremophor-containing agent ever became available in the US.

Brian Kay, an anesthesiologist from Derby in the UK, conducted the first clinical trial, with a formulation containing 2 % propofol in 16 % Cremophor EL and 8 % ethyl alcohol, while visiting George Rolly's department in Ghent, Belgium in 1977 [29]. Kay was a quick worker and three days later he telephoned ICI to report that he had already studied 22 patients. Induction of anesthesia was rapid and smooth, and recovery prompt. However, two unexpected results were obtained: first, anesthetic potency appeared to be greater than had been anticipated, with 1.0 mg/kg being an effective dose in these nominally unpremedicated patients. The one page record forms provided by Kay provided limited information and many years later when I approached George Rolly requesting a copy of the anaesthetic record of the first patient to receive propofol, I discovered that these patients had in fact been premedicated with fentanyl and droperidol. Second, several patients reported pain on injection into the smaller veins of the hand. As the pain was thought to relate to the free aqueous concentration of propofol in the preparation, the propofol concentration was decreased to 1 %. Because it was no longer needed to solubilize the propofol, the alcohol was also removed. Benefit from these maneuvers was confirmed in further clinical studies. A dose of 2.0 mg/kg induced anesthesia with this second formulation.

An important step forward occurred with our development of an animal model in pigs, in which Cremophor produced an anaphylactoid response resembling that seen in patients [30]. Cremophor EL or Cremophor-containing anesthetics produced no effect on first administration, but a second injection given 1–2 weeks later produced an anaphylactoid response in almost 100 % of test animals. In this model, a synthetic polyoxyethylene/polyoxypropylene surfactant (Synperonic PE39/70) made by ICI produced no adverse response. This was one of about 100 alternative solubilizing agents that we examined, and agents with satisfactory pharmaceutical properties were taken forward for animal testing in a cascade of tests. Although rats and dogs tolerated the Synperonic formulation well, in 30-day toxicology tests, histological evaluation detected minor, unexplainable hepatic changes. Human studies were never conducted with the formulation.

Clinical studies continued with the Cremophor formulation in Europe, in more than 1,000 patients, until several anaphylactoid reactions were encountered, and studies were halted. Cremophor was thought to be responsible for these reactions. Because the clinical profile continued to look promising, a decision was taken in 1981 to develop an emulsion formulation of propofol. Two years of study were required to identify constituents for a final suitable preparation. A formulation containing soybean oil with purified egg phosphatide was selected, and a formulation with these materials containing 1% propofol produced less pain in rats than did the Cremophor formulation [31]. The emulsion formulation did not alter the anesthetic properties, and did not produce an anaphylactoid response in pigs.

Ron Stark (an enthusiastic and well-organized ICI physician) coordinated the clinical evaluation of the emulsion formulation, and I was transferred to the Medical Department at ICI to assist with the international trials. The first study began in July 1983, and a full clinical evaluation, including repetition of dose finding and pharmacological compatibility studies, was completed by the end of 1984. Many anesthesiologists were involved in clinical trials and it is difficult to single out individuals. In the UK most of the major academic centers took part in studies with the Belfast department led by the late John Dundee prominent in early induction studies, while the Bristol department with Cedric Prys-Roberts and John Sear investigated continuous infusion techniques for maintenance of anesthesia. In Germany, Alfred Doenicke in Munich, and Juergen Schuttler in Bonn were early investigators. Elizabeth Gepts in Brussels and Frederique Servin in Paris, working in collaboration with Ian Cockshott at ICI performed pharmacokinetic studies. Patrick Ravussin in Switzerland and Hugo Van Aken, at that time in Belgium, conducted studies relevant to neuroanaesthesia.

The first regulatory approval was obtained in 1986 and I had the pleasure of participating, together with John Dundee from Belfast, in the first launch meetings, in Auckland and Rotorua, New Zealand, in May of that year. Clinical trials in the US followed the European development program. One of the first of these was done in Chicago by Bob Fragen, who had used the drug while on sabbatical leave in Holland. Paul White in St Louis studied its use in outpatient anesthesia. As opportunities in maintenance of anesthesia were further explored, Steve Shafer at Stanford, Jerry Reves and Peter Glass at Duke, and Carl Hug and Peter Sebel at Emory, became involved. Propofol received FDA approval in 1989.

With further clinical trials, approvals were extended to long-term maintenance, sedation for local-regional anesthesia and intensive care, use in children and use in specialized areas such as neuroanesthesia. In most countries a 2% formulation was introduced to limit the fat load associated with prolonged use for anesthesia or sedation. In the US, some instances of misuse of the standard formulation in an effort to economize, led to bacterial contamination and several cases of postoperative fever. A modified formulation containing 0.005% ethylenediamine-tetraacetate (EDTA) to limit bacterial growth (if accidental bacterial contamination occurred) was introduced, first in the US in 1997. Sodium

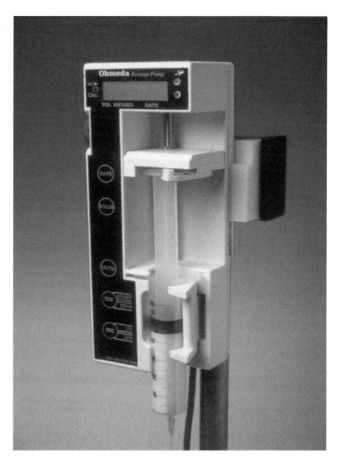

Fig. 66.5 The Ohmeda 9000 infusion pump produced by BOC Health Care in the UK in 1990 was the first of a new generation of computer controllable syringe drivers with the ability to deliver a maximum infusion rate of 200 ml/h and 'bolus' rates of 300, 600 or 1200 ml/h. (Courtesy of JB Glen)

metabisulphite was tested by Zeneca, but did not prevent bacterial growth at the pH specified in the formulation of Diprivan. However, by altering the pH specification, a bacteriostatic effect was achieved and a generic propofol formulation containing this additive was developed by Gensia Sicor and marketed by Baxter in the US.

In combination with opioids, propofol is now frequently used to produce total intravenous anesthesia (TIVA). An initial barrier to the wider use of propofol for maintenance of anesthesia by infusion was the lack of suitable equipment. Volumetric pumps were bulky and not ideal for a one or two-hour procedure. Most syringe pumps available in 1986 had a maximum delivery rate of 99 ml/h. The Ohmeda 9000 pump (Fig. 66.5) was the first of a new generation of syringe pumps with an extended dynamic range, a range sufficient to allow induction as well as maintenance of anesthesia by infusion [32]. Similar devices followed from Graseby Medical, Cardinal Health, and Fresenius-Kabi in Europe, Terumo in Japan and Bard, Medex and Baxter in the US.

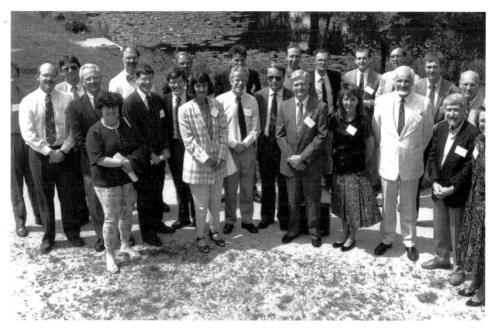

Fig. 66.6 Delegates invited to attend a workshop on 'Target Controlled Titration in Intravenous Anaesthesia, co-sponsored by ICI Pharmaceuticals and Janssen Pharmaceutica in Holland in 1992 included Academicians from the US (Julie Barr, Peter Glass, Carl Hug, Christina Mora, Jerry Reves, David Watkins, Steve Shafer, Don Stanski), from the UK (Michael Halsey, Cedric Prys-Roberts, Gavin Kenny, Martin White), from Germany (Juergen Schuttler), from Belgium (Elisabeth Gepts, Alain D'Hollander), from France (Frederique Servin), from Australia (David Crankshaw, Laurie Mather), from South Africa (Johan Coetzee), and a representative of the FDA in the US (Dan Spyker). (Courtesy of JB Glen, who organized the workshop)

Many infusion schemes were proposed for maintenance of anesthesia, one of the most popular being the Bristol scheme where infusion was successively decreased from 10 to 8 to 6 mg/kg/h to accommodate decreasing redistribution of propofol [33]. In 1981, Helmut Schwilden, a mathematician and anesthesiologist at the University of Bonn, introduced the concept of target-controlled infusion (TCI), whereby a pharmacokinetic model is incorporated into the pump software, and the pump controls the infusion rate, to achieve a desired target drug concentration. After extensive discussions with academic groups with an interest in this area (Fig. 66.6), ICI (now Zeneca) decided in 1993 to commercialize the system developed by Gavin Kenny and Martin White in Glasgow. The clinical utility of this approach, and their system, had been demonstrated, and Zeneca conducted an extensive 3-year program which involved software design and validation, regulatory discussions, the development of delivery performance specifications and clinical trials [34]. Following completion of this program, approval for the administration of propofol by Diprifusor TCI was obtained in the UK in 1996. This technique, which facilitates titration of propofol during maintenance of anesthesia or sedation, is now available in most countries of the world, but not to date in the US. See Chapters 26 and 33 for more details on the history of TCI.

Educational Support by Industry

For more than a half century, industry in the US and elsewhere has supported education of members of the anesthesia community. This has taken the form of grants for educational purposes, as support of speakers dedicated to conveying information concerning a specific device or drug, and as distribution of educational materials and at times support for publication of proceedings of meetings, the subject of which may be a specific pharmaceutical or device. Support might underwrite a meeting or construction of written or electronic resources such as the books and videos produced for the Distinguished Professors Programs, underwritten by Baxter Healthcare. These might consume hundreds of thousand of dollars—for example the program that resulted in the textbook Eger wrote with James Eisenkraft and Richard Weiskopf on the Pharmacology of Inhaled Anesthetics [35], and the video that accompanied the book. Teaching programs in the US and abroad, particularly student nurse anesthetist programs, have used tens of thousands of copies of the book and associated DVD. As noted earlier, industry contributed to the organization and funding of FAER and continues financial support of the WRSA, APSF, and the AANA Research Foundation.

There is an obvious self-interest, of promotion by industry in the support of programs that focus attention on the virtues of products and devices. Selection of materials and speakers may create an unbalanced presentation of information. Industry has been accused of "buying" members of the anesthesia community by providing gifts, sometimes trivial handouts such a pens or flash drives, and sometimes far fancier attractions such as a meeting at a fancy resort. But one member of industry (private communication) suggests that there are positive reasons for industry's support of clinicians. By partnering with specialists, industry can better appreciate the decision-making processes of clinicians and better appreciate their frustrations and unmet needs. Such an appreciation enables a more effective approach to those issues over the long haul. I think steps taken to safeguard against favoritism as a result of commercial incentives to customers have merit. But I also believe that ways will be found to get a company's message to customers for it has an incentive to do so. Anesthetists may be safeguarded against undue influence from such messages because they immediately see the effects of products on patients.

Regardless of where the truth lies, there has been an increasing concern by educational institutions, professional societies, and government organizations that industry's "educational" ventures distort the process of selecting the best drug for individual patients. Sometimes the response to these concerns was "I can't be bought by a gift of a pen or a book bag or even a one time trip to Miami." But that may not be true. When someone is nice to you, you may wish to return the favor, even for something as trivial as a pen or book bag. The salesman has become your friend, and friends help friends. Evidence suggests that repeated contact from, and advertising by, pharmaceutical companies can affect physician choice.

The resulting advocacy by those opposed to such support is sometimes farcical. One of the editors of this book (LJS) was at an ASA meeting and as Editor of Anesthesiology, was carrying a huge volume of material for discussion at various ASA business meetings. He was and is adamantly opposed to industry providing gifts and anesthetists accepting them. Still, he found himself in need of a book bag to carry materials and despite his principled position, accepted a book bag from a vendor advertising the merits of the vendor's offerings. LJS arrived with his materials in the book bag, having concealed his indiscretion by turning the bag inside out. Unfortunately, another one of the editors of this book (EIE) saw LJS carrying the bag. EIE has far fewer scruples than LJS and has never since missed an opportunity to tease LJS for his fall from grace.

Over the past decade, the voices arguing that educational support by industry distorts the selection of drugs and devices have prevailed. Gone are the pens and most book bags. Gone are the free lunches. Speakers underwritten by industry cannot now speak at universities, and pharmaceutical representatives are now banned from distributing "educational materials" at most teaching institutions. Some departments of anesthesia forbid residents to attend industry sponsored dinners or meetings. Pharmaceutical companies have responded to the pressures by scripting the material that can be used by speakers that they support.

One can debate whether more has been lost than gained in this process, but the purpose of this book is to tell a story, not to judge. I (RL) remember standing on a balcony overlooking the commercial exhibits at the San Francisco convention center, with an unnamed ASA officer. He said he thought the ASA needed to allocate more break time for the exhibits because more education was going on there than at the scientific sessions. Correct or incorrect, I am sure what he said was not for attribution.

At present, the focus of industry on educational support in the US has markedly diminished. In part this has resulted from the pressures brought to bear on industry by academic institutions and the implied threat of regulatory action by government agencies. In part, it results from the loss of patented positions and thus the loss of an incentive to compete with a privileged product. And the rise in generic competition has decreased the amount of "discretionary funds that industry has available to support educational ventures.

These perceptions and changes may differ from those in other parts of the world. Since the mid 1980s, Australia-New Zealand has had an Anaesthesia Industry Liaison Committee of representatives from the specialty and industry. The committee oversees involvement of the industry in major scientific meetings, assuring the achievement of mutually agreed objectives, including ensuring that exhibitors are reasonably treated (e.g., have adequate space near to delegates). One result is that morning and afternoon tea breaks and lunches are held in the exhibition space. This relationship has been an effective one, one built on the principle that industry and the specialty are in the same business and can learn from and educate each other. (personal communication, Rod N. Westhorpe).

Some Conclusions

The profit motive that drives and enables industry has been part of the history of anesthesia from its beginning. Dreams of financial gain animated Morton's demonstration of the anesthetic effects of ether. Without that incentive, the discovery of anesthesia would have been delayed.

We have presented exemplars of historical and ongoing contributions of industry to the advancement of anesthesia. In concert with clinicians, industry has supplied the specialty with anesthetics and anesthetic adjuvant drugs and the means to deliver and analyze them. Anesthetists have expressed their needs and worked with industry to generate these new and better products. Industry has recognized a responsibility beyond the supply of better products. It has materially advanced the specialty by its support of societies, foundations, and national and local educational ventures. It has been and is a symbiotic relationship in which everyone wins, especially the patient.

References

1. Fenster J. Ether Day: the strange tale of America's greatest medical discovery and the haunted men who made it. New York: Harper Collins; 2001.
2. Stephens HW. The Texas City Disaster, 1947. Austin: University of Texas Press;1997. p. 100.

3. Jacob AK, Kopp SL, Bacon DR, Smith HM. The history of anesthesia. In: Barash PG, Cullen BF, Stoelting RK, Cahalan M, Stock MC, editors. Clinical anesthesia. Philadelphia: Wolters Kluwer, Lippincott Williams & Wilkins. 2009. pp. 3–26.

4. Suckling CW. Some chemical and physical factors in the development of Fluothane. Br J Anaesth. 1957;29:466–72.

5. Raventos J. The action of Fluothane—a new volatile anaesthetic. Br J Pharmacol. 1956;11:394–410.

6. Summary of the National Halothane Study. Possible association between halothane anesthesia and postoperative hepatic necrosis. Report by Subcommittee on the National Halothane Study of the Committee on Anesthesia, National Academy of Science. JAMA. 1966;197:775–88.

7. Krantz JC Jr, Carr CJ, Lu G, Bell FK. Anesthesia. XL. The anesthetic action of trifluoroethyl vinyl ether. J Pharmacol Exp Ther. 1953;108:488–95.

8. Terrell RC, Speers L, Szur AJ, Treadwell J, Ucciardi TR. General anesthetics. 1. Halogenated methyl ethyl ethers as anesthetic agents. J Med Chem. 1971;14:517–9.

9. Speers L, Szur AJ, Terrell RC, Treadwell J, Ucciardi TR. General anesthetics. 2. Halogenated methyl isopropyl ethers. J Med Chem. 1971;14:593–5.

10. Terrell RC, Speers L, Szur AJ, Ucciardi TR, Vitcha JF. General anesthetics. 3. Fluorinated methyl ethyl ethers as anesthetic agents. J Med Chem. 1972;15:604–6.

11. Eger EI II, Smuckler EA, Ferrell LD, Goldsmith CH, Johnson BH. Is enflurane hepatotoxic? Anesth Analg. 1986;65:21–30.

12. Linde HW, Lamb VE, Quimby CW Jr, Homi J, Eckenhoff JE. The search for better anesthetic agents: clinical investigation of ethrane. Anesthesiology. 1970;32:555–9.

13. Stoelting RK, Blitt CD, Cohen PJ, Merin RG. Hepatic dysfunction after isoflurane anesthesia. Anesth Analg. 1987;66:147–53.

14. Douglas HJ, Eger EI II, Biava CG, Renzi C. Hepatic necrosis associated with viral infection after enflurane anesthesia. N Engl J Med. 1977;296:553–5.

15. Fisher NA, Iwata RT, Eger EI II, Smuckler EA. Hepatic necrosis associated with herpes virus after isoflurane anesthesia. Anesth Analg. 1985;64:1131–3.

16. Reiz S, Balfors E, Sorensen MB, Ariola S Jr, Friedman A, Truedsson H. Isoflurane—a powerful coronary vasodilator in patients with coronary artery disease. Anesthesiology. 1983;59:91–7.

17. Brodeur P. Annals of chemistry, "A Compelling Intuition". The New Yorker 1975: November 14, p. 122.

18. Corbett TH. Cancer and congenital anomalies associated with anesthetics. Ann N Y Acad Sci. 1976;271:58–66.

19. Eger EI II, White AE, Brown CL, Biava CG, Corbett TH, Stevens WC. A test of the carcinogenicity of enflurane, isoflurane, halothane, methoxyflurane, and nitrous oxide in mice. Anesth Analg. 1978;57:678–94.

20. Eger EI II. Partition coefficients of I-653 in human blood, saline, and olive oil. Anesth Analg. 1987;66:971–3.

21. Strum DP, Eger EI II. Partition coefficients for sevoflurane in human blood, saline, and olive oil. Anesth Analg. 1987;66:654–6.

22. Eger EI II, Johnson BH. Rates of awakening from anesthesia with I-653, halothane, isoflurane, and sevoflurane: a test of the effect of anesthetic concentration and duration in rats. Anesth Analg. 1987;66:977–82.

23. Eger EI II. Stability of I-653 in soda lime. Anesth Analg. 1987;66:983–5.

24. Eger EI II, Johnson BH. MAC of I-653 in rats, including a test of the effect of body temperature and anesthetic duration. Anesth Analg. 1987;66:974–6.

25. Holaday DA, Smith FR. Clinical characteristics and biotransformation of sevoflurane in healthy human volunteers. Anesthesiology. 1981;54:100–6.

26. Wallin RF, Regan BM, Napoli MD, Stern IJ. Sevoflurane: a new inhalational anesthetic agent. Anesth Analg. 1975;54:758–65.

27. Kohn LT, Corrigan JM, Donaldson MS. To err is human: building a safer health system. Washingon: National Academy Press (Institute of Medicine); 2000.

28. James R, Glen JB. Synthesis, biological evaluation, and preliminary structure-activity considerations of a series of alkylphenols as intravenous anesthetic agents. J Med Chem. 1980;23:1350–7.

29. Kay B, Rolly G. I.C.I. 35868, a new intravenous induction agent. Acta Anaesthesiol Belg. 1977;28:303–16.

30. Glen JB, Davies GE, Thomson DS, Scarth SC, Thompson AV. An animal model for the investigation of adverse responses to i.v. anesthetic agents and their solvents. Br J Anaesth. 1979;51:819–27.

31. Glen JB, Hunter SC. Pharmacology of an emulsion formulation of ICI 35 868. Br J Anaesth. 1984;56:617–26.

32. Stokes DN, Peacock JE, Lewis R, Hutton P. The Ohmeda 9000 syringe pump. The first of a new generation of syringe drivers. Anaesthesia. 1990;45:1062–6.

33. Roberts FL, Dixon J, Lewis GT, Tackley RM, Prys-Roberts C. Induction and maintenance of propofol anaesthesia. A manual infusion scheme. Anaesthesia. 1988;43(Suppl):14–7.

34. Glen JB. The development of 'Diprifusor': a TCI system for propofol. Anaesthesia. 1998;53(Suppl 1):13–21.

35. Eger EI II, Eisenkraft JB, Weiskopf RB. The pharmacology of inhaled anesthetics. Chicago: Healthcare Press; 2002. pp. 1–327.

The History of the Anesthetist as a Perioperative Physician

67

Marlene R. Meyer and Jeanine P. Wiener-Kronish

Summary

This essay provides exemplars contributing to the evolution of anesthesia from empiricism and technical skill to a present focus on evidence based medicine.

John Snow (1813–1858) fathered modern epidemiology. He devised principles used to assess anesthetic depth, and made vaporizers that reliably controlled ether and chloroform vaporization. His analysis of anesthesia-associated deaths provided the first perioperative outcome study.

Arthur Guedel (1883–1956) revived Snow's signs of anesthetic depth, and with Waters constructed the modern oral-pharyngeal airway.

In 1927, *Ralph Waters* (1894–1979) initiated the first academic department of anesthesia based on research, teaching, and administration.

John Lundy (1894–1973) developed the anesthesia department at the Mayo Clinic, helped establish the American Board of Anesthesiology, created the first blood bank, and encouraged the AMA to recognize anesthesia as a specialty.

Gertie Marx (1912–2004) brought modern anesthesia into the labor ward. She championed epidural anesthesia, providing maternal pain relief while minimizing the risks of newborn aspiration and death from deep sedation.

John Bonica's (1917–1994) articles and textbook inspired new techniques for treating pain. In 1960, he initiated a multi-modal approach to pain management.

Bjørn Ibsen's (1915–2007) use of artificial ventilation to support breathing during Copenhagen's 1952 polio epidemic, led to today's Intensive Care Units.

Peter Safar (1924–2003) promoted closed-chest cardiopulmonary resuscitation. He established the first residency in intensive care medicine (ICM).

In 1952, *Henry Beecher* (1904–1976) suggested the use of placebo controls in human studies. His 1954 study showed the lethality of unantagonized muscle relaxants. In 1966, he developed principles of informed consent for patient care and human experimentation. In 1968, he used brain death to define death, itself.

Charles Robson (1884–1969) was the first pediatric anesthesiologist, serving as chief of Anesthesia at Toronto's Hospital for Sick Children from 1919 to 1950.

In 1953, *Virginia Apgar* (1909–1974) published the "Apgar Score" that became the international standard used to assess a newborn's physical status.

Goran Haglund (1915–2007) used Ibsen's approach to manage the 1952 polio epidemic in Sweden, developing the paradigm leading to pediatric ICUs. He also designed a pediatric ventilator.

Introduction

Today's anesthesiologist assesses the perioperative risk of patients who are to undergo anesthesia. This has become complicated, given the increasing diversity and severity of illnesses, the increasing extremes of patient age, and the myriad procedures requiring anesthesia care. This risk assessment requires acquisition of pertinent information about the patient and their medical history, and additional investigation where necessary to guide the care plan.

At times the anesthesiologist may be called in consultation and at other times may seek consultation from other medical

M. R. Meyer (✉)
Department of Anesthesia, Massachusetts General Hospital, Boston, MA, USA
e-mail: meyer.donovan@rcn.com

J. P. Wiener-Kronish
Department of Anesthesia, Critical Care and Pain Medicine, Massachusetts General Hospital, Harvard Medical School, Boston, MA, USA
e-mail: jwiener-kronish@partners.org

E. I Eger II et al. (eds.), *The Wondrous Story of Anesthesia*, DOI 10.1007/978-1-4614-8441-7_67, © Edmond I Eger, MD 2014

specialists. With the needed information in place the anesthesiologist discusses the anesthetic plan with the patient and their family. The discussion will include explanation of risks and benefits, describing the post-procedure care, answering the patient's questions, and obtaining their consent to the plan. The anesthesiologist as a perioperative physician plans the pre-operative medical management, intra-and immediate post-operative care, pain management and, when indicated, intensive care or other interventional therapy.

Anesthesia as a medical specialty had humble beginnings. A surgeon might ask anyone to "give ether". In Britain and the antipodes such "etherizers" might give chloroform and be called "chloroformists". The more than century-long evolution from etherizers to physicians practicing a medical specialty required the acquisition of scientific thinking and the development of a considerable body of knowledge, culminating in today's anesthesiologist as a perioperative physician who supplies more than anesthesia.

Many contributed to this evolution. A few individuals created the basis for the specialty and led the anesthesiologist beyond the operating room to further benefit patients. This essay will describe notable individuals or exemplars whose interests, expertise, and leadership created diverse models of patient care. They may apply to special patients (e.g., children, parturients, patients having suffered a heart attack), areas within hospitals (Intensive Care Units, Post Anesthetic Care Units), new services (blood banking, pain management, preoperative assessment clinics), or a consideration of ethics in medicine (informed consent, when is a patient dead?) Such individuals moved the specialty from empiricism and technical skill to a present focus on evidence based medicine extending the reach of anesthesia far beyond the operating room. We will use the ground-breaking contributions of "exemplars" to explore the development of the practice of anesthesia from "etherizer" to anesthesiologist and perioperative physician.

In the Beginning....

Anesthesia is the only medical specialty that can claim a "birth date". On 16 October 1846 William Morton demonstrated the anesthetic properties of sulfuric ether before an audience in the surgical amphitheater of the Massachusetts General Hospital, prompting the surgeon, John Collins Warren, to exclaim, "Gentlemen, this is no humbug." [1] One of the men organizing the demonstration, Henry Bigelow, fearing the results could not be reliably replicated, observed a series of cases demonstrating the anesthetic properties of ether before publishing the news in the 18 November 1846 issue of the Boston Medical and Surgical Journal [2].

The reports of sulphuric ether's anesthetic properties spread from Boston to England through letters, newspaper clippings, and a copy of the *Boston Medical and Surgical Journal* article brought by Edward Warren (brother of John Collins Warren) to an American physician-scientist living in London, Francis Boott [1792–1863] [3] Edward Warren departed Boston on 3 December, aboard the paddle steamer "Acadia". Boott received the news on 18 December, the day after the Acadia made port.

Boott quickly sent the letter and the newspaper report to the *Lancet* and with his neighbor, dentist James Robinson, experimented with the new agent. On 19 December Robinson and Boott gave the first anesthetic in England at Boott's home. Soon after, other demonstrations were given. On 28 December, Boott and Robinson gave another demonstration in Boott's home. Present was the physician-scientist, John Snow [4, 5].

John Snow [1813–1858], the First and Greatest Anesthesiologist, Laid the Foundations for the Safe Delivery of Clinical Anesthesia

During his remarkable career, Snow published more than 100 articles, books, and pamphlets while carrying on a busy medical practice in Victorian England [6]. He was a "complete physician", outstanding in every aspect. Through meticulous record keeping and a keen analytical mind, he proved that cholera spread via contaminated water, doing this before the discovery of bacteria or the existence of the idea of "infection". This work is popularly known as the "Broad Street Pump" story. Snow's studies led him to conclude that the Broad Street well was the source of the contagion, and he helped quell the epidemic by advising removal of the handle of its pump. It is a foundation study in the fields of epidemiology and public health [7].

Not only did Snow "father epidemiology", he was also the first specialist anesthesiologist. At the time of his death at age 45 from a stroke (autopsy showed renal disease), he had given more than 5,000 anesthetics, all the while continuing his general medical and obstetric practice and undertaking research. His casebooks served as the basis for his publications and testify to his keen powers of observation.

His origins were humble. Snow's father could only afford a private primary school education for his son (there were no public schools). Snow served a series of apprenticeships, first qualifying as an apothecary, then as a surgeon. Finances forced him to take classes one by one until he completed the requirements needed to take the examination to become a physician. Perhaps it was fortunate that he could not attend a "proper" university. By avoiding the "philosopher" theories of medicine, his mind remained open to scientific discoveries.

Snow avidly attended medical meetings, presented papers, and debated medical issues. Being "well known" in London medical circles, on 28 December 1846 he was among the friends Boott invited for a demonstration of "The Yankee Dodge", as the surgeon Robert Liston called ether. Liston was the first surgeon to operate on an "etherized" patient at the London University Hospital, doing so on 19 December 1846 [7].

Because of his exposure to obstetrics and the associated problem of asphyxia of the newborn, Snow developed an interest in respiratory physiology. He did not accept the varieties of treatments and theories used to resuscitate the newborn. Practices such as immersing the infant in cold water, warm water, or even electrical stimulation were among the methods advocated. In 1841, he published an elegant article describing the components needed to successfully resuscitate the "stillborn" child. Included in this publication were the results of his experimentation, using diverse animal subjects to validate his recommendations for successful resuscitation [8].

With this insight into the physiology of respiration, he had the tools to conduct experiments using first ether and then chloroform. Both drugs, liquids with low boiling points, became gases (vapors) when exposed to air at room temperature. Inhalation of these vapors produced the state soon called "anesthesia", a state freeing the patient from pain.

After seeing the ether demonstration, Snow devised experiments to reliably demonstrate the effects of ether in all test species, including himself. In a lecture given on 17 May 1847, he provided the first scientific analysis of the physiology and pharmacology of ether, presenting a basis for its safe administration as an anesthetic. He devised a vaporizer that minimized variations in the delivered concentration of the inhaled anesthetic, especially those due to changes in the temperature of the liquid. The principles he applied are those found in modern vaporizers. In 18 articles "On narcotism by the inhalation of vapors" published in the *London Medical Gazette* [1848–1851] he provided a guide for the safe administration of both ether and chloroform to alleviate the pain of surgery. He described physical signs to guide the "etherizer" or "chloroformist" that might prevent lethal overdosing.

His fame as an "anaesthetist" with a busy obstetric anesthesia practice caused Queen Victoria to seek his services for the birth of Prince Leopold in 1853. This muted early objections to painless labor [9].

Reports of deaths associated with chloroform appeared within weeks of its introduction for anesthesia. Snow analyzed the causes of these deaths. In one patient he had anesthetized with chloroform, autopsy showed a "fatty heart," but no observation to suggest anesthetic overdose [10]. The patient was known to have had heart disease. In his preoperative assessment of the patient's fitness for anesthesia, Snow had expressed reservations concerning the patient's ability to withstand the effects of anesthesia and surgery but proceeded because the patient had previously undergone the procedure without difficulty.

Snow's analysis provided one of the first models of perioperative care. He had assessed the patient's medical status, provided care, and studied the cause of the patient's death. He determined that the anesthetic drug was probably not the sole cause of death. Snow had recognized the risk the patient brought to the procedure and had informed the patient of the risk. Snow's sudden death in 1858 left a great void.

The Last Half of the Nineteenth Century: Little is Demanded of Anesthesia

The discovery of anesthesia was such a colossal advance that it took nearly a century for surgery to catch up, and there was little need for advances in anesthesia until that happened. Some viewed specialization in medicine—a practice solely devoted to anesthetic delivery—to be a form of quackery. In major cities, a few physicians chose to focus their practices on surgery or obstetrics. Rarely did a physician become interested in anesthesia.

In Britain, medical students, dentists, and physicians administered anesthesia. The practice in the US was a step lower, and porters (orderlies) and secretaries sometimes gave anesthesia. Soon after the introduction of ether, nurses were recruited to administer it. Nurse anesthetists, along with nurse midwifes, were the pioneers in advance practice nursing.

Surgeons supervised the administration of anesthesia well into the twentieth century, even when the anesthetist was a physician. As surgery progressed, becoming more complex and technically demanding, the surgeon needed to focus on the procedure, leaving management of intra-operative and immediate postoperative care to the anesthetist.

The Twentieth Century: The Age of Science and Medicine

Many individuals contributed to the tools and techniques, and to the intellectual growth of anesthesiology. The focus of this essay is the evolution of anesthesia as it became a "medical specialty". The individuals we have selected represent those who either laid the foundations for the clinical practice and academic basis of anesthesiology, or brought the anesthesiologist out of the operating room. They provided care before and beyond this boundary.

The pace of scientific discovery during the twentieth Century rapidly added to the understanding of diseases. Application of scientific principles led to the development of effective medications. The practice of anesthesia benefited from improved methods of anesthetic delivery, new technologies for monitoring, and new drugs. By 1939 the knowledge and technical skills required to practice anesthesia prompted the

American Medical Association to recognize anesthesiology as a medical specialty [11].

The pace of change accelerated after World War I and then further after World War II. By the end of the twentieth Century, anesthesiology had itself given rise to sub-specialization in obstetrics, pediatrics, cardiothoracics, neurosurgery, intensive care, and pain management.

Arthur Guedel [1883–1956]. The Motorcycle Anesthesiologist

The "artists" of anesthesia catalogued patients' responses to anesthetics and incorporated their perceptions into an organized representation for their private use. There was a need for a system that could be easily learned and remembered, a system that could be broadly applied by diverse etherizers. Guedel supplied this, unknowingly reviving observations made by Snow. In the era before Index Medicus, PubMed, and Google, retrieving information from old publications was a tedious and difficult task not routinely undertaken. Old discoveries were often lost and then rediscovered.

Guedel began his career as a general practitioner, becoming fascinated by anesthesia during his internship, when his training required him to administer anesthetics. He built an extensive anesthesia practice before serving with the American Expeditionary Forces in France during World War I.

In France, he found himself confronted by soldiers with massive injuries requiring surgery. His responsibilities required him to move quickly from field hospital to field hospital in order to guide the delivery of ether by a wide range of etherizers. The motorcycle became his favored mode of transportation, giving rise to his fame as the motorcycle anesthesiologist.

As the only anesthesiologist in his region, he needed to quickly train nurses, secretaries, orderlies and others to safely administer ether anesthesia. Using observations from almost a decade of anesthesia practice, he devised a chart of the signs and stages of ether anesthesia, and trained personnel to follow it. The steps in the progression of patient responses as anesthesia deepened became known as Guedel's stages. The safety record resulting from the use of this guide proved its value. First published in 1920, [12] the guide quickly became the universal standard for conducting ether anesthesia. Others added details to the guide.

Guedel returned to private practice and later became an "academic" anesthesiologist. He invented several airway devices during his career, always looking for better ways to care for patients [13]. His oropharyngeal airway is used today.

The idea of connecting a drug dose to a predictable response was poorly understood in the early twentieth century. Anesthesia was "dangerous" when administered by unskilled people. Guedel's stages of anesthesia (the depth of anesthe-

sia) express the neurological and cardiovascular changes reflecting "doses" of ether. Like Snow, Guedel used easily observed physiologic changes to construct a dose-response relationship applicable to all patients. By using his clinical observations he created a useful tool for the safe administration of inhaled ether. It became one of the elements that led to the establishment of anesthesia as a specialty within the practice of medicine.

Unfortunately, the introduction of new inhaled anesthetic drugs presented a problem: Guedel's signs and stages for ether did not directly translate for different anesthetics. How did one quantify the correct concentration to administer when each drug produced its own profile of observable changes? In addition, opioids and sedative drugs used in conjunction with the inhaled drugs changed the observable signs.

The ability to measure the exact dose present in the patient's central nervous system and know the dose required to safely proceed with surgery would improve patient care. Edmond Eger [1930-] described the method for assessing the amount of volatile anesthetic drug needed to produce a crucial clinical endpoint, MAC (the minimum alveolar concentration required to suppress movement in response to a noxious stimulus such as surgery in 50% of subjects) in 1965 [14].

MAC provided a standard applicable to all inhaled anesthetics. It quantified Snow's qualitative findings. Using MAC, Eger's group and other investigators compared the relative effects of all commonly used anesthetics on the physiologic responses to clinically relevant anesthetic concentrations. With this information, and the breath-by-breath analysis of anesthetic concentration provided by present technology, today's anesthesiologist has the knowledge needed to administer the exact dose required by each patient throughout the surgical procedure.

Ralph Waters [1894–1979]. Father of the Academic Specialty of Anesthesia

Waters transformed the art of anesthetic administration into a scientific medical specialty. With Henry Beecher, Waters is acknowledged as the father of modern academic anesthesia in the US. He began medical practice, including occasional surgery, in 1913. He and his fellow surgeons aided each other by administering anesthesia. As a medical student and intern he taught himself to administer ether—to be an anesthetist, the term used for anyone who provided anesthesia.

By 1916 he decided to limit his practice to anesthesia. Over the next decade, he progressively increased contacts and friendships with anesthetic pioneers and those interested in respiratory physiology. In the 1920s, the new medical school at the University of Wisconsin changed the paradigm for medical education by creating full time clinical professors. In 1927, the university invited Waters to become the first full time professor of anesthesia. His academic appointment gave him entree to an academic milieu that allowed the development of anesthesiology as a medical specialty, a specialty devoted to patient care that was based on scientific principles.

Underlying Waters' approach to anesthesiology was his belief that an understanding of the science of medicine was essential for competency in a physician. Waters was uncompromising in his scientific integrity [15]. His interests in respiratory physiology raised questions that he believed could best be answered in a medical school where there was collaboration between basic scientists and clinical faculty.

John Snow was Waters' hero. Writing a biographical paper on Snow in 1936, he concluded that "We need not hesitate to say that John Snow was and remains the greatest anaesthetist as well as the first". Like his hero, he investigated methods for resuscitation [16]. He advocated tracheal intubation for cases of difficult airway management, and mouth to mouth respiration during resuscitation.

He had a prolific career, authoring many scientific papers and encouraging residents and staff in their academic development. Through his example and generous spirit he literally created the next generation of academic anesthesiologists. He led the way in professionalizing anesthesiology [17]. His protégés called themselves the "Aqua-Alumni".

John Lundy [1894–1973]. Developer of the Recovery Room, Blood Banking, Anesthetic Certification, and New Anesthetics

Lundy practiced anesthesia before it became a medical specialty. He sensed the limitations in those pursuing a career in anesthesia at the time: "There was a tendency for only those physicians who were incompetent in general practice or in other branches to limit themselves to the practice of anesthesia." [18] His life contributed mightily to changing that tendency.

Lundy met William Mayo in 1924 at a meeting in Seattle. Lundy's enthusiasm and knowledge of anesthesia so impressed Mayo that he invited Lundy to establish an anesthesia department at the Mayo Clinic. Before this appointment, nurses provided all anesthesia under the direction of surgeons. Mayo saw the opportunity to relieve surgeons of this responsibility.

Lundy championed anesthesia education, developed regional anesthesia, and created the first blood bank. The latter achievement occurred at a time when donors were called to contribute blood on an "as needed" basis. Venous access could be technically difficult because of the type of needles available in the1930s, and it was common for the vein to be exposed surgically, the venous "cut-down". Most transfu-

sions at the Mayo Clinic occurred in the operating rooms. Lundy had established his professional credentials as an expert in intravenous fluid administration, and had the technical expertise to procure and administer blood.

In 1934, citrated blood was occasionally kept in the icebox for as long as 14 days. It was noted that this "stored" blood could be infused safely. Lundy was put in charge of transfusions in 1934, and set up a system for the storage of citrated blood in the laboratory of WC MacCarty at the Mayo Clinic. Thus the Blood Bank was born. He also worked on techniques for the rapid infusion and freezing of blood [19].

In 1929, he formed the Anaesthesia Travel Club, one of the forerunners of the professional societies for promoting education and exchange of information. Lundy lobbied the American Medical Association for recognition of anesthesia as a specialty within the Association, and in 1939 the AMA recognized anesthesia as a section within the Association [20, 21].

He contributed to the clinical introduction of thiopental sodium, a drug administered intravenously for general anesthesia, as well as the anesthetic gas, cyclopropane. He championed the use of local anesthetics and techniques for regional anesthesia [22]. He pioneered the concept of "balanced anesthesia", the combined use of intravenous drugs, such as thiopental and opioids, with inhaled anesthetics.

He created a specialized section within the department of anesthesia that managed ventilators and supplied techniques for supplementing inspired oxygen [23]. In 1942, Lundy opened the world's first post anesthesia recovery room, now called the Post Anesthesia Care Unit, or PACU. This development recognized that surgery and anesthesia created conditions that could lead to adverse outcomes. Prevention of such outcomes required close observation in a specialized area near the operating suite by specially trained nurses. The anesthesiologist became the responsible physician for directing patient care in the PACU.

Gertie Marx [1912–2004]. The Grande Dame of Obstetric Anesthesia

Although Nathan Keep anesthetized Fanny Appleton (Mrs. Henry Wadsworth) Longfellow in 1847, [24] and Snow famously anesthetized Queen Victoria in 1853, [7] for their deliveries, prejudice against using anesthesia in obstetrics remained well into the mid-twentieth Century. Despite these well-publicized demonstrations, the benefits of analgesia for the ordinary woman in labor were not routinely available until the 1960s–1970s.

Marx was the "Grande Dame" of obstetric anesthesia [25]. Nazism forced her to leave Germany once she had completed medical school at the University of Bern, Switzerland. She immigrated to the US in 1937, obtaining a rotating internship at New York Beth Israel Hospital only after a male candidate chose not to attend. Originally planning a career in pediatrics, she discovered anesthesia while an intern.

At the time, laboring women might receive no anesthesia, heavy sedation, or general anesthesia, all choices potentially detrimental to mother and child. Marx championed epidural anesthesia because it provided pain relief for the mother while minimizing the risks of aspiration and possible death from deep sedation. In addition, the small amount of local anesthetic absorbed from the epidural space did not depress the newborn's respiration. Some thought epidural anesthesia would delay labor and thereby increase the incidence of Caesarean sections. Marx proved these critics wrong, winning the gratitude of mothers worldwide [26].

Marx's relentless efforts also changed the care of pregnant patients by introducing the anesthesiologist into the obstetric care team. Her clinical research in regional anesthesia improved patient care, increasing the use of epidural anesthesia during labor and for the management of post-operative pain. She is an exemplar because she brought anesthesia beyond the operating room into the labor ward.

John Bonica [1917–1994]. Founder of the Multidisciplinary Chronic Pain Clinic and Pain as a Subspecialty

After completing his residency in anesthesia during World War II, Bonica joined the US Army and was placed in charge of the anesthesia service at Fort Lewis, Washington. During his service, he supervised the anesthesia care of over 10,000 soldiers. He taught himself regional anesthesia techniques, something that had been absent from his anesthesia residency. He noted that regional anesthesia sometimes relieved both acute and chronic pain, stimulating a lifelong interest in the alleviation of pain.

After the war, Bonica became director of anesthesia at the Tacoma, Washington Hospital in 1947. There, he founded the first residency with formal training in regional anesthesia. In 1960, he assumed the Chair at the University of Washington, establishing a balanced program of general and regional techniques that stressed patient care and clinical research. His numerous articles and his massive textbook on pain inspired new techniques for treating pain. Perhaps his greatest contribution was the initiation of a multi-modal approach to pain management. On assuming the Chair, he founded a clinic that focused the combined efforts of anesthesiologists, neurologists, surgeons, psychologists, and physical therapists on pain management. It was a revolutionary concept that is now used worldwide [27].

Ironically, pain was no stranger to Bonica. He worked his way through school as a professional wrestler, and the resulting physical insults left him crippled with pain at the end of his life.

Most anesthesia residencies now have a pain clinic and a consultant service to manage perioperative pain. Because of Bonica's vision, the anesthesiologist-pain specialist takes the practice of anesthesia well beyond the operating room.

Bjørn Ibsen [1915–2007]. Father of Intensive Care Medicine

Wars and epidemics in the twentieth Century conspired to advance anesthesia practice and patient care. Ibsen completed medical school at the University of Copenhagen in January 1942, anticipating a career in thoracic surgery. Although Germany occupied Denmark in April of that year, Ibsen managed to continue his training and earned a prize in biochemistry in 1944 [28].

At the end of World War II, the tattered European economies offered few openings for research. Henry Beecher seized this opportunity to recruit eager young European physicians seeking research training. Ibsen went to the Massachusetts General Hospital in 1949 as an assistant resident for a year-long course, returning to Denmark in 1950 [29].

Although the Danish government established departments of anesthesia to care for "patients during the operation and postoperatively", [30] Ibsen could not secure a permanent appointment. He was working as a free-lance anesthesiologist when a devastating polio epidemic struck in 1952 [30]. Among Copenhagen's population of just over a million, 3,000 had polio; 1250 had some paralysis and 345 required respiratory support [31].

The (Blegdam) Fever Hospital, the hospital caring for most of these patients, was overwhelmed, and standard practices produced dismal results. Based on his work with Beecher and his experiences managing ventilation outside of the operating room, Ibsen proposed long term controlled or assisted ventilation for patients with impaired swallowing or respiration. He was invited to apply his suggestions, in particular a plan to ensure proper oxygenation while keeping the level of carbon dioxide within tolerable limits. To do this he created a cadre of specialized care providers, coordinating care within one space [32]. His plan dramatically improved survival, relative to the medical paradigm that had focused on diagnosis and causal therapy. His model corrected the physiological disturbance that the illness created.

Ibsen's genius created a collaborative team that worked in an integrated setting separated from the general medical patient population. This innovative concept was soon applied to patients with complex medical and surgical problems. Ibsen's creation, the Intensive Care Unit (ICU), now exists in all major medical centers. Today, anesthesia training includes intensive care rotations and opportunities for additional training and subspecialty certification.

Peter Safar [1924–2003] Invents CPR

Perhaps the Prophet Elijah performed the earliest successful resuscitation when he revived a dead boy, "putting his mouth upon the child's mouth." [Bible, 2 Kings 4:34]. Similarly, Peter Safar created a simple algorithm that could restore cardio-respiratory function and could be taught to the general public, increasing its life-saving potential.

Nominated three times but never awarded the Nobel Prize in Medicine, Safar was a prolific writer, educator, and consummate clinician. His passion was to "save the hearts and brains of those too young to die". Safar graduated from the University of Vienna, immigrated to the US in 1949, and completed an anesthesia residency at the University of Pennsylvania in 1952.

Most of us know that CPR stands for cardiopulmonary resuscitation—Safar's consuming interest. In 1956, Safar began his studies of unexpected sudden death, and in 1961, demonstrated that closed chest cardiac massage without ventilation described by Kowenhoven et al in 1960 [33] did not provide adequate tidal volume and recommended that "closed-chest cardiac massage should be preceded and accompanied by pulmonary ventilation". [34] The techniques were simple to learn and were widely taught to the public. In the 2000s, the timing and even the application of artificial ventilation became more complex than suggested by Safar. Resuscitation now began with chest compression followed by opening the airway and might or might not then be followed by artificial ventilation [35].

Safar pioneered the role of the anesthesiologist in emergency medicine, developed the first intensive care unit in the US, and established the first residency-training program for intensive care medicine. He made intensive care medicine a medical sub-specialty in anesthesia.

Henry Beecher [1904–1976]. Ethicist and Scientific Leader

Born Harry Unangst, Beecher was a scientist-clinician. Although his first loves were physiology and chemistry, he enrolled in Harvard Medical School, graduating with honors in 1932. He completed two years of training in the department of surgery at Massachusetts General Hospital, after which Edward Churchill, the chairman of the department of surgery, selected Beecher to develop the anesthesia department, at that time a division of surgery. He was sent to Denmark to work in the laboratory of the Nobel Laureate, August Krogh. On his return in 1936, he was appointed Anesthestist-In-Chief at the Massachusetts General Hospital. In 1941, Beecher became the Henry Isaiah Dorr Professor of Anesthesia Research, the first endowed chair in anesthesia in the US [36].

He is one of very few chairmen appointed to lead a department of anesthesia who had no specific training in anesthesia. His research contributions are considerable, including one of the first important outcome studies, his investigation of nearly 600,000 patients that showed the dangers of the use of curare, used to provide muscle relaxation in the absence of reversal of residual neuromuscular blockade at the end of surgery [37].

Patients must give their consent to receive medical care. What information did the patient need to know in order to give consent? In the 1940s, the traditional idea that "the doctor knows best" limited the information provided to patients concerning options, risks and benefits. The decision to treat was, in fact, the physician's. The patient's choice of a specific physician implied acceptance of the proposed care.

The Nuremburg trials documented human experimentation that horrified the medical community, but that community was reluctant to examine its own practices. Beecher's landmark publication in 1966 [38] revealed the systematic failure to tell patients the details of proposed treatments, including risks or benefits or the unproven nature of some proposed remedies.

Physicians must now obtain a patient's informed consent before embarking on a care plan. The once common practice of relying on a combined surgical and anesthesia consent form obtained by the surgeon, or the use of documents stating only the name of the operation and that anesthesia was provided, were clearly insufficient. Beecher's work expanded and codified the anesthesiologist's responsibility to educate each patient about the anesthesia plan and to obtain consent.

Beecher's protégé, Ibsen, raised a crucial problem that Beecher attacked: when was a patient dead? By the 1960s, ICU physicians could mechanically support respiration and maintain circulation with drug therapy and mechanical devices. How did one know if such a patient was alive or dead? The answer to the question required a consensus definition of the word "death". In 1968, a panel of physicians and ethicists led by Beecher published the "Harvard Criteria for Brain Death". [39] "Death" shifted from cessation of breathing and absence of cardiac activity to loss of discernable brain function and absence of the possibility of regaining function. Beecher's work in ethics and his credentials as a respected scientist added credence to the Committee's report and its acceptance by medical and legal communities, world-wide.

Beecher created a world class research program but is best remembered for two monumental contributions: the development of the principles of informed consent for patient care and human experimentation, and the definition of brain death as a criterion for determining a patient's demise.

Charles Robson [1884–1969]. First to Lead a Pediatric Department of Anesthesia; Advocate for Anesthesia in Infants

Children received anesthesia as early as 1842 when Crawford Long gave ether to a "Negro boy". Snow had extensive experience anesthetizing children, correctly identifying physiologic differences between children and adults. Advances in technology and measurements a century later supported Snow's observations and deductions [40]. Despite Snow's genius and guidance, anesthesia for children remained risky. Equipment used in anesthetic practice was poorly adapted for children, especially younger ones. Slowly, during the 1930s, surgical techniques and knowledge of pediatric physiology progressed, and it was recognized that the safe pursuit of complex surgical procedures on ill children required an anesthesia care team approach.

Robson was the first anesthesiologist to devote his practice exclusively to pediatric care. He graduated from McGill University School of Medicine in 1913. After a one-year internship at Montreal General Hospital, he joined the Canadian Expeditionary Forces during World War I where he developed his anesthesia skills, becoming the senior ranked anaesthetist. On returning to civilian life, he was appointed chief of the Department of Anaesthesia at the Hospital for Sick Children, Toronto, where he served from 1919–1950.

Snow's observations notwithstanding, the differences between the physiology of the developing child and the adult were not well understood when Robson began his career as a pediatric anesthesiologist. He used his keen powers of observation and inventiveness to develop equipment and airway management techniques appropriate for the differences in the anatomy and physiology found in children. He believed that infants experienced pain and required anesthesia for surgical procedures, a view that many of his contemporaries did not share. He championed better ways of approaching the frightened child. He pioneered the use of tracheal intubation during surgery in infants [40]. He was the first to recognize the importance of fasting a for few hours before surgery to lessen the risk of aspiration during anesthesia.

Virginia Apgar [1909–1974]. Care of the Newborn

Worldwide, "the Apgar" means the tool used to assess a newborn's physical status at birth. Few know the origin of the term and Apgar's remarkable story. She is a select member of a fraternity of physicians whose names are part of the vocabulary of medicine.

Although a gifted musician and athlete, Apgar chose medicine as a career while still a young child. Coming of age in the Great Depression, she worked her way through college

and medical school, aided by scholarships and loans from family members [41]. After graduating fourth in her class from the College of Physicians and Surgeons at Columbia in 1933, she was accepted into the surgical training program at Columbia Presbyterian Hospital.

Although the chairman of the department of surgery, Allen Whipple was convinced of Apgar's talent, he believed that prejudice against women in surgery would hinder her capacity to earn a living as a surgeon. After she completed three years of surgical residency, he persuaded her to take up anesthesia. Perhaps because it paid poorly and attracted few men, there was no bias against women in the practice of anesthesia [42]. Being in debt and with dim prospects of financial success as a surgeon, Apgar followed his advice. Her training was typical for the time. She worked with nurse anesthetists for a year, learning the art of anesthesia delivery, and then spent a year with Waters in Wisconsin learning the science. She continued her anesthesia training under Emory Rovenstine at Bellevue Hospital in New York.

On returning to Columbia in 1938, she was appointed director of anesthesia in the department of surgery. In this role, she laid the groundwork for a subsequent department of anesthesia. She educated medical students to facilitate their later recruitment as anesthesia residents. She provided patient care beyond anesthesia and contributed to the development of an anesthesia research program.

One morning, during the anesthesia breakfast discussions that she held each day, a question by a medical student prompted the birth of the Apgar Score: "How do you evaluate a newborn baby?" "Easy", she replied, jotting down five things to assess. Legend has it that she wrote these observations on a napkin for the student. She rushed off to start her day in the obstetric unit. During that day she thought about what she had written from a scientific perspective, and recruited colleagues to validate her observations. The rest is history. The five things were skin color, pulse, reflex irritability, muscle tone, and respiration, each scored as 0, 1, or 2 (best).

The Apgar Score was published in 1953 [43]. Its enormous value lay in its simplicity (it required no technology and was easy to learn and apply), and in its considerable predictive value (e.g., a value of 5 indicated an infant in trouble).

Later in her career, Apgar became involved with the problem of birth defects. Leaving Columbia in 1959, she went to Johns Hopkins University and earned her PhD in public health. She became the director of the division of congenital malformations for the National Foundation, also known as the March of Dimes, helping it refocus its activity after vaccines had solved the ravages of polio in the US. Apgar received the ASA Distinguished Service Award in 1961 and was posthumously honored by the United States Postal Service with a stamp bearing her image in 1994.

Goran Haglund [1915–2007]. Pediatric Intensive Care

The man who created modern anesthesiology in Sweden, Torsten Gordh, trained under Waters at the University of Wisconsin, returning shortly before the World War II blockade of Sweden. After the war, anesthesiologists interested in additional training turned to Waters' protégés in the US.

After completing medical school at the University of Lund, followed by two years of training in surgery and anesthesia, Haglund went to the US in 1949. He worked under the direction of Allen Conroy, one of the "aqua alumni" at the University of Chicago. On returning to Sweden in 1950, Haglund was one of three anesthesiologists in Gothenburg. In 1951 he accepted an appointment to the Children's Hospital [44].

His experiences in the US led him to conclude that problems with respiration and circulation in critically ill patients were better managed if the patients were concentrated in one location. The surgeons agreed to try his idea. Then the polio epidemic struck Sweden as it had Denmark [45]. The epidemic and its management fostered the development of the care paradigm that would underlie the pediatric intensive care unit [46].

Because there was no equipment designed for respiratory support for children, he constructed a ventilator of his own design [44]. By 1955 his plans for a pediatric intensive care unit were fully implemented. The pediatric anesthesiologist thus joined his anesthesia colleagues who were in the early phase of developing the subspecialty of intensive care medicine, extending their scope of practice beyond the operating room.

Besides his busy clinical practice, research, and teaching duties, Haglund was renowned for his classical education and knowledge of music. In addition to his many talents he possessed a fine sense humor. For several years, he and a friend hosted a popular Swedish radio program that showcased their humor and knowledge.

There are Many Exemplars

Our essay cited some of the most famous exemplars of the anesthesiologist as a perioperative physician, noting the contributions of each. We could have detailed the lives of many more. Meyer Saklad, for example, who devised the ASA Physical Status and was instrumental in the evolution of the American Board of Anesthesiology certification examination. Or Ellison (Jeep) Pierce whose leadership led to the formation of the Anesthesia Patient Safety Foundation. Or Lee Fleisher [47–51], who has influenced guideline development with the American College of Cardiology and the American Heart Association. He has worked with Medicare [CMS] as a member of the team involved with the surgical care improvement project [SCIP initiative]. Through Fleisher's efforts, anesthesiologists are now integrated into healthcare reform and quality initiatives. Or Michael Roizen [52, 53, 54], who found that the results of a patient's history and physical examination could obviate the need for (and cost of) many specific preoperative tests. He expanded preoperative assessment to include all of medical and wellness assessment, leading to his present career focused on improving wellness in patients. Or Daniel Sessler and Harriet Hopf (among others) who showed that what we do to our patients in the operating room—how much oxygen we deliver and how well we maintain our patient's temperature, whether we use epidural analgesia—can affect the postoperative well-being of our patients and can affect the incidence of infection or healing of wounds [55–57]. And Emory Rovenstine, much as Ralph Waters, was instrumental in the explosive growth in anesthesia, particularly academic anesthesia [58]. And John Severinghaus, developer of the blood gas electrodes we use every day [59]. There are many more anesthesiologists whose contributions reach beyond the operating room and the delivery of anesthesia, but space limitations force us to those we have chosen for detailed examination, exemplars of the exemplars.

Reprise

Diethyl ether was synthesized in the 1200s, rediscovered in the 1500s, and first publically used for anesthesia in humans in 1846. The demonstration of anesthesia occurred when society had evolved sufficiently to promote progress in surgery and science. What began as an act of administering a drug grew into a specialized branch of medical science called anesthesiology.

John Snow, the first and perhaps greatest anesthesiologist, set a standard of practice that we admire today. He was devoted to providing the best care for all of his patients, combining clinical observations with scientific experimentation to validate his observations. His care of a patient began with a pre operation assessment of the patient's ability to "survive" the planned surgery and anesthesia. He monitored the patient's responses to anesthesia, made adjustments to anesthetic doses accordingly, and remained with the patient until the patient was judged fit to be cared for by others. When necessary, Snow investigated intra operative fatalities to determine if the anesthetic was the cause of the death.

The generations of men and women who followed Snow, added to the knowledge and skills necessary to be an anesthesiologist. Many anesthesia departments include "Perioperative Medicine" in their title, denoting their expanded roles in patient care. Departments of Perioperative Medicine consist of individuals trained as "anesthesiologists" but whose training and interests extend beyond those focused on the traditional care of patients in the operating room. These expanded roles include preoperative assessment and testing intended to determine a patient's fitness for surgery, and intraoperative care of patients of all ages, sizes, complexity and illness. They include immediate and long-term care in PACUs and ICUs, acute pain management for surgical patients, and out-of-hospital pain management for patients with chronic pain (e.g., consequent to cancer or orthopedic problems). The perioperative physician offers educational assistance to nurses, other medical and non-medical professionals, including those delivering hospice care and home health infusion therapy. Finally, the increasingly diverse roles played by the perioperative physician include direction for institutions in the increasingly important and complex area of health care management and financing.

In a sense there is no perioperative physician since no individual can embrace all the functions that might be undertaken. But there can be Departments of Anesthesia and Perioperative Medicine that contain individuals whose combined talents provide the diverse functions of the perioperative physician.

References

1. Fenster JM. Ether day: the strange tale of America's greatest medical discovery and the haunted men who made it. New York: HarperCollins; 2001. p. 75.
2. Bigelow HJ. Surgical anaesthesia: addresses and other papers. Boston: Little, Brown, and Co; 1900. pp. 3–16.
3. Library of the Gray Herbarium Archives, Harvard University: Francis Boott (1792–1863) Papers. www.huh.harvard.edu/libraries/archives/BOOTT/html. Accessed 14 Dec 2010.
4. Ellis RH. The introduction of ether anaesthesia to Great Britain. 1. How the news was carried from Boston, Massachusetts to Gower Street, London. Anaesthesia. 1976;31:766–77.
5. Ellis RH. The introduction of ether anaesthesia to Great Britain. 2. A biographical sketch of Dr. Francis Boott. Anaesthesia 1977;32:197–208.
6. The John Snow archive and research companion: Snow's works. http://johnsnow.matrix.msu.edu. Accessed 14 Dec 2010.
7. Vinten-Johansen P, Brody N, Rachman S, Rip M, Zuck D. Cholera, chloroform, and the science of medicine: a life of John Snow. Oxford: Oxford University Press; 2003. p. 4, 242.
8. Snow J. On asphyxia, and on the resuscitation of still-born children. Lond Med Gaz. 1841;29:222–7.
9. Snow J. Death from chloroform in a case of fatty degeneration of the heart. Med Times Gaz. 1852;5:361–2.
10. Pernick MS. A calculus of suffering: pain, professionalism and anesthesia in nineteenth-century America. New York: Columbia University Press; 1985. p. 28.
11. Larson MD, Arthur E. Guedel Memorial Anesthesia Center: Guedel's anesthetic depth chart, Jone J. Wu, and Noel A. Gillespie. CSA Bulletin. 2008;57:85–9.
12. Guedel AE. Third-stage ether anesthesia: a sub-classification regarding the significance of the position and movements of the eye. Am J Surg. 1920;34(Suppl):53–7.
13. California Pacific Medical Center [Internet]. Pioneers: Arthur E. Guedel, MD, 1883–1956, Electronic Archives. www.cpmc.org/professionals/hslibrary/collections/guedel/guedelbio.html. Accessed 14 Dec 2010.
14. Eger EI 2nd, Saidman LJ, Brandstater B. Minimum alveolar concentration: a standard of anesthetic potency. Anesthesiology. 1965;26:756–63.
15. Steinhaus JE. The investigator and his "uncompromising scientific honesty." ASA Newsletter 2001;65(9):7–9.
16. Boulton TB. Ralph Waters' visit to Great Britain in 1936. ASA Newsletter 2001;65(9):13–16.
17. Caton D. Ralph M. Waters, M.D., and professionalism in anesthesiology: a celebration of 75 years. Anesthesiology. 2003;98:286.
18. Lundy JS. Factors that influenced the development of anesthesiology. Anesth Analg. 1946;25:38–43.
19. Rabbitts JA, Bacon DR, Nuttall GA, Moore SB. Mayo Clinic and the origins of blood banking. Mayo Clin Proc. 2007;82:1117–8.
20. Dr. John Silas Lundy. Can J Anaesth. 1973;20:595–6.
21. Lennon R, Lennon RL, Bacon DR. The anaesthestists' travel club: an example of professionalism. J Clin Anesth. 2009;21:137–42.
22. Nelson CW. Dr John S. Lundy and the 75th anniversary of anesthesiology at Mayo. Mayo Clin Proc. 1999;74:650.
23. Ellis TA 2nd, Narr BJ, Bacon DR. Developing a specialty: J. S. Lundy's three major contributions to anesthesiology. J Clin Anesth. 2004;16:226–9.
24. Calhoun CC. Longfellow: a rediscovered life. Boston: Beacon; 2004. p 189.
25. Finster M. Gertie F. Marx, M.D. (1912–2004): the "mother of OB anesthesia." ASA Newsletter. 2004;68:35.
26. Lenzer J. Gertie Marx. BMJ. 2004;328:586.
27. Leibeskind JC. The relief of pain and suffering, history of medicine collection [on line]. Louis M. Darling Biomedical Library, University of California, Los Angeles.
28. Richmond C. [Obituary] Bjørn Ibsen. BMJ. 2007;335:674.
29. Trubuhovich RV. Bjorn Ibsen: commemorating his life, 1915–2007. Crit Care Resus. 2007;9:398–403.
30. Lassen HC. The epidemic of poliomyelitis in Copenhagen, 1952. Proc R Soc Med. 1954;47:67–71.
31. Ibsen B. Intensive therapy: background and development. 1966. Int Anesthesiol Clin. 1999 (Winter);37:1–14.
32. Peter Safar. http://en.wikipedia.org/wiki/Peter_Safar. Accessed 15 Dec 2010.
33. Kouwenhoven WB, Jude JR, Knickerbocker GG. Closed-chest cardiac massage. JAMA. 1960;173:1064–7.
34. Safar P, Brown TC, Holtey WJ, Wilder RJ. Ventilation and circulation with closed-chest cardiac massage in man. JAMA. 1961;176:574–6.
35. 2010 American Heart Association Guidelines for CPR.
36. Lowenstein E, McPeek B, editors. Enduring contributions of Henry K. Beecher to medicine, science, and society. Int Anesthesiol Clin. 2007;45(4)135–55 and 2008;46(1)157–249.
37. Beecher HK, Todd DP. A study of the deaths associated with anesthesia and surgery: based on a study of 599,548 anesthesias in ten institutions 1948–1952, inclusive. Ann Surg. 1954;140:2–35.
38. Beecher HK. Ethics and clinical research. N Engl J Med. 1966;274:1354–60
39. A definition of irreversible coma. Report of the ad hoc committee of the Harvard Medical School to examine the definition of brain death. JAMA. 1968;205:337–40.
40. Costarino AT Jr, Downes JJ. Pediatric anesthesia historical perspective. Anesthesiol Clin North Am. 2005;23:573–95.
41. www.speakersontour.com, Virginia Apgar: Science and Technology.
42. Calmes SH. Virginia Apgar, M.D.: at the forefront of obstetric anesthesia. ASA Newsletter. 1992;56:9–12.
43. Apgar V. A proposal for a new method of evaluation of the newborn infant. Curr Res Anesth Analg. 1953;32:260–7.

44. Ekstrøm-Jodal B (MD, PhD Professor). The Queen Silvia Children's Hospital, University of Gothenburg, personal letter dated 10 January 2010.

45. Haglund G, Werkmaster I, Ekstrøm-Jodal B, McDougall DH. The pediatric emergency ward. In: Stetson JB, Swyer PR, editors. Neonatal intensive care. St. Louis: WH Green; 1976. p. 73–87.

46. Haglund G. The emergency clinic principle and reality, Beretning FRA Nordisk Anaesthesiologik Forenings 4 Kongress I Helsinki 1956, pp. 39–41.

47. Fleisher LA, Rosenbaum SH, Nelson AH, Barash PG. The predictive value of preoperative silent ischemia for postoperative ischemic cardiac events in vascular and nonvascular surgery patients. Am Heart J. 1991;122:980–6.

48. Fleisher LA, Beattie C. Current practice in the preoperative evaluation of patients undergoing major vascular surgery: a survey of cardiovascular anesthesiologists. J Cardiothorac Vasc Anesth. 1993;7:650–4.

49. Fleisher LA, Rosenbaum SH, Nelson AH, Jain D, Wackers FJ, Zaret BL. Preoperative dipyridamole thallium imaging and ambulatory electrocardiographic monitoring as a predictor of perioperative cardiac events and long-term outcome. Anesthesiology. 1995;83:906–17.

50. Poldermans D, Bax JJ, Kertai MD, Krenning B, Westerhout CM, Schinkel AF, Thomson IR, Lansberg PJ, Fleisher LA, Klein J, van Urk H, Roelandt JR, Boersma E: Statins are associated with a reduced incidence of perioperative mortality in patients undergoing major noncardiac vascular surgery. Circulation. 2003;107:1848–51.

51. Eagle KA, Brundage BH, Chaitman BR, Ewy GA, Fleisher LA, Hertzer NR, Leppo JA, Ryan T, Schlant RC, Spencer WH 3rd, Spittell JA Jr, Twiss RD, Ritchie JL, Cheitlin MD, Gardner TJ, Garson A Jr, Lewis RP, Gibbons RJ, O'Rourke RA, Ryan TJ. Guidelines for perioperative cardiovascular evaluation for noncardiac surgery. Report of the American College of Cardiology/American Heart Association Task Force on practice guidelines (Committee on Perioperative Cardiovascular Evaluation for Noncardiac Surgery). J Am Coll Cardiol. 1996;27:910–48.

52. Roizen MF, Parsa PS. Anaesthesia and medical disease. Curr Opin Anaesthesiol. 2000;13:317–9.

53. Roizen MF, Roach KW. Wellbeing in the workplace. BMJ. 2010;340:c1743. doi: 10.1136/bmj.c1743.

54. Govinda R, Kasuya Y, Bala E, Mahboobi R, Devarajan J, Sessler DI, Akça O. Early postoperative subcutaneous tissue oxygen predicts surgical site infection. Anesth Analg. 2010;111:946–52. Epub 2010 July 2.

55. Gottschalk A, Ford JG, Regelin CC, You J, Mascha EJ, Sessler DI, Durieux ME, Nemergut EC. Association between epidural analgesia and cancer recurrence after colorectal cancer surgery. Anesthesiology. 2010;113:27–34.

56. Busch HJ, Eichwede F, Födisch M, Taccone FS, Wöbker G, Schwab T, Hopf HB, Tonner P, Hachimi-Idrissi S, Martens P, Fritz H, Bode Ch, Vincent JL, Inderbitzen B, Barbut D, Sterz F, Janata A. Safety and feasibility of nasopharyngeal evaporative cooling in the emergency department setting in survivors of cardiac arrest. Resuscitation 2010;81:943–9. Epub 2010 Jun 2.

57. Hunt TK, Hopf HW. High inspired oxygen fraction and surgical site infection. JAMA 2009;302:1588–9.

58. Hershey SG: The Rovenstine inheritance—a chain of leadership. Emery A. Rovenstine Memorial Lecture on the occasion of the annual meeting of the American Society of Anesthesiologists. Anesthesiology 1983;59:453–8.

59. Severinghaus JW: Gadgeteering for health care: the John W. Severinghaus lecture on translational science. Anesthesiology 2009;110:721–8.

Index

μ-Opioid receptor, 586, 590, 592, 645, 651
β-endorphin, 590, 814

A

Abbott, G., 18, 22, 171, 613
Accreditation Council for Graduate Medical Education (ACGME), 121, 264, 492, 843
Acetylene, 63, 378, 382–384
Acta Anaesthesiologica Scandinavia (AAS), 154, 417, 423, 427, 452
Acute lung injury (ALI), 566
Acute myocardial infarction, 589, 840
Acute respiratory distress syndrome (ARDS), 115, 566, 780, 782
Addiction, 44, 128, 129, 175, 219–225, 238, 642, 695, 861
Addiction to cocaine, 44, 129, 175, 695, 861
Adriani, J., 281, 459, 466, 467, 665, 666
ADU vaporizer, 710
Advanced Textbook on Traditional Chinese Medicine and Pharmacology, 346
Advisory Board for Medical Specialties (ABMS), 57, 121, 232, 489
Air embolism, 100, 882
Airway management, 125, 380, 723–741, 786, 804, 893, 927, 930
Alfentanil, 112, 124, 399, 530–533, 641–651
Ambulatory surgery, 77, 95, 100, 121, 125, 129, 132, 139, 144, 153, 163, 609, 633–639, 799–808, 911
American Association of Anesthetists (AAA), 41, 55, 56, 60, 188, 231, 245, 251, 486, 487
American Association of Nurse Anesthetists (AANA), 54, 56, 107, 122, 220, 223, 261, 278
American Board of Anesthesiology (ABA), 57, 80, 81, 107, 108, 121, 122, 197, 246, 459–469, 491
American Board of Surgery (ABS), 57, 232, 259, 261, 280, 460, 474, 491
American College of Anesthesiology (ACA), 107, 412, 462
American College of Surgeons (ACS), 197, 214, 239, 491, 863
American Hospital Association (AHA), 107, 121, 264, 280, 474, 492
American Medical Association (AMA), 33, 55, 57, 81, 121, 126, 177, 189, 196, 212, 245, 508, 546, 926, 927
American Medical Graduates (AMGs), 94, 95
American Medical Women's Association (AMWA), 195, 196
American Osteopathic Association (AOA), 267
American Society of Anesthesiologists (ASA), 42, 55, 56, 69, 81, 107, 120, 127, 141, 189, 193, 212, 213, 225, 229–240, 245, 276, 324, 368, 448, 462, 486, 522, 548, 805, 913
American Society of Anesthesiology's Physical Status Classification, 461, 931
American Society of Critical Care Anesthesiologists (ASCCA), 239
American Society of Obstetricians and Gynecologists (ACOG), 866
American Society of Regional Anesthesia (ASRA), 112, 239, 260, 862
American Society of Veterinary Anesthesiology (ASVA), 301
Aminoamide local anesthetics, 89, 865
Anaesthesia and Intensive Care (journal), 197, 303, 318, 453
Anaesthesia Incident Monitoring Study (AIMS), 127, 128, 546, 549

Anaesthesia (journal), 450
Anaesthesiologica Scandinavica (journal), 427, 452
Anaesthetic pollution, 115, 384, 557, 565, 775, 777, 778
Anaesthetic Research Society, 96, 398
Andrews, E., 45, 63, 520, 616, 703, 705, 713
Anesthesia & Analgesia (journal), 60, 156, 197, 247, 249–255, 353, 855 HOW CAN WE HAVE THIS AND NOT HAVE ANAESTHESIA AND ANESTHESIOLOGY CALLED OUT?
Anesthesia breathing systems, see Breathing systems
Anesthesia Crisis Resource Management (ACRM), 494
Anesthesia during WWI, 53, 273, 274, 378, 485, 486
Anesthesia during WWII, 54, 194, 195, 232, 279–281, 364, 489, 490, 631, 707, 816
Anesthesia masks, 30, 31, 38, 42, 46, 48, 52, 71–74, 84, 113, 171, 333, 337–340, 371, 381–386, 615, 617, 704–718, 723, 725, 830, 887–895
Anesthesia in American Civil War, 23, 37, 40, 170, 271
Anesthesia machines, 43, 46, 54, 63–69, 113–115, 128, 135, 312, 317, 326, 338, 340, 347, 349, 381–383, 394, 410, 420, 422, 437, 520, 521, 545, 546, 703–714, 768, 906, 907, 913
Anesthesia Memorial Foundation (AMF), 235
Anesthesia Patient Safety Foundation (APSF), 127, 238, 250, 545, 551, 819, 913, 931
Anesthesia Quality Institute, 240
Anesthesia simulation, 90, 128, 136, 143, 155, 238, 240, 385, 469, 483, 493–496, 506, 547, 552
Anesthesia subspecialties in Europe, 497–504
Anesthésie et Analgésie (journal), 60, 366, 448
Anesthesiology (journal), 60, 193, 197, 211, 232, 248, 251, 447, 448, 450, 453, 456, 604,
Anesthetic agents (volatile), 64, 65, 83, 97, 105, 109–117, 135, 136, 146, 170, 186, 229, 277, 285, 475, 486, 572, 573, 576, 601–604, 609–626, 704, 708, 720, 878, 881, 883, 911–916
Anesthetic neurotoxicity, 255, 699–701
Annales Françaises d'Anesthésie et de Réanimation (AFAR) (journal), 366
Anoci-association, see Crile, anoci-association
Antibiotics, 53, 69, 145, 178, 889
Antisepsis, 39, 40, 53, 163, 170, 173, 181, 800, 877, 889
Aoyagi, T., 117, 126, 412, 522, 546, 756, 757
Apgar, V., 55, 58, 88, 100, 192–196, 201, 364, 561, 853, 855, 856, 930
Aprotinin, 577–580
Artificial ventilation, 9, 68, 80, 208, 273, 362, 382, 409, 419, 423, 426, 437, 501, 516, 560, 672, 675, 724, 730, 735, 736, 747, 761–769, 772, 774, 787, 791, 896, 929
ASA Preceptorship program, 94, 95, 236, 489
Association of American Medical Colleges (AAMC), 107, 237, 492
Association of Anaesthetists of Great Britain and Ireland (AAGBI), 54, 62, 300, 394, 498
Association of Canadian University Departments of Anesthesia (ACUDA), 326
Association of University Anesthesiologists (AUA), 81, 82, 235

Printed in the United States of America